Cambridge Handedicine
Second edition

Wholly ... ned *Cambridge Handbook of Psycho*... ...ssible, one-stop resource for health ... broadcasters specializing in health-... ...rsity of Sussex and Kenneth Wallsto...

The ... international interdisciplinary cast of authors have reconceptualized ... dropped and its most useful elements revised and incorporated into rel... ...ng the many new topics added throughout are: diet and health, ethnicity and health, clinical interviewing, mood assessment, communicating risk, medical interviewing, diagnostic procedures, organ donation, IVF, MMR, HRT, sleep disorders, skin disorders, depression and anxiety disorders.

No one interested in healthcare issues, promotion and care should be without this book.

Susan Ayers is Senior Lecturer in Health Psychology at the University of Sussex.

Andrew Baum is Professor of Pyschiatry and Psychology at the University of Pittsburgh School of Medicine, and Deputy Director for Cancer Control and Supportive Sciences at the University of Pittsburgh Cancer Institute.

Chris McManus is Professor of Psychology and Medical Education at University College London.

Stanton Newman is Professor of Health Psychology at the Centre for Behavioural and Social Sciences in Medicine, University College London.

Kenneth Wallston is Professor of Psychology in Nursing at the Vanderbilt University Medical Center, Nashville.

John Weinman is Professor of Psychology as applied to Medicine, Health Psychology Section, Institute of Psychiatry, King's College London, London.

Robert West is Professor of Health Psychology, Department of Epidemiology and Public Health, University College London.

From reviews of the first edition:

'The new Cambridge Handbook is simply indispensable.... The book will find a wide market. No clinical psychologist is going to want to be without it. Perhaps more important, many doctors will continue to dip into it from time to time, since one of the book's virtues is to be written in a generally jargon free manner, accessible to all health professionals. Journalists from the better papers will use it frequently, since it gives a quick synopsis of the current state of play on a vast range of topics which are rarely absent from the health pages. Finally, journal editors will find it a valuable address book when they need referees for the ever increasing flow of research papers in this fascinating field'. Simon Wessely, *Psychological Medicine*

'This book is a rich mine of information for the general practitioner.... The day I received it a student came to ask me for advice about essays. Putting the "encyclopaedic handbook" to its first test, we looked up a few keywords. There was a chapter on each one. Bite-size morsels of information, easily digestible, comprehensive. I shall certainly keep this book within easy reach for future reference'. Caroline Selai, *Journal of the Royal Society of Medicine*

'Easy to read; a practical book'. *Journal of Pediatric Endocrinology and Metabolism*

Cambridge Handbook of
Psychology, Health and Medicine

Second edition

Susan Ayers

Andrew Baum

Chris McManus

Stanton Newman

Kenneth Wallston

John Weinman

Robert West

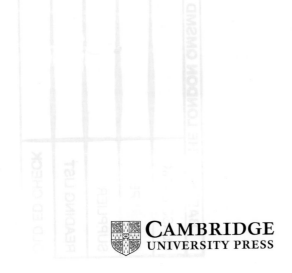

CAMBRIDGE
UNIVERSITY PRESS

CAMBRIDGE UNIVERSITY PRESS

Cambridge, New York, Melbourne, Madrid, Cape Town, Singapore, São Paulo

Cambridge University Press
The Edinburgh Building, Cambridge CB2 8RU, UK
Published in the United States of America by Cambridge University Press, New York

www.cambridge.org
Information on this title: www.cambridge.org/9780521879972

First published 2007

Printed in Malaysia by Imago

A catalogue record for this publication is available from the British Library

Library of Congress Cataloging-in-Publication data

Cambridge handbook of psychology, health, and medicine / [edited by]
Susan Ayers . . . [et al.]. -- 2nd ed.
p.;cm.
Includes bibliographical references and index.
ISBN-13   978-0-521-60510-6   (pbk.)
ISBN-10   0-521-60510-5   (pbk.)
1. Medicine and psychology—Handbooks, manuals, etc. I. Ayers, Susan, 1964-.
II. Title: Handbook of psychology, health, and medicine.
[DNLM: 1. Psychology, Medical—Handbooks. 2. Behavioral Medicine—Handbooks.
WB 39 C178 2007]
R726.5.C354 2007
616.001′9–dc22

2006028358

ISBN-13 978-0-521-60510-6 paperback
ISBN-13 978-0-521-87997-2 hardback

Contents

Section II Psychological assessment

Section III Psychological intervention

Section IV Healthcare practice

Part II Medical topics

Contributors

Leif Edvard Aarø, Research Centre for Health Promotion (HEMIL), University of Bergen, Christies gt 13, N-5015 Bergen, Norway

Charles Abraham, Psychology Department, University of Sussex, Brighton BN1 9QH, UK

Sarah Afuwape, Cancer Research UK Psychosocial Group, Institute of Psychiatry, King's College London, Adamson Centre for Mental Health, St. Thomas' Hospital, London SE1 7EH, UK

Michael Ainette, Albert Einstein College of Medicine, Yeshiva University, Jack and Pearl Resnick Campus, 1300 Morris Park Avenue, Belfer 1301, Bronx, NY 10461, USA

Beth Alder, Napier University, Room G4, Canaan Lane Campus, 74 Canaan Lane, Edinburgh EH9 2TB, UK

Robert Allan, Weill Medical College, Cornell University, New York Presbyterian Hospital, New York, USA

John Allen, HIV Medicine, Royal Free Hospital, Pond Street, London NW3 2QG, UK

Barbara Andersen, Department of Psychology, The Ohio State University, 149 Psychology Building, 1885 Neil Avenue, Columbus, OH 43210-1222, USA

Gerhard Andersson, Department of Behavioural Sciences, Linköping University, SE-581, 83 Linköping, Sweden

Michael Antoni, Department of Psychology, University of Miami, P.O. Box 248185, Coral Gables, FL 33124-0751, USA

Heather Ashton, School of Neurosciences, Division of Psychiatry, Royal Victoria Infirmary, Leazes Wing, University of Newcastle-upon-Tyne, Newcastle-upon-Tyne NE1 4LE, UK

Susan Ayers, Psychology Department, University of Sussex, Brighton BN1 9QH, UK

Peter Ayton, City University, Northampton Square, London EC1 0HB, UK

Elizabeth Bachen, Psychology Department, Mills College, Room 505, 5000 MacArthur Blvd, Oakland, CA 94613, USA

Albert Bandura, Department of Psychology, Stanford University, Building 420, Jordan Hall, Stanford, CA 94305, USA

Hugh Barr, Centre for Community Care and Primary Health, University of Westminster, 115 New Cavendish Street, London WIM 8JS, UK

Lisa Feldman Barrett, Department of Psychology, Boston College, 427 McGuinn Building, Chestnut Hill, MA 02467, USA

Christopher Bass, Department of Psychological Medicine, John Radcliffe Hospital, Oxford OX3 9DU, UK

Andrew Baum, Pittsburgh Cancer Institute, University of Pittsburgh Medical Center, 3600 Forbes Avenue, Suite 405, Pittsburgh, PA 15213-3412, USA

Paul Bennett, Nursing, Health and Social Care Research Centre, University of Cardiff, East Gate House 4th Floor, 35-43 Newport Road, Cardiff, CF24 0AB, UK

Yael Benyamini, Bob Shapell School of Social Work, Tel Aviv University, Tel Aviv 69978, Israel

John Berry, Psychology Department, Queen's University, Kingston, Ontario, K7L 3N6, Canada

Erin Bigler, Psychology Department, Brigham Young University, Salt Lake City, Utah, USA

Felicity Bishop, Complementary Medical Research Unit, Aldermoor Health Centre, Aldermoor Close, Southampton SO16 5ST, UK

Maurice Bloch, 2329 West Mall, Vancouver, BC V6T 1Z4, Canada

Sandra Boersma, Clinical & Health Psychology, Leiden University, Leiden, The Netherlands

Richard Boles, Clinical Child Psychology Program, University of Kansas, 2009 Dole Human Development Center, 1000 Sunnyside Avenue, Lawrence, KS 66045-7555, USA

Roger Booth, School of Medical Sciences, The University of Auckland, Private Bag 92019, Auckland, New Zealand

Robert Bor, HIV Medicine, Royal Free Hospital, Pond Street, London NW3 2QG, UK

Ron Borland, Victoria Health Centre for Tobacco Control, 1 Rathdowne Street, Carlton, VIC 3050, Australia

Peter Bower, National Primary Care Research and Development Centre, University of Manchester, Williamson Building, Oxford Road, Manchester M13 9PL, UK

Ann Bowling, Department of Primary Care & Population Sciences, University College London, London NW3 2PF, UK

Clare Bradley, Psychology Department, Royal Holloway, University of London, Egham, Surrey TW20 0EX, UK

Elizabeth Broadbent, Department of Psychological Medicine, The University of Auckland, Private Bag 92019, Auckland, New Zealand

Ronald Brown, Department of Pediatrics & Health Professions, Medical University of South Carolina, Charleston, SC 29425, USA

Kevin Browne, School of Psychology, University of Birmingham, Edgbaston, Birmingham B15 2TT, UK

Kelly Brownell, Department of Psychology, Yale University, New Haven, CT 06520, USA

Michael Bruch, Cognitive-Behavioural Psychotherapy Unit, Department of Mental Health Sciences, University College London, Wolfson Building, Riding House Street, London W1W 7EY, UK

Emily Buckley, Centre for Health Psychology, Staffordshire University, Mellor Building, College Road, Stoke on Trent ST4 2DE, UK

Tasha Burwinkle, Department of Anesthesiology, University of Washington, P. O. Box 356540, Seattle, WA 98195, USA

Ruth Cairns, Academic Department of Psychological Medicine, Institute of Psychiatry, King's College London, Weston Education Centre, Cutcombe Road, London SE5 9RJ, UK

Jo-anne Carlyle, Group Analytic Practice, Tavistock Clinic, 120 Belsize Lane, London NW3 5BA, UK

Timothy Carmody, 116-A VAMC, University of California, San Francisco, USA

Kristen Carpenter, Department of Psychology, The Ohio State University, 1885 Neil Avenue, Columbus, OH 43210-1222, USA

Adam Carrico, Department of Psychology, University of Miami, P.O. Box 248185, Coral Gables, FL 33124-0751, USA

Julie Carter, Centre for International Health and Development, Institute of Child Health, University College London, 30 Guilford Street, London WC1N 1EH, UK

Martin Cartwright, Health Care Evaluation Group, Department of Epidemiology and Public Health, University College London, 1-19 Torrington Place, London WC1E 6BT, UK

Ineke Pit-ten Cate, Developmental Brain Behaviour Unit, School of Psychology, University of Southampton, Highfield, Southampton S017 1BJ, UK

Trudie Chalder, Academic Department of Psychological Medicine, Institute of Psychiatry, King's College London, Weston Education Centre, Cutcombe Road, London SE5 9RJ, UK

Nancy Chiaravalloti, Kessler Medical Rehabilitation Research and Education Corporation, 1199 Pleasant Valley Way, West Orange, NJ 07052, USA

Chris Code, School of Psychology, University of Exeter, Washington Singer Laboratories, Exeter EX4 4QG, UK

Jay Cohen, Department of Psychology, Wayne State University, Detroit, MI 48202, USA

Sheldon Cohen, Department of Psychology, Baker Hall, Room 335-D, Carnegie Mellon University, Pittsburgh, PA 15213, USA

Brent Collett, University of Washington School of Medicine, Children's Hospital & Regional Medical Center, Outpatient Child & Adolescent Psychiatry & Behavioral Medicine

Mark Conner, School of Psychology, University of Leeds, Leeds LS2 9JT, UK

Tamlin Conner, University of Connecticut Health Center, 263 Farmington Avenue, Connecticut 06030, USA

Frances Cook, Michael Palin Centre for Stammering Children, Finsbury Health Centre, Pine Street, London EC1 0LP, UK

Elizabeth Coombes, Psychology Service BSMHT, University of Birmingham and Cancer Centre, Queen Elizabeth Hospital, 208 Monyhull Hall Road, Kings Norton, Birmingham B30 3QJ, UK

Alethea Cooper, Cardiothoracic Centre, St. Thomas' Hospital, 6th Floor, East Wing, Lambeth Palace Road, London SE1 7EH, UK

Penelope Cream, Royal Free Hospital, Pond Street, London NW3 2QG, UK

Peggy Dalton, 20 Cleveland Avenue, London W4 1SN, UK

Gerald Davison, Psychology Department, University of Southern California, SGM 538, Mail Code 1061, Los Angeles, CA 90089, USA

John DeLuca, Kessler Medical Rehabilitation Research and Education Corporation, 1199 Pleasant Valley Way, West Orange, NJ 07052, USA

Jennifer Devlen, Department of Psychology, Dickinson College, P.O. Box 1773, Carlisle, PA 17013-2896, USA

†**Frederick Dirbas**, Division of Surgical Oncology, Department of Surgery, Stanford University, Palo Alto, California, USA

Kim Dixon, Pain Prevention and Treatment Program, Duke University Medical Center, Durham, NC 27708, USA

Suzanne Dobbinson, Victoria Health Centre for Tobacco Control, 1 Rathdowne Street, Carlton, VIC 3050, Australia

Elizabeth Dormandy, Department of Psychology, Health Psychology Section, Institute of Psychiatry, King's College London, 5th Floor, Thomas Guy House, Guy's Campus, London SE1 9RT, UK

James Dornan, Royal Jubilee Maternity Service, Royal Group of Hospitals, Grosvenor Road, Belfast BT12 6BA, UK

Angela Liegey Dougall, Department of Psychology, University of Pittsburgh, Pittsburgh, PA 15260, USA

Laura Dreer, Department of Psychology, University of Alabama at Birmingham, 415 CH, 1530 3rd Avenue South, Birmingham AL 5294-1170, USA

Andrew Eagle, CNWL NHS Mental Health Trust, Pall Mall Mental Health Centre, 150 Barlby Road, London W10 6BS, UK

Robert Edelmann, Roehampton University, Erasmus House, Rochampton Lane, London SW15 5PU, UK

Robert Edwards, Department of Psychiatry and Behavioral Sciences, Center for Mind-Body Research, Johns Hopkins University School of Medicine, 600 N. Wolfe Street, Meyer 1-108, Baltimore, MD 21287, USA

Susan Eisen, Center for Health Quality, Outcomes and Economics Research, Edith Nourse Rogers Memorial Veterans Hospital, 200 Springs Road (152), Bedford, MA 01730, USA

James Elander, Psychology Department, University of Derby, Kedleston Road, Derby DE22 1GB, UK

Bjørn Ellertsen, The Reading Centre, University of Stavanger, N-4036 Stavanger, Norway

Sandra Elliott, South London and Maudsley NHS Trust, Adamson Centre, St. Thomas' Hospital, Lambeth Palace Road, London SE1 7EH, UK

Timothy Elliott, Department of Educational Psychology, Texas A&M University, College Station, 4225 TAMU, TX 77845, USA

Jason Ellis, Psychology Department, University of Surrey, Guildford Surrey, GU2 7XH, UK

Mark Emberton, Institute of Urology and Nephrology, University College London, 48 Riding House Street, London W1W 7EY, UK

Ruth Epstein, Royal National Throat, Nose and Ear Hospital, 330 Gray's Inn Road, London WC1X 8DA, UK

Paul Estabrooks, Kaiser Permanente-Colorado, Clinical Research Unit, P.O. Box 378066, Denver, CO 80237-8066, USA

Sara Faithfull, European Institute of Health and Medical Sciences, University of Surrey, Stag Hill, Guildford GU2 7TE, UK

Giovanni Fava, Department of Psychology, University of Bologna, Bologna, Italy

Rosalie Ferner, Department of Neurology, Guy's Hospital, St. Thomas' Street, London SE1 9RT, UK

Robin Fiore, Department of Philosophy, Florida Atlantic University, 777 Glades Road, Boca Raton, P.O. Box 3091 FL 33431-0991 USA

Baruch Fischhoff, Department of Engineering and Public Policy, Department of Social and Decision Sciences, Carnegie Mellon University, Pittsburgh, USA

Raymond Fitzpatrick, Nuffield College, University of Oxford, New Road, Oxford OX3 7LF, UK

Robert Frank, College of Public Health and Health Professions, Department of Clinical and Health Psychology, University of Florida, Gainesville, FL 32610-0185, USA

David French, School of Sports & Exercise Sciences, University of Birmingham, Edgbaston, Birmingham B15 2TT, UK

Irene Frieze, Department of Psychology, University of Pittsburgh, 3329 Sennott Square Pittsburgh, PA 15260, USA

Raymond Gaeta, Stanford University, 300 Pasteur Drive, Stanford, CA 94305, USA

Robert Gatchel, University of Texas at Arlington, 701 S. Nedderman Drive, Arlington, TX 76019, USA

Gary Geffken, Department of Psychiatry, University of Florida, P.O. Box 100234, Gainesville, FL 32610, USA

Russell Glasgow, Kaiser Permanente-Colorado, 335 Road Runner Road, Penrose, CO 81240, USA

Claire Glasscoe, Royal Liverpool Children's Hospital-Alder Hey, Child Mental Health Unit, 1st Floor, Mulbery House, Eaton Road, Liverpool L12 2AP, UK

Laura Goldstein, Department of Psychology, Institute of Psychiatry, King's College London, De Crespigny Park, London SE5 8AF, UK

Michael Gossop, Addiction Sciences Building, Institute of Psychiatry, De Crespigny Park, London SE5 8AF, UK

Benjamin Gottlieb, Department of Psychology, College of Social and Applied Human Sciences, University of Guelph, Guelph, ON N1G 2W1, Canada

John Green, Department of Clinical Health Psychology, St. Mary's Hospital, Clarence Wing, London W2 1PD, UK

Mary Gregerson, Family Therapy Institute of Alexandria, 220 South Washington Street, Alexandria, VA 22314-2712, Canada

Richard Griffiths, School of Clinical Sciences, University of Liverpool, Duncan Building, Daulby Street, Liverpool L69 3GA, UK

Konstadina Griva, Centre for Behavioural and Social Sciences in Medicine, University College London, 2nd Floor, Wolfson Building, 48 Riding House Street, London W1N 8AA, UK

Beth Grunfeld, Section of Health Psychology, Department of Psychology, Institute of Psychiatry, King's College London, Denmark Hill, London SE5 8AF, UK

Peter Hajek, Department of Human Science and Medical Ethics, Barts and The London, Queen Mary's School of Medicine and Dentistry, University of London, Turner Street, Whitechapel, London E1 2AD, UK

Angela Hall, Department of Medical and Health Care Education, St. George's, University of London, Cranmer Terrace, London SW17 0RE, UK

Catherine Hamilton-Giachritsis, School of Psychology, University of Birmingham, Edgbaston, Birmingham B15 2TT, UK

Ainsley Hardy, Centre for Child and Family Research, Department of Social Sciences, Loughborough University, Loughborough, Leicestershire LE11 3TU, UK

Clare Harries, Department of Psychology, University College London, 1-19 Torrington Place, London WC1E 6EA, UK

Jane Harrington, Centre for Behavioural and Social Sciences in Medicine, Royal Free and University College Medical School, Wolfson Building, 48 Riding House Street, London W1N 8AA, UK

Tirril Harris, Socio-Medical Research Group, Department of Social Psychiatry, HSRD, Institute of Psychiatry, St. Thomas' Hospital Campus, Lambeth Palace Road, London SE1 7EH, UK

Siobhan Hart, Colchester General Hospital, Turner Road, Colchester CO4 5JL.

Jennifer Haythornthwaite, Department of Psychiatry and Behavioral Sciences, Center for Mind-Body Research, Johns Hopkins University School of Medicine, 600 N. Wolfe Street, Mayer 1-108, Baltimore, MD 21287, USA

Michael Heap, Wathwood Hospital RSU, Gipsy Green Lane, Wath-upon-Dearne, Rotherham, S63 7TQ, UK

Barbara Hedge, South Devon Healthcare NHS Foundation Trust, Torbay Hospital, Torquay TQ2 7AA, UK

Kenneth Heller, Department of Psychology, Indiana University, 1101 E. 10th Street, Bloomington, IN 47405-7007, USA

Peter Hepper, School of Psychology, David Keir Building, Queen's University, Northern Ireland, Belfast BT7 1NN, UK

Martin Herbert, Exeter University, Exeter, Devon EX4 4QJ, UK

Sari Holmes, Department of Medical and Clinical Psychology, Uniformed Services University of the Health Sciences, 4301 Jones Bridge Road, Bethesda, MD 20814, USA

David J. de L. Horne, Psychology Service BSMHT, University of Birmingham and Cancer Centre, Queen Elizabeth Hospital, 208 Monyhull Hall Road, Kings Norton, Birmingham B30 3QJ, UK

Rob Horne, Centre for Behavioural Medicine, The School of Pharmacy, University of London, Mezzanine Floor, BMA House, Tavistock Square, London WC1H 9JP, UK

Gerry Humphris, Bute Medical School, University of St Andrews, St Andrews, Fife KY16 9TS, UK

Myra Hunter, Department of Psychology, Institute of Psychiatry, King's College London SE1, 7EH, UK

Staffan Hygge, Laboratory of Applied Psychology, Centre for Built Environment, University of Gävle, Gävle, SE-801 76, Sweden

Marjan Jahanshahi, Sobell Department of Motor Neuroscience and Movement Disorders, Institute of Neurology, University College London, Queen Square, London WC1N 3BG, UK

Katherine Joekes, Clinical and Health Psychology, Leiden University, Leiden, The Netherlands

Ine Baug Johnsen, The Reading Centre, University of Stavanger, N-4036 Stavanger, Norway

Marie Johnston, School of Psychology, Williams Guild Building, University of Aberdeen, Aberdeen AB24 2UB, Scotland, UK

Beth Jones, Department of Epidemiology and Public Health, Yale University School of Medicine, 60 College Street, P. O. Box 208034, New Haven, CT 06520-8034, USA

Christina Jones, School of Clinical Sciences, University of Liverpool, Duncan Building, Daulby Street, Liverpool L69 3GA, UK

Ad Kaptein, Medical Psychology LUMC, Leiden University, P.O. Box 9555, 2300 RB, Leiden, The Netherlands

Narinder Kapur, Neuropsychology Department, R3 Neurosciences, Box 83, Addenbrooke's Hospital, Cambridge CB2 2QQ, UK

Stanislav Kasl, Department of Epidemiology and Public Health, Yale University School of Medicine, 60 College Street, P. O. Box 208034, New Haven, CT 06520-8034, USA

Joel Katz, Department of Psychology and School of Kinesiology and Health Science, York University, 4700 Keele Street, BSB 232, Toronto, ON M3J 1P3, Canada

Francis Keefe, Pain Prevention and Treatment Program, Duke University Medical Center, Durham, NC 27708, USA

Stephen Kellett, Barnsley Primary Care NHS Trust, Barnsley HX70 6RS, UK

David Kennedy, Northumbria University, Newcastle upon Tyne, NE1 8ST, UK

Paul Kennedy, University of Oxford, Isis Education Centre, Warneford Hospital, Oxford OX3 7JX, UK

Dianna Kenny, School of Behavioural & Community Health Sciences, University of Sydney, C42, P.O. Box 170, Lidcombe, NSW 1825, Australia

Jane Kidd, Warwick Medical School, University of Warwick, Coventry CV4 7AL, UK

Karen Hye-cheon Kim, University of Health Behavior and Health Education Department, University of Arkansas for Medical Sciences, Little Rock, AR 72205-7199, USA

Christie King, F. Spellacy & Associates, 1005 Balmoral Road, Victoria, B.C. V8T 1A7, Canada

Irving Kirsch, University of Hull, Hull HU6 7RX, UK

Amber Koblitz, Psychology Department, North Dakota State University, 115D Minard Hall, Fargo, ND 58105, USA

Harold Koenig, Duke University Medical Center, Geriatric Research, Education and Clinical Center, Durham, North Carolina, USA

Gerjo Kok, Department of Experimental Psychology, University of Maastricht, P.O. Box 616, 6200 MD Maastricht, The Netherlands

Willem Kop, Division of Cardiology, University of Maryland Medical Center, 22 South Grezene Street-S3B04, Baltimore, MD 21201, USA

David Krantz, Department of Medical and Clinical Psychology, Uniformed Services University of the Health Sciences, 4301 Jones Bridge Road, Bethesda, MD 20814, USA

Jeffrey Labban, Department of Psychiatry and Behavioral Sciences, Duke University Medical Center, Durham, NC 27710, USA

Brian Lakey, Department of Psychology, Wayne State University, Detroit, MI 48202, USA

Melissa Lamar, Department of Psychology, Institute of Psychiatry, King's College London, Box P077, De Crespigny Park, London SE5 8AH, UK

Andrea Lee, College of Public Health and Health Professions, Department of Clinical and Health Psychology, University of Florida, Gainesville, FL 32610-0185, USA

Christina Lee, School of Psychology, The University of Queensland, St. Lucia, QLD 4072, Australia

Stephen Lepore, Temple University, 1700 No. Broad Street, Suit 304, Philadelphia PA 19122, USA

Eva Leslie, Cancer Prevention Research Centre, School of Population Health, The University of Queensland, Brisbane, Australia

David Lester, Center for the Study of Suicide, RR41, 5 Stonegate Court, Blackwood, NJ 08012-5356, USA

Naomi Lester, Department of Psychology, Bastyr University, 14500 Juanita Dr. NE, Kenmore, WA 98028-4966, USA

Elaine Leventhal, Department of Medicine, Robert Wood Johnson Medical School, University of Medicine and Dentisitry of New Jersey, CAB 2300, New Brunswick, NJ 08901, USA

Howard Leventhal, Institute for Health, Health Care Policy and Aging Research, Rutgers, The State University of New Jersey, New Brunswick, NJ 08901, USA

Robert Lewin, Health Sciences Research, 2nd Floor, Seebohm Building, University of York, Heslington, YO10 5DD, UK

George Lewith, Complementary Medicine Research Unit, Aldermoor Health Centre, University of Southampton, Aldermoor Close, Southampton SO16 5ST, UK

Patricia Loft, Health Psychology Department, The University of Auckland, Private Bag 92019, Auckland, New Zealand

James Maddux, Department of Psychology, George Mason University, Fairfax, VA 22030, USA

Esther Maissi, Department of Psychological Medicine, King's College London, Weston Education Centre, 10 Cutcombe Road, London SE5 9RJ, UK

Sharon Manne, Population Science Division, Fox Chase Cancer Center, 333 Cottman Avenue, Philadelphia, PA 11911-2497, USA

Antony Manstead, School of Psychology, Cardiff University, Cardiff CF10 3AT, UK

Ivana Marková, Department of Psychology, University of Stirling, Stirling FK9 4LA, Scotland, UK

Anna Marsland, Department of Psychology, University of Pittsburgh, 603 Old Engineering Hall, 4015 O'Hara Street, Pittsburgh, PA 15260, USA

Theresa Marteau, Psychology Department, Health Psychology Section, Institute of Psychiatry, King's College London, 5th Floor, Thomas Guy House, Guy's Campus, London Bridge, London SE1 9RT, UK

Christina Maslach, University of California, Berkeley, 200 California Hall, CA 94720-1500, USA

Kevin McCaul, Psychology Department, North Dakota State University, 115D Minard Hall, Fargo, ND 58105, USA

Robert McCrae, National Institute on Aging, NJH, DNHS, Gerontology Research Center, 5600 Nathan Shock Drive, Baltimore, MD 21224-6825, USA

Hannah McGee, Department of Psychology, Royal College of Surgeons in Ireland, Mercer Building, Merser Street Lower, Dublin 2, Ireland

Maureen McHugh, Psychology Department, Indiana University of Pennsylvania, Uhler Hall 204, Indiana, PA 15705, USA

Dan McKenna, Royal Jubilee Maternity Service, Royal Group of Hospitals, Grosvenor Road, Belfast BT12 6BA, UK

Frank McKenna, Department of Psychology, University of Reading, Earley Gate, Reading RG6 6AL, UK

Laurence McKenna, Royal National Throat, Nose and Ear Hospital, Gray's Inn Road, London WC1X 8DA, UK

Kirstie McKenzie-McHarg, National Perinatal Epidemiology Unit, University of Oxford, Old Road Campus, Oxford OX3 7LF, UK

Chris McManus, Department of Psychology, University College London, Gower Street, London WC1E 6BY, UK

Brian McMillan, School of Psychology, University of Leeds, Leeds LS2 9JT, UK

Nicki Mead, National Primary Care Research and Development Centre, University of Manchester, Williamson Building, Oxford Road, Manchester M13 9PL, UK

Geraldine Meechan, Health Psychology Department, The University of Auckland, Private Bag 92019, Auckland, New Zealand

Ronald Melzack, Department of Psychology, McGill University, Stewart Biology Building, Room W8/1, 1205 Dr. Penfield Avenue, Montreal, Quebec, H3A 1B1, Canada

Anne Miles, Department of Epidemiology and Public Health, University College London, Gower Street, London WC1E 6BT, UK

Keith Millar, Section of Psychological Medicine, University of Glasgow, Gartnavel Royal Hospital, 1055 Great Western Road, Glasgow G12 0XH, Scotland, UK

Antonio Millet, Division of Breast Diseases, Department of Obstetrics and Gynecology, Valencia School of Medicine, Spain

Heather Mohay, School of Psychology and Counselling, Queensland University of Technology, Beams Road, Carseldine, QLD-4034, Australia

Bernice Moos, Centre for Health Care Evaluation Veterans Affairs Health Care System, 795 Willow Road, Menlo Park, CA 94025, USA

Rudolf Moos, Centre for Health Care Evaluation Veterans Affairs Health Care System, 795 Willow Road, Menlo Park, CA 94025, USA

Stephen Morley, Academic Unit of Psychiatry, School of Medicine, University of Leeds, 15 Hyde Terrace, Leeds LS2 9LT, UK

Patricia Morokoff, Department of Psychology, Chafee Social Science Center, University of Rhode Island, Kingston, RI 02881

Jennifer Morse, Western Psychiatric Institute and Clinic, Room E-1135, 3811 O'Hara Street, Pittsburgh, PA 15213, USA

Rona Moss-Morris, School of Psychology, University of Southampton, Highfield Southampton, SO17 1BJ, UK

Kathleen Mulligan, Centre for Behavioural and Social Sciences in Medicine, University College London, 2nd Floor, Wolfson Building, 48 Riding House Street, London W1N 8AA, UK

Stanton Newman, Centre for Behavioural and Social Sciences in Medicine, University College London, Charles Bell House, 63-73 Riding House Street, London W1W 7EJ, UK

David Nias, Psychology Section, Barts and The London, Queen Mary's School of Medicine and Dentistry, University of London, London, E1 2AD, UK

Lorraine Noble, University College London, Academic Centre for Medical Education, Holborn Union Building, Archway Campus, Highgate Hill, London N19 5LW, UK

Carl Noe, Baylor Research Institute, Baylor University Medical Center, 3434 Live Oak Street 125, Dallas, TX 75204, USA

Amanda O'Brien, Kessler Medical Rehabilitation Research and Education Corporation, 1199 Pleasant Valley Way, West Orange, NJ 07052, USA

Catherine O'Leary, South Thames Cleft Service, 12th Floor Guy's Tower, Guy's Hospital, St. Thomas' Street, London SE1 9RT, UK

Jane Ogden, Department of Psychology, School of Human Sciences, University of Surrey, Guildford GU2 7XH, UK

Neville Owen, Cancer Prevention Research Centre, School of Population Health, The University of Queensland, Brisbane, Australia

Glynn Owens, Department of Psychology, The University of Auckland (Tamaki Campus), New Zealand

Colin Murray Parkes, 21 South Road, Chorleywood, Hertfordshire WD3 5AS, UK

Katharine Parkes, Department of Experimental Psychology, University of Oxford, Oxford OX1 3UD, UK

Andy Parrott, Department of Psychology, University of Wales Swansea, Swansea SA2 8PP, UK

James Pennebaker, Department of Psychology, The University of Texas at Austin, University Station, A 8000, Austin, TX 78712-0187, USA

Lisa Caitlin Perri, Pain Prevention and Treatment Program, Duke University Medical Center, Durham, NC 27708, USA

Keith Petrie, Health Psychology Department, The University of Auckland, Private Bag 92019, Auckland, New Zealand

Claire Phillips, Centre for Appearance Research, University of the West of England, Frenchay Campus, Coldharbour Lane, Bristol BS16 1QY, UK

John Pimm, Vale of Aylesbury Primary Care Trust, Community Neurological Rehabilitation Service, Rayners Hedge, Croft Road, Aylesbury, Buckinghamshire, UK

Deborah Polk, Department of Dental Public Health and Information Management, University of Pittsburgh, School of Dental Medicine, 381 Salk Hall, 3501 Terrace street, Pittsburgh, PA 15261, USA

Donna Posluszny, University of Pittsburgh Medical Center, 200 Lothrop Street, Pittsburgh, PA 15213-2582, USA

Jane Powell, Psychology Department, Goldsmiths College, University of London, Room 309, Whitehead Building, New Cross, London SE14 6NW, UK

Rachael Powell, Health Psychology, University of Aberdeen, 3rd Floor, Health Sciences Building, Foresterhill, Aberdeen AB25 2ZD, Scotland, UK

Michael Preece, Nutrition, Metabolism, Endocrinology & Dermatology Unit, Institute of Child Health, London WC1N 1EH, UK

Linda Pring, Psychology Department, Goldsmiths College, University of London, New Cross, London SE14 6NW, UK

Lyn Quine, Department of Psychology, Centre for Research in Health Behaviour, University of Kent, Canterbury, Kent CT2 7NP, UK

Klaus Rabe, Department of Pulmonary Medicine, Leiden University Medical Centre (LUMC), P.O. Box 9600, 2300 RC Leiden, The Netherlands

Amir Raz, Department of Child & Adolescent Psychiatry, Columbia University and the New York State Psychiatry Institute

Charles Reynolds III, Western Psychiatric Institute and Clinic, Room E-1135, 3811 O'Hara Street, Pittsburgh, PA 15213, USA

Lisa Reynolds, Health Psychology Department, The University of Auckland, Private Bag 92019, Auckland, New Zealand

Lena Ring, Department of Pharmacy, Uppsala University, BMC, Box 580, Mercer Street Lower, 751 23 Uppsala, Sweden

Kathryn Robb, Cancer Research UK Health Behaviour Unit, Department of Epidemiology and Public Health, University College London, 2-16 Torrington Place, London WC1E 6BT, UK

Katherine Roberts, Department of Health & Behavior Studies, Teachers College, Columbia University, Box 114, 525 W. 120th Street, New York NY 10027, USA

Michael Roberts, Clinical Child Psychology Program, University of Kansas, 2009 Dole Human Development Center, 1000 Sunnyside Avenue, Lawrence, KS 66045-7555, USA

Richard Rogers, Department of Psychology, Terril Hall 365, University of North Texas, P.O. Box 311277, Denton, Texas 76203, USA

Rachel Rowe, National Perinatal Epidemiology Unit, University of Oxford, Old Road Campus, Oxford OX3 7LF, UK

Meredith Rumble, Department of Psychiatry and Behavioral Sciences, Duke University Medical Center, Box 3159, Durham, NC 27710, USA

Nichola Rumsey, School of Psychology, Frenchay Campus, University of the West of England, Bristol BS16 1QI, UK

Jenny Rusted, Psychology Department, University of Sussex, Brighton BN1 9QH, UK

David Sam, Department of Psychological Science, University of Bergen, Bergen N-5015, Norway

Michael Sayette, Psychology Department, University of Pittsburgh, SENSQ 0000, Pittsburgh, PA 15260, USA

Graham Scambler, Centre for Behavioural and Social Sciences in Medicine, Wolfson Building, University College London, London W1W 7EY, UK

Jeanne Schaefer, Centre for Health Care Evaluation Veterans Affairs Health Care System, 795 Willow Road, Menlo Park, CA 94025, USA

Stephen Scheidt, Weill Medical College, Cornell University, 520 E. 70th Street - STARR-4, New York, USA

Andrew Scholey, Northumbria University, Newcastle upon Tyne, NE1 8ST, UK

Henk Schut, Research Institute for Psychology & Health, Utrecht University, Utrecht, The Netherlands

David Scott, Royal National Throat, Nose and Ear Hospital, Gray's Inn Road, London WC1X 8DA, UK

Suzanne Scott, Health Psychology Section, Institute of Psychiatry, King's College London, Thomas Guy House, London SE1 9RT, UK

Cristina Shafer, Institute for Health, Health Care Policy and Aging Research, Rutgers, The State University of New Jersey, New Brunswick, WJ 08901 USA

David Shaffer, Department of Psychology, University of Georgia, Athens, GA 30602-3013, USA

Lion Shahab, Cancer Research UK Health Behaviour Unit, Department of Epidemiology and Public Health, University College London, 2–16 Torrington Place, London WC1E 7HN, UK

Heather Shaw, Oregon Research Institute, 1715 Franklin Boulevard, Eugene, OR 97403, USA

Paschal Sheeran, Department of Psychology, University of Sheffield, Sheffield S10 2TN, UK

Lorraine Sherr, Department of Primary Care and Population Science, Royal Free and University College Medical School, Rowland Hill Street, London NW3 2PF, UK

Shoshana Shiloh, Department of Psychology, Tel Aviv University, Tel Aviv 69978, Israel

Jonathan Silverman, Clinical Skills Unit, School of Clinical Medicine, University of Cambridge, Box 111, Addenbrooke's Hospital, Hills Road, Cambridge CB2 2SP, UK

Alice Simon, Cancer Research UK Health Behaviour Unit, Department of Epidemiology and Public Health, University College London, 2-16 Torrington Place, London WC1E 6BT, UK

Laura Simonelli, Department of Psychology, The Ohio State University, 1885 Neil Avenue Mall, Columbus, OH 43210-1222, USA

Ellen Skinner, Psychology Department, Portland State University, P.O. Box 751, Portland, OR 97207-0751, USA

Pauline Slade, Clinical Psychology Unit, Department of Psychology, University of Sheffield, S10 2UR, UK

Richard Slatcher, The University of Texas at Austin, 1 University Station, A 8000, Austin, TX 78712-0187, USA

Christopher Smith, Albert Einstein College of Medicine, Yeshiva University, 1300 Morris Park Avenue, Bronx, NY 10461, USA

Nicoletta Sonino, Department of Statistical Science, University of Padova, Padova, Italy

Kym Spathonis, Cancer Prevention Research Centre, School of Population Health, The University of Queensland, Brisbane, Australia

Matthew Speltz, Department of Psychiatry Behavioral Sciences, University of Washington School of Medicine, Children's Hospital & Regional Medical Center, Seattle, WA 98195, USA

Meagan Spence, Department of Health Psychology, The University of Auckland, Private Bag 92019, Auckland, New Zealand

Stacie Spencer, Department of Psychology, University of Pittsburgh, Pittsburgh, PA, 15260, USA

Ulrich Stangier, Friedrich-Schiller-Universität Jena, Fiir Psychologie, Humboldt-Street 11, Jena 07743, Germany

Annette Stanton, Department of Psychology, University of California, 1285 Franz Hall, Box 951563, UCLA, Los Angeles, CA 90095-1653, USA

Liz Steadman, Department of Applied Social Sciences, Canterbury Chirst Church University, North Holmes Road, Canterbury, Kent, CT1 1QU, UK

Christine Stephens, School of Psychology, Massey University, Private Bag 11-222, Palmerston North, New Zealand

Andrew Steptoe, Department of Epidemiology and Public Health, University College London, 1-19 Torrington Place, London WC1E 6EA, UK

Robert Sternberg, The School of Arts and Sciences, Tufts University, Ballou Hall, 3rd Floor, Medford MA 02155, USA

Jim Stevenson, School of Psychology, University of Southampton, Highfield Southampton SO17 1BJ, UK

Eric Stice, Oregon Research Institute, 1715 Franklin Boulevard, Eugene, OR 97403, USA

Stephanie Stone, Johns Hopkins University, 1119 Taylor Road Street, Baltimore, MD 21154, USA

Eric Storch, Department of Psychiatry, University of Florida, College of Medicine, G-030 HDG, Gainesville, FL 32610-0234, USA

Margaret Stroebe, Research Institute for Psychology & Health, Utrecht University, Utrecht, The Netherlands

Wolfgang Stroebe, Research Institute for Psychology & Health, Utrecht University, Utrecht, The Netherlands

Jan Stygall, Centre for Behavioural and Social Sciences in Medicine, University College London, 2nd Floor, Wolfson Building, 48 Riding House Street, London W1N 7EY, UK

Valerie Sutherland, Sutherland Bradely Associates, SO1 UKNals, RHQ AFNORTH, BFPO 28

Stephen Sutton, Institute of Public Health, University of Cambridge, Forvie Site, Robinson Way, Cambridge CB2 2SR, UK

Christine Temple, Developmental Neuropsychology Unit, Department of Psychology, University of Essex, Wivenhoe Park, Colchester CO4 3SQ, UK

Jennifer Thomas, Department of Psychology, Yale University, New Haven, CT 06520, USA

Ingela Thuné-Boyle, Department of Mental Health Sciences, University College London, Royal Free Hospital School of Medicine, Rowland Hill Street, London NW3 2PF, UK

Janet Treasure, Department of Academic Psychiatry, 5th Floor, Thomas Guy House, Guy's Campus, London SE1 9RT, UK

Michele Tugade, Department of Psychology, Vassar College, 124 Raymond Avenue, Poughkeepsie, NY 12604, USA

Dennis Turk, Department of Anesthesiology, University of Washington, P. O. Box 356540, Seattle, WA 98195, USA

Jeremy Turk, Department of Clinical Developmental Sciences, St. George's, University of London, London SW17 0RE, UK

Julie Turner-Cobb, Department of Psychology, University of Bath, Bath BA2 7AY, UK

Jane Ussher, School of Psychology, Bankstown Campus, University of Western Sydney, Locked Bag 1797, Pennith South DC, NSW 1797, Australia

Michael Ussher, Department of Community Health Sciences, St. George's Hospital Medical School, University of London, Cranmer Terrace, London, SW17 0RE, UK

Gerard van Galen, Nijmegen Institute for Cognition and Information, P.O. Box 904, NL 6500 HE NIJMEGEN, The Netherlands

Kristen van Kessel, Department of Health Psychology, The University of Auckland, Private Bag 92019, Auckland, New Zealand

Isidro Villanueva, Department of Psychology, Arizona State University, Tempe, AZ 85287-1104, USA

Charles Vincent, Department of Surgery and Anaesthetics, Imperial College School of Medicine, 10th Floor,

Queen Elizabeth the Queen Mother, St. Mary's Campus, London SW7 2AZ, UK

Claus Vögele, School of Human and Life Sciences, Roehampton University, Whitelands College, Holybourne Avenue, London SW15 4JD, UK

Janelle Wagner, Department of Pediatrics & Health Professions, Medical University of South Carolina, Charleston, South Carolina, USA

Kenneth Wallston, 421, Godchaux Hall, Vanderbilt University Medical Center, Nashville, TN37205, USA

Sandra Waters, Pain Prevention and Treatment Program, Duke University Medical Center, Durham, NC 27708, USA

John Weinman, Health Psychology Section, Institute of Psychiatry, King's College London, 5th Floor, University of London, Thomas Guy's House, London Bridge, London SE1 9RT, UK

Robert West, Cancer Research UK Health Behaviour Unit, Department of Epidemiology and Public Health, University College London, 2nd Floor, 2-16 Torrington Place, London WC1E 6BT, UK

Thomas Whelan, Nursing and Health Sciences, Monash University, Caulfield, MLB, Australia

Amanda C. de C. Williams, Department of Clinical Health Psychology, University College London, Gower Street, London WC1E 6BT, UK

Anne Williams, Napier University, Canaan Lane Campus, Edinburgh EH9 2TD, UK

Gail Williamson, Department of Psychology, University of Georgia, Athens, GA 30602-3013, USA

Thomas Wills, Albert Einstein College of Medicine, Yeshiva University, Jack and Pearl Resnick Campus, 1300 Morris Park Avenue, Belfer 1301, Bronx, NY 10461, USA

Barbara Wilson, MRC Cognition and Brain Sciences Unit, Addenbrooke's NHS Trust, Box 58, Elsworth House, Cambridge CB2 2QQ, UK

Gerhard Winneke, Heinrich-Heine-Universität Düsseldorf, Auf'm Hennekamp 50, D-40225 Düsseldorf, Germany

Emma Witt, Department of Health Psychology, The University of Auckland, Private Bag 92019, Auckland, New Zealand

Maria Woloshynowych, Department of Surgery and Anaesthetics, Imperial College School of Medicine, Queen Elizabeth the Queen Mother, St. Mary's Campus, London SW7 2AZ, UK

Alison Woodcock, Psychology Department, Royal Holloway, University of London, Egham, Surrey TW20 0EX, UK

Julia Woodward, Duke University Medical Center, Raleigh, North Carolina, USA

Linda Worrall, Communication Disability in Ageing Research Centre and Division of Speech Pathology, School of Health and Rehabilitation Sciences, The University of Queensland, Brisbane, Queensland 4072, Australia

Michael Worrell, Psychology Department, Royal Holloway, University of London, 7a Woodfield Road, London W9 2NW, UK

Peggilee Wupperman, Guthrie Annex, 1-137, Department of Psychology, University of Washington, USA

Lucy Yardley, Department of Psychology, University of Southampton, Southampton SO9 5NH, UK

Alex Zautra, Department of Psychology, Arizona State University, Tempe, AZ 85287-1104, USA

Preface

Health psychology is an established field, with an impact on many aspects of medical training, practice and research. Although there are some very good textbooks and handbooks of health psychology available, these are directed primarily at psychologists working in health-related areas. There has been a need for a comprehensive reference text suitable for medical practitioners who wish to be appraised of ways in which psychology can help them in their work. Such a book should also provide a unique resource for undergraduate and postgraduate medical education.

This book is intended as a comprehensive handbook for medical practitioners and health professionals, and for psychologists who work with health professionals. It will also be of interest to undergraduates undertaking psychology, medicine and other health-related courses, and to postgraduate students on MSc and PhD courses.

The book is in two parts.

Part I: Psychology, health and illness is in four sections and reviews the main theories and findings in psychology as applied to medicine, covering (i) psychological aspects of health and illness, (ii) psychological assessment, (iii) psychological intervention and (iv) psychological factors associated with the practice of healthcare.

Part II: Medical topics examines psychological theories and findings relevant to particular medical conditions, investigations, treatments and prophylaxes.

It will be apparent that the decision to place some chapters in Part II rather than Part I is a matter of judgement. In general, the decision was made on whether the topic appeared to cut across a range of illnesses or treatments. However, if the reader cannot find a topic in Part II, he or she is quite likely to find material relevant to it in Part I.

This is primarily a reference text and therefore it is expected that readers will seek out particular chapters for particular purposes. For this reason the chapters within each section are arranged alphabetically and the titles phrased in encyclopaedic language.

Inevitably there is some overlap between chapters dealing with related topics because each chapter is self-contained and we have tried to keep to a minimum the need for movement back and forth between entries.

Clinical practitioners will probably wish to use the book by looking up entries in Part II that are of interest, gaining further background information or clarification of concepts from Part I. Teachers will probably focus mostly on chapters in Part I as basic reading for courses on psychology as applied to medicine, using material from Part II as supplementary reading to show how basic principles can be applied.

Although we have attempted to make the book as comprehensive as possible, it would be unrealistic to imagine that a single text could encompass the whole field adequately. It must also be the case that there are topics that have not been addressed at all. However, we have tried to make the coverage as broad as possible, and keep such gaps to a minimum. For added depth of coverage, the extensive reference lists should be an invaluable resource.

This second edition has been a long time in gestation and the editors are deeply indebted to the contributors for their efforts in producing what we believe are some very fine chapters and for their patience. We believe that the effort has been worthwhile and that the result has been worth waiting for. We hope that the contributors and the readers will agree.

Finally, special thanks are due to Dr Katherine Joekes for her editorial assistance.

Susan Ayers
Andrew Baum
Chris McManus
Stanton Newman
Kenneth Wallston
John Weinman
Robert West

Part I

Psychology, health and illness

Psychological aspects of health and illness

Adolescent lifestyle

Leif Edvard Aarø
University of Bergen

Definitions

Leading organizations in the field of disease prevention and health promotion, such as the World Health Organization (Headquarters in Geneva, Switzerland) and the Centers for Disease Control (Atlanta, USA), have since the early 1980s used healthy lifestyles as a label for a cluster of behaviours known to reduce the risk of injury, morbidity and mortality and increase the chances of good health and well-being. Health-related behaviours (health-enhancing or health-compromising) include eating habits, physical exercise, smoking, alcohol use, use of illegal addictive substances, sexual practices, risk-taking in traffic, work etc., use of safety devices (for instance wearing safety helmets when biking), sleeping habits, oral hygiene and personal hygiene. Examples of health-related behaviours which are relevant only to specific ethnic groups are exposure to the sun in order to obtain a more tanned skin among Caucasians, or use of skin-whitening creams among ethnic groups with dark skin colours.

The concept of lifestyle is also used in other contexts. In the field of marketing, analysis of consumer lifestyles means examining the way people live (their activities, interests, values and opinions) in order to better tailor marketing efforts to specific target groups.

According to Elliott (1993):

... a lifestyle has been defined as a distinctive mode of living that is defined by a set of expressive, patterned behaviors of individuals occurring with some consistency over a period of time.

It should be evident from this definition that the lifestyle construct is not meant to capture the totality of a person's behaviour. There are three aspects that make lifestyles more specific: their consistency or relative stability over time, their interrelatedness (being patterned), and the meaning they convey to others as well as oneself (expressiveness). Health-related lifestyles refer to behaviours that have been shown by epidemiological and other health research to predict disease or health. A related term, 'risk-taking behaviour', refers to behaviour patterns which are volitional and which increase risk of disease of injury (Irvin, 1990).

The lifestyle concept is less accepted as a term in developing countries. In Lalonde's classic report on 'The health of Canadians' (Lalonde, 1974) the definition of lifestyle that was suggested implied that lifestyles are the result of choices made by individuals. The lifestyle of an individual is seen as the result of an aggregate of decisions made by the person him- or herself, decisions over which the person has considerable control. Environmental and social factors have, however, been shown to exert a powerful influence on health behaviours, even in affluent societies, and factors over which the individual person has limited or no control are obviously of even higher importance in developing countries (Eaton et al., 2004).

When defining 'adolescence', several criteria are relevant, for instance secondary sex characteristics, cognitive abilities, social criteria or simply age. According to Adams et al. (1994), adolescence covers the age-groups 11–20, and distinction is made between early adolescence (11–14), middle adolescence (15–17) and late adolescence (18–20). There is no global consensus regarding the definition of adolescence. The World Health Organization defines adolescence as the period from 10 to 19 years of age.

Defining adolescence as a period covering such a wide age-range may seem particularly relevant for affluent societies of the West. During recent decades, however, it has become clear that a transitional stage between childhood and adulthood is evident in most societies of the world. This expanded, more-distinct transitional period includes longer schooling, earlier puberty, later marriage, removal from full-time labour, and greater separation from the world of adults (Larson & Wilson, 2004). During this period of life, through a complex interplay between biological, physiological, psychological, social, societal and cultural factors, lifestyles are shaped.

Health behaviour change during adolescence

During adolescence a number of health-compromising behaviours emerge. When entering adolescence, children are normally spontaneously physically active, and there is hardly any use of tobacco, alcohol or other addictive substances. When leaving adolescence, a substantial proportion of adolescents are physically inactive, have started smoking, and some have started using illegal addictive substances. The sexual debut usually takes place during adolescence, and being sexually active without adequate protection against unwanted pregnancies and sexually transmitted diseases, including HIV/AIDS, represents a serious threat to health and wellbeing.

According to a report from the World Health Organization international study on Health Behaviour in School-Aged Children (HBSC), the proportion of smokers increases during early adolescence (Currie et al., 2004). At age 11 the average proportion of smokers (smoking daily or weekly) across all samples (35 countries) is 2%, at age 13 it is 8%, and at age 15 it is 24%. The differences between boys and girls for all countries combined (mainly European countries plus Canada and the United States) were negligible. Corresponding figures for weekly alcohol consumption are 5, 12 and 29%. More boys than girls used alcohol weekly at age 15 (34 and 24% respectively).

This chapter was prepared while the author was visiting scholar at the Department of Psychology, Stanford University, Palo Alto, California, USA. Grants were provided by the Norwegian Research Council and the University of Bergen, Faculty of Psychology.

Prochaska *et al.* (2001) have developed a screening instrument which defines 'moderate-to-vigorous physical activity' (MVPA). Their definition was applied to data from the HBSC study. The proportion of young people meeting the MVPA guidelines on physical activity was (across all samples) 38% at age 11 and 29% at age 15; in other words there is a marked decrease with age that most likely continues across the remaining years of adolescence as well as into early adulthood (Stephens *et al.*, 1984). Food habits were also covered by the HBSC survey. The proportion of adolescents who eat fruit daily decreases from 38% among 11 year olds to 29% among the 15 year olds (Currie *et al.*, 2004).

Thuen *et al.* (1992) have shown that use of safety equipment (seat belts, bicycle helmets, reflectors, life jackets) drops dramatically during early adolescence, and the proportion involved in behaviour associated with elevated risks of accidents and injuries increases.

It must be kept in mind, however, that a majority of young people never become regular smokers, heavy drinkers or drug addicts, and a substantial proportion of young adults remain physically active and continue eating healthy food throughout and after the adolescent years. During adolescence the basis for a lifelong health-enhancing lifestyle may be established.

The effects of health-compromising behaviours during adolescence can be short-term as well as long-term. Drink driving increases the risk of dramatic and fatal accidents, and represents a major short-term threat to young people's health and lives. Daily smoking may lead to coronary heart disease and lung cancer, but these effects usually become visible only after many years of exposure. The importance of promoting healthy lifestyles among adolescents therefore to some extent depends on the stability of such behaviours. The higher the stability, the more important it is to promote healthy lifestyles at a young age.

Jessor *et al.* (1991) have studied the stability of problem behaviours from adolescence to adulthood, and conclude that there is considerable stability and continuity. They claim that 'the adolescent is parent of the young adult'.

Although few research projects have focused on the stability and change of physical activity from childhood to adolescence, there is one study which concludes that the level of physical activity in childhood and adolescence to some extent predicts the level of physical activity later in life (Anderssen *et al.*, 1996). Other studies of longitudinal tracking of behaviours (physical activity, food preference and smoking behaviour), have provided convincing evidence that behaviours established during early adolescence do predict behaviours measured during late adolescence and beyond (Klepp, 1993; Kelder *et al.*, 1994; Telama *et al.*, 1997). Substantial tracking has also been found for body mass index over an 18 years' age span (from 15 to 33 years) (Kvaavik *et al.*, 2003).

The promotion of healthy lifestyles among young people is obviously important, not only because of its short-term impact on health and wellbeing, but also because of its consequences for health-related behaviours later in life.

Clusters of health behaviours

A number of studies have examined to what extent health behaviours are intercorrelated, and to what extent these correlations reflect underlying clusters or dimensions. Analyses from the international study on Health Behaviour in School-Aged Children indicated two such underlying dimensions: (a) addictive and risk-taking behaviours and (b) health-enhancing behaviours (Nutbeam *et al.*, 1991; Aarø *et al.*, 1995). The correlation between the two factors was negative and estimates varied from approximately −0.40 to −0.50. Within these two 'second order factors', sub-clusters of health-related behaviours could also be identified. Røysamb *et al.* (1997) identified factors at three levels, a multidimensional level with a number of specific factors, a few-dimensional level with three broad factors, and finally a general factor encompassing the three broad factors. The three broad factors were 'High action', 'Addiction' and 'Protection'.

The addictive dimension corresponds well with Richard Jessor's 'problem behaviours' (Jessor & Jessor, 1977; Jessor, 1984). He claims that a number of health-related behaviours reflect a 'syndrome', or an underlying tendency to behave defiantly and unconventionally. He includes such behaviours as use of alcohol, marijuana and tobacco, and he maintains that these are associated with a higher likelihood of involvement in other types of risk behaviour, such as precocious sexual activity, aggression and delinquency. Jessor maintains that for these behaviours the pattern of associations with a number of personality and social environmental correlates is essentially the same.

Health-enhancing behaviours, which in some studies form a second factor, include physical activity, consumption of healthy food, oral hygiene, use of safety devices (seat belts, reflectors, etc.) and use of vitamins. The diffusion of innovation processes, which have been described by Everett Rogers, may serve as a framework for explaining why such behaviours are intercorrelated (Rogers, 2003). If we assume that health-education and health-promotion activities reach and influence health behaviours in certain individuals and certain groups to a larger extent than in other individuals and other groups, correlations among a range of health-enhancing behaviours tend to emerge.

Intercorrelations and clusters of intercorrelations among health-behaviour variables imply that they do not exist as independent and unique domains. Their interrelatedness indicates the usefulness of the notion of 'lifestyles'. It may be argued that such intercorrelations indicate similarities in the processes underlying different health behaviours. Furthermore, intercorrelations between health behaviours imply overlap in target groups across behavioural risk factors, and support the notion of a more integrated and holistic approach to health promotion among adolescents (Nutbeam *et al.*, 1991).

Predictors and correlates of health behaviours

A number of conceptual models and theories are relevant in order to identify factors and processes that influence health-related behaviours. The mainstream of health behaviour research is dominated by social cognition models (Rutter & Quine, 2002; Conner & Norman, 2005). A group of experts at a meeting organized by the National Institute of Health (NIH) came to the conclusion that the most important predictors were intentions, skills, environmental constraints, anticipated outcomes (or attitudes), social norms, self efficacy, self-standards and emotions (Fishbein *et al.*, 2001). They did not reach consensus regarding any specific theoretical or conceptual model by which these factors could be arranged into a single causal system. Among the most influential theories are Social Cognitive Theory (Bandura, 1986) and the Theory of Planned Behaviour (Ajzen, 1988). Ajzen assumes that a specific behaviour is determined to a large extent by intentions to perform the behaviour, and that such intentions are influenced by personal attitudes to the behaviour, subjective norms and perceived behavioural control. Rather than simply assuming that such factors as attitudes and perceived behavioural control are predictors, while behaviours are outcomes, we must suppose that there is an ongoing and continuous process of reciprocal determinism (Bandura, 1986). Bandura sees behaviours as shaped by an ongoing process of interrelationships with personal and environmental factors. Key concepts in Bandura's analyses of health behaviours are goals (proximal and distal), outcome expectations and self-efficacy (Bandura, 1998; 2005).

Although the major determinants of health-related lifestyles among adolescents are social, some personality characteristics have been shown to be consistently associated with 'problem behaviours'. Jessor claims that in the personality system, the main characteristics of proneness to problem behaviour include placing a lower value on academic achievement and lower expectations of academic achievement (Jessor, 1984). The sensation-seeking personality trait (Zuckermann, 1979) has been shown to correlate with such problem behaviours as smoking, alcohol consumption, number of lifetime sex partners and experience of casual sex (Kraft & Rise, 1994).

The cross-cultural relevance of theories and conceptual models for prediction of health behaviours developed in western countries has repeatedly been questioned (Campbell, 2003). Jessor et al. (2003), in a study of predictors of problem behaviours among adolescents in the United States and China, came to the conclusion that although the levels of problem behaviours may be different, the same set of predictors (protective factors and risk factors) seem to be relevant in these two widely different societies and cultures. The relevance of social cognition models in an African context is currently being examined in a large-scale multi-site study of sexual and reproductive behaviours (Aarø et al., 2006).

Structural and demographic factors

Health-compromising lifestyles are to a large extent a product of the modern world. Physical inactivity is fostered by modern means of transport and by passive exposure to TV channels, DVD movies, internet use and PC games. Widespread use of addictive substances may reflect a weakening of social norms and the deterioration of social networks. Broken families and family problems may lead to reduced parental control over food habits, sleeping habits and use of addictive substances.

Changes in health behaviours do not take place at the same speed and simultaneously in all groups. In the industrialized countries the use of tobacco first became widespread among men and among high-status groups. Presently, high-status groups have reduced their use of tobacco substantially. Low-status groups are falling behind, and in many countries the prevalence of regular smokers in low-status segments of the population is 3–4 times higher than among those belonging to high-status segments (Ferrence, 1996). Similar processes can be observed for other health behaviours. Belonging to high-status groups means that you are also more

likely to be physically active, to eat healthy food and to wear seat belts, just to mention some examples.

Since health behaviours of adolescents are closely related to those of their parents, similar socioeconomic inequalities may exist for adolescents as well. Adolescents are in a process of transition from having their socioeconomic status defined by their parents' education, income and jobs towards having their socioeconomic status defined by their own position in the societal structure. Several studies have reported rather moderate or weak associations between parents' level of education and offspring's health behaviours (Friestad & Klepp, 2006). Problems with obtaining valid and reliable measurements of parents' level of education may have contributed to reducing the strength of associations. Adolescents' relationship to school and education has sometimes been used as an indicator of their socioeconomic position. Friestad & Klepp (2006) found consistent associations between educational aspirations and composite measures of health behaviour (low aspirations predicting high scores on health-compromising behaviours and low scores on health-enhancing behaviours). Nutbeam et al. (1988; 1993) found strong associations between school alienation and use of addictive substances (tobacco and alcohol). This indicates that a socioeconomic gradient in lifestyles also exists for adolescents. Researchers have concluded that health-related behaviours to some extent carry over from one generation to the next, and that a process of social reproduction of socioeconomic inequalities in lifestyles can be demonstrated (Wold, 1989; Ketterlinus et al., 1994). Other researchers have found empirical support for adolescent lifestyles being predictive of future socioeconomic status (Koivusilta et al., 1999).

Health behaviours are also influenced by such factors as advertising, legislation (including bans on advertising), price and availability of products. Increasing the price of tobacco products leads to a decrease in consumption, and this decrease is higher among adolescents than among adults. Among adults the price elasticity is probably close to −0.5. A price elasticity of −0.5 means that increasing the price by 10% leads to a 5% reduction in consumption. The price elasticity is particularly high among young people. In one study it was shown to be −1.40 among 12–17 year olds (Warner, 1986).

The effects of tobacco advertising and the effects of banning such advertising on smoking habits of adolescents have been debated. The tobacco industry has aggressively defended their right to market legal products, while health authorities, health professionals and non-governmental organizations have argued that bans on all kinds of tobacco advertising are necessary in order to reduce smoking among adolescents. An increasing body of research gives both theoretical and empirical evidence for a causal relationship between advertising and use of tobacco, and it is likely that 'the dynamic tobacco market represented by children and adolescents' is the main target of tobacco sales promotion (Rimpelä et al., 1993). Braverman & Aarø (2004), in a study among adolescents, found that even low levels of exposure to tobacco marketing was associated with stronger expectations of future smoking, after controlling for present smoking habits and important social predictors of smoking. Longitudinal studies have consistently shown that exposure to tobacco advertising is associated with increased risk that adolescents will start to smoke (Lovato et al., 2003). It is reasonable to assume that effectively enforced bans on advertising contribute to reducing smoking among adolescents. In order to make the healthy choices the easiest ones, the prices of healthy products should be kept low, the prices of unhealthy products should be high, and for young people in particular, the availability of unhealthy products like alcohol and cigarettes should be limited as much as possible.

Health-behaviour interventions

Health-behaviour interventions targeting adolescents take place in the mass media, schools and communities. Examples of programmes that have not proven effective are numerous. There are also, however, examples of well-designed and research-based interventions that have had substantial effects. Kirby & Coyle (1997) reviewed 35 evaluations of school-based sexual education programmes, and found that a few programmes had contributed to delaying the onset of intercourse, reduced the frequency of intercourse, reduced number of sexual partners, or increased the use of condoms or other contraceptives. For the majority of the programmes, however, no statistical effects on risk-taking behaviours were observed. Thomas (2002) reviewed 76 randomized controlled trials of school-based interventions to prevent smoking. Among interventions based on the social influence approach, which has been regarded as the most effective approach to smoking prevention among adolescents, half of the studies showed statistically significant effects of the interventions. Jøsendal et al. (2005) found that a three-year programme based on the social-influence model reduced the prevalence of smoking by about 30%. Positive results have also been found for school-based interventions to reduce drug use (Faggiano et al., 2005).

There is less strong evidence for positive effects of mass-media and community-based interventions (Sowden & Arblaster, 1998; Sowden et al., 2003). This does not necessarily mean that such interventions are ineffective. Planning and conducting studies with strong research designs and demonstrating significant effects of interventions is much easier in schools than in most other settings. In addition, programmes which have no visible immediate effects on behaviour, may contribute to raising awareness, and changing beliefs, attitudes and social norms, and they may lead to increased support for restrictive and societal measures. Such indicators of change may, in the long term, trigger processes that are just as important for behaviour change in populations as programmes that succeed in bringing about immediate effects on behaviour.

Adolescents in developing countries

Among 1.2 billion adolescents worldwide, about 85% live in developing countries, and this proportion is increasing. Also, in the developing world, health-compromising lifestyles are gradually becoming a threat to health, and in developing countries such behaviours become more prevalent during adolescence. Research has shown that increasing production and consumption of alcohol is taking place in both rural and urban areas in Africa (Maula et al., 1988). Parallel with the reduction in tobacco smoking in Western Europe and North America, effective marketing contributes to increasing the prevalence of smoking in developing countries and in Eastern Europe (World Bank, 1999).

Eide & Acuda (1996) in a study from Zimbabwe showed that cultural influences from industrialized countries are accompanied by introduction of forms of alcohol use which are less well regulated by rituals and social norms than the use of traditional beverages. Young people with a 'western' cultural orientation have alcohol preferences which are different from those with a more traditional cultural orientation, and their consumption is higher. Similar cultural influences may operate on a variety of health behaviours, and the introduction of a 'modern' lifestyle may lead to a gradual increase in diseases which used to be typical of western countries. This adds health burdens and economic burdens to nations which are already confronted with infectious diseases (including the AIDS pandemic) and overwhelming health problems caused by poverty, poor housing, malnutrition, inadequate sanitation and lack of clean water.

REFERENCES

Aarø, L. E., Laberg, J. C. & Wold, B. (1995). Health behaviours among adolescents: towards a hypothesis of two dimensions. *Health Education Research*, **10**(1), 83–93.

Aarø, L. E., Flisher, A. J., Kaaya, S. et al. (2006). Promoting sexual and reproductive health in early adolescence in South Africa and Tanzania: development of a theory- and evidence-based intervention programme. *Scandinavian Journal of Public Health*, **34**(2), 150–8.

Adams, G. R., Gullotta, T. P. & Markstrom-Adams, C. (1994). *Adolescent Life Experiences*, (3rd edn). Pacific Grove, California: Brooks/Cole.

Ajzen, I. (1988). *Attitudes, personality, and behaviour*. Buckingham: Open University Press, UK.

Anderssen, N., Jacobs, D. R., Sidney, S. et al. (1996). Change and secular trends in physical activity patterns in young adults: a seven-year longitudinal follow-up in the Coronary Artery Risk Development in Young Adults Study (CARDIA). *American Journal of Epidemiology*, **143**(4), 351–62.

Bandura, A. (1986). *Social foundations of thought & action. A social cognitive theory.* Englewood Cliffs, New Jersey: Prentice-Hall.

Bandura, A. (1998). Health promotion from the perspective of social cognitive theory. *Psychology and Health*, **13**, 623–49.

Bandura, A. (2005). Health promotion by social cognitive means. *Health Education and Behavior*, **13**, 623–49.

Braverman, M. T. & Aarø, L. E. (2004). Adolescent smoking and exposure to tobacco marketing under a tobacco advertising ban: findings from 2 Norwegian national samples. *American Journal of Public Health*, **94**(7), 1230–8.

Campbell, C. (2003). *'Letting them die' – Why HIV/AIDS prevention programmes fail*. Oxford: The International African Institute.

Conner, M. & Norman, P. (2005). *Predicting Health Behaviour*, (2nd edn). Maidenhead, UK: Open University Press.

Currie, C., Roberts, C., Morgan, A. et al. (2004). *Young people's health in context*. Copenhagen: World Health Organization for Europe. (Health Policy for Children and Adolescents, No. 4.)

Eaton, L., Flisher, A. J. & Aarø, L. E. (2004). Unsafe sexual behavior in South African youth. In Djamba, Y. K. (Ed.). *Sexual behavior of adolescents in contempary sub-Saharan Africa*. Lewiston, New York: Edwin Mellen Press, pp. 65–109.

Eide, A. H. & Acuda, S. W. (1996). Cultural orientation and adolescents' alcohol use in Zimbabwe. *Addiction*, **91**(6), 807–14.

Elliott, D. S. (1993). Health enhancing and health-compromising lifestyles. In Millstein, S., Petersen, A. C. & Nightingale, E. O. (Eds.). *Promoting the health of adolescents. New directions for the twenty-first century.* New York: Oxford University Press, pp. 119–45.

Faggiano, F., Vigna-Taglianti, F. D., Versino, E., Zambon, A., Borracino, A. & Lemma, P. (2005). School-based prevention for illicit drugs' use. *Cochrane Database of Systematic Reviews,* **2005**(2), CD003020.

Ferrence, R. (1996). Using diffusion theory in health promotion. *Canadian Journal of Public Health,* **87**(Suppl. 2), S24–7.

Fishbein, M., Triandis, H. C., Kanfer, F. H., Becker, M., Middlestadt, S. E. & Eichler, A. (2001). Factors influencing behavior and behavior change. In Baum, A., Revenson, T. A. & Singer, J. E. (Eds.). *Handbook of health psychology.* Mahwah, New Jersey: Lawrence Erlbaum Associates.

Friestad, C. & Klepp, K.-I. (2006). Socioeconomic status and health behaviour patterns through adolescence: results from a prospective cohort study in Norway. *European Journal of Public Health,* **16**(1), 41–7.

Irvin, C. E. Jr. (1990). The theoretical concept of at-risk adolescents. *Adolescent Medicine: State of the Art Reviews,* **1**, 1–14.

Jessor, R. & Jessor, S. L. (1977). *Problem behavior and psychosocial development: a longitudinal study of youth.* New York: Academic Press.

Jessor, R. (1984). Adolescent development and behavioral health. In Matarazzo, J. D., Weiss, S. M., Herd, J. A., Miller, N. E. & Weiss, S. M. (Eds.). *Behavioral health: a handbook of health enhancement and disease prevention.* New York: Wiley, pp. 69–90.

Jessor, R., Donovan, J. E. & Costa, F. M. (1991). *Beyond adolescence. Problem behavior and young adult development.* New York: Cambridge University Press.

Jessor, R., Turbin, M. S., Costa, F. M., Dong, Q., Zhang, H. & Wang, C. (2003). Adolescent problem behavior in China and the United States: a cross-national study of psychosocial protective factors. *Journal of Research on Adolescence,* **13**(3), 329–60.

Jøsendal, O., Aarø, L. E., Torsheim, T. & Rasbash, J. (2005). Evaluation of the school-based smoking prevention program "BE smokeFREE". *Scandinavian Journal of Psychology,* **46**, 189–99.

Kelder, S. H., Perry, C. L., Klepp, K.-I. & Lytle, L. L. (1994). Longitudinal tracking of adolescent smoking, physical activity, and food choice behaviors. *American Journal of Public Health,* **84**(7), 1121–6.

Ketterlinus, R. D., Lamb, M. E. & Nitz, K. A. (1994). Adolescent nonsexual and sex-related problem behaviors: their prevalence, consequences, and co-occurrence. In Ketterlinus, R. D. & Lamb, M. E. (Eds.). *Adolescent problem behaviors.*

Issues and research. Hillsdale: New Jersey: Lawrence Erlbaum Associates.

Kirby, D. & Coyle, K. (1997). School-based programs to reduce sexual risk-taking behavior. *Children and Youth Services Review,* **19**(5/6), 415–36.

Klepp, K.-I. (1993). The Oslo Youth Study: a 12 year follow-up study of a school-based health education program. *HEMIL report,* **1993**(2), 94–106.

Koivusilta, L. K., Rimpelä, A. H. & Rimpelä, M. K. (1999). Health-related lifestyle in adolescence – origin of social class differences in health? *Health Education Research,* **14**, 339–55.

Kraft, P. & Rise, J. (1994). The relationship between sensation seeking and smoking, alcohol consumption and sexual behavior among Norwegian adolescents. *Health Education Research,* **9**(2), 193–200.

Kvaavik, E., Tell, G. S. & Klepp, K.-I. (2003). Predictors and tracking of body mass index from adolescence into adulthood: follow-up of 18 to 20 years in the Oslo Youth Study. *Archives of Pediatrics and Adolescent Medicine,* **157**(12), 1212–18.

Lalonde, M. (1974). *A new perspective on the health of Canadians.* Ottawa, Canada: Ministry of Health and Welfare.

Larson, R. & Wilson, S. (2004). Adolescence across place and time. Globalization and the changing pathways to adulthood. In Lerner, R. M. & Steinberg, L. (Eds.). *Handbook of Adolescent Psychology,* (2nd edn). Hoboken, New Jersey: Wiley, pp. 299–330.

Lovato, C., Linn, G., Stead, L. F. & Best, A. (2003). Impact of tobacco advertising and promotion on increasing adolescent smoking behaviours. *Cochrane Database of Systematic Reviews,* **2003**(4), CD003439.

Maula, J., Lindblad, M. & Tigerstedt, C. (1988). *Alcohol in developing countries. Proceedings from a meeting in Oslo, Norway, August 7–9, 1988.* Helsinki: Nordic Council for Alcohol and Drug Research. (NAD Publication No 18).

Nutbeam, D., Aarø, L. E. & Catford, J. (1988). Understanding children's health behaviour: the implications for health promotion for young people. *Social Science and Medicine,* **29**(3), 317–25.

Nutbeam, D., Aarø, L. E. & Wold, B. (1991). The lifestyle concept and health education with young people. Results from a WHO international survey. *World Health Statistics Quarterly,* **44**(2), 55–61.

Nutbeam, D., Smith, C., Moore, L. & Bauman, A. (1993). Warning! Schools can damage your health: alienation from school and its impact on health behaviour. *Journal of Paediatrics and Child Health,* **29**(1), 25–30.

Prochaska, J. J., Sallis, J. F. & Long, B. (2001). A physical activity screening measure for use with adolescents in primary care. *Archives of Paediatrics and Adolescent Medicine,* **155**, 554–9.

Rimpelä, M. K., Aarø, L. E. & Rimpelä, A. H. (1993). The effects of tobacco sales promotion on initiation of smoking. *Scandinavian Journal of Social Medicine, Supplementum,* **49**, 1–23.

Rogers, E. M. (2003). *Diffusion of innovations* (5th edn). New York: The Free Press.

Rutter, D. & Quine, L. (2002). *Changing health behaviour: intervention and research with social cognition models.* Buckingham, UK: Open University Press.

Røysamb, E., Rise, J. & Kraft, P. (1997). On the structure and dimensionality of health-related behaviour in adolescents. *Psychology and Health,* **12**, 437–52.

Sowden, A. J. & Arblaster, L. (1998). Mass media interventions for preventing smoking in young people. *Cochrane Database of Systematic Reviews,* **1998**(4), CD001006.

Sowden, A., Arblaster, L. & Stead, L. (2003). Community interventions for preventing smoking in young people. *Cochrane Database of Systematic Reviews,* **2003**(1), CD001291.

Stephens, T., Jacobs, D. R. & White, C. C. (1984). A descriptive epidemiology of leisure-time physical activity. *Public Health Reports,* **100**(2), 147–58.

Telama, R. *et al.* (1997). Physical activity in childhood and adolescence as predictor of physical activity in young adulthood. *American Journal of Preventive Medicine,* **13**(4), 317–23.

Thomas, R. (2002). School-based programmes for preventing smoking. *Cochrane Database of Systematic Reviews,* **2002**(2), CD001293.

Thuen, F., Klepp, K.-I. & Wold, B. (1992). Risk-seeking and safety-seeking behaviours: a study of health-related behaviours among Norwegian school children. *Health Education Research,* **7**(2), 269–76.

Warner, K. E. (1986). Smoking and health implications of a change in the federal cigarette excise tax. *Journal of the American Medical Association,* **255**(8), 1028–32.

Wold, B. (1989). *Lifestyles and physical activity. A theoretical and empirical analysis of socialization among children and adolescents.* Doctoral thesis. Bergen: University of Bergen, Research Centre for Health Promotion.

World Bank (1999). *Curbing the epidemic – governments and the economics of tobacco control.* Washington, DC: The World Bank.

Zuckerman, M. (1979). *Sensation seeking. Beyond the optimal level of arousal.* London: Lawrence Erlbaum Associates.

Age and physical functioning

Gail M. Williamson and David R. Shaffer
University of Georgia

Over the life span, the human body increasingly functions less efficiently. Skin wrinkles and sags; hair thins and turns grey; muscle mass and strength are more difficult to maintain; joints deteriorate; aerobic capacity and cardiac output decrease; the immune system becomes less responsive; visual and auditory acuity decline – and this is just a partial list. Faced with these changes, it is not surprising that many people dread growing old because they believe ageing portends losses in functional capacities and the enjoyable aspects of life. This chapter highlights the demographic realities of an ageing population, debunks some of the myths about age and physical functioning and summarizes research on the factors that promote successful ageing.

There is no doubt that the population of many western countries is 'greying'[1]. Average life expectancy in the US in 1900 was 47 years; today, it is closer to 76 years. Over two-thirds of people now live to at least age 65 (a three-fold increase from 1900). Furthermore, the fastest growing segment of the population is in the category over age 85 – 4% in 1900 to more than 10% today (e.g. US Department of Health and Human Services [DHHS], 1992; Volz, 2000). The first wave of the 76 million baby boomers born in the USA between 1946 and 1964 will approach traditional retirement age in 2010 (Binstock, 1999); in less than 30 years, there will be twice as many people 65 years of age and older, comprising 20% or more of the total population (e.g. Hobbs, 1996). By 2050, the number of centenarians (those over age 100) in the USA may be as high as 4.2 million (Volz, 2000).

The common view of old people is that they are physically disabled (e.g. Center for the Advancement of Health [CAH], 1998; Palmore, 1990; Rowe & Kahn, 1998), but an important truth is that most adults over age 65 are remarkably healthy and active. Rates of disability, even among the very old (i.e. those over age 95), are steadily declining. Only 5.2% of older adults in the USA live in nursing homes and similar facilities, a decrease of 1.1% since 1982 (CAH, 1998). In 1994, 73% of adults 78–84 years of age reported no disabling conditions and among the 'oldest old' (i.e. those over age 85), fully 40% had no functional disabilities (Manton *et al.*, 1995). Changing health status and attitudes have led to age 65 no longer being considered 'old' (Kiyak & Hooyman, 1999).

Along with increasingly widespread public knowledge and acceptance of the behavioural aspects of chronic illness, advances in medical technology forecast less age-related functional decline for current and future generations (DHHS, 1992). Through medical and psychological research, we know that the human body is remarkably forgiving (CAH, 1998) and that it is never too late to begin a healthful lifestyle. For example, regardless of duration of smoking and magnitude of tobacco consumption, after five years of abstinence, ex-smokers have about the same risk for heart disease as those who never smoked. The same is true for a variety of other risk factors, including obesity and a sedentary lifestyle. Thus, people, both young and old, bear some responsibility for their health status; the 'use it or lose it' adage about sexual functioning applies to other aspects of physical functioning as well. However, in addition to the inevitable physical decrements that accompany ageing, numerous psychosocial factors influence wellbeing in old age.

Physical, mental and social wellbeing are intertwined, and ageing successfully depends, to a large extent, on effective coping in all of these domains. In terms of the association between physical and mental health, physical illness and depression are closely, perhaps inextricably, linked, and the direction of causality remains a subject of considerable debate (see Williamson *et al.*, 2000a). With their age-related decrements in physical functioning, one might assume, as Rowe & Kahn (1998, p. 106) alleged, that 'depression is ... terribly prevalent in older people', but evidence is overwhelmingly to the contrary. In fact, clinically diagnosable depression is less prevalent in older than younger adults (e.g. Rybash *et al.*, 1995; Schulz & Ewen, 1993). Rather, elders often cope more effectively with stressful life events than do younger adults (McCrae, 1989). The prevailing explanation is that, over the life course, experiences and successes in coping with a variety of stressors build adaptive attitudes and beliefs that generalize to coping with new stressors (see Williamson & Dooley, 2001). Being able to find satisfying replacements for activities that have been given up may be as beneficial as not having to give up activities at all (Benyamini & Lomranz, 2004). Individuals who are able to continue engaging in valued activities cope well with life changes, avoid becoming depressed, and are physically healthier. They are also those who have high levels of social and personal resources.

One of the strongest and most consistent findings in health psychology research is that social support has powerful effects on both psychological and physical wellbeing (e.g. Cohen & McKay, 1983; Cohen & Wills, 1985) (see 'Social Support and Health'). It is true that social network losses occur over the life span through death, relocation and retirement, but even among very old people, new relationships are formed to replace lost ones (Rowe & Kahn, 1998).

---

[1] Most of the data reported in this chapter are based on trends in the population of the United States. All industrialized countries are facing similar situations, however, and emerging nations may soon be dealing with even more extreme increases in the proportions of older adults in their populations (e.g. Hendricks, Hatch & Cutler, 1999). We have chosen to focus on US-based data, but the conditions in other countries are either highly analogous to, or even more critical than, indicated in this chapter.

Using data from the MacArthur Foundation Study of Ageing in America indicating that social networks remain remarkably stable in size throughout the life span, with the number of close relationships among non-institutionalized older adults equaling those of younger people, Rowe & Kahn (1998, pp. 159–60) concluded that '... the common view of old age as a prolonged period of demanding support from an ever-diminishing number of overworked providers *is wrong*' [emphasis added].

Today's ageing adults also have other social advantages. Many are utilizing technology and cyberspace to stay in touch with family members and friends via email. Baby boomers are more likely than their younger counterparts to access internet information and support from a wide spectrum of people who share their needs and concerns (Kiyak & Hooyman, 1999). Another important way to maintain social contact after retirement is through activities outside the home. When given the opportunity, large numbers of seniors are eager to do voluntary work or take on low-paid part-time jobs (e.g. working in fast-food restaurants and bagging groceries). Moreover, relative to previous cohorts, current and future generations will be more advantaged in the employment domain as they age. Not only are attitudes about older employees becoming more favorable, but also, because of post-baby boom declines in birth rates, the number of employable adults will decrease relative to the number of new jobs (DHHS, 1992; Kiyak & Hooyman, 1999). Consequently, older workers will become more valued and sought after, and those who do not feel ready to retire will be less likely to be compelled to do so. The standard retirement age is rising, based on observations that, in terms of health and life expectancy, age 70 today is roughly the equivalent of age 65 in the 1930s when Social Security was established in the USA (e.g. Chen, 1994). Although most individuals who have adequate (or better) financial resources will retire at the usual time or follow the trend toward early retirement (e.g. Quinn & Burkhauser, 1990), physically healthy elders will be able to choose whether or not they will continue to work.

The point here is that the sense of personal control is critical. People who feel in control, who can make choices about the important aspects of their lives, are both physically and psychologically healthier than are those who perceive that they lack personal control (e.g. Peterson et al., 1988; Taylor, 1983; Taylor & Brown, 1988). Older adults are not unique in this respect. Regardless of age, people are motivated to exercise personal control (e.g. Schulz & Heckhausen, 1996). Although fully resolving the problems that go along with getting older (e.g. declines in health status) may not be possible, those who adapt well will shift their focus from actively trying to change the situation to managing stress-related emotional reactions by, for example, accepting the situation and continuing to function as normally as possible, thus maintaining a sense of personal control. Today's trend toward less stigmatization of older adults offers seniors more choices, as do other societal changes. For example, economic prosperity has created financial security for many current and future older Americans, enabling them to exercise control over how they spend their retirement years.

Closely tied to the benefits of maintaining a sense of control is a substantial literature on the importance of being able to continue valued activities. Continuity in social roles and personal identities appears to be a critical factor in ageing successfully (e.g. Atchley, 1989; Benyamini & Lomranz, 2004; Calderon, 2001; Ogilvie, 1987;

Zimmer et al., 1995). In response to earlier research (e.g. Parmelee et al., 1991; Williamson & Schulz, 1992), Williamson and colleagues devised the Activity Restriction Model of Depressed Affect (ARMDA), defining activity restriction as the inability to continue normal activities (self-care, care of others, doing household chores, going shopping, visiting friends, working on hobbies, sports and recreation, going to work and maintaining friendships). The ARMDA proposes that activity restriction mediates the association between stress and mental health. In other words, major life stressors (e.g. age-related health problems) lead to poorer mental health outcomes because they disrupt normal activities. An extensive programme of research supports this model (Walters & Williamson, 1999; Williamson, 2000; Williamson & Dooley, 2001; Williamson & Schulz, 1992, 1995; Williamson et al., 1994; Williamson & Shaffer, 2000; Williamson et al., 1998; Williamson et al., 2000b; also see Benyamini & Lomranz, 2004; Zeiss et al., 1996).

As a comprehensive conceptualization of the physical illness–mental health association, the ARMDA posits that losses in physical functioning are not the only contributors to activity restriction. Rather, individual differences are important factors as well. For example, older adults tolerate similar levels of pain better than younger adults do (Cassileth et al., 1984; Foley, 1985; Williamson & Schulz, 1992), a phenomenon most commonly attributed to the increased exposure to pain and disabling conditions that older people encounter. Indeed, less experience with pain and comprising health conditions is a better predictor of more activity restriction than is chronological age (Walters & Williamson, 1999; Williamson & Schulz, 1995; Williamson et al., 1998). Thus, old age does not necessarily foster activity restriction and depression.

As noted previously, another important individual difference is social support. People with stronger social support networks cope better with all types of stressful life events (e.g. Mutran et al., 1995; Oxman & Hull, 1997), and routine activities are facilitated by supportive others (e.g. Williamson et al., 1994). For example, disabled elders will attend church and visit friends more often if other people help with walking, transportation and words of encouragement. However, social support, to a large extent, depends on personality variables (e.g. Williamson & Dooley, 2001). Those with more supportive social ties, less activity restriction and lower levels of depressed affect also have more socially desirable, proactive personality characteristics (e.g. Abend & Williamson, 2002; Williamson, 1998, 2000).

Dispositionally, some people cope in maladaptive ways across all situations throughout their lives. In contrast, there are those who consistently face the situation, rationally evaluate possible solutions, seek help and information as appropriate and, if all else fails, accept that the problem has occurred, deal with their emotional reactions (often with help from others) and make every effort to resume life as usual (e.g. Williamson, 2002). Indeed, research indicates that numerous personality traits influence adjustment to major life stressors, including the declines in physical functioning associated with advancing age. To give just a few examples, people low in dispositional optimism do not cope effectively or adjust well to stress (e.g. Abend & Williamson, 2002; Carver et al., 1993) and are more vulnerable to activity restriction (Williamson, 2002). High levels of neuroticism are related to a maladaptive coping style (e.g. McCrae & Costa, 1986) that may include foregoing pleasurable activities. When faced with disrupting life events, individuals who are less agentically oriented and do not have a strong sense of mastery will have more difficulty finding ways to avoid restricting their rewarding activities (e.g. Femia *et al.*, 1997; Herzog *et al.*, 1998). In addition, those who are low in the dispositional predilection to hope for positive outcomes are less likely to conceptualize ways to continue (or replace) valued activities or to persist in their efforts to do so, particularly when pathways to achieving these goals are blocked (e.g. Snyder, 1998). Although research in this area is in its infancy, personality factors should not be ignored, particularly when the goal is to identify those who are at risk for restricting their activities, adapting poorly to declines in physical functioning and in need of early intervention.

Clinical implications

In the ARMDA, coping with stress is posited to be a complex, multifaceted process that is influenced by numerous factors (see also 'Coping'). With increasing age, decline in physical functioning may mean that coping successfully requires replacing previously adaptive strategies with ones better suited to the individual's own physical limitations. Therefore, worthwhile interventions could focus on helping elders shift from problem-focused to emotion-focused coping mechanisms (e.g. Costa & McCrae, 1993; Schulz & Heckhausen, 1996), but there may be better options.

Specifically, by acknowledging that depressed affect is a function of restricted activities, interventions can be designed to reduce both activity restriction and depression. Efforts to increase activity might take three (and, probably, several more) forms. First, by taking into account both personality and social factors, practitioners should be able to target the individuals most at risk for activity restriction and depression. Second, they should carefully consider the multiple reasons that activities have become restricted and design their interventions accordingly. Third, because finding satisfactory replacements for lost activities promotes wellbeing (Benyamini & Lomranz, 2004; Searle *et al.*, 1995), programmes should be targeted toward identifying manageable activities and available resources that engage ageing adults in pastimes which meet their specific interests and needs.

Social support, like personality traits and experience with illness, interacts with physical functioning to influence normal activities. With more supportive social support networks, activity restriction can be reduced (Williamson *et al.*, 1994). Maintaining usual activities, in turn, reduces the possibility of negative emotional responses and further decrements in health and functioning. Thus, identifying community-residing older adults with deficits in social support is a good starting point for intervention (see 'Social Support Intervention'). Before intervening, however, we need to specify which aspects of social support are absent or most distressing and target treatment accordingly (Oxman & Hull, 1997). Some older people may be depressed simply because they do not have enough social interaction. Others may have concrete needs for assistance that are not being met (e.g. getting out of bed or grocery shopping). Still others may be exposed to exploitative or abusive behaviour (Cohen & McKay, 1983; Suls, 1982; Williamson *et al.*, 2000*b*; Wortman, 1984).

Conclusion and directions for future research

No solution is in sight for the fact that, with age, physiological systems slow down (e.g. Birren & Birren, 1990; Whitbourne, 2005), but the best option appears to be remaining active for as long as possible. Traditional attitudes and the projected increase in elderly people have led scholars, commentators and policy-makers to conclude that society is about to be overwhelmed by people who are disabled and require constant care. With fewer children per capita than previous generations, a major concern is that as the baby boomers age, there will be fewer adult children available to provide care, creating a demand for formal care that may severely (if not, impossibly) tax societal resources. As with any major demographic shift, there are problems to be addressed. Substantial numbers of older adults will be disabled, socially isolated and depressed, but the same is true for other age groups as well.

On the other hand, research indicates that, more than ever before, ageing adults are and will be physically, psychologically and socially healthy. Older adults are remarkably skilled in making gradual lifestyle changes to accommodate diminishing physical abilities (e.g. Williamson & Dooley, 2001). Simply directing them towards the numerous resources available to elders (e.g. senior centre activities) can help some, but others may need psychological intervention to help them make adjustments that maximize their ability to remain engaged with life. From accumulating evidence, it is now clear that people consistently become depressed in the wake of physical illness and disability largely because these circumstances disrupt their ability to go about life as usual (see Williamson, 1998, 2002, for reviews). Lack of experience, less social support and personality variables all contribute to the ability to cope with major life changes (e.g. Walters & Williamson, 1999; Williamson, 1998, 2002; Williamson & Schulz, 1992, 1995; Williamson *et al.*, 1998).

In their acclaimed book, *Successful ageing*, Rowe and Kahn (1998) proposed that there are three components of successful ageing: (1) avoiding disease; (2) engagement with life; and (3) maintaining high cognitive and physical function. These factors are closely aligned with and, perhaps, subsumed in the ARMDA. First, avoiding disease is largely a function of routine activities. Physical exercise and temperance in detrimental behaviours (e.g. smoking, drinking alcohol, eating a high fat diet) are, under ideal circumstances, routine activities that promote better physical health, less disability and greater longevity (e.g. Cohen *et al.*, 1993; McGinnis & Foege, 1993). Second, 'engagement with life' (Rowe & Kahn, 1998) is virtually synonymous with continuing valued activities. People who feel engaged with life are those who are involved in personally meaningful activities, but what qualifies as 'meaningful' will vary according to each person's history. In the ARMDA, it is postulated that continuing to be involved in personally relevant activities (whether intellectual, physical, or social) is what matters most.

Finally, Rowe and Kahn (1998) advocated maintaining high levels of physical (and cognitive, see 'Age and Cognitive Functioning') functioning as the third key to ageing successfully. When confronted with age-related declines in physical functioning, the telling factor may well be the extent to which a semblance of normal activities can continue or be replaced in a satisfactory fashion (e.g. Benyamini and Lomranz, 2004). What does this mean when, for example, disability precludes playing several sets of tennis every day? If this activity was driven by love of the sport, then the ageing tennis addict can still participate by watching matches or, even better, by coaching others in the finer aspects of playing the game.

The ARMDA, like other stress and coping models (e.g. Lazarus & Folkman, 1984), implies that the causal path is unidirectional – e.g. that age-related declines in physical functioning cause activity restriction which, in turn, causes negative affect. Without doubt, this is an inadequate representation. Consider pain and depression as an example. Depression can result from the inability to deal with chronic pain. Conversely, substantial research suggests that depression fosters higher levels of reported pain (e.g. Lefebvre, 1981; Mathew *et al.*, 1981; Parmelee *et al.*, 1991). As clinicians have long known, being depressed causes people to forego many of their previous activities. In fact, one of the better behavioural treatments for depression is to motivate patients to become more socially and physically active (e.g. Herzog *et al.*, 1998). In a reciprocal fashion, for both physiological and psychological reasons, inactivity also increases level of experienced pain (e.g. Williamson & Dooley, 2001).

Controlled experimental studies will help clarify previous results by showing that strategies designed to increase activity level will, in fact, improve wellbeing. In addition, identifying differences between people who will tolerate discomfort in order to continue engaging in meaningful activities and those who will not voluntarily make such efforts under similar levels of discomfort will bring us closer to successful intervention programmes.

Contrary to common belief, growing old in the twenty-first century is not likely to be an onerous experience for many people. Those who age well feel in control of at least some of the important aspects of their lives and maintain (often with the help of others) the activities they value most. The association between decrements in physical functioning and adjustment is multifaceted and complex. In addition, because they vary as widely as their younger counterparts, lumping older adults into a homogenous group is inappropriate.

At this point, we know relatively little about what really happens when people are faced with the decrements in physical functioning that accompany growing old. Consequently, there are no easy answers about the best ways to intervene. Nevertheless, the ARMDA provides a foundation for intervention and further research. If people can continue to engage in at least some of their valued activities, they should be physically and psychologically healthier and depend less on others for assistance. Indeed, ageing well appears to revolve around maintaining participation in valued, meaningful activities despite losses in physical functioning.

REFERENCES

Abend, T. A. & Williamson, G. M. (2002). Feeling attractive in the wake of breast cancer: optimism matters, and so do interpersonal relationships. *Personality and Social Psychology Bulletin*, **28**, 427–36.

Atchley, R. C. (1989). The continuity theory of normal aging. *Gerontologist*, **29**, 183–90.

Benyamini, Y. & Lomranz, J. (2004). The relationship of activity restriction and replacement with depressive symptoms among older adults. *Psychology and Aging*, **19**, 362–6.

Binstock, R. H. (1999). Challenges to United States policies on aging in the new millennium. *Hallym International Journal of Aging*, **1**, 3–13.

Birren, J. E. & Birren, B. A. (1990). The concepts, models, and history in the psychology of aging. In J. E. Birren & K. W. Schaie (Eds.). *Handbook of the Psychology of Aging* (3rd edn.) (pp. 3–20). San Diego: Academic Press.

Calderon, K. S. (2001). Making the connection between depression and activity levels among the oldest-old: a measure of life satisfaction. *Activities, Adaptation and Aging*, **25**, 59–73.

Carver, C. S., Pozo, C., Harris, S. D. *et al.* (1993). How coping mediates the effect of optimism on distress: a study of women with early stage breast cancer. *Journal of Personality and Social Psychology*, **65**, 375–90.

Cassileth, B. R., Lusk, E. J., Strouse, T. B. *et al.* (1984). Psychosocial status in chronic illness: a comparative analysis of six diagnostic groups. *New England Journal of Medicine*, **311**, 506–11.

Center for the Advancement of Health (1998). Getting old: a lot of it is in your head. Facts of Life: an Issue Briefing for Health Reporters, 3.

Chen, Y. P. (1994). 'Equivalent retirement ages' and their implications for Social Security and Medicare financing. *Gerontologist*, **34**, 731–5.

Cohen, S. & McKay, G. (1983). Interpersonal relationships as buffers of the impact of psychosocial stress on health. In A. Baum, S. E. Taylor & J. E. Singer (Eds.). *Handbook of psychology and health, Vol. 4*, (pp. 253–67). Hillsdale, NJ: Erlbaum.

Cohen, S., Tyrrell, D. A. J., Russell, M. A. H., Jarvis, M. J. & Smith, A. P. (1993). Smoking, alcohol consumption, and susceptibility to the common cold. *American Journal of Public Health*, **83**, 1277–83.

Cohen, S. & Wills, T. A. (1985). Stress, social support, and the buffering hypothesis. *Psychological Bulletin*, **98**, 310–57.

Costa, P. T. & McCrae, R. R. (1993). Personality, defense, coping, and adaptation in older adulthood. In E. M. Cummings, A. L. Greene & K. K. Karraker (Eds.). *Life span developmental psychology: perspectives on stress and coping* (pp. 277–93). Hillsdale, NJ: Erlbaum.

Femia, E. E., Zarit, S. H. & Johansson, B. (1997). Predicting change in activities of daily living: a longitudinal study of the oldest old in Sweden. *Journal of Gerontology*, **52**, 294–302.

Foley, K. M. (1985). The treatment of cancer pain. *New England Journal of Medicine*, **313**, 84–95.

Hendricks, J., Hatch, L. R. & Cutler, S. J. (1999). Entitlements, social compacts, and the trend toward retrenchment in U.S. old-age programs. *Hallym International Journal of Aging*, **1**, 14–32.

Herzog, A. R., Franks, M. M., Markus, H. R. & Holmberg, D. (1998). Activities and well-being in older age: effects of self-concept and educational attainment. *Psychology and Aging*, **13**, 179–85.

Hobbs, F. B. (1996). *65+ in the United States*, U.S. Bureau of the Census, current population reports. Washington, DC: US Government Printing Office.

Kiyak, H. A. & Hooyman, N. R. (1999). Aging in the twenty-first century. *Hallym International Journal of Aging*, **1**, 56–66.

Lazarus, R. S. & Folkman, S. (1984). *Stress, appraisal and coping.* New York: Springer.

Lefebvre, M. F. (1981). Cognitive distortion and cognitive errors in depressed psychiatric and low back pain patients. *Journal of Consulting and Clinical Psychology*, **49**, 517–25.

Manton, K. G., Stallard, E. & Corder, L. (1995). Changes in morbidity and chronic disability in the U.S. elderly population: evidence from the 1982, 1984, and 1989 National Long Term Care Surveys. *Journal of Gerontology*, **50**, 194–204.

Mathew, R., Weinman, M. & Mirabi, M. (1981). Physical symptoms of depression. *British Journal of Psychiatry*, **139**, 293–6.

McCrae, R. R. (1989). Age differences and changes in the use of coping mechanisms. *Journal of Gerontology*, **44**, 161–4.

McCrae, R. R. & Costa, P. T., Jr. (1986). Personality, coping, and coping effectiveness in an adult sample. *Journal of Personality*, **54**, 385–405.

McGinnis, J. M. & Foege, W. H. (1993). Actual causes of death in the United States. *Journal of the American Medical Association*, **270**, 2207–12.

Mutran, E. J., Reitzes, D. C., Mossey, J. & Fernandez, M. E. (1995). Social support, depression, and recovery of walking ability following hip fracture surgery. *Journal of Gerontology*, **50**, 354–61.

Ogilvie, D. M. (1987). Life satisfaction and identity structure in late middle-aged men and women. *Psychology and Aging*, **2**, 217–24.

Oxman, T. E. & Hull, J. G. (1997). Social support, depression, and activities of daily living in older heart surgery patients. *Journal of Gerontology*, **52**, 1–14.

Palmore, E. (1990). Ageism: positive and negative. New York: Springer.

Parmelee, P. A., Katz, I. R. & Lawton, M. P. (1991). The relation of pain to depression among institutionalized aged. *Journal of Gerontology*, **46**, 15–21.

Peterson, C., Seligman, M. E. P. & Vaillant, G. E. (1988). Pessimistic explanatory style is a risk factor for physical illness: a thirty-five-year longitudinal study. *Journal of Personality and Social Psychology*, **55**, 23–7.

Quinn, J. F. & Burkhauser, R. V. (1990). Work and retirement. In R. Binstock & L. K. George (Eds.). *Handbook of Aging and The Social Sciences* (3rd edn.) (pp. 307–23). San Diego: Academic Press.

Rowe, J. W. & Kahn, R. L. (1998). *Successful aging*. New York: Pantheon Books.

Rybash, J. M., Roodin, P. A. & Hoyer, W. J. (1995). *Adult Development and Aging* (3rd edn.). Madison, WI: Brown and Benchmark.

Schulz, R. & Ewen, R. B. (1993). *Adult Development and Aging: Myths and Emerging Realities* (2nd edn.). New York: MacMillan.

Schulz, R. & Heckhausen, J. (1996). A life-span model of successful aging. *American Psychologist*, **51**, 702–14.

Searle, M. S., Mahon, M. J., Iso-Ahola, S. E., Sdrolias, H. A. & van Dyck, J. (1995). Enhancing a sense of independence and psychological well-being among the elderly: a field experiment. *Journal of Leisure Research*, **27**, 107–24.

Snyder, C. R. (1998). A case for hope in pain, loss, and suffering. In J. H. Harvey, J. Omarza & E. Miller (Eds.). *Perspectives on loss: a sourcebook* (pp. 63–79). Washington, DC: Taylor and Francis.

Suls, J. (1982). Social support, interpersonal relations, and health: benefits and liabilities. In G. S. Saunders & J. Suls (Eds.). *Social psychology of health and illness* (pp. 255–77). Hillsdale, NJ: Erlbaum.

Taylor, S. E. (1983). Adjustment to threatening events: a theory of cognitive adaptation. *American Psychologist*, **38**, 1161–73.

Taylor, S. E. & Brown, J. D. (1988). Illusion and well-being: a social psychological perspective on mental health. *Psychological Bulletin*, **103**, 193–210.

US Department of Health and Human Services. (1992). *Healthy people 2000: Summary report*. Washington, DC: US Government Printing Office.

Volz, J. (2000). Successful aging: the second 50. *Monitor on Psychology*, **31**, 24–8.

Walters, A. S. & Williamson, G. M. (1999). The role of activity restriction in the association between pain and depressed affect: a study of pediatric patients with chronic pain. *Children's Health Care*, **28**, 33–50.

Whitbourne, S. K. (2005). *Adult Development and Aging: Biopsychosocial Perspectives* (2nd edn.). Hoboken, NJ: John Wiley and Sons.

Williamson, G. M. (1998). The central role of restricted normal activities in adjustment to illness and disability: a model of depressed affect. *Rehabilitation Psychology*, **43**, 327–47.

Williamson, G. M. (2000). Extending the Activity Restriction Model of Depressed Affect: evidence from a sample of breast cancer patients. *Health Psychology*, **19**, 339–47.

Williamson, G. M. (2002). Aging well: Outlook for the 21st century. In C. R. Snyder & S. J. Lopez (Eds.). *The handbook of positive psychology* (pp. 676–86). New York: Oxford University Press.

Williamson, G. M. & Dooley, W. K. (2001). Aging and coping: the activity solution. In C. R. Snyder (Ed.). *Coping with stress: effective people and processes* (pp. 240–58). New York: Oxford University Press.

Williamson, G. M. & Schulz, R. (1992). Pain, activity restriction, and symptoms of depression among community-residing elderly. *Journal of Gerontology*, **47**, 367–72.

Williamson, G. M. & Schulz, R. (1995). Activity restriction mediates the association between pain and depressed affect: a study of younger and older adult cancer patients. *Psychology and Aging*, **10**, 369–78.

Williamson, G. M. & Shaffer, D. R. (2000). The Activity Restriction Model of Depressed Affect: antecedents and consequences of restricted normal activities. In G. M. Williamson, D. R. Shaffer & P. A. Parmelee (Eds.). *Physical illness and depression in older adults: a handbook of theory, research, and practice*. New York: Plenum.

Williamson, G. M., Shaffer, D. R. & Parmelee, P. A. (Eds.) (2000a). *Physical illness and depression in older adults: a handbook of theory, research, and practice*. New York: Plenum Publishing.

Williamson, G. M., Shaffer, D. R. & Schulz, R. (1998). Activity restriction and prior relationship history as contributors to mental health outcomes among middle-aged and older caregivers. *Health Psychology*, **17**, 152–62.

Williamson, G. M., Shaffer, D. R. & The Family Relationships in Late Life Project. (2000b). Caregiver loss and quality of care provided: pre-illness relationship makes a difference. In J. H. Harvey & E. D. Miller (Eds.). *Loss and trauma: general and close relationship perspectives*. Philadelphia: Brunner/Mazel.

Williamson, G. M., Schulz, R., Bridges, M. & Behan, A. (1994). Social and psychological factors in adjustment to limb amputation. *Journal of Social Behaviour and Personality*, **9**, 249–68.

Wortman, C. B. (1984). Social support and the cancer patient. *Cancer*, **53**, 2339–60.

Zeiss, A. M., Lewinsohn, P. M., Rohde, P. & Seeley, J. R. (1996). Relationship of physical disease and functional impairment to depression in older adults. *Psychology and Aging*, **11**, 572–81.

Zimmer, Z., Hickey, T. & Searle, M. S. (1995). Activity participation and well-being among older people with arthritis. *Gerontologist*, **35**, 463–71.

Age and cognitive functioning

David R. Shaffer and Gail M. Williamson
University of Georgia

Ageing and cognitive functioning: an overview

Attitudes about ageing reflect many negative stereotypes about the intellectual prowess of our senior citizens (Center for the Advancement of Health, 1998). Are older people as cognitively deficient as is commonly assumed? Are they significantly less capable than middle-aged or younger adults of profiting from classroom instruction, solving everyday problems such as remembering to turn off the oven after removing a roast, or learning to operate such new technologies as computers, DVD players, or ATM machines?

Study of the abilities to learn, remember, and solve problems has a long history in psychology and is arguably the most thoroughly investigated aspect of adult development and ageing (Siegelman & Rider, 2003). One reason for this emphasis is that cognitive functioning in adulthood has so many important implications for the quality of ordinary people's lives. Furthermore, cognitive functioning can play a major role in how people feel about themselves as they age. Middle-aged adults occasionally claim that they have experienced a 'senior moment' after forgetting someone's name, their own telephone number, or a step in a well practiced procedure such as recording a programme on their VCR. Although such comments may be offered in a humorous light, they also may reflect a deep-seated concern that many middle-aged and older adults have about losing their memories (Whitbourne, 2005) (see 'Dementias').

Indeed, older adults have reasons for suspecting that their cognitive powers are declining. With age, there is a slowing of the rate at which we process information, a lessening of the amount of information that we can keep in mind to solve problems, and even a reduction in ability to inhibit distractions and focus on the most pertinent information for problem-solving, changes that many have attributed to an ageing nervous system (Gaeta et al., 2001; Persad et al., 2002; Salthouse, 1996). However, other researchers favour a contextualist approach to ageing and cognitive functioning. They are not convinced that there is a universal biological decline in basic learning, memory and problem-solving capabilities, noting instead that older people's cognitive performances depend very heavily on such individual characteristics as the person's goals, motivations, abilities, and health, characteristics of the task at hand and characteristics of the broader context in which the task is performed (Sigelman & Rider, 2003). In a word, older adults can compensate for many of their shortcomings, learn new things and learn them well (e.g. Schaie, 1996; Volz, 2000). Moreover, whether older adults believe that they can learn, remember and solve problems is crucial to their success in doing so (Artistico et al., 2003; Cavanaugh, 1996). In practical terms, the contextualists believe that ageing adults bear some responsibilities for preventing (or slowing) cognitive decline by emphasizing their strengths and expertise and continuing to engage in cognitively challenging activities (Williamson, 2002).

Research on cognitive ageing

Age and intelligence

When people think about intelligence, they have an idea that it represents a person's ability to think and solve problems. Psychological definitions of intelligence come close to this simple idea of intelligence-as-mental-ability. Spearman (1927) conceptualized intelligence as a general factor (g) that influences performance on all mental tests. By contrast, Thurstone (1938) argued that intelligence is comprised of seven 'primary mental abilities' (PMAs): verbal meaning, word fluency, number, spatial relations, general reasoning, perceptual speed, memory) that were said to be separate, distinct and cover all possible aspects of intelligence. More recently, Cattell (1963, 1971) claimed that the PMAs can be clustered into two basic sets of abilities. 'Fluid intelligence' refers to the ability to solve abstract problems that are free of cultural influences (e.g. word fluency, reasoning, spatial relations). By contrast, 'crystallized intelligence' refers to the ability to solve problems that depend on knowledge acquired as a result of schooling or other life experiences (e.g. numerical reasoning, verbal meaning, tests of general knowledge).

Age-related changes in intellectual functioning were the focus of Schaie's (1983, 1996) Seattle Longitudinal Study. In 1956, participants aged 20–72 were tested to assess five PMAs and retested seven years later on the same abilities. In 1963, 1970, 1977 and 1984, new samples of 20–70-year-olds were given the same tests and retested periodically. This sequential study made it possible to determine how the performance of particular individuals changed over time (longitudinal comparisons) and to compare the performance of people of a particular age (e.g. 70 in 1956) with different cohorts of people who were the same age (70) in 1963, 1970, 1977 and 1984, thus providing ample information about different cohorts, as well as longitudinal data on some participants for as long as 28 years.

Several important findings emerged from this study. First, cohort effects implied that when an individual was born influences intellectual performances as much as does chronological age. Specifically, younger cohorts outperformed older cohorts on most tests. The only exception was numerical ability, on which older cohorts performed better than younger cohorts. Judging from these findings, young and middle-aged adults today can look forward to better intellectual functioning in old age than their grandparents.

Second, longitudinal data revealed that age-related patterns of performance vary for different abilities. Fluid intelligence declined earlier and more steeply than crystallized intelligence. Nevertheless, scores on fluid intelligence remained fairly stable until the late 60s, showing no meaningful decline until the late 70s and 80s. Indeed, a recent longitudinal study of relatively healthy 78–100-year-olds confirmed these patterns, revealing that the 'crystallized' ability of general knowledge did not show a meaningful decline until the 90s (Singer *et al.*, 2003). So adults may lose *some* of their 'fluid' abilities to grapple with novel problems by age 60–70 but will generally retain, well into old age, the crystallized abilities that support solving most practical problems.

One final message of the longitudinal studies: declines in intellectual abilities are not universal. Only 30–40% of the 81-year-olds in Schaie's (1994) study had experienced a significant decline in intellectual ability in the past seven years and declines among healthy participants, particularly in crystallized abilities, often are not pronounced until the mid-80s (Singer *et al.*, 2003). Furthermore, although few 81-year-olds in the Seattle study maintained all five mental abilities, almost all maintained at least one ability over time, and about half maintained four of the five abilities (Schaie, 1989). Clearly, individual variations in intellectual functioning among older adults are large, and anyone stereotyping elders as intellectually deficient is likely to be wrong most of the time.

Age and information processing

Information processing researchers regard human cognitive functioning as comparable to that of computers. 'Data' are entered into the brain through various sensory channels where they either disappear or are processed further. Should we attend to input, it passes into working memory (WM), a limited capacity store that holds information temporarily until we can operate on it. WM is where all conscious mental computations are thought to occur. For information in WM to be remembered for any length of time, it must be moved to long term memory (LTM), a relatively permanent store of information that represents what most people think of as memory. Finally, information in LTM must be retrieved to WM before it truly can be 'remembered' or used for some other purpose, such as problem-solving.

Age and processing speed

According to Salthouse's (1996) General Slowing Hypothesis, age-related declines in cognitive function are largely related to a general decrease in the speed of information processing within an ageing nervous system. Processing speed is assessed by reaction time tasks in which participants attend to and respond appropriately to information as quickly as possible. One example is the Digit Symbol Substitution Test (DSST), consisting of a reference table with a code illustrating how particular digits are paired with particular hieroglyphic symbols. Below are rows of boxes with a digit in the top section and an empty space in the bottom section of each box. One's score is the number of appropriate hieroglyphics inserted into the empty boxes in 90 seconds. The greater the number of correct symbol substitutions, the higher one's processing speed.

A recent review of 141 DSST studies that included more than 7000 adults aged 18–79 revealed a clear association between age and processing speed: 60–70-year-olds attained much lower scores on the DSST than did 18–30-year-olds (Hoyer *et al.*, 2004). These findings are consistent with a large body of data from studies employing other reaction time tasks indicating that processing speed peaks in early adulthood and then declines slowly over the adult years (Frieske & Park, 1999; Kail & Salthouse, 1994). Age-related sensory limitations (e.g. visual deficits), a gradual slowing of neural transmissions, or both, may underlie this decline in processing speed. If older adults have a sluggish 'computer' they may simply not be able to keep up with the processing demands of complex intellectual tasks to the point that they eventually evidence declines on tests of primary mental abilities.

Age and working memory

Another possible contributor to age-related declines in cognitive functioning is that WM capacity declines with age. Capacity of WM is assessed with memory-span tasks, measures of the number of unrelated and rapidly presented stimuli (e.g. digits) that one can recall when prompted to do so. WM capacity generally increases until middle age and slowly declines thereafter (Park *et al.*, 2002; Swanson, 1999). Moreover, adult WM capacity predicts performance on a wide variety of cognitive tasks (Engle *et al.*, 1999; Whitbourne, 2005). Older adults, it seems, require more limited WM space to carry out such basic processes as recognizing and storing stimuli, thus leaving less space for other purposes, such as reasoning or executing other cognitive operations. Indeed, differences between older and younger adults are most apparent on cognitive challenges that tax WM by requiring effortful thought or strategizing, and older adults struggle when they must devote a great deal of effort to carry out several activities at once. For example, trying to memorize a list of words (a mentally effortful activity requiring strategies such as rehearsal) while walking is much more difficult for older adults than for middle-aged or younger adults (Li *et al.*, 2001; Lindenberger *et al.*, 2000).

Age-related declines in WM functioning may be related to reduced processing speed. The older adult (who processes more slowly) may simply run out of time while performing WM tasks and be unable to complete the computations necessary to solve problems or attend to and store new input relevant to the task at hand (Salthouse, 1996).

An alternative explanation for the increasing inefficiency of WM in older adults stems from Hasher and Zack's Inhibitory Deficit Hypothesis (Hasher *et al.*, 1999). According to this view, efficient use of WM requires an individual to inhibit task-irrelevant information by preventing it from entering WM or by removing from WM information that is no longer of use. Consistent with this model, older adults are more likely than middle-aged or younger ones to activate irrelevant information and are less efficient at suppressing such information once it enters WM (Bowles & Salthouse, 2003; Hedden & Park, 2001; Malstrom & LaVoie, 2002). Thus, 'mental clutter' may overwhelm WM, resulting in a decline in WM capacity with age and interfering with retrieval of task-relevant material from LTM necessary for efficient problem solving. Cognitive neuroscientists have identified deficits in prefrontal cortical regions of the brain that suggest a biological basis for the inhibitory deficiencies of older adults (Braver *et al.*, 2001; Simensky & Abeles, 2002).

Age, learning and long-term memory

Older adults learn new material more slowly and sometimes do not learn it as well as young and middle-aged adults do, and they may not remember what they have learned so well (Howard *et al.*, 2004; Whitbourne, 2005). However, noticeable declines in learning and memory rarely occur until the late 60s, and the memory of 'young-old' adults (60–70 years) is more similar to that of 18–34-year-olds than to that of 71–82-year-olds (Cregger & Rogers, 1998). Moreover, not all older people experience noticeable learning and memory difficulties, and not all kinds of cognitive tasks cause older people difficulty.

Consider a sample of the weaknesses and, by implication, strengths of older adults. First, owing largely to the slowing of cognitive processing and reduction of WM capacity, older adults may need to go through new material more times than younger adults to learn it equally well – or need more time to respond when memory is tested. Thus, they show larger learning and memory deficits on *timed* as compared with untimed tasks (Sigelman & Rider, 2003).

Second, older adults fare especially poorly compared with younger ones when material to be learned and remembered is abstract or unfamiliar and cannot be tied to their existing knowledge. By contrast, older adults often equal or exceed the performance of younger adults when practical challenges are more familiar to them than to their younger counterparts (Artistico *et al.*, 2003; Barrett & Wright, 1981). As we have noted, such crystallized abilities as vocabulary and general knowledge continue to build well into old age (Schaie, 1996; Verhaeghen, 2003) and are slow to decline (Singer *et al.*, 2003). So, for many everyday learning, memory, or problem-solving challenges, older adults, by virtue of their greater knowledge base, have expertise that may compensate for their slower processing and less efficient WM and permit them to equal or exceed the performance of younger counterparts. By contrast, these same information-processing limitations place them at a strong disadvantage, relative to younger adults, on abstract, unfamiliar, or seemingly meaningless cognitive tasks.

Similarly, older adults are likely to be at a disadvantage when challenges require unpracticed skills that they rarely use as opposed to skills that are well-practiced and automatized (i.e. applied without conscious mental effort). Thus, it is much easier for older adults to remember whether a sentence makes sense in the context of what they have just read (an automatized skill for readers) than to judge whether a specific sentence has appeared in a story (requiring effort and skills seldom used outside of school; Reder *et al.*, 1986).

One interesting idea about ageing and memory is the Environmental Support Hypothesis (ESH): age differences in memory are most apparent when tasks provide little context or support and demand high levels of effortful processing (Craik, 1994; Naveh-Benjamin *et al.*, 2002). For example, older adults do much worse than younger adults on tests of free recall of previously presented material but no worse (or only slightly worse) on tests of recognition memory, which simply require the participant to say whether or not an item has been presented before. According to ESH, these findings support the notion that recognition tasks provide more contextual support and require less effortful processing than recall tasks (Whitbourne, 2005).

Older adults are also more likely to be disadvantaged on tests of explicit memory, which require effortful cognitive processing to encode, store, and retrieve information (e.g. lists of words) than implicit memory, or recall of information acquired unintentionally and retrieved automatically. Even an 85-year-old might demonstrate excellent implicit memory about how to drive a car or tie his or her shoe (implicit procedural memory), but he/she may have a very difficult time, compared with a young adult, consciously learning and remembering the list of steps one must perform to successfully complete either operation (Mitchell & Bruss, 2003; Whitbourne, 2005).

Prospective memory (PM) is particularly relevant to older adults when it comes to health regimens. PM requires one to retrieve from LTM an intention to perform an action (e.g. taking prescribed medication at noon). Because PM requires effortful processing to form intentions and later retrieve and implement them, we might expect older adults to perform worse than younger ones on such challenges. This is precisely what one recent review of the literature found for all laboratory-based measures of PM. The caveat, however, was that older adults outperformed younger adults on simple, everyday PM challenges (Henry *et al.*, 2004). Older adults may be less challenged by meaningful real-world PM tasks if they develop strategies to compensate for the effort required to retrieve an intention by creating their own 'environmental supports' (e.g. a post-it note to go to the dentist at 2:00 p.m.).

Overall, these findings suggest that older adults seem to have more difficulty with tasks that are cognitively demanding – those that require speed, grappling with unfamiliar material, unexercised skills, and effortful strategizing to learn and remember – rather than implicit and automatic processes. Nonetheless, older adults often can compensate for their processing deficiencies by relying heavily on their crystallized knowledge (expertise) and other ploys (e.g. external memory aids) to cope quite successfully with most everyday cognitive challenges.

Explaining age-rated changes in cognition

Throughout, we have mentioned such factors as a gradual slowing of information processing, a lessening of WM capacity, and a growing inability to inhibit attending to irrelevant information, as well as (yet poorly understood) neurological and sensory correlates of these events, as likely contributors to age-related declines in intellectual skills and learning/memory performance. Yet, recall that there are tremendous individual differences in the cognitive functioning of older adults, and these variations provide some clues about factors influencing the rate at which cognitive functioning declines with age.

Health and cognitive functioning

Poor health is one of the best predictors of cognitive decline among older adults. Aside from the various forms of dementia that have a devastating impact on intellect and information processing, people with cardiovascular diseases or other chronic illnesses show steeper declines in mental abilities than their healthier peers. Indeed, one longitudinal study found that 78-year-olds with hypertension had more white matter abnormalities in the brain than disease-free age mates and that these abnormalities were associated with lower levels of functioning, even after controlling for levels of intellect participants displayed earlier in life (Deary *et al.*, 2003). Diseases often contribute to a rapid decline in intellectual and information-processing capabilities in the years immediately preceding death (Johansson *et al.*, 2004), a phenomenon often labeled 'terminal drop'. Maybe there is something to the saying 'Sound body, sound mind.' (See also 'Ageing and health').

Lifestyles and cognitive functioning

Cognitive declines among the oldest-old (those 85 and older) often are more closely related to biological than to environmental factors (Singer *et al.*, 2003). However, twin studies reveal that environmental factors are more important than genes and genetically influenced characteristics for predicting age-related cognitive declines of 70–84-year-olds (Johansson *et al.*, 2004; McGue & Christensen, 2002). What environmental factors might be implicated?

Schaie's Seattle study revealed that elders showing the largest intellectual declines were widows living unstimulating lifestyles, residing alone, engaging in few activities and remaining seemingly disengaged from life. By contrast, elders who maintained (or improved) their capabilities tended to have above average socioeconomic status and mentally active lifestyles. Similar relations between the intellectual complexity of elders' environments and maintenance of intellectual performance have been demonstrated in Chinese samples (Schaie *et al.*, 2001) and in a variety of other contexts (Whitbourne, 2005) (see 'Socioeconomic status and health').

Clearly, these findings are consistent with the 'use it or lose it' rule that is widely touted to people hoping to maintain their muscular or sexual prowess. Simply stated, we are likely to maintain our intellectual faculties longer if we exercise them. Even reading books, working crossword puzzles, or learning to operate new technologies can help build new skills or maintain old ones (Rogers *et al.*, 1996). Apparently, the nervous system remains plastic (changeable) over the life span, enabling elderly individuals to benefit from intellectual stimulation, maintain the skills most relevant to their everyday activities and compensate for the loss of unpracticed abilities (Schaie, 1966, 1983). By contrast, even eminent college professors are at risk of declining intellectual performance if their retirement activities are far less stimulating than their working lives (Christensen *et al.*, 1997).

Self-efficacy and cognitive functioning

Finally, older people may fare worse than younger adults on many cognitive challenges, particularly abstract laboratory tasks, because they feel less self-efficacious about their abilities. Yet, on tasks for which elders feel more efficacious, they work as hard as, or harder than, younger adults and post higher levels of performance (Artistico *et al.*, 2003).

The implication? Older adults who feel mentally efficacious are less likely to display meaningful learning, memory and intellectual deficiencies later in life (Cavanaugh, 1996). However, it is not necessarily adaptive for seniors to ignore signs of mental decline and assume that they can do anything; motivation to maintain cognitive skills may be critical. Schaie (1983, 1996), for example, reported that elders who were most concerned about and who overestimated their cognitive declines were the ones most likely to continue to engage in cognitively challenging activities that fostered maintaining their intellectual prowess over time (see 'Self-efficacy and health behaviour').

Conclusions and implications for intervention

Clearly, most older adults are not the mental incompetents that stereotypes about ageing suggest. With age, there are some undeniable losses in cognitive processes such as fluid intelligence, speed of processing, and WM capacity/efficiency. However, many healthy older adults, particularly those who feel mentally self-efficacious and who continue to engage in intellectually challenging activities learn to rely on their crystallized intellect and find ways to automatize cognitive processes to master everyday problems, thereby maintaining their cognitive prowess until very late in their lives.

The continuing plasticity of the ageing nervous system has prompted cognitive ageing researchers to design a variety of interventions to slow (or even reverse) declines in cognitive functioning. Early studies from the 1970s and 1980s revealed that, given practice and training in cognitive strategies, older adults could improve performance on such fluid intellectual abilities as spatial and inductive reasoning (e.g. Plemons *et al.*, 1978; Willis *et al.*, 1981; see also Saczynski *et al.*, 2002). Moreover, Schaie and Willis (1986; Schaie 1996) reported that about 40% of their 64–95-year-olds who had evidenced cognitive decline, through training, restored their performance levels of 14 years earlier, before decline set in, and these gains were still evident seven years later. Other investigators have shown clear training effects among older adults for such cognitive activities as memory and timed (speeded) tasks (Whitbourne, 2005).

Knowing why older adults struggle with particular challenges is the key to designing effective interventions. Liu and Park (2004), for example, reasoned that medical regimens presenting complex PM problems (e.g. remembering to monitor blood glucose four times daily) could be made easier for their 60–81-year-old participants if their intentions could be activated and implemented automatically rather than through effortful cognitive processes. In this study, some participants formulated a specific plan that tied monitoring to particular activities that would automatically activate the intention (e.g. monitor just before lunch, at mid-afternoon before walking the dog, just before dinner, just after the evening news). Others simply verbally rehearsed the intention to monitor at noon, 1:30 p.m., 6:00 p.m. and 7:30 p.m. A third group spent an equal amount of time deliberating the pros and cons of monitoring. Results revealed that participants whose intentions had been automatically linked to daily activities were twice as likely to follow the regimen as were those in the other two groups who had to expend substantial mental effort to form, retrieve and implement their intentions to monitor.

The larger messages? You can teach old dogs new tricks – and reteach them old tricks – in very little time. These interventions cannot restore cognitive function in elderly people with dementia or in old-old adults who have experienced significant neurological ageing. But they do attest to the plasticity of an otherwise healthy nervous system well into late life and the ability to maintain or improve cognitive functioning by reviving unused skills or finding ways to automatize the processes older adults can use to master everyday challenges.

Artistico, D., Cervone, D. & Pezzati, L. (2003). Perceived self-efficacy and everyday problem solving among young and older adults. *Psychology and Aging,* **18,** 68–79.

Barrett, T. R. & Wright, M. (1981). Age-related facilitation of recall following semantic processing. *Journal of Gerontology,* **36,** 194–9.

Bowles, R. P. & Salthouse, T. A. (2003). Assessing the age-related effects of proactive interference on working memory tasks using the Rasch model. *Psychology and Aging,* **18,** 608–15.

Braver, T. S., Barch, D. M., Keys, B. A. *et al.* (2001). Context processing in older adults: evidence for a theory relating cognitive control to neurobiology in healthy aging. *Journal of Experimental Psychology: General,* **130,** 746–63.

Cattell, R. B. (1963). Theory of fluid and crystallized intelligence: a critical experiment. *Journal of Educational Psychology,* **54,** 1–22.

Cattell, R. B. (1971). *Abilities: their structure, growth, and action.* Boston: Houghton Mifflin.

Cavanaugh, J. C. (1996). Memory self-efficacy as a moderator of memory change. In F. Blanchard-Fields & T. M. Hess (Eds.). *Perspectives on cognitive change in adulthood and aging* (pp. 488–507). New York: McGraw-Hill.

Center for the Advancement of Health (1998). *Getting old: a lot of it is in your head.* Facts of Life: An Issue Briefing for Health Reporters, 3.

Christensen, H., Korten, A. E., Jorm, A. F. & Henderson, A. (1997). Education and decline in cognitive performance: compensatory but not protective. *International Journal of Geriatric Psychiatry,* **12,** 323–30.

Craik, F. I. M. (1994). Memory changes in normal aging. *Current Directions in Psychological Science,* **3,** 155–8.

Cregger, M. E. & Rogers, W. A. (1998). Memory for activities for young, young-old and old adults: *Experimental Aging Research,* **24,** 195–201.

Deary, I. J., Leaper, S. A., Murray, A. D., Staff, R. T. & Whalley, L. J. (2003). Cerebral white matter abnormalities and lifetime cognitive change: a 67-year follow-up of the Scottish Mental Survey of 1932. *Psychology and Aging,* **18,** 140–8.

Engle, R. W., Tuholski, S. W., Laughlin, J. E. & Conway, A. R. A. (1999). Working memory, short-term memory, and general fluid intelligence: a latent variable approach. *Journal of Experimental Psychology: General,* **128,** 309–31.

Frieski, D. A. & Park, D. C. (1999). Memory for news in young and old adults. *Psychology and Aging,* **14,** 90–8.

Gaeta, H., Friedman, D., Ritter, W. & Cheng, J. (2001). An event-related potential evaluation of involuntary attentional shifts in young and older adults. *Psychology and Aging,* **16,** 55–68.

Hasher, L., Zacks, R. T. & May, C. P. (1999). Inhibitory control, circadian arousal, and age. In *attention and performance, XVII, cognitive regulation of performance: interaction of theory and application* (pp. 653–75). Cambridge, MA: MIT Press.

Hedden, T. & Park, D. C. (2001). Aging and interference in verbal working memory. *Psychology and Aging,* **16,** 666–81.

Henry, J. D., MacLeod, M. S., Phillips, L. H. & Crawford, J. R. (2004). A meta-analytic review of prospective memory and aging. *Psychology and Aging,* **19,** 27–39.

Howard, D. V., Howard, J. H. Jr., Japikse, K. *et al.* (2004). Implicit sequence learning: Effects of level of structure, adult age, and extended practice. *Psychology and Aging,* **19,** 79–82.

Hoyer, W. J., Stawski, R. S., Wasylyshyn, C. & Verhaeghen, P. (2004). Adult age and digit symbol substitution performance: A meta-analysis. *Psychology and Aging,* **19,** 211–14.

Johansson, B., Hofer, S. M., Allaire, J. C. *et al.* (2004). Change in cognitive capabilities in the oldest old: the effects of proximity to death in genetically related individuals over a 6-year period. *Psychology and Aging,* **19,** 145–56.

Kail, R. & Salthouse, T. A. (1994). Processing speed as a mental capacity. *Acta Psychologica,* **86,** 199–225.

Li, K. Z. H., Lindenberger, U., Freund, A. M. & Baltes, P. B. (2001). Walking while memorizing: age-related differences in compensatory behavior. *Psychological Science,* **12,** 230–7.

Lindenberger, U., Marsiske, M. & Baltes, P. B. (2000). Memorizing while walking: increase in dual-task costs from young adulthood to old age. *Psychology and Aging,* **15,** 417–36.

Liu, L. L. & Park, D. C. (2004). Aging and medical adherence: the use of automatic processes to achieve effortful things. *Psychology and Aging,* **19,** 318–25.

Malstrom, T. & LaVoie, D. J. (2002). Age differences in inhibition of schema-activated distractors. *Experimental Aging Research,* **28,** 281–98.

McGue, M. & Christensen, K. (2002). The heritability of level and rate-of-change in cognitive functioning in Danish twins aged 70 years and older. *Experimental Aging Research,* **28,** 435–51.

Mitchell, D. B. & Bruss, P. J. (2003). Age differences implicit memory: conceptual, perceptual, or methodological? *Psychology and Aging,* **18,** 807–22.

Naveh-Benjamin, M., Craik, F. I. M. & Ben-Shaul, L. (2002). Age-related differences in cued recall: effects of support at encoding and retrieval. *Aging, Neuropsychology, and Cognition,* **9,** 276–87.

Park, D. C., Lautenschlager, G., Hedden, T. *et al.* (2002). Models of visuospatial and verbal memory across the adult life span. *Psychology and Aging,* **17,** 299–320.

Persad, C. C., Abeles, N., Zacks, R. T. & Denbury, N. L. (2002). Inhibitory changes after age 60 and their relationship to measures of attention and memory. *Journals of Gerontology Series B: Psychological Sciences and Social Sciences,* **57,** 223–32.

Plemons, J. K., Willis, S. L. & Baltes, P. B. (1978). Modifiability of fluid intelligence in aging: a short-term longitudinal training approach. *Journal of Gerontology,* **33,** 224–31.

Reder, L. M., Wible, C. & Martin, J. (1986). Differential memory changes with age: exact retrieval versus plausible inference. *Journal of Experimental Psychology: Learning, Memory, and Cognition,* **12,** 72–81.

Rogers, W. A., Fisk, A. D., Mead, S. E., Walker, N. & Cabrera, E. F. (1996). Training older adults to use automatic teller machines. *Human Factors,* **38,** 425–33.

Saczynski, J. S., Willis, S. L. & Schaie, K. W. (2002). Strategy use in reasoning training with older adults. *Aging, Neuropsychology, and Cognition,* **9,** 48–60.

Salthouse, T. A. (1996). The processing-speed theory of adult age differences in cognition. *Psychological Review,* **103,** 403–28.

Schaie, K. W. (1983). The Seattle Longitudinal Study: a 21-year exploration of psychometric intelligence in adulthood. In K. S. Schaie (Ed.). *Longitudinal studies of adult psychological development* (pp. 64–135). New York: Guilford.

Schaie, K. W. (1989). The hazards of cognitive aging. *Gerontologist,* **29,** 484–93.

Schaie, K. W. (1994). The course of adult intellectual development. *American Psychologist,* **49,** 304–13.

Schaie, K. W. (1996). *Intellectual development in adulthood: the Seattle longitudinal study.* New York: Cambridge University Press.

Schaie, K. W., Nguyen, H. T., Willis, S. L., Dutta, R. & Yue, G. A. (2001). Environmental factors as a conceptual framework for examining cognitive performance in Chinese adults. *International Journal of Behavioral Development*, **25**, 193–202.

Schaie, K. W. & Willis, S. L. (1986). Can decline in adult intellectual functioning be reversed? *Developmental Psychology*, **22**, 223–32.

Sigelman, C. K. & Rider, E. A. (2003). *Life-Span Human Development* (4th edn.). Belmont, CA: Wadsworth.

Simensky, J. D. & Abeles, N. (2002). Decline of verbal memory performance with advancing age: the role of frontal lobe functioning. *Aging and Mental Health*, **6**, 293–303.

Singer, T., Verhaeghen, P., Ghisletta, P., Lindenberger, U. & Baltes, P. B. (2003). The fate of cognition in very old age: six-year longitudinal findings in the Berlin Aging Study (BASE). *Psychology and Aging*, **18**, 318–31.

Spearman, C. (1927). *The abilities of man.* New York: Macmillian.

Swanson, H. L. (1999). What develops in working memory: a life span perspective. *Developmental Psychology*, **35**, 986–1000.

Thurstone, L. L. (1938). *Primary mental abilities.* Chicago: University of Chicago Press.

Verhaeghen, P. (2003). Aging and vocabulary scores: a meta-analysis. *Psychology and Aging*, **16**, 332–39.

Volz, T. (2000). Successful aging: The second 50. *Monitor on Psychology*, **31**, 24–8.

Whitbourne, S. K. (2005). *Adult Development and Aging: Biopsychosocial Perspectives* (2nd edn.). New York: Wiley.

Williamson, G. M. (2002). Aging well: outlook for the 21st century. In Snyder C. R. & Lopez S. J. (Eds.). *The Handbook of Positive Psychology* (pp. 676–86). New York: Oxford University Press.

Willis, S. L., Blieszner, R. & Baltes, P. B. (1981). Intellectual training research in aging: modification of performance on the fluid ability of figural relations. *Journal of Educational Psychology*, **73**, 41–50.

Ageing and health

Elaine A. Leventhal

UMDNJ-Robert Wood Johnson Medical School

Although there have been many theories advanced to account for ageing with none gaining wide acceptance, some generalizations are agreed upon by most investigators. The life span is represented by growth and development and then decline or senescence (normal ageing) over time. These are not static stages but represent the continuously changing processes of the life cycle. Senescence results from declines in actual numbers of active metabolic cells and cellular functions because of the accumulation of environmental exposures and behaviours coupled with genetic vulnerabilities over time (Jazwinski, 1996; Kirkwood, 1996).

However, individuals also have an innate and unique genetic or biological plasticity that is coupled with adaptive or coping strategies for the management of ageing-related somatic changes. Thus ageing also produces increasing heterogeneity between individuals as they age. Coupled with this heterogeneity and particular health behaviours can be seen differential rates of decline and change among cells, tissues and organ systems, so that individuals will age at different rates with some biologically 'old' at 45, while others can be vigorous and 'young' at 75.

General ageing

Generally, with senescence, there is a quantitative loss of tissue mass as well as functional decline. An example of functional changes can be seen in the timing of circadian rhythms that affect temperature control, sleep patterns and the secretion of hormones such as cortisol, as well as growth hormone, the gonadotropins, thyrotrophin and melatonin. The significance of these latter changes is not yet well understood, yet it is interesting to speculate about them in the light of the reports from the MacArthur studies on successful ageing which showed that individuals with higher nocturnal secretion of cortisol and catecholamines, and higher systolic blood pressures were more likely to show greater declines in cognitive and physical function during the follow-up period of three years (Rowe & Kahn, 1998).

Of the organ systems, the normal kidney, lung and the skin age much more rapidly than the heart and liver in both sexes, while the musculoskeletal system and the gonads decline at different ages in males and females (Finch & Schneider, 1985; Kenney, 1989). There is an 80% decrease in overall muscle mass and an average of 35% increase as well as a significant redistribution of body fat. Fat deposition accumulates around and within the viscera while there is a loss of fat on the surface. Thus older people lose 'insulation' and are more sensitive to extremes of ambient temperature than are younger people.

Cardiovascular system

The age-related decline in the cardiovascular system may be critical for decreased tolerance for exercise and loss of conditioning, and the major factor contributing to feelings of agedness and overall decline in energy reserve. However, there is much more than heart and blood vessel deterioration in the loss of energy reserve. There is a gender-specific dependency as well, on the muscles and skeleton and the lungs. Changes occur in the heart chambers, and the blood vessels and valves. With time, the heart muscle thickens, the ventricular cavities become smaller and the amount of blood pumped per contraction decreases. Heart rate also slows with time as cells in the sinus node decline by up to 90%. The decrease in rate may be related to 'down regulation' or decreased responsiveness of adrenergic receptors on heart muscle even though synthesis and clearance of epinephrine does not change. Thus, the maximum heart rate in response to increased activity and responses to stress demands diminishes (Lakatta, 1987; Marin, 1995).

Blood vessels narrow and become more rigid contributing to the slow elevation in blood pressure with ageing in the absence of cardiovascular disease. Women appear to enjoy a slower rate of progression of cardiac disease before the menopause with a lower incidence of coronary artery disease in pre-menopausal women. (Anderson *et al.*, 1995). However, cardiovascular disease becomes the major killer of older post-menopausal women, can present with atypical symptoms and can be more lethal than in men often with delay in seeking care because of stereotypic or lay perceptions of what heart disease and acute attacks should feel like (see 'Symptom Perception' and 'Delay in Seeking Help').

Respiratory system

There is an even more rapid rate of functional decline in all parts of the respiratory system. This includes lung tissue as well as the chest cavity, with its muscles and the ribs and vertebral column. There is less work capacity as all the types of muscles age in bronchi, the diaphragm and chest wall. There are clear gender differences in thoracic cage ageing. This may result from bone and muscle mass losses that are greater in females and cause diminished exercise capacity as well as a greater vulnerability of and a greater possibility for immobilization. Within the lung itself, the alveolar or air sac septae are the exchange sites for the gases, oxygen and carbon dioxide. Old lungs have scattered areas of scarring and damage to the septae that interfere with gaseous exchange. These manifestations of 'senile' emphysema may limit the amount of exercise and energy that can be expended even more than functional changes in the cardiovascular system described previously (Rossi *et al.*, 1996).

Moreover, it is difficult to determine how much of the respiratory functional decline that is observed is age-related and how much is environmentally and behaviourally induced since most individuals are exposed to some degree of air pollution and cigarettes or other inhaled substances abuse exaggerates the ageing changes. Smoking produces scarring or fibrosis, increased secretions and an increased rate of chronic infection. The cough is less vigorous and clearance of foreign particles is slower and bronchitis and emphysema result.

Musculo-skeletal system

Skeletal ageing probably generates most of the common symptoms responsible for limitations of recreational activities and functions of daily living as well as restrictions in job related activities; the joint and muscle aches and stiffness attributed to 'getting old'.

Bones thin at a rate of 0.8–1.0%/yr over the lifespan for both men and women, but there is acceleration in the rate for females around the menopause, of between 8–10%/yr. Thus post-menopausal women are more vulnerable than males of the same age to pathologically thin bones or to osteoporosis which can cause fractures of the vertebral spine. While both men and women are at risk for fractures of the long bones, women are fracture prone 10 years earlier than men of the same cohort. (Kenny, 2000; Raiz, 1997). Smoking changes these fracture risk odds for men and women because cigarette smoking is also toxic for bone growth cells and is a major cause of osteoporosis in both male and female smokers.

Liver

The liver has remarkable regenerative capacity but undergoes modest decreases in weight and size. Hepatic blood flow shows a 1.5% fall/yr so that there will be a 50% reduction in flow over the lifespan. All ingested drugs as well as metabolites absorbed from the small intestine and stomach, pass through the liver; some are unchanged while most undergo metabolic detoxification by microsomal enzymes into water-soluble substances for renal excretion. With decreases in liver mass, losses in this critical enzymatic function (primarily Cytochrome P-450) are seen and, along with a decrease in blood flow, there is a decrease in the rate of Phase I biotransformation, particularly in men. These functional changes result in a prolongation in the half-life of many of the metabolites and drugs that are inactivated by the liver. Conjugation or Phase II remains largely unchanged.

Kidney

All kidney functions deteriorate with age because of a steady loss of nephrons over time. Thus there are declines in filtration, active tubular secretion and re-absorption and passive tubular diffusion. This decline in renal function has serious implications for drug prescribing patterns (Kenney, 1989; Finch & Schneider, 1985) since the kidneys serve as the major excretion site for metabolites and drugs after transformation through the liver and renal insufficiency or functional loss prolongs the body's exposure to drugs and toxic substances as well as digestive by-products.

Immune system

With increasing age, the total number of immune cells changes minimally, but the functional, or qualitative changes in immunity with age are much more notable than the quantitative ones.

Investigators in the field of physiological psychology have described complex and direct links between the central nervous system and the immune system. The neurohumorally mediated effects of stress on the immune system have also been well demonstrated in carefully controlled experiments with rodents and primates (Borysenko & Borysenko, 1982; Rosenberg *et al.*, 1982). Studies in humans have demonstrated similar effects, though it is impossible to achieve the same degree of control as in the animal studies. Health surveys have reported clusters of illness (from the common cold to cancer) occurring around the time of major life changes (Minter & Patterson-Kimball, 1978). Other studies have found strong correlations between loneliness and decreased proliferative responses of lymphocytes to mitogens, decreased natural killer cell activity and impaired DNA splicing and repair in lymphocytes (Glaser *et al.*, 1985). Healthy adults over the age of 60 years with a strong social support system (i.e. a close confidant/e) have significantly greater total lymphocyte counts, and stronger stimulus-induced responses than those without such a relationship (Thomas *et al.*, 1991). Persons experiencing the stress of care giving for a spouse with dementia have poorer antibody responses to influenza vaccination than matched control subjects, and their lymphocytes make less interleukin 1β and interleukin 2 when stimulated with virus in vitro (Kiecolt-Glaser *et al.*, 1996). These caregivers also display delayed wound healing after punch biopsy of the skin compared to non-care giving, age-matched controls (Kiecolt-Glaser *et al.*, 1995). The mechanisms that underlie such associations, and the modulating effects of age, are not fully understood but are clearly important for maintaining full independent function (see also 'Psychoneuroimmunology', 'Stress and Health' and 'Social Support and Health').

The nervous system

Given the complexity of the nervous system, it is to be expected that there will be significant variability in the functional changes that mirror anatomic changes of ageing. In general, these descriptions are based on cross-sectional studies and are thus open to criticism, but it appears that functions that change very minimally from ages 25 to 75 include: vocabulary, information accrual and comprehension and digit forward pass. There are subtle changes in hand two point discrimination, and minimal touch sensation loss in the fingers and toes. A greater than 20% decline is seen in 'dexterity areas' including hand- and foot-tapping and tandem stepping. Greater decrements are seen in the ability to rise from a chair; however, these tasks must reflect muscle as well as nervous system function and may be confounded by joint disease. Arthritic changes in the hands will produce difficulty in 'dexterous' activities such as cutting with a knife, zipping and buttoning. Thus, studies of function using ADL types of behaviour may significantly confound ageing with chronic illness.

Recent research has shown that there is much less neuronal loss than had previously been assumed, although brain weight declines significantly with age and blood flow is decreased by about 20% in the absence of vascular disease. In addition, decrements are seen in cerebral autoregulation. Cells disappear randomly throughout the cortex, but in other brain areas, there is clustered loss, i.e. the disproportionally greater loss of cells in the cerebellum, the locus ceruleus and the substantia nigra. The hypothalamus, pons and medulla have modest age-related losses (Anglade *et al.*, 1997). These may be responsible for the altered sleep patterns characteristic of the elderly, and disturbances of gait and balance. The alterations in sleep patterns are a source of much concern for up to 50%

of persons aged 60 and older with 12% of an epidemiological sample of persons over 65 reporting significant and chronic insomnia. Ageing individuals believe they sleep poorly and insist they are up all night long. Indeed they are frequently aroused, but the total amount of sleep that occurs during the night is essentially unchanged (see 'Sleep and Health'). Careful inquiries reveal that such persons are usually refreshed and rarely sleepy when they awake, even though their sleep patterns have changed. Up to half of community-dwelling elderly persons use either over-the-counter or prescription sleeping medications. Most studies suggest a greater prevalence of subjective sleep abnormalities and greater use of hypnotics by older women, and those that have been studied have been shown to have sleep aberrations on monitoring. On the other hand, older women appear to have better preservation of slow wave sleep than older men. (Fukuda, 1999). The problem that confronts the clinician becomes the seeking of sleeping or hypnotic potions. The excessive prescribing of hypnotic medications is common for older patients. Hypnotic drugs cannot increase locus ceruleus cell number or reverse age related sleep cycle changes but can increase vulnerability to confusion and delirium as well as addiction. Thus it may be inappropriate to prescribe hypnotics, except under times of extreme stress or during hospitalization or sickness. Non-pharmacologic interventions to facilitate good 'sleep hygiene' need to be utilized to treat a maladaptive response to normal ageing.

Myelin decreases primarily in the white matter of the cortex. (Saunders *et al.*, 1999; Mielke *et al.*, 1998; Sjobeck *et al.*, 1999). Apoptosis or programmed cell death may be responsible for brain neuron loss. (Sastry *et al.*, 1997). Although there is cellular dropout, new synapses continue to form throughout the life span. (Aamodt & Constantine-Paton, 1999). The number of spinal cord motor neurons remains essentially unchanged until the seventh decade, after which losses occur in the anterior horn cells (Cruz-Sanchez *et al.*, 1998). Vibratory and tactile thresholds decrease and the thermal threshold in the fingers goes up thereby decreasing sensory sensitivities.

In summary, there are significant organ and cell-specific biological changes that occur at different rates within and between ageing individuals. The ability to respond to stress becomes compromised, yet in the absence of significant chronic disease, functional independence can be maintained well into the ninth decade. Specific aspects of senescence are particularly relevant for the health psychologist who must appreciate the limited reserve of the older patients, the fragility of the immune response and the increased vulnerability to medications of all types and, in particular, to psychoactive drugs and yet appreciate the remarkable resiliency of the elderly 'survivor'.

See also 'Psychological Care of the Elderly'.

REFERENCES

Aamodt, S. M. & Constantine-Paton, M. (1999). The role of neural activity in synaptic development and its implications for adult brain function. *Advances in Neurology*, **79**, 133–44. (Review).

Anderson, R. N., Kochanek, K. D., Murphy, S. I. (1995). Report of final mortality statistics, 1995. *Monthly Vital Statistics Report.* Hyattsville, MD: National Center for Health Statistics. 1007; **45**(11 Supp 2).

Anglade, P., Vyas, S., Hirsch, E. C., Agid, Y. (1997). Apoptosis in dopaminergic neurons of the human substantia nigra during normal aging. *Histology and histopathology,* **12**(3); 603–10.

Borysenko, M. & Borysenko, J. (1982). Stress, behavior and immunity: animal models and mediating mechanisms. *General Hospital Psychiatry,* **4**; 59–67.

Cruz-Sanchez F. F., Moral A., Tolosa E., de Belleroche J. & Rossi M. L. (1998). Evaluation of neuronal loss, astrocytosis and abnormalities of cytoskeletal components of large motor neurons in the human anterior horn in aging. *Journal of Neuronal Transmission*, **105**(6–7); 689–701.

Finch, C. E. & Schneider E. L. (1985). *Handbook of Biology of Aging, Vol. 2* (2nd Edn.). Van Nostrand Reinhold: New York.

Fukuda, N. (1999). Gender difference of slow wave sleep in middle aged and elderly subjects. *Psychiatry and Clinical Neurosciences*, **53**(2); 151–3.

Jazwinski, S. M. (1996). Longevity, genes, and aging. *Science*. **273**(5271); 54–9.

Kiecolt-Glaser, J. K., Glaser, R., Gravenstein, S., Malarkey, W. B. & Sheridan, J. (1996). Chronic stress laters the immune response to influenza virus vaccine in older adults. *Proceedings of the National Academy of Sciences*, **93**; 3043–7.

Kiecolt-Glaser, J. K., Marucha, P. T., Malarkey, W. H. *et al.* (1995). Slowing of wound healing by psychological stress. *Lancet*. **346**; 1194–6.

Kiecolt-Glaser, J. K., McGuire, L., Robles, T. F. & Glazer, R. Psychoneuroimmunology: Psychological influences on immune function and health. *Journal of*

Consulting and Clinical Psychology, **70**; 537–47.

Glaser, R., Thorn, B. E., Tarr, K. L. *et al.* (1985). Effects of stress on methyltransferase synthesis: an important DNA repair enzyme. *Health Psychology*, **4**; 403–12.

Kenney, A. R. (1989). *Physiology of Aging: A Synopsis* (2nd edn.). Chicago: Year Book Medical Publishers, Inc.

Kenny, A. M. (2000). Osteoporosis. *Pathogenesis Rheumatic Disease Clinics of North America*, **26**(3); 569–91.

Kirkwood, T. B. L. (1996). Human Senescence. *Bioessays*, **18**(12); 1009–16.

Lakatta, E. G. (1987). Cardiovascular function and age. *Geriatrics*, **42**; 84–94.

Marin J. (1995). Age-related changes in vascular responses: a review. *Mechanisms of Ageing and Development*, **79**(2–3); 71–114.

Mielke, R., Kessler, J., Szelies, B. *et al.* (1998). Normal and pathological aging–findings of positron-emission tomography. *Journal of Neural Transmission*, **105**(8–9); 821–37.

Minter R. E. & Patterson-Kimball, C. (1978). Life events and illness onset: a review. *Psychosomatics*, **19**; 334–9.

Raiz, L. G. (1997). The osteoporosis revolution. *Annals of Internal Medicine*, **126**(6); 458–62.

Rosenberg, I. T., Coe, C. I. & Levine, S. (1982). Complement levels in the squirrel monkey. *Laboratory Animal Science*, **32**; 371–72.

Rossi, A., Ganassini, A., Tantucci, C. *et al.* (1996). Aging and the respiratory system, *Aging* (Milano). **8**(3); 143–161.

Rowe J. W. & Kahn R. L. (1998). *Successful Aging*. New York: Pantheon Press.

Sastry, P. S. & Rao, K. S. (2000). Apoptosis and the nervous system. *Journal of Neurochemistry*, **74**(1); 1–20.

Saunders, D. E., Howe, F. A., van den Boogaart, A., Griffiths, J. R. & Brown, M. M. (1999). Aging of the adult human brain: in vivo quantitation of metabolite content with proton magnetic resonance spectroscopy. *Journal of Magnetic Resonance Imaging*, **9**; 711–6.

Thomas, P. D., Goodwin, J. M. & Goodwin, J. S. D. (1985). Effect of social support on stress-related changes in cholesterol level, uric acid level and immune function in a elderly sample. *The American Journal of Psychiatry*, **142**; 735–7.

Architecture and health

Angela Liegey Dougall[1], Stacie Spencer[1] and Andrew Baum[2]

[1]University of Pittsburgh
[2]University of Pittsburgh Medical Center

Overview

Architecture can be considered in many ways, as art or aesthetic stimuli, as an expression of societal pride or aspiration, and as a way of structuring interior and exterior spaces to facilitate their use by human occupants. This latter function of architectural design has strong but modifiable effects on social behaviour and users' mood and productivity and, to some extent, design features also affect health and wellbeing. Too often, however, these important sources of influence are ignored or not recognized, despite repeated demonstrations of these effects. While much remains to be done, research has identified several architectural features that appear to be associated with mood and health. Design characteristics or the way space is structured, presence or absence of windows and illumination all appear to affect people. For some features, the relationship to health is indirect (e.g. small, crowded work spaces may result in stress that may in turn affect health) while for other features the relationship to health is more direct (e.g. eye strain from poor lighting, illness from exposure to fumes).

The structural design or arrangement of space imposes restrictions on behaviour. Doorways determine our access to a room and room dimensions restrict the kinds of behaviours that can take place inside a room. As a result, one of the most important goals when designing a building is to match the built environment with the needs of the individuals for whom the environment is designed. However, even under the best conditions, primary uses of a building may change and interior changes must be made to meet the current purposes. Flexibility may therefore supersede many desirable design characteristics, which may have negative effects on use. Regardless of circumstances, among its effects, the interior design of space has an impact on the perception of density and crowding, can impose excess interaction or isolation and has been associated with arousal and stress (see Baum & Paulus, 1987).

Three inter-related variables are important considerations in the design of space because of the potential for indirect influences on mood and health. These variables are the perception of density, privacy and control. Density is the ratio of the number of individuals within a space to the actual size of that space and is thus an expression of physical properties of the setting (Baum & Koman, 1976; Stokols, 1972). Density can increase when the absolute amounts of available space decrease, and such changes in spatial density reflect the negative effects of decreasing space. For example, as density increases, people may have to work harder to maintain privacy (Altman, 1975). As the number of people increases, regardless of how much space is available, social overload and stress are also likely (see 'Stress and Health'). This focus on social density reflects the subjective experience of frequent or unwanted interaction and is often not easy to change (Baum & Valins, 1979). The high social density environment may threaten the control an individual tries to maintain over privacy and regulation of social interactions. If density increases because the amount of available space decreases, stress associated with exposure to high social density environments where there is little privacy or control over social interaction can lead to negative health outcomes (Paulus *et al.*, 1978).

A series of studies carried out in the 1970s investigated the impact of architecturally determined differences in social density on behaviour in college dormitories. Long-corridor-type dormitories in which a large number of individuals were required to share a hallway, bathroom and lounge also required residents to interact with many individuals, often with people they disliked and/or did not know very well. Further, many interactions occurred at inconvenient times (Baum & Valins, 1977).

In comparison, suite-type dormitories structurally determined smaller groups and reduced the number of required interactions when using shared spaces usually three to five suite-mates (Baum & Valins). Residents of corridor dorms reported that they felt more crowded than did suite residents, despite living on halls with comparable densities and total numbers of residents. Associated with this, corridor residents exhibited lower thresholds for crowding and avoided social interaction outside the dormitory environment, reported lower feelings of control in shared spaces, were less likely to know how hallmates felt about them and were less willing to share information about themselves with other people living on the floor (Baum & Valins, 1977; Baum *et al.*, 1975). In comparison with suite residents, long-corridor residents were more competitive and reactive, and appeared to be more motivated to regulate social contacts in the first few weeks of dormitory residence. However, in as few as seven weeks, behaviour changed and residents became more withdrawn and exhibited symptoms of helplessness (Baum *et al.*, 1978). The effects of crowding were strong enough to generalize to non-dormitory settings (Baum & Valins, 1977). One of the basic conclusions of these studies of dormitories was that design and layout of interior residential space affects crowding stress and health under conditions of high physical density (Evans *et al.*, 2002). Research has continued to report evidence of mediation of social behaviour by architectural design. For example, Evans *et al.* (1996) studied mitigating effects of interior design on residential density using a measure called architectural depth (AD). They defined AD as the number of spaces one must pass through to get from one room in a residence to another, reflecting variety, complexity and privacy afforded by a residential environment. High AD (presumably high complexity, privacy and so on) was associated with less social withdrawal and buffering of residential crowding (Evans *et al.* 1996). Independently, residential density was associated with mental health and task performance, with higher density linked to poorer mental health and less task persistence (Evans *et al.*, 2001).

Similarly, a study of 2017 households in Thailand found that household crowding was associated with wellbeing (Fuller *et al.*, 1996). Objective crowding (measures of physical density) was inversely linked with wellbeing but perceived crowding showed stronger negative relationships, suggesting that factors which increase perceived stress also increase the negative impact of residential crowding.

High social density and loss of control have also been associated with self-report, behavioural and biochemical indices of stress. In studies of prison inmates, death rates and rates of psychiatric commitments were higher in years when prison population was higher (Paulus *et al.*, 1975). Paulus *et al.* (1975) also found that inmates living under high social density conditions had higher blood pressure. In another study of prison inmates, perceived crowding was associated with urinary catecholamine levels (Schaeffer *et al.*, 1988). Residents of low density cells (private cells) reported less crowding and exhibited lower urinary catecholamine levels than did residents of high density cells (open dormitories). Residents of high density cells that had been modified to reduce social density (cubicles within a dormitory) exhibited catecholamine levels comparable to the private-cell inmates. However, these inmates had the highest number of health complaints (Schaeffer *et al.*, 1988).

These studies suggest that design of residential space has far-ranging effects on residents and should be considered when designing new buildings. In the case of pre-existing buildings, modifications can be made to reduce the stress of crowding. Studies have shown that partitioning space can accommodate increases in spatial density without increasing effective social density (Desor, 1972). These changes should be aimed at increasing the perception of control over regulation of social experiences and supporting local control of shared spaces. Cubicles within dormitory-style prison housing increased regulatory control and were associated with catecholamine levels similar to that of private-cell inmates (Schaeffer *et al.*, 1988). Similarly, an architectural intervention, in which a long-corridor dormitory hall was bisected, resulted in greater confidence in residents' control over social interactions in the dormitory, less residential and non-residential social withdrawal, and less crowding stress compared with the non-bisected long-corridor residents (Baum & Davis, 1980).

These findings have implications for the design of other spaces in which large numbers of individuals must share areas and/or work together. For example, in work environments it is often too costly to provide private offices for every employee. Simply filling a large room with desks would not be a good alternative because of the resulting noise as well as inefficiency and decreased regulatory control over social interaction (see 'Noise: Effects on Health'). Such a design would be likely to decrease productivity, increase stress levels and increase the likelihood of negative health outcomes. Use of modular cubicles or other methods of breaking space up would provide the structure for increasing control over local spaces and productivity and prevent increases in distress associated with crowding.

Other architectural features also have important influences on behavioural health. Windows and illumination appear to be particularly important factors. As with the interior design of space, each of these features has an impact on perceptions and behaviours that may affect health. Windows are so important to individuals that the assignment to an office with a window is tied directly to office hierarchies. Big promotions often include a move to an office with a window. The importance of windowed offices is also demonstrated by findings indicating that people in windowless offices report less job satisfaction, less interest in their jobs and are less positive about the physical work conditions (e.g. appearance, light, temperature) (Finnegan & Solomon, 1981). People in windowless offices also use more visual materials (typically of nature scenes) than do occupants of windowed spaces to decorate their environments (Heerwagen & Orians, 1986). While there is little argument about whether windows are a desired feature, they are expensive, energy inefficient and are limited to exterior walls. In large office buildings, some windowless offices are inevitable. The reductions or changes in the views people have, the positive ambience of the setting, and other effects of having or not having windows appear to affect mood and health in dramatic ways.

For example, research suggests that windows are important in recovery from surgery and in intensive care units. Ulrich (1983, 1984) argues that natural views are associated with positive emotional states which may play a role in the reduction of stressful thoughts and recovery from surgery. In a study of patients recovering from a cholecystectomy procedure, Ulrich compared post-cholecystectomy patients who had a window view of trees with patients who had a window view of a brick wall. In comparison with the wall-view patients, patients with a natural view had fewer post-surgical complications, took fewer moderate and high doses and more weak doses of pain medication, were described by nurses as demonstrating fewer negative characteristics (e.g. being upset and crying, needing much encouragement), and stayed in the hospital for less time post-surgery. In a different study, Keep, James and Inman (1980) found that intensive care patients in windowless units had less accurate memories of the length of their stays and were not as well orientated during their hospitalization as intensive care patients in windowed units. Comparisons of 137 staff and 100 inpatients' responses to variable windows and views in hospital settings suggested that patients were more negatively affected by poorly windowed rooms than were staff (Verderber & Reuman, 1987). Discharged hospital patients identify several sources of satisfaction with hospital environments including interior design, privacy and ambient environmental features such as lighting and view (Harris et al., 2002). Others have proposed a different, overlapping set of elements of satisfaction in hospital settings, with factors such as attractiveness, privacy, safety, comforts and conveniences emerging as important in affording therapeutic effects of clinical spares (Grosenick & Hatmaker, 1999).

Windows are also related to illumination; they provide natural lighting and the extent and nature of illumination are important features of design on many different levels. The kind of illumination (incandescent, fluorescent), the brightness of illumination and the spectral range of the illumination, are all important characteristics of light and govern their effects on mood and behaviour. The cool white fluorescent lights used in public places are economical, energy efficient and maintenance free, but these lights produce only partial spectrum light waves and lack the spectrum of natural sunlight (Sperry, 1984). In comparison with exposure to full spectrum lights, exposure to cool white fluorescent lights for as little as four hours has been associated with increased lethargy, visual fatigue and decreased visual acuity (Maas et al., 1974). This is important in settings such as libraries and offices, where the majority of work is visual (Sperry, 1984). Over days and weeks, the cumulative effects of repeated exposure to cool white fluorescent lighting may result in job stress, chronic fatigue and poor vision. The use of lighting which includes the full spectrum may be preferable.

Architectural features such as the design of space, the presence of windows, and illumination affect social behaviour, mood and productivity, and appear to be associated with health (Devlin & Arneill, 2003). While these features are important to consider during the design of space, they are sometimes easy to modify in existing space. Partitions can be used to decrease social density while allowing increases in special density. Window views can be designed to include natural scenes and where a window looks onto another building or in offices in which a window does not exist, murals can be used to simulate natural scenes. Interior lighting can be chosen to maximize the full spectrum of available light. Research and intervention in the design or redesign of space with these features in mind will provide further evidence of the impact of the design of interior spaces and will provide new insights in to the complex but important interactions of behavioural, biological and environmental variables in determining health and wellbeing.

REFERENCES

Altman, I. (1975). *The environment and social behavior.* Monterey, CA: Brooks/Cole.

Baum, A., Aiello, J. R. & Calesnick, L. E. (1978). Crowding and personal control: social density and the development of learned helplessness. *Journal of Personality and Social Psychology*, **36**, 1000–11.

Baum, A. & Davis, G. E. (1980). Reducing the stress of high-density living: an architectural intervention. *Journal of Personality and Social Psychology*, **38**, 471–81.

Baum, A., Harpin, R. E. & Valins, S. (1975). The role of group phenomena in the experience of crowding. *Environment and Behavior*, **7**, 185–98.

Baum, A. & Koman, S. (1976). Differential response to anticipated crowding: of social density. *Journal of Personality and Social Psychology*, **34**, 526–36.

Baum, A. & Paulus, P. B. (1987). Crowding. In D. Stokols & I. Altman (Eds.). *Handbook of environmental psychology.* New York: Wiley.

Baum, A. & Valins, S. (1977). *Architecture and social behavior: psychological studies of social density.* Hillsdale, NJ: Lawrence Erlbaum Associates.

Baum, A. & Valins, S. (1979). Architectural mediation of residential density and control: social contact. *Advances in Experimental Social Psychology*, **12**, 131–75.

Desor, J. A. (1972). Toward a psychological theory of crowding. *Journal of Personality and Social Psychology*, **21**, 79–83.

Devlin, A. S. & Arneill, A. B. (2003). Health care environments and patient outcomes: A Review of the Literature. *Environment and Behavior*, **35**, 665–94.

Evans, G. W., Lepore, S. J. & Schroeder, A. (1996). The role of interior design elements in human responses to crowding. *Journal of Personality and Social Psychology*, **70**, 41–6.

Evans, G. W., Lercher, P. & Kofler, W. W. (2002). Crowding and children's mental health: the role of house type. *Journal of Environmental Psychology*, **22**, 221–31.

Evans, G. W., Saigert, S. & Harrid, R. (2001). Residential density and psychological health among children in low-income families. *Environment and Behavior*, **33**, 165–80.

Finnegan, M. C. & Solomon, L. Z. (1981). Work attitudes in windowed vs. windowless environments. *Journal of Social Psychology*, **115**, 291–2.

Fuller, T. D., Edwards, J. N., Vorakitphokatorn, S. & Sermsri, S. (1996). Chronic stress and psychological well-being: evidence from Thailand on household crowding. *Social Science and Medicine*, **42**, 265–80.

Grosenick, J. K. & Hatmaker, C. M. (2000). Perceptions of the importance of physical setting in substance abuse treatment. *Journal of Substance Abuse Treatment*, **18**, 29–39.

Harris, P. B., McBride, G., Ross, C. & Curtis, L. (2002). A place to heal: environmental sources of satisfaction among hospital patients. *Journal of Applied Social Psychology*, **32**, 1276–99.

Heerwagen, J. H. & Orians, G. H. (1986). Adaptations to windowlessness: a study of the use of visual décor in windowed and windowless offices. *Environment and Behavior*, **18**, 623–39.

Keep, P., James, J. and wellness medicine in the intensive therapy unit' 0000 *Anesthesia*, **35**, 257–62.

Maas, J. B., Jayson, J. K. & Kleiber, D. A. (1974). Effects of spectral difference in illumination on fatigue. *Journal of Applied Psychology*, **59**, 524–6.

Paulus, P., Cox, V., McCain, G. & Chandler, J. (1975). Some effects of crowding in a prison environment, *Journal of Applied Social Psychology*, **5**, 86–91.

Paulus, P., McGain, G. & Cox, V. (1978). Death rates, psychiatric commitments, blood pressure and perceived crowding as a function of institutional crowding. *Environmental Psychology and Non-Verbal Behavior*, **3**, 107–16.

Schaeffer, M. A., Baum, A., Paulus, P. B. & Gaes, G. G. (1988). Architecturally mediated effects of social density in prison. *Environment and Behavior*, **20**, 3–19.

Sperry, L. (1984). Health promotion and wellness medicine in the workplace: programs, promises, and problems. *Individual Psychology: Journal of Adlerian Theory, Research and Practice*, **40**, 401–11.

Stokols, D. (1972). On the distinction between density and crowding; some implications for future research. *Psychological Review*, **79**, 275–7.

Ulrich, R. S. (1983). Aesthetic and affective response to natural environment. *Human Behavior and Environment: Advances in Theory and Research*, **6**, 85–125.

Ulrich, R. S. (1984). View through a window may influence recovery from surgery. *Science*, **224**, 420–1.

Verderber, S. & Reuman, D. (1988). Windows, views, and health status in hospital therapeutic environments. *Journal of Architectural and Planning Research*, **4**, 120–33.

Attributions and health

Yael Benyamini[1], Howard Leventhal[2] and Elaine A. Leventhal[3]

[1]Tel Aviv University
[2]The State University of New Jersey
[3]UMDNJ-Robert Wood Johnson Medical School

People are often motivated to determine the causes of events: the more unexpected and disruptive the event, the more likely is the individual to ask, 'Why did this happen?' (Weiner, 1985). As the symptoms and diagnoses of illness are often unexpected and disruptive and may have threatening implications, we can expect health threats to stimulate preoccupation with questions of cause. As social psychologists suggested decades ago (Heider, 1958), causal, i.e. attributional, thinking can clarify the meaning of an event and define its long term implications. In this brief chapter we will address the following questions about the attributional facet of commonsense psychology: 1) do illnesses (symptoms and diagnoses) stimulate causal thinking, i.e. attributions, and when are these attributions most likely to be made? 2) how are attributions for health threats formed? 3) what kinds of attributions do people make? 4) what are the behavioural consequences of these attributions for the management of and adjustment to illness? 5) do attributions have long-term effects on health?

Unfortunately, a straightforward review of results for each of these questions would be difficult to complete as there is considerable disagreement among published findings. Existing reviews of the literature in this area have also resulted in conflicting conclusions regarding questions such as the relationship of attributions to adjustment. Hall *et al.* (2003) reviewed 65 studies and found little evidence of a relationship between attributions and outcomes. Roesch and Weiner (2001) reviewed 27 studies and found evidence of an indirect relationship of attribution with adjustment, mediated through ways of coping. We have therefore decided to begin by addressing a prior question: 'Where do attributions fit within the context of common-sense reasoning and adjustment to anticipated and current health threats?' The answer to this question assumes that the meaning of an attribution, and hence its consequences, will differ as a function of the context, i.e. disease model, in which it is made. Thus, we hope to provide a framework that will transform inconsistencies into an orderly set of moderated effects and illuminate areas in need of further research.

A model for understanding attributions

If attributions are important for clarifying meaning (Jones, 1990), it is critical to define the structure and content of the behavioural system within which attributions are made. Our 'common-sense model of self-regulation in response to health threats' (Leventhal *et al.*, 1980; Leventhal *et al.*, 1992; Leventhal *et al.*, this volume), provides one such framework (see 'Lay Beliefs about Health and Illness'). The constituents of the behavioural system as defined by this and similar models are the representation of an illness/ threat, a set of procedures for threat/illness management, and criteria for evaluating outcomes. Thus, the implication or meaning of an attribution will vary depending upon the question it addresses, i.e. is it an attribution about a symptom, e.g. is the symptom a manifestation of a particular disease or of some non-disease process?; is it an attribution about the cause of a disease, e.g. a virus, genetic factor, psychological factor, etc.?; is it an attribution about the coping procedures for disease management, e.g. why is it plausible that this procedure will be effective, who is responsible for performing the procedure, self or doctor?; or is it an attribution about the outcome of a treatment procedure, e.g. did the symptom/disease go away because of the treatment or fade on its own?

Different diseases have different models, differentiated by biology and culture. For example, the concrete experience and abstract meaning of illness representations will differ for hypertension, breast cancer and the common cold; hypertension is believed to be accompanied by heart pounding, warm face and headaches though it is actually asymptomatic (Meyer *et al.*, 1985); breast cancer can produce discolouration of the breast and palpable lumps, and the common cold is accompanied by a stuffy nose, headaches, sneezing and coughing. These models are further differentiated according to one's cultural background.

Abstract, cultural concepts of methods for controlling these diseases and their likely success also differ. For example, surgery is appropriate for cancer but not for the cold, and cultural expectations for the success of control (cure) are clearly poorer for breast cancer than for hypertension or the common cold. Finally, the facet of the representation that is salient at a given point in time, e.g. its symptoms or consequences, will reflect the history of the specific disease episode, e.g. is the episode at its beginning with only vague manifestations, or has it progressed to diagnosis, treatment, or recovery and rehabilitation? (Alonzo, 1980; Safer *et al.*, 1979). Additionally, it will reflect the personal and vicarious illness experiences of the individual in the past (Benyamini *et al.*, 2003). The motivation for question asking, the type of question asked, the answers to this question, i.e. the attribution that is made and its consequences, will vary as a function of these factors. With this understood, we can proceed to address our questions.

Attributions in response to illness threats: *are* they made?

Our self-regulation model suggests that questions are more likely to be asked and causal attributions formed at some points within a disease episode than at others, e.g. when trying to identify the nature of a symptom rather than when considering the consequences of a diagnosis or treatment, and for some rather than for all diseases, e.g. a life-threatening cancer in contrast to an innocuous cold.

Investigators have typically used direct questions, requesting either closed-ended or open-ended answers, to determine the type of attributions being made, rather than using open-ended approaches to find out whether they are being made at all. Thus, the typical approach assumes that people will attempt to probe the cause of their illness once it is diagnosed and the meaning of symptoms clarified (Rodin, 1978). Indeed, Taylor, Lichtman and Wood (1984) interviewed women who have been diagnosed with breast cancer and found that 95% of them were able to provide a causal attribution for their cancer. Similarly, only one of 29 subjects paralyzed as a result of serious accidents did not come up with a hypothesis respecting its cause (Bulman & Wortman, 1977). In their review of the literature, Turnquist *et al.* (1988) reported that 69 to 95% of individuals make causal attributions for their illness, and that the frequency of causal reporting is usually higher the more severe the diagnosis (e.g. cancer) and the longer the time since diagnosis. Although patients do not always report explicit causes for their illness, they view cause as one of the most important pieces of information from their physician at diagnosis (Greenberg *et al.*, 1984).

These findings clearly indicate that people generate hypotheses about the causes of their illness, but they do not address whether they do so without being prompted. Two studies that asked chronically ill patients (with arthritis, diabetes, hypertension or soon after a myocardial infarction) if they have ever thought why this had happened to them, found that roughly half of the sample had said that they had not (Lowery *et al.*, 1987; Lowery *et al.*, 1992). Another study reported that, when asked, almost all patients provided causes for arthritis-related symptoms and for ambiguous symptoms, but only patients with a past history of cancer were preoccupied with the cause: a much larger number of those who called the doctor did so in order to verify the cause (Benyamini *et al.*, 2003). Taken together, these findings question the validity of the assumption that causal search is universally initiated under the conditions of unexpectedness, uncertainty and threat that are posed by illness, at least for diseases and risks other than cancer. For cancer, attributions may serve a function in promoting the belief that recurrence can be prevented; but for arthritis, hypertension or diabetes, recurrence is not the issue, and for a myocardial infarction, soon after the event, it is recovery and not recurrence that troubles people. When taking into account the low utility in holding attributions for these diseases it is not surprising that studies have found lower preoccupation with causes in these cases.

Studies have also examined the strength and perceived importance of causal attributions for disease, and found that patients with severe conditions and patients perceiving the outcome of their illness to be a failure seem to hold their attributions with less conviction (Turnquist *et al.*, 1988). This also seems to have an adaptive value: as health status changes, people change their illness model to include causes that show more promise in terms of current and future management of the illness threat. Being highly committed to any specific cause sets a higher value on such changes. In sum, it is likely that the occurrence and strength of attributional processes depend on their contribution to one's coping with the health threat at question. A mere understanding of the types of attributions made provides little insight into these processes. As researchers and practitioners, it is more useful to first understand how these attributions are made.

Attributions in response to illness threats: how are they made?

Efforts have been made to identify the rules guiding the attributional process. Examples from studies of social cognition include factors such as the actor–observer bias, i.e. actors identify environmental factors as the causes for their actions while observers attribute these actions to the personal characteristics of the actor (Jones & Davis, 1965), and self-serving biases such as attributing failure to environmental factors and success to characteristics of the self (Fiske & Taylor, 1991). A recent study of causal attributions for myocardial infarction (MI) in patient and non-patient samples provided evidence that does not favor the actor-observer hypothesis (French et al., 2004). The data suggested that method effects account for differences in attributions, with the important distinction being that between attributions in general and attributions regarding a specific person's MI (self or other). Attributions of causes of the disease in general are important in order to explain public opinions or 'stereotypes' of the disease and they may impact upon policy decisions and attitudes (and stigma) towards certain patient populations. For example, causal attributions were related to the perception of greater consequences of diabetes when judging this disease in general, but not when judging it as personally relevant (Shiloh et al., 2002). However, when the focus is on patients' coping with a disease, attributions to a specific person's disease are important in order to understand how people adjust and how close ones, such as spouses, provide support to the patient (Benyamini et al., 2007).

As is the case with determining if people make attributions spontaneously, the method of questioning is a source of difficulty for identifying mental rules. A wide variety of methods has been used to assess attributions in prior studies, and each may create its own biases. For example, closed-ended methods included Q-sort of possible causes, attribution of percentage of blame to different factors, ratings of importance of different internal and external causes, and more. Open-ended questions also varied, especially in their focus on 'what caused your illness?', on 'why me?' or even more specifically on 'why me, instead of someone else?' By focusing on the specifics of the disease, the first approach may generate information on rules that are disease-specific, while the second may elicit thoughts and comparisons that generate rules relevant to one's life situation and disease development. When asked about the causes of their MI, patients may be answering the questions 'Why did it happen now? What triggered it?' while researchers typically ask about the patients' perceptions of the causes of the underlying disease (French et al., 2005). Even the 'Why me?' question is multi-layered, as Steensma (2003) suggested, ranging from a search for a more mechanistic explanation of the condition to unanswerable questions of injustice.

Initially, patients use heuristics to identify causes, which serve as 'working cognitions' that can be later modified according to the progress of the disease and the patient's knowledge about it. These include rules such as the symmetry rule, which is the need to find labels for symptoms and symptoms for labels (Leventhal et al., 1992); the stress–illness rule, or the tendency to attribute symptoms to stress in the presence of stressors (Cameron et al., 1995); and the age–illness rule, which is the tendency to attribute slow-developing, not too severe symptoms, to age (Leventhal et al., 1992) (see 'Aging and health behaviour'). The latter two rules result in attributions to non-disease sources, a tendency that is particularly noticeable in the early stages of illness episodes when symptoms are ambiguous. Thus, when the symptoms of a disease are mild and slow to develop, they can be interpreted as 'normal' or as unavoidable signs of ageing rather than as signs of disease (Kart, 1981; Prohaska et al., 1987). In a similar vein, ambiguous symptoms, the onset of which is associated with recent life stresses, e.g. examinations, family quarrels, etc. are likely to be attributed to stress rather than illness (Baumann et al., 1989; Cameron, et al., 1995). Both interpretations lead to delays in seeking professional care.

As patients become more knowledgeable over time regarding the causes of their disease, their answers may increasingly come to reflect medical and cultural views based on what they have heard from their physician and other sources rather than reflecting their own thoughts and mental operations. For example, 'Western' Israeli women with breast cancer mentioned a variety of physiological causes, reflecting a more rational–scientific attitude while more 'traditional' religious women either did not know or perceived the cause to be personal–emotional (Baider & Sarell, 1983), similar to the differences found between Western and Asian Canadian students (Armstrong & Swartzman, 1999).

There are some indications that patients who have little medical knowledge follow very simple causal rules in addressing attributional issues, such as 'causes should be temporally and spatially close to effects' (Taylor, 1982), and 'causes should resemble effects' (Salmon et al., 1996). These rules are especially in error for chronic diseases such as cancer which have lengthy developmental histories. Most studies have paid little attention to variations in the content of attributions associated with differences in socioeconomic status (Pill & Stott, 1982) and ethnic group membership. For example, minority respondents are more likely to view serious chronic illnesses as unpreventable and uncontrollable, because of the fatalistic themes sometimes present in their culture (Landrine & Klonoff, 1994; Pérez-Stable et al., 1992). Thus, the questions asked about illness and the rules of inference observed in subjects from various social backgrounds will reflect orientations general to the culture rather than rules specific to the person.

Attributions: types and consequences

Attributions of symptoms

Do women later diagnosed with cancer ask questions about the source of their symptoms early in the disease process? In a retrospective study of women diagnosed with cancer, participants were clearly motivated to find explanations for uncertain physiological signs and symptoms, and the strength of this motivation was related to the salience and the perceived personal consequences of these bodily reactions (Cacioppo et al., 1986). As symptoms do not advertise their underlying, disease cause, people are far from accurate in self-diagnoses. In addition, their evaluations of the perceived symptoms tend to be hedonically biased: many subjects in the Cacioppo et al. (1986) study found it much easier to accept a non-threatening explanation for unexpected symptoms and stopped searching for further explanations.

A disease attribution is no assurance, however, of appropriate action. Studies find mis-attribution due to both the inherent ambiguity of symptoms, e.g. cardiovascular symptoms can be confused with symptoms of gastro-intestinal disorders, and to fear-motivated defensiveness. While defensiveness seems more likely to occur for life-threatening diseases, its frequency varies with the type of disease. For example, data suggest that defensive avoidance is more likely for many cancers than for heart attacks: while both sets may be susceptible to 'safe' alternative interpretations, the symptoms of cancer are usually slower to develop, less disruptive of daily function, and, therefore, easier to misinterpret (Cacioppo et al., 1986). Attributions to the 'wrong' disease generate wrong meanings and inappropriate procedures for self-management. An interesting example of both misinterpretation and changing interpretation was reported by Matthews et al. (1983) in their study of delay in care-seeking following the onset of coronary symptoms by type A and type B males; the type A delayed longer than did type B individuals while symptoms were vague during the early phase of an attack, but were quicker to seek care once it became clear that they were having a MI (see also 'Symptom perception' and 'Delay in seeking help').

Attributions of disease cause

Researchers have tried to categorize attributions using either bottom-up or top-down approaches. The top-down ones arose from general attribution theories and led to the classification of causes according to several core dimensions, such as locus of causality (internal/external), controllability and stability (Roesch & Weiner, 2001). Bottom-up approaches strived to uncover the structure of attributions derived from empirical data. These approaches typically resulted in categories such as environmental, behavioural and hidden causes (Senior et al., 2000; Shiloh et al., 2002). These attributions often differ between patients and providers, with patients sometimes offering a more varied array of causes and providers a narrower biomedical one (Bar-On & Cristal, 1987), or the opposite, for example, as with low back pain patients who strive to establish a biomechanical explanation as a response to the clinicians' uncertainty of the cause, which leads to implications of a psychological explanation of the illness (May et al., 2000). The problem with both approaches is that they are attempts to simplify a complex phenomenon. Trying to uncover the dimensions that underlie the empirically derived structures also shows that while a central feature such as the controllability of the cause explains some of the variance in these attributions, it is far from being a sufficient explanation since more features are likely to be involved (Shiloh et al., 2002). There is also evidence that people perceive multiple causes of disease (Arefjord et al., 2002), which makes sense in the light of the accuracy of such a perception for many chronic diseases. Since attributions are not formed in a void but within the person's struggle to reconstruct a narrative which incorporates the illness into their lives and enables them to cope with it (Williams, 1984), one should not be surprised that a focus on specific attributions or a few generalized dimensions is insufficient to understand why attributions are formed and what are their effects.

Attributions of responsibility

Many studies have examined the extent to which people attribute disease to themselves. It is important to distinguish attributions of causes of the event from attributions of success or failure in controlling it and to recognize that internal attributions in contrast to external ones, can lead to quite different outcomes depending upon the model of the underlying condition. For example, diabetic children who held themselves responsible for symptomatic episodes when their diabetes was out of control were in better metabolic control than children attributing such episodes to external factors: self-control was superior to external control (Brown et al., 1991). By contrast, poorer adherence to diets was found among those moderately overweight women who attributed adherence failures to internal factors (Ogden & Wardle, 1990). The seeming contradiction in outcome reflects fundamental differences in the models of the underlying conditions. Whereas the cause of diabetes in children is perceived as external, it is a disease that one must act to control, the cultural view of obesity is that it is caused by the actor's failure of control (a perception that is contrary to medical findings, Garner & Wooley, 1991). Thus, holding the self responsible for failure episodes, an internal attribution, by diabetic children, implies temporary deficits in self- regulation rather than chronic deficiencies in self control, the inference for failure episodes among the overweight (see also 'Perceived control').

Another example showing that differences in models of treatment and disease can alter the meaning of an internal attribution was provided by the Hypertension Prevention Trial (Jeffery et al., 1990). They found that participants assigned to weight-loss groups were significantly more likely to blame themselves for adherence failures than participants assigned to a non-weight-loss intervention, e.g. a reduced sodium group, though there was no relationship between these attributions and health outcomes. Thus, even though it is presumed to be more difficult to adhere to diets for reducing sodium and increasing potassium than to diet for reductions in caloric intake, failure in the latter may lead to self-blame. This is because dieting to reduce caloric intake can be perceived as a weight loss issue that requires self-efficacy skills which have been shown to be deficient by the very presence of the hypertensive disorder.

Attributions and adjustment to illness

Two hypotheses have been tested respecting the relationship of attributions to adjustment. The first is that adjustment is better when attributions are made than when they are not made, and the second is that adjustment is better if specific types of attributions are made, e.g. to the self rather than to others or to controllable rather than to uncontrollable causes. Data on the first are inconsistent, several studies showing more depression, anxiety and feelings of helplessness among patients failing to make causal attributions for their conditions (Affleck et al., 1987; Lowery et al., 1983, 1985; DuCette & Keane, 1984), others showing lower levels of anxiety in the presence of denial and the absence of causal search (Lowery et al., 1992). These inconsistencies appear to be resolvable if, as suggested in our discussion of the commonsense framework, we postulate that different aspects of a disease problem may be salient at different points in time. Thus, three days after a MI (Lowery et al.,

1992) and soon after the occurrence of an accident (van den Bout *et al.*, 1988), the absence of causal search is related to lower levels of anxiety, while later in time the presence of causal attributions is related to lower levels of anxiety (Affleck *et al.*, 1987; Lowery *et al.*, 1983; Lowery & Jacobsen, 1985). As Suls and Fletcher (1985) suggested, engaging in causal search soon after an event may be maladaptive, though causal search at later time points plays a positive role by providing the meanings needed to motivate risk reduction and avoidance of recurrence.

Data on the second question, i.e. the relationship of specific types of attributions to adjustment, is also inconsistent (Hall *et al.*, 2003). Several studies pointed to relationships between attributions and health behaviour change (e.g. changing your diet if you believe your illness was caused by poor diet, etc.; De Valle & Norman, 1992) or healthcare utilization (Herschbach *et al.*, 1999) and turning to complementary and alternative medicine (Maskarinec *et al.*, 2001). Thus, attributions could lead to behaviour change but whether or not this is adaptive depends on the accuracy of these attributions.

Regarding the benefits or harm in self and other attributions, Turnquist *et al.* (1988) concluded in their review that attributions to 'others' tend to relate to poorer outcomes (as did Tennen & Affleck, 1990, in another review) and attributions to 'self' fail to relate clearly to either a beneficial or a detrimental outcome (see also Michela & Wood, 1986). The inconsistent findings for internal attributions could be due to at least two sets of factors. First, the distinction between internal and external cause has been coded in different ways by different investigators, and the meaning of an internal attribution could be different depending upon whether it is an attribution for the initial cause of illness or an attribution of responsibility for managing oneself in relation to treatment or rehabilitation. If an internal attribution is for self-management, it will be equivalent to the perception of internal control, which is usually coupled with events that are controllable, in contrast to external control, which is usually attributed to events that are uncontrollable. Several findings are consistent with this reasoning: e.g. Taylor *et al.* (1984) found that attributions of cancer patients for the disease were mostly unrelated to adjustment, while beliefs in control of treatment and rehabilitation by self and medical experts were both independently associated with better adjustment; DuCette and Keane (1984) found that patients were better adjusted if they had attributed their post-thoracic surgical performance to their own effort or to care from the staff; and, Gilutz *et al.* (1991) found that thoughts of self 'limits and strengths' were positively associated with rehabilitation 6 months post MI, while thoughts about 'fate and luck' were predictive of poor rehabilitation. It seems, therefore, that attributing the onset of an illness to an uncontrollable event, as opposed to personal responsibility due to bad habits, and attributing responsibility for treatment and rehabilitation to controllable, mostly internal though sometimes external factors, is the combination that results in the least emotional distress and the most optimistic view of the future health status. In other words, taking responsibility and asserting control over future recurrence while avoiding blame could be adaptive and people seem to do so whenever possible (French *et al.*, 2005; Tishelman, 1997).

Second, many of the studies of illness attributions were cross-sectional or at best retrospective. Thus, a note of caution is in order as reports of negative correlations of emotional distress with factors such as preoccupation with 'why me?', the absence of causal attributions, and/or the presence of a specific type of attribution, may only reflect distress in the face of deteriorating health (Macleod, 1999). Among women with newly diagnosed breast cancer, behavioural self-blame was correlated with concurrent distress whereas characterological self-blame predicted increased distress over time (Glinder & Compas, 1999). As health deteriorates, individuals may shift from internal attributions to attributions that are external and unstable, reflecting the realities of loss of control over the disease process. Lowery and Jacobsen (1985) have suggested that this shift, along with reduced conviction about any specific causal factor, was characteristic of chronically ill patients whose disease was no longer under control, with actual loss of control generating causal beliefs that are least emotionally upsetting, i.e. to factors implying that the failure to control the disease was unavoidable. Indeed, Lowery *et al.* (1992) suggested that patients may oscillate between preoccupation with and ignoring of causes, focusing on causes as they attempt to come to terms with illness and retreating to denial when anxiety levels are too high, and both the focus of attention and the rate of fluctuation may vary as a function of where they are in the disease and coping process. Given the capricious nature of chronic, life-threatening diseases, the most effective way of minimizing distress produced by lack of confirmation of expectations may be to consider alternative explanations and not commit strongly to any of them. This may explain why attributions show low consistency over time (Arefjord *et al.*, 2002) and why patients who perceive themselves as recovering rapidly attribute their recovery to more stable and personally controllable factors than patients who perceive themselves as recovering slowly (Brewer *et al.*, 2000).

Finally, it is essential to recognize that attributions and adjustment are likely to vary with different illnesses. Accident victims are faced with an irreversible disaster resulting from a one-time mistake; cancer patients are dealing with long treatments accompanied by fear of recurrence; the prognosis for breast cancer is far more optimistic than that for lung cancer; MI survivors experienced a serious trauma with a brief recovery period and lingering fear of recurrence; daily, lifetime coping is the concern for arthritics and diabetics, recurrence is not. If attributions affect adjustment via their impact on control, it is clear that attributions and control will have different meanings in each of these contexts, as perceived control can be helpful only when it can contribute to positive outcomes. When the disease prognosis is extremely unfavourable, e.g. for lung cancer, an internal attribution can induce control but control will have no effect on adjustment (Berckman & Austin, 1993).

Attributional styles and long-term effects on health

Individual differences in the types of attributions people form may be a function of more stable, dispositional tendencies, namely, attributional styles. Research has focused mainly on the pessimistic attributional style, or the tendency to perceive negative events as caused by internal, stable and global factors. This attributional style is considered to be characteristic of learned helplessness (Abramson, Seligman & Teasdale, 1978) and has been found to be related to depression (see Sweeney *et al.*, 1986 and Robins,

1988, for reviews; but see also Cochran & Hammen, 1985 for an alternative view) and to be a risk factor for illness, as Peterson *et al.* (1988) have found in a 35-year longitudinal study. A possible mediator for this effect may be the effect of pessimistic explanatory style on immune functions: this style has been found to be related to lowered immunocompetence, controlling for health status, depressive mood and other possible mediators (Kamen-Siegel, *et al.*, 1991).

Another dispositional difference which may be related to health outcomes was reported by Strube (1985), who found more internal, stable and global attributions for positive than for negative outcomes for all respondents, but this self-serving bias was more characteristic of Type A personalities than Type Bs. In general, Type As are more likely to form causal attributions, especially under high-stress conditions (Keinan & Tal, 2005) (see 'Hostility, Type A behaviour and coronary heart disease').

Conclusion

Attributions are important for the person forming them and for investigators of health and illness behaviours if they help us to predict and to understand the determinants of these behaviours and their consequences for treating and adjusting to disease.

Research arising from a social-psychological view of attributions does not necessarily capture the critical dimensions required for understanding attributions in the domain of health and illness. In the attribution literature, internal attributions have often been linked with control, and therefore were usually expected to be associated with more favorable outcomes, whereas external attributions have been linked with depression, illness and overall poorer adjustment. The majority of studies of attributional processes, however, are cross-sectional and involve a short time frame. Reviews of this area attempted to reach overall conclusions, which are difficult to formulate without taking into account the specific context that each disease creates, the subjective model of that disease, and the needs of the person in each stage of the disease. The formation of attributions is a dynamic process, which happens over time, and in which people negotiate certain explanations for their illnesses in ways that play a positive role in their self-perception and ability to cope. Studies in this domain can reveal the multiple meanings that can be assigned to attributions and their varied consequences. Thus, we should view the study of attributions in the health area as an opportunity for developing a more comprehensive and deeper view of the determinants of human behaviour rather than viewing it as a narrow area of applied research.

REFERENCES

Abramson, L.Y., Seligman, M.E.P. & Teasdale, J.D. (1978). Learned helplessness in humans: critique and reformulation. *Journal of Abnormal Psychology*, **87**(1), 49–74.

Affleck, G., Pfeiffer, C, Tennen, H. & Fifield, J. (1987). Attributional processes in rheumatoid arthritis patients. *Arthritis and Rheumatism*, **30**(8), 927–31.

Alonzo, A.A. (1980). Acute illness behavior: a conceptual elaboration and specification. *Social Science and Medicine*, **14**, 515–25.

Arefjord, K., Hallaraker, E., Havik, O.E. & Maeland, J.G. (2002). Illness understanding, causal attributions and emotional reactions in wives of myocardial infarction patients. *Psychology and Psychotherapy: Theory, Research and Practice*, **75**(1), 101–14.

Armstrong, T.L. & Swartzman, L.C. (1999). Asian versus Western differences in satisfaction with western medical care: the mediational effects of illness attributions. *Psychology and Health*, **14**, 403–16.

Baider, L. & Sarell, M. (1983). Perceptions and causal attributions of Israeli women with breast cancer concerning their illness: the effects of ethnicity and religiosity. *Psychotherapy and Psychosomatics*, **39**, 136–43.

Bar-On, D. & Cristal, N. (1987). Causal attributions of patients, their spouses and physicians, and the rehabilitation of the patients after their first myocardial

infarction. *Journal of Cardiopulmonary Rehabilitation*, **7**, 285–98.

Baumann, L., Cameron, L.D., Zimmerman, R. & Leventhal, H. (1989). Illness representations and matching labels with symptoms. *Health Psychology*, **8**, 449–69.

Benyamini, Y., McClain, C., Leventhal, E.A. & Leventhal, H. (2003). Living with the worry of cancer: health perceptions and behaviors of elderly people with self, vicarious, or no history of cancer. *Psycho-Oncology*, **12**(2), 161–72.

Benyamini, Y., Medalion, B. & Garfinkel, D. (2007). Patient and spouse representations of the patient's heart disease and their associations with received and provided social support and undermining. *Psychology and Health*.

Berckman, K.L. & Austin, J.K. (1993). Causal attribution, perceived control, and adjustment in patients with lung cancer. *Oncology Nursing Forum*, **20**(1), 23–30.

Brewer, B.W., Cornelius, A.E., Van Raalte, J.L. et al. (2000). Attributions for recovery and adherence to rehabilitation following anterior cruciate ligament reconstruction: a prospective analysis. *Psychology and Health*, **15**, 283–91.

Brown, R.T., Kaslow, N.J., Sansbury, L., Meacham, L. & Culler, F.L. (1991). Internalizing and externalizing symptoms and attributional style in youth with diabetes. *Journal of the American Academy*

of Child and Adolescent Psychiatry, **30**(6), 921–25.

Bulman, R.J. & Wortman, C.B. (1977). Attributions of blame and coping in the "real world": severe accident victims react to their lot. *Journal of Personality and Social Psychology*, **35**(5), 351–63.

Cacioppo, J.T., Andersen, B.L., Turnquist, D.C. & Petty, R.E. (1986). Psychophysiological comparison processes: interpreting cancer symptoms. In B. Andersen (Ed.). *Women with cancer: psychological perspectives*. Springer-Verlag: New York.

Cameron, L., Leventhal, E.A. & Leventhal, H. (1995). Seeking medical care in response to symptoms and life stress. *Psychosomatic Medicine*, **57**, 37–47.

Cochran, S.D. & Hammen, C.L. (1985). Perceptions of stressful life events and depression: a test of attributional models. *Journal of Personality and Social Psychology*, **48**(6), 1562–71.

De Valle, M.N. & Norman, P. (1992). Causal attributions, health locus of control beliefs and lifestyle changes among pre-operative coronary patients. *Psychology and Health*, **7**, 201–11.

DuCette, J. & Keane, A. (1984). "Why me?": an attributional analysis of a major illness. *Research in Nursing and Health*, **7**(4), 257–64.

Fiske, S.T. & Taylor, S.E. (1991). *Social Cognition* (2nd Edn.). New York: McGraw-Hill.

French, D. P., Maissi, E. & Marteau, T. M. (2005). The purpose of attributing cause: beliefs about the causes of myocardial infarction. *Social Science and Medicine*, **60**, 1411–21.

French, D. P., Marteau, T. M., Weinman, J. & Senior, V. (2004). Explaining differences in causal attributions of patient and non-patient samples. *Psychology, Health, and Medicine*, **9**(3), 259–72.

Garner, D. M. & Wooley, S. C. (1991). Confronting the failure of behavioral and dietary treatment for obesity. *Clinical Psychology Review*, **11**, 729–80.

Gilutz, H., Bar-On, D., Billing, E., Rehnquist, N. & Cristal, N. (1991). The relationship between causal attribution and rehabilitation in patients after their first myocardial infarction: a cross-cultural study. *European Heart Journal*, **12**(8), 883–8.

Glinder, J. G. & Compas, B. E. (1999), Self-blame attributions in women with newly diagnosed breast cancer: a prospective study of psychological adjustment. *Health Psychology*, **18**(5), 475–81.

Greenberg, L. W., Jewett, L. S., Gluck, R. S. et al. (1984). Giving information for a life-threatening diagnosis. *American Journal of Diseases of Children*, **138**, 649–53.

Hall, S., French, D. P. & Marteau, T. M. (2003). Causal attributions following serious unexpected negative events: a systematic review. *Journal of Social and Clinical Psychology*, **22**(5), 515–36.

Heider, F. (1958). *The psychology of interpersonal relations*. New York: John Wiley & Sons.

Herschbach, P., Henrich, G. & von Rad, M. (1999). Psychological factors in functional gastrointestinal disorders: characteristics of the disorder or of the illness behavior? *Psychosomatic Medicine*, **61**(2), 148–53.

Jeffery, R. W., French, S. A. & Schmid, T. L. (1990). Attributions for dietary failures: problems reported by participants in the hypertension prevention trial. *Health Psychology*, **9**(3), 315–29.

Jones, E. E. (1990). *Interpersonal perception*. New York: W.H. Freeman & Company.

Jones, E. E. & Davis, K. S. (1965). From acts to dispositions: the attribution process in person perception. In L. Berkowitz (Ed.). *Advances in experimental social psychology, Vol. 2* (pp. 219–66). New York: Academic Press.

Kamen-Siegel, L., Rodin, J., Seligman, M. E. & Dwyer, J. (1991). Explanatory style and cell–mediated immunity in elderly men and women. *Health Psychology*, **10**(4), 229–35.

Kart, C. (1981). Experiencing symptoms: attributions and misattributions of illness among the aged. In M. Haug (Ed.). *Elderly patients and their doctors* (pp. 70–8). New York: Springer.

Keinan, G. & Tal, S. (2005). The effects of Type A behavior and stress on the attribution of causality. *Personality and Individual Differences*, **38**, 403–12.

Landrine, H. & Klonoff, E. A. (1994). Cultural diversity in causal attributions for illness: the role of the supernatural. *Journal of Behavioral Medicine*, **17**(2), 181–93.

Leventhal, H., Diefenbach, M. & Leventhal, E. A. (1992). Illness cognition: using common sense to understand treatment adherence and affect cognition interactions. *Cognitive Therapy and Research*, **16**, 143–63.

Leventhal, H., Meyer, D. & Nerenz, D. (1980). The common sense representation of illness danger. In S. Rachman (Ed.). *Contributions to medical psychology, Vol. II* (pp. 7–30). New York: Pergamon Press.

Lowery, B. J. & Jacobsen, B. S. (1985). Attributional analysis of chronic illness outcomes. *Nursing Research*, **34**(2), 82–8.

Lowery, B. J., Jacobsen, B. S. & Murphy, B. B. (1983). An exploratory investigation of causal thinking of arthritics. *Nursing Research*, **32**(3), 157–62.

Lowery, B. J., Jacobsen, B. S. & McCauley, K. (1987). On the prevalence of causal search in illness situations. *Nursing Research*, **36**(2), 88–93.

Lowery, B. J., Jacobsen, B. S., Cera, M. A. et al. (1992). Attention versus avoidance: attributional search and denial after myocardial infarction. *Heart and Lung*, **21**(6), 523–8.

Macleod, M. D. (1999), Why did it happen to me? Social cognition processes in adjustment and recovery from criminal victimization and illness. *Current Psychology*, **18**(1), 18–31.

Maskarinec, G., Gotay, C. C., Tatsumura, Y., Shumay, D. M. & Kakai, H. (2001). Perceived cancer causes: use of complementary and alternative therapy. *Cancer Practice*, **9**(4), 183–90.

Matthews, K. A., Seigel, J. M., Kuller, L. H., Thompson, M. & Varat, M. (1983). Determinants of decisions to seek medical treatment by patients with acute myocardial infarction symptoms. *Journal of Personality and Social Psychology*, **44**, 1144–56.

May, C. R., Rose, M. J. & Johnstone, F. C. W. (2000). Dealing with doubt: How patients account for non-specific chronic low back pain. *Journal of Psychosomatic Research*, **49**, 223–5.

Meyer, D., Leventhal, H. & Gutmann, M. (1985). Common-sense models of illness: The example of hypertension. *Health Psychology*, **4**, 115–35.

Michela, J. L. & Wood, J. V. (1986). Causal attributions in health and illness. In P. C. Kendall (Ed.). *Advances in cognitive-behavioral research and therapy, Vol. 5* (pp. 179–235). New York: Academic Press.

Ogden, J. & Wardle, J. (1990). Control of eating and attributional style. *British Journal of Clinical Psychology*, **29**(Pt 4), 445–6.

Pérez-Stable, E. J., Sabogal, F., Otero-Sabogal, R., Hiatt, R. A. & McPhee, S. J. (1992). Misconceptions about cancer among Latinos and Anglos. *Journal of American Medical Association*, **268**(22), 3219–23.

Peterson, C., Seligman, M. E. P. & Vaillant, G. E. (1988). Pessimistic explanatory style is a risk factor for physical illness: a thirty-five-year longitudinal study. *Journal of Personality and Social Psychology*, **55**(1), 23–7.

Pill, R. & Stott, N. C. H. (1982). Concepts of illness causation and responsibility: some preliminary data from a sample of working class mothers. *Social Science and Medicine*, **16**, 43–52.

Prohaska, T. R., Keller, M. L., Leventhal, E. A. & Leventhal, H. (1987). Impact of symptoms and aging attribution on emotions and coping. *Health Psychology*, **6**, 495–514.

Robins, C. J. (1988). Attributions and depression: why is the literature so inconsistent? *Journal of Personality and Social Psychology*, **54**(5), 880–9.

Rodin, J. (1978). Somatophysics and attribution. *Personality and Social Psychology Bulletin*, **4**(4), 531–40.

Roesch, S. C. & Weiner, B. (2001). A meta-analytic review of coping with illness: do causal attributions matter? *Journal of Psychosomatic Research*, **50**, 205–19.

Safer, M., Tharps, Q., Jackson, T. & Leventhal, H. (1979). Determinants of three stages of delay in seeking care at a medical clinic. *Medical Care*, **17**, 11–29.

Salmon, P., Woloshynowych, M. & Valori, R. (1996). The measurement of beliefs about physical symptoms in English general practice patients. *Social Science and Medicine*, **42**(11), 1561–7.

Senior, V., Marteau, T. M. & Weinman, J. (2000). Impact of genetic testing on causal models of heart disease and arthritis: an analogue study. *Psychology and Health*, **14**, 1077–88.

Shiloh, S., Rashuk-Rosenthal, D. & Benyamini, Y. (2002). Illness attributions:

their structure and associations with other illness cognitions and perceptions of control. *Journal of Behavioral Medicine,* **25**, 373–94.

Steensma, D. P. (2003). Why Me? *Journal of Clinical Oncology,* **21**(9), 64s–6s.

Strube, M. J. (1985). Attributional style and the type A coronary–prone behavior pattern. *Journal of Personality and Social Psychology,* **49**(2), 500–9.

Suls, J. & Fletcher, B. (1985). The relative efficacy of avoidant and non-avoidant coping strategies: a meta analysis. *Health Psychology,* **4**, 249–88.

Sweeney, P. D., Anderson, K. & Bailey, S. (1986). Attributional style in depression: a meta–analytic review. *Journal of Personality and Social Psychology,* **50**(5), 974–91.

Taylor, S. (1982). Social cognition and health. *Personality and Social Psychology Bulletin,* **8**(3), 549–62.

Taylor, S., Lichtman, R. R. & Wood, J. (1984). Attributions, beliefs about control, and adjustment to breast cancer. *Journal of Personality and Social Psychology,* **46**(3), 489–502.

Tennen, H. & Affleck, G. (1990). Blaming others for threatening events. *Psychological Bulletin,* **108**(2), 209–32.

Tishelman, C. (1997). Getting sick and getting well: a qualitative study of aetiologic explanations of people with cancer. *Journal of Advanced Nursing,* **25**, 60–7.

Turnquist, D. C., Harvey, J. H. & Andersen, B. L. (1988). Attributions and adjustment to life–threatening illness. *British Journal of Clinical Psychology,* **27**(Pt 1), 55–65.

van den Bout, J., van Son–Schoones, N., Schipper, J. & Groffen, C. (1988). Attributional cognitions, coping behavior, and self–esteem in inpatients with severe spinal cord injuries. *Journal of Clinical Psychology,* **44**(1), 17–22.

Weiner, B. (1985). "Spontaneous" causal thinking. *Psychological Bulletin,* **97**(1), 74–84.

Williams, G. (1984). The genesis of chronic illness: Narrative re-construction. *Sociology of Health and Illness,* **6**(2), 175–200.

Childhood influences on health

Julie M. Turner-Cobb

University of Bath

Overview

Early social experience appears to be one of the most important psychological factors influencing health outcome in children. Social experience in childhood includes interactions with care givers (e.g. parents and childcare providers) and with peers (e.g. friends made at childcare or school). Of particular note in the classical psychology literature is the significance of parental attachment, especially that of the maternal bond. When applied directly to health, research initially focused on the psychopathological or mental health implications of maternal attachment or parental abuse. Indeed such developmental work has yielded a number of important findings. More recent research applying the influence on physical health of stressful experiences during childhood, has revealed some potential physiological indicators involved in this relationship, primarily that of the hormone cortisol. This chapter deals with the themes and debates surrounding this emerging literature, applying the social experiences in childhood to the health arena throughout childhood and across the lifespan. It is acknowledged that whilst there may be more broader issues influencing health during childhood, the stress response focus given here outlines a possible psychophysiological mediating mechanism through which such factors might influence health.

The relevance of cortisol to health

The basic premise behind the research discussed here is that early life experiences and individual differences can activate the stress response systems of the body to influence health outcomes across the lifespan. These two response systems, which work in conjunction with one another, are those of the hypothalamic-pituitary-adrenal (HPA) axis and the sympathetic-adrenomedullary system (SAM) (for more detail see 'Psychoneuroimmunology'). Measurement of cortisol, the end product of the HPA axis stress response system, is now considered a reliable indicator of increased physiological stress arousal (Kirschbaum & Hellhammer, 1989) (for more detail see 'Psychoneuroimmunology assessments'). Cortisol is important to health as it is linked to suppression of some parts of the immune response and an overall dysregulation of immune function (Kirschbaum & Hellhammer, 1989, 1994). Under normal conditions, cortisol reveals a circadian rhythm with a diurnal decline from awakening to evening levels (Smyth *et al.,* 1997) from approximately three months of age (Gunnar, 1992).

Allostasis and allostatic load

The theory of allostasis and associated allostatic load offer an explanatory link between psychosocial stress responses and health outcome across the lifespan. Allostatic load is the collective somatic burden or accumulated lifetime stress associated with repeated stress responses (Sterling & Eyer, 1988; McEwen, 1998). This theory has generated interest particularly in relation to adult research, for example Seeman *et al.* (2002) demonstrate the importance of positive social experiences in lowering allostatic load in various ages within the adult population. Yet there exists a comparative lack of direct developmental investigation of childhood experience, particularly noticeable given the focus of allostatic load on accumulated lifetime stress and hence its relevance to early life. Both noise and crowding are potential sources of allostatic load and both have been linked to raised cortisol levels in children (Johnston-Brookes et al., 1998; Haines et al., 2001).

Activation of the stress response system of the HPA axis in early childhood has been associated with a range of psychological factors and physiological alterations during childhood and adolescence. For example, family environments characterized by aggression and conflict (termed 'risky' families) have been associated with negative mental and physical outcomes (Repetti et al., 2002). One of the earliest areas of interest within the field of developmental psychology is that of maternal attachment and critical periods or 'windows' of time have been the focus of recent work linking maternal attachment with neuroimmunological consequences in animals and children (for a recent review see Coe & Lubach, 2003). Under experimental conditions, maternal separation in healthy nine-month-old children has been found to elicit HPA axis activation, as demonstrated by raised salivary cortisol levels in the presence of an unfamiliar sitter who responded only when the infant fussed or cried. (Gunnar et al., 1992). The importance of a positive social environment for neuroendocrine adjustment is demonstrated by the fact that this physiological effect was diminished to almost that of the no separation condition when the sitter offered a nurturing and stimulating environment, demonstrating. Furthermore, higher diurnal cortisol in adult men who experienced parental loss at an average age of 12 years demonstrates the long term neuroendocrine effects of early experience (Nicolson, 2004).

Cortisol and psychopathology in response to maltreatment and maternal attachment

Neuroendocrine alteration in response to severe maltreatment and subsequent psychopathological development, a number of different patterns of alteration in cortisol levels and diurnal regulation have been observed. Variation in morning cortisol in children is reported by Cichetti & Rogosch (2001); depending on type and severity of maltreatment, the most severely maltreated children showed significant elevations in morning cortisol levels. Some clinical research in children with PTSD symptoms, following trauma such as separation and loss, reports HPA axis alteration as evidenced by a raised cortisol profile (termed 'hypercortisolism') particularly in girls (Carrion et al., 2002). Yet in other experimental studies, sexual abuse in children has been significantly related to lower cortisol levels compared to controls (King et al., 2001). A similar pattern of lower cortisol levels and a flatter diurnal cortisol rhythm is seen in children rescued from orphanage maltreatment (Gunnar et al., 2001). Indeed, as Gunnar and Vazquez (2001) point out, the concept of hypocortisolism suppression of the HPA axis response resulting in low cortisol levels, may be manifested during childhood itself rather than being a delayed effect in adulthood, as initially believed. Differences in the direction of cortisol appear to reflect the type of maltreatment and timing of assessments following the experience. For example, what may initially show itself as high cortisol may subsequently, or following a repeated episode of abuse, reveal a low cortisol response e.g. as evidenced in Resnick et al.'s (1995) study of repeated rape.

Intergenerational stress transmission

As already alluded to above, the notion of intergenerational stress transmission pervades this literature. This notion was examined directly by Yehuda and colleagues (2001), in an investigation of adult children of Holocaust survivors with post traumatic stress disorder (PTSD). They report a lower mean 24-hour urinary cortisol level in those who experienced childhood emotional abuse, compared with controls (Yehuda et al., 2001). Later studies have also reported subsequently altered cortisol levels in adult survivors of child sexual abuse (Newport et al., 2004) and similar observations have been made in animal models of maltreatment (Mar Sanchez, 2001). Relating to this notion of intergenerational transmission, a literature is also developing which links heritability of cortisol, both genetic and social. From the genetic perspective, twin studies estimate the heritability of cortisol responses at 60% (Bartels et al., 2003). With regard to social influences, evidence clearly links cortisol with socioeconomic status e.g. morning cortisol levels in children with low SES status are significantly higher and this appears to be linked to mothers' level of depressive symptoms (Lupien et al., 2000).

Stress and cortisol in healthy children

As described above, the influence of social experience during childhood was originally examined in relation to specific groups of children deprived of normal social contact or suffering maltreatment in one form or another. Both naturalistic and experimental studies have explored adaptive physiological responses to stressful social experiences in such children. An area that has more recently emerged is the examination HPA axis activation in healthy children as a window for exploring the origins and adaptation and accumulated life stress.

That early experiences may contribute to a child's allostatic load and be linked to poorer health outcome in healthy children is revealed in a study by Bugental et al. (2003). This study examined HPA axis reactivity to physical punishment by their mothers in a group of toddlers from low SES families. They found that children whose mothers disciplined by use of frequent spanking/slapping, exhibited greater cortisol reactivity to the stress of experimental separation. Also, mothers who employed various forms of emotional unavailability, regardless of intention, had higher baseline cortisol levels.

Research focusing on the role of social interaction beyond the family, to encompass social relationships of peers and group interaction in naturalistic daycare settings has also yielded some notable findings. In keeping with increasing exposure of preschool age children to various forms of childcare outside the home brought about by changes in maternal occupational patterns, more recent research has examined the nature of the childcare experience and differential outcomes of varying levels of care quality. Both naturalistic and experimental research have studied the interplay between social experience and temperament within this context. Evidence is accumulating which reveals that negative emotional temperaments and poorer quality of preschool care are associated with altered physical stress responses (Dettling et al., 2000; Gunnar & Donzella, 2002; Crockenberg, 2003).

Cortisol disruption in the social context of preschool (under fives)

With regard to neuroendocrine disruption, a dysregulation of the diurnal pattern of cortisol which is reflected in the rate of decline from morning to evening levels and is particularly evidenced by an elevation in afternoon cortisol levels, has been reported in children attending full day preschool. In those children whose social skills are less well developed, alterations to this evening pattern are particularly prevalent (Dettling *et al.*, 1999; Watamura *et al.*, 2003). Assessing cortisol reactivity in response to starting preschool, Gunnar *et al.* (1997) note that it is the neuroendocrine adaptability that is important rather than simply the level of the response. These ideas as applied to healthy children in this context fit well with the person–environment interactional model of stress put forward by Lazarus and Folkman (1984) now well accepted in the adult stress literature. In understanding childhood influences on health this neuroendocrine 'window' provides an opportunity to examine these person-environment responses. Although Gunnar *et al.* (1997) report that more outgoing, socially competent children exhibited high cortisol response to the initial start of preschool, when followed up one term later, these children exhibit a low reactivity. Similarly, the importance of infant–mother attachment on cortisol levels during adaptation to daycare has been recently demonstrated (Ahnert *et al.*, 2004). These studies all point to the importance of adaptability rather than initial reactivity for health outcome.

In the light of this, evidence for direct pathways between temperament and cortisol reactivity has not always been clear. Recent evidence from Gunnar *et al.* (2003) points to the existence of an indirect pathway involving aggression and peer rejection. Further explanation of this is provided by Zimmerman and Stansbury (2004) in their experimental study using a stranger-approach scenario in three-year old children. They report cortisol rise in both shy and bold children with the level of the response predicted by degree of shyness. In the majority of the children the response was attenuated after termination of the stressor (Zimmermann & Stansbury, 2004). Providing further support for the idea of context-specific HPA axis activation during childhood experiences (Watamura *et al.*, 2003), the authors argue that it is the repeated triggering of the stress response rather than neuroendocrine activation itself which may be problematic for shy children, as they may perceive threat to a greater number of everyday events.

From the parental perspective, issues surrounding home-life-balance are also important to consider in relation to childhood influences on health, particularly as neuroendocrine sensitization effects following exposure to maternal stress during the first year of life have been reported in four-and-a-half-year olds (e.g. Adam & Gunnar, 2001; Essex *et al.*, 2002). As yet unpublished findings from our own laboratory have found that mother's occupational factors (e.g. maternal satisfaction with work, level of emotional exhaustion) interact with daycare experience to influence cortisol levels in preschool children. Furthermore, we have found these factors to take on even greater significance once the child has made the transition to school.

The implications of this developing field of research are enormous, with applications extending to include the effect of social experience on learning and on health outcomes. Social and physiological adaptation is required in order to cope with transitional life experiences, whether these are due to early maternal separation in the form of childcare, starting school, or the experience of competition and the need to achieve, brought about through the assessments and examinations now demanded throughout childhood and adolescence in the UK. Indeed, it has been argued that neuroendocrine patterns seen in infants in response to maternal separation may be mirrored in older children for different age-related stressors such as academic examinations (Gunnar *et al.*, 1992).

Physiological responsivity in school transition (rising fives onwards)

On this basis, school transition can be classified as a dynamic process. Whether or not the child has experienced preschool, it is likely to be experienced as novel and socially stressful, leading to an increase in HPA axis reactivity and potentially to immune suppression (Boyce *et al.*, 1995). Life transitions provide a naturalistic research opportunity to investigate adaptability to stress and the link to health outcomes. Work by Gunnar and colleagues (e.g. Gunnar *et al.*, 1997; Gunnar & Donzella, 2002; Gunnar *et al.*, 2003) supports the notion that school transition stress is generated predominantly by the need for social engagement and social competence within the new environment. In an assessment of physiological responsivity to socio-emotional adjustment in children entering kindergarten in the USA, Smider *et al.* (2002) report that higher cortisol levels at age four-and-a-half years predicted poorer behavioural adjustment to kindergarten at age six. Similarly, in four-year old preschool children, classroom observations have also linked social isolation with cortisol levels depending on the meaning of the isolation behaviour for the child (Sanchez-Martin *et al.*, 2001). Children retreating into social isolation due to anxiety and inadequate social interaction skills revealed higher cortisol levels compared with children showing social isolation as a result of avoidance of the stressful social behaviour who revealed lower cortisol responses (Sanchez-Martin *et al.*, 2001). When considering the influence of stress in children, this link between cortisol and the meaning of the social interaction has also been demonstrated in a longitudinal study of diurnal cortisol response during the first five days of a new school year (Bruce *et al.*, 2002). In a group of six- to seven-year-old children, compared with weekend days, a greater rate of change in cortisol was observed on school days and in particular for those children who scored high on surgency (extroversion); this greater rate of change was still apparent on day five of school (Bruce *et al.*, 2002). Whilst some inconsistencies in the direction of the temperament–cortisol relationships exist between this study and previous research (Davis *et al.*, 1999), both studies found that more surgent children showed greater cortisol responses to transition on the fifth day of the first week (Bruce *et al.*, 2002). Further evidence of the importance of individual differences in cortisol regulation is provided by experimental work examining self-competence in seven-year-olds (Schmidt *et al.*, 1999). In this respect, self-competence in novel/social situations is argued as reflecting the ability to regulate emotion and to elicit less fear of approach, the process itself increasing levels of self-competency (Schmidt *et al.*, 1999). Furthermore, parental expectations of the school transition experience have also been linked to morning cortisol levels (Quas *et al.*, 2002).

A further stream of research is emerging in respect of stress responses during school transition: namely the effect on learning. Firstly, chronic high levels of cortisol secretion have been linked to hippocampal damage in the brain (Sapolsky *et al.*, 1986) and associated reduction in cognitive functioning e.g. in memory and spatial impairments (McEwen, 1997). These effects however, are in response to chronic stress exposure but when acute stress under experimental conditions is considered, the effects on healthy individuals become less clear. For example, experimental studies examining hormonal responses to stress at both ends of the life spectrum, in the elderly and in young adults, have shown a modulatory rather than a 'unidirectional' effect of stress hormones on learning and memory (Lupien *et al.*, 2002). In young adults (mean age 23.1 years), morning cortisol levels have been reduced by the addition of the pharmacological agent metyrapone, leading to delayed memory impairments, yet when hydrocortisone was administered during the diurnal trough in cortisol, positive effects for word recognition tasks were observed (Lupien *et al.*, 2002). In a recent experimental laboratory-induced stress study of children aged approximately four- to seven-years old (mean age five years and three months), differential effects for cortisol and autonomic reactivity at two-week follow-up, with cortisol reactivity linked to poorer memory and autonomic reactivity conferred risk only when a non-supportive interviewer was employed (Quas *et al.*, 2004). Learning and memory outcomes need further consideration in respect of the psychophysiological effects of life transitions.

Assessment of acute physical health outcome

The study of psychosocial factors influencing the onset and duration of an upper respiratory infection (URI), or an episode of the common cold has linked higher levels of stress with increased susceptibility to infection in adults and in children. This has been reported under both experimental conditions (for example, Cohen *et al.*, 1991, 1995) and naturalistic conditions (for example, Graham, 1986; Turner Cobb & Steptoe, 1996, 1998; Cohen *et al.*, 2002). Implicated in these findings are a number of psychosocial resources, such as coping responses, social support and health-related behaviours which act as moderators and mediators of stress on health (for more detail see 'Common cold'). In this chapter it is sufficient to say that measurement of the onset and duration of the common cold is a simple and non-intrusive way to assess the immune impact of stressful events (Boyce *et al.*, 1995). As already noted, there is comparatively little research to date that has incorporated acute physical health outcomes as measures of ability to deal with naturalistic psychophysiological challenge in children. One study which stands out in this regard evaluated susceptibility to the common cold for the duration of the first 13 years of life (Ball *et al.*, 2002). Interestingly, the

authors report that those children who attended the larges scale day care centres, were found to be protected from the common cold at ages 6, 8 and 11 years although a higher infection rate was seen earlier in life at the age of two years (Ball *et al.*, 2002). This study however, did not specifically examine school transition and it failed to examine temperament directly, or in association with, mediating hormonal responses to the social situations encountered.

As the majority of the preschool and school transition research to date has been carried out in the United States, it is important to point out that some important differences in educational practice exist between the two countries which could influence interpretation of research. Cultural differences may provide insight into the psychophysiological stress process, the effects of which may be highlighted by variations in age of entry or style of education. Yet there is a lack of research directly assessing school and indeed life transition influences on health. These transitions have been explored in depth by educationalists and developmental psychologists resulting in numerous child welfare intervention programmes, yet the psychobiological adaptation has itself largely been ignored. At the transition to senior school stage, a particular challenge to and opportunity for psychoneuroimmunological research is provided, given physiological challenges naturally occurring at this time, in relation to cortisol and dehydroepiandrosterone (DHEA) (Goodyer *et al.*, 2001; Tornhage, 2002; Netherton *et al.*, 2004).

In summary

As detailed above, childhood influences on health are bound up with the psychophysiological activation of the HPA axis during development and subsequent functioning in respect of health across the lifespan. Research in the developmental health arena may further our understanding of crucial psychosocial factors and relevant developmental junctures for providing intervention. The studies cited attest to the fact that it is not just extreme cases of maltreatment that give rise to changes in HPA axis patterning but that such individual differences are also observed in healthy populations of children under both experimental and naturalistic conditions. These alterations may serve as early subtle indicators of, and contribute to, physical health outcomes in adulthood. In order to further understand these influences and their importance in both short- and long-term health, further longitudinal studies are called for which include measures not only of physical health outcome but also of learning and memory as indicators of potential health effects.

REFERENCES

Adam, E. K. & Gunnar, M. R. (2001). Relationship functioning and home and work demands predict individual differences in diurnal cortisol patterns in women. *Psychoneuroendocrinology*, **26**, 189–208.

Ahnert, L., Gunnar, M. R., Lamb, M. E. & Barthel, M. (2004). Transition to child care: associations with infant–mother attachment, infant negative emotion, and cortisol elevations. *Child Development*, **75**, 639–50.

Ball, T. M., Holberg, C. J., Aldous, M. B., Martinez, F. D. & Wright, A. L. (2002). Influence of attendance at day care on the common cold from birth through 13 years of age. *Archives of Pediatrics and Adolescent Medicine*, **156**, 121–6.

Bartels, M., de Geus, E. J. C., Kirschbaum, C., Sluyter, F. & Boomsma, D. I. (2003). Heritability of daytime cortiosl levels in children. *Behavior Genetics*, **33**, 421–33.

Boyce, W. T., Adams, S., Tschann, J. M. *et al.* (1995). Adrenocortical and behavioral predictors of immune responses to starting school. *Pediatric Research*, **38**, 1009–17.

Bruce, J., Davis, E. P. & Gunnar, M. R. (2002). Individual differences in children's cortisol response to the beginning of a new school year. *Psychoneuroendocrinology*, **27**, 635–50.

Bugental, D. B., Martorell, G. A. & Barraza, V. (2003). The hormonal costs of subtle forms of infant maltreatment. *Hormones and Behavior*, **43**, 237–44.

Carrion, V. G., Weems, C. F., Ray, R. D. et al. (2002). Diurnal salivary cortisol in pediatric posttraumatic stress disorder. *Biological Psychiatry*, **51**, 575–82.

Cicchetti, D. & Rogosch, F. A. (2001). Diverse patterns of neuroendocrine activity in maltreated children. *Development and Psychopathology*, **13**, 677–93.

Coe, C. L. & Lubach, G. R. (2003). Critical periods of special health relevance for psychoneuroimmunology. *Brain, Behaviour and Immunity*, **17**, 3–12.

Cohen, S., Doyle, W. J., Skoner, D. P. et al. (1995). State and trait negative affect as predictors of objective and subjective symptoms of respiratory viral infections. *Journal of Personality and Social Psychology*, **68**, 159–69.

Cohen, S., Hamrick, N., Rodriguez, M. et al. (2002). Reactivity and vulnerability to stress-associated risk for upper respiratory illness. *Psychosomatic Medicine*, **64**, 302–10.

Cohen, S. T., Tyrell, D. A. J. & Smith, A. P. (1991). Psychological stress and susceptibility to the common cold. *New England Journal of Medicine*, **325**, 606–12.

Crockenberg, S. C. (2003). Rescuing the baby from the bathwater: how gender and temperament (may) influence how child care affects child development. *Child Development*, **74**, 1034–8.

Davis, E. P., Donzella, B., Krueger, W. K. & Gunnar, M. R. (1999). The start of a new school year: individual differences in salivary cortisol response in relation to child temperament. *Developmental Psychobiology*, **35**, 188–96.

Dettling, A. C., Gunnar, M. R. & Donzella, B. (1999). Cortisol levels of young children in full-day childcare centers: relations with age and temperament. *Psychoneuroendocrinology*, **24**, 519–36.

Dettling, A. C., Parker, S. W., Lane, S., Sebanc, A. & Gunnar, M. R. (2000). Quality of care and temperament determine changes in cortisol concentrations over the day for young children in childcare. *Psychoneuroendocrinology*, **25**, 819–36.

Essex, M. J., Klein, M. H., Cho, E. & Kalin, N. H. (2002). Maternal stress beginning in infancy may sensitize children to later stress exposure: effects on cortisol and behavior. *Biological Psychiatry*, **52**, 776–84.

Goodyer, I. M., Park, R. J., Netherton, C. M. & Herbert, J. (2001). Possible role of cortisol and dehydroepiandrosterone in human development and psychopathology. *British Journal of Psychiatry*, **179**, 243–9.

Graham, N. M. H., Douglas, R. M. & Ryan, P. (1986). Stress and acute respiratory infection. *American Journal of Epidemiology*, **124**, 389–401.

Gunnar, M. R. (1992). Reactivity of the hypothalamic-pituitary adrenal system to stressors in normal infants and children. *Pediatrics*, **90**, 491–7.

Gunnar, M. R. & Donzella, B. (2002). Social regulation of the cortisol levels in early human development. *Psychoneuroendocrinology*, **27**, 199–220.

Gunnar, M. R., Larson, M. C., Hertsgaard, L., Harris, M. L. & Brodersen, L. (1992). The stressfulness of separation among nine-month-old infants: effects of social context variables and infant temperament. *Child Development*, **63**, 290–303.

Gunnar, M. R., Morison, S. J., Chisholm, K. & Schuder, M. (2001). Salivary cortisol levels in children adopted from Romanian orphanages. *Development and Psychopathology*, **13**, 611–28.

Gunnar, M. R., Sebanc, A. M., Tout, K., Donzella, B. & van Dulmen, M. M. (2003). Peer rejection, temperament, and cortisol activity in preschoolers. *Developmental Psychobiology*, **43**, 346–58.

Gunnar, M. R., Tout, K., deHaan, M., Pierce, S. & Stansbury, K. (1997). Temperament, social competence, and adrenocortical activity in preschoolers. *Developmental Psychobiology*, **31**, 65–85.

Gunnar, M. R. & Vazquez, D. M. (2001). Low cortisol and a flattening of expected daytime rhythm: potential indices of risk in human development. *Development and Psychopathology*, **13**, 515–38.

Haines, M. M., Stansfeld, S. A., Job, R. F. S., Berglund, B. & Head, J. (2001). Chronic aircraft noise exposure, stress responses, mental health and cognitive performance in school children. *Psychological Medicine*, **31**, 265–77.

Johnston-Brookes, C. H., Lewis, M. A., Evans, G. W. & Whalen, C. K. (1998). Chronic stress and illness in children: the role of allostatic load. *Psychosomatic Medicine*, **60**, 597–603.

King, J. A., Mandansky, D., King, S., Fletcher, K. E. & Brewer, J. (2001). Early sexual abuse and low cortisol. *Psychiatry and Clinical Neurosciences*, **55**, 71–4.

Kirschbaum, C. & Hellhammer, D. H. (1989). Salivary cortisol in psychobiological research: an overview. *Neuropsychobiology*, **22**, 150–69.

Kirschbaum, C. & Hellhammer, D. H. (1994). Salivary cortisol in psychoneuroendocrine research: recent developments and applications. *Psychoneuroendocrinology*, **19**(4), 313–33.

Lazarus, R. S. & Folkman, S. (1984). *Stress, appraisal and coping*. New York: Springer.

Lupien, S., King, S., Meaney, M. J. & McEwen, B. S. (2000). Child's stress hormone levels correlate with mother's socioeconomic status and depressive state. *Biological Psychiatry*, **48**, 976–80.

Lupien, S. J., Wilkinson, C. W., Briere, S. et al. (2002). The modulatory effects of corticosteroids on cognition: studies in young human populations. *Psychoneuroendocrinology*, **27**, 401–16.

Mar Sanchez, M. (2001). Early adverse experience as a developmental risk factor for later psychopathology: evidence from rodent and primate models. *Development and Psychopathology*, **13**, 419–50.

McEwen, B. S. (1997). Hormones as regulators of brain development: life-long effects related to health and disease. *Acta Pediatrica Supplement*, **422**, 41–4.

McEwen, B. S. (1998). Stress, adaptation, and disease. Allostasis and allostatic load. *Annals of New York Academy of Sciences*, **840**, 33–44.

Netherton, C., Goodyer, I., Tamplin, A. & Herbert, J. (2004). Salivary cortisol and dehydroepiandrosterone in relation to puberty and gender. *Psychoneuroendocrinology*, **29**, 125–40.

Newport, D. J., Heim, C., Bonsall, R., Miller, A. H. & Nemeroff, C. B. (2004). Pituitary-adrenal responses to standard and low-dose dexamethasone suppression tests in adult survivors of child abuse. *Biological Psychiatry*, **55**, 10–20.

Nicolson, N. A. (2004). Childhood parental loss and cortisol levels in adult men. *Psychoneuroendocrinology*, **29**, 1012–18.

Quas, J. A., Bauer, A. & Boyce, W. T. (2004). Physiological reactivity, social support, and memory in early childhood. *Child Development*, **75**, 797–814.

Quas, J. A., Murowchick, E., Bensadoun, J. & Boyce, W. T. (2002). Predictors of children's cortisol activation during the transition to kindergarten. *Developmental and Behavioral Pediatrics*, **23**, 304–13.

Repetti, R. L., Taylor, S. E. & Seeman, T. E. (2002). Risky families: family social environments and the mental and physical health of offspring. *Psychological Bulletin*, **128**, 330–66.

Resnick, H. S., Yehuda, R., Pitman, R. K. & Foy, D. W. (1995). Effect of previous trauma on acute plasma cortisol level following rape. *American Journal of Psychiatry*, **152**, 1675–77.

Sanchez-Martin, R. J., Cardas, J., Ahedo, L. et al. (2001). Social behavior, cortisol, and sIgA levels in preschool children. *Journal of Psychosomatic Research*, **50**, 221–7.

Sapolsky, R. M., Krey, L. C. & McEwen, B. S. (1986). The neuroendocrinology of stress and aging: the glucocorticoid cascade hypothesis. *Endocrine Reviews*, **7**, 284–301.

Schmidt, L. A., Fax, N. A., Sternberg, E. M. *et al.* (1999). Adrenocortical reactivity and social competence in seven-year-olds. *Personality and Individual Differences*, **26**, 977–85.

Seeman, T. E., Singer, B. H., Ryff, C. D., Dienberg Love, G. & Levy-Storms, L. (2002). Social relationships, gender, and allostatic load across two age cohorts. *Psychosomatic Medicine*, **64**, 395–406.

Smider, N. A., Essex, M. J., Kalin, N. H. *et al.* (2002). Salivary cortisol as a predictor of socioemotional adjustment during kindergarten: a prospective study. *Child Development*, **73**, 75–92.

Smyth, J. M., Ockenfels, M. C., Gorin, A. A. *et al.* (1997). Individual differences in the diurnal cycle of cortisol. *Psychoneuroendocrinology*, **22**, 89–105.

Sterling, P. & Eyer, J. (1988). Allostasis: a new paradigm to explain arousal pathology. In S. Fisher & J. Reason (Eds.). *Handbook of life stress, cognition and health* (pp. 629–49). New York: Wiley.

Tornhage, C.-J. (2002). Reference values for morning salivary cortisol concentration: healthy school-aged children. *J Pediatr Endocrinol Metab*, **15**, 197–204.

Turner-Cobb, J. M. & Steptoe, A. (1996). Psychosocial stress and susceptibility to upper respiratory tract illness in an adult population sample. *Psychosomatic Medicine*, **58**, 404–12.

Turner-Cobb, J. M. & Steptoe, A. (1998). Psychosocial influences on upper respiratory infectious illness in children.

Journal of Psychosomatic Research, **45**, 319–30.

Watamura, S. E., Donzella, B., Alwin, J. & Gunnar, M. R. (2003). Morning-to-afternoon increases in cortisol concentrations for infants and toddlers at child care: age differences and behavioral correlates. *Child Development*, **74**, 1006–20.

Yehuda, R., Halligan, S. L. & Grossman, R. (2001). Childhood trauma and risk for PTSD: Relationship to intergenerational effects of trauma, parental PTSD, and cortisol excretion. *Development and Psychopathology*, **13**, 733–53.

Zimmermann, L. K. & Stansbury, K. (2004). The influence of emotion regulation, level of shyness, and habituation on the neuroendocrine response of three-year-old children. *Psychoneuroendocrinology*, **29**, 973–82.

Children's perceptions of illness and death

Richard E. Boles and Michael C. Roberts

University of Kansas

Psychologists have long attempted to gain an understanding of how children view the world and its components. A particular interest within paediatric psychology has been children's perceptions of such environmental components as medical events; personnel, and procedures; diseases; and death (Roberts, 2000). In order to effectively change the environment in ways to create more positive perceptions, it becomes paramount to know, in fact, how children perceive chronic illness and death. Psychologists have investigated what have been variously called children's knowledge, attitudes, attributions, understanding, conceptions and perceptions of health-related events, issues and concepts. Similarly, clinicians have sought to understand children's perceptions of diseases such as asthma or cystic fibrosis in order to design interventions and explanations for those with such conditions. Additionally, perceptions of siblings and peers about children with chronic illness and disease have been examined in order to enhance their acceptance and development of social relationships. Finally, clinical investigators have assessed children's views of medication and the causes of disease in order to influence adherence to treatment regimens. The following selective review highlights children's perceptions regarding chronic illness and death, explicating theoretical and conceptual considerations, peer and sibling relationships, medication issues and clinical implications.

Theories of children's perceptions and attitudes

Several theoretical frameworks have been developed or modified within which to conceptualize children's perceptions and understanding of chronic illness and death. The Health Belief Model (HBM) has been widely used to conceptualize adults' motivations to adopt health-enhancing behaviours (Rosenstock, 1974). In general, research has been supportive of the HBM with adults (see 'The Health Belief Model'). However, noticeably less research has investigated the applicability of HBM with children (e.g. DePaola *et al.*, 1997). A somewhat similar theoretical model, Protection Motivation Theory (PMT), has been advanced as a more comprehensive and adaptable model. PMT postulates that preventive health behaviour results from the cognitive mediational processes of threat appraisal and coping appraisal. As with HBM, PMT relies on cognitive perceptions and has been supported by considerable research with adults; although PMT concepts have been extended to children (e.g. Knapp, 1991), support for the extension remains limited. Thus, with both HBM and PMT frameworks, the downward extension of adult-oriented theories to children has not been sufficient, just as it has not been for other aspects of health and clinical psychology.

Models that have incorporated a more developmental approach have been advanced with regard to children's perceptions of phenomena in paediatrics. For example, many of these formulations have relied upon Piaget's concepts in which increasingly sophisticated cognitive development leads directly to positive changes in children's health conceptions, beyond the predictive ability of simply looking at child age (e.g. Berry *et al.*, 1993). Often, research studies have not been organized by a particular theoretical framework. These studies have been guided more by pragmatic considerations or questions of 'what are children's beliefs and perceptions?' and 'what influences children's conceptions?'. These have been valuable for explicating children's beliefs and as heuristics for developing theories and interventions to help children and families. The following sections summarize the research studies into children's conceptions of various paediatric phenomena.

Children's conceptions of illness and death

Early work into children's conceptualizations and perceptions of illness and death was conducted with healthy children. For example, Nagy (1951) determined that preschool children (3–5 years) were relatively unsophisticated in their causal explanations of illness. Slightly older children explained illness as a result of infections (6–7 years) and exposure to germs (8–10 years), while children ages 11–12 years understood multiple causes of illness. Potter and Roberts (1984), in an application of Piagetian constructs, determined that preoperational children (ages 2–7 years) perceived themselves as more vulnerable to contagion.

Investigations into healthy children's disease conceptions have examined perceptions of AIDS in terms of contagion, vulnerability, attitudes toward persons with AIDS, etc. Children and adolescents, for example, have limited understanding of AIDS and possess a variety of conceptions of the disease not commensurate with professional knowledge (but probably not unlike what adults know and believe). Walsh and Bibace (1991) found that children's conceptions of AIDS followed developmental progressions related to cognitive development and are similar to their understanding of other illnesses. The importance of developmental factors has been revealed when considering children's AIDS knowledge. For instance, older children with more AIDS knowledge show more mature illness conceptualizations when compared with children who have less knowledge (De Loye *et al.*, 1993). Zimet, *et al.* (1991) determined that knowing somebody with AIDS lowered adolescents' social anxiety about interacting with a person with AIDS, but had no effect on perceptions of personal vulnerability.

Researchers have also studied relatively abstract concepts such as the development of concepts about death and personal mortality. Nagy (1948; as cited in Willis, 2002) proposed that children understand death as occurring in a progression across 3 stages. Stage 1 is a simplistic belief by children ages 3 to 5 years old) that death is nothing more than individuals not being present at that time. In Stage 2, children (ages 5 to 9 years old) may think that death is completely avoidable. Finally, during Stage 3, children (ages 9 and 10 years old) begin to recognize that death is permanent, unavoidable and omnipresent.

When considering a child's ability to conceptualize death, cognitive development is considered a key influential characteristic (Koocher & MacDonald, 1992). For example, infants and nonverbal toddlers are thought not to make inferences of causality between disease and treatment process. As toddlers become older they may often attribute negative events and outcomes to events far from reality and show evidence of magical thinking. However, as children begin grade school, they begin to understand that death is permanent, irreversible and not simply a form of sleep (Koocher & MacDonald, 1992). Similarly, Reilly *et al.* (1983) found belief in personal mortality beginning in children at about the age of six years. Death is a fairly abstract concept, but apparently death-related experiences facilitate acquisition and increased understanding of death concepts. Similarly, experiences with chronic illness also appear to facilitate children's understanding of the aetiology of illness, although more definitive investigations are needed to determine which features of experience create facilitating effects.

Children's perceptions of peers with illness or disorders

The paediatric psychology research previously noted considered children's perceptions of health and illness in general. Even when specific to a disease such as AIDS or cancer, the interest has been relatively focused on their conceptions in the abstract. A large body of literature has developed into how children view, interact with and hold attitudes about those individuals who may have an illness or disorder. Knowledge of children's understanding about conditions of disability can assist all parties during integration of children with chronic diseases into the classroom. Furthermore, professionals have realized the importance of children's understanding of illness in order to facilitate communication about illnesses and improve interactions among children (see 'Breaking bad news').

Several studies have found that children hold more negative attitudes about peers who are different, namely, who are mentally retarded, visually, hearing or speech impaired and physically impaired. Across perceived conditions, younger children and girls tend to hold more prosocial behaviours and empathy than do older children and boys (e.g. Gray & Rodrigue, 2001). When considering peer acceptance of disabled or non-disabled children, healthy children often indicate a preference for non-disabled peers. In contrast, hypothetical peers diagnosed with cancer were rated by children as equal in social image and acceptance when compared to healthy hypothetical peers, suggesting a diagnosis of cancer is not necessarily socially undesirable.

Peer perceptions have a potentially large impact during peer interactions. For instance, an increasingly higher number of children who are HIV-positive will be attending school, where many peers (and teachers) may worry about such close proximity or have a stigmatizing view of individuals with AIDS. When assessing the factors that affected the acceptance of hypothetical peers with AIDS, there is more support for increased peer acceptance when informing children about how HIV is *not* transmitted (e.g. the myth of drinking from a water fountain) compared with providing information about the modes of transmission (Maieron *et al.*, 1996). These findings may be the result of children's higher frequency of myth behaviours as opposed to behaviours that are likely to lead to HIV transmission, such as sex or drug sharing.

Cole *et al.* (1996) also used vignettes of hypothetical ill peers to elicit children's views about disease perceptions. Interestingly, they found that the type of disease and the impact on physical interactive activity did not have a significant effect on peer acceptance; however, older children reported greater acceptance of chronically ill children. In general, regardless of methodology, perceptions about peers with physical, medical, or psychological disorders tend to be more negative than those about peers without disorders and show age or developmental relationships.

Children's perceptions of medication for chronic illness

In studying perceptions of specific phenomena in paediatrics, the importance of knowing children's knowledge and attitudes about medication and treatment regimens has been demonstrated in several reports (see 'Hospitalization in Children'). Practitioners have asserted that attitudes and beliefs about treatment and its components influence the acceptance, the adherence and the outcome of health care interventions.

For example, DePaola, et al. (1997) examined the perceptions of children and their mothers regarding the most common prescribed medical treatment for asthma: at-home medication use. Providing modest support for the application of the Health Belief Model to children, this study revealed that when children disliked a medication, so did the parent. Additionally, when children perceived benefits to the medication, parents did also. Overall, these perceptions were shown to be related to the severity of the children's asthma and mother and child perceptions were significantly correlated. While these findings support similar previous correlational research, it is important to note that the directionality of influence is unknown; it is more likely that a bidirectionality of influence exists between child and parent perceptions of medical phenomena. Furthermore, McNeal et al. (2000) found similar perception complexities in the perceptions of mothers and their children diagnosed with attention deficit/hyperactive disorder (ADHD) regarding medication treatments. Attitudes about treatment such as these influence communication, information seeking and adherence. Thus, studies support the view that parents do have an important relationship with and influence on their children's health beliefs and behaviours.

Clinical implications

Recognizing that children and adults generally perceive people with physical and behaviour disorders as less acceptable than those without disorders, health care and educational professionals have attempted a variety of interventions to influence the perceptions and improve acceptance and understanding. These interventions are often envisioned to have positive effects for the child with a disorder (e.g. illness, physical handicap, or behavioural problems) in understanding their own situation and improving regimen compliance, lessening anxiety and enhancing adjustment. Children with chronic health disorders generally report having more adjustment problems when compared with various control groups. However, only a minority of children with chronic illness appear maladjusted, supporting the finding that there is an increased vulnerability for maladjustment but is not the most likely outcome (Eiser, 1990). Although research on the perceptions of chronic illness and the effects on adjustment has grown substantially in recent years,

much more conceptually driven research is still needed (see Wallander & Varni, 1998).

Currently, little empirical evidence exists regarding interventions designed to facilitate children's understanding and adjustment to death. In general, guidelines suggest that parents and service providers use a developmentally based approach to provide an appropriate healthy model of emotional behaviour, minimizing euphemistic speech, being concrete and engaging in activities which promote self-expression, such as art, music, or writing pretend letters to those who died (e.g. Willis, 2002). Clearly, more investigations are needed in order to fully understand best practices with regard to children's perceptions and adjustment to death.

In addition, children without health problems could better understand their peers or siblings who may have chronic illnesses. For example, AIDS educators should provide curricula that specifically address misconceptions on transmission, focusing on the day-to-day behaviours such as sharing toys with a child who has AIDS. Additionally, peers of children with chronic illness who are at risk for negative psychological effects will be likely to benefit from interventions which focus on accurate information sessions, support groups and attention to internalizing behaviours, such as anxiety and depression.

Finally, knowledge and attitudes about medication acceptance and adherence to treatment regimens are likely to be favourably enhanced by addressing misunderstandings about the particular benefits and drawbacks of individual medications. Moreover, interventions that provide information on side-effects, reasons for dosage (and changes in dosage) should also be considered for both parents and children with chronic illness.

Conclusion

Research into children's conceptions of illness, their perceptions of peers with disorders, and their comprehension of medical treatments, is useful for understanding children's development and their views of the world. Interventions to improve each of these aspects often follow from this understanding. Paediatric psychology, having the qualities of both basic and applied research, has given important attention to both in studying children's perceptions and understanding of paediatrics.

Future investigations are greatly needed to enhance understanding of the key variables associated with children's perceptions of chronic illness and death that can be utilized for the development of effective psychological interventions for key related issues, such as maladjustment and poor medication adherence. Specifically, theoretically derived models incorporating a developmental perspective are needed to provide an adequate framework to empirically test more complex models (Wallander & Varni, 1998). Additionally, methodologies and measurement procedures should include perspectives for perceptions across various chronic illnesses in order to identify common characteristics, as well as including under-studied populations, such as minorities and economically disadvantaged groups. Finally, interventions, based on both maladaptive and adaptive perceptions of chronic illness and death, can be developed and evaluated in relation to psychological adjustment.

REFERENCES

Berry, S. L., Hayford, J. R., Ross, C. K., Pachman, L. M. & Lavigne, J. V. (1993). Conceptions of illness by children with juvenile rheumatoid arthritis: a cognitive developmental approach. *Journal of Pediatric Psychology, 18*, 83–97.

Cole, K. L., Roberts, M. C. & McNeal, R. E. (1996). Children's perceptions of ill peers: effects of disease, grade, and impact variables. *Children's Health Care, 25*, 107–15.

De Loye, G. J., Henggeler, S. W. & Daniels, C. M. (1993). Developmental and family correlates of children's knowledge and attitudes regarding AIDS. *Journal of Pediatric Psychology, 18*, 209–19.

DePaola, L. M., Roberts, M. C., Blaiss, M. S., Frick, P. J. & McNeal, R. E. (1997). Mothers' and children's perceptions of asthma medication. *Children's Health Care, 26*, 265–83.

Eiser, C. (1990). Psychological effects of chronic disease. *Journal of Child Psychology and Psychiatry, 3*, 85–98.

Gray, C. C. & Rodrigue, J. R. (2001). Brief report: Perceptions of young adolescents about a hypothetical new peer with cancer: an analog study. *Journal of Pediatric Psychology, 26*, 247–52.

Knapp, L. (1991). Effects of type of value appealed to and valence of appeal on children's dental health behavior. *Journal of Pediatric Psychology, 16*, 675–86.

Koocher, G. P. & MacDonald, B. L. (1992). Preventive intervention and family coping with a child's life-threatening or terminal illness. In T. J. Akamatsu, M. A. Parris Stephens, S. E. Hobfoll & J. H. Crowther. (Eds.). *Family health psychology* (pp. 67–86) Washington: Hemisphere.

Maieron, M. J., Roberts, M. C. & Prentice-Dunn, S. (1996). Children's perceptions of peers with AIDS: assessing the impact of contagion information, perceived similarity, and illness conceptualization. *Journal of Pediatric Psychology, 21*, 321–33.

McNeal, R. E., Roberts, M. C. & Barone, V. J. (2000). Mothers' and children's perceptions of medication for children with attention-deficit hyperactivity disorder. *Child Psychiatry and Human Development, 30*, 173–87.

Nagy, M. (1948). The child's theory concerning death. *Journal of Genetic Psychology, 73*, 3–27.

Nagy, M. H. (1951). Children's ideas of the origin of illness. *Health Education Journal, 9*, 6–12.

Potter, P. & Roberts, M. (1984). Children's perceptions of chronic illness: the roles of disease symptoms, cognitive development, and information. *Journal of Pediatric Psychology, 9*, 13–27.

Reilly, T. P., Hasazi, J. E. & Bond, L. A. (1983). Children's conceptions of death and personal mortality. *Journal of Pediatric Psychology, 8*, 21–31.

Roberts, M. C. (2000). Pediatric psychology. In A. E. Kazdin (Ed.). *Encyclopedia of psychology* (pp. 79–82). Washington, DC: American Psychological Association and Oxford University Press.

Rosenstock, I. M. (1974). The health belief model and preventive health behavior. *Health Education Monographs, 2*, 354–86.

Wallander, J. L. & Varni, J. W. (1998). Effects of pediatric chronic physical disorders on child and family adjustment. *Journal of Child Psychology and Psychiatry 39*, 29–46.

Walsh, M. E. & Bibace, R. (1991). Children's conceptions of AIDS: a developmental analysis. *Journal of Pediatric Psychology, 16*, 273–85.

Willis, C. A. (2002). The grieving process in children: strategies for understanding, educating, and reconciling children's perceptions of death. *Early Childhood Education Journal, 29*, 221–6.

Zimet, G. D., Hillier, S. A., Anglin, T. M., Ellick, E. M., Krochuk, D. P. & Williams, P. (1991). Knowing someone with AIDS: the impact on adolescents. *Journal of Pediatric Psychology, 16*, 287–94.

Coping with bereavement

Margaret Stroebe, Henk Schut and Wolfgang Stroebe

Utrecht University

Over the course of a lifespan, most people will be confronted with the loss of a close relationship: if attachments have been formed, one is likely to have to suffer the consequences of separation. The term 'bereavement' refers to the situation of a person who has recently experienced the loss of someone significant in their lives through that person's death (see 'Coping with death and dying'). The loss of a family member – such as a parent, partner, sibling or child – are typical examples, although the death of other important relationships – such as a meaningful friendship, classmate or good neighbour – may also be significant. Bereavements evoke grief, which can be defined as a primarily emotional (affective) reaction to the loss through death of a loved one. Affective reactions include yearning and pining and intense feelings of distress over the loss of the deceased person. Grief also incorporates diverse psychological and physical manifestations. The former type of manifestation includes cognitive and social-behavioural reactions such as self-blame and withdrawal from others. The latter includes physiological/somatic reactions, such as head- and stomach ache, and increased vulnerability to diseases. Sometimes mourning is used interchangeably with grief. However, there are good reasons to define mourning as the social expressions or acts expressive of grief that are shaped by the practices of a given society or cultural group. It is worth noting that researchers following the psychoanalytic tradition often use the term 'mourning' rather than 'grief' to denote the psychological reaction to bereavement.

41

The impact of bereavement

Bereavement leaves many people feeling heart-broken, fearful, uncertain about how to go about their changed lives, and terribly lonely, even when surrounded by others. Most bereaved persons gradually accommodate to their loss, however, and manage to find pleasure in their lives again over the course of time (though many bereaved persons say they 'get used to' rather than 'get over' a loss). At the same time, it is important to recognize that bereaved persons are at elevated risk of developing mental and physical health problems, which may persist long after the loss has occurred (Parkes, 1972/1996; Stroebe & Stroebe, 1987). A minority of individuals are vulnerable to complications in the grieving process itself, for example, chronic grief, which is characterized by protracted grief and prolonged difficulty in normal functioning (Bowlby, 1980). The risk of mortality, though small in terms of the absolute numbers of bereaved persons at elevated risk, is also higher than rates for non-bereaved persons of equivalent age and gender. This 'broken heart' effect pertains across different types of relationships, including spouses and parents who have lost a child (Li *et al.*, 2003; Stroebe & Stroebe, 1993). Not surprisingly, then, bereaved people quite often feel in need of consultations with their general practitioners or seek support from other health care institutions such as the various volunteer and professional counselling or therapy intervention services (Schut *et al.*, 2001) (see 'Counselling').

Given the diversity in bereaved persons' reactions to their loss, it becomes important to establish who is at risk of the diverse detrimental effects. Bereavement researchers have come to use the term 'risk factors', to signify the identification of situational and personal characteristics likely to be associated with increased vulnerability across the spectrum of poor bereavement outcome variables (W. Stroebe & Schut, 2001). For example, high risk subgroups have been identified – admittedly with differing levels of empirical robustness – according to sociodemographic variables (e.g. male gender among spouses; younger rather than older age in general), causes and circumstances of bereavement (e.g. sudden death; child loss), personal factors (e.g. a history of mental disturbance; personality characteristics/relationship difficulties) and concurrent circumstances during bereavement (e.g. economic difficulties that have come about as a result of the death).

Coping with bereavement

It is also important to examine the different ways that people cope with bereavement. Why is it that some persons manage to cope, while others remain devastated by their experience and fail to adapt well? Do these good- versus poor-outcome bereaved people go about their grieving in different ways? Can others help a grieving person to cope with loss? Who needs help with coping? More fundamentally, what is the nature of adaptive coping, and what scientific understanding has been reached on this topic?

Classic theoretical approaches

For most of the twentieth century it was generally believed that to get over the loss of a loved one it was necessary to do one's 'grief work'. Grief work refers to the cognitive process of confronting the reality of a loss through death, of going over the events that occurred before and at the time of death, and of focusing on memories and working towards detachment from the deceased. The grief work concept was fundamental to the psychoanalytic perspective, formulated by Freud (1917/1957) in 'Mourning and Melancholia', and was subsequently influential not only in major theories of grief, but also in the development of principles and guidelines for bereavement counselling and therapy. Yet, is it enough to say that people who are 'doing their grief work' are coping effectively? In the latter decades of the last century, doubts were raised on a number of levels (Bonanno, 2001; Stroebe, 1992; Wortman & Silver, 1987, 1989). First, the concept of grief work lacks specification. For example, it is difficult to distinguish yearning and pining, which are part of grieving but which are associated with negative outcome (Nolen-Hoeksema, 2001), from grief work, which comprises a constructive confrontation with the reality of loss, one that would then lead to positive outcome. Second, empirical studies have failed to confirm that confronting and working through a loss leads to better outcomes than not doing so, or that avoiding confrontation is necessarily detrimental to adaptation. Third, different 'recipes' for grieving could be found in different cultures, including ones that called for suppression of emotions of grief, a clearly different strategy that was not apparently associated with particularly bad outcomes (Wikan, 1988). Finally, attention has been drawn to two further features of the grieving process itself: it is a complex, dynamic process calling for adaptation to many different life changes, all of which need to be addressed but which cannot be attended to all at the same time: the grief work notion does not cater explicitly for this complexity. Grieving is also exhausting: a person cannot do grief work unremittingly, 'dosage' is necessary, so we need to be aware of the need for emotion regulation and to extend our theoretical modelling to incorporate a more dynamic perspective.

Contemporary theoretical appraches

Contemporary theoretical perspectives postulate finer-grained strategies of adaptive coping with bereavement. Coping is nowadays generally understood to encompass 'the person's cognitive and behavioural efforts to manage (reduce, minimize, master or tolerate) the internal and external demands of the person-environment transaction that is appraised as taxing or exceeding the resources of the person' (Folkman *et al.*, 1986, p. 572). Bereaved people use certain ways of coping to manage the stressful situation that follows bereavement, and the associated negative emotions. 'Adaptive strategies' would then be those that actually lead to a reduction in the negative psychosocial and physical health consequences of bereavement and/or to a lowering of grief. Such definitions may seem straightforward, but it is important to note the difficulties in assessing adaptive coping (see W. Stroebe, 2000). Different strategies may be more effective at different times or for coping with different aspects of bereavement; a strategy may be useful short-term but harmful long-term; it may positively affect physical health but increase distress. Methodologically too, many of the empirical studies that have been conducted to assess effective coping have shortcomings. For example, assessments are not conducted longitudinally (coping strategies need to be assessed at a first measurement point, to predict outcome at a second), and sometimes have even been conducted retrospectively. Furthermore, definitions of coping strategies or styles often include outcome as well as process variables. For example, some of the scales used to assess emotion-focused coping contain items that confound coping strategy with coping outcome (e.g. including questions about distress or low self-esteem among those on controlling emotions).

Toward identification of (mal)adaptive processes

A number of quite diverse theoretical approaches can be drawn on to identify principles of (in)effective coping with bereavement (for a review, see M. Stroebe & Schut, 2001*a*). These perspectives range from general stress and trauma theories, to general theories of grief, to models of coping which are specific to bereavement. Each approach has generated empirically testable hypotheses (although far more research is needed to explore the effectiveness of proposed strategies). In addition to elaborating on the grief work process in general, stress and trauma theories have examined processes involving emotion-versus problem-focused coping, confrontation–avoidance strategies, cognitive regulation, the efficacy of communication with others about the loss and the role of revision of assumptions that have been shattered, or making sense and finding meaning in the loss.

General grief-related theories also built on the grief work notion to include examinations of the transformation in the relationship to the deceased and trajectories of adaptation, for example, in terms of psychosocial transitions (e.g. Parkes, 1993) or attachment and recovery processes (Bowlby, 1980; Rubin & Malkinson, 2001). Similarly, Weiss (1988) defined three specific adaptive tasks involved in coming to terms with loss; cognitive acceptance, emotional acceptance and identity change.

Models of coping with bereavement have suggested a number of quite specific processes of (mal)adaptive coping. The best among these studies have adopted well controlled, longitudinal designs. For example, Nolen-Hoeksema (2001) has provided evidence that a ruminative coping style is maladaptive. Rumination was defined as engaging in thoughts and behaviours that maintain one's focus on one's negative emotions and on the possible causes and consequences of those emotions. Rumination was found to prolong distress and to make it more difficult for bereaved people to solve the problems they face following their loss. On the other hand, suppression of grief-related distress has also been shown to be maladaptive (Folkman *et al.*, 1996), although there may be benefits to controlling the emotion of grief (Fraley & Bonanno, 2004; Stroebe & Schut, 1999). Future research needs to tease out precisely when and for whom confronting versus avoiding grief is beneficial versus harmful.

Following a different line of approach, Folkman (2001) adapted cognitive stress theory (Lazarus & Folkman, 1984) to the special characteristics of bereavement, in an effort to derive specific predictions about coping following this particular life event. A key element of Folkman's model was the inclusion of positive indicators of adjustment and delineation of processes which support the positive indicators. Again, longitudinal evidence was provided to show that the co-occurrence of positive with negative affect was not only a correlate, but that positive affect actually had adaptational significance in the coping process: 'The coping processes that generate positive affect and the positive affect itself appear to help sustain renewed problem- and emotion-focused coping efforts in dealing with the chronic stressful condition' (Folkman, 2001, p. 571).

Not only intra- but also interpersonal coping variables have been suggested in theories of adaptation to bereavement, with examinations ranging from studies of bereaved families' interactions, biography reconstruction in family groups, and incremental grief processes dependent on (a)symmetry and (in)congruence within bereaved family groups (M. Stroebe & Schut, 2001*a*; Winchester-Nadeau, 2001). Looking more specifically at interpersonal processes, investigators have examined the role of disclosure and of types of social support (emotional, instrumental, companionship, etc.) from others as assisting coping with bereavement. Following the extensive work of Pennebaker and colleagues (for a review see Pennebaker & Keough, 1999) which has demonstrated the efficacy of diary writing and spoken disclosure in adjustment to stressful life events, one would expect these manipulations to help in bereavement, which, after all, is frequently considered the most stressful event of all (see 'Emotional expression and health'). Surprisingly, results have been very mixed, with the best-designed studies failing to find any benefits of disclosure among bereaved samples (M. Stroebe *et al.*, 2002). Similarly disappointing have been studies of social support, including the provision of professional support in the form of counselling or therapy. These have also failed to show beneficial effects among samples of normally bereaved individuals. Only in cases of high risk or where there are existing complications (e.g. prior psychological disturbance) has intervention from others been shown to attenuate grief and reduce symptomatology in general (Jordan & Neimeyer, 2003; Schut *et al.*, 2001). Social support has simply been shown to help all people – irrespective of whether or not they were bereaved – but not to buffer the bereaved in particular against the negative consequences of loss (Stroebe, Stroebe, Abakoumkin & Schut, 1996). It seems that the emotional loneliness experienced on the loss of a loved person cannot, then, be assuaged by others, though others may be able to help with tasks arising through the loss. Furthermore, professionals need to channel their intervention toward the most vulnerable among the bereaved.

The dual process model of coping with bereavement

Taken together, we see that many kinds of adaptive tasks have been identified – and some empirically-researched – deriving from very different theoretical approaches. Is it possible to develop an integrative model of coping with bereavement that incorporates many of the elements of these approaches and, most importantly, enables one to incorporate the coping processes that have been identified as (mal)adaptive into a single framework? Two integrative models have been proposed, namely, the Four Component Model by Bonanno and Kaltman (1999) and the Dual Process Model of Coping with Bereavement (DPM) by Stroebe and Schut (1999). Bonanno and Kaltman's model is a broader bereavement model, for example, it includes risk factors, while the DPM focuses more narrowly on the adaptiveness of the coping process itself. Bonanno and Kaltman adopt an emotion theory perspective, while the DPM draws more broadly and explicitly on the earlier theoretical approaches described above. The two approaches are largely compatible. Here we focus on the DPM.

The DPM comprises an attempt to integrate existing ideas into a single framework to enable prediction of adaptive coping and to overcome the shortcomings of the grief work model described earlier. The DPM defines two broad types of stressor, to cover the range of diverse stressors that grieving people have to deal with, namely, those that are loss- versus restoration-oriented. 'Loss oriented stressors' are those that have to do with the bereaved person's concentration on and processing of some aspect of the loss experience itself. The focus of attachment theory on the nature of the lost relationship would be consistent with this, as would the integration of grief work (grief work is indeed an important part of grieving). 'Restoration-orientation' refers to the focus on the secondary stressors that are also consequences of bereavement. Cognitive stress theory is applicable here: it assumes that a range of sub-stressors may occur (e.g. worries about making ends meet, being able to master the tasks previously undertaken by the deceased). Both orientations are sources of upset and stress, and are involved in the coping process. Both are attended to in varying degrees (according to individual and cultural variations). Thus, one can speak of 'tasks' of grieving but these tasks are more extensive than described previously (see Worden, 1982/1991/2002).

Given that cognitive processes of confrontation–avoidance have been identified as central in coping with bereavement, it is important to integrate an emotion regulation process into the model. Indeed this is also necessitated by the postulation of the two types of stressor, and because of the conceptualization of the grieving process as a dynamic and fluctuating phenomenon. The DPM specifies a dynamic coping process of oscillation, a regulatory process that distinguishes this model from others. It is proposed that a bereaved person will alternate between coping with loss- and restoration-oriented stressors. At times the person will confront and dwell on aspects of loss (or restoration) and at other times avoid them. Oscillation between the two types of stressor is necessary for adaptation. We noted too that grieving is arduous: for successful coping to take place there also, then, needs to be 'time off'. We maintain that it is actually beneficial to the coping process itself to have respite from confronting either type of stressor for a while. What emerges, then, is a more complex regulatory process of confrontation and avoidance than that described and investigated in other models. The structural components of the DPM are depicted in Figure 1.

Clearly, it is also necessary to represent a broader range of cognitive processes in the model including meanings, assumptions and types of expression associated with good versus poor adaptation. Drawing on the cognitive process models of positive versus negative (re)appraisal described earlier, the DPM provides an analysis of cognitions related to the confrontation–avoidance process. Following the previous research outlined above, there are good reasons to argue the need for oscillation between positive and negative affect – in relationship not only to loss- but also to restoration-stressors – as integral to the coping process. For example, persistent negative affect is maladaptive, although negative affect is part of grieving, while somewhat conversely, positive affect sustains the grieving process, but if positive states are maintained relentlessly, grieving is neglected. To illustrate, a chronic griever would be likely to attend relentlessly to negative aspects associated with loss, dwelling on the deceased, failing to take comfort in positive features and ignoring the tasks of restoration that need attending to (or taking a respite from grieving to do pleasant things). Such pathways as these have been integrated within the DPM (Stroebe & Schut, 2001b).

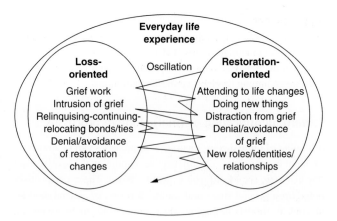

Fig 1 Dual Process Model of coping with bereavement.

Further empirical testing of the DPM is needed, although studies are beginning to find supportive results for some of the parameters (Stroebe, Schut & Stroebe, 2005). Although not a direct test, results of the study by Schut et al. (1997) are indicative. It is known that women – at least in traditional western societies – tend to be more emotion-focused and men more problem-focused in their coping. In a blind assignment, Schut offered two types of intervention for bereaved men and women who suffered high levels of persisting distress approximately a year after their bereavement. One type was focused more on emotions, the other on problems. Interestingly, the bereaved women, who were typically more focused on their emotions (loss-orientation), benefited more from the problem-focused intervention, while the bereaved men, more focused on dealing with things through problem (restoration) orientation, benefited most by confronting their emotions.

Conclusions

There are good reasons for arguing the importance of further development and testing of scientific models of coping with bereavement, such as the one illustrated above. Theories provide a sound basis for methodical testing of the validity of assumptions that people have about coping with bereavement: do we need to 'give sorrow words' or 'keep grief within', as the poets disparately claim? Without a systematic analysis it is difficult to ascertain which of these assumptions is correct (we have suggested that neither is; that it is not really that simple!) or, even more importantly, to know whether people's beliefs about what is best for grieving people, are actually correct. Theories are also important for the development of assessment instruments to investigate (mal)adaptive coping with bereavement: 'A rational, theory-driven strategy should be preferred over inductive, empirical approaches which run the risk of coincidental solutions' (Heck & de Ridder, 2001, p. 460). Finally, theoretical approaches to coping with bereavement, backed up by sound empirical testing, should not only teach us more about the nature of grief and grieving, but also enable us to answer questions about effective coping more precisely, and thereby improve understanding of those who suffer extremely from the loss of a significant person in their lives.

REFERENCES

Bonanno, G. (2001). Grief and emotion: a social-functional perspective. In M. S. Stroebe, R. O. Hansson, W. Stroebe & H. Schut (Eds.). *Handbook of bereavement research: consequences, coping, and care* (pp. 493–515). Washington, DC: American Psychological Association Press.

Bonanno, G. & Kaltman, S. (1999). Toward an integrative perspective on bereavement. *Psychological Bulletin*, **125**, 760–76.

Bowlby, J. (1980). *Attachment and loss: Vol. 3. Loss: sadness and depression.* New York: Basic Books.

Folkman, S. (2001). Revised coping theory and the process of bereavement. In M. S. Stroebe, R. O. Hansson, W. Stroebe & H.A.W. Schut (Eds.). *Handbook of bereavement research: consequences, coping and care* (pp. 563–84). Washington, DC: American Psychological Association Press.

Folkman, S., Lazarus, R. S., Gruen, R. J. & de Longis, A. (1986). Appraisal, coping, health status and psychological symptoms. *Journal of Personality and Social Psychology*, **50**, 571–9.

Folkman, S., Chesney, M., Collette, L., Boccelari, A. & Cooke, M. (1996). Post-bereavement depressive mood and its prebereavement predictors in HIV+ and HIV– gay men. *Journal of Personality and Social Psychology*, **70**, 336–48.

Fraley, C. & Bonanno, G. (2004). Attachment and loss: a test of three competing models on the association between attachment-related avoidance and adaptation to bereavement. *Personality and Social Psychology Bulletin*, **30**, 878–90.

Freud, S. (1917/1957). Mourning and melancholia. In J. Strachey (Ed. & Trans.). *Standard edition of the complete psychological works of Sigmund Freud* (pp. 152–70). London: Hogarth Press, 1957.

Heck, G. van & de Ridder, D. (2001). Assessment of coping with loss: dimensions and measurement. In M. S. Stroebe, R. O. Hansson, W. Stroebe & H. Schut (Eds.). *Handbook of bereavement research: consequences, coping and care* (pp. 449–69). Washington, DC: American Psychological Association Press.

Jordan, J. & Neimeyer, R. (2003). Does grief counseling work? *Death Studies*, **27**, 765–86.

Lazarus, R. S. & Folkman, S. (1984). *Stress, appraisal, and coping.* New York: Springer.

Li, J., Precht, D., Mortensen, B. & Olsen, J. (2003). Mortality in parents after death of a child in Denmark: a nationwide follow-up study. *The Lancet*, **361**, 363–7.

Nolen-Hoeksema, S. (2001). Ruminative coping and adjustment to bereavement. In M. S. Stroebe, R. O. Hansson, W. Stroebe & H. Schut (Eds.). *Handbook of bereavement research: consequences, coping and care* (pp. 545–62). Washington DC: American Psychological Association Press.

Parkes, C. M. (1972/1996). *Bereavement: studies of grief in adult life.* Harmondsworth: Penguin/London: Routledge.

Parkes, C. M. (1993). Bereavement as a psychosocial transition: processes of adaptation to change. In M. S. Stroebe, W. Stroebe & R. O. Hansson (Eds.). *Handbook of bereavement: theory, research, and intervention* (pp. 91–101). New York: Cambridge University Press.

Pennebaker, J. W. & Keough, K. A. (1999). Revealing, organizing, and reorganizing the self in response to stress and emotion. In R. J. Contrada & R. D. Ashmore (Eds.). *Self, social identity, and physical health: interdisciplinary explorations* (pp. 101–21). Oxford: Oxford University Press.

Rubin, S. & Malkinson, R. (2001). Parental responses to loss across the life cycle: clinical and research perspectives. In M. Stroebe, R. O. Hansson, W. Stroebe & H. Schut (Eds.). *Handbook of bereavement research: consequences, coping, and care* (pp. 219–40). Washington, DC: American Psychological Association Press.

Schut, H., Stroebe, M. S., de Keijser, J. & van den Bout, J. (1997). Intervention for the bereaved: gender differences in the efficacy of grief counselling. *British Journal of Clinical Psychology*, **36**, 63–72.

Schut, H., Stroebe, M. S., van den Bout, J. & Terheggen, M. (2001). The efficacy of bereavement interventions: Determining who benefits. In: M. S. Stroebe, R. O. Hansson, W. Stroebe, & H. Schut (Eds.). *Handbook of bereavement research: consequences, coping and care* (pp. 705–38). Washington: American Psychological Association Books.

Stroebe, M. S. (1992). Coping with bereavement: a review of the grief work hypothesis. *Omega: Journal of Death and Dying*, **26**, 19–42.

Stroebe, M. S. & Schut, H. (1999). The Dual Process Model of coping with bereavement: rationale and description. *Death Studies*, **23**, 197–224.

Stroebe, M. S. & Schut, H. (2001*a*). Models of coping with bereavement: a review. In M. Stroebe, R. O. Hansson, W. Stroebe & H. Schut. (Eds.). *Handbook of bereavement research: consequences, coping, and care* (pp. 375–404).

Stroebe, M. S. & Schut, H. (2001b). Meaning making in the Dual Process Model. In R. Neimeyer (Ed.). *Meaning reconstruction and the experience of loss* (pp. 55–73). Washington: American Psychological Association Press.

Stroebe, M. S., Schut, H. & Stroebe, W. (2005). Attachment in coping with bereavement: A theoretical integration. *Review of General Psychology*, **9**, 48–66.

Stroebe, M. S. & Stroebe, W. (1993). The mortality of bereavement: A review. In M. S. Stroebe, W. Stroebe & R. O. Hansson (Eds.). *Handbook of bereavement: theory, research, and intervention* (pp. 175–95). New York: Cambridge University Press.

Stroebe, M. S., Stroebe, W., Schut, H., Zech, E. & van den Bout, J. (2002). Does disclosure of emotions facilitate recovery from bereavement? Evidence from two prospective studies. *Journal of Consulting and Clinical Psychology*, **70**, 169–78.

Stroebe, W. (2000). *Social psychology and health.* Milton Keynes, UK: Open University Press.

Stroebe, W. & Stroebe, M. S. (1987). *Bereavement and health.* New York: Cambridge University Press.

Stroebe, W. & Schut, H. (2001). Risk factors in bereavement outcome: A methodological and empirical review. In M. Stroebe, R. O. Hansson, W. Stroebe & H. Schut (Eds.). *Handbook of bereavement research: Consequences, coping, and care* (pp. 349–71). Washington, DC: American Psychological Association Press.

Stroebe, W., Stroebe, M. S., Abakoumkin, G. & Schut, H. (1996). The role of loneliness and social support in adjustment to loss: a test of attachment versus stress theory. *Journal of Personality and Social Psychology*, **70**, 1241–9.

Weiss, R. S. (1988). Loss and recovery. *Journal of Social Issues*, **44**, 37–52.

Wikan, U. (1988). Bereavement and loss in two Muslim communities: Egypt and Bali compared. *Social Science and Medicine*, **27**, 451–60.

Winchester-Nadeau, J. (2001). Meaning-making in family bereavement: a family systems approach. In M. S. Stroebe, R. O. Hansson, W. Stroebe & H. Schut (Eds.). *Handbook of bereavement research: consequences, coping, and care* (pp. 329–47). Washington, DC: American Psychological Association Press.

Worden, W. (1982/1991/2002). *Grief counseling and grief therapy: a handbook for the health care practitioner.* New York: Springer.

Wortman, C. & Silver, R. (1987). Coping with irrevocable loss. In G. van den Bos &

B. Bryant (Eds.). *Cataclysms, crises, and catastrophes: psychology in action* (pp. 189–235). Washington, DC: American Psychological Association Press.

Wortman, C. & Silver, R. (1989). The myths of coping with loss. *Journal of Consulting and Clinical Psychology,* **57**, 349–57.

Coping with chronic illness

Keith J. Petrie and Lisa Reynolds

The University of Auckland

The increase in chronic illness

Chronic illness is now the predominant disease pattern in most developed countries. Advances in medicine have transformed many previously deadly infectious diseases, such as tuberculosis, pneumonia and influenza into treatable conditions and some have disappeared almost completely. The resulting improved longevity of populations has meant a growth in the burden caused by chronic conditions such as cancer, heart disease, stroke and diabetes. Chronic illnesses often strike in middle- and older-age-groups and bring with them considerable difficulties in adjustment and coping which can severely compromise patients' quality of life. While chronic diseases do kill, most people diagnosed with a chronic illness will live for many years with their condition. Understanding and improving the process of coping with a chronic illness has become an important area of health care.

Adjustments required

The initial psychological adjustments following the diagnosis of a chronic disease generally involve issues related to a loss of function. Individuals at the stage of diagnosis confront the reality that their state of health and function of their body have changed, and are likely to remain impaired. The speed with which individuals confront this loss can be strongly influenced by the nature of the illness. With some chronic illnesses, such as heart disease which is diagnosed following a myocardial infarction, awareness of the presence of the disease is usually sudden. In other chronic illnesses, such as arthritis, the patient may be aware of their disease long before a formal diagnosis is made.

Dealing with the ongoing demands of a chronic illness often requires the learning of new skills and adjustments to daily lifestyle. Patients need to cope with the symptoms of their condition and the requirements of medical treatment, which may mean learning new techniques for managing symptoms or administering therapy and coping with daily life disruption from both symptoms and treatment. Many illnesses, such as insulin-dependent diabetes and end-stage renal disease, require

patients to learn specific techniques for controlling symptoms, such as dialysis in the case of renal disease. Furthermore, an active awareness and monitoring of bodily function may be necessary in diseases like diabetes, where patients are often required to provide 95% or more of their daily care to avoid medical crises (Anderson *et al.,* 1995) (see 'Self-management' and 'Adherence to treatment').

Maintaining intimate and social relationships and developing effective working relationships with medical staff are other important adaptive tasks of living with a chronic illness. Chronic illness can put a strain on these social support networks. Relationships with healthcare staff can be a major source of difficulty in the management of chronic illness. The issue of patient autonomy versus independence from healthcare professionals is often an ongoing problem in long-term treatment programmes. Spouses, in particular, bear a large proportion of the stresses and burdens engendered by the illness. Tasks that the patient normally completed around the home before developing the illness but can no longer manage, need to be assumed by a spouse or other family member. Sometimes this creates feelings of guilt and inadequacy on the part of the patient and feelings of extra pressure and resentment on the part of members of the patient's family.

The restriction in social and other previously pleasurable activities is often an outcome of living with a chronic illness. This change, along with the emotional demands of integrating a new view of the self that includes the chronic illness, result in difficulties in affect regulation and an increased risk of adjustment and emotional disturbances. Individuals with chronic illness are more likely to be depressed than those who do not have a chronic condition, and this relationship has been found to be strongest amongst those who develop chronic illnesses early in life (Schnittker, 2005). However only a minority of patients develop clinical levels of emotional disturbance and this is more common among patients who experience greater levels of pain and disability. Emotional problems, such as depression, often interfere with the adoption and maintenance of rehabilitation programmes and seem to worsen prognosis in many conditions. It is important to note, however, that the emotional response to chronic illness is highly variable and not all the emotional consequences of chronic illness are negative. The few studies that have investigated positive outcomes, also known as 'benefit finding' (e.g. Carver & Antoni, 2004, Sears *et al.*, 2003), report that individuals have found an increased value in close relationships, greater meaning in day-to-day activities and a greater compassion towards others with difficulties.

The coping process

How well patients adjust to chronic illness can be explained in part by their individual coping responses. 'Coping' is the cognitive, behavioural and emotional ways that people manage stressful situations. Coping has been previously conceptualized by researchers as a trait which is stable across situations, or alternatively, as a process that is strongly influenced by situational factors. However, Lazarus and Folkman's (1984) transactional model has had the largest impact on the current conceptualization of coping with chronic illness. This model sees the patients' coping responses being determined by both their appraisal of the degree of threat posed by an illness, and the resources seen as being available to help them cope in the situation. Coping responses in this model are divided into emotion-focused and problem-focused strategies. The function of problem-focused coping is to actively alter the stressful situation in some way, while emotion-focused coping is directed at regulating the patient's emotional response to a stressor.

Each response can be potentially adaptive or maladaptive depending on the situation. Some emotion-focused strategies show positive benefits across illnesses. Reframing the illness in a positive light, acceptance of the disease, and utilizing social support appear to be adaptive coping strategies across many chronic illnesses. Other emotion-focused strategies such as disengaging from the situation by giving up or avoiding thinking about the illness have generally been related to increased distress and disability (Carver *et al.*, 1993; Dunkel-Schetter *et al.*, 1992; Felton *et al.*, 1984). Problem-focused strategies, which in theory should have a greater adaptive potential, have frequently failed to demonstrate a strong relationship to outcome in chronic illness. However, seeking information about the illness and planning seem to be two strategies that do have the most consistent relationship with positive outcomes (Felton *et al.*, 1984). These strategies seem to have the greatest effect when the stressor is appraised by the patient as controllable (Folkman *et al.*, 1993). The lack of a strong relationship between problem-focused strategies and positive outcomes in chronic illness may be due to a mismatch between situations which are not amenable to change or control and the use of problem-focused strategies by the individual. In such circumstances emotion-focused strategies may be more useful, and recently interventions have been developed for patients with chronic illness to more accurately match the coping strategy to the characteristics of the situation. Such interventions seem to result in reducing the psychological distress associated with managing a chronic illness (Chesney *et al.*, 2003).

Influences on coping

The severity and nature of the disease does not seem to have a consistent relationship to patient coping and adjustment to chronic illness, whereas the coping process is strongly affected by both psychological and social influences. An important influence is the patient's own subjective understanding of their illness. Leventhal *et al.* (1980) have proposed that cognitive illness representations direct both coping strategies and emotional responses to an illness in a parallel process that feeds back to influence the patient's own illness model. For example, a patient who attributes her hypertension to stress caused by work and who subsequently gives up her job only to find that this has made no difference to her level of blood pressure, may revise her view of the cause of the hypertension. Evidence suggests that particular illness models may be associated with more functional coping strategies and that illness representations may have a critical role in influencing adjustment to a range of common chronic illnesses such as heart disease, cancer and diabetes. In people who have recently had a myocardial infarction, beliefs about cause, timeline, controllability and consequences have been shown to be related to time taken returning to work and attendance at cardiac rehabilitation (Petrie *et al.*, 1996; Cooper *et al.*, 1999) and patients' drawings of perceived damage on their hearts predict recovery better than do medical indicators of damage (Broadbent *et al.*, 2004).

Social and partner support also plays an important role in adjustment to chronic illness. A number of studies have shown social support to be related to better disease outcomes and psychological adjustment in a variety of illnesses (see 'Social support and health'). A large follow-up study of chronically ill patients found social support was beneficial for health over time and this effect was strongest in older patients (Sherbourne *et al.*, 1992). Social support has been associated with better metabolic control in diabetes patients (Akimoto *et al.*, 2004), as well as improved outcomes in breast cancer (Waxler-Morrison *et al.*, 1991), kidney failure (Dimond, 1979) and heart disease (Case *et al.*, 1992). There may also be a gender difference in the way social support operates. In people with heart disease, the protective effects of social support have been less consistent for women. In addition, support can sometimes be too intrusive and people can be deluged with help or conflicting advice causing negative effects on the outcome of chronic illness (e.g. Garrity, 1973). In HIV patients, social conflict has been found to have a stronger association with coping than has perceived support (Fleishman *et al.*, 2000).

The exact nature of the benefits which accrue from social support in the context of chronic illness is not clear. Improved adherence to treatment and better health habits associated with higher levels of social support are likely to be important factors. The role of family and friends noticing changes in the patient's health that need attention may also reduce treatment delay if the illness worsens and the patient needs medical assistance. It seems that patients' perceptions of what actions are helpful are influenced by the social role of the provider. Esteem and emotional support are seen as most helpful when they come from spouses or family (Dakof & Taylor, 1990). Some researchers have suggested that the benefits of social support may not, in fact, derive from its positive aspects but rather from the absence of upsetting or conflictual relationships that interfere with successful function (Coyne & Bolger, 1990).

As well as the critical role of illness perceptions and social support, there is evidence that a number of individual difference variables also influence the coping process. The age of the person, their educational background and personality traits such as optimism can act to influence coping with chronic illness (Carver *et al.*, 1993; Felton *et al.*, 1984). Factors related to the disease itself in terms of its stage, physical characteristics and symptomotology are also important. It is apparent that each chronic illness is made up of a large number of stressors, and patients may apply different coping responses to each of these illness-related problems (Cohen *et al.*, 1986).

Coping interventions

A number of successful intervention strategies have recently been developed for patients suffering from chronic illness. These programmes vary in their focus from being strictly information-based to teaching specific skills which help to address problems faced by the patient. Kate Lorig has developed an intervention based around improving patients' self-efficacy and self-management techniques. It has been adopted in a number of countries as a way of improving the management of chronic illness (Donaldson, 2003). The Chronic Disease Self-Management Programme, also known as the Expert Patient Programme, uses trained patients as leaders of patient groups and draws on the findings of patients' own experience. The groups, which are also being trialled over the internet, focus on improving patients' ability to interpret changes in the disease and its consequences. Group sessions also aim to improve patients' use of medication and utilization of medical and community support as well as pain control and managing the emotional consequences of the illness. The programme encourages patients to set goals and identify effective feedback. Research shows participants experience improved physical activity, reduced symptoms and have significantly less need for medical treatment in comparison with control groups (Lorig *et al.*, 1999).

Mike Antoni and his colleagues at the University of Miami have developed a group cognitive behavioural intervention (see Behaviour therapy and Cognitive behaviour therapy) for a number of chronic illness groups including HIV-infected individuals, men with prostate cancer and women diagnosed with early-stage breast cancer. This programme, which is adapted for each specific illness group, provides information on the stress response and various coping strategies best matched to deal with specific stressors. Imagery and progressive muscle relaxation techniques (see Relaxation training) are taught to help patients deal with personal stress. Cognitive behavioural techniques are employed to modify maladaptive appraisals and interpersonal social skills are taught to improve the utilization of social support networks. Results from clinical trials show that the intervention increased the incidence of reporting by patients that breast cancer had impacted positively on their lives (Antoni *et al.*, 2001), improved quality of life in men recovering from treatment of prostate carcinoma (Penedo *et al.*, 2004) and improved the use of effective coping and reduced mood disturbance in HIV-infected individuals (Antoni *et al.*, 2001).

While the results from intervention studies provide impressive support for developing coping skills as a treatment, it is difficult to separate the non-specific factors that occur in these group interventions from the specific effects of enhancing coping skills. These group treatment programmes incorporate other aspects such as psychological support and education with the teaching of coping strategies, and further research needs to be done to ascertain the specific benefits of coping training. Intervention studies are a valuable method of testing the coping skills model and they provide a useful way of investigating coping processes over time.

Coping with chronic illness has become an important area for research and intervention in health psychology. Research in this area is likely to become even more important in the future as the large numbers of individuals suffering from such diseases continue to grow. The diagnosis of a chronic illness typically brings with it a number of complex problems, emotional difficulties and changes in lifestyle. The patient's own understanding of the illness and the levels of appropriate social support available to them are key factors in promoting successful long-term coping. Interventions that develop coping strategies and improve the matching of problem-focused or emotion-focused strategies with the situational context seem to provide a promising avenue to improve the quality of life for patients living with a chronic illness.

REFERENCES

Akimoto, M., Fukunishi, I., Kanno, K. *et al.* (2004). Psychosocial predictors or relapse among diabetes patients: a 2-year follow-up after inpatient diabetes education. *Psychosomatics*, **45**, 343–49.

Anderson, R.M., Arnold, M.S., Funnell, M.M. *et al.* (1995). Patient empowerment: results of a randomized controlled trial. *Diabetes Care*, **18**, 943–49.

Antoni, M.H., Lehman, J.M., Kilbourn, K.M. *et al.* (2001). Cognitive–behavioral stress management intervention decreases the prevalence of depression and enhances benefit finding among women under treatment for early-stage breast cancer. *Health Psychology*, **20**, 20–32.

Broadbent, E., Petrie, K.J., Ellis, C.J., Ying, J. & Gamble, G. (2004) A picture of health – myocardial infarction patients' drawings of their hearts and subsequent disability: a longitudinal study. *Journal of Psychosomatic Research*, **57**, 583–7.

Carver, C.S., Pozo, C., Harris, S.D. *et al.* (1993). How coping mediates the effect of optimism on distress: a study of women with early stage breast cancer. *Journal of Personality and Social Psychology*, **65**, 375–90.

Carver, C.S. & Antoni, M.H. (2004). Finding benefit in breast cancer during the year after diagnosis predicts better adjustment 5 to 8 years after diagnosis. *Health Psychology*, **23**, 595–8.

Case, R.B., Moss, A.J., Case, N., McDermott, M. & Eberly, S. (1992). Living alone After myocardial infarction: impact on prognosis. *The Journal of the American Medical Association*, **267**, 515–19.

Chesney, M.A., Chambers, D.B., Taylor, J.M., Johnson, L.M. & Folkman S. (2003). Coping effectiveness training for men living with HIV: results from a randomized clinical trial testing a group-based intervention. *Psychosomatic Medicine*, **65**, 1038–46.

Cohen, F., Reese, L. B., Kaplan, G. A. & Roggio, R. E. (1986). Coping with the stresses of arthritis. In R. W. Moskowitz & M. R. Haug (Eds.). *Arthritis in the elderly*. New York: Springer.

Cooper, A., Lloyd, G., Weinman, J. & Jackson, G. (1999). Why patients do not attend cardiac rehabilitation: role of intentions and illness beliefs. *Heart*, **82**, 234–6.

Coyne, J. C. & Bolger, N. (1990). Doing without social support as an explanatory concept. *Journal of Social and Clinical Psychology*, **9**, 148–58.

Dakof, G. A. & Taylor, S. E. (1990). Victims perceptions of social support: what is helpful from whom? *Journal of Personality and Social Psychology*, **58**, 80–9.

Dimond, M. (1979). Social support and adaptation to chronic illness: the case of maintenance hemodialysis. *Research in Nursing and Health*, **2**, 101–8.

Donaldson, L. (2003). Expert patients usher in a new era of opportunity for the NHS. *British Medical Journal*, **326**, 1279–80.

Dunkel-Schetter, C., Feinstein, L. G., Taylor, S. E. & Falke, R. L. (1992). Patterns of coping with cancer. *Health Psychology*, **11**, 79–87.

Felton, B. J., Revenson, T. A. & Hinrichsen, G. A. (1984). Stress and coping in the explanation of psychological adjustment among chronically ill adults. *Social Science and Medicine*, **18**, 889–98.

Fleishman, J. A., Sherbourne, C. D., Crystal, S. *et al.* (2000). Coping, conflictual social interactions, social support, and mood among HIV-infected persons. *American Journal of Community Psychology*, **28**, 421–53.

Folkman, S., Chesney, M., Pollack, L. & Coates, T. (1993). Stress, control, and depressive mood in human immunodeficiency virus-positive and -negative gay men in San Francisco. *The Journal of Nervous and Mental Disease*, **181**, 409–16.

Garrity, T. F. (1973). Vocational adjustment after first myocardial infarction: comparative assessment of several variables suggested in the literature. *Social Science and Medicine*, **7**, 705–17.

Lazarus, R. S. & Folkman, S. (1984). *Stress, appraisal, and coping*. New York: Springer.

Leventhal, H., Meyer, D. & Nerertz, D. (1980). The common–sense representations of illness danger. In S. Rachman (Ed.). *Medical psychology* 2 (pp. 7–30). New York: Guilford Press.

Lorig, K. R., Sobel, D. S., Stewart, A. L. *et al.* (1999). Evidence suggesting that a chronic disease self-management program can improve health status while reducing hospitalization: a randomized trial. *Medical Care*, **37**, 5–14.

Penedo, F. J., Dahn, J. R., Molton, I. *et al.* (2004). Cognitive-behavioral stress management improves stress-management skills and quality of life in men recovering from treatment of prostate carcinoma. *Cancer*, **100**(1), 192–200.

Petrie, K. J., Weinman, J., Sharpe, N. & Buckley, J. (1996). Role of patients' view of their illness in predicting return to work and functioning after myocardial infarction: a longitudinal study. *British Medical Journal*, **312**, 1191–4.

Sears, S. R., Stanton, A. L. & Danoff-Burg, S. (2003). The yellow brick road and the emerald city: benefit finding, positive appraisal coping and posttraumatic growth in women with early-stage breast cancer. *Health Psychology*, **22**, 487–97.

Schnittker, J. (2005). Chronic illness and depressive symptoms in late life. *Social Science and Medicine*, **60**, 13–23.

Sherbourne, C. D., Meredith, L. S., Rogers, W. & Ware, J. E. (1992). Social support and stressful life events: age differences in their effects on health-related quality of life among the chronically ill. *Quality of Life Research*, **1**, 235–46.

Waxler-Morrison, N., Hislop, T. G., Mears, B. & Can, L. (1991). The effects of social relationships on survival with women with breast cancer: a prospective study. *Social Science and Medicine*, **33**, 177–83.

Weinman, J., Petrie, K. J. Moss–Morris, R. E. & Horne, R. (1996). The illness perception questionnaire: a new method for assessing the cognitive representation of disease. *Psychology and Health*, **11**, 431–45.

Coping with chronic pain

Naomi Lester[1], Francis J. Keefe[2], Meredith E. Rumble[2] and Jeffrey D. Labban[2]

[1]Bastyr University
[2]Duke University Medical Center

Chronic pain is a problem that affects millions of individuals every year. Much of chronic pain is associated with significant progressive degenerative disease. Such diseases include arthritis and cancer, and involve prolonged severe pain which may be only partially ameliorated through the use of analgesic medication. This chapter examines the ways in which individuals cope with chronic pain. We describe how pain coping is conceptualized and measured and discuss what has been learned about adaptive and maladaptive methods for coping with chronic pain. We conclude with an exploration of new directions for research in this area.

Coping with chronic pain

Coping has been defined as the process of managing stressful situations, either external or internal, that are viewed as taxing an individual's adaptive resources (Lazarus & Folkman, 1984). The ways in which individuals view or appraise potentially stressful situations is an important component of this process definition of coping. In chronic pain, the ways in which a patient views pain are particularly important in their reactions to pain. Individuals may view pain as unpredictable and feel very little control over pain flares. Conversely, they may view pain as a constant irritation but one that can often be dealt with successfully.

Coping with pain can be thought of as cognitions and behaviours that serve to manage or decrease the sensation of pain and distress caused by pain. Within this basic framework, researchers have formulated several models of pain-coping. We will discuss five such models – the problem/emotion-focused coping model; the active/passive coping model; the cognitive/behavioural coping model; the fear avoidance model; and the acceptance model.

The problem- and emotion-focused coping model

Using the Ways of Coping Checklist (WCCL; Folkman & Lazarus, 1980), Folkman and Lazarus have created a coping model that categorizes coping strategies as either problem-focused or emotion-focused. Table 1 lists sample items from the WCCL. Problem-focused efforts seek to alter the individual's relationship to a stressor. Emotion-focused coping serves to alter one's internal reactions to a stressor. For example, the chronic pain patient faced with the choice of engaging in an activity known to cause pain (say sitting in a cinema for a back pain patient) may use a problem-focused coping strategy such as having a friend pick up a video instead and/or an

Table 1. Items from the Ways of Coping Checklist

Problem-focused coping:
  Concentrated on something good that could come out of the whole thing
  Made a plan of action and followed it

Seeking social support:
  Talked to someone to find out about the situation
  Asked someone for advice and followed it

Wishful-thinking:
  Hoped a miracle would happen
  Wished I could change what happened

Self-blame:
  Realized that I brought the problem on myself
  Blamed myself

Avoidance:
  Went on as if nothing had happened
  Tried to forget the whole thing

emotion-focused strategy such as controlling their disappointment by thinking about some other pleasant activity.

The WCCL is a 42-item pencil and paper questionnaire. Individuals are asked to indicate a recent stressful experience and then answer each question. When this questionnaire is used in studies of chronic pain, respondents are usually asked to indicate a stressor associated with their pain condition. Some forms of the WCCL use a 'Yes/No' response format while others employ a scale on which respondents indicate the extent to which they use each coping strategy. There are several scoring methods for the WCCL. One which is frequently used (Vitaliano et al., 1985) adds questionnaire responses to form one problem-focused and four emotion-focused sub-scales. The emotion-focused sub-scales measure seeking social support, wishful thinking, self-blame and avoidance. The problem-focused scale contains items such as 'just took things one step at a time'. The emotion-focused scales are composed of such items as 'asked someone I respected for advice and took it', 'hoped a miracle would happen', 'blamed myself' and 'kept others from knowing how bad things were'.

Research examining the relationships between problem- and emotion-focused coping, and adjustment to chronic pain has been carried out in several groups of arthritis patients (Manne & Zautra, 1990; Parker et al., 1988; Regan et al., 1988). This research suggests that arthritis patients who rely on wishful thinking, and to a lesser extent, on blame and avoidance-coping strategies may experience more depression and greater physical disability

Table 2. Items from the Vanderbilt Pain Management Inventory

Active coping:
    Engaging in physical exercise or physical therapy
    Clearing your mind of bothersome thoughts or worries
Passive coping:
    Restricting or cancelling your social activities
    Taking medication for the purposes of immediate pain relief

than those who use fewer of these emotion-focused types of coping. In low back pain patients, Turner *et al.* (1987) found that individuals who relied on seeking social support reported lower pain levels than those who did not use this strategy. In the Turner *et al.* study, problem-focused coping did not relate to pain.

Comment

The problem- and emotion-focused coping model has three major advantages for understanding chronic pain coping. First, research has demonstrated that this coping model is valid not only for pain but for a wide range of stressful conditions (Lazarus & Folkman, 1984). Use of this model thus enables pain researchers to link their research to other recent studies in the literature on coping. Secondly, the questionnaire instrument used to asses problem/emotion-focused coping, the WCCL, is an established instrument which meets reasonable psychometric standards. Thirdly, the WCCL assesses a broad selection of coping strategies. Because of its breadth and utility for measuring both pain-coping and coping with other stressors, the WCCL may be used to compare the ways an individual copes with pain and the ways in which they cope with other stressors.

The active and passive coping model

Another category system, using the Vanderbilt Pain Management Inventory (VPMI; Brown & Nicassio, 1987), creates a model which classifies pain-coping strategies as either active or passive. Table 2 Lists sample items from the VPMI. In this classification system, active coping methods are those that require the individual to take some behavioural action to manage pain. An example of an active strategy would be doing muscle strengthening exercises in response to pain. Passive pain-coping strategies focus more on withdrawing or giving up instrumental control over pain. An example of a passive strategy would be the use of medications in response to pain.

The VPMI is an 18-item pencil and paper questionnaire. Respondents are asked to indicate the frequency with which they use each of the coping strategies when coping with pain of a moderate or higher level of intensity. The active coping scale of the VPMI is composed of items such as 'participating in leisure activities' and 'distracting your attention away from pain'. The passive coping scale contains items such as 'talking to others about how much your pain hurts' and 'taking medication for purposes of immediate pain relief'.

The VPMI has been used primarily in studies of arthritis patients. In one such study, Covic *et al.* (2000) investigated the relationship between coping, pain, perceived physical disability and depression in rheumatoid arthritis patients. These researchers found passive coping to uniquely predict higher levels of pain. Passive coping was also found to mediate the effects of pain, perceived physical disability and depression. Consistent results were also found in a study examining the relationships of coping and adjustment to rheumatoid arthritis (Strahl *et al.*, 2000). Results indicated that patients reporting the usage of passive coping also reported more impaired physical functioning. Though the internal reliability of both the active and passive coping scales of the VMPI has been demonstrated, the passive coping scale has been shown to be the more valid construct of the two and thus demonstrated more significant relationships (Snow-Turek *et al.*, 1996). However, reports of active coping have been shown to be associated with less pain, depression and functional disability (Brown & Nicassio, 1987).

Comment

The active/passive coping model is appealing because it is simple and straightforward. Treatment efforts based on this model seek to increase active adaptive coping and decrease passive maladaptive coping. The questionnaire instrument developed from this model (the VMPI) is a very brief instrument that enables one to quickly and reliably categorize a patient's coping strategies. One limitation of this model is that some of the strategies that are labelled as passive (e.g. taking medication) require an active effort on the part of the patient (Keefe *et al.*, 1992).

The cognitive and behavioural coping model

Using the Coping Strategies Questionnaire (CSQ: Rosenstiel & Keefe, 1983) to assess cognitive and behavioural coping, Keefe and colleagues have developed a third model of pain-coping. Table 3 Lists sample items from the CSQI. This system parcels coping strategies into a greater number of coping scales. Examples of these scales include, coping self-statements, ignoring pain sensations and catastrophizing about pain. The CSQ also assesses individuals' perceived ability to control and decrease their pain. Studies of patients with osteoarthritis, rheumatoid arthritis and low back pain have indicated that most people with chronic pain use combinations of these methods for coping with their pain (Keefe *et al.*, 1987, 1990, 1991).

The CSQ is a 48-item questionnaire that asks individuals to indicate the extent to which they use each coping strategy when they experience pain. The items are then totalled to create seven sub-scales: diverting attention, reinterpreting pain sensations, coping self-statements ignoring pain sensations, praying or hoping, catastrophizing and increasing behavioural activities. Two higher-order factors, coping attempts and pain control and rational thinking may be calculated from the CSQ responses. The CSQ also assesses respondents' perceived ability to control and decrease their pain.

Research using the CSQ been carried out in several different ways. Some studies have used the seven sub-scales to assess coping, others have used the two higher order factors, and still

Table 3. Items from the Coping Strategies Questionnaire

Diverting attention:
    I try to think of something pleasant
    I count numbers in my head or run a song through my mind

Reinterpreting pain sensations:
    I don't think of it as pain but rather as a dull or
        warm feeling
    I imagine that the pain is outside my body

Coping self statements:
    I tell myself to be brave and carry on despite the pain
    I tell myself that I can overcome the pain

Ignoring pain sensations:
    I don't pay any attention to the pain.
    I go on as it nothing happened

Praying or hoping:
    I pray to God that it won't last long
    I have faith in doctors that someday there will be a cure for
        my pain

Catastrophizing:
    It's awful and I feel that it overwhelms me
    I worry all the time about whether it will end

Increasing behavioural activity:
    I do something I enjoy, such as watching TV or
        listening to music
    I do something active, like household chores or projects

others have re-factored the questionnaire to form additional scales. The CSQ has also been used with a wide variety of pain conditions, including osteoarthritis (Keefe *et al.*, 2000), low back pain (Jensen *et al.*, 2003), rheumatoid arthritis (Covic *et al.*, 2003), fibromyalgia (Hassett *et al.*, 2000), and cancer-related pain (Wilkie & Keefe, 1991). Because of the wide variety of research with this instrument we will confine our description of findings to a more general level. In general, results have indicated that individuals who cope by trying to exert control over pain report less pain, depression and physical disability than those who make less use of this type of coping. Catastrophizing also appears to be a particularly maladaptive way to cope with chronic pain and individuals using this coping pattern appear to be more depressed and have greater functional disability. For example, Turner *et al.* (2002) found that greater catastrophizing was found to be significantly associated with greater pain-related disability and psychological distress in patients suffering from chronic pain after a spinal cord injury. Similarly, a longitudinal study focusing on pain and depression in rheumatoid arthritis patients (Covic *et al.*, 2003) found passive coping strategies, most notably catastrophizing, to be predictive of higher levels of pain and depression.

In examining other sub-scales, Turner *et al.* (2002) found that coping self-statements and ignoring pain were associated with greater psychological wellbeing. Similarly, Keefe and Williams (1990) found that patients who were referred to a pain management programme that endorsed more items from the coping self-statements sub-scale and who reported that they felt they could control and decrease pain, had lower depression.

Comment

The cognitive–behavioural model of coping has had a major impact on chronic pain assessment and treatment. The CSQ is now widely used in clinical pain assessment and in programmatic research examining the efficacy of cognitive-behavioural interventions (see 'Cognitive behaviour therapy'). The CSQ measures a variety of pain-coping strategies as well as identifying a patient's sense of efficacy for controlling pain. This emphasis on both coping and the appraisal of pain controllability fits well with theories of stress coping and provides additional information for the clinicians who are designing programmes to help patients cope more effectively.

The fear-avoidance model

Over the past decade, numerous studies have examined the utility of the fear-avoidance model in explaining adjustment to pain. The fear-avoidance model focuses on two behavioural coping responses to pain-related fear and anxiety: avoidance versus confrontation (Vlaeyen & Linton, 2000). An example of avoidance would be thinking that pain is a signal of damage to oneself and consequently trying to avoid all activities which are pain-related, whereas a more confrontational response would be engaging in activity appropriately considering some pain-related lifestyle changes. Within this model, avoidant responses are thought to lead to the maintenance or intensification of fear as well as to undesirable pain-related outcomes over time through several pathways, including an increase in negative appraisals of pain and its consequences, a decrease in normal activity leading to the disuse of the musculo-skeletal and cardiovascular system, little opportunity for disconfirmation of maladaptive beliefs about pain and its consequences to occur and more opportunity for mood disturbances to increase. This contrasts with confrontational responses, which are thought to lead to better adaptation to pain over time because individuals are engaged in activity and therefore have more opportunities to confront maladaptive beliefs about their pain, more reinforcers in their environment to regulate mood, and more physical activity to maintain functional ability (Vlaeyen & Linton, 2000).

Pain-related anxiety and fear have been assessed most frequently using one of two measures: 1) the Pain Anxiety Symptoms Scale (PASS; McCracken *et al.*, 1992) – a 40-item measure that was designed to assess cognitive anxiety, escape and avoidance, fearful appraisals and physiological anxiety in response to pain and 2) the Tampa Scale for Kinesiophobia (TSK; Kori *et al.*, 1990) – a 17-item measure that assesses fear of (re)injury due to movement. A growing body of research studies has examined pain-related anxiety and fear in patients with chronic low back pain (Crombez *et al.*, 1999; McCracken *et al.*, 1992; Picavet *et al.*, 2002; Verbunt *et al.*, 2003; Vlaeyen *et al.*, 1995), neck pain (Nederhand *et al.*, 2004) and acute low back pain (Fritz *et al.*, 2001; Swinkels-Meewisse *et al.*, 2003). One of the most consistent findings emerging from this literature is that patients scoring high on pain-related anxiety and fear measures report higher levels of disability and poorer performance on physical tasks such as lifting and carrying capacity and trunk extension and flexion exercises (Burns *et al.*, 2000; Crombez *et al.*, 1999; Fritz *et al.*, 2001; McCracken *et al.*, 1992; Nederhand *et al.*, 2004; Picavet *et al.*, 2002; Swinkels-Meewisse *et al.*, 2003; Verbunt *et al.*, 2003; Vlaeyen *et al.*, 1995). These findings are particularly impressive given that they have been obtained even after controlling for important variables which might explain adjustment to pain such as pain intensity and duration.

Comment

The consistency of findings emerging from studies of the fear–avoidance model is impressive. This model is clinically useful because it links well to exposure-based interventions (see 'Behaviour therapy'). These interventions teach patients to overcome pain-related anxiety and fear through graded exposure to a series of pain-related fears. Preliminary findings from studies using single case designs suggest such interventions are helpful in reducing pain-related anxiety, disability and increasing activity level in patients with chronic low back pain (Vlaeyen *et al.*, 2001; Vlaeyen *et al.*, 2002). Controlled studies are needed to test the efficacy of such interventions with larger samples of chronic pain patients. Future research also needs to examine the degree to which the fear avoidance–model is useful in understanding the adjustment to disease-related pain (e.g. pain due to arthritis or cancer.)

The acceptance model

Recently, there has been growing interest in acceptance as a pain coping approach (McCracken *et al.*, 2004). Interest in acceptance comes from the clinical observation that the lives of many patients having persistent pain are dominated by the struggle to control a problem that is in part uncontrollable. There is growing recognition that maladaptive efforts to control or avoid pain can exacerbate pain and lead to heightened suffering and disability (Asmundson *et al.*, 1999; McCracken *et al.*, 1996).

Recent studies of acceptance and persistent pain have utilized the Chronic Pain Acceptance Questionnaire (CPAQ; Geiser, 1992), a reliable and standardized measure which assesses two dimensions of acceptance: a) willingness to experience pain – the absence of attempts to reduce or avoid pain; and b) activity engagement – the extent to which a person actively pursues valued life activities. McCracken *et al.* (1998) found that patients who scored higher on this measure not only had significantly lower levels of pain-related anxiety and depression, but also had lower levels of disability. These findings regarding acceptance were particularly noteworthy in that they were apparent even after controlling for pain intensity. McCracken and Eccleston (2003) compared the predictive utility of the CPAQ and a commonly used pain coping measure (the Coping Strategies Questionnaire) and found that the CPAQ accounted for almost twice as much variance as coping variables in explaining pain, disability, depression, uptime and work status. Finally, a recent study found that acceptance of pain was predictive of fewer health care visits for pain and pain medication intake (McCracken *et al.*, 2004).

Comment

Although the acceptance model of coping with pain is relatively new, it appears to have promise in fostering our understanding of adjustment to pain. Recent promising findings regarding this model have generated renewed interest in acceptance-based intervention protocols, such as the mindfulness-based stress reduction protocol developed by Kabat-Zinn and his colleagues (1985). To date, no rigorous randomized clinical trial has been conducted to assess the efficacy of acceptance-based interventions for patients having persistent pain. Also, the utility of the acceptance model has largely been examined in patients having chronic pain syndromes (e.g. chronic low back pain) and the utility of this model for disease-related pain conditions is unknown.

General conclusions

Coping efforts which focus on thinking rationally about pain and taking concrete cognitive and behavioural steps to control pain seem to be the most efficacious methods for chronic pain management. Coping strategies which lead the individual to withdrawal or become passive when dealing with pain appear to be the least effective pain management techniques. Research has clearly shown that effective coping can help the chronic pain sufferer to manage pain and maintain higher levels of psychological health. Intervention and treatment programmes which help patients learn new ways of coping with pain have met with considerable success (Keefe *et al.*, 2004).

Our understanding of the ways in which individuals cope with chronic pain and relationships of coping to psychological, physical and behavioural adjustment is not complete. Research in this area is currently exploring the usefulness of new assessment methods such as daily coping diaries and interviews that ask patients to describe, in detail, the thoughts and behaviours which they engage in when coping with pain. In addition, research is now examining the relationships between pain and coping over longer periods of time. Some coping methods may not impact adjustment in the short term but may contribute to disease progression and quality of life over many years time. Chronic disease is now the leading cause of death for individuals in most industrialized nations (see 'Coping with chronic illness') and chronic pain plays a central part in many of these conditions. Future research in this area will help pain researchers and clinicians to design programmes to help individuals learn how to cope with chronic, painful disease.

Acknowledgements

Preparation of this chapter was supported, in part, by the following grants from the National Institutes of Health: NIAMS AR 46305, AR047218, P01 AR50245, NIMH MH63429; Cancer Institute grants: R21-CA88049-01, CA91947-01, National Institute of Neurological Diseases and Stroke grant: NS46422 and by support from the Arthritis Foundation and Fetzer Institute.

REFERENCES

Asmundson, G. & Norton, G. (1999). Beyond pain: the role of fear and avoidance in chronicity. *Clinical Psychology Review*, **19**, 97–119.

Brown, G. K. & Nicassio, P. M. (1987). The development of a questionnaire for the assessment of active and passive coping strategies for chronic pain patients, *Pain*, **31**, 53–65.

Burns, J., Mullen, J., Higdon, L., Wei, J. & Lansky, D. (2000). Validity of the pain anxiety symptoms scale (PASS): prediction of physical capacity variables. *Pain*, **84**, 247–52.

Covic, T., Adamson, B. & Hough, M. (2000). The impact of passive coping on rheumatoid arthritis pain. *Rheumatology*, **39**, 1027–30.

Covic, T., Adamson, B., Spencer, D. & Howe, G. (2003). A biopsychosocial model of pain and depression in rheumatoid arthritis: a 12-month longitudinal study. *Rheumatology*, **42**, 1287–94.

Crombez, G., Vlaeyen, J., Heuts, H. & Lysens, R. (1999). Pain-related fear is more disabling than pain itself: evidence on the role of pain-related fear in chronic back pain disability. *Pain*, **80**(1–2), 329–39.

Folkman, S. & Lazarus, R. S. (1980). An analysis of coping in a middle-aged community sample. *Journal of Health and Social Behavior*, **21**, 219–39.

Fritz, J., George, S. & Delitto, A. (2001). The role of fear-avoidance beliefs in acute low back pain: relationships with current and future disability and work status. *Pain*, **94**, 7–15.

Geiser, D. S. (1992). *A comparison of acceptance-focused and control-focused psychological treatments in a chronic pain treatment center*. Unpublished doctoral dissertation. Reno: University of Nevada.

Hassett, A. L., John, D. C., Sondra, J. P. & Leonard, H. S. (2000). The role of catastrophizing in the pain and depression of women with fibromyalgia syndrome. *Arthritis and Rheumatism*, **43**(11), 2493–500.

Jensen, M. P., Keefe, F. J., Lefebvre, J. C., Romano, J. M. & Turner, J. A. (2003). One- and two-item measures of pain beliefs and coping strategies. *Pain*, **104**, 453–69.

Kabat-Zinn, J., Lipworth, L. & Burney, R. (1985). The clinical use of mindfulness meditation for the self regulation of chronic pain. *Journal of Behavioral Medicine*, **8**, 163–90.

Keefe, F. J., Caldwell, D. S., Martinez, S. *et al.* (1991). Analyzing pain in rheumatoid arthritis patients: pain coping strategies in patients who have had knee replacement surgery. *Pain*, **46**, 153–60.

Keefe, F. J., Caldwell, D. S., Queen, K. T. *et al.* (1987). Pain coping strategies in osteoarthritis patients. *Journal of Consulting and Clinical Psychology*, **55**, 208–12.

Keefe, F. J., Caldwell, D. S., Williams, D. A. *et al.* (1990). Pain coping skills training in the management of osteoarthritic knee pain: a comparative study. *Behavior Therapy*, **21**, 49–62.

Keefe, F. J., Lefebvre, J. C., Egert, J. R. *et al.* (2000). The relationship of gender to pain, pain behavior, and disability in osteoarthritis patients: the role of catastrophizing. *Pain*, **87**, 325–34.

Keefe, F. J. & Williams, D. A. (1990). A comparison of coping strategies in chronic pain patients of different age groups. *Journal of Gerontology*, **45**, 161–65.

Keefe, F. J., Salley, A. N. & Lefebvre, J. C. (1992). Coping with pain: conceptual concerns and future direction. *Pain*, **51**, 131–4.

Keefe, F. J., Rumble, M., Scipio, C., Giordano, L. & Perri, L. (2004). Psychological aspects of persistent pain: current state of the science. *The Journal of Pain*, **5**(4), 195–211.

Kori, S., Miller, R. & Todd, D. (1990). Kinesiophobia: a new view of chronic pain behavior. *Pain Management*, **3**, 35–43.

Lazarus, R. S. & Folkman, S. (1984). *Stress, appraisal and coping*. New York: Springer Publishing Co.

Manne, S. L. & Zautra, A. J. (1990). Couples coping with chronic illness: women with rheumatoid arthritis and their healthy husbands. *Journal of Behavioral Medicine*, **13**, 327–42.

McCracken, L. M. (1988). Learning to live with the pain: acceptance of pain predicts adjustment in persons with chronic pain. *Pain*, **74**, 21–7.

McCracken, L. M., Carson, J. W., Eccleston, C. & Keefe, F. J. (2004). Acceptance and change in the context of chronic pain. *Pain*, **109**(1–2), 4–7.

McCracken, L. M. & Eccleston, C. (2003). Coping or acceptance: what to do about chronic pain? *Pain*, **105**, 197–204.

McCracken, L. M., Gross, R. T., Aikens, J. & Carnike, C. L. M. (1996). The assessment of anxiety and fear in persons with chronic pain: a comparison of instruments. *Behavior Research and Therapy*, **34**, 927–33.

McCracken, L. M., Vowels, K. E. & Eccleston, C. (2004). Acceptance of chronic pain: component analysis and a revised assessment method. *Pain*, **107**, 159–66.

McCracken, L., Zayfert, C. & Gross, R. (1992). The Pain Anxiety Symptoms Scale: development and validation of a scale to measure fear of pain. *Pain*, **50**, 67–73.

Nederhand, M., Ijzerman, M., Hermens, H., Turk, D. & Zilvold, G. (2004). Predictive value of fear avoidance in developing chronic neck pain disability: consequences for clinical decision making. *Archives of Physical Medicine and Rehabilitation*, **85**, 496–501.

Parker, J., McRae, C., Smarr, K. *et al.* (1988). Coping strategies in rheumatoid arthritis. *Journal of Rheumatology*, **15**, 1376–83.

Picavet, H., Vlaeyen, J. & Schouten, J. (2002). Pain catastrophizing and kinesiophobia: predictors of chronic low back pain. *American Journal of Epidemiology*, **156**, 1028–34.

Regan, C. A., Lorig, K. & Thoresen, C. E. (1988). Arthritis appraisal and ways of coping: scale development. *Arthritis Care and Research*, **3**, 139–50.

Rosenstiel, A. K. & Keefe, F. J. (1983). The use of coping strategies in chronic low back pain patients: relationships to patient characteristics and current adjustment. *Pain*, **17**, 34–44.

Snow-Turek, A. L., Norris, M. P. & Tan, G. (1996). Active and passive coping strategies in chronic pain patients. *Pain*, **64**, 455–62.

Strahl, C., Kleinknecht, R. A. & Dinnel, D. L. (2000). The role of pain anxiety, coping, and pain self-efficacy in rheumatoid arthritis patient functioning. *Behavior Research and Therapy*, **38**, 863–73.

Swinkels-Meewisse, I., Roelofs, J., Verbeek, A., Oostendorp, R. & Vlaeyen, J. (2003). Fear of movement/(re)injury, disability, and participation in acute low back pain. *Pain*, **105**, 371–9.

Turner, J. A., Clancy, S. & Vitalian, P. P. (1987). Relationships of stress, appraisal and coping, to chronic low back pain. *Behaviour Research and Therapy*, **25**(4), 281–8.

Turner, J. A., Jensen, M. P., Warms, C. A. & Cardenas, D. D. (2002). Catastrophizing is associated with pain intensity, psychological distress, and pain-related disability among individuals with chronic pain after spinal cord injury. *Pain*, **98**, 127–34.

Verbunt, J., Seelen, H., Vlaeyen, J., van der Heijden, G. & Knottnerus, J. (2003). Fear of injury and physical deconditioning in patients with chronic low back pain. *Archives of Physical Medicine and Rehabilitation*, **84**, 1227–32.

Vitaliano, P. P., Russo, J., Carr, J. E., Maiuro, R. S. & Becker, J. (1985). The ways of coping checklist: revision and psychometric properties. *Multivariate Behavioral Research*, **20**, 3–26.

Vlaeyen, J., Kole-Snijders, A., Boeren, R. & van Eek, H. (1995). Fear of movement/(re)injury in chronic low back pain and its relation to behavioral performance. *Pain*, **62**, 363–72.

Vlaeyen, J. & Linton, S. (2000). Fear-avoidance and its consequences in chronic musculoskeletal pain: a state of the art. *Pain*, **85**, 317–32.

Vlaeyen, J. W., de Jong, J., Geilen, M., Heuts, P. H. & van Breukelen, G. (2001). Graded in vivo exposure in the treatment of pain-related fear: a replicated single-case experimental design in four patients with chronic low back pain. *Behavior Research and Therapy*, **39**, 151–66.

Vlaeyen, J. W., de Jong, J., Geilen, M., Heuts, P. H. & van Breukelen, G. (2002). The treatment of fear of movement/(re)injury in chronic low back pain: further evidence on the effectiveness of exposure in vivo. *Clinical Journal of Pain*, **18**, 251–61.

Wilkie, D. J. & Keefe, F. J. (1991). Coping strategies of patients with lung cancer-related pain. *Clinical Journal of Pain*, **7**, 292–9.

Coping with death and dying

Colin Murray Parkes

Chorleywood, Hertfordshire

Death is, perhaps, the ultimate test which we face as patients, relatives and members of the caring professions. All of us have to cope with it and, no matter how experienced we become, the coping is seldom easy. Death is often a loss but it can also be a time of peaceful transition. It may represent failure or success, ending or beginning, disaster or triumph. We may try to improve our ways of caring but, whatever the circumstances, death must never become routine.

In recent years, the psychological care of the dying and the bereaved has improved greatly, largely thanks to the work of the Hospices and the various organizations, such as Cruse – Bereavement Care, which provide counselling to the bereaved. Hospices have always seen the unit of care as being the family, which includes the patient, rather than the patient with the family as an optional extra to be taken on if we have time.

The field is a large one and it will not be possible, in the space available here, to give more than an outline of some of the major issues or to review the scientific and clinical research which underlies the theory and practice which I shall describe. The interested reader will find this type of information in the books by Kauffman (2002) and by Kissane and Bloch (2002), also in my own books, Parkes (1996) and Parkes and Markus (1998). A more detailed examination of the theory and practice of the counselling of dying patients and their families is given by Parkes *et al.* (1996).

When people are coming close to death, the professionals may have little or no control over what is happening. Scientific medicine can help us to mitigate some of the pains of dying but, with all our knowledge, 100% of our patients will still die. Despite this, patients and their families continue to turn to us for help. To a large extent, we have replaced priests as the recognized authorities on death, a change of role with which most of us feel uncomfortable.

Death is a social event, it affects the lives of many people. In this circle of people, the patients are the centre of care as long as they are alive; but their troubles will soon be over, those of the family may just be beginning.

Whether or not we think of death as a transition for the patient, it is certainly a transition for the family. Their lives will never be the same again. Death tips the survivors into new situations, new roles, new dangers and new opportunities. They are often forced to learn new ways of coping at a time when overwhelming grief makes it hard for them to cope with old responsibilities, let alone new ones (see 'Coping with bereavement').

The traditional training of doctors and nurses does little to prepare us for the challenges of terminal and bereavement care. We are so preoccupied with saving life that we are at a loss to know what to do when life cannot be saved. Some of us deal with the problem by denying its existence; we insist on fighting for a cure until the bitter end. Sadly, the weapons that we employ too often impair the quality of the life that is left; the end, when it comes, is truly bitter.

Others acknowledge to themselves that the patient is dying but attempt to conceal it from the patient. If they succeed, the patient may die in 'blissful' ignorance, but they often fail. As the disease progresses, the patient looks in the mirror and realizes that somebody is lying. At a time when they most need to trust their medical attendants, they realize that they have been deceived. In either case, the family who survive are denied the opportunity to say 'goodbye', and to conclude any unfinished psychological business with the patient.

Of course, it is not only the professional staff who find it hard to cope with people who are dying; friends, workmates and family members are equally at a loss and they may deal with their own feelings of inadequacy by putting pressure on us to continue treatment long after it can do good or to collude with them in concealing the true situation from the patient. 'You won't tell him he's dying, will you doctor? It would kill him if he found out'. While such remarks may occasionally be justified, they are more likely to reflect the informant's own inability to cope with the truth rather than that of the patient.

In all our work with terminally ill patients and their families, we must consider three psychological problems that complicate the psychosocial transitions which they face. These are fear, grief and resistance to change.

The problem of fear

Fear is the natural response to any threat to our own life or to the lives of those we love. It has important biological functions in preparing our minds and bodies to fight or to flee. Our entire autonomic nervous system exists to support these ends. Among the many consequences of fear are hyperalertness to further dangers, increased muscular tension, increased cardiac rate and inhibition of digestive and other inessential vegetative functions. In the types of emergency that arose in the environment of evolution, these reactions ensured our survival, but they are seldom of much use to us today.

It would be highly inappropriate for a cancer patient who has been told the nature of his diagnosis to run away or to hit out at the doctor, yet he may have an impulse to do both things. The hyperalertness produced by fear may cause fearful people to imagine additional dangers where none exist. It may also impair their ability to pay attention to anything but the danger itself. If increased muscle tension goes on for long, the muscles begin to fatigue and to ache; such symptoms may themselves be misinterpreted as signs of cancer or whatever disease it is that the person dreads. Similarly, cardiac hyperactivity is often misinterpreted as a sign of heart disease, thereby increasing fear and setting up a vicious circle of escalating fear and symptoms.

All of us have our own ways of coping when we are afraid. Some of us become aggressive, seeking someone or something to blame in the hope that we can rectify the situation. Thus some patients, faced with worsening symptoms, respond by blaming them on the treatment. It is easier to fight a doctor than a cancer. Others use alcohol or other drugs in an attempt to find 'Dutch' courage, a habit which can give short-term relief but may cause fresh problems in the long run.

The logical response to danger is to seek help and, if doctors have failed to cure an illness, we should not be surprised or angry if the patient seeks for a cure from unorthodox practitioners. But cure is not the only thing that people need. Comfort of the non-verbal kind, that a mother can give to a frightened child, is just as welcome to the frightened adult and just as effective in reducing fear. Nurses, who are touching patients all the time, know how powerful a touch of the hand can be. Doctors are often bad at touching, avoiding physical contact with their patients as if the patient's fear might be infectious, which, of course, it is.

When somebody is dying, it is not only the patient who is likely to be afraid, it is everybody around them. This can produce another kind of vicious circle when frightened patients see their fear reflected in the eyes of the people around them. Although most healthy people, asked where they would want die, will say 'at home', the level of anxiety which sometimes surrounds a person who is dying at home often gives good reason to admit them to a hospital or hospice. As one person who had been admitted to a hospice said, 'It's safe to die here!'.

Since most people are afraid of dying, we tend to assume that we know why a dying person is afraid. It is tempting to say, 'I understand'. The truth is, none of us can know another's fear and many of the fears of terminally ill patients have nothing to do with death. Time and again patients have said to me, 'It's not being dead that frightens me, doctor, it's dying'. Most people in our society have not seen anybody die. Their image of death comes from the horror comics and other dramatic and often horrific portrayals of death, which sell newspapers and the like. When people learn about real deaths, it is often the deaths that have been badly handled that get talked about. To many people 'death' means 'agony' and it may come as a surprise to them to learn that, with proper care, pain need not be a problem.

The problem of grief

Grief is the normal reaction to any major loss and is not confined to bereavement. Illnesses such as cancers and AIDS tend to progress in steps. At each setback the patient is faced with another cluster of losses. Initially, the loss of security and body parts affected by the disease constitute the major losses but, in later stages of the illness, increasing disability may cause loss of mobility, occupation and an increasing range of physical functions. In the last phase, the patient faces the prospect of losing life itself and all the attachments that go with it.

Each new loss will tend to evoke intense feelings of pining and yearning for the object that is lost. The person experiences a strong need to cry aloud and to search for ways of retaining some or all of the lost object. A woman may intensely miss the breast that she has lost and find some solace in a good prosthesis or in reconstructive surgery. A man may long to return to work and surprise his workmates by arriving at his place of work despite severe debility. Patients in a hospital regularly pine to go home, and many will do so despite the problems that this may cause to their families.

It is important not to confuse normal grief with clinical depression. Grief is intermittent and, even within an hour or so, people who allow themselves to express grief will feel better, although the pangs will return. Depression, by contrast, is lasting and undermines sufferers, preventing them from doing the very things that would get them out of the slough of depression. The slowing down of thought and movement, and the feelings of worthlessness, which characterize clinical depression, contrast with the restlessness and pining of the grieving person. Other symptoms of depression – anorexia, loss of weight and early morning waking – also occur as part of grieving (particularly if the grief is caused by a debilitating illness).

Diagnosis is important because clinical depression requires, and will usually respond to, treatment with antidepressant medication. Given this help, people who are grieving and depressed often find that, as the depression gets better, they can grieve more easily.

Resistance to change

More problematic is the tendency to deny the reality of the diagnosis, or prognosis, or to avoid facing the implications of this. Many patients make it clear that they do not want to be told about their illness. This is most likely to happen if the doctors are themselves uncertain or are giving conflicting messages. Family members too may find it hard to accept the fact that a loved person's lifespan is very limited and may be more resistant to facing reality than the patient.

Denial is a defence against overwhelming anxiety, and may enable people to adjust more gradually to the massive changes that threaten their internal world. It is a basic assumption in the minds of most people that we know where we stand. This rather trite statement covers a major but under-rated fact that we can only relate to the world around us because we possess an internal model of that world by which we recognize the world that we meet and plan our behaviour accordingly. This applies at the level of everyday habits (getting up in the morning, walking across the room, laying two places for breakfast, etc.) and at the deeper level of finding meaning and direction in life (wanting to get up in the morning, eat breakfast, etc.).

Major losses render obsolete large sections of our internal world and require a process of restructuring at both levels of functioning. For a while, people who are faced with a discrepancy between the world that is, and the world that should be (on the basis of our experience up to now), continue to operate the old obsolete mode which is, after all, the only model they have. The amputee leaps out of bed and finds himself sprawling on the floor, the widow lays the table for two. Even more common are the habits of thought which lead into blind alleys ('When I get better, I shall go back to work' or 'I must ask my husband about that').

Each time we are brought up short by a discrepancy of this kind, we suffer another pang of grief, intense, painful pining for what we have lost. This forces us to take stock and to begin the long and difficult process of revising our assumptive world. This takes time and it takes even longer for us to revise the basic assumptions that give meaning to life, e.g. that we can find new sources of self-esteem without having to go to work each day, that life in a wheelchair can be quite tolerable or that a widow is not condemned to perpetual mourning.

Because we rely on the possession of an accurate internal model of the world to cope with the world and to keep us safe, we feel, and are, extremely vulnerable whenever we are faced with major discrepancies of this kind. More than at any other time, we need the understanding and protection of people close to us; small wonder that patients and family members grow closer to each other at times of threat and that many people would rather be at home than in a strange or impersonal hospital ward. For those without families, the support of doctors and nurses may be invaluable, but such patients may cling to the security of their home as if this were the only safe place in the world.

The psychosocial transition faced by the dying patient may be more frightening but is usually less complex than the transition faced by the patient's spouse. Having faced the facts of the illness, the patient has not got to learn new ways of coping, acceptance brings its own rewards and the patient will often find that family and other carers are happy to take over responsibility for managing the affairs which previously caused anxiety and stress in the patient's life. 'Don't you worry, we'll look after things now', can be very reassuring to someone who has never previously had the opportunity to 'let go'. Perhaps, because of this, patients who face their illness, and accept that there is nothing more to be done, often enter a peaceful state and achieve a relatively happy conclusion to their lives. They seem to come through the process of grieving more quickly and completely than their spouses who have to discover a new identity and who will often continue to grieve for years to come.

The problems that arise when we are faced with the need to change our basic assumptions about the world have been explored in more depth by Kauffman (2002).

Coping strategies

Many of the differences between the ways people cope with threats reflect the assumptions and coping strategies that have been found to minimize stress early in life. At times of threat, those who lack the confidence in their own resources may seek help of others, express clear signals of distress and cling inappropriately. Those who lack trust in others, on the other hand, may keep their problems to themselves, bottle up their feelings and blame health care providers or therapies for their symptoms. Their lack of trust makes it necessary for them to control us rather than be controlled by us. A few, who lack trust in themselves *and* others, may keep a low profile, turn in on themselves and become anxious and depressed (Parkes, 2006).

Some people may have learned that the one sure way of getting love and attention is to become sick. In later life they respond to threat by developing hypochondriacal symptoms or exaggerating the symptoms of organic illness. If the threat has been caused by an illness, the interaction of psychological and physical influences may be difficult to disentangle. These interactions have been explored, with sensitivity, by Wilkinson who stresses that we need to learn 'the music that the patient is dancing to, the form of their complaining' (Wilkinson, 2004).

Influencing the transition

All of these strategies reflect insecurity and will respond to reassurance and the creation of a 'secure base', a safe place and a secure relationship in which, little by little, the insecure person can begin to pay attention to and discuss the problems that make them insecure.

To those who lack self-esteem the most important thing we have to offer is our esteem for their true worth and potential. To those who lack trust in others we can show that we understand their suspicion and their need to be in control of us. We act as advisors rather than instructors and show that we accept that trust must be earned: it is not our right to be trusted.

Life-threatening illness can undermine the confidence and trust of us all and the process of revising one's internal model of the world is made easier if the issues are clear and if there is someone nearby who will keep us safe during the period of vulnerability. It follows that members of the caring professions can do a great deal to help people through these psychosocial transitions. Accurate information is essential to planning; hence the reaction of relief that is expressed by many patients when they are told they have cancer. It is easier to cope with the worst than to live in a state of planlessness.

Much has been written about the patient's right to know the truth about an illness, but we must respect his or her right to monitor the amount of new and painful information that he/she can cope with at any given time (see 'Breaking bad news'). It is just as wrong to tell people too much, too soon, as it is to tell them too little, too late. Patients who refuse to give consent to major surgery may just need a little time to call on the support of other family members before changing their mind. If we respond by threatening them with the dire consequences of their refusal, this may increase their anxiety and delay the final decision.

Similarly, we need to recognize that it takes time to break bad news. To impart the information to a person that they have cancer or AIDS is to inflict a major psychological trauma. No surgeon would think of operating without booking an operating theatre and setting aside sufficient time to do the job properly. The same should apply to all important communication between professional carers and the families we serve.

We need to know whose lives are going to be affected by the information we possess, to decide who should be invited to meet us and where the meeting should take place. This means that someone must draw a genogram, a family tree which identifies each relevant person in the patient's family. Having identified the key people, we must decide who is the best person to talk with them and whether they should be seen together or separately. (Some are so over-protective of each other that they will never ask questions that might cause distress unless they are seen on their own.)

People will remember, for the rest of their lives, the details of the occasions when important news was broken. Even the pictures on the wall are important, and there is a world of difference between the doctor who adopts a relaxed and supportive attitude in a pleasant home-like atmosphere and the busy, impersonal consultant who breaks bad news in a public ward, or in the sterile environment of a treatment room. The placing of chairs at the same level, and at an angle to each other so that human contact is possible and there are no desks or other barriers between us, helps to create the conditions in which communication is possible.

Before telling people what we think they need to know, we should find out what they already know, or think they know, about the situation and what their priorities are. If they use words like 'cancer' or 'death', we should check out that these words mean the same to them as they do to us. 'There are many kinds of cancer, what does the word mean to you?', 'Have you seen anyone die? How do you view death?' will often reveal considerable ignorance and open the door to positive reassurance and explanation. Too often, doctors fail to invite questions and miss the opportunity to help people with the issues that are concerning them most.

Members of the primary care team are in a position to provide continuity of care throughout the illness and bereavement, and are particularly important sources of support. They are likely to be familiar with the social context in which the illness has arisen, to know the family members who are most at risk of adjustment problems and to have a relationship of trust with them that will enable the team to see them through this turning point in their lives. The fact that the primary care team are providing long-term care means that they will often have more time and opportunities to help the family to work things out than other caregivers have.

Eventually the time may come when further active treatment aimed at curing symptoms will cause more problems than it solves. From now on, our concern is more with palliation than with cure and the need for psychosocial care will be greater than ever. The question will arise as to whether to refer the patient to a hospice or specialist home care team. Hospices have focused attention on the need for improved symptom control at the end of life. Although St Christopher's Hospice in Sydenham, the first of the modern style of hospice, was initially restricted to in-patients, the home care which is now provided by most hospices was not long to follow. More recently, support teams have been set up in many hospitals to enable some of the methods of care which have been developed in hospices to be provided in general hospitals, and most hospitals and primary care teams are now able to relieve pain and other distressing symptoms in the later stages of cancer. Less easy to provide is the psychosocial care, which not only relieves the mental suffering of the patient but can help those members of the family whose lives must change, because of the death, to achieve a smooth and satisfactory transition. It is a criticism of existing services in the United Kingdom that the excellent psychosocial and spiritual care which is provided by many (but not all) hospices is not more widely available, and is limited to the final phase of life.

Finally we must recognize that the care of the dying can be stressful for the professionals as well as those for whom they care. A good staff support system is essential and should include the recognition that, if it is all right for patients and their families to cry when they grieve, it should be all right for us too. The 'stiff upper lip' which makes it so hard to help some patients and family members is even more of a problem in doctors (see 'Psychological support for health professionals').

REFERENCES

Kauffman, J. (Ed.). (2002). *Loss of the assumptive world: a theory of traumatic loss.* New York: Brunner-Routledge.

Kissane, D. & Bloch, S. (2002). *Family focused grief therapy: a model of family centred care during palliative care and bereavement.* Buckingham, UK: Open University Press.

Parkes, C.M. (1996). *Bereavement: Studies of Grief in Adult Life* (3rd edn.). London: Tavistock/Routledge.

Parkes, C.M., Relf, M. & Couldrick, A. (1996). *Counselling in terminal care and bereavement.* London: British Psychological Society.

Parkes, C.M. & Markus, A. (Eds.). (1998). *Coping with loss: helping patients and their families.* London: BMJ Books.

Parkes, C.M. (2006). *Love and loss: the roots of grief and it's complications.* London & New York: Routledge.

Wilkinson, S.R. (2004). *Coping and complaining: attachment and the language of dis-ease.* London: Brunner-Routledge.

Coping with stressful medical procedures

Yael Benyamini

Tel Aviv University

Stressful medical procedures range from highly stressful ones, such as major surgery and chemotherapy, to simple procedures such as immunizations and blood tests. Though such procedures vary greatly in the degree of physical intrusiveness, pain and discomfort they cause, the stress experienced by patients results not only from these physical factors but also from the subjective meaning of the procedure for the patient and his/her resources for coping (Scott et al., 2001; Wallace, 1985) (see 'Abortion'; 'Coronary heart disease: surgery'; 'Chemotherapy' and 'Intimate examinations'). The physical aspects are interpreted within the subjective framework, which determines the extent of psychological reactions. Therefore, in order to understand how patients cope with these procedures and how to assist them in their effort, health care providers must understand both the objective and the subjective aspects of this experience.

Undergoing a medical procedure entails coping with the procedure itself and coping with the accompanying negative feelings (mainly anxiety). Such feelings are related to the context in which the procedure is carried out, for example, cancer as highly anxiety-provoking (Schou et al., 2004), infertility as a low-control situation (Terry & Hynes, 1998), coronary artery bypass surgery or transplant surgery, which elicit fears due to the uncertainty involved (Heikkila et al., 1999; Jalowiec et al., 1994). Negative feelings also arise from discrepancies between prior expectancies or pre-existing imaginings and the actual procedure (e.g. the difference between the expectation and the reality of giving birth, see Katz, 1993; Slade et al., 1993). Prior experiences also influence reactions to a stressful medical procedure, whether these are prior medical experiences as a child (Pate et al., 1996) or as an adult (for example, undergoing mammography among women who have had a lumpectomy; see Kornguth et al., 2000), recent life stress or even early traumatic experiences (such as the Holocaust; see Schreiber et al., 2004).

Procedures such as surgery require a recovery period. Anxiety related to the procedure can impede recovery from it. Studying the direct predictors or outcomes of such anxious reactions is insufficient (Kopp et al., 2003) since anxiety operates through a variety of behavioural and physiological mechanisms, within a personal and social context (Kiecolt-Glaser et al., 1998). Therefore, this chapter will first briefly review individual differences in coping with stressful procedures as well as the effects of the social and cultural context and then discuss ways to assist patients undergoing these procedures.

Individual differences in coping with medical procedures

Many studies have examined differences in coping styles. One of the most common distinctions is between an avoidant and an active or instrumental coping style. Typically, studies found avoidant coping with medical procedures and the physical and psychological distress they cause to be related with worse outcomes and active coping with better outcomes among adults (Rosenberger et al., 2004), and adolescents (LaMontagne et al., 2004). Moreover, a maladaptive spiral of distress and avoidant coping can evolve over time (Culver et al., 2002).

Another distinction is between attention focusing and distracting as ways of coping. Distraction by focusing on a specific stimulus could be helpful whereas simply attempting to ignore the situation could result in a rebound effect that leads to more intrusion later on (Fauerbach et al., 2002). Attention focusing has been found to be helpful in some studies (LaMontagne et al., 2000) and detrimental in others (Fauerbach et al., 2002). The inconsistencies may be due to the nature of the stressor with which patients coped: attention to an injury-related procedure could increase post-traumatic responses whereas attention to concrete aspects of a procedure aimed at healing an illness or removing a health threat could decrease such responses.

The attention/distraction distinction has also been studied as a personality disposition, typically labelled as monitoring versus blunting information-seeking style (Miller et al., 1988). In relation to medical procedures, research has shown that relaxation training led low monitors and high blunters to suffer from less surgical pain (Miro & Raich, 1999) and less anxiety due to cancer chemotherapy, possibly because relaxation is a distraction technique (Lerman et al., 1990) (see 'Relaxation training'). High monitors benefited from the provision of detailed information, such as viewing the contraction monitor during labour (Shiloh et al., 1998), and fared most poorly with no preparation at all (Gattuso et al., 1992). Other personality dispositions have also been associated with coping and outcomes of medical procedures (Kopp et al., 2003): Dispositional optimism was related to better recovery and lower rates of re-hospitalization following coronary artery bypass surgery (Scheier et al., 1989, 1999); internal locus of control moderated the relationship between coping strategies and long-term recovery from surgery for scoliosis among adolescents (LaMontagne et al., 2004).

Age differences in coping with medical procedures

Though many findings replicate across ages, there are indications that we need to consider children and adolescents separately (from each other and from adults) when attempting to understand and facilitate their coping with medical procedures. Children's conceptualization of pain, their appraisal of the situation and their ways of coping differ from those of adults (Rudolph, Dennig & Weisz, 1995) (see 'Children's perceptions of illness and death').

Children's approach-avoidance coping may be qualitatively different from adult's approach-avoidance (Bernard *et al.*, 2004) and they may need more preparation and training for coping with medical procedures (Peterson *et al.*, 1999). Their ability to cope at different ages is also a major factor in decisions regarding the best age for elective surgical procedures (Hagglof, 1999). Even within childhood, coping varies by age: older children, compared with younger ones, exhibited more vigilant coping that was related to quicker return to activities following surgery (LaMontagne *et al.*, 1996) and older adolescents' coping, compared with younger ones', was more strongly related to recovery from surgery (LaMontagne *et al.*, 2004). In addition, it is important to remember that children are greatly influenced by their parents' reactions to the situation and ways of coping with it (Salmon & Pereira, 2002). In light of the differences between adults and children in their reactions to procedures, there are also separate instruments that measure individual differences in coping with stressful medical procedures among adults (Krohne *et al.*, 2000) and among children and their parents (Blount *et al.*, 2001).

Gender differences in coping with medical procedures

Women report higher levels of fear than men in reaction to injections and blood sample collection, examinations and symptoms (e.g. Olatunji *et al.*, 2005) and report more pre-operation anxiety than men (Karanci & Dirik, 2003). Women and men often perceive stressful medical procedures differently, sometimes because they are experienced at a different age (for example, cardiac procedures, Hawthorne, 1994). Some procedures have different effects on women's and men's self and body image (Manderson, 1999), and coping with them could be differentially affected by social support in the two gender groups (Krohne & Slangen, 2005). Yet, there has been surprisingly little attention paid to these differences and their implications for planning interventions.

The social and cultural context

Coping with stressful medical procedures entails intensive contact with health care providers in a situation that often involves a lot of uncertainty. Different 'languages' are used in the culture of patients and the culture of providers when talking about health, illness and uncertainty (Becker & Nachtigall, 1991). Patients often interpret statistics and other information in ways that are biased so as to preserve their hopes, whereas doctors judge treatment success across the general patient population (Modell, 1989) (see 'Communicating risk' and 'Healthcare professional-patient communication').

This cultural clash can result in much frustration and feelings of being misled on the part of the patients and in similar feelings of frustration among providers in reaction to their patients' responses. The physician–patient cultural differences can be intensified if they occur within wider cultural gaps, such as a different ethnic or religious background. Sculptures of childbirth from traditional societies typically show several figures surrounding the woman at labour. Drawings of folk healers typically portray an encounter that takes place amidst a small crowd. These depictions of traditional medicine vastly differ from modern clinics and hospitals. The differences they portray can lead to misunderstandings and feelings of alienation and anxiety among immigrants and patients from more traditional families. In culturally sensitive issues, such as third-party assisted conception procedures (Blyth & Landau, 2004), it is especially important to be aware of ethical considerations that differ around the globe.

The family environment is also of utmost importance to the person coping with a stressful procedure. Family members typically offer a lot of encouragement and support while the patient undergoes the procedure and during initial recovery but may underestimate the length of time required for full recovery and the patient's needs during that time (Feigin *et al.*, 2000). In addition, family care givers have their own fears and therefore their own needs for information and reassurance (Nikoletti *et al.*, 2003). This is especially prominent for female spouses (Mahler & Kulik, 2002).

Finally, the immediate social context also plays a role. The opportunity for social comparison with someone who has already undergone the procedure can provide reassurance and useful information: pre-operative patients assigned to a room at the hospital with a post-operative patient showed less anxiety and a quicker recovery; patients with any roommate recovered faster than no-roommate patients, and cardiac patients assigned to a room with another cardiac patient were discharged sooner after bypass surgery compared with those assigned to a non-cardiac roommate (Kulik, Mahler & Moore, 1996).

Assisting patients coping with stressful procedures: what troubles them?

In order to plan interventions to assist patients, we need to understand the issues that bother them as they face a stressful medical procedure. The common-sense model of illness (Leventhal *et al.*, 1980, 1984) provides a useful framework to illustrate these issues. This model attempts to delineate the principles underlying lay people's perceptions of health threats (see 'Lay beliefs about health and illness'). Research has shown that these perceptions are mostly structured around five dimensions: the identity and symptoms of the health threat; its causes; the timeline; the degree of controllability; and the consequences. In relation to stressful medical procedures, these dimensions suggest that patients are troubled by the following concerns:

i) *Identity and symptoms* – patients focus on questions such as: What is happening to me? What am I supposed to feel? What will I feel?

ii) *Causes* – What caused my situation? Why do I need to undergo this procedure?

iii) *Timeline* – Is this an elective procedure or an emergency one? What happens before, during and after the procedure? How long will I have to wait for the procedure? How long will it take? How much time will it take me to return to my normal routine?

iv) *Controllability* – Is it mandatory that I undergo this procedure? What are the potential benefits and risks? Who is responsible for the decision to undergo this procedure? What are the alternatives? What information do I need in order to choose among them? How can I regain control and decrease helplessness? Is there anything I can do to increase the chances of success of the procedure and of quick recovery?

v) *Consequences* – How serious is my condition? How serious and intrusive is this procedure? What are the expected side-effects in the short and the long term?

Assisting patient coping with stress procedures: planning interventions

Successful interventions must be planned so that they address patients' concerns, as suggested above. A single intervention cannot cover all possible concerns and problems that could arise. Therefore, when planning (and evaluating) such interventions it is important first to characterize the population, the health problem and the context in which it is experienced. In the light of these characteristics, it is important to clearly define criteria for success: Is the goal to decrease anxiety? To lessen the side effects? To minimize patient problem behaviours? To facilitate recovery? To shorten the period of hospitalization? Many studies have evaluated interventions aimed at preparing patients so that they will cope more adaptively with stressful procedures. Their findings suggest several principles and essential components that should be included when planning and administering such interventions.

The provision of information is a necessary component of any intervention in this area. In order to determine which information will be provided and at what level of detail, one needs to consider this from the patient's viewpoint. Patients will need various types of information:

- factual/procedural (what will happen to you)
- behavioural (what do you need to do in preparation for the procedure and for the recovery period; how can you cope most effectively with the procedure itself and its side effects)
- sensory (what will you feel)
- emotional (which emotions will you feel)
- administrative (what do you need to do in order to set this up, receive reimbursement, etc.).

While all of these aspects should be addressed, it is also important to consider the level of detail that is beneficial to the patient: detailed information could 'overwhelm' the patient beyond his or her ability to process it and benefit from it and/or result in increased instead of decreased levels of anxiety. Therefore, for many procedures preparation should be a multi-stage effort. For example, patients undergoing surgery may have different concerns and need different types of information and support pre-operatively, post-operatively and pre-discharge (Gammon & Mulholland, 1996).

Preparation for procedures typically includes mostly verbal information. Providing this information in written form also allows patients to retain it for future reference (see 'Written communication'). The information need not be merely verbal: many hospitals and clinics have used videotapes or tours. It is not clear whether tours are effective for adults (Lynn-McHale *et al.*, 1997) and for children they are even more questionable (O'Byrne *et al.*, 1997). In touring a ward there may be less control over the stimuli to which patients are exposed whereas videotapes allow for pre-planned and well controlled exposure.

In providing information to patients, it is important to attend to the full timeline from the initial deliberation regarding whether to undergo the procedure until full recovery. Naturally, when preparing the patient and his/her family, providers tend to concentrate on alleviating the immediate distress from the procedure they are about to administer by focusing on the procedure itself and the time around it. This focus can lead to disregarding both the difficulties of decision-making and preparation for the procedure, and, even more importantly, the long-term effects. Inadequate preparation for the long-term recovery can result in later patient distress and misunderstanding within the family (Feigin *et al.*, 2000). Even procedures that end positively and are not considered by the health care system to have any long-term effects, such as biopsies that provide reassuring results, require thought about the after-effects: some patients, especially the less educated and the more anxious to begin with, are not easily reassured (Meechan *et al.*, 2005).

Ideally, the information provided should be tailored to the patient's characteristics and preferences. Patients vary greatly in the types of pre-operative information and support they preferred (Mitchell, 1997). Many studies have shown better outcomes when the information matched the patients' coping styles (e.g. Morgan *et al.*, 1998; Shiloh *et al.*, 1998). When children are the patients, it is especially important to provide developmentally appropriate information (Rasnake & Linscheid, 1989). For example, an explanation that 'you will be put to sleep before the procedure' leads them to think that they will feel the same as they do every night in bed. It does not prepare them for the very unnatural way of falling asleep through the use of anaesthetics, which could include a few quite terrifying moments in which everything swirls around them.

The main reason for providing information has always been to reduce anxiety. Information can reduce anxiety by decreasing uncertainty and helplessness and by enhancing feelings of control. Control can also be increased by other means: patients can be more involved in decision-making regarding the preferred procedure. They can be given control over aspects of the procedure and recovery, whenever possible (as in patient-controlled analgesia following surgery; Shiloh *et al.*, 2003). Patients who are more involved could improve the quality of preparation for procedures if they are assertive, ask questions, gather information, do their 'homework', and attend structured preparation sessions. However, it is important to remember that many patients expect to be obedient to medical and nursing staff when they undergo a procedure and they do not always understand that they can exercise active control, even when clearly instructed to do so (Peerbhoy *et al.*, 1998). Patients may also initially accept a more paternalistic approach but over time desire more active involvement in the choice of treatment (Cohen & Britten, 2003).

In addition to preparing the patients, it is important that they receive effective support from their family members and care givers. Negative support can hinder recovery more than positive support and other resources can improve it (Stephens *et al.*, 2002). Therefore, it is important to attend to the perceptions and misperceptions of the situation by the care givers and to provide information and training specifically to the care givers (Mahler & Kulik, 2002). With children, it is essential to train the parents so that they will boost their children's ability to cope effectively instead of increasing the children's distress (Manne *et al.*, 1992) as well as their own (Zelikovsky *et al.*, 2001).

Concluding comments

The difficulties of coping with stressful medical procedures and the positive effect of adequate preparation for these procedures have been documented for several decades. Since the 1980s sufficient evidence has accumulated showing that preparation interventions, which include not only 'technical' information, but also modeling and teaching coping strategies, improve both physical and psychological outcomes among adults (O'Halloran & Altmaier, 1995) and children (O'Byrne *et al.*, 1997) and are cost-effective. The type of intervention has often been found to be less important than the mere fact that some type of intervention was provided. Yet, many patients are not provided with any type of structured intervention aimed at supporting them in coping with stressful procedures.

This does not mean that they are not provided with any preparation at all: on the contrary, preparation always takes place because providers always give some information and patients always ask some questions. However, such non-structured preparation is much less effective and often not provided at the optimal timing or by the optimal person, as compared with planned and structured interventions.

To summarize, understanding the meaning of the procedure for the patient and his/her family and their specific concerns and planning interventions accordingly can greatly improve patients' coping efficacy and recovery outcomes, at a relatively low cost. Future research should further investigate ways of optimizing such interventions by tailoring them to the patients' subjective perceptions of the procedure and the health threat for which it is intended. In addition, future research should also examine gender differences in coping with stressful medical procedures.

REFERENCES

Becker, G. & Nachtigall, R. D. (1991). Ambiguous responsibility in the doctor-patient relationship: the case of infertility. *Social Science and Medicine*, **32**(8), 875–85.

Bernard, R. S., Cohen, L. L., McClellan, C. B. & MacLaren, J. E. (2004). Pediatric procedural approach – avoidance coping and distress: a multitrait-multimethod analysis. *Journal of Pediatric Psychology*, **29**(2), 131–41.

Blount, R. L., Bunke, V., Cohen, L. L. & Forbes, C. J. (2001). The child-adult medical procedure interaction scale-short form (CAMPIS-SF): validation of a rating scale for children's and adults' behaviors during painful medical procedures. *Journal of Pain and Symptom Management*, **22**(1), 591–9.

Blyth, E. & Landau, R. (Eds.). (2004). *Third party assisted conception across cultures: social, legal and ethical perspectives*. London: Jessica Kingsley Publishers.

Cohen, H. & Britten, N. (2003). Who decides about prostate cancer treatment? A qualitative study. *Family Practice*, **20**(6), 724–9.

Culver, J. L., Arena, P. L., Antoni, M. H. & Carver, C. S. (2002). Coping and distress among women under treatment for early stage breast cancer: comparing African Americans, Hispanics and non-Hispanic Whites. *Psycho-Oncology*, **11**(6), 495–504.

Fauerbach, J. A., Lawrence, J. W., Haythornthwaite, J. A. & Richter, L. (2002). Coping with the stress of a painful medical procedure. *Behaviour Research and Therapy*, **40**(9), 1003–15.

Feigin, R., Greenberg, A., Ras, H. *et al.* (2000). The psychosocial experience of women treated for breast cancer by high-dose chemotherapy supported by autologous stem cell transplant: a qualitative analysis of support groups. *Psycho-Oncology*, **9**(1), 57–68.

Gammon, J. & Mulholland, C. W. (1996). Effect of preparatory information prior to elective total hip replacement on post-operative physical coping outcomes. *International Journal of Nursing Studies*, **33**(6), 589–604.

Gattuso, S. M., Litt, M. D. & Fitzgerald, T. E. (1992). Coping with gastrointestinal endoscopy: self-efficacy enhancement and coping style. *Journal of Consulting and Clinical Psychology*, **60**(1), 133–9.

Hagglof, B. (1999). Psychological reaction by children of various ages to hospital care and invasive procedures. *Acta Paediatrica Supplement*, **88**(431), 72–8.

Hawthorne, M. H. (1994). Gender differences in recovery after coronary artery surgery. *Image – the Journal of Nursing Scholarship*, **26**(1), 75–80.

Heikkila, J., Paunonen, M., Virtanen, V. & Laippala, P. (1999). Gender differences in fears related to coronary arteriography. *Heart and Lung*, **28**(1), 20–30.

Jalowiec, A., Grady, K. L. & White-Williams, C. (1994). Stressors in patients awaiting a heart transplant. *Behavioral Medicine*, **19**(4), 145–54.

Karanci, A. N. & Dirik, G. (2003). Predictors of pre- and postoperative anxiety in emergency surgery patients. *Journal of Psychosomatic Research*, **55**(4), 363–9.

Katz, V. L. (1993). Two trends in middle-class birth in the United States. *Human Nature*, **4**(4), 367–82.

Kiecolt-Glaser, J. K., Page, G. G., Marucha, P. T., MacCallum, R. C. & Glaser, R. (1998). Psychological influences on surgical recovery. Perspectives from psychoneuroimmunology. *American Psychologist*, **53**(11), 1209–18.

Kopp, M., Bonatti, H., Haller, C. *et al.* (2003). Life satisfaction and active coping style are important predictors of recovery from surgery. *Journal of Psychosomatic Research*, **55**(4), 371–7.

Kornguth, P. J., Keefe, F. J., Wright, K. R. & Delong, D. M. (2000). Mammography pain in women treated conservatively for breast cancer. *Journal of Pain*, **1**(4), 268–74.

Krohne, H. W., de-Bruin, J. T., El-Giamal, M. & Schmukle, S. C. (2000). The assessment of surgery-related coping: the coping with surgical stress scale (COSS). *Psychology and Health*, **15**(1), 135–49.

Krohne, H. W. & Slangen, K. E. (2005). Influence of social support on adaptation to surgery. *Health Psychology*, **24**(1), 101–5.

Kulik, J. A., Mahler, H. I. & Moore, P. J. (1996). Social comparison and affiliation under threat: effects on recovery from major surgery. *Journal of Personality and Social Psychology*, **71**(5), 967–79.

LaMontagne, L. L., Hepworth, J. T. & Cohen, F. (2000). Effects of surgery type and attention focus on children's coping. *Nursing Research*, **49**(5), 245–52.

LaMontagne, L. L., Hepworth, J. T., Cohen, F. & Salisbury, M. H. (2004). Adolescents' coping with surgery for scoliosis: effects on recovery outcomes over time. *Research in Nursing & Health*, **27**(4), 237–53.

LaMontagne, L. L., Hepworth, J. T., Johnson, B. D. & Cohen, F. (1996). Children's preoperative coping and its effects on postoperative anxiety and return to normal activity. *Nursing Research*, **45**(3), 141–7.

Lerman, C., Rimer, B., Blumberg, B. *et al.* (1990). Effects of coping style and relaxation on cancer chemotherapy side effects and emotional responses. *Cancer Nursing*, **13**(5), 308–15.

Leventhal, H., Meyer, D. & Nerenz, D. R. (1980). The common sense representation of illness danger. In S. Rachman (Ed.). *Contributions to medical psychology, Vol. 2*, (pp. 17–30). New York: Pergamon.

Leventhal, H., Nerenz, D. R. & Steele, D. J. (1984). Illness representations and coping with health threats. In A. Baum, S. E. Taylor & J. E. Singer (Eds.). *Handbook of psychology and health, Vol. 4*, (pp. 219–52). Hillsdale, New Jersey: Erlbaum.

Lynn-McHale, D., Corsetti, A., Brady-Avis, E. et al. (1997). Preoperative ICU tours: are they helpful? *American Journal of Critical Care*, **6**(2), 106–15.

Mahler, H. I. & Kulik, J. A. (2002). Effects of a videotape information intervention for spouses on spouse distress and patient recovery from surgery. *Health Psychology*, **21**(5), 427–37.

Manderson, L. (1999). Gender, normality and the post-surgical body. *Anthropology and Medicine*, **6**(3), 381–94.

Manne, S. L., Bakeman, R., Jacobsen, P. B. et al. (1992). Adult–child interaction during invasive medical procedures. *Health Psychology*, **11**(4), 241–9.

Meechan, G. T., Collins, J. P., Moss-Morris, R. E. & Petrie, K. J. (2005). Who is not reassured following benign diagnosis of breast symptoms? *Psycho-Oncology*, **14**, 239–46.

Miller, S. M., Brody, D. S. & Summerton, J. (1988). Styles of coping with threat: implications for health. *Journal of Personality and Social Psychology*, **54**, 142–8.

Miro, J. & Raich, R. M. (1999). Preoperative preparation for surgery: an analysis of the effects of relaxation and information provision. *Clinical Psychology and Psychotherapy*, **6**(3), 202–9.

Mitchell, M. (1997). Patients' perceptions of pre-operative preparation for day surgery. *Journal of Advanced Nursing*, **26**(2), 356–63.

Modell, J. (1989). Last chance babies: interpretations of parenthood in an in vitro fertilization program. *Medical Anthropology Quarterly*, **3**, 124–38.

Morgan, J., Roufeil, L., Kaushik, S. & Bassett, M. (1998). Influence of coping style and precolonoscopy information on pain and anxiety of colonoscopy. *Gastrointestinal Endoscopy*, **48**(2), 119–27.

Nikoletti, S., Kristjanson, L. J., Tataryn, D., McPhee, I. & Burt, L. (2003). Information needs and coping styles of primary family caregivers of women following breast cancer surgery. *Oncology Nursing Forum*, **30**(6), 987–96.

O'Byrne, K. K., Peterson, L. & Lisa, S. (1997). Survey of pediatric hospitals' preparation programs: evidence of the impact of health psychology research. *Health Psycholology*, **16**(2), 147–54.

O'Halloran, C. M. & Altmaier, E. M. (1995). The efficacy of preparation for surgery and invasive medical procedures. *Patient Education and Counseling*, **25**, 9–16.

Olatunji, B. O., Arrindell, W. A. & Lohr, J. M. (2005). Can the sex differences in disgust sensitivity account for the sex differences in blood-injection-injury fears? *Personality and Individual Differences*, **39**, 61–71.

Pate, J. T., Blount, R. L., Cohen, L. L. & Smith, A. J. (1996). Childhood medical experience and temperament as predictors of adult functioning in medical situations. *Children's Health Care*, **25**(4), 281–98.

Peerbhoy, D., Hall, G. M., Parker, C., Shenkin, A. & Salmon, P. (1998). Patients' reactions to attempts to increase passive or active coping with surgery. *Social Science and Medicine*, **47**(5), 595–601.

Peterson, L., Crowson, J., Saldana, L. & Holdridge, S. (1999). Of needles and skinned knees: children's coping with medical procedures and minor injuries for self and other. *Health Psychology*, **18**(2), 197–200.

Rasnake, L. K. & Linscheid, T. R. (1989). Anxiety reduction in children receiving medical care: developmental considerations. *Journal of Developmental and Behavioral Pediatrics*, **10**(4), 169–75.

Rosenberger, P. H., Ickovics, J. R., Epel, E. S., D'Entremont, D. & Jokl, P. (2004). Physical recovery in arthroscopic knee surgery: unique contributions of coping behaviors to clinical outcomes and stress reactivity. *Psychology and Health*, **19**(3), 307–20.

Rudolph, K. D., Dennig, M. D. & Weisz, J. R. (1995). Determinants and consequences of children's coping in the medical setting: conceptualization, review and critique. *Psychological Bulletin*, **118**(3), 328–57.

Salmon, K. & Pereira, J. K. (2002). Predicting children's response to an invasive medical investigation: the influence of effortful control and parent behavior. *Journal of Pediatric Psychology*, **27**(3), 227–33.

Scheier, M. F., Matthews, K. A., Owens, J. F. et al. (1989). Dispositional optimism and recovery from coronary artery bypass surgery: the beneficial effects on physical and psychological well-being. *Journal of Personality and Social Psychology*, **57**(6), 1024–40.

Scheier, M. F., Matthews, K. A., Owens, J. F. et al. (1999). Optimism and rehospitalization after coronary artery bypass graft surgery. *Archives of Internal Medicine*, **159**, 829–35.

Schou, I., Ekeberg, O., Ruland, C. M., Sandvik, L. & Karesen, R. (2004). Pessimism as a predictor of emotional morbidity one year following breast cancer surgery. *Psycho-Oncology*, **13**(5), 309–20.

Schreiber, S., Soskolne, V., Kozohovitch, H. & Deviri, E. (2004). Holocaust survivors coping with open heart surgery decades later: posttraumatic symptoms and quality of life. *General Hospital Psychiatry*, **26**(6), 443–52.

Scott, S. R. H., Kent, G. & Rowlands, A. (2001). Psychological distress reported by patients undergoing limb reconstruction surgery: implications for psychological interventions. *Journal of Clinical Psychology in Medical Settings*, **8**(4), 301–5.

Shiloh, S., Mahlev, U., Dar, R. & Ben-Rafael, Z. (1998). Interactive effects of viewing a contraction monitor and information-seeking style on reported childbirth pain. *Cognitive Therapy and Research*, **22**(5), 501–16.

Shiloh, S., Zukerman, G., Butin, B. et al. (2003). Postoperative patient controlled analgesia (PCA): how much control and how much analgesia? *Psychology and Health*, **18**(6), 753–70.

Slade, P., MacPherson, S. A., Hume, A. & Maresh, M. (1993). Expectations, experiences and satisfaction with labour. *British Journal of Clinical Psychology*, **32**(4), 469–83.

Stephens, M. A., Druley, J. A. & Zautra, A. J. (2002). Older adults' recovery from surgery for osteoarthritis of the knee: psychosocial resources and constraints as predictors of outcomes. *Health Psychology*, **21**(4), 377–383.

Terry, D. J. & Hynes, G. J. (1998). Adjustment to a low-control situation: reexamining the role of coping responses. *Journal of Personality and Social Psychology*, **74**(4), 1078–92.

Wallace, L. M. (1985). Psychological adjustment to and recovery from laparoscopic sterilization and infertility investigation. *Journal of Psychosomatic Research*, **29**(5), 507–18.

Zelikovsky, N., Rodrigue, J. R. & Gidycz, C. A. (2001). Reducing parent distress and increasing parent coping-promoting behavior during children's medical procedure. *Journal of Clinical Psychology in Medical Settings*, **8**(4), 273–81.

Cultural and ethnic factors in health

John W. Berry[1] and David L. Sam[2]

[1]Queen's University
[2]University of Bergen

Introduction

Understanding how cultural and ethnic factors relate to health is very much an interdisciplinary enterprise: anthropology, biology, economics, history, medicine, nursing, psychiatry, psychology, rehabilitation and sociology have all participated in the study and application of their own concepts and findings to health. The focus of this chapter however, will be on the contributions of anthropology ('medical anthropology': see e.g. Brown, 1998; Foster & Anderson, 1978; Hahn, 1999; Helman, 2000), psychiatry ('trans-cultural psychiatry': see e.g. Kleinman, 1980; Murphy, 1981; Tseng, 2001; Yap, 1974) and psychology ('cross-cultural psychology': see, e.g. Dasen *et al.*, 1988). In particular, because of the placement of this chapter in the section on 'Psychology, health and illness', and the background of the authors, the approach will be from the perspective of cross-cultural health psychology (Kazarian & Evans, 2001; MacLachlan, 2001; MacLachlan & Mulatu, 2004).

The field of cross-cultural health psychology can be divided into two related domains. The earlier, more established, domain is the study of how cultural factors influence various aspects of health. This enterprise has taken place around the globe, driven by the need to understand individual and community health in the context of the indigenous cultures of the people being examined and served. The second, more recent and very active, domain is the study of the health of individuals and groups as they settle into, and adapt to, new cultural circumstances, as a result of their migration, and the persistence of their original cultures in the form of ethnicity. This enterprise has taken place in culturally plural societies where there is the need to understand and better serve an increasingly diverse population in multicultural societies (Berry, 1997a; Mulatu & Berry, 2001). This separation into work across cultures (internationally) and with ethnic groups within societies is a common one in the field of cross-cultural psychology more generally (Berry *et al.*, 2002). Despite this division, it is a common position that the methods, theories and findings derived from the international enterprise should inform the domestic enterprise. That is, immigrants and members of the ethnic communities should be understood and served in culturally informed ways, and not simply categorized and treated as 'minorities'.

Cultural domain

The broad, international and comparative work linking culture and health has been carried out by medical anthropology, trans-cultural psychiatry and cross-cultural health psychology. Much of this work has resulted from the collaboration of medical, social and behavioural scientists. The field is thus inherently an interdisciplinary one, and is concerned with all aspects of health; physical, social and psychological.

Three orientations

In this large and complex body of work, three theoretical orientations can be discerned; absolutism, relativism and universalism (Berry *et al.*, 2002).

The absolutist position is one that assumes that human phenomena are basically the same (qualitatively) in all cultures: 'honesty' is 'honesty' and 'depression' is 'depression', no matter where one observes it. From the absolutist perspective, culture is thought to play little or no role in either the meaning or display of human characteristics. Assessments of such characteristics are made using standard instruments (perhaps with linguistic translation) and interpretations are made easily, without alternative culturally based views taken into account.

In sharp contrast, the relativist approach is rooted in anthropology, and assumes that all human behaviour is culturally patterned. It seeks to avoid ethnocentrism by trying to understand people 'in their own terms'. Explanations of human diversity are sought in the ones that a cultural group gives to a phenomenon. Comparisons are judged to be problematic and ethnocentric and are thus virtually never made.

A third perspective, one that lies somewhat between the two positions, is that of universalism. Here it is assumed that basic human characteristics are common to all members of the species (i.e. constituting a set of biological givens), and that culture influences the development and display of them (i.e. culture plays different variations on these underlying themes). Assessments are based on the presumed underlying process, but measures are developed in culturally meaningful versions. Comparisons are made cautiously, employing a wide variety of methodological principles and safeguards, and interpretations of similarities and differences are attempted that take alternative culturally based meanings into account.

Intersection of culture and health

Perhaps the most comprehensive exposition of the way in which culture can influence health and disease was presented by Murphy (1982). He proposed that cultural factors can affect the following aspects: definition, recognition, symptomatology, prevalence and response (by society or healer).

Numerous studies have shown that the very concepts of health and disease are defined differently across cultures; this basic link between culture and health was recognized early (Polgar, 1962) and has continued up to the present time (Foster, 1997; Helman, 2000, Chapter 2). The concept of health has undergone rapid change in international thought, witness the World Health Organization's emphases on the existence of (positive) wellbeing, and not only on the absence of (negative) disease or disability. Of special interest here is the existence of 'culture-bound syndrome' that appears to be unique to one (or a few) cultures (American Psychiatric Association, 2000; Simons & Hughes, 1985).

Recognition of a condition as healthy or as a disease is also linked to culture. Some conditions such as trance are recognized as important curing (health-seeking) mechanisms in some cultures, but may be classified as psychiatric disorder in others (Ward, 1989). Similarly, the expression of a condition through the exhibition of various symptoms has also been linked to cultural norms (Zola, 1966). For example, it is claimed by many (e.g. Kleinman, 1982; Kirmayer, 1984) that psychological problems are expressed somatically in some cultures (e.g. Chinese) more than in other cultures (Tseng, 2001, Chapter 16).

Prevalence studies across cultures have produced very clear evidence that disease and disability are highly variable. From heart disease (Marmot & Syme, 1976; Prener et al., 1991), to depression and schizophrenia (Murphy, 1982; Siegert, 2001), cultural factors such as traditional diet, substance abuse and social relationships within the family all contribute to the prevalence of disease (World Health Organization, 2001, 2002).

The response by society generally (and by the healer) to ill health also varies across cultures. Acceptance or rejection of persons with particular diseases (such as leprosy or AIDS) has changed over time, and differs across cultures (Pick, 1998; Waxler, 1997). Healing practices, based on variations in medicines and beliefs about causations have wide variation in the treatment of both physical and psychological disorder (Haln, 1999; Murphy, 1981; Yap, 1974).

An attempt has been made to link culture to health, drawing upon some established conceptual distinctions in the behavioural sciences by Berry (1989). Figure 1 shows four categories of health phenomena and two levels of analyses (community/cultural and individual/psychological). Crossing the two dimensions produces eight areas in which information can be sought during the study of links between culture and individual health. The community level of work typically involves ethnographic methods to study the culture, and yields a general characterization of shared health concepts, values, practices and institutions in a society.

The individual level of work involves the psychological study of a sample of individuals from the society and yields information about individual differences (and similarities), which can lead to inferences about the psychological underpinnings of individual health beliefs, attitudes, behaviours and relationships.

The reason for taking cultural level health phenomena into account is so that the broad context for the development and display of individual health phenomena can be established; without an understanding of this background context, attempts to deal with individuals and their health problems may well be useless, even harmful. The reason for considering individual level health phenomena is that not all persons hold the same beliefs or attitudes, nor do they engage in the same behaviours and relationships; without an understanding of their individual variations from the general community situation, harm may well, again, be inflicted.

Examples of work in the eight areas of interest are common in the research and professional literature. At the cultural level, as we have already seen in relation to Murphy's ideas, the way in which a cultural group defines what is health and what is not, can vary substantially from group to group. These collective cognitive phenomena include shared conceptions, and categories, as well as definitions of health and disease. At the individual level, health beliefs and knowledge, while influenced by the cultural conceptions, can also vary from person to person. Beliefs about the causes of an illness or disability, or about how much control one has over it (both getting it and curing it) shows variations across individuals and cultures (Berry & Dalal, 1994). For example, in one community, the general belief is that if pregnant women eat too much (or even 'normally') there will be insufficient room for the fetus to develop; hence, under-eating is common, and prenatal malnutrition results, with an associated increase in infant disability. However, there are variations across individuals in this belief, with education, status and participation in public health programmes making a difference. In the fishing villages that line Lake Victoria in East Africa, the parasitic disease schistosomiasis is so prevalent that the bloody urine of young males during the full-bloom stage of the disease is considered a healthy sign of approaching manhood. There is no reason to seek medical attention for this ailment (Desowitz, 1981).

With regard to affective phenomena, the value placed on health is known to vary from culture to culture and within cultures across subgroups. For example, Judaic Law prescribes that health is given by God, and it is the responsibility of the individual to sustain it, the value placed on good health is thus a shared belief among practising Jews. However there is a significant variation in the acceptance of this across three Jewish groups; Orthodox Jews have been found to have the highest value, Reformed Jews have a lower value, and Secular Jews have an even lower value on health (Dayan, 1993). And within the three groups, there are further variations according to a number of personal and demographic factors.

Levels of analysis	Categories of health phenomena			
	Cognitive	Affective	Behavioural	Social
Community (cultural)	Health conceptions and definitions	Health norms and values	Health practices	Health roles and institutions
Individual (psychological)	Health knowledge and beliefs	Health attitudes	Health behaviours	Interpersonal relationships

Fig 1 Eight areas of interest in the relationship between culture and individual health.

Pain, in one form or the other is an inseparable part of everyday life, yet, not all social or cultural groups may respond to pain in exactly the same way. How people perceive and respond to pain, both in themselves and in others, is influenced by their cultural and social background (Halman, 2000). Zborowski (1952) examined the cultural component of the experience of pain among three groups of patients at a hospital in New York: Italian- and, Jewish-Americans and Protestant 'Old Americans' (of Anglo-Saxon background) and found vast variations. While the Italians and Jews were emotional in their response to pain, and exaggerated their pain experience, the two differed in their attitudes towards the pain. The Italians were more concerned about the immediacy of the pain experience and complained a lot. However, once they were given palliatives and the pain subsided, they quickly forgot about their suffering and returned to their normal behaviour. The Jewish patients on the other hand were more concerned about the implications of the pain to their health. Many of the Jews distrusted palliatives and were reluctant to accept them as they were anxious about 'side-effects', as well as being more concerned about the drug only relieving the pain and not the underlying disease. In contrast, the 'Old Americans' had a 'matter-of-fact' orientation towards pain. They were less emotional in reporting their pain and saw no point in exaggerating it, as it did not help anyone. It was also more common for them to withdraw from the society as a reaction to severe pain.

Health practices and behaviours also vary across cultures and individuals. For example, in respect of nutrition (Dasen & Super, 1988), what is classified as suitable food, and who can eat it are matters of cultural practice. Many high protein 'foods' are not placed in the food category (e.g. grubs, brains) and are avoided, while in other cultures they are an important part of the diet. Within these general cultural practices, however, individuals vary in what they can eat, depending on age, status or food factors related to clan membership. The social organization of health activities into instructions, and the allocation of roles (e.g. healer, patient) is also known to vary across cultures. In some cultures, religious or gender issues affect the role of healer (e.g. only those with certain spiritual qualities, or only males, may become a healer), while in others, the high cost of medical or other health professional training limits the roles to the wealthy. In some cultures, health services are widely available and fully integrated into the fabric of community life (e.g. Aversasturi, 1988; Folland et al., 2001) while in others doctors and hospitals are remote, mysterious and alien to most of the population. In the former case, individual patient–healer relationships may be collegial, in which a partnership is established to regain health, while in the latter, the relationship is likely to be hierarchical, involving the use of authority and compliance.

Psychosocial factors

A second approach to understanding individual health in a broader context has been through the conceptualization and measurement of psychosocial factors (World Health Organization, 1992). While these factors are not usually seen as 'cultural', a case can be made that all known psychosocial factors are also cultural factors, in the sense that they vary substantially across cultures. Hence, they have been treated as cultural variables, and can be understood in terms of

local cultural beliefs, values and behaviours. This position was advocated early (World Health Organization, 1982):

Psychosocial factors have been increasingly recognised as key factors in the success of health and social actions. If actions are to be effective in the prevention of diseases and in the promotion of health and well being, they must be based on an understanding of culture, tradition, beliefs and patterns of family interaction. (p. 4)

Most of these psychosocial factors (World Health Organization, 1992) are known to vary across cultures. For example, the psychosocial factor of specific behaviour patterns (such as the Type A/Type B distinction, or 'burnout') is probably one prevalent in western industrial cultures. Similarly, the influence of lifestyle (including a diet of 'fast foods'), is also likely to be a factor in some societies and not in others. A third psychosocial factor, that of problems of person–environment fit is obviously linked to culture (as a fundamental 'environment'). In particular, the acculturation problems of immigrants and refugees are identified by WHO: these are considered in detail in the next section.

The role of social inequality in health has been emphasized by Wilkinson (1996). It is the maldistribution of resources and wealth within a society, rather than the average level of wealth, that influences an individual's wellbeing. This inequality is often related to a person's cultural or ethnic background; being poor, especially combined with being a member of an oppressed cultural community, is bad for one's health (Desjarlais et al., 1995) (see 'Socioeconomic status and health').

Three of the psychosocial factors refer to excessive stress (relating to close social relations, to the work place, and to broader societal settings). Problems with family and friends are likely to vary according to family organization and type (monogamous/polygamous; endogamous/exogamous; nuclear/extended; matrilineal/patrilineal; matrilocal/patrilocal, etc.). Since these are core contrasts in the ethnographic literature, the type and extent of such problems is likely to be linked to their cultural variations. Similarly, the workplace (the hunt, the garden, the pasture, the factory, the office, the unemployment line), and broader social conditions (poverty, war, famine, imprisonment, being the victim of crime or racism) all vary from culture to culture.

Finally, in the WHO list of psychosocial factors, are the health hazards and protective factors that are present in one's social environment, including: on the one hand, malnutrition, unsafe settings where accidents are likely to occur, and iatrogenic factors and on the other, social support and health promotion programmes (see 'Health promotion').

The degree of cultural variation in the psychosocial factors is plausibly very high, but as yet the extent is not known. It is proposed that such cultural variations be the focus of concerted research.

Ethnic domain

When we focus on the health of culturally distinct groups and individuals, who live in culturally plural societies, we are dealing with the ethnic domain (Berry, 1997a). By 'ethnic' is meant those phenomena that are derived from fully independent cultures; ethnic groups operate with an evolving culture that flows from their original heritage culture, in interaction with the culture of the larger (dominant) society.

Approach to ethnicity

While ethnic groups are not full-scale or independent cultural groups, it is a working belief of cross-cultural psychology that all the methodological, theoretical and substantive lessons learned from working with cultural groups in the international enterprise should inform our work with ethnic groups (Berry, 1980). That is, we need to know about both their community health conceptions, values, practices and institutions and about how these are distributed as health beliefs, attitudes, behaviours and interpersonal relationships among individual members of the ethnic groups.

Put another way, we are not dealing with 'minorities' that are simply deviant from some 'mainstream', but with communities that deserve to have their health and health needs understood just as well as any other cultural community. In this sense, work on health in the ethnic domain does not differ in principle from work in the cultural domain. However, there is now an important new element, that of contact and possibly conflict, between cultural groups. This is the case in a number of respects: first, the health phenomena of ethnic individuals may be quite different from those of the larger society, and create misunderstanding, confusion and conflict between the two groups. Secondly, these conflicts may themselves generate health problems; and thirdly, the health services of the larger society may not be sufficiently informed, or sensitive, to enable them to deal with either the health problems that are linked to the heritage of the ethnic group, or those that have their roots in the conflict between the two groups in contact (Beiser *et al.*, 1988). Since the first of these issues is very similar to the discussion of the cultural domain, it will not be pursued further here. However, there is one important difference: when a health professional does not understand an individual's health needs while practising in another country, at least the individual may have recourse to an indigenous health system; when this lack of understanding occurs with respect to an ethnic individual, there may no longer be such an alternative service of health support. The second and third issues can be considered using the notions of acculturative stress, and multicultural health.

Acculturative stress

In the literature on the health and wellbeing of ethnic groups and individuals, there was an earlier assumption that the experience of culture contact and change will always be stressful, and lead to loss of health status. As is the case for other forms of stress (as one psychosocial factor), this assumption is no longer supported; to understand why there are variable outcomes to culture contact, the notions of acculturation strategies need to be introduced.

Acculturation was first identified as a cultural level phenomenon by anthropologists (e.g. Redfield *et al.*, 1936) who defined it as culture change resulting from contact between two autonomous cultural groups. Acculturation is also an individual level phenomenon, requiring individual members of both the larger society and immigrants to work out new forms of relationships in their daily lives. This idea was introduced by Graves (1967), who has proposed the notion of 'psychological acculturation' to refer to these new behaviours and strategies. One of the findings of much subsequent research in this area is that there are vast individual differences in how people attempt to deal with acculturative change (termed 'acculturation strategies'; see Berry, 2003; Berry & Sam, 1997). These strategies have three aspects. Their preferences ('acculturation attitudes'); how much change they actually undergo ('behavioural shifts'); and how much of a problem these changes are for them (the phenomenon of 'acculturative stress'; see Berry *et al.*, 1987).

Perhaps the most useful way to identify the various orientations which individuals may have towards acculturation is to note that two issues predominate in the daily life of most acculturating individuals. One pertains to the maintenance and development of one's ethnic distinctiveness in society, in which people decide how much their own cultural identity and customs are of value and should be retained. The other issue involves the desirability of interethnic contact, in which people decide whether relations with other groups in the larger society are of value and should be sought. These two issues are essentially questions of values, and may be responded to on a continuous scale, from positive to negative. When these two value dimensions are related to each other, four general acculturation strategies are defined. Each is considered to be an option available to individuals and to groups in plural societies, towards which people may hold attitudes; these are assimilation, integration, separation and marginalization.

When there is a negative orientation to the first issue, and a positive orientation to the second issue, the assimilation option is defined, namely, relinquishing one's cultural identity and moving into the larger society. This can take place by way of absorption of a non-dominant group into an established dominant group, as in the 'melting pot' concept.

The integration option (a positive orientation to both issues) implies the maintenance of the cultural integrity of the group, as well as the movement by the group to become an integral part of a larger societal framework. In this case, a large number of distinguishable ethnic groups results, all co-operating within a larger multicultural society (sometimes referred to as a 'mosaic').

When there are no relations desired with the larger society, and this is accompanied by a wish to maintain ethnic identity and tradition, another option is defined. Depending upon which group (the dominant or non-dominant) controls the situation, this option may take the form of either segregation or separation. When the pattern is imposed by the dominant group, classic segregation to 'keep people in their place' appears. On the other hand, the maintenance of a traditional way of life outside full participation in the larger society may derive from a group's desire to lead an independent existence, as in the case of separatist movements. In these terms, segregation and separation differ primarily with respect to which group or groups have the power to determine the outcome.

Finally, there is an option (a negative orientation to both issues) that is difficult to define precisely, possibly because it is accompanied by a good deal of collective and individual confusion and anxiety. It is characterized by being poised in psychological uncertainty between the two cultures, and by feelings of alienation and loss of identity. This option is marginalization, in which groups lose cultural and psychological contact with both their traditional culture and the larger society.

Inconsistencies and conflicts between various acculturation strategies are one of many sources of difficulty for acculturating individuals. Generally, when acculturation experiences cause problems for acculturating individuals, we observe increased levels of acculturative stress. In an overview of this area of research (Berry, 1997b), it was argued that stress may arise, but it is not inevitable. Or as Beiser et al. (1988) have phrased it: migrant status is a mental health risk factor; but risk is not destiny.

There are three concepts involved in understanding the roots of acculturative stress. First, acculturation occurs in a particular situation (e.g. an ethnic community), and individuals participate in and experience these changes to varying degrees; thus, individual acculturation experience may vary from a great deal to rather little. Secondly, stressors may result from this varying experience of acculturation; for some people, acculturative changes may all be in the form of stressors, while for others, they may be benign or even seen as opportunities. Thirdly, varying levels of acculturative stress and health problems may become manifest as a result of one's inability to cope with acculturation experience and stressors.

Results of studies of acculturative stress have varied widely in the level of difficulties found in acculturating groups and individuals. Early views were that cultural contact and change inevitably led to acculturative stress; however, current views (Berry & Sam, 1997) are that stress is linked to acculturation in a probabilistic way and the level of stress experienced will depend on a number of factors, such as host society prejudice, coping resources and strategies, education, acculturation strategies and national policies dealing with the issue of cultural diversity.

Research in a number of countries has typically revealed variations in, but sometimes no greater acculturative stress or mental health problems among, ethnic groups than in the general population (Beiser et al., 1988). However, stress is usually lower when integration is being sought (but is highest for marginalization); migration was voluntary, (i.e. for immigrants) rather than forced (i.e. for refugees); there is a functioning social support group (i.e. an ethnic community willing to assist during the settlement process); and when tolerance for diversity and ethnic attitudes in the larger society are positive (Berry, 1997b).

In summary, the health outcomes for acculturating individuals are highly variable, and depend on a variety of factors that are under the control of policy makers. Stress, with resultant poor health, can be avoided if certain steps are taken. One of these, to which we now turn, is the development of a pluralistic health care system, one that is knowledgeable about and sensitive to the health needs of ethnic groups and individuals.

Multicultural health

Essentially, the area of multicultural health involves research and action directed towards improving the level of understanding and quality of services available to ethnic groups and individuals who now live in culturally plural societies (Beiser et al., 1988; Mulatu & Berry, 2001).

The research component is driven by the work in the cultural domain and on acculturative stress, and should result in better understanding of the health, and health needs of ethnic groups. To many observers, it is obvious why this research should be undertaken: it is unethical to presume to provide health services to people one does not understand; it is inequitable to train health service providers to know the needs of only part of the population; and it is unjust (especially in countries with a tax-supported health system) to allocate all of the resources to assist only some of the people.

The action component is directed towards changing the health institutions of the larger society, and the beliefs, attitudes, behaviours and relationships of members of the larger society with respect to these issues. The same framework employed earlier to outline areas of interest in the relationship between culture and health can guide the actions that are required.

To provide one example (from Canada), there is a national organization which promotes the need for multicultural health, with active member organizations in every Province. It advocates curriculum change in all health education programmes, to more fully portray the role of culture and ethnicity in health; it provides in-service workshops on issues of ethnocentrism and racism and on the special needs of immigrants and refugees; and it promotes awareness in the ethnic communities of their rights to health and how to gain access to better healthcare.

Many of these and related activities are supported by governments, in recognition of the value, not only of pluralism, but of healthy pluralism. Experience in many countries suggests that diverse populations can be denied basic services such as health only to a certain extent, and only for a limited period, before social pathologies become manifest, and the health statuses of all members of society deteriorate further.

Conclusions

This chapter has ranged widely over a number of disciplines, across and within cultures, and from research to action advocacy. Despite this diversity, there is a set of core ideas: cultures vary in their understanding and treatment of health; individuals also vary both across and within cultures; this dual variation needs to be taken into account whether working internationally, or with ethnic groups domestically.

It is well understood that health and disease are complex phenomena, and that they are multidetermined. This chapter has necessarily added to this complexity by focusing on the role of cultural and ethnic factors, but it also has attempted to present a systematic overview of their relationships, in addition to a portrayal of what we already know, and what we should, but do not yet know and do. (see also 'Gender issues and health' and 'Lay beliefs about health and illness'.)

Acknowledgement

This article was prepared while the first author was a Visiting Scholar at the Research Centre for Health Promotion, and Department of Psychosocial Science, University of Bergen, Norway.

REFERENCES

American Psychiatric Association. (2000). *Diagnostic and Statistical Manual of Mental Disorders Text Revision (DSM-IV-TR)* (4th edn.). Washington, DC: APA.

Averasturi, L. G. (1988). Psychosocial factors in health: the Cuban model. In P. Dasen, J.W. Berry & N. Sartorius (Eds.). *Health and cross-cultural psychology: towards application* (pp. 291–7). London: Sage Publications.

Beiser, M., Barwick, C., Berry, J.W. *et al.* (1988). *After the door has been opened: report of task force on mental health issues affecting immigrants and refugees.* Ottawa, Canada: Health and Welfare, and Muticulturalism and Citizenship.

Berry, J.W. (1980). Social and cultural change. In H. C. Triandis & R. Brislin (Eds.). *Handbook of cross-cultural psychology, Vol. 5, Social.* Boston: Allyn & Bacon.

Berry, J.W. (1989). The role of cross-cultural psychology in understanding community-based health. In M. Peat (Ed.). *Community-based rehabilitation: social and practice.* Kingston, Canada: Queen's University School of Rehabilitation Therapy.

Berry, J.W. (1997*a*). Acculturation and health: theory and research. In S. S. Kazarian & D. Evans (Eds.). *Cultural clinical psychology.* New York: Oxford University Press.

Berry, J.W. (1997*b*). Immigration, acculturation and adaptation. *Applied Psychology: An International Review,* **46,** 5–68.

Berry, J.W. (2003). Conceptual approaches to acculturation. In K. Chun, P. Balls-Organista & G. Marin (Eds.). *Acculturation: advances in theory, measurement and applied research* (pp. 17–37). Washington DC: APA Books.

Berry, J.W. & Dalal, A. (1994). Disability attitudes, beliefs and behaviours: international study of community based rehabilitation. Kingston: International Centre for Community Based Rehabilitation.

Berry, J.W., Kim, U., Minde, T. & Mok, D. (1987). Comparative studies of acculturative stress. *International Migration Review,* **21,** 491–511.

Berry, J.W., Pooringa, Y. H., Segall, M. H. & Dasen, P. R. (2002). *Cross-cultural psychology: research and applications.* New York: Cambridge University Press.

Berry, J.W. & Sam, D. L. (1997). Acculturation and adaptation. In J.W. Berry, *et al.* (Eds.). *Handbook of cross-cultural psychology, Vol. 3, Social behaviour and applications* (pp. 291–326). Boston: Allyn & Bacon.

Brown, P. J. (Ed.). (1997). *Understanding and applying medical anthropology.* Mountain View, CA: Mayfield Publishing Company.

Dasen, P. R., Berry, J.W. & Sartorius, N. (1988). *Health and cross-cultural psychology: towards applications.* London: Sage Publications.

Dasen, P. & Super, C. (1988). The usefulness of cross-cultural approach in studies of malnutrition and psychological development. In. P. D. Dasen, J.W. Berry & N. Sartorius (Eds.). *Health and cross-cultural psychology: towards application* (pp. 112–41). London: Sage Publications.

Dayan, J. (1993). Health values, beliefs and behaviours of Orthodox, Reformed and Secular Jews. Unpublished M.A. thesis. Kingston, Canada: Queen's University.

Desjarlais, R., Eisenberg, L., Good, B. & Kleinman, A. (1995). *World mental health: problems and priorities in low-income countries.* Oxford: Oxford University Press.

Desowitz, R. S. (1981). New Guinea tapeworms and Jewish grandmothers. Tales of parasites and people. New York: Norton.

Folland, S., Goodman, A. C., Stano, Miron (2001). *The economies of health and health care.* Ripper Saddle River, NJ: Prentice Hall.

Foster, G. M. (1997). Disease aetiologies in non-Western medical systems. In P. J. Brown (Ed.). *Understanding and applying medical anthropology* (pp. 110–117). Mountain View, CA: Mayfield Publishing Company.

Foster, G. & Anderson, B. (1978). *Medical anthropology.* New York: Wiley.

Graves, T. (1967). Psychological acculturation in a triethnic community. *Southwestern Journal of Anthropology,* **23,** 337–50.

Hahn, R. R. A. (Ed.). (1999). *Anthropology in public health.* Oxford: Oxford University Press.

Helman, C. G. (1985). Psyche, soma and society: the social construction of psychosomatic disorders. *Culture, Medicine and Psychiatry,* **9,** 1–26.

Helman, C. G. (2000). *Culture, health and illness.* Oxford: Butterworth-Heinemann.

Kazarian, S. & Evans, D. R. (Eds.). (2001). *Handbook of cultural health psychology.* San Diego: Academic Press.

Kirmayer, L. (1984). Culture, affect and somatization. *Transcultural Psychiatric Review,* **21,** 139–58.

Kleinman, A. (1980). *Patients and healers in the context of culture.* Berkeley: University of California Press.

Kleinman, A. (1982). Neurasthenia and depression: a study of somatiztion and

culture in China. *Culture, Medicine and Psychiatry,* **6,** 117–90.

MacLachlan, M. (2001). *Culture and Health* (2nd edn.). Chichester: Wiley.

MacLachlan, M. & Mulatu, M. (2004). Culture and health. In C. Spielberger (Ed.). *Encyclopedia of applied psychology, Vol. 2* (pp. 167–78). San Diego: Elsevier

Marmot, M. & Syme, S. L. (1976). Acculturation and coronary heart disease in Japanese Americans. *American Journal of Epidemiology,* **104,** 225–47.

Mulatu, M. & Berry, J.W. (2001) Cultivating health through multiculturalism. In M. MacLachlan (Ed.). *Promoting health across cultures* (pp. 15–35), Chichester: Wiley.

Murphy, H. B. M. (1981). *Comparative psychiatry.* Berlin: Springer-Verlag.

Murphy, H. B. M. (1982). Culture and schizophrenia. In I. Al-Isa (Ed.). *Culture and psychopathology.* Baltimore: University Park Press.

Pick, S. (1998). Sexual and reproductive health education. In J. Adair, D. Belanger & K. Dion (Eds.). *Advances in psychological science, Vol. 1* (pp. 455–511), Hove: Psychology Press.

Polgar, S. (1962). Health and human behaviour: areas of common interest to social and medical sciences. *Current Anthropology,* **2,** 159–205.

Prener, A., Hojgaard-Nielson, N., Storm, H. & Hart-Hansen, J. P. (1991). Cancer in Greenland: 1953–1985. *Acta Pathologica, Microbiologica et Immunologica Scandinavia,* **99,** Suppl. 20.

Redfield, R., Linton, R. & Herskovits, M. J. (1936). Memorandum on the study of acculturation. *American Anthropologist,* **38,** 149–52.

Siegert, R. J. (2001). Culture, cognition and schizophrenia. In J. F. Schumarker & T. Ward. (Eds.). *Cultural cognition and psychopathology* (pp. 171–89). London: Praeger.

Simons R. & Hughes, C. (Eds.). (1985). *The culture-bound syndromes.* Dordrecht: Reidel.

Tseng, W. S. (2001). *Handbook of cultural psychiatry.* San Diego: Academic Press.

Ward, C. (Ed.). (1989). *Altered states of consciousness and mental health.* London: Sage.

Wexler, N. E. (1997). Learning to a leper: a case study in the social construction of illness. In P. J. Brown (Ed.). *Understanding and applying medical anthropology* (pp. 147–57). Mountain View, CA: Mayfield Publishing Company.

Wilkinson, R. (1996). *Unhealthy societies: the afflictions of inequality.* London: Routledge.

World Health Organization (1982). *Medium term programme.* Geneva: World Health Organization.

World Health Organization (1992). *The ICD.10 Classification of mental and behavioural disorders: clinical descriptions and diagnostic guidelines.* Geneva: World Health Organization.

World Health Organization (2001). *The world health report 2001.*

Mental health: new understanding, new hope. Geneva: World Health Organization.

World Health Organization (2002). *The world health report, 2002. Reducing risks, promoting healthy life.* Geneva: World Health Organization.

Yap, P. M. (1974). *Comparative psychiatry.* Toronto: University of Toronto Press.

Zborowski, M. (1952). Cultural components in response pain. *Journal of Social Issues,* **8**, 16–30.

Zola, I. (1966). Culture and symptoms: an analysis of patients' presenting symptoms. *American Sociological Review,* **31**, 615–30.

Delay in seeking help

Suzanne E. Scott

King's College London

Following the detection of a symptom, the majority of individuals do not seek professional help, but instead do nothing or self-medicate (Freer, 1980). Whilst these responses may play a useful role in limiting the burden on healthcare services for benign and minor conditions, a continuing and important issue is delay in seeking help for symptoms that are indicative of life-threatening diseases. The intention of this chapter is to summarize the theoretical approaches used to study and understand help-seeking behaviour, with particular reference to delay in seeking help for symptoms of cancer and myocardial infarction (as these have been the most widely researched areas), and finally to discuss the implications of this research.

Delay in help-seeking or 'patient delay' (Pack & Gallo, 1938) is the time taken from the detection of a symptom to the first consultation with a healthcare professional for that symptom. This is distinct from 'professional delay' (the time from the first consultation with a healthcare professional regarding a symptom to the receipt of a definitive diagnosis). The overall duration of delay has been divided in such a manner because an undifferentiated measure like 'total delay' (the time from the detection of a symptom to the receipt of a definitive diagnosis) may confound the effects of multiple factors that influence delay (Safer *et al.*, 1979). For instance, the factors that hinder a patient's decision to seek help following the self-discovery of a breast lump may be quite different from those that cause a delay in reaching a definitive diagnosis of breast cancer following the first consultation with a healthcare professional. As such, focusing on separate sub-stages such as 'patient delay' and 'professional delay' provides a more informative and meaningful insight into delay behaviour.

When comparing the time duration for patient and professional delay, it is patient delay that generally constitutes the majority of the overall delay time (Onizawa *et al.*, 2003; Pattenden *et al.*, 2002). Patient delay has been found to have important health-related consequences. For instance, with regard to sexually transmitted infections, prolonging the duration of the untreated infection will increase the probability of disease progression, its adverse sequelae (e.g. untreated chlamydia can lead to pelvic inflammatory disease, which in turn can cause infertility) and transmission to others (Hills *et al.*, 1993). Similarly, delay in seeking care for airborne diseases such as tuberculosis may be detrimental not only to the individual (due to the increasing severity of the illness over time) but also to the community, as ongoing transmission will continue until effective treatment is administered (Godfrey-Faussett *et al.*, 2002). Patient delay can also lead to a reduction in the efficacy of treatments. For instance, there is a strong relationship between the timing of thrombolytic therapy for myocardial infarction and its efficacy, with early treatment leading to less myocardial damage and reductions in morbidity and mortality (GISSI, 1986; Simoons *et al.*, 1986). Finally, although a link between patient delay and progression of disease has not been established for all cancer sites, the incidence of advanced stage cancer is frequently attributed to delay by patients in presenting to a healthcare professional. Studies with breast cancer patients indicate that patient delay of over 12 weeks is associated with increased tumour size, advanced stage disease at diagnosis and poor survival (Neave *et al.*, 1990; Rossi *et al.*, 1990). Regardless of these detrimental consequences, delay in seeking medical consultation is common (Facione, 1993; Mor *et al.*, 1990). Given the impact of patient delay it is important to understand the decision to seek help and identify the determinants of delay in seeking help.

Measurement of patient delay

Patient delay is typically studied retrospectively, using samples of patients who have recently sought help for the particular symptom or disease being studied. The use of this retrospective data obviously has its limitations with the possibility of error in recall, particularly for those patients with long delay periods. Nevertheless, analysing the decision to seek help using prospective methodology is not without its drawbacks. Studies examining 'hypothetical help-seeking' or intentions to seek help (i.e. if you noticed a breast lump, when would you seek help?) are problematic, as they do not take contextual and situational factors into account. Such factors are known to play an important role in the decision to seek help. For instance, Safer *et al.* (1979) found that having a recent competing problem (e.g. marriage or divorce) was associated with increased delay in seeking help. Similarly, Dignan *et al.* (1990) reported that mothers with cervical cancer prioritize looking after their child over seeking care for their own symptoms.

Finally, although analysing patient delay as a continuous variable can make greater use of the data, it is common for researchers to specify a duration of patient delay that is considered to be substantial (e.g. patient delay of three months or more) and compare 'delayers' to 'non-delayers'. It should be noted however, that these operational definitions are often arbitrary, in that they may be chosen without thought to their clinical relevance.

Reasons for delay behaviour

It is often assumed that individuals delay seeking medical attention following the self-discovery of symptoms because they fear the diagnosis, or are in denial. However, evidence for an association between fear or anxiety and patient delay is not conclusive (Facione, 1993). Recent research suggests that rather than those who delay seeking help being the most anxious or fearful upon finding symptoms, it is precisely this group who are more likely to seek help promptly (Meechan *et al.*, 2003; Nosarti *et al.*, 2000). Similarly, there is little evidence indicating that denial plays a major role in the delay to seek help (Fisher, 1967). In fact, individuals who delay seeking help often think a great deal about their symptoms and possible treatments and it may be the inability to cope or take action that prevents help-seeking rather than denial (Leventhal, 1970; Safer *et al.*, 1979). This is not to say that denial does not exist but, rather that when denial is evident, it seems to be short lived (see also 'Coping with stressful medical procedures').

In sum, the expanse of literature on help-seeking behaviour indicates that rather than simply denial or fear being responsible for patient delay, a complex matrix of factors influences the decision to seek help following the self-discovery of symptoms. There are three main approaches to the study of help-seeking behaviour, which together provide an understanding of patient delay. These approaches – predispositions, symptom appraisal and the influence of the healthcare system – are now discussed in turn.

Predispositions

The dispositional approach assumes that people have a fairly stable pattern of responses to illness. In this way, some people will nearly always avoid consultation with a healthcare professional, whereas others will be almost 'frequent attenders' at the primary healthcare centre. The dispositional approach seeks to identify differences in patterns of help-seeking and also to determine the reasons for their development. An example of the dispositional approach is the study of gender differences in help-seeking. In the United Kingdom, it has

been reported that compared with women, men are less likely to visit a doctor when they are ill and are less likely to report the symptoms of disease or illness (Department of Health, 2000). Women's rates of utilization of almost all healthcare services are higher than men's (OPCS, 1991) and men often do not seek help until a disease has progressed (Francome, 2000). Men and women also utilize different healthcare services. For instance, women are more likely to visit doctors, nurses, social workers, psychologists or physiotherapists whereas men are more likely to use accident and emergency services (Corney, 1990). However, in their review of men and their health help-seeking behaviour, Galdas *et al.* (2005) noted that there is a significant body of research that argues against gender as a determining factor in help-seeking behaviour and that variables such as occupation and socio-economic status are more important than gender alone.

The dispositional approach has rarely gone beyond description of basic socio-demographic factors or compared the reasons for the dispositional tendencies in seeking help (Mechanic, 1982). Thus, although the dispositional approach can inform us of *who* uses particular health services, it does not provide a full explanation of *why*. Furthermore, the same person with comparable symptoms but at varying times can choose to seek medical care on one occasion but not on another (Mechanic, 1978). Hence, the dispositional approach only offers a limited contribution to the understanding of help-seeking behaviour as the processes of responding to symptoms seems to be more dynamic than this approach suggests. (See also 'Personality and health').

Symptom appraisal

A way of understanding help-seeking behaviour that does focus on the processes leading to the decision to seek help is the symptom appraisal approach. This perspective considers the ways through which people identify and evaluate symptoms, the ways in which people make interpretations of the causes and implications of symptoms, and how these inferences are used in the decision to seek help. The symptom appraisal approach maintains that, following the detection of a symptom, an individual will continue to appraise and then decide whether a symptom means something is 'wrong' and it is this appraisal that will drive the decision of whether professional care is necessary (Safer *et al.*, 1979). Cacioppo *et al.* (1986) drew together theory and research from the fields of social and health psychology to form a general attribution framework that outlines the process of symptom appraisal. This 'Psychophysiological Comparison Theory' is based on two assumptions. Firstly, it is argued that people are motivated to maintain an understanding of their physiological condition because once symptoms are detected we almost automatically assign reasons for their presence. The second assumption notes that this symptom appraisal may not be accurate in terms of the physiological aetiology. For instance, a feeling of discomfort within the mouth may be appraised as a mouth ulcer whereas the discomfort is actually arising from a malignancy of the tongue (Scott *et al.*, 2006).

Based on the work of Safer *et al.* (1979), Anderson *et al.* (1995) proposed that symptom appraisal is the most important stage in the process of seeking medical attention, constituting approximately 60% of total delay. Evidence supporting this proposition comes from both the cancer and myocardial infarction literature.

Patients whose do not initially attribute their symptoms to cancer are more likely to delay than those whose do interpret their symptoms as indicative of cancer (de Nooijer *et al.*, 2001; Ramirez *et al.*, 1999). Similarly, recent research indicates that the belief that symptoms were those of a heart attack is a predictor of early arrival at hospital (Ruston *et al.*, 1998). Horne *et al.* (2000) found that patients with a mismatch between their expectations of a heart attack and their experiences of a heart attack had significantly longer delays than those whose experiences matched their expectations.

There are many factors that influence the symptom appraisal process. For instance, an individuals' past experience of symptoms can guide subsequent symptom appraisal. If a symptom is similar to one that previously turned out to be benign, the individual will be more likely to delay seeking help (Safer *et al.*, 1979). As well as using their own experiences, people can base their symptom interpretation on other people's experiences. The opinion of significant others is often sought prior to seeking help from healthcare professionals. In fact it is estimated that for every medical consultation there are approximately eleven 'lay' consultations usually involving a spouse or close friend (Scambler & Scambler, 1984). These consultations have a number of functions including confirmation that the problem is not trivial, recommendations for home remedies, advice to seek professional help and receipt of 'social permission' to seek care. It has been demonstrated that women with breast cancer who do not disclose the discovery of their symptoms to a significant other are more likely to delay seeking help than those who do make their discovery of a symptom known to others (Ramirez *et al.*, 1999). Timko (1987) notes that sometimes overt encouragement to seek help is not always necessary, as individuals who believe significant others want them to seek help are more likely to do so than those who believe others think they should wait. It should be recognized however, that although the result of consultation with their significant others may act as a trigger to seeking help, the 'lay referral network' (Friedson, 1961) may sometimes be just as erroneous in its symptom interpretation as the individual, and may recommend self-medication when professional attention is actually required.

The nature of the presenting symptoms also has an important role in the evaluation of symptoms. Strong sensory signals such as pain or bleeding lead to shorter appraisal delays (Safer *et al.*, 1979) yet many early symptoms of life-threatening conditions are often devoid of pain and discomfort. When discussing the symptoms of oral and oropharyngeal cancer (e.g. a soreness in the mouth, a red or white patch, persistent mouth ulcer), Guggenheimer *et al.* (1989) noted that they do not appear to be threatening to the patient as they are remarkably similar to those innocuous manifestations which the patient has experienced throughout his or her life. Hence the 'benign' nature of many symptoms does not initiate an immediate realization that the symptoms are indicative of something ominous and in need of professional attention. Demonstrating this point, in their study of delay in help-seeking for the symptoms of myocardial infarction, Horne *et al.* (2000) found that those patients who experienced 'typical' cardiac symptoms (e.g. chest pain, radiating pain, numbness, collapse) experienced shorter patient delay compared with those with more atypical symptoms (e.g. shortness of breath, nausea, vomiting, flu-like symptoms). In the same way, women with breast cancer whose first symptom is not a breast lump are more than four times more likely to delay than those whose first symptoms do include a lump (Burgess *et al.*, 1998). Finally, those symptoms which interfere with social or personal relations or activities act as triggers for help-seeking (Zola, 1973). For example, if symptoms interfere with an individual's ability to work they will spur the individual to seek the advice of a healthcare professional.

Whilst recognizing that symptom appraisal is a particularly important process in the decision to seek help, it must also be recognized that this process may not be sufficient to complete the process of seeking help. As Anderson *et al.*'s (1995) model of total patient delay suggests, seeking medical attention is a process that involves a number of stages, each governed by a distinct set of decisional and appraisal processes. Once a person has interpreted a symptom as a sign of illness, they will only seek help if they decide this illness requires medical attention ('illness delay'), act on this decision by making an appointment with a healthcare professional ('behavioural delay') and finally make it to the appointment and receive medical attention ('scheduling delay'). Therefore one must also look beyond symptom appraisal to gain a thorough understanding of help-seeking behaviour. (See also 'Symptom perception')

Influence of the healthcare system

The third approach used to study help-seeking behaviour focuses on understanding the influence of the healthcare system on people's decisions to seek help. This perspective purports that modifying the ways in which agencies and professionals are organized can tackle the problem of patients' delay in seeking help (Mechanic, 1982). However, compared with the other approaches used to understand patient delay, this approach has received relatively little attention. Andersen (1968) discussed the concept of 'enabling factors' such as the nature and accessibility of a source of healthcare which can assist or hinder help-seeking behaviour. In support of this notion, poor access to health services is known to influence the decision to seek help for symptoms of breast cancer (Facione, 1993). More recent research has expanded Andersen's work by defining the concept of 'access' and suggesting it is composed of several dimensions that include 'availability' (the volume of existing services), 'accessibility' (the location of the services in relation to the location of the patients) and 'affordability' to the patients (Penchansky & Thomas, 1981). The term 'access' also includes the 'accommodation' of the services, such as the opening hours of primary healthcare practices. This is particularly important given that a deterrent to prompt help-seeking is the inability to take the time off work in order to attend a healthcare professional (McClean & Reid, 1997). The way healthcare provision is perceived by individuals also influences healthcare use. For instance, perceptions that healthcare is rationed (e.g. due to the implementation of user charges and waiting lists for certain procedures) can impact on the way people use healthcare services such that they 'do not want to bother the doctor' with something that might prove to be trivial (Rogers *et al.*, 1999). Other barriers to healthcare include the nature of the doctor–patient relationship. The perceived closeness of this relationship has been shown to influence patient delay (Henderson, 1965) and patients' previous experiences with physicians have a significant impact on their subsequent medical help-seeking (Moore *et al.*, 2004). (See also 'Patient-centred healthcare')

Implications for interventions

As delayed help-seeking has detrimental consequences for the individual, the community and the cost of healthcare, it is vital that we understand who delays seeking help and the reasons for those delays, in order to tackle the problem of patient delay. This chapter has outlined the approaches used to study help-seeking behaviour and highlights the importance of psychosocial factors in the decision to seek help. The research on help-seeking behaviour has various implications, particularly with regard to the design of interventions aimed at reducing the duration of patient delay for conditions where patient delay has repercussions on morbidity and mortality.

Although it does not inform us as to why certain groups tend to seek help faster than others, the dispositional approach directs us to those patients who are more likely to delay seeking help. This data is useful in that it can be used to develop 'targeted' interventions to those who are (a) at risk of developing the particular disease and (b) more likely to delay seeking help for symptoms of that disease. This targeting is important as this will ensure that medical services are not overloaded by a large increase in help-seeking for benign symptoms among low-risk groups or 'waste' resources on those who are likely seek help appropriately anyway. However, this tactic can only succeed if there are clearly definable risk factors for the particular disease. For instance, such an approach could be useful for reducing patient delay for symptoms of oral cancer where the main risk factors are oral tobacco use and a high intake of alcohol.

The symptom appraisal approach emphasizes the importance of an individual's own evaluation of his or her symptom(s). Empirical evidence indicates that this process plays a major role in the decision to seek help. The misinterpretation of symptoms has implications for public education in that the importance of symptom appraisal can be used to guide the content of interventions to reduce patient delay. For instance, educational campaigns must detail the symptoms that are indicative of life-threatening conditions and hence require medical attention. However, because symptoms of serious ailments often mirror those of more common and benign conditions, there is the need not only to educate the public on the symptoms of conditions but also to show them a way of accurately evaluating symptoms when they occur. For instance, although chest pain is a symptom of myocardial infarction, only chest pain that lasts more than 15 minutes should be considered potentially indicative of myocardial infarction (Herlitz *et al.*, 1989). The application of a symptom appraisal based intervention is dependent on there being a clear connection between the disease in question and symptoms specific to that disease. For instance, this approach would be useful for reducing patient delay for early signs of breast cancer where symptoms include a breast lump, discharge and inversion of the nipple, yet less appropriate for delay for early stage prostate cancer where there is no clear link between symptoms and pre-metastatic disease (see also 'Health promotion').

Additionally, we should be aware that although knowledge about symptoms is an important variable in the appraisal of symptoms and the subsequent decision to seek help, this relationship is by no means definitive (Sheikh & Ogden, 1998). In turn, one must consider aspects of the healthcare system that may impact an individual's utilization of services. Here lies the importance of a good doctor–patient relationship, and affordable and available healthcare services, including consideration of opening hours and minimal waiting times. Furthermore, the introduction of additional services such as 'NHS direct' (a 24-hour nurse-led telephone service) has the potential for encouraging those in need of medical attention to seek the care they need, whilst reassuring those who do not need to visit a healthcare professional. Future research should assess the impact of these and other services (e.g. online health information) on the decision to seek help.

Despite the implications of the abundance of literature on help-seeking behaviour, there have been few theory-driven interventions to reduce patient delay. Future attempts should therefore focus on the psychosocial issues shown to be relevant to help-seeking behaviour and embrace the three approaches used to understand patient delay.

REFERENCES

Andersen, B. L., Cacioppo, J. T. & Roberts, D. C. (1995). Delay in seeking a cancer diagnosis: delay stages and psychophysiological comparison processes. *British Journal of Social Psychology*, **34**, 33–52.

Andersen, R. (1968). *A behavioral model of families' use of health services, Research Series No. 25*. Chicago: Centre for Health Administration Studies, University of Chicago.

Burgess, C. C., Ramirez, A. J., Richards, M. A. & Love, S. B. (1998). Who and what influences delayed presentation in breast cancer? *British Journal of Cancer*, **77**, 1343–48.

Cacioppo, J. T., Andersen, B. L., Turnquist, D. C. & Petty, R. E. (1986). Psychophysiological comparison processes: interpreting cancer symptoms. In B. L. Anderson. (Ed.). *Women with cancer: psychological Perspectives*. New York: Springer-Verlag.

Corney, R. H. (1990). Sex differences in general practice attendance and help-seeking for minor illness. *Journal of Psychosomatic Research*, **34**, 525–34.

de Nooijer, J., Lechner, L. & de Vries, H. (2001). A qualitative study on detecting cancer symptoms and seeking medical help; an application of Andersen's model of total patient delay. *Patient Education and Counselling*, **42**, 145–57.

Department of Health. (2000). *Press release: reference 2000/0187*. London: DoH.

Dignan, M., Michielutte, R., Sharp, P., Bahnson, J., Young, L. & Beal, P. (1990). The role of focus groups in health education for cervical cancer among minority women. *Journal of Community Health*, **15**, 369–75.

Facione, N. C. (1993). Delay versus help seeking for breast cancer symptoms: a critical review of the literature on patient and provider delay. *Social Science and Medicine*, **36**, 1521–34.

Fisher, S. (1967). Motivation for patient delay. *Archives of General Psychiatry*, **16**, 676–8.

Francome, C. (2000). *Improving men's health*. London: Middlesex University Press.

Freer, C. B. (1980). Self-care: a health diary study. *Medical Care*, **18**, 853–61.

Friedson, E. (1961). *Patients' view of medical practice*. New York: Russell Sage Foundation.

Galdas, P. M., Cheater, F. & Marshall, P. (2005). Men and health help-seeking behaviour: literature review. *Journal of Advanced Nursing*, 49, 616–23.

Godfrey-Faussett, P., Kaunda, H., Kamanga, J. *et al.* (2002). Why do patients with a cough delay seeking care at Lusaka urban health centres? A health systems research approach. *International Journal of Tuberculosis and Lung Disease*, 6, 796–805.

Gruppo Italiano per lo Studio della Stretochinasi nell'Infarto Miocardico (GISSI). (1986). Effectiveness of intravenous thrombolytic treatment in acute myocardial infarction. *Lancet*, 8478, 397–402.

Guggenheimer, J., Verbin, R. S., Johnson, J. T., Horkowitz, C. A. & Myers, E. N. (1989). Factors delaying the diagnosis of oral and oropharyngeal carcinomas. *Cancer*, 64, 932–5.

Henderson, J. G. (1965). Denial and repression as factors in the delay of patients with cancer presenting themselves to the physician. *Annals of the New York Academy of Sciences*, 125, 856–64.

Herlitz, J., Hartford, M., Blohm, M. *et al.* (1989). Effect of a media campaign on delay times and ambulance use in suspected acute myocardial infarction. *American Journal of Cardiology*, 64, 90–3.

Hills, S. D., Joesoef, R., Marchbanks, P. A. *et al.* (1993). Delayed care of pelvic inflammatory disease as a risk factor for impaired fertility. *American Journal of Obstetrics and Gynecology*, 168, 1503–9.

Horne, R., James, D., Petrie, K., Weinman, J. & Vincent, R. (2000). Patients' interpretation of symptoms as a cause of delay in reaching hospital during acute myocardial infarction. *Heart*, 83, 388–93.

Leventhal, H. (1970). Findings and theory in the study of fear communications. *Advances in Experimental Social Psychology* 5, 119.

McClean, H. L. & Reid, M. (1997). Use of gum services and information and views held by first time service users in a large UK city: implications for information provision. *International Journal of STD and AIDS*, 8, 154–8.

Mechanic, D. (1978). *Medical Sociology* (2nd edn.). New York: The Free Press.

Mechanic, D. (1982). The epidemiology of illness behaviour and its relationship to physical and psychological distress. In D. Mechanic. (Ed.). *Symptoms, illness behaviour and help-seeking*. New York: Prodist Press.

Meechan, G., Collins, J. & Petrie, K. J. (2003). The relationship of symptoms and psychological factors to delay in seeking medical care for breast symptoms. *Preventative Medicine*, 36, 374–8.

Moore, P. J., Sickel, A. E., Malat, J., Williams, D. & Alder, N. E. (2004). Psychosocial factors in medical and psychological treatment avoidance: the role of the doctor-patient relationship. *Journal of Health Psychology*, 9, 421–33.

Mor, V., Masterson-Allen, S., Goldber, R., Guaagnoli, E. & Wool, M. S. (1990). Pre-diagnostic symptom recognition and help seeking among cancer patients. *Journal of Community Health*, 15, 253–66.

Neave, L. M., Mason, B. H. & Kay, R. G. (1990). Does delay in diagnosis of breast cancer affect survival? *Breast Cancer Research and Treatment*, 15, 103–8.

Nosarti, C., Crayford, T., Roberts, J. V. *et al.* (2000). Delay in presentation of symptomatic referrals to a breast clinic: patient and system factors. *British Journal of Cancer*, 82, 742–8.

Onizawa, K., Nishihara, K., Yamagata, K., Yusa, H., Yanagawa, T. & Yoshida, H. (2003). Factors associated with diagnostic delay of oral squamous cell carcinoma. *Oral Oncology*, 39, 781–8.

Office of Population Censuses and Surveys (1991). *General Household Survey*. London: Her Majesty's Stationary Office.

Pack, G. T. & Gallo, J. S. (1938). The culpability for delay in the treatment of cancer. *American Journal of Cancer*, 33, 443.

Pattenden, J., Watt, I., Lewin, R. J. & Stanford, N. (2002). Decision making processes in people with symptoms of acute myocardial infarction: qualitative study. *British Medical Journal*, 324, 1006–9.

Penchansky, R. & Thomas, J. W. (1981). The concept of access: definition and relationship to consumer satisfaction. *Medical Care*, 19, 127–40.

Ramirez, A. J., Westcombe, A. M., Burgess, C. C. *et al.* (1999). Factors predicting delayed presentation of symptomatic breast cancer: a systematic review. *Lancet*, 353, 1127–31.

Rogers, A., Chapple, A. & Sergison, M. (1999). "If a patient is too costly they tend to get rid of you": the impact of people's perceptions of rationing on the use of primary care. *Health Care Analysis*, 7, 225–37.

Rossi, S., Cinini, C. Di Pietro, C. *et al.* (1990). Diagnostic delay in breast cancer: correlation with disease stage and prognosis. *Tumori*, 76, 559–62.

Ruston, A., Clayton, J. & Calnan, M. (1998). Patients' action during their cardiac event: qualitative study exploring differences and modifiable factors. *British Medical Journal*, 316, 1060–4.

Safer, M. A., Tharps, Q. J., Jackson, T. C. & Leventhal, H. (1979). Determinants of three stages of delay in seeking care at a medical clinic. *Medical Care*, 17, 11–29.

Scambler, G. & Scambler, A. (1984). The illness iceberg and aspects of consulting behaviour. In J.H.R. Fitzpatrick, S. Newman, G. Scambler & J. Thompson (Eds.). *The Experience of illness*. London: Tavistock Publications.

Scott, S. E., Grunfeld, E. A., Main, J. & McGurk, M. (2006). Patient delay in oral cancer: a qualitative study of patients' experiences. *Psycho-Oncology*, 15, 474–85.

Sheikh, I. & Ogden, J. (1998). The role of knowledge and beliefs in help seeking behaviour for cancer: a quantitative and qualitative approach. *Patient Education and Counselling*, 35, 35–42.

Simoons, M. L., Serruys, P. W., van de Brand, M. *et al.* (1986). Early thrombolysis in acute myocardial infarction: limitation of infarct size and improved survival. *Journal of the American College of Cardiology*, 7, 717–28.

Timko, C. (1987). Seeking medical care for a breast cancer symptom: determinants of intentions to engage in prompt or delay behavior. *Health Psychology*, 6, 305–28.

Zola, I. K. (1973). Pathways to the doctor – from person to patient. *Social Science and Medicine*, 7, 677–89.

Diet and health

Jane Ogden

University of Surrey

Diet and health

Diet influences health through a variety of pathways. This chapter will explore the nature of a healthy diet, how diet affects health and the theoretical perspectives which have been used to understand eating behaviour.

A healthy diet

Although the nature of a good diet has changed dramatically over the years, there is currently a consensus amongst nutritionists as to what constitutes a healthy diet (DOH, 1991). Current recommendations according to food groups are as follows:

- Fruit and vegetables: A wide variety of fruit and vegetables should be eaten and preferably five or more servings should be eaten per day.
- Bread, pasta, other cereals and potatoes: Plenty of complex carbohydrate foods should be eaten, preferably those high in fibre.
- Meat, fish and alternatives: Moderate amounts of meat, fish and alternatives should be eaten and it is recommended that the low fat varieties are chosen.
- Milk and dairy products: These should be eaten in moderation and the low fat alternatives should be chosen where possible.
- Fatty and sugary foods: Food such as crisps, sweets and sugary drinks should be eaten infrequently and in small amounts.

Other recommendations for a healthy diet include a moderate intake of alcohol (a maximum of 3–4 units per day for men and 2–3 units per day for women); the consumption of fluoridated water where possible; a limited salt intake of 6 g per day; eating unsaturated fats from olive oil and oily fish rather than saturated fats from butter and margarine and consuming complex carbohydrates (e.g. bread and pasta) rather than simple carbohydrates (e.g. sugar). It is also recommended that men aged between 19 and 59 require 2550 calories per day and that similarly aged women require 1920 calories per day although this depends upon body size and degree of physical activity (Department of Health, 1995). Diet is linked to health by influencing the onset of illness and as part of treatment and management once illness has been diagnosed.

Diet and health

Diet affects health through an individual's weight in terms of the development of eating disorders or obesity. Eating disorders are linked to physical problems such as heart irregularities, heart attacks, stunted growth, osteoporosis and reproduction (see 'Eating disorders'). Obesity is linked to diabetes, heart disease and some forms of cancer (see 'Obesity'). Research also suggests a direct link between diet and illnesses such as heart disease, cancer and diabetes. Much research has addressed the role of diet in health and, although at times controversial, studies suggest that foods such as fruits and vegetables, oily fish and oat fibre can be protective whilst salt and saturated fats can facilitate poor health.

Diet also has a role to play in treating illness once diagnosed. Obese patients are mainly managed through dietary-based interventions. Patients diagnosed with angina, heart disease or following a heart attack are also recommended to change their lifestyle with particular emphasis on stopping smoking, increasing their physical activity and adopting a healthy diet. Dietary change is also central to the management of both Type 1 and Type 2 diabetes. At times this aims to produce weight loss as a 10% decrease in weight has been shown to result in improved glucose metabolism (Wing et al., 1987). Dietary interventions are also used to improve the self-management of diabetes and aim to encourage diabetic patients to adhere to a more healthy diet (see 'Self-management' and 'Adherence to treatment').

Eating a healthy diet

A healthy diet therefore consists of high carbohydrate and low fat intake and links have been found between diet and both the onset of illnesses and their effective management. Research indicates, however, that many people across the world do not eat according to these recommendations. Data on children's diets indicate that children's diets in the western world do not match the recommendations for a healthy diet. Western children have been shown to eat too much fat and too few fruit and vegetables (see 'Adolescent lifestyle'). Therefore, dietary recommendations aimed at the western world in the main emphasize a reduction in food intake and the avoidance of becoming overweight. For the majority of the developing world, however, under-eating remains a problem resulting in physical and cognitive problems and poor resistance to illness due to lowered intakes of both energy and micronutrients. Recent data from the World Health Organization indicates that 54% of childhood mortality is caused by malnutrition, particularly that which is related to a deficit of protein and energy consumption. Research has also explored the diets of young adults. One large scale study carried out between 1989–1990 and 1991–1992 examined the eating behaviour of 16 000 male and female students aged between 18 and 24 from 21 European countries (Wardle et al., 1997). The results suggest that the prevalence of the fairly basic recommended healthy eating practices was low in this large sample of young adults, particularly in men. The results also provided insights into the different dietary practices across the different European countries. For example, countries such as Sweden, Norway, The Netherlands and Denmark ate the most fibre; Mediterranean countries such as Italy, Portugal and Spain ate the most fruit and England and Scotland ate the least; and salt consumption was highest in Poland and Portugal and lowest in Sweden, Finland and Iceland. Finally, research exploring the diets of the elderly indicates that, although many younger and non-institutionalized members of this group have satisfactory diets, many elderly people, particularly the older elderly, report diets which are deficient in vitamins, too low in energy and have poor nutrient content.

Research indicates that many people do not eat according to current recommendations. Much research has explored why people eat what they do. This chapter will describe developmental models, cognitive models and the role of weight concern in understanding eating behaviour.

Understanding eating behaviour

Developmental models

A developmental approach to eating behaviour emphasizes the role of exposure, social learning and associative learning.

Exposure

Human beings need to consume a variety of foods in order to have a balanced diet and yet show a fear and avoidance of novel foodstuffs termed 'neophobia'. Research has shown that mere exposure to novel foods can change children's preferences. For example, Birch and Marlin (1982) gave two-year-old children novel foods over a six-week period. One food was presented 20 times, one 10 times, one 5 times, whilst one remained novel and the results showed a direct relationship between exposure and food preference. Neophobia has been shown to be greater in males than females (both adults and children), to run in families (Hursti & Sjoden, 1997), to be minimal in infants who are being weaned onto solid foods but greater in toddlers, pre-school children and adults (Birch et al., 1998).

Social learning

Social learning describes the impact of observing other people's behaviour on one's own behaviour and is sometimes referred to as 'modelling' or 'observational learning'. An early study explored the impact of social suggestion on children's eating behaviours and arranged to have children observe a series of role models with eating behaviours different from their own (Duncker, 1938). The models chosen were other children, an unknown adult and a fictional hero. The results showed a greater change in the child's food preference if the model was an older child, a friend or the fictional hero. The unknown adult had no impact on food preferences. In another study, peer modelling was used to change children's preference for vegetables (Birch, 1980). The target children were placed at lunch for four consecutive days next to other children who preferred a different vegetable from themselves (peas versus carrots). By the end of the study the children showed a shift in their vegetable preference which persisted at a follow-up

assessment several weeks later. The impact of social learning has also been shown in an intervention study designed to change children's eating behaviour using video based peer modelling (Lowe et al., 1998). Parental attitudes to food and eating behaviours are also central to the process of social learning. For example, Klesges et al. (1991) showed that children selected different foods when they were being watched by their parents compared with when they were not, Olivera et al. (1992) reported a correlation between mothers' and children's food intakes for most nutrients in pre-school children, and likewise, Contento et al. (1993) found a relationship between mothers' health motivation and the quality of children's diets.

Associative learning

Associative learning refers to the impact of contingent factors on behaviour. In terms of eating behaviour, research has explored the impact of pairing food cues with aspects of the environment. Some research has examined the effect of rewarding eating behaviour as in 'if you eat your vegetables I will be pleased with you'. For example, Birch et al. (1980) gave children food in association with positive adult attention compared with more neutral situations. This was shown to increase food preference. Similarly a recent intervention study using videos to change eating behaviour reported that rewarding vegetable consumption increased that behaviour (Lowe et al., 1998). Rewarding eating behaviour seems to improve food preferences.

Other research has explored the impact of using food as a reward. For these studies, gaining access to the food is contingent upon another behaviour as in 'if you are well behaved you can have a biscuit'. Birch et al. (1980) presented children with foods either as a reward, as a snack or in a non-social situation (the control). The results showed that food acceptance increased if the foods were presented as a reward but that the more neutral conditions had no effect. This suggests that using food as a reward increases the preference for that food.

The relationship between food and rewards, however, appears to be more complicated than this. In one study, children were offered their preferred fruit juice as a means to be allowed to play in an attractive play area (Birch & Martin, 1982). The results showed that using the juice as a means to get the reward reduced the preference for the juice. Similarly, Lepper et al. (1982) told children stories about children eating imaginary foods called 'hupe' and 'hule' in which the child in the story could only eat one if he/she had finished the other. The results showed that the food that was being rewarded became the least preferred one. This finding has been supported by similar studies (Newman & Taylor, 1992). These examples are analogous to saying 'if you eat your vegetables you can eat your pudding'. Although parents use this approach to encourage their children to eat vegetables the evidence indicates that this may be increasing their children's preference for pudding even further as pairing two foods results in the 'reward' food being seen as more positive than the 'access' food.

The association between food and reward highlights a role for parental control over eating behaviour. Some research has addressed the impact of control as studies indicate that parents often believe that restricting children's access to food and forbidding them to eat food are good strategies to improve food preferences. Birch (1999) reviewed the evidence for the impact of imposing any form of parental control over food intake and argued that it is not only the use of foods as rewards which can have a negative effect of children's food preferences but also attempts to limit a child's access to foods. She concluded from her review that 'child feeding strategies that restrict children's access to snack foods actually make the restricted foods more attractive' (Birch, 1999, p.11).

Cognitive models of eating behaviour

A cognitive approach to eating behaviour focuses on an individual's cognitions and explores the extent to which cognitions predict and explain behaviour and most research has drawn upon social cognition models particularly the Theory of Reasoned Action (TRA) and the Theory of Planned Behaviour (TPB) (see 'Theory of planned behaviour'). Some research using a social cognitive approach to eating behaviour has focused on predicting the intentions to consume specific foods. For example, a series of studies has explored the extent to which cognitions relate to the intentions to eat biscuits, skimmed milk, organic vegetables and wholemeal bread (Sparks et al., 1992; Raats et al., 1995; Sparks & Shepherd, 1992). Much research suggests that behavioural intentions are not particularly good predictors of behaviour per se and studies have also used the TRA and the TPB to explore the cognitive predictors of actual behaviour. For example, Shepherd and Stockley (1985) used the TRA to predict fat intake and reported that attitude was a better predictor than subjective norms. Similarly, attitudes have also been found to be the best predictor of table salt use (Shepherd & Fairleigh, 1986), eating in fast food restaurants (Axelson et al., 1983), the frequency of consuming low fat milk (Shepherd, 1988) and healthy eating conceptualized as high levels of fibre and fruit and vegetables and low levels of fat (Povey et al., 2000). Research has also pointed to the role of perceived behavioural control in predicting behaviour particularly in relation to healthy eating (Povey et al., 2000). The social norms component of these models has consistently failed to predict eating behaviour.

Some studies have explored the impact of adding extra variables to the standard framework described within the social cognition models. For example, Shepherd and Stockley (1987) included a measure of nutritional knowledge, Povey et al. (2000) included additional measures of descriptive norms, and perceived social support and recent studies have explored the role of ambivalence in predicting eating behaviour (Sparks et al., 2001). The research in this area points to a consistently important role for attitudes towards a food and a role for an individual's beliefs about behavioural control. There is also some evidence that ambivalence may moderate the association between attitude and intention. However, there is no evidence for either social norms or other hypothesized variables.

A weight concern model of eating behaviour

Food is associated with many meanings such as a treat, a celebration, the forbidden fruit, a family get-together, being a good mother and being a good child (Ogden, 2003). Furthermore, once eaten, food can change the body's weight and shape, which is also associated with meanings such as attractiveness, control and success (Ogden, 2003). As a result of these meanings many women,

in particular, show weight concern in the form of body dissatisfaction, which often results in dieting. The impact of dieting, which has been termed 'restrained eating' on eating behaviour will now be described.

Restrained eating aims to reduce food intake and several studies have found that at times this aim is successful. Thompson et al. (1988) reported that in an experimental situation the restrained eaters consumed fewer calories than the unrestrained eaters after both the low and high preloads. This suggests that their attempts at eating less were successful. Similar results have been reported by Kirkley et al. (1988) using a food diary approach.

In opposition to these findings, however, several studies have suggested that higher levels of restrained eating are related to increased food intake. In particular, restraint theory has identified the disinhibition of restraint as characteristic of overeating in restrained eaters. The original study illustrating disinhibition (Herman & Mack, 1975) used a preload/taste test paradigm, and involved giving groups of dieters and non-dieters either a high calorie preload or a low calorie preload. The results indicated that whereas the non-dieters showed compensatory regulatory behaviour, and ate less after the high calorie preload, the dieters consumed more in the taste test if they had had the high calorie preload rather than the low calorie preload. This form of disinhibition or 'the what the hell effect' illustrates over-eating in response to a high-calorie preload. More general research has explored possible mechanisms for the over-eating shown by restrained eaters. These include the causal model of over-eating, cognitive shifts, mood modification, denial, escape theory and over-eating as relapse.

i) The causal analysis of over-eating

The causal analysis of eating behaviour was first described by Herman and Polivy who suggested that dieting and bingeing were causally linked and that 'restraint not only precedes overeating but contributes to it causally' (Herman & Polivy, 1988, p. 33). This suggests that attempting not to eat, paradoxically increases the probability of over-eating; the specific behaviour which dieters are attempting to avoid. The causal analysis of restraint represented a new approach to eating behaviour and the prediction that restraint actually caused over-eating was an interesting reappraisal of the situation. Wardle and Beales (1988) experimentally tested the causal analysis of over-eating and concluded that the over-eating shown by dieters is actually caused by attempts at dieting.

ii) Cognitive shifts

The over-eating found in dieters has also been understood in terms of shifts in the individual's cognitive set. Using experimental designs, research has highlighted two alternative cognitive shifts which seem to precipitate a state of over-eating. The first reflects a passive state involving 'motivational collapse' and a state of giving in to the overpowering drives to eat (Herman & Polivy, 1980) and the second reflects a more active state involving cognitions such as 'rebellious', 'challenging' and 'defiant' (Ogden & Greville, 1993). It has been argued that whilst at times over-eating may involve passively giving in to an overwhelming desire to eat, at other times the individual may actively decide to over-eat as a form of rebellion against self-imposed food restrictions.

iii) Mood modification

Dieters over-eat in response to lowered mood and researchers have argued that disinhibitory behaviour enables the individual to mask his or her negative mood with the temporarily heightened mood caused by eating. This has been called the 'masking hypothesis' and has been tested by empirical studies. For example, Polivy and Herman (1999) told female subjects that they had either passed or failed a cognitive task and then gave them food either ad libitum or in small controlled amounts. The results in part supported the masking hypothesis as the dieters who ate ad libitum attributed more of their distress to their eating behaviour than to the task failure. The authors argued that dieters may over-eat as a way of shifting responsibility for their negative mood from uncontrollable aspects of their lives to their eating behaviour.

iv) The role of denial

Cognitive research illustrates that thought suppression and thought control can have the paradoxical effect of making the thoughts that the individual is trying to suppress more salient (Wenzlaff & Wegner, 2000). This has been called the 'theory of ironic processes of mental control' (Wegner, 1994). For example, in an early study participants were asked to try not to think of a white bear but to ring a bell if they did (Wegner et al., 1999). The results showed that those who were trying not to think about the bear thought about the bear more frequently than those who were told to think about it. Similar results have been found for thinking about sex, mood and stigma (see Wenzlaff & Wegner, 2000). A decision not to eat specific foods or to eat less is central to the dieter's cognitive set. This results in a similar state of denial and attempted thought suppression and dieters have been shown to see food in terms of 'forbiddenness' and to show a preoccupation with the food that they are trying to deny themselves. Therefore, as soon as food is denied it simultaneously becomes forbidden and this translates into eating which undermines any attempts at weight loss.

v) Escape theory

Researchers have also used escape theory to explain over-eating (Heatherton & Baumeister, 1991; Heatherton et al., 1991). This perspective has been applied to both the over-eating characteristic of dieters and the more extreme form of binge eating found in bulimics and describes over-eating as a consequence of 'a motivated shift to low levels of self awareness' (Heatherton & Baumeister, 1991). It is argued that individuals prone to over-eating show comparisons with 'high standards and demanding ideals' (p. 89) and that this results in low self-esteem, self-dislike and lowered mood. It is also argued that inhibitions exist at high levels of awareness when the individual is aware of the meanings associated with certain behaviours. In terms of the over-eater, a state of high self-awareness can become unpleasant as it results in self-criticism and low mood. However such a state is accompanied by the existence of inhibitions. The individual is therefore motivated to escape from self-awareness to avoid the accompanying unpleasantness, but although such a shift in self-awareness may provide relief from self-criticism, it results in a reduction in inhibitions thereby causing over-eating. Within this analysis disinhibitory over-eating is indicative of a shift from high to low self-awareness and a subsequent reduction in inhibitions.

vi) Overeating as a relapse

Parallels exist between the under- and over-eating of the restrained eater and the behaviour of the relapsing smoker or alcoholic. The traditional biomedical perspective of addictive behaviours viewed addictions as being irreversible and out of the individual's control. It has been argued that this perspective encourages the belief that the behaviour is either 'all or nothing', and that this belief is responsible for the high relapse rate shown by both alcoholics and smokers (Marlatt & Gordon, 1985). Thus, the abstaining alcoholic believes in either total abstention or relapse, which itself may promote the progression from lapse to full-blown relapse. In the case of the restrained eater, it is possible that they too believe in the 'all or nothing' theory of excess which promotes the shift from a high calorie lapse to the 'what the hell' relapse characterized by disinhibition. These parallels have been supported by research suggesting that both excessive eating and alcohol use can be triggered by high risk situations and low mood (Grilo et al., 1989). In addition, the transition from lapse to relapse in both alcohol consumption and eating behaviour has been found to be related to the internal attributions (eg. 'I am to blame') for the original lapse (e.g. Ogden & Wardle, 1990).

In summary, diet relates to health both in terms of illness onset, prevention and treatment, however, many people do not always eat in accordance with current dietary recommendations. Psychological research has focused on three main theoretical perspectives to explain eating behaviour. A developmental approach emphasizes exposure and social and associative learning; a cognitive model emphasizes individuals' cognitions; and a weight concern model draws upon the literature relating to restrained eating and the causes of over-eating.

REFERENCES

Axelson, M. L., Brinberg, D. & Durand, J. H. (1983). Eating at a fast-food restaurant – a social–psychological analysis. *Journal of Nutrition Education*, 15, 94–8.

Birch, L. L. (1980). Effects of peer models' food choices and eating behaviors on preschoolers' food preferences. *Child Development*, 51, 489–96.

Birch, L. L. (1999). Development of food preferences. *Annual Review of Nutrition*, 19, 41–62.

Birch, L. L., Gunder, L., Grimm-Thomas, K. & Laing, D. G. (1998). Infant's consumption of a new food enhances acceptance of similar foods. *Appetite*, 30, 283–95.

Birch, L. L. & Marlin, D. W. (1982). I don't like it; I never tried it: effects of exposure on two-year-old children's food preferences. *Appetite*, 23, 353–60.

Birch, L. L., Zimmerman, S. & Hind, H. (1980). The influence of social affective context on preschool children's food preferences. *Child Development*, 51, 856–61.

Contento, I. R., Basch, C., Shea, S. et al. (1993). Relationship of mothers' food choice criteria to food intake of pre-school children: identification of family subgroups. *Health Education Quarterly*, 20, 243–59.

Department of Health (1991). *Dietary reference values for food energy and nutrients for the United Kingdom.*

(Report on health and social subjects no. 41). London: Her Majesty's Stationary Office.

Department of Health (1995). *Obesity: reversing an increasing problem of obesity in England. A report from the Nutrition and Physical activity task forces.* London: Her Majesty's Stationary Office.

Duncker, K. (1938). Experimental modification of children's food preferences through social suggestion. *Journal of Abnormal Social Psychology*, **33**, 489–507.

Grilo, C. M., Shiffman, S. & Wing, R. R. (1989). Relapse crisis and coping among dieters. *Journal of Consulting and Clinical Psychology*, **57**, 488–95.

Heatherton, T. F., Polivy, J. & Herman, C. P. (1991). Restraint, weight loss and variability of body weight. *Journal of Abnormal Psychology*, **100**, 78–83.

Heatherton, T. F. & Baumeister, R. F. (1991). Binge eating as an escape from self awareness. *Psychological Bulletin*, **110**, 86–108.

Herman C. P. & Polivy, J. A. (1988). Restraint and excess in dieters and bulimics. In K. M. Pirke & D. Ploog (Eds.). *The Psychobiology of Bulimia*. Berlin: Springer Verlag.

Herman, C. P., Polivy, J. & Saunders, W. B. (1980). Restrained eating. In A. J. Stunkard (Ed). *Obesity*. Philadelphia, London, Toronto.

Herman, P. & Mack, D. (1975). Restrained and Unrestrained Eating. *Journal of Personality*, **43**, 646–60.

Hursti, U. K. K. & Sjoden, P. O. (1997). Food and general neophobia and their relationship with self-reported food choice: familial resemblance in Swedish families with children of ages 7–17 years. *Appetite*, **29**, 89–103.

Kirkley, B. G., Burge, J. C., Ammerman, M. P. H. (1988). Dietary restraint binge eating and dietary behaviour patterns. *International Journal of Eating Disorders*, **7**, 771–78.

Klesges, R. C., Stein, R. J., Eck, L. H. *et al.* (1991). Parental influences on food selection in young children and its relationships to childhood obesity. *American Journal of Clinical Nutrition*, **53**, 859–64.

Laessle, R. G., Tuschl, R. J., Kotthaus, B. C. & Pirke, K. M. (1989). Behavioural and biological correlates of dietary restraint in normal life. *Appetite*, **12**, 83–94.

Lepper, M., Sagotsky, G., Dafoe, J. L. & Greene, D. (1982). Consequences of superfluous social constraints: effects on young children's social inferences and subsequent intrinsic interest. *Journal of Personality and Social Psychology*, **42**, 51–65.

Lowe C. F., Dowey, A. & Horne, P. (1998). Changing what children eat. In A. Murcott, (Ed.). *The nation's diet: the social science of food choice*, Addison Wesley Longman Ltd.

Marlatt, G. A. & Gordon, J. R. (1985). *Relapse prevention*. New York: Guilford Press.

Newman, J. & Taylor, A. (1992) Effect of a means-end contingency on young children's food preferences. *Journal of Experimental Psychology*, **64**, 200–16.

Ogden, J. (2003). *The psychology of eating: from healthy to disordered behaviour.* Blackwell: Oxford.

Ogden, J. & Greville, L. (1993). Cognitive changes to preloading in restrained and unrestrained eaters as measured by the Stroop task. *International Journal of Eating Disorders*, **14**, 185–95.

Ogden, J. & Wardle, J. (1990). Control of eating and attributional style. *British Journal of Clinical Psychology*, **29**, 445–6.

Olivera, S. A., Ellison, R. C., Moore, L. L. *et al.* (1992). Parent–child relationships in nutrient intake: the Framingham children's study, *American Journal of Clinical Nutrition*, **56**, 593–8.

Polivy, J. & Herman, C. P. (1999). The effects of resolving to diet on restrained and unrestrained eaters: a false hope syndrome. *International Journal of Eating Disorders*, **26**(4), 434–47.

Povey, R., Conner, M., Sparks, P., James, R. & Shepherd, R. (2000). The theory of planned behaviour and healthy eating: examining additive and moderating effects of social influence variables. *Psychology and Health*, **14**, 991–1006.

Raats, M. M., Shepherd R. & Sparks, P. (1995). Including moral dimensions of choice within ther structure of the theory of planned behavior. *Journal of Applied Social Psychology*, **25**, 484–94.

Shepherd, R. (1988). Belief structure in relation to low-fat milk consumption.

Journal of Human Nutrition and Dietetics, **1**, 421–8.

Shepherd, R. & Farleigh, C. A. (1986). Preferences, attitudes and personality as determinants of salt intake. *Human Nutrition: Applied Nutrition*, **40A**, 195–208.

Shepherd, R. & Stockley, L. (1987). Nutrition knowledge, attitudes, and fat consumption. *Journal of the American Dietetic Association*, **87**, 615–19.

Sparks, P., Hedderley, D. & Shepherd, R. (1992). An investigation into the relationship between perceived control, attitude variability and the consumption of two common foods. *European Journal of Social Psychology*, **22**, 55–71.

Sparks, P. & Shepherd, R. (1992). Self-identify and the theory of planned behavior: assessing the role of identification with green consumerism. *Social Psychology Quarterly*, **55**, 1388–99.

Sparks, P., Conner, M., James, R., Shepherd, R. & Povey, R. (2001). Ambivaleance about health-related behaviours: an exploration in the domain of food choice. *British Journal of Health Psychology*, **6**, 53–68.

Thompson, J. P., Palmer, R. L. & Petersen, S. A. (1988). Is there a metabolic component to counterregulation? *International Journal of Eating Disorders*, **7**, 307–19.

Wardle, J. & Beales, S. (1988). Control and loss of control over eating: an experimental investigation. *Journal of Abnormal Psychology*, **97**, 35–40.

Wardle, J., Steptoe, A., Bellisle, F. *et al.* (1997). Health dietary practices among European students. *Health Psychology*, **16**, 443–50.

Wegner, D. M. (1994). Ironic processes of mental control. *Psychological Review*, **101**, 34–52.

Wegner, D. M., Shortt, J. W., Blake, A. W. & Page, M. S. (1999). The suppression of exciting thoughts. *Journal of Personality and Social Psychology*, **58**, 409–18.

Wenzlaff, R. M. & Wegner, D. M. (2000). Thought suppression. *Annual review of Psychology*, **51**, 59–91.

Wing, R. R., Koeske, R., Epstein, L. H. *et al.* (1987). Long term effects of modest weight loss in Type II diabetic patients. *Archives of Internal Medicine*, **147**, 1749–53.

Disability

Timothy R. Elliott[1] and Laura Dreer[2]

[1]Texas A&M University
[2]University of Alabama at Birmingham

Disability has traditionally been defined by prevailing medical and legal systems across cultures. Less apparent have been social and technological contributions that substantially determine the experience of disability. The many and multidisciplinary definitions of disability in clinical, legal and academic life inadvertently compromise efforts to develop, sponsor and enact effective policy and service for persons who live with disabling conditions (Walkup, 2000).

Theoretical models of disability

The most pervasive definitions of disability have been provided by disciplines associated with healthcare delivery. Contemporary perspectives have evolved in response to the increase of chronic health conditions across societies generally, and from criticisms of the medical model that recognize the broader policy, psychological and socio-economic issues associated with the management of disabling conditions over time and throughout communities.

Medical model of disability

The medical model of disability is the traditional and predominant model. Essentially, healthcare services which flow from this model assume a 'find it and fix it' perspective: health problems are diagnosed and specialized services are prescribed to cure the problem (Kaplan, 2002). This perspective is most effective in the detection and treatment of acute health problems; so effective, in fact, that this model has guided the development and status of medical training, facilities and specialties. The medical model is also responsible for the rapid and effective response to the acute needs of persons with physical disabilities and other chronic health conditions, and the first initiatives to address issues of improved care, survival and quality of life can be attributed to professions who embraced the medical model. In the United States, medical definitions of disability provide the cornerstone for determining disability for legal and occupational purposes (and for determining eligibility for financial assistance; Chan & Leahy, 1999). This model places a clear and unambiguous premium on the diagnosis of a specific cause for a health problem, and on the expert delivery of a curative treatment. These treatments may include rehabilitative services and restorative training to enhance reintegration.

Despite the great benefits this model has endowed upon societies for decades, it has many practical limitations in contemporary applications. In the initial services provided to preserve life and allay acute problems following the onset of a physical disability (and for acute care needs for those living with disability) the value of the model is readily apparent. However, the model has difficulty accommodating the permanent and chronic trajectory of an incurable condition in which symptoms or impairments may be managed over the lifespan, and preventive and long-term changes in personal behaviour or to environmental constraints may be required for optimal health and quality of life (see 'Coping with chronic illness' and 'Quality of life'). The increasing number of persons with chronic health conditions across cultures is not adequately served by institutions which were designed to focus primarily on the delivery of acute, short-term conditions.

The medical model relies heavily on measures and tests of the disease process, and in this enterprise, the model places a lower value on the subjective report of quality of life and wellbeing, and by extension, to patient input concerning treatment options and recommendations for prescribed regimens. This is due, in part, to the occasional incongruence between subjective reports and objective indicators of disease activity. The successful diagnosis and treatment of acute conditions does not hinge solely on the accuracy or quality of patient input (see 'Disability assessment').

In fairness to the professions allied with the medical model, the measurement of functional ability (e.g. range of motion, impairment in activities of daily living, mobility) now characterizes studies of rehabilitation outcomes and occasionally these measures rely on participant self-report. These instruments still focus on residual deficits associated with the medical diagnosis, and with possible gains in response to the prescribed treatments for affected symptoms (Mermis, 2005).

The course of chronic disease and disability over the lifespan, however, is substantially influenced by behavioural and social mechanisms, and the medical model has limited capacity for assessing and making changes in these important domains. Additionally, the financial costs associated with chronic and disabling conditions have strained healthcare delivery systems grounded in this model. These costs have resulted in attempts to manage losses that include a decrease in available services to many persons with disability, and in a decrease in available insurance coverage for these individuals. Consequently, many persons with disability find greater impairment over time from systems which closely adhere to the medical model, as services are contingent upon reimbursement and the ability of specific programmes and their administrative systems to absorb financial losses incurred in providing services.

These issues have been addressed in contemporary revisions of the model by the Institute of Medicine. These revisions still rely on diagnostic categories but emphasize greater attention to the processes that place individuals at risk for disability (and secondary complications following disability) including biological, environmental, social, cultural and behavioural factors (Pope & Tarlov, 1991). The needs for active continuous and collaborative partnerships with the consumer, and for increased access to information and customized programmes of assistance are espoused to promote quality of life and optimal health (Institute of Medicine, 2001). In these important revisions of the model, greater emphasis is placed on behavioural and social factors in the ultimate health and wellbeing of persons living with disability.

The WHO model of disability

The limitations of the medical model have been familiar to advocates, consumers and other health care professions throughout the international community. An alternative perspective of disability was developed by the World Health Organization (WHO) in its seminal 1980 report, *International classification of impairments: disability and handicaps*. In this conceptualization, disability was construed across three separate levels of performance at the organ level (impairment), personal level (disability) and societal level (handicap). Although this was a distinct improvement over the medical model, it did not adequately address environmental issues that contribute to disablement and many consumers found the use of the term 'handicap' inappropriate (Heinemann, 2005).

In 2001, the WHO published the *International classification of functioning, disability, and health* (ICF; WHO, 2001). As depicted in Figure 1, the ICF used labels more appropriate to the disability experience and permitted separate ratings along dimensions of body structure and function/impairment at the organ level, activity (vs. activity limitation) at the person level and participation (vs. participation restriction) at the societal level. The scheme conceptualized environmental factors as important contributors of disability. It allows an analysis of disabling features across several dimensions and does not regard a specific medical diagnosis as a concept that determines disability. The WHO model has enjoyed support from many professions, advocates and consumer groups throughout the international community.

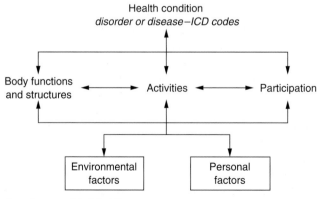

Fig 1 The ICF model of disability.

Alternative models

Several variations of the WHO model have been proposed by specific groups representing particular agencies (e.g. the 'new paradigm' of disability; the National Institute of Disability Research and Rehabilitation, 1999–2003) and from the disability studies literature (the social-constructionist view; Olkin, 1999). These models share a value on the civil rights of persons with disability, the need for access and opportunities for independent living and express a general disapproval of the medical model as a template for policy decisions concerning persons with disability. Disability is conceptualized in these models as a '... function of the person within the environment' (Brandt & Pope, 1997, p. 64). The individual is seen as the organizing core within these models, but impairments are defined and stipulated by the environmental and social contexts; indeed, the environment is construed as the '... major determinant of individual functioning' (Pledger, 2003, p. 281).

Yet these models do not clearly distinguish who qualifies as a person with a disability (or how disability is measured or determined), and they have yet to establish a distinct body of scholarship which systematically posits empirically testable and potentially falsifiable hypotheses that refine theory and advance knowledge (and, as such, lack essential properties required of scientific theories). In fact, some proponents appear to disregard the utility of theory and research in the psychological literature, generally, and construe psychological theory and scholarship as an embodiment of a medical model which conceptualizes disability as a pathological condition insensitive to the impact of environmental and social factors (see Olkin & Pledger, 2003).

Research evidence

Approximately 49.7 million people in the United States live with some type of long lasting condition or disability (U.S. Census Bureau, 2003). Of this number, 9.3 million (3.6%) have a sensory disability involving sight or hearing (see 'Blindness and visual disability' and 'Deafness and hearing loss'); 2.2 million (8.2%) have a condition limiting basic physical activities, such as walking, climbing stairs, reaching, lifting or carrying; 12.4 million (4.8%) live with a physical, mental or emotional condition causing difficulty in learning, remembering or concentrating; 6.8 million (2.6%) live with a physical, mental or emotional condition causing difficulty in dressing, bathing or getting around inside the home; 18.2 million of those aged 16 and older live with a condition that makes it difficult to go outside the home to shop or visit a doctor; and 21.3 million of those aged 16 to 64 live with a condition that affects their ability to work at a job or business. Disability rates escalate with age for both men and women (see 'Age and physical functioning') and 46.3% of people with any disability report more than one disabling condition. Persons between the ages of 16 and 64 are less likely to be employed if they are disabled and 8.7 million people with disabilities are poor (United States Census Bureau, 2003). These data are based on reports from only those persons who responded to the Census 2000 form and thus may significantly under-represent persons living with chronic disabilities in the United States. (See also 'Spinal cord injury').

Chronic health and disabling conditions are increasing throughout the world (World Health Organization, 2002). Within the next 15 years, it is estimated that chronic, disabling conditions and mental disorders will account for 78% of the global disease burden in developing countries (World Health Organization, 2002, p. 13). The disability experience can be influenced across cultures in terms of access to rehabilitative services; cultural stereotypes among service providers; differences in approaches to treating disabilities among different countries; service utilization and healthcare costs among different countries and cultures; disparities in the epidemiology of various disabilities at the international level; differences in governmental policies; collaborative efforts between healthcare providers and grassroots leaders; and differences in values and views of disability in various societies. Differences may also exist in cultural meanings attached to disability and quality of life, in attitudes and perceptions of disability, and the role of the family and society (Landrine & Klonoff, 1992; Murdick et al., 2004) (see 'Cultural and ethnic factors in health').

Many disabilities result from lifestyle factors which include unhealthy behaviours; consumption patterns; inadequate or improper prevention of disease, injuries and accidents and improper management of other chronic health conditions (World Health Organization, 2002). Well known health problems associated with disability include diabetes (American Diabetes Association, 2003), obesity (National Task Force on the Prevention and Treatment of Obesity, 2000), cardiovascular disease (Keil et al., 1989) and multiple visual impairments (Rudberg et al., 1993).

Costs of disability

Disability imposes serious economic consequences (World Health Organization, 2002). Direct and indirect costs associated with disability are expected to escalate with the increasing number of persons who will live with a disability over the next several decades (US Department of Health and Human Services, 2000). On average, persons with disabilities spend more than four times as much on medical care, services and equipment as their non-disabled counterparts (Max, Rice & Trupin, 1995). In general, higher healthcare costs are associated with chronic physical disability; secondary complications; loss in employment productivity; impaired quality of life; care and management of chronic disease and disability along with acute episodes of care associated with such conditions; and problems with psychosocial functioning (Hansen et al., 2002; Kessler et al., 2001; Tugwell, 2000).

Measuring disablement

Measuring different aspects of disability and outcomes associated with rehabilitation services has resulted in a number of empirically based instruments of disability which have advanced the science and practice of functional assessment and health services research (Heinemann, 2005; Mermis, 2005) (see 'Disability assessment'). These instruments are frequently used to 1) evaluate and quantify the extent of physical disability and capacity for self-care, 2) identify limitations for discharge and/or rehabilitation, 3) identify outcomes associated with rehabilitation interventions and 4) inform the identification of goals for rehabilitation. An example of one of the more widely used functional status measures is the Functional Independence Measure (FIM; Hamilton et al., 1987). The FIM was designed to rate the severity of disability and the outcomes of medical rehabilitation and has been successfully used with a variety of disabled populations.

The WHO models of disability spurred the development of instruments that measure several aspects of optimal adjustment and possible impairment (the Craig Handicap Assessment and Reporting Technique; Whiteneck et al., 1992) and the nature and extent of environmental factors (the Craig Hospital Inventory of Environmental Factors; CHIEF; Craig Hospital Research Department, 2001). Specifically, the CHIEF evaluates physical, environmental and architectural obstacles and other potential barriers (family, access to technology and information, employment issues, governmental policies, etc.).

Clinical implications

Clinical programmes for persons with disability vary according to the working models of disability. Medical perspectives traditionally place greater emphasis on the management of a specific diagnosis and related conditions (see 'Neuropsychological rehabilitation', 'pain management' and 'coronary heart disease: rehabilitation'); other health professions tend to focus their services on the individual with the disabling conditions and the persons who live with him or her, although many of these may recognize the need for policies that address environmental and social impediments. Consumers and their advocates are much more attuned to the demands and issues centred in the environmental and social context, with ensuing recommendations for alterations, accommodation and assistive devices that maximize independent functioning.

The WHO model of disability complements alternative models that represent advocacy and consumer perspectives. Thus, services that promote independent living with improved access to institutions, improve role functioning and mobility reduce disability across the dimensions in the WHO model. This also entails the effective and strategic provision and usage of assistive devices and enhanced computer technologies, and the removal of existing environmental barriers (Scherer, 2002).

Clinical services also benefit from the WHO model. Many legislated policies and services (e.g. vocational rehabilitation) have foundations in the medical model but also reflect advancements and the recognized need for technological assistance, improved access and adequate training and preparation to maximize functioning (Elliott & Jackson, 2005). Although acute medical rehabilitation maintains many characteristics associated with the medical model, service delivery systems and associated policies now urge greater attention to the necessity of collaborating partnerships with persons who live with a disabling condition and to increase community- and home-based services with ongoing access to information and support (Institute of Medicine, 2001; World Health Organization, 2002). Greater emphasis on health promotion for persons with disabling conditions will occur (Rimmer & Braddock, 2002).

Biopsychosocial models of health conditions permeate the psychological literature, generally, and these take into account the interactive effects of disease/disability parameters, psychosocial stressors and personal and environmental factors which account for varying degrees of adaptation. Biopsychosocial models of disability – usually developed to study adjustment associated with specific disability diagnoses (e.g. spinal cord injury, traumatic brain injury, multiple sclerosis) – proliferate in the rehabilitation psychology literature (see Frank & Elliott, 2000, for several examples). A recent conceptualization of adjustment following disability emphasizes the primacy of subjective, phenomenological appraisals of resources, stressors and contextual issues across diagnostic conditions (Elliott *et al.*, 2002). Appraisals of environmental assets and liabilities, functional abilities and activities are likely to influence self-reports of the dimensions stipulated in the WHO model of disability. Individual differences and other psychological characteristics usually account for greater variance in the prediction of adjustment among persons with disability than in any condition-specific variable (see 'Coping with chronic illness' and 'Coping with chronic pain').

Psychological interventions have demonstrated considerable impact in the treatment of specific adjustment issues among persons living with disability, and in enhancing role function in certain areas (e.g. return to work; Elliott & Jackson, in press; Elliott & Leung, 2005). The WHO model of disability offers tremendous opportunity for psychologists to further demonstrate the respectable utility and impact of research, service and interventions that are informed by psychological theory and expertise, and in this process, offer a more prominent role for psychology (Johnstone, 1997).

Conclusions

The WHO model of disability will emerge as the preferred perspective in the international community, due to its recognition of the many factors that determine the disability experience. This will inevitably increase conflict in western societies that subscribe to a medical model, as policy-makers will debate issues related to reimbursement, resource allocation and the development and management of institutions and service delivery programmes, generally. In these debates policy-makers will encounter influence from stakeholders who have invested in current systems.

Psychology has made important contributions within the traditional medical perspective of disability, and may exert a more influential role within the WHO framework. Psychological expertise in theory, measurement, research design and interventions can contribute to the development of informed, empirically driven and cost-effective health care delivery and policy formation. At times, however, tensions may occur as psychologists conduct theory-based and empirical studies which do not fit well within the medical model (e.g. the effectiveness of home-based interventions that promote wellness) or that seem to place greater weight on individual – rather than environmental – factors (e.g. individual characteristics that contaminate individual self-reports of environmental barriers, or that predict secondary complications and objective indicators of adjustment over time, independent of environmental and medical variables).

REFERENCES

American Diabetes Association (2003). Economic costs of diabetes in the U.S. in 2002. *Diabetes Care*, **26**, 917–32.

Brandt, E. N. & Pope, A. M. (Eds.). (1997). *Enabling America: assessing the role of rehabilitation science and engineering.* Washington, DC: National Academy Press.

Chan, F. & Leahy, M. (Eds.). (1999). *Health care and disability case management.* Lake Zurich, IL: Vocational Consultants Press.

Craig Hospital Research Department (2001). *Craig hospital inventory of environmental factors (CHIEF) Manual.* Englewood: Co. Craig Hospital, Colorado USA.

Elliott, T. & Jackson, W. T. (2005). Cognitive–behavioral therapy in rehabilitation psychology. In A. Freeman (Ed.). *Encyclopedia of cognitive behaviour therapy* (pp. 324–7). New York: Springer Science + Business Media, Inc.

Elliott, T., Kurylo, M. & Rivera, P. (2002). Positive growth following an acquired physical disability. In C. R. Snyder & S. Lopez (Eds.). *Handbook of positive psychology* (pp. 687–99). New York: Oxford University Press.

Elliott, T. & Leung, P. (2005). Vocational rehabilitation: history and practice. In W. B. Walsh & M. Savickas (Eds.). *Handbook of Vocational Psychology* (3rd edn.)

(pp. 319–43). New York: Lawrence Erlbaum Press.

Frank, R. G. & Elliott, T. (2000). *Handbook of rehabilitation psychology.* Washington, DC: American Psychological Association Press.

Hamilton, B. B., Granger, C. V., Sherwin, F. S., Zielezny, M. & Tashman, J. S. (1987). A uniform national data system for medical rehabilitation. In M. J. Fuhrer (Ed.). *Rehabilitation outcomes: analysis and measurement Vol. 10* (pp. 137–47). Baltimore: Brookes.

Hansen, M. S., Fink, P., Frydenberg, M. & Oxhoj, M. L. (2002). Use of health services, mental illness, and self-rated disability and health in medical inpatients. *Psychosomatic Medicine*, **64**, 668–75.

Heinemann, A. (2005). Putting outcome measurement in context: a rehabilitation psychology perspective. *Rehabilitation Psychology*, **50**, 6–14.

Institute of Medicine. (2001). *Crossing the quality chasm: a new health system for the 21st century.* Washington, DC: National Academy Press.

Johnstone, M. (1997). Representations of disability. In J. A. Weinman & K. J. Petrie, (Eds.). *Perceptions of health and illness: current research and*

applications (pp. 189–212). Amsterdam, Netherlands: Harwood Academic Publishers.

Kaplan, R. M. (2002). Quality of life: an outcomes perspective. *Archives of Physical Medicine and Rehabilitation*, **83**, Suppl. 2, S44–S50.

Keil, J. E., Gazes, P. C., Sutherland, S. E., Rust, P. F., Branch, L. G. & Tyroler, H. A. (1989). Predictors of physical disability in elderly blacks and whites of the Charleston Heart Study. *Journal of Clinical Epidemiology*, **42**, 521–29.

Kessler, R. C., Greenberg, P. E., Mickelson, K. D., Meneades, L. M. & Wang, P. S. (2001). The effects of chronic medical conditions on work loss and work cutback. *Journal of Occupational and Environmental Medicine*, **43**, 218–25.

Landrine, H. & Klonoff, E. A. (1992). Culture and health-related schema: a review and proposal for interdisciplinary integration. *Health Psychology*, **11**, 267–76.

Max, W., Rice, D. P. & Trupin, L. (1995). Medical expenditures for people with disabilities. *Disability Statistics Abstract, Number 12.* Washington, DC: US Department of Education, National Institute on Disability and Rehabilitation Research (NIDDR).

Mermis, B. J. (2005). Developing a taxonomy for rehabilitation outcome measurement. *Rehabilitation Psychology*, **50**, 15–23.

Murdick, N., Shore, P., Chittooran, M. M. & Gartin, B. (2004). Cross-cultural comparison of the concept of "otherness" and its impact on persons with disabilities. *Education and Training in Developmental Disabilities*, **39**, 310–16.

National Institute on Disability and Rehabilitation Research (1999). NIDRR long-range plan. *Federal Register*, 68578, Washington DC, USA.

National Task Force on the Prevention and Treatment of Obesity (2000). Overweight, obesity, and health risk. *Archives of Internal Medicine*, **160**, 898–904.

Olkin, R. (1999). *What psychotherapists should know about disability*. New York: Guilford Press.

Olkin, R. & Pledger, C. (2003). Can disability studies and psychology join hands? *American Psychologist*, **58**, 296–304.

Pledger, C. (2003). Discourse on disability and rehabilitation issues: opportunities for psychology. *American Psychologist*, **58**, 279–84.

Pope, A. M. & Tarlov, A. R. (Eds.). (1991). *Disability in America: toward a national agenda for prevention*. Washington, DC: National Academy Press.

Rimmer, J. H. & Braddock, D. (2002). Health promotion for people with physical, cognitive, and sensory disabilities: an emerging national priority. *American Journal of Health Promotion*, **16**, 220–4.

Rudberg, M. A., Furner, S. E., Dunn, J. E. & Cassel, C. K. (1993). The relationship of visual and hearing impairments to disability: an analysis using the longitudinal study of aging. *Journal of Gerontology*, **48**, M261–M265.

Scherer, M. (Ed.). (2002). *Assistive technology: matching device and consumer for successful rehabilitation*. Washington, DC: American Psychological Association.

Tugwell, P. (2000). Pharmacoeconomics of drug therapy for rheumatoid arthritis. *Rheumatology*, **39**(Suppl.), 43–7.

US Census Bureau. (2003). *Disability status: 2000*. US Department of Commerce: Economics and Statistics Administration, Washington DC, USA.

US Department of Health and Human Services. (2000). *Healthy people 2010*. Washington, DC: US Department of Health and Human Services.

Walkup, J. (2000). Disability, health care, and public policy. *Rehabilitation Psychology*, **45**, 409–22.

Whiteneck, G., Brooks, C., Charlifue, S. *et al.* (1992). *Guide for use of CHART: Craig hospital assessment and reporting technique*. Englewood, CO: Craig Hospital.

World Health Organization (1980). *International classification of impairments, disabilities, and handicaps: a manual of classification relating to the consequences of disease*. Geneva, Switzerland: WHO.

World Health Organization (2001). *International classification of functioning, disability, and health*. Geneva, Switzerland: WHO.

World Health Organization (2002). *Innovative care for chronic conditions: building blocks for action*. Geneva, Switzerland: WHO.

Emotional expression and health

Richard B. Slatcher and James W. Pennebaker

The University of Texas at Austin

A longstanding puzzle within psychology and psychosomatic medicine concerns the relationship between the expression of emotions and physical health. Descartes and Shakespeare suggested that not expressing powerful emotions could be unhealthy. Similarly, William James (1890) and Franz Alexander (1950) forcefully argued that inhibiting the expression of strong emotions over time could result in physical health problems through basic biological stress-related channels (see 'Psychoneuroimmunology' and 'Psychosomatics'). Despite these early hypotheses, there is still no overwhelming evidence to support the idea that the suppression of emotional expression is unhealthy and, conversely, that the open expression of emotions is beneficial.

Emotional expression has been viewed by our culture somewhat ambivalently. On the one hand, emotional expression is often viewed as rather uncivilized, as 'giving in' to passion (King & Emmons, 1990, p. 864). On the other hand, it is assumed that emotions usually should be let out, that the healthy end to an emotional response is emotional expression. This view is especially common in the psychological literature. From Breuer and Freud (1895/1966) to the present (e.g. Cole *et al.*, 1996; Pelletier, 1985) the inherent value of naturally expressing one's thoughts and feelings has been emphasized. Emotional expression is thus viewed as a somewhat unseemly but normal part of everyday life.

While emotional expression is a normative behaviour which is neither good nor bad per se, actively holding back emotion through inhibition may have negative health consequences. Much of the literature examining the links between emotional expression and health has focused on the consequences of inhibition (Cole *et al.*, 1996; Gross & Levenson, 1997; Traue & Deighton, 1999). The findings from these studies suggest that actively holding back thoughts, emotions or behaviours can be a form of stress that exacerbates a number of adverse biological processes, such as increased cortisol production and immune suppression (Traue & Deighton, 1999). By expressing emotions, one may be able to organize and assimilate previously inhibited thoughts and feelings, thus bypassing the need for further inhibition. Several correlational studies have hinted that such processes may be at work (Cole *et al.*, 1996; Gross & Levenson, 1997; Major & Gramzow, 1999).

Certain life events may be more likely than others to have deleterious health consequences because of their links to emotional expression. Those events that produce the most conflict are ones that are most difficult to share with others – sexual abuse, being fired from one's job, having a stigmatizing disease, marital infidelity and other potentially traumatic experiences (see 'Intimate partner violence' and 'Post-traumatic stress disorder'). Under such circumstances, individuals often try to inhibit thoughts and feelings about their experiences. Often, attempts at thought suppression may actually lead to an increase in thoughts about the very experience that they are trying to erase from memory (Wegner, 1984). Such inhibition, especially if it continues for extended periods of time, can exacerbate stress, and, in turn, lead to declines in immune system functioning and other markers of physical health.

In recent years there has been a rapid growth in research examining emotional expression and health, but a large number of questions remain unanswered. For example, to what extent does the expression of emotions bring about changes in people's psychological and social worlds? Are some people more likely then others to benefit from emotional expression? What are the cognitive, linguistic and social mechanisms that link emotional expression to health outcomes? One method that has been used to test the effects of emotional expression – expressive writing – is particularly relevant to our understanding of the links among upheavals, emotion, language and health. Included in this overview will be a discussion of some of the underlying processes that may help to explain some of the powerful effects associated with emotional expression.

Testing the relationship between emotional expression and health: expressive writing

There are a number of ways in which people are able to express their thoughts and emotions about important events in their lives. Beyond simple venting, perhaps most common is that people talk to others. This translation of an emotional experience into language is also the basis of expressive writing. In 1986, Pennebaker and Beall published the first expressive writing study. In that and subsequent studies, when people were asked to write about their emotional upheavals over a period of 3–4 days for 15–30 minutes per day, they exhibited improvements in physical health relative to controls who had been randomly assigned to write about superficial topics. The initial studies focused on physician visits to the student health centre as an outcome measure. Later studies expanded these findings to various health indicators, such as blastogenesis measures, CD4 counts, liver enzymes and other biological markers (Pennebaker, 1997). About 10 years ago, multiple labs around the world began testing the expressive writing intervention with generally positive results. Meta-analyses of the writing paradigm have suggested that this method produces positive effects for various markers of physical health (Smyth, 1998; Frattaroli, 2006).

In recent years, the number of expressive writing studies has grown exponentially. Multiple studies have examined the effectiveness of expressive writing in the treatment of AIDS, diabetes, cancer and other physical health problems. A wide variation of writing instructions have been tried across an enormous range of participant populations. As more studies have been conducted, we are now beginning to get a sense of some of the boundary conditions of writing.

Expressive writing is not a panacea. Although an early meta-analysis by Smyth (1998) found that the effect size of writing on objective health outcomes was 0.67, these effects were based on relatively healthy samples. More recent meta-analyses with medical samples suggest that effect sizes for clinical trials are smaller ($d = 0.21$) but still significant (Frisina *et al.*, 2004). Because virtually no writing studies could be classified as true RCTs, a recent Cochrane Report concluded that the use of writing as a medical intervention was still in the 'not proven' category (Meads, 2003). But since the Meads report was completed, several promising medical studies have been completed (e.g. Taylor *et al.*, 2003; Petrie *et al.*, 2004; Solano *et al.*, 2003).

Although the overall effect size of the intervention is modest several weeks or months afterwards, given its low cost and minimal adverse effects, the findings continue to be promising. The health benefits for writing are evident in measures of physical and mental health and hold up across samples of widely varying social class, ethnicity, language and cultures. It may be more effective for people dealing with more traumatic than expected upheavals and with events that happened several weeks or months after the event as opposed to immediately afterwards.

Why does expressive writing work? The search for mechanisms

While there is now solid evidence that disclosing emotional experiences can be healthy, one of the more intriguing aspects of this phenomenon has been trying to develop theories that best explain it. Over the years, theoretical views in this area have evolved tremendously. These theories are outlined briefly below.

Inhibitory processes

One of the first theories to explain the effectiveness of expressive writing dealt with inhibition. But direct tests of changes in inhibition following emotional disclosure have yielded disappointing results. For example, participants who claim that they have not previously disclosed their traumas have not differed in health outcomes versus those who have disclosed their traumas (Greenberg *et al.*, 1996). In addition, individuals have great difficulty answering (or even understanding) questions that ask them the degree to which they are actively inhibiting their thoughts, emotions or behaviours (Pennebaker *et al.*, 1988). Thus, at this point, the inhibition model is still unproven.

Cognitive processes

Another explanation for the effects of expressive writing is that the act of converting emotions and images into words changes the way a person cognitively organizes and thinks about an emotional experience. By integrating thoughts and feelings about an emotional experience, one can then construct a coherent narrative of that experience. Once this integration takes place, the event can be summarized, stored and forgotten more efficiently. Various cognitive models have focused on different facets of cognitive construction and narrative construction. Smyth and his colleagues (1999), for example, have assumed that emotional expression fundamentally organizes an upsetting experience. As an indirect test of this, the authors asked people to write about a trauma in either an organized or an unstructured way. Only the organized writing resulted in health and mood improvements.

Using a different analysis strategy of looking directly at the ways individuals express emotions, several researchers are now finding support for the idea that constructing a narrative over the course of writing about emotional topics helps individuals to better integrate the experience. Specifically, by looking at word usage (e.g. an increasing use of cognitive words over the days of writing), health improvements are efficiently predicted. These word patterns have now been reported in multiple studies (e.g. Campbell & Pennebaker, 2003; Klein & Boals, 2001).

Social integration

Emotional expression, by nature, is an inherently social actively. The ultimate purpose of language is to communicate ideas and thoughts with other people. When someone talks to other people about his or her experiences, it alerts them to the person's psychological state and, ultimately, allows him or her to remain socially tied to them. Conversely, people who have traumatic experiences and do not tell their friends are more likely to live in a detached, isolated state. Consistent with this approach, Rimé (1995) argues that disclosure in the first days or weeks after a trauma has the power to change the quality of a person's social network by bringing people closer together. Disclosure, then, serves as a force of social integration. Rimé suggests that even private disclosure (as well as with writing) helps free a person from the stress of a non-disclosed

event, which ultimately allows for greater social integration. This is consistent with many of the social integration ideas first suggested by Durkheim (1951) wherein mental health was viewed as the result of the relationship between individuals and their social worlds (see 'Social support and health').

Researchers are now examining the social effects of expressive writing. In one pilot study, Matthias Mehl and the second author asked 52 participants to wear a re-engineered tape recorder called the Electronically Activated Recorder (EAR) as a part of an expressive writing experiment (discussed in Pennebaker & Graybeal, 2001). After the writing manipulation, those in the expressive writing group changed how they interacted with others, exhibiting significant increases in interactions with others, use of self-references and the use of emotion words. Similarly, another recent study examined social interaction patterns before and after expressive writing among 95 bilingual participants whose first language was either Spanish or Korean (Kim, 2004). Compared with controls, those in the experimental condition increased in their amount of talking to others in the days following expressive writing. While social integration theory still has not been fully tested, these preliminary findings have been encouraging.

Conclusion

Expressive writing studies have yielded important new ways to think about how emotional expression can encourage mental and physical health improvements. The mechanisms underlying this effect are still unclear but, in all likelihood, there is no single mediating influence between expressive writing and health. Perceptual, cognitive, emotional, linguistic and social processes all undoubtedly contribute and influence each other. Rather than continuing the task of trying to learn which of these features contributes the most or is the most pivotal, future research should draw on all of these processes in trying to maximize the salutary effects of emotional expression.

REFERENCES

Alexander, F. (1950). *Psychosomatic Medicine*. New York: Norton.

Breuer, J. & Freud, S. (1966). *Studies on hysteria*. New York: Avon. (Original work published 1895).

Campbell, R. S. & Pennebaker, J. W. (2003). The secret life of pronouns: Flexibility in writing style and physical health. *Psychological Science*, **14**, 60–5.

Cole, S. W., Kemeny, M. E., Taylor, S. E. & Visscher, B. R. (1996). Elevated physical health risk among gay men who conceal their homosexual identity. *Health Psychology*, **15**, 243–51.

Durkheim, E. (1951). *Suicide*. New York: Free Press.

Frattaroli, J. (2006). Experimental disclosure and its moderators : a meta-analysis. *Psychological Bulletin*, **132**, 823–65.

Frisina, P. G., Borod, J. C. & Lepore, S. J. (2004). A meta-analysis of the effects of

written disclosure on the health outcomes of clinical populations. *The Journal of Nervous and Mental Disease*, **192**, 629–34.

Greenberg, M. A., Stone, A. A. & Wortman, C. B. (1996). Health and psychological effects of emotional disclosure: a test of the inhibition-confrontation approach. *Journal of Personality and Social Psychology*, **71**, 588–602.

Gross, J. J. & Levenson, R. W. (1997). Hiding feelings: the acute effects of inhibiting negative and positive emotion. *Journal of Abnormal Psychology*, **106**, 95–103.

James, W. (1890). *The principles of psychology*. New York: H. Holt and Co.

Kim, Y. (2004). Effects of expressive writing among Mexican and Korean bilinguals on social,physical, and mental well-being. Unpublished doctoral dissertation, University of Texas, Austin.

King, L. A. & Emmons, R. A. (1990). Conflict over emotional expression: psychological and physical correlates. *Journal of Personality and Social Psychology*, **58**, 864–77.

Klein, K. & Boals, A. (2001). Expressive writing can increase working memory capacity. *Journal of Experimental Psychology: General*, **130**, 520–33.

Major, B. & Gramzow, R. (1999). Abortion as stigma: cognitive and emotional implications of concealment. *Journal of Personality and Social Psychology*, **77**, 735–45.

Meads, C. (2003, October). *How effective are emotional disclosure interventions? A systematic review with meta-analyses*. Paper given at the 3rd International Conference on The (Non)Expression of Emotions in Health and Disease. Tilburg, NL.

Pennebaker, J. W. (1997). Writing about emotional experiences as a therapeutic process. *Psychological Science*, **8**, 162–6.

Pennebaker, J. W. & Beall, S. K. (1986). Confronting a traumatic event: toward an understanding of inhibition and disease. *Journal of Abnormal Psychology*, **95**, 274–81.

Pennebaker, J. W., Kiecolt-Glaser, J. & Glaser, R. (1988). Disclosure of traumas and immune function: health implications for psychotherapy. *Journal of Consulting and Clinical Psychology*, **56**, 239–45.

Pennebaker, J. W. & Graybeal, A. (2001). Patterns of natural language use: disclosure, personality, and social integration. *Current Directions in Psychological Science*, **10**, 90–3.

Pelletier, K. R. (1985). *Mind as healer, mind as slayer.* New York: Delacorte Press.

Petrie, K. J., Fontanilla, I., Thomas, M. G., Booth, R. J. & Pennebaker, J. W. (2004).

Effect of written emotional expression on immune function in patients with HIV infection: a randomized trial. *Psychosomatic Medicine*, **66**, 272–5.

Rimé, B. (1995). Mental rumination, social sharing, and the recovery from emotional exposure. In J. W. Pennebaker (Ed.). *Emotion, disclosure, and health* (pp. 271–91). Washington, DC: American Psychological Association.

Solano, L., Donati, V., Pecci, F., Persichetti, S. & Colaci, A. (2003). Post-operative course after papilloma resection: effects of written disclosure of the experience in subjects with different alexithymia levels. *Psychosomatic Medicine*, **65**, 477–84.

Smyth, J. M. (1998). Written emotional expression: effect sizes, outcome types, and moderating variables. *Journal of Consulting and Clinical Psychology*, **66**, 174–84.

Smyth, J. M., Stone, A. A., Hurewitz, A. & Kaell, A. (1999). Effects of writing about stressful experiences on symptom reduction in patients with asthma or rheumatoid arthritis: a randomized trial. *Journal of the American Medical Association*, **14**, 1304–9.

Taylor, L., Wallander, J., Anderson, D., Beasley, P. & Brown, R. (2003). Improving chronic disease utilization, health status, and adjustment in adolescents and young adults with cystic fibrosis. *Journal of Clinical Psychology in Medical Settings*, **10**, 9–16.

Traue, H. C. & Deighton, R. (1999). Inhibition, disclosure, and health: don't simply slash the Gordian knot. *Advances in Mind–Body Medicine*, **15**, 184–93.

Wegner, D. M. (1994). Ironic processes of mental control. *Psychological Review*, **101**, 34–52.

Expectations and health

James E. Maddux

George Mason University

The major health care challenge in the twenty-first century, as it was at the close of the twentieth century, will be motivating people to make changes in their own behaviour in ways that reduce the risk of health and medical problems and enhance health. These motivational efforts must consist not only of educating people about the positive and negative effects of various behaviours but also, and perhaps more importantly, persuading people that they indeed *can* change their behaviour and teaching them the skills for doing so. For this reason, understanding self-regulation – the capacity of people to think about the future, set goals, develop plans to attain these goals, and regulate their own behaviour based on these goals and plans – will be crucial to solving the health and medical problems of the twenty-first century (see 'Health-related behaviours').

Self-regulation consists of several key components, including setting goals, developing plans, monitoring progress towards goals and modifying one's plans and behaviours in reaction to perceived progress towards one's goals. At the heart of the ability to self-regulate is the ability to develop expectancies – to use past experience and knowledge to form beliefs about and predict future events (Olson *et al.*, 1996). The expectancy construct is among the most thoroughly investigated constructs in psychology. Expectancies

gained importance with the development of social learning theory, as originally developed by Rotter (1954) (see also Woodward, 1982). As social learning theory evolved, it became more explicitly cognitive, as in Bandura's (1986) social cognitive theory and Mischel's (1973) cognitive social learning theory and expectancies were given increasing importance. All of the major models of health behaviour are social cognitive models and feature expectancies as key concepts. Among these are the health belief model (Janz & Becker, 1984), protection motivation theory (Maddux & Rogers, 1983; Rogers, 1975), the theory of reasoned action/planned behaviour (Fishbein & Ajzen, 1975; Ajzen, 1988), (Bandura, 1977), precaution adoption theory (Weinstein, 1988), self-efficacy theory (Bandura, 1977) and the health action process approach (Schwarzer, 1992). These models essentially deal with the same social cognitive determinants while giving them different names and rearranging them in different ways (Maddux, 1993; Weinstein, 1993; Bandura, 2004) (see 'The Health belief model', 'Self-efficacy and health behaviour', 'Theory of planned behaviour').

The influence of expectancies on health behaviour can only be understood if placed in the context of a general model or theory that describes different types of expectancies, their relationships with each other and their relationships with non-expectancies variables. Fortunately, we do not have to examine every theory in detail to achieve a basic understanding of expectancies and behaviour. Regardless of their differences, these models share several basic principles and hypothesized processes about human behaviour.

The principle of reciprocal causation proposes that environmental events, cognition, emotion and behaviour are mutually interactive influences. People respond cognitively, emotionally, and behaviourally to environmental events, but through cognition they also exercise control over their own behaviour, which then influences not only the environment but also cognitive, emotional and biological states.

The principle of the centrality of cognitive construals proposes that people have powerful symbolizing capabilities which enable them to cognitively construe (construct or build) their worlds. These cognitive construals have the great influence over behaviour and emotions. People attempt to explain events which have occurred and to predict future events so that they can control them. People develop expectancies about their ability to exercise those competencies under specific conditions, and expectancies about the consequences of exercising those competencies in certain situations. These explanations and expectancies greatly influence how people behave. The capacity for cognition also includes the capacity for consciousness, self-awareness, and self-reflection. People observe their own behaviours, thoughts, and feelings. They evaluate their ongoing behaviour based on how well it is working to accomplish their situational aims and objectives.

These cognitive abilities provide people with the tools for self-regulation or self-management. People envision goals and develop plans to attain those goals. They create incentives which motivate and guide their behaviour. They develop standards for their ongoing behaviour, evaluate their behaviour against these standards and then make strategic choices about their behaviour based on these standards.

The principle of the social embeddedness of the self proposes that people define themselves largely by what they think about, how they feel about and how they behave toward other people. The individual's behaviour is influenced and shaped by other people and by what the individual expects other people to think, feel and do in response to his or her behaviour. The most important learning is social learning – what people learn from other people about how to think, feel and behave. The most important cognitions are social cognitions – explanations and predictions about the behaviours, thoughts, and feelings of other people. 'Self' and 'personality' are perceptions (accurate or not) of one's own and others' patterns of social cognition, emotion and action as they occur in patterns of situations. Thus, self and personality are inextricably embedded in social contexts.

Expectancies and health behaviour

Various expectancy theories have proposed a wide variety of expectancies and an even wider variety of labels for the various types of expectancies. Research has linked each of these expectancies in significant ways to health behaviour.

Behaviour–outcome expectancy

A behaviour–outcome expectancy (as it was termed by Mischel, 1973) is a belief about the contingency between a specific behaviour and a specific outcome (result, consequence) or set of outcomes in a particular situation. Other names include expectancy for behaviour reinforcement sequence (Rotter, 1954), outcome expectancy (Bandura, 1977), means–end belief (Kirsch, 1995), action–outcome expectancy (Heckhausen, 1977), response–stimulus expectancy (Bolles, 1972), response–reinforcer association (Rescorla, 1987) and, simply, expectancy (Vroom, 1964). The theory of reasoned action (Fishbein & Ajzen, 1975) and the theory of planned behaviour (Ajzen, 1988) include behaviour–outcome expectancy in the assessment of two major predictors of behavioural intentions – attitudes towards the behaviour and social norms regarding the behaviour. Both constructs are assessed by asking people what outcomes they expect to result from the behaviour in question and how much importance (value) they place on those outcomes (Bandura, 2004). (See also 'Perceived control'.)

Behaviour–outcome expectancies influence health behaviour because people make decisions about their health behaviour based partly on their beliefs about the possible consequences of certain behaviours – such as the belief that using condoms will help prevent sexually transmitted diseases or the belief that regular exercise will help prevent heart disease (Bandura, 2004; Maddux, 1993).

Two kinds of behaviour–outcome expectancies can be distinguished based on two different kind of outcomes: environmental events and non-volitional responses such as a emotional reactions, sexual arousal and pain. A behaviour–stimulus expectancy (or response–stimulus expectancy; Kirsch, 1999) is the expectancy that a behaviour will lead to an environmental event. A behaviour–response expectancy (or response–response expectancy; Kirsch, 1999) is the expectancy that a behaviour will lead to a non-volitional response. Both types are important in understanding health behaviour. People who exercise to reduce risk of heart disease want to prevent these illnesses because they are painful, debilitating and possibly deadly. In addition, the major desired outcomes which lead people to exercise regularly are feelings of physical and psychological wellbeing, and among the major 'costs' associated with exercise are non-volitional responses such as fatigue, discomfort and pain.

Health behaviours are also influenced by social expectations – that is, by how people expect other people to respond (e.g. expected approval or disapproval). Major changes in a person's health behaviour, especially changes in lifestyle such as dietary changes and adopting an exercise regimen, can greatly affect other people, especially friends and family members. Expectancies for approval and support from close others can greatly facilitate behaviour change while expectancies for disapproval and resistance can discourage its initiation and maintenance. Thus, effectively changing sexual behaviour, substance use or abuse, diet and exercise can often depend heavily on a person's ability to manage close relationships and the emotions inherent in these relationships. These social expectancies are examples of behaviour–stimulus expectancies (see 'Social support and health').

Bandura offers an alternative way of categorizing behaviour–outcome expectancies relevant to health behaviour (Bandura, 2004). Physical behaviour–outcome expectancies pertain to the pleasurable and aversive outcomes of the behaviour (behaviour–response expectancies) and to material losses and benefits (behaviour–stimulus expectancies). Social behaviour–outcome expectancies pertain to the social approval and disapproval of other people regarding the behaviour. Finally, self-evaluative expectancies are concerned with one's own positive and negative reactions to one's health behaviour and health status (e.g. self-approval/disapproval; self-satisfaction/dissatisfaction). These self-evaluative expectancies can be viewed as either behaviour–response expectancies or behaviour–stimulus expectancies, depending on the extent to which one believes that self-evaluative reactions are within volitional control.

Stimulus–outcome expectancy

Stimulus–outcome expectancies are expectancies that certain events signal the possible occurrence of other events (Mischel, 1973; Bolles, 1972; Rotter, 1954; Vroom, 1964; Heckhausen, 1977). For example, a siren predicts the appearance of a police car, fire engine or ambulance; the worsening of a smoker's cough may be viewed as a predictor of lung disease; or the presence of a lump in a breast may be viewed as a sign of breast cancer.

Stimulus–outcome expectancies can be divided into two types based on the distinction between environmental events and non-volitional responses. A 'stimulus–stimulus expectancy' (Kirsch, 1999) is the expectancy that a stimulus signals the probable occurrence of an external environmental event (e.g. a dark cloud predicts rain). A 'stimulus–response expectancy' (Kirsch, 1999) is the expectancy that a stimulus signals the probable occurrence of a non-volitional response (e.g. watching a sad movie might make one cry). Both types of expectancies can influence health behaviour. I may decide not to go running this evening because I believe that the clouds I see predict rain soon (stimulus–stimulus expectancy). A diabetic may avoid regularly testing his or her level of insulin because he finds the procedure painful (stimulus–response expectancy).

Expectancies and outcome value

The power of expectancies over behaviour depends directly on the importance or value (positive or negative) which people place on what they expect. Outcome value is the value or importance attached to specific outcomes in specific situations (Rotter, 1982; Mischel, 1973; McClelland, 1985). Outcomes can be either (external) stimulus events or (internal) non-volitional responses. An outcome can be valued because we wish to attain it (money, better health) or because we wish to avoid it (e.g. paint, fatigue, cancer, obesity). In most social cognitive models of health behaviour, such as protection–motivation theory (e.g. Maddux & Rogers, 1983; Rogers, 1975) and the health belief model (e.g. Janz & Becker, 1984), the perceived severity of the health threat is an outcome value (Maddux, 1993). In the theory of reasoned action/planned behaviour, outcome value is evident in the assessment of attitudes and social norms because both are measured as the product of

behaviour–outcome expectancies and the value of those expected outcomes. The values of outcomes are not static but can change over time. For example, people often begin exercise programmes for the expected physical health and appearance benefits, but over time mood enhancement and social benefits become increasingly important incentives (Hsiao & Thayer, 1998). The importance of outcome value in numerous health-related behaviours has been demonstrated by a considerable body of research (e.g. Strecher et al., 1997; Rogers & Prentice-Dunn, 1997).

Self-efficacy expectancy

A self-efficacy expectancy is a belief in one's ability to perform a specific behaviour or set of behaviours under specific conditions and to 'mobilize the motivation, cognitive resources, and courses of action to exercise control' (Bandura, 1990, p. 316) over a specific task demanded in a specific situation. Self-efficacy expectancies are not competencies. Competencies are what people know about the world and what they are capable of doing in the world (Mischel, 1973). Self-efficacy beliefs are beliefs (accurate or not) about one's competencies and one's ability to exercise these competencies in certain domains and situations. Self-efficacy beliefs are not intentions to behave or intentions to attain particular goals. Intentions are what people say they are committed to doing or accomplishing, not what they believe they accomplish. Self-efficacy expectancies are not causal attributions. Casual attributions are explanations for events, including one's own behaviour and its consequences. Self-efficacy beliefs can influence causal attributions and vice versa because beliefs about competencies can influence explanations of success and failure and because explanations for success and failure will, in turn, influence perceptions of competence (Bandura, 1997). Finally, self-efficacy expectancies are not traits – they are beliefs about the ability to coordinate skills and abilities to attain desired goals in particular domains and circumstances. Self-efficacy beliefs can generalize from one situation or task to another, depending on the similarities between the task demands and the skills and resources required for meeting those demands (e.g. Samuels & Gibb, 2002), but self-efficacy in a specific domain does not emanate from a general sense of efficacy. Measures of traits, such as optimism and perceived control, seem to predict behaviour only to the extent to which they overlap with the measurement of self-efficacy (Dzewaltowski et al., 1990). In addition, measures of global efficacy beliefs have been developed (e.g. Sherer et al., 1982; Tipton & Worthington, 1984) and are used frequently in research, but generally they do not predict behaviour as well as domain-specific self-efficacy measures.

Self-efficacy expectancies influence health behaviour in several ways. First, they influence the health-related goals which people set for themselves. People who feel more self-efficacious set more challenging goals for their health. Second, they influence people's reactions to the inevitable setbacks which occur when people try to alter long-standing habits or adopt new, healthier habits. People with stronger self-efficacy expectancies are more like to be resilient and persistent in the face of barriers to change than are people with weaker self-efficacy beliefs, partly because they are less likely to experience the debilitating self-doubt and despondency that so often results from encountering barrier and setbacks.

Research on self-efficacy has greatly enhanced our understanding of how and why people adopt healthy and unhealthy behaviours and of how to change behaviours which affect health (Bandura, 1997; Maddux *et al.*, 1995; O'Leary & Brown, 1995). All of the major theories of health behaviour noted previously (protection motivation theory; health belief model, theory of reasoned action/planned behaviour; precaution adoption model; health action process approach) include self-efficacy as a key component. Research indicates that self-efficacy beliefs are crucial to successful change and maintenance of virtually every behaviour crucial to health – including exercise, diet, stress management, safe sex, smoking cessation, overcoming alcohol abuse, compliance with treatment and prevention regimens and detection behaviours such as breast self-examinations (Bandura, 2004, 1997; Maddux *et al.*, 1995; Maddux & Gosselin, 2003).

Self-efficacy beliefs not only influence behaviour, but they also influence a number of biological processes which, in turn, influence health and disease (Bandura, 1997). Self-efficacy beliefs affect the body's physiological responses to stress, including the immune system (Bandura, 1997; O'Leary & Brown, 1995) and the physiological pathways activated by physical activity (Rudolph & McAuley, 1995). Lack of perceived control over environmental demands can increase susceptibility to infections and hasten the progression of disease (Bandura, 1997). Self-efficacy beliefs also influence the activation of catecholamines, a family of neurotransmitters important to the management of stress and perceived threat, along with the endogenous painkillers referred to as endorphins (Bandura, 1997; O'Leary & Brown, 1995).

Self-efficacy expectancy is similar to perceived behavioural control, as defined in the theory of planned behaviour (Ajzen, 1988). Both involve beliefs that an individual has the resources and opportunities to execute a behaviour or attain a goal. However, the lack of clarity in the definition and measurement of both self-efficacy expectancy and perceived behaviour control raises some questions. In research, perceived behavioural control has been measured as perceived control over the behaviour and as perceived control over goal attainment (e.g. Ajzen & Madden, 1986; Madden *et al.*, 1992; Schifter & Ajzen, 1985). These are different constructs.

A common source of confusion is the relationship between self-efficacy expectancy and intentions. Sometimes when people say 'I can't' they are referring to beliefs about lack of skills and abilities; at other times they are referring to beliefs about lack of ability to manage discomfort and distress and expressing their resulting unwillingness to do something that may be a simple motor task. This distinction is particularly important in situations in which performing a behaviour may lead to involuntary aversive reactions such as fear, pain or discomfort – situations in which the individual has strong response expectancies for aversive outcomes (Kirsch, 1999). When people anticipate aversive outcomes (e.g. fear or pain) and are not willing to engage in behaviour that may produce those outcomes, their linguistic habit is to say they cannot perform the behaviour (low self-efficacy) rather than they will not perform it. Measures of willingness may simply be measures of intention as employed in the theory of reasoned action. Therefore, in situations in which fear or pain is anticipated, measures of perceived ability to perform the behaviour (self-efficacy) may be measures of intention to perform the behaviour. This intention is determined primarily by the strength of the person's response expectancies. The mislabelling of intention and perceived ability may occur in other important domains in which people are asked to engage in behaviours that may lead to immediate discomfort, such as dieting, exercising or violating personal norms (Baker & Kirsch, 1991). In situations involving anticipated pain, discomfort or emotional distress (e.g. picking up a snake, asking an attractive person for a date, running a marathon), measures of self-efficacy expectancy for the simple motor behaviours involved in these complex tasks (grasping, talking, running) are strongly influenced by response expectancies and thus are largely equivalent to measures of willingness and intention (Kirsch, 1995). Self-efficacy expectancy for the complex performances (including self-efficacy for coping with disturbing thoughts, anxiety, pain) are not the equivalent of willingness and intention.

Expectancies for proximal versus distal outcomes

One of the major obstacles to changing from an unhealthful behaviour to a healthful behaviour is the conflict between expectancies for proximal (immediate) and distal (future) consequences and in particular the power that expectancies for proximal consequences exert over behaviour. Many unhealthful 'lifestyle' behaviours (e.g. eating and drinking too much, unsafe sex, smoking) are unhealthful only in the long run but are immediately pleasurable and gratifying. Likewise, changing from unhealthful to healthful behaviour (e.g. starting an exercise programme, giving up tasty high fat foods) almost always involves great effort and often results in initial pain or discomfort. This conflict between expectancies makes if difficult for people to adopt safer sexual practices, quit smoking, eat and drink less and exercise regularly. Sex, smoking, eating ice cream, and watching TV in bed are immediately pleasurable and gratifying, while the costs of these behaviours exist only in the imagined and indefinite future. Likewise, giving up these behaviours involves immediate loss of pleasure and an increase in discomfort.

Conclusions

The most important influences on health will continue to be the decisions which people make about healthy and unhealthy behaviour in their daily lives. For this reason it is essential that healthcare professionals become more concerned with teaching people skills for the self-regulation of health behaviour (see 'Cognitive behaviour therapy', 'Health promotion', 'Motivational interviewing', 'Physical activity interventions', 'Self-management', and 'Stress management'). Expectancies are key components of all theories of health behaviour and self-regulation. A complete understanding of the role of expectancies in health behaviour depends on a clearer understanding of the broader social cognitive perspective and the relationships among expectancies and other social cognitive constructs. Research has found that a number of different types of expectancies influence health behaviour in important ways. Self-efficacy expectancies – expectancies about one's ability to engage in certain health-related behaviours – are probably the most important and influential expectancies.

Understanding of the influence of expectancies on health behaviour depends on understanding important similarities among the behaviours which influence health. Certainly, each health problem and health behaviour presents a unique challenge. For example, efforts to convince middle-aged people to exercise regularly will differ in important ways from efforts to convince sexually active teenagers to use condoms. Despite these differences, however, the processes or mechanisms that explain changes in these behaviours are the same. The expected consequences of exercising or not exercising differ from the expectancies for condom use or non-use, but for both behaviours expectancies for the outcomes

of these behaviours (outcome expectancies) are important determinants. Likewise, convincing older adults that they are capable of engaging in regular exercise and convincing teenagers that they are capable of either abstaining from sex or negotiating safe sex with a partner will require different strategies. In both cases, however, beliefs about personal ability and control (self-efficacy expectancies), will be crucial determinants of success. For this reason, we do not need different expectancies or expectancy-based theories for different health-related behaviours such as specific theories to explain safe and unsafe sexual behaviour, smoking, eating behaviour, and so on. The proliferation of behaviour-specific or problem-specific theories is a waste of intellectual resources and a barrier to theory development and refinement.

REFERENCES

AbuSabha, R. & Achterberg, C. (1997). Review of self-efficacy and locus of control for nutrition- and health-related behavior. *Journal of the American Dietetic Association*, **97**, 1122–33.

Ajzen, I. (1988). *Attitudes, personality, and behavior.* Chicago: Dorsey Press.

Ajzen, I. & Madden, T. J. (1986). Prediction of goal-directed behavior: attitudes, intentions, and perceived behavioral control. *Journal of Experimental Social Psychology*, **22**, 453–74.

Baker, S. L. & Kirsch, I. (1991). Cognitive mediators of pain perception and tolerance. *Journal of Personality and Social Psychology*, **61**, 504–10.

Bandura, A. (1977). Self efficacy: toward a unifying theory of behavior change. *Psychological Review*, **84**, 191–215.

Bandura, A. (1986). *Social foundations of thought and action.* New York: Prenctice-Hall.

Bandura, A. (1990). Some reflections on reflections. *Psychological Inquiry*, **1**, 101–5.

Bandura, A. (1997). *Self-efficacy: the exercise of control.* New York: Cambridge University Press.

Bandura, A. (2004). Health promotion by social cognitive means. *Health Education and Behavior*, **31**(2), 143–64.

Baum, W. M. & Heath, J. L. (1992). Behavioral explanations and intentional explanations in psychology. *American Psychologist*, **47**, 1312–17.

Bolles, R. C. (1972). Reinforcement, expectancy, and learning. *Psychological Review*, **79**(5), 394–409.

Bryan, A. D., Aiken, L. S. & West, S. G. (1997). Young women's condom use: the influence of acceptance of sexuality, control over the sexual encounter, and perceived susceptibility to common STDs. *Health Psychology*, **16**, 468–79.

Dawson, K. A. & Brawley, L. R. (2000). Examining the relationship between exercise goals, self-efficacy, and overt behavior with beginning exercisers. *Journal of Applied Social Psychology*, **30**, 315.

Deci, E. L. & Ryan, R. M. (1995). Human autonomy: the basis for true self-esteem. In M. H. Kernis (Ed.). *Efficacy, agency, and self-esteem* (pp. 31–49). New York: Plenum.

Dzewaltowski, D. A., Noble, J. M. & Shaw, J. M. (1990). Physical activity participation: social cognitive theory versus the theories of reasoned action and planned behavior. *Journal of Sport and Exercise Psychology*, **12**, 388–405.

Eagly, A. H. & Chaiken, S. (1993). *The psychology of attitudes.* New York: Harcourt, Brace, Jovanovitch.

Ewart, C. K. (1995). Self-efficacy and recovery from heart attack: implications for a social-cognitive analysis of exercise and emotion. In J. E. Maddux (Ed.). *Self-efficacy, adaptation, and adjustment: theory, research, and application* (pp. 203–26). New York: Plenum.

Fishbein, M. & Ajzen, I. (1975). Belief, attitude, intention, and behavior: an introduction to theory and research. Reading, MA: Addison-Wesley.

Heckhausen, H. (1977). Achievement motivation and its constructs: a cognitive model. *Motivation and Emotion*, **1**, 283–329.

Holman, H. R. & Lorig, K. (1992). Perceived self-efficacy in self-management of chronic disease. In R. Schwarzer (Ed.). *Self-efficacy: thought control of action* (pp. 305–24). Washington, DC: Hemisphere.

Hsiao, E. T. & Thayer, R. E. (1998). Exercising for mood regulation: the importance of experience. *Personality and Individual Differences*, **24**, 829–36.

Janz, N. K. & Becker, M. H. (1984). The Health Belief Model: a decade later. *Health Education Quarterly*, **11**, 1–47.

Kirsch, I. (1985). Response expectancy as a determinant of experience and behavior. *American Psychologist*, **40**, 1189–202.

Kirsch, I. (1995). Self-efficacy and outcome expectancies: a concluding commentary. In J. E. Maddux (Ed.). *Self-efficacy, adaptation, and adjustment: theory, research and application* (pp. 331–45). New York: Plenum Press.

Kirsch, I. (1999) (Ed.). *How expectancies shape behavior.* Washington, DC: American Psychological Association.

Madden, T. J., Ellen, P. S. & Ajzen, I. (1992). A comparison of the theory of planned behavior and the theory of reasoned action. *Personality and Social Psychology Bulletin*, **1**, 3–9.

Maddux, J. E. (1993). Social cognitive models of health and exercise behavior: an introduction and review of conceptual issues. *Journal of Applied Sport Psychology*, **5**, 116–40.

Maddux, J. E., Brawley, L. & Boykin, A. (1995). Self-efficacy and healthy decision-making: protection, promotion, and detection. In J.E. Maddux (Ed.). *Self-efficacy, adaptation, and adjustment.* New York: Plenum Press.

Maddux, J. E., DuCharme, K. A. (1997). Behavioral intentions in the theories of health behavior. In D. Gochman (Ed.). *Handbook of health behavior research.* New York: Plenum Press.

Maddux, J. E. & Gosselin, J. T. (2003). Self-efficacy. In M. R. Leary & J.P. Tangney (Eds.) *Handbook of self and identify.* New York: Guilford.

Maddux, J. E. & Rogers, R. W. (1983). Protection motivation and self-efficacy: a revised theory of fear appeals and attitude change. *Journal of Experimental Social Psychology*, **19**, 469–79.

Maddux, J. E. (1999). Expectancies and the social cognitive perspective: basic principles, processes, and variables. In I. Kirsch (Ed.). *How expectancies shape behavior* (pp. 17–39). Washington, DC: American Psychological Association.

McClelland, D. C. (1985). How motives, skills, and values determine what people do. *American Psychologist*, **40**(7), 812–25.

Mischel, W. (1973). Toward a cognitive social learning reconceptualization of personality. *Psychological Review*, **80**(4), 252–84.

O'Leary, A. & Brown, S. (1995). Self-efficacy and the physiological stress response. In J.E. Maddux (Ed.). *Self-efficacy, adaptation, and adjustment: theory, research and application* (pp. 227–48). New York: Plenum.

Olson, J. M., Roese, N. J. & Zanna, M. P. (1996). Expectancies. In E. T. Higgins & A. W. Kruglanski (Eds.). *Social psychology: handbook of basic principles* (pp. 211–38).

Rescorla, R. A. (1987). A Pavlovian analysis of goal-directed behavior. *American Psychologist*, **42**, 119–29.

Rogers, R. W. (1975). A protection motivation theory of fear appeals and attitude change. *Journal of Psychology*, **91**, 93–114.

Rogers, R.W. & Prentice-Dunn, S. (1997). Protection motivation theory. In D. S. Gochman (Ed.). *Handbook of health behavior research: I: Personal and social determinants* (pp. 113–32). New York: Plenum.

Rotter, J. B. (1954). *Social learning and clinical psychology.* Englewood Cliffs, NJ: Prentice-Hall.

Rotter, J. B. (1982). *The development and application of social learning theory: selected papers.* New York: Praeger.

Rotter, J. B. (1990). Internal versus external control of reinforcement: a case history of a variable. *American Psychologist*, **45**(4), 489–93.

Rudolph, D. L. & McAuley, E. (1995). Self-efficacy and salivary cortisol responses to acute exercise in physically active and less active adults. *Journal of Sport and Exercise Psychology*, **17**, 206–13.

Samuels, S. M. & Gibb, R. W. (2002). Self-efficacy assessment and generalization in physical education courses. *Journal of Applied Social Psychology.* **32**, 1314–27.

Schifter, D. B. & Ajzen, I. (1985). Intention, perceived control, and weight loss: an application of the theory of planned behavior. *Journal of Personality and Social Psychology*, **49**, 843–51.

Schwarzer, R. (1992). Self-efficacy in the adoption and maintenance of health behaviors: theoretical approaches and a new model. In R. Schwarzer (Ed.). *Self-efficacy: thought control of action* (pp. 217–44). Washington, DC: Hemisphere.

Sherer, M., Maddux, J. E., Mercandante, B. *et al.* (1982). The self-efficacy scale: construction and validation. *Psychological Reports*, **51**, 633–71.

Strecher, V. J., Champion, V. L. & Rosenstock, I.M. (1997). The health belief model and health behavior. In D. Gochman (Ed.). *Handbook of health behavior research I: Personal and social determinants* (pp. 71–92). New York: Plenum.

Tipton, R. M. & Worthington, E. L. (1984). The measurement of generalized self-efficacy: a study of construct validity. *Journal of Personality Assessment*, **48**, 545–8.

Vroom, V. H. (1964). *Work and motivation.* New York: Wiley.

Weinstein, N. D. (1988). Testing four competing theories of health-protective behavior. *Health Psychology*, **7**, 324–33.

Weinstein, N. D. (1993). Testing four competing theories of health-protective behavior. *Health Psychology*, **12**, 324–33.

Williams, S. L. (1995). Self-efficacy, anxiety, and phobic disorders. In J. E. Maddux (Ed.). *Self-efficacy, adaptation, and adjustment: theory, research and application* (pp. 69–107).

Woodward, W. R. (1982). The "discovery" of social behaviorism and social learning theory, 1870–1980. *American Psychologist*, **37**, 396–410.

Gender issues and women's health

Jane M. Ussher

University of Western Sydney

The legacy of early critiques of women's health

Thirty years ago Women's Health was a field fighting for recognition in a world dominated by androcentric research, theory and clinical intervention. Today it is a rich and vibrant body of work, spanning many diverse disciplines. The health of women is now firmly on the agenda of the World Health Organization, government and research funding bodies, providers of health services and educators. Researchers, theorists and social activists continue to move knowledge and practice forwards, improving service provision for women, at the same time as we reach a greater understanding of 'what women want' regarding their health.

Yet it hasn't always been this way. The last few decades of the twentieth century have seen the publication of a number of groundbreaking studies and critical polemics which highlighted the paucity of knowledge about the health and wellbeing of women. They documented how women's bodies, women's minds, and by extension, women's lives have historically been marginalized, ignored or dealt with in a detrimental way by mainstream health professions. Whole disciplines such as medicine, psychology and psychiatry were subjected to critical scrutiny. It was argued that women's mental health was defined in relation to man as the norm, and inevitably found wanting as a result. Femininity was pathologized, with mental health treatments merely serving as vehicles of social control, pushing women back into patterns of behaviour and social roles which were sources of distress and despair in the first place. It was argued that the reproductive body was positioned as a site of illness, irrationality and weakness, used as an excuse for excluding women from an equal place along side men. Or it was positied as a site of medical and psychological intervention, over which women had no choice or control. It was also argued that there was a dearth of knowledge about the normal aspects of reproduction, as psychological and medical research focussed on and reinforced the notion of reproduction as site of deviancy or debilitation, framing the female body within a narrow scientific gaze (Showalter, 1987; Sayers, 1982; Ussher, 1989).

It became clear that vast areas of health research excluded women altogether. For example, work on mid-life concentrated on men, with Erickson's male model of mid-life developmental changes being extrapolated unquestioningly to women, much as Kohlberg's theories of moral development had also been (Gilligan, 1982). Both theories found women lacking. Their deviation from a male norm was deemed deficiency, not difference. Many major clinical trials on heart disease excluded women altogether, as did early research on AIDS. In research on cancer, there has been a focus on the breast and genitals, even though lung cancer surpasses breast cancer as a cause of death for women. Research on all other forms of cancer in women is rare, or gender differences are not analysed when women are included in clinical trials. Research on alcohol use, or on drug use, has also focused almost solely on men until recently – despite the fact that significant numbers of women experience substance abuse, as well as problems from prescribed psycho-active drugs (Lee, 1998; Stanton & Gallant, 1995) (see 'Alcohol abuse' and 'Drug dependencies'). Even when women *are* included in health research, it is only as a narrow and specific group, for in the main the focus has been on middle-class, able-bodied, heterosexual, white women.

These early critiques which focused on the marginalization or exclusion of women's health issues have provided an important legacy for current research, theory and practice. They have highlighted the way in which 'woman' has been constructed in quite specific ways by health professions and researchers. They have documented the way in which women have historically been excluded from shaping the agenda as researchers, clinicians and policy makers, and how this has had a significant impact on the development of knowledge and professional practice in the arena of women's health (Ehrenriech & English, 1979). These critiques provided the foundations for the current field of Women's Health, setting an example and an agenda, simultaneously. Today, in disciplines as disparate as psychology, sociology, cultural studies, women's studies, social work, nursing, anthropology, psychiatry and medicine, scholars and researchers have brought their considerable energies to bear on the question of women's health and a rapidly growing literature on the subject is the result (Lee, 1998). This chapter will examine the gender issues in mental health, as an example of the debates and theoretical issues in this field.

Women's mental health

The existence of gender differences in mental health problems is a well established phenomenon. Prior to puberty, boys are over represented in significantly greater numbers (by a factor of approximately 4:1) in the whole gamut of psychological or behavioural problems experienced by children. For example, prior to the age of eight, boys predominate in a range of behavioural and psychological disorders, including bedwetting/soiling, feeding and appetite problems, sleep problems, over-activity and restlessness, including reading and writing difficulties, autism, hyperactivity and anti-social behaviour (Crown & Lee, 1999). However, after puberty the situation is reversed. Estimates of the ratio of women to men suffering from disorders such as depression, anxiety and eating disorders range from 6:1–5:3. Community surveys, hospital admissions and statistics on outpatient treatment (both medical and psychological) all concur: women are represented in far greater numbers than men (Bebbington, 1996). The only exceptions are in the diagnosis of schizophrenia, where there are no clear gender differences and of alcoholism, where men dominate. For decades, researchers have searched for the factors underlying this gender difference, claiming that if we can explain it, we will have the key to understanding mental health problems per se. Numerous competing biological, psychological and social aetiological theories have been put forward as a result.

Aetiological theories of childhood mental health and behavioural problems predominantly focus on issues other than gender. Whilst differential rates of diagnosis between boys and girls are acknowledged in discussions of incidence and prevalence, in the main, research and clinical intervention has concentrated on non-gender specific theories. These include factors such as teratogens or perinatal trauma, parental attachment, separation and hospital admission, family discord and divorce, maternal depression, bereavement, school effects, social deprivation and social class, temperament or cognitive factors, such as absence of theory of mind as an explanation for autism (Rutter & Hersov, 1987). Any analysis of differential patterns of problems between boys and girls invariably attributes them to biological differences between the male and female fetus, infant or child, which are said to produce developmental differences between boys and girls that make them more vulnerable in the early years. For example, recent explanations for gender differences in autism posited this problem as being due to sex differences in the brain (Baron-Cohen, 2003).

In the field of adult mental health, biomedical accounts have historically dominated, providing the basis for the widespread use of biomedical interventions, in particular psychotropic drug use. The attribution of symptomatology to 'synaptic events', such as noradrenalin, 5-HT, serotonin, dopamine and acetetycholine neurotransmitters can clearly be applied equally to men and women. The biological explanation for sex differences is seen to be 'female hormones', particularly oestrogen and progesterone, which lead to depression associated with the reproductive life cycle: Premenstrual syndrome (PMS), postnatal depression (PND) or menopausal problems (Studd, 1997).

However, in recent years, the majority of researchers and clinicians have moved away from a strictly biological model, acknowledging instead the role of psychosocial factors in women's mental health. Social or environmental factors which have been reported to be associated with higher reporting of mental health problems include marital status, with married women reporting higher rates of problems than single women or married men; caring roles, with women looking after small children or elderly relatives being at higher risk; employment status, with work generally providing a protective factor, particularly for working-class women; absence of social support and economic or social power; gender role socialization, which leads to depressogenic attributional styles, and an emphasis on affiliation rather than achievement, leading to vulnerability when relationships are under threat; multiple role strain and conflict, as well as the devaluation of traditional feminine roles; and sexual violence or abuse, in adulthood or childhood (Brown *et al.*, 1986; Baker, 2002; Stoppard & McMullen, 2003). Psychological theories which have been put forward include cognitive vulnerability, specifically the greater likelihood of women to attribute problems to internal, stable and global factors; coping styles; and perception of control (Bebbington, 1998). Psychodynamic theories, including object relations theory and Freudian theory, have been influential in psychotherapeutic circles, as well as in many recent feminist critiques, but have had less impact on mainstream research and practice (see 'Psychodynamic psychotherapy').

Alternative models of conceptualizing, researching, and, if necessary, treating symptomatology have also been developed from within a broadly social constructionist perspective (Stoppard, 1999). Social constructionists challenge the realist assumptions of traditional biomedical and psychological research, arguing instead that subjectivity, behaviour and the very definition and meaning of what constitutes 'health' and what constitutes 'illness' is constructed within social practices and rules, language, relationships and roles: it is always shaped by culture and history (Burr, 1995). Many of the now numerous feminist critiques of women's mental health problems and of the treatment of women within the mental health professions, could be placed under a broad social constructionist umbrella. Feminist critics have argued that misogynistic assumptions about gender roles and normal femininity are used to diagnose and treat women who deviate as 'mad'; that assumptions about the proper position of women within the institution of heterosexuality are used to prescribe notions of normality; that the age-old practice of locating distress or deviancy in the womb (or in reproductive hormones) reinforces notions of woman as more animalistic or biologically driven than man, as well as dismissing all legitimate anger or discontent as the result of 'raging hormones'; and that social and political inequalities, which understandably produce symptoms of distress, are ignored (Ussher, 1991, 2006: Chesler, 1998). This has lead to critical feminist analyses of mental health research and treatment; to a deconstruction of the very concept of 'mental illness'; and, more recently, to the development of women-centred research and therapy.

However, one of the main problems is that in adopting a social constructionist perspective, or in arguing that 'mental illness' exists entirely at a discursive level, we are implicitly denying the influence of biology or genetics, or we may appear to relegate the body to a passive subsidiary role, which has meaning or interpretation imposed upon it (Yardley, 1997). Other material aspects of women's lives may also be negated in a discursive analysis: the influence of age, social class, power, economic factors, ethnicity, sexual identity, personal relationships and social support or a prior history of sexual abuse, amongst other factors. Equally, within a social constructionist or discursive approach the 'reality' of mental health problems may appear to be denied; 'mental illness' can appear to be conceptualized as merely a social label or category. What is needed is a move towards a material–discursive–intrapsychic analysis, where material, discursive and intrapsychic aspects of experience can be examined without privileging one level of analysis above the other.

A material–discursive–intrapsychic analysis of women's mental health

'Material–discursive' approaches have recently been developed in a number of areas of psychology, such as sexuality, reproduction and mental or physical health (Ussher, 1997*b*; Yardley, 1997). This is as a result of both a frustration with mainstream psychology, which has tended to adopt a solely materialist standpoint, thus serving to negate discursive aspects of experience, and dissatisfaction with the negation of the material aspects of life in many discursive accounts. However, the intrapsychic is often left out of material–discursive approaches, for the reason that it is seen as individualistic or reductionist. Equally, when intrapsychic factors are considered (for example in psychoanalytic or cognitive theorizing) they are invariably conceptualized separately from either material or discursive factors. It is time that all three levels together are incorporated into academic theory and practice, in order to provide a multidimensional analysis of women's lives, of mental health and illness as discursive categories and of the mental health symptoms many women experience. So what is meant by a material–discursive–intrapsychic approach?

The level of materiality

To talk of materiality is to talk of factors which exist at a corporeal, a societal or an institutional level; factors which are traditionally at the centre of bio-medical or sociological accounts. This would include biological factors associated with psychological symptomatology; material factors which institutionalize the diagnosis and treatment of mental health problems as 'mental illness' or 'madness'; gender inequalities and inequalities in heterosexual relationships, legitimating masculine power and control. The latter would encapsulate economic factors which make women dependent on men; presence or absence of accommodation which allows women in destructive relationships to leave; support for women of a legal, emotional and structural kind, which allows protection from further harassment or abuse; and the fact that women take on the primary caring role in relationships, at both a physical and psychological level. It would include issues of social class which lead to expectations of 'normal' behaviour for women and men, and which are implicated in educational or employment opportunities available to both, as well as in the way individuals are treated by external institutions such as social services or the mental health professions. The fact of whether children are present in the relationship or not (or are in custody battles withheld), and the material consequences of being married (or not) are also part of this level of analysis. Equally, previous history of sexual violence or abuse is partly a material event; as is family history – the number of siblings, parental relationships and factors such as parental divorce or separation from parents in childhood. There are also many material consequences of experiencing or being treated for mental health problems, in terms of physical or psychological vulnerability, as well as powerlessness at an economic or societal level. The social isolation which can be a consequence of mental health problems, or which can act to exacerbate its effects is also partly a material issue. Sex, ethnicity and sexuality are also associated with materiality – with the reproductive body, with gendered or sexual behaviour and with physical appearance.

The level of the discursive

To focus on the 'discursive' is to look to social and linguistic domains – to talk, to visual representation, to ideology, culture, and power. What is arguably of most relevance here is the discursive construction of mental illness or madness, of medical or psychological expertise, and the discursive construction of gender, as well as the analysis of the relationship between representations of 'woman' and 'man', and constructions of the particular leads social roles adopted by individual women and men.

As was outlined above, many critics have argued that mental health and illness can be conceptualized as social categories created by a process of expert definition. In this view, it is a discursively constructed label, based on value-laden definitions of normality. What is deemed 'mental illness' in one context, at one point in time, is deemed normal at another (Foucault, 1967). For example, it is the model of normal selfhood that underpins late twentieth century Western notions of mental health, where stability of affect is held up as the norm, and consistent happiness the ideal we should aspire to, which is used to categorize women (and men) as suffering from a mental health problem. Any deviation from this stable norm is deemed illness, a state to be avoided or cured. To illustrate that this is an historical and cultural construct, we only have to look to the model of the self that underpins Eastern models of mental health, such as that found in Buddhist meditation and psychotherapy. Here the illusion of a core consistent 'me', that is always positive and good, is directly confronted (Epstein, 1995). Rather than eradicate 'symptoms', this model would suggest that through the practice of mindfulness, an appreciation of the temporally based dimension of self is arrived at, by paying attention to bodily based experiences and sensations as they occur. There is no reaction or judgement of these experiences or sensations, merely a witnessing of them, leading to awareness that feelings are rarely constant. There is an acceptance of fluctuation and change, but this is not posited as pathological, as needing psychiatric diagnosis or 'cure'.

Equally, within a discursive account, rather than femininity being seen as pre-given or innate, here it is seen as something which is performed or acquired. In the process of becoming 'woman', it is argued that women follow the various scripts of femininity which are taught to them through the family, through school and through the myriad representations of 'normal' gender roles in popular and high culture, as well as in science and the law (Ussher, 1997a). The taking up of the archetypal feminine position, within what has been described as a heterosexual matrix (Butler, 1990), has been seen to put women at risk for mental health problems, as it is a role which requires self-sacrifice, self-denigration and a stifling of independence and desire (O'Grady, 2004). The dominance of phallocentric scripts of femininity is one of the explanations put forward for why women stay in unhappy, neglectful or violent relationships and arguably one of the explanations for why women internalize marital or family difficulties as depression. Women are taught to gain happiness through relationships, invariably with men. They are also taught that it is their fault if they can't (Jack, 1991). At the same time, a number of feminist critics have argued that the discursive construction of madness and femininity are closely aligned, thus to be a 'woman' is to be at risk of being positioned as 'mad', particularly if one steps out of line by being violent, sexual or in some other way contravening the feminine role (Chesler, 1998).

The level of the intrapsychic

Intrapsychic factors are those which operate at the level of the individual and the psychological: factors which are traditionally the central focus of psychological analyses of women's mental health problems, outlined above. This would include analyses of the way in which women blame themselves for problems in relationships, and psychological explanations for why this is so, incorporating factors such as low self-esteem, depression, the impact of previous neglect or abuse, guilt, shame, fear of loss or separation and the idealization of both heterosexuality and of men (Baker, 2002). It would include an analysis of psychological defences, such as repression, denial, projection or splitting, as mechanisms for dealing with difficulty or psychological pain. For example, we see evidence of splitting in the way women see themselves, or their man, as 'all good' or 'all bad', with no acknowledgement that everyone can exhibit both positive and negative characteristics at the same time; or in the way women blame themselves, or their bodies, for problems which they experience (Ussher, 2006). It would also include women's internalization of the idealized fantasy of motherhood and of the expectations of being 'woman' in a heterosexual social sphere (Mauthner, 2000). The fear women experience in relation to the threat of violence or abuse in relationships, or in society as a whole, is also an important factor (Yodanis, 2004).

Conclusion

The field of mental health is one where there are clear gender differences between men and women. A number of unidimensional theories have been put forward to explain these gender differences. However, a multifactorial approach which acknowledges a connection between material, discursive and intrapsychic factors is the most appropriate. Mental health problems are thus phenomena experienced by individual women at a material, discursive and an intrapsychic level; we cannot disentangle one from the other. The meaning of mental health to women, and to the experts who research and treat it, has to be understood in relation to the specific historical and cultural contexts in which they are positioned, the material factors impacting on individual women's lives, and the intrapsychic factors which impact upon individual women's experience and negotiation of 'symptoms'. As researchers, clinicians and theorists, we need to move to a position where we can take each of these levels of experience on board, without privileging one above the other. Thus the role of hormones, the endocrine system or physiological arousal, as well as the influence of social stressors, age or economic factors, can be acknowledged and studied in analyses of the aetiology of mental health problems. The existence of symptoms would also be acknowledged, whether they are psychological or physical, as would the existence of psychological or material factors which might ameliorate symptoms. However, these symptoms or material factors are not conceptualized as independent entities which exist separately from the historical or cultural context in which the woman lives. They are always positioned within discourse, within culture. 'Mental health problems' are therefore always a product of the symbiotic relationship between material, discursive and intrapsychic factors: one level of analysis cannot be understood without the other. (See also 'Men's health'.)

REFERENCES

Baker, C.D. (2002). *Female survivors of sexual abuse*. London: Routledge.

Baron-Cohen, S. (2003). *The essential difference: the truth about the male and female brain*. London: Perseus.

Bebbington, P. (1996). The origins of sex differences in depressive disorder: bridging the gap. *International Review of Psychiatry*, **8**, 295–332.

Bebbington, P.E. (1998). Sex and depression, *Psychological Medicine*, **28**, 1–8.

Brown, G.W., Andrews, B., Harris, T.O. & Adler, Z. (1986). Social support, self-esteem and depression. *Psychological Medicine*, **16**, 813–31.

Burr, V. (1995). *An introduction to social constructionism*. London: Routledge.

Butler, J.P. (1990). *Gender trouble: feminism and the subversion of identity*. New York: Routledge.

Chesler, P. (1998). *Women and Madness*. New York: Doubleday.

Crown, S. & Lee, A. (1999). *The handbook of child and adolescent clinical psychology: a contextual approach*. London: Routledge.

Ehrenriech, B. & English, D. (1979). *For her own good: 150 years of expert advice for women*. London: Pluto Press.

Epstein, M. (1995). Thoughts without a thinker: Buddhism and psychoanalysis, *Psychoanalytic Review*, **82**, 391–406.

Foucault, M. (1967). *Madness and civilisation: A history of insanity in the age of reason*. London: Tavistock.

Gilligan, C. (1982). *In a different voice: psychological theory and women's development*. Cambridge, MA: Harvard University Press.

Jack, D.C. (1991). *Silencing the self: women and depression*. Cambridge, MA: Harvard University Press.

Lee, C. (1998). *Women's heath: psychological and social persepctives*. London: Sage.

Mauthner, N. (2000). Feeling low and feeling really bad about feeling low. Women's experience of motherhood and post-partum depression, *Canadian Psychology*, **40**, 143–61.

O'Grady, H. (2004). *Women's relationships with themselves: gender, Foucault, therapy*. London: Routledge.

Rutter, M. & Hersov, L. (1987). *Child and adolescent psychiatry: modern approaches*. London: Blackwell.

Sayers, J. (1982). *Biological politics: feminist and anti-feminist perspectives*. London: Tavistock.

Showalter, E. (1987). *The female malady: women, madness and english culture 1830–1940*. London: Virago.

Stanton, A.L. & Gallant, S. (1995). *The psychology of women's health. Progress and challenges in research and application*. Washington, DC: Amercian Psychological Association.

Stoppard, J. (1999). *Women's depression: a social constructionist account*, London: Routledge.

Stoppard, J. & McMullen, L.M. (2003). *Situating sadness. Women and depression in social context*. New York: New York University Press.

Studd, J. (1997). Depression and the menopause, *British Medical Journal*, **314**, 977.

Ussher, J.M. (1989). *The psychology of the female body*. Florence, KY, US: Taylor and Francis/Routledge.

Ussher, J.M. (1991). *Women's madness: misogyny or mental illness?* Amherst, MA, US: University of Massachusetts Press.

Ussher, J.M. (1997*a*). *Fantasies of femininity: reframing the boundaries of sex*. London: Penguin.

Ussher, J.M. (1997*b*). *Body talk: the material and discursive regulation of sexuality, madness and reproduction*. London: Routledge.

Ussher, J.M. (2006). *Managing the monstrous feminine: regulating the reproductive body*. London: Routledge.

Yardley, L. (1997). *Material discourses in health and illness*. London: Routledge.

Yodanis, C.L. (2004). Gender inequality, violence against women and fear. *Journal of Interpersonal Violence*, **19**, 655–75.

The health belief model[1]

Charles Abraham[1] and Paschal Sheeran[2]

[1]University of Sussex
[2]University of Sheffield

Development of the health belief model (HBM)

In the 1950s US public health researchers began developing psychological models designed to enhance the effectiveness of health education programmes (Hochbaum, 1958). Demographic factors such as socio-economic status, gender, ethnicity and age were known to be associated with preventive health behaviours and use of health services (Rosenstock, 1974), but these factors could not be modified through health education. Thus the challenge was to develop effective health education targeting modifiable, individual characteristics that predicted preventive health behaviour and service usage.

Beliefs provided an ideal target because they are enduring individual characteristics which influence behaviour and are potentially modifiable. Beliefs may also reflect different socialization histories arising from demographic differences while, at the same time, differentiating between individuals from the same background. If persuasive methods could be used to change beliefs associated with health behaviours and such interventions resulted in health behaviour change then this would provide a theory-based technology of health education.

An expectancy–value model was developed in which events believed to be more or less likely were seen to be positively or negatively evaluated by the individual. In particular, the likelihood of experiencing a health problem, the severity of the consequences of that problem, the perceived benefits of any particular health behaviour and its potential costs were seen as core beliefs guiding health behaviour (see 'Expectations and health').

Rosenstock (1974) attributed the first health belief model (HBM) research to Hochbaum's (1958) studies of the uptake of tuberculosis X-ray screening. Hochbaum found that perceived susceptibility to tuberculosis and the belief that people with the disease could be asymptomatic (so that screening would be beneficial) distinguished between those who had and had not attended for chest X-rays. Similarly, a prospective study by Kegeles (1963) showed that perceived susceptibility to the worst imaginable dental problems and awareness that visits to the dentist might prevent these problems were useful predictors of the frequency of dental visits over the next three years. Haefner and Kirscht (1970) took this research one step further and demonstrated that a health education intervention designed to increase participants' perceived susceptibility, perceived severity and anticipated benefits resulted in a greater number of check-up visits to the doctor compared with controls over the following eight months. Thus, by the early 1970s a series of studies suggested that these key health beliefs provided a useful framework for understanding and changing health behaviour.

Structure of the HBM

The HBM focuses on two aspects of individuals' representations of health and health behaviour: threat perception and behavioural evaluation. Threat perception comprises two key beliefs, namely, perceived susceptibility to illness or health problems and anticipated severity of the consequences of illnesses. Behavioural evaluation also includes two distinct sets of beliefs, those concerning the benefits or efficacy of a recommended health behaviour and those concerning the costs of or barriers to enacting the behaviour. In addition, the model proposes that cues to action can activate health behaviour when appropriate beliefs are held. These 'cues' include a diverse range of triggers including individual perceptions of symptoms, social influence and health education campaigns. Finally, an individual's general health motivation or 'readiness to be concerned about health matters' was included in later versions of the model (e.g. Becker *et al.*, 1977). There are, therefore, six distinct constructs specified by the HBM. As Figure 1 indicates, there are no clear guidelines on how to operationalize the links these constructs so the model has usually been operationalized as a series of up to six separate independent variables which can be used to predict health behaviours.

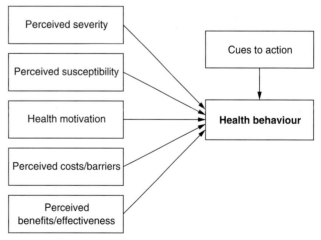

Fig 1 The Health Belief Model.

---

[1] This chapter is based on a more detailed chapter; Abraham, C. & Sheeran, P. (in press, 2005). Health Belief Model. In M. Conner & P. Norman (Eds.) *Predicting health behaviour: research and practice with social cognition models* (2nd edn.). Buckingham, UK: Open University Press.

Research using the HBM to predict health-related behaviour

The HBM has been applied to the prediction of an impressively broad range of health behaviours among a wide range of populations. Three broad areas can be identified: (a) preventive health behaviours, which include health-promoting (e.g. diet, exercise) and health-risk (e.g. smoking) behaviours as well as vaccination and contraceptive practices; (b) sick role behaviours, particularly adherence to recommended medical regimens; and (c) clinic use, which includes physician visits for a variety of reasons (for a review see Abraham & Sheeran, 2005).

Most HBM studies have employed cross-sectional designs, although Janz and Becker's (1984) review found that 40% of HBM studies were prospective. Prospective studies are important because simultaneous measurement of health beliefs and (especially self-reported) behaviour may be subject to memory and social desirability biases and does not permit causal inferences (Field, 2000). Most studies have used self-report measures of behaviour but some have used physiological measures (e.g. Bradley *et al.*, 1987), behavioural observations (e.g. Hay *et al.*, 2003) or medical records (e.g. Orbell *et al.*, 1995) as outcome measures. While the majority of measures of health beliefs employ self-completion questionnaires, structured face-to-face (e.g. Volk & Koopman, 2001) and telephone (e.g. Grady *et al.*, 1983) interviews have also been employed. Use of random sampling techniques is commonplace and specific representation of low-income and minority groups is also evident (e.g. Becker *et al.*, 1974).

There have been two quantitative reviews of predictive research using the HBM with adults (see Gochman & Parcel, 1982 for review of applications involving children). These reviews adopted different strategies in quantifying findings from research studies. Janz and Becker's (1984) review employed a vote count procedure showing the percentage of times the four main HBM constructs were statistically significant correlates or predictors (in the expected direction) across 46 studies. Across all studies, the significance ratios are very supportive of HBM predictions. Susceptibility was significant in 81% of studies, severity in 65%, benefits in 78% and barriers in 89%. Moreover, the results were also supportive of the model when only the prospective studies (N = 18) were included. The ratios were 82%, 65%, 81% and 100% for susceptibility, severity, benefits and barriers-based, respectively. Results showed that barriers were the most reliable predictor of behaviour, followed by susceptibility and benefits, and finally, severity.

Unfortunately, limitations of the vote count procedure suggest caution in interpreting Janz and Becker's results. The significance ratios only reveal how often HBM components were significantly associated with behaviour, not how large the effects of HBM measures were on behaviour. Moreover, significance ratios give equal weighting to findings from studies with large and small numbers of participants and do not differentiate between bivariate relationships between a HBM construct and behaviour and multivariate associations.

Harrison *et al.*'s (1992) meta-analytic review of the HBM addressed these methodological issues. Harrison and colleagues originally identified 234 published empirical tests of the HBM. Of these, only 16 studies (i.e. 6.8%) measured all four major components and included reliability checks. This underlines the extent to which operationalizations of the HBM have failed to measure all constructs or provide psychometric tests of measures. The meta-analysis involved converting associations between HBM constructs and behaviour measures, in each study, into a common effect size, namely Pearson's *r*. A weighted average of these effect sizes was then computed for each component (see Rosenthal, 1984). Across all studies, the average correlations between HBM components and behaviour were 0.15, 0.08, 0.13 and 0.21 for susceptibility, severity, benefits and barriers, respectively. While these correlations are all statistically significant, they are small in effect sizes terms; individual constructs accounting for only 0.5% to 4% of the variance in behaviour, across studies. Unlike Janz and Becker (1984), Harrison *et al.* found that HBM components had different associations in cross-sectional versus longitudinal designs. Both benefits and barriers had significantly larger effect sizes in prospective than in retrospective research, whereas in the case of severity, the effect size was significantly larger in retrospective studies.

These two quantitative reviews of the susceptibility, severity, benefits and barriers constructs suggest that these variables are very often found to be significant predictors of health-related behaviours but that their effects are small. However, a number of caveats are important. First, the effects of individual health beliefs should be combined and the combined effect may be greater than the sum of individual effects. Second, Harrison *et al.* (1992) adopted very strict criteria for inclusion in their review and the effect sizes they obtained are based on findings from only 3515 respondents. Finally, Harrison *et al.* point out that their effect sizes also show considerable heterogeneity, which suggests that design or measurement differences across studies or different conceptualizations of the constructs influenced the results. Overall then, while tests of the predictive utility of the four main HBM constructs are supportive, poor operationalizations of the model and failure to check both the reliability and the validity of constructs have been significant drawbacks in many studies applying the HBM.

Cues to action and health motivation have been relatively neglected in empirical tests of the HBM. Neither Janz and Becker (1984) nor Harrison *et al.* (1992) included these components because of the paucity of relevant studies. One reason for researchers' failure to operationalize these components may be the lack of clear construct definitions. Cues to action can include a wide range of experiences and so has been operationalized differently by different researchers. For example, Grady *et al.* (1983) found significant associations between the numbers of family members with breast/other cancers and participation in a breast self-examination teaching programme. These authors did not, however, refer to these measures as 'cues to action', while an almost identical variable in Keesling and Friedman's (1987) study of skin cancer prevention was conceptualized in this way.

Measurements of health motivation have generally comprised just a single item, usually expressing general 'concern' about health, though a small number of researchers have developed psychometric scales (e.g. Champion, 1984). Bivariate relationships between health motivation and health behaviour are generally small but statistically significant (e.g. Ali, 2002), with some non-significant exceptions (Umeh & Rogan-Gibson, 2001). Findings from multivariate analyses are mixed, with some studies finding positive relationships (e.g. Ali, 2002) and others finding no association (e.g. King, 1982).

HBM measurement issues

Failures to operationalize the HBM in its entirety may be partly due to the lack of clear guidelines on how HBM constructs should be defined and measured (see Abraham & Sheeran, 2005 for further discussion). For example, there have been suggestions that susceptibility and severity could be combined to form the concept 'threat', and similarly, that benefits and barriers should be subtracted from one another rather than treated as separate constructs (Becker & Maiman, 1975). Consequently, some researchers have used a threat index rather than measure susceptibility and severity separately (e.g. Kirscht et al., 1976) This appears to violate the expectancy–value structure of the HBM and can be seen as an inferior, and perhaps incorrect, operationalization of the model (see Feather, 1982). Moreover, it has been suggested that perceived susceptibility may only become important once perceived severity reaches a certain threshold and that, after that, perceived severity has no further influence on decision-making (Weinstein, 1988). To operationalize this idea Lewis (1994) suggested that threat could be measured using the following equation.

$$threat = susceptibility + (susceptibility \times severity)$$

Similarly, some researchers have combined benefits and barriers in a single index (e.g. Gianetti et al., 1985). This practice raises theoretical and empirical issues. At a theoretical level, Weinstein (1988) suggests that there is a qualitative difference between benefits and barriers, at least in hazard situations, which means that they should be treated as distinct constructs. For example, while barriers relating to taking exercise or giving up salt are certain and concrete (e.g. time and effort, loss of pleasure), the benefits in terms of avoiding hypertension are more hypothetical. At an empirical level, the benefits construct may comprise distinct components, namely the efficacy of the behaviour in achieving an outcome (sometimes called 'response efficacy') as well as possible psychosocial benefits such as social approval. Similarly, the barriers construct may comprise both physical limitations (e.g. ability or expense) and psychological costs associated with its performance (e.g. distress). It seems unlikely that a single index could adequately represent these different outcome expectancies. An empirical approach to resolving this issue is to employ factor and reliability analyses to assess whether, and which, benefits and barriers can be legitimately combined, from a psychometric perspective (e.g. Abraham et al., 1992).

Do HBM measures mediate the effects of demographic factors on health behaviour?

When the HBM was developed it was hoped that the effects of demographic factors such as socio-economic status (SES) could be accounted for, or mediated by (Baron & Kenny, 1986), variation in individuals' beliefs. However, few studies have tested this proposition and available evidence is mixed. Cummings et al. (1979) found that SES was not related to health beliefs, though both SES and beliefs were significantly related to inoculation behaviour in bivariate analyses. Orbell et al. (1995), on the other hand, found that perceived susceptibility and barriers entirely mediated the effects of social class upon uptake of cervical screening.

Direct (i.e. unmediated) effects were, however, obtained for both marital status and sexual experience. Salloway et al. (1978) obtained both direct and indirect effects for occupational status, sex and income and an indirect effect of education upon appointment-keeping at an inner city hypertension clinic. Further research is needed to determine the impact of SES upon health beliefs and behaviour and to discriminate between the effects of cognitions and the effects of factors such as financial constraints, culture of poverty/network effects and health system/provider behaviour barriers on health-related behaviours (Rundall & Wheeler, 1979).

Extending the HBM

Recognizing limitations of the HBM, Rosenstock (1974) suggested that a more comprehensive model of cognitive antecedents could reveal how health beliefs are related to other psychological stages in decision-making and action. King (1982) demonstrated how this might be achieved by 'extending' the HBM in a study of screening for hypertension. She included measures of individuals' causal understanding of high blood pressure derived from 'attribution theory' (Kelley, 1967), which she theorized as determinants of health beliefs that, in turn, prompted intention formation (Fishbein & Ajzen, 1975). Using a prospective design, King found that eight measures, including intention, could correctly classify 82% of respondents as either attenders or non-attenders. Her results showed that measures of perceived severity, perceived benefits and the extent to which respondents identified one or many causes of high blood pressure, accounted for 18% of the variance in behavioural intention, which, in turn, was the best single predictor of attendance. This study is noteworthy because it combined constructs from a number of theories (attribution theory, the HBM and the theory of reasoned action) and created a new model that simultaneously explored the cognitive foundations of health beliefs and sketched a mechanism by which they might generate action (see 'Theory of planned behaviour').

Rosenstock, Strecher and Becker (1988) acknowledged the importance of Bandura's (e.g. 1977) research by proposing that 'self-efficacy' (the belief that one can successfully perform a behaviour) be added to the HBM (see 'Self-efficacy and health behaviour'). Subsequent studies have tested the predictive utility of an extended HBM, including self-efficacy, and generally confirmed that self-efficacy is a useful additional predictor (e.g. Hay et al., 2003). Unfortunately, unlike King (1982), Rosenstock et al. (1988) offered no new theoretical formulation specifying interactions between beliefs and self-efficacy. This may have been short-sighted because subsequent research indicated that key HBM constructs have indirect effects on behaviour as a result of their effect on perceived control and intention which may, therefore, be regarded as more proximal determinants of action For example, Schwarzer's (1992) 'health action process approach' combines constructs from the HBM with those from other social cognitive models. In this model, susceptibility and severity beliefs are construed as antecedents of anticipated consequences (outcome expectancies) and strength of intention while intention and self-efficacy are identified as the most proximal antecedents of action.

Using the HBM to change health behaviour

Accurate prediction is an indicator of veridical explanation. As Sutton (1998, p. 1317) observed, 'models that do not enable us to predict behaviour are unlikely to be useful as explanatory models' Consequently, considerable effort has been invested in testing the predictive utility of the HBM. However, the model was originally conceived of as a tool to improve health education and so shape health behaviour and it has inspired researchers interested in behaviour change interventions for decades (e.g. Haefner & Kirscht, 1970). We have noted limitations in the predictive utility of the HBM and these findings suggest concomitant limitations in the effectiveness of behaviour-change interventions that target HBM-specified beliefs. Nonetheless, HBM constructs are correlated with a range of health-related behaviours and changing these beliefs may prompt behaviour change (whether or not this involves simultaneous changes in cognitions not specified by the HBM – e.g. intention and self-efficacy). (See 'Health promotion').

Abraham and Sheeran (2005) report a review of evaluations of HBM-based, behaviour-change interventions and highlight 17 such evaluations. Some of these were derived directly from the HBM (e.g. Carmel et al., 1996) whereas others drew upon HBM and other social cognition models in order to target a broader range of cognitions (e.g. Strecher et al., 1994). Some took the form of educational presentations to groups in classes or workshops (e.g. Abood et al., 2003) and/or involved the distribution of leaflets or booklets (e.g. Carmel et al., 1996) whereas others were delivered at an individual level (referred to variously as 'educational' or 'counseling' interventions), and often involved assessment of the recipient's current beliefs before new information and persuasive arguments were presented (e.g. Champion, 1994, Jones et al., 1998). Such interventions are tailored to the individual's cognitions. Computer-generated, individually tailored letters have also been used (Strecher et al., 1994). All of the interventions relied on information provision and verbal persuasion as means to change HBM-specified beliefs. Thirteen of the 17 evaluations found evidence of behaviour change. This is encouraging but, because these evaluations were not selected on the basis of methodological rigour, conclusions regarding effectiveness need be examined on a study-by-study basis.

Jones et al. (1988) provide a good illustration of an evaluation of an HBM-based behaviour change intervention. These researchers report a randomized controlled trial (RCT) of an intervention designed to persuade patients using hospital emergency services to make and keep follow-up appointments with their own doctor. The sample comprised 842 patients with 11 presenting problems (chest pain, hypertension, asthma, otitis media, diabetes, urinary tract infection, headache, urethritis [men], vaginitis [women], low back pain and rash) which did not require hospitalization. An intervention for individual patients was developed. This involved assessment of patients' HBM-specified beliefs and delivery of protocol-based, condition-specific educational messages to target beliefs that were not accepted by recipients. The intervention was designed to increase the patients' perceived susceptibility to illness complications, perceived seriousness of the complications, and benefits of a follow-up referral appointment in terms of avoiding further complications. It was delivered by a research nurse during required nursing care. Four intervention conditions were tested: (i) a routine care, control group, (ii) the individual, nurse-delivered hospital intervention, (iii) the hospital intervention combined with a follow-up telephone call (iv) a follow up telephone call without the hospital intervention. Only 33% of the control group patients scheduled a follow-up appointment whereas 76% of the hospital intervention group, 85% of the telephone intervention group and 85% of the combined intervention did so. Twenty four percent of the control group kept a follow-up appointment compared to 59% in the hospital intervention group, 59% in the telephone intervention group and 68% in the combination group. Thus, the combination intervention worked most effectively. Jones et al. did not conduct a cost-effectiveness analysis, but noted that the telephone intervention alone might be the most effective practical intervention when costs such as staff training and staff time are taken into account.

Abraham and Sheeran (2005) identified a number of shortcomings in HBM intervention evaluations. Evaluation designs have been limited due to the lack of appropriate control groups, lack of randomization to conditions, samples that do not support generalization, and short-term follow-ups. Moreover, the HBM, like other social cognition models, specifies targets for cognition change but does not describe processes responsible for belief change. It is possible to combine models like the HBM with cognition change theories such as cognitive dissonance theory (Festinger, 1957; see Stone et al., 1994, for an empirical example) in order to design interventions with theory-based targets and theory-based intervention techniques. However, this approach is not typical of HBM-based interventions. Consequently, the selection of intervention techniques (as opposed to cognition targets) is often not, or not explicitly, theory-based. In addition, interventions usually comprise a variety of techniques making it unclear which particular technique (or combinations of techniques) are crucial to effectiveness. Finally, in order to establish whether an intervention generates behaviour change because it alters target beliefs, it is necessary both to measure cognitions and behaviour pre- and post-intervention and to conduct mediation analysis (Baron & Kenny, 1986). However, mediation analysis is rarely reported in HBM-inspired intervention evaluations. Consequently, even when HBM-inspired interventions are effective in changing behaviour, it is unclear whether such effects are due to changes in HBM-specified beliefs. In summary, although the HBM has inspired the development of effective behaviour change interventions, the lack of programmatic experimental work means that we are unable to identify a series of belief-changing techniques and, in most cases, unable to say whether effective HBM-inspired interventions work because they change HBM-specified beliefs.

Conclusions

The HBM has provided a useful theoretical framework for investigators of the cognitive determinants of a wide range of behaviours for more than 30 years. The model's common-sense constructs are easy for non-psychologists to assimilate and are easy to operationalize in self-report questionnaires. The HBM has focused researchers' and health care professionals' attention on modifiable psychological prerequisites of behaviour and provided a basis for practical interventions across a range of behaviours. Research to date has, however, predominantly employed cross-sectional correlational designs and further prospective experimental studies are required to clarify the causal direction of belief–behaviour relationships. The proposed mediation of socioeconomic influences on health behaviour by health beliefs also remains unclear.

The HBM has inspired researchers to develop interventions found to be effective in changing health behaviour. However, given the heterogeneity of evaluation designs, intervention techniques, target behaviours and populations, it is likely that reviews focusing on interventions designed to change particular behaviours for particular populations will be most informative. For example, in a review of 63 interventions designed to increase mammography use, Yabroff and Mandelblatt (1999) found that four theory-based interventions drawing upon the HBM (e.g. Champion, 1994) increased mammography utilization, on average, by 23% compared to usual care. This is an impressive finding. The review also indicated that theory-based cognitive interventions which did not involve interpersonal interaction (e.g. those distributing letters or videos) were not effective. Meta-analyses of this kind can identify types of intervention and modes of intervention delivery that are effective in changing specified health behaviours. This information could then be used to design experimental studies that isolate particular techniques and combinations of techniques and measure potential mediators, including pre- and post-intervention beliefs.

REFERENCES

Abraham, C. & Sheeran, P. (2005). Health belief model. In M. Conner & P. Norman (Eds.). *Predicting Health Behaviour: Research and Practice with Social Cognition Models* (2nd edn.). Buckingham, UK: Open University Press.

Abraham, C., Sheeran, P., Spears, R. & Abrams, D. (1992). Health beliefs and the promotion of HIV-preventive intentions amongst teenagers: a Scottish perspective. *Health Psychology*, **11**, 363–70.

Abood, D. A., Black, D. R. & Feral, D. (2003). Smoking cessation in women with cardiac risk: a comparative study of two theoretically based therapies. *Journal of Nutrition Education and Behavior*, **35**, 260–7.

Ali, N. S. (2002). Prediction of coronary heart disease preventive behaviors in women: a test of the Health Belief Model. *Women and Health* **35**, 83–96.

Bandura, A. (1977). Self-efficacy: towards a unifying theory of behavioural change. *Psychological Review*, **84**, 191–215.

Baron, R. & Kenny, D. A. (1986). The moderator–mediator variable distinction in social psychological research: conceptual, strategic, and statistical considerations. *Journal of Personality and Social Psychology*, **51**, 1173–82.

Becker, M. H., Drachman, R. H. & Kirscht, P. (1974). A new approach to explaining sick-role behaviour in low income populations. *American Journal of Public Health*, **64**, 205–16.

Becker, M. H., Haefner, D. P., Kasl, S. V. *et al.* (1977). Selected psychosocial models and correlates of individual health-related behaviors. *Medical Care*, **15**, 27–46.

Becker, M. H. & Maiman, L. A. (1975). Sociobehavioural determinants of compliance with health and medical care recommendations. *Medical Care*, **13**, 10–24.

Bradley, C., Gamsu, D. S. & Moses, S. L. (1987). The use of diabetes-specific perceived control and health belief measures to predict treatment choice and efficacy in a feasibility study of continuous subcutaneous insulin infusion pumps. *Psychology and Health*, **1**, 133–46.

Carmel, S., Shani, E. & Rosenberg, L. (1996). Skin cancer protective behaviors among the elderly: explaining their response to a health education program using the health belief model. *Educational Gerontology*, **22**, 651–68.

Champion, V. L. (1984). Instrument development for health belief model constructs. *Advances in Nursing Science*, **6**, 73–85.

Champion, V. L. (1994). Strategies to increase mammography utilization. *Medical Care*, **32**, 118–29.

Cummings, K. M., Jette, A. M. & Brock, B. M. (1979). Psychological determinants of immunization behaviour in a swine influenza campaign. *Medical Care*, **17**, 639–49.

Feather, N. T. (1982). *Expectations and actions: expectancy-value models in psychology.* Hillsdale, NJ: Erlbaum.

Festinger, L. (1957). *A theory of cognitive dissonance.* Stanford, CA: Standford University Press.

Field, A. (2000). *Discovering statistics: using SPSS for windows.* London: Sage.

Fishbein, M. & Ajzen, I. (1975). *Belief, attitude, intention and behavior: an introduction to theory and research.* Reading, MA: Addison-Wesley.

Fishbein, M., Triandis, H. C., Kanfer, F. H. *et al.* (2001). *Factors influenceing behaviour and behaviour change.* In A. Baum, T. A. Revenson & J. E. Singer (Eds.). *Handbook of health psychology* (pp. 3–17). Mahwah, NJ: Lawerence Erlbaum Associates.

Gianetti, V. J., Reynolds, J. & Rihen, T. (1985). Factors which differentiate smokers from ex-smokers among cardiovascular patients: a discriminant analysis. *Social Science and Medicine*, **20**, 241–5.

Gochman, D. S. & Parcel, G. S. (Eds.). (1982). Children's health beliefs and health behaviours. *Health Education Quarterly*, **9**, 104–270.

Grady, K. E., Kegeles, S. S., Lund, A. K., Wolk, C. H. & Farber, N. J. (1983). Who volunteers for a breast self-examination program? Evaluating the bases for self-selection. *Health Education Quarterly*, **10**, 79–94.

Haefner, D. P. & Kirscht, J. P. (1970). Motivational and behavioural effects of modifying health beliefs. *Public Health Reports*, **85**, 478–84.

Harrison, J. A., Mullen, P. D. & Green, L. W. (1992). A meta-analysis of studies of the health belief model with adults. *Health Education Research*, **7**, 107–16.

Hay, J. L., Ford, J. S., Klein, D. *et al.* (2003). Adherence to colorectal cancer screening in mammography-adherent older women. *Journal of Behavioral Medicine*, **26**, 553–76.

Hochbaum, G. M. (1958). *Public participation in medical screening programs: a socio-psychological study.* Public Health Service Publication No. **572**. Washington, DC: United States Government Printing Office.

Janz, N. & Becker, M. H. (1984). The health belief model: a decade later. *Health Education Quarterly*, **11**, 1–47.

Jones, S. L., Jones, P. K. & Katz, J. (1988). Health belief model intervention to increase compliance with emergency department patients. *Medical Care*, **26**, 1172–84.

Keesling, B. & Friedman, H. S. (1987). Psychological factors in sunbathing and sunscreen use. *Health Psychology*, **6**, 477–93.

Kegeles, S. S. (1963). Why people seek dental care: a test of a conceptual framework. *Journal of Health and Human Behaviour*, **4**, 166.

Kelley, H. H. (1967). Attribution theory in social psychology. In D. Levine (Ed.). *Nebraska symposium on motivation.*

Lincoln: University of Nebraska Press, 192–241.

King, J. B. (1982). The impact of patients' perceptions of high blood pressure on attendance at screening: an extension of the health belief model. *Social Science and Medicine*, **16**, 1079–91.

Kirscht, J. P., Becker, M. H. & Eveland, P. (1976). Psychological and social factors as predictors of medical behaviour. *Journal of Medical Care*, **14**, 422–31.

Lewis, K. S. (1994). *An examination of the health belief model when applied to diabetes mellitus.* Unpublished Doctoral Dissertation, University of Sheffield.

Orbell, S, Crombie, I. & Johnston, G. (1995). Social cognition and social structure in the prediction of cervical screening uptake. *British Journal of Health Psychology*, **1**, 35–50.

Rosenstock, I. M. (1974). Historical origins of the health belief model. *Health Education Monographs*, **2**, 1–8.

Rosenthal, R. (1984). *Meta-analysis procedures for social research.* Beverly Hills, CA: Sage.

Rosenstock, I. M., Strecher, V. J. & Becker, M. H. (1988). Social learning theory and the health belief model. *Health Eduction Quarterly*, **15**, 175–83.

Rundall, T. G. & Wheeler, J. R. (1979). The effect of income on use of preventive care: an evaluation of alternative explanations. *Journal of Health and Social Behaviour*, **20**, 397–406.

Salloway, J. C., Pletcher, W. R. & Collins, J. J. (1978). Sociological and social psychological models of compliance with prescribed regimen: in search of a synthesis. *Sociological Symposium*, **23**, 100–21.

Schwarzer, R. (1992). Self-efficacy in the adoption and maintenance of health behaviours: theoretical approaches and a new model. In R. Schwarzer (Ed.). *Self-efficacy: thought control of action* (pp. 217–42). Washington, DC: Hemisphere.

Stone, J., Aronson, E., Crain, A. L., Winslow, M. P. & Fried, C. B. (1994). Inducing hypocrisy as a means of encouraging young adults to use condoms. *Personality and Social Psychology Bulletin*, **20**, 116–28.

Strecher, V. J., Kreuter, M., DenBoer, D. J. *et al.* (1994). The effects of computer-tailored smoking cessation messages in family practice settings. *Journal of Family Practice*, **39**, 262–70.

Sutton, S. (1998). Predicting and explaining intentions and behavior: how well are we doing? *Journal of Applied Social Psychology*, **15**, 1317–38.

Umeh, K. & Rogan-Gibson, J. (2001). Perceptions of threat, benefits, and barriers in breast self-examination amongst young asymptomatic women. *British Journal of Health Psychology*, **6**, 361–72.

Volk, J. E. & Koopman, C. (2001). Factors associated with condom use in Kenya: a test of the health belief model. *AIDS Education and Prevention.* **13**, 495–508.

Weinstein, N. D. (1988). The precaution adoption process. *Health Psychology*, **7**, 355–86.

Yabroff, K. R. & Mandelblatt, J. S. (1999). Interventions targeted towards patients to increase mammography use. *Cancer Epidemiology Biomarkers and Prevention*, **8**, 749–57.

Health-related behaviours: common factors

Timothy P. Carmody

University of California

Introduction

Any behaviour that affects a person's health status, either positively or negatively, is considered to be a health-related behaviour. Daily habits involving diet, exercise, safety practices and substance use are not only related to the prevention of disease, but also affect the management of chronic illness and degree of disability (Fries, 2002). It is difficult to imagine any activity or behaviour that does not affect our health in some way, either directly or indirectly.

Common health-related behaviours include diet, exercise, smoking, alcohol use, safety practices and participation in health screening examinations such as testing for cholesterol levels, breast and prostate cancer (Fishbein *et al.*, 2001). Among the health-related behaviours most often encouraged in health promotion programmes is regular physical exercise because of its positive impact on health, disease prevention, psychological wellbeing and overall longevity (Johnson, 2003). Regular physical activity is associated with lower death rates for adults of any age, even when only moderate levels of physical activity are performed (Center for Disease Control, 1999).

Regular physical activity decreases the risk of death from heart disease, lowers the risk of developing diabetes, reduces the risk of colon cancer and helps reduce blood pressure (Center for Disease Control, 1999). In 1999, only 65% of adolescents engaged in the recommended amount of physical activity. Even more disappointing, in 1997, only 15% of adults performed the recommended amount of physical activity, and 40% of adults engaged in no leisure time physical activity (Center for Disease Control, 1999). (See 'Adolescent lifestyle', 'Age and physical functioning', and 'Phsyical activity interventions').

In the United States, over 1.7 million Americans die from heart disease, diabetes, cancer, asthma or stroke (US Public Health Service, 2000). These chronic diseases account for 75% of the $1.4 trillion that the United States spends on health care (US Public Health Service, 2000). Over 125 million Americans live with one of these chronic diseases and millions of new cases are diagnosed each year (US Public Health Service, 2000). Smoking, exercise, diet and alcohol use contribute to the development of most of these major causes of morbidity and mortality in the industrialized world (McGinnis & Forge, 1993; Smith *et al.*, 2004). However, there are other behaviours that affect health, which are less obvious to the general public. These latter behaviours pertain to the ways in which people cope with stress and negative emotions (Adler & Matthews, 1994). For example, the way that a person expresses anger may be associated with the development or acceleration of coronary heart disease (CAD) and neoplasms in some individuals (e.g. Adler & Matthews, 1994; Eysenck, 1988; Sparagon et al., 2001) (see 'Hostility, Type A and coronary heart disease'). Similarly, engaging in a pleasurable activity can be health related when such behaviour helps an individual to manage pain, stress or depressed mood.

Whereas behavioural experts have traditionally emphasized the importance of health-related behaviours and methods of behaviour change at the individual level, there is a growing trend to embrace a population-based approach and public health perspective (Smith et al., 2004). Some health-related behaviours (e.g. health screening, diet modification, smoking cessation, drug abuse or safe sex practices) have such an impact on the health of entire populations that they have become the focus of public health education campaigns aimed at promoting health and preventing disease in school, work and community settings (Orleans, 2000; Smith et al., 2004). Such health education campaigns are aimed either at healthy people to promote health maintenance and disease prevention or they target individuals who are already afflicted with illnesses or diseases in order to enhance the quality of their lives, reduce level of disability, delay death or prevent further deterioration. (See 'Community-based interventions'.)

Probably the most important public health education campaign of the past decade has been the worldwide effort to reduce behavioural risk factors associated with HIV infection and autoimmune disorder (AIDS) (Kelly & Kalichman, 2002). Early AIDS prevention efforts focused on safe sex practices and elimination of needle sharing among heroin addicts (Carey et al., 2004). More recent health education campaigns are aimed at promoting adherence to complex antiretroviral combination medication therapies (e.g. Tucker et al., 2004).

In the United States, the Healthy People 2010 campaign (US Public Health Service, 2000) was created as a comprehensive, nationwide approach to health promotion and disease prevention and was designed to serve as a roadmap for improving the health of all people in the United States during the first decade of the twenty-first century. Like the preceding Healthy People 2000 initiative, Healthy People 2010 is committed to the single, overarching purpose of promoting health and preventing illness, disability and premature death (US Public Health Service, 2000). An important goal of the Healthy People 2010 campaign is to eliminate health disparities among segments of the population, including differences that occur by gender, race or ethnicity, education or income, disability, geographic location or sexual orientation (US Public Health Service, 2000). (See 'Cultural and ethnic factors in health' and 'Socioeconomic status and health').

To determine the need for, and effectiveness of, such health education campaigns, public health assessment and surveillance surveys have been developed to monitor health-related behaviours or lifestyle patterns in representative samples. For instance, Walker et al. (1987) developed the Health-Promoting Lifestyle Profile (HPLP) which assesses six dimensions of health-related behaviours: self-actualization, health responsibility, exercise, nutrition, interpersonal support and stress management. Likewise, Sugarman et al.

(1992) described the Behavioral Risk Factor Surveillance System, a data set based on telephone surveys conducted by state departments of public health in co-ordination with the Center for Disease Control (CDC) to assess progress toward the health objectives for the United States.

Changing demographics of health-related behaviours

The demographics of health-related behaviours have undergone significant change in recent decades (Whitfield et al., 2002). As the average age of the world's population has increased, particularly in industrialized countries, there have been age-related increases in the prevalence of the major causes of morbidity and mortality (e.g. CAD, diabetes, hypertension, cancer, renal disease) and the role that behaviour plays in the prevention, development, and management of these diseases in older adults (Wilcox & King, 1999).

It is well known that the prevalence of chronic diseases and the health-related behaviours associated with those diseases varies across ethnic and cultural groups and socio-economic status (SES) (Whitfield et al., 2002). There has been an increasing recognition of disparities in the prevalence of chronic diseases and health-related behaviours among ethnic, cultural and SES groups (Landrine & Klonoff, 2001). Health disparities related to ethnicity, culture, SES and ageing point to the importance of understanding the effects of contextual factors on health status and health-related behaviours. For example, morbidity and mortality from colorectal cancer is higher among African Americans than other population groups in the United States (American Cancer Society, 2003). Income and education levels are associated with differences in the occurrence of illness and death, including heart disease, diabetes, obesity, elevated blood lead level and low birth weight (US Public Health Service, 2000). It is well known that higher income permits increased access to medical care, enables people to afford better housing and live in safer neighbourhoods, and increases the opportunity to engage in health-promoting behaviours.

The executive summary of the recent report on healthcare disparities (US Department of Health and Human Services, 2003) described the following:

- Minorities are more likely to be diagnosed with late-stage breast cancer and colorectal cancer compared with whites.
- Patients of lower socio-economic position are less likely to receive recommended diabetic services and more likely to be hospitalized for diabetes and its complications.
- When hospitalized for acute myocardial infarction, Hispanics are less likely to receive optimal care.
- Many racial and ethnic minorities and persons of lower socio-economic position are more likely to die from HIV. Minorities also account for a disproportionate share of new AIDS cases.
- The use of physical restraints in nursing homes is higher among Hispanics and Asian/Pacific Islanders compared with non-Hispanic whites.
- Blacks and poorer patients have higher rates of avoidable hospital admissions (i.e. hospitalizations for health conditions that, in the presence of comprehensive primary care, rarely require hospitalization).

Common dimensions of health-related behaviours

Health-related behaviours vary in terms of their duration, frequency, and manner of impact on health (i.e. positive versus negative; direct versus indirect; immediate versus long term). Some health-related behaviours are single actions that occur at a certain point in time and usually involve only one primary decision. Participating in a health screening examination (e.g. mammography, cholesterol, etc.) is an example of this type of health-related behaviour. Other health-related behaviours are long-term habits or patterns of behaviour that continue over an extended period of time and usually involve many decisions. Smoking, physical exercise, dietary habits, Type A behaviour and adherence to complex antiretroviral medication regimens are examples of these long-term health-related behaviours (Smith *et al.*, 2004). Many health-related behaviours such as smoking and alcohol use are not only long-term habits but are also addictive behaviours, characterized by the complex biopsychosocial determinants of obsessive chemical dependence.

Health-related behaviours that affect health in a positive way are sometimes referred to as health-protective behaviours. Examples of health-protective behaviours include eating a low fat diet, engaging in regular physical exercise, using sunscreen, wearing seat belts and engaging in safe sex practices (e.g. wearing condoms). Likewise, some health behaviours have a negative or deleterious effect on health (e.g. eating a high fat diet, sedentary lifestyle, substance abuse and stress-inducing behaviours). Still other health-related behaviours can have both a positive and negative impact on our health. For instance, dietary restraint can facilitate weight loss, but also can result in a restraint–disinhibition pattern of problematic 'yo-yo' dieting, weight fluctuation, alcohol use and cigarette smoking associated with health risk (Copeland & Carney, 2003; Herman & Polivy, 1980; Lowe, 1993; Stewart *et al.*, 2000).

Behaviour can influence health either directly or indirectly through its impact on other behaviours. Some health-related behaviours have a direct impact on physical health. Cigarette smoking is an example of this kind of health-risk behaviour (US Public Health Service, 1990, 2000). Other behaviours have an indirect impact on health by way of their association with other behaviours or lifestyle patterns, which in turn have a direct impact on health. For instance, according to one theory, hostility increases coronary risk because of its association with other coronary risk behaviours such as smoking (Scherwitz & Rugulies, 1992; Smith & Christensen, 1992; Smith & Ruiz, 2002). Drug abuse and heavy drinking are examples of health-risk behaviours that have both a direct and indirect impact on health, for example, among individuals infected with HIV by way of their association with non-adherence to antiretroviral medications (Tucker *et al.*, 2004).

Health-related behaviours also vary in terms of the timing of their impact on health. Some behaviours have an immediate impact on health (e.g. accidentally cutting a finger with a knife), others have a long-term effect (e.g. high fat diet, sedentary lifestyle) and still other actions have both immediate and long-term impact on health (e.g. cigarette smoking, dietary restraint, use of sunscreen, regular physical exercise).

Another common feature of health-related behaviours is that they often co-occur. For example, it is well known that alcohol, smoking and coffee consumption are inter-related (Carmody *et al.*, 1985; Istvan & Matarazzo, 1984). Most of the empirical research has shown a robust association between smoking and alcohol use, and between smoking and coffee consumption. However, there is a dearth of research investigating the co-occurrence of all three of these behaviours (Istvan & Matarazzo, 1984). Similarly, health-protective behaviours can interact with health-risk behaviours. For instance, exercise may provide a healthy substitute for smoking. Some health-related behaviours may become cues for other behaviours (e.g. a cocktail and a cigarette). In some cases, stopping one health-related behaviour may even lead to the onset of another (e.g. quitting smoking leading temporarily to overeating). Likewise, expectancies regarding the relationship between health-related behaviours can influence decisions regarding engaging in those behaviours. For example, Copeland and Carney (2003) found that women who were higher in dietary restraint and disinhibition reported stronger beliefs in the appetite and weight control properties of cigarettes and were more likely to smoke than those who were lower in dietary restraint and disinhibition. Similarly, Stewart *et al.* (2000) found that chronic dieting among female college students appeared to be related to a heavy alcohol use (see 'Diet and health').

Given the interactions among health-related behaviours, public health experts have debated whether or not to target multiple behaviours for change concurrently (Prochaska *et al.*, 2004). This debate has emerged in the treatment of tobacco use among alcohol-dependent smokers (Joseph *et al.*, 2003). It has also appeared in studies of health behaviour change aimed at reducing cardiovascular risk. Prochaska and Sallis (2004) compared an intervention that targeted physical activity and nutrition with a second intervention which targeted physical activity alone. Increases in physical activity were similar for the two intervention groups, but dietary change was minimal for the intervention that targeted nutrition in addition to physical activity.

Common determinants of health-related behaviours

Common psychosocial and environmental factors are involved in the development, maintenance and modification of health-related behaviours. The psychosocial determinants of health-related behaviours include cognitive factors (i.e. attitudes, beliefs, expectancies, intentions), individual differences involved in learning and decision-making processes (e.g. hardiness, optimism, locus of control), socio-cultural variables (i.e. influences of family, friends, healthcare providers) and environmental factors (e.g. stressful events, poverty, access to recreational facilities). (See 'Expectations and health', 'Personality and health', 'Social support and health', and 'Life events and health'.) At a recent workshop sponsored by the National Institute of Mental Health (NIMH), a panel of experts identified eight variables involved in the execution of any deliberate behaviour: intention, environmental constraints, skills, anticipated outcomes, norms, self-standards, emotion and self-efficacy (Fishbein *et al.*, 2001). However, these experts were not able to come to a consensus regarding a single causal model linking these variables to behaviour, causal ordering or strength of inter-relationships among these variables.

Psychosocial and environmental determinants can be categorized in terms of their chronological proximity to a particular health-related behaviour. Determinants which are more distant from the health-related behaviour include biological vulnerabilities, developmental characteristics, early learning history and other cognitive, social and background variables. More immediate psychosocial precipitants which cue or trigger particular health behaviours also include cognitive, social or environmental factors. Generally, intentions are viewed as most proximal to a specific health-related behaviour (Fishbein *et al.*, 2001).

The initiation, maintenance and modification of long-term health-related behaviours often involve classical (respondent) conditioning, operant and social learning factors such as stimulus control, modelling, positive reinforcement and punishment (Dragoi *et al.*, 2003; Fishbein *et al.*, 2001; Skinner, 1953). Classical conditioning has been shown to be involved in the development of addictive behaviours (e.g. Niaura *et al.*, 1988) and dietary behaviour patterns (e.g. Rozin, 1984). As learned behaviours, health-related behaviours have cues and consequences that influence the occurrence of these behaviours. According to operant learning theory, immediate consequences tend to exert a more powerful influence on behaviour than long-term consequences (Skinner, 1953). Research has shown that the most effective methods for changing health-related behaviours are based on the principles of respondent and operant learning (Bandura, 1986; Epstein *et al.*, 2004). These include self-monitoring, goal specification, stimulus control, self-reinforcement and behavioural rehearsal.

Health-related behaviours also have various cognitive determinants. Some of the cognitive factors thought to be involved in the initiation, maintenance and modification of various health-related behaviours include attributions, expectations, intentions, attitudes and core beliefs (Fishbein *et al.*, 2001). Attitudes have been conceptualized as including both cognitive and affective components. Intentions are usually considered to be the most immediate influence on behaviour as people make rational use of information available to them (Ajzen & Fishbein, 1980). Beliefs and attributions about the determinants of health and expectations about one's ability to control health play important roles in the learning and decision-making processes involved in the development and modification of health-related behaviours (Bandura, 1986, 1997). Expectations about one's ability to accomplish certain behaviours (i.e. self-efficacy expectations) are thought to be important determinants of health-related behaviour (Bandura, 1986, 1997). Self-efficacy has been studied in relation to several health-related behaviours, including diet, smoking, alcohol use, weight control and physical exercise (i.e. Bandura, 1982, 1986, 1997).

Health-related behaviours have also been studied from a personality or individual difference perspective. For example, optimism has been positive associated with health-protective behaviours (McGregor *et al.*, 2004; Scheier & Carver, 1987). Likewise, hardiness (Britt *et al.*, 2001; Funk, 1992; Kobasa, 1979), which has been conceptualized as involving challenge, commitment and control, has been shown to be positively associated with health. Both of these individual difference variables have been investigated in relation to their buffering effects on stress. Type A behaviour pattern (Friedman, 1992; Matthews, 1982; Smith & Ruiz, 2002; Sparagon *et al.*, 2001), health-protection motivation (Prentice-Dunn & Rogers, 1986), dispositional sense of coherence (Antonovsky, 1990; Hoge & Bussing, 2004), sensation-seeking (Zuckerman *et al.*, 1980), introversion–extraversion (Eysenck, 1970) and health locus of control (Strickland, 1989). These individual differences involve patterns of behaviour which are themselves health-related. Likewise,

personality traits may have a moderating effect on other lifestyle risk factors (e.g. Denollet, 1993). The relationships between personality, behaviour and health are complex and largely remain to be elucidated in future multifactorial and longitudinal research.

Health-related behaviours are also influenced by social and cultural factors. For example, peer pressure is a primary factor leading to onset of smoking behaviour in adolescents (Mills & Noyes, 1984). Social support can be an important factor in the development and modification of all forms of addictive behaviours. Social factors can play a role in maintenance of health-risk behaviours (e.g. specific forms of substance abuse) as well as health-protective behaviours (e.g. Kaplan & Toshima, 1990). For example, social support has been shown to be an important factor in smoking cessation and the prevention of smoking relapse (Carmody, 1990). Since social skills can be helpful in eliciting and maintaining social support, such behaviours can also be viewed as health-related.

Ethnic and cultural factors also affect the determinants of health-related behaviours (e.g. Pick *et al.*, 2003). For example, Vaughan *et al.* (2004) compared Hispanic and White mothers regarding paediatric injuries. White mothers reported more injuries among younger children. Among Hispanic mothers, preference for and use of English language were associated with more reported injuries. Their results indicated that risky behaviours, mother's judgement about child compliance and stressful life events were better predictors of injuries than housing quality. However, in the Hispanic group, stress and child temperament explained injury differences between more- and less-acculturated Hispanic families but only partially accounted for differences between White mothers and less-acculturated Hispanics.

Stress has been shown to have a direct impact on the autonomic nervous, neuroendocrine, cardiovascular and immune systems (Selye, 1980). Stress is also associated with health-related behaviours. The manner in which an individual copes with stressful situations can be considered to be a health-related behaviour (Hoge & Bussing, 2004; Lazarus & Folkman, 1984). Stress can also have an indirect effect on health by disrupting health-protective lifestyle patterns. For instance, adolescents who are in more distress are more likely to experiment with addictive drugs and develop chemical dependencies (Mills & Noyes, 1984). Similarly, depression has been associated with difficulty in quitting cigarette smoking (Carmody, 1990; Hitsman *et al.*, 2003; Kassel, Stroud & Paronis, 2003). In fact, stress is the most commonly reported trigger for relapse among chemical-dependent individuals (Marlatt & Gordon, 1985; Shiffman & Waters, 2004) (see 'Stress and health').

Environmental determinants of health-related behaviours include all aspects of an individual's physical surroundings and life circumstances, including exposure to information available to electronic and printed media, proximity to health care and health education resources and access to facilities conducive to engaging in health-protective behaviours such as physical exercise. Socioeconomic status (SES) has generally been regarded as an important determinant of health-related behaviours and overall health status. For example, health-risk factors such as obesity and cigarette smoking tend to be more prevalent among individuals from lower SES backgrounds (US Public Health Service, 1988). The mechanisms involved in determining the association between SES and health are yet to be elucidated (Adler *et al.*, 1994). Legal, economic and regulatory factors also influence health-related behaviours.

For instance, in California and elsewhere in the United States, health economists and policy experts (e.g. Glanz, 1993) have examined the impact of various taxation and other regulatory practices on exposure to environmental tobacco smoke (ETS).

Theories of health-related behaviours

Numerous theories of motivation, learning and decision-making have been applied to the study of health-related behaviours. These theories have been helpful in guiding research aimed at enhancing our understanding of health-related behaviours and developing more effective behaviour-change strategies. However, behavioural scientists have only just begun to apply their theories and methods of studying human behaviour to the fields of health promotion and disease management.

The most widely researched theories of health-related behaviour include: the health belief model (e.g. Kirscht, 1988), subjective expected utility theory (e.g. Sutton, 1982), conflict theory of decisional balance (Janis & Mann, 1968; Velicer et al., 1985), protection–motivation theory (Prentice-Dunn & Rogers, 1986), transtheoretical stages of change model (Prochaska & DiClemente, 1984), theory of reasoned action (Ajzen & Fishbein, 1980), theory of planned behaviour (Ajzen, 1988), and behavioural economics theory (Epstien & Saelens, 2000). (See 'The health belief model', 'Theory of planned behaviour', 'Self-efficacy and health behaviour' and 'Transactional model of behaviour change'.) Each of these theories emphasizes the role of attitudes and beliefs regarding the health consequences of particular behaviours as determinants of health-related decision-making and behaviour. The influence of significant others is also acknowledged as a source of information about subjective norms. These theories are based on the notion that people are rational and that they typically engage in a process of weighing the pros and cons of engaging in any behaviours that affect their health. Traditionally, they have emphasized perceptions of risk but not beliefs about non-risk issues such as self-esteem which also influence decision-making regarding health-related behaviours (Weinstein, 1993).

Most of these theories of health-related decision-making aim toward predicting a single decision (Weinstein, 1993). In contrast, dynamic models assume that the adoption of health behaviours is a dynamic process involving more than one decision rule and usually consisting of several steps or stages (e.g. Prochaska & DiClemente, 1984; Prochaska et al., 1994). An example of such a dynamic model is the transtheoretical stages of change model (Prochaska & DiClemente, 1984) which includes the following stages in the modification of any health-related behaviour: precontemplation (not thinking about change), contemplation (thinking about change in the next six months), action (overt change) and maintenance (continuation of changed behaviour beyond six months). According to this model, specific behaviour-change processes and decision rules tend to be associated with different stages. This transtheoretical model of change has been applied to a variety of addictive behaviours (e.g. smoking, compulsive eating, alcohol use) as well as health-protective behaviours (e.g. weight control, physical exercise, pain management) (e.g. Armitage et al., 2004; Prochaska et al., 1988; Prochaska et al., 1994; Segan, Borland & Greenwood, 2004).

Prochaska et al. (1994) studied the stages of change and decisional balance variables in relation to 12 health-related behaviours: smoking cessation, quitting cocaine, weight control, high-fat diets, adolescent delinquent behaviours, safe sex, condom use, sunscreen use, radon gas exposure, physical exercise, mammography screening and physicians' preventive practices with smokers. Their results supported the applicability of the transtheoretical model of change (Prochaska & DiClemente, 1984) and demonstrated commonalities in terms of the stages of change and decisional balance factors across these 12 health-related behaviours.

Behavioural economics theory (Epstien & Saelens, 2000) focuses on the way in which individuals make decisions about the allocation of time among available behavioural alternatives. This theory has recently been applied to the reduction of sedentary behaviour in obese children by increasing opportunities for more physical activity. In one study (Epstein et al., 2004), significant reductions in percent overweight were observed for obese children participating in treatment programmes in which reduction of sedentary behaviour was promoted either by stimulus control or reinforcement procedures.

The relationship between health risk perception and health-related behaviours is complex (Sjoberg, 2003). For example, people tend to evaluate health risks for themselves differently from risks for others (Sjoberg, 2003). Beliefs about risks associated with certain health-damaging behaviours may not necessarily be associated with the absence of those health-risk behaviours. In a recent survey of health behaviours in young adults in eight countries throughout Europe (Steptoe & Wardle, 1992), the results showed that respondents who engaged in more drinking and smoking behaviour were as aware of the negative consequences of these health-damaging behaviours as people who did not engage in these addictive behaviours. Across the countries surveyed in this study, few relationships were observed between health-risk behaviours and risk awareness. In contrast, beliefs about the positive effects of health-protective behaviours (e.g. eating a low fat diet) were strongly associated with the prevalence of those positive health behaviours.

Since adherence to medical regimen involves behaviour that impacts health, theories of adherence have been useful in furthering our understanding of the psychosocial and environmental determinants of health-related behaviours (see 'Adherence to treatment'). Leventhal and Cameron (1987) summarized five theories of adherence which focused on biomedical, behavioural, communication, decision-making and self-regulatory factors. They advocated for an integration of these theories in adherence research that addresses the patient's history of illness, perceptions, coping strategies and habitual versus reasoned determinants of behaviour change.

Summary and conclusions

I have argued that most of our behaviour is health-related in the sense that most of our actions affect our health, either directly or indirectly. Some behaviours have multiple effects on our health, some positive and some negative. Common psychosocial and environmental factors influence the learning and decision-making processes involved in the initiation, maintenance and modification of health-related behaviours. These include cognitive, socio-cultural, environmental, ethnic/racial and individual difference factors. There has been an increased focus on health disparities related to cultural, ethnic and SES factors, the investigation of the primary factors underlying these disparities, and the development of strategies for eliminating these disparities.

Long-term patterns of health-related behaviours usually involve various respondent conditioning and operant learning factors that influence multiple decision-making processes. Moreover, health-related behaviours often interact both in terms of their impact on lifestyle and health. These behaviours evolve in a dynamic process that involves many decisions and multiple cognitive, social and environmental determinants. Different sets of psychosocial determinants may be critical at different stages in the development and modification of a particular health-related behaviour.

Several theories have guided and facilitated empirical analysis of contextual and psychosocial determinants of health-related behaviours and processes of change. Nevertheless, behavioural scientists have only just begun to apply these theories and methods of studying human behaviour to the field of health-related behaviours. Initial successes have been achieved in such areas as smoking cessation, adherence to prescribed medications, regular physical exercise and fitness, safe sex practices, stress management and modification of CAD lifestyle risk factors. However, further theory-based research is needed to enhance our ability to understand, predict and modify health-related behaviours. Among the most promising theoretical approaches are cognitive social learning theory (Bandura, 1986, 1997) and the transtheoretical model of change (Prochaska & DiClemente, 1984) which attempts to integrate key constructs from several theoretical models in order to develop a more comprehensive understanding of health-related behaviours and enhance our ability to promote health-protective behaviour change.

REFERENCES

Adler, N. E., Boyce, T., Chesney, M. A. *et al.* (1994). Socioeconomic status and health: the challenge of the gradient. *American Psychologist*, **49**, 15–24.

Adler, N. E. & Matthews, K. A. (1994). Health psychology: why do some people get sick and some stay well? *Annual Review of Psychology*, **45**, 229–59.

Ajzen, I. (1988). *Attitudes, personality and behavior*. Milton Keynes, UK: Open University Press.

Ajzen, I. & Fishbein, M. (1980). *Understanding attitudes and predicting behavior*. Englewood Cliffs, NJ: Prentice-Hall.

American Cancer Society (2003). *Cancer facts and figures*. Atlanta: Author.

American Dietetic Association (2004). Position of the American Dietetic Association and Dietitians of Canada: nutrition and women's health. *Journal of the American Dietetic Association*, **104**, 984–1001.

Antonovsky, A. (1990). Personality and health: testing the sense of coherence model. In H. S. Friedman (Ed.). *Personality and disease* (pp. 155–77). New York: Wiley.

Armitage, C. J., Sheeran, P., Conner, M. & Arden, M. A. (2004). Stages of change or changes of stage? Predicting transitions in transtheoretical model stages in relation to healthy food choice. *Journal of Consulting and Clinical Psychology*, **72**, 491–9.

Bandura, A. (1982). Self-efficacy mechanism in human agency. *American Psychologist*. **37**, 122–42.

Bandura, A. (1986). *Social foundations of thought and action*. Englewood Cliffs, NJ: Prentice-Hall.

Bandura, A. (1997). *Self-efficacy: the exercise of control*. New York: Freeman.

Britt, T. W., Adler, A. B. & Bartone, P. T. (2001). Deriving benefits from stressful events: the role of engagement in meaningful work and hardiness. *Journal of Occupational Health Psychology*, **6**, 53–63.

Carey, M. P., Carey, K. B., Maisto, S. A. *et al.* (2004). Reducing HIV-risk behavior among adults receiving outpatient psychiatric treatment: results from a randomized controlled trial. *Journal of Consulting and Clinical Psychology*, **72**, 252–68.

Carmody, T. P. (1990). Preventing relapse in the treatment of nicotine addiction: current issues and future directions. *Journal of Psychoactive Drugs*, **22**, 211–38.

Carmody, T. P., Brischetto, C. S., Matarazzo, J. D., O'Donnell, R. P. & Connor, W. E. (1985). Co-occurrent use of cigarettes, alcohol, and coffee in healthy community-living men and women. *Health Psychology*, **4**, 323–35.

Center for Disease Control and Prevention (1999). *Promoting physical activity: a guide for community action*. U.S. Department of Health and Human Services, National Center for Chronic Disease Prevention and Health Promotion, Division of Nutrition and Physical Activity.

Copeland, A. L. & Carney, C. E. (2003). Smoking expectancies as mediators between dietary restraint and disinhibition and smoking in college women. *Experimental and Clinical Psychopharmacology*, **11**, 247–51.

Denollet, J. (1993). Biobehavioral research on coronary heart disease: where is the person? *Journal of Behavioral Medicine*, **16**, 115–41.

Dragoi, V., Staddon, J. E. R., Palmer, R. G. & Buhusi, C. V. (2003). Interval timing as an emergent learning property. *Psychological Review*. **110**, 126–44.

Epstein, L. H., Paluch, R. A., Kilanowski, C. K. & Raynor, H. A. (2004). The effect of reinforcement or stimulus control to reduce sedentary behavior in the treatment of pediatric obesity. *Health Psychology*, **23**, 371–80.

Epstein, L. H. & Saelens, B. E. (2000). Behavioral economics of obesity: food intake and energy expenditure. In W. K. Bickel & R. E. Vuchinich (Eds.). *Reframing health behavior change with behavioral economics* (pp. 293–311). Mahwah, NJ: Erlbaum.

Eysenck, H. J. (1970). *The Structure of Human Personality* (3rd edn.). London: Methuen.

Eysenck, H. J. (1988). Behaviour therapy as an aid in the prevention of cancer and coronary heart disease. *Scandinavian Journal of Behavior Therapy*, **17**, 171–87.

Fishbein, M., Triandis, H.C., Kanfer, F. H. *et al.* (2001). Factors influencing behavior and behavior change. In A. Baum, T. A. Revenson & J. E. Singer (Eds.). *Handbook of health psychology* (pp. 3–18). Mahwah, NJ: Lawrence Erlbaum Associates.

Friedman, H. S. (Ed.). (1992). *Hostility, coping, and health*. Washington, DC: American Psychological Association.

Fries, J. F. (2002). Reducing disability in older age. *Journal of the American Medical Association*, **288**, 3164–66.

Funk, S. C. (1992). Hardiness: a review of theory and research. *Health Psychology*, **11**, 335–45.

Glanz, S. A. (1993, December). *Tobacco industry response to passive smoking*. Paper presented at a meeting of the Tobacco-related Diseases Research Program, San Francisco.

Herman, C. P. & Polivy, J. (1980). Restrained eating. In A. J. Stunkard (Ed.). *Obesity* (pp. 208–25). Philadelphia: Saunders.

Hitsman, B., Borrelli, B., McChargue, D. E., Spring, B. & Niaura, R. (2003). History of depression and smoking cessation outcome: a meta-analysis. *Journal of Consulting and Clinical Psychology*, **71**, 657–63.

Höge, T. & Büssing, A. (2004). The impact of sense of coherence and negative affectivity on the work stressor-strain relationship. *Journal of Occupational Health Psychology*, **9**, 195–205.

Istvan, J. & Matarazzo, J.D. (1984). Tobacco, alcohol, and caffeine use: a review of their interrelationships. *Psychological Bulletin*, **95**, 301–26.

Janis, I.L. & Mann, L., (1968). A conflict-theory approach to attitude change and decision making. In A. Greenwald, T. Brook & T. Ostrom. (Eds.). *Psychological foundations of attitudes* (pp. 327–60). New York: Academic Press.

Johnson, N.G. (2003). Psychology and health: research, practice, and policy. *American Psychologist*, **58**, 670–7.

Joseph, A., Willenbring, M., Nugent, S. & Nelson, D. (2003). Timing of alcohol and smoking cessation study. Paper presented at Annual Meeting of the Society for Research on Nicotine and Tobacco, New Orleans.

Kaplan, R.M. & Toshima, M.T. (1990). Social relationships in chronic illness and disability. In I.G. Sarason, B.R. Sarason & G.R. Pierce (Eds.). *Social support: an interactional perspective*. New York: Wiley.

Kassel, J.D., Stroud, L.R. & Paronis, C.A. (2003). Smoking, stress, and negative affect: correlation, causation, and context across stages of smoking. *Psychological Bulletin*, **129**, 270–304.

Kelly, J.A. & Kalichman, S.C. (2002). Behavioral research in HIV/AIDS primary and secondary prevention: recent advances and future directions. *Journal of Consulting and Clinical Psychology*, **70**, 626–39.

Kirscht, J.P. (1988). The health belief model and predictions of health actions. In D. Gochman (Ed.). *Health behavior* (pp. 27–41). New York: Plenum Press.

Kobasa, S.C. (1979). Stressful life events, personality, and health: an inquiry into hardiness. *Journal of Personality and Social Psychology*, **37**, 1–11.

Landrine, H. & Klonoff, E.A. (2001). Cultural diversity and health psychology. In A. Baum, T.A. Revenson & J.E. Singer (Eds.). *Handbook of health psychology* (pp. 851–91). Mahwah, NJ: Erlbaum.

Lazarus, R.S. & Folkman, S. (1984). *Stress, appraisal, and coping*. New York: Springer.

Leventhal, H. & Cameron, L. (1987). Behavioral theories and the problem of compliance. *Patient Education and Counseling*, **10**, 117–38.

Lowe, M.R. (1993). The effects of dieting on eating behavior: a three-factor model. *Psychological Bulletin*, **114**, 100–21.

Marlatt, G.A. & Gordon, J.R. (1985). *Relapse prevention*. New York: Guilford Press.

Matthews, K.A. (1982). Psychological perspectives on the Type A behavior pattern. *Psychological Bulletin*, **91**, 293–323.

McGinnis, J.M. & Foege, W.H. (1993). Actual causes of death in the United States. *Journal of Consulting and Clinical Psychology*, **270**, 2207–12.

McGregor, B.A., Bowen, D.J., Ankerst, D.P. *et al.* (2004). Optimism, perceived risk of breast cancer, and cancer worry among a community-based sample of women. *Health Psychology*, **23**, 339–44.

Mills, C.J. & Noyes, H.L. (1984). Patterns and correlates of initial and subsequent drug use among adolescents. *Journal of Consulting and Clinical Psychology*, **52**, 231–43.

Niaura, R.S., Rohsenow, D.J., Binkoff, J.A. *et al.* (1988). Relevance of cue reactivity to understanding alcohol and smoking relapse. *Journal of Abnormal Psychology*, **97**, 133–52.

Orleans, C.T. (2000). Promoting the maintenance of health behavior change: recommendations for the next generation of research and practice. *Health Psychology*, **19**(Suppl. 1), 76–83.

Pick, S., Poortinga, Y.H. & Givaudan, M. (2003). Integrating intervention theory and strategy in culture-sensitive health promotion programs. *Professional Psychology: Research and Practice*, **34**, 422–9.

Prentice-Dunn, S. & Rogers, R.W. (1986). Protection motivation theory and preventive health: beyond the health belief model. *Health Education Research*, **1**, 153–61.

Prochaska, J.J. & Sallis, J.F. (2004). A randomized controlled trial of single versus multiple health behavior change: promoting physical activity and nutrition among adolescents. *Health Psychology*, **23**, 314–18.

Prochaska, J.O. & DiClemente, C.C. (1984). *The transtheoretical approach: crossing traditional boundaries of change*. Homewood, IL: J. Irwin.

Prochaska, J.O., Velicer, W.F., DiClemente, C.C. & Fava, J. (1988). Measuring processes of change: applications to the cessation of smoking. *Journal of Consulting and Clinical Psychology*, **56**, 520–8.

Prochaska, J.O., Velicer, W.F., Rossi, J.S. *et al.* (1994). Stages of change and decisional balance for 12 problem behaviors. *Health Psychology*, **13**, 39–46.

Prochaska, J.O., Velicer, W.F., Rossi, J.S. *et al.* (2004). Multiple risk expert systems interventions: impact of simultaneous stage-matched expert system interventions for smoking, high-fat diet, and sun exposure in a population of parents. *Health Psychology*, **23**, 503–16.

Rozin, H.P. (1984). The acquisition of food habits and preferences. In J.D. Matarazzo, S.M. Weiss, J.A. Herd, N.E. Miller & S.M. Weiss (Eds.). *Behavioral health: a handbook of health enhancement and disease prevention* (pp. 590–607). New York: Wiley.

Scheier, M.F. & Carver, C.S. (1987). Dispositional optimism and physical well-being: the influence of generalized outcome expectancies on health. *Journal of Personality*, **55**, 169–210.

Scherwitz, L. & Rugulies, R., (1992). Lifestyle and hostility. In H.S. Friedman (Ed.). *Hostility, coping, and health* (pp. 77–98). Washington, DC: American Psychological Association.

Segan, C.J., Borland, R. & Greenwood, K.M. (2004). What is the right thing at the right time? Interactions between stages and processes of change among smokers who make a quit attempt. *Health Psychology*, **23**, 86–93.

Selye, H. (1980). The stress concept today. In I.L. Kutash, L.B. Schlesinger *et al.* (Eds.). *Handbook on stress and anxiety* (pp. 127–9). San Francisco: Jossey-Bass.

Shiffman, S. & Waters, A.J. (2004). Negative affect and smoking lapses: a prospective analysis. *Journal of Consulting and Clinical Psychology*, **72**, 192–201.

Sjoberg, L. (2003). Neglecting the risks: the irrationality of health behavior and the quest for *La Dolce Vita*. *European Psychologist*, **8**, 266–78.

Skinner, B.F. (1953). *Science and human behavior*. New York: Macmillan.

Smith, T.W. & Christensen, A.J. (1992). In H.S. Friedman (Ed.). *Hostility, coping, and health* (pp. 33–48). Washington, DC: American Psychological Association.

Smith, T.W., Orleans, C.T. & Jenkins, C.D. (2004). Prevention and health promotion: decades of progress, new challenges, and an emerging agenda. *Health Psychology*, **23**, 126–31.

Smith, T.W. & Ruiz, J.M. (2002). Psychosocial influences on the development and course of coronary heart disease: current status and implications for research and practice. *Journal of Consulting and Clinical Psychology*, **70**, 548–68.

Sparagon, B., Friedman, M., Breall, W.S. *et al.* (2001). Type A behavior and coronary atherosclerosis. *Atherosclerosis*, **156**, 145–9.

Steptoe, A. & Wardle, J. (1992). Cognitive predictors of health behaviour in contrasting regions of Europe. *British Journal of Clinical Psychology*, **31**, 485–502.

Stewart, S. H., Angelopoulos, M., Baker, J. M. & Boland, F. J. (2000). Relations between dietary restraint and patterns of alcohol use in young adult women. *Psychology of Addictive Behaviors*, **14**, 77–82.

Strickland, B. R. (1989). Internal–external control expectancies: from contingency to creativity. *American Psychologist*, **44**, 1–12.

Sugarman, J. R., Warren, C. W., Oge, L. & Helgerson, S. D. (1992). Using the behavioral risk factor surveillance system to monitor year 2000 objectives among American Indians. *Public Health Reports*, **107**, 449–56.

Sutton, S. R. (1982). Fear arousing communications: a critical examination of theory and research. In J. R. Eiser (Ed.). *Social psychology and behavioral medicine* (pp. 303–38). New York: Wiley.

Tucker, J. S., Orlando, M., Burnam, M. A. *et al.* (2004). Psychosocial mediators of antiretroviral nonadherence in HIV-positive adults with substance use and mental health problems. *Health Psychology*, **23**, 363–70.

US Department of Health and Human Services (2003). National healthcare disparities report. Rockville, MD: Agency for Healthcare Research and Quality.

US Public Health Service (1988). *The surgeon general's report on nutrition and health*. Washington, DC: US Department of Health and Human Services.

US Public Health Service (1990). *The health consequences of smoking: a report of the surgeon general* (CDC Report No 89–8411). Rockville, MD: US Department of Health and Human Services.

US Public Health Service (2000). *Health people 2010: understanding and improving health*. Washington, DC: US Department of Health and Human Services.

Vaughan, E., Anderson, C., Agran, P. & Winn, D. (2004). Cultural differences in young children's vulnerability to injuries: a risk and protection perspective. *Health Psychology*, **23**, 289–98.

Velicer, W. F., DiClemente, C. C., Prochaska, J. O. & Brandenburg, N. (1985). Decisional balance measure for assessing and predicting smoking status. *Journal of Personality and Social Psychology*, **48**, 1279–89.

Vounis, N., Soran, H. & Farook, S. (2004). The prevention of Type 2 diabetes mellitus: recent advances. *Quarterly Journal of Medicine*, **97**, 451–5.

Walker, S. N., Schrist, K. R. & Pender, N. J. (1987). The health-promoting lifestyle profile: development and psychometric characteristics. *Nursing Research*, **36**, 76–81.

Weinstein, N. D. (1993). Testing four competing theories of health-protective behavior. *Health Psychology*, **12**, 324–33.

Whitfield, K. E., Weidner, G., Clark, R. & Anderson, N. B. (2002). Sociodemographic diversity and behavioral medicine. *Journal of Consulting and Clinical Psychology*, **70**, 463–81.

Wilcox, S. & King, A., (1999). Health behavior and aging. In W. R. Hazzard, J. P. Blass, W. H. Ettinger, J. B. Halter & J. G. Ouslander (Eds.). *Principles of geriatric medicine and gerontology* (pp. 287–302). New York: McGraw-Hill.

Zuckerman, M., Buschbaum, M. & Murphy, D. (1980). Sensation-seeking and its biological correlates. *Psychological Bulletin*, **88**, 187–214.

Hospitalization in adults

Rachael Powell and Marie Johnston

University of Aberdeen

Introduction

Hospitalization occurs when symptoms of illness can no longer be tolerated in the individual's domestic environment, when technical investigations need to be performed or when treatments requiring specific equipment or 24-hour patient monitoring are to be undertaken. One might therefore expect that, at least for a substantial minority, hospitalization would be viewed as a source of relief or reassurance, or would hold out the possibility of offering a better understanding of symptoms or even resolution of symptoms. However, in the psychological literature, it is primarily conceptualized as a source of stress. Additionally, discharge from hospital is seen as a stressful time and Ley (1988) has reported high levels of depression in patients in the period following discharge.

This chapter discusses the stressors faced by hospitalized adults and emotional and cognitive responses to hospitalization. The role of health professionals in meeting the needs of hospitalized adults is considered and the impact of adult hospitalization on family members is examined.

Stressors

The Hospital Stress Rating Scale (Volicer & Bohannon, 1975) describes 49 'events' associated with being in hospital which may be stressful. These events were ranked by 261 medical and surgical patients from the most to the least stressful. The most stressful, thinking you might lose your sight, relates to the threat of illness as does the fourth, knowing that you have a serious illness. Illness course was also identified as an area of concern in chronic bronchitis and emphysema patients by Small and Graydon (1993). Several of Volicer and Bohannon's (1975) high-ranking stressors concern lack of information or poor communication ('not being told what your diagnosis is' (ranking: 6), 'not knowing for sure what illness you have (7), 'not knowing the results or reasons for your treatments' (9) and 'not having your questions answered by staff' (13)). Major sources of stress in hospital are the investigations and treatments, which may involve pain and uncertainty of outcome (e.g. 'knowing you have to have an operation' (18)) and other studies have found that anticipating painful treatments and procedures is a source of apprehension or distress for the great majority of patients. Other items relate to being away from family and home, e.g. 'missing your spouse' (12) or 'being hospitalized far away from home' (17) or to being in a new environment which lacks privacy and is shared by other people who are ill and receiving treatment (Lucente & Fleck, 1972). Volicer and Bohannon found a high degree of consensus between medical and surgical patients (see also 'Coping with stressful medical procedures' and 'Surgery').

Emotional state

Given the range of perceived stressors, investigation into the emotional state of patients is a logical progression. Many studies use scales that have been developed specifically to measure patients' anxiety about hospitalization but others use scales that have been used to measure mood or distress in other situations and populations. These latter scales have usually been extensively developed and validated and allow comparison of hospitalized patients with normal mood levels, with people undergoing other kinds of threat or with patients who have mood disorders. An important consideration is whether the scale confuses symptoms of the patient's illness or the effects of treatment with somatic mood effects; for example, patients may report feeling lethargic because of thyroid disorder or the after-effects of anaesthesia rather than as a feature of depressed mood. Some scales, such as the Hospital Anxiety and Depression Scale (HADS, Zigmond & Snaith, 1983) have been developed to either separate or omit such somatic items. The HADS has been shown to be reasonably successful in this (Johnston et al., 2000) (see also 'Mood assessment').

Numerous studies show evidence of high levels of psychological distress in hospitalized patients when compared with normal populations, including high rates of clinical emotional disorder. For example, surgical patients assessed on the day prior to surgery show levels of anxiety that, on average, fall between normal levels and levels reported by psychiatric patients with diagnosed anxiety disorder, but are similar to those found in students prior to examinations. Anxiety levels continue to be high after surgery (Johnston, 1980), suggesting that the anxiety is caused not only by the threat of surgery but also by the ongoing discomforts and uncertainties. It is important that staff are aware of and can address emotional state for both the patients' psychological and physical wellbeing. Munafò and Stevenson (2001), for example, found pre-surgical anxiety to consistently predict post-operative outcome. In recent years, the area of psychoneuroimmunology has made great progress in identifying associations between psychological and physical health and has been found to be relevant to patient outcomes after surgery. For example, Broadbent et al. (2003) found pre-surgical perceived stress to predict levels of interleukin-1, a cytokine involved in the inflammatory response, in wound fluid collected post-operatively for patients undergoing hernia repair (see 'Surgery').

Cognitions

When the concerns of hospital patients have been examined, it is clear that they have significant worries which are unrelated to the hospital environment, often concerning the welfare of their family at home in the patient's absence or even ongoing everyday worries irrelevant to health and the hospital (Johnston, 1988). Hospital worries may be related to both their medical condition and its treatment. While research has tended to focus on worries about treatment procedures, patients are more likely to be concerned about treatment outcomes or the outcome of the disease whether or not treatment is possible.

Hospitalized patients' concerns are not limited to the hospitalization period itself: Small and Graydon (1993) found that being able to manage their own homes and self-care post-discharge were the most commonly expressed concerns in a small sample of patients with chronic bronchitis and/or emphysema. Leech (1982) found a sense of control to be considered important by 95% of their sample of pre-operative patients with arterial occlusive disease. Only 42% perceived themselves to be in control but, for 82%, it was control over their future rather than lack of control caused by imposed hospital routines that was important. Hence, to some extent, worries are inevitable because of the unpredictable nature of these outcomes, but this is exacerbated by the lack of information available to patients or appropriate coping skills. Studies of psychological preparation for surgical procedures demonstrate that changing cognitions by the provision of information or enhancing the patient's ability to tolerate the uncertainties can reduce the negative effects of the experience (Doering et al., 2000; Johnston & Vögele, 1993).

Individual differences

People who are anxious by disposition are more likely to be highly anxious in the hospital situation than people low in trait anxiety. Hospital and the associated health problems would appear to provide the threatening situations which elicit this underlying personality. People with high levels of anxiety may also use different coping strategies in dealing with the situation (see 'Personality and health').

Coping strategies can be divided into problem-focused and emotion-focused strategies, the former attempting to reduce the impact of stress by removing the source, while the latter aim to minimize the emotional impact without necessarily dealing with the source. It has been suggested that some patients having surgery may try to deal with the threats by using an avoidant strategy which includes minimizing the dangers and directing one's attention to other matters, and such patients would tend to have low scores on tests of anxiety. Initially, it was proposed by Janis (1958) that such a strategy would result in poor outcomes for patient as they would fail to do the necessary cognitive preparation, or 'work of worrying', and as a result would find the post-operative period unexpectedly harsh. Janis proposed that patients with low and high anxiety scores would do badly post-operatively and that a moderate level of anxiety was necessary to achieve optimal preparation. However, empirical studies have not found support for this hypothesis and instead patients having low levels of pre-operative anxiety or those using avoidant coping strategies have done well post-operatively; it would appear that avoidant coping is adaptive for stressors of relatively short duration (DeGroot et al., 1997; Suls & Fletcher, 1985).

Factors which influence responses to hospitalization may be different in children or in elderly people (see 'Hospitalization in children'). Those with particular clinical conditions may also have different issues to contend with. For example, hospital staff on a surgical ward may have difficulty in ascertaining the level of support necessary for a disabled patient or the supervision and support required by a psychiatric patient.

Roles of health professionals in meeting needs

Psychological preparation

While little work has been done to prepare adult patients for hospitalization per se, there is now very strong evidence that psychological preparation for surgery can result in better outcomes (Johnston & Vögele, 1993). A variety of methods have been used including:

- behavioural instruction: teaching techniques such as breathing and relaxation;
- procedural information: giving patients information about the procedures they will undergo;
- sensory information: giving patients information about the sensations they will experience;
- cognitive coping: teaching methods of re-interpreting apparent threats in a more positive light, using distraction etc.

All of these methods have been shown to be effective. They have been found to improve a wide variety of important outcomes including:

- anxiety
- pain
- pain medication
- behavioural recovery
- physiological indices
- length of stay.

Thus, benefits are not confined to benefits in psychological functioning, but include outcomes of physiological significance and outcomes that affect health care costs.

Surgical patients have also been found to benefit by spending the pre-operative period with patients who have already had the operation they are about to undergo (Kulik & Mahler, 1987). This study suggests that there is considerable potential for improving patient care by organizational as well as direct patient care interventions.

Interventions have also been designed for patients undergoing non-surgical procedures. Such procedures differ from the typical surgical procedure in that the patient is conscious and may be required to co-operate to ensure an efficient and effective procedure. For example, in cardiac catheterization the patient must respond to instructions for breath holding and coughing. Ludwick-Rosenthal and Neufeld (1993) found cardiac catheterization took less time for participants in a high-information group than for those in a low-information group. Sensory information and cognitive coping procedures have also been found to be effective (Kendall & Epps, 1990).

There has been some concern that psychological preparation might be damaging for patients using avoidant coping strategies as the preparation might disrupt the patient's coping. While there is some evidence to support this view, a study by Shipley et al. (1978) suggests that the problem can be overcome by giving adequate preparation. Patients awaiting a stressful medical procedure saw a preparatory videotape either once or three times. Those with an avoidant coping style showed higher levels of anxiety during the endoscopy compared with a control group who saw an irrelevant control video, but only when they had seen the video once; they showed neither detrimental nor beneficial effects when they had seen it three times. Patients with attention coping styles showed benefit whether the video was shown once or three times. Thus the more thorough preparation resulted in benefits without the damaging side-effects for the avoidant copers. Ludwick-Rosenthal and Neufelt (1993) found information seekers receiving low-level information prior to cardiac catheterization showed higher behavioural anxiety than avoiders receiving low information or seekers receiving high information. Differences between information avoiders and seekers in the high-information condition were non-significant. See also 'Behaviour therapy', 'Cognitive behaviour therapy', 'Relaxation training' and 'Stress management'.

Communication and information

Patients in hospital depend on staff for their care and treatment, for information about their treatment and progress, and for meeting their basic needs when the patient is severely disabled or restricted even temporarily as in the case of surgical patients. While patients may be diffident about asking for information and the ethos of the hospital may imply that the 'good patient' takes a more passive role, studies have consistently shown that patients are dissatisfied with the amount of information they receive (Ley, 1988). Information provision and support should not be limited to hospitalization itself: D'Angelica et al. (1998) found that patients undergoing surgery for pancreatic cancer were satisfied with information provided before surgery and while in hospital, but 27% of patients had unanswered questions about diagnosis and treatment at the time of the survey (mean 13 months post-surgery). Healthcare professionals should be aware that patient satisfaction at the time of contact may not reflect the information needed by patients in the long term.

Doctors and nurses have been wary of giving information which might be misinterpreted or which might alarm the patient, but even in serious illness such as cancer, over 90% of patients want to know about their diagnosis and treatment (Reynolds et al., 1981). Tamburini et al. (2003) found cancer patients' most commonly reported need to be the desire to receive more information both about future conditions and about their diagnosis. In patients with motor neurone disease, a disease which is progressively disabling, incurable and eventually terminal, lacking palliative treatments, the majority of patients have been found to report positive aspects to being given the diagnosis (Johnston et al., 1996). In contrast, patients resent finding out important information by indirect means such as overhearing professional conversations.

Healthcare professionals may lack the skills to identify patients' concerns or to communicate effectively (Ley, 1988). Nurses underestimate patients' pain and are poor at identifying which patients are worried about particular matters. Courses to develop communication skills are now an integral part of the training of doctors and nurses in many colleges.

Professionals may also fail to communicate effectively because communicating bad news or talking to very ill patients is particularly stressful (Parks, 1985). Doctors and nurses are observed to have high levels of stress and may even demonstrate burnout. See also 'Healthcare professional–patient communication' and 'Written communication'.

Family members and significant others

Any individual patient is part of a social network and their hospitalization is likely to impact on friends and relatives who are concerned about the patient's well-being and treatment. Delva *et al.* (2002) found the anxiety levels of relatives of critical care patients to be high: less than 10% of people in 'normal' situations are as anxious or more anxious than these relatives. Titler *et al.* (1991) found feelings of vulnerability to be widely reported by spouses and children of critical care patients and high levels of anxiety and depression have been reported in partners of myocardial infarction patients (Johnston *et al.*, 1999).

For the adult patient population, effects of hospitalization are likely to be particularly severe as adults are often caregivers and/or bread-winners, supporting other family members both emotionally and practically. Hospitalization of an adult can lead to the disruption of home routines and altered relationships (Titler *et al.*, 1991). Children's lifestyle patterns may also be disrupted, leading to decreased school attendance and reduced time with friends (Titler *et al.*, 1991).

Relatives must cope not only with increased pressures resulting from the need to cover the patient's role but also take on the visiting role, finding the time to visit the patient who may be hospitalized at some distance from the family home. Lifestyle changes reported by adult visitors of intensive care patients include fewer hours' sleep and poorer sleep quality, changes in eating patterns and low energy levels (Van Horn & Tesh, 2000). Changes in family roles or responsibilities were reported by 56%.

A number of studies included items assessing the perceived needs of relatives or significant others. Consistently, the need for information emerges as highly important (Delva *et al.*, 2002; Hickey, 1990; Van Horn & Tesh, 2000). It would appear that addressing these informational needs may have a positive impact on the anxiety of significant others. Raleigh *et al.* (1990) assessed the anxiety levels of patients and 'significant others' (relatives or friends accompanying the patients) before and after a pre-operative class for cardiac surgery patients. Prior to the class, the significant others were significantly more anxious than the patients. This anxiety was found to have reduced significantly after the class, with no difference being found between significant others and patients post-test.

Johnston *et al.* (1999) found a cardiac counselling and rehabilitation programme given to both myocardial infarction patients and their partners resulted in lower levels of partner anxiety than a control group up to 12 months later.

Patient welfare is likely to benefit from looking after relatives as healthy family members will be better able to support them both during hospitalization and at discharge. Patients may also be less distressed if their relatives are coping well: in a small experimental study Doerr and Jones (1979) found that patients visited by family members prepared with information about the coronary care unit showed decreased anxiety compared with patients visited by family members without such preparation. The authors concluded that prepared family members transferred less anxiety. It could be, however, that these better informed visitors were more able to fulfil the patients' information needs. Information may also improve the post-hospitalization support given to patients by family members. Johnston *et al.* (1999) successfully improved the knowledge about myocardial infarction of patients and partners. In this study, the majority of partners were women who were likely to have had some control over the patients' diets and so their improved understanding of heart disease had the potential to influence patient health. Taylor *et al.* (1985) found wives who personally performed the same level of treadmill test as their husbands three weeks after the husbands had suffered myocardial infarction perceived the patient's efficacy to be higher than wives who did not perform the task. The combined efficacy perceptions of patients and their wives was consistently found to predict patients' cardiovascular functioning at 11 and 26 weeks, indicating the importance of attending to efficacy perceptions of partners as well as patients when enabling patient recovery. See also 'Social support' and 'Social support interventions'.

Conclusion

Adult patients face a range of stressors on hospitalization which can result in distress and worry and patients may not always employ optimal coping strategies. Some of these stressors, such as illness and having a new environment to contend with, are unavoidable consequences of hospitalization. Others, such as concerns relating to inadequate psychological preparation, insufficient information or poor communication can be addressed with beneficial outcomes. Preparing patients adequately for procedures can be beneficial both for the patient in terms of psychological and physiological outcomes and also for healthcare institutions as healthcare costs may be reduced. The welfare of family members should also be considered by hospital staff. Providing relatives with adequate information and support will not only aid their coping but also benefit the patient as better informed relatives appear to more successfully support the patient.

REFERENCES

Broadbent, E. A., Petrie, K. J., Alley, P. G. & Booth, R. J. (2003). Psychological stress impairs early wound repair following surgery. *Psychosomatic Medicine*, **65**, 865–9.

D'Angelica, M., Hirsch, K., Ross, H., Passik, S. & Brennan, M. F. (1998). Surgeon–patient communication in the treatment of pancreatic cancer. *Archives of Surgery*, **133**(9), 962–66.

DeGroot, K. I., Boeke, S., Bonke, B. & Passchier, J. (1997). A revaluation of the adaptiveness of avoidant and vigilant coping with surgery. *Psychology and Health*, **12**, 711–17.

Delva, D., Vanoost, S., Bijttebier, P., Lauwers, P. & Wilmer, A. (2002). Needs and feelings of anxiety of relatives of patients hospitalized in intensive care units: Implications for social work. *Social Work in Health Care*, **35**(4), 21–40.

Doering, S., Katzlberger, F., Rumpold, G. et al. (2000). Videotape preparation of patients before hip replacement surgery reduces stress. *Psychosomatic Medicine,* **62**(3), 365–73.

Doerr, B. & Jones, J. (1979). Effect of family preparation on the state anxiety level of the CCU patient. *Nursing Research,* **28**(5), 315–16.

Hickey, M. (1990). Family needs in critical care. *Heart & Lung,* **19**(4), 401–15.

Janis, I. (1958). *Psychological Stress.* New York: Wiley.

Johnston, M. (1980). Anxiety in surgical patients. *Psychological Medicine,* **10**, 145–52.

Johnston, M. (1988). Impending Surgery. In S. Fisher & J. Reason (Eds.). *Handbook of life stress, cognition and health* (pp. 79–100). New York, NY: John Wiley & Sons Inc.

Johnston, M., Earll, L., Mitchell, E., Morrison, V. & Wright, S. (1996). Communicating the diagnosis of motor neurone disease. *Palliative Medicine,* **10**(1), 23–34.

Johnston, M., Foulkes, J., Johnston, D. W., Pollard, B. & Gudmundsdottir, H. (1999). Impact on patients and partners of inpatient and extended cardiac counseling and rehabilitation: a controlled trial. *Psychosomatic Medicine,* **61**(2), 225–33.

Johnston, M., Pollard, B. & Hennessey, P. (2000). Construct validation of the hospital anxiety and depression scale with clinical populations. *Journal of Psychosomatic Research,* **48**(6), 579–84.

Johnston, M. & Vögele, C. (1993). Benefits of psychological preparation for surgery: a meta-analysis. *Annals of Behavioral Medicine,* **15**, 245–56.

Kendall, P. C. & Epps, J. (1990). Medical treatments. In M. Johnston & L. Wallace (Eds.). *Stress and medical procedures.* Oxford: Oxford University Press.

Kulik, J. A. & Mahler, H. I. M. (1987). Effects of preoperative room-mate assignment on preoperative anxiety and recovery from coronary by-pass surgery. *Health Psychology,* **6**, 525–43.

Leech, J. (1982). Psychosocial and physiologic needs of patients with arterial occlusive disease during the preoperative phase of hospitalization. *Heart and Lung,* **11**(5), 442–9.

Ley, P. (1988). *Communicating with patients.* London: Croom Helm.

Lucente, F. E. & Fleck, S. (1972). A study of hospitalisation anxiety in 408 medical and surgical patients. *Psychosomatic Medicine,* **34**, 304–12.

Ludwick-Rosenthal, R. & Neufelt, R. W. J. (1993). Preparation for undergoing an invasive medical procedure: Interacting effects of information and coping style. *Journal of Consulting and Clinical Psychology,* **61**(1), 156–64.

Munafò, M. R. & Stevenson, J. (2001). Anxiety and surgical recovery. Reinterpreting the literature. *Journal of Psychosomatic Research,* **51**(4), 589–96.

Parks, K. R. (1985). Stressful episodes reported by first year student nurses: a descriptive account. *Social Science and Medicine,* **20**, 945–53.

Raleigh, E. H., Lepczyk, M. & Rowley, C. (1990). Significant others benefit from pre-operative information. *Journal of Advanced Nursing,* **15**(8), 941–5.

Reynolds, P. M., Sanson-Fisher, R., Poole, A. & Harker, J. (1981). Cancer and communication: information given in an oncology clinic. *British Medical Journal,* **282**, 1449–51.

Shipley, R. H., Butt, J. H., Horwitz, B. & Farbry, J. E. (1978). Preparation for a stressful medical procedure: effect of amount of stimulus pre-exposure and coping style. *Journal of Consulting and Clinical Psychology,* **46**, 499–507.

Small, S. P. & Graydon, J. E. (1993). Uncertainty in hospitalized patients with chronic obstructive pulmonary disease. *International Journal of Nursing Studies,* **30**(3), 239–46.

Suls, J. & Fletcher, B. (1985). The relative efficacy of avoidant and nonavoidant coping strategies: A meta-analysis. *Health Psychology,* **4**, 249–88.

Tamburini, M., Gangeri, L., Brunelli, C. et al. (2003). Cancer patients' needs during hospitalisation: a quantitative and qualitative study. *BioMed Central Cancer,* **3**(12).

Taylor, C. B., Bandura, A., Ewart, C. K., Miller, N. H. & DeBusk, R. F. (1985). Exercise testing to enhance wives' confidence in their husbands' cardiac capability soon after clinically uncomplicated acute myocardial infarction. *American Journal of Cardiology,* **55**(6), 635–8.

Titler, M. G., Cohen, M. Z. & Craft, M. J. (1991). Impact of adult critical care hospitalization–perceptions of patients, spouses, children, and nurses. *Heart and Lung,* **20**(2), 174–82.

Van Horn, E. & Tesh, A. (2000). The effect of critical care hospitalization on family members: stress and responses. *DCCN - Dimensions of Critical Care Nursing,* **19**(4), 40–9.

Volicer, B. J. & Bohannon, M. W. (1975). A hospital stress rating scale. *Nursing Research,* **24**, 352–9.

Zigmond, A. S. & Snaith, R. P. (1983). The hospital anxiety and depression scale. *Acta Psychiatrica Scandinavia,* **67**, 361–70.

Hospitalization in children

Thomas Whelan

Monash University

Every year vast numbers of children are admitted to hospital. For example, more than 1 in 10 preschoolers in England (MacFaul & Werneke, 2001) and over 2 million children under 15 years in America (Popovic & Hall, 2001) have a hospital stay each year. Indeed, it has been estimated that around half of the population in many countries will have at least one hospital admission during childhood (Schmidt, 1997).

Recent advances in medical treatment have meant that an increasing number of children are treated on an outpatient or day surgery basis. As a consequence, a high proportion of child patients who remain in hospital have complicated or chronic conditions. A further result of improvements in medical practice is that compared with previous decades, children are far more likely to survive birth trauma, severe injuries or illnesses. In the case of childhood cancer, the five-year survival rates have increased from less than 30% in the 1960s to nearly 80% in the late 1990s (Smith & Hare, 2004). Nonetheless, there remains a high emotional cost for children and their parents as many of these patients undergo repeated hospitalizations and prolonged, demanding treatment.

Hospitalized children and their parents have to cope with a variety of stressors. These include factors directly relevant to the illness or injury, such as physical discomfort, loss of autonomy, absences from school, the effects of medication and changes in family interactions. In addition, aspects related to the hospital itself can provoke anxiety including the strange surroundings; separations from family and friends; and unusual, often painful, medical procedures.

Not surprisingly, children have been reported to show a variety of negative behavioural and emotional reactions at some point during a stay in hospital. These have ranged from temporary distress to chronic depression, and have included agitated behaviour, anxiety, withdrawal, enuresis, phobia, altered sleep patterns and appetite problems (Connolly et al., 2004; Papaqkostas et al., 2003; Peterson & Mori, 1988). For some children these reactions last long after they leave hospital (Quinton & Rutter, 1976), although for most the effects appear to subside in the weeks soon after discharge (Thompson & Vernon, 1993).

Notwithstanding that most children experience difficulty; some reportedly show behavioural improvements either during or after a stay in hospital (Kotiniemi et al., 1996). Such improvements might be due to the hospital environment being more nurturing than home, the successful treatment of a condition that has been adversely influencing behaviour or a sense of mastery at having managed a difficult experience (Schmidt, 1997; Wright, 1995).

Given the wide variability in the nature and extent of children's responses to hospitalization, over recent decades investigators have focused on examining the factors that influence these reactions. Such research assists in the identification of those who are vulnerable to poor adjustment and leads to the development of individualized interventions to help child patients to cope. Some of the important factors include previous medical experience, developmental status, severity of the illness or procedure, coping style and parental responses.

Influencing factors

Previous medical experience

A child's history of contacts with hospitals and other medical settings has been found to influence responses to subsequent hospital admissions (Yap, 1988). That is, a greater frequency or longer duration of hospitalization can increase the likelihood of negative reactions to following admissions. This is not surprising, as regular hospital admissions and longer stays are likely to be associated with factors such as more serious health conditions and higher levels of medical intervention.

A child's adaptation to illness and hospitalization can also be influenced indirectly through their perception of the experiences of other family members. Healthy children with a history of family

experience of hospitalization, whether this relates to siblings (Murray, 2000) or parents (Eiser & Eiser, 1990), have been found to be more likely to harbour increased concerns about illness and its consequences.

Developmental status

The extent of negative reactions to illness in children appears to be related to levels of development. Young children, those under six or seven years, are more likely to report anxieties and exhibit greater behavioural distress in medical situations than older children (Dahlquist et al., 1994; Melamed & Ridley-Johnson, 1988). Even so, each developmental period has vulnerabilities that influence how stressors are perceived and responses are manifested (Vessey, 2003). Thus, older children still experience negative behavioural reactions to hospitalization.

Bibace and Walsh (1980) attempted to classify children's understanding of health and illness according to phases of development. They suggested that children's concepts of illness can be ordered in a systematic manner, comparable to the stages of cognitive development proposed by Piaget (1952). Although there has been argument regarding the nature of the developmental stages (e.g. Eiser et al., 1990), the notion that there is a developmental trend in children's concepts of illness has been supported by other investigators. Generally, younger and less cognitively developed children offer less complex and more flawed explanations for illness (O'Dougherty & Brown, 1990), are less likely to understand the causes of pain (Bush, 1987), are less able to understand medical procedures and hospitalization (Eiser & Patterson, 1984), are less likely to seek out information about impending medical procedures (Peterson & Toler, 1986), but are more likely than older children to have frightening and guilty misconceptions regarding hospitalization and surgery (Redpath & Rogers, 1984). As well, younger children are likely to exhibit more symptoms of distress when pain and illness occur (Rudolph et al., 1995), have more externally oriented locus of control beliefs about illness (Sanger et al., 1988), and engage in fewer coping behaviours during medical procedures (Manne et al., 1993).

While these differences in children's cognitive abilities and related perceptions have been clearly identified, contemporary investigators (e.g. Rushforth, 1999) caution against an exclusive focus on what younger child patients are unable to do or understand. Such a perspective can lead to the assumption that a child of a certain age is unable to comprehend a particular concept and therefore should not be informed about a condition or its treatment. As noted by Rushforth (1999), even very young children have the ability to achieve a sophisticated level of understanding of their illness experience provided the information is given in a manner and form that is relevant to their level of understanding (see 'Children's perceptions of illness and death').

Illness severity

Other factors that influence the reactions of child patients and their families to hospitalization and surgery relate to the nature of the child's condition and the procedures included in the treatment. In terms of the child's condition, Rennick et al. (2002) found that the best predictor of psychological distress six weeks after hospital discharge was the number of invasive procedures (e.g. chest tube insertion, rectal temperature) that the child experienced. As might be predicted, mothers are more likely to experience distress when a child is hospitalized with a serious condition, such as pneumonia or concussion, than with a moderately serious condition, such as bronchitis (Berenbaum & Hatcher, 1992). Similarly, Roskies *et al.* (1975) reported that emergency admissions were more stressful for parents than were less urgent hospitalizations.

However, as O'Dougherty and Brown (1990) observed, estimations of a child's likely reaction to illness or medical procedures cannot be predicted simply by the severity of illness or the nature of the treatment. Even relatively minor treatments, such as immunizations (Hatcher *et al.*, 1993) and same-day hospital procedures (Faust *et al.*, 1991) can be extremely stressful for children and their parents. It appears that more important than the actual illness or its treatment is how the experience is perceived by the patient and his or her family.

Coping style

Research dealing with the reactions of adult and child patients to aversive medical procedures has highlighted the role of personal styles of coping (e.g. Montagne, 2000). Although there are a variety of coping styles, there is usually a dominant pattern characterized by approach or avoidance behaviours. Patients who predominantly approach, variously classified as 'sensitizers', 'vigilants' or 'active copers', seek out information, consider it, and attempt to prepare themselves for the procedure. Whereas more avoidant patients, labelled as 'repressors', 'deniers' or 'avoiders', tend to reject information, deny stress and attempt to focus on thoughts unrelated to the medical intervention (Martelli *et al.*, 1987; Myers, 1995).

As with adult patients, studies with children have indicated consistently that being at the active end of the active–avoidant scale is associated with more beneficial behaviours (see review by Rudolph *et al.*, 1995). Active copers have been found to be more co-operative with hospital staff and to have higher tolerance for pain (Siegel, 1981), to be less distressed following surgery (Hubert *et al.*, 1988) and to show more adaptive responses prior to medical procedures (Peterson & Toler, 1986).

Nonetheless, the research to date suggests there is not a definitive one-to-one correspondence between a child's coping style and his or her adjustment. According to LeRoy *et al.* (2003), the critical dimension appears to be the extent to which a child has a plan for dealing with a procedure. For example, behaviours associated with positive adjustments include active information seeking and exploration of the medical setting, but might also include deliberate avoidance or distraction (see also 'Hospitalization in adults').

Parental responses

A crucial factor in a child's response to medical events is the reaction of his or her parents. Mothers and fathers of child patients have reported experiencing a range of negative reactions to their child being in hospital. In fact, Ogilvie (1990) indicated that parents often perceive their own anxiety as greater than that of the child. This has been supported by the observation of Thompson and her colleagues (1996) that when children were undergoing assessments for lung transplantations, the parents were far more likely to indicate clinically significant levels of distress. The anxiety of parents might not always be obvious, even when it is extreme.

As several investigators (e.g. Boyer & Barakat, 1996) have noted, parents can conceal or play down their concern, perhaps in order to present a 'brave face' for their child.

The impact of their child's hospitalization can affect parents long after discharge. Investigations (e.g. Board & Ryan-Wenger, 2002) have suggested that the diagnosis and subsequent treatment of children with serious conditions can precipitate symptoms of post-traumatic stress in their parents. One study of child survivors of cancer has shown that up to two years after treatment, parents were three times more likely than the child patients to report severe post-traumatic stress (Kazak *et al.*, 1997) (see also 'Post-traumatic stress disorder').

When a parent expresses negative reactions to the child's illness or hospitalization, this is likely to impact on the child's ability to cope (DuHamel *et al.*, 2004; Melnyk & Feinstein, 2001). Studies across a variety of medical situations have indicated that when a mother's anxiety is high her child's co-operative behaviour decreases and the child is likely to show increased anxiety. Alternatively, a child's co-operative behaviour increases and anxiety decreases when the mother's anxiety is low (Cameron *et al.*, 1996; Mabe *et al.*, 1991).

In an effort to understand how this communication of emotion takes place, a range of specific parental behaviours have been investigated. Behaviours with a more emotive emphasis have been linked with children's poorer responses to the stress of hospitalization and medical procedures. This includes rejection, over-indulgence, over-protection (Carson *et al.*, 1991), agitation (Bush *et al.*, 1986), non-involvement (Wells & Schwebel, 1987), reinforcement of complaining or of illness behaviour (Gidron *et al.*, 1995), and criticizing or apologizing to the child (Blount *et al.*, 2003). Alternatively, parenting behaviours encouraging a child's active coping, such as the use of information, positive reinforcement, humour or distraction have been found to be associated with the child engaging in more adaptive responses (Bush *et al.*, 1986; Vance & Eiser, 2004). Blount *et al.* (1990) found that when parents varied their behaviour to suit different phases of the procedure (e.g. using distraction during anticipatory phases and encouraging the child to breathe during painful phases), children were more likely to have lower levels of distress.

Clearly, reducing parental anxiety is an important goal for healthcare professionals. It has long been recognized that better communication between parents and caregivers, and emotional support of parents can reduce their child's anxiety both before and during medical procedures. Unfortunately, while researchers have focused on the influence of the mother–child dyad on children's reactions to hospitalization, little examination has been directed to father–child or sibling–child interactions. In addition, investigations of factors that enable families to achieve positive changes would be of value. For example, researchers have suggested that a child's illness and hospitalization can provide opportunities for parents and siblings to enhance their understanding of illness, increase their sense of competence in caring, expand their social networks to include families with similar concerns to their own, and strengthen family coping behaviours (Kotiniemi *et al.*, 1996; Perrin, 1993).

Children's coping with medical events

After some 50 years of research, there is a greater awareness of the specific needs of child patients. As a consequence, a variety of strategies have been developed to help children and their parents to cope. These methods have ranged from broad-based approaches that affect large groups of patients to more individualized interventions.

Hospital setting and policies

One area where there has been widespread change is in hospital practices related to parent access. Until the 1960s, children endured extended separation from their parents as reflected in the following visiting regulations.

Patients are not allowed visitors unless they have been in the hospital for a period of 4 weeks, after which time only the parents or guardians (no friends or relatives are allowed) are permitted to visit on each alternate Sunday in each month, between the hours of 2 p.m. and 3.30 p.m. Parents or guardians of patients dangerously ill are allowed to visit as often as the Doctors consider necessary.[1]

Today, typically hospitals have unrestricted access in that parents can remain with their child overnight, be present during medical procedures while the child is conscious and participate in the daily care of their child. Clearly, these family centred practices are preferable to the previous restrictions. To be of real benefit, however, they have to be adequately supported. For example, in order for parents to stay overnight they require suitable facilities and parents who choose to be present during difficult procedures need effective preparation to enable them to direct their full attention to caring for their child.

Another broad-based strategy to help children to cope involves consideration of the hospital environment, such as the design and layout of facilities, and the use of visual displays. Surprisingly, this area has received little attention from researchers in the psychological literature. Generally, efforts to make the environment more familiar and home-like are beneficial. The availability of play areas and materials is important so that children can have spaces where they are free from medical procedures, can express themselves and find enjoyment.

Of course, the continued development of medical treatments that minimize pain is essential to children's coping, as is providing child patients with appropriate levels of pain medication (Ellis *et al.*, 2002). Where possible, affording children with the opportunity to participate in decision-making regarding their care and treatment can help them to gain a sense of control over a situation that might otherwise be overwhelming (Kuther, 2003).

Not surprisingly, children's coping with medical events is influenced by the nature of the interactions they have with health professionals. In order to assist children, staff need to be aware of the potential effects of hospitalization and of factors that can influence a child's vulnerability to maladaptive reactions. Most importantly, staff need to be willing and able to invest time in attending to children's emotional as well as their physical needs (Wright, 1995).

Psychological techniques

A wide range of more individualized psychological techniques has been developed to help child patients and their parents cope with difficult medical events (see reviews by Melnyk *et al.*, 2004;

Powers, 1999). Outcome studies have indicated that these approaches result in specific benefits to child patients and their families, including reduced anxiety and fewer problem behaviours. Most strategies can be classified into three groupings: information provision; modelling; and cognitive behavioural techniques (Whelan & Kirkby, 1998).

The types of information that can be offered to patients can be categorized as procedural (i.e. what will happen to the child), sensory (i.e. what the child will see, hear and feel) and behavioural (i.e. what the child can do). Providing such information is thought to reduce anxiety by clarifying expectations and encouraging a sense of control (Wallace, 1984). The effective provision of information is particularly important for child patients given their potential for having distorted beliefs about impending medical events (Cohen *et al.*, 2001). Information can be provided to children through a variety of formats including written material, instruction from hospital staff, hospital tours and play therapy (see also 'Written communication').

The modelling technique is based on the research of Bandura and his associates (e.g. Bandura & Menlove, 1968) who demonstrated the efficacy of using vicarious processes to reduce children's fears about a variety of stressors. In a hospital setting, this involves exposing the child to fearful events in an upcoming procedure through a model (a peer in a film, a storybook character or a toy figure). Seeing the model demonstrate effective coping enables the child to prepare his or her own adaptive behaviours. A wide range of benefits have been reported for child patients (and their parents) who have undergone modelling-based preparation (Melamed & Ridley-Johnson, 1988). These benefits, however, are influenced by variables such as a child's age (Melamed *et al.*, 1976), the timing of preparation (Melamed *et al.*, 1976), previous hospitalization (Melamed *et al.*, 1983) and parental presence during preparation programmes (Robinson & Kobayashi, 1991) (see also 'Behaviour therapy').

In recent decades, investigations of treatments to help children deal with distress related to medical events have focused on cognitive behavioural techniques (Powers, 1999). This approach includes a variety of components that have the advantage of assisting children with distress both before and during medical procedures. Typical components have included breathing exercises and other forms of relaxation and refocusing (e.g. blowing bubbles, playing with toys, reading pop-up books, practising progressive muscle relaxation), imagery and coping statements. Coaching (i.e. prompting the child to engage in coping skills) by the parent or medical staff during the procedure has also been a typical aspect of treatments. Other common elements include reinforcement for using coping skills and behavioural rehearsal (Powers, 1999) (see also 'Cognitive behavioural therapy' and 'Relaxation training').

Although there appears to be widespread recognition of the value of psychological preparation among health professionals, unfortunately, often the most effective interventions are not available for children and their parents (Koetting O'Byrne *et al.*, 1997; Whelan & Kirkby, 1995). In a survey of 123 pediatric hospitals in North America, Koetting O'Byrne *et al.* (1997) found that the most common types of preparation offered were those likely to be less effective, such as hospital tours, printed materials and narrative preparation. Only half of the hospitals studied reported that they taught coping techniques and 48% used films in preparation for surgery. In addition, it appears that such programmes have

[1] Policy statement of the Royal Children's Hospital 1947, Melbourne, Australia

been vulnerable to financial restrictions at times of economic stringency. This is despite empirical evidence that structured preparation programmes provide substantial financial advantages through shorter hospital stays, reduced post-surgery complications and decreased medication usage (Groth-Marnat & Edkins, 1996). Given the desirability of preparation programmes in terms of reductions in stress for families and economic savings, future investigations should provide further cost–benefit analyses, and just as importantly, investigate ways to best communicate these findings to health institutions.

Conclusion

Much has been learnt about the psychological impact of hospitalization and illness on children. Even so, recent changes in hospital practices have meant that this research needs to be updated. For example, compared with the previous decade, today there are shorter hospital stays, more invasive procedures completed in outpatient settings, different staffing patterns, more children treated outside paediatric units and greater expectations that parents will be involved in patient care (Vessey, 2003). As yet, the full impact of these changes is not understood. Given the increasing funding and resource pressures faced by hospitals, along with advances in medical technology, it is likely that there will be further changes. As cautioned by Wright (1995), in order to continue the gains of efforts to minimize the adverse consequences of hospitalization, any subsequent modifications need to be considered in terms of the possible effects on children's behaviour.

A salient weakness with much of the literature on hospitalization in children has been a failure to adopt theoretical frameworks. The reactions of children cannot be explained by examining contributing factors in isolation from one another. In the future, it is important that investigations determine how variables interact to produce children's responses (Vessey, 2003). Similarly, there has been a failure to evaluate psychological interventions within clearly developed theoretical contexts. As a result, the processes by which the strategies have exerted their effects have been poorly understood. It is hardly surprising that in clinical settings the usual approach has been to provide '... a smorgasbord of intervention techniques' (Ludwick-Rosenthal & Neufeld, 1988, p. 326) with the assumption that one or more features of the treatment will facilitate a child's adjustment. Investigations that provide a clearer identification of the effective components of interventions are more likely to produce cost-effective treatments. Such research could include an examination of factors that moderate the effects of interventions (e.g. age or temperament) on child and parent outcomes. Furthermore, specific treatments could be developed for specialist patient groups, such as the substantial numbers of children who are emergency admissions or health system 'veterans' with multiple hospital stays.

Finally, much of the research on the effects of hospitalization on children has been conducted in developed nations that have relatively well resourced health systems. Few studies have been reported from developing countries. Investigations are required to determine the special requirements of hospitalized children in these nations and to develop culturally relevant models of care.

REFERENCES

Bandura, A. & Menlove, F. L. (1968). Factors determining vicarious extinction of avoidance behavior through symbolic modeling. *Journal of Personality and Social Psychology*, **8**, 99–108.

Berenbaum, J. & Hatcher, J. (1992). Emotional distress of mothers of hospitalized children. *Journal of Pediatric Psychology*, **17**, 359–72.

Bibace, R. & Walsh, M. E. (1980). Development of children's concepts of illness. *Pediatrics*, **66**, 912–17.

Blount, R. L., Piira, T. & Cohen, L. L. (2003). Management of pediatric pain and distress due to medical procedures. In M. C. Roberts (Ed.). *Handbook of Pediatric Psychology* (3rd edn.) (pp. 216–33). New York: Guilford Press.

Blount, R., Sturges, J. & Powers, S. (1990). Analysis of child and adult behavioral variations by phase of medical procedure. *Behavior Therapy*, **21**, 33–48.

Board, R. & Ryan-Wenger, N. (2002). Long-term effects of pediatric intensive care unit hospitalization on families with young children. *Heart and Lung*, **31**, 53–66.

Boyer, B. A. & Barakat, L. P. (1996). Mothers of children with leukemia: self-reported

and observed distress and coping during painful pediatric procedures. *American Journal of Family Therapy*, **24**, 227–41.

Bush, J. P. (1987). Pain in children: a review of the literature from a developmental perspective. *Psychology and Health*, **1**, 215–36.

Bush, J. P., Melamed, B. G., Sheras, P. L. & Greenbaum, P. (1986). Mother–child patterns of coping with anticipatory medical stress. *Health Psychology*, **5**, 137–57.

Cameron, J. A., Bond, M. J. & Pointer, S. C. (1996). Reducing the anxiety of children undergoing surgery: parental presence during anaesthetic induction. *Child Health*, **32**, 51–6.

Carson, D. K., Council, J. R. & Gravley, J. E. (1991). Temperament and family characteristics as predictors of children's reactions to hospitalization. *Developmental and Behavioral Pediatrics*, **12**, 141–7.

Cohen, L. L., Blount, R. L., Cohen, R. J., Mc Clellan, C. B., Bernard, R. S. & Ball, C. M. (2001). Children's expectations and memories of acute distress: the short and long-term efficacy of pain management

interventions. *Journal of Pediatric Psychology*, **26**, 367–74.

Connolly, D., McClowry, S., Hayman, L., Mahony, L. & Artman, M. (2004). Posttraumatic stress disorder in children after cardiac surgery. *The Journal of Pediatrics*, **144**, 480–4.

Dahlquist, L. M., Power, T. G., Cox, C. N. & Fernbach, D. J. (1994). Parenting and child distress during cancer procedures: a multidimensional assessment. *Children's Health Care*, **23**, 149–66.

DuHamel, K. N., Manne, S., Nereo, N. *et al.* (2004). Cognitive processing among mothers of children undergoing bone marrow/stem cell transplantation. *Psychosomatic Medicine*, **66**, 92–103.

Eiser, C. & Eiser, J. R. (1990). The effects of personal and family hospital experience on children's health beliefs, concerns and behavior. *Social Behavior*, **5**, 307–14.

Eiser, C., Eiser, J. R. & Jones, B. A. (1990). Scene schemata and scripts in children's understanding of hospital. *Child: Care, Health and Development*, **16**, 303–17.

Eiser, C. & Patterson, D. (1984). Children's perceptions of hospital: a preliminary study. *International Journal of Nursing Studies*, **21**, 45–50.

Ellis, J. A., O'Connor, B. V., Cappelli, M. *et al.* (2002). Pain in hospitalized pediatric patients: how are we doing? *Clinical Journal of Pain*, **18**, 262–9.

Faust, J., Olson, R. & Rodriguez, H. (1991). Same-day surgery preparation: reduction of pediatric patient arousal and distress through participant modeling. *Journal of Consulting and Clinical Psychology*, **59**, 475–8.

Gidron, Y., McGrath, P. J. & Goodday, R. (1995). The physical and psychosocial predictors of adolescents' recovery from oral surgery. *Journal of Behavioral Medicine*, **18**, 385–99.

Groth-Marnat, G. & Edkins, G. (1996). Professional psychologists in general health care settings: a review of the financial efficacy of direct treatment interventions. *Professional Psychology–Research and Practice*, **27**, 161–74.

Hatcher, J. W., Powers, L. L. & Richtsmeier, A. J. (1993). Parental anxiety and response to symptoms of minor illness in infants. *Journal of Pediatric Psychology*, **18**, 397–408.

Hubert, N. C., Jay, S. M., Saltoun, M. & Hayes, M. (1988). Approach-avoidance and distress in children undergoing preparation for painful medical procedures. *Journal of Clinical Child Psychology*, **17**, 194–202.

Kazak, A. E., Barakat, L. P., Meeske, K. *et al.* (1997). Post-traumatic stress, family functioning, and social support in survivors of childhood leukemia and their mothers and fathers. *Journal of Consulting and Clinical Psychology*, **65**, 120–9.

Koetting O'Byrne, K., Peterson, L. & Saldana, L. (1997). Survey of pediatric hospitals' preparation programs: evidence of the impact of health psychology research. *Health Psychology*, **16**, 147–54.

Kotiniemi, L. H., Ryhanen, P. T. & Moilanen, I. K. (1996). Behavioural changes following routine ENT operations in two-to-ten-year-old children. *Paediatric Anaesthesia*, **6**, 45–9.

Kuther, T. L. (2003). Medical decision-making and minors: issues of consent and assent. *Adolescence*, **38**, 343–58.

LeRoy, S., Elixson, E. M., O'Brien, P. *et al.* (2003). Recommendations for preparing children and adolescents for invasive cardiac procedures: a statement from the American Heart Association Pediatric Nursing Committee of the Council on Cardiovascular Nursing in collaboration with the Council on Cardiovascular Diseases of the Young. *Circulation*, **108**, 2550–64.

Ludwick-Rosenthal, R. & Neufeld, R. W. J. (1988). Stress management during noxious medical procedures: an evaluative review of outcome studies. *Psychological Bulletin*, **104**, 326–42.

Mabe, A., Treiber, F. A. & Riley, W. T. (1991). Examining emotional distress during pediatric hospitalization for school-aged children. *Children's Health Care*, **20**, 162–9.

MacFaul, R. & Werneke, U. (2001). Recent trends in hospital use by children in England. *Archives of Disorders in Childhood*, **85**, 203–7.

Manne, S. L., Bakeman, R., Jacobsen, P. & Redd, W. H. (1993). Children's coping during invasive medical procedures. *Behavior Therapy*, **24**, 143–58.

Martelli, M. F., Auerbach, S. M., Alexander, J. & Mercuri, L. G. (1987). Stress management in the health care setting: matching interventions with patient coping styles. *Journal of Consulting and Clinical Psychology*, **55**, 201–7.

Melamed, B. G., Dearborn, M. & Hermez, D. A. (1983). Necessary conditions for surgery preparation: age and previous experience. *Psychosomatic Medicine*, **45**, 517–25.

Melamed, B. G., Meyer, R., Gee, C. & Soule, L. (1976). The influence of time and type of preparation on children's adjustment to hospitalization. *Journal of Pediatric Psychology*, **1**, 31–7.

Melamed, B. G. & Ridley-Johnson, R. (1988). Psychological preparation of families for hospitalization. *Developmental and Behavioral Pediatrics*, **9**, 96–102.

Melnyk, B. M. & Feinstein, N. F. (2001). Mediating functions of maternal anxiety and participation in care on young children's posthospital adjustment. *Research in Nursing and Health*, **24**, 18–26.

Melnyk, B. M., Small, L. & Carno, M. A. (2004). The effectiveness of parent-focused interventions in improving coping/mental health outcomes of critically ill children and their parents: an evidence base to guide clinical practice. *Pediatric Nursing*, **30**, 143–8.

Montagne, L. (2000). Children's coping with surgery: a process-oriented perspective. *Journal of Pediatric Nursing*, **15**, 307–12.

Murray, J. S. (2000). Understanding sibling adaptation to childhood cancer. *Issues in Comprehensive Pediatric Nursing*, **23**, 39–47.

Myers, L. B. (1995). ''It won't happen to me'': repressive coping style and optimism about health. *Proceedings of the British Psychological Society*, **3**, Special Group in Health Psychology, Annual Conference Sheffield University, 7–9 Sept. 1994.

O'Dougherty, M. & Brown, R. T., (1990). The stress of childhood illness. In L.E. Arnold (Ed.). *Childhood stress* (pp. 325–49). New York: Wiley.

Ogilvie, L. (1990). Hospitalization of children for surgery: the parent's view. *Children's Health Care*, **19**, 49–56.

Papaqkostas, K., Moraitis, D., Lancaster, J. & McCormick, M. S. (2003). Depressive symptoms in children after tonsillectomy. *International Journal of Pediatric Otorhinolaryngology*, **67**, 127–32.

Perrin, E. C. (1993). Children in hospitals. *Developmental and Behavioral Pediatrics*, **14**, 50–2.

Peterson, L. & Mori, L. (1988). Preparation for hospitalisation. In D.K. Routh (Ed.). *Handbook of paediatric psychology* (pp. 460–91). New York: Guilford Press.

Peterson, L. & Toler, S. M. (1986). An information seeking disposition in child surgery patients. *Health Psychology*, **5**, 343–58.

Piaget, J. (1952). *The origins of intelligence in children*. New York: International Universities Press.

Popovic, J. & Hall, M. (2001). *1999 National hospital discharge survey*. Hyattsville, MD: National Center for Health Statistics.

Powers, S. W. (1999). Empirically supported treatments in pediatric psychology: procedure-related pain. *Journal of Pediatric Psychology*, **24**, 131–45.

Quinton, D. & Rutter, M. (1976). Early hospital admissions and later disturbances of behavior: an attempted replication of Douglas' findings. *Developmental Medicine and Child Neurology*, **18**, 447–59.

Redpath, C. C. & Rogers, M. C. (1984). Healthy young children's concepts of hospitals, medical personnel, operations, and illness. *Journal of Pediatric Psychology*, **9**, 29–40.

Rennick, J. E., Johnston, C. C., Dougherty, G., Platt, R. & Ritchie, J. A. (2002). Children's psychological responses after critical illness and exposure to invasive technology. *Journal of Developmental and Behavioral Pediatrics*, **23**, 133–49.

Robinson, P. J. & Kobayashi, K. (1991). Development and evaluation of a presurgical preparation program. *Journal of Pediatric Psychology*, **16**, 193–212.

Roskies, E., Bedard, P., Gaureau-Guilbault, H. & Lafourtune, D. (1975). Emergency hospitalization of young children: some neglected psychological considerations. *Medical Care*, **13**, 570–81.

Rudolph, K. D., Dennig, M. D. & Weisz, J. R. (1995). Determinants and consequences of children's coping in the medical setting: conceptualization, review, and critique. *Psychological Bulletin*, **118**, 328–57.

Rushforth, H. (1999). Practitioner review: communication with hospitalised children: review and application of research pertaining to children's understanding of health and illness. *Journal of Child Psychology and Psychiatry*, **40**, 683–91.

Sanger, M. S., Sandler, H. K. & Perrin, E. C. (1988). Concepts of illness and perception of control in healthy children and in children with chronic illnesses. *Journal of Developmental and Behavioral Pediatrics*, **9**, 252–6.

Schmidt, L. R. (1997). Hospitalization in children. In A. Baum, S. Newman, J. Weinman, R. West & C. McManus (Eds.). *Cambridge handbook of psychology, health & medicine* (pp. 124–7). Cambridge, UK: Cambridge University Press.

Siegel, L. J. (1981, March). *Naturalistic study of coping strategies in children facing medical procedures.* Paper presented at the meeting of the Southeastern Psychological Association, Atlanta.

Smith, M. & Hare, M. L. (2004). An overview of progress in childhood cancer survival. *Journal of Pediatric Oncology Nursing*, **21**, 160–4.

Thompson, R. H. & Vernon, D. T. A. (1993). Research on children's behavior after hospitalization: a review and synthesis. *Developmental and Behavioral Pediatrics*, **14**, 28–35.

Thompson, S. M., DiGirolamo, A. M. & Mallory, G. B. Jr. (1996). Psychological adjustment of pediatric lung transplantation candidates and their parents. *Journal of Clinical Psychology in Medical Settings*, **3**, 303–17.

Vance, Y. & Eiser, C. (2004). Caring for a child with cancer – a systematic review. *Pediatric Blood Cancer*, **42**, 249–53.

Vessey, J. A. (2003). Children's psychological responses to hospitalization. *Annual Review of Nursing Research*, **21**, 173–201.

Wallace, L. M. (1984). Psychological preparation as a method of reducing the stress of surgery. *Journal of Human Stress*, **10**, 62–79.

Wells, R. D. & Schwebel, A. I. (1987). Chronically ill children and their mothers: predictors of resilience and vulnerability to hospitalization and surgical stress. *Journal of Developmental and Behavioral Pediatrics*, **8**, 83–9.

Whelan, T. A. & Kirkby, R. J. (1995). Children and their families: psychological preparation for hospital intervention. *Journal of Family Studies*, **1**, 130–41.

Whelan, T. A. & Kirkby, R. J. (1998). Advantages for children and their families of psychological preparation for hospitalisation and surgery. *Journal of Family Studies*, **4**, 35–51.

Wright, M. C. (1995). Behavioural effects of hospitalization in children. *Journal of Paediatric Child Health*, **31**, 165–7.

Yap, J. N. (1988). The effects of hospitalization and surgery on children: a critical review. *Journal of Applied Developmental Psychology*, **9**, 349–58.

Hostility and Type A behaviour in coronary artery disease

Willem J. Kop[1] and David S. Krantz[2]

[1]University of Maryland Medical Center
[2]Uniformed Services University of the Health Sciences

Historical perspective and early research

Systematic research on behavioural patterns related to increased risk of coronary artery disease (CAD) and its clinical manifestation as myocardial infarction was initiated by Friedman and Rosenman in the 1950s. The Type A Behaviour Pattern (TABP) was documented to be predictive of future myocardial infarction. TABP is defined as: 'an action-emotion complex that can be observed in any person who is aggressively involved in a chronic, incessant struggle to achieve more and more in less and less time, and if required to do so, against the opposing efforts of other things or persons ...' (Friedman & Rosenman, 1959). Later research (reviewed below) has documented that hostility may be the 'toxic' component of TABP. Type A behaviour is characterized by an excessive competitive drive, impatience, hostility and vigorous speech characteristics. The complement of TABP was called Type B behaviour and was described as the relative absence of Type A characteristics.

The early reports by Friedman, Rosenman and co-workers have resulted in numerous epidemiological and experimental investigations on the relationship between TABP and manifestations of coronary artery disease. In the 1960s and 1970s, most epidemiological studies supported the association between TABP and risk of future coronary artery disease (CAD) in men and women. The magnitude of these associations was comparable to that of traditional risk factors for CAD and also independent of these factors, such as hypertension and elevated lipid levels. One major study in this area was the Western Collaborative Group Study (WCGS) in which 3200 males were followed up for 8.5 years (Rosenman *et al.*, 1975). It was observed that individuals with Type A behaviour were more than twice as likely to suffer CAD disease than their Type B counterparts. Another important study was the Framingham Heart Study (Haynes *et al.*, 1980), where Type A behaviour was found to be predictive of CAD among men with white-collar professions and in women working outside the home. These findings led a review committee of the National Heart, Lung, and Blood Institute to construe Type A behaviour as a risk factor for CAD in middle-aged US citizens (The review panel on coronary-prone behaviour and coronary heart disease (NHLBI), 1981). Later studies, however, failed to show an association between TABP and clinical coronary disease (for review see Matthews & Haynes, 1986) (Matthews & Haynes, 1986). These negative findings have contributed to deconstructing the TABP, examining its culprit aetiological mechanisms and searching for components of TABP that did predict adverse CAD outcomes.

Evidence suggested that 'hostility' is the 'toxic' component of TABP (e.g. (Helmer *et al.*, 1991)). Similar to TABP, hostility is defined as a psychological trait. Hostility is characterized by a negative attitudinal set, a cynical view of the world, an antagonistic style and the presence of negative expectations as to the intentions of other people (Siegman & Smith, 1994). The attitudinal trait of hostility is distinct from anger, which is an emotional state and often leads to aggressive behaviour. Type A behaviour and hostility relate to anger in the sense that thus-affected individuals experience an elevated number of anger experiences. Therefore, Type A behaviour, hostility and trait anger share common characteristics, but they are also independent to a considerable degree (Smith *et al.*, 2004; Kawachi *et al.*, 1998). However, equivocal results in the TABP/ hostility literature have remained and may depend in part on whether or not the assessment tools incorporate behavioural observations, rather than measuring self-reported personality traits (see also 'Personality and health').

Assessment of Type A behaviour and hostility

A Structured Interview (SI) was developed to improve Type A behaviour assessments. The SI interrupts and challenges the interviewee to evoke behavioural responses such as vigorous speech and competition of control over the conversation. Apart from the behavioural observations, the SI also enables content analysis of the answers. Because the clinical assessment of overt and non-verbal behaviour is an essential part of this technique, special training is required to administer and score the SI. In addition, Friedman and colleagues also developed a scoring technique based on videotaped TABP interviews.

As alternative assessment procedures, several self-administrated questionnaires have been developed (e.g. the Jenkins Activity Survey (JAS: (Jenkins *et al.*, 1971); Bortner Type A scale ((Bortner, 1969); and the Framingham Type A scale (Haynes *et al.*, 1980)). Because Type A questionnaires rely solely on self-report, only modest correlations are observed between the SI and self-report questionnaires (Engebretson & Matthews, 1992).

Hostility is most commonly assessed with the Cook–Medley Hostility Inventory (Cook & Medley, 1954). The Cook–Medley scale is a 50-item self-report questionnaire derived from the Minnesota Multiphasic Personality Inventory. Several papers report on subfactors that may comprise the Cook-Medley questionnaire, of which 'cynicism', 'aggressive responding', and 'hostile affect' appear to have the strongest relationships with CAD (Barefoot *et al.*, 1989). Also, other questionnaires are available to assess hostility (e.g. the Buss–Durkee Hostility Scale; (Buss & Durkee, 1957)).

A better alternative for the assessment of hostility as CAD risk factor is based on interview analysis of the Structured Interview (initially developed to assess TABP). Two interview-based measures of hostility exist: the Potential for Hostility, and the Interpersonal Hostility Assessment Technique (IHAT (Haney *et al.*, 1996; Brummett *et al.*, 2000)). The IHAT includes four components: irritation, indirect challenge, direct challenge and hostile withhold/evade. Irritation is scored for irritated tone, impatience or exasperation with the interview or interviewer, arousal while re-experiencing negative life events, condescension or snide remarks, harsh generalizations and punched words with angry emphasis. Indirect and direct challenges refer to indirectly versus explicitly challenging the questions or the interviewer. Hostile withholding/evading refers to respondents' avoidance or refusal to answer a question. The total IHAT ratings tend to be positively skewed, and approximately 10% CAD of patients show no hostile behaviours. Total IHAT ratings are associated with aforementioned SI-based clinical ratings of Potential for Hostility ($r = 0.32$). IHAT scores are stable over a four-year period (intraclass $r = 0.69$), reflecting the trait-nature of hostility.

Many studies show that questionnaire- and interview-based measures of hostility share common variance, but classifications of individuals may vary considerably. This is, as in the aforementioned methods of TABP assessment, likely to be caused by the fact that the SI classification is dependent on behavioural observations such as speech characteristics, whereas the Cook–Medley depends on self-reports of a cynical or a hostile demeanor.

Equivocal results obtained in Type A behaviour and hostility research

The Multiple Risk Factor Intervention Trial (MRFIT) and a subsequent longer follow-up analysis of the WCGS revealed the most compelling evidence against the association between TABP and subsequent manifestations of CAD. In the MRFIT study (Shekelle *et al.*, 1985), both the SI and the JAS were administered in high-risk men, and neither was associated with future cardiac disease. Ragland and Brand (Ragland, 1989) reported on the recurrence of myocardial infarction in men who participated in the WCGS and who survived their first myocardial infarction. Unexpectedly, Type A behaviour was found to be protective in this sample. Thus, the predictive value of Type A behaviour in populations with elevated risk of coronary disease remains controversial. Furthermore, since 1979, virtually no positive reports have been published that support the relationship between questionnaire-assessed Type A behaviour and CAD. Recent reviews also suggest that the contribution of hostility is relatively low compared with other psychosocial risk factors such as depression and social isolation (Hemingway & Marmot, 1999) (Myrtek, 2001; Miller *et al.*, 1996) (see also 'Social support and health').

The question could be raised as to whether hostility and TABP are still important constructs for cardiovascular health. The answer to this question is probably confirmative, although the emphasis has definitely changed in the past 10 years (see (Riska, 2000). There are several reasons why it remains important to consider hostility and TABP in behavioural medicine. First, methodological issues are important in the interpretation of the studies with negative results. Studies that revealed negative findings regarding TABP and prediction of future cardiac disease investigated 'high-risk' populations. Because Type A behaviour may be related to the presence and persistence of several coronary risk factors and adverse health behaviour (e.g. smoking, unhealthy diet, etc.), this may attenuate the observed covariate-adjusted association between TABP and cardiac disease in high-risk populations. Second, several negative studies included patients who participated in treatment trials (either pharmacological or behaviour modification), which may have biased recruitment and reduced the magnitude of the associations observed between TABP and cardiac disease. Recent developments in informed consent procedures, which include more time and are inconsistent with a hostile attitude, may have further enhanced this bias. Third, hostility and TABP may be associated with specific non-survival of first cardiac events. That is, Type A persons who suffer their first myocardial infarction may be less likely to survive this incident than Type Bs. If this is correct, then study samples that are limited to survivors of myocardial infarction do not include the high-risk Type A individuals. Finally, the original description of TABP had a primary behavioural observational perspective without a consistent aetiological theory. The inclusion of personality traits as theoretical perspective has resulted in negative findings and deconstruction of the TABP concept. As reviewed below, quantification of the behavioural aspects of hostility and TABP is likely to reveal important novel information in CAD pathophysiology and risk stratification.

Hostility and Type A behaviour as related to coronary disease

Measures of hostility derived from the Structured Interview are predictive of severity of coronary artery disease in samples where global Type A behaviour was not similarly predictive (Dembroski et al., 1989). On the other hand, the Cook–Medley questionnaire does not unequivocally predict severity of CAD see (Siegman & Smith, 1994). One study (Siegman, Dembroski & Ringel, 1987) suggests the particular importance of the behavioural manifestation of hostility in the relationship with CAD severity.

Several longitudinal studies have addressed the predictive value of hostility in the development of clinical manifestations of CAD. SI-assessed hostility predicts cardiac events in initially healthy subjects and in patients at high risk of coronary disease who were participants in the Recurrent Coronary Prevention Project (RCPP; (Friedman et al., 1986)) and the MRFIT study (Dembroski et al., 1989). A recent analysis of the MRFIT data confirmed the role of interview-based hostility on cardiac events (Matthews et al., 2004).

The Cook–Medley questionnaire has yielded mixed results in follow-up studies of healthy individuals. This may partially result from the particular circumstances in which participants completed the inventories (often as part of a job or university selection procedure), and the use of very long follow-up durations (frequently more than 20 years). Apparently, the behavioural component of hostility – which is more likely to be detected by the SI – is an essential feature in the elevated risk of cardiac end-points (Siegman & Smith, 1994). It is noteworthy that both cross-sectional studies and longitudinal studies support the notion that the relationship between hostility and coronary artery disease is most evident among individuals younger than 60 years of age. This may reflect the fact that younger hostile persons encounter provocative situations more often than older individuals.

Psychobiological mechanisms

Acute psychological stressors result in elevations in heart rate, blood pressure, increases in blood lipids and catecholamines and also in platelet activity and blood clotting factors. The primary mechanism accounting for associations between TABP/hostility and CAD involves increased physiological response to environmental stressors among hostile individuals (Williams, Jr. et al., 1991; Krantz et al., 1988). For example, in a recent study we documented that hostility, particularly hostile affect, was associated with endothelial dysfunction during a mental challenge task (Gottdiener et al., 2003).

High blood pressure may promote damage to the coronary vessel wall, especially at sites where turbulence in coronary blood flow exists (e.g. branching points). In the setting of this mild coronary injury, deposition of lipids may occur which further enhances vascular damage. The progression of CAD is determined by an intermittent process of gradual coronary atherosclerosis combined with blood clot formation and degradation that may finally develop into coronary obstruction and, consequently, clinical manifestations of coronary disease. Inflammatory processes are likely to play an important role in this process. Different disease stages are associated with characteristic pathophysiological processes, which can be affected by psychological factors via neuroendocrine and autonomic nervous system pathways (Kop et al., 1994).

A series of animal studies by Kaplan, Manuck and colleagues, found that high dominant male monkeys (macaques) in socially unstable circumstances showed more coronary atherosclerosis at necropsy (Kaplan et al., 1982). In other studies, this research group established that individual differences in the consequences of aggressive behaviour can be explained in part by the psychosocial context in which these behaviours are displayed.

As for Type A behaviour and hostility in humans, several reports support the contention that psychobiological over-reactivity is characteristic of hostile individuals, particularly when these individuals are exposed to situations that elicit hostile behaviour. Thus, prolonged exposure to elevated stress responses in blood pressure, heart rate, catecholamines, blood clotting factors and inflammatory processes may account for the elevated risk of disease progression in hostile individuals.

It is conceivable that the consequences of a chronic hostile attitude are not limited to physiological changes that promote CAD, but also involve psychological repercussions of hostility. Glass proposed a psychological model in which Type A individuals were hypothesized to experience a state of frustration and exhaustion, a 'prodromal depression', preceding myocardial infarction (Glass, 1977). The basic assertion was that Type A individuals exert intense efforts to control stressful events. These active coping attempts eventually extinguish and lead to frustration and psychological exhaustion. This notion provides a model accounting for why Type A behaviour and hostility may interact with constructs such as depression and exhaustion, which are also factors that may affect the progression of coronary artery disease (Carney et al., 1988; Kop et al., 1994). We have found that trait anger and exhaustion have additive effects in predicting clinical events after coronary percutaneous interventions (Mendes de Leon et al., 1996) (see also 'Psychoneuroimmunology' and 'Stress and health').

Modification of hostility and Type A behaviour

Positive effects of behaviour modification in CAD patients have been reported in several investigations. The majority of these studies have been directed at reducing Type A behaviour. Because hostility appears to be a significant feature of Type A, these studies are applicable to strategies aiming at modifying hostility. Type A and hostile persons may be more prone to develop CAD because of (a) an overall increased cardiovascular reactivity, and (b) frequent exposure to conditions in which anger occurs. In addition, TABP/hostility is related to a reduced availability of stress-decreasing resources such as social support, which partly results from the antagonistic behaviours portrayed by hostile individuals. In general, intervention studies indicate that control over angry emotional experiences can be enhanced by 'behavioural' approaches (e.g. addressing issues such as patience when driving, taking sufficient time for daily meals), whereas the hostile attitude might be altered using 'cognitive' strategies (i.e. managing unreasonable expectations and ideas) (Kop, 2004).

In general, hostility interventions are conducted in a group setting consisting of approximately 10 participants. First, an attempt is made to gain insight into the triggers of anger-provoking incidents. Usually, participants are asked to self-monitor their behaviour to determine the circumstances in which anger or irritation occurs. Second, new strategies to cope with aggravating situations are introduced, such as learning to voluntarily insert a delay between the provoking incident and the reaction to it. At later stages of the intervention, a cognitive approach is taken, where unrealistic beliefs and expectations are addressed and modified. This may eventually result in opportunities to address provoking situations in a 'problem-solving' way.

The efficacy of these interventions is supported in a number of studies. For example, in the RCPP the number of re-appearing myocardial infarctions was significantly lower in patients who received Type A intervention (7.2% versus 13.2%, during three years of follow-up (Friedman et al., 1986). A substantial decrease in Type A behaviour occurred far more often in a Type A treatment group than in a control group. Moreover, patients who were successful in considerably decreasing their Type A behaviour, suffered a re-infarction four times less than those who failed to do so (Mendes de Leon et al., 1991). Recent clinical applications of these interventions incorporate various components of 'negative affectivity' in cardiac rehabilitation programmes, including depressive symptoms, exhaustion and anxiety (for review see (Kop, 2004).

Recent trends and future research

The study of hostility and TABP has received increasing international attention. Population trend analyses suggest that TABP not only decreases with progressing age, but also that population trends display an overall reduction in TABP (Kojima et al., 2004; Smith & Sterndorff, 1993). These trends may reflect changes in global socio-economic patterns and changes in public health that have addressed components of TABP as a target (for an excellent Foulcaudian perspective see (Riska, 2000). Increased attention for negative emotions and TABP in the workplace (Brummett et al., 2000) and

assessment of Type A and its biobehavioural cardiovascular risk factors in children and young adults (e.g. (Raikkonen, Matthews & Salomon, 2003) may have additionally contributed to this decrease.

Assessment and treatment of hostility, TABP and other psychosocial risk factors in women have received increasing scientific attention (Eaker, 1998). Some evidence suggests an interaction between TABP and the use of hormone replacement in postmenopausal women (Chaput et al., 2002). Hostility may also differentially affect men versus women in acute responses to social challenge (Smith & Gallo, 1999) (see 'Gender issues and women's health'). Despite potential differences in biopsychological pathways, prospective studies indicate that hostility is predictive of adverse cardiovascular health outcomes in post-menopausal women. More research is needed, however, to examine the interaction between gender with race and ethnicity in determining associations between psychosocial factors and cardiovascular disease.

Results indicate that psychological interventions are capable of reducing negative emotions and antagonistic behaviour patterns. However, evidence is not consistent as to whether these psychological improvements lead to a reduction of cardiovascular risk. Further studies are needed to investigate the biological and health behaviour concomitants of hostility. For example, it has been suggested that a relative depletion of the neurotransmitter serotonin is characteristic of hostile individuals. This deficiency has also been purported for other psychological measures associated with CAD, of which depression is the most well established. Some evidence supports the role of genetic factors in both hostility and its biological correlates e.g. (Sluyter et al., 2000). It may therefore be that a combined behavioural and pharmacological approach proves to be successful in ameliorating hostility. In the prevention of CAD-related events, hostility may not be the primary target for intervention because its modest predictive value for adverse cardiovascular outcomes (Myrtek, 2001; Miller et al., 1996). The assessment and treatment of the behavioural component of hostility and TABP appears to be more important than their underlying personality dimensions. These psychological measures need to be evaluated from a sociocultural perspective that may change over time. Nonetheless, interventions that reduce hostile behaviours and attitudes may enhance both quality of life and alter concurrent psychological CAD risk factors such as acute stress responses and depressive symptoms in individuals at risk of coronary disease.

See also 'Coronary heart disease: impact', 'Coronary heart disease: cardiac psychology', 'Coronary heart disease: rehabilitation' and 'Coronary heart disease: surgery'.

Acknowledgement

We thank Micah Stretch for his assistance in the preparation of this manuscript.

REFERENCES

Barefoot, J. C., Dodge, K. A., Peterson, B. L., Dahlstrom, W. G. & Williams, R. B. (1989). The Cook–Medley hostility scale: item content and ability to predict survival. *Psychosomatic Medicine*, **51**, 46–57.

Bortner, R. W. (1969). A short rating scale as a potential measure of pattern A behaviour. *Journal of Chronic Diseases*, **22**, 87–91.

Brummett, B. H., Maynard, K. E., Haney, T. L., Siegler, I. C. & Barefoot, J. C. (2000). Reliability of interview-assessed hostility ratings across mode of assessment and time. *Journal of Personality Assessment*, **75**, 225–36.

Buss, A. H. & Durkee, A. (1957). An inventory for assessing different kinds of hostility. *Journal of Consulting Psychology*, **21**, 343–9.

Carney, R. M., Rich, M. W., Freedland, K. E. et al. (1988). Major depressive disorder predicts cardiac events in patients with coronary artery disease. *Psychosomatic Medicine*, **50**, 627–33.

Chaput, L. A., Adams, S. H., Simon, J. A. et al. (2002). Hostility predicts recurrent events among postmenopausal women with coronary heart disease. *American Journal of Epidemiology*, **156**, 1092–9.

Cook, W. W. & Medley, D. M. (1954). Proposed hostility and pharisaic virtue scales for the MMPI. *Journal of Applied Psychology*, **38**, 414–18.

Dembroski, T. M., MacDougall, J. M., Costa, P. T., Jr. & Grandits, G. A. (1989). Components of hostility as predictors of sudden death and myocardial infarction in the Multiple Risk Factor Intervention Trial. *Psychosomatic Medicine*, **51**, 514–22.

Eaker, E. D. (1998). Psychosocial risk factors for coronary heart disease in women. *Cardiology Clinics*, **16**, 103–11.

Engebretson, T. O. & Matthews, K. A. (1992). Dimensions of hostility in men, women, and boys: relationships to personality and cardiovascular responses to stress. *Psychosomatic Medicine*, **54**, 311–23.

Friedman, M. & Rosenman, R. (1959). Association of specific overt behavior pattern with blood and cardiovascular findings: blood cholesterol level, blood clotting time, incidence of arcis senilis and clinical coronary artery disease. *Journal of American Medical Association*, **169**, 1286–96.

Friedman, M., Thoresen, C. E., Gill, J. J. et al. (1986). Alteration of Type A behavior and its effect on cardiac recurrences in post myocardial infarction patients: summary results of the recurrent coronary prevention project. *American Heart Journal*, **112**, 653–5.

Glass, D. (1977). *Behavior pattern, stress and coronary disease*. Hillsdale, NJ: Lawrence Erlbaum.

Gottdiener, J. S., Kop, W. J., Hausner, E. et al. (2003). Effects of mental stress on flow-mediated brachial arterial dilation and influence of behavioral factors and hypercholesterolemia in subjects without cardiovascular disease. *American Journal of Cardiology*, **92**, 687–91.

Haney, T. L., Maynard, K. E., Houseworth, S. J. et al. (1996). Interpersonal hostility assessment technique: description and validation against the criterion of coronary artery disease. *Journal of Personality Assessment*, **66**, 386–401.

Haynes, S. G., Feinleib, M. & Kannel, W. B. (1980). The relationship of psychosocial factors to coronary heart disease in the Framingham Study. III. Eight-year incidence of coronary heart disease. *American Journal of Epidemiology.*, **111**, 37–58.

Helmer, D. C., Ragland, D. R. & Syme, S. L. (1991). Hostility and coronary artery disease. *American Journal of Epidemiology*, **133**, 112–22.

Hemingway, H. & Marmot, M. (1999). Psychosocial factors in the aetiology and prognosis of coronary heart disease: systematic review of prospective cohort studies. *British Medical Journal*, **318**, 1460–7.

Jenkins, C. D., Zyzanski, S. J. & Rosenman, R. H. (1971). Progress toward validation of a computer-scored test for the Type A coronary-prone behavior pattern. *Psychosomatic Medicine*, **33**, 193–202.

Kaplan, J. R., Manuck, S. B., Clarkson, T. B. et al. (1982). Social status, environment, and atherosclerosis in cynomolgus monkeys. *Arteriosclerosis*, **2**, 359–68.

Kawachi, I., Sparrow, D., Kubzansky, L. D. et al. (1998). Prospective study of a self-report type A scale and risk of coronary heart disease: test of the MMPI-2 type A scale. *Circulation*, **98**, 405–12.

Kojima, M., Nagaya, T., Takahashi, H., Kawai, M. & Tokudome, S. (2004). A chronological decrease in Type A behavior patterns among Japanese male workers in 1995–1999. *Journal of Occupational Health*, **46**, 171–4.

Kop, W. J. (2004). Psychological interventions in patients with coronary heart disease. In L. C. James & R. Folen (Eds.). *The primary care consultant: the next frontier for psychologists in hospitals and clinics* (chapter. 4, pp. 61–81). American Psychological Association, Division 38 (Health Psychology) Book Series. Washington, DC: American Psychological Association.

Kop, W. J., Appels, A. P., Mendes de Leon, C. F., de Swart, H. B. & Bar, F. W. (1994). Vital exhaustion predicts new cardiac events after successful coronary angioplasty. *Psychosomatic Medicine*, **56**, 281–7.

Krantz, D. S., Contrada, R. J., Hill, D. R. & Friedler, E. (1988). Environmental stress and biobehavioural antecedents of coronary heart disease. *Journal of Consulting and Clinical Psychology*, **56**, 333–41.

Matthews, K. A., Gump, B. B., Harris, K. F., Haney, T. L. & Barefoot, J. C. (2004). Hostile behaviors predict cardiovascular mortality among men enrolled in the multiple risk factor intervention trial. *Circulation*, **109**, 66–70.

Matthews, K. A. & Haynes, S. G. (1986). Type A behavior pattern and coronary disease risk. Update and critical evaluation. *American Journal of Epidemiology*, **123**, 923–60.

Mendes de Leon, C. F., Kop, W. J., de Swart, H. B., Bar, F. W. & Appels, A. P. (1996). Psychosocial characteristics and recurrent events after percutaneous transluminal coronary angioplasty. *American Journal of Cardiology*, **77**, 252–5.

Mendes de Leon, C. F., Powell, L. H. & Kaplan, B. H. (1991). Change in coronary-prone behaviors in the recurrent coronary prevention project. *Psychosomatic Medicine*, **53**, 407–19.

Miller, T. Q., Smith, T. W., Turner, C. W., Guijarro, M. L. & Hallet, A. J. (1996). A meta-analytic review of research on hostility and physical health. *Psychological Bulletin*, **119**, 322–48.

Myrtek, M. (2001). Meta-analyses of prospective studies on coronary heart disease, type A personality, and hostility. *International Journal of Cardiology*, **79**, 245–51.

Ragland, D. R. (1989). Type A behavior and outcome of coronary disease letter; Comment. *New England Journal of Cardiology*, **319**, 1480–1.

Raikkonen, K., Matthews, K. A. & Salomon, K. (2003). Hostility predicts metabolic syndrome risk factors in children and adolescents. *Health Psychology*, **22**, 279–86.

Riska, E. (2000). The rise and fall of Type A man. *Social Science and Medicine*, **51**, 1665–74.

Rosenman, R. H., Brand, R. J., Jenkins, D. et al. (1975). Coronary heart disease in Western Collaborative Group Study. Final follow-up experience of 8 1/2 years. *Journal of American Medical Association*, **233**, 872–7.

Shekelle, R. B., Hulley, S. B., Neaton, J. D. et al. (1985). The MRFIT behavior pattern study. II. Type A behavior and incidence of coronary heart disease. *American Journal of Epidemiology*, **122**, 559–70.

Siegman, A. W., Dembroski, T. M. & Ringel, N. (1987). Components of hostility and the severity of coronary artery disease. *Psychosomatic Medicine*, **49**, 127–35.

Siegman, A. W. & Smith, T. W. (1994). *Anger, hostility, and the heart*. New York: Lawrence Earlbaum Associates.

Sluyter, F., Keijser, J. N., Boomsma, D. I. *et al.* (2000). Genetics of testosterone and the aggression–hostility–anger (AHA) syndrome: a study of middle-aged male twins. *Twin Research*, **3**, 266–76.

Smith, D. F. & Sterndorff, B. (1993). Coronary-prone behavior may be declining in Danish men and women. *Scandinavian Journal of Psychology*, **34**, 379–83.

Smith, T. W. & Gallo, L. C. (1999). Hostility and cardiovascular reactivity during marital interaction. *Psychosomatic Medicine*, **61**, 436–45.

Smith, T. W., Glazer, K., Ruiz, J. M. & Gallo, L. C. (2004). Hostility, anger, aggressiveness, and coronary heart disease: an interpersonal perspective on personality, emotion, and health. *Journal of Personality*, **72**, 1217–70.

The review panel on coronary-prone behavior, and coronary heart disease (NHLBI) (1981). Coronary-prone behavior and coronary heart disease: a critical review. *Circulation*, **63**, 1199–215.

Williams, R. B., Jr., Suarez, E. C., Kuhn, C. M., Zimmerman, E. A. & Schanberg, S. M. (1991). Biobehavioural basis of coronary-prone behavior in middle-aged men. Part I: evidence for chronic SNS activation in Type As. *Psychosomatic Medicine*, **53**, 517–27.

Lay beliefs about health and illness

Howard Leventhal[1], Yael Benyamini[2] and Cristina Shafer[1]

[1]The State University of New Jersey
[2]Tel Aviv University

Risky behaviours promote and healthy behaviours reduce disease risks

The evidence is clear: risky behaviours can lead to health crises and healthy behaviours can delay and avoid health crises. Cigarette smoking increases the probability of multiple types of cancer in addition to lung cancer, including cancers in organs as far from the mouth and lungs as the cervix. Cigarette smoking also greatly increases the likelihood of cardiovascular disease. Yet lung cancer has now exceeded breast cancer as a cause of death among women. Obesity is a risk factor for a broad range of diseases (Thompson & Wolf, 2001) and we are facing an epidemic of Type 2 diabetes, formally seen among the elderly and now increasingly diagnosed among teenagers (Mokdad *et al.*, 2001). The epidemic is occurring in spite of the clear evidence that weight loss and exercise can reduce the risk of diabetes. A multi-centre trial with over 3000 participants, each of whom was at high risk for becoming diabetic, found that exercise and dietary changes resulted in a 58% reduction in the number of individuals becoming diabetic whilst medication resulted in a 31% reduction relative to a control group receiving placebo (Knowler *et al.*, 2002). In short, despite knowledge of risk many people smoke, eat unhealthy, high fat, high calorie foods and are physically inactive. Knowledge of risk does not translate into risk avoidant behaviour (see also 'Health related behaviours').

Adherence is poor

Is the failure to adhere to recommended and effective preventive, disease-controlling and curative behaviour due to lack of intentions (Ajzen & Fishbein, 1980) or due to a failure of confidence in one's ability to perform the required action? (Bandura, 1986) (see 'Theory of planned behaviour' and 'Self-efficacy and health behaviour').

As many as half of the patients whom clinicians encounter on a daily basis are partially or completely non-adherent to the recommended treatment for hypertension; to the use of medication that reduces the frequency and intensity of asthma attacks (Halm *et al.*, 2006); to the use of medication that lowers blood sugar levels and to recommendations to take preventive measures including avoiding risky behaviours to prevent diabetes or control its complications (Phillips *et al.*, 2001). Many who fail to adhere fully to medically prescribed treatment are fully capable of forming intentions to act and acquiring the skills needed to follow through and adhere to 'alternative' or complementary treatments (Astin, 1998). Whether one is old or young, a graduate degree in biology or psychology is not essential for taking a diuretic each morning to control blood pressure or using a corticosteroid inhaler once a day to control the pulmonary inflammation which is a source of vulnerability to attacks of asthma. An important set of questions remains to be addressed concerning why people do not adhere to treatment to prevent and control illness threats when the behaviours recommended are well within their mental and physical competencies. Unfortunately, many investigators who use measures of intentions and efficacy to predict behaviour offer little practical or theoretical guidance as to how intentions or efficacy are created in adherent patients and which factors are involved when intention and efficacy are present but unrelated to action; both types of information are important for behavioural intervention. Correlations of behavioural measures with intention and/or efficacy are insufficient evidence for causation and insufficient guides for intervention; i.e. correlation should not be confused with causation (Pedhazur, 1997) (see 'Adherence to treatment').

Social learning and self-management

Historically, social learning models have provided the main source of guidance for creating and testing behavioural interventions.

The pioneering work of Lorig and colleagues (Lorig *et al.*, 2001) has shown that identifying and creating motivational resources and performance skills improves patient management of chronic illnesses. Social learning approaches and cognitive behavioural models were the basis for the highly effective behavioural interventions used in the diabetes prevention trial (Knowler *et al.*, 2002). Although the behavioural intervention was highly effective and exceeded the efficacy of the drug Metformin in deterring the transition from risk to diabetes, it had a serious downside; it was extremely intensive. Altering participant's lifestyles required as many as 16 lengthy face-to-face contacts and multiple phone contacts with well trained change agents. The cognitive behavioural treatment effective for the initiation and maintenance of the life style changes, i.e. alterations in eating and exercise patterns, effective for avoiding diabetes onset were clearly too expensive to implement within the current healthcare system. Is there a short cut? Is there a way of educating and teaching patients with 'less that is more'? (see also 'Behaviour therapy' and 'Cognitive behaviour therapy').

Common-sense and self-management

Clinicians who listen carefully to what their patients say and examine patient responses in focus groups, report that many patients may see little reason for adhering to treatment. Why, patients ask, should they take a hypertension medication when they feel perfectly fine? And why should they inhale a corticosteroid when the papers are filled with stories about the risk of steroids for athletes? These actions make no sense given patients' perceptions and beliefs about their health status, the diseases they supposedly have and the benefits and risks of treatment.

The beliefs people hold about specific diseases and treatments are based upon a combination of what they hear from people around them, their understanding and misunderstanding of what practitioners tell them, their observations of other persons, and their perceptions and experience with their own physical and emotional states. These beliefs form a repertory of 'common-sense' knowledge; they are beliefs that are supported by social consensus and information from practitioners and the individual's repository of experience and ongoing perceptions of illness symptoms, duration, causes, efforts at control and consequences (Leventhal *et al.*, 1980, 2003). As Festinger (1954) proposed decades ago, social information is less likely to persuade when the recipient of the message believes they have objective evidence to back their own beliefs. You cannot convince me that I am holding a sheet of paper if the sheet is a shiny, metallic grey, is difficult to bend and impossible to tear. Similarly, you will have a hard time convincing me that I have a disease called hypertension if I have no symptoms and feel perfectly well (Meyer, Leventhal & Gutmann, 1985), or that I have asthma when I have no symptoms and am not having an attack (Halm *et al.*, 2006). Also, does it make sense to use a prescribed medication to treat a condition or illness that currently I do not have? My common-sense representation of my somatic status does not call for medication.

Representations of illness and treatment

Studies have identified five domains of illness representations that form a base for initiating, maintaining and evaluating the efficacy of preventive or treatment behaviours (Leventhal *et al.*, 1980): the identity of the illness (its symptoms and label), its time-line (acute or chronic), its cause (genes, exposure to virus, etc.), control (can it be prevented, cured or controlled?; Lau & Hartmann, 1983) and consequences (pain, dysfunction, economic and social losses). Treatments also have representations. Treatment representations can be described by summary features, that is they can be perceived as necessary and/or as sources of side effects and risk (Horne, 2003), and they can also be represented in greater detail in the five domains; e.g. their identity or names and symptoms (surgery has wound-healing pain), time frames (antidepressants take weeks to alter mood), causal routes of action (surgery removes tumours), consequences (weeks of debilitation), and control (effectiveness for preventing, curing or controlling a disease).

The factors in each of the domains are represented in both abstract and in concrete, experiential form, my illness has an abstract label (hypertension) and concrete symptoms (nervousness, warm face, etc.), my anti-depressant has an abstract time frame (weeks to improve mood) and a concrete time line (I can feel the {side} effects of the medication within hours), and my illness has consequences that I can verbalize or literally see as vivid images in my mind's eye (Gibbons & Gerrard, 1997). The abstract and concrete levels of the factors comprizing the representations need not be consistent with one another. For example, both patients and non-patients attribute symptoms to conditions that are asymptomatic (more patients do so than do non-patients); warm faces, nervous tension, heart beating, etc. are misperceived as symptoms of chronic elevations of resting levels of blood pressure (hypertension) although resting levels are asymptomatic (Baumann *et al.*, 1985) (see also 'Symptom perception'). Adherence to treatment for hypertension is higher among patients who perceive treatment as having a positive effect (reducing) on their symptoms; patients are less likely to adhere when they do not perceive these benefits (Meyer *et al.*, 1985).

Heuristics give meaning to somatic experience

The speed and ease with which events (symptoms, functional changes) are labelled (a cold, asthma), evaluated (benign, life-threatening) and affectively responded to can obscure the many heuristics or rules-of-thumb involved in the evaluative process. Symmetry, the bi-directional process of labelling symptoms and finding symptoms when labelled, appears to be a fundamental feature in the formation of representations whether these be representations about illness or treatments. For example, when given false feedback suggesting their blood pressure is elevated, non-hypertensive undergraduates report the same symptoms and reduced health status as reported by hypertensive patients (Bauman *et al.*, 1985; Croyle, 1990), and absence due to sickness was more frequent among aware hypertensives and among falsely aware hypertensives who perceived a high symptom level, compared with both normotensives and unaware hypertensives (Melamed, Froom & Green, 1997). Heuristics facilitate decision making when dealing with ambiguous and highly salient cues (symptoms, pain) and the emotional distress that may arise in the context of ambiguity and limited information. Heuristics such as symptom pattern (chest pain or pressure is the symptom pattern for heart attack and is perceived to be more typical of men), location (breathlessness is a problem of the lungs not the heart), duration (after three days it may be serious), and novelty (never had it before – better it check it out), provide provisional 'diagnostic meanings' and suggest the need for seeking care (Woloshynowych, Valori & Salmon, 1998). More complex heuristics that are involved in decisions as to whether symptoms are a sign of illness or a non-illness condition include the age-illness heuristics (mild, chronic symptoms are likely to be seen as signs of age not illness), and the stress-illness heuristics (when under high stress symptoms are likely seen as indicators of stress not illness). The full meaning of a symptom and/or illness evolves over time and the evolution is speeded by the success or failure in the control of symptoms by self selected or medically recommended treatments (see 'Self-management').

Social factors shape representations of disease and preventive and treatment behaviours

Social influences play a critical role in health behaviours for the prevention, treatment and control of disease. Social factors can operate by creating or moderating the impact of more specific health beliefs, and they can have direct effects on health behaviours. Social comparisons are involved in the interpretation of symptoms and decisions to seek medical care; (Lau & Hartman, 1983), multiple studies find that virtually all elderly individuals discuss symptoms with other persons and virtually all people seeking medical care have been told to do so by someone (Cameron, Leventhal & Leventhal, 1993). Social comparisons reinforce beliefs about exposures to pathogens, reinforce the interpretation and meanings assigned to symptoms with specific patterns and can increase uncertainty and concerns about novel symptoms (Taylor, 1983). Comparison can also provide reassurance of the safety of needed and potentially threatening treatments such as bypass surgery by minimizing the emotional distress associated with threat-induced images of surgical mutilation and pain (Kulik & Mahler, 1987). Consistent with the basic premise of the common-sense model and with the multitude of studies of observational learning (Bandura, 1969), information from individuals who have experienced treatment and struggled with disease, communicates the lived experience of the source. For example, misconceptions about cancer are more prevalent among Latinos than Anglos, in part because they fit a Latino fatalistic cultural theme (Pérez-Stable et al., 1992).

Putting it all together

Many data analytic tools such as multiple regression analysis tend to emphasize the contribution of single factors to specific behavioural and health outcomes. Studies report the effect of particular personal beliefs and/social influences on action, the effect of each factor is assessed independent of the contribution of others. Conceptual models however, make clear the need for further integration. Qualitative studies suggest that people develop integrative narratives of their illnesses, which transcend the details of the illness experience and dynamically combine a wealth of information from somatic cues, mass media and input from their practitioners (Docherty and McColl, 2003; Hunt et al., 1989). Theoreticians have proposed that specific beliefs have beneficial effects on preventive and treatment behaviours when the set is consistent or coherent

(Moss-Morris et al., 2002; Antonovsky, 1993) or generates a sense of overall competence or self-efficacy for behavioural management (Bandura, 1986). The common sense model identifies several types of coherence or consistency that are important for preventive and treatment actions.

Coherence: Abstraction bind concrete experience

Concrete experiences are tied to specific points in time, they are time bound. For example, a patient interviewed in hospital reported experiencing "fatigue two days ago, breathlessness a few hours later, a collapse on the floor at home, a day later, and the panic of inability to breathe and walk, an hour before appearing at the hospital emergency department for treatment"; these were perceived to be distinct, separate events as they were not understood to be indicators of congestive heart failure, CHF (Horowitz et al., 2004). Because the experiences are not bound together by a common concept, the patient did not seek care when she collapsed and did not see the collapse as a sign that she would soon need emergency treatment. The patient suffering from CHF was hospitalized because she did not see the connections among these experiences and did not attend to or treat the milder chronic symptoms to avoid later collapse. Appropriate linkages are critical for symptom management and inappropriate linkages risky. This idea is critical for prevention as well as for treatment. It is fine to feel good, but feelings are sensitive to many factors and they do not necessarily indicate good health. One can feel relaxed and 'high' after exercising, vigorous exercise can be an antidote to depression and have health benefits. However, one can also feel relaxed and high while inhaling a cigarette, an antidote to depression with a health risk.

Coherence among representations

A second aspect of coherence is the fit between the representation of a disease threat and the representations of the behaviours selected for prevention and control. If stress is perceived as the cause of hypertension, stress reduction rather than medication makes more sense and lowering stress will be supported as an effective means of controlling hypertension as it will result in the reduction of psychophysiological symptoms that are perceived to be signs of elevated blood pressure. Little effort is needed to retrieve examples of 'good fit' ranging from rubbing sore muscles, salving a rash or drinking a household remedy to deal with stomach cramps and gas. Each focuses behaviour on the location and presumed cause of the symptoms, signs and physical distress.

Coherence and the selection of indicators

Common-sense representations of illnesses and preventive and treatment behaviours are control systems. Coherence in a system that is bi-level, i.e. abstract and concrete, requires a sense of 'good fit' at each level and between levels. Coherence at the perceptual or concrete level requires evidence that behaviour affects a perceptual cue, e.g. symptoms, taste, momentary moods and emotions of satisfaction and/or satiation, etc. Satisfaction of goal attainment at the concrete level may not produce movement toward goals at the abstract level. Selection of appropriate concrete cues, where somatic cues exist, or transferring monitoring from somatic to external indicators (from symptoms to objective readings of blood sugar or blood pressure) is critical for insuring that movement at the perceptual level will achieve abstract goals.

Coherence among illness/treatment representations, the self and social context

Two sets of questions need to be addressed concerning the fit among representations of illness threats and procedures for prevention and control with representations of the self and representations of the social context (Gibbons & Gerrard, 1997). Strategies for resource management that have been acquired over the life span, such as conservation of resources or "use it or lose it (exercise)" are perceived to be essential for preserving function. These strategies will affect the perception of how best to approach management of specific illness threats (Leventhal & Crouch, 1997). Belief that conservation is critical to avoid recurrence of heart attack encourages non-adherence to active rehabilitation programmes and hypervigilance and over-utilization of medical care in response to chest complaints (Aikens *et al.*, 1999). The perceived vulnerabilities and strengths of the self, based upon perceived resemblances of the self and specific others and their vulnerabilities, will moderate the interpretive process. Finally, cultural beliefs provide specific ways of interpreting the meaning or identity of somatic complaints including their causes, consequences, time frames and modes of control. These broader beliefs interact with and moderate the interpretation and meanings of somatic experiences and affect the selection of practitioners to assist in prevention and control.

Techniques for studying coherence are not well understood or developed. It is clear that we have a lot to do and much to learn. Forward movement will require new methods for describing representations, heuristics and action and interventions designed to influence particular factors in the landscape of beliefs presumed to affect health behaviours and health outcomes. Forward movement will require close collaboration among psychologists, physicians, cell biologists and other social scientists as well as the design of studies that create and translate findings from the clinical setting to the laboratory and back again.

REFERENCES

Aikens, J. E., Michael, E., Levin, T. & Lowry, E. (1999). The role of cardioprotective avoidance beliefs in noncardiac chest pain and associated emergency department utilization. *Journal of Clinical Psychology in Medical Settings*, **6**(4), 317–32.

Ajzen, I. & Fishbein, M. (1980). *Understanding attitudes and predicting social behaviour*. Englewood Cliffs, NJ: Prentice-Hall.

Antonovsky, A. (1993). The structure and properties of the Sense of Coherence scale. *Social Science and Medicine*, **36**, 725–33.

Astin, J. A. (1998). Why patients use alternative medicine: results of a national study. *Journal of the American Medical Association*, **279**, 1548–53.

Bandura, A. (1969). *Principles of behaviour modification*. New York: Holt, Rinehart, & Winston.

Bandura, A. (1982). Self-efficacy mechanism in human agency. *American Psychologist*, **37**, 122–7.

Bandura, A. (1986). Self-efficacy mechanism in physiological activation and health-promoting behaviour. In. J. Madden, J. S. Matthysse & J. Barchas (Eds.). *Adaptation, learning and affect* (pp. 1–51). New York: Raven Press.

Baumann, L. J. & Leventhal, H. (1985). "I can tell when my blood pressure is up, can't I?" *Health Psychology*, **4**, 203–18.

Cameron, L., Leventhal, E. A. & Leventhal, H. (1993). Symptom representations and affect as determinants of care seeking in a community dwelling adult sample population. *Health Psychology*, **12**, 171–9.

Croyle, R. T. (1990). Biased appraisal of high blood pressure. *Preventive Medicine*, **19**, 40–4.

Docherty, D. & McColl, M. A. (2003). Illness stories: themes emerging through narrative. *Social Work in Health Care*, **37**(1), 19–39.

Festinger, L. (1954). A theory of social comparison processes. *Human Relations*, **7**, 183–201.

Fishbein, M. & Ajzen, I. (1975). *Beliefs, attitudes, intention, and behaviour: an introduction to theory and research*. Reading, MA: Addison-Wesley.

Gibbons, F. X. & Gerrard, M. (1997). Health images and their effects on health behaviour. In B. P. Buunk & F. X. Gibbons (Eds.). *Health coping and well being* (pp. 63–94). Mahwah, NJ: Lawrence Erlbaum Associates, Inc.

Halm, E., Mora, P., & Leventhal, H. (2006). No Symptoms, no asthma: the acute episodic disease belief is associated with poor self-management among inner-city adults with persistent asthma. *Chest*, **129**, 573–80.

Horne, R. (2003). Treatment perceptions and self-regulation. In L. D. Cameron, Linda & H. Leventhal (Eds.). *The self regulation of health and illness behaviour* (pp. 138–54). London: Routledge Taylor & Francis Group.

Horowitz, C. R., Rein, S. B. & Leventhal, H. (2004). A story of maladies, misconceptions and mishaps: effective management of heart failure. *Social Sciences and Medicine*, **58**, 631–43.

Hunt, L. M., Jordan, B. & Irwin, S. (1989). Views of what's wrong: diagnosis and patients' concepts of illness. *Social Science and Medicine*, **28**, 945–56.

Knowler, W. C., Barrett-Connor, E., Fowler, S., Hamman, R. F., Lachin, J. M., Walker, E. A., & Nathan, D. M. (2002). Reduction in the incidence of type 2 diabetes with lifestyle intervention or metformin. *The New England Journal of Medicine*, **346**(6), 393–403.

Kulik, J. A. & Mahler, H. I. (1987). Effects of preoperative roommate assignment on preoperative anxiety and recovery from coronary-bypass surgery. *Health Psychology*, **6**, 525–43.

Lau, R. R. & Hartman, K. A. (1983). Common sense representations of common illnesses. *Health Psychology*, **2**, 167–85.

Leventhal, H., Brissette, I. & Leventhal, E. A. (2003). The common sense model of self-regulation of health and illness. In L. D. Cameron & H. Leventhal (Eds.). *In the self-regulation of health and illness behaviour* (pp. 42–61). London: Routledge Taylor & Francis Group.

Leventhal, E. A. & Crouch, M. (1997). Are there differences in perceptions of illness across the lifespan? In K. J. Petrie & J. Weinman (Eds.). *Perceptions of health and illness: current research and applications* (pp. 77–102). London: Harwood Academic.

Leventhal, H., Meyer, D. & Nerenz, D. (1980). The common sense representation of illness danger. In. S. Rachman (Ed.). *Contributions to medical psychology* (pp. 7–30). New York: Pergamon Press.

Lorig, K. R., Ritter, P., Stewart, A. L. et al. (2001). *Chronic disease self-management program medical Care*, **39**, 1217–23.

Melamed, S., Froom, P. & Green, M. S. (1997). Hypertension and sickness absence: the role of perceived symptoms. *Journal of Behavioural Medicine*, **20**(5), 473–87.

Meyer, D., Leventhal, H. & Gutmann, M. (1985). Common-sense models of illness: the example of hypertension. *Health Psychology*, **4**, 115–35.

Miller, C. D., Ziemer, D. C. & Barnes, C. S. (2001). Clinical Inertia. *Annals of Internal Medicine*, **135**, 825–34.

Mokdad, A. H., Bowman, B. A., Ford, E. S. et al. (2001). The continuing epidemics of obesity and diabetes in the U.S. *Journal of the American Medical Association*, **286**, 1195–200.

Moss-Morris, R., Weinman, J., Petrie, K. J. et al. (2002). The revised illness perception questionnaire (IPQ-R). *Psychology and Health*, **17**, 1–16.

Pedhauzer, E. J. (1997). *Multiple Regression in Behavioural Research: Explanation and Prediction* (3rd edn.). New York: Harcourt.

Pérez-Stable, E. J., Sabogal, F., Otero-Sabogal, R., Hiatt, R. A. & McPhee, S. J. (1992). Misconceptions about cancer among Latinos and Anglos. *JAMA*, **268**(22), 3219–23.

Phillips, L. S., Branch, W. T., Cook, C. B. et al. (2001). Clinical Inertia. *Annals of Internal Medicine*, **135**, 825–34.

Salmon, P., Woloshynowych, M. & Valori, R. (1996). The measurement of beliefs about physical symptoms in English general practice patients. *Social Science and Medicine*, **42**(11), 1561–7.

Taylor, S. E. (1983). Adjustment to threatening life events: a theory of cognitive adaptation. *American Psychologist*, **38**, 1161–73.

Taylor, S. E., Buunk, B. & Aspinwall, L. (1990). Social comparison, stress, and coping, *Personality and Social Psychology Bulletin*, **16**,(1), 74–89.

Thompson, D. & Wolf, A. M. (2001). The medical-care cost burden of obesity. *Obesity Reviews*, **2**(3), 189–97.

Weinman, J. & Horne, R. (1996). The illness perception questionnaire: a new method for assessing the cognitive representation of illness. *Psychology and Health*, **11**, 431–45.

Woloshynowych, M., Valori, R. & Salmon, P. (1998). General practice patients' beliefs about their symptoms. *British Journal of General Practices*, **48**, 885–90.

Life events and health

Tirril Harris

St. Thomas' Hospital Campus

Introduction

The notion of life events adversely affecting health is deeply embedded in popular consciousness. However among theorists there have been interesting variations. Some early thinkers pursued general theories involving homeostasis, viewing disease in terms of 'illness as a whole'. The best known were Cannon's (1932) fight–flight reaction and Selye's (1956) general adaptation syndrome. These detailed a number of biological responses to environmental demands, presenting them as an orchestrated pattern, almost regardless of the specific nature of these demands. These generalized patterns included responses which were easy to measure in early psychological laboratories, such as heart rate or sweating, and this may partly have accounted for the interest shown in this model of illness. Others pursued theories involving more specificity, believing that particular disorders arise from specific circumstances. During the 1950s this was accepted by followers of Franz Alexander and the school of psychosomatic medicine. Another example was Flanders Dunbar's influential set of ideas that specific personality types were more vulnerable to certain illnesses (Dunbar, 1954). The specificity considered nearly always involved the person's underlying attitude rather than the specific way the environment impinged in the form of a life event. However more recent research has suggested the value of examining the latter in relation to particular health outcomes and this chapter aims to convey this perspective (see also 'Personality and health' and 'Stress and health').

Life events, difficulties and meaning

One important difference between various perspectives on stress involves what may be called their conceptual level of stress analysis. Five such levels can be distinguished:

i) Microunit: incidents such as insults, which in aggregate amount to an experience at the next level, such as an estrangement.

ii) Unit: the basic life event of most research instruments – an estrangement, house-move, job-change, or death.

iii) Specific qualities of units: what type of event? a loss, humiliation, danger, frustration, challenge, or intrusion? Would it induce guilt or fatigue in most people?

iv) General qualities of units: less specific characteristics such as positive/negative, severely versus mildly unpleasant.

v) Person's summary score (not all instruments): where scores are allotted individuals may be characterized in terms of their total experience – say of severely unpleasant events – during a given period.

Level (i), the incident level, is usually identified with the Hassles and Uplifts scale (Kanner *et al.*, 1981). While the distinction between hassles and uplifts suggests the positive/negative distinction at level (iv), many studies looking at health outcomes with this instrument ignore the effects at level (ii) and it thus becomes difficult to interpret how much stress a person is under at level (v). In other words by concentrating attention on altercations with parking attendants and troubles getting computers to function, this instrument is in danger of missing the impact of more serious experiences such as children leaving home. Most instruments however do operate from level (ii), although the location of inclusion thresholds varies between them. The earliest measure, the Schedule of Recent Experiences (SRE: Holmes & Rahe, 1967) sees life events as anything involving significant change/readjustment, but leaves the estimate of this significance entirely to the respondent: the latter has the ultimate say as to whether a 'serious illness' or a 'loss of someone close' has occurred. This allows bias to creep into the data (collected according to a checklist of 67 events), as the more anxious respondents will define as 'serious' illnesses which more sanguine personalities will consider only minor (say a bout of bronchitis), and respondents who have become depressed look back and redefine their neighbour who has moved to Australia as 'very close', while those who have not suffered depressive onset may continue to feel friendly but not romanticize the degree of closeness of the relationship before the move (Brown, 1974).

The SRE then moves straight up to level (v). Each event on the checklist has been allotted a 'typical life-change unit score' from 0 (no change/distress likely) to 100 (maximum change/distress). Scores for each experience are then summed to give each individual a total score, and this, rather than the occurrence of more specific experiences, is the most frequently used measure employed in analyses of the SRE's impact on health outcomes. Another major disadvantage of this approach is its failure to deal with the meaning of events for individuals: a planned first pregnancy in a secure marital and financial situation has a totally different meaning from an unplanned pregnancy for a single parent where there are already three children, cramped housing and a shortage of money, but both would get the same 'pregnancy' score on the checklist system.

Approaches to stress measurement such as the Life Experiences Survey (Sarason et al., 1978) or the Life Events Inventory (Tennant & Andrews, 1976) which do consider level (iv) can, of course, take account of the difference in the 'undesirability' between two such pregnancies. But they usually leave it entirely to the respondent to define 'undesirable', and here again there are dangers of bias in that sick and well sub-groups may well vary systematically in their self-defined threshold for this. One approach, the Life Events and Difficulties Schedule or LEDS (Brown & Harris, 1978) attempts to capture such variations in the 'context' of the pregnancy without specifically taking account of the actual emotional appraisal of the individual concerned. For this *contextual* method of rating a judgement is made by the investigator about the likely meaning of each event for the person concerned, on the basis of what most people would feel in such a situation, given biography, prior plans and current circumstances, but ignoring what he/she reports as the actual response. Based on a semi-structured face-to-face interview, obtaining a full coherent account of any relevant incident, the interviewer uses a set of previously developed rules embodied in training manuals to decide which of 68 different types of possible event or ongoing difficulty can be included as having occurred during a defined period (level ii). The verbal interview and the detailed manuals permit an assessment of key stressors which often involve secrets and lies, unbiased by respondent appraisal. They also give the LEDS three other advantages:

a) an ability denied to simple questionnaires to deal more precisely with the relative timing of stressor and onset/exacerbation of disorder, by allowing cross-questioning and backtracking during the interview; relating symptoms to each other, and to events such as National Holidays (as well, of course, as to other stressful events under study).

b) a wealth of narrative material which supplements specific probes designed to make distinctions at level (iii) as well as at level (iv), and thus allows analysis by specific sub-types of unpleasant event. This permits exploration within the debate outlined earlier between general and specific theories of the impact of stress on health.

c) a check on various types of investigator bias, along with control over respondent biases, through manuals with extensive lists of precedents and through consensus meetings with other research workers who are unaware of the subject's symptoms and reactions. This also ensures high rates of inter-rater reliability (Tennant et al., 1979; Parry et al., 1981).

More recently a number of other instruments have adopted this type of contextual interview approach (Dohrenwend et al., 1990: Brugha & Cragg, 1990; Sandberg et al., 1993; Costello et al., 1998) or systematized the approach already employed (Paykel, 1997; Wethington et al., 1996). Because of these advantages the remainder of this chapter will concentrate on findings using this contextual approach (see also 'Stress assessment').

Vulnerability to the impact of life events and difficulties

Reference to the multi-factorial nature of illness aetiology has become like grace before meals, often repeated but rarely followed through. Research still tends to focus on one factor while paying lip service to the others. It will be argued here that the impact of life events on health can only be understood in the light of knowledge about what makes some people more likely than others to become ill after particular types of stressor. In other words without an understanding of vulnerability, understanding of the relationship between stress and health will remain limited.

Early work with the LEDS in Camberwell, London in the late 1960s focused on depressive disorder. Parallel findings in patient and random community female samples identified 'severe events and major difficulties' as factors provoking onset of depression. These *provoking agents* constitute only a small minority of all stressors recorded by the LEDS instrument and largely involved interpersonal crises, such as discoveries of partners' infidelities, children's stealing or estrangements from former good friends or family, but depression was also linked with more material stressors such as threats of eviction or unemployment. It was noteworthy that events such as house moves, not rated severe because they involved only hassle and were only mildly unpleasant, were not associated with depression. Nor were events which were severe in the short but not the long term, such as a child with a threatened diagnosis of meningitis which turned later out to be migraine. Although extremely distressing during the first few days, such 'non-severe' events were, by definition, largely resolved by the end of two weeks.

A thorough exploration of the background and social network variables suggested that four 'vulnerability factors' might be at work. Two of them involved lack of supportive relationships, the first with a partner currently, the second in the past – loss of mother by death or long-term separation before age 11. The other two – lack of employment and household containing three or more children – were closely linked with current roles, suggesting that women trapped at home were more vulnerable (see also 'Socioeconomic status and health' and 'Social support and health'). Speculation on the common theme uniting these four factors suggested they were all likely to be associated with an intrapsychic state such as poor self-esteem or low mastery. This would cause minor feelings of depression (likely in anyone experiencing such events) to generalize into the full-blown clinical state (for detailed discussion see Brown & Harris, 1978). Subsequent findings offered five types of confirmation concerning this intrapsychic mediator:

1) In a later sample self-esteem was deliberately measured at first interview and at follow up those who had shown *negative self evaluation* were nearly three times more likely than the rest to become clinically depressed after a provoking agent (Brown *et al.*, 1986).

2) Further exploration of the nature of the provoking agents revealed that it was really losses involving humiliation/entrapment that played the key role, echoing the theme of low self image/powerlessness (Brown *et al.*, 1995: Broadhead and Abbas, 1998: Abbrev Kendler *et al.*, 2003).

3) 'Fresh start' events found to precede depressive remission (Brown *et al.*, 1992; Leenstra *et al.*, 1995) seem to represent the opposite process, a sense of renewed self-worth, power and hope.

4) The well known doubling of rates of depression among women has been related to differing types of severe events involving their greater entrapment in domestic roles as compared with men (Nazroo *et al.*, 1996).

5) The contribution of the third and fourth vulnerability factors seemed to change with alterations in women's roles by the year 2000. With increasing proportions of women in the labour force, though part-time employment is still protective, full-time work no longer is, especially for single mothers (Brown & Bifulco, 1990). Moreover the greater availability of contraception that is free and easier to use, of legal abortion and of nursery places means that having as many as three children is no longer associated with lesser mastery (i.e. of fertility), with being trapped at home nor with depression (Brown, personal communication 2000).

This brief account of the historical development of the LEDS perspective on depression shows how increasing refinement from the side of vulnerability – the move from gross demographic factors such as lack of employment or supportive partner to the allied low self-esteem – can lead to increasing specificity in the nature of the life events seen as critical: from 'severe' in level (iv), to 'humiliation' in level (iii), a type of stress even more likely to resonate with negative self-evaluation than would non-humiliating losses such as adult

children emigrating because of promotion, or markedly reduced family income because of employer's bankruptcy leading to job loss.

Specificity of life-event stress resonates with specificity of vulnerability to produce specific illnesses

The LEDS has now been used to investigate a range of disorders, both psychiatric and somatic, and while there is no space here to go into details it may be of use to highlight particular causal chains which seem to have been identified.

a) Humiliation/entrapment, low self-esteem and depression (see above).

b) Danger, vigilance and anxiety disorder (Finlay Jones, Chapter 3 in Brown & Harris, 1989).

c) Intrusiveness, sensitivity to criticism and schizophrenia (Awaiting further confirmation, Brown & Harris, 1989, chapter 16, p. 451).

d) Pudicity (or events involving sexual shame) and restricting anorexia nervosa (Schmidt *et al.*, 1997).

e) Goal-frustration, striving stubbornness and peptic ulcer disease (Craig, Chapter 9 in Brown & Harris, 1989).

f) Goal-frustration/work difficulties, irascibility/type-A and myocardial infarction (Neilson *et al.*, in Brown & Harris, 1989, Chapter 12).

g) Challenge, dedication and secondary amenorrhea (Harris in Brown & Harris, 1989, Chapter 10).

h) Conflict over speaking out, punctiliousness and functional dysphonia (Andrews & House in Brown & Harris, 1989, Chapter 13).

i) Severe events and functional illness: abdominal pain, menorrhagia and somatization: A number of LEDS studies suggest that the old distinction between functional and organic disorder still has some value. In one early study with patients undergoing appendectomy, pathologists' reports on the appendices were only consulted long after the life events had been rated (Creed in Brown & Harris, 1989, Chapter 8). This lends all the greater credibility to his finding that the same type of severe events associated with depressive onset were more than twice as common in the nine months before appendectomy for those without appendicitis as for both those with acute inflammation and those in a community comparison group. The author suggested that pain in the absence of inflammation may form part of a cluster of psychiatric symptoms in response to a more severely threatening event, as may increases in gut motility (also invoked to account for functional abdominal pain). Further research with a range of gastrointestinal disorders confirmed this perspective (Craig, op. cit). Again those without signs of tissue damage showed a raised proportion with at least one of the severe events associated with depression, while those with other 'organic' conditions resembled the community comparison group. A similar patterning was found for functional menorrhagia, although here the high number with depression meant that a large number of these severe events were humiliations and losses (Harris, op. cit). One study of somatization took particular care to distinguish somatizers with functional somatic symptoms from other mixed physical/psychiatric cases (Craig *et al.*, 1993). Its findings not only confirmed the picture of preceding severe depressogenic-type events but also highlighted another parallel with depression – a high rate of neglect by parent figures in childhood. However, as children, somatizers in addition, and more often than pure psychiatric cases, had experience of either their own or their parents' physical illness. The authors suggest that these produced the somatizers' particular form of coping with the loss of hope consequent upon the provoking event, namely presenting with a physical symptom, which might have become their habitual way to elicit care and support.

Severe events have also been implicated in the development of such 'organic' conditions as multiple sclerosis (Grant in Brown & Harris, 1989, Chapter 11), stroke (House *et al.*), diabetes mellitus (Robinson & Fuller, 1985) and disease progression in HIV infection (Evans *et al.*, 1997). The evidence for their role in onset/relapse of breast cancer is contradictory (Ramirez *et al.*, 1989), (Barraclough *et al.*, 1992; Chen *et al.*, 1995; Geyer, 1991; Protheroe *et al.*, 1999) (see also 'Psychosomatics').

These findings also suggest that depression may mediate between the occurrence of severe events and the onset of somatic illness, but that this could operate in at least two different ways. First, even though there is no organic tissue damage, it may render people more likely to interpret themselves as ill along the following lines:

Events and difficulties ————————Psychiatric Caseness
———————— Increased sensitivity to physical abnormality/pain without gross organic damage

Second, the results on multiple sclerosis and breast cancer suggest the possibility of a chain of the following kind:

Provoking agent ————————Depression of at least borderline–case level ————————Disorders consequent on decreased immunological competence

Both of these pathways might be seen as characterized by a measure of 'disengagement' from usual functioning. In other instances, anxiety, anger, and tension may operate as mediating factors, and these might be considered disorders of 'overengagement', such as

ulcers, heart disease and even secondary amenorrhea (see also 'Coronary heart disease: cardiac psychology').

These diagrams highlight the need to specify the intervening physiological mechanisms serving to relate the emotional meaning of the stress experienced to the biochemistry of the disease. Henry and Stephens (1977) have counterposed the pituitary–adreno–cortical (PAC) and the sympatho–adreno–medullary (SAM) systems, relating the former to conservation–withdrawal (like 'disengagement') and the latter to the fight–flight complex of reactions to stress (more like over-engagement). Calloway and others (1984) reported higher levels of urinary-free cortisol in those of their depressed patients who had undergone a severe event before illness onset, though other reports of basal salivary cortisol in those with recent life events have been conflicting (confirmatory by Strickland *et al.*, 2002; negative by Harris *et al.*, 2000, who did however find higher baseline morning cortisol predicted depressive onset independently of other psychosocial factors). Changes in corticosteroid levels may have 'extensive and complex effects upon the immune system' (Stein *et al.*, 1981), suggesting that studies of physical illness resulting from disorders of immune function should pursue hypotheses involving humiliation, loss, low self-esteem and depressive response (see also 'Psychoneuroimmunology').

In summary, the specificity perspective on life events and health promises to encourage a multi-factorial approach, in which data on life events, meaning and psychosocial vulnerability should be collected alongside detailed physiological data.

Acknowledgements

The life events research described was originally conceived by Professor George Brown, and largely supported by the Medical Research Council. I am indebted to all the members of the research team who have participated in the data collection over the last 20 years, to Laurie Letchford and Sheila Williams for work with the computer and to all those who have taken the trouble to respond to our questions by telling of such painful and private experiences.

REFERENCES

Alexander, F. (1950). *Psychosomatic medicine*. New York: Norton.

Barraclough, J., Pinder, P., Cruddas, M., Osmond, C., Taylor, I. & Perry, M. (1992). Life events and breast cancer prognosis, *British Medical Journal*, **304**, 1078–81.

Broadhead, J. & Abas, M. (1998). Life events, difficulties and depression among women in an urban setting in Zimbabwe. *Psychological Medicine*, **28**, 29–38.

Brown, G. W. (1974). Meaning, measurement, and the stress of life events. In B. S. Dohrenwend & B. P. Dohrenwend (Eds.). *Stressful life events: their nature and effects*. USA: John Wiley and Sons.

Brown, G. W., Andrews, B., Harris, T. O., Adler, Z. & Bridge, L. (1986). Social support, self-esteem and depression. *Psychological Medicine*, **16**, 813–31.

Brown, G. W. & Bifulco, A. (1990). Motherhood, employment and the development of depression: a replication of a finding? *British Journal of Psychiatry*, **156**, 169–79.

Brown, G. W. & Harris, T. (1978). *Social origins of depression: a study of psychiatric disorder in women*. London: Tavistock Press & New York: Free Press.

Brown, G. W. & Harris, T. O. (1989), *Life events and illness*. New York: Guilford & London: Unwin Hyman.

Brown, G. W., Harris, T. O. & Hepworth, C. (1995). Loss, humiliation and entrapment among women developing depression: a patient and non-patient comparison. *Psychological Medicine*, **25**, 7–21.

Brown, G. W., Lemyre, L. & Bifulco, A. T. (1992). Social factors and recovery from anxiety and depressive disorders: a test of the specificity hypothesis. *British Journal of Psychiatry*, **161**, 44–54.

Brugha, T. S. & Cragg, D. (1990). The list of threatening experiences: the reliability and validity of a brief life events questionnaire. *Acta Psychiatrica Scandinavica*, **82**, 77–81.

Calloway, S. P., Dolan, R. J., Fonagy, P., De Souza, F.V.A. & Wakeling, A. (1984). 'Endocrine changes and clinical profiles in depression: 1. The dexamethasone suppression test'. *Psychological Medicine*, **14**, 749–58.

Cannon, W. B. (1932). *The Wisdom of the Body* (2nd edn.). New York: Norton.

Chen, C. C., David, A. S., Nunnerley, H. *et al.* (1995). Adverse life events and breast cancer: case-control study. *British Medical Journal*, **311**, 1527–30.

Costello, E., Angold, A., March, J. & Fairbank, J. (1998). Life events and posttraumatic stress: the development of a new measure for children and adolescents. *Psychological Medicine*, **28**, 1275–88.

Craig, T. K. J., Boardman, A. P., Mills, K., Daly-Jones, O. & Drake, H. (1993). The South London somatisation study I: longitudinal course and influence of early life experiences. *British Journal of Psychiatry*, **163**, 579–88.

Dohrenwend, B. P., Link, B. G., Kern, R. & Markowitz, J. (1990). Measuring life events: the problem of variability within event categories. *Stress Medicine*, **6**, 179–89.

Dunbar, H. F. (1954). *Emotions and bodily changes: a survey of literature on psychosomatic interrelationships.* New York: Columbia University Press.

Evans, D. L., Leserman, J., Perkins, D. O. *et al.* (1997). Severe life stress as a predictor of early disease progression in HIV infection. *American Journal of Psychiatry*, **154**, 630–4.

Geyer, S. (1991). Life events prior to manifestation of breast cancer: a study concerning eight years before diagnosis. *Journal of Psychosomatic Research*, **35**, 355–63.

Harris, T. O., Borsanyi, S., Messari, S. *et al.* (2000). Morning cortisol as a risk factor for subsequent major depressive disorder in adult women. *British Journal of Psychiatry*, **177**, 505–10.

Henry, J. P. & Stephens, P. M. (1977). *Stress, health and the social environment. A sociobiological approach to medicine.* New York: Springer Verlag.

Holmes, T. H. & Rahe, R. H. (1967). The Social Readjustment Rating Scale. *Journal of Psychosomatic Research*, **11**, 213–18.

House, A., Dennis, M., Mogridge, L., Hawton, K. & Warlow, C. (1990). Life events and difficulties preceding stroke. *Journal of Neurology, Neurosurgery and Psychiatry*, **53**, 1024–8.

Kanner, A. D., Coyne, J. C., Schaefer, C. & Lazarus, R. S. (1981). Comparison of two methods of stress measurement: daily hassles and uplifts versus major life events. *Journal of Behavioral Medicine*, **4**, 1–39.

Kendler, K. S., Hettema, J. M., Butcra, F., Gardner, C. O. & Prescott, C. A. (2003). Life event dimensions of loss, humiliation entrapment and danger in the prediction of onsets of depression and generalized anxiety. *Archives of General Psychiatry*, **60**, 789–96.

Lleenstra, A. S., Ormel, J. & Giel, R. (1995) Positive life change and recovery from anxiety and depression. *British Journal of Psychiatry*, **166**, 333–43.

Nazroo, J. Y., Edwards, A. C. & Brown, G. W. (1996). Gender differences in the onset of depression following a shared life event: a study of couples. *Psychological Medicine*, **27**, 9–19.

Parry, G., Shapiro, D. A. & Davies, L. (1981). Reliability of life event ratings: an independent replication. *British Journal of Clinical Psychology*, **20**, 133–4.

Paykel, E. S. (1997). The interview for recent life events. *Psychologicial Medicine*, **27**, 301–10.

Protheroe, D., Turvey, K., Horgan, K. *et al.* (1999). Stressful life events and difficulties and onset of breast cancer: case-control study. *British Medical Journal*, **319**, 1027–30.

Ramirez, A., Craig, T.K.J., Watson, J. P., Fentiman, I. S., North, W. R. S. & Rubens, R. (1989). Stress and the relapse of breast cancer. *British Medical Journal*, **298**, 291–3.

Robinson, N. & Fuller, J. H. (1985). The role of life events and difficulties in the onset of diabetes mellitus. *Journal of Psychosomatic Research*, **29**, 583–91.

Sandberg, S., Rutter, M., Giles, S. *et al.* (1993). Assessment of Psychological experiences in childhood: methodological issues and some illustrative findings. *Journal of Child Psychology and Psychiatry*, **34**, 879–97.

Sarason, I., Jonson, J. H. & Siegel, J. M. (1978). Assessing the impact of life changes: development of the life experiences survey. *Journal of Consulting and Clinical Psychology*, **46**, 932–46.

Schmidt, U. H., Tiller, J. M., Andrews, B., Blanchard, M. & Treasure, J. (1997). Is there a specific trauma precipitating onset of an eating disorder? *Psychological Medicine*, **27**, 523–30.

Selye, H. (1956). *The stress of life.* New York: McGraw-Hill.

Stein, M., Keller, S. & Schleifer, S. (1981). The hypothalamus and the immune response. In H. Weiner, M. A. Hofer & A. J. Stunkard (Eds.). *Brain, behaviour, and bodily disease.* New York: Raven Press.

Strickland, P. L., Deakin, J. F. W., Percival, C., *et al.* (2002). Bio-social origins of depression in the community: interactions between social adversity, cortisol and serotonin neurotransmission, *British Journal of Psychiatry*, **180**, 168–73.

Tennant, C. & Andrews, G. (1976). A scale to measure the stress of life events. *Australian and New Zealand Journal of Psychiatry*, **10**, 27–32.

Tennant, C., Smith, A., Bebbington, P. & Hurry, J. (1979). The contextual threat of life events: the concept and its reliability'. *Psychological Medicine*, **9**, 525–8.

Wethington, E., Brown, G. W. & Kessler, R. C. (1996). Interview measures of life events. In L. Gorden, S. Cohen & R. C. Kessler (Eds.). *Measuring stress: a guide for health and social scientists.* Oxford: Oxford University Press.

Men's health

Christina Lee[1] and R. Glynn Owens[2]

[1]The University of Queensland
[2]The University of Auckland

Why men's health?

Research in psychology, health and medicine has traditionally focused on men, to the neglect of women, but in the process men have tended to be treated as if they were 'standard human beings', and the effects of the gendered nature of society on men's health have been ignored. This chapter takes the view that a social perspective on men's health needs to focus on gender: what, other than biology, does it mean to be a man in contemporary society, and how might social and cultural expectations of masculinity affect men's behaviour, their relationships and their physical and emotional health? Systemic gender inequities in income, social responsibilities, social power and access to resources are as influential on men's lives and health as they are on women's (see also 'Gender issues and women's health').

Contemporary men are, to varying degrees, caught between the demands of two sets of social expectations, neither of which is readily compatible with contemporary reality (e.g. Copenhaver & Eisler, 1996). Theorists of masculinity argue for the existence of multiple 'masculinities' reflecting the lives of men from varied ethnic backgrounds, social classes and sexual orientations (e.g. Connell, 1995; Mac an Ghaill, 1996). In this chapter, we concentrate on two main social constructions of how men should behave. We contrast the traditionally dominant model of 'hegemonic masculinity' – that model of masculinity which society privileges as 'true' maleness – with modern, egalitarian perspectives on men's 'new' gender roles.

'Hegemonic masculinity' refers to the traditional, patriarchal view of men's behaviour: a man is characterized by toughness, unemotionality, physical competence, competitiveness and aggression. By contrast, modern views of gender relations downplay differences between the sexes, recognizing that many gendered aspects of life are arbitrary, and prescribing that men should find more egalitarian ways of living. This apparently more equitable and permissive model of gender is also problematic, in that it neglects economic, cultural and social forces, ignoring the fact that individual choices are rarely free of constraint.

We argue that neither of these prescriptive masculinities is easy to achieve, that their incompatibilities mean that however a man chooses to lead his life will in some sense be 'wrong', and that one result of this tension is damage to men's health. This emphasis on gender means that a focus on specific illnesses and risk factors is less important than an analysis which deals with the social nature of gender. From a social science point of view, what is important is not that men get prostate cancer and women get breast cancer: it is that men's and women's lives, the contexts within which they experience health and illness, are very different from each other.

Health behaviours and health service use

One of the best established gender differences in health is that men's life expectancy averages three years less than women's (Population Reference Bureau, 2003). However, the size of the gender gap varies between regions. In Eastern Europe, men's life expectancy is 11 years less than women's, while in countries such as Afghanistan, Pakistan and Nepal, it is equal to or greater than women's. This suggests a need to look beyond essential biological differences to explain differences in life expectancy.

Males are certainly biologically weaker than females, as is demonstrated by consistently higher neonatal death rates among males than females. But other causes of death have more complex explanations. For example, coronary heart disease is a leading cause of death for both men and women (e.g. Australian Bureau of Statistics, 2000), but men die younger than women. Explanations exist at biological, behavioural and sociocultural levels. At a biological level, men lack the protective effect of

oestrogen (Dubbert & Martin, 1988). But at the same time, hegemonic masculinity encourages men to adopt attitudes and behaviours which increase risk of coronary heart disease. These include hostile and competitive social relationships, high fat, high alcohol diets and other harmful attitudes and behaviours, chosen at least in part because they enable enactment of a 'male script' (Helgeson, 1995).

The evidence that men lead less healthy lifestyles than women is well established, but is rarely interpreted from a perspective that acknowledges the social pressures on men to conform to unhealthy gender-based stereotypes. Men who make less than optimal health choices are seen as individually responsible. This has led to lack of efforts to improve men's health behaviours, and an assumption that such efforts will be unsuccessful (Courtenay, 1998).

Hegemonic models of gender position a concern for one's health as feminine; men are 'naturally' unresponsive to pain and unconcerned with minor symptoms (Petersen, 1998). Surveys across countries and age groups demonstrate that men engage in more health-damaging behaviours and women in more health-protective behaviours (e.g. Courtenay *et al.*, 2002; Stronegger *et al.*, 1997; Uitenbroek *et al.*, 1996) (see 'Health-related behaviours').

Men make less use of health care and screening services than women, even when gynaecological services are accounted for (e.g. Stoverinck *et al.*, 1996), are slower to acknowledge symptoms of illness (e.g. Gijsbers van Wijk *et al.*, 1999), and are more likely to be 'sent' by their spouse (e.g. Seymour-Smith *et al.*, 2002). This is particularly the case for psychological services; boys are more likely than girls to be taken to a psychologist by parents, but men are less likely than women to seek psychological services for themselves (Jorm, 1994).

Men know less about health than women, and cultural institutions position women as responsible for men's health. Lyons and Willott (1999), for example, have analysed the way in which popular media direct information about men's health towards women, reinforcing the notion that men are incapable of caring for their own health. Loss of a partner, whether through divorce (Umberson, 1992) or widowhood (Clayton, 1990), is associated with more negative changes in health behaviours for men than for women (Byrne *et al.*, 1999). Women's culturally determined willingness to take care of men's health may appear to benefit men but in fact serves to reduce their freedom to make lifestyle choices.

Young men are disproportionately at risk of injury and accidental death (Smith, 1993); they have low levels of health-promoting behaviour and high rates of risky behaviours. Courtenay (1998) has argued that young men should not be dismissed as wilfully negligent of their health, but that social influences should be acknowledged in gender-specific health interventions to help young men make the transition to adulthood safely (see 'Adolescent lifestyle').

Risky behaviour

The major sex differences in death rates are not in disease but in accidents and violence. Hegemonic models of masculinity encourage men to expose themselves to danger, reflecting cultural constructions which regard these characteristics as superior despite their obvious capacity to harm (Petersen, 1998).

Injuries are significant public health problem (Krug *et al.*, 2000) but social discourse constructs accidental injuries as isolated incidents, rather than the result of gendered patterns of behaviour. Gender differences in risk of accidental injury or death are apparent from early childhood. Several national surveys (e.g. Danseco *et al.*, 2000; Lam *et al.*, 1999) show that boys are twice as likely as girls to be injured or killed in accidents. Adult men are around three times as likely to die from injuries than are women (e.g. Li & Baker, 1996), and these death rates are paralleled by rates of morbidity, hospitalization and disability (e.g. Gardiner *et al.*, 2000).

The excess of men in accidental injury and death statistics is observable whether one focuses on occupational (e.g. Gerberich *et al.*, 1998; Wong *et al.*, 1998), traffic-related (Li & Baker, 1996; Li *et al.*, 1998) or sporting and recreational (e.g. Williams *et al.*, 1998) settings. But in each area of activity, men's higher rates of injury are explicable not by individual men's carelessness but by men's higher exposure to risk. When one accounts for gender differences in exposure, the differences disappear. Thus, it is not the risk behaviours of individual men that require understanding, but the social forces which lead to gender differences in choice of occupation and recreational activity.

Suicide is around four times as common among males than among females at all age groups in all western countries (e.g. Lee *et al.*, 1999), although this gender difference does not appear in Asian countries (e.g. Yip, 1998). Lee *et al.* (1999) showed that suicide rates are highest among migrant, indigenous, gay and other minority men. Marginalization, poverty and social isolation appear to affect men more strongly and negatively than they do women (e.g. Taylor *et al.*, 1998), possibly because such experiences are seen as indicating men's failure to fulfil traditional role expectations of being protector and provider. Higher rates of suicide among men, and young men in particular, are related to higher levels of use of alcohol and other drugs (e.g. Lester, 1995) and risk-taking more generally (Langhinrichsen-Rohling *et al.*, 1998) (see also 'Alcohol abuse' and 'Suicide').

Social roles and health

There is no men's literature that parallels the extensive research on multiple roles in women's lives (e.g. Repetti *et al.*, 1989). Research on social roles has focused on the difficulties faced by women who combine paid work, domestic labour, care of children and care giving for frail or elderly family members (e.g. Doress-Worters, 1994; Lundberg, 1996). By contrast, there appears to be an assumption that men have only one role, that of paid worker, that any other roles are secondary and can be abandoned at any time, and that all men have a full-time unpaid helper who manages all other aspects of their lives. Such assumptions, obviously, do not reflect reality, and many men experience stress and stress-related illness as a result of conflict between social expectations and the reality of their personal and family lives (e.g. Duxbury & Higgins, 1994; Milkie & Peltola, 1999).

A central tenet of hegemonic masculinity is the assumption that a 'real' man will have a full-time, permanent job that supports his family financially (Price *et al.*, 1998). This myth is no longer tenable, but continues to influence both men's and women's concepts of successful masculinity. Men who do not conform to this stereotype are stigmatized and often find it difficult to avoid low self-esteem (e.g. Willott & Griffin, 1997); while the job market has changed, there is an assumption that men without full-time permanent employment are somehow responsible for this. Several studies of the impact on men and their families of systemic unemployment have demonstrated negative effects on men's health, self-esteem and relationships with their families (e.g. Davis, 1993; Dixon, 1998; Lobo & Watkins, 1995) (see 'Stigma').

Unpaid domestic labour is primarily a female activity (e.g. Baxter, 1997). Fathers who do contribute to household labour are most likely to involve themselves with childcare (e.g. Deutsch *et al.*, 1993). Men in role-reversed households enjoy this role but find it difficult, both to define and to carry out (Grbich, 1995; Smith, 1998). Men's active involvement in family life tends to lead to better relationships with their partners and children (e.g. Bailey, 1994; Brody, 1999). However, both broader social structures and individual gender socialization make an equitable approach to parenting and to household labour extremely difficult to put into practice (Smith, 1998).

The majority of men have positive views about fatherhood and family life. Men, like women, generally grow up with the expectation that they will have children (Grewal & Urschel, 1994) and are frequently distressed if they find they are infertile (Webb & Daniluk, 1999). It is argued (e.g. Hawkins *et al.*, 1993) that a closer involvement by fathers in parenting leads to more positive personal development among men, as well as a closer match between men's and women's adult life trajectories, which maintains the quality of their marital relationship (e.g. Kalmijn, 1999).

There is little research that examines the emotional effects on men of becoming fathers, with the focus tending to be on the effect on children of the presence or absence of a father figure in the home (e.g. Clarke-Stewart *et al.*, 2000). The evidence suggests that the majority of parents, both fathers and mothers, find the transitions associated with new parenthood to be challenging and difficult. Ballard *et al.* (1994) found that 9% of fathers were depressed six weeks after the birth, and 5% at six months. Fathers are at greatest risk of depression if their partners have received a diagnosis of depression, while fathers' adjustment problems, like mothers', are strongly related to lack of social support and high levels of economic and work-related pressure (Zelkowitz & Milet, 1997).

Just under half of all first marriages will end in divorce, and the rate for second and subsequent marriages is even higher (e.g. Thompson & Amato, 1999). Divorce and separation are initiated by women more often than by men (Stevens & Gardner, 1994). Men are less likely than women to be emotionally prepared for separation, and divorced men experience worse physical health and have less healthy lifestyles than married men, but this may be explained by pre-existing differences in variables such as alcohol use and aggressiveness, which predispose men towards relationship breakdown (Cheung, 1998). Men who want to continue to maintain a relationship with their own children face structural and systemic barriers (Pasley & Minton, 1997). Negotiating satisfactory roles and relationships as non-custodial parents, stepfathers and single fathers is a challenge for which there are few successful role models (Pasley & Minton, 1997).

Other issues

The field of men's health covers an enormous range of topics (see Lee & Owens, 2002*a*,*b*), and space does not permit a consideration even of some of the most important. These include men's sexuality and sexual behaviour, both for heterosexual men and for those with alternative sexual orientations or preferences. They also include issues relating to body image, including eating disorders and the non-medicinal use of steroids. Other topics are the roles and reactions of men in issues surrounding contraception, fertility problems, miscarriage and abortion. There are also issues surrounding criminality and assault, both as perpetrators and as victims. Another area is the particular challenges faced by men leading gay or other alternative lifestyles, and gendered issues surrounding ageing, retirement, frailty, family care giving, widowerhood and facing death are also important.

Conclusion

The purpose of this chapter has been to present an argument for a particular perspective on men and their health: that of focusing on socially constructed concepts of gender and the impacts that these have on individual men's behavioural choices and thus on their health. This may be contrasted with a more traditional, reductionist and 'piecemeal' approach to men's health: the identification of specific, isolated topics to be investigated individually without attention to the social or cultural context.

Strategies to improve men's health can only be developed if gendered differences in behavioural choices are taken seriously, and the underlying differences in men's and women's social worlds adequately explored. This chapter has attempted to demonstrate that men are affected by a sexist and heterosexist society, and by the stereotypes promoted by hegemonic and prescriptive notions of masculinity. Men's choices are further constrained by a social context that values them for their economic productivity rather than for their ability to sustain positive relationships. Research on men's health needs to take these issues into account. Men's lives need to be examined in context, with an awareness of the diversity of men's experiences, in order to develop an inclusive and socially relevant understanding of men's health.

REFERENCES

Australian Bureau of Statistics. (2000). *Deaths, Australia 1999* (Cat no. 3302.0). Canberra, Australia: Australian Bureau of Statistics.

Bailey, W. T. (1994). A longitudinal study of fathers' involvement with young children: infancy to age 5 years. *Journal of Genetic Psychology*, **155**, 331–9.

Ballard, C. G., Davis, R., Cullen, P. C., Mohan, R. N. & Dean, C. (1994). Prevalence of postnatal psychiatric morbidity in mothers and fathers. *British Journal of Psychiatry*, **164**, 782–8.

Baxter, J. (1997). Gender equality and participation in housework: a cross-national perspective. *Journal of Comparative Family Studies*, **28**, 220–47.

Brody, L. R. (1999). *Gender, emotion, and the family*. Cambridge, MA: Harvard University Press.

Byrne, G. J. A., Raphael, B. & Arnold, E. (1999). Alcohol consumption and psychological distress in recently widowed older men. *Australian and New Zealand Journal of Psychiatry*, **33**, 740–7.

Cheung, Y. B. (1998). Can marital selection explain the differences in health between married and divorced people? From a longitudinal study of a British birth cohort. *Public Health*, **112**, 113–17.

Clarke-Stewart, K. A., Vandell, D. L., McCartney, K. *et al.* (2000). Effects of parental separation and divorce on very young children. *Journal of Family Psychology*, **14**, 304–26.

Clayton, P. J. (1990). Bereavement and depression. *Journal of Clinical Psychiatry*, **51**(suppl.), 34–8.

Connell, R. W. (1995). *Masculinities*. Sydney, Australia: Allen and Unwin.

Copenhaver, M. M. & Eisler, R. M. (1996). Masculine gender role stress: a perspective on men's health. In P. Kato *et al.* (Eds.). *Handbook of diversity issues in health psychology* (pp. 219–35). New York: Plenum Press.

Courtenay, W. H. (1998). College men's health: an overview and a call to action. *Journal of American College Health*, **46**, 279–90.

Courtenay, W. H., McCreary, D. R. & Merighi, J. R. (2002). Gender and ethic differences in health beliefs and behaviours. *Journal of Health Psychology*, **7**, 219–32.

Danseco, E. R., Miller, T. R. & Spicer, R. S. (2000). Incidence and costs of 1987–1994 childhood injuries: demographic breakdowns. *Pediatrics*, **105**(2), E27.

Davis, D. L. (1993). When men become "women": gender antagonism and the changing sexual geography of work in Newfoundland. *Sex Roles*, **29**, 457–75.

Deutsch, F. M., Lussier, J. B. & Servis, L. J. (1993). Husbands at home: predictors of paternal participation in childcare and housework. *Journal of Personality and Social Psychology*, **65**, 1154–66.

Dixon, P. (1998). Employment factors in conflict in African American heterosexual relationships: some perceptions of women. *Journal of Black Studies*, **28**, 491–505.

Doress-Worters, P. B. (1994). Adding elder care to women's multiple roles: a critical review of the caregiver stress and multiple roles literatures. *Sex Roles*, **31**, 597–616.

Dubbert, P. & Martin, J. (1988). Exercise. In E. A. Blechman, K. D. Brownell (Eds.). *Handbook of behavioral medicine for women*, New York: Pergamon.

Duxbury, L. & Higgins, C. (1994). Interference between work and family: a status report on dual-career and dual-earner mothers and fathers. *Employee Assistance Quarterly*, **9**, 55–80.

Gardiner, J. P., Judson, J. A., Smith, G. S., Jackson, R. & Norton, R. N. (2000). A decade of intensive care unit trauma admissions in Auckland. *New Zealand Medical Journal*, **113**, 327–30.

Gerberich, S. G., Gibson, R. W., French, L. R. *et al.* (1998). Machinery-related injuries: regional rural injury study-I (RRIS-I). *Accident Analysis and Prevention*, **30**, 793–804.

Gijsbers van Wijk, C. M., Huisman, H. & Kolk, A. M. (1999). Gender differences in physical symptoms and illness behavior. A health diary study. *Social Science and Medicine*, **49**, 1061–74.

Grbich, C. F. (1995). Male primary caregivers and domestic labour: involvement or avoidance? *Journal of Family Studies*, **1**, 114–29.

Grewal, R. P. & Urschel, J. D. (1994). Why women want children: a study during phases of parenthood. *Journal of Social Psychology*, **134**, 453–5.

Hawkins, A. J., Christiansen, S. L., Sargent, K. P. & Hill, E. J. (1993). Rethinking fathers' involvement in child care: a developmental perspective. *Journal of Family Issues*, **14**, 531–49.

Helgeson, V.S. (1995). Masculinity, men's roles, and coronary heart disease. In D.F. Sabo, F. Donald, D.F. Gordon *et al.* (Eds.). *Men's health and illness: gender, power, and the body*. Thousand Oaks, CA: Sage.

Jorm, A. F. (1994). Characteristics of Australians who reported consulting a psychologist for a health problem: an analysis of data from the 1989–90 National Health Survey. *Australian Psychologist*, **29**, 212–15.

Kalmijn, M. (1999). Father involvement in childrearing and the perceived stability of marriage. *Journal of Marriage and the Family*, **61**, 409–21.

Krug, E. G., Sharma, G. K. & Lozano, R. (2000). The global burden of injuries. *American Journal of Public Health*, **90**, 523–6.

Lam, L. T., Ross, F. I. & Cass, D. T. (1999). Children at play: the death and injury pattern in New South Wales, Australia, July 1990–June 1994. *Journal of Paediatrics and Child Health*, **35**, 572–7.

Langhinrichsen-Rohling, J., Lewinsohn, P., Rohde, P. *et al.* (1998). Gender differences in the suicide-related behaviors of adolescents and young adults. *Sex Roles*, **39**, 839–54.

Lee, C. & Owens, R. G. (2002a). *The psychology of men's health*. Buckingham, UK: Open University Press.

Lee, C. & Owens, R. G. (2002b). Issues for a psychology of men's health. *Journal of Health Psychology*, **7**, 209–10.

Lee, C. J., Collins, K. A. & Burgess, S. E. (1999). Suicide under the age of eighteen: a 10-year retrospective study. *American Journal of Forensic Medicine and Pathology*, **20**, 27–30.

Lester, D. (1995). The association between alcohol consumption and suicide and homicide rates: a study of 13 nations. *Alcohol and Alcoholism*, **30**, 465–8.

Li, G. & Baker, S. P. (1996). Exploring the male-female discrepancy in death rates from bicycling injury: the decomposition method. *Accident Analysis and Prevention*, **28**, 537–40.

Li, G., Baker, S. P., Langlois, J. A. & Kelen, G. D. (1998). Are female drivers safer? An application of the decomposition method. *Epidemiology*, **9**, 379–84.

Lobo, F. & Watkins, G. (1995). Late career unemployment in the 1990s: its impact on the family. *Journal of Family Studies*, **1**, 103–11.

Lundberg, U. (1996). Influence of paid and unpaid work on psychophysiological stress responses of men and women. *Journal of Occupational Health Psychology*, **1**, 117–30.

Lyons, A. C. & Willott, S. (1999). From suet pudding to superhero: representations of men's health for women. *Health*, **3**, 283–302.

Mac an Ghaill, M. (Ed.). (1996). *Understanding masculinities: social relations and cultural arenas*. Buckingham, UK: Open University Press.

Milkie, M. A. & Peltola, P. (1999). Playing all the roles: gender and the work-family balancing act. *Journal of Marriage and the Family*, **61**, 476–90.

Pasley, K. & Minton, C. (1997). Generative fathering after divorce and remarriage: beyond the "disappearing dad." In A. J. Hawkins, D. C. Dollahite *et al.* (Eds.). *Generative fathering: beyond deficit perspectives*. Thousand Oaks, CA: Sage.

Petersen, A. (1998). *Unmasking the masculine: "men" and "identity" in a sceptical age*. London: Sage.

Population Reference Bureau. (2003). *2003 World Population Datasheet*. Washington, DC: PRB (http://www.prb.org/).

Price, R. H., Friedland, D. S. & Vinokur, A. D. (1998). Job loss: hard times and eroded identity. In J.H. Harvey (Ed.). *Perspectives on loss: a sourcebook*. Philadelphia, PA: Brunner/ Mazel.

Repetti, R. L., Matthews, K. A. & Waldron, I. (1989). Employment and women's health. *American Psychologist*, **44**, 1394–401.

Seymour-Smith, S., Wetherell, M. & Phoenix, A. (2002). "My wife ordered me to come!" A discursive analysis of doctors' and nurses' accounts of men's use of general practitioners. *Journal of Health Psychology*, **7**, 253–68.

Smith, C. D. (1998). "Men don't do this sort of thing": a case study of the social isolation of househusbands. *Men and Masculinities*, **1**, 138–72.

Smith, D. W. E. (1993). *Human longevity*. Oxford: Oxford University Press.

Stevens, G. & Gardner, S. (1994). *Separation anxiety and the dread of abandonment in adult males*. Westport, CT: Praeger Publishers/Greenwood Publishing Group.

Stoverinck, M. J., Lagro-Janssen, A. L. & Weel, C. V. (1996). Sex differences in health problems, diagnostic testing, and referral in primary care. *Journal of Family Practice*, **43**, 567–76.

Stronegger, W. J., Freidl, W. & Rasky, E. (1997). Health behaviour and risk behaviour: socioeconomic differences in an Austrian rural county. *Social Science and Medicine*, **44**, 423–6.

Taylor, R., Morrell, S., Slaytor, E. & Ford, P. (1998). Suicide in urban New South Wales, Australia 1985–1994: socio-economic and migrant interactions. *Social Science and Medicine*, **47**, 1677–86.

Thompson, R. A. & Amato, P. R. (Eds.). (1999). *The postdivorce family: children, parenting, and society*. Thousand Oaks, CA: Sage.

Uitenbroek, D. G., Kerekovska, A. & Festchieva, N. (1996). Health lifestyle behaviour and socio-demographic characteristics: a study of Varna, Glasgow and Edinburgh. *Social Science and Medicine*, **43**, 367–77.

Umberson, D. (1992). Gender, marital status and the social control of health behavior. *Social Science and Medicine*, **34**, 907–17.

Webb, R. E. & Daniluk, J. C. (1999). The end of the line: infertile men's experiences of being unable to produce a child. *Men and Masculinities*, **2**, 6–25.

Williams, J. M., Wright, P., Currie, C. E. & Beattie, T. F. (1998). Sports related injuries in Scottish adolescents aged 11–15. *British Journal of Sports Medicine*, **32**, 291–6.

Willott, S. & Griffin, C. (1997). "Wham bam, am I a man?": Unemployed men talk about masculinities. *Feminism and Psychology*, **7**, 107–28.

Wong, T. Y., Lincoln, A., Tielsch, J. M. & Baker, S. P. (1998). The epidemiology of ocular injury in a major US automobile corporation. *Eye*, **12**, 870–4.

Yip, P. S. (1998). Suicides in Hong Kong and Australia. *Crisis*, **19**, 24–34.

Zelkowitz, P. & Milet, T. H. (1997). Stress and support as related to postpartum paternal

Noise: effects on health

Staffan Hygge

University of Gävle

Noise: nature and measurement

Noise is often defined as unwanted sound or sounds that have an adverse effect on humans. What is sweet music for one person may be noise to someone else. Thus, noise is a psychological construct influenced both by physical and psychosocial properties.

Sound is created by the rapidly changing pressure of air molecules at the eardrum. A single tone, such as that from a tuning fork, can be depicted as a fixed wavelength sinusoidal pressure distribution across time. The number of pressure cycles per second, measured in hertz (Hz), is the basis for the sensation of pitch. A healthy young ear is sensitive to sounds between approximately 20 Hz and up to 20 kHz. The amplitude of the sine wave is perceived as loudness. To accommodate the wide dynamic power range of the human ear a logarithmic magnitude scale for sounds has been introduced. Its unit is the decibel (dB). Adding two independent sound sources of the same dB-level will yield a sum that is $\approx$3 dB higher than one of them alone. The subjective effect of a change in 3 dB amounts to a just perceptible change. A change of around 10 dB is needed to experience the sound as twice as loud.

The hearing threshold for pure tones is lowest in the frequency range 500–4000 Hz, which also is the range where human speech has its maximum energy content. In order to compensate for the ear's frequency sensitivity, and to make units that are comparable across the audible frequency range, standardized weighting curves or filters have been defined for sound level meters (see Fig. 1).

The A-filter, which is the most commonly used filter, is intended to mirror hearing thresholds. The B- and C-filters were made to mirror the ear's sensitivity to intermediate and high intensities, and the D-filter was designed to penalize sounds in the frequency ranges important for human speech. When the low frequency components of a sound dominate, such as in HVAC-noise, dBA underestimates perceived noise.

Several indices have been suggested to represent fluctuating sounds across time. A simple one is that of maximum level, L_{max}, which can be combined with a number index for how many times a certain L_{max}-level has been exceeded. The L_p-measure, as in L_1 and L_{50}, states the percentage of time a certain value (in dB, dBA etc.) is exceeded. The equivalent continuous sound pressure level, L_{eq}, is the average constant level across the time period that represents

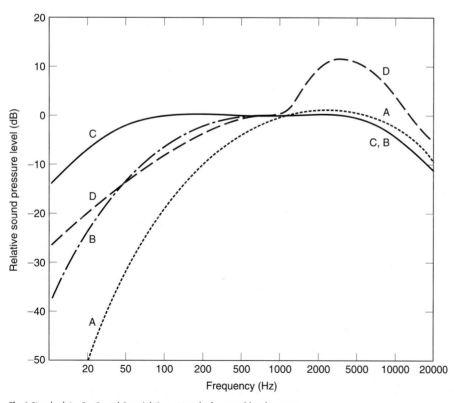

Fig 1 Standard A-, B-, C- and D-weighting networks for sound level meters.

the total energy of the fluctuating variable sound. L_{eq}-levels are commonly used for codes and regulations and can be weighted to dBA, dBB etc. Because of its logarithmic nature the L_{eq}-measure is strongly influenced by high peak values, but very insensitive to increases in background sound levels.

Many other indices have been proposed (cf. Kryter, 1985). These include attempts to incorporate masking, critical bands, rise-time, predictability, fluctuations and the design of ratio-scales for the measurement of annoyance and perceived loudness.

Auditory health effects

Hearing impairment

Prolonged exposure to intense sounds results in noise-induced hearing loss. Three types of noise induced hearing losses can be distinguished: (1) temporary threshold shifts (TTS); (2) permanent threshold shifts (PTS); and (3) acoustic trauma. TTS show an increase with SPL-levels and exposure time, starting at about 70 dB for noise in the frequency bands around 4 kHz and about 75 dB for bands around 250 Hz when the noise is present for several hours. TTS is reversible but requires silent periods to recover. PTS is the effect of prolonged exposure to high intensity sounds with insufficient silent recovery periods in between. The effect to the inner ear is the irreversible destruction of hair cells. To reduce the risk of PTS most western countries have restricted sound exposure in the work environment to 85 or 90 dBA for eight hours a day, five working days a week for several years when no hearing protection is worn. However, that is not a decision purely guided by the concern to avoid hearing loss, since it has been estimated that around 10% of those so exposed to 85 dBA will accrue a hearing loss. The figure is estimated to drop to 4% if the levels are reduced to 80 dBA. Thus, converging evidence suggests exposure levels of around 75 dBA will be safe from the point of hearing impairment, temporary or permanent.

Noise-induced acoustic trauma involves very short exposure to very intense sounds, such as riveting, gunfire, explosives, toy pistols and clicking toys. These impulse sounds are treacherous because of their short duration, which falls short of the integration time of the brain, but not of the inner ear. Thus, their perceived loudness is much lower than the damage caused to the hair cells in the inner ear.

Degree of hearing impairment is assessed by audiometry, which normally consists of measuring hearing thresholds for pure tones in the frequency range 500–8000 Hz. The resulting audiograms are evaluated against standardized age-corrected audiograms for unimpaired hearing. Hearing impairment caused by broadband noise often starts in the frequency range 3000–6000 Hz, with a downward spread to 500–1000 Hz as the impairment grows worse. A slight impairment in the 3000–6000 Hz range does not much affect speech comprehension in an otherwise silent environment. However, when the frequency ranges from 2000 Hz and downwards is affected, speech comprehension is markedly reduced. Hearing impaired persons and persons who do not fully master the language spoken may need up to a 10 dB better signal-to-noise ratio than normal hearing persons to understand speech.

During recent decades, noisy leisure activities rather than industrial work noise, have become more important as contributors to hearing impairment. In particular guns and rifles, explosives, chain-saws, lawn-mowers, snow mobiles, water scooters, loud concert and disco music and certain toys with loud click sounds may cause hearing impairment by itself or by blocking recovery from TTS accrued at work (see 'Deafness and hearing loss').

Non-auditory health effects

The World Health Organization defines health as the state of complete physical, mental and social wellbeing, not merely as an absence of disease and infirmity. Therefore, the health effects of noise include a broader array of adverse effects than damage to organs and tissue.

Stress reactions and cardiovascular disorders

Noise has often been implicated as a contributing cause to the development of stress reactions and cardiovascular disorders. Correlational studies report higher systolic or diastolic blood pressure (BP) or elevated stress hormone levels in hearing-impaired or noise-exposed industrial workers (Evans & Cohen, 1987). Children and adults chronically exposed to aircraft noise have been found to have higher BPs and elevated levels of stress hormones compared with controls matched on sociodemographic characteristics (Cohen et al., 1986). Correlational and cross-sectional studies suffer from methodological flaws, primarily from possible selection bias and inability to rule out other possible causes for the stress reactions and cardiovascular disorders, such as a hazardous chemical environment and other stress inducing work-related factors. Experimental studies, which for practical and ethical reasons must be restricted to acute rather than chronic noise effects, show noise effects on several non-specific physiological measures associated with stress reactions, including BP, heart rate, stress hormone output and vasoconstriction. These reactions habituate to a large extent and thus it is not clear how they can build up to a chronic effect (Evans & Cohen, 1987). However, stress reactions to chronic noise exposure have been shown in an experimental study by Peterson et al. (1981). Rhesus monkeys were exposed to loud noise for nine months. BPs increased by one third and high BP-levels were maintained for a one-month follow-up period after noise cessation.

It is probably fair to conclude that chronic exposure to high intensity noise increases the risk of cardiovascular problems. Because of this and of fairly well controlled studies where noise has also been shown to increase secretion of stress hormones (Stansfeld & Lercher, 2003), also in children, it can be claimed that noise plays a role in a general stress response. Since detailed dose-response relationships are not fully specified this conclusion must be restricted to high-intensity noise at this point (see also 'Stress and health'). With regard to other medical symptoms reportedly linked to noise, e.g. ulcers, miscarriage, weight at birth, consumption of medication, visits to doctors, infectious diseases, the evidence is still too meagre to be conclusive (Cohen et al., 1986).

Mental health

Since noise affects annoyance and prolonged annoyance may cause mental problems, it has been argued that noise may impair mental health. Studies on mental health or mental hospital admissions around Heathrow airport in London, Schiphol in Amsterdam and the different airports in Los Angeles, give correlational support for such claims. However, in most of these cases critics have shown that stringent and proper controls for sociodemographic variables diminish the correlations between noise levels and various indices of mental health. Thus, the results are conflicting and there is as yet no solid empirical basis for arguing a strong direct effect of noise on mental health (Stansfeld & Lercher, 2003).

Sleep

Sleep and sleep quality is among the most noise-sensitive human activities. From laboratory studies is has been concluded that 20–35% of normal and self-reported noise sensitive persons have problems falling asleep, change sleep stage or are awakened by a number of peaks as low as 50 dBA (Öhrström, 1993). There seems to be some agreement that peak levels below 40 dBA or equivalent noise levels below 35 dBA L_{eq}, do not have much effect on sleep. However, field studies indicate much less noise induced sleep disturbance (Griefahn & Schuette, 2003), which partly may be due to less refined sleep recording techniques in the field.

People who are drowsy or sleeping have difficulties in actively identifying and recognizing sounds, and consequently they have a problem in adapting or habituating to sounds. Children change sleep stages less often than adults because of noise and are less easily awakened than adults, but the opposite is true for the elderly. Effects of sleep deprivation on task performance the next day vary with the difficulty of the task, but no conclusive dose response relationships can be stated at this time (see 'Sleep and health' and 'Sleep disorders').

Performance and cognition

The traditional findings from laboratory noise studies are that fairly high noise levels (80–90 dB in intermittent bursts) are needed to show effects on attention, signal-detection, vigilance, short term-memory etc. (see reviews by Broadbent, 1983; Jones, 1990; Smith, 1993; Hygge, Jones & Smith, 1998). However, recent studies, both in the laboratory and in the field, have changed that picture both by scrutinizing the nature of the disturbing sound and by introducing more cognitively demanding tasks (reading, memory). Further, during the last decade noise impacts on children's cognition have been a focus of attention.

In experiments on speech-like noise and short-term memory serial recall, a set of 7–9 digits or letters is presented visually at a fixed rate. A rehearsal period is inserted between the presentation of the last item in the set and a prompt to reproduce the series in correct order. Speech in the rehearsal period, even devoid of semantic content such as a foreign tongue, or vocals in a song, interferes with recall, but broadband noise does not (see overviews by Jones & Macken, 1993; Jones & Morris, 1992). The effect is stable across sound levels ranging down to around 50 dBA, and has been shown to extend to a range of non-speech sounds that have speech-like

level fluctuations (Hughes & Jones, 2003). However, the serial nature of the memory task seems to be crucial. The effects of irrelevant speech on more cognitive tasks such as proofreading and understanding are not as marked and are less consistent.

Classroom experiments of recall memory in children aged 12–14 years one week after a 15-minute learning session in noise (Hygge, 2003) showed impairment from aircraft and road traffic noise at 66 dBA L_{eq} and from aircraft noise at 55 dBA L_{eq}. No impairment was found from exposure to train noise and verbal noise, nor did any of the noise sources affect long-term recognition. In a larger study of noise effects on many different memory tasks, with children, young adults, middle aged and older teachers (Boman et al., 2005) it was shown that language-based memory for texts was more sensitive to noise impairment than other memory tasks, that road traffic noise and irrelevant speech was about equally harmful, and that the relative noise impairment was roughly equal across age groups.

The results from these laboratory studies fit nicely with findings from field studies of children living in the vicinity of some European airports. In a longitudinal prospective study around the old and new airports in Munich (Hygge et al., 2002), noise-exposed children at the old airport were found to improve their initially lower cognitive performance in memory and reading compared with that of the control group after the airport closed down. At the new airport, the reverse was true. Before the opening of the new airport, there were no differences in reading and memory tasks between the prospective noise-exposed group and their quiet control group, but after the new airport had opened the noise-exposed children started to lag behind their controls. In a cross-sectional comparison between three European airports, Stansfeld et al. (2005) found similar effects of aircraft noise exposure, but not for road traffic noise exposure.

The vulnerability of language acquisition and mastery, memory and reading to noise exposure, particularly in children, fits in well with findings from other cross-sectional studies of school achievement and cognitive performance in noisy and less noisy areas (Evans & Lepore, 1993).

In a well known series of experiments, Glass and Singer (1972) reported performance after-effects on the number of times their subjects attempted to solve insoluble geometric puzzles and proofreading errors. The noise they used was a mixture of office machines and foreign languages presented in aperiodic bursts in intensity ranges from 60–108 dBA depending on experiment. Their main findings were that the noise had deleterious effects on post-noise behaviour when the noise was uncontrollable or unpredictable by the subjects. The introduction of perceived control by making the noise predictable or controllable eliminated the adverse noise effect even when compared with a silent control group. These adverse effects of uncontrollable and unpredictable noise have been replicated in several studies for various types of noise, as well as for stressors other than noise (Cohen, 1980). Thus, research on the after-effects of noise points to psychological coping mechanisms that may be basic and central to others stressors as well.

Social behaviour

In the laboratory, noise has consistently interacted with anger in provoking aggression as measured by the delivery of electric shocks to a confederate of the experimenter (Cohen & Spacapan, 1984). That is, the presence of noise at the time of aggression is not by itself sufficient for increased aggression, but when the subject is made angry the presence of noise adds to the aggression shown. For helping behaviour, a mixture of experimental studies in the field and the lab show less helping when exposed to noise. However, the noise effect on helping is not as consistent and marked as that on aggression.

Theoretical accounts of the noise effects

There are detailed and well documented empirical findings of how physical energy of a certain intensity, frequency composition, duration, onset-time etc. causes certain amounts of hearing impairment, but there is no good comprehensive theory as to why and how.

Stress theories adapted to explain noise effects have two sides to them. One side explores the physiological effects, the other the psychological outcomes. The physiological theories have pointed to the roles played by epinephrine and norepinephrine secretion in the activation of the sympathetic–adrenal medullary system, and to hormone output from the pituitary–adrenocortical axis (Evans & Cohen, 1987). Psychological stress theories such as Lazarus (1966) view the person's psychological appraisal of a stimulus as threatening as a first stage, followed by a stage where the individuals evaluate their resources to cope with the threat. If they perceive that they can cope, no stress response occurs, but they may later reappraise their coping ability. If they do not perceive that they can cope or are uncertain, stress is experienced (see 'Stress and health').

Psychological theories of the performance effects of noise have relied primarily on two constructs: arousal and informational load. Arousal refers to nonspecific brain activity signifying different levels of general alertness. The Yerkes–Dodson law (Kahneman, 1973) of arousal and performance assumes an inverted U-relationship between performance and arousal. Too high or too low arousal, with reference to the optimum level, impairs performance, but the exact optimal level depends on the difficulty of the task and individual skill in carrying out the task. Arousal theory and the inverted U-hypothesis suffer from several shortcomings (Hockey & Hamilton, 1983), including the multidimensionality of the construct and the problem of finding data-independent locations of the optimum level. On the other hand it is a convenient theoretical vehicle to accommodate combined and interactive effects of many different stressors, noise just being one.

Another line of theorizing (Smith, 1989) has emphasized a dominant strategy selection, and reduced efficiency in the control processes while working in noise. In information overload models (Cohen *et al.*, 1986), an emphasis is put on shrinking cognitive capacity as a result of attention allocation during noise and stress exposure, and the individual's adaptation to demands on information processing. One implication of this theory is that cumulative cognitive fatigue effects should show up as residuals also after the cessation of the noise, as in after-effects of non-controllable noise. Another important implication of the model is that both noise itself as a stressor plus individual efforts to cope with the noise can create adverse effects. Recently, there has also been some theoretical advancement into the area of noise and its effects on memory structure (Enmarker, Boman & Hygge, 2006).

Further reading

For more detailed accounts of noise, noise measurement, the effects on people and theories see relevant sections and references in Cohen *et al.* (1986), Jones and Chapman (1984), Kryter (1985), Smith & Jones (1992) and Tempest (1985). For a very good text on noise and noise effects, accessible on the Internet, see Berglund & Lindvall (1995).

REFERENCES

Berglund, B. & Lindvall, T. (Eds.). (1995). Community noise. *Archives of the Center for Sensory Research*, 2, 1–195. (Document prepared for the World Health Organization, WHO, URL: http://www.nonoise.org/library/whonoise/whonoise.htm).

Boman, E., Enmarker, I. & Hygge, S. (2005). Strength of noise effects on memory as a function of noise source and age. *Noise & Health*, **7**, 11–26.

Broadbent, D. E. (1983). Recent advances in understanding performance in noise. In G. Rossi (Ed.). *Proceedings of the 4th international congress on noise as a public health problem, Vol. 2* (pp. 719–38). Milan: Centro Ricerche e Studi Amplifon.

Cohen, S. (1980). Aftereffects of stress on human performance and social behavior: a review of research and theory. *Psychological Bulletin*, **88**, 82–108.

Cohen, S., Evans, G. W., Stokols, D. & Krantz, D. S. (1986). *Behavior, health, and environmental stress.* New York: Plenum Press.

Cohen, S. & Spacapan, S. (1984). The social psychology of noise. In D. M. Jones & A. J. Chapman (Eds.). *Noise and society.* London: Wiley.

Enmarker, I., Boman, E. & Hygge, S. (2006). Structural equation models of memory performance across noise conditions and age groups. *Scandinavian Journal of Psychology*, **47**, 449–60.

Evans, G. E. & Cohen, S. (1987). Environmental stress. In D. Stokols & I. Altman (Eds.). *Handbook of environmental psychology* (pp. 571–610). New York: Wiley.

Evans, G. W. Lepore, S. J. (1993). Nonauditory effects of noise on children: a critical review. *Children's Environments*, **10**, 31–51.

Glass, D. C. & Singer, J. E. (1972). *Urban stress: experiments on noise and social stressors.* New York: Academic Press.

Griefahn, B. & Schuette, M. (2003). Noise and sleep: present state (2003), and further needs. In R. G. de Jong, T. Houtgast, E.A.M. Franssen & W. F. Hofman (Eds.). *Proceedings of the 8th international congress of international congress on noise as a public health problem* (pp. 183–184). Delft: Foundation ICBEN 2003.

Hockey, R. & Hamilton, P. (1983). The cognitive patterning of stress states. In R. Hockey (Ed.). *Stress and fatigue in human performance* (pp. 331–62). New York: Wiley.

Hughes, R. W. & Jones, D. M. (2003). Indispensable benefits and unavoidable costs of unattended sounds for cognitive functioning. *Noise and Health*, **6**, 63–76.

Hygge, S. (2003). Classroom experiments on the effects of different noise sources and sound levels on long-term recall and recognition in children. *Applied Cognitive Psychology*, **17**, 895–914.

Hygge, S., Evans, G. W. & Bullinger, M. (2002). A prospective study of some effects of aircraft noise on cognitive performance in school children. *Psychological Science*, **13**, 469–74.

Hygge, S., Jones, D. M. & Smith, A. P. (1998). Recent developments in noise and performance. In N. Carter & R.F.S. Job (Eds.). *Noise Effects '98 – proceedings of the 7th international congress on noise as a public health problem, Vol. 1* (pp. 321–8). Sydney, Australia: National Capital Printing ACT.

Jones, D. M. (1990). Progress and prospects in the study of performance in noise. In B. Berglund & T. Lindvall (Eds.). *Noise as a public health problem, Vol. 4: new advances in noise research*. Part 1 (pp. 383–400). Stockholm: Swedish Council for Building Research.

Jones, D. M. & Chapman, A. J. (Eds.). (1984). *Noise and society*. London: Wiley.

Jones, D. M. & Macken, W. J. (1993). Irrelevant tones produce an irrelevant speech effect: implications for coding in phonological memory.

Journal of Experimental Psychology: Learning, Memory and Cognition, **19**, 369–81.

Jones, D. M. & Morris, N. (1992). Irrelevant speech and cognition. In D. M. Jones & A. P. Smith (Eds.). *Factors affecting human performance: Vol. 1*. The physical environment (pp. 29–54). London: Academic Press.

Kahneman, D. (1973). *Attention and effort*. Englewood Cliffs, NJ: Prentice Hall.

Kryter, K. (1985). *The Effects of Noise on Man* (2nd edn.). New York: Academic Press.

Lazarus, R. S. (1966). *Psychological stress and coping processes*. New York: McGraw-Hill.

Öhrström, E. (1993). Research on noise and sleep since 1988: Present state. In M. Vallet (Ed.). *Noise as a public health problem. Proceedings of the 6th international congress, Vol. 3* (pp. 331–8). Arcueil, France: Inrets.

Peterson, E. A., Augenstein, J. S., Tanis, D. C. & Augenstein, D. G. (1981). Noise raises blood pressure without impairing auditory sensitivity. *Science*, **211**, 1450–52.

Stansfeld, S. A., Berglund, B., Clark, C. *et al.* (2005). Aircraft and road traffic noise and children's cognition and health: a cross-sectional study. *Lancet*, **365**, 1942–49.

Stansfeld, S. & Lercher, P. (2003). Non-auditory physiological effects of noise: five year review and future directions. In R. G. de Jong, T. Houtgast, E.A.M. Franssen & W. F. Hofman (Eds.). *Proceedings of the 8th international congress of international congress on noise as a public health problem* (pp. 84–90). Delft: Foundation ICBEN 2003.

Smith, A. (1989). A review of the effects of noise on human performance. *Scandinavian Journal of Psychology*, **30**, 185–206.

Smith, A. P. (1993). Recent advances in the study of noise and human performance. In M. Vallet (Ed.). *Noise as a public health problem. Proceedings of the 6th international congress, Vol. 3* (pp. 293–300). Arcueil, France: Inrets.

Smith, A. P. & Jones, D. M. (1992). Noise and performance. In D. M. Jones & A. P. Smith (Eds.). *Factors affecting human performance: Vol. 1. The physical environment* (pp. 1–28). London: Academic Press.

Tempest, W. (Ed.). (1985). *The noise handbook*. London: Academic Press.

Pain: a multidimensional perspective

Dennis C. Turk and Tasha Burwinkle

University of Washington

Pain has been the focus of philosophical speculation and scientific attention since earliest recorded times. Yet, despite its history, advances in knowledge of neurophysiology and biochemistry, and the development of potent analgesic medications and sophisticated invasive modalities that have evolved, pain relief remains elusive. On average fewer than 50% of patients obtain at least a 30% reduction in pain following treatment with potent medications, pain reduction following rehabilitation averages around 30% (Turk, 2002*a*). Pain remains a perplexing and challenging problem for pain sufferers, their significant others, healthcare providers and society.

Although pain is an almost universal experience, there is little consensus even with regard to how to define it. Historical debates have raged back to the time of the ancient philosophers as to whether pain was a purely sensory or uniquely affective phenomenon. Arguments have persisted and the conceptualization of pain has more than philosophical consequences; it will affect how pain is assessed and how and even whether pain is treated.

One factor that has contributed to the debate about what pain is relates to the fact that it is a subjective experience. Unlike temperature, there is no 'pain thermometer' to determine the extent of pain that an individual has or should have. The only way to know how

D.C. Turk and T. Burwinkle

much pain someone has is to ask them and to make inferences from observation of their behaviours (see 'Pain assessment'). Another difficulty with understanding and treating pain is that it is associated with many diseases and may result from diverse sources of pathology. Moreover, the report of pain is common even in the absence of definitive physical pathology.

Another factor that has contributed to confusion relates to differential characteristics of pain. For example, pain is frequently viewed along a time continuum; acute pain, defined by its relatively brief duration (e.g. days), to sub-acute pain (e.g. months), to chronic (years) (Turk & Okifuji, 2001). Other specific variations or classifications are noted. People with migraine have episodes of severe pain that may last for hours interspersed with periods where the individual is pain free – recurrent acute pain. Pain is also associated with malignancies. This is a unique category due to the special meaning attributed to potentially lethal conditions although the mechanisms involved may be no different then those involved with other pain syndromes (Turk, 2002a).

Other distinctions are made between pain associated with neurological damage (neuropathic pain), musculoskeletal perturbations (nociceptive pain) and visceral pain having components of both (Woolf & Mannion, 1999).

The distinction between those whose symptoms are attributed to physiological in contrast to psychological factors (psychogenic) has a long history. Sub-groups of patients based on type of onset, for example, traumatic versus idiopathic have also been discussed (Turk et al., 1996).

The ways of classifying subtypes of pain and pain sufferers are important because they illustrate the differential contributions of affective, cognitive and behavioural, as well as sensory factors. The transient pain associated with a time-limited procedure (e.g. needle injection) is not likely to generate the same degree of emotional arousal as pain such as the chronic pain associated with cancer. Patients with acute pain may be aware of the cause of the pain and expect resolution in a known timeframe; whereas for patients with chronic back pain, the cause may be unknown, the time course is indefinite and treatments are inadequate. Interpretations of the meaning of the pain and expectancies for the future will influence behavioural responses; and it has been shown to influence physiology associated with the transduction of sensory information which is interpreted as pain (e.g. Flor et al., 1985) as well as neurotransmitters (Bandura et al., 1987).

Focus on chronic pain

For the person experiencing chronic pain, there is a continuing quest for relief that often remains elusive, leading to feelings of helplessness, hopelessness and depression. Significant others share the frustration as pain persists in their loved one with no end in sight. Healthcare providers share these feelings of frustration as patients' reports of pain continue despite the provider's best efforts. On a societal level, pain creates a significant burden in lost productivity and disability benefits. Third-party payers are confronted with escalating medical and disability costs and experience irritation when patients remain disabled despite extensive and

Table 1. Pain: magnitude of the problem

Prevalence of chronic pain

- Almost 1 in 5 adult Americans (30 million) experience chronic pain (Joranson & Lietman, 1994)
- Thirty-one million Americans have low back pain at any given time (Jensen et al., 1994)
- Over 11 million American suffer from recurring episodes of migraine headaches (Stewart et al., 1991)
- One in four Americans (23%) experience joint pain daily or every few days (Arthritis Foundation, 2002)
- 46% of women and 37% of men experience pain daily (Arthritis Foundation, 2002)
- Back pain ranks 6th among all reasons for office-based physician visits, accounting to 17.4 million visits (23% of all visits) per year (Cherry et al., 2001)
- Approximately 23 million Americans suffer from CLBP (Latham & Davis, 1994), and it is responsible for 40% of all visits to orthopaedists and neurosurgeons (Cavanaugh & Weinstein, 1994)

Costs of chronic pain

- Annual direct costs associated with migraine in the US have been estimated at $1 billion, while indirect costs amount to $13 billion (1993 prices) (Hu et al., 1999)
- Patients with rheumatoid arthritis are estimated to incur over $14 billion (2000 prices) in medical expenditures and work loss (Lubeck, 2001)
- The costs of low back pain are estimated to be $50 billion yearly (Back Pain Patient Outcomes Assessment Team, 1994)
- Costs attributed to chronic pain (e.g. treatment, lost work days) are $215 billion per year in the United States (American Academy of Orthopaedic Surgeons, 1999)

Workdays lost due to chronic pain

- Clinic-based patients with migraine lose 19.5 workday equivalents per year (Gerth et al., 2001)
- Among US workers, everyday pain accounts for 50 million sick days per year (Louis Harris and Associates, 1996)
- More than 1 million Americans were out of work in 1999 because of musculoskeletal pain (National Research Council, 2001)

expensive treatment and rehabilitation efforts. In short, pain is a major health problem in society that affects millions of people and costs billions of dollars (Table 1).

With such astronomical figures, it is easy to lose sight of the incalculable human suffering accompanying chronic pain for both pain sufferers. The emotional distress that is prevalent may be attributed to a variety of factors, including inadequate or maladaptive coping resources; iatrogenic complications; overuse of medication; disability; financial difficulties; litigation; disruption of usual activities; inadequate social support and sleep disturbance. Moreover, the experience of 'medical limbo' – that is the presence of a painful condition which eludes diagnosis and which carries the implication of either psychiatric causation or malingering, on the one hand, or an undiagnosed life-threatening disease on the other – is in itself the source of significant stress which can initiate, exacerbate and maintain emotional distress.

In sum, chronic pain is a demoralizing situation that confronts the person not only with the stress created by pain but with a cascade of ongoing stressors that compromise all aspects of the life of the sufferer. Living with chronic pain requires considerable emotional resilience, tends to deplete emotional reserves and taxes not only the pain sufferer but also the capacity of significant others to provide support (see 'Coping with chronic pain').

Alternative conceptualizations

In order to understand the basis for the current treatment of pain, it is useful to consider several alternative conceptualizations. These can be loosely grouped into single factor models that focus on a particular cause of the symptoms (i.e. the biomedical, psychogenic, motivational and behavioural models) and multidimensional models that emphasize the contributions of a range of factors that influence patients' experiences and reports of pain (i.e. Gate Control Theory and the biopsychosocial model).

Biomedical model

The biomedical (sensory) conceptualization of pain dates back thousands of years and is based on a simple linear view that predicated on a close correspondence between a biological state and symptom perception. From this perspective, the extent of pain severity is presumed to be proportionate to the amount of tissue damage. As a consequence, treatment consists of eliminating the physical cause of the patient's pain or disrupting the putative pain pathways.

There are several perplexing features of persistent pain that do not fit cleanly within the biomedical model. A particular conundrum is the fact that pain may be reported even in the absence of identified physical pathology, such as is the case of back pain. Conversely up to 35% of people with observed pathological processes remain asymptomatic (e.g. Jensen et al., 1994). It has been suggested that the presence of pain may alter the peripheral and central nervous systems such that they become hypersensitive to normally non-noxious stimuli or it may lower the threshold for noxious stimuli to be perceived as painful (Woolf & Mannion, 1999). Methods for detecting the underlying mechanisms involved in humans are not well established and the postulated changes in the nervous system remain to be demonstrated (Terman & Bonica, 2001).

Psychogenic model

As is frequently the case in medicine, when physical explanations prove inadequate, psychological alternatives are imputed. If the pain reported is 'disproportionate' objective physical pathology or if the complaint is recalcitrant to 'appropriate' treatment, then it is assumed that psychological factors must be involved. Several variants of psychogenic aetiologic models have been proposed. For example, a postulate of a 'pain-prone' personality (Engel, 1959) suggests that persistent complaints occur in people who are predisposed to experience pain due to maladaptive child-rearing practices, physical or sexual abuse and longstanding personality characteristics.

Based on the psychogenic perspective, assessment of chronic pain patients is directed towards identifying the psychopathological tendencies that instigate and maintain pain. Treatment is geared towards helping patients achieve 'insight' into the psychological contributors (e.g. Basler et al., 2002). Empirical evidence to support this model is scarce. In fact, evidence suggests although emotional distress is prevalent in chronic pain patients (M. Sullivan &

Turk, 2001), the emotional distress observed more typically occurs in response to pain and not as a causal agent (e.g. Fishbain et al., 1997) and may resolve once pain is adequately treated (Wallis et al., 1997). Furthermore, there is no evidence demonstrating that insight-oriented psychotherapy successfully reduces symptoms for the majority of patients with chronic pain. The psychogenic model is silent on the observation that a substantial majority of people who have been exposed to potentially destructive and traumatic childhood experiences never develop chronic pain syndromes.

Motivational model

The motivational perspective, ascribed to by many third-party payers, suggests that a pain complaint in the absence of physical pathology indicates that the patient is intentionally seeking secondary gains (malingering, exaggerating) such as attention or financial compensation (Fishbain, 1994). In this case, treatment consists of denial of disability payments that is believed to resolve symptom complaints. There is scant evidence, however, to support this claim (Mendelson, 1982).

Classical (respondent) conditioning

In the classical or 'respondent conditioning' model, if a painful stimulus is repeatedly paired with a neutral stimulus, the neutral stimulus will come to elicit a pain response. For example, a patient who received a painful treatment from a physical therapist (PT) may become conditioned to experience a negative emotional response to the presence of the PT and to any stimulus associated with painful stimuli. The negative emotional reaction may instigate muscle tensing, thereby exacerbating pain, and further reinforcing the association between the PT and pain. Fear of movement has been reported to be more disabling than the pain itself (Crombez et al., 1999).

Treatment based on this model consists of repeatedly engaging in behaviour (e.g. exposure) that produces progressively less pain than was predicted (corrective feedback), which is then followed by reductions in anticipatory fear and anxiety associated with the activity (i.e. desensitization) (Vlaeyen et al., 1995). In this way, patients progressively increase their activity, despite fear of injury and discomfort associated with the use of deconditioned muscles.

Operant conditioning

The operant conditioning model (Fordyce, 1976) proposes that when an individual is exposed to a stimulus that causes tissue damage, the immediate response is withdrawal and attempts to escape. This may be accomplished by observable behaviours such as avoidance of activity believed to cause or exacerbate pain, help-seeking and so forth. The operant model does not concern itself with the initial cause of pain. Rather, it considers pain an subjective experience that may be maintained even after the physical cause of pain has resolved. The operant model focuses on expressions of pain ('pain behaviours' – e.g. limping).

According to the operant model, positive reinforcement (e.g. attention from others, avoidance of undesirable or feared activities) may maintain the pain behaviours even in the absence of nociception itself. In this way, respondent behaviours that occur following an acute injury may be maintained by reinforcement.

The behavioural principle of stimulus generalization is also important as patients may come to avoid more and more activities that they believe are similar to those that previously evoked pain. Reduction of activity leads to greater physical deconditioning, to more activities eliciting pain and consequently to greater disability. Moreover, it is likely that the deconditioning resulting from reinforced **in**activity can result directly in increased noxious sensory input. Muscles that were involved in the original injury generally heal rapidly but due to under-use of these muscles, they become weakened and subject to noxious stimulation when called into action. Studies have provided evidence that supports the underlying assumptions of the operant model (e.g. Keefe *et al.*, 1992). The operant model has, however, been criticized as inadequate (e.g. Schmidt *et al.*, 1989).

A fundamental problem with the operant approach in practice is the emphasis on pain behaviour rather than pain per se because observed behaviours are then used as the basis to infer something about the internal state of the individual – that the behaviours are communications of pain (Turk & Matyas, 1992). In this case, however, there is no way of determining whether the behaviour results from pain or from a structural abnormality. Limping, for example, from the operant perspective, is viewed as a pain behaviour; however, this is an inference. It is possible that limping is the result of physical pathology and has no direct association with pain. (See also 'Behaviour therapy'.)

Social learning model

According to the social learning model, the acquisition of pain behaviours occurs through observational learning. Children, for example, learn how others respond to pain. Based on these 'models', they may be more or less likely to ignore or over-respond to symptoms they experience (Craig, 1986). Expectancies and actual behavioural responses to painful stimulation are based, at least partially, on prior social learning history. Even physiological responses may be conditioned during observation of others in pain (Vaughan & Lanzetta, 1980).

Incompleteness of common models

The models briefly described are not wrong; rather they are incomplete. The inadequacies of these models have initiated attempts to reformulate thinking about pain. Healthcare providers, lay people and third-party payers have long considered pain as being synonymous with physical pathology. It is important, however, to make a distinction between nociception, pain and suffering.

'Nociception' refers to the peripheral sensory stimulation in nerves that conveys information about tissue damage. This information is capable of being perceived as pain. 'Pain', because it involves conscious awareness, selective abstraction, appraisal, ascribed meaning and experience, is best viewed as a perceptual process. 'Suffering' includes interpersonal disruption, psychological distress and a myriad of other factors associated with perception of the impact of pain on one's life and future (Turk & Fernandez, 1997). From this description, it should be apparent that there is no direct link between nociception, pain and suffering. Rather, the extent of pain and suffering is associated with an interpretive process.

The variability of people's responses to nociceptive stimuli and treatment is more understandable when we consider that pain is a personal experience influenced by attention, anxiety, prior learning history, the meaning and other physiological and environmental factors, as well as physical pathology (Turk & Monarch, 2002). Biomedical factors, in the majority of cases, appear to instigate the initial report of pain. Over time, however, psychosocial and behavioural factors may serve to maintain and exacerbate levels of pain, and influence adjustment and disability. Following on from this view, pain that persists over time should not be viewed as either solely physical or psychological; rather, the experience of pain is maintained by an interdependent set of biomedical, psychosocial and behavioural factors.

Gate control model

The gate control model contradicts the notion that pain is either somatic or psychogenic, rather it postulates that both factors have potentiating and moderating effects. Melzack and his colleagues (Melzack & Casey, 1968; Melzack & Wall, 1965) emphasize the modulation of pain by peripheral and central nervous system processes. Prior to this formulation, psychological processes were largely dismissed as reactions to pain. Melzack and Casey (1968) differentiated three systems related to the processing of nociceptive stimulation –motivational–affective, cognitive–evaluative and sensory–discriminative – all thought to contribute to the subjective experience of pain.

After the gate control model was first described in 1965, no one could try to explain pain exclusively in terms of peripheral factors. However, the physiological details of the gate control model have been challenged (e.g. Price, 1987). Nevertheless, it has had a substantial impact on basic research and in generating treatment modalities.

Biopsychosocial model

Although the gate control model introduced the role of psychological factors in the maintenance of pain symptoms, it focused primarily on neurophysiology. The biopsychosocial model, by extension, adds in cognitive, affective and behavioural components of pain and it views illness as a dynamic and reciprocal interaction between biological, psychological and sociocultural variables which shape the person's response to pain (Turk & Monarch, 2002).

The biopsychosocial model is unique, in that it takes into consideration the influence of higher order cognitions. It accepts that people are active processors of information, and that behaviour, emotions, and even physiology are influenced by interpretations of events, rather than solely by physiological factors. People with chronic pain may therefore have negative expectations about their own ability and responsibility to exert any control over their pain. Moreover, pain sufferers' behaviours elicit responses from significant others that can reinforce both adaptive and maladaptive modes of thinking, feeling and behaving.

The biopsychosocial model has led to the development of treatment interventions based on a cognitive–behavioural perspective (Turk, 2002b). According to this perspective, patient's attitudes, beliefs and unique schema filter and interact reciprocally with emotional factors, sensory phenomenon and behavioural responses. Moreover, patients' behaviours elicit responses from significant others that can reinforce both adaptive and maladaptive modes of thinking, feeling and behaving.

Similar to the operant model of chronic pain, the most important focus of the cognitive-behavioural perspective is on the pain sufferer, rather than on only symptoms or pathophysiology. Unlike the operant model, however, the cognitive–behavioural perspective places a great deal of emphasis on people's idiosyncratic beliefs, appraisals and coping repertoires, as well as sensory, affective and behavioural contributions, in the formation of pain perceptions.

For chronic pain sufferers, certain ways of thinking and coping are believed to influence the perception of nociception, the distress associated with it, or factors that may increase nociception directly. Pain that is interpreted as signifying ongoing tissue damage or life-threatening illness is likely to produce considerably more suffering and behavioural dysfunction than pain that is viewed as being the result of a minor injury, although the amount of nociceptive input in the two cases may be equivalent.

In addition to triggering or aggravating nociception directly, psychological factors also have indirect effects on pain and disability. Chronic pain sufferers can develop ways of thinking and coping that in the short-term seem adaptive, but in the long-term serve to maintain the chronic pain condition and result in greater disability. As noted, because the fear of pain is aversive, the anticipation of pain is a strong motivator for avoidance of situations or behaviours that are expected to produce nociception. Moreover, the belief that pain signals harm further reinforces avoidance of activities believed to cause pain and increase physical damage. Through the process of stimulus generalization, more and more activities are avoided to prevent exacerbation of pain. The undesirable result of this avoidance is greater physical deconditioning and increased disability.

Inactivity may also lead to preoccupation with the body and pain and these attentional changes increase the likelihood of amplifying and distorting pain symptoms and perceiving oneself as being disabled. At the same time, the pain sufferer limits opportunities to identify activities that build flexibility, endurance and strength without the risk of pain or injury. Moreover, distorted movements and postures used to avoid pain can cause further pain unrelated to the initial injury. Avoidance of activity, although it is a seemingly rational way to manage a pain problem, can play a role in facilitating nociception and disability when maintained for extended periods (Vlaeyen et al., 1995).

When chronic pain sufferers develop negative expectations about their own ability to exert control over their pain, these expectations instantiate feelings of distress when 'uncontrollable' pain interferes with participation in activities. Pain sufferers frequently terminate efforts to develop new strategies to manage pain and instead turn to passive coping strategies such as inactivity and self-medication to reduce emotional distress and pain. They also absolve themselves of personal responsibility for managing their pain and instead rely on significant others including healthcare providers. Those who feel little personal control over their pain are also likely to 'catastrophize' about the impact of pain-flare episodes and situations that might initiate or exacerbate pain. Catastrophizing includes over-evaluating

Table 2. Characteristics of treatments based on the Cognitive–Behavioural perspective

- Problem-oriented
- Behaviourally focused
- Time-limited
- Educational
- Collaborative (patient and health care provider work together)
- Make use of in-clinic and home practice to identify problems and consolidate skills
- Emphasize maintenance and generalization

and over-reacting in a negative, maladaptive manner, as if even relatively small problems were major catastrophes (Sullivan et al., 2001). Catastrophizing has been related to greater pain, disability and emotional distress independent of physical pathology (Severeijns et al., 2001).

Thus, pain sufferers often develop negative, maladaptive appraisals about their condition and personal efficacy in controlling their pain. Problems associated with pain reinforce their experience of distress, inactivity and over-reaction to nociceptive stimulation. In contrast, persons who believe that they are able to control the situations that contribute to pain flare-ups are more resourceful and are more likely to develop strategies (the self-management strategies described below) that are effective in limiting the impact of painful episodes and thus are able to reduce the impact of the pain problem.

To summarize, the cognitive–behavioural perspective takes a broad view of pain that focuses on the person and not just the symptom. Persistent pain, like any chronic disease, extends over time and affects all domains of the person's life. Rather than focusing on cognitive and affective contributions to the perception of pain in a static fashion, as in the gate control model, or exclusively on behavioural responses and physical pathology as the sensory and operant conceptualizations, respectively, do, the cognitive–behavioural conceptualization posits the interaction of ongoing physical, cognitive, affective and behavioural factors (Turk, 2002b).

The cognitive–behavioural perspective offers a heuristic way of thinking about people who suffer from chronic pain. There has been a growing body of evidence supporting the efficacy of treatment based on the cognitive–behavioural perspective for diverse chronic pain syndromes (Morley et al., 1999); however, there is wide diversity of the specific techniques incorporated with treatment. Table 2 lists features that appear to be consistent across the different treatment protocols that can be ascribed to the cognitive–behavioural perspective and Table 3 the targets of intervention (Turk, 2002b). The methods used to accomplish these vary. (See also 'Cognitive behavioural therapy' and 'Pain management'.)

Summary and concluding comments

The unidimensional models of pain that focus on only one aspect of pain, whether it be sensory, affective or behavioural, seem inadequate to explain such a complex phenomenon. More recently

Table 3. Targets of Cognitive-Behavioural treatment

- Reconceputalization of patients' views of their problems (pain and others) from overwhelming to manageable (Combat demoralization)
- Convince patients that the skills necessary for responding to problems more adaptively will be included in the treatment (Enhance motivation and outcome efficacy)
- Change patients views of themselves from passive, reactive, and helpless to active, resourceful, and in control (Foster self-efficacy)
- Ensure that patients learn how to monitor their thoughts, feelings, behaviour, and physiological reactivity and learn the interrelationships among these (Break-up maladaptive patterns)
- Teach patients how to and when to use necessary overt and covert behaviours required for more adaptive responding (Skills training)
- Encourage patients to attribute success to their own efforts
- Anticipate problems and discuss these and ways to cope with them (Facilitate maintenance and generalization)

---

attempts to integrate the range of medical–physical, psychosocial and behavioural factors within a broad multidimensional framework

have been made and a body of research appears to support the appropriateness of these conceptual models, at least in chronic pain.

Patients all come to treatment with diverse sets of attitudes, beliefs and expectancies. Research suggests that the importance of addressing these subjective factors is likely to influence how patients present themselves and respond to treatments offered. Viewing all patients with the same medical diagnosis as similar is likely to prove unsatisfactory. It would seem prudent to (1) attempt to identify pain patients' idiosyncratic beliefs, (2) identify the environmental contingencies of reinforcement, (3) address those beliefs and environmental relationships that are maladaptive, and (4) match treatment interventions both to physical characteristics of the diagnosis and also to relevant psychosocial and behavioural ones (Turk, 1990).

(See also 'Coping with chronic pain', 'Pain assessment', 'Pain management', 'Amputation and phantom limb pain', 'Back pain', 'Non-cardiac chest pain', and 'Pelvic pain').

REFERENCES

American Academy of Orthopaedic Surgeons (1999). Musculoskeletal conditions in the United States. *American Academy of Orthopaedic Surgeons Bulletin,* **27**, 34–6.

Arthritis Foundation (2002). Pain factsheet: speaking of pain – how to talk to your doctor about pain. Retrieved July 19, 2004 from http://www.arthritis.org/conditions/speakingofpain/factsheet.asp.

Back Pain Patient Outcomes Assessment Team (BOAT). (1994). In MEDTEP Update, *Vol. 1 Issue 1.* Rockville, MD: Agency for Health Care Policy and Research.

Bandura, A., O'Leary, A., Taylor, C. B., Gauthier, J. & Gossard, D. (1987). Perceived self-efficacy and pain control: opioid and nonopioid mechanisms. *Journal of Personality and Social Psychology,* **53**, 563–71.

Basler, S. C., Grzesiak, R. C. & Dworkin, R. H. (2002). Integrating relational psychodynamic and action-oriented psychotherapies: treating pain and suffering. In D. C. Turk, & R. J. Gatchel, (Eds.). *Psychological approaches to pain management: a practitioner's handbook* (pp. 94–127). New York: Guilford Press.

Cavanaugh, J. M. & Weinstein, J. N. (1994). Low back pain: epidemiology, anatomy, and neurophysiology. In P. D. Wall & R. Melzack (Eds.). *Textbook of Pain* (3rd edn.) (pp. 441–56). New York: Churchill Livingstone.

Cherry, D., Burt, C. & Woodwell, D. (2001). National ambulatory medical care survey: 1999 summary. *Division of Healthcare Statistics,* **204**, 322.

Craig, K. D. (1986). Social modeling influences: pain in context. In R. A.

Sternbach (Ed.). *The Psychology of Pain* (2nd edn.) (pp. 67–95). New York: Raven Press.

Crombez, G., Vlaeyen, J. W. S., Heuts, Ph. H. & Lystens, R. (1999). Pain-related fear is more disabling than pain itself: evidence on the role of pain-related fear in chronic back pain disability. *Pain,* **80**, 329–39.

Engel, G. L. (1959). 'Psychogenic' pain and the pain-prone patient. *American Journal of Medicine,* **26**, 899–918.

Fishbain, D. A. (1994). Secondary gain concept: definition problems and its use in medical practice. *American Pain Society Journal,* **3**, 264–73.

Fishbain, D. A., Cutler, R., Rosomoff, H. L. & Steele-Rosomoff. (1997). Chronic pain-associated depression: antecedent or consequence of chronic pain? A review. *Clinical Journal of Pain,* **13**, 116–37.

Flor, H., Turk, D. C. & Birbaumer, N. (1985). Assessment of stress-related psychophysiological responses in chronic pain patients. *Journal of Consulting and Clinical Psychology,* **35**, 354–64.

Fordyce, W. E. (1976). *Behavioral methods for chronic pain and illness.* St Louis: C.V. Mosby.

Gerth, W. C., Carides, G. W., Dasbach, E. J., Visser, W. H. & Santanello, N. C. (2001). The multinational impact of migraine symptoms on healthcare utilization and work loss. *Pharmacoeconomics,* **19**, 197–206.

Hu, X. H., Markson, L. E., Lipton, R. B., Stewart, W. F. & Berger, M. L. (1999). Burden of migraine in the United States: disability and economic costs. *Archives of Internal Medicine,* **159**, 813–18.

Jensen, M., Brant-Zawadzki, M., Obuchowski, N., Modic, M. T., Malkasian, D. & Ross, J. S. (1994). Magnetic resonance imaging of the lumbar spine in people without back pain. *The New England Journal of Medicine,* **331**, 69–73.

Joranson, D. E. & Lietman, R. (1994). *The McNeil national pain study.* New York: Louis Harris and Associates.

Keefe, F. J., Dunsmore, J. & Burnett, R. (1992). Behavioral and cognitive–behavioral approaches to chronic pain: recent advances and future directions. *Journal of Consulting and Clinical Psychology,* **60**, 528–36.

Latham, J. & Davis, B. D. (1994). The socioeconomic impact of chronic pain. *Disability and Rehabilitation,* **16**, 39–44.

Louis Harris and Associates (1996). *Pain and absenteeism report.* Retrieved August, 2, 2002 from http://208.153.7.104/resources/reports/related_news_0301.html.

Lubeck, P. A. (2001). Review of the direct costs of rheumatoid arthritis. *Pharmacoeconomics,* **19**, 811–18.

Melzack, R. & Casey, K.L. (1968). Sensory, motivational and central control determinants of pain: a new conceptual model. In D. Kenshalo (Ed.). *The skin senses* (pp. 423–43). Springfield, IL: Thomas.

Melzack, R. & Wall, P. D. (1965). Pain mechanisms: a new theory. *Science,* **50**, 971–9.

Mendelson, G. (1982). Not 'cured by a verdict.' *Medical Journal of Australia,* **2**, 132–4.

Morley, S., Eccleston, C. & Williams, A. (1999). Systematic review and meta-analysis of randomized controlled trials of cognitive–behavioural therapy and behavior therapy for chronic pain in adults, excluding headache. *Pain,* **80**, 1–13.

National Research Council (2001). *Musculoskeletal disorders and the workplace.* Washington, DC: National Academy Press.

Price, D. D. (1987). *Psychological and neural mechanisms of pain.* New York: Raven Press.

Schmidt, A. J. M., Gierlings, R. E. H. & Peters, M. L. (1989). Environment and interoceptive influences on chronic low back pain behavior. *Pain,* **38**, 137–43.

Severeijns, R., Vlaeyen, J. W. S., van den Hout, M. A. & Weber, W. E. J. (2001). Pain catastrophizing predicts pain intensity, disability, and psychological distress independent of level of physical impairment. *Clinical Journal of Pain,* **17**, 165–72.

Stewart, W. F., Lipton, R. B., Celentano, D. D. & Reed, M. L. (1991). Prevalence of migraine headache in the United States. Relation to age, income, race, and other sociodemographic factors. *Journal of the American Medical Association,* **267**, 64–9.

Sullivan, M. D. & Turk, D. C. (2001). Psychiatric illness, depression, and psychogenic pain. In J. D. Loeser, S. D. Butler, C. R. Chapman & D. C. Turk, (Eds.). *Bonica's Management of Pain* (3rd edn.) (pp. 483–500). Philadelphia: Lippincott, Williams, & Wilkins.

Sullivan, M. J. L., Thorn, B., Haythornthwaite, J. A. *et al.* (2001). Theoretical perspectives on the relation between catastrophizing and pain. *Clinical Journal of Pain,* **17**, 52–64.

Terman, G. W. & Bonica, J. J. (2001). Spinal mechanisms and their modulation. In J. D. Loeser, S. D. Butler, C. R. Chapman & D. C. Turk (Eds.) *Bonica's Management of Pain* (3rd edn.) (pp. 73–152). Philadelphia: Lippincott Williams & Wilkins.

Turk, D. C. (1990). Customizing treatment for chronic pain patients: who, what and why. *Clinical Journal of Pain,* **6**, 225–70.

Turk, D. C. (2002*a*). Clinical effectiveness and cost effectiveness of treatments for chronic pain patients. *Clinical Journal of Pain,* **18**, 355–65.

Turk, D. C. (2002*b*). A Cognitive-Behavioral perspective on treatment of chronic pain patients. In: D. C. Turk & R. J. Gatchel (Eds.). *Psychological approaches to pain management* (pp. 138–58). New York: The Guilford Press.

Turk, D. C. & Fernandez, E. (1990). On the putative uniqueness of cancer pain: do psychological principles apply? *Behavior Research and Therapy,* **28**, 1–13.

Turk, D. C. & Fernandez, E. (1997). Cognitive–behavioral management strategies for pain and suffering. *Current Review of Pain,* **1**, 99–106.

Turk, D. C. & Matyas, T. A. (1992). Pain-related behaviors > communications of pain. *American Pain Society Journal,* **1**, 109–111.

Turk, D. C. & Monarch, E. S. (2002). Biopsychosocial perspective on chronic pain. In D. C. Turk & R. J. Gatchel (Eds.). *Psychological approaches to pain management: a practitioner's handbook* (pp. 3–29). New York: Guilford Press.

Turk, D. C. & Okifuji, A. (2001). Pain terms and taxonomies of pain. In J. D. Loeser, S. D. Butler, C. R. Chapman & D. C. Turk (Eds.). *Bonica's Management of Pain* (3rd edn.) (pp. 17–25). Philadelphia: Lippincott Williams & Wilkins.

Turk, D. C., Okifuji, A., Starz, T. W. & Sinclair, J. D. (1996). Effects of type of symptom onset on psychological distress and disability in fibromyalgia syndrome patients. *Pain,* **68**, 423–30.

Vaughan, K. B. & Lanzetta, J. T. (1980). Vicarious instigation and conditioning of facial expressive and autonomic responses to a model's expressive display of pain. *Journal of Personality and Social Psychology,* **38**, 909–23.

Vlaeyen, J. W., Kole-Snijders, A. M., Boeren, R. B. & van Eck, H. (1995). Fear of movement/(re)injury in chronic low back pain and its relation to behavioral performance. *Pain,* **62**, 363–72.

Wallis, B. J., Lord, S. M. & Bogduk, N. (1997). Resolution of psychological distress of whiplash patients following treatment by radiofrequency neurotomy: a randomised, double-blind, placebo-controlled trial. *Pain,* **73**, 15–22.

Woolf, C. J. & Mannion, R. J. (1999). Neuropathic pain: aetiology, symptoms, mechanisms, and management. *Lancet,* **353**, 1959–64.

Perceived control

Kenneth A. Wallston

Vanderbilt University Medical Center

Perceived control (also referred to as an internal locus of control orientation, perceived personal control, perceived competence, self-efficacy or a sense of mastery) has been defined as the belief that one can determine one's own internal states and behaviour, influence one's environment and/or bring about desired outcomes (Wallston, Wallston, Smith & Dobbins, 1987). If people say that things are under their control, they are saying that they are able to determine or influence important events or situations (Walker, 2001), including their own actions or those of other people.

Perceived control has long been 'recognized as a central concept in the understanding of the relationships between stressful experience, behaviours and health. Experimental investigations indicate that control over aversive stimulation has profound effects on autonomic, endocrine and immunological responses, and may influence the pathological processes implicated in the development of cardiovascular disease, tumour rejection and proliferation, and the acquisition of gastrointestinal lesions' (Steptoe & Appels, 1989).

It is critical to understand the distinction between actual control – the objective responsiveness of an event to influence by human or other factors – and perceived control which might bear little correspondence to reality. The mental and physical health benefits which have been associated with control have been related more to the subjective perception that control exists than to the objective determination of that control. A person's wellbeing is a function of the degree to which they feel in control, not how much they are in control. Actual (or veridical) control may be sufficient to lead to a perception of control, but it is not necessary. Perceived control in the absence of actual control has been termed 'illusory' control (Glass & Singer, 1972; Taylor & Brown, 1988; Taylor, 1989): it is the perception (or illusion) of control that mediates the health effects, not the actual control itself.

Primary and secondary control

Rothbaum, Weisz & Snyder (1982) distinguished between two types of control. In primary control, individuals directly influence their outcomes by acting upon the environment or situation to make it conform to their individual needs. In secondary control, individuals change themselves to better conform to the situation in order to compensate for the inability to engage in primary control. According to Rothbaum *et al.* (1982), there are many sub-types of secondary control:

- predictive control – adjusting one's expectancies based on knowledge of what will occur
- illusory control – taking credit for the control even when it is not there

- vicarious control – aligning oneself with powerful other entities who exercise control
- interpretive control – deriving meaning from otherwise uncontrollable situations.

Heckhausen & Schulz (1995) built their lifespan theory of control upon the typology of primary versus secondary control, but added two other dimensions: functional versus dysfunctional and veridical versus illusory. In their view, primary control has functional primacy over secondary control. They argue that the major function of secondary control is to minimize losses in, maintain and expand existing levels of primary control. At each period of the life course, individuals experience different opportunities and constraints leading to shifts and trade-offs between primary and secondary control strategies.

The distinction between primary and secondary control nicely matches Lazarus and Folkman's (1984) distinction between problem-focused and emotion-focused coping. Compas and his colleagues have taken this one step further by distinguishing between primary control coping and secondary control coping, both of which lead to better outcomes than disengagement coping (see Connor-Smith & Compas, 2004). One function of coping, whether by acting directly on the environment or on one's own reactions to events, is to maintain or regain a sense of control. There is a reciprocal causal relationship between perceived control and coping behaviours; a sense of control leads to effective coping behaviours (and, thus, to the outcomes of those behaviours). At the same time, engaging in effective coping behaviours increases one's sense of control.

Locus of control and related constructs

One conceptualization which has received a great deal of attention in the perceived control literature is 'locus of control' (Rotter, 1966). 'Locus' refers to the place (or origin) of the control. When using this conceptualization, the target of control (Wallston *et al.*, 1987) is one's outcomes (or reinforcements). An internal locus of control orientation is where one believes one's outcomes (or reinforcements) are controlled by one's own actions or one's enduring characteristics, such as one's personality. When people believe their outcomes (or reinforcements) are determined by the actions of other people, they have an external locus of control orientation. The belief that outcomes/reinforcements are determined by fate, luck, chance or other random events has also been classified as an external locus of control orientation.

A related, but different, perceived control construct is 'self-efficacy' (Bandura, 1977, 1997). As originally set forth by Bandura, self-efficacy is the belief that one 'can do' a particular behaviour in a particular situation. It is possible to believe that one's actions are responsible for one's outcomes – an internal locus of control – without believing that one can act in such a manner as to optimize one's outcomes. Bandura originally intended self-efficacy to be both behaviour-specific and situation-specific, but others have broadened the construct to make it generalizable to many behaviours in many situations. This broadened construct has been termed generalized self-efficacy (Schwarzer, 1992), mastery (Pearlin & Schooler, 1978) or perceived competence (Wallston, 2001a;b). The lack of perceived control has been termed helplessness (Seligman, 1975). By whatever name it is called, the belief that one is capable of taking effective action increases the likelihood that the action will occur (see also 'Self-efficacy and health behaviour').

Perceived control of one's health

When the outcome in question is health or health status, perceptions of control are either referred to as perceived health competence (Smith *et al.*, 1995) or health locus of control (see Wallston, 2001a;b; 2004). Perceived health competence is positively related to internal health locus of control (Smith *et al.*, 1995), but the correlation is only moderately positive indicating that the two constructs are differentiated. Perceived health competence is unidimensional: the more competent one feels, the greater the perceived control of one's health and the more positive the health outcomes (Smith *et al.*, 1995). Health locus of control, on the other hand, is multidimensional (Wallston *et al.*, 1978): an internal health locus of control orientation is usually orthogonal to (i.e. independent of) an external health locus of control orientation, especially powerful others' externality. It is possible to believe that control of one's health is simultaneously due to one's own actions as well as to the actions of other people, such as family members, friends or healthcare providers. It is even possible to hold those beliefs alongside the belief that one's health is due to fate, luck or chance. Thus, the relationship of health locus of control beliefs to perceived control of one's health is complex, as is the relationship of health locus of control beliefs to outcomes.

Measurement of control beliefs relevant to health

Forms A and B of the Multidimensional Health Locus of Control (MHLC) scales (Wallston *et al.*, 1978) consist of three, 6-item, Likert scales assessing one internal and two external HLC belief dimensions (powerful others and chance). These original MHLC scales were designed to assess locus of control beliefs about one's health in general. The two forms, A and B, were meant to be 'equivalent', although, over the years, Form A was more likely to be used with 'healthy' respondents, while Form B was more likely to be administered to patients. Form C of the MHLC (Wallston *et al.*, 1994) also consists of 18 items, but was designed to be made condition-specific. Thus, by substituting for the word 'condition' in each item, Form C can be turned into a measure of one's locus of control beliefs regarding any given medical condition (such as diabetes, arthritis, cancer, HIV infection, etc.). With Form C, the powerful others external dimension is split

into two independent dimensions: doctors and other people. More recently, Wallston and his colleagues (Wallston *et al.*, 1999) developed the God Locus of Health Control (GLHC) subscale to assess a different external dimension – the belief that one's health is controlled by God or a higher power. The 6-item GLHC subscale can either be administered by itself or can be integrated into the existing MHLC scales.

Derived from the generalization of Bandura's construct of self-efficacy, the Perceived Health Competence Scale (PHCS; Smith *et al.*, 1995) is an 8-item assessment of an individual's belief that he or she can do whatever is necessary to bring about good health. There are many other measures of control-related beliefs other than the MHLC and PHC scales including a number of disease-specific locus of control and behaviour-specific self-efficacy measures (see Wallston, 1989; 2001a;b; 2004; Walker, 2001). There are even disease-specific self-efficacy measures such as the arthritis self-efficacy scales (Lorig *et al.*, 1989).

A unifying theory of control

Jan Walker (2001) has recently developed a theory of control, based on her research and clinical experience with chronic pain patients, which unifies a number of control-related constructs and findings. Among the propositions in Walker's theory are the following:

- control (i.e. the attainment of desired outcomes in a given situation) may be achieved through the actions of self or other
- perceived control is influenced by past history of control and lack of control
- perceived control is associated with confidence and optimism
- external control (by others) is a type of instrumental social support
- instrumental support is maladaptive if it usurps personal control and leads to dependence
- emotional and informational support enhance a sense of control
- perceived personal control and perceived social support should be viewed as complementary variables in relation to control, but personal control is preferable to social support because it is more reliable and sustainable
- perceived certainty and perceived predictability are sufficient but not necessary conditions for perceived controllability
- perceived uncontrollability is associated with fear, anxiety and/or depression
- sense of control may be bolstered by spiritual beliefs (represented by belief in an external source of support)
- positive and negative emotions associated with confidence, optimism, fear, anxiety and depression reflect the degree of perceived control available from any source (self, others or spiritual) at a particular point in time.

Altering perceived control

Most forms of health care, disease prevention and patient education are designed to give patients a greater sense of control over their health (Wallston, 2004). The effectiveness of all forms of coaching and teaching is probably mediated by an increase in control-related beliefs. In helping individuals hone their skills, coaches (and/or teachers and/or healthcare providers) help alter both actual and perceived control which, at least theoretically, leads to better performance and outcomes. Providing patients with greater control over some aspect of their healthcare delivery by giving them increased information about what will happen to them and why (thereby decreasing uncertainty), or giving them choices over some aspects of their care (thereby increasing decisional control), has been shown to lead to lower distress and faster recovery (Wallston, 1989). Shapiro & Austin (1998) developed an integrated approach to psychotherapy, health and healing which they termed 'control therapy'. One outcome of this type of therapy, as well as with a number of cognitive–behavioural therapies, is to increase individuals' sense of control.

REFERENCES

Bandura, A. (1977). Self-efficacy: toward a unifying theory of behaviour change. *Psychological Bulletin*, **84**, 191–215.

Bandura, A. (1997). *Self-efficacy: the exercise of control.* New York: W. H. Freeman.

Connor-Smith, J. K. & Compas, B. E. (2004). Coping as a moderator of relations between reactivity to interpersonal stress, health status, and internalizing problems. *Cognitive Therapy and Research*, **28**, 347–68.

Glass, D. C. & Singer, J. E. (1972). Behavioural aftereffects of unpredictable and uncontrollable aversive events. *American Scientist*, **60**, 457–65.

Heckhausen, J. & Schulz, R. (1995). A life-span theory of control. *Psychological Review*, **102**, 284–304.

Lazarus, R. S. & Folkman, S. (1984). *Stress, appraisal, and coping.* New York: Springer-Verlag.

Lorig, K., Chastain, R., Ung, E., Shoor, S. & Holman, H. (1989). Development and evaluation of a scale to measure the perceived self-efficacy of people with arthritis. *Arthritis and Rheumatism*, **32**, 37–44.

Pearlin, L. I. & Schooler, C. (1978). The structure of coping. *Journal of Health and Social Behaviour*, **19**, 2–21.

Rothbaum, F., Weisz, J. R. & Snyder, S. S. (1982). Changing the world and changing the self: a two-process model of perceived control. *Journal of Personality and Social Psychology*, **42**, 5–37.

Rotter, J. B. (1966). Generalized expectancies for internal vs. external control of reinforcement. *Psychological Monographs: General and Applied*, **80**, 1–28.

Schwarzer, R. (Ed.). (1992). *Self-efficacy: thought control of action.* Washington, DC: Hemisphere.

Seligman, M. E. P. (1975). *Helplessness.* San Francisco: Freeman.

Shapiro, D. H., Jr. & Astin, J. A. (1998). *Control therapy: an integrated approach to psychotherapy, health, and healing.* New York: Wiley.

Sinclair, V. G., Wallston, K. A., Dwyer, K. A., Blackburn, D. S. & Fuchs, H. (1998). Effects of a cognitive–behavioural intervention for women with rheumatoid arthritis. *Research in Nursing and Health*, **21**, 315–26.

Smith, M. S., Wallston, K. A. & Smith, C. A. (1995). The development and validation of the Perceived Health Competence Scale. *Health Education Research: Theory and Practice*, **10**, 51–64.

Stein, M. J., Wallston, K. A. & Nicassio, P. M. (1988). Factor structure of the Arthritis Helplessness Index. *Journal of Rheumatology*, **15**, 427–32.

Steptoe, A. & Appels, A. (Eds.). (1989). *Stress, personal control, and health.* Brussels, Luxembourg: Wiley.

Taylor, S. E. & Brown, J. D. (1988). Illusion and well-being: a social psychological perspective on mental health. *Psychological Bulletin*, **103**, 193–210.

Taylor, S. E. (1989). *Positive illusions: creative self-deception and the healthy mind.* New York: Basic Books.

Walker, J. (2001). *Control and the psychology of health.* Buckingham, UK: Open University Press.

Wallston, K.A. (1989). Assessment of control in health care settings. In A. Steptoe & A. Appel (Eds.). *Stress, personal control and health* (pp. 85–105). Chicester, England: Wiley.

Wallston, K. A. (1992). Hocus-pocus, the focus isn't strictly on locus: Rotter's social learning theory modified for health. *Cognitive Therapy and Research*, **16**, 183–99.

Wallston, K.A. (2001a). Control beliefs. In N. J. Smelser & P. B. Baltes (Eds.). *International encyclopedia of the social and behavioural sciences.* Oxford, England: Elsevier Science.

Wallston, K.A. (2001b). Conceptualization and operationalization of perceived control. In A. Baum, T. Revenson & J. E. Singer (Eds.). *The handbook of health psychology* (pp. 49–58). Mahwah, NJ: Erlbaum.

Wallston, K. A. (2004). Control and health. In N. Anderson (Ed.). *Encyclopedia of health & behaviour, Vol. 1* (pp. 217–9). Thousand Oaks, CA: Sage.

Wallston, K. A., Malcarne, V. L., Flores, L. *et al.* (1999). Does God determine your health? The God Locus of Health Control scale. *Cognitive Therapy and Research*, **23**, 131–42.

Wallston, K. A., Stein, M. J. & Smith, C. A. (1994). Form C of the MHLC Scales: a condition-specific measure of locus of control. *Journal of Personality Assessment*, **63**, 534–53.

Wallston, K. A., Wallston, B. S. & DeVellis, R. (1978). Development of the multidimensional health locus of control (MHLC) scales. *Health Education Monographs*, **6**, 160–70.

Wallston, K. A., Wallston, B. S., Smith, S. & Dobbins, C. J. (1987). Perceived control and health. *Current Psychological Research and Reviews*, **6**, 5–25.

Personality and health

Stephanie V. Stone[1] and Robert R. McCrae[2]

[1]Johns Hopkins University
[2]National Institute of Aging

The ways in which personality and health interact are myriad and complex. Does personality predispose us to certain diseases? Does disease lead to changes in personality? The original formulation of psychosomatic medicine sought a direct link between personality and health – anxiety and hypertension, depression and cancer – and was largely unfruitful. Current research seeks to clarify how personality is associated with health-related behaviours like smoking and exercise, which put people at risk for disease. By elucidating the link between personality and health behaviours, the field makes substantive contributions to both patient treatment and public health prevention and intervention programmes aimed at reducing the incidence and prevalence of disease.

Personality as traits

For most of history, scholars and laypersons alike viewed human beings as rational creatures with propensities, abilities and beliefs that guided their conduct. Early in the twentieth century, this view was supplanted by psychoanalysis and behaviourism which characterized personality in radically different ways: for psychoanalysts, the essence of the person was in unconscious and often irrational processes; for behaviourists, the person was no more than a collection of learned responses to environmental reinforcements. Contemporary research has in turn rejected these two extreme views of personality and returned to a more commonsense approach, in which familiar traits such as persistence and sociability are seen as important determinants of behaviour.

It does not follow, however, that personality psychology is nothing but common sense. It is only common sense to believe that old age leads to depression and social withdrawal, that raising the standard of living will make everyone happier, that parental discipline is the most important determinant of character. But none of these beliefs happens to be true (McCrae & Costa, 2003). In considering the 'commonsense' effects of personality on physical health, a healthy skepticism is sensible.

The remainder of this chapter focuses on current conceptions of individual differences in traits and some of their broad implications for health and medicine. For a discussion of alternative approaches to personality, consult Pervin & John (1999).

The nature of traits

Personality traits can be defined as 'dimensions of individual differences in tendencies to show consistent patterns of thoughts,

feelings, and actions' (McCrae & Costa, 2003, p. 25). One patient, for example, may be friendly and talkative and eager to communicate with the physician, whereas another may be reserved and volunteer little information. These behavioural differences may be due in part to past experience with physicians who encouraged or discouraged a personal relationship. But they are also likely in part to reflect pervasive characteristics of the patient, individual differences in the personality dimension of 'Extraversion'. Extraverts tend to be sociable, energetic and enthusiastic whether they are at home, at work, at a party or in the hospital.

The definition of traits calls attention to several of their important characteristics. First, the word 'dimension' implies a continuous distribution of traits in the population. Although it is convenient to talk about 'introverts' and 'extraverts', in fact most people have an intermediate level of extraversion. All personality traits approximate a normal, bell-shaped distribution. Second, the word 'tendencies' highlights the fact that the influence of traits is probabilistic; even the most well-adjusted person is occasionally anxious or depressed; even the most conscientious person occasionally fails to complete a task. As a consequence, personality traits usually cannot be inferred from a single behaviour or a single interaction: instead, personality assessment requires the search for consistent patterns across many times and situations. Third, personality traits cut across the academic distinctions between cognitive, affective and behavioural domains: they are inferred not merely from overt behaviour, as habits would be, but also from patterns of thoughts and feelings.

The structure of traits

The English language has well over 4000 adjectives to describe personality traits and personality psychologists have developed hundreds of scales to measure traits they consider to be important. For decades, the sheer number of traits made systematic research difficult. If a researcher wished to discover the traits associated with, say, hypertension or arthritis, which should be measured? Short of assessing all 4000, research was bound to be hit-or-miss. When different researchers chose to measure different traits, how could their results be compared?

If all 4000 words referred to completely different traits, there would be no easy solution to those problems. But in fact there is great redundancy among trait terms and formal psychological constructs. The terms 'assertive', 'bossy', 'controlling', 'dominant' and 'exacting' all refer to similar, if not identical, attributes. These similarities can be used to organize a trait taxonomy that reflects the structure of personality.

Table 1. Examples of adjectives and questionnaire scales defining the five factors[a]

Factor name	Definer Adjective	NEO-PI-R scale[b]
Neuroticism (or Negative Affectivity vs. emotional Stability)	Anxious Self-pitying Tense Touchy Unstable Worrying	Anxiety Angry hostility Depression Self-consciousness Impulsiveness Vulnerability
Extraversion (or Surgency, dominance vs. introversion	Active Assertive Energetic Enthusiastic Outgoing Talkative	Warmth Gregariousness Assertiveness Activity Excitement-seeking Positive emotions
Openness to Experience (or Intellect, culture vs. conventionality)	Artistic Curious Imaginative Insightful Original Wide interests	Fantasy Aesthetics Feelings Actions Ideas Values
Agreeableness (or Love, friendly compliance vs. Antagonism)	Appreciative Forgiving Generous Kind Sympathetic Trusting	Trust Straightforwardness Altruism Compliance Modesty Tender-mindedness
Conscientiousness (or Dependability, will to achieve vs. Undirectedness)	Efficient Organized Planful Reliable Responsible Thorough	Competence Order Dutifulness Achievement striving Self-discipline Deliberation

[a]Adapted from McCrae & John, 1992.
[b]Scales are facet scales from the Revised NEO Personality Inventory.

In the past decade it has become clear that personality traits can be described in terms of five very broad dimensions of personality. Table 1 lists some of the adjectives and personality questionnaire scales that define each dimension of the Five-Factor Model. These dimensions constitute the highest level of a hierarchy; within each of the five it is possible and sometimes important to make distinctions. Anxiety and depression, for example, are both definers of Neuroticism, and people who are anxious are frequently depressed as well. But the two traits are also distinguishable both conceptually and empirically, and psychotherapists often find that distinction very important.

Development and life course of personality

One of the most surprising findings of recent years has come from studies of the behaviour genetics of personality. Monozygotic twins, whether raised together or apart, strongly resemble each other in personality. Children who are raised in the same family but who are biologically unrelated show little or no resemblance in personality. The conclusion seems to be that personality traits are more influenced by heredity than by child-rearing practices (Plomin & Daniels, 1987) – a finding that both psychoanalysts and behaviourists would

have difficulty explaining. Developmentalists have known for years that certain temperamental traits, like activity level and distress-proneness, appear to be biologically based, and these temperaments are clearly linked to the two dimensions of 'extraversion' and 'neuroticism'. But 'openness', 'agreeableness' and 'conscientiousness' seem to be equally influenced by genetics.

This does not mean that the individual's personality is fixed at infancy, and that adult character can be read from infant behaviour. There are many changes from infancy through adolescence and personality changes continue throughout the twenties. From college to middle-age, both men and women tend to become less emotional and excitable, and more altruistic and organized. These declines in neuroticism and extraversion and increases in agreeableness and conscientiousness seem to summarize much of what is meant by maturity. After age 30, personality changes little. In particular, old age is not marked by increasing depression, social withdrawal, conservativism or crankiness.

Personality is also stable in another sense: individual differences are preserved. That is, those individuals who score highest on a personality trait at one time also tend to score highest at a later time – even over intervals of 30 years (Costa & McCrae, 1992). People who are well-adjusted, imaginative and persistent at age 30 are likely to be well-adjusted, imaginative and persistent at age 80. This fact is crucial to an understanding of adult development: it means that people's basic tendencies are highly predictable over long periods of time. One implication is that people can plan rationally for their own future by taking into account their current values, motivations and interests. Another implication is that once adequately assessed, personality trait information will retain its utility for behavioural medicine. Like sex, race and education, personality traits might be considered basic background information which could be included in an individual's medical record.

The five factors and their relevance to medical practice

Historically, personality traits were of interest to physicians chiefly because they were thought to predispose individuals to particular diseases. Different personality patterns were believed to be contributing causes to hypertension, ulcer, asthma and other so-called psychosomatic disorders. Today there are continuing research efforts in psychophysiology (Stough et al., 2001) and psychoneuroimmunology (Miller et al., 1999) that try to establish a biological link between personality and health (see 'Psychosomatics' and 'Psychoneuroimmunology'). However, most of the classical psychosomatic theories have not been supported by empirical research, and many others are the subject of ongoing controversy. But there is no doubt that traits influence health-related behaviours (Carmody et al., 1999), including risky behaviours (Vollrath & Torgersen, 2002); the ways patients perceive (Goodwin & Engstrom, 2002) and cope with illness (Bosma et al., 2004); and how they interact with health care providers (Eaton & Tinsley, 1999), and comply with medical advice (Courneya et al., 2002) (see 'Adherence to Treatment', 'Coping with Chronic Illness', 'Health-related Behaviours' and 'Symptom Perception').

In this section we discuss the five major personality factors in greater detail and suggest ways in which knowledge of personality traits might help health care providers.

Neuroticism

Modern psychiatric nomenclature no longer recognizes a category of neuroses, but personality psychologists still use the term 'Neuroticism' to describe a basic dimension of personality (see Table 1 for some alternative labels). Individuals who score high on this dimension are prone to experience a wide variety of negative emotions, such as fear, shame and guilt. External stressors and internal drives often overwhelm them, leading them to feel helpless and act impulsively. They are prone to unrealistic thinking and have a poor self-image. Low scorers on this dimension are calm and hardy, resilient in the face of stress.

Although neuroticism – even at very high levels – is a dimension of normal personality rather than a psychiatric disorder, it is associated with increased risk for a wide variety of psychiatric disorders (Zonderman et al., 1993). Neuroticism is also related to somatic distress. Individuals who are chronically anxious and depressed make more somatic complaints (De Gucht et al., 2004). They may be more sensitive to their internal states, or more prone to interpret physiological sensations as signs of illness, or more likely to remember and report symptoms. At an extreme level, this is recognizable as hypochondriasis, but even moderate levels of neuroticism are associated with moderate increases in somatic complaints. This phenomenon complicates medical diagnosis, which depends heavily on patient reports of medical history and symptoms. Patients who are very high in neuroticism may over-report symptoms, but their self-reports cannot be ignored – after all, even hypochondriacs get sick. Conversely, patients who are very low in neuroticism may minimize symptoms and fail to seek appropriate care.

Does neuroticism actually cause disease? Certainly, acute emotional reactions have physiological consequences, and individuals high in neuroticism have more frequent distressing emotional reactions. Although it is reasonable to hypothesize that the long-term effect of these physiological disturbances would include organic disease, a number of large-scale studies have failed to show any direct link between neuroticism and mortality or morbidity from cancer or coronary disease. There is evidence, however, that neuroticism affects health behaviours which are in turn risk factors for disease. In a five-year observational study, covert hostility, an aspect of neuroticism, predicted both being overweight and weight cycling (Carmody et al., 1999). In a large-scale community sample, beer consumption was positively related to neuroticism (McGregor et al., 2003).

Extraversion

Extraversion includes both interpersonal and temperamental aspects. Interpersonally, extraverts are warm and friendly, enjoying conversation and having close personal relationships; they also enjoy the sheer social stimulation of crowds of strangers. Extraverts are assertive and easily take on leadership roles. Temperamentally, extraverts are characterized by a need for excitement, high levels of energy and activity and cheerful optimism; they laugh easily. Introverts, although they may have perfectly adequate social skills, prefer to avoid crowds and tend to be serious in mood and measured in their pace of activity. Contrary to popular belief, introverts are not necessarily introspective or deep thinkers, nor are extraverts necessarily well-adjusted.

The characteristics that define extraversion are readily observed, and this dimension is the one which is most easily noticed by the health care provider. Most obviously, extraverts are talkative. This fact is of particular significance in view of the fact that 'talk is the main ingredient in medical care' (Roter & Hall, 1992, p. 3). How much and what is said in a medical interview depends upon many factors (Beisecker & Beisecker, 1990), including the physician's own level of extraversion. For example, Mechanic (1978) has suggested that family practitioners are more sociable than hospital doctors, and their interactions with patients are correspondingly more warm and personal. While interpersonal warmth may be appreciated by extraverted patients, introverts may prefer to maintain their distance and focus attention on the medical problem. Physicians may need to make extra effort to elicit information from these patients who are less likely to volunteer it.

While the interpersonal aspects of extraversion may be the most apparent to clinicians, there is growing interest in its relation to health via health-related behaviours. Courneya et al. (2002) reported that extraversion predicted exercise adherence in cancer survivors. In a longitudinal study by Kressin et al. (1999), extraversion predicted oral self-care behaviour.

Openness to experience

Individuals who are open to experience prefer novelty, variety and ambiguity in a variety of areas. They are imaginative and creative, with an active fantasy life, and they are responsive to beauty in art and nature. They are keenly aware of their own inner states, including emotional ambivalence. Open men and women are innovative and willing to try new approaches and they have a high degree of intellectual curiosity. They are liberal and unconventional in their political and social views. Closed individuals, by contrast, are conservative, conventional and down-to-earth; they prefer symmetry and simplicity and tend toward black-and-white thinking. They are reluctant to change either their behaviours or their views. Open individuals tend to be somewhat better educated than closed individuals, but openness should not be confused with intelligence.

Although openness is not strictly speaking an interpersonal domain of personality, it affects social interaction and is therefore relevant to clinical practice. Openness is an important predictor of how mothers communicate with paediatricians about their babies (Eaton & Tinsley, 1999). In the mental health setting, clinicians find that differences in openness are important determinants of the patient's view of therapy (Miller, 1991). Closed patients are likely to prefer conventional medical treatment; they tend to assume that doctors are the authorities and believe what they are told. Open patients may be less compliant: they may want more information than is normally provided, ask for second opinions and perhaps even research the topic themselves. They are more willing to consider innovative and non-traditional therapies and it seems likely that they make disproportionate use of alternative medicine. Acupuncture, aromatherapy and hypnosis are more appealing to open than to closed patients.

Agreeableness

Like extraversion, agreeableness is primarily an interpersonal dimension. Agreeable people are prosocial: they trust others and are themselves candid and straightforward; they try to help others and are sympathetic in attitudes. Antagonistic people are more self-centred, suspicious and devious. They may be arrogant and quarrelsome. Although agreeableness is socially desirable and agreeable people are more popular with their peers, there are also advantages to being disagreeable. Antagonistic individuals are competitive and proud of their tough-mindedness.

Early studies that sought to identify the so-called toxic component of the Type A behaviour pattern found that individuals who were rude, condescending and willing to express their anger directly to others – that is, who were low in agreeableness – were at higher risk of developing coronary heart disease (Dembroski *et al.*, 1989). More recent research indicates that health behaviours may mediate this association: antagonism, especially when coupled with low conscientiousness, predicts poor health behaviours (Martin *et al.*, 1999).

Antagonistic patients present other problems for healthcare providers: they are mistrustful, demanding and manipulative and often non-compliant (Auerbach *et al.*, 2002). Physicians not surprisingly find such patients unlikeable and such patients are frequently dissatisfied with their medical treatment (Roter & Hall, 1992). Extremely agreeable patients are well liked and generally satisfied, but may be too compliant for their own good – they are unlikely to adopt the consumerist perspective which some patient advocates recommend.

Conscientiousness

The final dimension of the Five-Factor Model is conscientiousness, a cluster of traits that encompass both self-restraint (order, dutifulness and deliberation) and active pursuit of goals. High scorers on measures of this dimension are hardworking, persistent and highly motivated; low scorers are easy-going and somewhat disorganized, and lack a clear direction in their life. At best, highly conscientious people are purposeful and effective; at worst, they are driven to perfectionism and neglect their personal life for the sake of their work.

In a recent meta-analysis of 194 cross-sectional studies, conscientiousness significantly (negatively) predicted a wide array of health risk behaviours including excessive alcohol use, unhealthy eating, risky driving, risky sex, suicide, tobacco use and violence (Bogg & Roberts, 2004). In another study, conscientiousness predicted not only wellness behaviours (e.g. exercise, taking vitamins), but also accident control (e.g. learning first aid), and low traffic risk-taking (Booth-Kewley & Vickers, 1994). Conscientiousness is a prospective predictor of exercise behaviour (Conner & Abraham, 2001), and conscientious people are also the most likely to adhere faithfully to prescribed medical regimens (Christensen & Smith, 1995). They have the self-discipline and prudence to follow the advice that public service announcements offer. Not surprisingly, conscientious individuals live longer (Martin & Friedman, 2000).

Patients who are very low in conscientiousness present a problem to the healthcare system. Regimens that are distasteful or that require organization or effort are likely to be abandoned. Ideally, treatments would be designed to take into account the patient's level of conscientiousness. For example, a rigorous exercise programme might be best for a high scorer, whereas a more passive drug therapy might be more realistic for a low scorer. Where patient efforts are essential, health care providers should make special efforts to motivate and monitor patients low in conscientiousness. External support, e.g. reminder calls, may help these patients comply with treatment.

Behaviour and health: practical considerations

Understanding personality is vital for health care providers. For clarity, we have discussed each of the five domains of personality separately, but in reality they all operate concurrently in the patient. While this adds to the complexity of assessment, it also has positive implications for treatment, because it allows clinicians to focus on patients' strengths to design treatments that are maximally effective. For example, if a patient is both antagonistic and conscientious, he probably would not exercise to please his doctor, but might if medical advice were framed as a challenge.

The stability of personality is a double-edged sword for practitioners. To the extent that personality predisposes patients to engage in health-injurious behaviours, personality may be viewed as a lifelong risk factor for disease. But stability of personality also gives the physician a reliable basis for interacting with the patient and formulating treatment strategy.

Personality traits are not easily changed, but fortunately, it is not the traits themselves but the behaviours they predispose toward that are problematic for health. Although it is helpful to understand the patient at the level of broad dispositions, the goals of treatment are best framed in terms of modifications to specific behaviours.

REFERENCES

Auerbach, S. M., Clore, J. N., Kiesler, D. J. et al. (2002). Relation of diabetic patients' health-related control appraisals and physician–patient interpersonal impacts to patients' metabolic control and satisfaction with treatment. *Journal of Behavioral Medicine*, 25, 17–31.

Beisecker, A. E. & Beisecker, T. D. (1990). Patient information-seeking behaviors when communicating with doctors. *Medical Care*, 28, 19–28.

Bogg, T. & Roberts, B. W. (2004). Conscientiousness and health-related behaviors: a meta-analysis of the leading behavioral contributors to mortality. *Psychological Bulletin*, 130(6), 887–919.

Booth-Kewley, S. & Vickers, R. R. Jr. (1994). Associations between major domains of personality and health behavior. *Journal of Personality*, 62, 281–98.

Bosma, H., Sanderman, R. & Scaf-Klomp, W. (2004). Demographic, health-related and psychosocial predictors of changes in depressive symptoms and anxiety in late middle-aged and older persons with fall-related injuries. *Psychology and Health*, 19, 103–15.

Carmody, T. P., Brunner, R. L. & St. Jeor, S. T. (1999). Hostility, dieting, and nutrition attitudes in overweight and weight-cycling men and women. *International Journal of Eating Disorders*, 26, 37–42.

Christensen, A. J. & Smith, T. W. (1995). Personality and patient adherence: Correlates of the Five-Factor Model in renal dialysis. *Journal of Behavioral Medicine*, 18, 305–12.

Conner, M. & Abraham, C. (2001). Conscientiousness and the Theory of Planned Behavior: toward a more complete model of the antecedents of intentions of behavior. *Personality and Social Psychology Bulletin*, **27**, 1547–61.

Costa, P. T. Jr. & McCrae, R. R. (1992). Trait psychology comes of age. In T. B. Sonderegger (Ed.). *Nebraska symposium on motivation: psychology and aging* (pp. 169–204). Lincoln, NE: University of Nebraska Press.

Courneya, K. S., Friedenreich, C.M, Sela, R. A., Quinney, H. A. & Rhodes, R. E. (2002). Correlates of adherence and contamination in a randomized controlled trial of exercise in cancer survivors: an application of the theory of planned behavior and the five factor model of personality. *Annals of Behavioral Medicine*, **24**, 257–68.

De Gucht, V., Fischler, B. & Heiser, W. (2004). Personality and affect as determinants of medically unexplained symptoms in primary care: a follow-up study. *Journal of Psychosomatic Research*, **56**, 279–85.

Dembroski, T. M., MacDougall, J. M., Costa, P. T. Jr. & Grandits, G. (1989). Components of hostility as predictors of sudden death and myocardial infarction in the Multiple Risk Factor Intervention Trial. *Psychosomatic Medicine*, **51**, 514–22.

Eaton, L. G. & Tinsley, B. J. (1999). Maternal personality and health communication in the pediatric context. *Health Communication*, **11**, 75–96.

Goodwin, R. & Engstrom, G. (2002). Personality and the perception of health in the general population. *Psychological Medicine*, **32**, 325–32.

Kressin, N. R., Spiro, A., Bossé, R. & Garcia, R. I. (1999). Personality traits and oral self-care behaviors: longitudinal findings from the Normative Aging Study. *Psychology and Health*, **14**, 71–85.

Martin, L. R. & Friedman, H. S. (2000). Comparing personality scales across time: an illustrative study of validity and consistency in life-span archival data. *Journal of Personality*, **68**, 85–110.

Martin, R., Wan, C. K., David, J. P. *et al.* (1999). Style of anger expression: relation to expressivity, personality, and health. *Personality and Social Psychology Bulletin*, **25**, 1196–207.

McCrae, R. R., & Costa, P. T., Jr. (2003). *Personality in Adulthood: A Five-Factor Theory Perspective* (2nd edn.). New York: Guilford.

Mc Crae, R. R. & John, O. P. (1992). An introduction to the five-factor model and its applications. *Journal of Personality*, **60**, 175–215.

McGregor, D., Murray, R. P. & Barnes, G. E. (2003). Personality differences between users of wine, beer and spirits in a community sample: the Winnipeg Health and Drinking Survey. *Journal of Studies on Alcohol*, **64**, 634–40.

Mechanic, D. (1978). *Medical sociology* (2nd edn.). New York: Free Press.

Miller, G. E., Cohen, S., Rabin, B., Skoner, D. P. & Doyle, W. J. (1999). Personality and tonic cardiovascular, neuroendocrine, and immune parameters. *Brain, Behavior and Immunity*, **13**, 109–23.

Miller, T. (1991). The psychotherapeutic utility of the Five-Factor Model of personality: a clinician's experience. *Journal of Personality Assessment*, **57**, 415–33.

Pervin, L. A. & John, O. P. (Eds.). (1999). *Handbook of Personality: Theory, & Research* (2nd edn.). New York: Guilford.

Plomin, R. & Daniels, D. (1987). Why are children in the same family so different from one another? *Behavioral and Brain Sciences*, **10**, 1–16.

Roter, D. L. & Hall, J. A. (1992). *Doctors talking with patients/patients talking with doctors: improving communication in medical visits.* Westport, CT: Auburn House.

Stough, C., Donaldson, C. & Scarlata, B. (2001). Psychophysiological correlates of the NEO-PI-R openness, agreeableness and conscientiousness: preliminary results. *International Journal of Psychophysiology*, **41**, 87–91.

Vollrath, M. & Torgersen, S. (2002). Who takes health risks? A probe into eight personality types. *Personality and Individual Differences*, **32**, 1185–97.

Zonderman, A. B., Herbst, J. H., Schmidt, C., Jr., Costa, P. T., Jr. & McCrae, R. R. (1993). Depressive symptoms as a non-specific, graded risk for psychiatric diagnoses. *Journal of Abnormal Psychology*, **102**, 544–52.

Physical activity and health

Neville Owen, Kym Spathonis and Eva Leslie

The University of Queensland

Introduction

Participation in physical activity is associated with significant benefits to health, most importantly in the prevention of Type 2 diabetes, cardiovascular disease and some cancers (Bauman *et al.*, 2002; United States Department of Health and Human Services [USDHHS], 1996). In this chapter, we provide an overview of research on health-enhancing physical activity in adults. We provide brief examples of epidemiological studies on the relationships of physical activity to health outcomes: we also consider descriptive studies of adult populations on levels of participation. Our focus is on physical activity as a set of behaviours: we describe research findings on the 'determinants' of physical activity and describe the theories of health behaviour that are now widely used in understanding and influencing physical activity.

Physical activity exercise and fitness

The terms, 'physical activity', 'exercise' and 'fitness' are sometimes used interchangeably and at times incorrectly (Sallis & Owen, 1999).

'Physical activity' refers to any bodily movement, but generally to the movements of groups of large muscles (particularly of the legs and arms) that result in significant increases in metabolic energy expenditure, above the resting level. Regularly taking part in such activities is associated with better health outcomes. Physical activity can be performed at a wide range of intensities: walking or other moderate-intensity activities such as swimming at a low, moderate or brisk pace; vigorous endurance activities (for example, jogging or running, walking fast uphill, riding a bicycle fast or in hilly terrain); and activities that increase strength and/or flexibility (for example, weight training, calisthenics or strenuous occupational or domestic tasks such as heavy lifting or carrying). 'Exercise' is physical activity done with the explicit purpose of improving or maintaining physical fitness or health. Exercise can be performed at a variety of intensities, although it usually involves more vigorous activities. Nevertheless, walking at a moderate intensity can be exercise, if it is done for the purpose of improving fitness or health.

Physical fitness is a physiological state, not a behaviour. It is thus not interchangeable with the terms 'physical activity' or 'exercise', which refer to sets of behaviours and to their contexts or purposes. Psychological fitness (personal resiliency or 'hardiness') can be associated with physical fitness. While psychological fitness is distinct from physical activity or fitness, for some individuals or groups (for example, athletes or those who are living with a chronic illness), the relationship between these two domains of health and well-being will be strong.

A behavioural epidemiology framework for physical activity and health

Sallis & Owen (1999) propose five main phases of 'behavioural epidemiology' research, as they may be applied to physical activity and health:

1. *Establish the links between physical activity and health:* This phase is complex, because different types and amounts of physical activity are related to different health benefits and risks. Once epidemiological and other studies document the associations between the relevant behaviour and health outcomes, research in the subsequent phases has strong foundations.
2. *Accurately measure physical activity:* The measurement of physical activity, particularly in large population studies and in the evaluation of interventions, is an ongoing challenge, but high quality measures are essential for all types of research. Many studies rely on self-report data, but more objective measurement tools are being developed and validated.
3. *Identify factors that influence physical activity:* Describing the characteristics of those who are most and least active can be helpful in deciding which groups are most in need of interventions. The potentially modifiable factors that are identified can then be targeted for change in exercise counselling, programmes or public campaigns.
4. *Develop and evaluate interventions to promote physical activity:* The majority of adults in the populations of industrialized nations are not sufficiently physically active for health benefits. Effective, evidence-based intervention programmes need to be developed and tested systematically.
5. *Translate research into policy and practice:* Each phase of the behavioural epidemiology framework is intended to build upon the previous phase or phases, so that evidence-based approaches may be adopted more widely and with confidence.

Understanding and influencing physical activity for individuals, groups, communities and whole populations is a new and important interdisciplinary area. Health psychology experts in the physical activity field work closely with exercise physiologists, physical educators, epidemiologists and other social and biomedical scientists (Sallis *et al.*, 2000).

Health psychology has much to offer. Psychological theories and methods are used in clinical and community settings to guide health practitioners in assisting individuals to become more physically active. They are used to inform the development of large-scale interventions for communities and populations (Marcus *et al.*, 1998). Psychological theories underpin ecological models of health behaviour (Owen *et al.*, 2004; Sallis & Owen, 1997, 2002). These provide a conceptual basis for the environmental and policy initiatives which will be needed to bring about population-wide increases in physical activity (Sallis *et al.*, 1998).

Phases 3 and 4 of the behavioural epidemiology framework (identifying factors that influence physical activity; developing and evaluating interventions to promote physical activity) are where health psychology has made particularly strong contributions. These have been in the development of conceptual models, in measurement and other research methods and in developing a plethora of practical programmes. These two phases of research and application form the main focus of our chapter.

Physical activity and population health outcomes

There is a substantial body of evidence suggesting that regularly taking part in physical activities of moderate intensity (for example, recreational walking or cycling) can have significant health-protective benefits (Bauman *et al.*, 2002; USDHHS, 1996). In the 1980s and early 1990s, the strongest evidence for physical activity and health benefits was in the area of heart-disease prevention. More recent reviews support the earlier recommendations on physical activity and health and continue to emphasize participation in moderate-intensity activities (particularly walking) on most days of the week for 30 minutes or more: this criterion is intended to be realistic and optimal for achieving health benefits in sedentary adult populations (Bauman, 2004). Higher volumes and intensities of activity and specific types of activity such as strength training have additional health benefits (Bauman *et al.*, 2002; USDHHS, 1996).

Epidemiological studies and controlled trials conducted in recent years reinforce the broader preventive benefits and the range of specific disease outcomes that may be postponed or amended, by being physically active on a regular basis. This is seen clearly in the case of Type 2 diabetes. There is recent compelling evidence from controlled trials that regular physical activity has a key role in the prevention of Type 2 diabetes in high-risk groups. For example, in a study conducted in Finland, intensive nutritional counselling and endurance exercise advice given to people with impaired glucose tolerance resulted in a significantly lower rate of progression to diabetes, compared with a control group.

The decrease in risk was related to the degree of lifestyle change (Tuomilehto *et al.*, 2001) (see 'Diabetes').

Physical activity also contributes to a reduced risk of developing some cancers, particularly colon and breast cancer (International Agency for Research on Cancer [IARC], 2002). There is a reduction in risk of colon cancer with increasing levels of activity, particularly more intense activities. Recent reviews highlight the potential for physical activity to reduce the risk of breast cancer, with indications of a 20–40% risk reduction in both pre- and post-menopausal women (Thune & Furberg, 2001). Physical activity has an independent effect on colon and breast cancer risk in addition to its role in preventing unhealthy weight gain (IARC, 2002).

The increasing population prevalence of inactivity is an important contributor to what is now being characterized as an 'obesity epidemic' (Erlichman *et al.*, 2002). Physically active persons are less likely to gain weight over the course of their adult lives. Findings from a range of cross-sectional studies have shown lower weight, body mass index or skin-fold measures among people with higher measured fitness and higher levels of habitual physical activity; however, prospective studies have shown less consistent relationships (Erlichman *et al.*, 2002) (see 'Obesity').

Over half of the adult population in most industrialized countries is, however, insufficiently physically active for health benefits (USDHHS, 1996). For example, recent data on trends in physical activity participation in Australia in the late 1990s (Bauman *et al.*, 2002; Bauman *et al.*, 2003) suggest that the rate of participation in physical activity by adults had declined by 6% between 1997 and 1999. Less than 50% of adult Australians achieved the recommended 150 minutes (30 minutes on at least five days of the week) of at least moderate-intensity activity. Similar findings have emerged in population surveys in the UK (Hillsdon *et al.*, 2001).

Public policies and programmes to encourage physical activity are being pursued seriously in many developed countries and elsewhere (Bauman *et al.*, 2002; USDHHS, 1996). Yet, the majority of the adult population of many industrialized countries is not engaging in the level of activity needed to accrue worthwhile health benefits. Thus, there is much that needs to be done, in research and in practice, to increase participation in physical activity. Effective interventions which can change the personal, social and environmental factors related to physical inactivity are needed.

Identifying factors that influence physical activity

The published research on physical activity is replete with findings from cross-sectional investigations of the associations between physical activity and a range of personal, social and environmental factors.

en used in the
incorrectly to
surveys) that
rather than
02). While
not identify cause-and-effect relationships, they do help to generate hypotheses for further study and can illuminate the relevance (or otherwise) of particular theoretical constructs.

Table 1. Summary overview of the new evidence from studies of the correlates of physical activity, published since 1998 (based on the review by Trost *et al.*, 2002)

Demographic and biological factors
- Marital status (married; −)
- Overweight or obesity (−)

Psychological, cognitive and emotional factors
- Self-efficacy for physical activity (+)
- Barriers to physical activity (lack of time; −)

Behavioural attributes and skills
- Past physical activity behaviour or 'habit' (+)
- Healthy diet (+)
- Smoking (−)

Socio-cultural factors
- Social support (++)

Physical environment factors
- Exercise equipment at home (+)
- Perceived access to facilities (+)
- Satisfaction with recreational facilities (+)
- Neighbourhood safety (+)
- Hilly terrain (+)
- Frequently observe others exercising (+)
- Enjoyable scenery (+)
- Urban location (−)

− mixed or weak evidence of negative association; −− strong negative association; + mixed or weak evidence of positive association; ++ strong positive association.

Sallis & Owen (1999, Chapter 7) examined the personal, social and environmental factors associated with adults' participation in physical activity. Six classes of correlates of activity were identified: demographic and biological factors; psychological, cognitive and emotional factors; behavioural attributes and skills; socio-cultural factors; physical environment factors; and physical activity characteristics.

The overall pattern of findings suggests that individual-level attributes such as socioeconomic status and perceived self-efficacy demonstrate the strongest and most consistent associations with physical activity. Fewer consistent positive or negative associations were found in relation to behavioural attributes and personal skills, sociocultural influences and physical environmental influences.

In a more recent review, Trost *et al.* (2002) reported further evidence on associations between these six classes of attributes and being physically active, engaging in particular activities or conducting higher volumes of activity (see Table 1).

Several of the correlates of physical activity listed in Table 1 are associated with constructs from theoretical models of health behaviour. These correlates, for example, include self-efficacy, perceived barriers, past exercise habits and environmental attributes. The relevant theoretical models from health psychology, as we will illustrate below, have been particularly influential in the development of physical activity interventions.

Theories of physical activity behaviour and their applications

Theoretical models of health behaviour (see Glanz *et al.*, 2002) have been applied to research on the factors which can influence physical activity and to the development and evaluation of interventions (see Godin, 1994; Marcus et al., 1998; Owen et al., 2004; Sallis & Owen, 1997, 2002; Spence & Lee, 2003).

Social–cognitive theory

Social–Cognitive Theory (SCT) has been widely used in developing interventions to influence physical activity, often in combination with constructs such as stages of change and the Transtheoretical Model (TTM; Marcus, Owen et al., 1998). SCT has been particularly helpful in expanding the understanding of factors that influence physical activity participation, beyond individual-level factors. Theories focusing more on intra-personal processes (for example, attitudes, intention, beliefs) such as the Theory of Planned Behaviour and the Theory of Reasoned Action, have been applied to understanding the determinants of physical activity behaviour, with modest but, in many cases, significant predictive power (Godin, 1994).

Social–cognitive Theory proposes that personal, behavioural and environmental factors operate as reciprocal interacting determinants (Bandura, 1986). Studies of the correlates of physical activity and intervention trials based on SCT have focused on the individual's ability to control her or his own behaviour (or 'self-efficacy') and on how changes in the individual, the environment, or in both can produce changes in behaviour.

Bandura (1986) identifies four main sources of influences on self-efficacy: mastery of accomplishments (learning new skills and building confidence through successful new experiences); social modelling (learning new skills by observing others); social persuasion (being convinced by others of the desirability of new activities and their outcomes); and the interpretation of physiological states (in the case of physical activity, this might include, for example, interpreting the physical signs of exertion generally, or learning to feel comfortable with increased heart rate and respiration changes) (see 'Self-efficacy and health').

The transtheoretical model

The TTM (also know as the 'Stages of Change' model; Prochaska & DiClemente, 1983) has formed the theoretical basis for a number of cross-sectional studies and intervention trials on physical activity. According to the TTM, five stages of motivational readiness for physical activity may be identified (Marcus & Simpkin, 1994).

In the initial stage (precontemplation), individuals do not intend to take action to become more physically active in the foreseeable future. However, as the individual becomes more aware of the costs and benefits of engaging more regularly in physical activity, he/she progresses to the second stage (contemplation). As the individual takes steps to engage in physical activity (preparation), the development of behavioural plans and skills may assist him/her to become active. The fourth stage (action) occurs when an individual starts to become active, and the fifth stage (maintenance) is when the individual is able to continue activity on a regular basis for six months and beyond. Both the fourth and the fifth stages of behavioural change often require individuals to employ both cognitive and behavioural strategies to assist in avoiding relapse (dropping out of regular physical activity), or in re-engaging in activity following relapse (see 'Transtheoretical model of behaviour change').

Interventions derived from SCT and the TTM

Interventions targeting self-efficacy and decision-making (key constructs from SCT and the TTM) have accumulated significant support from research trials (Sallis & Owen, 1999). These interventions emphasize building confidence about being physically active (enhancing self-efficacy). They also use specific techniques such as goal setting, completing 'decisional balance' protocols (explicitly listing and considering both the advantages and disadvantages of trying to be more active), relapse prevention training (skills in resuming being more active after time out), stimulus control (how to identify environmental factors that can prompt and remind one to be more active) and social support (help and encouragement from others).

Methods based on such behavioural techniques have a long history of being used in combined ways in physical activity interventions. For example, Martin et al. (1984) conducted a series of cognitive–behavioural intervention trials with sedentary adults. They found that attendance at exercise sessions was significantly improved by frequent personalised praise and feedback from instructors, and flexible goal setting. Overall, the interventions based on SCT produced attendance rates of 80% or greater, while a control group with the most basic programme had attendance of around 50%. In another intervention study, McAuley et al. (1993) randomly assigned middle-aged, sedentary adults to a self-efficacy enhancing programme or to a standard walking programme. Following the intervention, those in the efficacy-enhancement group were walking almost 50% more than were those in the control group. These two examples provide an example of how specific and combined SCT-based components can contribute to at least short-term successes of physical activity interventions which are delivered face-to-face in structured settings.

Other evidence however, suggests that most people prefer to be active on their own – either at home or in their local neighbourhood (Booth et al., 1997). This is in contrast to using structured facilities such as gyms or fitness centres. Attending a clinic, a fitness facility or leisure centre, a class or group is inconvenient for many people: it may be more difficult for some to actually get to the site of the class than it is to engage in the physical activity elsewhere. There is a modest but consistent body of research to suggest that mass media campaigns targeting those in early stages of motivational readiness for physical activity can result in significant increases in slogan and message content recall, and have significant, but small and short-term impacts on behaviour (Bauman et al., 2001; Marcus et al., 1998).

Trials of 'mediated' interventions based on the TTM have used print and Internet delivery methods (Bock et al., 2001; Marcus et al., 1998). These interventions aim to match the main elements of the programme to the individual's stage of motivational readiness for change. However, the task of matching interventions to a person's level of motivational readiness for change must take into account that some people are not yet ready to change their behaviour but may be ready to make changes in their thinking about behaviour (Marcus & Forsyth, 2003). For example, programmes for precontemplators may focus on enhancing particular aspects of knowledge;

programmes for those in the action stage may, for example, focus on social support and injury prevention.

There is promising new evidence for the potential of physical activity programs that can be delivered via telephone and the Internet (Napolitano *et al.*, 2003). However, the trials of Internet-delivered programmes conducted thus far have dealt with small numbers of self-selected participants. A recent Australian trial compared print versus Internet delivery of a stage-targeted programme (Marshall *et al.*, 2003). It identified major challenges in the recruitment and retention of participants. For website-delivered programmes, there remains limited evidence to support their efficacy in changing behaviour, except in trials with small numbers of motivated participants.

While the new mediated approaches do show considerable promise, it is not realistically possible to engage all sedentary or insufficiently active adults in structured, formal physical activity programmes (whether face-to-face or mediated). It may also be unreasonable to expect large proportions of the population to make motivationally driven personal behaviour changes, if these efforts are not fully supported by the relevant environmental circumstances (see also 'Physical activity interventions').

Understanding environmental influences on physical activity: ecological models of health behaviour

Sallis & Hovell (1990) proposed a model of physical activity behaviour based on Social Learning Theory (an earlier version of SCT), which used a combination of personal, cognitive, social and environmental factors to explain patterns of physical activity. A key element of the Sallis and Hovell (1990) model was its emphasis on the role of environmental settings and supports. Specifically, environments that lack resources, or impose barriers may act to reduce the probability that the choice to be active will be made. As we will illustrate below, Sallis and Hovell's focus on the role of the physical environment has been developed within 'ecological' models of physical activity behaviour.

Sallis & Owen (1997, 1999, 2002) and Spence & Lee (2003) have proposed an ecological approach to understanding the determinants of physical activity behaviour, and have highlighted the distinction between social and physical environmental influences. Within the physical environment, natural environment factors such as the weather or climate; and built environment factors, such as urban design or availability of facilities can influence physical activity behaviour (Saelens *et al.*, 2003).

Ecological models can provide frameworks for considering the multiple levels (personal, social, environmental) on which physical activity determinants exert their influences (Sallis & Owen, 1997, 2002; Spence & Lee, 2003). The explicit emphasis on attributes of the physical environment in a complex, multi-level network of causality is a key feature of ecological models of physical activity (Owen *et al.*, 2000; Sallis & Owen, 1997, 2002). In public health advocacy and community initiatives, Sallis and Owen's (1997, 2002) ecological model has been used to highlight the interactions of social and organizational factors with environmental attributes and the communication media initiatives that can prompt personal choices to be active (Matsudo *et al.*, 2004).

The 'behaviour settings' construct, drawn from ecological psychology (Barker, 1968) is a key to understanding the role of environmental determinants of physical activity (Owen *et al.*, 2000). Behaviour settings are the physical and social contexts in which behaviours occur, some being supportive of activity and others being discouraging or prohibiting of activity (Wicker, 1979).

Because cognitive–social theories (particularly SCT and the TTM) have been the predominant influences in behavioural studies of physical activity (Godin, 1994), the field has been shaped by assumptions that choices to be active or inactive are conscious, deliberate choices – consequent upon attitudes, intentions, self-efficacy and other cognitive mediators of behavioural change (Owen *et al.*, 2004). However, social–cognitive models do identify a strong role for environmental influences under some circumstances. For example, Bandura (1986) has argued that when behaviour is strongly facilitated or constrained by attributes of the environment in which it takes place (and plausibly this often is likely to be so for physical activity), direct environmental influences would be the predominant class of determinants.

Differences in physical activity between communities that have different environmental attributes have been observed – residents of 'traditional' communities, characterized by higher population density, higher street connectivity and mixed land use ('high walkable'), report significantly more walking and cycling for transport, than do residents of low population density, poorly-connected and single land use ('low walkable') neighbourhoods (Saelens *et al.*, 2003). Overall, there was an average difference between high- and low-walkable communities of approximately 15–30 minutes more walking per week for residents of high-walkable neighbourhoods.

The evidence from behavioural and public health research has recently been reviewed (Humpel *et al.*, 2002; Owen *et al.*, 2004) and a number of environmental attributes associated with being physically active have been identified (see Table 1). Even if relatively small amounts of the variation in physical activity are ultimately explained by the influence of environmental variables, it is the case that whole communities can be impacted by any change to make the environment more supportive of physical activity (Giles-Corti & Donovan, 2002). The effects of many small effects across communities could accumulate, to result in substantial support for individual behaviour change, which should lead to broader changes across whole populations.

Conclusions

Health psychology research and interventions to influence physical activity are rapidly developing areas, stimulated by a strong and growing body of evidence on the major health benefits of being habitually active. Health psychologists have contributed significantly to the knowledge base and to developing, refining and applying the theories that are now widely used in the physical activity field. We have used a behavioural epidemiology framework, to highlight those dimensions of research on physical activity and health (understanding determinants, developing theoretical models, designing interventions), within which health psychology has particularly important contributions to make.

It seems likely that future conceptual and practical advances will come from the blending together of the best of what is known about motivational approaches, with an ecological perspective.

Our understanding of the relevant determinants will become more definitive and theories of physical activity behaviour will be refined. It thus should be possible to design and implement interventions that will strongly mobilize the personal, social and environmental factors which can help people to initiate and maintain the relevant behavioural changes.

REFERENCES

Bandura, A. (1986). *Social foundations of thought and action*. Englewood Cliffs, NJ: Prentice-Hall.

Barker, R. G. (1968). *Ecological psychology*. Stanford, CA: Stanford University Press.

Bauman, A. E. (2004). Updating the evidence that physical activity is good for health: an epidemiological review 2000–2003. *Journal of Science and Medicine in Sport*, **7**(Suppl. 1), 6–19.

Bauman, A., Armstrong, T., Davies, J. *et al.* (2003). Trends in physical activity participation and the impact of integrated campaigns among Australian adults, 1997–1999. *Australian and New Zealand Journal of Public Health*, **27**, 76–9.

Bauman, A., Bellew, B., Brown, W. & Owen, N. (2002). *Getting Australia active. Towards better practice for the promotion of physical activity*. Melbourne, Australia: National Public Health Partnership.

Bauman, A. E., Bellew, B., Owen, N. & Vita P. (2001). Impact of an Australian mass media campaign targeting physical activity in 1998. *American Journal of Preventive Medicine*, **21**, 41–7.

Bauman, A. E., Sallis, J. F., Dzewaltowksi, D. A. & Owen, N. (2002). Towards a better understanding of the influences on physical activity: the role of determinants, correlates, causal variables, mediators, moderators and confounders. *American Journal of Preventive Medicine*, **23**(Suppl. 2), 5–14.

Bock, B. C., Marcus, B. M., Pinto, B. M. & Forsyth, L. H. (2001). Maintenance of physical activity following an individualised motivationally tailored intervention. *Annals of Behavioral Medicine*, **23**, 79–87.

Booth, M., Bauman, A., Owen, N. & Gore, C. J. (1997). Physical activity preferences, preferred sources of assistance, and perceived barriers to increased activity among physically-inactive Australians. *Preventive Medicine*, **26**, 131–7.

Erlichman, J., Kerbey, A. L. & James, P. T. (2002). Physical activity and its impact on health outcomes. Paper 2: Prevention of unhealthy weight gain and obesity by physical activity: an analysis of the evidence. *Obesity Reviews*, **3**, 273–87.

Giles-Corti, B. & Donovan, R. J. (2002). Socioeconomic status differences in recreational physical activity levels and real and perceived access to a supportive physical environment. *Preventive Medicine*, **35**, 601–11.

Glanz, K., Lewis, F. M. & Rimer, B. K. (Eds.). (2002). *Health Behavior and Health Education: Theory, Research, and Practice* (3rd edn.). San Francisco: Jossey-Bass.

Godin, G. (1994). Social–cognitive models. In R. K. Dishman (Ed.). *Advances in exercise adherence* (pp. 113-36). Champaign IL: Human Kinetics.

Hillsdon, M., Cavill, N., Nanchahal, K., Diamond, A. & White, I. R. (2001). National level promotion of physical activity: results from England's ACTIVE for LIFE campaign. *Journal of Epidemiology and Community Health*, **55**, 755–61.

Humpel, N., Owen, N. & Leslie, E. (2002). Environmental factors associated with adults' participation in physical activity: a review. *American Journal of Preventive Medicine*, **22**, 188–99.

International Agency for Research on Cancer. (2002). *IARC Handbooks of cancer prevention, volume 6 – weight control and physical activity*. Oxford: Oxford University Press.

Marcus, B. H., Bock, B. C., Pinto, B. M. *et al.* (1998). Efficacy of an individualized, motivationally-tailored physical activity intervention. *Annals of Behavioral Medicine*, **20**, 174–80.

Marcus, B. H. & Forsyth, L. H. (2003). *Motivating people to be physically active*. Champaign, IL: Human Kinetics.

Marcus, B. H., Owen, N., Forsyth, L. H. Cavill, N. A. & Fridinger, F. (1998). Interventions to promote physical activity using mass media, print media and information technology. *American Journal of Preventive Medicine*, **15**, 362–78.

Marcus, B. H. & Simkin, L. R. (1994). The transtheoretical model: applications to exercise behavior. *Medicine and Science in Sports and Exercise*, **11**, 1400–4.

Marshall, A. L., Leslie, E. R., Bauman, A. E., Marcus, B. H. & Owen, N. (2003). Print versus website physical activity programs: a randomized trial. *American Journal of Preventive Medicine*, **25**, 88–94.

Martin, J. E., Dubbert, P. M., Kattell, A. D. *et al.* (1984). Behavioral control of exercise in sedentary adults: studies 1 through 6. *Journal of Consulting and Clinical Psychology*, **52**, 795–811.

Matsudo, S. M., Matsudo, V. R., Andrade, D. R. *et al.* (2004). Physical activity promotion: experiences and evaluation of the Agita Sao Paulo program using the ecological mobile model. *Journal of Physical Activity and Health*, **1**, 81–97.

McAuley, E., Lox, C. & Duncan, T. E. (1993). Long-term maintenance of exercise, self-efficacy, and physiological change in older adults. *Journal of Gerontology: Series B. Psychological Sciences and Social Sciences*, **48**, 218–24.

Napolitano, M. A., Fotheringham, M., Tate, D. *et al.* (2003). Evaluation of an internet-based physical activity intervention: a preliminary investigation. *Annals of Behavioral Medicine*, **25**, 92–9.

Owen, N., Humpel, N., Leslie, E., Bauman, A. & Sallis, J. F. (2004). Understanding environmental influences on walking: review and research agenda. *American Journal of Preventive Medicine*, **27**, 67–76.

Owen, N., Leslie, E., Salmon, J. & Fotheringham, M. J. (2000). Environmental determinants of physical activity and sedentary behavior. *Exercise and Sport Sciences Reviews*, **28**, 153–8.

Prochaska, J. O. & DiClemente, C. C. (1983). Stages and processes of self-change of smoking: toward an integrative model of change. *Journal of Consulting and Clinical Psychology*, **51**, 390–5.

Saelens, B. E., Sallis, J. F. & Frank, L. D. (2003). Environmental correlates of walking and cycling: findings from the transportation, urban design, and planning literatures. *Annals of Behavioral Medicine*, **25**, 80–91.

Sallis, J. F., Bauman, A. & Pratt, M. (1998). Environmental and policy interventions to promote physical activity. *American Journal of Preventive Medicine*, **15**, 379–97.

Sallis, J. F. & Hovell, M. F. (1990). Determinants of exercise behavior. In J. O. Holloszy & K. B. Pandolf (Eds.). *Exercise and sports sciences reviews Vol. 18* (pp. 307–30). Baltimore: Williams and Wilkins.

Sallis, J. F. & Owen, N., (1997). Ecological models. In K. Glanz, F. M. Lewis & B. K. Rimer (Eds.). *Health Behavior and Health Education: Theory, Research, and Practice* (2nd edn.). (pp. 403–24) San Francisco: Jossey-Bass.

Sallis, J. F. & Owen, N. (1999). *Physical activity and behavioral medicine.* Thousand Oaks, CA: Sage.

Sallis, J. F. & Owen, N., (2002). Ecological models of health behavior. In K. Glanz, F. M. Lewis & B. K. Rimer (Eds.). *Health Behaviour and Health Education: Theory, Research, and Practice* (3rd edn.). (pp. 462–84). San Francisco: Jossey-Bass.

Sallis, J. F., Owen, N. & Fotheringham, M. J. (2000). Behavioral epidemiology: a systematic framework to classify phases of research on health promotion and disease prevention. *Annals of Behavioral Medicine,* **22,** 294–8.

Spence, J. & Lee, R. (2003). Toward a comprehensive model of physical activity. *Psychology of Sport and Exercise,* **4,** 7–24.

Thune, I. & Furberg, A. S. (2001). Physical activity and cancer risk: dose-response and cancer, all sites and site-specific. *Medicine and Science in Sports and Exercise,* **33** (Suppl. 6), S530–S50.

Trost, S. G., Owen, N., Bauman, A. E., Sallis, J. F. & Brown, W. (2002). Correlates of adults participation in physical activity: review and update. *Medicine and Science in Sports and Exercise,* **34,** 1996–2001.

Tuomilehto, J., Lindstrom, J., Eriksson, J. G. *et al.* (2001). Prevention of Type 2 diabetes mellitus by changes in lifestyle among subjects with impaired glucose tolerance. *New England Journal of Medicine,* **344,** 1343–50.

United States Department of Health, & Human Services (USDHHS) (1996). Physical activity and health: a report of the Surgeon General. Atlanta: USDHHS.

Wicker, A. W. (1979). *An introduction to ecological psychology.* Monterey, CA: Brooks/Cole.

Placebos

Irving Kirsch

University of Hull

Overview

A placebo is a sham treatment that may be used clinically to placate a patient or experimentally to establish the efficacy of a drug or other medical procedure. The placebo effect is the effect produced by administering a placebo. In addition, active medications may produce placebo effects as well as drug effects and these may be additive. In this case, the placebo effect is that portion of the treatment effect that was produced psychologically, rather than through physical means.

Typically, placebos are physically inert substances which are identical in appearance to an active drug. Occasionally, active substances are used as placebos. Active placebos have side-effects that mimic those of the drug being investigated, but do not possess the physical properties hypothesized to produce the beneficial treatment effect. Active placebos are used to prevent patients from using the sensory cues provided by side effects to deduce the condition to which they have been randomized.

Placebo effects are not limited to drug treatments. Any medical procedure can have effects due to the physical properties of the treatment and effects due to its psychological properties. Just as the effects of the physical properties of a medication can be tested by comparing its effects to those of a sham medication, so too the physically produced effects of other medical procedures can be established by comparison with sham procedures (e.g. sham surgery). For example, real and sham surgery have been compared in the treatment of angina (Cobb *et al.,* 1959; Dimond *et al.,* 1960) and osteoporosis of the knee (Moseley *et al.,* 2002). In both cases, the effects appear to be due to the psychological properties of the treatment, rather than to the surgical procedures themselves.

Four notable and controversial issues currently occupy the attention of researchers investigating the placebo effect. The first is whether placebos are capable of producing psychological or physical effects. The second concerns the mechanisms by which these effects are produced. The third involves the search for a placebo responder. The fourth issue relates to attempts to extend the placebo construct beyond the bounds of physical medicine and into the arena of psychotherapy.

Research evidence

Are placebos effective?

The term placebo is Latin and means 'I shall please'. This reflects the historical use of placebos to placate patients whose complaints could not otherwise be treated. It also indicates a belief that while the placebos might please patients, they are not likely to produce real benefits.

During the 1950s, the possibility that placebo treatment might have genuine effects became more widely recognized, and the use of placebo controls in medical research became common. In case after case, medicines and treatment procedures that had been 'proven' effective in clinical trials were found to be no more effective than treatment by placebo. Though the mechanism of placebo-induced change was a mystery, medical researchers began to suspect that many effects previously attributed to specific treatments were in fact placebo effects. It was suggested that placebos could reduce the frequency of asthma attacks, relieve hay fever, suppress coughs, alleviate tension and anxiety, cure headaches, reduce pain, prevent colds and alleviate cold symptoms, cure ulcers, inhibit symptoms of withdrawal from narcotics, alter gastric function, control the blood sugar levels of diabetics, reduce enuresis, lessen the severity of arthritis, reduce the frequency and severity of angina attacks and reverse the growth of malignant tumours (Beecher, 1961; Honigfeld, 1964a, 1964b; Klopfer, 1957; Volgyesi, 1954). These data led to the concept of 'the powerful placebo' (Beecher, 1955).

The response to a medication is not the same thing as the effect of that medication. This is because there are many reasons by which a person might get better. One is the natural history of the disease. People get better from many conditions (e.g. the common cold) regardless of whether they are treated or not. Sometimes there is spontaneous remission in disorders that aren't always self-healing (e.g. depression or cancer). There is also the statistical problem of regression towards the mean, i.e. when you re-assess something, people who scored at the extremes will tend to display scores closer to the mean. Finally, the response to a medication includes the placebo effect. Placebos are intended to control for all these sources of improvement. Thus, the drug effect is assumed to be the difference between the response to medication and the response to placebo.

Analogously, a distinction can be drawn between the placebo response and the placebo effect. The placebo response is the change observed following placebo administration. In addition to the placebo effect, it includes the changes due to the natural history of the disorder, spontaneous remission and regression to the mean. For this reason, the placebo effect is best evaluated via comparisons with a no-treatment control condition. However, this is rarely done in medical research, where the interest is in evaluating treatment effects rather than placebo effects.

In an effort to evaluate placebo effects, Hróbjartsson and Gøtzsche (2001) reported a meta-analysis of treatments in which response to placebo was compared to changes observed in a no-treatment control condition. Finding a small but significant 'placebo effect', along with significant heterogeneity outcomes, the authors concluded that they had 'found little evidence in general that placebo had powerful clinical effects' (Hróbjartsson & Gøtzsche, 2001, pp. 1594–5). This widely cited meta-analysis has sparked an intense debate concerning the purported power of placebo.

Critics of the Hróbjartsson and Gøtzsche (2001) meta-analysis have noted a number of shortcomings. First, they included treatments for a wide variety of conditions, including the common cold, alcohol abuse, smoking, poor oral hygiene, herpes, infertility, mental retardation, marital discord, faecal soiling, Alzheimer's disease, carpal tunnel syndrome and other 'undiagnosed ailments'. It is likely that some of these conditions are responsive to placebo treatment and others not, hence the significant heterogeneity of outcomes reported by Hróbjartsson and Gøtzsche. As noted by Wampold et al. (in press), 'aggregating without regard to

consideration of heterogeneity of disorders and their amenability to placebo action does not allow for detection of a placebo effect should it exist'.

Wampold et al. (2005) reanalyzed the studies in the Hróbjartsson and Gøtzsche (2001) data set after classifying them by the degree to which the disorder was deemed by independent raters to be amenable to placebo treatment and by the adequacy of the experimental design. Disorders like insomnia, chronic pain and depression were deemed to be amenable to placebo treatment, whereas disorders like anemia and bacterial infection were deemed to be not amenable to placebo treatment. Design adequacy involved on such factors as random assignment and the placebo being indistinguishable from the active treatment. The results of this meta-analysis indicated a significant placebo effect in well-designed studies of conditions deemed amenable to placebo treatment, but no placebo effect in well-designed studies for conditions that had been deemed to not be amenable to placebo treatment. A particularly interesting finding in this meta-analysis was that there was no significant drug/placebo difference for conditions deemed amenable to placebo treatment.

These are not the only data indicating a powerful placebo effect. Although there are relatively few clinical trials of medications that include no-treatment control conditions, a number of experimental studies have been designed to investigate the effects of placebos. Numerous studies not included in Hróbjartsson and Gøtzsche's (2001) meta-analysis have shown that placebo analgesics, tranquilizers, stimulants and alcohol produce effects beyond those observed in untreated control conditions (see studies cited in Kirsch, 1997). In addition, a meta-analysis of published clinical trials of antidepressant medication indicated a change of 1.16 standard deviations on measures of depression following administration of placebo antidepressants, compared with a change of 0.37 standard deviations among untreated controls (Kirsch & Sapirstein, 1998). These data indicate a placebo effect size of 0.79 standard deviations. This is a powerful effect by any standard.

Just as inclusion of a placebo control is only one method of evaluating the effects of medical treatments, the inclusion of a no-treatment control group is only one method of evaluating the placebo effect. Medical treatment effects can be inferred when different doses of the same drug produce different effects or when a particular treatment is found to be significantly more effective than an alternative treatment. Similarly, placebo effects can be inferred when different placebos or apparent doses of the same placebo produce significantly different effects or when the effects of a placebo vary as a function of the information provided to the person to whom it is administered. Effects of this sort have been reported in a number of studies. For example:

- Asthmatic patients have been shown to exhibit bronchoconstriction after inhaling a placebo described as a bronchoconstrictor and brochodilation after inhaling a placebo described as a bronchodilator (Luparello et al., 1968; McFadden et al., 1969; Neild & Cameron, 1985; Spector et al., 1976).
- Placebo morphine is considerably more effective than placebo Darvon, which in turn is more effective than placebo aspirin (Evans, 1974). In each case, the placebo is about half as effective as the pharmacologically active drug. Similarly, placebos produce more pain relief when given after a more potent drug than they do

when given after a less potent drug (Kantor *et al.*, 1966). Thus, the effectiveness of a placebo pain reliever varies as a function of its believed effectiveness.

- Placebo and active analgesics are more effective when presented with a well-known brand name (Branthwaite & Cooper, 1981).
- Placebo injections are more effective than placebo pills (de Craen *et al.*, 2000).
- The colour of a placebo can influence its effects (reviewed in de Craen *et al.*, 1996). When administered without information about whether they are simulants or depressives, blue placebo pills produce depressant effects, whereas red placebos induce stimulant effects (Blackwell *et al.*, 1972). Patients report falling asleep significantly more quickly after taking a blue capsule than after taking an orange capsule (Luchelli *et al.*, 1978). Red placebos seem to be more effective pain relievers than white, blue or green placebos (Huskisson, 1974; Nagao *et al.*, 1968).
- The magnitude of the placebo response has been shown to vary as a function of the dose that the person is asked to consume (de Craen *et al.*, 1999; Kirsch & Weixel, 1988).
- Finally, Benedetti and colleagues (Benedetti *et al.*, 2003) developed a methodology for assessing the placebo effect without the use of placebos. Participants gave permission to receive a medication with or without foreknowledge of the onset of administration. Medication was subsequently administered intravenously, in some cases with the patient's knowledge and in other cases without any signal. Using this methodology, they found that substantial proportions of the effects of morphine on pain, stimulation of the subthalamic nucleus in Parkinsonian patients, and beta–blockers (propranolol) and muscarinic antagonists (atropine) on heart rate were due to the placebo effect. In addition, they reported that the effect of diazepam on postoperative anxiety was entirely a placebo effect, as hidden infusions of diazepam were totally ineffective in reducing postoperative anxiety.

Taken together, these data provide ample documentation of the presence of a placebo effect.

Psychological mechanisms underlying the placebo effect

Classical conditioning

How is it that an inert substance can produce psychological and physical changes? Currently, the two most popular explanations of the placebo effect are classical conditioning and response expectancy. Classical conditioning is a phenomena discovered by the Russian physiologist, Ivan Pavlov, at the beginning of the twentieth century. In classical conditioning, a stimulus (called an unconditional stimulus) that automatically elicits a response (called an unconditional response) is paired repeatedly with a neutral stimulus (called a conditional stimulus). After a number of such pairings, the conditional stimulus acquires the capacity to evoke a response (called a conditioned response). Generally, the conditional response is the same as the unconditional response, only weaker. In some cases, however, it appears to be the opposite of the unconditional response, in which case it may be referred to as a compensatory response.

As applied to placebo effects, conditioning theory posits the following sequence of events. Active medications are unconditional stimuli and the therapeutic responses they elicit are unconditional responses. The pills, capsules and injections by means of which the medications are delivered are conditional stimuli. Because these conditional stimuli are repeated paired with the active medications that produce the therapeutic benefits, they acquire the capacity to elicit these benefits as conditional responses.

Conditioning theory appears capable of explaining many placebo effects, but there are also some problems with this explanation. For one thing, the conditional response to morphine is an increase in sensitivity to pain (Siegel, 1983). However, the effect of placebo morphine is a reduction in pain sensitivity. Therefore, it cannot be due to classical conditioning. In fact, it seems to override the conditioning effect. Another problem with the conditioning model of placebo effects is that it does not account well for the existence of placebo effect throughout the history of medicine. Most of the substances that were used as medications before the twentieth century (e.g. turpentine, crushed glass, worms, spiders, furs, feathers, crocodile dung, lizard's blood, frog's sperm, pig's teeth, rotten meat, fly specs, powdered stone, iron filings and human sweat) are now recognized to have been placebos. Because they do not automatically produce therapeutic benefits, they cannot have functioned as unconditional stimuli for placebo effects.

Response expectancy

Response expectancies are anticipation of automatic subjective responses (e.g. changes in pain, anxiety, depression). According to Kirsch (1985), response expectancies tend to elicit the expected response. Thus, the anticipation of anxiety makes people anxious, the belief than one will stay depressed forever is very depressing, and the anticipation of changes in pain alters the perception of pain. More generally, subjective experience appears to be due to a mix of external and internal factors. It is shaped partially by external stimuli and partially by the person's beliefs, expectations and interpretations of those stimuli. As applied to the placebo effect, expectancy theory asserts that placebos produce their effects by changing people's expectations. A placebo antidepressant, for example, leads people to expect a change in their depression, and that expectation makes them feel less depressed. A shortcoming of expectancy theory is that it does not easily account for the physical effects of placebos (see also 'Expectations and health').

Research on conditioning and expectancy

Evidence in support of the classical conditioning model of placebo effects was reported by Voudouris *et al.* (1985; 1989; 1990). They reported an enhanced placebo effect following a series of conditioning trials during which the intensity of a pain stimulus was surreptitiously lowered when paired with placebo administration. They also showed that this conditioning effect was greater than that of a verbal expectancy manipulation. From a cognitive perspective, however, conditioning trials are themselves expectancy manipulations. So what was demonstrated in these studies can be interpreted as indicating that experiential manipulations (i.e. conditioning trials) are more effective than verbal manipulations in altering expectancies, a finding that had previously been reported by expectancy theorists (Wickless & Kirsch, 1989).

Montgomery and Kirsch (1997) conducted an empirical comparison of stimulus substitution and response expectancy interpretations of conditioned placebo effects. In addition to replicating the conditioning procedure used by Voudouris *et al.* (1985; 1989; 1990), Montgomery included an informed paring conditioning group and an extinction control group. The informed pairing condition differed from the usual conditioning group in that subjects were told that the stimulus intensity was being lowered during conditioning trails. If the conditioning effect is a direct consequence of CS–US pairings, it should not be blocked by informing subjects of the manipulation. Conversely, if the conditioning effect is mediated by expectancy, nondeceptive pairings should fail to produce conditioning. Consistent with the expectancy interpretation, an increase in the placebo effect was obtained only when subjects were deceived into thinking that the intensity of the pain stimulus had been held constant. Furthermore, changes in pain reduction were accompanied by corresponding changes in expected pain reduction, indicating that the effect of the conditioning trials was mediated by expectancy.

It is important to note that conditioning theory and expectancy theory are not mutually exclusive. Specifically, classical conditioning may be one of the means by which expectancies are altered. Thus, if an active drug (the US) repeated elicits a particular therapeutic benefit (the UR), it will also lead people to expect that benefit when they think they are taking the drug, and that expectation might produce the placebo effect (the CR). Indeed, it is now widely accepted that classical conditioning works by producing representations (i.e. expectancies) about the consequences of conditional stimuli (Kirsch, Lynn, Vigorito & Miller, 2004).

Individual differences in placebo responding: the search for a placebo responder

There is considerable variation in response to placebo. Some participants may show a strong response, some a weak one and some no response at all. This has led researchers to search for the personality correlates of placebo responding. However, after more than a half century of research, 'the virtually unanimous conclusion among those reviewing the placebo literature is that there is no such thing as the placebo responder' (see review by Brody & Brody, 2000).

The conclusion that there is no such thing as a placebo responder is based on the failure to find reliable personality correlates of the placebo response. However, a failure to find correlates does not necessarily mean that placebo responding is not a personality trait. For example, the search for stable correlates of hypnotic suggestibility has been largely unsuccessful and the few correlates that have been found account for only a tiny proportion of the variance (Kirsch & Council, 1992). Nevertheless, hypnotic responding itself seems to be exceptionally stable, with test re-test correlations as high as 0.75 even with a 25-year interval between testing (Piccione *et al.*, 1989). Thus, hypnotic suggestibility appears to be a stable trait without many stable personality correlates. It is conceivable that this is the case for placebo responding as well, which is also, after all, a form of suggestibility.

Attempts to find correlates of the placebo response could succeed only if there is some reliability in the placebo response. However, it is also possible that there is no such thing as a placebo responder and that placebo response is inherently unreliable. Data in support of this hypothesis were reported in an early but very influential study on the prevention of nausea (Wolf *et al.*, 1957). Participants were successively given placebo treatments for nausea, following which ipecac was administered. Response was defined as blocking the emetic effects of ipecac. This procedure was repeated seven times. Wolf *et al.* reported that response to earlier trials failed to predict response to subsequent trials. On the very last trial, for example, those who had been consistent placebo responders on the previous six trials were no more likely to respond to the placebo than those who had been consistent non-responders.

Although the Wolf *et al.* (1957) study supports the widespread conclusion that there is no such thing as a reliable placebo responder, there are a number of reasons for doubting this conclusion. First, it is not clear whether participants were informed that they might be receiving placebo on at least some trials. If so, they might have anticipated a crossover. In this case, success on a trial might lead them to think that they had received the active medication, rendering it more likely that a subsequent trial would be a placebo trial. This might counteract their tendency to respond to the subsequent trials. A second problem is that there were only 35 participants in the Wolf *et al.* (1957) study. Thus, the power was low for detecting a significant relationship. Third, because there was no no-treatment control condition and ipecac does not always produce nausea, it is possible that the non-occurrence of nausea on some trials was not always due to placebo administration.

Placebo psychotherapy

Given the importance of placebo effects in medical interventions, it was only natural that researchers began to question the degree to which the effects of psychological interventions might be placebo effects. To answer that question, studies were designed to include placebo psychotherapies, the effects of which can be compared to the genuine treatment (e.g. Paul, 1966). At first glance, this strategy seems reasonable, but, in fact, it is very problematic (Kirsch, 1978). There are both practical and conceptual problems with attempts to extend the placebo concept from the medical setting to the psychotherapeutic setting. Practically, it cannot be done; conceptually, it makes no sense to try.

The practical problem

In medical research, the purpose of using a placebo is to control for the psychologically produced effects of a particular treatment. To do this, it is important that the placebo have the same psychological properties as the treatment it is replacing. With pills and injections, this is easy. All that is needed is to omit the active ingredient. Thus, the placebo is the same size, shape, colour, taste and smell as the active medication. It is also provided with the same label and information.

With psychological treatments, constructing a matching placebo is impossible. By definition, a psychological treatment has no active physical properties. All of its ingredients are psychological. If a psychological treatment contained the same psychological properties as the real treatment (i.e. if the therapist used the same words and procedures), it would no longer be a placebo or a control condition of any other kind. Instead, it would be the treatment.

As a result, procedures used as placebos in psychotherapy research are usually very different than the psychotherapies to which they are being compared. Among the procedures used as 'placebos' in psychotherapy research are the following: listening to stories, reading books, attending language classes, viewing films, participating in 'bull' sessions, playing with puzzles, sitting quietly with a silent therapist and discussing current events (see Prioleau *et al.*, 1983). Indeed, simply being placed on a waiting list has been labelled a placebo (e.g. Sloane *et al.*, 1975).

The conceptual problem

Following the medical model, it has become common to partition the response to psychotherapy as due to specific and non-specific factors, the latter being thought of as placebo effects. In medical research, that partition is unproblematic. Specific effects are those due to the chemical properties of the medication (or physical properties of a surgical intervention), whereas non-specific effects are those due to the psychological properties of the intervention. In psychotherapy research, the situation is altogether different. We do not need placebo controls to determine whether the physical properties of the treatment have an effect. We know the answer to that question without doing any studies at all, and that answer is no. Most psychotherapies do not have physically active properties. Their substance is words, and it is clearly not the sound of the words that are having an effect. Rather, it is their meaning. Moerman and Jonas (Moerman & Jonas, 2002) have defined the placebo effect as a patient's response to the meaning of a treatment. In this sense, most psychotherapy is a placebo by definition. That is, it is a treatment that is effective because of its psychological properties rather than its physical properties.

There are some treatment characteristics which are common to most psychotherapies and these are often referred to as placebo factors. Common factors include the establishment of a therapeutic relationship, discussion of the presenting problem; cognitive restructuring; and the provision of warmth, empathy, positive regard and response-contingent reinforcement, all of which might thus be labelled 'placebo factors'. Conversely, the specific rationale provided to clients about how the treatment works varies from treatment to treatment. So this would not be a placebo factor. It is worthwhile to examine the degree to which the effects of various psychotherapies are due to common factors, and comparative effect sizes suggest that this may account for a substantial proportion of treatment effects (Smith *et al.*, 1980; Wampold, 2001). However, this does not mean that psychotherapy is a placebo. Rather, it indicates the conceptual problem of applying the placebo concept to psychotherapy.

Clinical implications

Clinical use of placebos is relatively common. A survey of physicians and nurses, 60% acknowledged giving patients placebos (Nitzan & Lichtenberg, 2004). Given clinical benefits that are sometimes substantial and coupled with low rates of side-effects, it is not surprising that health providers would want to use them. Galvanizing the placebo effect may be especially useful in disorders like depression, in which placebos are almost effective as active medications (Kirsch *et al.*, 2002; Kirsch, Scoboria & Moore, 2002) and in which the medications pose serious side effect risks (Healy, 2003; Healy & Whitaker, 2003). The problem, however, is to find a way to capitalize on the placebo effect without deception. One way of doing this is to look for alternative treatments (e.g. physical exercise as a treatment for depression) which have been shown to provide benefit without incurring significant risk. The effects of these alternative treatments may also be largely due to the placebo effect, but this has not yet been demonstrated, and the side-effect profile may render these alternatives preferable. A second way to elicit the placebo effect without deception is to prescribe psychotherapy for disorders amenable to psychological treatment. In the case of depression, for example, meta-analyses indicate that psychotherapy is as effective as medication, possibly with the added benefit of a lower relapse rate (Hollon *et al.*, 1991).

The placebo effect may also enhance the benefits of an effective active treatment (Benedetti *et al.*, 2003). For that reason, clinicians should be careful about how they present the treatments they are administering or prescribing. Two different quantitative dimensions along which placebos can vary are the subjective probability or confidence that a change will occur and the magnitude of the expected change (Kirsch & Weixel, 1988). If too large a change is expected, a negative placebo effect may occur. For that reason, inculcation of high levels of confidence for initially subtle improvement may be optimal.

Conclusions

Placebos can affect a wide variety of conditions, and their effects can be substantial, in some cases coming close to duplicating the effects of active medications. These effects are specific to the type of placebo administered. Thus, placebo stimulants produce arousal, placebo sedatives produce sedation and so on. In addition, placebo effects can be observed in healthy volunteers. Thus, placebo effects cannot be fully explained by such factors as hope, faith or the therapeutic relationship. The effects of placebos seem to be mediated by response expectancies, and these can be produced or modified by classical conditioning. There is some evidence that placebo effects and drug effects are additive. This suggests the advisability of maximizing the placebo component of treatment, by inculcating realistically positive outcome expectations.

REFERENCES

Beecher, H. K. (1955). The powerful placebo. *Journal of the American Medical Association*, **159**(17), 1602–6.

Beecher, H. K. (1961). Surgery as placebo: a quantitative study of bias. *Journal of the American Medical Association*, **176**, 1102–7.

Benedetti, F., Maggi, G., Lopiano, L. *et al.* (2003). Open versus hidden medical treatments: the patient's knowledge about a therapy affects the therapy outcome. *Prevention & Treatment, 6, Article 1*. Available on the World Wide Web: http://journals.apa.org/prevention/volume6/pre0060001a.html.

Blackwell, B., Bloomfield, S. S. & Buncher, C. R. (1972). Demonstration to medical students of placebo responses and non-drug factors. *The Lancet, 19*, 1279–82.

Branthwaite, A. & Cooper, P. (1981). Analgesic effects of branding in treatment of headaches. *British Medical Journal (Clin Res Ed), 282*(6276), 1576–8.

Brody, H. & Brody, D. (2000). *The placebo response: how you can release the body's inner pharmacy for better health*. New York: Cliff Street Books/HarperCollins Publishers.

Cobb, L., Thomas, G. I., Dillard, D. H., Merendino, K. A. & Bruce, R. A. (1959). An evaluation of internal-mammary artery ligation by a double blind technique. *New England Journal of Medicine, 260*, 1115–8.

de Craen, A. J. M., Moerman, D. E., Heisterkamp, S. H. *et al.* (1999). Placebo effect in the treatment of duodenal ulcer. *British Journal of Clinical Pharmacology, 48*, 853–60.

de Craen, A. J. M., Roos, P. J., de Vries, A. L. & Kleijnen, J. (1996). Effect of colour of drugs: systematic review of perceived effect of drugs and their effectiveness. *British Medical Journal, 313*, 1624–6.

de Craen, A. J. M., Tijssen, J. G. P., de Gans, J. & Kleijnen, J. (2000). Placebo effect in the acute treatment of migraine: subcutaneous placebos are better than oral placebos. *Journal of Neurology, 247*, 183–8.

Dimond, E. G., Kittle, C. F. & Crockett, J. E. (1960). Comparison of internal mammary ligation and sham operation for angina pectoris. *American Journal of Cardiology, 5*, 483–6.

Evans, F. J. (1974). The placebo response in pain reduction. *Advances in Neurology, 4*, 289–96.

Healy, D. (2003). Lines of evidence on the risks of suicide with selective serotonin reuptake inhibitors. *Psychotherapy and Psychosomatics, 72*(2), 71–9.

Healy, D. & Whitaker, C. (2003). Antidepressants and suicide: risk–benefit conundrums. *Journal of Psychiatry and Neuroscience, 28*(5), 331–7.

Hollon, S. D., Shelton, R. C. & Loosen, P. T. (1991). Cognitive therapy and pharmacotherapy for depression. *Journal of Consulting and Clinical Psychology, 59*, 88–99.

Honigfeld, G. (1964*a*). Non-specific Factors in Treatment. I. Review of Placebo Reactions and Placebo Reactors. *Diseases of the Nervous System, 25*, 145–56.

Honigfeld, G. (1964*b*). Non-specific Factors in Treatment. II. Review of Social–Psychological Factors. *Diseases of the Nervous System, 25*, 225–39.

Hróbjartsson, A. & Gøtzsche, P. C. (2001). An analysis of clinical trials comparing placebo with no treatment. *New England Journal of Medicine, 344*, 1594–602.

Huskisson, E. (1974). Simple analgesics for arthritis. *British Medical Journal*, 196–200.

Kantor, T. G., Sunshine, A., Laska, E., Meisner, M. & Hopper, M. (1966). Oral analgesic studies: pentazocine hydrochloride, codeine, aspirin, and placebo and their influence on response to placebo. *Clinical Pharmacology and Therapeutics, 7*(4), 447–54.

Kirsch, I. (1978). The placebo effect and the cognitive-behavioral revolution. *Cognitive Therapy and Research, 2*(3), 255–64.

Kirsch, I. (1985). Response Expectancy as a Determinant of Experience and Behavior. *American Psychologist, 40*(11), 1189–202.

Kirsch, I. (1997). Specifying nonspecifics: psychological mechanisms of placebo effects. In Harrington, A. (Ed.). *The placebo effect: an interdisciplinary exploration* (pp. 166–86). Cambridge, MA: Harvard University Press.

Kirsch, I. & Council, J. R. (1992). Situational and personality correlates of hypnotic responsiveness. In Nash, M. R. & Fromm, E. (Ed.). *Contemporary hypnosis research* (pp. 267–91). New York, NY: Guilford Press.

Kirsch, I., Lynn, S. J., Vigorito, M. & Miller, R. R. (2004). The role of cognition in classical and operant conditioning. *Journal of Clinical Psychology, 60*(4), 369–92.

Kirsch, I., Moore, T. J., Scoboria, A. & Nicholls, S. S. (2002). The emperor's new drugs: an analysis of antidepressant medication data submitted to the U.S. Food and Drug Administration. *Prevention and Treatment, 5*. Available on the World Wide Web: http://www.journals.apa.org/prevention/volume5/pre0050023a.html.

Kirsch, I. & Sapirstein, G. (1998). Listening to Prozac but hearing placebo: a meta-analysis of antidepressant medication. *Prevention and Treatment, 1, Article 0002a*, Available on the World Wide Web: http://www.journals.apa.org/prevention/volume1/pre0010002a.html.

Kirsch, I., Scoboria, A. & Moore, T. J. (2002). Antidepressants and placebos: secrets, revelations, and unanswered questions. *Prevention and Treatment*. Available on the World Wide Web: http://www.journals.apa.org/prevention/volume5/pre0050033r.html.

Kirsch, I. & Weixel, L. J. (1988). Double-blind versus deceptive administration of a placebo. *Behavioral Neuroscience, 102*(2), 319–23.

Klopfer, B. (1957). Psychological variables in human cancer. *Journal of Protective Techniques, 21*(4), 331–40.

Luchelli, P. E., Cattaneo, A. D. & Zattoni, J. (1978). *European Journal of Clinical Pharmacology, 13*, 153–5.

Luparello, T., Lyons, H. A., Bleecker, E. R. & McFadden, E. R., Jr. (1968). Influences of suggestion on airway reactivity in asthmatic subjects. *Psychosomatic Medicine, 30*(6), 819–25.

McFadden, E. R., Jr., Luparello, T., Lyons, H. A., Bleecker, E. & Bleecker, E. R. (1969). The mechanism of action of suggestion in the induction of acute asthma attacks: influences of suggestion on airway reactivity in asthmatic subjects. *Psychosomatic Medicine, 31*(2), 134–43.

Moerman, D. E. & Jonas, W. B. (2002). Deconstructing the placebo effect and finding the meaning response. *Annals of Internal Medicine, 136*, 471–6.

Montgomery, G. H. & Kirsch, I. (1997). Classical conditioning and the placebo effect. *Pain, 72*(1–2), 107–13.

Moseley, J. B., O'Malley, K., Petersen, N. J. *et al.* (2002). A controlled trial of arthroscopic surgery for osteoarthritis of the knee. *New England Journal of Medicine, 347*, 81–8.

Nagao, Y., Komia, J., Kuroanagi, K., Minaba, Y. & Susa, A. (1968). Effect of the color of analgesics on their therapeutic results. *Shikwa Gakuho, 68*, 139–42.

Neild, J. E. & Cameron, I. R. (1985). Bronchoconstriction in response to suggestion: its prevention by an inhaled anticholinergic agent. *British Medical Journal (Clin Res Ed), 290*(6469), 674.

Nitzan, U. & Lichtenberg, P. (2004). Questionnaire survey on use of placebo. *British Medical Journal, 329*(7472), 944–6.

Paul, G. L. (1966). *Insight vs. desensitization in psychotherapy*. Stanford, CA: Stanford University Press.

Piccione, C., Hilgard, E. R. & Zimbardo, P. G. (1989). On the degree of stability of measured hypnotizability over a 25-year period. *Journal of Personality and Social Psychology, 56*, 289–95.

Prioleau, L., Murdock, M. & Brody, N. (1983). An analysis of psychotherapy versus placebo studies. *Behavioral and Brain Sciences, 6*, 275–310.

Siegel, S. (1983). Classic conditioning, drug tolerance, and drug dependence. In W. Schmidt (Ed.). *Research advances in alcohol and drug problems Vol. 7* (pp. 207–46). New York: Plenum.

Sloane, R. B., Staples, F. R., Cristol, A. H., Yorkston, N. J. & Whipple, K. (1975). *Psychotherapy versus behavior therapy.* Cambridge, MA: Harvard University Press.

Smith, M. L., Glass, G. V. & Miller, T. I. (1980). *The benefits of psychotherapy.* Baltimore, MD: John Hopkins University Press.

Spector, S., Luparello, T. J., Kopetzky, M. T. *et al.* (1976). Response of asthmatics to methacholine and suggestion. *American Review of Respiratory Disease*, **113**(1), 43–50.

Volgyesi, F. A. (1954). "School for patients", hypnosis therapy and psycho prophylaxis. *British Journal of Medical Hypnotism*, **5**, 8–17.

Voudouris, N. J., Peck, C. L. & Coleman, G. (1985). Conditioned placebo responses. *Journal of Personality and Social Psychology*, **48**, 47–53.

Voudouris, N. J., Peck, C. L. & Coleman, G. (1989). Conditioned response models of placebo phenomena: further support. *Pain*, **38**, 109–16.

Voudouris, N. J., Peck, C. L. & Coleman, G. (1990). The role of conditioning and verbal expectancy in the placebo response. *Pain*, **43**, 121–8.

Wampold, B. E. (2001). *The great psychotherapy debate: models, methods, and findings.* Mahwah, NJ: Lawrence Erlbaum Associates.

Wampold, B. E., Minami, T., Tierney, S. C., Baskin, T. W. & Bhati, K. S. (in press). The Placebo Is Powerful: Estimating Placebo Effects in Medicine and Psychotherapy from Randomized Clinical Trials. *Journal of Clinical Psychology*.

Wickless, C. & Kirsch, I. (1989). Effects of verbal and experiential expectancy manipulations on hypnotic-susceptibility. *Journal of Personality and Social Psychology*, **57**(5), 762–8.

Wolf, S., Doering, C. R., Clark, M. L. & Hagans, J. A. (1957). Chance distribution and the placebo "reactor." *Journal of Laboratory and Clinical Medicine*, **49**, 837–41.

Psychoneuroimmunology

Elizabeth Bachen[1], Sheldon Cohen[2] and Anna L. Marsland[3]

[1]Mills College
[2]Carnegie Mellon University
[3]University of Pittsburgh

Introduction

Stressful life events have been linked to a range of immune-related disorders, including autoimmune diseases, infectious diseases and cancer. Some of the most compelling evidence for stress and disease associations stems from viral challenge studies, in which volunteers are exposed to a cold or influenza virus and then monitored in quarantine for the development of infection and illness. These studies find that individuals with more life stress, as measured by a higher number of recent stressful life events, higher perceived stress and more negative affect are more likely to develop colds than individuals with lower levels of stress (Cohen *et al.*, 1991), and that stressful events lasting a month or more are better predictors of developing colds than those of a briefer duration (Cohen *et al.*, 1998). In addition, individuals who are more sociable and have a diverse social network are less likely to develop a cold (Cohen *et al.*, 2003; Cohen *et al.*, 1997), possibly because such factors may be able to decrease the frequency of stressful life events or buffer deleterious effects of stress.

In addition to disease outcomes, stressful life events may also delay the healing of wounds. Recent studies have shown that long-term care givers who were caring for a severely ill family member experienced greater emotional distress and took nine days longer to heal a dermal punch biopsy wound than age- and income-matched controls (Kiecolt-Glaser *et al.*, 1995). Similar findings were observed in dental students, whose punch biopsy wounds healed 40% more slowly during an examination period than during vacation (Marucha *et al.*, 1998). Such decrements in wound repair may have important implications with regard to surgical recovery and clinical wound repair. Broadbent *et al.* (2003) found that in patients undergoing a hernia operation, those with greater perceptions of stress and worry prior to operation had a more painful, poorer and slower recovery. Among patients at a wound clinic, Cole-King & Harding (2001) found that the healing of leg ulcers was delayed in individuals with higher levels of anxiety and depression (see also 'Life events and health' and 'Stress and health').

Potential mechanisms linking stress and immune disease

One means by which stress may lead to increased susceptibility to disease is by altering the function of the immune system. This hypothesis is one of the central concerns of the field of psycho-neuroimmunology (PNI) which attempts to elucidate the relations between psychosocial factors, nervous, endocrine and immune

Table 1. Cells of the immune system

Cell type	Function
White blood cells (WBCs)/Leukocytes	Respond to antigens such as bacteria or viruses and altered host cells such as tumour or infected cells; include lymphocytes and phagocytes
Lymphocytes	Subset of WBCs that include T- and B-lymphocytes and NK cells; functions described below
T-helper lymphocytes	Enhance immune responses by stimulating T-cell replication and activating antibody production by B-lymphocytes
T-suppressor lymphocytes	Inhibit immune responses
T-cytotoxic lymphocytes	Destroy virus-, parasite- and tumour-infected cells; reject transplanted tissue
B-lymphocytes	Produce antibodies
NK cells	Destroy virally infected and tumour cells
Phagocytes	Subset of WBCs that include basophils, eosinophils, neutrophils, monocytes and macrophages; ingest and destroy antigens

systems and health. How stress may influence the immune system is not entirely clear. Stress may alter immune responses through the adoption of coping behaviours, such as smoking or drinking alcohol, that are known to compromise immunity (Kiecolt-Glaser & Glaser, 1988). Alternatively, stress may directly influence immune function through the activation of neuroendocrine pathways that lead to the release of various hormones and neurotransmitters, such as cortisol and catecholamines. Sympathetic nerve fibres innervate lymphoid organs, and immune cells, which migrate between lymphoid organs and the peripheral bloodstream, contain receptors for numerous hormones and neurotransmitters that are produced during stress (Plaut, 1987).

In PNI research, the most commonly measured component of the immune system is the immune cells, which are collectively known as white blood cells (WBCs) or leukocytes. While there are many types of leukocytes, each with distinct functions, such cells are interdependent and perform their functions in an orchestrated fashion to achieve immunocompetence. Table 1 lists the different types of immune cells and their primary functions.

Leukocytes also produce substances called cytokines. Cytokines which are produced by a subset of T-helper cells, called Th1 cells, include IL-2, TNFβ and INFγ. These cytokines selectively activate T-cytotoxic cells and NK cells and thus promote cellular immunity. Cytokines produced by Th2 helper-cells include IL-4, IL-5, IL-6 and IL-13; they selectively activate B-cells and induce antibody production, thus promoting humoral immunity. For a description of measurements of immunocompetence in PNI research see the chapter on 'Psychoneuroimmunology assessments'.

Psychological stress and immunity

A substantial literature in both humans and animals supports associations between immunologic changes and psychological and physical forms of stress (for a recent review, see Segerstrom & Miller, 2004). While the most frequently reported consequence of stressful events is the suppression of immune responses, other research suggests that some forms of stress may be able to both enhance and suppress aspects of the immune response by altering patterns of cytokine secretion (Marshall et al., 1998). Because the cytokines of Th1 and Th2 cells antagonize each other, a suppression of one response may result in enhanced production of the other.

Naturalistic stressors and immunity

Academic stressors

Some of the most commonly examined stressors in relation to immunologic status have been examinations and other forms of academic stress. Indeed, several indices of immunosuppression have been observed among medical students during final exams. Compared to test-free periods, students undergoing exams have shown decrements in lymphocyte response to mitogenic stimulation, reduced NK cell activity, alterations in T-cell populations, increased plasma levels of circulating antibodies and changes in cytokine production (Kennedy et al., 1988; Marshall et al., 1998). Increased levels of circulating antibodies to Epstein–Barr and other herpes viruses have also been observed during examination periods, indicating, perhaps, the reactivation of latent virus by either direct neuroendocrine influences or weakened immunocompetence.

Several studies have found that some individuals are more susceptible to immune alterations during exams than others. For example, the largest immunologic changes were found to occur in students with the highest levels of overall life stress, anxiety, loneliness or tendency to ruminate about stressful events (Glaser et al., 1992; Kiecolt-Glaser et al., 1984; Marshall et al., 1998; Workman & La Via, 1987). Personality styles associated with greater positive affect and adaptive coping strategies may attenuate stress-related immune alterations. Segerstrom et al. (1998) observed that optimistic first-year law students had higher levels of T-helper cells and NK cell cytoxicity during their first semester of law school than did pessimistic students (see 'Personality and health').

While most studies support an effect of immune suppression from examination stress, other recent findings suggest that exams and other brief naturalistic stressors may increase Th2 cell-mediated humoral immunity and macrophage activity, and concurrently decrease Th1 cell-mediated cellular immunity. In a recent meta-analytic review of the PNI field, Segerstrom and Miller (2004) found that examinations are often associated with increases in IL-6 and IL-10, and decreases in IFN-γ. The decreased Th1 cytokine production is consistent with observed decreases in T-cell proliferative responses and NK cell activity, and increased antibody production to latent viruses. It is also possible that an increase in humoral activity during stress might contribute to an increased incidence of type-2-mediated conditions, such as allergic/asthmatic reactions and heightened autoimmune activity (Marshall et al., 1998).

Bereavement

The loss of an intimate relationship from either death or divorce has also been associated with altered immunity, including suppression of lymphocyte responses to mitogenic stimulation, reduced NK cell activity and changes in T-cell sub-populations. Early investigations found lowered mitogenic lymphocyte proliferation in bereaved subjects following the loss of a spouse (Bartrop *et al.*, 1977) and that the degree of immune change was related to the severity of depressive response before and after the loss (Irwin *et al.*, 1987). In men infected with the human immunodeficiency virus (HIV), the death of an intimate partner or close friend has been found to result in lowered NK cell activity and proliferative responses to PHA compared with nonbereaved, HIV-infected men (Goodkin *et al.*, 1996; Kemeny *et al.*, 1995). Findings relating bereavement to numbers of T-helper (CD4) cells in HIV-positive men have been mixed, with some studies showing no relationship (Goodkin *et al.*, 1996; Kemeny *et al.*, 1995), and others linking bereavement to an enhanced CD4 decline (Kemeny & Dean, 1995) (see 'Coping with bereavement').

Separation, divorce and marital conflict

Separation, divorce and marital conflict have similarly been associated with immune alterations. Kiecolt-Glaser, Glaser, and colleagues found that recently separated or divorced women demonstrated lower percentages of circulating NK and T-helper cells, decreased proliferative responses to PHA and Con A, and higher antibodies to Epstein–Barr virus than a comparison group of married persons (see Kennedy *et al.*, 1988). Higher antibody levels to latent viruses were also found in separated or divorced men and couples reporting poorer marital quality (Kennedy *et al.*, 1988). Finally, studies from this research group have found that marital conflict that includes hostile interactions may evoke fairly persistent immune changes, even when couples report being happily married (Kiecolt-Glaser *et al.*, 1993; Kiecolt-Glaser *et al.*, 1997). In a study of newly-wed couples, those who exhibited more hostile or negative behaviours during a brief conflict resolution task were found to exhibit greater declines in functional immune measures 24 hours later (Kiecolt-Glaser *et al.*, 1993). Similar results were found in couples who had been married an average of 42 years (Kiecolt-Glaser *et al.*, 1997).

Other prolonged stressful events

Immunologic changes accompany other prolonged stressors, as well, such as long-term unemployment, occupational stress and care giving for a terminally ill patient. In an examination of the immune-related effects of care giving for a family member with Alzheimer's Disease, Kiecolt-Glaser and colleagues found that caregivers exhibited lower percentages of total lymphocytes and T-helper cell subsets, and higher antibody titers to Epstein Barr virus (Kiecolt-Glaser *et al.*, 1987). In addition, care givers demonstrated lower antibody responses to both influenza virus and pneumococcal pneumonia vaccines compared with age-matched controls (Glaser *et al.*, 2000; Kiecolt-Glaser *et al.*, 1996; Vedhara *et al.*, 1999). In two of these studies, fewer care givers achieved the four-fold increase in antibody titre (used as a marker of vaccination success) than did controls (Kiecolt-Glaser *et al.*, 1996; Vedhara *et al.*, 1999). Given the increased morbidity and mortality among the elderly after exposure to influenza viruses, such findings may be of clinical importance. Finally, there is evidence that chronic stress and depression may contribute to the greater production of cytokines (Anisman & Merali, 2002) or a dysregulated cytokine response to vaccination (Glaser *et al.*, 2003). Higher levels of plasma IL-6 were observed in a group of care givers compared to individuals who were anticipating a housing relocation or community controls (Lutgendorf *et al.*, 1999). In older adults receiving an annual influenza vaccination, those with more depressive symptoms showed an increase in plasma IL-6 by two weeks after vaccination, whereas there was little change in adults reporting few or no symptoms of depression. Such findings suggest that depressed mood may be related to an amplified and prolonged inflammatory response after vaccination (Glaser *et al.*, 2003).

Both job stress and long-term unemployment have been linked to lowered lymphocyte reactivity to PHA (Arnetz *et al.*, 1987). In contrast to stress and burnout at work, a high sense of personal accomplishment at work may be associated with higher numbers of peripheral lymphocytes, particularly T-cell subsets (Bargellini *et al.*, 2000).

Traumatic events

Fewer studies have examined immunologic changes associated with exposure to extreme traumatic stressors, such as natural disasters, and accidental and deliberate man-made traumatic events. Such studies, however suggest that immune alterations may persist for long periods of time, particularly if symptoms of rumination, anxiety or post-traumatic stress disorder (PTSD) result. In an early study, persistent distress over the nuclear accident at Three Mile Island was associated with higher latent antibody levels and enumerative immune alterations in community residents more than six years after the accident (McKinnon *et al.*, 1989). Symptoms of PTSD were also related to lower NK cell cytotoxicity in residents of neighbourhoods that were damaged by Hurricane Andrew and this effect appeared to be mediated by the development of sleep disturbances associated with the trauma (Ironson *et al.*, 1997).

Two studies have investigated immune alterations in released male prisoners of war and women living in a refugee camp during the Bosnian and Croatian wars (Dekaris *et al.*, 1993; Sabioncello *et al.*, 2000). Both studies found higher numbers of activated lymphocytes in these individuals, compared with laboratory staff controls, along with an increase in proliferating lymphocytes in the female refugees (Sabioncello *et al.*, 2000). Although neither study included assessments for PTSD, other research suggests that the development of PTSD following war and other catastrophic events may be associated with elevated serum IL-6 and IL-1β concentrations (Maes *et al.*, 1999; Spivak *et al.*, 1997), and NK cell activity (Laudenslager *et al.*, 1998). In addition, there is preliminary evidence that veterans with current PSTD or anxiety mount greater cutaneous delayed hypersensitivity test reactions than do veterans without PTSD, suggesting that exposure to disasters and the development of PTSD may be associated with enhanced cell-mediated immunity (Boscarino & Chang, 1999). Despite the methodological difficulties in this area, these findings remain interesting because they counter evidence that chronic stress suppresses immune functions. These disparate results may be due, in part, to a dysregulation of the HPA axis in PTSD, whereby persistent activation of the HPA axis and enhanced negative feedback of this system lead to lower plasma and urinary cortisol concentrations (Yehuda et al., 1990).

Taken together, most studies involving stress and immunity indicate that psychological stressors are associated with changes in immune functions. The most consistent alterations include reduced NK cell activity and lymphocyte proliferation to PHA and Con A, and increased antibody levels to latent herpes viruses. Changes in percentages or absolute numbers of lymphocyte populations are also frequently reported stress-related immune responses, although these changes are weaker and not as reliable across studies (Segerstrom & Miller, 2004). Preliminary studies also suggest that brief forms of stress may lead to cytokine changes that promote a shift from cellular (Th1) immunity to humoral (Th2) immunity and that traumatic events such as disasters might be linked to enhanced immune function, perhaps in the context of post-traumatic stress disorder and diminished cortisol levels.

Short-term laboratory stressors and immunity

During the last decade, many laboratory studies have been conducted to examine stress-immune interactions. Such investigations are advantageous because they approximate the effects of transient daily life stressors and provide a means to investigate potential endocrine mechanisms underlying associated immunological changes. A number of standardized laboratory stressors have been used in these experiments, including challenging computer tasks, mental arithmetic, electrical shocks, loud noise, unsolvable puzzles, graphic films depicting combat surgery, marital discussions involving conflict and mood manipulation tasks. Exposure to these stressors has been shown to evoke a variety of enumerative immune changes, the most consistent of which are increases in the numbers of circulating NK cells and T-suppressor/cytotoxic lymphocytes, and a decrease in the ratio of T-helper to T-suppressor cells. Decreases in lymphocyte mitogenesis and increased NK cell activity are also commonly reported (for a review, see Kiecolt-Glaser et al., 1992). Less is known about cytokine responses to acute psychological stressors, but preliminary reports indicate that such tasks can evoke increases in serum levels and mitogen-induced production of certain cytokines, such as IL-6 and TNF-α (Kunz-Ebrecht et al., 2003; Steptoe et al., 2001), although negative findings have also been reported (Heesen et al., 2002).

The data suggest that most of the immunologic changes following acute stress are rapid and transient, occurring as early as 5 minutes from stressor onset (Herbert et al., 1994). One exception to this rapid response may be stress-induced alterations in serum cytokine levels, which, in some cases, may not be detectable until 45 minutes post-stress (Kunz-Ebrecht et al., 2003; Steptoe et al., 2001). The duration of immunological reactions to acute mental stress may also depend on the parameter in question. Changes in cell redistribution return to baseline within 15 minutes of stressor termination (Brosschot et al., 1992), whereas changes in immune function may persist for at least 90 minutes after challenge (Zakowski et al., 1992).

There is now a great deal of evidence that acute immune responses to psychological stress are largely mediated by activation of the sympathetic nervous system. The most direct evidence for sympathetic mediation is derived from the observation that changes in cellular immune function under stress are ameliorated by the prior administration of an adrenoceptor antagonist (Bachen et al., 1995). Consistent with these findings, studies have also shown that individuals who demonstrate the greatest sympathetic reactions to brief mental stress (as indicated by heightened cardiovascular and catecholamine responses) also produce the greatest immunologic changes (Manuck et al., 1991).

The extent to which individuals differ in their sympathetic, endocrine and immunological responses to stress may have implications for their susceptibility to stress-related illnesses. Recently, investigations have demonstrated that sympathetic and immunologic reactions to brief psychological stress may predict antibody responses to vaccines. Marsland et al. (2001) found that medical students who demonstrated the greatest decline in lymphocyte proliferation to PHA following laboratory stress also had the poorest antibody response to a hepatitis B vaccination programme. Cacioppo (1994) also found that sympathetic activation predicted response to an influenza vaccination, with a measured T-cell response declining more quickly in individuals who showed greater cardiac sympathetic activation following a mental task. Similarly, Burns et al. (2002) found that individuals who responded to acute stress with a larger cardiac output (reflecting heightened cardiac activation mediated by beta-adrenergic processes), exhibited lower antibody titres to hepatitis B vaccination, compared with those demonstrating a smaller cardiac output. How concomitant changes in other stress-related substances, such as cortisol may influence antibody responses to vaccines is currently unclear, but it is noteworthy that positive relationships between the magnitude of sympathetic and cortisol responses to acute stress have been reported (Cacioppo et al., 1994).

Implications and future directions

Stressors of various types do induce a wide range of immunologic alterations in humans. It is through such changes in immune system functioning that stressors may ultimately be linked to subsequent disease. Before these firm conclusions can be reached, however, several gaps in our knowledge of stress-immune-disease relationships must be empirically addressed. Apart from the experimental studies on susceptibility to colds and wound healing in the PNI field, few studies have measured health outcomes. For example, no studies examining the effects of stress on antibody responses to vaccines have included an assessment of vaccine efficacy in terms of disease incidence and severity (Burns et al., 2003). The importance of measuring health outcomes is highlighted by the fact that immune responses of stressed persons generally fall within normal ranges and thus it remains unclear if the nature and magnitude of immunologic change found in PNI research bears relevance to increased disease susceptibility.

Additional research that focuses on populations that may be most susceptible to the influence of stress is also needed. Older people are known to have greatly increased morbidity and mortality from infectious illness and immune alterations associated with ageing include decreases in proliferative responses to mitogens, natural killer cell activity, antibody production and phagocytic activity (Scapagnini, 1992) as well as increases in IL-6 production (Cohen, 2000). Stress-related immune alterations may have more important consequences for individuals with already compromised immune systems, such as the elderly or those with autoimmune disorders or HIV-infection (Kiecolt-Glaser & Glaser, 1987).

There is little empirical evidence defining the roles of health behaviours and other mechanisms in evoking immunologic changes to stress. Preliminary evidence indicates that sleep disturbances following stress may play an important mechanistic role (Ironson et al., 1997). Interactive effects between health practices and other variables may also be important to consider, especially for behavioural changes that are moderate. For example, Jung et al. (1999) found that mild to moderate levels of cigarette smoking were associated with lower NK cell activity, but only in individuals who were also depressed. Further research on neuroendocrine influences on immune alterations during naturalistic stress is also needed, but is complicated by regulatory processes that accompany prolonged stress, such as negative feedback systems, receptor down-regulation and shifts in circadian rhythms. Despite these complexities, naturalistic studies do suggest that both the sympathetic nervous system and HPA axis play important roles in modulating immune function during stress (Burns et al., 2002; Goodkin et al., 1996; Mckinnon et al., 1989; Vedhara et al., 1999).

In conclusion, during the last 30 years, PNI research has made great strides in identifying relationships between psychological stressors and altered functioning in the immune system. This remains one of the most promising pathways through which stress may alter host resistance to disease onset or exacerbation. Carefully designed prospective studies, measuring all three aspects of the stress-immune-disease model are needed to more fully understand these associations.

REFERENCES

Anisman, H. & Merali, Z. (2002). Cytokines, stress, and depressive illness. *Brain, Behavior, and Immunity*, **16**, 513–24.

Arnetz, B. B., Wasserman, J., Petrini, B. et al. (1987). Immune function in unemployed women. *Psychosomatic Medicine*, **49**, 3–12.

Bachen, E. A., Manuck, S. B., Cohen, S. et al. (1995). Adrenergic blockade ameliorates cellular immune responses to stress in humans. *Psychosomatic Medicine*, **57**, 366–72.

Bargellini, A., Barbieri, A., Rovesti, S. et al. (2000). Relation between immune variables and burnout in a sample of physicians. *Occupational and Environmental Medicine*, **57**, 453–7.

Bartrop, R., Lazarus, L., Luckhurst, E., Kiloh, L. G. & Penny, R. (1977). Depressed lymphocyte function after bereavement. *Lancet*, **i**, 834–6.

Boscarino, J. A. & Chang, J. (1999). Higher abnormal leukocyte and lymphocyte counts 20 years after exposure to severe stress: research and clinical implications. *Psychosomatic Medicine*, **61**, 278–386.

Broadbent, E., Petrie, K. J., Alley, P. G. & Booth, R. J. (2003). Psychosocial stress impairs early wound repair following surgery. *Psychosomatic Medicine*, **65**, 865–9.

Brosschot, J. F., Benschop, R. J., Godaert, G. L., Heijnen, C. J. & Balieux, R. E. (1992). Effects of experimental psychological stress on distribution and function of peripheral blood cells. *Psychosomatic Medicine*, **54**, 394–406.

Burns, V. E., Carroll, D., Ring, C. & Drayson, M. (2003). Antibody response to vaccination and psychosocial stress in humans: relationships and mechanisms. *Vaccine*, **21**, 2523–34.

Burns, V. E., Ring, C., Drayson, M. & Carroll, D. (2002). Cortisol and cardiovascular reactions to mental stress and antibody status following hepatitis B vaccination: a preliminary study. *Psychophysiology*, **39**, 361–8.

Cacioppo, J. T. (1994). Social neuroscience – Autonomic, neuroendocrine, and immune-responses to stress. *Psychophysiology*, **31**, 113–28.

Cohen, H. J. (2000). In search of the underlying mechanisms of frailty: editorial. *The Journals of Gerontology Series A: Biological Sciences and Medical Sciences*, **55**, M706–8.

Cohen, S., Doyle, W. J., Skoner, D. P., Rabin, B. S. & Gwaltney, J. M. (1997). Social ties and susceptibility to the common cold. *Journal of the American Medical Association*, **24**, 1940–4.

Cohen, S., Doyle, W. J., Turner, R., Alper, C. M. & Skoner, D. P. (2003). Sociability and susceptibility to the common cold. *Psychological Science*, **14**, 389–95.

Cohen, S., Frank, E., Doyle, W. J. et al. (1998). Types of stressors that increase susceptibility to the common cold in healthy adults. *Health Psychology*, **17**, 214–23.

Cohen, S., Tyrrell, D. A. & Smith, A. P. (1991). Psychological stress and susceptibility to the common cold. *The New England Journal of Medicine*, **325**, 606–12.

Cole-King, A. & Harding, K. G. (2001). Psychological factors and delayed healing in chronic wounds. *Psychosomatic Medicine*, **63**, 216–20.

Dekaris, D., Sabioncello, A., Mazuran, R. et al. (1993). Multiple changes of immunologic parameters in prisoners of war. *Journal of the American Medical Association*, **270**, 595–9.

Glaser, R., Kiecolt-Glaser, J. K., Bonneau, R. H. et al. (1992) Stress-induced modulation of the immune response to recombinant hepatitis B vaccine. *Psychosomatic Medicine*, **54**, 22–9.

Glaser, R., Robles, T. F., Sheridan, J., Malarkey, W. B. & Kiecolt-Glaser, J. K. (2003). Mild depressive symptoms are associated with amplified and prolonged inflammatory responses after influenza virus vaccination in older adults. *Archives of General Psychiatry*, **60**, 1009–14.

Glaser, R., Sheridan, J. F., Malarkey, W. B., MacCallum, R. C. & Kiecolt-Glaser, J. K. (2000). Chronic stress modulates the immune response to a pneumococcal pneumonia vaccine, *Psychosomatic Medicine*, **62**, 804–7.

Goodkin, K., Feaster, D. J., Tuttle, R. et al. (1996). Bereavement is associated with time-dependent decrements in cellular immune function in asymptomatic human immunodeficiency virus Type 1-seropositive homosexual men. *Clinical and Diagnostic Laboratory Immunology*, **3**, 109–18.

Heesen, C., Schulz, H., Schmidt, M. et al. (2002). Endocrine and cytokine responses to acute psychological stress in multiple sclerosis. *Brain, Behavior, and Immunity*, **16**, 282–7.

Herbert, T. B., Cohen, S., Marsland, A. L., Bachen, E. A., Rabin, B. S., Muldoon, M. F. & Manuck, S. B. (1994). Cardiovascular reactivity and the course of immune response to an acute psychological stressor. *Psychosomatic Medicine*, **56**, 337–44.

Ironson, G., Wynings, C., Schneiderman, N. et al. (1997). Posttraumatic stress symptoms, intrusive thoughts, loss, and immune function after Hurricane Andrew. *Psychosomatic Medicine*, 59, 128–41.

Irwin, M., Daniels, M., Smith, T. L., Bloom, E. & Weiner, H. (1987). Impaired natural killer cell activity during bereavement. *Brain Behavior, and Immunity*, 1, 98–104.

Jung, W. & Irwin, M. (1999). Reduction of natural killer cytotoxic activity in major depression: interaction between depression and cigarette smoking. *Psychosomatic Medicine*, 61, 263–70.

Kemeny, M. E. & Dean, L. (1995). Effects of AIDS-related bereavement on HIV progression among New York City gay men. *AIDS Education and Prevention*, 7, 36–47.

Kemeny, M. E., Weiner, H., Duran, R. *et al.* (1995). Immune system changes after the death of a partner in HIV-positive gay men. *Psychosomatic Medicine*, 57, 547–54.

Kennedy, S., Kiecolt-Glaser, J. K. & Glaser, R. (1988). Immunological consequences of acute and chronic stressors: mediating role of interpersonal relationships. *British Journal of Medical Psychology*, 61, 77–85.

Kiecolt-Glaser, J. K., Cacioppo, J. T., Malarkey, W. B. & Glaser, R. (1992). Acute psychological stressors and short-term immune changes: what, why, for whom, and what extent? *Psychosomatic Medicine*, 54, 680–5.

Kiecolt-Glaser, J. K., Garner, W., Speicher, C. *et al.* (1984). Psychosocial modifiers of immunocompetence in medical students. *Psychosomatic Medicine*, 46, 7–14.

Kiecolt-Glaser, J. K. & Glaser, R. (1988). Methodological issues in behavioral immunology research with humans. *Brain, Behavior and Immunity*, 2, 67–78.

Kiecolt-Glaser, J. K., Glaser, R., Cacioppo, J. T., MacCallum, R. C., Snydersmith, M., Kim, C. & Malarkey, W. B. (1997). Marital conflict in older adults: endocrinological and immunological correlates. *Psychosomatic Medicine*, 59, 339–49.

Kiecolt-Glaser, J.K, Glaser, R., Gravenstein, S., Malarkey, W. B. & Sheridan, J. (1996). Chronic stress alters the immune response to influenza virus vaccine in older adults. *Proceedings of the National Academy of Sciences, USA*, 93, 3043–7.

Kiecolt-Glaser, J. K., Glaser, R., Shuttleworth, E. *et al.* (1987). Chronic stress and immunity in family caregivers of Alzheimer's disease victims. *Psychosomatic Medicine*, 49, 523–35.

Kiecolt-Glaser, J. K., Malarkey, W. B., Chee, M. *et al.* (1993). Negative behavior during marital conflict is associated with immunological down-regulation. *Psychosomatic Medicine*, 55, 395–409.

Kiecolt-Glaser, J. K., Marucha, P. T., Malarkey, W. B., Mercado, A. M. & Glaser, R. (1995). Slowing of wound healing by psychological stress. *Lancet*, 346, 1194–6.

Kunz-Ebrecht, S. R., Mohamed-Ali, V., Feldman, P. J., Kirschbaum, C. & Steptoe, A. (2003). Cortisol responses to mild psychological stress are inversely associated with proinflammatory cytokines. *Brain, Behavior, and Immunity*, 17, 373–83.

Laudenslager, M. L., Aasal, R., Adler, L. *et al.* (1998). Elevated cytotoxicity in combat veterans with long-term post-traumatic stress disorder: preliminary observations. *Brain, Behavior, and Immunity*, 12, 74–9.

Lutgendorf, S. K., Garand, L., Buckwalter, K. C. *et al.* (1999). Life stress, mood disturbance, and elevated interleukin-6 in healthy older women. *The Journals of Gerontology Series A: Biological Sciences and Medical Sciences*, 54, M434–9.

Maes, M., Lin, A., Delmeire, L. *et al.* (1999). Elevated serum interleukin-6 (IL-6) and IL-6 receptor concentrations in posttraumatic stress disorder following accidental man-made traumatic events. *Biological Psychiatry*, 45, 833–9.

Manuck, S. B., Cohen, S., Rabin, B. S., Muldoon, M. F. & Bachen, E. A. (1991). Individual differences in cellular immune response to stress. *Psycholocical Science*, 2, 111–15.

Marshall, G. D., Agarwall, S. K., Lloyd, C. *et al.* (1998). Cytokine dysregulation associated with exam stress in healthy medical students. *Brain, Behavior, and Immunity*, 12, 297–307.

Marsland, A. L., Cohen, S., Rabin, B. S. & Manuck, S. B. (2001). Associations between stress, trait negative affect, acute immune reactivity, and antibody response to hepatitis B injection in healthy young adults. *Health Psychology*, 20, 4–11.

Marucha, P. T., Kiecolt-Glaser, J. K. & Favagehl, M. (1998). Mucosal wound healing is impaired by examination stress. *Psychosomatic Medicine*, 60, 362–5.

McKinnon, W., Weisse, C. S., Reynolds, C. P., Bowles, C. A. & Baum, A. (1989). Chronic stress, leukocyte subpopulations, and humoral response to latent viruses. *Health Psychology*, 8, 389–402.

Plaut, M. (1987). Lymphocyte hormone receptors. *Annual Review of Immunology*, 5, 621–69.

Sabioncello, A., Kocijan-Hercigonja, D., Rabatic, S. *et al.* (2000). Immune, endocrine, and psychological responses to civilians displaced by war. *Psychosomatic Medicine*, 62, 502–8.

Scapagnini, U. (1992). Psychoneuroendocrinoimmunology: the basis for a novel therapeutic approach in aging. *Psychoneuroendocrinology*, 17, 411–20.

Segerstrom, S. C. & Miller, G. E. (2004). Psychological stress and the human immune system: a meta-analytic study of 30 years of inquiry. *Psychological Bulletin*, 130, 601–30.

Segerstrom, S. C., Taylor, S. E., Kemeny, M. E. & Fahey, J. L. (1998). Optimism is associated with mood, coping, and immune change in response to stress. *Journal of Personality and Social Psychology*, 74, 1646–55.

Spivak, B., Shohat, B., Mester, R. *et al.* (1997). Elevated levels of serum interleukin-1β in combat-related posttraumatic stress disorder *Biological Psychiatry*, 42, 345–8.

Steptoe, A., Willemsen, G., Owen, N., Flower, L. & Mohamed-Ali, V. (2001). Acute mental stress elicits delayed increases in circulating inflammatory cytokine levels. *Clinical Science*, 101, 185–92.

Vedhara, K., Cox, N. K., Wilcock, G.K. *et al.* (1999). Chronic stress in elderly carers of dementia patients and antibody response to influenza vaccination, *Lancet*, 353, 627–31.

Workman, E. A. & La Via, M. F. (1987). Immunological effects of psychological stressors: a review of the literature. *International Journal of Psychosomatics*, 34, 35–40.

Yehuda, R., Soutwick, S. M., Nussbaum, G. *et al.* (1990). Low urinary cortisol excretion in patients with post-traumatic stress disorder. *Journal of Nervous and Mental Disorders*, 187, 366–9.

Zakowski, S. G., McAllister, C. G., Deal, M. & Baum, A. (1992). Stress, reactivity, and immune function in healthy men. *Health Psychology*, 11, 223–32.

E. Bachen *et al.*

Psychosomatics

Christopher Bass

John Radcliffe Hospital

Introduction and historical overview

The term 'psychosomatic' was first used in the early nineteenth century by Heinroth to mean 'belonging to the body and the mind' (Bynum, 1983). Psychosomatic conceptions were much older than this however. Plato observed that the ability of the 'physicians of Hellas' to cure disease was limited because they disregarded 'the Whole, which ought to be studied also, for the part can never be well unless the whole is well' (Plato (transl) See Padis, 1952). The term 'psychosomatic' is a modern designation for that holistic view of man and medicine which has its roots in ancient Greece. Throughout the nineteenth century it was widely accepted that psychological factors could play a part in the aetiology of physical illness.

The term has been used in a number of different ways in the last hundred years however. In the first half of the twentieth century three psychosomatic schools emerged and competed for prominence: the psychoanalytic, the psychophysiological and the psychobiological (holistic, biopsychosocial). The development of these three schools, which proved difficult to integrate, will be briefly described.

The psychoanalytical school, led by Alexander, focused on the postulated psychogenesis of a handful of somatic disorders of unknown cause such as bronchial asthma, rheumatoid arthritis, ulcerative colitis, essential hypertension, neuro-dermatitis, thyrotoxicosis and peptic ulceration. Alexander (1950) proposed that emotional changes in human beings were accompanied by physiological changes which led in turn to pathological physical changes: once physical pathology was established, psychological factors could help to maintain or aggravate it or to trigger relapse. For Alexander, a specific 'emotional constellation', one consisting of an unconscious conflict, defences against it, and emotions engendered by it, would elicit specific vegetative responses, which could lead to a specific bodily disorder. This led to the belief that a physical condition produced in this way would improve if the psychological disturbance improved, either spontaneously or as a result of psychological treatment.

Alexander's theories came to connote for many people nothing but the psychological causation of bodily disorders, and this psychological reductionism fell into disfavour after the 1950s. The other psychosomatic schools, the psychophysiological and the psychobiological, have gained prominence over the last 50 years, as the psychoanalytical school's influence has faded away. The psychophysiological school, derived from the work of Pavlov on the conditioned reflex and of Canon on the physiological concomitants of emotions, such as fear and rage, was prominently represented by Wolff, who postulated the contributory role of psychological stress on in the occurrence, course and outcome of a wide range of diseases. Wolff and his colleagues examined the mediating physiological mechanisms that occur following one's exposure to personally meaningful information. That whole area of research has flourished subsequently under the label of psychophysiology.

The psychobiological school was derived from the work of Adolf Meyer. Led by Flanders Dunbar, this school was most explicitly holistic in its orientation. Dunbar, who founded the American Psychosomatic Society, published a substantial survey of her own and other clinicians' observations in the book 'Emotions and Bodily Changes' (Dunbar, 1954). She emphasized the need for a comprehensive, biopsychosocial approach to the study and management of all patients and not just those called 'psychosomatic'. She was one of the pioneers of liaison psychiatry, and also emphasized the need for preventive medicine and stressed the important role played by psychosocial factors in disease development and prevention.

In its modern usage the term 'psychosomatic' has come to connote holistic. This refers to a set of assumptions about mind and body, the role of psychosocial factors in health and disease and the place of these factors in medical management.

Recent definitions of the term psychosomatic emphasize the mind-body relationship as follows:

1. *Involving or concerned with the interdependence of mind and body*
2. *(Medicine) designating, pertaining or relating to illnesses having both physical and mental components, usually involving a physical condition caused or aggravated by mental or emotional disorder (Shorter Oxford English Dictionary, 2001).*

Psychosocial factors are believed to be involved, to a greater or lesser extent, in every disease and episode of illness. All disease is assumed to be multicausal, which is to say it is the result of a complex interplay of biological, psychological and social variables.

Recent developments

Since the 1970s theories have been less dogmatic. A key publication by Engel in 1977 proposed the biopsychosocial approach to illness. Subsequent research has focused on a number of broad areas that are not mutually exclusive. They include psychophysiological mechanisms; the impact of life events and difficulties on illness; the physical manifestations of psychological illness; the psychological consequences of physical illnesses; and the effect of psychological treatments. These five areas will be discussed below. The word 'psychosomatic' now appears in five leading journals, and both general hospital (liaison) psychiatry and health psychology have developed as major areas of clinical practice and research over the last two decades. A recent updated database of key references in this field has been published by Strain *et al.* (2003).

Psychophysiological research

A major purpose psychological physiological research has been to detect the physiological mechanisms and pathways between the perception of personally meaningful stimuli or information by the individual and the consequent changes in the functions of his or her various organs or tissues. Every sick person is exposed to personally meaningful information, such as remarks from doctors, which have the potential to affect mood or behaviour and in turn elicit changes in physiological functions. These may be therapeutic or deleterious. The most commonly researched psychosocial variable has been emotional stress.

The two main biological systems involved in the stress response are the sympathetic nervous system and hypothalamic–pituitary–adrenal system (HPA axis). The normal role of the sympathetic nervous system is to mediate the unconscious regulation of basic bodily functions. In a stressful situation it is also the chief mediator of the bodies' immediate alarm reaction – the so-called fight-or-flight response.

Disturbed regulation of the HPA axis can also occur in response to long lasting arousal. Regulatory disturbances in the HPA axis have been suggested to play a role in certain illnesses. For example, the lack of response to stimulation of the HPA axis results in low plasma cortisol levels: as a consequence normal activation does not take place when the HPA axis activated artificially. A subgroup of patients with chronic fatigue syndrome and fibromyalgia show these characteristic patterns (Parker *et al.*, 2001).

Other studies have shown that a person's psychological state may induce, presumably through neuroendocrine mechanisms, changes in the immune system that would facilitate the development of neoplasia. The field of psychoneuroimmunology has recently been the subject of a major review (Reiche *et al.*, 2004) (see 'Stress and health' and 'Psychoneuroimmunology').

Arising from the work of Dunbar in the 1950s a number of investigators examined the links between certain personality and behavioural characteristics and the development of coronary heart disease (CHD). Despite two decades of research effort the 'Type A' behaviour pattern turned out not to be aetiologically relevant, and a meta-analysis of the body of research on the physical health consequences of hostility concluded that the psychological trait of hostility – cynical mistrust, anger and aggression – is a risk factor for not only CHD but also for virtually physical illness (Miller *et al.*, 1996) (see 'Hostility, Type A behaviour and coronary heart disease' and 'Personality and health').

One of the most potent (and most frequently investigated) stressors in contemporary life is work. Occupational stress has become very topical, and is also a legitimate field of research (Wainwright & Calnan, 2002). It has been demonstrated that certain occupational characteristics are more likely to lead to adverse outcomes than others. For example, many jobs involving high degrees of effort but providing lower levels of reward – in terms of remuneration, job security and prospects for promotion – are at higher risk of developing several of the biological precursors of heart attack, such as raised cholesterol level and blood pressure. Job strain and effort – reward imbalance have also been found to be associated with high health risk behaviours and psychological illness (Marmot and Bartley, 2002).

This research in occupational stress has emphasized that being unsure of your ability to control a stressor appears to make matters worse. Uncontrollable stressors carry a higher risk of provoking psychological depression than equally severe but controllable stressors. For example, when animals are subjected to severe and uncontrollable stressors they can develop a mental state called learned helplessness, which bears many of the hallmarks of clinical depression in humans (Seligman, 1986). Marmot has extended this work and recently argued that low social standing is seen not only as a condition of material deprivation but also an indicator of people's capability to control life and fully participate in society (psychosocial disadvantage). As a person's position in the social hierarchy decreases, the less likely he or she is to have full control over life and opportunities for full participation in society. Marmot (2004) has made a forceful case showing that low control over life and social disengagement are the most powerful explanatory factors for the social gradient of health: people who are lower in the hierarchy tend to have worse health and shorter life expectancy.

Control has multiple ramifications for mental and physical wellbeing (Breier *et al.*, 1987). For instance, it helps people to deal with chronic pain. A person who feels he/she is in control of pain and of their life will be consistently better able to cope with prolonged high levels of pain than one who feels helpless. Research has confirmed that boosting patients' sense of control helps in the management of pain. This is an important practical issue for cancer patients and others suffering from chronic pain (Morley *et al.*, 1999) (see 'Coping with chronic pain' and 'Self-efficacy and health').

Life events and difficulties

The notion that we are at increased risk of falling ill when exposed to a lot of disruptive change or emotional turmoil is not a new one. Early studies of absenteeism indicated that employees with unsettled personal lives tended to suffer frequent bouts of illness and take more sick leave from work.

The formulation of the concept of stressful 'life events' has led to thousands of research projects which have investigated the relationships between life events and health. Methodological problems bedevilled this work, which is essentially retrospective in nature and influenced by the perception and interpretation of the significance and meaning of events by individuals.

George Brown and his colleagues in London have been pioneers in this research endeavour and have developed a methodology that attempts to circumvent these difficulties (Brown & Harris, 1989). In a key early study they demonstrated that the link between severe life events and the onset of organic illness was likely to be mediated by the occurrence of a psychiatric (affective) disturbance (Murphy & Brown, 1980). Subsequent research, using the Life Events and Difficulties Schedule (LEDs) has shown that life events can have a very important role not only as precipitants but also as formative causes of a wide range of illnesses. For example, important links have been established between life events and the onset of a number of physical disorders such as multiple sclerosis and stroke. In the recent INTERHEART study, in which patients were recruited from 52 countries, the presence of a range of psychosocial stressors was associated with increased risk of myocardial infarction (Rosengren *et al.*, 2004). A range of functional somatic syndromes such as functional dysphonia, chronic fatigue syndrome and functional gastrointestinal disorders have also been shown to be related to stressful life events (see Hatcher & House, 2003, for a recent account of this field) (see also 'Life events and health').

In addition to major life events, such as bereavement and unemployment, more mundane 'hassles of everyday life' and 'chronic ongoing difficulties' have also been shown to have an impact on health. Indeed, because these mundane problems are such a frequent occurrence, their cumulative influence on health may be more pervasive than the effects of rarer, but more traumatic life events (Bennett et al., 1998).

Physical manifestations of psychological disorder

Patients who report physical symptoms with no identifiable cause have attracted considerable interest and controversy; not least because there is no consensus on how these disorders should be described. For many years patients with unexplained symptoms were said to have a 'psychosomatic' illness. However, this term is now considered to be potentially misleading when used to describe these patients, as it implies that the symptoms necessarily have a purely psychogenic origin, which is not always the case. An alternative term, 'somatisation', has been coined to describe a putative process by which some people experience and communicate psychological distress as physical symptoms, but this description presumes that psychological problems are being avoided and that the physical symptoms are 'all in the mind'. To avoid the artificial separation of the mind and body, terms such as 'medically unexplained symptom' and 'functional somatic symptoms' have been used. None of these terms is satisfactory, but it has been shown recently that patients with these disorders prefer the term 'functional' to other descriptions (Stone et al., 2002).

Clusters of chronic medically unexplained symptoms can appear to form symptom syndromes, and so are sometimes given diagnostic labels such as irritable bowel syndrome, chronic fatigue syndrome or fibromyalgia, depending on the symptoms and the medical specialty to which the patient is referred. The results of a recent observational study suggest that substantial overlap exists across diverse symptom syndromes. Indeed, the overlap between such syndromes is so great that they are better seen as a single underlying disorder (Nimnuan et al., 2001).

In adults, medically unexplained symptoms prompt almost half of all primary care consultations, but are shown to have an organic origin in only about 10–15% of patients who were followed for one year. In general hospitals these patients are responsible for 30–50% of presentations in outpatient departments: these patients are difficult to manage, costly and often the victims of iatrogenic illness if they are not identified and treated promptly. These disorders have attracted considerable attention (Mayou et al., 1995) and have been the subject of numerous treatment studies in the general hospital. Cognitive behaviour therapy (CBT) is widely advocated for these patients, and in a systematic review of 31 controlled studies (29 randomized) physical symptoms improved in 71% of studies, psychological distress decreased in 38% and functional status improved in 47% (Kroenke & Swindle, 2000). Group CBT also helps patients with medically unexplained symptoms, and hypnosis has also shown benefits (see 'Cognitive behaviour therapy'). Regrettably, there are insufficient clinical psychologists in general hospitals available to provide appropriate treatment for these patients, who are an enormous burden on healthcare resources.

Table 1. Determinants of the occurrence of psychiatric disorder among physically ill patients

The physical disease as a cause of:
Symptomatic psychiatric disorder
Threat to normal life
Disability
Pain

Nature of the treatment
Side-effects
Mutilation
Demands for self-care

Factors in the patient
Psychological vulnerability
Social circumstances
Other life stresses

Reactions of others
Family
Employers
Doctors

Psychological consequences of physical illness

Organic mental disorder may occur in the course of many serious physical illnesses or surgical procedures, especially among the elderly. Delirium, dementia and other organic disorders associated with specific medical conditions have been described by Lishman (1998). This section is concerned with emotional disorders consequent upon physical illness.

Certain factors increase the risk of serious psychiatric disorders developing in the physically ill. Patients are more vulnerable if they have had a previous psychiatric disorder or a life-long inability to deal with adversity, or if they have a disturbed home life or an otherwise unsatisfactory social background. Furthermore, certain kinds of physical illness are more likely to provoke serious psychiatric consequences. These include life-threatening illnesses, and illnesses requiring lengthy and unpleasant treatment such as radiotherapy or renal dialysis or mutilating treatment such as mastectomy (see 'Coping with chronic illness').

In the physically ill, the commonest psychiatric disorders are emotional disorders, which occur in 10–30% of patients with severe physical illnesses. Most of these emotional disorders can be diagnosed as adjustment disorders, whilst specific anxiety and affective disorders are also common. Other conditions that are less frequent are somatoform disorders and paranoid disorders. The many psychological symptoms that can be caused directly by physical illness are shown in Table 1.

Depressive and anxiety disorders precipitated by physical illness or injury may be regarded as being mediated by the meaning of the illness for the patient, rather than as a direct manifestation of cerebral dysfunction. Significant depression has been found in approximately 20–25% of unselected medical inpatients, but its prevalence has been reported as much higher immediately following myocardial infarction, and in patients suffering from rheumatoid arthritis, Parkinsonism or carcinoma of the pancreas. It is important to diagnose mood disorder in patients with physical illnesses because the psychiatric complications may adversely effect patients' prognosis and interfere with rehabilitation and timely return to work.

Furthermore, depression is associated with an approximately 50% increase in medical costs of chronic medical illness, even after controlling for severity for physical illness. Increasing evidence suggest that both the depressive symptoms and a major depression may be associated with increased morbidity and mortality from such illnesses as diabetes and heart disease. The adverse effect of major depression on health habits, such as smoking, diet, over-eating and sedentary lifestyle, its maladaptive effect on adherence to medical regimens, as well as direct adverse physiological effects (i.e. decreased heart rate variability, increase adhesiveness of platelets) may explain this association within morbidity and mortality (Katon, W. J. 2003).

In the last two decades there has been considerable interest in the psychosocial and psychopathological effects on modern medical and surgical technology, for example, transplantation surgery, chronic dialysis, intensive care units and long-term parenteral nutrition. More recent surgery for obesity has become a safer and more 'evidence based' procedure (Buchwald et al., 2004) with improved outcomes. The recent clamour for cosmetic and plastic surgical procedures in patients with body image disorders has resulted in psychiatric casualties. As a consequence a need for pre-operative psychological assessment has increased, placing extra demands on psychological resources that often cannot be met (Grossbart & Sarwer, 2003).

Therapeutic research

Interventions in this field are usually directed towards modifying selected psychological variables; behavioural, cognitive or emotional. Therapeutic studies can be divided into two groups, which are not mutually exclusive: (a) those that employ psychotropic medication and (b) those that employ psychological methods.

a. *Drug therapy*. Hypnotic and anxiolytic drugs are valuable for short periods when distress is severe, for example, during treatment in hospital. The indications for antidepressants are probably the same as those for patients who are not physically ill, although the older tricyclic antidepressants have drawbacks because of their side-effects. In a recent randomized, double-blind, placebo-controlled trial, Sertraline was found to be a safe and effective treatment in patients with recent myocardial infarction or unstable angina and without other threatening medical conditions (Glassman et al., 2002).

b. *Psychological treatments*. Behaviour medication and biofeedback have been used for many years for the relief of a wide range of symptoms such a urinary incontinence, tension headache, various other painful disorders and, more recently, chronic constipation (Bassotti et al., 2004). This field of behavioural medicine demonstrates that physiological and pathophysiological functions can be modified by manipulation of psychological variables, a demonstration predictable from psychosomatic assumptions discussed earlier (see 'Behaviour therapy' and 'Biofeedback').

Psychological interventions have also been used in the rehabilitation of a wide variety of physical disorders such as stroke and myocardial infarction. Although there is no evidence to support the routine use of pharmaco- or psychotherapeutic treatment for depression after stroke, the evidence for behavioural treatment after myocardial infarction is more positive (Mayou et al., 2002).

Weinman and his colleagues showed that patients' initial perceptions of illness are important determinants of different aspects of recovery after myocardial infarction. Furthermore, they predict overall functioning and number of visits to the outpatient clinic in patients with chronic obstructive pulmonary disease. More recently Petrie et al. (2002) showed that an in-hospital intervention designed to alter patients' illness beliefs and perceptions about their heart attack resulted in improved functional outcome. This is clearly a key area for future research in cardiac rehabilitation (see 'Coronary heart disease: rehabilitation').

The usefulness of Cognitive behaviour therapy in medically unexplained symptoms – the so-called 'functional' disorders – has already been mentioned. Similar approaches have been used to treat patients with chronic pain, especially in the setting of multidisciplinary pain clinics (Morley et al., 1999) (see 'Cognitive behaviour therapy' and 'Pain management').

Developments since 2001

In March 2003 the American Board of Medical Specialties unanimously approved the creation of a seventh psychiatric sub-specialty, 'psychosomatic medicine', which defines all those working in consultation liaison psychiatry and general hospital psychiatry.

This title should not seem surprising, given the appearance of the word 'psychosomatic' in four of the five leading journals that serve the sub-specialty and the names of professional associations. This followed two decades of lobbying among US psychiatrists (and similar informal discussions among UK psychiatrists) and has been reviewed by McIntyre (2002).

A word of caution is in place however. In a recent article Stone et al. (2004) explored the ways in which the word 'psychosomatic' was used in US and UK newspaper articles. They carried out a survey of all articles published in 14 US and UK newspapers between 1996 and 2002. The survey was limited to broadsheet newspapers. The authors found that 'psychosomatic' had a pejorative meaning, such as 'imaginary' or 'made up', in 34% of the articles in which the meaning could be judged. Most commonly, 'psychosomatic' was used to describe a problem that was psychological or in which the mind affects the body (56%) rather than a reciprocal interaction (5%). The authors concluded that although the term 'psychosomatic medicine' is the new name for the seventh sub-specialty of psychiatry, more needed to be done to educate the media about its actual meaning to make it attractive to patients.

Conclusion

Like hysteria, the word 'psychosomatics' continues to be widely used and has outlived its obituaries. The concept of psychosomatic medicine has become more widely accepted and is recognized as not only a reaction against mind-body dualism, but also as an organized field of scientific enquiry. In a clinical sense it represents an approach to the patient that recognizes the important relationship between psychological factors and bodily function, both in health and disease.

REFERENCES

Alexander, F. (1950). *Psychosomatic medicine*. New York: Norton.

Bassotti, G., Christolini, F., Sietchping-Nzepa, F. *et al.* (2004). Biofeedback for pelvic floor dysfunction in constipation. *British Medical Journal*, **328**, 393–6.

Bennett, E. J., Tennant, C., Piesse, C., Badcock, C. & Kellow, J. (1998). Level of chronic life stress predicts clinical outcome in irritable bowel syndrome. *Gut*, **43**, 256–61.

Breier, A., Albus, M., Pickar, D., Zahn, T. P., Wolkowitz, O. M. & Paul, S. M. (1987). Controllable and uncontrollable stress in humans: alterations in mood and neuroendocrine and psychophysiological function. *The American Journal of Psychiatry*, **144**(11), 1419–25.

Brown, G. & Harris, T. (Eds.). (1989). *Life events and illness*. London: Guildford Press.

Buchwald, H., Avidor, Y., Braunwald, E. *et al.* (2004). Bariatric surgery: a systematic review and meta-analysis. *Journal of the American Medical Association*, **292**, 1724–37.

Bynum, W. F. (1985). Psychiatry in its historical context. In Shepherd, M. & Zangwill, O. L. (Eds.). *Handbook of psychiatry. Vol 1*. Cambridge: Cambridge University Press.

Dunbar, F. (1954). *Emotions and bodily changes*. New York: Columbia University Press.

Engel, G. (1977). The need for a new medical model: a challenge for biomedicine. *Science*, **196**, 129–36.

Glassman, A. H., O'Connor, C. M., Califf, R. M. *et al.* (SADHEART Group) (2002). Sertraline treatment of major depression in patients with acute unstable angina. *Journal of the American Medical Association*, **288**, 701–9.

Grossbart, J. & Sarwer, D. (2003). Psychosocial issues and their relevance to the cosmetic surgery patient. *Seminars in Cutaneous Medicine and Surgery*, **22**, 136–47.

Hatcher, S. & House, A. (2003). Life events, difficulties and dilemmas in the onset of chronic fatigue syndrome: a case control study. *Psychological Medicine*, **33**, 1185–92.

Katon, W. J. (2003). Clinical and health services relationships between major depression, depressive symptoms, and general medical illness. *Biological Psychiatry*, **54**(3), 216–26.

Kroenke, K. & Swindle, R. (2000). Cognitive behavioural therapy for somatisation and symptom syndrome: a critical review of controlled clinical trials. *Psychotherapy and Psychosomatics*, **69**, 205–15.

Lishman (1998). *Organic Psychiatry. The Psychological Consequences of Cerebral Disorder* (3rd edn.). Oxford: Blackwells.

Marmot, M. (2004). *Status syndrome: how your social standing directly affects your health and life expectancy*. London: Bloomsbury.

Marmot, M. & Bartley, M. (2002). Social class and coronary heart disease. In S. A. Stansfields & M. Marmot. (Eds.). *Stress and the heart. Psychosocial pathways to coronary heart disease*, (pp. 5–19). London: BMJ Books.

Mayou, R., Bass, C. & Sharpe, M. (Eds.). (1995). *Treatment of functional somatic symptoms*. Oxford: Oxford University Press.

Mayou, R. A., Thompson, D., Clements, A. *et al.* (2002). Guideline-based early rehabilitation after myocardial infarction. A pragmatic randomised controlled trial. *Journal of Psychosomatic Research*, **52**(2), 89–95.

McIntyre, J. S. (2002). A new subspecialty. *The American Journal of Psychiatry*, **159**, 1961–3.

Miller, T. Q., Smith, T., Turner, C., Guijarro, M. & Hallet, A. (1996). A meta-analytic review of research on hostility and physical health. *Psychological Bulletin*, **119**, 322–48.

Morley, S., Eccleston, C. & Williams, A. (1999). Systematic review and meta-analysis of randomised controlled trials of cognitive behavioural therapy and behaviour therapy for chronic pain in adults, excluding headache. *Pain*, **80**, 1–13.

Murphy, E. & Brown, G. (1980). Life events, psychiatric disturbance and physical illness. *British Journal of Psychiatry*, **136**, 326–38.

Nimnuan, C., Rabe-Hesketh, S. Wessely, S. & Hotopf, M. (2001). How many functional somatic syndromes? *Journal of Psychosomatic Research*, **51**, 549–57.

Padis, N. (1952). Plato and psychosomatic medicine. *Transaction & Studies of the College of Physicians of Philadelphia*, **19**, 127–9.

Parker, A., Wessely, S. & Cleare, A. (2001). The neuroendocrinology of chronic fatigue syndrome and fibromyalgia. *Psychological Medicine*, **31**, 1331–45.

Petrie, K., Cameron, L., Ellis, C., Buick, D. & Weinman, J. (2002). Changing illness perceptions after myocardial infarction: an early intervention randomised controlled trial. *Psychosomatic Medicine*, **64**, 580–6.

Reiche, E., Nunes, S. & Morimoto, H. (2004). Stress, depression, the immune system, and cancer. *Lancet Oncology*, **10**, 617–25.

Rosengren, A., Hawken, S., Ounpuu, S. *et al.* (2004). Association of psychological risk factors with risk of acute myocardial infarction in 11, 119 cases and 13,648 controls from 52 counties (in INTERHEART study): case-control study. *Lancet*, **364**, 953–62.

Seligman, M. (1986). Learned helplessness in children: a longitudinal study of depression, achievement, and explanatory style. *Journal of Personal and Social Psychology*, **51**(2), 435–42.

Stone, J., Wojcik, W., Durrance, D. *et al.* (2002). What should we say to patients with symptoms unexplained by disease? The "number needed to offend". *British Medical Journal*, **325**, 1449–50.

Stone, J., Colyer, M., Feltbower, S., Carson, A. & Sharpe, M. (2004). "Psychosomatic": a systematic review of its meaning in newspaper articles. *Psychosomatics*, **45**, 287–90.

Strain, J., Strain, J., Mustafa, S. *et al.* (2003). Consultation – Liaison Psychiatry literature database (2003 update). *General Hospital Psychiatry*, **25**, 377–478.

Wainwright, D. & Calnan, M. (2002). *Work stress: the making of a modern epidemic*. Buckingham, UK: Open University Press.

Quality of life

Lena Ring

Uppsala University

Human beings continually strive to create meaning in their lives and they struggle to achieve happiness by pursuing the things that they value (Diener *et al.*, 2003). Speculation about how to achieve 'the good life' or 'good quality of life' (QoL) is probably as old as humankind. According to Socrates: 'You should put the highest value, not on living, but on living well'. However, it is only in recent decades that there has been a growing interest in assessing QoL in healthcare (SAC, 2002) and conceptualizations of QoL in healthcare have been heavily influenced by earlier developments in the measurement of functional health status in medicine and the evolution of social indicators in the social sciences (Prutkin & Feinstein, 2002).

The concept of QoL began to appear in the social science literature in the 1920s (Wood-Dauphinee, 1999). The development of population indices was influenced by the social indicators movement, which emphasized the need to focus on social factors that influence satisfaction (Erickson, 1974; Andrews & Withey, 1976; Campbell, 1976). Most of these early measures were based on experts' ratings of objective phenomena such as the distribution of income. Later studies assessed subjective indicators such as satisfaction with income and satisfaction with life, using measures such as Cantril's self-anchoring scale, Bradburn's Scale of Affect Balance and Campbell and Converse's Human Meaning of Social Change Scale (Cantril, 1965; Bradburn, 1969; Campbell and Converse, 1972). Traditionally, medicine had focused on objective outcomes, such as mortality and morbidity assessed by clinical and laboratory indicators. In order to provide a comprehensive assessment of the benefits and costs of a treatment, a broader range of measures, such as QoL instruments, was proposed (Wood-Dauphinee, 1999). However, early measures such as the Karnofsky scale (Karnofsky & Burchenal, 1948) were based on 'experts' assessments of patients' functional status. It is now generally accepted that the patient is in the best position to assess his/her own QoL as proxies generally underestimate patients' QoL. Agreements between patient and proxy assessments are highest for physical aspects and lowest for psychological aspects of QoL, but proxies' ratings are consistently higher when the proxy is a relative compared to a member of the healthcare team (Wilson *et al.*, 2000) (see 'Health status assessment' and 'Quality of life assessment').

Patient QoL is increasingly measured as an adjunct to more traditional clinical outcomes and 'quality of life' has been a key term in MEDLINE since 1977. This reflects an increasing acceptance of a holistic approach to health that is more in keeping with a bio-psychosocial model than the traditional biomedical model of disease (Engel, 1977). This change is due, in part, to the ageing of populations with a resulting increase in the prevalence of chronic and degenerative diseases. Since there are few curative treatments available, maintaining or improving QoL may be the most realistic goals. Kozma *et al.* (Kozma, Reeder *et al.*, 1993) have proposed what they call the Economic, clinical, and humanistic outcomes (ECHO) model of health outcomes, that involves assessing interventions in terms of economic, clinical and humanistic (QoL) outcomes. By measuring such a range of such outcomes, a comprehensive picture, known as the 'balloon effect', of the impact of interventions on the healthcare system can be formulated. If only one outcome is assessed, we do not know how the rest of the balloon will react following an intervention or treatment. For example, a particular treatment regimen might save on drug costs but lead ultimately to an increase in hospitalization (Gunter, 1999).

Impressive developments in medical technology and knowledge, combined with budgetary restrictions, have increased the demand for evidence-based healthcare and have highlighted the need to enumerate outcomes for all medical decisions both at the policy level and at the level of individual treatment planning (Zou *et al.*, 2004). The development of more broadly based assessments is relevant here since such measures can contribute to the assessment of treatment efficacy and side effects resulting in more informed treatment planning (Claridge & Fabian, 2005).

The health goals of many governments and international organizations are to improve QoL. For example, the World Health Organization's goal for 'The Healthy Cities Project' is to improve all citizens' health and QoL. The European Commission's 'Quality of Life and Management of Living Resources Programme' is targeted at enhancing the QoL of all European citizens. In the US, the primary goal of 'Healthy People 2010' is to increase life expectancy and improve QoL. Several professional associations also focus increasingly on QoL as an important outcome. In pharmacy, for example, the definition of pharmaceutical care is 'the responsible provision of drug therapy for the purpose of achieving definite outcomes that improve the patient's quality of life' (Hepler & Strand, 1990). A number of scientific organizations, such as The International Society for Quality of Life Research (ISOQoL; http://www.isoqol.org) and the Cochrane Collaboration Health Related QoL Methods Group (http://www.cochrane-hrqol-mg.org) focus on the scientific measurement of QoL.

QoL assessment

The past two decades have seen a dramatic increase in the development of measures of QoL and hundreds of measures now exist (Bowling, 2001); The QOLID database; www.qolid.org). Many current QoL measures are based on population indices of happiness and wellbeing or on functional capacity and performance indices

(Prutkin & Feinstein, 2002). Only about 20% of measures are generic, 10% utility based and 1% individualized (Garratt *et al.*, 2002). Most are disease-, population- or domain-specific and many have been developed originally for use in oncology, cardiology and rheumatology. Most measures consist of multi-item scales but single-item, visual analogue scales might provide a valid and reliable alternative (de Boer *et al.*, 2004). Some authors have introduced shorter versions of their instruments (Coste *et al.*, 1997). Many of these measures are now widely used in clinical trials and some are also used in clinical practice and in population-based studies (see 'Quality of life assessment').

Clinical trials

QoL is now widely used as either a primary or a secondary endpoint in clinical trials and the range of applications of QoL measurements in clinical trials continues to expand. Even if the primary purpose of a treatment regimen is to increase survival, QoL outcomes are relevant. For example, Gridelli *et al.* (Gridelli *et al.*, 2004) found that Docetaxel administered weekly was more satisfactory for lung cancer patients than when administered every third week. Comparable increases in survival were found with both regimens, but the weekly treatment was associated with increased QoL and with fewer adverse events. QoL assessments are also relevant when comparing treatments regarding dose, administration form etc. Diel *et al.* (Diel, Body *et al.*, 2004) found that a higher dose of ibandronate increased QoL (physical, emotional, social and global) and decreased pain for patients with breast cancer and bone metastases. Weiss *et al.* (Weiss, Nguyen *et al.*, 2005) found a novel betamethasone valerate foam for treating stasis dermatitis, not only to be clinically superior to placebo, but also to be associated with improved QoL. QoL measures are particularly important for evaluating long-term preventive therapies such as blood pressure and cholesterol lowering drugs. In a now classic study, Croog *et al.* (Croog *et al.*, 1986) demonstrated that, whereas captopril, propranolol and methyl-dopa all showed satisfactory and comparable efficacy and safety profiles in patients with hypertension, QoL was significantly enhanced by captopril only.

The application of QoL outcomes in clinical trials is a complex and developing field. The outcomes of such studies have begun to be considered by regulatory authorities such as the FDA but it is generally agreed that significant further development is required before the weight accorded to such outcomes is similar to that accorded to the more traditional indicators of efficacy and safety (Willke *et al.*, 2004).

Clinical practice

QoL assessments have primarily been used for research purposes in clinical trials but have had relatively little impact on clinical practice, even though monitoring patients' QoL in clinical practice is likely to achieve better treatment outcomes. Patients are often unsatisfied with the quality of communication with, and the amount of information they receive from, their healthcare providers (Glimelius *et al.*, 1995) (see '*Patient satisfaction*'). Acute, medical problems are often attended to, while chronic problems and psychosocial aspects of care and treatment receive

less attention (Fallowfield *et al.*, 2001). Both patients and physicians often wish that these aspects of treatment could be given more attention (Detmar *et al.*, 2000). Even though patients and physicians are willing to discuss physical aspects of the condition, each expects the other to initiate discussion of psychosocial issues (Detmar *et al.*, 2000). Systematically monitoring patients' QoL might help to individualize care, enhance patient–physician communication, inform clinical decision-making and improve patient outcomes especially QoL itself. QoL information could enhance the clinical interview which tends to focus primarily on physical symptoms and it could serve as the basis for joint doctor patient decision-making about treatment options. Some studies have explored the possibility of improving the care of patients by using systematic and continuing QoL assessments in clinical practice (Greenhalgh & Meadows, 1999; Espallargues *et al.*, 2000). Improvements in patient–physician communication were found, but the impact on patient satisfaction was limited. Intervention studies in cancer patients have shown that providing patient-specific QoL information to the physician and the patient before an appointment is an effective means of improving patient–provider communication (Detmar *et al.*, 2002) (see 'Healthcare professional–patient communication').

If QoL measures are to become a routine feature of clinical practice, they must be easy to use, highly reliable, valid and sensitive to change. Many current measures fail to meet these criteria (McHorney & Tarlow, 1995). Previous studies in clinical practice have used standardized QoL instruments, although it has been suggested that more individualized instruments might be preferable (Greenhalgh & Meadows, 1999). One approach might be to use individualized quality of life (IQoL) instruments (O'Boyle *et al.*, 2005). Developments in information technology mean that computer-administered instruments can now be used to overcome some of the difficulties of administration and scoring in clinical practice (Velikova *et al.*, 2002).

Population studies

As early as the 1920s, QoL issues were included in political debate when discussing the potential impact on people's lives of policy decisions (Pigou, 1920). However, it was only after the Second World War that attention was focused on evaluating the QoL of whole populations. Around this time, the World Health Organization introduced a new definition of health which included physical, emotional and social wellbeing (World Health Organization, 1948). Subsequently, the social indicators movement emphasized the need to examine the distribution of health and wellbeing in different populations and to monitor change in relation to national goals (Michalos, 1980). For example, studies of QoL in general populations examined the influence of education, health, family and personal life, work, environment and finances on wellbeing (Andrews & Withey, 1976; Campbell, 1976).

Today, national health interview surveys (HIS) are common in Europe, the USA, Canada and Australia (Aromaa *et al.*, 2003). Most studies include self-assessed health, general mental health and physical disability as measures of wellbeing. Other initiatives such the International Quality of Life Assessment (IQOLA) project collect QoL data to obtain national reference norms for the SF-36

(Ware & Gandek, 1998). The IQOLA project has found a significant impact of chronic conditions on physical health and a moderate impact on mental health across the countries studied (Alonso *et al.*, 2004). The World Health Organization Quality of Life Assessment (WHOQoL) has been designed to assess QoL cross-culturally and to reflect the WHO's commitment to a holistic view of health (Skevington *et al.*, 2004). Diener and colleagues (Diener *et al.*, 2003) have focused on assessing subjective wellbeing in many different countries and have demonstrated substantial differences between cultures. It is proposed that these differences might be due to individual factors such as personality, genetic make-up, attitude and expectations as well as more global factors such as cultural norms, GNP and political systems.

Research in health economics that incorporates measures of both quantity and quality of life might help in realizing better population health. Governments must often make policy decisions about the allocation of limited resources and reliable data on the impact of such decisions on QoL may lead to more informed choices. Some health economists have argued for the use of combined economic and QoL measures such as the QALY as an aid to decision making in resource allocation (Drummond, O'Brien *et al.*, 1999).

Some future challenges for QoL research

Interpretability

The results of QoL assessments require interpretation since the meaning of QoL scores is neither intuitive nor exclusively causally related to biological factors. Interpretation of scale scores requires more than just a consideration of statistical significance. It requires demonstration of clinical relevance. Different concepts of clinical significance have been proposed (Marquis *et al.*, 2004). 'Distribution-based interpretations' are based on the statistical distribution of the results and the effect size is the most commonly used measure here. This refers to the magnitude of change compared to the variability in stable subjects. It is also possible to compare or '*anchor*' scores to clinical status or other meaningful criteria such as life events or global ratings. Content-, construct- or criterion-based interpretations involve examining the content of the measure using qualitative and quantitative methods, examining the relationship between or among scales or examining how the scale relates to external variables such as job loss or utilization of healthcare. Norm-based interpretations compare scores for a particular group with large population-based samples.

Cultural issues

Although the meaning of QoL can differ across cultures, it may be possible to develop measures that can capture at least some elements of QoL across all cultures (WHO, 1998). The cross-cultural adaptation of an instrument involves both assessment of conceptual and linguistic equivalence and evaluation of measurement properties (Bowden & Fox-Rushby, 2003). However, cultures also differ markedly in their cognitive systems and beliefs about the world. Social differences affect not only beliefs about specific aspects of the world but also beliefs about the nature of cognitive processes themselves. For example, happiness, as opposed to perceived norms about whether one should be satisfied or not, correlates significantly more strongly with life satisfaction in more individualistic nations such as North America and Western Europe than in more collectivist cultures such as China and India (Suh *et al.*, 1998). Latin Americans are among the happiest and East Asians are among the least happy based on this characterization of happiness (Diener *et al.*, 2003). It appears that East Asians weigh the worst areas of their lives when computing their life satisfaction while Latin Americans may be rooted in cultural norms supporting a belief that life in general is good (see also 'Cultural and ethnic factors in health').

Computerized adaptive testing (CAT)

Computerized Adaptive Testing (CAT) is a new method designed to make surveys much shorter, more precise and less expensive. In contrast to traditional surveys where the same questions are asked of everyone regardless of their answers, CAT surveys make it possible to individualize each assessment so that only the most relevant and informative questions are asked of each person at their particular level of health. Associated with CAT is the emerging statistical approach of item response theory (IRT), which is used instead of the 'classical' psychometric approach for constructing and calibrating generic and disease-specific HRQoL measures (Ware, 2003).

Cognitive aspects of survey methodology (CASM)

QoL assessments, although apparently simple, require sophisticated cognitive processing. Respondents are typically required to understand complex, abstract questions, retrieve information from long-term memory, aggregate that information and apply frequency judgements, magnitude estimation and decision heuristics in selecting which response category to endorse. There is growing interest in applying Cognitive Aspects of Survey Methodology (CASM) techniques to existing instruments to investigate whether the cognitive processes employed by respondents, in reading, comprehending and interpreting questions and in formulating and providing answers vary across cultures or with respect to other respondent characteristics. CASM provides techniques such as cognitive interviewing and linguistic analysis that help to elucidate the cognitive mechanisms underlying responses (McColl *et al.*, 2003).

Response shift

People with severe diseases often report QoL equal or superior to less severely ill people or healthy people and consistent disparities arise between clinical measures and patients' own evaluations. These findings reflect the dynamic nature of QoL, increasingly known as response shift (Schwartz & Sprangers, 2000). Response shift refers to a change in the meaning of one's evaluation of a construct as a result of a change in one's internal standards of measurement, a change in one's values or a redefinition of the construct. In repeated measures studies, a response shift may mask or exaggerate a treatment effect where the measures are patient reported outcomes (PROs) such as QoL. It can also be argued that achieving a response shift may be a reasonable therapeutic aim in helping patients adapt to health-related challenges.

This is in line with current suggestions in the positive psychology literature for using well-being therapy (Fava & Ruini, 2003).

Conclusion

The application of QoL assessment in healthcare has grown rapidly over the past decade. The concept and measurement of QoL entered medical research from two different sources, i.e. medical assessment of functional health status and developments in social indicators research. QoL assessments in healthcare are used mainly in clinical trials, clinical practice and in population-based studies. Exciting new developments in QoL research include, *inter alia*, the application of computer adaptive testing technology (CAT), item response theory (IRT), cognitive aspects of survey methodology (CASM) and response shift analysis. The major challenge to the field is to develop a level of sophistication, interpretation and cross-cultural validity that allows QoL information to become an important part of routine clinical practice making possible an evidence-based approach to holistic patient care.

Acknowledgement

This chapter was completed while the author, Dr Lena Ring, was EU Marie Curie Research Fellow at the Department of Psychology, Royal College of Surgeons in Ireland.

REFERENCES

Alonso, J., Ferrer, M., Gandek, B. *et al.* (2004). Health-related quality of life associated with chronic conditions in eight countries: results from the International Quality of Life Assessment (IQOLA) Project. *Quality of Life Research*, **13**(2), 283–98.

Andrews, F. M. & Withey, S. B. (1976). *Social indicators of well-being: American perspectives on life quality.* New York: Plenum.

Aromaa, A., Koponen, P., Tafforeau, J. *et al.* (2003). Evaluation of health interview surveys and health examination surveys in the European Union. *European Journal of Public Health*, **13**(3 Suppl), 67–72.

Bowden, A. & Fox-Rushby, J. A. (2003). A systematic and critical review of the process of translation and adaptation of generic health-related quality of life measures in Africa, Asia, Eastern Europe, the Middle East, South America. *Social Science & Medicine*, **57**(7), 1289–306.

Bowling, A. (2001). *Measuring disease.* Buckingham, UK: Open University Press.

Bradburn, N. M. (1969). *The structure of psychological well-being.* Chicago: Aldine.

Campbell, A. (1976). *The quality of American life.* New York: Russell Sage Foundation.

Campbell, A. & Converse, P. E. (1972). *The human meaning of social change.* New York: Russell Sage Foundation.

Cantril, H. (1965). *The patterns of human concern.* New Brunswick, NJ: Rutgers University Press.

Claridge, J. A. & Fabian, T. C. (2005). History and development of evidence-based medicine. *World Journal of Surgery*, **14**, 14.

Coste, J., Guillemin, F., Pouchot, J. *et al.* (1997). Methodological approaches to shortening composite measurement scales. *Journal of Clinical Epidemiology*, **50**(3), 247–52.

Croog, S. H., Levine, S., Testa, M. A. *et al.* (1986). The effects of antihypertensive therapy on the quality of life. *New England Journal of Medicine*, **314**(26), 1657–64.

de Boer, A. G., van Lanschot, J. J., Stalmeier, P. F. *et al.* (2004). Is a single-item visual analogue scale as valid, reliable and responsive as multi-item scales in measuring quality of life? *Quality of Life Research*, **13**(2), 311–20.

Detmar, S. B., Aaronson, N. K., Wever, L. D. *et al.* (2000). How are you feeling? Who wants to know? Patients' and oncologists' preferences for discussing health-related quality-of-life issues. *Journal of Clinical Oncology*, **18**(18), 3295–301.

Detmar, S. B., Muller, M. J., Schornagel, J. H. *et al.* (2002). Health-related quality-of-life assessments and patient–physician communication: a randomized controlled trial. *Journal of American Medical Association*, **288**(23), 3027–34.

Diel, I. J., Body, J. J., Lichinitser, M. R. *et al.* (2004). Improved quality of life after long-term treatment with the bisphosphonate ibandronate in patients with metastatic bone disease due to breast cancer. *European Journal of Cancer*, **40**(11), 1704–12.

Diener, E., Oishi, S. & Lucas, R. E. (2003). Personality, culture, and subjective well-being: emotional and cognitive evaluations of life. *Annual Review of Psychology*, **54**, 403–25. Epub 2002 Jun 10.

Drummond, M. F., Brien, B. O. *et al.* (1999). *Methods for the evaluation of health care programmes* (2nd edn.). New York: Oxford University Press Inc.

Engel, G. L. (1977). The need for a new medical model: a challenge for biomedicine. *Science*, **196**(4286), 129–36.

Erickson, R. (1974). Welfare as a planning goal. *Acta Sociologica*, **17**, 32–43.

Espallargues, M., Valderas, J. M. & Alonso, J. (2000). Provision of feedback on perceived health status to health care professionals: a systematic review of its impact. *Medical Care*, **38**, 175–86.

Fallowfield, L., Ratcliffe, D., Jenkins, V. *et al.* (2001). Psychiatric morbidity and its recognition by doctors in patients with cancer. *British Journal of Cancer*, **84**, 1011–5.

Fava, G. A. & Ruini, C. (2003). Development and characteristics of a well-being enhancing psychotherapeutic strategy: well-being therapy. *Journal of Behavior Therapy and Experimental Psychiatry*, **34**(1), 45–63.

Garratt, A., Schmidt, L., Machintosh, A. *et al.* (2002). Quality of life measurement: bibliographic study of patient assessed health outcome measures. *British Medical Journal*, **324**(7351), 1417.

Glimelius, B., Hoffman, K., Graf, W. *et al.* (1995). Cost-effectiveness of palliative chemotherapy in advanced gastrointestinal cancer. *Annals of Oncology*, **6**(3), 267–74.

Greenhalgh, J. & Meadows, K. (1999). The effectiveness of the use of patient-based measures of health in routine practice in improving the process and outcomes of patient care: a literature review. *Journal of Evaluation in Clinical Practice*, **5**, 401–16.

Gridelli, C., Gallo, C., Di Maio, M. *et al.* (2004). A randomised clinical trial of two docetaxel regimens (weekly vs 3 week) in the second-line treatment of non-small-cell lung cancer. The DISTAL 01 study. *British Journal of Cancer*, **91**(12), 1996–2004.

Gunter, M. J. (1999). The role of the ECHO model in outcomes research and clinical practice improvement. *American Journal of Managed Care*, **5**(4), 217–24.

Hepler, C. D. & Strand, L. M. (1990). Opportunities and responsibilities in pharmaceutical care. *American Journal of Hospital Pharmacy*, **47**(3), 533–43.

Karnofsky, D. A. & Burchenal, J. H. (1948). The clinical evaluation of chemotherapeutic agents in cancer. In C. M. Macleod (Ed.). *Evaluation of chemotherapeutic agents*. New York: Columbia University Press.

Kozma, C. M., Reeder, C. E. & Schulz, R. M. (1993). Economic, clinical, and humanistic outcomes: a planning model for pharmacoeconomic research. *Clinical Therapeutics*, **15**(6), 1121–32; discussion 1120.

Marquis, P., Chassany, O. & Abetz, L. (2004). A comprehensive strategy for the interpretation of quality-of-life data based on existing methods. *Value in Health*, **7**(1), 93–104.

McColl, E., Meadows, K. & Barofsky, I. (2003). Cognitive aspects of survey methodology and quality of life assessment. *Quality of Life Research*, **12**(3), 217–18.

McHorney, C. A. & Tarlow, A. R. (1995). Individual patient monitoring in clinical practice: are available health status surveys adequate? *Quality of Life Research*, **4**, 293–307.

Michalos, A. C. (1980). *North American social report, Vol.1: foundations, population and health*. Dordrecht: Oxford University Press.

O'Boyle, C., Höfer, S. Ring, L. (2005). Individualized Quality of Life. In P. Fayers & R. D. Hays (Eds.). *Assessing the quality of life in clinical trials* (2nd edn., pp. 225–42). Oxford: Oxford University Press, 225–42.

Pigou, A. C. (1920). *The economics of welfare*. London: MacMillan.

Prutkin, J. M. & Feinstein, A. R. (2002). Quality-of-life measurements: origin and pathogenesis. *The Yale Journal of Biology and Medicine*, **75**(2), 79–93.

SAC (2002). Assessing health status and quality-of-life instruments: attributes and review criteria. *Quality of Life Research*, **11**(3), 193–205.

Schwartz, C. E. & Sprangers, M. (Eds.). (2000). *Adaptation to changing health. Response shift in quality of life research*. Washington, DC: American Psychological Association.

Skevington, S. M., Sartorius, N. & Amir, M. (2004). Developing methods for assessing quality of life in different cultural settings. The history of the WHOQOL instruments. *Social Psychiatry and Pschiatric Epidemiology*, **39**(1), 1–8.

Suh, E., Diener, E., Oishi, S. *et al.* (1998). The shifting base of life satisfaction judgements across cultures: emotions versus norms. *Journal of Personality and Social Psychology*, **74**(2), 482–93.

Velikova, G., Brown, J. M., Smith, A. B. *et al.* (2002). Computer-based quality of life questionnaires may contribute to doctor–patient interactions in oncology. *British Journal of Cancer*, **86**(1), 51–9.

Ware, J. E., Jr. (2003). Conceptualization and measurement of health-related quality of life: comments on an evolving field. *Archives of Physical Medicine and Rehabilitation*, **84**(4 Suppl 2), S43–51.

Ware, J. E. Jr. & Gandek, B. (1998). Overview of the SF-36 Health Survey and the International Quality of Life Assessment (IQOLA) project. *Journal of Clinical Epidemiology*, **51**(11), 903–12.

Weiss, S. C., Nguyen, J., Chon, S. *et al.* (2005). A randomized controlled clinical trial

assessing the effect of betamethasone valerate 0.12% foam on the short-term treatment of stasis dermatitis. *Journal of Drugs in Dermatology*, **4**(3), 339–45.

Willke, R. J., Burke, L. B. & Erickson, P. (2004). Measuring treatment impact: a review of patient-reported outcomes and other efficacy endpoints in approved product labels. *Controlled Clinical Trials*, **25**(6), 535–52.

Wilson, I. B. (2000). Clinical understanding and clinical implications of response shift. In C. E. Schwartz & M. A. G. Sprangers (Eds.). Adaptation to changing health. Response shift in quality of life research (pp. 159–73). Washington, D.C: American Psychological Association.

Wood-Dauphinee, S. (1999). Assessing quality of life in clinical research: from where have we come and where are we going? *Journal of Clinical Epidemiology*, **52**(4), 355–63.

World Health Organization (1948). *Official record of the World Health Organization*. Geneva: WHO.

World Health Organization (1998). The World Health Organization Quality of Life Assessment (WHOQOL): development and general psychometric properties. *Social Science and Medicine*, **46**(12), 1569–85.

Zou, K. H., Fielding, J. R. & Ondategui-Parra, S. *et al.* (2004). What is evidence-based medicine? *Academic Radiology*, **11**(2), 127–33.

Religion and health

Karen Hye-cheon Kim[1] and Harold G. Koenig[2]

[1]University of Arkansas for Medical Sciences
[2]Duke University Medical Center and Geriatric Research, Education and Clinical Center, VA Medical Center

Religion is an influential force in today's society. Over 4 billion worldwide identify themselves with a religious group (Bedell, 1997). In the USA alone, recent polls report that 93% believe in God, 30–42% of adults (72 million) attend religious services weekly and 85% report that religion is at least fairly important in their own lives (DDB Needham Worldwide, 2000; Gallup Poll, 2001). Religion is not only an influential force but a growing force as well. In the late twentieth century came the rise of religious fundamentalism (Sherket & Ellison, 1999), the awakening of new religious movements and the expansion of other older movements such as

Mormonism and Pentecostalism (Chaves, 1994). Religious beliefs about political issues and the family also continue to influence the cultural milieu. Since religion is deeply interwoven in social life, could not religion also influence health?

Research on the religion–health relationship has not only arisen from recognizing religion's continuing influence on private and public life, but also from the changing nature of medical institutions. The impersonal nature of medical treatment, burgeoning healthcare costs and the realization of science's limitations through medical mistakes have moved medical professionals and researchers to consider and examine other avenues for health promotion and treatment (Koenig *et al.*, 2001).

Religion and medicine were virtually one and the same entity before the fourteenth century, but the divide between them grew after the 1500s, resulting after the Enlightenment in the clash between the two disciplines seen today (Koenig *et al.*, 2001). However, recent research on religion's connection to health has prompted a renegotiation of this relationship.

In this chapter, we will examine religion's relationship with physical health and with mental health. We will then discuss potential mechanisms through which religion may be connected to health. Finally, we will discuss the implications this research field has on medical practice and public health. Given that most research on religion and health has been conducted in the United States (Koenig *et al.*, 2001), the content of this chapter will be based largely on conceptualizations and studies of religion and health from a Judaeo-Christian framework.

Religion and physical health

Mortality

Over 100 studies have examined religion's relationship with mortality, including longitudinal investigations (Koenig, 2001*a*). Several aspects of religiosity have been consistently related to lower mortality, including self-reported religious attendance and mortality. In a 28-year longitudinal study of 5286 adults, frequent religious service attenders had a 23–36% lower mortality rate than infrequent attenders (Strawbridge *et al.*, 1997). In another study, those who never attended religious services exhibited 1.87 times the risk of death during a nine-year period compared with those who attended religious services more than once a week (Hummer *et al.*, 1999). Longitudinal studies examining religion's relationship with mortality have reported an average 30% reduction in mortality in healthy subjects after controlling for important confounders (Powell *et al.*, 2003). Regarding religious denomination, Seventh-Day Adventists, Mormons, the Amish, and to a lesser extent, Jews, have lower mortality rates than the general population (Koenig, 2001*a*).

Although the evidence suggests that religion (particularly religious attendance) is related to lower mortality, a few studies have reported the opposite (Koenig, 2001*a*). Patients experiencing religious struggles (i.e. believing that God does not love them, has abandoned them, is punishing them or does not have the power to help them) had a 19–28% higher mortality during a 2-year follow-up period (Pargament *et al.*, 2001). Thus, religion's relationship with mortality may depend on what aspect of religion is assessed in relation to health.

Cardiovascular disease

Studies examining religion's relationship with cardiovascular disease have reported less heart disease and lower cardiovascular mortality among the more religiously involved (Koenig, 2001*a*; Mueller *et al.*, 2001; Powell *et al.*, 2003). In two longitudinal studies following large American adult samples, religious attendance was related to lower rates of death from cardiovascular disease, even after adjusting for age, gender, education, ethnicity, health status

and social contacts (Hummer *et al.*, 1999; Oman *et al.*, 2002). The relationship of religious denomination membership with cardiovascular disease is more mixed, with some studies reporting higher rates of cardiovascular disease in some religious groups and lower rates in others (Friedlander *et al.*, 1986; Medalie *et al.*, 1973; Goldbourt *et al.*, 1993).

Regarding religion's relationship with stroke, few studies have been conducted. One six-year longitudinal study reported a positive relationship between religious attendance and lower stroke incidence (Colantonio *et al.*, 1992). Those who attended religious services once or twice per year or more were 14% less likely to have a stroke during the follow-up period. Controlling for mediating factors such as blood pressure helped to explain this effect.

Cancer

Numerous studies have compared the risk of cancer and mortality rates from cancer by religious denomination (Koenig, 2001*a*). Most consistently, Mormons and Seventh-Day Adventists have a lower risk of mortality from cancer than the general population (Phillips *et al.*, 1980; Berkel & deWaard, 1983; Enstrom, 1989). A handful of studies, however, have examined the relationship of general religious activity with cancer. National representative samples of American adults followed from one to three decades have reported a positive relationship between religious attendance and lower cancer mortality (Hummer *et al.*, 1999; Oman *et al.*, 2002). These relationships between religion and cancer mortality, however, became insignificant when demographics, health behaviours and prior health status were controlled. Studies examining religion's relationship with cancer progression have reported few significant relationships (Powell *et al.*, 2003).

Hypertension

Different aspects of religion have been positively related to lower blood pressure and less hypertension, particularly lower diastolic blood pressure (Koenig, 2001*a*; Mueller *et al.*, 2001). Most of these studies are cross-sectional, but two are prospective in design (Koenig *et al.*, 1998*a*; Timio *et al.*, 1997). In one of the largest of these studies, cross-sectional results at baseline indicated that participants who attended religious services and engaged in private religious practices (e.g. prayer and frequent Bible studying) had a 40% lower likelihood of having high diastolic blood pressure (90mm Hg or higher), even after adjusting for known risk factors for hypertension (Koenig *et al.*, 1998*a*).

Other studies of physical health

The literature on religion's relationship with disability is less clear. Two well-controlled longitudinal studies in the elderly have reported no relationship between religion (religious attendance, depth of religiousness) and disability development (Colantonio *et al.*, 1992; Goldman *et al.*, 1995). However, a well-controlled prospective study from Yale University reported a significant association of religious attendance and lowered risk for disability over 6 to 12 years of follow-up (Idler & Kasl, 1997). On the other hand, a few studies have reported religion's relationship with greater body weight

(Ferraro, 1998; Kim *et al.*, 2003), which may influence health (see 'Obesity').

Religion and mental health

Although the relationship between religion and physical health remains controversial, associations with mental health are more consistent.

Psychological well-being

A review of religion's relationship with psychological well-being reported that 79 of 100 studies found significant positive correlations (Koenig, 2001*b*). These positive associations between religion and well-being have been reported in a variety of samples, including groups of varying ages and religions (i.e. Christian, Jewish and Muslim) (Koenig *et al.*, 2001). Some longitudinal studies examining religion's relationship with well-being have reported significant relationships cross-sectionally (Graney, 1975; Willits & Crider, 1988), but not over time. However, at least half a dozen longitudinal studies have found significant positive relationships between religious involvement and well-being when studied over time (Koenig *et al.*, 2001).

Depression

Numerous studies have documented a lower rate of depression and faster recovery from depression among the more religious (Koenig, 2001*b*; McCullough & Larson, 1999; Mueller *et al.*, 2001). This relationship between religion and depression has been documented in several methodologically sophisticated studies. In a one-year longitudinal study of medically ill older patients, those reporting higher intrinsic religiosity experienced faster remission from depression (Koenig *et al.*, 1998b). This relationship remained significant after controlling for confounders. Of eight clinical trials, five reported that depressed subjects receiving a religious intervention recovered faster than subjects in control groups or those receiving secular interventions (Koenig, 2001*b*).

Anxiety

A majority of prospective cohort studies and clinical trials have reported religion's association with less anxiety (Koenig, 2001*b*; Mueller *et al.*, 2001). In one clinical trial, Muslim subjects randomly assigned to religious psychotherapy experienced lower anxiety than those receiving medications and supportive psychotherapy alone (Razali *et al.*, 1998). Cross-sectional studies examining religion's relationship with anxiety have reported mixed results; thus religion may not only influence anxiety but those who are anxious may turn to religion as well.

Other studies of mental health

Studies examining religion's relationship with psychotic symptoms and disorders are sparse and mixed, with some reporting religion's relationship with fewer psychotic symptoms or disorders (Koenig, 2001*b*; Verghese *et al.*, 1989), greater psychotic symptoms (Neeleman & Lewis, 1994) or no relationship (Cothran & Harvey, 1986; Lindgren & Coursey, 1995).

The literature on religion's relationship with suicide is clearer. A majority of studies, including those with prospective designs, have reported relationships between different aspects of religion (attendance, self-reported importance, belief in God, religious upbringing) and less suicide or more negative attitudes towards suicide (Koenig, 2001*b*; Mueller *et al.*, 2001).

A majority of studies examining religion's relationship with delinquency or crime have also reported inverse relationships, particularly among younger persons (Koenig, 2001*b*). Studies utilizing national samples have reported a positive relationship between different aspects of religion (attendance, importance) and lower delinquency among high school students (Stark, 1996; Wallace & Forman, 1998).

A small number of studies have also examined religion's relationship with body image and dieting, reporting mixed results (Kim, 2006; Kim, 2007; Wechsler *et al.*, 1981).

How is religion related to health?

Health behaviours

Religion's social sanctions against smoking, drinking and high-risk behaviours are possible mechanisms for its relationship with positive physical outcomes (Ellison & Levin, 1998; Sherkat & Ellison, 1999). A substantial number of studies confirm that more religious persons are less likely to abuse and use alcohol, drugs and cigarettes. These have included longitudinal studies and randomized trials, with different conceptualizations of religion (denomination, attendance, salience, upbringing) (Koenig *et al.*, 2001; Mueller *et al.*, 2001). Religion is also associated with lower high-risk sexual practices, extra-marital affairs and numbers of sexual partners among young adults (Koenig, 2001*b*) (see 'Sexual risk behaviour').

Theological teachings about the body and certain dietary restrictions may also serve to promote positive health behaviours, such as healthier nutrition and increased physical activity (Shatenstein & Ghadirian, 1998; Kim *et al.*, 2004). In contrast, religious teachings may also discourage adherents from obtaining appropriate medical care, which may serve to hinder health (Chatters, 2000).

Social support and networks

Religion provides adherents with social resources by increasing opportunities to enlarge and enhance social networks through religious services and other events (Chatters, 2000). Meaningful relationships may also be encouraged through religious doctrine's emphases on the virtue of caring and supporting others in need. Social support and network mechanisms through religion may also negatively affect health. Social relationships could be sources of distress and deterring from group norms could lead to negative emotions such as guilt and shame, which may hinder health (Chatters, 2000) (see 'Social support and health').

Stress and coping

Religious teachings, beliefs and behaviours (e.g. prayer) may enable adherents to counter and cope with stress (Mickley *et al.*, 1995). The similar ideologies, world-views and values which congregants share may also promote the formation of meaningful relationships, which enables stress to be interpreted and tackled from a base of shared values and world outlooks (Ellison and Levin, 1998). This support in times of chronic and acute stress may help to buffer the negative relationship of stress with health (Sherkat & Ellison, 1999). However, religious coping may also be maladaptive. Utilizing negative religious coping, where one is struggling with one's faith, may contribute to poorer health outcomes (Pargament *et al.*, 2001) (see 'Stress and health').

Other psychosocial mechanisms

Religion provides meaning and understanding with regard to metaphysical questions and those questions related to why things happen (Musick *et al.*, 2000). Having this framework of understanding may serve to positively effect health. Embedded in religion's role of providing metaphysical meaning are theological teachings about worth which may also serve to promote health. Believing that one has a relationship with a divine being who loves personally and unconditionally may serve as a source of meaning and self-esteem (Ellison & Levin, 1998; Sherkat & Ellison, 1999).

Religion may also increase self-efficacy and perceived control. 'Doing' religion through supporting others could give participants a sense of achievement. Further, communicating with a deity through prayer, meditation and song offers a means through which the believer can petition for changes in circumstances that would otherwise seem beyond their control (Ellison & Levin, 1998; Sherkat & Ellison, 1999) (see 'Perceived control' and 'Self-efficacy and health').

However, some religious beliefs may engender feelings of shame and guilt, leading to negative self-esteem (Chatters, 2000). Religious struggle, including feeling punished by God, may also serve to decrease self-esteem (Pargament *et al.*, 2001). Thus negative aspects of religion may work concomitantly with other forms of religiousness to affect health.

Immune and neuroendocrine function and biological pathways

Religion may be related to health in part through influencing immune and neuroendocrine function. Several recent studies have reported religion's significant correlation with several immune function parameters, including higher T helper/inducer cell (CD4) counts (Woods *et al.*, 1999), greater numbers of white blood cells, greater total lymphocyte counts (Sephton *et al.*, 2001) and lower levels of an inflammatory marker (Interleukin-6) (Sephton *et al.*, 2000). Religion has also been linked with lower levels of cortisol, a biological measure of stress (Ironson *et al.*, 2002; Sephton *et al.*, 2000) (see 'Psychoneuroimmunology').

Implications

Physicians have struggled over the role religion should play in their work. Religion can be a sensitive topic that elicits a range of highly charged beliefs, attitudes and emotions from both doctor and patient. Unlike the traditional practice of medicine, religion is also seen as highly subjective and personal, which brings ethical concerns. Given these apprehensions, however, physicians see religion's role in the lives of many of their patients, and consequently realize that for some, health is beyond physical and mental and may in fact involve the spiritual as well. Taking a brief spiritual history of a patient would inform the physician as to whether faith is playing a role in their patient's health. If faith is playing a role, understanding the relationship between religion and health would enable the physician to encourage better health through a patient-centred approach, which can include referrals to chaplains or other pastoral counsellors as needed (Koenig, 2002).

Understanding the relationship between religion and health would not only enable medical professionals to be more knowledgeable in interacting with some patients, but would also enable public health professionals to more sensitively collaborate with religious communities. Religious communities have been the sites for several successful public health interventions (Lewis & Green, 2000; Resnicow *et al.*, 2001). Thus better understanding religion's relationship with various health outcomes may lead to the creation of more effective faith-based interventions. Being aware of how different aspects of religion can promote both positive and negative health outcomes could also inform programme makers in the creation of health promotion materials.

The study of religion and health is an ancient discipline that has been re-awakened in its present form. This new form has materialized itself in the empirical study of religion's relationship with health: Is there a connection? If so, how is religion connected to health? Future studies utilizing sophisticated methodological designs will be needed to elucidate direction of causality. Future work will also need to more accurately capture the complex, multi-dimensional nature of religion by including measures of religion other than religious attendance. Examining religion's relationship with health in a framework other than a predominately U.S. Judaeo-Christian one will also be needed to fully understand the religion–health connection. Thus in its current form, the work of religion and health is only beginning. However, in other ways the study of religion and health has been an ongoing one in that it asks questions that we have all asked ourselves at one point or another: Is there an unseen that affects what is seen? What is the exact nature of the world that we live in? Is there something bigger than the self that has an influence on life? Thus in this sense, the study of religion and health is nothing new, but rather an ancient question that has not only intrigued many generations past but will continue to intrigue many generations to come.

REFERENCES

Bedell, K. B. (1997). *Yearbook of American and Canadian Churches 1997*. Nashville: Abingdon Press, pp. 252–8.

Berkel, J. & deWaard, F. (1983). Mortality pattern and life expectancy of Seventh-Day Adventists in the Netherlands.

International Journal of Epidemiology, **12**, 455–9.

Chatters, L. M. (2000). Religion and health: public health research and practice. *Annual Review of Public Health*, **21**, 335–67.

Chaves, M. (1994). Secularization as declining religious authority. *Social Forces*, **72**(3), 749–74.

Colantonio, A., Kasl, S. V. & Ostfeld, A. M. (1992). Depressive symptoms and other psychosocial factors as predictors of stroke in the elderly. *American Journal of Epidemiology*, **136**, 884–94.

Cothran, M. M. & Harvey, P. D. (1986). Delusional thinking in psychotics: correlates of religious content. *Psychological Reports*, **58**, 191–9.

DDB Needham Worldwide (2000). DDB Needham Worldwide, 303 East Wacker Drive, Chicago, IL 60601–5282.

Ellison, C. G. & Levin, J. S. (1998). The religion–health connection: evidence, theory, and future directions. *Health Education and Behavior*, **25**, 700–20.

Enstrom, J. E. (1989). Health practices and cancer mortality among active California Mormons. *Journal of the National Cancer Institute*, **81**, 1807–14.

Ferraro, K. F. (1998). Firm believers? Religion, body weight, and well-being. *Review of Religious Research*, **39**(3), 224–44.

Friedlander, Y., Kark, J. D. & Stein, Y. (1986). Religious orthodoxy and myocardial infarction in Jerusalem – a case control study. *International Journal of Cardiology*, **10**, 33–41.

Goldbourt, U., Yaari, S. & Medalie, J. H. (1993). Factors predictive of long-term coronary heart disease mortality among 10,059 male Israeli civil servants and municipal employees. *Cardiology*, **82**, 100–21.

Goldman, N., Korenman, S. & Weinstein, R. (1995). Marital status and health among the elderly. *Social Science and Medicine*, **40**, 1717–30.

Graney, M. J. (1975). Happiness and social participation in aging. *Journal of Gerontology*, **30**, 701–6.

Hummer, R. A., Rogers, R. G., Nam, C. B. & Ellison, C. G. (1999). Religious involvement and U.S. adult mortality. *Demography*, **36**, 273–85.

Idler, E. L. & Kasl, S. (1997). Religion among disabled and nondisabled persons: II. Attendance at religious services as a predictor of the course of disability. *Journal of Gerontology*, **52B**(6), 306–16.

Ironson, G., Solomon, G. F., Balbin, E. G. *et al.* (2002). The Ironson–Woods Spirituality/Religiousness Index is associated with long survival, health behaviors, less distress, and low cortisol in people with HIV/AIDS. *Annals of Behavioral Medicine*, **24**, 34–48.

Kim, K. H. (2006). Religion, body satisfaction and dieting. *Appetite*, May; **46**(3), 285–96.

Kim, K. H. (2007). Religion, weight perception, and weight control behavior. Jan; **8**(1), 121–31.

Kim, K. H. & Sobal, J. (2004). Religion, fat-intake, and physical activity. *Public Health Nutrition* **7**(6), 773–81.

Kim, K. H., Sobal, J. & Wethington, E. (2003). Religion and body weight. *International Journal of Obesity*, **27**, 469–77.

Koenig, H. G. (2002). An 83-year-old woman with chronic illness and strong religious beliefs. *Journal of the American Medical Association*, **288**(4), 487–93.

Koenig, H. G. (2001*a*). Religion and medicine IV: religion, physical health, and clinical implications. *International Journal of Psychiatry in Medicine*, **31**(3), 321–36.

Koenig, H. G. (2001*b*). Religion and medicine II: religion, mental health, and related behaviors. *International Journal of Psychiatry in Medicine*, **31**(1), 97–109.

Koenig, H. G., Cohen, H. J., George, L. K. *et al.* (1997). Attendance at religious services, interleukin-6 and other biological parameters of immune function in older adults. *International Journal of Psychiatry in Medicine*, **27**, 233–50.

Koenig, H. G., George, L. K., Hays, J. C. *et al.* (1998*a*). The relationship between religious activities and blood pressure in older adults. *International Journal of Psychiatry in Medicine*, **24**, 122–30.

Koenig, H. G., George, L. K. & Peterson, B. L. (1998*b*). Religiosity and remission of depression in medically ill older patients. *American Journal of Psychiatry*, **155**, 536–42.

Koenig, H. G., McCullough, M. E. & Larson, D. B. (2001). *Handbook of religion and health*. New York: Oxford University Press.

Lewis, R. K. & Green, B. L. (2000). Assessing the health attitudes, beliefs, and behaviors of African Americans attending church: a comparison from two communities. *Journal of Community Health*, **25**(3), 211–24.

Lindgren, K. N. & Coursey, R. D. (1995). Spirituality and serious mental illness: a two-part study. *Psychosocial Rehabilitation Journal*, **18**(3), 93–111.

McCullough, M. E. & Larson, D. B. (1999). Religion and depression: a review of the literature. *Twin Research*, **2**, 126–36.

Medalie, J. H., Kahn, H. A., Neufled, H. N., Riss, E. & Goldbourt, U. (1973). Five-year myocardial infarction incidence II. Association of single variables to age and birthplace. *Journal of Chronic Diseases*, **26**, 329–49.

Mickley, J. R., Carson, V. & Soeken, K. L. (1995). Religion and adult mental health: state of the science in nursing. *Issues in Mental Health Nursing*, **16**(4), 345–60.

Mueller, P. S., Plevak, D. J. & Rummans, R. A. (2001). Religious involvement, spirituality, and medicine: implications for clinical practice. *Mayo Clinic Proceedings*, **76**, 1225–35.

Musick, M. A., Traphagan, J. W., Koenig, H. G. & Larson, D. B. (2000). Spirituality in physical health and aging. *Journal of Adult Development*, **7**(2), 73–86.

Neeleman, J. & Lewis, G. (1994). Religious identity and comfort beliefs in three groups of psychiatric patients and a group of medical controls. *International Journal of Social Psychiatry*, **40**, 124–34.

Oman, D., Kurata, J. H., Strawbridge, W. J. & Cohen, R. D. (2002). Religious attendance and cause of death over 31 years. *International Journal of Psychiatry in Medicine*, **32**, 69–89.

Pargament, K. I., Koenig, H. G., Tarakeshwar, N. & Hahn, J. (2001). Religious struggle as a predictor of mortality among medically ill elderly patients: a two-year longitudinal study. *Archives of Internal Medicine*, **161**, 1881–5.

Phillips, R. L., Garfinkel, L., Kuzma, J. W. *et al.* (1980). Mortality among California Seventh-Day Adventists for selected cancer sites. *Journal of the National Cancer Institute*, **65**, 1097–107.

Powell, L. H., Shahbi, L. & Thoresen, C. E. (2003). Religion and spirituality: linkages to physical health. *American Psychologist*, **58**, 36–52.

Razali, S. M., Hasanah, C. I., Aminah, K. & Subramaniam, M. (1998). Religious–sociocultural psychotherapy in patients with anxiety and depression. *Australian and New Zealand Journal of Psychiatry*, **32**, 867–972.

Resnicow, K., Jackson, A., Wang, T. *et al.* (2001). A motivational interviewing intervention to increase fruit and vegetable intake through Black Churches: results of the Eat for Life Trial. *American Journal of Public Health*, **91**(10), 1686–93.

Sephton, S. E., Sapolsky, R. M., Kraemer, H. C. & Spiegel, D. (2000). Dirunal cortisol rhythm as a predictor of breast cancer. *Journal of the National Cancer Institution*, **92**, 994–1000.

Shatenstein, B. & Ghadirian, P. (1998). Influences on diet, health behaviours and their outcome in select ethnocultural and religious groups. *Nutrition*, **14**, 223–30.

Sherkat, D. E. & Ellison, C. G. (1999). Recent developments and current controversies in the sociology of religion. *Annual Review of Sociology*, **25**, 363–94.

Stark, R. (1996). Religion as a context: hellfire and delinquency one more time. *Sociology of Religion*, **57**, 163–73.

Strawbridge, W. J., Cohen, R. D., Shema, S. J. & Kaplan, G. A. (1997). Frequent attendance at religious services and mortality over 28 years.

American Journal of Public Health, **87**(6), 957–61.

The Roper Center for Public Opinion Research, Gallup Poll (2001). United States. Storrs, CT: Author.

Timio, M., Lippi, G., Venanzi, S. *et al.* (1997). Blood pressure trend and cardiovascular events in nuns in a secluded order: a 30-year follow-up study. *Blood Pressure*, **6**, 81–7.

Verghese, A., John, J. K., Rajkumar, S. *et al.* (1989). Factors associated with the course and outcome of schizophrenia in India: results of a two-year multi-centre follow-up study. *British Journal of Psychiatry*, **154**, 499–503.

Wallace, J. M. & Forman, T. A. (1998). Religion's role in promoting healthy and reducing the risk among American youth. *Health Education and Behavior*, **25**, 721–41.

Wechsler, H., Rohman, M. & Solomon, L. (1981). Emotional problems and concerns of New England college students. *American Journal of Orthopsychiatry*, **51**, 719–23.

Willits, F. K. & Crider, D. M. (1988). Religion and well-being: men and women in the middle years. *Review of Religious Research*, **29**, 281–94.

Woods, T. E., Antoni, M. H., Ironson, G. H. & Kling, D. W. (1999). Religiosity is associated with affective and immune status in symptomatic HIV-infected gay men. *Journal of Psychosomatic Research*, **46**, 165–76.

Risk perception and health behaviour

Baruch Fischhoff

Carnegie Mellon University

Introduction

Health depends, in part, on deliberate decisions. Some are private, such as deciding whether to wear bicycle helmets and seat belts, follow safety warnings, use condoms and fry (or broil) food. Other decisions involve societal issues, such as whether to protest about the siting of an incinerator or halfway house, vote for fluoridation and 'green' candidates or support sex education.

Sometimes, single choices have large effects on health risks (e.g. buying a car with airbags, taking a dangerous job, getting pregnant). At other times, the effects of individual choices are small, but accumulate over multiple decisions (e.g. repeatedly ordering broccoli, wearing a seat belt or using the escort service in parking garages). Yet other times, choices intended to reduce health risks achieve nothing or the opposite (e.g. responding to baseless cancer scares, subscribing to quack treatments).

In order to make health decisions wisely, individuals must understand the risks and benefits associated with alternative courses of action. They also need to understand the limits to their own knowledge and to the advice proffered by various experts. This chapter considers how to describe people's beliefs about health risk issues, as a step toward designing (and evaluating) interventions designed to improve their choice. A fuller account would also consider the roles of emotion, personality, culture and social processes (Lerner & Keltner, 2000).

Framing health-risk decisions

Any study of decision-making faces four strategic choices (Fischhoff, 2005):

a. *Does it begin with a formal analysis of the decision?* With cancer, for example, those decisions could include whether to rely on breast self-examination, get a genetic test, take an experimental treatment or reduce sunbathing. The focal outcomes might include health effects, as well as changes in psychological wellbeing, personal relationships, insurability and family finances. The probabilities of these outcomes might be assessed with meta-analyses or expert judgement. The outcomes might be evaluated by conversion to a common unit (e.g. dollars, Quality Adjusted Life Years (QALYs)) or by the decision makers' preferences. Researchers who skip the formal analysis implicitly assume that they know both how people's choices will affect their lives and how people feel about those effects. Some decisions pose very familiar choices, hence need little formal analysis; others are novel, complex and uncertain – challenging any researchers' intuitions (Hastie & Dawes, 2002).

b. *Does the research adopt a persuasive stance?* Health researchers often hope to identify choices needing improvement. Those choices could be evaluated in terms of either 'rationality' or 'optimality'. The former criterion asks whether people have followed the internal logic of their beliefs and values. The latter asks whether people have done the best thing. The two standards could differ if people's beliefs or values are deemed wrong. If people have the wrong facts, then the remedy might be communicating the risks of current behaviours and the risk-reduction benefits of alternative ones. Having the wrong values might mean enjoying short-term pleasures (food, sex, thrills) too much and carrying about negative long-term consequences too little – even after knowing just what they entail. Trying to change what matters to people means presuming to know what is good for them. Adopting a persuasive stance means determining that people cannot be trusted to understand the facts and reach a rational conclusion. Its legitimacy depends on whether its targets acknowledge these limits (as might happen with complex, time-constrained choices or ones not worth thinking about).

c. *Do interventions seek to improve specific choices or confer general mastery of the decision-making domain?* Any (non-fatal) choice is but one in a sequence. It may be revisited (e.g. 'should I stay the course [with a lifestyle change or drug treatment]?'). It may create new choices (e.g. 'should I reveal my test result?'). It may change the person involved (e.g. facing future choices with regret or pain). Broadening the context can make choices clearer – or overwhelm decision makers with detail. Efficiently manipulating behaviour, time after time, may undermine the chances for sustained, informed change. People may think in terms of individual choices, not realizing how risks and benefits mount up through repeated exposure.

d. *Which individual differences should be considered?* People's circumstances (e.g. health, social support, financial resources, sensitivity to medication) and values (e.g. time horizon, tolerance for ambiguity, concern for others) may vary, so that people in ostensibly the same situation may face very different choices. A full account would also consider differences in the decision-making processes that they favour (e.g. reflecting their need for technical mastery, desire for autonomy, emotional resilience) and their social context (e.g. cultural expectations, shared decision making, safety net). People may also vary in their health literacy or in their decision-making competence (Parker & Fischhoff, 2005). The importance of all these factors varies. An effect can be robust and theoretically informative without having practical impact.

Quantitative assessment

Estimating the size of risks

A common presenting symptom in experts' complaints about lay decision making is that 'they do not realize how small (or large) the risk is'. Where that is the case, the mission of health communication is conceptually simple (if technically challenging): transmit credible risk estimates. Research suggests that lay risk estimates are, indeed, subject to bias (Kahneman *et al.*, 1982; Slovic, 1987).

In one early study (Lichtenstein *et al.*, 1978), subjects judged the annual number of deaths in the US from each of 30 causes (e.g. botulism, tornados, motor vehicle accidents), using one of two response modes. One task presented pairs of causes; subjects chose the more frequent, then estimated the ratio of the frequencies. The second task had subjects directly estimate the death tolls, after being told the answer for one cause (an anchor), in order to give an order-of-magnitude feeling for what numbers were appropriate. The study reached several seemingly robust conclusions.

a. *Estimates of relative frequency were quite consistent across response mode.* Thus, subjects seemed to have a moderately well-articulated internal risk scale, which they could express even with these unfamiliar tasks.

b. *Direct estimates were influenced by the anchor.* Subjects told that 50 000 people die annually from car accidents produced estimates that were two to five times higher than those produced by subjects told that 1000 die from electrocution.

Thus, they had a weak feel for absolute frequency, leaving them sensitive to the implicit cues in how questions are posed.

c. *Subjects' mean estimates varied less than the statistical estimates.* The overall trend was over-estimating small frequencies and underestimating large ones. However, the anchoring effect means that absolute estimates are method dependent, making the compression of lay estimates the more fundamental result.

d. *Some causes of' death consistently received higher estimates than others of equal statistical frequency.* They tended to involve disproportionately visible risks (e.g. homicide vs. asthma), consistent with estimating frequency by events' availability, while failing to realize how fallible that index is (Gilovich *et al.*, 2002).

e. *Subjects also assessed the probability of having chosen the more frequent of the paired causes of death.* They tended to be overconfident (e.g. choosing correctly only 75% of the time when 90% confident of having done so) – a special case of the general tendency to be inadequately sensitive to the extent of one's knowledge (Yates, 1989).

One recurrent obstacle to assessing or improving risk estimates is using verbal quantifiers such as 'very likely' or 'rare'. Such terms can mean different things to different people in one situation and to the same person in different contexts (e.g. likely to be fatal vs. likely to rain) (Wallsten *et al.*, 1986). The patterns in the 'causes of death' study could only be observed because it elicited quantitative estimates. As mentioned, though, with unfamiliar tasks, responses reflect the cues that people infer from task details, like anchors (Poulton, 1994; Schwarz, 1999). For example, Woloshin *et al.* (2000) evaluated a response mode using a linear scale for probabilities from 1–100% and a four-order log scale for probabilities from 0–1%. The responses that it elicited were at least as reliable and trustworthy as judgements evoked by other methods. However, it also elicited lower probabilities than a linear 0–100% scale. Presumably, the log-linear scale both made it easier to express small values *and* suggested that they might be appropriate. The opposite was true for the linear scale. If people knew just what they wanted to say, then the response mode would not matter. However, that need not be the case with the novel, often obscure tasks generated by researchers – or presented by life.

Evaluating the accuracy of lay estimates requires credible statistical estimates, for comparison purposes. Performance might be different (poorer?) for risks whose magnitude is less certain than those in public health statistics. Furthermore, laypeople may not see population risks as personally relevant, when assessing their own risk. Many studies have found that people see themselves as facing less risk than average others (which could be true for only half the population) (Weinstein, 1987). Such an optimism bias could prompt unwitting risk-taking (e.g. because warnings seem more relevant to other people). It could reflect both cognitive processes (e.g. the greater availability of ones' own precautions) and motivational ones (e.g. wishful thinking). The bias appears similarly in adults and adolescents, despite the common belief that teens' risk-taking is fuelled by a unique perception of invulnerability (Quadrel *et al.*, 1993).

These studies measure health risk perceptions under the assumption that people define 'risk' as 'probability of death'. However, in scientific practice, the meaning of 'risk' can vary by analysis. It might be expected loss of life expectancy or the expected probability of death. The former definition places a premium on deaths of young people, who lose more life when they die prematurely. Thus, disagreements about the size of risks can reflect both different views of the facts and different definitions of 'risk'. Without a shared definition of 'risk', researchers and respondents may be talking about different things (see 'Communicating risk').

Investigators have examined the correlations between quantitative judgements of 'risk' and various subjective features (e.g. voluntariness, scientific uncertainty, controllability). Looking at correlations among ratings of the features (Slovic, 1987), they have found a recurrent picture, with two or three dimensions of risk, emerging similarly across elicitation method, subject population (e.g. experts vs. laypeople), and risk domain. Core concepts underlying these dimensions include how well a risk seems to be understood and how much of a feeling of dread it evokes. The locations of individual hazards in this 'risk space' may vary by person, in ways related to their preferred risk management policies (e.g. how tightly a risk should be regulated). Characterizing risks in multi-attribute terms allow individuals to decide what matters to them (Florig et al., 2001). The British government has recently proposed characterizing risks in terms of these risk dimensions, complementing economic measures (HM Treasury, 2005).

Qualitative assessment

Event definitions

Scientific estimates of a risk's magnitude require detailed specification of the conditions under which it is to be observed. When researchers ask about risks without providing these needed details, they make it very hard to provide sensible answers. In order to respond correctly, subjects must first guess the question, and then know the answer to it. Consider, for example, a survey asking, 'How likely do you think it is that a person will get the AIDS virus from sharing plates, forks or glasses with someone who has AIDS?' Any simple aggregation of responses assumes that all subjects have spontaneously assigned the same value to each missing detail – and that the investigator knows what subjects have decided. For example, what did they infer about the kind of sharing (e.g. eating from the same bowl, using utensils that have been through a dishwasher) and about how frequently it occurs?

The inferences that subjects make, when reading between the lines, in order to complete the event definition, reveal their beliefs about the processes involved. For example, we asked teens to think aloud as they judged the probabilities of deliberately ambiguous events (e.g. getting into an accident after drinking and driving, getting AIDS through sex) (Fischhoff, 1996). These teens wanted to know the 'dose' involved with most risks (e.g. how much drinking, how much driving), when it was not stated. However, they seldom asked about the amount of sex, when asked about the risks of pregnancy and the risks of HIV transmission. They seemed to believe that a person either is or is not sensitive to the risk, regardless of the amount of the exposure. Morrison (1985) concluded that many sexually active adolescents explain not using contraceptives with variants of, 'I thought I (or my partner) couldn't get pregnant'.

Mental models of risk processes

These intuitive theories of how risks accumulate were a byproduct of research intended to improve the elicitation and communication of quantitative probabilities. Often, however, people are not poised to decide anything, hence need no estimates. Rather, they just want to know how a risk works, for the sake of warranted self-efficacy or to give quantitative estimates intuitive credibility ('How could the experts say that the risk is so small [or big]?' 'How could they be so sure about their predictions?'). The term 'mental model' is often applied to lay theories that are well enough elaborated to generate predictions.

If these mental models contain critical bugs, then they can lead to erroneous conclusions, even when people are otherwise well informed. For example, not knowing that repeated sex increases the associated risks could undermine much other knowledge. Morgan et al. (2001) found that many people know that radon is a colourless, odourless, radioactive gas posing some health risk. Unfortunately, people also associate radioactivity with permanent contamination, a widely publicized property of high-level radioactive waste that is not shared by radon. Not realizing that the major radon byproducts have short half-lives, homeowners might not even bother to test (believing that there was nothing that they could do, should a problem be detected). Leventhal and Cameron (1987) demonstrated how misunderstanding the physiology and phenomenology of maladies (e.g. hypertension) can reduce compliance with treatment regimes.

Creating communications

The design process

The first step in designing communication is to select the information that they should contain (Fischhoff, 1992). Poorly chosen information can both waste recipients' time and be seen as wasting it. Recipients may be judged unduly harshly if they are uninterested in information that seems (and perhaps is) only vaguely relevant to their choices.

In health decisions, like any others, not all facts are equally important. Even with well-formulated questions, it is easy enough to create a test of knowledge that any person will pass – or fail. A necessary precursor to assessing, or improving, health risk knowledge is explicitly identifying the critical factors creating and controlling a risk. Identifying people's existing beliefs must use procedures sufficiently open-ended to allow naïve mental models and formulations to emerge, beyond those presumed by researchers. The research should, for example, allow detecting the 'false fluency' of people using terms, without a functional understanding of their meaning (e.g. 'safe sex'; McIntyre & West, 1992).

Interventions can then focus on the most critical gaps. That could mean adding missing concepts, correcting mistakes, strengthening correct beliefs and de-emphasizing peripheral ones. It should concentrate on critical 'bugs' in recipients' beliefs, cases where they confidently hold incorrect beliefs that could lead to inappropriate actions (or, where they lack enough confidence in correct beliefs to act on them). The identification of those facts can be formalized by value-of-information analysis, determining the sensitivity of decisions to various facts. In one application, we considered the facts critical to patients considering carotid endarterectomy (scraping out an artery leading to the brain, in order to reduce stroke risk) (Fischhoff, 1999). Although many things might go wrong, we found that only a few would change many patients' optimal choice. Focusing on those few facts best fulfils the duty of informed consent. It also frames the analysis of whether people understand enough to avoid paternalistic interventions.

Once information has been selected, it must be presented comprehensibly. That means considering both the terms that people use for understanding individual concepts and the mental models they use for integrating them. It means exploiting research into text comprehension, showing that (a) comprehension improves when text has a clear structure, (b) critical information is best remembered when it appears at the highest level of a clear hierarchy and (c) readers benefit from 'adjunct aids', such as highlighting, advanced organizers (showing what to expect), and summaries (Kintsch, 1986) (see 'Written communication').

Misdirected communications can prompt wrong decisions, create confusion, provoke conflict and cause undue alarm or complacency. Indeed, poor communications can have greater public health impact than the risks that they attempt to describe. When that is true, it should be no more acceptable to release an untested communication than an untested drug. Because communicators' intuitions about recipients' risk perceptions cannot be trusted, there is no substitute for empirical validation.

A case study, using a behavioural decision research approach

Young people hear a lot about how to reduce risks from sexually transmitted infections (STIs), especially HIV/AIDS. Nonetheless, the rates of STIs (and unplanned pregnancies) remain high. As a result, some adults despair of informational approaches, favouring manipulative ones. However, the 'failed' messages have seldom been based on normative analyses of teenagers' choices and informational needs. Rather, educators decided what teenagers needed to know, then tried to present it engagingly. A common criticism of campaigns, like 'Just Say 'No', is that they oversimplify the normative analysis, by ignoring the full set of concerns held by teenagers.

In a normative analysis of the 'facts of life' needed for effective decision making, we identified the intertwined cognitive, affective,

social and physiological processes shaping STI risks (Fischhoff *et al.*, 1998). We found that most current messages focus on a subset of these factors. That focus has been rewarded: teenagers know many of those details. However, the repetition of familiar facts may create an unwarranted feeling of 'knowing it all'.

Moreover, teenagers, mastery of some facts is shaky, while other critical facts are missing from their mental models. Some of these omissions are deliberate. For example, although it is not hard to explain why oral and anal sex are risky, few US schools allow such 'explicit' explanations. Social constraints on discussion with adults may contribute to the confusion of many teenagers about how to use condoms or terms like 'safe sex'. Other omissions reflect topics outside health educators' usual concerns. For example, few are familiar with the research showing that teenagers (like adults) tend to think about the outcomes of single actions, rather than the results of repeating those actions (e.g. having sex, driving fast) (Downs *et al.*, 2006; Fischhoff, 1996).

Our prescriptive work has focused on filling such gaps in teens' mental models, as well as giving them a more realistic feeling for how much they know. It has also recognized that information means little unless teens feel empowered to use it. As a result, we created an interactive DVD for young women, conveying critical facts (about diseases, condoms, etc.), while also showing how to make and implement choices about sexual relations. Although the DVD's goals were determined from a behavioural decision research perspective, it draws broadly on behavioural research (e.g. self-efficacy theory). In a randomized control trial, the DVD increased STI knowledge and self-reported condom use, while decreasing condom problems and chlamydia reinfection rates (Downs *et al.*, 2004).

Conclusion

Communicating risks can be as complicated as assessing them. Research in this area is fortunate in being able to draw on well-developed literatures in such areas as cognitive, health and social psychology, survey research, psycholinguistics, psychophysics and behavioural decision theory. It needs those resources for dealing with unfamiliar topics, surrounded by uncertainty, without stable vocabularies, and difficult, threatening tradeoffs.

REFERENCES

Downs, J. S., Bruine de Bruin, W., Murray, P. J. & Fischhoff, B. (2006). Specific STI knowledge may be acquired too late. *Journal of Adolescent Health*, **38**, 65–7.

Downs, J. S., Murray, P. J., Bruine de Bruin, W. et al. (2004). An interactive video program to reduce adolescent females' STD risk: a randomized controlled trial. *Social Science and Medicine*, **59**, 1561–72.

Fischhoff, B. (1992). Giving advice: decision theory perspectives on sexual assault. *American Psychologist*, **47**, 577–88.

Fischhoff, B. (1996). The real world: what good is it? *Organizational Behavior and Human Decision Processes*, **65**, 232–48.

Fischhoff, B. (1999). Why (cancer) risk communication can be hard. *Journal of the National Cancer Institute Monographs*, **25**, 7–13.

Fischhoff, B. (2005). Decision research strategies. *Health Psychology*, 21(4), S9–16.

Fischhoff, B., Downs, J. & Bruine de Bruin, W. (1998). Adolescent vulnerability: a framework for behavioural interventions. *Applied and Preventive Psychology*, **7**, 77–94.

Florig, H. K. et al. (2001). A deliberative method for ranking risks. *Risk Analysis*, **21**, 913–22.

Gilovich, T., Griffin, D. & Kahneman, D. (Eds.). (2002). *Judgment under uncertainty: extensions and applications*. New York: Cambridge University Press.

Hastie, R. & Dawes, R. M. (2002). *Rational choice in an uncertain world*. Thousand Oaks, CA: Sage.

HM Treasury (2004). *The management of risks: principles and concepts*. London: Author.

HM Treasury (2005). *Managing risks to the public*. London: Author.

Kahneman, D., Slovic, P. & Tversky, A. (Eds.). (1982). *Judgement under uncertainty: heuristics and biases.* New York: Cambridge University Press.

Kintsch, W. (1986) Learning from text. *Cognition and Instruction*, **3**, 87–108.

Lerner, J. S. & Keltner, D. (2002). Fear, anger and risk. *Journal of Personality and Social Psychology*, **89**, 146–59.

Lerner, J. S. & Keltner, D. (2000). Beyond valence: toward a model of emotion-specific influences on judgement and choice. *Cognition and Emotion*, **14**, 473–493.

Leventhal, H. & Cameron, L. (1987). Behavioural theories and the problem of compliance. *Patient Education and Counseling*, **10**, 117–38.

Lichtenstein, S., Slovic, P., Fischhoff, B., Layman, M. & Combs, B. (1978). Judged frequency of lethal events. *Journal of Experimental Psychology: Human Learning and Memory*, **4**, 851–78.

McIntyre, S. & West, P. (1992), What does the phrase "safer sex" mean to you? *AIDS*, **7**, 121–6.

Morgan, M. G., Fischhoff, B., Bostrom, A. & Atman, C. (2001). *Risk communication: the mental models approach.* New York: Cambridge University Press.

Morrison, D. M. (1985) Adolescent contraceptive behavior: a review. *Psychological Bulletin*, **98**, 538–8.

Parker, A. & Fischhoff, B. (2005). Decision-making competence: external validity through an individual-differences approach. *Journal of Behavioral Decision Making*, **18**, 1–27.

Poulton, E. C. (1994). *Behavioural decision making.* Hillsdale, NJ: Lawrence Erlbaum.

Quadrel, M. J., Fischhoff, B. & Davis, W. (1993) Adolescent (in)vulnerability. *American Psychologist*, **48**, 102–16.

Schwarz, N. (1999). Self-reports: How the questions shape the answers. *American Psychologist*, **54**, 93–105.

Slovic, P. (1987). Perceptions of risk. *Science*, **236**, 280–5.

Wallsten, T. S., Budescu, D. V., Rapoport, A., Zwick, R. & Forsyth, B. (1986). Measuring the vague meanings of probability terms. *Journal of Experimental Psychology*, **115**, 348–65.

Weinstein, N. (1987). *Taking care: understanding and encouraging self-protective behavior.* New York: Cambridge University Press.

Woloshin, S., Schwartz, L. M., Byram, S., Fischhoff, B. & Welch, H. G. (2000). A new scale for assessing perceptions of chance. *Medical Decision Making*, **20**, 298–307.

Yates, J. F. (1989). *Judgment and decision making.* Englewood Cliffs, NJ: Prentice-Hall.

Self-efficacy in health functioning

Albert Bandura

Stanford University

We are witnessing a divergent trend in the field of health. On the one hand, we are pouring massive resources into medicalizing the ravages of detrimental health habits. On the other hand, the conception of health is shifting from a disease model to a health model. It emphasizes health promotion rather than disease management.

Health promotion should begin with goals not means. If health is the goal, biomedical interventions are not the only means to it. The quality of health is heavily influenced by lifestyle habits. This enables people to exercise some control over their health. To stay healthy, people should exercise, reduce dietary fat, refrain from smoking, keep blood pressure down and develop effective ways of managing stressors. By managing their health habits, people can live longer, healthier and retard the process of ageing. Self-management is good medicine. If the huge benefits of these few habits were put into a pill it would be declared a scientific milestone in the field of medicine.

Current health practices focus heavily on the medical supply side. The growing pressure on health systems is to reduce, ration and curtail health services to contain escalating health costs. The days for the supply side health system are limited. People are living longer. This creates more time for minor dysfunctions to develop into chronic diseases requiring costly treatments.

Social cognitive approaches focus on the demand side. They promote effective self-management of health habits that will keep people healthy through their life span. The mounting demand for health care will force societies to change the balance of efforts from disease care to health promotion.

Effective self-management of health behaviour is not a matter of will. It requires development of self-regulatory skills on how to influence one's own motivation and behaviour (see 'Self-management'). Among the mechanisms of self-regulation, none is more central or pervasive than beliefs of personal efficacy. This core belief is the foundation of human motivation, wellbeing and accomplishments. Unless people believe they can produce desired effects by their actions they have little incentive to act or to persevere in the face of difficulties. Whatever other factors serve as guides and motivators, they are rooted in the core belief that one has the power to effect changes by one's actions.

Efficacy beliefs affect every phase of personal change: whether people even consider changing their health habits; whether they enlist the motivation and perseverance needed to succeed should they choose to do so; their vulnerability to relapse; success in recovering control after a setback; how well they maintain the habit changes they have achieved (Bandura, 1997). Perceived efficacy is the common pathway through which diverse psychosocial influences affect health functioning.

There are two major ways in which people's belief in their personal efficacy affects their health. At the more basic level, such beliefs act on biological systems that mediate health and illness.

At the second level, they operate by direct control over habits that affect health and the rate of biological ageing.

Biological effects of perceived coping efficacy

Many of the biological effects of beliefs of personal efficacy arise in the context of coping with stressors. Stress has been implicated as an important contributor to many physical dysfunctions (Krantz, Grunberg & Baum, 1985; O'Leary, 1990) (see 'Stress and health'). Controllability is a key organizing principle regarding the nature of stress effects. It is not stressful life conditions per se, but the perceived inability to manage them which produces the detrimental biological effects (Bandura, 1991; Maier, Laudenslager & Ryan, 1985; Shavit & Martin, 1987).

In social cognitive theory, stress arises from perceived inefficacy to exercise control over aversive threats and taxing environmental demands (Bandura, 1986). If people believe that they can deal effectively with potential environmental stressors, they are not perturbed by them. But, if they believe that they cannot control aversive events, they distress themselves and impair their level of functioning. The causal impact of beliefs of controlling efficacy on biological stress reactions is clearly verified in experimental studies in which people are exposed to stressors under perceived inefficacy and after their beliefs of coping efficacy are raised to high levels through guided mastery experiences (Bandura, 1997). Exposure to stressors without perceived efficacy to control them activates autonomic, catecholamine and endogenous opioid systems. After people's perceived coping efficacy is strengthened, they manage the same stressors without experiencing any distress, autonomic agitation or activation of stress-related hormones.

The types of biochemical reactions that accompany a weak sense of coping efficacy are involved in the regulation of the immune system. Hence, exposure to uncontrollable stressors tends to impair the function of the immune system in ways that can increase susceptibility to illness (Kiecolt-Glaser & Glaser, 1987; Maier et al., 1985; Shavit & Martin, 1987). Lack of behavioural or perceived control over perturbing conditions increases susceptibility to bacterial and viral infections, contributes to the development of physical disorders, and accelerates the rate of progression of disease (Schneiderman et al., 1992) (see 'Psychosomatics').

Most human stress is activated in the course of developing competencies. Stress activated in the process of acquiring coping efficacy may have different physiological effects from stress experienced in aversive situations with no prospect of ever achieving any self-protective efficacy. Indeed, stress aroused while gaining coping mastery over threatening situations can enhance different components of the immune system (Bandura, 1991). Providing people with the means for managing acute and chronic stressors increases immunological functioning. This has substantial evolutionary benefits given the prevalence of stressors in everyday life. If stressors only impaired immune function, people would be bedridden much of the time if not deceased.

The field of health has been heavily preoccupied with the physiologically debilitating effects of stressors. Self-efficacy theory also acknowledges the physiologically strengthening effects of mastery over stressors. A growing body of research verifies the physiological toughening by successful coping (Dienstbier, 1989).

Self-efficacy in self-management of health behaviour

As previously noted, people can exercise some measure of control over their health by managing their lifestyle habits. This requires development of motivational and self-regulatory skills (Bandura, 2004). Effective self-management operates through a set of psychological subfunctions that provide the motivators, guides and supports for personal change. People have to monitor their health behaviour and the circumstances under which it occurs, set proximal goals to motivate themselves and guide their behaviour, create incentives for themselves and enlist social supports to sustain their efforts.

Habit changes are of little consequence unless they endure. Maintenance of habit change requires instilling a resilient sense of efficacy as well as imparting skills. Experience in exercising control over troublesome situations and setbacks serve as efficacy builders (Marlatt et al., 1995). This is an important aspect of self-management. If people are not fully convinced of their personal efficacy, they rapidly abandon the skills they have been taught when they fail to get quick results or suffer reverses. Once equipped with self-regulatory skills and a resilient sense of efficacy, people are better able to adopt behaviours that promote health and to eliminate those that impair it.

To improve the quality of health of a nation requires intensifying health promotion efforts and restructuring health delivery systems to make them more productive. Efficacy-based models have been devised combining knowledge of self-regulation of health habits with computer-assisted implementation. This self-management model provides effective health-promoting services in ways that are individualized, intensive, highly convenient and cost effective (Bandura, 2004). By linking the interactive aspects of the self-management model to the Internet, one can vastly expand its availability to people wherever they may live, at whatever time they may choose to use it.

The weight of disease is shifting from acute to chronic maladies. Biomedical approaches are ill-suited for chronic diseases because they are devised mainly for acute illness. The self-management of chronic diseases is another example where self-regulatory and self-efficacy theories provided guides for the development of cost-effective models with high social utility.

The treatment of chronic disease must focus on self-management of physical conditions over time. Holman and Lorig (1992) devised a generic self-management program in which patients are taught pain control techniques and proximal goal setting combined with self-incentives as motivators to increase level of activity. They are also taught problem-solving and self-diagnostic skills, and how to take greater initiative for their health care in dealing with health systems. This approach retards the biological progression of diseases, raises perceived efficacy, reduces pain, decreases the use of medical services and improves the quality of life.

Impact of prognostic judgements on efficacy beliefs and health outcomes

Much of the work in the health field is concerned with diagnosing maladies, forecasting the likely course of physical disorders and prescribing remedies. Medical prognostic judgements involve probabilistic inferences from knowledge of varying quality and inclusiveness about the multiple factors governing the course of a given disorder. One important issue regarding medical prognosis concerns the range of determinants included in the prognostic models. Because psychosocial factors account for some of the variability in the course of health functioning, inclusion of self-efficacy determinants in prognostic models enhances their predictive power (Bandura, 2000).

Prognostic judgments are not simply inert forecasters of a natural course of a disease. Prognostic expectations can affect patients' beliefs in their self-efficacy. Therefore, diagnosticians not only foretell, but may partly influence, the course of recovery from disease. Prognostic expectations are conveyed to patients by attitude, word and the type and level of care provided them. People are more likely to be treated in enabling ways under positive expectations than under negative ones. Differential care that promotes in patients different levels of personal efficacy and skill in managing health-related behaviour can exert stronger impact on the trajectories of health functioning than simply conveying prognostic information. Prognostic expectations can alter patients' sense of efficacy and behaviour in ways that confirm the original expectations. The self-efficacy mechanism operates as one important mediator of such self-confirming effects.

Socially-oriented approaches to health

The quality of health of a nation is a social matter not just a personal one. It requires changing the practices of social systems that impair health rather than just changing the habits of individuals. Vast sums of money are spent annually in advertising and marketing products and promoting lifestyles detrimental to health. With regard to injurious environmental conditions, some industrial and agricultural practices inject carcinogens and harmful pollutants into the air we breathe, the food we eat and the water we drink, all of which take a heavy toll on health. Vigorous economic and political battles are fought over environmental health and where to set the limits of acceptable risk.

We do not lack sound policy prescriptions in the field of health. What is lacking is the collective efficacy to realize them. People's beliefs in their collective efficacy to accomplish social change by perseverant group action play a key role in the policy and public health approach to health promotion and disease prevention (Bandura 1997; Wallack et al., 1993). Such social efforts take a variety of forms. They raise public awareness of health hazards, educate and influence policymakers, devise effective strategies for improving health conditions, and mobilize public support to enact policy initiatives (see 'Health promotion').

REFERENCES

Bandura, A. (1986). *Social foundations of thought and action: a social cognitive theory.* Englewood Cliffs, NJ: Prentice-Hall.

Bandura, A. (1991). Self-efficacy mechanism in physiological activation and health-promoting behavior. In J. Madden, IV (Ed.). *Neurobiology of learning, emotion and affect*, (pp. 229–69). New York: Raven.

Bandura, A. (1997). *Self-efficacy: the exercise of control.* New York: Freeman.

Bandura, A. (2000). Psychological aspects of prognostic judgments. In R. W. Evans, D. S. Baskin & F. M. Yatsu (Eds.). *Prognosis of neurological disorders* (2nd edn.). (pp. 11–27). New York: Oxford University Press.

Bandura, A. (2004). Health promotion by social cognitive means. *Health Education and Behavior*, **31**, 143–64.

Dienstbier, R. A. (1989). Arousal and physiological toughness: implications for mental and physical health. *Psychological Review*, **96**, 84–100.

Holman, H. & Lorig, K. (1992). Perceived self-efficacy in self-management of chronic disease. In R. Schwarzer (Ed.). *Self-efficacy: thought control of action*, (pp. 305–23) Washington, DC: Hemisphere.

Kiecolt-Glaser, J. K. & Glaser, R. (1987). Behavioural influences on 8 immunme functions: evidence for the interplay between stress and health. In T. Field, P. M. McCabe & N. Schneiderman (Eds.). *Stress and coping across development, Vol. 2*, (pp. 189–206). Hillsdale, NJ: Erlbaum.

Krantz, D. S., Grunberg, N. E. & Baum, A. (1985). Health psychology. *Annual Reviews in Psychology*, **36**, 349–83.

Maier, S. F., Laudenslager, M. L. & Ryan, S. M. (1985). Stressor controllability, immune function, and endogenous opiates. In F. R. Brush & J. B. Overmier (Eds.). *Affect, conditioning, and cognition: essays on the*

determinants of behaviour (pp. 183–201). Hillsdale, NJ: Erlbaum.

Marlatt, G. A., Baer, J. S. & Quigley, L. A. (1995). Self-efficacy and addictive behavior. In A. Bandura (Ed.). *Self-efficacy in changing societies*, (pp. 289–315). New York: Cambridge University Press.

O'Leary, A. (1990). Stress, emotion, and human immune function. *Psychological Bulletin*, **108**, 363–82.

Schneiderman, N., McCabe, P. M. & Baum, A. (Eds.). (1992). *Stress and disease process: perspectives in behavioral medicine.* Hillsdale, NJ: Erlbaum.

Shavit, Y. & Martin, F. C. (1987). Opiates, stress, and immunity: animal studies. *Annals of Behavioral Medicine*, **9**, 11–20.

Wallack, L., Dorfman, L., Jernigan, D. & Themba, M. (1993). *Media advocacy and public health: power for prevention.* Newbury Park, CA: Sage.

Sexual risk behaviour

Lorraine Sherr

Royal Free and University College Medical School

Sex and risk – strange bedfellows

It is strange that the concept of sexual behaviour – the most normal and human of behaviours – should be considered in the same context as 'risk', which relates to extreme, out of the norm and potentially danger invoking behaviours. Yet the concept of sexual risk behaviour has been well established. Sexual risk and the underlying related issues are of great importance in the pursuance and sustaining of health.

What is meant by risk?

There are a number of theories which try to encapsulate the concept of risk and risk behaviour (see 'Risk perception'). Generally, risk behaviour can be divided into two forms, namely (1) risk exposure and (2) risk seeking. Risk exposure concerns the situational variables associated with risk, often, but not always, not under the direct control of the individual. Risk seeking encompasses all behaviours where there is some active planning or behaviour to seek out risk. However, it may also include an absence of behaviour, which may result in risk. So for example the non-use of contraception may be seen as a risky behaviour, where inactivity or the failure to behave is the core risk determinant. Whilst seeking unprotected sex with a casual partner may be a more active risk-seeking behaviour, where the action (rather than the inaction) is at the core of the risk exposure.

There is also a difference between risk seeking and risk exposure. Many acts may be potentially risky, but the actual risk is unknown. For example unprotected sex may result in a pregnancy, but it may not.

When is sexual behaviour risky?

It is difficult to gather a precise definition of when sexual behaviour is risky. If it is related to consequence, the same consequences may be risky for some individuals and not for others. Pregnancy as an outcome may be desired and then considered as not risky. On the other hand it may not be desired, and then sexual behaviour resulting in a pregnancy is risky – despite the same outcome. So it is clear that outcomes in themselves cannot be the only definition of risk. Exposure to sexually transmitted diseases and infections is an area where the concepts of risk and sex are clearly associated. Much research in relation to HIV infection, HIV prevention and the promotion of 'safer sex' has emerged since the beginning of the HIV epidemic in the late 1980s. Such literature explores individual, couple and social levels of behaviour, safety and risk (see 'HIV and AIDS').

A working hypothesis for risky sexual behaviour is associated with undesirable outcome. Although this provides a helpful working definition, it also depends on whose desires are to be considered. Given that sexual behaviour affects couples, groups, families and societies, the desires of one element may not necessarily coincide with the desires of another. Sexual behaviour, risk reporting and coding is complex (Cleland et al., 2004) and there is a wide debate on the efficacy of research, the reliability of measurement and the difficulties in recording and verifying sexual behaviour as well as risk (Ankrah, 1989; Catania et al., 1990; Frank, 1994; Sheeran and Abraham, 1994; Huygens et al., 1996; Weinhardt et al., 1998; Fenton et al., 2001).

A number of areas of research will be briefly outlined where issues of sex and risk are studied. Sexual risk is associated with pregnancy, contraception, sexual behaviour, sexual health and sexually transmitted infections (STIs). HIV infection and AIDS is one of the most studied areas of risk associated with sexual behaviour.

Sexual debut

The recent National Survey of Sexual Attitudes and Lifestyles (Natsal) studies in the UK have provided detailed evidence of sexual behaviour patterns (Wellings et al., 2001). In this national survey (1990 $n = 18\,867$; 2000 $n = 11\,161$), it was found that by the age of 25, 95% of men and 98% of women had experienced heterosexual intercourse. Birth cohort data from the two successive studies show a downward turn of age at first intercourse over time, with recordings of 20 years for men and 21 for women for those born in 1930s, 17 for both men and women for those born in the 1970s and 16 for both men and women for those born in the 1980s. These figures vary in different countries and cultures.

Early age of sexual debut is seen as a marker for risk, or potential risk, in a number of studies. Early age of sexual debut was associated with increased risk of pregnancy in the under 18-year age group. Age itself may not be the only risk associated with early sexual debut, but contraceptive use may be a clearer indication of potential risk exposure.

Pregnancy-related risk

Pregnancy is both a desired and undesired outcome of sex. The risk in this context relates to the biological risk as well as the psychosocial risk associated with conception. Thus failure to conceive (infertility) has a set of psychological risks associated with it, while on the other hand, unplanned conception or conception in association with a set of correlates is often categorized (rightly or wrongly) as risky. Age (too young or too old) has been seen as a risk, but this may often mask public attitude rather than outcome. For example young age is often measured in terms of the maternal age, rather than couple age. Youth may be a surrogate marker for unplanned pregnancy or economic hardship. These other factors may be the drivers of risky outcomes rather than simple age. Similarly, older age and risk is studied. Biological risk (such as higher prevalence of genetic conditions) may be associated with older age – but again maternal rather than paternal age is usually measured. Possible confounders also exist in this literature where people with difficulties in conceiving may be disproportionately represented in older age groups. Furthermore studies have shown that if one focuses on negative outcomes then biased views are enhanced. Positive outcomes have been well established with both younger and older parenthood (Sherr, 1995).

In a systematic review of sexual risk and teenage pregnancy, Mead and Ickovics (2005) have shown that behaviours which lead to teenage pregnancy also place young women at risk for STDs and repeat pregnancy.

Sexual behaviour risk

There are a number of components of sexual behaviour risk which have been described, studied and the target of intervention studies. Caution is needed to ensure that the indicators of risk actually match true risk behaviour (Slaymaker, 2004).

• *Sexual health*

There has been an increased focus of attention in the area of sexual health. The rates of sexually transmitted infections have driven health services to enhance provision and broaden interventions. In the British National Survey of Sexual Attitudes and Lifestyles (Natsal) Fenton *et al.* (2005) noted that numbers and type of partners remained the dominant risk factors associated with STIs in the UK. Mercer *et al.* (2003) noted a high degree of sexual problems (34.8% men and 53.8% women reported some form of problem in the NATSAL survey). Johnson *et al.* (2001) examined changes in sexual behaviour over time in two consecutive national surveys and found an increase in partner numbers, new partners, paying for sex and generally pointed out that gains from increased condom use were offset by increased partner change. Sangani *et al.* (2004) have shown in an overview that there is a clear link between STI and HIV infections. They further noted that there is some evidence that STI interventions can affect HIV and vice versa (see 'Sexually transmitted infections').

• *HIV and AIDS*

The HIV epidemic runs unabated (see 'HIV and AIDS'). Some countries have managed to exhibit a downturn of new infections. The advent of new treatments, antiretroviral drugs, enhanced adherence to these treatments, HIV prevention initiatives and global strategies have all contributed to the efforts to contain the spread of HIV. Yet new infections occur rapidly, illness and death rates are still dramatic and emerging problems of drug resistance virus, orphaned children and an AIDS weariness in the public eye are all current challenges. Sexual risk in the presence of HIV remains the major factor for exposure. Risk behaviours are described as unprotected sex with a partner of unknown or discordant serostatus. A steady increase in such behaviours has been reported over time in a large number of population based studies (Elford *et al.*, 2004; Dodds *et al.*, 2004).

• *Contraceptive risk*

The availability and uptake of contraception is a major factor in behavioural management of sexual risk. However, there has been some tension in the literature given concerns that the provision of contraception may increase risk by promoting sexual behaviours and that abstinence policies may be preferable. In a recent review (Bennett and Assefi, 2005), there was clear evidence that abstinence only programmes were not as effective as contraceptive promotion for avoidance of teenage pregnancies.

Holmes *et al.* (2004) showed in a systematic review that condoms were effective in both HIV and STI prevention (see 'Contraception').

• *Unprotected sex risk*

In HIV, Creese *et al.* (2002) showed the cost efficacy of interventions in Africa. Bollinger *et al.* (2004) provide a clear matrix on the complexity of interventions and their potential efficacy. The advent of HIV, the upsurge of incidence of sexually transmitted infections as well as avoidance of unwanted pregnancies has resulted in a mass of studies looking at condom use. In general there have been a multitude of condom prevention programmes with varying degrees of success. Barriers to condom use are associated with individual factors (such as motivation, personal appraisal, willingness, experience, knowledge), couple factors (such as negotiation, trust, sustained condom use) and community factors (such as availability, social norms, endorsement, social meaning and the conflict between condoms and the desire for reproduction). The data is more complex, given that it is not simply condom use that is important, but sustained condom use. Partial or sporadic condom use may provide some protection, but is not complete. Social power and normative support can influence condom use (Albarracin *et al.*, 2004).

• *Sexual partner risk*

Choice of sexual partners has been studied as potential risk. Furthermore, a number of studies have explored risk for groups where choice is not active and coercion, relationship imperatives or social need have limited such choice. Clearly sexual networking raises the potential for risk exposure. A number of studies have examined strategies used to limit such risk, such as

- Negotiated safety where partners enter into negotiated agreements regarding sexual partners and risk,
- Age selection where some partners preferentially choose sexual partners from certain age groups in an attempt to ameliorate risk. This has a two-sided effect where it may decrease risk for one partner, but enhance risk for the other.
- Couple interventions. These have particularly examined discordant couples in relation to HIV infection where one member is negative and the other positive. A number of psychological interventions in the form of behavioural counselling have been effective. Additional biomedical resources, such as sperm washing techniques for those wanting to conceive have been shown to be protective for the negative partner.
- Social level factors must not be overlooked. HIV widowhood or orphanhood is associated with a period of increased risk.

Mobility, migration and economic hardship are also well established contributors to elevated risk exposure.

- Forced sex and rape have immediate as well as long-term consequences. Rape survivors are at elevated risks of infection, unwanted pregnancies and mental health problems.

• *Sexual behaviour and emotional relationships*

Sexual behaviour is intricately bound up with emotional relationships. Thus risk cannot be confined to physical or biological risk, but must also examine emotional risk and the social environment in which sexual behaviour as well as sexual risk is conducted. Studies have provided insight into a range of sexual behaviours, with an understanding of a number of concepts. The literature on sexual deviance explores the normative and non-normative practices and consequences for individuals. The literature on sexual abuse provides complex understanding of the experience, triggers and ramification of sexual abuse. Responses to sexual abuse and subsequent risks have been well documented. There is a broad literature which studies the relationship between sex, drugs and alcohol. Some studies show how risk and risk behaviours cluster, while others look at causative links between drug use, alcohol use and sexual risk.

The advent of impotence treating drugs such as sildenafil (Viagra) may have implications for safe sexual behaviour and HIV prevention (Sherr *et al.*, 2000). Studies have shown that the use of such compounds is not necessarily associated with increased risk behaviour, but have also highlighted the use of the internet for access to such compounds for reasons of stigma and shame. This opens up the whole area of health education and prescription associated counselling and the ways in which new technologies need to be adapted to accommodate such need.

• *Sexual risk mediators*

There are a number of factors which mediate sexual risk, such as gender, culture, age, economics and social environment. Sexual risk is not equivalent between the genders.

• *Theoretical explanations and sexual risk*

It is complicated to understand what constitutes a sexual risk, how this is measured and operationalized in studies. This is compounded by the subsequent need to understand associations and links between individual and situational factors and such risk. Psychological understanding of sexual risk in HIV has concentrated on social and or cognitive models (see for example *Theory of Planned Behaviour*, Ajzen, 1991), with applications that have looked at relationships, negotiations and normative influences (see, for e.g. van der Ven *et al.*, 2002; Crawford *et al.*, 2001; Davidovich *et al.*, 2000). Personality theory provides a line of understanding (see for example studies looking at personality clusters and risk) or risk judgements (see, for example, Weinstein, 1980, 1984, 1989; Weinstein & Lachendro, 1982; McKenna, 1993). Integrated concepts have also been explored, such as the notion that risk evaluation affects planned behaviour or personality (Elford, Bolding & Sherr, 2002; Elford, Bolding, Maguire & Sherr, 1999; International Collaboration on HIV Optimism, 2002).

Risk reduction has been addressed in some theories. Three major approaches include Social Learning theory, Social Influence Theory and Cognitive Behavioural Theory. These theories indicate that risk reduction requires a number of stages such as:-

- Information handling
- Identification of social pressure and peer influence
- Prepare for and anticipate risk situations
- Create positive behavioural norms
- Skill acquisition for coping and acting under pressure
- Testing

There are many tests available to monitor and measure outcome. The process of such testing may play a role in risk identification, reduction and management. For example a test for HIV has long been available. The process of HIV testing has been expanded to include a basic minimum of counselling in preparation for testing and on receipt of test results. Such counselling has a role to play not only in risk identification and emotional preparation, but also in future risk reduction.

In pregnancy, routine antenatal care may include elements of risk identification and management. High levels of abuse in pregnant women have been monitored in studies in the US, Canada and the UK. Antenatal discussion has a role to play in disclosure and management. Sexual and physical abuse in pregnancy is associated with negative mental health as well as physical outcomes.

• *Myths and Sexual risk*

As well as an extensive literature understanding sexual risk, there are also a number of myths and misunderstandings surrounding the concept. Some of these will be briefly set out.

Optimism and HIV risk

It was generally believed that optimism over the new HIV treatments would be associated with enhanced sexual risk. This could be understood in two ways – optimism around treatment which reduced the 'seriousness' of HIV infection or optimism around infectivity which reduced the likelihood of infection after risk exposure. Clearly this raised a worrying concept. However, studies have shown that the absolute levels of optimism are actually low, and realism is the better descriptor of the post antiretroviral treatment mood. Amongst the optimistic, cross-sectional studies have shown associations with risk. However, more thorough longitudinal studies have shown increases in risk behaviour among both the optimistic and non-optimistic, thus cautioning against blanket presumptions.

The inherent appeal of risk

Another problem is the literature is the presumption that risk is aversive. There is good evidence to show that there is an inherent appeal of risk. This may vary by factors such as personality, situation or age. Thus health promotion that labels risk may have a 'boomerang' effect whereby it enhances the appeal rather than decreases the appeal of certain behaviours.

Gender and power

Some studies make presumptions about power. This is often seen in relation to women who are construed in many studies as lacking in power. However, a careful examination of female behaviour, especially in the HIV context, shows that a power analysis is a very gender-biased analysis and that concepts such as compassion, commitment and reliability may better explain such female behaviour.

Cognitive factors

A clear understanding of cognitions, how they work and how they affect behaviour may provide some insight into decision-making, information appraisal and risk behaviour. Information is selectively recalled. Memory plays a key role in decision-making. Information and understanding are necessary but not sufficient factors in behaviour change.

Psychological interventions

Any understanding of sexual risk requires some insight into whether such risks can be understood, predicted, avoided, modified or are open to change (Abraham *et al.*, 1998). A number of theories have provided insight into risk behaviour (Albarracin *et al.*, 2001) and have formed the basis for intervention studies (Fishbein, 2000).

Kamb *et al.* (1998) carried out a definitive randomized controlled trial intervention in STD clinics across the USA showing how various counselling interventions were related to significant risk behaviour

decreases at multiple follow-up. Elwy *et al.* (2002) carried out a systematic review of effectiveness of interventions to prevent STIs and HIV in heterosexual men. Successful interventions were invariably comprised of multiple component interventions. Bennett and Assefi (2005) provided a systematic review of interventions to prevent teenage pregnancy and showed that much of the decrease was associated with increased contraceptive use rather than sexual abstinence.

Conclusion

Sexual risk is a complex phenomenon. Yet there is a high burden of ill health, emotional challenge and social consequence associated with the outcomes of sexual risk behaviours. Sexually transmitted infections, unwanted pregnancies, HIV infection and AIDS are all consequences of sexual risk that require urgent attention. Psychological understanding can aide in formulating the problems, measuring the behavioural components, providing interventions and ameliorating the effects of such risk.

REFERENCES

Abraham, C., Sheeran, P. & Orbell, S. (1998). Can social cognitive models contribute to the effectiveness of HIV-preventive behavioural interventions? A brief review of the literature and a reply to Joffe (1996; 1997) and Fife-Schaw (1997). *British Journal of Medical Psychology*, **71** (Pt 3), 297–310.

Ajzen, I. (1991). The theory of planned behavior. *Organizational Behavior and Human Decision Processes*, **50**, 179–211.

Albarracin, D., Johnson, B. T., Fishbein, M. & Muellerleile, P. A. (2001). Theories of reasoned action and planned behavior as models of condom use: a meta-analysis. *Psychology Bulletin*, **127**(1), 142–61.

Albarracin, D., Kumkale, G. T. & Johnson, B. T. (2004) Influences of social power and normative support on condom use decisions: a research synthesis. *AIDS Care*, **16**(6), 700–23.

Ankrah, E. M. (1989). AIDS: methodological problems in studying its prevention and spread. *Social Science and Medicine*, **29**, 265–76.

Bennett, S. E. & Assefi, N. P. (2005). School-based teenage pregnancy prevention programs: a systematic review of randomized controlled trials. *Journal of Adolescent Health*, **36**(1), 72–81.

Bollinger, L., Cooper-Arnold, K. & Stover, J. (2004). Where are the gaps? The effects of HIV-prevention interventions on behavioral change. *Studies in Family Planning*, **35**(1), 27–38.

Catania, J. A., Gibson, D. R., Chitwood, D. D. Coates, T. J. (1990). Methodological problems in AIDS behaviour research: influences on measurement error and

participation bias in studies of sex behaviour. *Psychology Bulletin*, **108**, 339–62.

Cleland, J., Boerma, T., Carael, M. & Weir, S. S. (2004). Monitoring sexual behaviour in general populations: a synthesis of lessons of the past decade. *Sexually Transmitted Infections*, December 1, 2004; **80**(Suppl. 2), ii1–7.

Crawford, J. M., Rodden, P., Kippax, S. & Van de Ven, P. (2001). Negotiated safety and other agreements between men in relationships: risk practice redefined. *International Journal of STD and AIDS*, **12**, 164–70.

Creese, A., Floyd, K., Alban, A. & Guinness, L. (2002). Cost-effectiveness of HIV/AIDS interventions in Africa: a systematic review of the evidence. *Lancet*, **359**(9318), 1635–43.

Davidovich, U., De Wit, J.B.F. & Stroebe, W. (2000). Assessing sexual risk behaviour of young gay men in primary relationships: the incorporation of negotiated safety and negotiated safety compliance. *AIDS*, **14**, 701–6.

Dodds, J. P., Mercey, D. E., Parry, J. V. & Johnson, A. M. (2004). Increasing risk behaviour and high levels of undiagnosed HIV infection in a community sample of homosexual men. *Sexually Transmitted Infections*, **80**(3), 236–40.

Elford, J., Bolding, G. & Sherr, L. (2002). High-risk sexual behaviour increases among London gay men between 1998 and 2001: what is the role of HIV optimism? *AIDS*, **16**, 1537–44.

Elford, J., Bolding, G., Maguire, M. & Sherr, L. (1999). Sexual risk behaviour among gay men in a relationship. *AIDS*, **13**, 1407–11.

Elford, J., Bolding, G., Davis, M., Sherr, L. & Hart, G. (2004). *Trends in sexual behaviour among London homosexual men 1998–2003: implications for HIV prevention and sexual health promotion. Sexually Transmitted Infections*, **80**(6), 451–4.

Elwy, A. R., Hart, G. J., Hawkes, S. & Petticrew, M. (2002). Effectiveness of interventions to prevent sexually transmitted infections and human immunodeficiency virus in heterosexual men: a systematic review (2002). *Archieves of Internal Medicine*, **162**(16), 1818–30.

Fenton, K. A., Johnson, A. M., McManus, S. et al. (2001). Measuring sexual behaviour: methodological challenges in survey research. *Sexually Transmitted Infections*, **77**, 84–92.

Fishbein, M. (2000). The role of theory in HIV prevention. *AIDS Care*, **12**(3), 273–8.

Fenton, K. A., Mercer, C. H., Johnson, A. M., Byron, C. L., McManus, S., Erens, B., Copas, A. J., Nanchahal, K., Macdowall, W. & Wellings, K. (2005). Reported sexually transmitted disease clinic attendance and sexually transmitted infections in Britain: prevalence, risk factors, and proportionate population burden. *Journal of Infectious Diseases*, **191** (Suppl. 1), S127–38.

Frank, O. (1994). International research on sexual behaviour and reproductive health: a brief review with reference to methodology. *Annu Rev Sex Res*, **5**, 1–49.

Holmes, K. K., Levine, R. & Weaver, M. (2004). Effectiveness of condoms in preventing sexually transmitted infections. *Bulletin of World Health Organisation*, **82**(6), 454–61.

Huygens, P., Kajura, E., Seeley, J. *et al.* (1996). Rethinking methods for the study of sexual behaviour. *Social Science and Medicine*, **42**, 221–31.

Johnson, A. M., Mercer, C. H., Erens, B. *et al.* (2001). Sexual behaviour in Britain: partnerships, practices, and HIV risk behaviours. *Lancet*, **358**(9296), 1835–42.

Kamb, M. L., Fishbein, M., Douglas, J. M. Jr. *et al.* (1998). Efficacy of risk-reduction counseling to prevent human immunodeficiency virus and sexually transmitted diseases: a randomized controlled trial. Project RESPECT Study Group. *Journal of American Medical Association*, **280**(13), 1161–7.

Mckenna, F. P. (1993). It won't happen to me-unrealistic optimism or illusion of control. *British Journal of Psychology*, **84**, 39–50.

Meade, C. S. & Ickovics, J. R. (2005). Systematic review of sexual risk among pregnant and mothering teens in the USA: pregnancy as an opportunity for integrated prevention of STD and repeat pregnancy. *Social Science and Medicine*, **60**(4), 661–78.

Mercer, C. H., Fenton, K. A., Johnson, A. M., Wellings, K., Macdowall, W., Mc Manus, S., Nanchahal, K. & Erens, B. (2003). Sexual

function problems and help seeking behaviour in Britain: national probability sample survey. *British Medical Journal*, **327**(7412), 426–7.

Sangani, P., Rutherford, G., Wilkinson, D. (2004). Population-based interventions for reducing sexually transmitted infections, including HIV infection. *Cochrane Database of Systematic Reviews*, **2**, CD001220.

Sheeran, P. & Abraham, C. (1994). Measurement of condom use in 72 studies of HIV-preventive behaviour: a critical review. *Patient Education and Counselling*, **24**, 199–216.

Sherr, L. (1995). *The psychology of pregnancy and childbirth*. Oxford: Blackwell Scientific Publications.

Sherr, L., Bolding, G., Maguire, M. & Elford, J. (2000). Viagra use and sexual risk behaviour among gay men in London. *AIDS*, **14**(13), 2051–3.

Slaymaker, E. (2004). A critique of international indicators of sexual risk behaviour. *Sexually Transmitted Infections*, **80** (Suppl. 2), ii13–21.

Van De Ven, P., Rawstorne, P., Crawford, J. & Kippax, S. (2002). Increasing proportions of Australian gay and homosexually active men engage in

unprotected anal intercourse with regular and with casual partners. *AIDS Care – Psychological and Socio-Medical Aspects of AIDS/HIV*, **14**, 335–41.

Weinhardt, L. S., Forsyth, A. D., Carey, M. P. *et al.* (1998). Reliability and validity of self-report measures of HIV-related sexual behavior: progress since 1990 and recommendations for research and practice. *Archieves of Sexual Behaviour*, **27**, 155–80.

Weinstein, N. D. (1980). Unrealistic optimism about future life events. *Journal of Personality and Social Psychology*, **39**, 806–20.

Weinstein, N. D. (1984). Why it won't happen to me – perceptions of risk factors and susceptibility. *Health Psychology*, **3**, 431–57.

Weinstein, N. D. (1989). Optimistic biases about personal risks. *Science*, **246**, 1232–3.

Weinstein, N. D. & Lachendro, E. (1982). Egocentrism as a source of unrealistic optimism. *Personality and Social Psychology Bulletin*, **8**, 195–200.

Wellings, K., Nanchahal, K., Macdowall, W. *et al.* (2001). Sexual behaviour in Britain: early heterosexual experience. *Lancet*, **358**(9296), 1843–50.

Sleep and health

Jason Ellis

University of Surrey

Introduction

Where much has been written about sleep from a clinically disordered perspective, only relatively recently, with the direct and indirect costs of an increasingly demanding 24-hour society being realized, has the concept of sleep entered the arenas of health psychology and behavioural medicine. Moreover, the reported neglect of discussions regarding sleep, beyond the use of hypnotics within doctor–patient interactions, coupled with an increasing understanding of sleep as a modifiable health behaviour has led to calls for sleep being placed high on the health psychologists' agenda. To this end, researchers have uncovered reciprocal links between the quality, quantity and timing of sleep, as both a subjective and objective

phenomenon, and numerous health and social outcomes. This chapter explores those links, focusing on the relationship between sleep need, sleep regulation and circadian rhythmicity, whilst examining the influence of human behaviour on these relationships.

What is sleep?

Sleep is an active process consisting of two stages, rapid eye movement sleep (REM) and non rapid eye movement sleep (NREM) (of which there are four sub-stages). Although not discrete, each stage of sleep can be characterized physiologically by different frequencies and amplitudes in brain-wave activity and together they make up what is known as sleep architecture. In Stage 1 the body enters a transitional period between sleep and wakefulness from which awakening is easy. Electroencephalographic (EEG) activity changes from a rhythmic pattern of alpha waves (8–13 cycles per second and below 50 microvolts) to mixed frequency, lower voltage brainwave activity, eventually leading to the official onset of sleep or Stage 2 sleep. Stage 2 is characterized by the presence of 'sleep spindles' (bursts in EEG activity above 11.5 cycles per second for more than 0.5 seconds) and 'K-complexes' (high voltage, short duration waveforms) as well as reduced muscle tension and slow rolling eye movements. Stages 3 and 4, also known as Slow Wave Sleep (SWS), are deeper, involving progressively higher voltage (an amplitude of 75 microvolts is usual) and slower brainwave activity (i.e. delta activity of less than 4 cycles per second), limited eye movements and muscle tension. During this time it is usual to have sleep spindles accompanying delta waves. The final stage of sleep, REM, is similar to Stage 1 sleep, being characterized by low voltage, mixed frequency electroencephalographic activity without sleep spindles and K-complexes. However, REM differs from Stage 1 sleep in that muscle tension is nonexistent, indicating that the body is in a state of paralysis and only the eyes and respiratory system are active. It is during REM that dream activity is believed to take place, although recent research suggests people can also dream in NREM. There are many theories as to the purpose of REM and consequently dreams. Traditional explanations for REM, such as the voiding of unwanted thoughts or reversed learning, have shown little empirical validity, whereas the suggestion that REM sleep is a period whereby information obtained throughout the day is assimilated into existing neural templates appears most credible and fits well within the existing literature (Jouvet, 1998).

An important feature of the K-complex (also known as an 'arousal'), found predominately in NREM sleep, is that it can create nocturnal awakening. Normally, an arousal is approximately 10–15 seconds in duration and the sleeper is briefly awoken but unable to remember the event in the morning. However, arousals may increase in quantity and duration in response to internal (e.g. upper airway obstruction) or external (e.g. noise) stimuli.

Sleep throughout the lifespan

Marked changes in sleep architecture occur throughout the lifespan, with newborn infants requiring approximately 15 hours of sleep each day and entering sleep through REM then cycling between REM and NREM on a 50–60 minute cycle. After infancy, children enter sleep through NREM and this pattern continues throughout the lifespan. The time spent in SWS is at a peak in young children then begins to decrease during late adolescence. A young adult's sleep comprises 75% NREM sleep and 25% REM on a 90-minute cycle, although most deep sleep occurs during the first third of the night. The typical progression of sleep throughout the lifespan (excluding neonates) is a movement through NREM stages 2–4 (only the first cycle includes full Stage 1 sleep) then a reversal through stages 4–2 before the onset of REM sleep, then the cycle begins again. Over the course of a night there will be approximately 4–6 complete sleep cycles with the later sleep cycles comprising longer REM periods and shorter NREM periods.

The ageing process has marked effects on specific aspects of sleep architecture, pertinent to sleep-onset-latency (initiating sleep) and sleep maintenance (staying asleep) (Dijk et al., 2001). Compared with the sleep of a young adult, researchers suggest an overall sleep efficiency of between 70–75% in older adults (Bliwise, 2000). However, when sleep disorders such as periodic limb movements (PLMs) and sleep disordered breathing are controlled for, this difference is approximately 80–85% (McCall et al., 1992). Additionally, whereas arousal rates during sleep are calculated at approximately 10 per hour in young adults (Anderson & Waters, 1998), this increases to approximately 23–27 arousals per hour in the older adult population (Boselli et al., 1998). SWS also changes with ageing, reducing from 18% of total sleep time at age 20 to between 5–10% for those between 60 and 80 years old (Hume et al., 1998) (see 'Ageing and health behaviour').

Sleep need and sleep regulation

Although inter- and intra-individual differences in quantity of sleep need exist (e.g. short sleep durations are associated with extraversion), as do significant discrepancies between sleep need and actual sleep durations achieved, there appears a consensus that approximately 7–7.5 hours a night is typical, with larger deviations being associated with an increasing risk of mortality. Additionally, sleeping less than 4 hours a night has been associated with a 2.8 times higher mortality from cancer in men and 1.5 in women (Kripke et al., 1979). More recently, associations between shorter sleep durations and obesity have been found in young adults (Hasler et al., 2004) even after controlling for other obesity-related factors such as family history of obesity and levels of physical exercise. In this instance Spiegel et al. (2005) suggest that reduced leptin levels (leptin is a hormone which is receptive to caloric intake and communicates energy needs to the brain), as a result of reduced sleep, may be responsible through alterations in appetite regulation.

Overall, sleep durations are considered in alignment with sleep needs if the individual reports feeling refreshed and alert throughout the day. However, perceived sleep needs are also prone to change due to affective state. During stressful periods, such as exam periods, and in depression-related disorders, longer sleep durations are preferred and as such a greater discrepancy between actual sleep need and sleep durations can develop and become problematic (Ellis & Fox, 2004; McCann & Stewin, 1988). Moreover, studies have shown sleep architecture is disrupted by anxiety, resulting in less SWS and an increase in Stage 1 sleep (Fuller et al., 1997). It is argued however that regularity in sleep scheduling, especially waking time, is a major determinant of sleep satisfaction and sleep regulation in itself is maintained through a continual interplay between the ANS, the homeostatic drive for sleep and the circadian rhythm.

Autonomic nervous system balance

Sleep regulation is largely tied to the balance between the sympathetic and parasympathetic branches of the ANS and it is during the transition through the NREM stages that parasympathetic dominance increases until full dominance is reached within REM. Conversely, during the latter phases of sleep, the sympathetic branch of the ANS begins to dominate as evidenced by the increase in HPA secretory activity. Both exogenous (e.g. excessive heat or noise) and endogenous factors (e.g. pain or anxiety), through activation of the sympathetic branch of the ANS, can inhibit sleep initiation or evoke an arousal during sleep. Additionally, it has been shown that individual differences in refractory periods, following ANS activation, can also affect sleep regulation and ANS activation is also prone to conditioning.

Homeostatic drive for sleep

Just as homeostatic mechanisms govern the relationship between hunger and food intake, sleep and the specific ultradian stages of sleep (i.e. NREM stages), are regulated by a homeostatic drive. The homeostatic drive increases the need for sleep based upon the timing and duration of the last sleep episode and declines once sleep has been initiated. In these instances the hypothalamic system creates the motivation to sleep and attempts to balance any discrepancies between sleep need and sleep durations accrued, by mobilizing sleep promoting behaviours (e.g. feelings of tiredness).

Daytime napping for longer than 20 minutes has been related to adverse changes in the sleep–wake cycle through reducing the homeostatic drive for sleep, whereas physical activity relates to an increase in the homeostatic drive. This is particularly relevant when considering as many as 80% of older healthy adults nap during the day (Wauquier *et al.*, 1992) and levels of physical activity are also low in this population.

Sleep deprivation

It is important to note that although a third of the population report sleepiness as a result of chronic sleep deprivation, sleep deprivation studies (both partial sleep and total sleep deprivation) as models of sleep deprivation should be examined cautiously. Experimental manipulations of sleep are prone to both experimenter and participant motivation, as blinded studies are difficult to perform. Additionally, most sleep deprivation studies tend to involve a strict regulation of waking activities, therefore creating an unnatural environment. With these points in mind, researchers concur that sleep deprivation reduces psychomotor performance, cognitive functioning and memory, resulting in deteriorations in mood, although the effects of sleep loss on mood have been shown to be moderated by personality characteristics such as neuroticism (Blagrove & Akehurst, 2001) (see 'Personality and health'). Other studies have shown the adverse effects of sleep deprivation on medical decision-making and levels of witness suggestibility.

Another feature of sleep deprivation is intrusive NREM sleep episodes during periods of wakefulness, the most common of which are known as microsleeps. Microsleeps manifest for between 15–30 seconds and attention to the environment and motor functioning reactivity are significantly reduced, making them potentially dangerous (e.g. whilst driving). Similarly, REM sleep may also intrude on the waking experience during a prolonged sleep deprivation, manifesting in the form of hallucinations.

Sleep loss also has consequences on the immune system, with even a minor sleep deprivation leading to acute reductions in natural killer cell, T-Cell and monocyte functioning, impairing the host defence mechanism and increasing susceptibility to pathogens. For example, Bergmann and colleagues (1994) found that natural carcinoma cells were attacked with only 40–50% efficiency after a period of sleep deprivation in rats. Additionally, Spiegel *et al.* (1999) suggest that the increases in sympathetic nervous system activity and higher evening cortisol concentrations, following sleep deprivation, are comparable to those of older adults, thus increasing susceptibility to premature age-related chronic conditions such as hypertension. Furthermore, Van Cauter investigated the relationship between sleep deprivation and glucose tolerance. She found that a relatively short period of sleep deprivation (i.e. 96 hours) led to glucose metabolisms resembling those seen in the primary stages of diabetes (Scheen & Van Cauter, 1998; Van Cauter *et al.*, 1998).

The effects of sleep loss can be quickly reversed. A recovery period between one and three days, irrespective of the amount of sleep debt accrued is usual with the recovery sleep comprising largely of REM and SWS. Additionally, levels of arousal on awakening can have a great impact on subjective measures of sleepiness, so having to attend to the environment quickly may ameliorate the immediate effects of sleep loss.

Circadian rhythms

The circadian pacemaker is the 24-hour body clock that influences chronobiological changes, endocrine changes and Body Core Temperature (BCT) through the suprachiasmatic nuclei (SCN), with BCT being one of the best markers of circadian rhythmicity. Located in the anterior of the hypothalamus, the two SCN, containing approximately 10 000 neurons each help regulate the circadian rhythm through an interplay between the optic nerves and the pineal gland. Signals from the optic nerves pass through the SCN and on to the pineal gland, regulating the production or inhibition of melatonin (melatonin is a hormone which reduces body temperature, aiding sleep onset). Darkness signals the pineal gland to release melatonin into the bloodstream whereas light inhibits its proliferation. Studies with blind people demonstrate that melatonin is still regulated to a 24-hour cycle by the pineal gland in the absence of light signals; however, the timing of the circadian rhythm is usually disrupted. Melatonin release is increased by selective serotonin re-uptake inhibitors and antipsychotic drugs but significantly reduced by benzodiazepines and caffeine.

During a normal 24-hour sleep–wake schedule, several hormones, tied to the circadian rhythm, are also secreted. Growth hormone and prolactin are released during SWS and testosterone blood levels peak during REM sleep. Similarly, although sleep-independent, several hormone secretions are aligned to the circadian rhythm. Cortisol secretion, in response to adrenocorticotrophic hormone (ACTH), rises toward the end of the sleep and is at its peak upon waking.

Studies in time-free environments (e.g. caves) suggest a slightly longer natural circadian rhythm than 24 hours and without environmental cues such as food intake, bright light exposure and physical activity (zeitgebers), the circadian rhythm can desynchronize. If the circadian rhythm becomes desynchronized (arrhythmicity), dysfunctional chronobiological changes such as lowered melatonin release occur and a significant discrepancy between the BCT and circadian rhythm develops. BCT increases at night are associated with nocturnal wakefulness and physiological activation, particularly in older adults (Lushington *et al.*, 2000). As the body ages, the SCN, begins to deteriorate, leaving the body clock to rely increasingly upon zeitgebers to monitor the sleep–wake cycle (Duffy et al., 1996). Two additional factors which can disrupt the endogenous harmony of the circadian rhythm are shift work and transmeridian flight.

Rotating shift work has been widely associated with gastrointestinal dysfunction and cardiovascular disease, although poor eating habits and the timing of food intake (i.e. the timing of gastric juice secretion) may moderate these relationships. Another possible explanation for the ill effects experienced through rotating shift work is the gradual adaptation in cortisol secretion timing, which may take weeks to adjust to a change in routine. The least disruptive shift rotation is one that occurs slowly and follows a natural circadian cycle (i.e. earlies . . . lates . . . nights . . . off). However, the adverse effects of shift work can be further exacerbated by an existing illness (diabetes or epilepsy particularly) and coping with shift work is in itself affected by the timing and types of work undertaken. Shifts of 12 hours or more that involve handling harmful substances, heavy physical activity or critical monitoring are more deleterious. Similarly, shift work with few breaks or with breaks of a short duration are more harmful.

The daytime sleep after a night shift tends to be shorter and contain reduced Stage 2 and REM sleep and increased Stage 1 sleep. Additionally, being 'on-call' during the night, even if not awoken, tends to create an expectancy fragmentation in normal sleep architecture. Overall, the circadian pacemaker of the night shift worker is in continual opposition to environmental zeitgebers and therefore the circadian rhythm remains arrhythmic. Another important factor to consider is the socio-domestic consequences of shift work. Although evening shift work results in little circadian dysregulation, complexities within family role functioning, social isolation and marital disharmony are commonly reported and are reflected in the high rates of divorce amongst evening shift workers (see 'Shift work and health').

In terms of transmeridian flight, desynchronization between the circadian pacemaker and cues from the external environment create phase-delay (westward travel) or phase-advance (eastward travel) in the circadian rhythm. Both phase-delay and phase-advance result in 'jet lag', the physical manifestations of which include lethargy, disorientation, loss of appetite and sleep disturbances the following night. Several factors, such as number of time zones crossed and age (50+) mediate the level of 'jet-lag' experienced and eastward travel has been shown to be more deleterious, requiring a longer recovery period. However, individual differences in experiences of jet lag do exist with approximately one third of people unaffected by transmeridian flight and another third highly susceptible.

In cases of circadian arrhythmicity, due to transmeridian flight, deterioration in the SCN or shift-work, controlled release of melatonin has been shown to reinitialize the circadian rhythm (Garfinkle et al., 1995) although the long-term consequences of self-administered melatonin remain undetermined.

Other sleep disrupting factors

Where it appears that variation in sleep and circadian routines adversely affects sleep architecture, several drugs can also have a significant impact on sleep through the Central Nervous System (CNS), the most common of which are caffeine, nicotine and alcohol.

Caffeine has a plasma half-life of approximately three to four hours (although significant individual differences exist) and is an antagonist to adenosine receptors within the CNS. Doses of caffeine, between 100mg–500mg, significantly delay sleep onset, resulting in less total sleep time and reduced SWS and REM sleep. Caffeine is found in many foods and drinks (one cup of tea contains 25–50 mg; instant coffee 60–80 mg) and most OTC analgesics contain high levels of occult (non-identified) caffeine. Similarly, with a half-life of approximately one to two hours, in large doses, nicotine inhibits nicotinic synapses within the CNS, resulting in CNS stimulation and reductions in total sleep time and REM as well as delays in the onset of sleep. Further compounding the relationship between nicotine and sleep is the finding that one of the main symptoms reported during smoking cessation is sleep disturbance (see 'Tobacco use').

Although alcohol promotes the initiation of sleep and has been shown to increase total sleep time, through depression of the cent nervous system, the sleep obtained changes quite dramatically. REM sleep is suppressed whilst blood alcohol levels are high but a rebound in REM sleep occurs (to the cost of SWS) when blood alcohol levels reduce. The diuretic effect of alcohol as well as the increased time spent in REM creates frequent nocturnal awakenings. An additional problem exists in that frequent use of alcohol to sleep creates a tolerance and more alcohol is needed to obtain its sedative effects, creating dependence (see 'Alcohol abuse').

Conclusions

Although research has begun to draw associations between the quantity, quality and timing of sleep episodes and health and social outcomes, the full extent of the relationship between sleep and health still remains largely uncovered. With causal studies of the relationships between sleep functioning and psychological and physical health outcomes in their infancy many more studies are needed to progress our understanding of sleep and its correlates in the real world. What is known is that complex interrelationships exist between the homeostatic drive for sleep, the circadian rhythm and the autonomic nervous system in order to maintain sleep homeostasis and it is our behaviour and the conditions within our society which challenge these systems, increasingly beyond tolerable levels.

REFERENCES

Anderson, T. W. & Waters, W. F. (1998). Frequency of spontaneous, transient arousals in normals, sleep apnea, periodic limb movement disorder and insomnia. Sleep, 21, 76.

Bergmann, B. M., Everson, C. A., Kushida, C. A. et al. (1994). Sleep deprivation in the rat V: energy use and mediation. Sleep, 12, 31–41.

Blagrove, M. & Akehurst, L. (2001). Personality and the modulation of effects of sleep loss on mood and cognition. Personality and Individual Differences, 30, 819–28.

Bliwise, D. L. (2000). Normal Aging. In
M. H. Kryger, I. Roth & W. C. Dement
(Eds.). *Principles and practice of sleep
medicine* (3rd edn.) (Chapter 3). New York:
W.B Saunders.

Boselli, M., Parrino, L., Smerieri, A. &
Terzano, M. G. (1998). Effects of age on
EEG arousals in normal sleep. *Sleep*, **21**,
351–7.

Dijk, D. J., Duffy, J. F. & Czeisler, C. A. (2001).
Age-related increase in awakenings:
impaired consolidation of Non-REM sleep
at all circadian phases. *Sleep*, **24**(5), 565–77.

Duffy, J. F., Kronauer, R. E. & Czeisler, C. A.
(1996). Phase shifting human circadian
rhythms: influence of sleep timing, social
contact and light exposure. *Journal of
Physiology*, **495**, 289–97.

Ellis, J. & Fox, P. (2004). Promoting mental
health in students: is there a role for sleep?
*Journal of the Royal Society for the
Promotion of Health*, **124**(3), 129–33.

Fuller, K. H., Waters, W. F., Binks, P. G. &
Anderson, T. (1997). Generalized anxiety
and sleep architecture: a
polysomnographic investigation. *Sleep*, **20**
(5), 370–6.

Garfinkle, D., Laudon, M., Nof, D. &
Zisapel, N. (1995). Improvement of sleep
quality in elderly people by controlled-
release melatonin. *The Lancet*, **346**, 541–4.

Hasler, G., Buysse, D. J., Klaghofer, R. *et al.*
(2004). The association between short
sleep duration and obesity in young
adults: a 13-year prospective study. *Sleep*,
27(4), 661–6.

Hume, K. I., Van, F. & Watson, A. (1998).
A field study of age and gender differences
in habitual adult sleep. *Journal of Sleep
Research*, **7**, 85–94.

Jouvet, M. (1998). Paradoxical sleep as a
programming system. *Journal of Sleep
Research*, **6**, 61–77.

Kripke, D. F., Simons, R. N., Garfinkle, L. &
Hammond, E. C. (1979). Short and long
sleep and sleeping pills: is increased
mortality associated? *Archives of General
Psychiatry*, **36**, 103–16.

Lushington, K., Dawson, D. & Lack, L.
(2000). Core body temperature is elevated
during constant wakefulness in elderly
poor sleepers. *Sleep*, **23**(4), 504–10.

McCall, W. V., Erwin, C. W., Edinger, J. D.,
Krystal, A. D. & Marsh, G. R. (1992).
Ambulatory polysomnography:
technical aspects and normative values.
Journal of Clinical Neurophysiology, **9**(1),
68–77.

McCann, S. J. H. & Stewin, L. L. (1988).
Worry, anxiety, and preferred length of
sleep. *Journal of Genetic Psychology*,
149(3), 413–18.

Scheen, A. J. & Van Cauter, E. (1998). The
roles of time of day and sleep quality in
modulating glucose regulation: clinical
implications. *Hormone Research*, **49**(3–4),
191–201.

Spiegel, K., Leproult, R. & Van Cauter, E.
(1999). Impact of sleep debt on metabolic
and endocrine function. *The Lancet*, **354**,
1435–9.

Spiegel, K., Leproult, R., L'Hermite-
Baleriaux, M. *et al.* (2005). Leptin levels
are dependent on sleep duration:
relationships with sympathovagal balance,
carbohydrate regulation, cortisol, and
thyrotropin. *The Journal of Clinical
Endocrinology and Metabolism*, **89**(11),
5762–71.

Van Cauter, E., Polonsky, K. S. & Scheen,
A. J. (1998). Roles in circadian rhythmicity
and sleep in human glucose regulation.
Endocrine Review, **18**(5), 716–38.

Wauquier, A., Van Sweden, B., Lagaay,
A. M., Kemp, B. & Kamphuisen, H. A. C.
(1992). Ambulatory monitoring of
sleep–wakefulness patterns in health
elderly males and females (>88 years): the
'senieur' protocol. *Journal of the American
Geriatrics Society*, **40**, 109–14.

Social support and health

Thomas A. Wills and Michael G. Ainette

Albert Einstein College of Medicine

Social support and health

This chapter discusses the relation of social support to health outcomes. We consider approaches to the conceptualization of social
support and discuss findings on the relation of social support to
onset, progression or recovery from chronic illnesses which are
major sources of mortality. An emphasis is on understanding
physiological and behavioural mechanisms through which social
support is related to health status. In a final section we summarize
developments in this area, note current debates and suggest
directions for clinical research.

Conceptualization and measurement of social support

There are two major approaches to conceptualizing social variables
related to health. The structural approach focuses on assessing the
structure of a person's network of social connections. In a typical
network assessment the respondent is asked to name persons with
whom he/she has a connection, typically including questions about
spouse, family, friends, neighbours and workmates. Network assessments may also include questions about membership of community
organizations (e.g. churches, professional or service organizations,
fraternal organizations) and participation in sports, cultural

activities and leisure/recreational activities. A score for network size is based on the total number of connections a person has; a score for social integration is based on the total number of different roles a person has in the community; and a score termed 'social participation' is based on the total amount of participation in activities that involve other people. These indices are taken to represent the extent of a person's integration in the community (Cohen, Underwood & Gottlieb, 2000).

The functional approach to support measurement focuses on asking questions about the extent to which a person would have supportive functions available if needed. The supportive functions typically assessed include emotional support, the availability of persons with whom one can talk about problems and receive sympathy, understanding and reassurance. Instrumental support is the availability of persons who can provide relevant goods and services, for example assistance with household tasks, child care or transportation and loaning money or tools when needed. Informational support is having people available who can provide useful advice and guidance and information about community resources or contacts. Assessments of social companionship ask whether there are persons available to do things with for a range of leisure activities. These indices represent the extent to which a person has available social resources that would be useful for coping with problems (see 'Social support assessment').

Models of support effects

A conceptual theme in social support research is whether having good support serves to reduce the impact of stressors. If a support index shows comparable effects for persons with a low stress level and a high stress level, this is termed a main-effect process and suggests that the operation of support does not depend on the person's stress level. An alternative model suggests that support will be particularly beneficial for persons experiencing a high level of stress. This is termed the 'buffering model' because having high support serves to reduce (buffer) the impact of stress and this process implies that support helps people to cope better with stressors. Prior studies of health outcomes indicated that main effects were typically observed for structural measures of support (e.g. network size), whereas buffering effects were observed for functional measures, particularly emotional support (Cohen & Wills, 1985).

Social support and health: findings

Support and mortality

In prospective studies with mortality as the criterion variable, the researchers assess a sample of participants at a baseline point, obtaining structural and/or functional support measures and indexing demographic or behavioural variables that could be correlated with support. The sample is then followed over time and mortality status is determined some years later. At present over 80 such studies have been conducted; almost all show significant beneficial effects of support on mortality from diseases including cardiovascular disease and cancer. On average, persons with low support have two to three times greater risk of mortality compared to those with high support (Uchino, 2004). Studies have been conducted with large population-based samples in various areas of the USA and Europe, and effects of social support are found to be independent of variables such as age and gender. Protective effects have been found for all structural indices (network size, social integration and social participation) and recent studies have found effects on mortality for functional measures including emotional and instrumental support (Wills & Filer, 2001). The prospective studies have typically found effects of support on mortality with control for indices of substance use (e.g. cigarette smoking) and preventive health behaviours (e.g. diet and exercise), but also have noted that persons with higher support tend to have a more health-promoting lifestyle. This suggests that the effect of social support on health status may be at least partly attributable to these other factors, but possible mechanisms of support effects have not generally been tested in studies of mortality.

In recent years, studies have shown similar effects of social support in other national populations; for example, studies conducted in Hong Kong and Japan showed that higher social participation predicted lower rates of mortality. Differences in support effects as a function of social/cultural variables such as socio-economic status, ethnicity and individualistic vs. collectivist cultures have been investigated to some extent, but the amount of research is limited and there remains a need for further exploration of this question (Uchino, 2004). Research has also extended the concept of individual social support to supportiveness at the community level, defined as feelings of mutual trust, cohesion and responsibility among community residents and termed 'social capital'. For example, Kawachi et al. (1997) analyzed state-level indices of social trust and civic engagement from survey data collected in 39 states in the USA, and results showed that states with higher social capital had lower age-adjusted mortality rates.

Support and disease progression

Longitudinal studies have linked social support to disease progression for several conditions including cardiovascular disease and cancer (Helgeson et al., 1998). For example, Angerer et al. (2000) found emotional support was related to less progression of coronary artery disease over a 2-year period, as assessed by angiography. A 9-year study of patients with HIV examined effects of life events and social support and found that persons with higher functional support showed slower disease progression as indexed by both CD4 cell counts and clinical diagnoses (Leserman et al., 2002).

Support and recovery from illness

Research has also shown measures of social support related to recovery from illness. In these studies, participants who have a major health problem (e.g. myocardial infarction) are identified through clinic or hospital settings: an interview including a support assessment is conducted and the participants are then followed over time to determine their outcomes. Results have shown that persons with larger social networks or more functional support are more likely to recover from an episode of serious illness. For example, a study by Williams et al. (1992) examined a large sample of patients identified by an angiography clinic as having advanced coronary artery disease and followed them over a 10-year period; results showed that a compound support index was related to longer survival time, controlling for household income and for a comprehensive index of medical risk at baseline. Effects for recovery from illness were also found by Berkman *et al.* (1992) in a community sample of older persons for whom data on support were available from several time points before and after the illness. Among persons who had been hospitalized for a myocardial infarction, emotional support predicted lower likelihood of mortality over a 6-month period, controlling for demographics and prior medical status. Recent studies of medical patients have been consistent with prior findings, showing measures of social participation and confidant availability related to lower likelihood of new disease episodes or mortality (e.g. Brummett *et al.*, 2001; Dickens *et al.*, 2004).

Buffering effects

Many studies have shown buffering effects of social support for psychological outcomes: negative life events have less effect on depression/anxiety among persons with high support, compared with those with low support (Cohen & Wills, 1985). Buffering effects have also been demonstrated in several studies with mortality as the outcome. For example, Rosengren *et al.* (1993) found that life stress had a strong effect on mortality among men with low emotional support, but stress had little effect for men with high emotional support. Falk *et al.* (1992) found that men with high job stress and low emotional support had a disproportionate risk of all-cause mortality, compared with those with high stress and high support. This study also found a buffering effect for a structural measure, social participation.

Relations to physiological indices

Several studies have tested relations of social support to physiological indices which are relevant for cardiac disease and other illnesses. Studies using ambulatory monitoring have shown social support related to blood pressure in daily situations; for example, Linden *et al.* (1993) conducted a day of ambulatory blood pressure monitoring with college students and found that women higher in available support showed lower aggregated systolic blood pressure in daily life. In a 9-year longitudinal study of a middle-aged female cohort, Raikkonen *et al.* (2001) found that decreases in functional support over time were related to development of hypertension. A study of women in Sweden investigated several risk factors and

found higher functional support related to lower levels on all four elements of the metabolic syndrome (central obesity, hypertension, dislipidemia and elevated blood glucose), which presents a substantial risk for heart disease (Horsten *et al.*, 1999). With regard to cancer, a study of participants from a screening program found a composite social support measure related to lower levels of prostate-specific antigen, which has been linked to prostate cancer (Stone, Mezzacappa, Donatone & Gonder, 1999).

Mechanisms of support effects

Because of accumulated findings on health effects of social support, research has shifted in recent years towards studying how these effects occur (Berkman *et al.*, 2000). While social networks or social support could be related to health status without involving any other processes, it is plausible that social variables have effects on intermediate processes that then influence a person's health status, a process termed 'mediation' (Wills & Cleary, 1996). The mediator could be a psychological process (e.g. perceived control), a behavioural process (e.g. smoking) or a physiological process (e.g. stress reactivity). Figure 1 illustrates a direct effect from a social variable to a physical effect (path a or path d), and an indirect effect from a social variable to a physical effect through a mediator (paths be or ce). For example, low support could be related to cigarette smoking, which would then have effects on lung and arterial cells so as to increase risk for disease. We discuss three plausible mechanisms for mediated effects as follows:

Reactivity and inflammatory processes

Support could be related to risk for cardiovascular disease through a stress-reactivity mechanism. Several studies have tested whether having support reduces autonomic reactivity (i.e. increase in heart rate and blood pressure) under stressful conditions and whether social support has relations to other cardiovascular parameters (Rozanski *et al.*, 1999). Studies in laboratory settings show that having support available is related to less reactivity under stress, whereas negative social interactions predict greater reactivity under stress (Uchino, 2004). Such studies suggest a mechanism for why social support is related to blood pressure in various settings, because persons with higher autonomic reactivity are posited

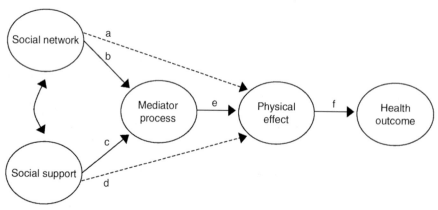

Fig 1 Theoretical model of relation of social network structure and social support functions to health outcome, with indirect relation through mediator process or direct pathway to physical effect.

to be more likely to develop hypertension (cf. Horsten *et al.*, 1999; Raikkonen *et al.*, 2001). Studies in field settings have also shown measures of loneliness or social support related to levels of C-reactive protein (Schnorpfeil *et al.*, 2003) and fibrinogen (e.g. Steptoe *et al.*, 2004), which reflect inflammatory processes in risk for heart disease (see 'Stress and health').

Immune system functioning

A mechanism has been outlined in which social support may influence susceptibility to infectious diseases and cancer through effects on immune system functioning. Studies with animal models and human subjects have previously linked social affiliation and perceived support to immune-function indices such as greater T-cell proliferation and higher levels of natural killer (NK) cells (Kiecolt-Glaser *et al.*, 2002). Current research has continued these trends. For example, a study of a workplace sample found, controlling for a number of potential confounders, that persons with more supportive social networks had higher levels of NK cells (Steptoe *et al.*, 2004). Support measures have also been linked to levels of cytokines such as interleukin-2 and -6, and to tumour angiogenesis factors such as Vascular Endothelial Growth Factor (VEGF). For example, a study of patients with malignant tumours found that persons with greater social wellbeing had lower levels of VEGF (Lutgendorf *et al.*, 2002). It has been suggested that support operates through enhancing emotional status, because several studies have found larger networks and higher functional support related to lower levels of cortisol, a marker for negative affect (Steptoe *et al.*, 2004; Turner-Cobb *et al.*, 2000) (see 'Psychoneuroimmunology').

Behavioural mechanisms

Social support could also influence health status through relations to behavioural processes. One plausible process is substance use, as a number of studies have shown that persons with higher support are less likely to smoke cigarettes and engage in heavy drinking (Wills & Filler 2001). It has also been suggested that social control processes linked to social support could encourage persons to maintain a healthier diet, to exercise regularly and to get adequate sleep, all of which are protective factors against several diseases (Berkman *et al.*, 2000; Steptoe *et al.*, 2004). In addition, a substantial body of research has found that persons with more support from friends and family show better adherence to medical treatment regimens, a process that could reduce disease recurrence and enhance recovery from illness (DiMatteo, 2004).

Developments, debates and clinical implications

In summary, research has shown that persons with larger social networks or higher levels of functional support enjoy better health status. This protective effect has been demonstrated across a variety of national populations and has been found for persons of different age, gender and social standing. The field has expanded conceptually to include community-level measures of social capital. In addition to main effects for support, stress-buffering effects have been demonstrated in a number of studies. Prior distinctions between structural and functional aspects of support have become less clear, as measures of network size and social participation have shown buffering effects for mortality as an outcome, while studies of emotional support and relationship satisfaction have shown these related to lower mortality rates. Thus a prior emphasis on social networks as a health-protective factor has expanded to include consideration of how structural and functional approaches can be merged so as to better understand the role of social factors in health status (Berkman *et al.*, 2000; Cohen, 2004).

Recent developments

A recent development in the area is research designed to investigate mechanisms of how support is related to health, through studying physiological and behavioural processes that may mediate the protective effect of social support. Though mechanisms have not typically been tested in studies of mortality (Uchino, 2004), recent studies have examined relevant intermediate processes. This research has shown support measures related to autonomic reactivity and immune-system functioning and has also shown social support to be related to several behavioural processes. These findings are suggestive in helping explain the linkage of social variables to individuals' health status.

While the field has advanced in this regard, the role of positive or negative affect in support effects is not well studied; the relative importance of stress-dampening mechanisms and effects on immune system function is not known; mediation through behavioural mechanisms has not been studied in detail and it is possible that part of the protective effect of social networks does not involve any of these processes (i.e. a direct effect). We lack comparative studies to clarify which of the intermediate processes are most relevant in accounting for the health effects of social support, using analyses that test directly for mediation. Though many pieces of evidence are available, achieving this larger aim will require studies that link social and physiological assessments and examine intermediate processes over longitudinal periods sufficient to show whether support has direct effects or mediated effects on outcomes. Analytic approaches such as structural equation modelling can help to clarify such questions (Wills & Cleary, 1996).

Debates

Although many findings on the role of social support for disease onset and recovery from illness are well established, there is ongoing discussion about interventions designed to improve health through increasing social support. In recent years, studies have been conducted to investigate whether support can be increased through working directly with indigenous supporters (e.g. family and relatives), or through adding what is termed grafted support: formal psychotherapy or professionally-led support groups. While studies typically show that social support interventions enhance mental health and quality-of-life indices (Hogan, Linden & Najarian, 2002), effects on health outcomes have been mixed; there have been null effects for psychotherapy interventions with heart disease patients, and for cancer patients some possible negative effects of peer support groups have been noted (Helgeson *et al.*, 2001). It is now recognized that the technical issues for conducting support interventions are not well understood, and explicating these issues is a focus of current research (see 'Social support interventions').

A specific debate concerns the role of support interventions for increasing survival time among cancer patients. Earlier studies had shown that patients who participated in support-group interventions had longer survival times, but some recent studies have reported that support improved quality of life but had no effect on survival. The promise of the positive findings has been balanced against the null results, and the reasons for the differing results are debated at present (see Palmer, Coyne, Spiegel & Giese-Davis, 2004).

Clinical implications

A large body of research has shown that social ties can be a protective factor, making individuals less vulnerable to disease and more resilient in the face of negative life events. An implication for health professionals is that social relationships existing in the community can be important for assisting the treatment effort, or in the case of negative interactions, making it more difficult for individuals to benefit from treatment.

Though the technology of conducting support interventions is still developing, researchers agree that health professionals can adopt an expanded view of physician–patient relationships through thinking about the patient's social network as well as the patient him- or herself. Health professionals can make systematic efforts to reach out to social network members so as to inform them (as well as the patient) about treatment procedures and educate them about how to help maintain treatments, using home visits, telephone calls or more recently, Internet communications. Learning how to enlist the beneficial effects of social networks in the treatment process is a question for both psychology and medicine and interdisciplinary research should be productive for discovering the best ways to accomplish this goal.

Acknowledgements

This work was supported by a Research Scientist Development Award K02 DA00252 from the National Institute on Drug Abuse (TAW) and by a Minority Fellowship from the American Psychological Association (MGA).

REFERENCES

Angerer, P., Siebert, U., Kothny, W. et al. (2000). Impact of social support, cynical hostility, and anger expression on progression of coronary atherosclerosis. *Journal of the American College of Cardiology*, **36**, 1781–8.

Berkman, L. F., Glass, T., Brissette, I. & Seeman, T. E. (2000). From social integration to health. *Social Science and Medicine*, **51**, 843–57.

Berkman, L. F., Leo-Summers, L. & Horwitz, R. I. (1992). Emotional support and survival after myocardial infarction: a prospective, population-based study of the elderly. *Annals of Internal Medicine*, **117**, 1003–9.

Brummett, B. H., Barefoot, J. C., Siegler, I. E. et al. (2001). Characteristics of socially isolated patients with coronary artery disease who are at elevated risk for mortality. *Psychosomatic Medicine*, **63**, 267–72.

Cohen, S., (2004). Social relationships and health. *American Psychologist*, **59**, 676–84.

Cohen, S., Underwood, L. G. & Gottlieb, B. H. (Eds.) (2000). *Social support measurement and intervention: a guide for health and social scientists.* New York: Oxford University Press.

Cohen, S. & Wills, T. A. (1985). Stress, social support, and the buffering hypothesis. *Psychological Bulletin*, **98**, 310–57.

Dickens, E. N., McGowan, L., Percival, C. et al. (2004). Lack of a close confidant predicts further cardiac events after myocardial infarction. *Heart*, **90**, 518–22.

DiMatteo, M. R. (2004). Social support and patient adherence to medical treatment: a meta-analysis. *Health Psychology*, **23**, 207–18.

Falk, A., Hanson, B. S., Isacsson, S.-O. & Ostergren, P.-O. (1992). Job strain and mortality in elderly men: social network, support, and influence as buffers. *American Journal of Public Health*, **82**, 1136–9.

Helgeson, V. S., Cohen, S. & Fritz, H. (1998). Social ties and cancer. In J. Holland (Ed.). *Psycho-oncology* (pp. 99–109). London: Oxford University Press.

Helgeson, V. S., Cohen, S., Schulz, R. & Yasko, J. (2001). Group support interventions for people with cancer: benefits and hazards. In A. Baum & B. L. Andersen (Eds.). *Psychosocial interventions for cancer* (pp. 269–86). Washington, DC: American Psychological Association.

Hogan, B. E., Linden, W. & Najarian, B. (2002). Social support interventions: do they work? *Clinical Psychology Review*, **22**, 381–440.

Horsten, M., Mittleman, M. A., Wamala, S. P., Scheck-Gustafsson, K. & Orth-Gomer, K. (1999). Social relations and the metabolic syndrome in middle-aged Swedish women. *Journal of Cardiovascular Risk*, **6**, 391–7.

Kawachi, I., Kennedy, B. P., Lochner, K. & Prothrow-Stith, D. (1997). Social capital, income inequality, and mortality. *American Journal of Public Health*, **87**, 1491–8.

Kiecolt-Glaser, J. K., McGuire, L., Robles, T. F. & Glaser, R. (2002). Emotions,

morbidity, and mortality: new perspectives from psychoneuroimmunology. *Annual Review of Psychology*, **53**, 83–107.

Leserman, J., Petitto, J. M., Gu, H. et al. (2002). Progression to AIDS, a clinical AIDS condition and mortality: psychosocial and physiological predictors. *Psychological Medicine*, **32**, 1059–73.

Linden, W., Chambers, L., Maurice, J. & Lenz, J. W. (1993). Sex differences in social support, self-deception, hostility, and ambulatory cardiovascular activity. *Health Psychology*, **12**, 376–80.

Lutgendorf, S. K., Johnsen, E. L., Cooper, B. et al. (2002). Vascular endothelial growth factor and social support in patients with ovarian carcinoma. *Cancer*, **95**, 808–15.

Palmer, S. C., Coyne, J. C., Spiegel, D. & Giese-Davis, J. (2004). Examining the evidence that psychotherapy improves the survival of cancer patients. *Biological Psychiatry*, **56**, 61–4.

Raikkonen, K., Matthews, K. A. & Kuller, L. H. (2001). Trajectory of psychological risk and incident hypertension in middle-aged women. *Hypertension*, **38**, 798–802.

Rosengren, A., Orth-Gomer, K., Wedel, H. & Wilhelmsen, L. (1993). Stressful life events, social support, and mortality in men born in 1933. *British Medical Journal*, **307**, 1102–5.

Rozanski, A., Blumenthal, J. A. & Kaplan, J. (1999). Impact of psychological factors on the pathogenesis of cardiovascular disease. *Circulation*, **99**, 2192–217.

Schnorpfeil, P., Noll, A., Schulze, R. et al. (2003). Allostatic load and work conditions. *Social Science and Medicine,* **57**, 647–56.

Steptoe, A., Owen, N., Kunz-Ebrecht, S. R. & Brydon, L. (2004). Loneliness and neuroendocrine, cardiovascular, and inflammatory stress responses in middle-aged men and women. *Psychoneuroendocrinology,* **29**, 593–611.

Stone, A. A., Mezzacappa, E. S., Donatone, B. A. & Gonder, M. (1999). Stress and social support associated with prostate-specific antigen levels in men. *Health Psychology,* **18**, 482–6.

Turner-Cobb, J. M., Sephton, S. E., Koopman, C., Blake-Mortimer, J. & Spiegel, D. (2000). Social support and salivary cortisol in women with metastatic breast cancer. *Psychosomatic Medicine,* **62**, 337–45.

Uchino, B. N. (2004). *Social support and physical health: Understanding the health consequences of relationships.* New Haven, CT: Yale University Press.

Williams, R., Barefoot, J., Califf, R. *et al.* (1992). Prognostic importance of social resources among patients with CAD.

Journal of the American Medical Association, **267**, 520–4.

Wills, T. A. & Cleary, S. D. (1996). How are social support effects mediated? A test for parental support and adolescent substance use. *Journal of Personality and Social Psychology,* **71**, 937–52.

Wills, T. A. & Filer, M. (2001). Social networks and social support. In A. Baum, T. A. Revenson & J. E. Singer (Eds.). *Handbook of health psychology* (pp. 209–34). Mahwah, NJ: Erlbaum.

Socioeconomic status and health

Lion Shahab

University College London

Background

Although the influence of wealth, status and power on health has been documented across different cultures for centuries (Liberatos, Link & Kelsey, 1988), it was not until the nineteenth century that more systematic scientific evidence emerged showing that those who were more affluent lived longer and healthier (e.g. by Villermé (1840) in France, Chadwick (1842) in Britain and Virchow (1848) in Germany). However, with the advance of bacteriology in the late nineteenth century and the ensuing dominance of the biomedical paradigm of health and illness, considerations of socioeconomic status (SES) in relation to health were largely put aside and confined to its role as a control variable (House, 2002).

With the realization of the limits of modern medicine, interest in social epidemiology and medical sociology grew again during the second half of the twentieth century (Bloom, 2002) and so did the output of research looking at SES, in particular poverty, and health. These early studies assumed a threshold effect of SES on health (Adler & Ostrove, 1999, see Figure 1); increases in income were thought to improve health only beneath, not above, a given 'poverty line'. As discussed below, however, emerging evidence showed the picture to be far more complex than this.

Main observations

Socioeconomic status as used in research is a conglomeration of various concepts which centre around indicators of desirable social and material attributes. How it is operationalized depends both on theoretical orientations as well as practical limitations and most studies tend to estimate SES either by educational attainment, income, occupation or a combination of these (Kaplan & Keil, 1993). Irrespective of the actual SES measure used, the last 50 years have produced a number of consistent 'big' findings about the association between SES and health (Young, 2004).

The most ubiquitous feature of this association is its shape. What has been found in virtually all studies is a 'gradient' effect (Adler *et al.*, 1994) rather than a threshold effect (Figure 1), which holds across various countries (Braveman & Tarimo, 2002), different ethnic groups within countries (e.g. Davey-Smith *et al.*, 1996) and gender (e.g. Bosma *et al.*, 1997). Stepwise increase in SES is accompanied by:

- Stepwise improvement of standardized mortality rates (e.g. Marmot, Shipley & Rose, 1984), disease progression (Lynch *et al.*, 1998) and life expectancy (e.g. Guralnik *et al.*, 1993)
- Stepwise reduction of infant mortality (e.g. Maher & Macfarlane, 2004), chronic disease (e.g. Townsend, 1974) and psychiatric disorder morbidity (e.g. Dohrenwend & Schwartz, 1995)
- Stepwise increase in self-reported good physical (Figure 2) and mental (Figure 3) health (e.g. Hemingway *et al.*, 1997).

The only notable exception to this rule is the differential incidence of neoplastic diseases, some of which follow the social gradient (e.g. lung cancer, Mao *et al.*, 2001) whereas others do not (e.g. breast cancer, Devesa & Diamond, 1980).

Additional features of the SES–health relationship include the existence of ethnic differences that hold within each different social class; non-white populations tend to have worse health indices than white populations along the social spectrum (Pamuk *et al.*, 1998).

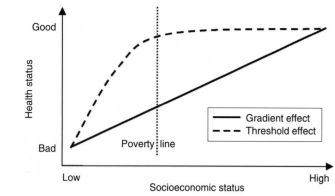

Fig 1 Relationship between SES and health.

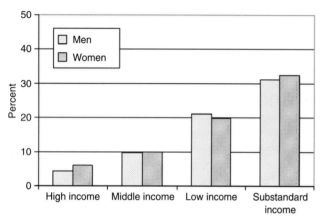

Fig 2 Fair or poor health by family income and sex, United States 1995. Adapted from: Pamuk *et al.*, 1998.

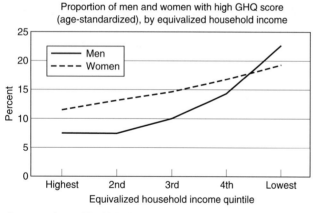

Fig 3 General mental health by family income and sex, England, 2003. *Source:* Health Survey for England, 2003.

There is considerable evidence for the influence of SES on health at all stages of the life cycle; the social gradient is found from childhood (e.g. Case, Lubotsky & Paxon, 2002) through to old age (e.g. House *et al.*, 1994). Of particular importance for health across the lifespan is childhood SES. Although health is modified by changes in SES throughout life (Blane, 1999), the social class of origin influences health risks independent of risks associated with the class of destination (e.g. Bartley & Plewis, 1997).

It is worth noting that the health gap between the rich and poor is widening. Both in the UK (Macintyre, 1997) and in the USA (Pappas, Queen, Hadden & Fisher, 1993), there is ample evidence for an increase in health disparities between different socioeconomic groups despite overall improvement in general health. A similar widening of health inequalities has also been observed between countries. For instance, over the last 30 years life expectancy rose in Western Europe whereas it declined in Eastern Europe (Bobak & Marmot, 1996).

Cross-cultural research into population health has unearthed another aspect of the social gradient. Although it is clear that a nation's health depends on its wealth, what may be equally important is how this wealth is distributed within socio-economic hierarchies. More egalitarian countries such as Sweden tend to have better overall health indices than other wealthy countries with greater social inequalities such as the USA (Daniels, Kennedy & Kawachi, 2000 but see Mackenbach *et al.*, 1997) (see 'Cultural and ethnic factors in health').

Lastly, the association between SES and health seems to persist even after controlling for a wide range of possible determinants (Lantz *et al.*, 1998). This implies that there may be direct causal pathways from SES to health. How then, can one explain the link between socio-economic status and health?

Causal explanations

The reasons offered for socioeconomic inequalities in health are diverse and multifaceted. The seminal Black Report, produced by the UK Department of Health's Working Group on Health Inequalities in 1980, suggested three possible explanations for the observed association.

Artefact

First of all, the association may be an artefact of the way that both SES and health are assessed. In fact, despite the suggestion that findings may be affected by the methods used to estimate SES (e.g. Oakes & Rossi, 2003), the consensus is that the consistency of findings across different measures strongly implies that the relationship cannot be artefactual (e.g. Blane, 1997).

Social selection

Secondly, the report proposed that social selection may explain differentials in health by SES. This view implies that health determines SES and not vice versa (see next section). Whether people change their socio-economic position with reference to their parents (intergenerational) or to themselves at an earlier point in life (intragenerational) depends on their health status. While there is evidence for the effect of ill health on downward and good health on upward inter- and intragenerational social mobility, this effect is estimated to be only very moderate in size and therefore not sufficient to explain the SES–health associations (van de Mheen *et al.*, 1999).

Yet it is also possible that a less direct selection pathway could account for socioeconomically determined health differences. One could argue that some individual qualities, such as cognitive ability, coping styles, physical and mental fitness etc. influence success in life and health simultaneously, thereby making social mobility dependent on determinants of health rather than health itself (Goldman, 2001). This approach may indeed have more explanatory scope than the direct selection hypothesis, especially with regards to the possible contribution of genetic factors to the SES–health relationship through personal attributes (Mackenbach, 2005) (see 'Personality and health').

Social causation

It is, however, the third explanation provided by the Black Report, which accounts for most (40–70%, Marmot *et al.*, 1991) of the observed social gradient – the impact of socioeconomically conditioned determinants on health. In particular, material, behavioural,

psychosocial and biological factors have been identified as providing distal and more proximate causal pathways from SES to health (e.g. see Figure 4 for a comprehensive theoretical model of the various determinants of health).

Material factors

The main thrust of health inequalities is likely to derive from material and economic inequalities. People in lower socioeconomic positions have to put up with worse living conditions; they are more often exposed to toxic waste, air and water pollution, crowding, ambient noise and generally poor housing quality, all of which are linked to ill health (Evans & Kantrowitz, 2002). Furthermore, these living environments are more conducive to unhealthy lifestyles, featuring a higher concentration of alcohol outlets and a lack of stores selling healthy foods (e.g. Macintyre, Maciver & Sooman, 1993). People with lower income also experience more risky and physically demanding working environments (Lucas, 1974).

In addition, there is evidence of restricted access to, and less effective utilization of, medical care by patients from lower SES (e.g. Field & Briggs, 2001), in part due to the physical environment (e.g. lack of transportation, Takano & Nakamura, 2001).

The influence of economically determined access to health care alone, however, cannot explain the social gradient (Adler *et al.*, 1993), as material differences do not explain the subtle graduation of health indices detected even at the higher end of SES.

Behavioural factors

Behavioural factors related to medical care provide additional insights into this association. Differential health outcomes across different socioeconomic groups may be a result of both differences in doctor–patient communication (Willems *et al.*, 2005) and varying compliance with medical advice. For instance, unsatisfactory adherence to a prescribed medication regime predicts health deterioration and is more common in less well educated people likely to be lower down the socioeconomic scale (Goldman & Smith, 2002)

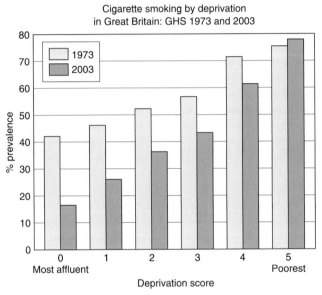

Fig 4 Smoking prevalence in the UK by SES.
Source: Jarvis & Wardle, 2005.

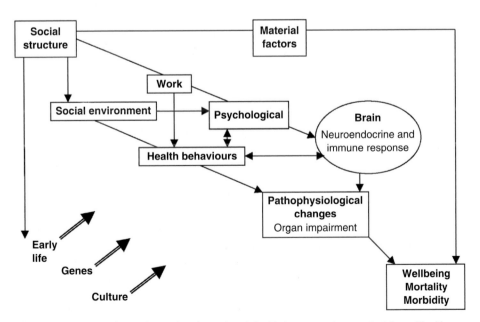

Fig 5 Model of pathways that mediate and moderate the relationship between socioeconomic status and health.
Source: Brunner & Marmot, 1999.

(see 'Adherence to treatment'). However, although possibly explaining some of the SES–health relationship, this is unlikely to be the whole story since the social gradient is evident even before the need to seek medical treatment.

A more obvious explanation relates to behaviours which determine health status directly. For instance, cigarette smoking is strongly linked to socio-economic status and exhibits a gradient very similar to that of health and SES (see Figure 5). What is more, the gap in smoking prevalence between social groups has substantially increased over the last 30 years. Thus health behaviours such as smoking may account not only for health differentials across the whole social spectrum but also explain the observed widening of health differences between socio-economic groups (Jarvis & Wardle, 2005). This proposition is corroborated by evidence of comparable gradient relationships with SES in a variety of other health behaviours. People in lower SES are less likely to be physically active (e.g. Helmert et al., 1989), are more likely to overeat and be obese (e.g. Helmert, Mielck & Classen, 1992), as well as to consume alcohol to excess (e.g. Davey-Smith et al., 1996).

However, even when these various behavioural factors are controlled for in analysis, the social gradient is reduced not eliminated (e.g. Marmot et al., 1984). Perhaps psychosocial factors can further elucidate causal pathways from SES to health.

Individual psychosocial factors

One of the most prevalent psychosocial determinants of health is stress. Empirical studies show that people of lower SES are more consistently exposed to chronic stress (Turner et al., 1995), which in turn is associated with poorer physical and mental health (e.g. Avison & Turner, 1988). Variation in chronic stress may also explain some of the ethnic differences in health that are found along the social gradient. For instance, discrimination as a stressor has been related to hypertension, a precursor of cardiovascular disease (Krieger & Sidney, 1996). There is additional evidence that being higher up in the socio-economic hierarchy reduces the risk of exposure to negative life events (Mcleod & Kessler, 1990), which may induce acute (Theorell, 2005) and chronic illnesses (Cohen & Williamson, 1991).

Social support is a psychosocial factor proposed to moderate the relationship between SES and health. Social support appears to buffer the impact of stress on health, and is associated with socio-economic status both in terms of social network size and participation (Thoits, 1995). Other coping resources important to the social gradient include 'sense of control'. Higher perceived control over life circumstances is more prevalent in people of higher SES and this is related to improved health outcomes (Lachman & Weaver, 1998) (see 'Perceived control'). In accordance with the demand-control model (Karasek, 1979), low perceived job control has been associated with both lower SES and increased cardiovascular disease risk in the UK Whitehall II study and, furthermore predicted sickness absence when it was accompanied by high work demands (North et al., 1993). Psychosocial work characteristics may also partially explain the inverse association of depression, itself a risk factor for coronary heart disease (Booth-Kewley & Friedman, 1987), with SES (Stansfeld, Head & Marmot, 1998).

It appears that those exposed to most hardship are also those who have the least resources (both in economic and psychosocial terms) to cope with it. But it is not only at the individual level of explanation that it is possible to discern reasons for the reported observations on health and SES.

Population psychosocial factors

Research shows that residents of low-income neighbourhoods show lower collective efficacy; that is they perceive less social cohesion and social control, which may not only affect physical wellbeing (e.g. reduction in physical activity outside the home) but also mental health (Cohen et al., 2003). These population effects are not only restricted to low-income neighbourhoods; rather they appear to be related to income inequalities in the social environment. Greater inequality is associated with lower collective efficacy but also greater hostility (a risk factor for coronary heart disease, see Dembroski et al., 1989) (see 'Hostility, Type A behaviour and coronary heart disease') and violence (Wilkinson, 1999). Indeed, neighbourhood effects account for a large proportion of health outcomes (Pickett & Pearl, 2001).

Wilkinson has argued that social ordering may have a direct effect on health through the effects of social anxiety, which arises from fear of rejection and negative evaluations by others. Shame and social anxiety are intimately linked to social comparison, a process at least partly based on socio-economic position (Sennett & Cobb, 1973). Social anxiety is an innate mechanism that fosters social inclusion by diverting conflict in social relationships (Leary & Kowalski, 1995). However, increased social inequalities lead to intolerable and chronic anxiety which may result in frustration and aggression. Thus in societies with narrower income differences and therefore lower social anxiety, the quality of social interaction is postulated to be better and overall health superior.

Of course all the factors cited so far, be they material, behavioural or psychosocial, at the individual or population level, are themselves interrelated. For example, adopting a healthier lifestyle like giving up smoking – usually a difficult process – may be particularly difficult for people whose lives are already more prone to stressful episodes due to work strain and neighbourhood effects, which deplete their coping resources. In addition, people of lower SES, as a result of economic constraints, would find themselves in an environment that promotes smoking both physically (access to more stores selling cigarettes) and socially (greater acceptance of smoking habit, e.g. Curry et al., 1993) (see 'Tobacco use').

Biological factors

All of the above determinants, at least within a biomedical model (for a more sociological explanation see Young, ibid. for instance), are thought to influence health through proximal biological factors. For example, as a result of damage to arterial walls and a decrease in HDL cholesterol, smoking leads to atherosclerosis, which is linked to cardiovascular disease morbidity (e.g. Brischetto et al., 1983).

More generally, Seeman and McEwan (1999) suggest that stress (in the broadest sense of the word), which is caused by various material, behavioural and psychosocial health determinants, elevates the activity of physiological systems and over time leads to 'wear and tear' of these. Life experiences but also genetic predisposition contribute to 'allostatic load', i.e. stress-induced damage. In the short run, the human body is well equipped to deal with stressors through the action of hormonal stress mediators in the hypothalamic–pituitary–adrenal axis and sympathetic adrenal medullary response system. However, constant insults delivered to this system decrease the efficiency with which it is turned on and off (as captured by the concept of 'reactivity') and the resultant bodily changes lead to poor health and illness (see 'Stress and health'). The assessment of allostatic load by secondary outcome measures such as fibrinogen has produced gradients equal to those for disease morbidity and mortality (Markowe et al., 1985) and their inclusion as control variables has even been shown to reduce SES risk differences to non-significance (e.g. Lynch et al., 1996).

Current and future directions

This biological perspective lends support to the emerging field of life course epidemiology (Kuh et al., 2003), which proposes the study of long-term effects across the life span. It is evident that no single pathway is responsible for the observed health differentials and this approach is able to integrate different causal descriptions into a coherent whole, forming a conceptual framework for the multitude of explanatory levels (see Figure 5) that bear upon individual and population health. It allows for a better understanding of the temporal influence on health, such as the impact of childhood SES on adult health. As mentioned earlier, numerous studies have found that both the social and physical environment in childhood partly determines a child's mental and physical ability as well as biological and behavioural patterns later in life (e.g. Rahkonen et al., 1997).

The life course approach can thus account for cumulative risk (as implied by 'allostatic load') but also for the independent and interactive influence on health exerted by biological and social factors (Kuh et al., 2003). Lastly, it allows for an exploration of the reciprocal nature of the relation between environmental and genetic determinants on health (Mackenbach, ibid).

Others, however, argue for a paradigm shift to a sociological (critical realist) perspective as offering a better approach for explaining socioeconomic health differentials (e.g. Scambler & Higgs, 2001).

Either way, with the development of novel frameworks comes the demand for appropriate methodology to do justice to the investigation of issues as complex as those involved in social epidemiology. More sophisticated multilevel analytical approaches rather than simple regression analyses are required in order to disentangle the various dynamic forces that affect health outcomes (Merlo, 2003). This also highlights the need for better measures of social status in order to preclude the possibility of producing spurious relationships in increasingly intricate analyses (Oakes & Rossi, 2003).

Whatever the outcome of future research, health inequalities are not immutable (Whitehead, 1990). Rather they represent a social injustice that is unlikely to be alleviated by anything other than wide-ranging public policies, which promote a more egalitarian society and aim directly at reducing socioeconomic inequalities (Link & Phelan, 1995).

REFERENCES

Adler, N. E., Boyce, T., Chesney, M. A., Cohen, S., Folkman, S., Kahn, R. L. & Syme, S. L. (1994). Socioeconomic status and health. The challenge of the gradient. *American Psychologist*, **49**(1), 15–24.

Adler, N. E., Boyce, W. T., Chesney, M. A., Folkman, S. & Syme, S. L. (1993). Socioeconomic Inequalities in Health – No Easy Solution. *JAMA – Journal of the American Medical Association*, **269**(24), 3140–5.

Adler, N. E. & Ostrove, J. M. (1999). Socioeconomic status and health: what we know and what we don't. *Annals of the New York Academy of Sciences*, **896**, 3–15.

Avison, W. R. & Turner, R. J. (1988). Stressful life events and depressive symptoms – disaggregating the effects of acute stressors and chronic strains. *Journal of Health and Social Behavior*, **29**(3), 253–64.

Bartley, M. & Plewis, I. (1997). Does health-selective mobility account for socioeconomic differences in health? Evidence from England and Wales, 1971 to 1991. *Journal of Health and Social Behavior*, **38**(4), 376–86.

Black, D., Morris, J. N., Smith, C. & Townsend, P. (1980). *Inequalities in health: report of a research working group.* London, UK: Department of Health and Social Security.

Blane, D. (1997). Inequality and social class. In G. Scambler (Ed.). *Sociology as Applied to Medicine*, (4th edn.) (pp. 103–20). London, UK: Bailliere Tindall.

Blane, D. (1999). The life course, the social gradient, and health. In M. Marmot & R. G. Wilkinson (Eds.). *Social Determinants of Health*, (1st edn.) (pp. 64–80). New York: Oxford University Press.

Bloom, S. W. (2002). *The word as scalpel: a history of medical sociology.* New York: Oxford University Press.

Bobak, M. & Marmot, M. (1996). East–West mortality divide and its potential explanations: proposed research agenda. *BMJ – British Medical Journal*, **312**(7028), 421–5.

Booth-Kewley, S. & Friedman, H. S. (1987). Psychological predictors of heart- disease – a quantitative review. *Psychological Bulletin*, **101** (3), 343–62.

Bosma, H., Marmot, M. G., Hemingway, H., Nicholson, A. C., Brunner, E. & Stansfeld, S. A. (1997). Low job control and risk of coronary heart disease in Whitehall II (prospective cohort) study. *BMJ – British Medical Journal*, **314**(7080), 558.

Braveman, P. & Tarimo, E. (2002). Social inequalities in health within countries: not only an issue for affluent nations. *Social Science and Medicine*, **54**(11), 1621–35.

Brischetto, C. S., Connor, W. E., Connor, S. L. & Matarazzo, J. D. (1983). Plasma-lipid and lipoprotein profiles of cigarette smokers from randomly selected families – enhancement of hyperlipidemia and depression of high-density lipoprotein. *American Journal of Cardiology*, **52**(7), 675–80.

Brunner, E. & Marmot, M. (1999). Social organisation, stress, and health. In M. Marmot & R. G. Wilkinson (Eds.). *Social Determinants of Health*, (1st edn.) (pp. 17–43). New York, US: Oxford University Press.

Case, A., Lubotsky, D. & Paxon, C. H. (2002). Economic status and health in childhood: the origins of the gradient. *American Economic Review*, **92**(5), 1308–34.

Chadwick, E. (2000). *Report of the sanitary condition of the labouring population of Great Britain (1842).* London, UK: Routledge/Thoemmes.

Cohen, D. A., Farley, T. A. & Mason, K. (2003). Why is poverty unhealthy? – Social and physical mediators. *Social Science and Medicine*, **57**(9), 1631–41.

Cohen, S. & Williamson, G. M. (1991). Stress and infectious disease in humans. *Psychological Bulletin*, **109**(1), 5–24.

Curry, S. J., Wagner, E. H., Cheadle, A. et al. (1993). Assessment of community-level influences on individuals' attitudes about cigarette-smoking, alcohol-use, and consumption of dietary-fat. *American Journal of Preventive Medicine*, **9**(2), 78–84.

Daniels, N., Kennedy, B. & Kawachi, I. (2000). Justice is good for our health. In J. Cohen & J. Rogers (Eds.). *Is inequality bad for our health?* Boston, MA: Beacon Press.

Davey-Smith, G., Neaton, J. D., Wentworth, D., Stamler, R. & Stamler, J. (1996). Socioeconomic differentials in mortality risk among men screened for the Multiple Risk Factor Intervention Trial: I. White men. *American Journal of Public Health*, **86**(4), 486–96.

Davey-Smith, G., Wentworth, D., Neaton, J. D., Stamler, R. & Stamler, J. (1996). Socioeconomic differentials in mortality risk among men screened for the Multiple Risk Factor Intervention Trial: II. Black men. *American Journal of Public Health*, **86**(4), 497–504.

Dembroski, T. M., Macdougall, J. M., Costa, P. T. & Grandits, G. A. (1989). Components of hostility as predictors of sudden death and myocardial infarction in the Multiple Risk Factor Intervention Trial. *Psychosomatic Medicine*, **51**(5), 514–22.

Department of Health. (2003). *Health survey for England, 2003*. London, UK: The Stationery Office.

Devesa, S. S. & Diamond, E. L. (1980). Association of breast cancer and cervical cancer incidences with income and education among whites and blacks. *Journal of the National Cancer Institute*, **65**(3), 515–28.

Dohrenwend, B. P. & Schwartz, S. (1995). Socioeconomic status and psychiatric disorders. *Current Opinion in Psychiatry*, **8**(2), 138–41.

Evans, G. W. & Kantrowitz, E. (2002). Socioeconomic status and health: the potential role of environmental risk exposure. *Annual Review of Public Health*, **23**, 303–31.

Field, K. S. & Briggs, D. J. (2001). Socio-economic and locational determinants of accessibility and utilization of primary health-care. *Health and Social Care in the Community*, **9**(5), 294–308.

Goldman, D. P. & Smith, J. P. (2002). Can patient self-management help explain the SES health gradient? *Proceedings of the National Academy of Sciences of the United States of America*, **99**(16), 10929–34.

Goldman, N. (2001). Social inequalities in health disentangling the underlying mechanisms. *Annals of the New York Academy of Sciences*, **954**, 118–39.

Guralnik, J. M., Land, K. C., Blazer, D., Fillenbaum, G. G. & Branch, L. G. (1993).

Educational status and active life expectancy among older blacks and whites. *New England Journal of Medicine*, **329**(2), 110–16.

Helmert, U., Herman, B., Joeckel, K. H., Greiser, E. & Madans, J. (1989). Social-class and risk-factors for coronary heart disease in the Federal Republic of Germany – Results of the baseline survey of the German Cardiovascular Prevention Study (GCP). *Journal of Epidemiology and Community Health*, **43**(1), 37–42.

Helmert, U., Mielck, A. & Classen, E. (1992). Social inequities in cardiovascular disease risk factors in East and West Germany. *Social Science and Medicine*, **35**(10), 1283–92.

Hemingway, H., Nicholson, A., Stafford, M., Roberts, R. & Marmot, M. (1997). The impact of socioeconomic status on health functioning as assessed by the SF-36 questionnaire: the Whitehall II Study. *American Journal of Public Health*, **87**(9), 1484–90.

House, J. S. (2002). Understanding social factors and inequalities in health: 20th century progress and 21st century prospects. *Journal of Health and Social Behavior*, **43**(2), 125–42.

House, J. S., Lepkowski, J. M., Kinney, A. M., Mero, R. P., Kessler, R. C. & Herzog, A. R. (1994). The social stratification of aging and health. *Journal of Health and Social Behavior*, **35**(3), 213–34.

Jarvis, M. J. & Wardle, J. (2005). Social patterning of individual health behaviours: the case of cigarette smoking. In M. Marmot & R. G. Wilkinson (Eds.). *Social Determinants of Health*, 2nd edn. New York: Oxford University Press.

Kaplan, G. A. & Keil, J. E. (1993). Socioeconomic factors and cardiovascular disease: a review of the literature. *Circulation*, **88**(4 Pt 1), 1973–98.

Karasek, R. A. (1979). Job demands, job decision latitude, and mental strain – implications for job redesign. *Administrative Science Quarterly*, **24**(2), 285–308.

Krieger, N. & Sidney, S. (1996). Racial discrimination and blood pressure: The CARDIA study of young black and white adults. *American Journal of Public Health*, **86**(10), 1370–8.

Kuh, D., Ben Shlomo, Y., Lynch, J., Hallqvist, J. & Power, C. (2003). Life course epidemiology. *Journal of Epidemiology and Community Health*, **57**(10), 778–83.

Lachman, M. E. & Weaver, S. L. (1998). The sense of control as a moderator of social class differences in health and well-being.

Journal of Personality and Social Psychology, **74**(3), 763–73.

Lantz, P. M., House, J. S., Lepkowski, J. M. *et al.* (1998). Socioeconomic factors, health behaviors, and mortality: results from a nationally representative prospective study of US adults. *JAMA – Journal of the American Medical Association*, **279**(21), 1703–8.

Leary, M. R. & Kowalski, R. M. (1995). *Social anxiety*. New York: Guilford Press.

Liberatos, P., Link, B. G. & Kelsey, J. L. (1988). The measurement of social class in epidemiology. *Epidemiologic Reviews*, **10**, 87–121.

Link, B. G. & Phelan, J. (1995). Social conditions as fundamental causes of disease. *Journal of Health and Social Behavior*, **35**(Special Issue), 80–94.

Lucas, R. E. B. (1974). Distribution of job characteristics. *Review of Economics and Statistics*, **56**(4), 530–40.

Lynch, J. W., Everson, S. A., Kaplan, G. A., Salonen, R. & Salonen, J. T. (1998). Does low socioeconomic status potentiate the effects of heightened cardiovascular responses to stress on the progression of carotid atherosclerosis? *American Journal of Public Health*, **88**(3), 389–94.

Lynch, J. W., Kaplan, G. A., Cohen, R. D., Tuomilehto, J. & Salonen, J. T. (1996). Do cardiovascular risk factors explain the relation between socioeconomic status, risk of all-cause mortality, cardiovascular mortality, and acute myocardial infarction? *American Journal of Epidemiology*, **144**(10), 934–42.

Macintyre, S. (1997). The Black Report and beyond: what are the issues? *Social Science and Medicine*, **44**(6), 723–45.

Macintyre, S., Maciver, S. & Sooman, A. (1993). Area, class and health – should we be focusing on places or people? *Journal of Social Policy*, **22**, 213–34.

Mackenbach, J. P. (2005). Genetics and health inequalities: hypotheses and controversies. *Journal of Epidemiology and Community Health*, **59**(4), 268–73.

Mackenbach, J. P., Kunst, A. E., Cavelaars, A. E. J. M. *et al.* (1997). Socioeconomic inequalities in morbidity and mortality in western Europe. *Lancet*, **349**(9066), 1655–9.

Maher, J. & Macfarlane, A. (2004). Inequalities in infant mortality: trends by social class, registration status, mother's age and birthweight, England and Wales, 1976–2000. *Health Statistics Quarterly*, **Winter (24)**, 14–22.

Mao, Y., Hu, J. F., Ugnat, A. M., Semenciw, R. & Fincham, S. (2001). Socioeconomic status and lung cancer risk

L. Shahab

in Canada. *International Journal of Epidemiology*, **30**(4), 809–17.

Markowe, H. L. J., Marmot, M. G., Shipley, M. J. *et al.* (1985). Fibrinogen – a possible link between social class and coronary heart disease. *BMJ – British Medical Journal*, **291**(6505), 1312–14.

Marmot, M. G., Davey Smith, G. D., Stansfeld, S. *et al.* (1991). Health inequalities among British civil servants – the Whitehall II Study. *Lancet*, **337**(8754), 1387–93.

Marmot, M. G., Shipley, M. J. & Rose, G. (1984). Inequalities in death – specific explanations of a general pattern? *Lancet*, **1**(8384), 1003–6.

Mcewen, B. S. & Seeman, T. (1999). Protective and damaging effects of mediators of stress – elaborating and testing the concepts of allostasis and allostatic load. *Annals of the New York Academy of Sciences*, **896**, 30–47.

Mcleod, J. D. & Kessler, R. C. (1990). Socioeconomic status differences in vulnerability to undesirable life events. *Journal of Health and Social Behavior*, **31**(2), 162–72.

Merlo, J. (2003). Multilevel analytical approaches in social epidemiology: measures of health variation compared with traditional measures of association. *Journal of Epidemiology and Community Health*, **57**(8), 550–2.

North, F., Syme, S. L., Feeney, A., Head, J., Shipley, M. J. & Marmot, M. G. (1993). Explaining socioeconomic differences in sickness absence – the Whitehall II Study. *BMJ – British Medical Journal*, **306**(6874), 361–6.

Oakes, J. M. & Rossi, P. H. (2003). The measurement of SES in health research: current practice and steps toward a new approach. *Social Science and Medicine*, **56**(4), 769–84.

Pamuk, E., Makue, D., Heck, K., Reuben, C. & Lockner, K. (1998). *Socioeconomic status and health chartbook: health, United States, 1998.* Hyattsville, MD, US: National Center for Health Statistics.

Pappas, G., Queen, S., Hadden, W. & Fisher, G. (1993). The increasing disparity in mortality between socioeconomic groups in the United States, 1960 and 1986. *New England Journal of Medicine*, **329**(2), 103–9.

Pickett, K. E. & Pearl, M. (2001). Multilevel analyses of neighbourhood socioeconomic context and health outcomes: a critical review. *Journal of Epidemiology and Community Health*, **55**(2), 111–22.

Rahkonen, O., Lahelma, E. & Huuhka, M. (1997). Past or present? Childhood living conditions and current socioeconomic status as determinants of adult health. *Social Science and Medicine*, **44**(3), 327–36.

Scambler, G. & Higgs, P. (2001). 'The dog that didn't bark': taking class seriously in the health inequalities debate. *Social Science and Medicine*, **52**(1), 157–9.

Sennett, R. & Cobb, J. (1973). *The hidden injuries of class.* New York: Knopf.

Stansfeld, S. A., Head, J. & Marmot, M. G. (1998). Explaining social class differences in depression and well-being. *Social Psychiatry and Psychiatric Epidemiology*, **33**(1), 1–9.

Takano, T. & Nakamura, K. (2001). An analysis of health levels and various indicators of urban environments for Healthy Cities Projects. *Journal of Epidemiology and Community Health*, **55**(4), 263–70.

Theorell, T. (2005). Life events before and after the onset of a premature mycardial infarction. In B. S. Dohrenwend & B. P. Dohrenwend (Eds.). *Stressful life events: their nature and effects*, (pp. 101–17). New York: Wiley.

Thoits, P. A. (1995). Stress, coping, and social support processes – where are we – what next? *Journal of Health and Social Behavior*, **35**(Special Issue), 53–79.

Townsend, P. (1974). Inequality and the health service. *Lancet*, **1**(7868), 1179–90.

Turner, R. J., Wheaton, B. & Lloyd, D. A. (1995). The epidemiology of social stress. *American Sociological Review*, **60**(1), 104–25.

van de Mheen, H., Stronks, K., Schrijvers, C. T. & Mackenbach, J. P. (1999). The influence of adult ill health on occupational class mobility and mobility out of and into employment in The Netherlands. *Social Science and Medicine*, **49**(4), 509–18.

Villermé, R. L. (1840). *Tableau de l'etat physique et moral des ouvriers employés dans les manufactures de coton, de laine et de soie, Vol. 2.* Paris: Renouard.

Virchow, R. (1985). Report on the typhus epidemic in Upper Silesia (1848). In L. J. Rather (Ed.). *Collected essays on public health and epidemiology*, (pp. 205–319). Madison, WI: Watson Publishing International.

Whitehead, M. (1990). *The concepts and principles of equity and health.* Copenhagen: World Health Organization.

Wilkinson, R. G. (1999). Health, hierarchy, and social anxiety. *Annals of the New York Academy of Sciences*, **896**, 48–63.

Willems, S., De Maesschalck, S., Deveugele, M., Derese, A. & De Maeseneer, J. (2005). Socio-economic status of the patient and doctor-patient communication: does it make a difference? *Patient Education and Counseling*, **56**(2), 139–46.

Young, F. W. (2004). Socioeconomic status and health: the problem of explanation and a sociological solution. *Social Theory and Health*, **2**, 123–41.

Stigma

Robert West[1] and Ainsley Hardy[2]

[1]University College London
[2]Loughborough University

Stigma involves a negative evaluation of and associated lowering of respect for individuals because of some personal characteristic, which may be physical or behavioural. For a review see Major & O'Brien (2005). It may arise from violation of moral precepts, fear of contamination, pity, perception of reduced competence, disgust or any of a number of different evaluations. It can be 'enacted' in the sense that non-sufferers treat the stigmatized individual differently or 'felt' in the sense that the individual feels embarrassed or shamed

R. West and A. Hardy

regardless of what others do or feel (see Scambler, 1998). It can vary in intensity and clearly has no fixed boundaries. Thus people can feel and be stigmatized even by virtue of their age.

Stigma as a phenomenon is important in medical practice partly because of medical conditions that arouse it and partly because of other characteristics that influence the way that medical conditions are addressed. Thus, mental illness carries a degree of stigma and that affects the degree to which patients seek help and the kind of help that is provided. However, poverty, age or lack of education can also be stigmatized and that can affect the treatment people receive for conditions such as heart disease.

Stigma can arise from a variety of aspects of medical conditions. Stigma is associated with disfigurement arising from the condition itself (Papathanasiou et al., 2001) or its treatment (Devins et al., 1994), a reduction in perceived competence such as intellectual impairment (Rasaratnam et al., 2004) or even hearing loss (Hetu, 1996), behaviours that appear bizarre such as 'tics' (Davis, Davis et al., 2004), frightening such as epileptic fits (Chaplin et al., 1998) or dangerous such as delusional behaviours (Brady & McCain, 2004), conditions that are considered to have been brought about in part as a result of actions that are considered immoral as in AIDS (Duffy, 2005), conditions that reflect adversely on a person's social position as can occur in the case of tuberculosis and poverty (Jaramillo, 1998), conditions that affect body parts that are considered 'private' or 'dirty' such as urological conditions and faecal incontinence (Go et al., 2002; Norton, 2004) or conditions that reflect adversely on a patient's strength of character such as obesity (Seidell, 1998) and drug dependence (Joseph et al., 2000) or conditions that are judged to be at least partly self-inflicted (Ritson, 1999).

There are clear differences in stigmatization of medical conditions across countries and cultures. For example one study found differences in stigmatization of epilepsy across different European countries (Baker et al., 2000). Another reported that 'supernatural' explanations of epilepsy can protect individuals from stigmatization (Peng, 1983). Male infertility appears to be particularly stigmatized in countries where ability to produce children is highly prized (Inhorn, 2004).

The effects of stigmatization are obvious, both in terms of self-esteem and psychological wellbeing of sufferers of stigmatized conditions and in terms of how they are treated by the clinical community and society at large (e.g. Fabrega, 1991; MacLeod & Austin, 2003; Puhl & Brownell, 2003). These effects have been well documented in terms of delay in treatment-seeking, resources devoted to care, the individual clinician's approach to care and the systems in place for managing the care process. What is less obvious is the effect on the diagnosis or cause of death that is recorded (King, 1989). Neither is it so well appreciated that stigma can attach to the relatives of afflicted individuals. For example, the stigma attached to suicide in Taiwan has been found to have important effects on the surviving relatives (Tzeng & Lipson, 2004). Stigma can also lead to reluctance to disclose diagnoses to patients. It has been reported that clinicians are often reluctant to disclose a diagnosis of 'borderline personality disorder' to patients for fear of the affect this may have on the patient (Lequesne & Hersh, 2004).

In terms of reducing the adverse effects of stigmatization of medical conditions, clearly legislation has some role to play in reducing overt discrimination but this need not influence attitudes. It is important for all clinicians to be aware of the potential felt or enacted stigma associated with a wide range of conditions, to recognize their own feelings about particular conditions and in multicultural societies to be acutely aware of cultural differences that may influence presentation of and response to different conditions. Disclosure can be enhanced by use of written forms or even computer-administered interviews, possibly because of the greater sense of anonymity (Newman et al., 2002). It is generally believed that stigma can, in many cases be combated at both an individual and population level by improved education and it appears that increased media exposure to stigmatized conditions such as disfigurement or epilepsy can lessen the adverse emotional reactions through a process of 'normalization' (e.g. Joachim & Acorn, 2000). Counselling is one obvious approach to helping patients to overcome felt or enacted stigma (e.g. Galletti & Sturniolo, 2004) but there has been little research into its effectiveness. An innovative approach is the use of websites to change the way that people view conditions such as depression (Griffiths et al., 2004).

One aspect of stigma that is not widely considered is the intentional or unintentional effects that public health campaigns can have (Guttman & Salmon, 2004). At least part of the reduction in smoking prevalence in some countries can be attributed to a decrease in its social acceptability. It may be argued that this kind of social pressure can be extended in the cause of public health though the cost would obviously be high for individuals who cannot or do not want to conform to the new social values.

REFERENCES

Baker, G. A., Brooks, J. et al. (2000). The stigma of epilepsy: a European perspective. *Epilepsia*, **41**(1), 98–104.

Brady, N. & McCain, G. C. (2004). Living with schizophrenia: a family perspective. *Online Journal of Issues in Nursing*, **10**(1), 7.

Chaplin, J. E., Wester, A., Tomson, T. et al. (1998). Factors associated with the employment problems of people with established epilepsy. *Seizure*, **7**(4), 299–303.

Davis, K. K., Davis, J. S. et al. (2004). In motion, out of place: the public space(s) of Tourette Syndrome. *Social Science and Medicine*, **59**(1), 103–12.

Devins, G. M., Stam, H. J. et al. (1994). Psychosocial impact of laryngectomy mediated by perceived stigma and illness intrusiveness. *Canadian Journal of Psychiatry*, **39**(10), 608–16.

Duffy, L. (2005). Suffering, shame, and silence: the stigma of HIV/AIDS. *The Journal of the Association of Nurses in AIDS Care: JANAC*, **16**(1), 13–20.

Fabrega, H., Jr. (1991). The culture and history of psychiatric stigma in early modern and modern Western societies: a review of recent literature. *Comprehensive Psychiatry*, **32**(2), 97–119.

Galletti, F. & Sturniolo, M. G. (2004). Counseling children and parents about epilepsy. *Patient Education and Counseling*, **55**(3), 422–5.

Go, V. F., Quan, V. M., Zehilman, J. M., Moulton, L. H. & Celentano, D. D. (2002). Barriers to reproductive tract infection (RTI) care among Vietnamese women: implications for RTI control programs. *Sexually Transmitted Diseases*, **29**(4), 201–6.

Griffiths, K. M., Christensen, H. et al. (2004). Effect of web-based depression literacy and cognitive-behavioural therapy interventions on stigmatising attitudes to depression: randomised controlled trial. *British Journal of Psychiatry: The Journal of Mental Science*, **185**, 342–9.

Guttman, N. & Salmon, C. T. (2004). Guilt, fear, stigma and knowledge gaps: ethical issues in public health communication interventions. *Bioethics*, **18**(6), 531–52.

Hetu, R. (1996). The stigma attached to hearing impairment. *Scandinavian Audiology Supplementum*, **43**, 12–24.

Inhorn, M. C. (2004). Middle Eastern masculinities in the age of new reproductive technologies: male infertility and stigma in Egypt and Lebanon. *Medical Anthropology Quarterly*, **18**(2), 162–82.

Jaramillo, E. (1998). Pulmonary tuberculosis and health-seeking behaviour: how to get a delayed diagnosis in Cali, Colombia. *Tropical Medicine and International Health: TM & IH*, **3**(2), 138–44.

Joachim, G. & Acorn, S. (2000). Living with chronic illness: the interface of stigma and normalization. *Canadian Journal of Nursing Research*, **32**(3), 37–48.

Joseph, H., Stancliff, S. & Langrod, J. (2000). ''Methadone maintenance treatment (MMT): a review of historical and clinical issues.'' *The Mount Sinai Journal of Medicine*, **67**(5–6), 347–64.

King, M. B. (1989). AIDS on the death certificate: the final stigma. *British Medical Journal*, **298**(6675), 734–6.

Lequesne, E. R. & Hersh, R. G. (2004). Disclosure of a diagnosis of borderline personality disorder. *Journal of Psychiatric Practice*, **10**(3), 170–6.

MacLeod, J. S. & Austin, J. K. (2003). Stigma in the lives of adolescents with epilepsy: a review of the literature. *Epilepsy and Behavior*, **4**(2), 112–7.

Major, B. & O'Brien, L. T. (2005). The social psychology of stigma. *Annual Review of Psychology*, **56**, 393–421.

Newman, J. C., Des Jarlais, D. C., Turner, C. F., Gribble, J., Cooley, P. & Paone, D. (2002). The differential effects of face-to-face and computer interview modes. *American Journal of Public Health*, **92**(2), 294–7.

Norton, C. (2004). Nurses, bowel continence, stigma, and taboos. *Journal of Wound, Ostomy, and Continence Nursing*, **31**(2), 85–94.

Papathanasiou, I., MacDonald, L., Whurr, R. & Jahanshahi, M. (2001). Perceived stigma in spasmodic torticollis. *Movement Disorders*, **16**(2), 280–5.

Peng, K. L. (1983). A Malay cultural explanation for epilepsy. *The Australian and New Zealand Journal of Psychiatry*, **17**(4), 397–9.

Puhl, R. & Brownell, K. D. (2003). Ways of coping with obesity stigma: review and conceptual analysis. *Eating Behaviors*, **4**(1), 53–78.

Rasaratnam, R., Crouch, K. Regan, A. (2004). Attitude to medication of parents/primary carers of people with intellectual disability. *Journal of Intellectual Disability Research*, **48**(Pt 8), 754–63.

Ritson, E. B. (1999). Alcohol, drugs and stigma. *International Journal of Clinical Practice*, **53**(7), 549–51.

Scambler, G. (1998). Stigma and disease: changing paradigms. *Lancet*, **352**(9133), 1054–5.

Seidell, J. C. (1998). ''Societal and personal costs of obesity.'' *Experimental and Clinical Endocrinology of Diabetes*, **106** (Suppl. 2), 7–9.

Tzeng, W. C. & Lipson, J. G. (2004). The cultural context of suicide stigma in Taiwan. *Qualitative Health Research*, **14**(3), 345–58.

Stress and health

Susan Ayers[1] and Andrew Steptoe[2]

[1]University of Sussex
[2]University College London

The concept of stress is used in a variety of disciplines such as physiology, engineering and sociology. The concept originated in physics where stress is defined as external force applied to a system, and strain is the change in the system that is due to the applied force. In psychology and behavioural medicine the study of stress has moved beyond simple definitions towards identifying the processes of stress and mediating factors. Thus in psychology and medicine the term 'stress' covers a wide range of research that concentrates on different aspects of the stress process. For example, much medical stress research does not consider psychological factors and concentrates on physical stress responses, such as the impact of physical exercise on blood volume depletion. There are therefore conflicting views on how useful the concept of stress is. On the one hand some believe the concept is so widely misused and poorly defined that it is no longer useful and should be abandoned (e.g. Kasl, 1983). On the other hand, stress can be seen as an important construct that has the potential to unify different disciplines and help us understand the relationship between mind and body.

Stress is therefore a complex and multifaceted construct with many component parts. At a basic level, it is useful to distinguish between stressors, which are internal or external factors that cause 'stress responses', which can be physical, behavioural, cognitive or affective; and chronic strain, which is the negative impact of the stress process on the person. Current psychological models of stress emphasize the role of appraisal as central in determining a stress response.

When considering the link between stress and health it is important to acknowledge the breadth of the concept of health also. Physical health outcomes vary widely and psychosocial stress is likely to play a different role in different health outcomes – both in terms of varying clinical impact and the processes or mechanisms

S. Ayers and A. Steptoe

underlying this. Add to this the role of stress in psychological health and it is apparent that we need to acknowledge many different possible pathways between stress and health, such as physiological, psychological and behavioural. For example, the mechanisms by which stress may exacerbate an asthma attack are likely to be very different to the mechanisms by which stress may affect symptoms of depression or disability.

In this chapter we will look briefly at some of the conceptual issues and problems that arise in stress research, then examine current transactional theories of stress, before considering the link between stress and health and the possible pathways between stress and health. This chapter is an abbreviated version of a more detailed chapter we have written elsewhere (see Steptoe & Ayers, 2004).

Conceptual problems

As the concept of stress is amorphous and widely used in different disciplines, it is a challenge to try to unify conceptual understanding and research findings from different areas. In order to do this we need to rely on more complex models of stress and its components. However, this often results in somewhat artificial distinctions. For example, psychosocial stressors are numerous and can be classified in a number of different ways. It is possible, for instance, to distinguish between external objective events such as natural disasters, and internal subjective experiences like role conflict or not achieving one's goals. Then there are inter-personal stressors such as conflict at work, and macrosocial stressors like high unemployment, socioeconomic inequality and war. Stressors vary on many dimensions, including duration and severity and these dimensions have also been used to define various categorical systems.

A common distinction is made between acute life events such as the death of a relative or job loss, chronic stressors such as family conflict or looking after a disabled relative and less severe daily hassles such as problems travelling to work. Further stressor categories such as role strain and traumatic stress are also sometimes used. One of the advantages of identifying acute life events is that they can be pinpointed in time and are relatively easy to define. This makes it possible to analyse the temporal sequence between life experiences and illness onset and life event methods have proved especially useful in psychiatric research. As far as physical illness is concerned, chronic stressors are frequently more important, since they elicit long-term disturbances in behavioural and biological processes which contribute to the development of disease.

These categorizations have a number of conceptual and measurement problems. First, the distinction between different categories of stressor is not always clear. For example, an apparently acute event, such as divorce, is usually preceded by the chronic stress of a difficult relationship and can lead to further chronic stressors, such as financial difficulties. Secondly, there are conceptual limitations to many of the categories. For example, whether a stressor is perceived as traumatic varies between individuals, therefore classifying an event as a 'traumatic stressor' confuses subjective response with the event. Related to this is a third problem, which is that it is difficult to measure stressors without some reference to stress responses (see 'Stress assessment'). Measures of daily hassles include items such as 'trouble relaxing' and 'not enough personal energy', which are arguably symptoms of strain rather than stressors. Finally, there are instances where non-events, such as a lack of stimulation, are stressful.

Theories of stress

Psychological theories of stress have arisen from two different sources – those that try to account for normal stress processes and those that look specifically at psychological stress disorders, such as post-traumatic stress disorder. These theories of normal and abnormal stress processes have developed largely independently of each other. In this chapter we concentrate on theories of normal stress responses.

The study of normal stress processes initially led to theories that concentrated on aspects of the stress process, such as the stressor (e.g. life events approach) or the physical stress response (e.g. Selye, 1956) (see 'Life events and health' and 'Psychosomatics'). Current interactional or transactional theories of stress emphasize individual differences in perceived stress and the importance of psychological processes – particularly cognitive appraisal. The interactional approach to stress proposes that the interplay between environmental stimuli and the person is critical in determining stress responses. An example of an interactional approach is the person–environment fit model in occupational psychology, in which stress arises when people are exposed to environments with which they are unfamiliar, or which do not suit their skills and capacity (French et al., 1982).

The transactional approach goes beyond the interactional approach by positing that the various factors involved in stress influence each other and act as both independent and dependent variables. The dominant transactional model was developed by Richard Lazarus and his colleagues, who defined stress as 'a particular relationship between the person and the environment that is appraised by the person as taxing or exceeding his or her resources' (Lazarus & Folkman, 1984, p. 19). Cognitive appraisal is central to this model. Lazarus suggests that when an event occurs individuals go through three stages of appraisal. The first stage is primary appraisal, where the demands of the event on the individual are evaluated. The second stage is secondary appraisal, where people evaluate the resources they have available to cope with the demands. Available resources can be environmental (such as economic factors, social factors, the presence of others) or personal (such as previous experience with this type of event, self-efficacy, self-esteem, repertoire of coping strategies). It should be apparent that these resources also influence primary appraisal. For example, an academic examination will be appraised as less demanding by a student with a thorough knowledge of the subject and plenty of time to revise (good resources to cope). On the other hand, the examination will be appraised as more demanding by a student with little knowledge of the subject and little time to revise (poor resources to cope). Thus primary and secondary appraisal do not necessarily occur in a linear and sequential fashion, but influence each other and may occur in parallel. Recent research suggests that this may vary according to level of demands, and that perceived personal resources are more likely to influence appraisals of stress under low levels of demand (Guillet et al., 2002).

As a result of this process, an event can be evaluated as irrelevant, i.e. not relevant to the individual's wellbeing; benign-positive, i.e. positive and/or non-threatening; or stressful. According to this model, stressful appraisals can be further broken down into those that involve harm or loss, challenge or threat, although these categories are not mutually exclusive. For example, physical assault can involve appraisals of both immediate harm and future threat of recurrence. These ideas have been incorporated into theories of abnormal stress responses, such as anxiety disorders, where appraisal of continued threat is thought to be important in the development of the disorder (e.g. Ehlers & Clark, 2000). According to the transactional approach, when demands are appraised as exceeding resources coping strategies are applied in an effort to change the situation, or the response to that situation. The process is iterative, with the situation being reappraised after coping attempts have been made, often leading to further coping efforts.

This model has stimulated a substantial amount of research, much of which supports the role of appraisal in modulating subjective and physiological stress responses. For instance, Lazarus and others have carried out a series of experiments in which people are shown gruesome films, having been randomized to different types of appraisal or cognitive orientation, such as reminding them that the film is acted (denial of reality), that film is real but shown for educational purposes (intellectualization). People assigned to denial or intellectualization appraisals have smaller physiological and subjective responses to the film compared with controls (e.g. Steptoe & Vögele, 1986). Non-experimental research also supports a role for appraisal in adaptation to stressors. Pakenham & Rinaldis (2001) found that strong appraisals of challenge, controllability and weak appraisals of threat were predictive of better psychological adjustment to HIV/AIDS, as measured by depression, global distress, social adjustment and subjective health status.

However, the model has been criticized on a number of points, many of which question the central role allocated to cognitive appraisal processes (Zajonc, 1984). The difficulty of measuring appraisal as part of a dynamic process means it is hard to distinguish appraisal from cognitive processes that are part of the stress response itself. There are undoubtedly situations where conscious appraisal does not take place and people react quickly to hazards, such as when avoiding accidents. The model has also been criticized for being limited to the psychological level of analysis, without consideration of physical, social and cultural influences. It has little to say about the nature of stress responses themselves and how they interact. Nevertheless, transactional models have greatly increased understanding of individual differences in the stress process, and the role of cognitive factors in integrating experience of the environment with the social and psychological responses which the person brings to bear on the situation.

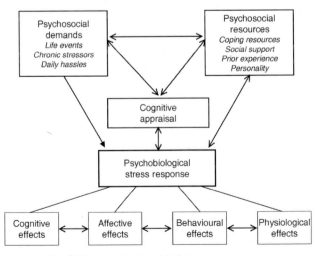

Fig 1 An outline of the transactional model of stress.

Figure 1 is a simple schematic of a transactional framework that attempts to bring together the factors that are relevant to the stress process. This framework begins with the assumption that stress responses are stimulated by potential or actual threats or challenges to the integrity or survival of the person (Weiner, 1992). Psychosocial stressors may be anticipated, may be real or imaginary and may involve understimulation as well as overstimulation. The appraisal of these aversive experiences depends in part on the psychosocial resources that the individual brings to bear on the situation. These resources include coping responses, prior experience of similar situations in the past and social supports. Appraisal is also influenced by personality and temperament. The multidimensional stress response arises when adaptive capacity is exceeded. The pattern of stress response varies over time, depending on whether exposure to the threat is acute or chronic, and whether there is habituation or sensitization to the situation. There is also a close interplay between the components of the stress response and the coping process. For example, an increase in cigarette smoking has been frequently observed as part of the stress response (Jarvis, 2002). At the same time, a large proportion of smokers state that smoking helps relieve tension, so smoking is partly a coping response. Smoking may alter the cognitive response to stress by increasing alertness and aiding mental concentration, so it can be viewed as partly adaptive. However, smoking also augments physiological stress responses and health risks, so it has maladaptive consequences as well.

It is evident from this framework that stress is a process and not a state and that it involves a fully interactive rather than a linear system. A major challenge in health research is teasing out the interplay between these elements.

Links between stress and health

The influence of stress processes on health and risk of disease is studied from a variety of perspectives using animal models, epidemiological survey techniques, clinical investigations and laboratory experiments. There are two broad approaches to studying these effects in humans. The first is to assess the impact of particular categories of potentially stressful conditions and the second is to investigate the aetiology of specific diseases. Many studies have shown that stress and morbidity are associated, but this does not necessarily mean that stress plays a causal role. There are a number of difficulties in establishing a definitive link. Firstly, the diseases in which stress is implicated are typically multifactorial, with a range of genetic, biological and environmental determinants. It is not a case of a disease being due either to stress or to other factors, but of stress processes contributing to aetiology to a variable extent in different people and different conditions. This can make it difficult to identify an independent role of stress. Much clinical research on stress and health is cross-sectional, so inferences about causality cannot be drawn. Indeed, no single type of scientific investigation is sufficient. Rather, it is necessary to integrate evidence from several sources – animal experiments, prospective epidemiological surveys, clinical investigations and laboratory experiments.

Secondly, there are a number of moderators of the stress response that need to be taken into account. Stressor characteristics, such as duration and severity are important determinants of the psychobiological response. In addition to this, characteristics such as controllability, predictability and novelty have been shown elicit greater emotional, behavioural and physiological responses. For example, a wide range of animal and human studies has shown that uncontrollable stressors elicit greater corticosteroid and catecholamine responses, increase tendencies to gastric lesions and reduce immune defences (Steptoe & Appels, 1989). Coping responses and social support are also important moderators of the stress response (see 'Psychoneuroimmunology' and 'Social support and health'), as are individual differences. For example, Taylor *et al.* (2000) put forward an argument, largely based on animal models, that females have different physiological and behavioural responses to stress. They posit that the well documented fight–flight response is more likely in males whereas females are more likely to show a tend–befriend response.

Thirdly, the impact of stress processes on health is not all mediated through direct biological responses. As noted earlier, behavioural responses also contribute. An elegant example of behavioural mediation comes from studies of the development of high blood pressure in air traffic controllers. Air traffic control is a stressful occupation, with persistent high demands and need for rapid decision-making, which carries great responsibility. It was established 30 years ago that air traffic controllers have increased risk of hypertension compared with workers in similar environments doing other jobs (Cobb & Rose, 1973). It was supposed that this was due to persistent activation of the sympathetic nervous system. But DeFrank *et al.* (1987) showed that the occurrence of high blood pressure was preceded by marked increases in alcohol consumption, and that this mediated the link between work stress and morbidity. Research has since established that stress is associated with a range of risky health behaviours, such as poor diet, less exercise and increased smoking (e.g. Ng & Jeffery, 2003), which suggests that behavioural responses to stress are likely to contribute to the relationship between stress and health.

A fourth problem in establishing causal links between stress and disease is the wide variation in individual responsivity. How is it that two people have similar life experiences, yet one becomes ill while the other remains healthy? Why do some people contract infectious illness while others experience increased risk of coronary heart diseases when faced with chronic stressors? Some of this variation is due to the interplay of demands and resources outlined in Figure 1. But in addition, it is necessary to consider individual vulnerability factors. This has lead to the diathesis–stress model, a version of which is summarized in Figure 2. The outcome of the stress process

depends on constitutional and biological risk factors that determine whether the individual remains healthy or develops coronary heart disease, musculoskeletal pain, shows exacerbation of autoimmune diseases or other adverse effects. For example, a recent longitudinal study found that the association between stressors and depression is moderated by a polymorphism in the serotonin transporter gene (Caspi *et al.*, 2003).

The diathesis–stress model enables us to account for individual vulnerability and therefore differences in health outcome. In addition, it is important to recognize that stress can act in a number of different ways to influence the onset or progression of disease. For example, Steptoe (1998) outlines four ways in which psychosocial stress may act on disease. In the first instance, stress may be causal in disease, such as chronic stress resulting in damage to arterial walls and hence aiding the development of atherosclerosis. Secondly, stress may trigger an episode of disease, such as a sudden stressor triggering a heart attack, although this is unlikely unless there is some underlying pathology in the first instance. Thirdly, stress may disrupt or exacerbate existing pathology or symptoms, hence affecting the course or prognosis of the disease. Fourthly, stress may inhibit physical defence systems. For example, chronic stress may deplete the immune system, which increases vulnerability to infection.

Conclusion

Psychosocial stress and its link with health is a complex and multifactorial process. Transactional models of stress account for individual differences in perceived stress and in stress responses. The diathesis–stress model explains how individual vulnerability interacts with stress to result in a range of different health outcomes. The complexity of psychosocial stressors and individual variability in both stress responses and health outcomes makes it difficult to establish a definitive link between stress and health. The processes through which stress may affect health can be psychobiological or behavioural, and stress may act in various ways to influence the onset and progression of illness. However, there is a wealth of evidence demonstrating an association between stress and health and research in the areas of psychophysiology and psychoneuroimmunology is critical in understanding the physiological processes which may mediate between perceived stress and physical health (see 'Psychoneuroimmunology').

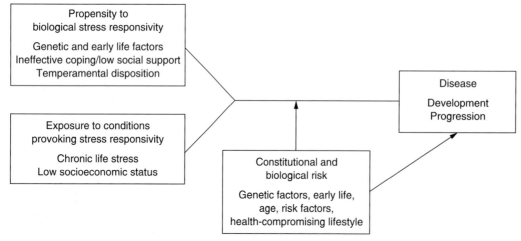

Fig 2 Diatheisis-stress model: pathways linking stress with disease.

Acknowledgement

This chapter is based on material from: Steptoe, A. & Ayers, S. Stress and health. Chapter 7, in: In S. Sutton, A. Baum & M. Johnston (Eds.) *The Sage Handbook of Health Psychology*. London: Sage Publications Inc. The material is reproduced with the kind permission of Sage Publications Inc.

REFERENCES

Caspi, A., Sugden, D., Moffitt, T. E. *et al.* (2003). Influence of life stress on depression: moderation by a polymorphism in the 5-HTT gene. *Science,* **301**(5631), 386–9.

Cobb, S. & Rose, R. M. (1973). Hypertension, peptic ulcer and diabetes in air traffic controllers. *Journal of the American Medical Association,* **224**, 489–92.

DeFrank, R. S., Jenkins, C. D. & Rose, R. M. (1987). A longitudinal investigation of the relationships among alcohol consumption, psychosocial factors, and blood pressure. *Psychosomatic Medicine,* **49**, 236–49.

Ehlers, A. & Clark, D. (2000). A cognitive model of posttraumatic stress disorder. *Behaviour Research and Therapy,* **38**, 319–45.

French, J. R. P., Caplan, R. D. & Van Harrison, R. (1982). *The mechanisms of job stress and strain.* Chichester: John Wiley and Sons.

Guillet, L., Hermand, D. & Mullet, E. (2002). Cognitive processes involved in the appraisal of stress. *Stress and Health,* **18**, 91–102.

Jarvis, M. (2002). Smoking and stress. In S. A. Stansfeld & M. G. Marmot (Eds.). *Stress and the heart* (pp. 150–7). London: BMJ Books.

Kasl, S. (1983) Pursuing the link between stressful life experiences and disease: a time for reappraisal. In C. I. Cooper (Ed.). *Stress research.* New York: Mentor Books.

Lazarus, R. S. & Folkman, S. (1984) *Stress, appraisal and coping.* New York: Springer Publishing Company.

Ng, D. M. & Jeffery, R. W. (2003). Relationships between perceived stress and health behaviours in a sample of working adults. *Health Psychology,* **22**(6), 638–42.

Pakenham, K. I. & Rinaldis, M. (2001). The role of illness, resources, appraisal, and coping strategies in adjustment to HIV/AIDS: the direct and buffering effects. *Journal of Behavioral Medicine,* **24**, 259–79.

Selye, H. (1956) *The stress of life.* New York: McGraw-Hill.

Steptoe, A. (1998). Psychophysiological bases of disease. In M. Johnston & D. Johnston (Eds.). *Comprehensive clinical psychology, Vol. 8*: Health psychology. New York: Elsevier Science.

Steptoe, A. & Appels, A. (Eds.). (1989). *Stress, personal control and health.* Chichester: John Wiley.

Steptoe, A. & Ayers, S. (2004). Stress and health. In S. Sutton, A. Baum & M. Johnston (Eds.). *The Sage handbook of health psychology.* London: Sage Publications Inc.

Steptoe, A. & Vögele, C. (1986). Are stress responses influenced by cognitive appraisal? An experimental comparison of coping strategies. *British Journal of Psychology,* **77**, 243–55.

Taylor, S. E., Klein, L. C., Lewis, B. P. *et al.* (2000). Biobehavioral responses to stress in females: tend-and-befriend, not fight-or-flight. *Psychological Review,* **107**, 411–29.

Weiner, H. (1992). *Perturbing the organism: the biology of stressful experience.* Chicago: University of Chicago Press.

Zajonc, R. B. (1984). On the primacy of affect. *American Psychologist,* **39**, 117–23.

Symptom perception

Elizabeth Broadbent and Keith J. Petrie

The University of Auckland

Introduction

Experiencing physical symptoms is very common. General population surveys show most people experience some form of symptom like headaches, aching joints and muscles or upper respiratory complaints two to three times a week (Dunnell & Cartwright, 1972; Hannay, 1978; Kroenke & Spitzer, 1998). Studies also show that rates of symptom reporting differ across various demographic groups. For instance, females generally report more symptoms than males, unemployed people more than employed, people living alone more than people living with a few others (Pennebaker & Epstein,

1983). These findings suggest that there is more to the reporting of symptoms than just underlying changes in physiology.

Understanding the factors that influence the perception of symptoms is important because symptom reporting forms such a central part of most medical encounters and diagnosis. The (mis)perception of symptoms typically forms the basis of delay in seeking treatment, the overuse of medical services and the inappropriate use of medication. Symptom perception is also important in determining responses in chronic illnesses. People with diabetes or asthma, for example, must regularly manage their illness by monitoring their symptoms and responding with self-medication and

E. Broadbent and K.J. Petrie

behavioural responses. This chapter explores the psychological processes involved in the perception and reporting of physical symptoms.

How accurately do people perceive symptoms?

People are generally accurate when perceiving extreme symptoms or bodily states that need attention immediately. For example, individuals can almost always tell when they need sleep, need to eat or to urinate. More ambiguous symptoms such as heart rate or blood pressure have not evolved in such a way that they dictate behaviours. Peoples' reports of such symptoms have generally been shown to be poorly related to objective markers of their physiology in laboratory studies (Pennebaker, 1984). For example, although some individuals are more accurate than others, on average participants are unable to accurately report their heart rate during several differing tasks (Pennebaker, 1984). There is some evidence that accuracy improves in naturalistic settings, with one study showing that diabetics are better at estimating their blood glucose levels at home than when blood glucose is artificially manipulated in a hospital setting (Cox *et al.*, 1985). Asthmatics rely on symptom perceptions to self-medicate, yet 60% of asthma patients have been shown to be unreliable in detecting changes in their lung function under normal daily conditions (Kendrick *et al.*, 1993). Other studies show that while 90% of hypertensive patients believe they are able to tell when their blood pressure is up by monitoring their symptoms, such as heart beat and face-warming (Meyer *et al.*, 1985), the bulk of evidence suggests the contrary (Baumann & Leventhal, 1985; Brondolo *et al.*, 1999; Meyer *et al.*, 1985). Part of the reason why symptom reports are poorly related to objective measures of physiology may simply be that we are more hard-wired to notice large or abnormal changes in physiological functioning rather than more subtle or graduated changes. Other reasons for the disparity involve the psychological process concerned with noticing and interpreting symptoms.

Noticing symptoms

The extent to which we notice symptoms depends on how much attention we pay to our bodily states. Studies have demonstrated that people report more symptoms in boring rather than in interesting environments. This finding can be explained by the competition of cues theory which proposes individuals have a limited capacity to process stimuli and internal (bodily) and external (environmental) cues compete for attention (Pennebaker, 2000). When we are engaged in a cognitively engaging and demanding activity, such as playing sport, our attention is focused on external cues and we are less likely to attend to our bodies. When we are in less interesting situations, such as sitting in a boring lecture or movie, we become more aware of our bodies and notice more symptoms. In fact, higher teaching evaluations of lecturers has been related to lower frequency of students coughing during class (Pennebaker, 1980). Thus the extent to which we notice symptoms depends on how stimulating we find the environment. Two interesting experiments have shown that the provision of external cues can improve jogging speed and reduce symptom reports (Pennebaker & Lightner, 1980). Participants were found to run faster on a cross-country

course than on an oval running track, and joggers on a treadmill who listened to distracting sounds reported less fatigue and fewer symptoms than joggers who listened to an amplification of their own breathing. As this study shows, the more we focus internally, the more we notice symptoms. This characteristic has been exploited by most parents to distract young children when they fall over and injure themselves. Ironically in clinical conditions, the social isolation and disability that often accompanies chronic illnesses and pain conditions intensify the noticing of patients' symptoms and pain (see 'Coping with chronic illness' and 'Pain management').

In most situations individuals use a combination of both external and internal information to determine their current bodily state. However, it seems that high symptom reporters have a strong tendency to make use of external cues to determine internal body states. In a study where high and low symptom reporters were shown neutral and gruesome slides and asked to estimate their heart rate, high symptom reporters reported their heart beat increased markedly in response to the more grisly slides although their actual heartbeat showed little change (Pennebaker, 1981).

Studies also suggest that men and women may differ in the prominence they give to internal and external cues. Research shows men tend to rely more on internal physiological cues as sources of information, whereas women rely more on external contextual cues (Roberts & Pennebaker, 1995). In laboratory conditions, where external cues are not available, women tend to be less accurate than men, and correlations between symptoms and blood pressure readings are higher for men than for women (Pennebaker *et al.*, 1982). In the real world, accuracy does not tend to differ between men and women because internal and external cues are both available.

Individuals potentially have a large amount of somatic information available but we screen out all but the information that is most salient, relevant and potentially threatening. Our cognitive schema, can guide which information we attend to and cause us to interpret the information in a way that is consistent with the activated schema. Changing the cognitive schema can manipulate the type of somatic information attended to, causing individuals to selectively look for and encode information consistent with that particular schema. For example, when individuals have been labelled with a fictitious illness they are more likely to report symptoms consistent with their knowledge of that illness than individuals who are told they do not have the 'illness' (Croyle & Sande, 1988).

The process of attending to schema consistent information can happen very quickly. For example, the effect of someone vigorously scratching their back and arms when seated next to you, means you are much more aware of itchy areas on your skin and likely to also start scratching. Similarly, one person yawning at a dinner table can cause others to yawn almost instantaneously.

More dramatic examples of the effect of schemas on symptom perception are medical students' disease and mass psychogenic illness. As many as a third of medical students report an incident where they fear they may have the disease they have been recently studying. Mass psychogenic illness incidents represent the same process on a far grander scale. Typically, a dramatic or highly visible illness in one individual sets off a rapid escalation of similar cases. Usually the incident occurs in the context of a closed social setting such as a school or factory and sometimes following a triggering event such as an unusual smell. The most common symptoms in such incidents are nausea, headache, tight chest, dizziness and fainting. Colourful examples of mass psychogenic illness appear throughout history (Bartholomew, 1994).

Expectations about experiencing symptoms are also an important determinant of symptom reporting, particularly after the administration of drugs. Placebo controlled trials have shown individuals tend to amplify symptoms they expect and minimize symptoms they do not anticipate (see 'Placebos'). A study of patients suffering from food allergies found a quarter of patients developed allergic symptoms following injection with saline when it was described as an allergen (Jewett et al., 1990). Similarly, in a study of aspirin for treatment of unstable angina, the participant information form at two study centres listed gastrointestinal irritation as a possible side effect, but the third centre did not. Six times as many patients withdrew from the study because of gastrointestinal distress in the centres mentioning this symptom than the centre that did not (Myers et al., 1987). Expectations of symptoms in response to medication seem to operate by priming individuals to notice any unusual symptoms and to interpret these sensations in the context of a reaction to treatment (see 'Expectations and health').

Interpreting symptoms

There is some evidence that people may hold symptom attribution styles, or a tendency to attribute symptoms along one of three dimensions: somatic (e.g. something wrong with the body), psychological (e.g. due to being upset) or normalizing (e.g. room too hot) (Robbins & Kirmayer, 1991). These styles are related to past experiences of illness and predict clinical symptom presentation, with somatic attributers more likely to present with somatic symptoms and psychological attributers more likely to present with psychosocial symptoms than the other groups. Past experience of illness may provide a schema for the interpretation and attribution of new symptoms.

Causal attributions for symptoms can have far-reaching consequences on health behaviours, including adherence, restriction of activities and presentation to the doctor. A recent study found that HIV patients who attributed their symptoms to medication side effects were more likely to be non-adherent to their medication regime than those who believed the symptoms were due to other factors such as disease progression (Siegel et al., 1999). Those who did not experience a reduction in symptoms after starting their medication and believed that this indicated their medication was not working were also more likely to be non-adherent. In a community sample of people with fatigue, those who attributed their fatigue to myalgic encephalomyelitis were found to be more handicapped and to restrict their activities more at follow-up than those who attributed their fatigue to either psychological or social factors (Chalder et al., 1996) (see 'Attributions and health').

Our responses to symptoms depend on how we interpret them. Most symptoms are transient and benign and the majority of individuals respond by waiting, doing nothing or self-medicating (Freer, 1980). One diary study showed that while symptoms were recorded on 38% of the days in the study medical care was only sought for 5% of those symptoms. So, how do we decide if our chest pain is a pulled muscle or a heart attack?

As symptoms are common and mostly benign, individuals often judge the seriousness of symptoms through the use of simple heuristics and how their symptoms match to the prototypes they hold for various common illnesses. If symptoms appear quickly and are accompanied by pain and restrict activities, symptoms are more likely to be judged as serious and requiring medical attention. People develop prototypes of illnesses based on their own previous experiences as well as knowledge gained from the media and other sources. When people experience a symptom they try to identify which illness they have by matching the symptom to their lay prototype of an illness. This match strongly influences coping strategies and help-seeking behaviour. For example, heart attack patients who experience symptoms consistent with their mental picture of a heart attack (most typically this includes chest pain and sudden collapse) present to hospital earlier than patients whose symptoms vary from their preconceived ideas of a heart attack and may be a closer match to their ideas about indigestion (e.g. upset stomach, nausea) (Perry et al., 2001). Similarly, patients who experience a breast lump present to a doctor more quickly than those who experience other breast symptoms, because a lump is more consistent with their picture of breast cancer (Meechan et al., 2003). Thus symptom interpretation can contribute to delay in seeking medical care in the areas of breast cancer and myocardial infarction and strongly influence prognosis (FTT Group, 1994; Richards et al., 1999). A better understanding of this psychological process has the potential to improve interventions designed to reduce delay and significantly influence patterns of mortality (Petrie & Weinman, 2003) (see 'Delay in seeking help').

The influence of emotions

Emotions play a strong role in symptom reporting. Considerable research has been conducted on the role of negative mood, trait negative affectivity and anxiety on symptom reporting and help-seeking behaviour. Negative moods have been shown to consistently trigger symptoms and health care actions such as taking medicines, seeking medical advice and restricting activity (Verbrugge, 1985). Following induction of a negative mood, healthy participants report more aches and pains and greater perceived vulnerability to health events (Salovey & Birnbaum, 1989). Research has shown that high trait negative affect is closely linked to higher symptom reports without any consistent relationship to objective health status (Costa & McCrae, 1987). Individuals high in negative affect are characterized by a tendency to experience a range of distressing negative emotions such as anxiety and depression. Individuals scoring high on trait negative affect have been shown to report two to three times as many symptoms as individuals low on negative affect (Costa & McCrae, 1980).

Evidence suggests that negative affect influences both noticing and interpretive processes. In situations framed as non-threatening, the accuracy of symptom perception has been shown to be similar between individuals high and low in negative affect, but in situations framed as threatening accuracy decreases in individuals high in negative affect and increases in individuals low in negative affect (van den Bergh et al., 2004). High negative affect has been associated with hypervigilance and increased scanning for impending trouble, which seems increase the extent to which people notice symptoms and attribute these symptoms to an illness.

Those high in negative affect are more schema-driven in determining their somatic states and tend make more negative interpretations than other individuals regarding common symptoms (Affleck et al., 1992). This is supported by a recent study examining symptoms following vaccination. A week following the vaccination participants high in negative affect attributed a far wider range of general symptoms to the effects of the vaccination than did low negative affect participants (Petrie et al., 2004). Similarly, high trait negative affect was associated with higher rates of symptom complaints following exposure to a respiratory virus regardless of whether individuals had objective evidence of a cold (Feldman et al., 1999).

A number of patients who generally do not have significant medical illness consistently seek medical care, consuming a large amount of health care resources in terms of primary care and specialist appointments, hospital admissions and laboratory and other investigations (Smith et al., 1986). These frequent attenders of health services tend to be high in trait anxiety (Banks et al., 1975). Those who use healthcare services extensively are also less likely to make normalizing attributions for common somatic symptoms than are other people (Sensky et al., 1996).

Conclusions

Psychological processes strongly influence symptom perception and reporting. Future research in the psychology of physical symptoms is likely to improve our understanding of the links between symptoms and health care behaviour. Furthermore, psychological interventions offer a way to change individuals' symptom perception to improve their functioning and alter their health behaviours. For example, a diabetes training programme on the recognition of symptoms, inaccurate symptom beliefs and external influences on blood glucose levels has been shown to improve patients' recognition of hypoglycaemic and hyperglycaemic episodes, estimations of blood glucose levels and metabolic control (Cox et al., 1988; Cox et al., 1989; Cox et al., 1991). Another intervention, which trained somatization syndrome patients in both biological and psychological aspects of somatoform symptoms, reduced their number of somatoform symptoms, general psychopathology, anxiety, depression, subjective health status, life satisfaction and visits to the doctor (Bleichhardt et al., 2004) (see 'Psychosomatics').

REFERENCES

Affleck, G., Tennen, H., Urrows, S. & Higgins, P. (1992). Neuroticism and the pain mood relation in rheumatoid arthritis: insights from a prospective daily study. Journal of Consulting and Clinical Psychology, 60, 119–26.

Banks, M. H., Beresford, S. A., Morrell, D. C., Waller, J. J. & Watkins, C. J. (1975). Factors influencing demand for primary medical care in women aged 20–44 years: a preliminary report. International Journal of Epidemiology, 4, 189–95.

Bartholomew, R. E. (1994). Tarantism, dancing mania and demonopathy: The anthro-political aspects of "mass psychogenic illness." Psychological Medicine, 24, 281–306.

Baumann, L. J. & Leventhal, H. (1985). "I can tell when my blood pressure is up, can't I?" Health Psychology, 4, 203–18.

Bleichhardt, G., Timmer, B. & Rief, W. (2004). Cognitive–behavioural therapy for patients with multiple somatoform symptoms – a randomised controlled trial in tertiary care. Journal of Psychosomatic Research, 56, 449–54.

Brondolo, E., Rosen, R. C., Kostis, J. B. & Schwartz, J. E. (1999). Relationship of physical symptoms and mood to perceived and actual blood pressure in hypertensive men: a repeated-measures design. Psychosomatic Medicine, 61, 311–18.

Chalder, T., Power, M. J. & Wessely, S. (1996). Chronic fatigue in the community: "A question of attribution." Psychological Medicine, 26, 791–800.

Costa, P. T. & McCrae, R. R. (1980). Somatic complaints in males as a function of age and neuroticism: a longitudinal analysis. Journal of Behavioral Medicine, 3, 245–57.

Costa, P. T. & McCrae, R. R. (1987). Neuroticism, somatic complaints, and disease: is the bark worse than the bite? Journal of Personality, 55, 299–316.

Cox, D. J., Carter, W. R., Gonder-Frederick, L., Clarke, W. & Pohl, S. (1988). Training awareness of blood glucose in IDDM patients. Biofeedback and Self-Regulation, 13, 201–17.

Cox, D. J., Clarke, W. L., Gonder-Frederick, L. et al. (1985). Accuracy of perceiving blood glucose in IDDM. Diabetes Care, 8, 529–36.

Cox, D. J., Gonder-Frederick, L., Julian, D., Carter, W. R. & Clarke, W. (1989). Effects and correlates of blood glucose awareness training among patients with IDDM. Diabetes Care, 12, 313–18.

Cox, D. J., Gonder-Frederick, L., Julian, D. et al. (1991). Intensive versus standard glucose awareness training (BGAT) with insulin-dependent diabetes: mechanisms and ancillary effects. Psychosomatic Medicine, 53, 453–62.

Croyle, R. T. & Sande, G. N. (1988). Denial and confirmatory search: paradoxical consequences of medical diagnosis. Journal of Applied Social Psychology, 18, 473–90.

Dunnell, K. & Cartwright, A. (1972). Medicine takers, prescribers, and hoarders. London: Routledge.

Feldman, P. J., Cohen, S., Doyle, W. J., Skoner, D. P. & Gwaltney, J. M. Jr. (1999). The impact of personality on the reporting of unfounded symptoms and illness.

Journal of Personality and Social Psychology, 77, 370–78.

Freer, C. B. (1980). Self-care: a health diary study. Medical Care, 18, 853–61.

FTT Group (1994). Indications for fibrinolytic therapy in suspected acute myocardial infarction: collaborative overview of early mortality and major morbidity results from all randomised controlled trials of more than 1000 patients. Lancet, 343, 311–22.

Hannay, D. R. (1978). Symptom prevalence in the community. Journal of the Royal College of General Practitioners, 28, 492–9.

Jewett, D. L., Fein, G. & Greenberg, M. H. (1990). A double-blind study of symptom provocation to determine food sensitivity. New England Journal of Medicine, 323, 429–33.

Kendrick, A. H., Higgs, C. M., Whitfield, M. J. & Laszlo, G. (1993). Accuracy of perception of severity of asthma: patients treated in general practice. BMJ, 307, 422–4.

Kroenke, K. & Spitzer, R. L. (1998). Gender differences in the reporting of physical and somatoform symptoms. Psychosomatic Medicine, 60, 150–5.

Meechan, G., Collins, J. & Petrie, K. J. (2003). The relationship of symptoms and psychological factors to delay in seeking medical care for breast symptoms. Preventive Medicine, 36, 374–78.

Meyer, D., Leventhal, H. & Gutmann, M. (1985). Common-sense models of illness: the example of hypertension. Health Psychology, 4, 115–35.

Myers, M. G., Cairns, J. A. & Singer, J. (1987). The consent form as a possible source of side effects. *Clinical Pharmacology Therapy*, **42**, 250–3.

Pennebaker, J. W. (1980). Perceptual and environmental determinants of coughing. *Basic & Applied Social Psychology*, **1**, 83–91.

Pennebaker, J. W. (1981). Stimulus characteristics influencing estimation of heart rate. *Psychophysiology*, **18**, 540–8.

Pennebaker, J. W. (1984). Accuracy of symptom perception. In A. Baum, S. E. Taylor & J. E. Singer (Eds.). *Handbook of psychology and health: social psychological aspects of health*. Hillsdale, N.J.: L. Erlbaum Associates.

Pennebaker, J. W. (2000). Psychological factors influencing the reporting of physical symptoms. In A. A. Stone, J. S. Turkkan, C. A. Bachrach, J. B. Jobe, H. S. Kurtzman & V. S. Cain (Eds.). *The science of self-report: implications for research and practice*. London: Lawrence Erlbaum Associates.

Pennebaker, J. W. & Epstein, D. (1983). Implicit psychophysiology: effects of common beliefs and idiosyncratic physiological responses on symptom reporting. *Journal of Personality*, **51**, 468–96.

Pennebaker, J. W., Gonder-Frederick, L., Stewart, H., Elfman, L. & Skelton, J. A. (1982). Physical symptoms associated with blood pressure. *Psychophysiology*, **19**, 201–10.

Pennebaker, J. W. & Lightner, J. M. (1980). Competition of internal and external information in an exercise setting. *Journal of Personality and Social Psychology*, **39**, 165–74.

Perry, K., Petrie, K. J., Ellis, C. J., Horne, R. & Moss-Morris, R. (2001). Symptom expectations and delay in acute myocardial infarction patients. *Heart*, **86**, 91–2.

Petrie, K. J., Moss-Morris, R., Grey, C. & Shaw, M. (2004). The relationship of negative affect and perceived sensitivity to symptom reporting following vaccination. *British Journal of Health Psychology*, **9**, 101–11.

Petrie, K. J. & Weinman, J. (2003). More focus needed on symptom appraisal. *Journal of Psychosomatic Research*, **54**, 401–3.

Richards, M. A., Smith, P., Ramirez, A. J., Fentiman, I. S. & Ruben, R. D. (1999). The influence on survival of delay in the presentation of symptomatic breast cancer. *British Journal of Cancer*, **79**, 858–64.

Robbins, J. M. & Kirmayer, L. J. (1991). Attributions of common somatic symptoms. *Psychological Medicine*, **21**, 1029–45.

Roberts, T. A. & Pennebaker, J. W. (1995). Gender differences in perceiving internal state: toward a his-and-hers model of perceptual cue use. In M. P. Zanna (Ed.). (1995). *Advances in experimental social psychology*. California, USA: Academic Press.

Salovey, P. & Birnbaum, D. (1989). Influence of mood on health-relevant cognitions. *Journal of Personality and Social Psychology*, **57**, 539–51.

Sensky, T., MacLeod, A. K. & Rigby, M. F. (1996). Causal attributions about common somatic sensations among frequent general practice attenders. *Psychological Medicine*, **26**, 641–6.

Siegel, K., Schrimshaw, E. W. & Dean, L. (1999). Symptom interpretation and medication adherence among late middle-aged and older HIV-infected adults. *Journal of Health Psychology*, **4**, 247–57.

Sigerist, H. E. (1943). *Civilization and disease*. New York: Cornell University Press.

Smith, G. R. Jr., Monson, R. A. & Ray, D. C. (1986). Patients with multiple unexplained symptoms. Their characteristics, functional health, and health care utilization. *Archives of Internal Medicine*, **146**, 69–72.

van den Bergh, O., Winters, W., Devriese, S. et al. (2004). Accuracy of respiratory symptom perception in persons with high and low negative affectivity. *Psychology and Health*, **19**, 213–22.

Verbrugge, L. M. (1985). Triggers of symptoms and health care. *Social Science and Medicine*, **20**, 855–76.

Theory of planned behaviour

Stephen Sutton

University of Cambridge

The theory of planned behaviour (TPB; Ajzen, 1991, 2002*b*), an extension of the theory of reasoned action (TRA; Ajzen & Fishbein, 1980; Fishbein & Ajzen, 1975), is widely used to study the cognitive determinants of health behaviours (Conner & Sparks, 2005; Sutton, 2004). It has several advantages over other 'social cognition models': (1) it is a general theory, and it can be argued that general theories should be preferred to health- or behaviour-specific theories for reasons of parsimony (Stroebe, 2000); (2) the constructs are clearly defined and the causal relationships between the constructs clearly specified; (3) there exist clear recommendations for how the constructs should be operationalized (Ajzen, 2002*a*); and (4) meta-analyses of observational studies show that the TPB accounts for a useful amount of variance in intentions and behaviour (but see the discussion of variance explained in Sutton, 2004).

According to the theory, behaviour is determined by the strength of the person's intention to perform that behaviour and the amount of actual control that the person has over performing the behaviour (Figure 1). According to Ajzen (2002*b*), intention is 'the cognitive representation of a person's readiness to perform a given behaviour, and ... is considered to be the immediate antecedent of behaviour',

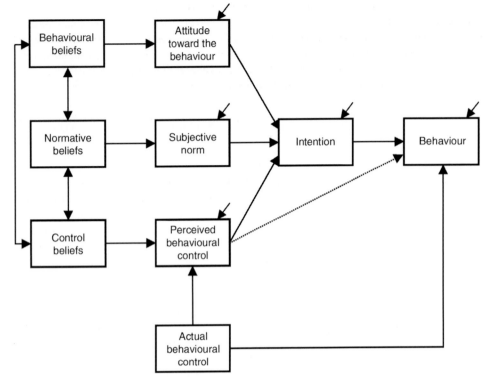

Fig 1 The Theory of Planned Behaviour. The small, unlabelled arrows represent other, unspecified causes of the endogenous variables.

and actual behavioural control '... refers to the extent to which a person has the skills, resources and other prerequisites needed to perform a given behaviour'. Figure 1 also shows an arrow from perceived behavioural control to behaviour. 'Perceived behavioural control' refers to the person's perceptions of their ability to perform the behaviour. It is similar to Bandura's (1986) construct of self-efficacy (see 'Perceived control' and 'Self-efficacy and health'). Indeed Ajzen (1991) states that the two constructs are synonymous. Perceived behavioural control is assumed to reflect actual behavioural control more or less accurately, as indicated by the arrow from actual to perceived behavioural control in Figure 1. To the extent that perceived behavioural control is an accurate reflection of actual behavioural control, it can, together with intention, be used to predict behaviour.

The strength of a person's intention is determined by three factors: (a) their attitude toward the behaviour, that is, their overall evaluation of performing the behaviour; (b) their subjective norm, that is, the extent to which they think that important others would want them to perform it; and (c) their perceived behavioural control.

Attitude toward the behaviour is determined by the total set of accessible (or salient) behavioural beliefs about the personal consequences of performing the behaviour. Specifically, attitude is determined by $\sum b_i e_i$, where b_i is belief strength and e_i is outcome evaluation. Similarly, subjective norm is determined by the total set of accessible normative beliefs, that is, beliefs about the views of important others. Specifically, subjective norm is determined by $\sum n_j m_j$, where n_j is belief strength and m_j is motivation to comply with the referent in question. Finally, perceived behavioural control is determined by accessible control beliefs, that is, beliefs about the presence of factors that may facilitate or impede performance of the behaviour. Specifically, perceived behavioural control is determined

by $\sum c_k p_k$, where c_k is belief strength (the perceived likelihood that a given control factor will be present) and p_k is the perceived power of the control factor (the extent to which the control factor will make it easier or more difficult to perform the behaviour).

The 'principle of correspondence' (Ajzen & Fishbein, 1977; Fishbein & Ajzen, 1975) or 'compatibility' (as it was renamed by Ajzen, 1988) states that, in order to maximize predictive power, all the variables in the theory should be measured at the same level of specificity or generality. This means that the measures should be matched with respect to the four components of action, target, time and context. The rationale given for the principle is a pragmatic one: it improves prediction. Presumably, however, there is also a theoretical rationale for the principle, namely that, by measuring the TPB variables at the same level of specificity, we are matching cause and effect (Sutton, 1998).

Although the TPB holds that all behaviours are determined by the same limited set of variables, each behaviour is also substantively unique, in two senses (Fishbein, 2000). First, for a given population or culture, the relative importance of attitude, subjective norm and perceived behavioural control may vary across different behaviours. For example, some behaviours may be influenced mainly by attitude, whereas other behaviours may be influenced mainly by subjective norm. Ogden (2003) points out that many studies using the TPB find no role for one or other of the three putative determinants of intention and therefore that the theory 'cannot be tested'. However, this represents a misunderstanding of the TPB. If at least one of the components is found to predict intention in a given study, this is consistent with the TPB. Nevertheless, it is a weakness of the theory that it does not specify the conditions under which intention will be mainly influenced by attitude, subjective norm or perceived behavioural control.

The second sense in which each behaviour is substantively unique is that, for a given population or culture, the behavioural, normative and control beliefs that underlie attitude, subjective norm and perceived behavioural control respectively may also differ for different behaviours. In the same way, for a given behaviour, the relative importance of attitude, subjective norm and perceived behavioural control and the content of the underlying beliefs, may vary across different cultures or populations.

The TPB is a general theory. In principle, it can be applied to any target behaviour without needing to be modified. For example, in applying the theory to a health-related behaviour, there should be no need to add a variable representing risk perceptions. If beliefs about the health risks of the behaviour (or its effect on reducing risk) are salient to a substantial proportion of the target population, this should emerge in an elicitation study that uses open-ended questions to elicit accessible beliefs (Ajzen, 2002a; Ajzen & Fishbein, 1980; for an example of an elicitation study, see Sutton et al., 2003).

Like other theories of health behaviour, the TPB is a causal model and should be treated as such (Sutton, 2002a, 2004). It says, for instance, that if you hold constant a person's subjective norm, perceived behavioural control and actual behavioural control and you change their attitude toward the behaviour, this will lead to a change in their intention (assuming that attitude is a determinant of intention for the behaviour in question in this target group), and this in turn will lead to a change in their probability of performing the behaviour (assuming that the person's intention is stable and that the behaviour is at least partly under their control).

The TPB is often depicted without actual control in the path diagram and, to date, has always been tested without measuring actual control. In this case, the direct path from perceived behavioural control to behaviour is causally ambiguous (Sutton, 2002a, 2002b). In particular, if we observe an independent predictive effect of perceived behavioural control on behaviour in an observational study in which actual control is not measured, this may be due partly to a causal effect of perceived behavioural control on behaviour and partly to a correlation induced by actual behavioural control influencing both perceived behavioural control and behaviour (Sutton, 2002a, 2002b). More generally, failing to measure and control for the effects of actual behavioural control will lead to biased estimates of the causal effects of perceived behavioural control and intention on behaviour, unless it can be assumed that perceived control is an accurate reflection of actual control (i.e. that perceived and actual control are perfectly correlated and this correlation arises from a direct causal effect of actual on perceived control).

Although Figure 1 shows an arrow going directly from actual control to perceived control, this is inconsistent with the theory's assumption that the effects of any variable on perceived control must be mediated by control beliefs. The absence of arrows, either one- or two-headed, between actual control and behavioural and normative beliefs respectively can be interpreted as indicating zero correlations and no direct causal influence in either direction. However, to date, Ajzen has not discussed these possible relationships. If actual control were related to one or both of these variables, again this would have implications for the interpretation of regression analyses from which actual control was omitted.

The theory predicts an interaction between perceived behavioural control and intention on behaviour. Ajzen (2002b) states it as

follows: 'Conceptually, perceived behavioural control is expected to moderate the effect of intention on behaviour, such that a favourable intention produces the behaviour only when perceived behavioural control is strong'. He also notes that 'In practice, intentions and perceptions of behavioural control are often found to have main effects on behaviour, but no significant interaction' (see also Conner & Armitage, 1998). This interaction derives from an interaction between intention and actual control (and so would be predicted to occur only in situations in which perceptions of control are accurate). In particular, intention is expected to have a stronger influence on behaviour the greater the degree of actual control the person has over the behaviour. For simplicity, this interaction is not shown in Figure 1.

The TPB is often described as a deliberative processing model. However, although some decisions may involve conscious deliberation and careful weighing up of pros and cons, in many cases the processes involved in the formation and modification of beliefs, attitudes and intentions may be largely automatic (Ajzen & Fishbein, 2000; Fishbein & Ajzen, 1975). A person's attitude toward a particular behaviour may be automatically updated when new information about the behaviour is received, and this attitude may be automatically elicited and guide behaviour in relevant situations. (However, although it seems plausible that automatic processes control the formation and change of beliefs, attitudes and intentions, for most health-related behaviours it seems less plausible to suggest that behaviour itself is automatically elicited.)

How well does the theory perform?

Table 1 summarizes the findings from meta-analyses of observational studies of the TPB in terms of the multiple correlation (R) and its square (which can be interpreted as the proportion of variance explained) for predicting intention and behaviour. With the exception of Ajzen (1991), all the meta-analyses explicitly or by implication restricted the analysis of prediction of behaviour to prospective studies in which intention and perceived behavioural control were measured at time 1 and behaviour was measured at time 2.

The findings for both intention and behaviour show reasonable consistency. For intention, the multiple correlations range from 0.59 to 0.71 (between 35% and 50% of variance explained). Prediction of behaviour was lower, as expected, with the multiple correlations ranging between 0.51 and 0.59 (between 26% and 35% of the variance explained). All the effect sizes in Table 1 are 'large' in terms of Cohen's (1992) guidelines.

Godin and Kok (1996) found differences between different kinds of behaviours with respect to how well the theory predicted intentions and behaviour. For example, for behaviour, the theory worked better in studies of HIV/AIDS-related behaviours than in studies of 'clinical and screening' behaviours. However, these results were based on small numbers of studies and possible confounds such as sample characteristics and differences in how the TPB variables were measured were not examined. Godin and Kok's review needs to be updated and extended.

Extensions of the TPB

There have been numerous attempts to extend the TPB by adding variables such as anticipated regret, moral norm and self-identity

Table 1. Summary of findings from meta-analyses of the theory of planned behaviour

	Effect size[a]					
	Predicting intention (BI) from AB, SN and PBC			Predicting behaviour from BI and PBC		
Meta-analysis	k[b]	R	R^2	k	R	R^2
Ajzen (1991)	19	.71	.50	17	.51	.26
Godin & Kok (1996)[c]	76	.64	.41	35	.58	.34
Sheeran & Taylor (1999)[d]	10	.65	.42	–	–	–
Albarracín et al. (2001)[d]	23	.71	.50	23	.53	.28
Armitage & Conner (2001)	154	.63	.39	63	.52	.27
Hagger et al. (2002)[e]	49	.67	.45	35	.52	.27
Trafimow et al. (2002)[f]						
PBC as Perceived difficulty	11	.66	.44	9	.59	.35
PBC as Perceived control	11	.59	.35	9	.58	.34

[a]Effect sizes are given in terms of the multiple correlation (R) and R^2.
[b]k is the number of datasets.
[c]Restricted to studies of health-related behaviours.
[d]Restricted to studies of condom use.
[e]Restricted to studies of physical activity.
[f]Restricted to studies that included measures of both 'perceived difficulty' and 'perceived control'.

(Conner & Armitage, 1998). For the sake of parsimony and theoretical coherence, candidate variables should be provisionally accepted as official components of the theory only if a number of conditions are satisfied. First, there should be sound theoretical reasons for believing that a given candidate variable influences intention or behaviour independently of the existing variables, that is, that the variable has a direct causal effect on intention or behaviour. In some cases, it is possible that the proposed additional variable is already captured by one of the existing variables.

Second, in order to retain the existing structure of the TPB, the proposed new variable should have an expectancy-value basis like attitude, subjective norm and perceived behavioural control; in other words, the new variable should be determined by accessible beliefs that are specific to the target behaviour. This would seem to rule out some variables, for example self-identity. This also means that the expectancy-value basis of descriptive norm (the belief that significant others are or are not performing the target behaviour), which Ajzen (2002a) has proposed as a sub-component of subjective norm in the latest version of the theory, needs to be specified. This requirement, that any additional variable is homologous in structure to the existing variables, also implies that including too many additional variables in the theory would make it unwieldy to use in practice. Furthermore, additional open-ended questions for eliciting accessible beliefs would need to be devised for use in

pilot studies. This has not yet been done for descriptive norm (Ajzen, 2002a).

Third, measures of a proposed new variable should be shown to have discriminant validity with respect to measures of the existing components, in other words to be measuring something different from measures of the existing variables (see 'Health cognition assessment').

Finally, the new variable should be shown to predict intention and/or behaviour independently of the existing components in studies in which the latter are well measured in accordance with published recommendations. It is likely that there are many false positive findings in the literature because the existing components are not always optimally measured. Of course, if the aim is simply to improve the predictive power of the theory rather than to specify additional determinants of intention, only the last of the requirements set out above is relevant.

External variables

The TPB, like other social cognition models, does not rule out other causes of behaviour. Many other factors such as socio-demographic, cultural and personality factors may influence behaviour, but these are assumed to be distal factors, in other words to be farther removed from the behaviour than the proximal factors specified by the theory. Thus, the TPB divides the determinants of behaviour into two classes: a small number of proximal determinants, which are specified by the theory (i.e. are internal to the theory); and all other causes, which are left unspecified but which are assumed to be distal and to influence behaviour only via their effects on the proximal determinants. In this sense, the TPB is sometimes said to be 'sufficient'.

A strategy for guiding future research on the determinants of health behaviour is to continue to use the TPB as a model of the proximal determinants of a given behaviour and to specify external factors that are hypothesized to influence the components of the theory or to influence behaviour directly, that is to develop theories that relate external factors to the theory's components. In effect, this is extending the causal model representing the TPB to the left, specifying the more distal causes of a particular behaviour and the mechanisms by which they influence the components of the theory and behaviour (Sutton, 2004).

Intervention studies

The TPB has direct implications for behaviour change interventions. According to the theory, changing behaviour requires changing either (1) the accessible beliefs that underlie attitude, subjective norm and perceived behavioural control or (2) actual behavioural control or (3) both (Sutton, 2002b). As Hobbis and Sutton (2005) point out, with the possible exception of Project RESPECT (Fishbein et al., 2001), there have so far been few successful examples of effective TRA- or TPB-based interventions. In their systematic review, Hardeman et al. (2002) identified seven studies in which the TPB was used to develop the intervention and the effectiveness of the intervention was evaluated in a randomized controlled trial with a behavioural outcome. Of these, four showed at least one positive change in the intervention group compared with the control group and the other three showed mixed effects. Although these findings seem encouraging at first glance, Hardeman *et al.* note a number of problems with these studies. In particular, in most cases it was not possible to identify which components of the theory were being targeted in the intervention. Furthermore, only one study (Brubaker & Fowler, 1990) reported a mediation analysis to test the extent to which the intervention effect on behaviour was mediated by the components of the theory. This study deserves further discussion as Fishbein and Ajzen (2005) cite it as a 'success'. The study compared three conditions: a persuasive message based on the TPB that was designed to modify participants' beliefs about the consequences of performing testicular self-examination (TSE); a persuasive message that was not based on the TPB; and a no-message control condition. There were significant differences in self-reported behaviour at one week and four weeks after the intervention. The mediation analysis (which combined the two message conditions) suggested that the effect of exposure to a message on intention and behaviour was partly mediated by the TPB variables, though the most important mediator was actually 'TSE knowledge', which is not a component of the theory.

Conclusions

The TPB provides fairly consistent prediction of intentions and, to a lesser extent, behaviour, across a range of different behaviours including health-related behaviours. However, the vast majority of studies have used observational designs; the causal predictions of the theory should be tested in randomized experiments (Sutton, 2002*a*). The theory has not so far fulfilled its promise as the basis for developing effective health behaviour interventions.

Acknowledgement

This chapter is based partly on Sutton (2004).

REFERENCES

Ajzen, I. (1988). *Attitudes, personality, and behavior*. Buckingham, UK: Open University Press.

Ajzen, I. (1991). The theory of planned behavior. *Organizational Behavior and Human Decision Processes*, **50**, 179–211.

Ajzen, I. (2002*a*). *Constructing a TpB questionnaire: conceptual and methodological considerations*. Retrieved September 1, 2004, from http://www.people.umass.edu/aizen

Ajzen, I. (2002*b*). *The theory of planned behavior*. Retrieved September 1, 2004, from http://www.people.umass.edu/aizen

Ajzen, I. & Fishbein, M. (1977). Attitude–behavior relations: A theoretical analysis and review of empirical research. *Psychological Bulletin*, **84**, 888–918.

Ajzen, I. & Fishbein, M. (1980). *Understanding attitudes and predicting social behavior*. Englewood Cliffs, NJ: Prentice-Hall.

Ajzen, I. & Fishbein, M. (2000). Attitudes and the attitude–behavior relation: Reasoned and automatic processes. *European Review of Social Psychology*, **11**, 1–33.

Albarracín, D., Johnson, B. T., Fishbein, M. & Muellerleile, P. A. (2001). Theories of reasoned action and planned behavior as models of condom use: a meta-analysis. *Psychological Bulletin*, **127**, 142–61.

Armitage, C. J. & Conner, M. (2001). Efficacy of the theory of planned behaviour: a meta-analytic review. *British Journal of Social Psychology*, **40**, 471–99.

Bandura, A. (1986). *Social foundations of thought and action: a social cognitive theory*. New York: Prentice-Hall.

Brubaker, R. G. & Fowler, C. (1990). Encouraging college males to perform testicular self-examination: evaluation of a persuasive message based on the revised theory of reasoned action. *Journal of Applied Social Psychology*, **17**, 1411–22.

Cohen, J. (1992). A power primer. *Psychological Bulletin*, **112**, 155–9.

Conner, M. & Armitage, C. J. (1998). Extending the theory of planned behavior: a review and avenues for further research. *Journal of Applied Social Psychology*, **28**, 1429–64.

Conner, M. & Sparks, P. (2005). The theory of planned behaviour and health behaviour. In M. Conner & P. Norman (Eds.). *Predicting Health Behaviour: Research and Practice with Social Cognition Models* (2nd edn.) (pp. 170–222). Buckingham, UK: Open University Press.

Fishbein, M. (2000). The role of theory in HIV prevention. *AIDS Care*, **12**, 273–8.

Fishbein, M. & Ajzen, I. (1975). *Belief, attitude, intention, and behavior: an introduction to theory and research*. Reading, MA: Addison-Wesley.

Fishbein, M. & Ajzen, I. (2005). Theory-based behavior change interventions: comments on Hobbis and Sutton. *Journal of Health Psychology*, **10**, 27–31.

Fishbein, M., Hennessy, M., Kamb, M., Bolan, G. A., Hoxworth, T., Iatesta, M., Rhodes, F., Zenilman, J. M. & Project RESPECT Study Group (2001). Using intervention theory to model factors influencing behavior change: Project RESPECT. *Evaluation and the Health Professions*, **24**, 363–84.

Godin, G. & Kok, G. (1996). The theory of planned behavior: a review of its applications to health-related behaviors. *American Journal of Health Promotion*, **11**, 87–98.

Hagger, M. S., Chatzisarantis, N. L. D. & Biddle, S. J. H. (2002). A meta-analytic review of the theories of reasoned action and planned behavior in physical activity: predictive validity and the contribution of additional variables. *Journal of Sport and Exercise Psychology*, **24**, 3–32.

Hardeman, W., Johnston, M., Johnston, D. W. *et al.* (2002). Application of the theory of planned behaviour in behaviour change interventions: a systematic review. *Psychology and Health*, **17**, 123–58.

Hobbis, I. C. A. & Sutton, S. (2005). Response to invited commentaries: the opportunity for integration remains. *Journal of Health Psychology*, **10**, 37–43.

Ogden, J. (2003). Some problems with social cognition models: a pragmatic and conceptual analysis. *Health Psychology*, **22**, 424–8.

Sheeran, P. & Taylor, S. (1999). Predicting intentions to use condoms: a meta-analysis and comparison of the theories of reasoned action and planned behavior. *Journal of Applied Social Psychology*, **29**, 1624–75.

Stroebe, W. (2000). *Social Psychology and Health* (2nd edn.). Buckingham, UK: Open University Press.

Sutton, S. (1998). Predicting and explaining intentions and behaviour: how well are we doing? *Journal of Applied Social Psychology*, **28**, 1317–38.

Sutton, S. (2002a). Testing attitude–behaviour theories using non-experimental data: an examination of some hidden assumptions. *European Review of Social Psychology*, **13**, 293–323.

Sutton, S. (2002b). Using social cognition models to develop health behaviour interventions: problems and assumptions. In D. Rutter & L. Quine (Eds.). *Changing health behaviour: intervention and research with social cognition models*

(pp. 193–208). Buckingham, UK: Open University Press.

Sutton, S. (2004). Determinants of health-related behaviours: Theoretical and methodological issues. In S. Sutton, A. Baum & M. Johnston (Eds.). *The Sage handbook of health psychology* (pp. 94–126). London: Sage.

Sutton, S., French, D.P., Hennings, S.J. *et al.* (2003). Eliciting salient beliefs in research on the theory of planned

behaviour: the effect of question wording. *Current Psychology*, **22**, 234–51.

Trafimow, D., Sheeran, P., Conner, M. & Finlay, K.A. (2002). Evidence that perceived behavioural control is a multidimensional construct: Perceived control and perceived difficulty. *British Journal of Social Psychology*, **41**, 101–21.

Transtheoretical model of behaviour change

Stephen Sutton

University of Cambridge

Stage theories of health behaviour assume that behaviour change involves movement through a set of discrete stages, that different factors influence the different stage transitions and that interventions should be matched to a person's stage (Sutton, 2005; Weinstein *et al.*, 1998).

The transtheoretical model (TTM; Prochaska & DiClemente, 1983; Prochaska *et al.*, 1992, 2002; Prochaska & Velicer, 1997) is the dominant stage model in health psychology and health promotion. It was developed in the 1980s by a group of researchers at the University of Rhode Island. The model has been used in a large number of studies of smoking cessation, but it has also been applied to a wide range of other health behaviours (Prochaska *et al.*, 1994). Although it is often referred to simply as the stages of change model, the TTM includes several different constructs: the 'stages of change', the 'pros and cons of changing' (together known as 'decisional balance'), 'confidence and temptation' and the 'processes of change'. The TTM was an attempt to integrate these different constructs drawn from different theories of behaviour change and systems of psychotherapy into a single coherent model; hence the name transtheoretical (for example, see 'Health belief model', 'Self-efficacy and health behaviour' and 'Theory of planned behaviour').

The stages of change provide the basic organizing principle. The most widely used version of the model specifies five stages: precontemplation, contemplation, preparation, action and maintenance. The first three stages are pre-action stages and the last two stages are post-action stages (although preparation is sometimes defined partly in terms of behaviour change). People are assumed to move through the stages in order, but they may relapse from action or maintenance to an earlier stage. People may cycle through the stages several times before achieving long-term behaviour change.

The pros and cons are the perceived advantages and disadvantages of changing one's behaviour. Confidence is similar to Bandura's (1986) construct of self-efficacy. It refers to the

confidence that one can carry out the recommended behaviour across a range of potentially difficult situations. The related construct of temptation refers to the temptation to engage in the unhealthy behaviour across a range of difficult situations. Finally, the processes of change are the covert and overt activities that people engage in to progress through the stages. The Rhode Island group has identified 10 such processes that appear to be common to a number of different behaviours: five experiential processes and five behavioural processes.

In stage theories, the transitions between adjacent stages are the dependent variables, and the other constructs are variables that are assumed to influence these transitions – the independent variables. The processes of change, the pros and cons of changing and confidence and temptation are all independent variables in this sense. Descriptions of the TTM to date have not specified the causal relationships among these variables.

Measures

The most commonly used method of measuring stages of change is the staging algorithm, in which a small number of questionnaire items is used to allocate participants to stages in such a way that no individual can be in more than one stage. Table 1 shows a staging algorithm for smoking that has been used in a large number of studies since it was first introduced by DiClemente *et al.* (1991). Precontemplation, contemplation and preparation are defined in terms of current behaviour, intentions and past behaviour (whether or not the person has made a 24-hour quit attempt in the past year), whereas action and maintenance are defined purely in terms of behaviour; ex-smokers' intentions are not taken into account.

This algorithm has a logical flaw: a smoker cannot be in the preparation stage unless he or she has made a recent quit attempt.

Table 1. TTM staging algorithm for adult smoking, from http://www.uri.edu/research/cprc/measures.htm

---

Are you currently a smoker?

- Yes, I currently smoke
- No, I quit within the last 6 months (Action Stage)
- No, I quit more than 6 months ago (Maintenance Stage)
- No, I have never smoked (Non-smoker)

(For smokers only) In the last year, how many times have you quit smoking for at least 24 hours?

(For smokers only) Are you seriously thinking of quitting smoking?

- Yes, within the next 30 days (Preparation Stage; if they have one 24-hour quit attempt in the past year – refer to previous question … if no quit attempt then Contemplation Stage)
- Yes, within the next 6 months (Contemplation Stage)
- No, not thinking of quitting (Precontemplation Stage)

Thus, a smoker can never be 'prepared' for his or her first quit attempt (Sutton, 2000*a*).

A problem with most staging algorithms is that the time periods are arbitrary. For instance, action and maintenance are usually distinguished by whether or not the duration of behaviour change exceeds six months. Changing the time periods would lead to different stage distributions. The use of arbitrary time periods casts doubt on the assumption that the stages are qualitatively distinct, that is, that they are true stages rather than pseudo-stages (Bandura, 1997; Sutton, 1996).

Staging algorithms and measures of the TTM independent variables for a number of different health behaviours are given on the Rhode Island group's website (http://www.uri.edu/research/cprc/measures.htm).

Evidence

Weinstein *et al.* (1998) specified four research designs that can be used to test predictions from stage theories: cross-sectional studies comparing people in different stages; examination of stage sequences; longitudinal prediction of stage transitions; and experimental studies of matched and mismatched interventions. This section will focus on TTM studies that have used the last two of these designs because in principle they provide the strongest tests of the model. We also consider intervention studies that have compared TTM-based stage-matched interventions with generic, nonmatched interventions or no-intervention control conditions. See Sutton (2000*b*) for a discussion of the analysis and interpretation of cross-sectional data on stages of change, and Rosen (2000) and Marshall and Biddle (2001) for meta-analyses of cross-sectional studies on the TTM.

Longitudinal prediction of stage transitions

Longitudinal data can be used to test whether different theoretically relevant variables predict stage transitions among people in different baseline stages. To date, 11 prospective studies have used the TTM variables to predict stage transitions, all in the domain of smoking cessation. Two of these (DiClemente *et al.*, 1985; Prochaska *et al.*, 1985) used an old staging algorithm and an early

version of the TTM. They were reviewed by Sutton (2000*a*). Nine more recent studies were reviewed by Sutton (2006): De Vries and Mudde (1998); Dijkstra and De Vries (2001); Dijkstra *et al.* (2003); Hansen (1999); Herzog *et al.* (1999); Segan *et al.* (2002, 2006*a*, 2006*b*); Velicer *et al.* (1999).

These nine studies found some evidence that different predictors are associated with different stage transitions. However, there were few consistent findings, providing little support for the TTM. Most of the studies used relatively long follow-up periods (at least six months). Future studies should use shorter follow-up periods to minimize the likelihood of missing stage transitions (with the proviso that at least six months is required to detect the transition from action to maintenance).

Experimental match–mismatch studies

The strongest evidence for a stage theory would be to show consistently in randomized experimental studies that stage-matched interventions are more effective than stage-mismatched interventions in moving people to the next stage in the sequence. Only three studies to date have compared matched and mismatched interventions within the framework of the TTM or closely related models (Blissmer & McAuley, 2002; Dijkstra *et al.*, 1998; Quinlan & McCaul, 2000).

Dijkstra *et al.* (1998) compared the effectiveness of individually tailored letters designed either to increase the pros of quitting and reduce the cons of quitting (outcome information) or to enhance self-efficacy or both. Smokers were categorized into four stages of change: preparers (planning to quit within the next month); contemplators (planning to quit within the next six months); precontemplators (planning to quit within the next year or in the next five years); and immotives (planning to quit sometime in the future but not in the next five years, to smoke indefinitely but cut down or to smoke indefinitely without cutting down). The sample size for the main analyses was 1100.

Dijkstra *et al.* (1998) hypothesized that immotives would benefit most from outcome information only, preparers from self-efficacy enhancing information only and the other two groups from both types of information. Thus, counter-intuitively, precontemplators and contemplators were predicted to benefit from the same kind of information. However, the study showed only weak evidence for a beneficial effect of stage-matched information. In respect of the likelihood of making a forward stage transition, assessed at 10-week follow-up, there were no significant differences between the three types of information among smokers in any of the four stages. However, preparers who received the self-efficacy-enhancing information only were significantly more likely to have quit smoking for seven days at follow-up than preparers in the outcome information only condition. Combining immotives and precontemplators, the percentage of smokers who made a forward stage transition did not differ significantly between those who received stage-matched and stage-mismatched information. Among contemplators and preparers combined, the percentage who made a forward stage transition and the percentage who quit for seven days were higher among those who received the stage-matched information than among those who received the stage-mismatched information, but these comparisons were only marginally significant (*p* < 0.10). It is not clear why the researchers combined the stages in this way (immotives and precontemplators; contemplators and preparers), given the hypothesis of the study.

Quinlan and McCaul (2000) compared a stage-matched intervention, a stage-mismatched intervention and an assessment-only condition in a sample of 92 college-age smokers in the precontemplation stage. The stage-matched intervention consisted of activities designed to encourage smokers to think more about quitting smoking. The stage-mismatched intervention consisted of action-oriented information and activities intended for smokers who are ready to quit smoking. At one month, 30 participants had progressed to contemplation, one participant had progressed to preparation and 5 participants had progressed to action. Contrary to the hypothesis, a greater percentage of participants in the stage-mismatched condition (54%) progressed than in the stage-matched (30%) or assessment-only (35%) conditions; however, this difference was not significant. Significantly more smokers in the stage-mismatched condition tried to quit smoking than in the stage-matched condition.

Finally, in a study of physical activity, Blissmer and McAuley (2002) randomly assigned 288 university staff to four conditions, including: (1) stage-matched materials (personalized, stage-appropriate covering letter plus stage-matched manuals) delivered via campus mail on a monthly basis; and (2) stage-mismatched materials delivered in the same way. After 16 weeks, 40.4% of the matched group had progressed one or more stages compared with 31.8% of the mismatched group. This difference was in the predicted direction but did not approach significance at the 0.05 level (Sutton, 2005). A limitation of the study, which the authors acknowledge, is that 57% of participants were in the action or maintenance stage at baseline, and the short follow-up period would have prevented those who had recently entered the action stage from progressing to maintenance.

Considered together, these three experimental studies of matched and mismatched interventions found little or no evidence for the stage model predictions.

Intervention studies

Three reviews have summarized the evidence on the effectiveness of TTM-based stage-matched interventions compared with generic, non-matched interventions or no-intervention control conditions (Bridle et al., 2005; Riemsma et al., 2003; Spencer et al., 2002). The second and third of these reviews were restricted to smoking cessation interventions. Both Bridle et al. (2005) and Riemsma et al. (2003) concluded that there was limited evidence for the effectiveness of stage-based interventions, but Spencer et al. (2002) reached a more positive conclusion.

However, all these reviews included studies that were not proper applications of the TTM. For an intervention to be labelled as TTM-based, it should (1) stratify participants by stage and (2) target the theory's independent variables (pros and cons, confidence and temptation, processes of change), focusing on different variables at different stages. Not surprisingly, the interventions that come closest to a strict application of the TTM are those developed by the Rhode Island group. The group's studies of TTM-based smoking cessation interventions have yielded mainly positive findings (e.g. Pallonen et al., 1998; Prochaska et al., 1993; Prochaska, Velicer, Fava, Rossi et al., 2001; Prochaska, Velicer, Fava, Ruggiero et al., 2001). By contrast, adaptations of these interventions evaluated by other research groups in the UK and Australia have yielded mainly negative results (Aveyard et al., 1999, 2001, 2003; Borland et al., 2003; Lawrence et al., 2003).

None of these studies speaks directly to the validity or otherwise of the TTM. Process analyses demonstrating that TTM-based interventions do indeed influence the variables they target in particular stages and that forward stage movement can be explained by these variables have not been published to date.

Conclusions

The TTM has been very influential and has popularized the idea that behaviour change involves movement through a series of discrete stages. It has also stimulated the development of innovative interventions. However, the model cannot be recommended in its present form. Fundamental problems with the definition and measurement of the stages need to be resolved. Although a cursory glance at the huge literature on the TTM gives the impression of a large body of mainly positive findings, a closer examination reveals that there is remarkably little supportive evidence. It would be helpful if the Rhode Island group presented a fuller specification of the model that (1) stated which variables influence which stage transitions and (2) specified the causal relationships among the pros and cons, confidence and temptation and processes of change. It would also be helpful if the group addressed the detailed critiques of the TTM by, among others, Carey et al. (1999), Joseph et al. (1999), Littell & Girvin (2002), Rosen (2000) and Sutton (1996, 2000a, 2001), and responded to Weinstein and colleagues' (1998) exposition of the conceptual and methodological issues surrounding stage theories.

To date, research on stage theories has been dominated by the TTM. However, partly in response to the problems that have been identified with this model, alternative stage theories are beginning to attract attention and hold promise for future research and practice. These include the precaution adoption process model (Weinstein & Sandman, 1992, 2002) and the 'perspectives on change' model developed by Borland and colleagues (Borland, 2000; Borland et al., 2004; Segan et al., 2006a).

Acknowledgement

This chapter is based partly on Sutton (2005).

REFERENCES

Aveyard, P., Cheng, K. K., Almond, J. et al. (1999). Cluster randomized controlled trial of expert system based on the transtheoretical ("stages of change") model for smoking prevention and cessation in schools. British Medical Journal, **319**, 948–53.

Aveyard, P., Griffin, C., Lawrence, T. & Cheng, K. K. (2003). A controlled trial of an expert system and self-help manual intervention based on the stages of change versus standard self-help materials in smoking cessation. Addiction, **98**, 345–54.

Aveyard, P., Sherratt, E., Almond, J. et al. (2001). The change-in-stage and updated smoking status results from a cluster-randomized trial of smoking prevention and cessation using the transtheoretical model among British adolescents. *Preventive Medicine*, **33**, 313–24.

Bandura, A. (1986). *Social foundations of thought and action: a social cognitive theory*. New York: Prentice-Hall.

Bandura, A. (1997). The anatomy of stages. *American Journal of Health Promotion*, **12**, 8–10.

Blissmer, B. & McAuley, E. (2002). Testing the requirements of stages of physical activity among adults: the comparative effectiveness of stage-matched, mismatched, standard care, and control interventions. *Annals of Behavioral Medicine*, **24**, 181–9.

Borland, R. (2000). The Steps to Stop Program: Underlying theory and structure of the advice provided. Unpublished manuscript.

Borland, R., Balmford, J. & Hunt, D. (2004). The effectiveness of personally tailored computer-generated advice letters for smoking cessation. *Addiction*, **99**, 369–77.

Borland, R., Balmford, J., Segan, C., Livingston, P. & Owen, N. (2003). The effectiveness of personalized smoking cessation strategies for callers to a Quitline service. *Addiction*, **98**, 837–46.

Bridle, C., Riemsma, R. P., Pattenden, J. et al. (2005). Systematic review of the effectiveness of health interventions based on the transtheoretical model. *Psychology and Health*, **20**, 283–301.

Carey, K. B., Purnine, D. M., Maisto, S. A. & Carey, M. P. (1999). Assessing readiness to change substance abuse: a critical review of instruments. *Clinical Psychology Science and Practice*, **6**, 245–66.

De Vries, H. & Mudde, A. N. (1998). Predicting stage transitions for smoking cessation applying the attitude–social influence–efficacy model. *Psychology and Health*, **13**, 369–85.

DiClemente, C. C., Prochaska, J. O., Fairhurst, S. K. et al. (1991). The process of smoking cessation: An analysis of precontemplation, contemplation, and preparation stages of change. *Journal of Consulting and Clinical Psychology*, **59**, 295–304.

DiClemente, C. C., Prochaska, J. O. & Gibertini, M. (1985). Self-efficacy and the stages of self-change of smoking. *Cognitive Therapy and Research*, **9**, 181–200.

Dijkstra, A. & De Vries, H. (2001). Do self-help interventions in health education lead to cognitive changes, and do cognitive changes lead to behavioural change? *British Journal of Health Psychology*, **6**, 121–34.

Dijkstra, A., De Vries, H., Roijackers, J. & van Breukelen, G. (1998). Tailored interventions to communicate stage-matched information to smokers in different motivational stages. *Journal of Consulting and Clinical Psychology*, **66**, 549–57.

Dijkstra, A., Tromp, D. & Conijn, B. (2003). Stage-specific psychological determinants of stage transition. *British Journal of Health Psychology*, **8**, 423–37.

Hansen, J. (1999). The stages and processes of change for smoking cessation: testing the transtheoretical model. *Dissertation Abstracts International*, **59**(9–B): 5083.

Herzog, T. A., Abrams, D. B., Emmons, K. M., Linnan, L. & Shadel, W. G. (1999). Do processes of change predict smoking stage movements? A prospective analysis of the transtheoretical model. *Health Psychology*, **18**, 369–75.

Joseph, J., Breslin, C., & Skinner, H. (1999). Critical perspectives on the transtheoretical model and stages of change. In J. A. Tucker, D. M. Donovan & G. A. Marlatt (Eds.). *Changing addictive behavior: bridging clinical and public health strategies* (pp. 160–90). New York: Guilford.

Lawrence, T., Aveyard, P., Evans, O. & Cheng, K. K. (2003). A cluster randomised controlled trial of smoking cessation in pregnant women comparing interventions based on the transtheoretical (stages of change) model to standard care. *Tobacco Control*, **12**, 168–77.

Littell, J. H. & Girvin, H. (2002). Stages of change: a critique. *Behavior Modification*, **26**, 223–73.

Marshall, S. J. & Biddle, S.J.H. (2001). The transtheoretical model of behavior change: a meta-analysis of applications to physical activity and exercise. *Annals of Behavioral Medicine*, **23**, 229–46.

Pallonen, U. E., Velicer, W. F., Prochaska, J. O. et al. (1998). Computer-based smoking cessation interventions in adolescents: description, feasibility, and six-month follow-up findings. *Substance Use and Misuse*, **33**, 935–65.

Prochaska, J. O. & DiClemente, C. C. (1983). Stages and processes of self-change of smoking: toward an integrative model of change. *Journal of Consulting and Clinical Psychology*, **51**, 390–95.

Prochaska, J. O., DiClemente, C. C. & Norcross, J. C. (1992). In search of how people change: applications to addictive behaviors. *American Psychologist*, **47**, 1102–14.

Prochaska, J. O., DiClemente, C. C., Velicer, W. F., Ginpil, S. & Norcross, J. C. (1985). Predicting change in smoking status for self-changers. *Addictive Behaviors*, **10**, 395–406.

Prochaska, J. O., DiClemente, C. C., Velicer, W. F. & Rossi, J. S. (1993). Standardized, individualized, interactive, and personalized self-help programs for smoking cessation. *Health Psychology*, **12**, 399–405.

Prochaska, J. O., Redding, C. A., & Evers, K. E. (2002). The transtheoretical model and stages of change. In K. Glanz, B. K. Rimer & F. M. Lewis (Eds.). *Health Behavior and Health Education: Theory, Research, and Practice* (3rd edn., pp. 99–120). San Francisco: Jossey-Bass.

Prochaska, J. O. & Velicer, W. F. (1997). The transtheoretical model of health behavior change. *American Journal of Health Promotion*, **12**, 38–48.

Prochaska, J. O., Velicer, W. F., Fava, J. L., Rossi, J. S. & Tsoh, J. Y. (2001). Evaluating a population-based recruitment approach and a stage-based expert system intervention for smoking cessation. *Addictive Behaviors*, **26**, 583–602.

Prochaska, J. O., Velicer, W. F., Fava, J. L. et al. (2001). Counselor and stimulus control enhancements of a stage-matched expert system intervention for smokers in a managed care setting. *Preventive Medicine*, **32**, 23–32.

Prochaska, J. O., Velicer, W. F., Rossi, J. S. et al. (1994). Stages of change and decisional balance for 12 problem behaviors. *Health Psychology*, **13**, 39–46.

Quinlan, K. B. & McCaul, K. D. (2000). Matched and mismatched interventions with young adult smokers: testing a stage theory. *Health Psychology*, **19**, 165–71.

Riemsma, R. P., Pattenden, J., Bridle, C. et al. (2003). Systematic review of the effectiveness of stage based interventions to promote smoking cessation. *British Medical Journal*, **326**, 1175–7.

Rosen, C. S. (2000). Is the sequencing of change processes by stage consistent across health problems? A meta-analysis. *Health Psychology*, **19**, 593–604.

Segan, C. J., Borland, R. & Greenwood, K. M. (2002). Do transtheoretical model measures predict the transition from preparation to action in smoking cessation? *Psychology and Health*, **17**, 417–35.

Segan, C. J., Borland, R. & Greenwood, K. M. (2006a). Can transtheoretical model measures predict relapse from the action stage of change among ex-smokers who quit after calling a quitline? *Addictive Behaviors*, **31**, 414–28.

Segan, C.J., Borland, R. & Greenwood, K. M. (2006b). Do transtheoretical model measures predict forward stage transitions among smokers calling a quitline? Manuscript submitted for publication.

Spencer, L., Pagell, F., Hallion, M. E. & Adams, T. B. (2002). Applying the transtheoretical model to tobacco cessation and prevention: a review of the literature. *American Journal of Health Promotion*, **17**, 7–71.

Sutton, S. (2000*a*). A critical review of the transtheoretical model applied to smoking cessation. In P. Norman, C. Abraham & M. Conner (Eds.). *Understanding and changing health behaviour: from health beliefs to self-regulation* (pp. 207–25). Reading, UK: Harwood Academic Press.

Sutton, S. (2000*b*). Interpreting cross-sectional data on stages of change. *Psychology and Health*, **15**, 163–71.

Sutton, S. (2001). Back to the drawing board? A review of applications of the transtheoretical model to substance use. *Addiction*, **96**, 175–86.

Sutton, S. (2005). Stage theories of health behaviour. In M. Conner & P. Norman (Eds.). *Predicting health behaviour: research and practice with social cognition models* (2nd edn., pp. 223–75). Buckingham, UK: Open University Press.

Sutton, S. (2006). Do the transtheoretical model variables predict stage transitions? A review of the longitudinal studies. Manuscript in preparation.

Sutton, S. R. (1996). Can "stages of change" provide guidance in the treatment of addictions? A critical examination of Prochaska and DiClemente's model. In G. Edwards & C. Dare (Eds.). *Psychotherapy, psychological treatments and the addictions* (pp. 189–205). Cambridge, UK: Cambridge University Press.

Velicer, W. F., Norman, G. J., Fava, J. L. & Prochaska, J. O. (1999). Testing 40 predictions from the transtheoretical model. *Addictive Behaviors*, **24**, 455–69.

Weinstein, N. D., Rothman, A. J. & Sutton, S. R. (1998). Stage theories of health behavior: conceptual and methodological issues. *Health Psychology*, **17**, 290–9.

Weinstein, N. D. & Sandman, P. M. (1992). A model of the precaution adoption process: evidence from home radon testing. *Health Psychology*, **11**, 170–80.

Weinstein, N. D. & Sandman, P. M. (2002). The precaution adoption process model. In K. Glanz, B. K. Rimer & F. M. Lewis (Eds.). *Health Behavior and Health Education: Theory, Research, and Practice* (3rd edn., pp. 121–43). San Francisco: Jossey-Bass.

Unemployment and health

Stanislav V. Kasl and Beth A. Jones

Yale University School of Medicine

Introduction

In this chapter we intend to provide an assessment of the research literature on unemployment and health. We draw on our somewhat more recent and much more detailed review of this research (Kasl & Jones, 2000), as well as on some key or trendsetting studies that have been published in the last few years.

In orienting the reader to this topic, we begin with a few general observations on recent research trends and themes:

1. There continues to be a strong and sustained interest in the topic of unemployment and health, both in the USA and, even more so, in Western Europe.

2. The boundaries of the topic have enlarged, reflecting the impact of changes in the economies of many industrial countries. Specifically, there is a growing interest in the impact of job insecurity, downsizing and involuntary part-time employment (e.g. Ferrie, Shipley *et al.*, 2003; Friedland & Price, 2003; Kivimaki *et al.*, 2003). In fact, the old dichotomy of working vs. unemployed is being replaced by a continuum which includes in-between categories of sub-optimal employment (Grzywacz & Dooley, 2003). This newly complex domain of research has generated its own glossary to help readers understand the concepts being investigated (Bartley & Ferrie, 2000).

3. There is a commendable trend toward more sophisticated study designs. This includes, above all, longitudinal data analyzed with multivariate techniques which allow reasonable controls for potential confounders. Thus the concerns centering on the question of 'causation or selection?' (i.e. does the observation of poorer physical and/or mental health reflect the impact of unemployment or does it, instead, denote the influence of prior characteristics of the individuals who later become unemployed?), which were highlighted at the beginning of our chapter in the first edition of this handbook, no longer seem as salient. However, these concerns remain pertinent since the studies of the impact of unemployment on health are based on a variety of observational (non-experimental) designs.

Some conceptual and methodological issues

Unemployment studies are often conducted from the perspective of classical occupational epidemiology: the exposure variable is operationalized rather simply, such as working vs. unemployed, secure vs. insecure employment, downsized vs. not. Length of exposure may be sometimes incorporated as well. In contrast, conceptualizations that centre on the meaning of work and on the impact work can have on individuals and their families tend to be rich and complex. For example, Jahoda (1992) suggests that a job, aside from meeting economic needs, has additional 'latent functions': a) imposes time structure on the day; b) implies regularly shared experiences and contacts with others; c) links an individual to goals and purposes which transcend his/her own; d) defines aspects of personal status and identity; e) enforces activity. Similarly, Warr (1987) discusses a number of environmental features of work which he postulates are responsible for psychological wellbeing: opportunity for control, skill use, interpersonal contact, external goal and task demands, variety, environmental clarity, availability of money, physical security and valued social position. In addition, for some individuals, job loss may represent the termination of exposures, such as work stress or specific work hazards, which themselves may be adverse influences on health. The implication of such formulations is that the experience of job loss and unemployment is likely to be multi-faceted and involve different intervening processes, moderating influences and outcomes. At minimum, one should try to separate the effects of economic hardships from the other effects of being without a job, a distinction which many studies do not address. The unemployment experience may also affect sub-groups of individuals differently. For example, age (and stage of the life cycle) is an important consideration: the unemployment experience is likely to be different for a) a young person completing his/her education and unable to find a job, versus b) a young worker with unclear career goals, and in his/her first job which s/he finds unsatisfying, versus c) a middle-aged head of household, with dependents at home, losing a long-held job made obsolete by new technology, versus d) an elderly worker, in poor health and close to retirement, in a job which is physically demanding.

Studies which are designed to capture the complexity of theoretical formulations about the meaning of the job loss experience are relatively rare and most often deal with mental health outcomes. For example, a Michigan study (Price, Choi & Vinokur, 2002) examined several steps in the mediating mechanisms leading from exposure to poor health and functioning, including financial strain and reduction in personal control.

With regard to study design methodologies, it is self-evident that except for controlled randomized intervention programmes (e.g. Price, 1992), all unemployment studies have been observational (non-experimental). However, important distinctions among study designs need to be recognized. The strong observational designs have included: a) studies of factory closures in which all employees lose their jobs and are then followed for health status changes (Morris & Cook, 1991); b) longitudinal follow-up studies of employed and unemployed individuals on whom baseline health status data allow for statistical adjustments of possible selection biases (e.g. Morris, Cook & Shaper, 1994); and c) follow-up studies of unemployed individuals in which the benefits of re-employment can be examined and adjusted for selection biases. Weak designs have included: a) longitudinal follow-ups of employed and unemployed persons on whom baseline data are too limited (e.g. age and education only) to adequately control for many possible selection factors; and b) cross-sectional comparisons in which selection factors can rarely be separated from causation. Retrospective accounts of reasons for job loss (i.e. whether or not it is health-related) allow for some control of selection biases, but their adequacy is difficult to assess.

We should also note the existence of a hybrid design in which data on individuals are supplemented with ecological information on economic indicators for the community or the region (e.g. Turner, 1995). This is a strong design, particularly when longitudinal data are collected. Specifically, it enables one to answer two additional questions: a) Do changes in community level of unemployment impact on the health and wellbeing of those who remain employed? b) Do the levels of community unemployment moderate the impact on the unemployed, e.g. is the impact on the individual unemployed person greater when the community level of unemployment is high than when it is low? A recent report (Beland, Birch & Stoddart, 2002) failed to show a contextual effect, either as a main effect or as a moderator and the authors emphasized the importance of the multi-level modelling approach as the proper strategy for examining ecological effects.

Finally, we wish to mention one additional approach which has a long history in unemployment research (see Kasl, 1982): the analysis of aggregate ('ecologic' or 'macroeconomic') data in which annual fluctuations in some economic indicator, often the nationwide percentage of the labor force that is unemployed, are related to annual changes in some outcome, such as total mortality, cause-specific mortality, alcohol consumption and acts of domestic violence (e.g. Brenner, 1987). At present, these business cycle analyses are seen as rather controversial, often involving data analyses which are difficult to follow and understand. For example, recent data from Germany (Neumayer, 2004) show that when one controls for state-specific effects, aggregate mortality rates are lower in recessions; opposite (i.e. expected) results are obtained if one fails to control for state-specific effects.

Impact of unemployment on mortality and morbidity

There are some eight to ten epidemiologic studies which have examined the relationship between unemployment and mortality during the last decade (see Kasl & Jones, 2000, for more detail). Studies using data for Great Britain, Sweden, Finland, Denmark and Italy are in agreement in demonstrating an excess mortality associated with unemployment. The excess may be as high as 50%–100%, but is reduced to about 20%–30% by adjustments for confounders which reflect pre-existing characteristics. When those who became unemployed for health reasons are excluded, aspects of social class are stronger confounders than baseline health (usually assessed with limited data) and lifestyle habits (see 'Socioeconomic status and health'). Men and women appear to show comparable impact, as do wives of unemployed men. Younger persons seem to be at risk for greater impact, while occupational groupings do not suggest much variation in impact. Cause-specific analyses suggest that suicides, accidents, violent deaths and alcohol-related deaths tend to be especially elevated, but do not explain all of the excess mortality.

It is noteworthy that the one study which used US data but otherwise similar methodology (Sorlie & Rogot, 1990), failed to detect any impact of unemployment on mortality. This discrepancy with the European data is not easily explained, particularly since it is believed that the 'social net' protecting the unemployed is stronger in these European countries than in the USA.

Overall, the conclusion that unemployment increases the risk of total mortality is prudent but not unassailable. Selection factors are clearly present as contributory influences, and fully controlling for them has not yet been possible.

Studies of unemployment and morbidity introduce potentially a new concern not applicable to mortality studies: the procedure for measuring health status outcomes. There are at least two concerns: 1) The influence of psychological distress on some measures could be substantial: that is, measured physical symptoms and complaints could be due to the distress rather than some underlying physical condition, or psychological distress could lower the threshold for reporting existing physical symptoms. 2) Measures based on seeking and/or receiving care could indicate differences in illness behaviour rather than underlying illness. In addition, it may be occasionally simply too difficult to determine what is being measured. Thus in a nicely designed prospective study of closure of a sardine factory in Norway (Westin, 1990), the rates of disability pension observed over a 10-year follow-up period were higher, compared with rates at a nearby 'sister factory' which stayed open. While these pensions are 'granted for medical conditions only', it is still difficult to know what exactly is being assessed and what health status differences would have been observed with other types of measurements.

There is reasonable agreement from several longitudinal studies (see Kasl & Jones, 2000 for more detail) that the job loss experience has a negative impact on health, though the precise nature of this impact is difficult to pinpoint. For example, in a Canadian study of GE factory closure (Grayson, 1989) former employees reported on a survey a high number of ailments. However, the elevated rates were for such a wide range of conditions that the authors suggested that the results indicate higher levels of stress which produce 'a series of symptoms that people mistake for illness itself'. (see 'Stress and health' and 'Symptom perception'). A British study of factory closure examined the impact on general practice consultation rates (Beale & Nethercott, 1988). Comparisons of rates were made both before vs. after factory closure as well as changes over time among cases vs. controls. The factory closure was clearly associated with increased rates of consultation, referrals and visits to the hospital. More refined analyses revealed that illnesses which were indicative of relatively 'chronic' conditions (i.e. those with previous high rates of consulting) were the ones which showed the increase. Thus it is not clear if these conditions were exacerbated by the factory closure, or if there was simply an increased rate of consulting, without any underlying clinical changes.

A number of other reports, based both on longitudinal and cross-sectional data, have offered confirmatory evidence regarding an adverse impact of unemployment on morbidity. The range of outcome variables is quite wide - hospital admissions, medical consultations, use of prescribed drugs, reports of chronic conditions, disability days, activity limitations and somatic symptoms. The difficulty is that these studies typically show a selected impact rather than a uniform one across all indices examined and little consistency emerges across studies when one tries to identify those variables which are particularly sensitive to the job loss experience.

While most of the studies address the impact of unemployment in middle-aged workers, we are now beginning to see also studies of workers in their last decade of employment. For example, Gallo and colleagues (Gallo, Bradley, Siegel et al., 2000; Gallo, Bradley, Falba et al., 2004) have shown that older workers (50+) experiencing involuntary job loss may be at greater risk for depression, disability, stroke and (possibly) myocardial infarction, compared with those who continued being employed. Those who chose to retire after losing their jobs were excluded from analysis. This suggests that being in the later stages of the life cycle does not protect older workers from the adverse effects of job loss seen among middle-aged workers.

Studies of unemployment among those in their late teens and early twenties have been mostly cross-sectional reports on various behavioural and physiological outcomes (Kasl & Jones, 2000). However, now we are beginning to see such studies being converted into longitudinal follow-ups; for example, a 14-year follow-up of a Swedish cohort (Hammarstrom & Janlert, 2002) shows that early unemployment among young men and women can contribute to adult health problems such as higher levels of symptoms and unhealthy lifestyles.

Impact of unemployment on biological and behavioural risk factors

The biological variables which have been examined in relation to unemployment include: a) indicators of 'stress' reactivity, such as serum cortisol, which do not have a well documented relationship to specific diseases; b) a very diverse set of indicators of immune functioning which are linked to possible disease outcomes theoretically rather than empirically; and c) risk factors for specific diseases, typically cardiovascular disease, where the presumption is that a chronic impact on these due to unemployment translates into higher risk for clinical disease (Kasl & Jones, 2000).

Studies using neuroendocrine variables or indicators of immune functioning find broad support for the conclusion that these biological parameters are sensitive to some aspect of the unemployment experience. Specifically, the findings strongly suggest the presence of anticipation effects (i.e. before job loss has taken place) and short-term elevations, but generally do not demonstrate the continually elevated levels with continued unemployment. It appears that in these unemployment studies these biological parameters exhibit acute reactivity, but chronic effects suggestive of increased risk of future disease are not usually demonstrated (see 'Psychoneuroimmunology').

Investigations of cardiovascular risk factors in relation to unemployment reveal that the threat of unemployment (i.e. holding a job with an insecure future) may be associated with higher levels of risk factors, particularly total serum cholesterol and low density lipoproteins. Otherwise, the results suggest a pattern somewhat similar to the neuroendocrine findings. For example, analyses of blood pressure and serum cholesterol changes from a Michigan study of plant closure (Kasl & Cobb, 1980) revealed a substantial sensitivity of these variables to the experience of anticipating the closing of the plant, losing the job and going through a period of unemployment and finding a new job. However, these were acute effects reflecting specific transitions. Men who continued to be unemployed did not stay at higher levels of risk factors but their risk factor level declined even in the absence of finding a new job.

There are also studies of very young adults which suggest the possibility that cardiovascular risk factors may not be sensitive to unemployment in this age group. It is not clear, however, if this is an age effect per se, or if the unemployment experience so close to the end of formal schooling is different from unemployment later in the life cycle.

There are several reports which are concerned with the impact of unemployment on health habits and behavioural risk factors. The typical variables examined include cigarette smoking, alcohol consumption, body weight and physical exercise (Kasl & Jones, 2000). Cigarette smoking tends to be relatively stable, while body weight shows an impact in some studies (i.e. an increase) but not in others. Alcohol consumption has been of great interest, but the picture is distinctly a mixed one (e.g. Hammarstrom, 1994). Many studies fails to show an increase, though one well designed longitudinal study showed an increase in the diagnosis of clinically significant alcohol abuse attributable to being laid off (Catalano et al., 1993). That same study also showed that employed persons working in communities with high unemployment rates were at a reduced risk of becoming alcohol abusers. It is worth noting that some of the examined health habits are also likely to represent selection factors; that is, there is evidence that higher levels of smoking and heavy drinking predict a greater likelihood of subsequent unemployment.

Impact of unemployment on mental health and wellbeing

There is little doubt that unemployment has a negative impact on mental health and wellbeing (Kasl & Jones, 2000). This conclusion, however, does not preclude or pre-empt a second one, namely that selection dynamics often play a role as well. Still, moving beyond these broad generalizations, in order to formulate additional more specific conclusions, becomes difficult because the evidence is less consistent and/or less complete.

Longitudinal studies strongly support the expectation that unemployment will have an adverse impact on (sub-clinical) symptoms of poor mental health (e.g. Warr et al., 1988); it is unlikely that the impact is also on overt diagnosable clinical disorder. Longitudinal studies also generally (but not always) demonstrate that becoming re-employed is associated with a reduction in symptoms (e.g. Kessler et al., 1988; Warr et al., 1988). In general, it would appear that depressive symptoms are the most sensitive indicator of impact of unemployment. However, because symptom checklists tend to be very inter-correlated, often similar finding are obtained with other scales such as anxiety or psycho-physiological symptoms. Other types of impact have been described, such as lower self-confidence and higher externality (one's life is beyond one's control); self-esteem may be impacted only on items which reflect self-criticism (Warr et al., 1988).

The considerable literature on the psychological impact of unemployment permits some additional observations:

1. Findings on young adults generally show a similar negative impact but also point to the considerable importance of the nature of the first (or early job): symptoms of distress may be highest among dissatisfied workers, lowest among satisfied workers and the unemployed at intermediate levels.
2. Evidence for possible gender differences in impact is inconclusive, but there is some suggestion that women may be less likely to benefit (i.e. reduction of symptoms) from the unemployment-to-re-employment transition than men. Among wives of husbands who have been laid off, symptoms do go up, but with some delay. We have no studies of impact of wives' layoff on husbands.

3. Evidence for rural–urban differences is limited but fairly suggestive: the impact on symptoms of distress may be weaker in the rural setting, but rural workers are more likely to miss aspects of work and work-linked activities (Kasl & Cobb, 1982).
4. The magnitude, duration and time course of impact are not easily linked to duration of unemployment in the many studies, suggesting that adaptive processes may attenuate or alter the impact.
5. Financial difficulties and additional life events are two likely mediators of impact of unemployment on mental health.
6. Buffers which moderate the impact include high levels of social support, participation in social–leisure activities, absence of psychiatric history and high sense of mastery over life's important outcomes, and high self-esteem. High work commitment aggravates the negative impact of becoming unemployed, but among those going from unemployment or re-employment, high work commitment enhances the degree of recovery.

Impact of job insecurity, downsizing and under-employment

As we noted in the introduction, the old dichotomy of working vs. unemployed is being replaced by a continuum which includes in-between categories of sub-optimal employment (Grzywacz & Dooley, 2003), such as experiencing the threat of job loss, working in a downsized company, and being involuntarily underemployed. We conclude this chapter with some of the emerging evidence of the impact of these employment situations.

There are several recent prospective investigations of the effects of job insecurity (e.g. Ferrie et al., 2002; Ferrie et al., 2003; Lee et al., 2004) which suggest that: a) the loss of job security negatively affects self-reported health and psychological symptoms, particularly as this becomes a chronic situation of insecurity; b) financial insecurity is the by-product of job insecurity which has the strongest negative impact; c) removal of the threat of insecurity does not fully re-establish pre-threat levels; d) impact on specific diseases, such as coronary heart disease, is only partially demonstrated. Temporary employment, which is another facet of job insecurity, appears to be associated with increased mortality while moving from temporary to permanent employment is protective (Kivimaki et al., 2003).

Studies of downsizing (e.g. Kivimaki et al., 2003; Kivimaki et al., 2001; Kivimaki et al., 2000) suggest that there are broad negative effects on health and wellbeing, including sickness absences and musculo-skeletal symptoms. These effects seem to be mediated by increases in job demands and job insecurity, reduction in job control and changes in social relations at work. In short, downsizing seems to lead to profound changes in the work setting which increase some of the familiar work stressors and reduce social buffers.

The concept of 'underemployment' has just recently begun to gather investigators' attention. The September 2003 issue of the *American Journal of Community Psychology* is devoted to this topic (Dooley & Catalano, 2003) and Friedland and Price (2003) present some of the evidence on health impact from a longitudinal study. Support is provided for the general conclusion that health and wellbeing of under-employed workers is poorer than for those who are adequately employed. However, types of underemployment – hours, income, skills and status – have somewhat different effects and effects also differ by the indicator of health that is used.

Clearly, the recent changes in the economies of most industrial countries have added to our old concerns – adverse health impact of physical exposures, of work stressors and of unemployment – some new concerns that reflect the adverse impact of insecurity, downsizing, and under-employment.

REFERENCES

Bartley, M. & Ferrie, J. (2000). Glossary: unemployment, job insecurity, and health. *Journal of Epidemiology and Community Health*, **55**, 776–81.

Beale, N. & Nethercott, S. (1988).The nature of unemployment morbidity. 2. Description. *Journal of the Royal College of General Practitioners*, **38**, 200–2.

Beland, F., Birch, S. & Stoddart, G. (2002). Unemployment and health: contextual-level influences on the production of health in populations. *Social Science and Medicine*, **55**, 2033–52.

Brenner, M. H. (1987). Economic change, alcohol consumption, and heart disease mortality in nine industrialized countries. *Social Science and Medicine*, **25**, 119–32.

Catalano, R., Dooley, D., Wilson, G. & Hough, R. (1993). Job loss and alcohol abuse: a test using data from the Epidemiologic Catchment Area Project. *Journal of Health and Social Behavior*, **34**, 215–25.

Dooley, D. & Catalano, R. (2003). Introduction to underemployment and its social costs. *American Journal of Community Psychology*, **32**, 1–7.

Ferrie, J. E., Shipley, M. J., Stansfeld, S. A. & Marmot, M. G. (2002). Effects of chronic job insecurity on self reported health, minor psychiatric morbidity, physiological measures, and health related behaviours in British civil servants: the Whitehall II study. *Journal of Epidemiology and Community Health*, **56**, 450–4.

Ferrie, J. E., Shipley, M. J., Stansfeld, S. A., Smith, G. D. & Marmot, M. (2003). Future uncertainty and socioeconomic inequalities in health: the Whitehall II study. *Social Science and Medicine*, **57**, 637–46.

Friedland, D. S. & Price, R. H. (2003). Underemployment: consequences for the health and well-being of workers. *American Journal of Community Psychology*, **32**, 33–45.

Gallo, W. T., Bradley, E. H., Falba, T. A. *et al.* (2004). Involuntary job loss as a risk factor for subsequent myocardial infarction and stroke: findings from the Health and Retirement Survey. *American Journal of Industrial Medicine*, **45**, 408–16.

Gallo, W. T., Bradley, E. H., Siegel, M. & Kasl, S. V. (2000). Health effects of involuntary job loss among older workers: a prospective study. *Occupational and Environmental Medicine*, **58**, 811–17.

findings from the Health and Retirement Survey. *Journal of Gerontology*, **55**, S131–40.

Grayson, J. P. (1989). Reported illness after CGE closure. *Canadian Journal of Public Health*, **80**, 16–9.

Grzywacz, J. G. & Dooley, D. (2003). "Good jobs" to "bad jobs": replicated evidence of an employment continuum from two large surveys. *Social Science and Medicine*, **56**, 1749–60.

Hammarstrom, A. & Janlert, U. (2002). Early unemployment can contribute to adult health problems: results from a longitudinal study of school leavers. *Journal of Epidemiology and Community Health*, **56**, 624–30.

Hammarstrom, A. (1994). Health consequences of youth unemployment – review from a gender perspective. *Social Science and Medicine*, **38**, 699–709.

Jahoda, M. (1992). Reflections on Marienthal and after. *Journal of Occupational and Organizational Psychology*, **65**, 355–8.

Kasl, S. V. (1982). Strategies of research on economic instability and health. *Psychological Medicine*, **12**, 637–49.

Kasl, S. V. & Cobb, S. (1980). The experience of losing a job. Some effects on cardiovascular functioning. *Psychotherapy and Psychosomatics*, **34**, 88–109.

Kasl, S. V. & Cobb, S. (1982). Variability of stress effects among men experiencing job loss. In L. Goldberger & S. Breznitz (Eds.). *Handbook of stress* (pp. 445–65). New York: The Free Press.

Kasl, S. V. & Jones, B. A. (2000). The impact of job loss and retirement on health. In L. F. Berkman & I. Kawachi (Eds.). *Social epidemiology* (pp. 118–36). New York: Oxford University Press.

Kessler, R. C., Turner, J. B. & House, J. S. (1988). Effects of unemployment on health in a community survey: main, modifying, and mediating effects. *Journal of Social Issues*, **44**, 69–85.

Kivimaki, M., Vahtera, J., Elovainio, M., Pentti, J. & Virtanen, M. (2003). Human costs of organizational downsizing: comparing health trends between leavers and stayers. *American Journal of Community Psychology*, **32**, 57–67.

Kivimaki, M., Vahtera, J., Ferrie, J. E., Hemingway, H. & Pentti, J. (2001). Organisational downsizing and musculoskeletal problems in employees: a prospective study. *Occupational and Environmental Medicine*, **58**, 811–17.

Kivimaki, M., Vahtera, J., Pentti, J. & Ferrie, J. E. (2000). Factors underlying the effect of organizational downsizing on health of employees: longitudinal cohort study. *British Medical Journal*, **320**, 971–5.

Kivimaki, M., Vahtera, J. *et al.* (2003). Temporary employment and risk of overall and cause-specific mortality. *American Journal of Epidemiology*, **158**, 663–8.

Lee, S., Colditz, G. A., Berkman, L. F. & Kawachi, I. (2004). Prospective study of job insecurity and coronary heart disease. *Annals of Epidemiology*, **14**, 24–30.

Morris, J. K. & Cook, D. G. (1991). A critical review of the effect of factory closures on health. *British Journal of Industrial Medicine*, **48**, 1–8.

Morris, J. K., Cook, D. G. & Shaper, A. G. (1994). Loss of employment and mortality. *British Medical Journal*, **308**, 1135–9.

Neumayer, E. (2004). Recessions lower (some) mortality rates: evidence from Germany. *Social Science and Medicine*, **58**, 1037–47.

Price, R. H. (1992). Impact of preventive job search intervention on likelihood of depression among unemployed. *Journal of Health and Social Behavior*, **33**, 158–67.

Price, R. H., Choi, J. N. & Vinokur, A. D. (2002). Links in the chain of adversity following job loss: how financial strain and loss of personal control lead to depression, impaired functioning, and poor health. *Journal of Occupational Health and Psychology*, **7**, 302–12.

Sorlie, P. D. & Rogot, E. (1990). Mortality by employment status in the National Longitudinal Mortality Study. *American Journal of Epidemiology*, **132**, 983–92.

Turner, J. B. (1995). Economic context and the health effects of unemployment. *Journal of Health and Social Behavior*, **36**, 213–29.

Warr, P. B. (1987) *Unemployment and mental health*. Oxford: Clarendon Press.

Warr, P. B., Jackson, P. & Banks, M. (1988). Unemployment and mental health: some British studies. *Journal of Social Issues*, **44**, 47–68.

Westin, S. (1990). The structure of a factory closure: individual responses to job-loss and unemployment in a 10-year controlled follow-up study. *Social Science and Medicine*, **31**, 1301–11.

Section II

Psychological assessment

Brain imaging and function

Erin D. Bigler

Brigham Young University

Brain imaging and function

Until the advent of computerized tomography (CT) in the 1970s, it was impossible to non-invasively image the brain (Eisenberg, 1992). However, once introduced, CT imaging rapidly advanced the technology of brain imaging and today remains one of the cornerstone technologies, especially for the assessment of acute neurologic symptom onset (i.e. a stroke) or injury.

Simultaneous with the development of CT imaging were tremendous improvements in computer technology, with faster processors and increased memory capacity. This provided the backdrop for essentially all other improvements that have occurred in brain imaging, once the breakthrough technology of CT imaging had been introduced. The physics and mathematics behind CT technology also became the inspiration for applying the principles of nuclear magnetic resonance (NMR) to human brain imaging. NMR principles had long been known and were, in fact, the basis for the Nobel Prize in Physics in 1952, but essentially had only been applied to physics and engineering (Eisenberg, 1992). In the 1970s researchers realized that radio frequency (RF) waves could reflect differences in biological tissues, such as the brain, since atoms within the molecules that form grey matter of the brain would 'resonate' differently in response to a pulsed magnetic field than those within white matter or cerebrospinal fluid. Detecting these differences in emitted RF waves – following the application of brief, pulsed, but very strong magnetic fields – could then be reconstructed to create an image of the brain (or any other biological tissue). We now refer to this as magnetic resonance imaging or MRI. As with CT imaging, the image resolution was initially limited but now image quality mimics gross anatomy.

Not only does MRI have the capability to approximate gross anatomy, it also has been shown to have many properties that permit multiple ways to analyze the brain image. For example, MRI-based diffusion tensor imaging (DTI) permits the detailing of brain pathways as well as indexes of the health of brain tissue. MRI spectroscopic analysis, referred to as magnetic resonance spectroscopy (MRS), provides a method to assess chemical composition of brain tissue. For example, certain levels of N-acetylaspartate (NAA), which can be readily determined with MRS techniques, are considered markers of neuronal injury. Such findings may be particularly important in anoxic and degenerative disorders (Gimenez et al., 2004).

Taking from CT technology, another aspect of brain imaging developed out of what was originally nuclear medicine: these techniques provide methods of measuring functions of the brain. The early standards of 'functional neuroimaging' (Bigler, 1996a,b; Bigler & Orrison, 2003; Orrison et al., 1995) consisted of single photon emission computed tomography (SPECT) and positron emission tomography (PET). Both of these methods utilize radioactive compounds referred to as radiopharmaceuticals. These are injected into the blood stream and the imaging methods capitalize on detecting the uptake of the radiopharmaceutical as a measure of brain function.

Another method of functional imaging, however, utilizes MRI technology which in turn permits the preciseness of anatomical detail from MRI. This technology is referred to as functional magnetic resonance imaging or fMRI, actually localizing brain regions that activate to a particular stimulus or that may deviate from normal in a particular disease or disorder. The main principle in fMRI is the detection of subtle differences in what is referred to as the blood oxygen level dependent (BOLD) signal, which is an indirect reflection of haemodynamic flow and oxygen utilization (see Papanicolaou, 1998).

The oldest non-invasive way to record activity from the brain was electroencephalography (EEG), which dates back to developments early in the previous century, but not really put into widespread clinical application until the early 1950s. In the past, EEG methods would not have been considered a form of brain imaging, but in the last two decades EEG recordings have been integrated with various neuroimaging methods and are very much considered part of contemporary neuroimaging. While a distinctly separate technology from EEG, magnetoencephalography (MEG) is often discussed in the same context as EEG, in large part because the original recording montage was similar to EEG (see Papanicolaou, 1998). However, in MEG what is being recorded are minute changes in magnetic field potentials. Based on the superconducting quantum interference device (SQUID), ultrasensitive detection of subtle magnetic flux within the brain is possible without the spatial limitations that restrict how many brain regions can be monitored by EEG. As with EEG, MEG can be integrated with three-dimensional (3-D) MRI to assist in demonstrating where changes or differences in the MEG reside within the brain.

Some select examples of brain imaging techniques will be presented in the next section. There are numerous excellent texts that more comprehensively review the various brain imaging techniques described in this chapter, as well as others, and their application in the study of brain–behaviour relationships (Orrison, 2000; Osborn, 1994; Osborn et al., 2004). The reader should keep in mind how rapidly this field has expanded, especially in the last decade, and the broad application of brain imaging techniques to the study of human behaviour has really just begun. Along these lines neuroimaging is now becoming a critical part of evaluation and treatment for neuropsychiatric disorders (Etkin et al., 2005).

Examples of neuroimaging in normal and pathological states

CT Imaging

Figure 1(A) shows CT imaging in a case of traumatic brain injury. Currently, CT scanning is the imaging of choice for acute assessment of brain injury, because it is fast, detects most types of major pathological conditions and does not have the same restrictions of MRI with regards to use with life-saving devices (i.e. since MRI is based on applying a powerful magnetic field, any device that has magnetic properties, such as a heart pacemaker are not compatible with performing an MRI). CT imaging is particularly adept at detecting skull anatomy and pathology, but anatomic resolution is limited, and detailed neuroanatomical research is typically better served by MRI technology.

MRI

Contemporary MRI provides exquisite detail of brain anatomy, as shown in Figure 1(B). MRI capitalizes on a straightforward biological fact of brain tissue: brain tissue can be compartmentalized into three main categories – white matter comprised of mainly myelinated axons; grey matter comprised of cell bodies; and Cerebral Spinal Fluid (CSF) filled spaces, which also house part of the cerebrovasculature. Particularly evident in MRI imaging, there are two basic premises in interpreting findings which are shown in Figure 1(B): (1) symmetry of bilateral brain structures and, (2) similarity of normal brain structures, in other words the 'normalcy' of how one brain compares to another. Because of the clarity of isolating brain tissue with MRI techniques, 3-D reconstruction of the brain can be routinely achieved, as shown in Figure 1(E), (F) and (G), which can depict normal brain anatomy and/or pathology.

Functional neuroimaging

Functional neuroimaging refers to a variety of imaging methods that provide some inference about underlying activity or function of a particular brain region. There are numerous functional neuroimaging methods, but the most common are functional MRI or fMRI (Rorden & Karnath, 2004), single photon emission tomography

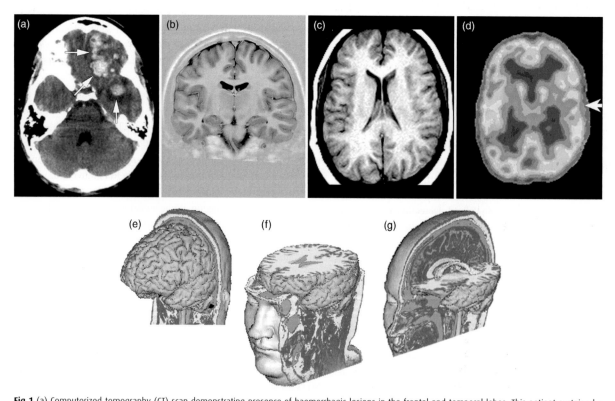

Fig 1 (a) Computerized tomography (CT) scan demonstrating presence of haemorrhagic lesions in the frontal and temporal lobes. This patient sustained a significant brain injury in a fall down a flight of stairs. CT imaging is based on tissue density where the darker the image, the less dense the tissue and oppositely, the whiter the image the more dense the tissue. That is why the skull shows white since bone has the greatest density. The haemorrhagic lesions also show white (see arrows), because as blood coagulates, it becomes denser. Note the clarity that CT has in detecting the haemorrhage. (b) Coronal section of a healthy brain using contemporary magnetic resonance imaging (MRI) showing the clarity of anatomical detail that can be achieved. Such level of clarity permits precision in studying anatomical relationships with behaviour. (c) Magnetic resonance imaging (MRI) axial view of the brain with a section through the level of the lateral ventricles in a case of anoxic brain injury that shows no structural abnormalities; however, (d) Positron emission tomography (PET) imaging shows reduced activity in the mid-left hemisphere (see arrow). This illustration nicely shows that even when structural imaging using MRI may appear normal, the functional imaging can reveal various abnormalities. (e, f and g) Using thin section magnetic resonance imaging (MRI), as in (b), the human brain can be reconstructed in any plane and sectioned in any perspective. Note that all three models of this healthy brain are on the same level with the brain in the same location for all, only the section removed is different. (e) represents a left frontal oblique revealing part of the brain, with the posterior part still imbedded in the skull. (f) and (g) represent variations on left frontal oblique views of the brain in situ. Obviously, from such illustrations it is evident that three-dimensional (3-D) reconstruction of the brain can be achieved for any brain structure or region of interest.

(SPECT), positron emission tomography (PET), quantitative electro-encephalography (qEEG) and magnetoencephalography (MEG); see also Orrison *et al.*, and Papanicolaou books on functional brain imaging (Orrison *et al.*, 1995; Papanicolaou, 1998). MRI is based on the 'signal' detection of radiofrequency waves from the head and how they react when a strong magnet field is pulsed. fMRI capitalizes on that technology where the detection of differences in the blood oxygen level detection (BOLD) MRI signal indicates level of activity or engagement of a particular brain region. Both PET and SPECT depend on the detection of some type of a radiopharmaceutical that has been introduced into the body. At rest, the brain should exhibit general uniform levels of activation and both PET and SPECT can detect changes from the baseline that reflect either areas of increased or decreased activity of a particular brain region. qEEG is essentially a computerized analysis of brain electrophysiology that can be presented in a holistic montage to view brain activity and MEG is somewhat similar, but is dependent on very small magnetic fields associated with neural cells and how they may change from baseline.

As an example of functional neuroimaging, the case shown in Figure 1(C) had an MRI of normal appearance, yet when PET imaging is integrated with the MRI as in Figure 1(D) it is clearly evident that a large area that looks 'normal' on MRI is not functioning normally. This case is a nice example that normal-appearing brain tissue does not necessarily mean normal function.

Future directions

Faster processing and higher field strength will undoubtedly improve the capability of MRI. For example, MRI techniques are being developed for what is referred to as in vivo microscopy (Bilgen, 2004). This technique provides exquisite detail that has the potential to show such things as cellular layering in the cerebral cortex. Advances are also being made in the development of neurotransmitter ligands to study drug interactions and drug/brain/behaviour interactions using various MRI technologies (see Jenkins *et al.*, 2004). Similar statements can be made about the other imaging methods where developments in computer technology will undoubtedly improve all aspects of functional neuroimaging as well.

Conclusions

Contemporary neuroimaging techniques provide a breadth of methods for studying in vivo brain–behaviour relationships. MRI resolution is currently on par with gross anatomic inspection of the brain. Three-dimensional image analyses permit the study of structural brain regions from any perspective, as well as the framework for either directly studying activation patterns with fMRI techniques, or for integrating other functional neuroimaging methods such as MEG, EEG or PET. Functional neuroimaging techniques have been rapidly improving; these improvements permit the study of brain activation patterns in normal and abnormal conditions with the goal of better understanding the neurobiological basis of human behaviour. Such discoveries will have particular relevance not only for assessing but also for treating a broad spectrum of neurological and neuropsychiatric disorders.

Acknowledgements

Supported in part by the Ira Fulton Foundation. The technical assistance of Tracy Abildskov and Craig Vickers and the editorial assistance of Jo Ann Petrie are gratefully acknowledged.

REFERENCES

Bigler, E. D. (1996a). *Handbook of human brain function: Neuroimaging I. Basic science.* New York: Plenum Press.

Bigler, E. D. (1996b). *Handbook of human brain function: Neuroimaging II. Clinical applications.* New York: Plenum Press.

Bigler, E. D. & Orrison, J. W. W. (2003). Neuroimaging in sports-related brain injury. In M. Collins, M. Lovell, J. T. Barth *et al.* (Eds.). *Sports-related traumatic brain injury: an international perspective* (pp. in press). Lisse, The Netherlands: Swets & Zeitlinger Publishers.

Bilgen, M. (2004). Simple, low-cost multipurpose RF coil for MR microscopy at 9.4 T. *Magnetic Resonance in Medicine,* **52**(4), 937–40.

Eisenberg, R. L. (1992). *Radiology: an illustrated history.* St. Louis: Mosby Year Book, Inc.

Etkin, A., Pittenger, C., Polan, H. J. & Kandel, E.R. (2005). Toward a neurobiology of psychotherapy: basic science and clinical applications. *Journal of Neuropsychiatry and Clinical Neurosciences,* **17**(2), 145–58.

Gimenez, M., Junque, C., Narberhaus, A. *et al.* (2004). Medial temporal MR spectroscopy is related to memory performance in normal adolescent subjects. *Neuroreport,* **15**(4), 703–7.

Jenkins, B.G., Sanchez-Pernaute, R., Brownell, A. L., Chen, Y. C. & Isacson, O. (2004). Mapping dopamine function in primates using pharmacologic magnetic resonance imaging. *Journal of Neuroscience,* **24**(43), 9553–60.

Orrison, W. W. (2000). *Neuroimaging.* Philadelphia: W.B. Saunders Company.

Orrison, W. W., Lewine, J. D., Sanders, J. A. & Hartshorne, M. F. (1995). *Functional Brain Imaging* (1st edn.). St. Louis, MO: Mosby.

Osborn, A. G. (1994). *Diagnostic neuroradiology.* St. Louis, MO: Mosby.

Osborn, A. G., Blaser, S. & Salzman, K. (2004). *Diagnostic imaging: Brain – Top 250 diagnoses.* Philadelphia: W.B. Saunders Company.

Papanicolaou, A. C. (1998). *Fundamentals of functional brain imaging.* Lisse: Swets & Zeitlinger.

Rorden, C. & Karnath, H. O. (2004). Using human brain lesions to infer function: a relic from a past era in the fMRI age? *Nature Reviews. Neuroscience,* **5**(10), 813–19.

Communication assessment

Linda Worrall

The University of Queensland

This chapter outlines how a speech and language therapist might assess communication disability. It firstly describes the different approaches to communication and communication disability, and then uses a biopsychosocial approach using the World Health Organization's International Classification of Functioning, Disability and Health (World Health Organization, 2001) as a conceptual framework for communication disability assessment. The different types and purposes of assessment for speech and language therapists are outlined and examples of communication assessments are provided throughout. The description of communication disabilities and assessments is by necessity brief and avoids the use of profession-specific terms. Readers are referred to texts by Haynes and Pindzola (1998) or Ruscello (2001) for more detailed information on communication disability assessment.

The study of communication and communication disabilities is often interdisciplinary involving audiologists, neuropsychologists, psycholinguists, sociolinguists, linguists, neurologists, physiologists, neurophysiologists, otolaryngologists and speech and language therapists, to name a few. In most countries of the world, however, it is the responsibility of speech and language therapists to provide services to people with communication disabilities. While hearing impairment is also a communication disability, audiologists have the expertise to assess this area. Speech and language therapists view communication holistically and may use a modality approach (verbal, nonverbal or written) to communication, a linguistic approach (phonetic, phonological, semantic, syntactical and pragmatic), or an information processing or psycholinguistic approach (e.g. input and output modular systems). When speech and language therapists wish to examine communication disability more broadly, they are often interested not only in the impairment, but also the effects that the impairment has on their client's life. The World Health Organization's International Classification of Functioning, Disability and Health (ICF; World Health Organization, 2001) is increasingly becoming the conceptual framework of the profession, with several countries adopting the framework in their scope of practice documents (Threats & Worrall, 2004). In simple ICF terms, speech and language therapists consider voice, speech, fluency, language and swallowing impairments. They then consider the effects of these impairments of the activities and participation in everyday life. They also consider how the environment and the client's own personal factors contribute to their communicative functioning. All of these constructs are considered in the assessment process.

Assessments are conducted by speech and language therapists for a number of reasons: diagnosis, determination of severity, prognosis and therapy planning (Rosenbek *et al.*, 1989) and outcome measurement (Frattali, 1998). It is unusual that any one assessment will fulfil all these requirements. Speech and language therapists will therefore use different types of assessment (standardized testing, ecological observations, therapy as assessment, client self-report scales, goal attainment scaling and simple outcome ratings) to meet their needs. This paper will however focus on commercially available standardized communication assessments.

There has been considerable debate in the literature about whether speech and language therapists should assess (and treat) impairments only or whether functional or social model approaches should be a clinician's first option (e.g. Duchan, 2001; Worrall, 2001). Generalization and priorities in goal setting have also been issues in this debate with some authors challenging the assumption that the rehabilitation process must begin with efforts to lessen the impairment (with the assumption that this will generalise to everyday life) with compensatory efforts to minimize the activity limitations and participation restrictions attempted after that. The biopsychosocial approach to disability espoused in the ICF suggests that contextual factors are important components of human functioning and assessing or treating the impairment in isolation at any stage of the rehabilitation process ignores a vital part of disability – that the impairment is not the sole source of the disability. Emerging from this debate has been the discussion of the role of the client in goal-setting and ultimately assessment and intervention. Collaborative decision-making has become a professional value that is being embraced by speech and language therapists and is influencing many aspects of the why, when, where and how communication assessment occurs. Collaborative decision-making with communicatively disabled clients brings its own set of challenges. The emergence of client-centred healthcare in many parts of the world and legislation that protects the rights of people with disabilities is mandating collaboration with clients with communication disabilities, no matter how severe the communication disability may be (see 'Disability' and 'Disability assessment').

The following sections describe the primary components of communication from a speech and language therapist's perspective. Using the ICF terminology, the different impairments that contribute to a communication disability are outlined. Examples of health conditions that may cause the impairment are provided. A review of the impairment-based measures is made and, where available, measures of activity limitation or participation restriction, environmental and personal factors are described. Evidence-based practice is a mainstay of speech and language therapy practice. Evidence-based practice issues in communication assessment primarily relate to the psychometric properties of the assessments and therefore are contained within the technical manuals of individual assessments.

Voice

Impairments of the voice include structural or functioning problems of the vocal tract. Vocal nodules, spastic dysphonia, vocal fold paralysis and laryngectomy following laryngeal cancer are all examples of impairments of the voice (see 'Voice disorders'). Voice assessment at the impairment level is often a mixture of perceptual voice analysis which uses the clinician's ear to listen to the pitch, volume and quality of the voice (e.g. Laver, 1980; Oates & Russell, 1998, 2003; Pindzola, 1987) and acoustic or physiological measures which measure the performance of the vocal tract using instruments such as the Visipitch or the Computerized Speech Laboratory (www.kayelemetrics.com). Many modern hospitals have established voice clinics which have videolaryngoscopy and other imaging techniques that allow clinicians to view, record and measure the functioning of the vocal tract, particularly the all-important vocal folds.

Assessments such as the Voice Activity and Participation Profile (Ma & Yiu, 2001) and the Voice Handicap Index (Jacobson et al., 1997) are being used to assess the impact of the voice impairment of the lives of the clients.

Speech

Speech impairments are a result of structural or functioning problems of the total speech production mechanism and while it includes the vocal tract (and hence includes impairments of the voice), the term speech impairment is predominantly focused on articulatory problems which occur in the oral region. Speech impairments in children include articulation disorders or sound production impairments which are an 'inability to produce a perceptually acceptable version of a phone in isolation or in any phonetic context' (Dodd, 1995; p. 54) and phonological disorders (impairment of rules of sound production, such as final-consonant deletion, which can cause speech to be unintelligible) and can be caused by health conditions such as cleft palate, developmental verbal dyspraxia or congenital hearing impairment. Dodd (1995) distinguishes between three types of phonological disorder; a delayed phonological disorder in which the phonological processes are normal but typical of younger child; consistent deviant phonological disorder which has one or a number of disordered rules; and an inconsistent phonological disorder whereby 10 or more words (of 25 given) are produced differently on two out of three occasions and this is associated with phonological planning deficit. There is some debate about whether phonological disorders in children are speech or language impairments since the phonological rules impaired in this type of disorder are a part of the language processing system (Crystal & Varley, 1993). In adults, speech impairments may result after surgery for cancer of the tongue or result from neurological conditions such as stroke, brain injury, Parkinson's disease or multiple sclerosis which affect the muscles of speech.

Assessment of speech impairment in children uses oromotor examinations (e.g. St Louis & Ruscello, 2000) and articulation tests which allow phonological analysis if required (e.g. Goldman & Fristoe, 1986) while in adults, speech impairments such as dysarthria or verbal dyspraxia are assessed using tools specifically designed for that purpose such as the Frenchay Dysarthria Assessment (Enderby, 1983) and the Apraxia Battery for Adults (Dabul, 1979). Physiological measures such as electropalatography (e.g. Dent, 2001) are also becoming more widespread. Commercially available assessments of speech that examine the impact of the speech impairment on everyday life are not so common (Beukelman, Mathy & Yorkston, 1998; Enderby, 2000).

Fluency

An impairment of fluency includes both stuttering and cluttering. While stuttering is relatively well known, cluttering is not so identifiable, but consists of rapid unintelligible bursts of speech. Authors such as Gillam et al. (2000) and Crystal and Varley (1993) consider that fluency is as an aspect of speech, therefore stuttering is a type of speech impairment (see 'Stuttering').

Many children progress through a phase of normal dysfluency that does not result in chronic stuttering behaviour (Onslow & Packman, 1999). There are assessments for young children, school-aged children, adolescents and adults (see Haynes & Pindzola, 1998). Assessment at the impairment level typically includes counts of repetitions, prolongations, percentage of syllables stuttered and speaking rates. There are also assessments of avoidance behaviour and attitudes towards communication but as Yaruss (2002) and Blood and Conture (1998) note, there has been little development of stuttering measures at the activity limitation/participation restriction level.

Language

Language impairment is possibly the most complex part of communication to assess. Language is considered to be a central function, most commonly centred in the dominant hemisphere of the brain with receptive language being processed in the posterior region around Wernicke's area and expressive language being processed in the anterior region around Broca's area. Language impairments are acquired from brain damage in these areas through stroke (aphasia), traumatic brain injuries, or degenerative conditions such as dementia. In developing children, language impairment may be associated with developmental delay or may be seen in otherwise normal children who have a specific language impairment which can affect their communication from an early age and their education upon entering school. There may also be disruptions or disorders to the language system in conditions such as autism or Rett's syndrome. An impairment of literacy or written language use (reading and writing) has a lay term of 'dyslexia' but is viewed by speech and language therapists as a phonological awareness disorder.

There has been ongoing debate about the co-existing roles of cognition and language in many health conditions that result in a language impairment, but in general it has been recognized that some health conditions where there is generalized brain damage (e.g. traumatic brain injury, dementia), the term that should be used is cognitive–language or cognitive–communication disorder, rather than aphasia (a term used to describe focal lesions). However, even when there is localized damage in aphasia, there has been debate about the coexistence of cognitive problems and their impact on language (see 'Aphasia'). Speech and language therapists seeking to separate cognition and language impairments in their clients typically use specially constructed assessments which assess cognition without a language load (e.g. Helm Estabrooks, 2001).

Assessment of language impairment in adults is mostly through aphasia tests such as the Western Aphasia Battery (Kertesz, 1982) and the Boston Diagnostic Aphasia Examination (Goodglass *et al.*, 2001). Tests that use a psycholinguistic model of processing include the Psycholinguistic Assessment of Language Processing in Aphasia (Kay *et al.*, 1997) and the Comprehensive Aphasia Test (Swinburn *et al.*, 2004). There are specific tests for single modalities such as reading (e.g. LaPointe & Horner, 1998) or specific linguistic constructs such as semantics (e.g. Kaplan *et al.*, 1983) syntax (e.g. Bishop, 2003) or pragmatics (e.g. Prutting & Kirschner, 1987). The effects on everyday life of the language impairment in adults may be measured by numerous assessments which include the American Speech Language Hearing Association Functional Assessment of Communication for Adults (Frattali *et al.*, 1995), the Communication Activities of Daily Living (Holland *et al.*, 1999), the Communicative Effectiveness Index (Lomas *et al.*, 1989) and the Stroke and Aphasia Quality of Life Scale-39 (Hilari *et al.*, 2003).

In children, language impairment is gauged through a myriad of assessments. Goldstein and Gierut (1998) list almost 100 language assessments for children and adolescents. One of the most popular assessments is the Clinical Evaluation of Language Fundamentals, 4th edition (Semel *et al.*, 2003). Goldstein and Gierut also note that there are few commercially available measures of activity limitation or participation restriction for children with language impairment. Clinicians mostly rely on observational coding and ecological inventories to report the effect of language impairment on communicative activity limitations.

Conclusion

This chapter has described voice, speech, fluency and language impairments from a speech and language therapist's perspective. Standardized assessments of the impairments, activity limitations and participation restrictions that form part of the communication disability have also been described. It is clear that while assessment at the impairment level is well developed, there remains much to be done to assess the consequences of voice, speech, fluency and language impairments in everyday life. Whether standardized assessment is the most appropriate method of evaluating everyday communication is debatable. Further research into the viability and acceptability of alternative methods using more ecological methods is required.

The assessment of contextual factors, both environmental and personal, that impact on an individual with a communication disability is also not well researched. Some speech and language therapists have developed services that seek to dismantle barriers to participation for people with a communication disability. In London, Connect – Communication Disability Network (www.ukconnect.org) is an excellent example of such a service. While appropriate evidence about the effectiveness of this service is yet to emerge, this is one of the exciting service developments in speech and language therapy. In an effort to develop appropriate communication assessment methods for evaluating their service, this group has pioneered methods that fully value the client and their opinions in the assessment process (see http://www.ukconnect.org/research/index.html?rate_scale). This is the new direction for communication assessment.

REFERENCES

Beukelman, D. R., Mathy, P. & Yorkston, K. (1998). Outcomes measurement in motor speech disorders. In C. M. Frattali (Ed.). *Measuring outcomes in speech-language pathology* (pp. 334–53). New York: Thieme.

Bishop, D. (2003). *Test for reception of grammar, Version 2*. London: Harcourt Assessment.

Blood, G. W. & Conture, E. G. (1998). Outcome measurement issues in fluency disorders. In C. M. Frattali (Ed.). *Measuring outcomes in speech-language pathology* (pp. 387–405). New York: Thieme.

Crystal, D. & Varley, R. (1993). *Introduction to Language Pathology* (3rd edn.). London: Whurr Publishers.

Dabul, B. (1979). *Apraxia battery for adults*. Tigard, OR: C. C. Publications.

Dent, H. (2001). Electropalatography: a tool for psycholinguistic therapy. In J. Stackhouse & B. Wells (Eds.). *Children's speech and literacy difficulties: identification and intervention*. London: Whurr Publishers.

Dodd, B. (1995). *The differential diagnosis and treatment of children with speech disorder*. London: Whurr.

Duchan, J. F. (2001). Impairment and social views of speech-language pathology: clinical practices re-examined. *Advances in Speech Language Pathology*, 3(1), 37–45.

Enderby, P. M. (1983). *Frenchay dysarthria assessment*. Austin, TX: Pro-Ed.

Enderby, P. M. (2000). Assessment and treatment of functional communication in dysarthria. In L. E. Worrall & C. M. Frattali (Eds.). *Neurogenic communication disorders: a functional approach* (pp. 247–61). New York: Thieme.

Frattali, C. M. (Ed.). (1998). *Measuring outcomes in speech-language pathology*. New York: Thieme.

Frattali, C., Thompson, C. K., Holland, A. L., Wohl, C. B. & Ferketic, M. K. (1995). *American speech-language-hearing association assessment of functional communication skills for adults*. Rockville, MD: American Speech-Language-Hearing Association.

Gillam, R. B., Marquardt, T. P. & Martin, F. N. (2000). *Communication sciences and disorders: from science to clinical practice*. San Diego, CA: Singular-Thomson Learning.

Goldman, R. & Fristoe, M. (1986). *Goldman–fristoe test of articulation*. Circle Pines, MN: American Guidance Service.

Goldstein, H. & Gierut, J. (1998). Outcomes measurement in child language and phonological disorders. In C. M. Frattali (Ed.). *Measuring outcomes In speech-language pathology* (pp. 406–37). New York: Thieme.

Goodglass, H., Kaplan, E. & Barresi, B. (2001). *Boston Diagnostic Aphasia Examination* (3rd edn.). Philadelphia, Lippincott: Willliams & Wilkins.

Haynes, W. O. & Pindzola, R. H. (1998) *Diagnosis and Evaluation in Speech Pathology* (5th edn.). Boston, MA: Allyn and Bacon.

Helm Estabrooks, N. (2001). *Cognitive Linguistic Quick Test*. San Antonio, TX: Psych Corp.

Hilari, K., Byng, S., Lamping, D. L. *et al.* (2003). Stroke and aphasia quality of life scale-39 (SAQOL-39): evaluation of acceptability, reliability, and validity. *Stroke*, **34**, 1944–50.

Holland, A. L., Frattali, C. & Fromm, D. (1999). *Communication Activities of Daily Living* (2nd edn.). Austin, TX: Pro-Ed.

Jacobson, B. H., Johnson, A., Grywalski, C. *et al.* (1997). The voice handicap index (VHI): development and validation. *American Journal of Speech Language Pathology*, **6**(3), 66–70.

Kaplan, E. F., Goodglass, H. & Weintraub, S. (1983). *The Boston Naming Test* (2nd edn.). Philadelphia: Lea and Febiger.

Kay, J., Lesser, R. & Coltheart, M. (1997). *Psycholinguistic assessments of language processing in aphasia*. Hove, UK: Psychology Press.

Kertesz, A. (1982). *Western aphasia battery*. New York: Grune and Stratton.

LaPointe, L. L. & Horner, J. (1998). *Reading Comprehension Battery for Aphasia* (2nd edn.). Austin, TX: Pro-Ed.

Laver, J. (1980). *The phonetic description of voice quality*. New York: Cambridge University Press.

Lomas, J., Pickard, L., Bester, S. *et al.* (1989). The communicative effectiveness index: development and psychometric evaluation of a functional communication measure for adult aphasia. *Journal of Speech and Hearing Disorders*, **54**, 113–24.

Ma, E. P. & Yiu, E. M. (2001). Voice activity and participation profile: assessing the impact of voice disorders on daily activities. *Journal of Speech, Language, and Hearing Research*, **44**(3), 511–24.

Oates, J. & Russell, A. (1998). Learning voice analysis using an interactive multi-media package: development and preliminary evaluation. *Journal of Voice*, **12**(4), 500–12.

Oates, J. & Russell, A. (2003). *A sound judgement*. Melbourne, Australia: La Trobe University.

Onslow, M. & Pachman, A. (Eds.). (1999). *The hand book of early shuttering intervention*. San Diego, CA: Singular Publishing Group.

Pindzola, R. H. (1987). *The voice assessment protocol for children and adults*. Austin, TX: Pro-Ed.

Prutting, C. A. & Kirchner, D. M. (1987). A clinical appraisal of the pragmatic aspects of language. *Journal of Speech and Hearing Disorders*, **52**(2), 105–19.

Ruscello, D. (Ed.). (2001). *Tests and measurement in speech-language pathology*. Boston, MA: Butterworth–Heinemann.

Rosenbek, J. C., LaPointe, L. L. & Wertz, R. T. (1989). *Aphasia: a clinical approach*. Austin, TX: Pro-Ed.

Semel, E., Wiig, H. & Secord, W. (2003). *Clinical Evaluation of Language fundamentals* (4th edn.). San Antonio, TX: Psych Corp.

St Louis, K. O. & Ruscello, D. M. (2000). *Oral Speech Mechanism Screening Examination (OSMSE)*. (Rev. ed.). Austin, TX: Pro-Ed.

Swinburn, K., Porter, G. & Howard, D. (2004). *The Comprehensive Aphasia Test*. Hove, UK: Psychology Press.

Threats, T. T. & Worrall, L. E. (2004). Classifying communication disability using the ICF. *Advances in Speech Language Pathology*, **6**(1), 53–62.

World Health Organization (2001). *International classification of functioning, disability and health*. Geneva: Author.

Worrall, L. (2001). The social approach: another new fashion in speech-language pathology? *Advances in Speech-Language Pathology*, **3**(1), 51–4.

Yaruss, J. S. (2002). Facing the challenge of treating stuttering in the schools. *Seminars in Speech and Language*, **23**(3), 153–7.

Coping assessment

Ellen A. Skinner

Portland State University

Introduction

When adversity strikes, when mental and physical functioning and health are at risk, humans 'fight back'. Humans come with and develop a set of adaptive processes that gives them the potential to fend off disaster, to reshape challenges and to transform stressful experiences into psychological growth. Coping describes some of these adaptive processes (Coelho *et al.*, 1974; White, 1974). Researchers agree that how people cope makes a material difference to the impact which stressful life events (including illnesses and chronic medical conditions) will have on them, both concurrently and long-term. However, the nature of these coping processes and how to assess them remain issues of hot contention.

Overview of the field

In early work, coping and defending were conceptualized as indicators of ego maturity; hence, coping was assessed by clinicians using extensive interviews (e.g. Haan, 1977; Valliant, 1986). As it became uncoupled from ego psychology, coping was seen as a manifestation of personality traits; hence, dispositional coping styles were assessed by questionnaires that tapped one or two dimensions of coping, such as sensitization versus repression. (For historical overviews, see Lazarus, 1993; Lazarus & Folkman, 1984; Murphy, 1974; Parker & Endler, 1996; Skinner, 2003; Snyder, 1999.)

Starting in the late 1970s, transactional, contextual and process-oriented views of coping appeared, which dominate the field today (Lazarus & Folkman, 1984; Moos & Billings, 1982;

Pearlin & Schooler, 1978). From this perspective, coping depicts the ways an individual deals with a specific stressor in a particular context, as the transaction unfolds over time. How people cope is shaped, not only by personal factors, but also by the stressors they are facing, the social resources available, and especially by their appraisals of the meaning of the stressful encounter (see 'Stress and health').

However, stressors (such as illnesses) are not single discrete traumatic events. Instead they represent a series of new, ongoing and cumulative demands (e.g. the disease's symptoms, course, treatment, side effects and prognosis, as well as social, emotional and physical consequences and reactions). Hence, when constructing patterns of coping, individuals are not only seeking effective actions, they must also defend high priority goals, manage emotions and maintain relationships. A repertoire of ways of coping is needed to deal with these sometimes contradictory demands. For example, in coping with a medical condition, it is important to acquire information in order to create an effective treatment plan. However, facing the facts can also be overwhelming. Strategies, such as minimization or focusing on the positive, are needed to keep distress within manageable levels (see 'Coping with chronic illness' and 'Coping with stressful medical procedures').

Moreover, coping is a dynamic process, consisting of episodes or bouts of dealing with these multiple different facets of stressors. Within a coping episode, ways of coping can change or cycle, depending on how the transaction unfolds. If a coping strategy proves to be ineffective, it may be replaced by an alternative strategy, or induce a fall into helplessness. Across episodes, coping itself evolves as new stressors are encountered, as appraisals are recalibrated and as resources are added or depleted. Coping depicts an active effortful struggle to continually (re)balance opposing demands, to recover from setbacks and to prepare for future challenges.

Overview of assessment

At present, it would be warranted to describe the state of assessment in the field of coping as chaotic and confusing. An enormous number of coping assessments, perhaps hundreds, are in use. Assessments have been created for adults, children, adolescents and the elderly. They measure ways of coping with stress in general, with stressful events in specific domains (such as work or health), with specific traumatic events (e.g. crime victimization or loss of a loved one), or they require participants to identify a single recent stressful event and describe how they actually coped with it. In a recent review, we identified over 100 assessments, tapping over 400 ways of coping (Skinner *et al.*, 2003). Researchers attempting to select an assessment of coping can justifiably feel bewildered, not only by the sheer number of measures available, but also by the wide range of strategies assessed and the heterogeneity of items used to assess them. Critiques of coping assessments abound (e.g. Beehr & McGrath, 1996; Cohen, 1987; Coyne & Gottlieb, 1996; Schwarzer & Schwarzer, 1996; Sommerfield, 1996; Stone *et al.*, 1992).

However, confusion in assessment is not based solely on operational issues. The solution is not as simple as comparing psychometrics and selecting the best questionnaire, checklist, interview,

or observational system. Confusion, to some extent, reflects a growing recognition of the complexity of the phenomena itself. The challenge to researchers is to capture coping in a way that does justice to its conceptual richness. Coping is not a simple construct. It does not reflect a single set of self-perceptions or a unidimensional group of behaviours. Coping is a complex higher-order organizational construct that reflects the functioning of a multi-level interactional system unfolding over time. That is why coping is so critical to human adaptation. That is also why it is so difficult to assess (see also 'Stress assessment').

Researchers creating (or selecting) a measurement scheme must grapple with three inter-related facets of coping: (1) coping encompasses a profile of changing ways of dealing with demands, current and future; (2) although coping describes an individual's actions, it emerges from a system and is diagnostic of the entire coping system, of which the individual is just a part; and (3) coping is a multi-level process that takes place across several time scales. Each of these facets is explained briefly and its implications for assessment considered. The presumption is that researchers and practitioners who understand the complex underlying nature of coping will be better prepared to capture and study it meaningfully in empirical investigations and to recognize and respond to it meaningfully in their clients and patients.

Coping as a profile

In order to be adaptive, a coping response must be suited to the demands it was created to deal with as well as the circumstances and resources available at the time. As a result, the number of potential coping responses in virtually unlimited. Researchers have dealt with this issue by grouping coping responses into 'ways' of coping; among the most common are problem-solving, avoidance, seeking social support, distraction, direct action, aggression, self-blame, escape, social withdrawal, religion, positive cognitive restructuring, emotional expression, information-seeking, acceptance, wishful thinking, rumination and worry, denial and focus on the positive.

Each of these ways of coping has a set of questionnaire items, a checklist entry and/or a set of coding criteria for open-ended interviews or observations. For example, problem-solving might be tapped by items like 'I made a plan of action and followed it', cognitive restructuring by items like 'I think about the good things I am learning from the situation', rumination by items like 'I can't stop thinking about how I am feeling', social withdrawal would include 'I avoided being with people' and catastrophizing would include 'I feel like I can't stand it any more'.

In terms of specific ways of coping, the best assessments in the field today have been constructed using confirmatory factor analysis. Researchers identify a set of items (usually five or six in number) tapping each target way of coping, and then examine the extent to which each set is unidimensional and can be distinguished from each other set. Using this strategy, researchers have created unidimensional, reliable (internally consistent) and distinct indicators of a wide variety of ways of coping. These represent state-of-the-art assessments.

However, no encounter with stress can be dealt with by a single way of coping. Also, although there is consensus on the best strategies for measuring single ways of coping, there is no agreement about how many (and which) strategies should be included in comprehensive assessments of coping. In our review of systems for classifying ways of coping, we note that, of the 100 schemes identified, no two included the same set of ways of coping: some included as few as 2 or 3, others tapped 20 to 30 (Skinner *et al.*, 2003). The problem is widespread disagreement over what constitute core or central ways of coping.

Several distinctions have been suggested as higher-order categories to encompass multiple ways of coping (for a complete list see Rudolph *et al.*, 1995 or Skinner *et al.*, 2003). The most common are 'approach versus avoidance' and 'problem- versus emotion-focused' coping. Despite the contributions both of these distinctions have made to the field, neither is useful as a higher-order category of coping (Skinner *et al.*, 2003). Approach and avoidance are not good higher-order categories because both include potentially adaptive and maladaptive ways of coping. Emotion-focused and problem-focused coping are not good higher-order categories because all ways of coping have implications for both problem-solving and emotional reactions (Lazarus & Folkman, 1984).

Families of coping

In recent years, researchers have turned to the notion of higher-order families of ways of coping to organize the hundreds of ways of coping identified in previous research (Skinner *et al.*, 2003). A family includes a variety of ways of coping that all serve the same functions in dealing with stress. For example, if problem-solving is considered part of a family, it could include other ways of coping that serve the same functions, such as strategizing, planning, repair, direct attempts, instrumental action and decision-making.

We have identified a dozen core families of coping based on action types (see Table 1; Skinner *et al.*, 2003). Although there is not complete consensus that these are the core categories of coping, several are not particularly controversial, such as problem-solving, seeking support and escape/avoidance. Some represent the dominant ways of coping in specific domains, for example, information-seeking in the health domain, and negotiation in dealing with interpersonal stressors. Some reflect reactions to stress that have been studied extensively outside the field of coping, such as helplessness (Seligman, 1975) and dependency (M.M. Baltes, 1997).

Several reflect cutting edge ideas in the field of coping. For example, ways of coping have been identified that serve to direct attention away from the distressing features of a situation and toward more positive thoughts and activities. Referred to as accommodation (Brandtstädter & Renner, 1990) or secondary control coping, this family includes positive thinking, cognitive restructuring, focus on the positive and distraction. It is structurally distinct from escape (Ayers *et al.*, 1996) and, unlike denial, does not interfere with effective action.

Another family includes ways of coping that focus attention toward the negative features of a stressful situation. The best understood way of coping in this family is rumination (Nolen-Hoeksema, 1998), a risk factor for depression. Sometimes referred to as submission, surrender, or involuntary engagement, this family also includes

ways of coping such as perseveration and intrusive thoughts. Unlike constructive expression of emotions, however, these ways of coping exacerbate distress and interfere with problem-solving.

Families of coping as adaptive processes

In order to understand their functions in adapting to stress, these twelve families can be organized as three sets of four tightly connected pairs and their opposites, as depicted in Table 1. In one set, problem solving is closely connected with information-seeking and these are considered to be opposites of helplessness and escape. These four families help people coordinate their actions with the contingencies in the environment in order to produce desired or prevent undesired outcomes. Problem solving identifies effective actions and information seeking locates new contingencies.

A second set of four families is organised around support seeking, which is considered to be tightly connected to self-reliance, and the opposites of delegation and social isolation. These four families help people coordinate their reliance on others with the social resources that are available in order to stay connected to others. Support seeking allows the individual to access social resources whereas self-reliance preserves resources for later use and protects others from the burdens of stress.

The third set of four families is organized around negotiation, which is closely connected to accommodation, and the opposites of surrender and opposition. These families help people coordinate their preferences with available options in order to reach high priority goals. Accommodation allows an individual to adjust to the options that are currently available and negotiation may lead to the creation of more options.

Comprehensive coping profiles

The idea of twelve families of coping linked to higher-order adaptive processes provides a framework for assessment. It implies that any measure of coping, no matter the domain, developmental level, or time frame, should consider including ways of coping from each family. Although, as mentioned previously, some families may be more commonly studied in conjunction with particular stressors, this framework allows researchers to consider the use of less common strategies, such as information seeking for interpersonal problems (e.g. 'I asked my friend why she got so mad at me') or the use of negotiation with medical conditions (e.g. 'I decided that even if I couldn't walk, I could still get around in a wheelchair').

The specific ways of coping selected from each family will depend on their appropriateness for the target event and age group. For example, young children accommodate to unchangeable negative events using behavioural distraction whereas older children can use cognitive strategies, such as focus on the positive. Moreover, an indicator of 'stressfulness' can be drawn from the idea of the twelve families. An event would be more stressful to the extent that it eliminates an entire family of coping from use. So, for example, certain medical conditions are more stressful because little is known about their cause or treatment (eliminating information-seeking).

Most importantly, this framework makes clear the tenability of the notion of coping profiles, meaning that coping cannot be described by a single dimension, no matter how important, but instead should

Table 1. Families of coping organized according to their adaptive processes

Family of Coping	Family function in adaptive process	Adaptive process	Also implicated
Problem-solving Strategizing Instrumental action Planning	Adjust actions to be effective	Coordinate actions and contingencies in the environment	Watch and learn Mastery Efficacy
Information-Seeking Reading Observation Asking others	Find additional contingencies		Curiosity Interest
Helplessness Confusion Cognitive interference Cognitive exhaustion	Find limits of actions		Guilt Helplessness
Escape Cognitive avoidance Behavioural avoidance Denial Wishful thinking	Escape non-contingent environment		Drop and roll Flight Fear
Self-reliance Emotion regulation Behaviour regulation Emotional expression Emotion approach	Protect available social resources	Coordinate reliance and social resources available	Tend and befriend Pride
Support Seeking Contact seeking Comfort seeking Instrumental aid Spiritual support	Use available social resources		Proximity-seeking Yearning Other alliance
Delegation Maladaptive help-seeking Complaining Whining Self-pity	Find limits of resources		Self-pity Shame
Isolation Social withdrawal Concealment Avoiding others	Withdraw from unsupportive context		Duck and cover Freeze Sadness
Accommodation Distraction Cognitive restructuring* Minimization Acceptance	Flexibly adjust preferences to options	Coordinate preferences and available options	Pick and choose Secondary control
Negotiation Bargaining Persuasion Priority-setting	Find new options		Compromise
Submission Rumination Rigid perseveration Intrusive thoughts	Give up preferences		Disgust Rigid perseverance
Opposition Other-blame Projection Aggression	Remove constraints		Stand and fight Anger Defiance

be characterized by a range of ways of coping, which can best be organized according to these twelve families. The use of these twelve families allows researchers to select meaningfully from among the hundreds of ways of coping which they encompass, but also to consider how the families work together with each other (as synergistically positive or as antagonistic opposites) and how they function in service of higher-order adaptive processes.

Coping as a system

Researchers are slowly coming to grips with the notion that coping reflects the functioning of an entire system. The simplest implication of this view is that it is not possible to understand coping by looking only at coping itself. Coping actions emerge from a coping system, the elements of which have been pretty well identified. They include the coping individual as well as the stressor, the person's appraisals, the personal and social resources and liabilities in the situation and the history of outcomes of previous coping efforts.

Because ways of coping emerge from (and are diagnostic of) this entire system, there has been controversy about how to interpret their meaning. When coping was considered a manifestation of ego processes or of personality, maladaptive coping indicated an immature person or a neurotic personality. As coping came to be seen as situation-specific, no ways of coping could be considered 'maladaptive': they were all suited to their particular demands and contexts.

However, considering coping as a system reveals a third alternative. On the one hand, some ways of coping are maladaptive, as recognized by any parent, teacher, spouse, or friend. These are ways of coping, such as helplessness, rumination, or exploding, which are detrimental in the long run, or developmentally maladaptive, because they weaken the coping system, robbing it of social and personal resources and consolidating liabilities, such as low self-efficacy or exhausted friends. On the other hand, these are not 'wrong' ways of coping or individual flaws; instead they are the result of a coping system that is overwhelmed. This can happen when personal vulnerabilities are high, when social resources are low, or when the stressor is simply too great.

If formal or informal interventions are to be effective in improving coping, then information about the entire coping system must be assessed (Skinner & Edge, 1998). Parents or doctors who see individuals falling into helplessness or stuck in cycles of rumination, can recognize the problem, but without understanding the rest of the system (including the range of stressors, other demands, the individual's appraisals and his or her social and personal resources and liabilities), it is not possible to make changes to the system that will allow the person to cope more adaptively. Simply telling someone to 'pull themselves together' or to 'stop stewing about it' can place additional burdens (e.g. self-regulatory demands or self-blame) on an already overtaxed system.

Coping as a multi-level process

Coping takes place on many levels and over many time scales (Beehr & McGrath, 1996). When dealing with complex long-term demands

(such as a chronic illness or a child who is emotionally disturbed), people may eventually develop a network of coping that incorporates all these levels. At the highest level, they may work out an overall structure for handling the demands, a kind of proactive coping (Aspinwall & Taylor, 1997), such as a plan of diet, medication, exercise and relaxation for a chronic illness, or a plan of individualized education, homework and sleep schedules for an emotionally disturbed child. At the next level, they may develop and practice routines for dealing with reoccurring stressors (e.g. flare-ups or outbursts), allowing them to be handled with minimum effort and attention (Coyne & Gottlieb, 1996).

They may accrue a buffer of time, credit, or social support to aid them in dealing with crises (Taylor et al., 2000). They may also discover ways of coping that help them recover from failures and setbacks (Heckhausen & Schulz, 1995). Finally, they can work toward a pattern of daily coping that allows them to monitor global conditions, but to focus awareness away from the negative features of the situation and onto its genuine positive aspects (Folkman & Moskowitz, 2000).

To capture these holistic multilevel processes of coping, cutting edge research has turned (back) to the use of detailed open-ended interviews (e.g. Folkman, 1997; Murphy & Moriarity, 1976). As stated by Moos, more than 30 years ago:

Full understanding can only come with detailed intensive study, either through interviews or through naturalistic observations of the actual day-to-day processes by which adaptation occurs. (Moos, 1974, p. 335)

Moreover, reflecting the idea that coping is a changing profile of responses to multiple varying stressors over time, new methods for assessment have been developed in which participants report their coping every day, or even multiple times a day, using a daily diary format (e.g. Stone & Neale, 1984; Tennen et al., 2000). These methods, if they are expanded to tap the entire coping system, promise assessments that can capture the dynamics of coping.

When intervening into a coping system, practitioners should consider all these levels. For example, early in the course of treatment, it might be necessary to gather information about the condition (e.g. using daily diaries) in order to determine the factors that trigger a flare-up, even though focusing on the condition may increase distress. After structures have been set up, coping strategies can be promoted that direct attention away from the condition and toward positive experiences. It should be noted that the time frame for creating such an adaptive network of coping might be months or even years.

Conclusion

From their entry into the field of psychology, conceptualizations of coping as an adaptive process have held the promise of contributing to our understanding of how people are able to deal with adversity and why they sometimes succumb to its pressures. As assessments become more organized around families of coping which are connected to adaptive processes and begin to reflect coping as a profile of responses that emerge from an entire system of coping that itself unfolds on multiple levels and time scales, research on coping may better fulfil that promise.

Aspinwall, L. G. & Taylor, S. E. (1997). A stitch in time: self-regulation and proactive coping. *Psychological Bulletin, 121*, 417–36.

Ayers, T. S., Sandler, I. N., West, S. G. & Roosa, M. W. (1996). A dispositional and situational assessment of children's coping: testing alternative models of coping. *Journal of Personality, 64*, 923–58.

Baltes, M. M. (1997). *The many faces of dependency.* New York: Cambridge University Press.

Beehr, T. A. & McGrath, J. E. (1996). The methodology of research on coping: conceptual, strategic, and operational-level issues. In M. Zeidner & N. S. Endler (Eds.). *Handbook of coping: theory, research, applications* (pp. 65–82). New York: Wiley.

Brandtstädter, J. & Renner, G. (1990). Tenacious goal pursuit and flexible goal adjustment: explication and age-related analysis of assimilative and accommodative strategies of coping. *Psychology and Aging, 5*(1), 58–67.

Coelho, G. V., Hamburg, D. A. & Adams, J. E. (Eds.). (1974). *Coping and adaptation.* New York: Basic Books.

Cohen, F. (1987). Measurement of coping. In S. V. Kasl & C. L. Cooper (Eds.). *Stress and health: issues in research methodology* (pp. 283–305). New York: Wiley.

Coyne, J. C. & Gottlieb, B. H. (1996). The mismeasure of coping by checklist. *Journal of Personality, 64*, 959–91.

Folkman, S. (1997). Using bereavement narratives to predict well-being in gay men whose partners died of AIDS: four theoretical perspectives. *Journal of Personality and Social Psychology, 72*, 851–4.

Folkman, S. & Moskowitz, J. T. (2000). Positive affect and the other side of coping. *American Psychologist, 55*, 647–54.

Haan, N. (1977). *Coping and defending: processes of self-environment organization.* New York: Academic Press.

Heckhausen, J. & Schulz, R. (1995). A life-span theory of control. *Psychological Review, 102*, 284–304.

Lazarus, R. (1993). Coping theory and research: past, present, and future. *Psychosomatic Medicine, 55*, 234–47.

Lazarus, R. S. (2000). Toward better research on stress and coping. *American Psychologist, 55*, 665–73.

Lazarus, R. S. & Folkman, S. (1984). *Stress, appraisal, and coping.* New York: Springer.

Moos, R. H. (1974). Psychological techniques in the assessment of adaptive behavior. In G. V. Coelho, D. A. Hamburg & J. E. Adams (Eds.). *Coping and adaptation* (pp. 334–99). New York: Basic Books.

Moos, R. H. & Billings, A. G. (1982). Conceptualizing and measuring coping resources and coping processes. In L. Goldberger & S. Breznitz (Eds.). *Handbook of stress: theoretical and clinical aspects* (pp. 212–30). New York: Free Press.

Murphy, L. B. (1974). Coping, vulnerability, and resilience in childhood. In G. V. Coelho, D. A. Hamburg & J. E. Adams (Eds.). *Coping and adaptation* (pp. 47–68). New York: Basic Books.

Murphy, L. & Moriarity, A. (1976). *Vulnerability, coping, and growth: from infancy to adolescence.* New Haven: Yale University Press.

Nolen-Hoeksma, S. (1998). Ruminative coping with depression. In J. Heckhausen & C. S. Dweck (Eds.). *Motivation and self-regulation across the life span* (pp. 237–56). Cambridge, UK: Cambridge University Press.

Parker, J. A. & Endler, N. S. (1996). Coping and defense: a historical overview. In M. Zeidner & N. S. Endler (Eds.). *Handbook of coping* (pp. 3–23). New York: Wiley.

Pearlin, L. I. & Schooler, C. (1978). The structure of coping. *Journal of Health and Social Behavior, 19*, 2–21.

Ptacek, J. T., Smith, R. E., Espe, K. & Rafferty, B. (1994). Limited correspondence between daily coping reports and retrospective coping recall. *Psychological Assessment, 6*, 41–9.

Roth, S. & Cohen, L. (1986). Approach, avoidance, and coping with stress. *American Psychologist, 41*, 813–19.

Rudolph, K. D., Dennig, M. D. & Weisz, J. R. (1995). Determinants and consequences of children's coping in the medical setting: conceptualization, review, and critique. *Psychological Bulletin, 118*, 328–57.

Schwarzer, R. & Schwarzer, C. (1996). A critical survey of coping instruments. In M. Zeidner & N. S. Endler (Eds.), *Handbook of coping: theory, research, applications* (pp. 107–32). New York: Wiley.

Seligman, M. E. P. (1975). *Helplessness: on depression, development, and death.* San Francisco: Freeman.

Skinner, E. A. (2003). Coping across the lifespan. In N. J. Smelser & P. B. Baltes (Eds.-in-Chief), N. Eisenberg (Vol. Ed.). *International encyclopedia of the social and behavioral sciences.* Elsevier: Oxford, UK.

Skinner, E. A. & Edge, K. (1998). Reflections on coping and development across the lifespan. *International Journal of Behavioral Development, 22*, 357–66.

Skinner, E., Edge, K., Altman, J. *et al.* (2003). Searching for the structure of coping: a review and critique of category systems for classifying ways of coping. *Psychological Bulletin, 129*, 216–69.

Snyder, C. R. (Ed.). (1999). *Coping: the psychology of what works.* New York: Oxford University Press.

Sommerfield, M. R. (1996). On the use of checklist measures of coping in studies of adaptation to cancer. *Journal of Psychosocial Oncology, 14*, 21–40.

Stone, A. A. & Neale, J. M. (1984). New measure of daily coping: development and preliminary results. *Journal of Personality and Social Psychology, 46*, 892–906.

Stone, A. A., Greenburg, M. A., Kennedy-Moore, E. & Newman, M. G. (1991). Self-report, situation-specific coping questionnaires: what are they measuring? *Journal of Personality and Social Psychology, 61*(4), 648–58.

Stone, A. A., Kennedy-Moore, E., & Newman, M. G., Greenburg, M. A. & Neale, J. M. (1992). Conceptual and methodological issues in current coping assessments. In B. Carpenter (Ed.). *Personal coping: theory, research, and application* (pp. 15–29). Westport, CT: Praeger.

Taylor, S. E., Klein, L. C., Lewis, B. P. *et al.* (2000). Biobehavioral responses to stress in females: tend-and-befriend, not fight-or-flight. *Psychological Review, 107*, 411–29.

Tennen, H., Affleck, G., Armeli, S. & Carney, M. A. (2000). A daily process approach to coping: linking theory, research, and practice. *American Psychologist, 55*, 626–36.

Valliant, G. E. (1986). *Empirical studies of ego mechanisms of defense.* Washington, DC: American Psychiatric Association.

White, R. W. (1974). Strategies of adaptation: an attempt at systematic description. In G. V. Coelho, D. A. Hamburg & J. E. Adams (Eds.). *Coping and adaptation* (pp. 47–68). New York: Basic Books.

Diagnostic interviews and clinical practice

Richard Rogers[1] and Peggilee Wupperman[2]

[1]University of North Texas
[2]University of Washington

Traditional assessments of mental disorders provide highly individualistic evaluations of the patients' presenting problems, recent stressors and salient symptoms. Such individualized assessments, while rich in detail, lack the necessary standardization for reliable diagnoses. As a result, traditional assessments are often marred by inaccuracies, most notably in missed diagnoses and misdiagnoses (Rogers, 2003). To improve diagnostic reliability, healthcare professionals should augment traditional evaluations with more standardized assessments that include structured interviews. Following a review of current diagnostic predicaments, the chapter examines the role of structured interviews in improving clinical practice.

Diagnostic predicaments

The assessment of mental disorders within the primary care system has not kept pace with diagnostic advances. As a result, diagnoses are often a hit-or-miss proposition. Consider for the moment the comparatively straightforward diagnosis of major depression. Tiemens et al. (1999) found the majority of patients with major depression went undiagnosed and untreated by primary care physicians. This finding is very consistent. Lowe et al. (2004) found that 60% of cases with major depression were missed diagnoses in primary health care. Even when the diagnosis was broadened to include any depressive disorder, the accuracy did not improve (i.e. 59% missed diagnoses). Misdiagnosis of major depression was also common. When these physicians did diagnose major depression, they were inaccurate in 62% of the cases. These worrisome results extend beyond major depression to a range of Axis I disorders (see Christensen et al., 2003; Spitzer et al., 1994).

Many healthcare professionals take comfort in the availability and expertize of mental health specialists. Research data suggest this may be a false comfort. When traditional psychiatric evaluations are compared with standardized assessments, several important findings are suggested. First and foremost, traditional evaluations typically are not comprehensive; they often miss co-morbidity, overlooking additional Axis I and Axis II disorders (see Zimmerman & Mattia, 1999). Probably because of comorbidity, Shear et al. (2000) found clinicians in outpatient practice overlooked most anxiety disorders (94.7%). Second, traditional evaluations tend to neglect uncommon diagnoses. In reviewing 500 traditional evaluations, Zimmerman and Mattia (1999) found that body dysmorphic and somatoform disorders were almost never diagnosed; these results are markedly discrepant with 500 standardized assessments from the same setting.

The subjectivity of traditional evaluations makes them susceptible to biases. North et al. (1997) studied diagnoses in an outpatient care programme for homeless persons. We interpret their results as suggesting the possibility of diagnostic bias. Their traditional evaluations appeared to over-diagnose antisocial personality disorder by 100% and under-diagnose depression by 60%. Such biases may also extend to cultural issues. As carefully reviewed by Baker and Bell (1999), clinicians tend to overdiagnose schizophrenia and under-diagnose depression in African American patients. While not eliminating biases, systematic assessments ensure that standardized questions and clinical ratings are applied methodically, irrespective of circumstances or cultural background.

Overview of structured interviews

Healthcare professionals must grapple with diagnostic predicaments outlined above. Treatment of mental disorders cannot be optimally effective without accurate multiaxial diagnoses. Fortunately, structured interviews can provide the verifiable reliability and diagnostic accuracy required for modern healthcare practices. This section begins with a simple overview of terminology.

The term, 'structured interview', applies to all standardized interviews that provide verbatim clinical inquiries and quantify responses based on explicitly delineated criteria. Structured interviews are subdivided into 'fully-structured' and 'semi-structured' formats (Rogers, 2003). Fully-structured interviews standardize all inquiries and do not permit clinician-initiated probes. In contrast, most standardized interviews are semi-structured: clinicians are obliged to ask verbatim questions and probes. In occasional cases of ambiguity, they augment these verbatim inquiries with their own individualized (i.e. non-standard) questions. Semi-structured interviews sacrifice a small degree of standardization in order to achieve greater clarification of clinical data.

What can be accomplished with structured interviews? In an enumerated format, we outline their five chief advantages:

1. *Comprehensiveness.* Structured interviews ensure that clinical inquiries provide complete coverage of diagnoses or other clinical constructs. For example, Psychopathy Checklist-Revised

(PCL-R; Hare, 2003) guarantees that major elements of psychopathy are systematically evaluated.

2. *Standardization.* The hallmark of structured interviews is the systematization of clinical inquiries and concomitant ratings. In particular, variations in the recording of valuable clinical data are minimized. This uniformity of data allows practitioners to make direct comparisons needed in documenting the course of the disorder or response to specific treatments. For example, the Schedule of Affective Disorders and Schizophrenia (SADS; Spitzer & Endicott, 1978a) anchors gradations of symptom severity with specific criteria.

3. *Level of measurement.* Traditional interviews yield idiosyncratic information at the nominal (i.e. presence or absence) level of measurement. In contrast, the carefully constructed ratings of structured interviews typically provide an ordinal (i.e. greater or lesser severity) level of measurement that reliably distinguishes levels of impairment. For example, the Structured Interview for DSM-IV Personality Disorders (SIDP-IV; Pfohl *et al.*, 1995) provides four levels for Axis II symptoms: (1) not present, (2) sub-threshold (i.e. some but insufficient evidence of the trait), (3) present and (4) strongly present (i.e. causing impairment or subjective distress).

4. *Non-pejorative enquiries.* Clinicians must exercise considerable sensitivity and professional judgement when asking patients with mental disorders to disclose the nature of their symptoms and impairment. Structured interviews are tested clinically, if not empirically, to ensure that their inquiries do not offend patients but promote mutual respect and self-disclosure. For example, the SIDP-IV asks indirect questions about social relationships rather than intrusive probes into avoidant and borderline characteristics.

5. *Reliability.* Empirically validated assessment methods require a formal investigation of reliability (i.e. the consistency of observations across time and different clinicians). Structured interviews can be rigorously tested to ensure they have sufficient reliability for the assessment of diagnoses and salient symptoms. Rogers (2001) systematically reviewed reliability data for Axis I and Axis II structured interviews.

Seminal research by Ward and his colleagues offers insights into the advantages of structured interviews. In examining diagnostic disagreements, they found that most discrepancies (62.5%) occurred among experienced psychiatrists because they used different standards for evaluating symptoms of mental disorders. They found that most of the remaining disagreements (32.5%) resulted from differences in clinical inquiries used by individual psychiatrists. Structured interviews with standardized ratings seek to minimize differences based on both clinical inquiries and diagnostic criteria.

Despite these advantages, structured interviews can be misused in health care settings. The most common risk is a routinization of the assessment, whereby clinicians become bound to the protocol and insensitive to human elements of the interactive process. With proper training, this risk is easily avoidable. The goal of structured interviews is a natural and unforced flow of clinical inquiries. With practice, the formal structure should become unobtrusive. While faithful to the standardization, clinicians can remain empathetic and genuinely interested in the patient's responses.

Diagnostic models and healthcare practice

Modern healthcare faces formidable challenges as many public and private agencies struggle with cost containment and even the unspoken rationing of services. To succeed, diagnostic interviews must take into account these uninviting realities. Therefore, we propose two diagnostic approaches. First, the 'augmented clinical practice' essentially re-tools the clinical assessment but requires a minimum expenditure of professional resources. Second, the 'multiaxial-diagnostic model' provides a sophisticated assessment of Axis I and Axis II disorders. Each model is introduced and examined separately.

Augmented clinical practice

Many healthcare facilities have only limited access to highly trained psychologists and psychiatrists. Despite high patient loads, primary care settings want to avoid the current diagnostic predicaments. For mental disorders, current data suggest that missed diagnoses and misdiagnoses significantly outnumber accurate diagnoses in primary care practices. When faced with high demand and limited resources, we recommend the augmented clinical practice approach.

The overriding goal of augmented clinical practice is simply to maximize diagnostic accuracy for common Axis I disorders. Two structured interviews are clinically useful for this endeavour: the Mini International Neuropsychiatic Interview (MINI; Sheehan *et al.*, 1997) and the SADS-Change Version (SADS-C; Spitzer & Endicott, 1978b). Each interview has a separate goal: the MINI targets common Axis I disorders, while the SADS-C focuses on salient symptoms which often require clinical intervention.

The MINI

The MINI (Sheehan *et al.*, 1997) is a brief Axis I interview, approximately 15 minutes in length which is conducted by healthcare staff who need only modest training in mental disorders. Despite its brevity, the MINI provides surprisingly good coverage of common Axis I disorders. It addresses the following diagnostic categories: (a) mood disorders (i.e. major depression, dysthymia and mania), (b) anxiety disorders (i.e. panic disorder, agoraphobia, social phobia, simple phobia, generalized anxiety disorder, obsessive–compulsive disorder and post-traumatic stress disorder), (c) psychotic disorders (i.e. general screen but no specific diagnoses), (d) eating disorders (i.e. anorexia and bulimia nervosa) and (e) substance abuse disorders (i.e. alcohol abuse, alcohol dependence, drug abuse and drug dependence).

Validation research (see Sheehan *et al.*, 1998) has examined its results in relationship to both the DSM-IV and ICD-10 using the Structured Clinical Interview for DSM-IV Disorders (SCID) and the Composite International Diagnostic Interview (CIDI). Research demonstrates a moderately high agreement with more extensive structured interviews; median kappas were 0.67 with SCID-based diagnoses and 0.63 with CIDI-based diagnoses.

The MINI was fully intended to be an international measure, easily accessible to healthcare professionals. It was simultaneously

Table 1. An overview of commonly-used Axis I and Axis II interviews

Feature	Axis I structured interviews			Axis II structured interviews		
	SADS	SCID	CIDI	SIDP-IV	IPDE	SCID-II
DSM-IV	Partial	Yes	Yes	Yes	Yes	Yes
ICD-10	No	No	Yes	No	Yes	No
Diagnostic reliability	Excellent	Good	Good	Sufficient	Good	Sufficient
Gradations of symptoms	3 to 6	2 or 3	2	4	3	3
Level of training	High	Moderate	Moderate	Moderate	Moderate	Low
International research	Limited	Limited	Extensive	Limited	Extensive	Limited

validated in English and French. Further efforts are underway to provide translations in 30 different languages. As an important feature for cost containment, the MINI is available free of charge and can be downloaded from the internet at http://www.medical-outcomes.com.

The MINI appears to be an ideal measure for minimising missed diagnoses and misdiagnoses. When potential diagnoses are identified, either a mental health specialist or physician knowledgeable in mental disorders should confirm the diagnosis and recommend the treatment regimen.

The SADS-C

The SADS-C (Spitzer & Endicott, 1978b) addresses 36 key symptoms of mental disorders which are often the focus of clinical intervention. While evaluating cardinal symptoms of mood, anxiety and psychotic disorders, the SADS-C does not provide sufficient coverage for formal diagnoses. Instead, it targets these salient symptoms and alerts healthcare professionals to potential diagnoses.

The SADS-C has impressive reliability and validity (Rogers et al., 2003). With a moderate level of training, healthcare staff can learn to administer this brief measure (10–20 minutes) and achieve high levels of reliability for individual symptoms and sub-scales. Importantly, research (see Rogers, 2001) has demonstrated the usefulness of the SADS-C to evaluate critical changes in clinical status. Therefore, the SADS-C can provide a vital role in primary health care in relapse prevention and identifying new episodes of mental disorders.

Multiaxial-diagnostic model

The sophisticated assessment of mental disorders requires a systematic evaluation of Axis I and Axis II diagnoses. Some healthcare settings have the professional resources to place a premium on accurate diagnoses, including complex differential diagnoses. Towards this goal, the multiaxial-diagnostic model systematically evaluates disorders, syndromes and salient symptoms affecting the patients' functioning.

Rogers (2001) provides a comprehensive examination of Axis I and Axis II interviews, including their clinical applications and validation. This chapter selects three Axis I and three Axis II interviews

that are widely used in clinical practice. It distills information on their development and updates data on their validation. The three Axis I interviews include the SADS (Spitzer & Endicott, 1978a), the Structured Clinical Interview for DSM-IV Disorders (SCID; First et al., 1997, 2002), and the Composite International Diagnostic Interview (CIDI; World Health Organization, 1997). The three Axis II interviews are comprised of the SIDP-IV (Pfohl et al., 1995), the International Personality Disorder Examination (IPDE; Loranger, 1999) and the Structured Clinical Interview for DSM-IV Axis II Personality Disorders (SCID-II; First et al., 1994). These six structured interviews provide healthcare professionals with an array of well-validated diagnostic measures which are clinically applicable to a broad range of settings.

Axis I interviews vary substantially in their diagnostic coverage (see Table 1). For example, the SADS opted for an in-depth examination of mood and psychotic disorders addressing symptoms and associated features in considerable detail. In contrast, the SCID has chosen a much broader coverage of DSM-IV disorders but sacrificed symptom severity and associated features. Finally, the CIDI has the broadest coverage but focuses primarily on the presence and absence of Axis I symptoms.

Table 1 summarizes the salient features of Axis I and Axis II interviews. This table and the following discussion should assist health care professionals in identifying the appropriate structured interviews for their setting and populations. We begin with a review of the SADS, a classic measure with contemporary applications.

The SADS

The SADS is an extensive semi-structured Axis I interview that relies heavily on the training of interviewers in order to achieve impressive inter-rater and test-retest reliabilities. The SADS is distinguished from other Axis I interviews by the natural flow of its questions and its sophisticated rating of symptom severity. As a result, interviewers need advanced training in diagnostic interviews and supervized experience with the SADS.

The SADS focuses on depth rather than breadth. In addition to inclusion criteria, it evaluates clinical characteristics and associated features of mood and psychotic disorders. As a result, it provides rich description of the patient's functioning rather than a checklist format found with some Axis I interviews.

The SADS is especially suited for assessing Axis I symptomatology and measuring its severity. The SADS should be given strong consideration in clinical settings where it is hoped that hope to achieve the following objectives:

- *Clinical management of critical symptoms.* In conjunction with the SADS-C, the SADS can measure the severity of symptoms and their changes in severity across time.
- *Diagnoses for discrete episodes.* The SADS allow the experienced interviewer to focus on current and past episodes in reliably establishing the course of specific disorders.
- *Extensive use in medical settings.* Clinical research has demonstrated the usefulness of the SADS in assessing co-morbidity and mental disorders in medical populations (Rogers *et al.*, 2003).
- *Reliability on both diagnostic and symptom levels.* For specialized applications in healthcare settings, it is imperative to assess diagnoses and concomitant symptoms with a high level of reliability. The SADS has unprecedented reliability (Rogers, 2001). Even for individual symptoms, the median intra-class coefficients tend to exceed 0.70. For current diagnoses, most studies (see Rogers, 2001) produce exceptional inter-rater reliabilities (i.e. >0.85 for median kappas or ICCs).

The SADS does have several drawbacks. Internationally, few studies have formally investigated the effects of language and cultural issues on its validity. In addition, the SADS does not correspond perfectly with DSM-IV; SADS-based diagnoses will occasionally need to be augmented with several additional inquiries to match DSM-IV inclusion criteria.

The SCID

The SCID was developed expressly for the evaluation of DSM symptoms and disorders. With an emphasis on diagnostic simplicity, its questions often parallel the inclusion criteria for DSM-IV. With an emphasis on efficiency, many screening questions are used to reduce the administration time. As a result, the SCID provides comprehensive coverage of common Axis I diagnoses. By design, however, it de-emphasizes the assessment of individual symptoms and does not provide gradations of symptom severity.

The SCID should be selected in health care settings that place a premium on broad diagnostic coverage and reliability. The SCID requires comparatively less training than the SADS and conveniently addresses specific diagnoses in a sequential manner. Several versions of the SCID are available. A major limitation of the current SCID-Clinical Version (SCID-CV) is the absence of a subclinical level; interviewers are forced to rate symptoms as present or absent.

The classic reliability study by Williams, Gibbon *et al.* (1992) produced worrisome results for the SCID including highly variable agreement on such common disorders as depression and substance abuse. Fortunately, more recent research (e.g. Zimmerman & Mattia, 1999) has produced much more consistent and positive results. Because it de-emphasizes symptoms, the SCID should not be used to establish symptom reliability.

Researchers have an exceptional opportunity to utilize an expanded SCID, namely the SCID-I Research Version (SCID-RV; First *et al.*, 2002), which utilizes a sub-clinical gradation and offers comprehensive diagnostic coverage. For example, the SCID-RV provides extensive coverage of somatoform disorders, including somatisation and body dysmorphic disorders. Importantly, the SCID-RV can be tailored to individual studies. For a reasonable charge, it is available on disk and can even be sent as an email attachment (website: http://www.scid4.org/orderfrm.htm). Naturally, researchers will need to establish diagnostic reliability for their tailored versions of the SCID-RV.

In summary, the SCID-CV is a well validated efficient interview that can be effectively used in both mental health and medical settings. It efficiently provides broad diagnostic coverage with good reliability. Its research counterpart, the SCID-RV, provides broader diagnostic coverage and more refined clinical ratings.

The CIDI

The CIDI is a composite Axis I interview that combines all the items from the Diagnostic Interview Schedule (DIS; Robins *et al.*, 1989) with selected items from the Present State Examination (PSE; Wing *et al.*, 1998). This exhaustive measure evaluates Axis I disorders for both DSM and ICD diagnoses. With its cross-cultural perspective, the CIDI was translated into more than a dozen languages.

Establishment of the CIDI reliability and validity is complicated by (a) its complex array of symptom questions and ratings, (b) use of distinct versions with different content, (c) use of two diagnostic systems (DSM and ICD) and (d) many different language translations. Nevertheless, studies of diagnostic reliability have produced mixed (Rogers, 2001) to very positive results (see Wittchen, 1994). For validity studies, the CIDI relies heavily on DIS research with moderately good convergence.

The CIDI appears to be a good choice as an Axis I interview in countries where both DSM and ICD systems are used. It provides a functional bridge across diagnostic systems. The CIDI offers rich clinical descriptions with generally reliable Axis I diagnoses.

Axis II interviews

Personality disorders are often overlooked by traditional interviews. Fortunately, three structured interviews (see Table 1) are readily available with strong psychometric properties. In the subsequent paragraphs, the comparative strengths of each Axis II interview are underscored.

The SIDP has been validated with a broad range of inpatient and outpatient populations. It is ideally suited for assessing comorbidity in patients with Axis I disorders. Its topical organization (e.g. activities, relationships and emotions) flows naturally and facilitates patients' participation. With moderately good reliability, the SIDP has been used extensively in treatment outcome studies. The hallmark of the SIDP is its clear diagnostic boundaries, producing 'pure' personality disorders (i.e. single diagnosis) in approximately half of the patients evaluated.

The IPDE is composed of separate versions to evaluate DSM and ICD personality disorders. Like the SIDP, it is topically organized to promote patient cooperation. Patients with Axis I disorders can be evaluated with the IPDE, although it has not been sufficiently tested with psychotic disorders or severe depression. The IPDE has moderately good reliability for both symptoms and diagnoses Given its extensive research with dimensional diagnoses, the IPDE produces very reliable results in measuring the level of personality traits. The hallmark of the IPDE is its international applications to different cultures, languages and diagnostic systems.

The SCID-II is an efficient Axis II interview organized by diagnosis rather than relevant topics. Used in conjunction with a written screen, interviewers can rapidly assess probable personality disorders. This emphasis on efficiency detracts from the natural flow of questions and can be experienced as repetitive because questions on the SCID-II parallel those on the screen. The hallmark of the SCID-II is its efficiency in minimising the number of inquiries and facilitating rapid diagnoses.

Concluding remarks

Traditional evaluations are fraught with diagnostic errors, namely missed diagnoses and misdiagnoses. Recent advances in structured interviews have brought much-needed standardization to clinical inquiries and concomitant ratings. As a result, Axis I and Axis II interviews produce reliable and valid diagnoses widely applicable across healthcare settings.

REFERENCES

Baker, F. M. & Bell, C. C. (1999). Issues in the psychiatric treatment of African Americans. *Psychiatric Services*, **50**, 362–8.

Christensen, K. S., Toft, T., Frostholm, L. et al. (2003). The FIP study: a randomized, controlled, trial of screening and recognition of psychiatric disorders. *British Journal of General Practice*, **53**, 758–63.

First, M. B., Spitzer, R. L., Gibbon, M., Williams, J. B. W. & Benjamin, L. (1994). *The structured clinical interview for DSM-IV Axis II personality disorders (SCID-II)* (Version 2.0). New York: Biometrics Research, New York State Psychiatric Institute.

First, M. B., Spitzer, R. L., Williams, J. B. W. & Gibbon, M. (1997). *Structured clinical interview of DSM-IV disorders–clinician version (SCID-CV)*. Washington, DC: American Psychiatric Association.

First, M. B., Spitzer, R. L., Williams, J. B. W. & Gibbon, M. (2002). *Structured clinical interview of DSM-IV disorders–research version (SCID-RV)*. Washington, DC: American Psychiatric Association.

Hare, R. D. (2003). *Manual for the Revised Psychopathy Checklist* (2nd edn.). Toronto: Multi-Health Systems.

Loranger, A. W. (1999). *International personality disorder Examination (IPDE) manual*. Odessa, FL: Psychological Assessment Resources.

Lowe, B., Spitzer, R. L., Gräfe, K. et al. (2004). Comparative validity of three screening questionnaires for DSM-IV depressive disorders and physician's diagnoses. *Journal of Affective Disorders*, **78**, 131–40.

North, C. S., Pollio, D. E., Thompson, S. J. et al. (1997). A comparison of clinical and structured interview diagnoses in a homeless mental health clinic. *Community Mental Health Journal*, **33**, 531–43.

Pfohl, B., Blum, N. & Zimmerman, M. (1995). *The structured interview for DSM-IV personality: SIDP-IV*. Iowa City: University of Iowa.

Robins, L. N., Helzer, J. E., Cottler, L. B. & Goldring, E. (1989). *NIMH diagnostic interview schedule, version III – revised*. St. Louis: Washington University School of Medicine.

Rogers, R. (2001). *Handbook of diagnostic and structured interviewing*. New York: Guilford Publications.

Rogers, R. (2003). Standardizing DSM-IV diagnoses: The clinical applications of structured interviews. *Journal of Personality Assessment*, **81**, 220–5.

Rogers, R., Jackson, R. L. & Cashel, M. L. (2003). SADS: Comprehensive assessment of mood and psychotic disorders. In M. Hersen, M. J. Hilsenroth & D. J. Segal (Eds.). *The handbook of psychological assessment. Vol. 2. Personality assessment* (pp. 144–52). New York: Wiley.

Shear, M. K., Greeno, C., Kang, J. et al. (2000). Diagnosis of nonpsychotic patients in community clinics. *American Journal of Psychiatry*, **157**, 581–7.

Sheehan, D. V., Lecrubier, Y., Sheehan, K. H. et al. (1998). The mini international neuropsychiatric interview (MINI): the development and validation of structured diagnostic psychiatric interview for DSM-IV and ICD-10. *Journal of Clinical Psychiatry*, **59**(Suppl. 20), 22–33.

Sheehan, D. V., Lecrubier, Y., Sheehan, K. H. et al. (1997). The validity of the mini international neuropsychiatric interview (MINI) according to the SCID-P and its reliability. *European Psychiatry*, **12**, 232–41.

Spitzer, R. L. & Endicott, J. (1978a). *Schedule of Affective Disorders and Schizophrenia* (3rd edn.). New York: Biometrics Research.

Spitzer, R. L. & Endicott, J. (1978b). *Schedule of affective disorders and schizophrenia – change version*. New York: Biometrics Research.

Spitzer, R. L., Williams, J. B. W., Gibbon, M. & First, M. B. (1990). *Structured clinical interview for DSM-III-R personality disorders (SCID-II)*. Washington, DC: American Psychiatric Press.

Spitzer, R. L., Williams, J. B. W., Kroenke, K. et al. (1994). Utility of a new procedure for diagnosing mental disorders in primary care: the PRIME-MD 1000 study. *Journal of the American Medical Association*, **272**, 1749–56.

Tiemens, B. G., VonKorff, M. & Lin, E. H. B. (1999). Diagnosis of depression by primary care physicians versus a structured diagnostic interview. *General Hospital Psychiatry*, **21**, 87–96.

Ward, C. H., Beck, A. T., Mendelson, M., Mock, J. E. & Erbaugh, J. K. (1962). The psychiatric nomenclature. *Archives of General Psychiatry*, **7**, 198–205.

Williams, J. B. W., Gibbon, M., First, M. B. et al. (1992). The structured clinical interview for DSM-III-R (SCID): II. Multisite test-retest reliability. *Archieves of General Psychiatry*, **49**, 630–6.

Wing, J. K., Sartorius, N. & Ustun, T. B. (1998). *Diagnosis and clinical measurement in psychiatry: a reference manual for SCAN/PSE-10*. Cambridge, UK: Cambridge University Press.

Witchen, H. U. (1994). Reliability and validity studies of the WHO Composite international diagnostic interview: a critical review. *Journal of Psychiatric Research*, **28**, 57–84.

World Health Organization (1997). *The composite international diagnostic interview* (Version 2, 12 month). Geneva: author.

Zimmerman, M. & Mattia, J. I. (1999). Psychiatric diagnosis in clinical practice: Is comorbidity being missed? *Comprehensive Psychiatry*, **40**, 182–91.

Disability assessment

Raymond Fitzpatrick

University of Oxford

The concept of disability

Disability is a broad and sometimes contentious term. It provides an apparently neutral method of describing limitations and difficulties that individuals may have of functioning in their environment. However to individuals with disabilities, and to organizations that represent them, the term 'disability' appears unnecessarily negative with implications of deviance and abnormality. A plethora of approaches to disability span those that at one extreme define disability as inherent properties of individuals, through to the other extreme that considers disability a harmful social construction which labels and oppresses particular minorities.

Fundamental changes to how we view disability are revealed in the evolution of the World Health Organization's thinking about health and disease. In 1980 it produced what was at the time considered a progressive and enlightened International Classification of Impairments, Disabilities and Handicaps (ICIDH). The ICIDH schema defines impairment as any loss or abnormality of psychological, physiological or anatomical structure or function. Impairment therefore refers to failure at the level of organs or systems of the body, with impairment usually arising from disease. Disability refers to any restriction or lack of ability to perform an activity in the manner considered normal. The emphasis is therefore on things that individuals cannot do. Handicap is any disadvantage for an individual, resulting from impairment or disability that limits the fulfilment of a role for that individual. It refers to the social disadvantages that may follow from disease. A simple example might be that osteoarthritis (disease) results in poorly functioning hips or knees (impairment). This impairment results in reduced mobility (disability), in turn resulting in loss of work and social contact (handicap).

Two sets of criticisms were frequently expressed about ICIDH. Firstly it was viewed as too biomedical and reductionist, because it viewed all the problems of individuals with disabilities as stemming from inherent aspects of their disease, rather than, for example, societal approaches to disability. Secondly the emphasis upon 'disability' and 'handicap' was excessively negative reinforcing unhelpfully pessimistic views of disability. The WHO therefore introduced a new classification system: the International Classification of Functioning, Disease and Health, or ICF (WHO, 2001).

The ICF model is more interactive (rather than linear) with four key elements: (i) body functions and structures (e.g. memory function, structure of the nervous system), (ii) activities and participation (e.g. self care, social and community life), (iii) environmental factors (products and technology for communication, immediate family) and (iv) personal factors (age, gender). Health is another contextual factor similar to environment and personal factors but not considered necessarily of primary causal importance. Overall the language is neutral, causes are not unilinear from disease and the emphasis is upon the scope for positive activities and participation. Another key shift is that the new WHO model is applicable to all individuals in a population (viewing activities and participation as a continuum), rather than focusing on a minority of 'disabled'. Overall disability is considered an umbrella term for all of the interactions between the four elements just described rather than a property of individuals. This new WHO schema offers potentially a more thorough and coherent approach to disability; however at present it is largely a theoretical formulation and sustained effort will be required to operationalise it in terms of the measurement systems described in the remainder of this chapter (see also 'Disability').

Population surveys in both the UK and the USA have reached rather similar estimates of the prevalence of disability amongst adults – approximately 14% being considered disabled due to ill health. Arthritis, blindness, stroke, coronary heart disease and bronchitis are the disorders most responsible for disability.

Principles of assessment

Until recently assessment of disability focused almost exclusively upon a core of issues; the extent to which the individual can operate independently in terms of a range of important functions. To some degree assessment has begun to include broader issues such as handicap. More recently, assessment has also incorporated issues raised by the WHO's paradigm shift towards participation. As assessment includes such broader domains, it inevitably becomes more multidimensional since, for example, disability in one dimension will not necessarily predict high levels of problem in another dimension.

Two levels of functioning are commonly distinguished; basic and instrumental activities of daily living (ADL). Basic ADL functions are those that are essential for self-care such as bathing, dressing and feeding. Instrumental ADL are those activities such as doing laundry, shopping, housekeeping, getting around in public, activities that are necessary for someone to maintain a level of independent living. Problems with instrumental ADL (IADL) are far more common than for basic ADL, so that estimates of the prevalence of disability are very much influenced by whether the broader range of IADLs are included.

Purposes of assessment

Assessment of disability may serve a number of different purposes. It is essential to be quite clear about the purpose to which any given measure is to be put. A particular measure of disability may, for example, be very useful as a population survey instrument for estimating the prevalence of disability in a population, but not perform well as a measure of outcome in clinical trials.

The earliest applications of measures to assess disability were in the context of hospital decisions about how to allocate nursing care to patients of greatest dependency and need. They now have a broader range of application in helping health professionals' assessments of their patients. In a typical study of such applications, Wagner and colleagues (1997) set out to improve the care of patients with epilepsy by providing evidence about patients' disability to their doctors, with the data on disability provided by patients themselves by completing a health status measure. Doctors were unaware of the information so provided and in 13% of consultations the new information resulted in a change of therapy. Both patients and doctors generally find it helpful and appropriate that the doctor is aware of the broader impact of their health problems. However to date systematic reviews suggest that, although providing health professionals with evidence about their patients' disability and broader aspects of health is considered important, it does not change the management of their patients sufficiently to significantly impact upon ultimate health outcomes (Greenhalgh & Meadows, 1999).

Another use of measures of disability is to track trends in populations in order to assess progress in public health and identify barriers to progress at the level of the population as a whole rather than selected sub-groups receiving interventions. Thus, the US Department of Health and Human Services uses a simple set of core questions in population surveys, for example, respondents' self-ratings of health and judgements of number of days in month that health prevented the respondent from performing usual activities (Centers for Disease Control and Prevention, 2000). These simple measures identify differences in health between states, poorer health and higher disability levels in sections of the United States with less education and trends over time in population disability.

Prognosis

A related use of disability assessments is in the prediction of future problems, either in terms of increased risk of deterioration in health or indeed mortality, or in terms of increased demands on the healthcare system. There is substantial evidence that such assessments play that role. For example, Keysor and colleagues (2004) administered a simple, short measure of self-reported health status, the Health Assessment Questionnaire to over 1400 patients with rheumatoid arthritis recruited from clinics from 11 cities across the United States. Higher levels of disability reported in the questionnaire at baseline proved to be a significant predictor of mortality in a ten-year follow-up of mortality.

Measures of outcome

Disability measures may be used to assess the progress of patients over time, and by extension to assess outcomes of healthcare in quality assurance, evaluation studies or clinical trials. For example, Messier and colleagues (2004) carried out a randomized controlled trial to examine whether long-term exercise or dietary weight loss

would be effective in reducing pain and disability in obese individuals with osteoarthritis. The principle outcome measure was self-reported physical function as assessed by Western Ontario and McMaster Universities' Osteoarthritis Index (WOMAC). Modest weight loss combined with moderate exercise proved to have a significantly greater beneficial effect on disability than either intervention alone or a control group in standard care. The scope for finding real benefit from novel interventions, whether drugs or complex interventions is quite modest and self-reported disability measures offer an attractive way of identifying such small but worthwhile gains.

Measurement requirements

The measurement properties required for disability assessments are the same as for all other health status and psychometric instruments. Assessments need to be reliable, valid, sensitive to change, acceptable, relevant and practical to use. However a proliferation of disability instruments has occurred in which the majority of instruments have not been evaluated against such criteria. Test–retest reliability is one key component of measures, but for observer-based measures of disability, inter-rater reliability is also of importance. There are no 'gold-standard' criteria against which to measure validity. Instead, a battery of approaches should be used that includes the important stage of informal examination of whether the content of measures is appropriate to the intended use and encompasses all relevant dimensions. More formal assessment of validity involves construct validity by comparing results with other related measures or predictive validity in which scores are examined against subsequent health status or healthcare use.

Sensitivity to change requires particular attention. It cannot be assumed that, because an instrument has been shown to be valid in terms of distinguishing degrees of severity of disability between patients that it will also be sensitive to change over time in disability within patients. For example, the standard American Rheumatism Association (ARA) functional classification distinguishes just four levels of disability, ranging from 'complete functional capacity' to 'largely or wholly incapacitated'. There is a substantial amount of change that can occur to patients in degree of disability whilst remaining within a single grade of the ARA scale. Such broad categories can therefore understate the effects of healthcare interventions. Similarly in Parkinson's disease, the Hoehn and Yahr scale distinguishes between just five levels of severity. When patients are asked to judge disability themselves in measures repeated over time, changes are identified that are not detected by the more broad categories of Hoehn and Yahr (Fitzpatrick et al., 1997). Increasing attention is now given to identifying the smallest change in a disability measure that would be meaningful to the patient or of statistical significance, in order to improve the clinical interpretability of change scores for instruments, either in terms of individual patient care or results from trials. The evidence with regard to disability assessment in Parkinson's disease is that similar change scores emerge as meaningful whether the criterion is based on patient judgement of what is meaningful or on statistical criteria (Fitzpatrick et al., 2004).

A problem that can limit the sensitivity to change of disability measures derives from so-called 'ceiling' and 'floor' effects. Instruments may not leave scope for patients to express further improvement or deterioration beyond the items included in the instrument. A common way of identifying possible floor and ceiling effects is by the proportion of scores falling at the extremes of an instrument. Thus Mao and colleagues (2002) compared three measures of balance in patients who had a stroke. The instruments differed in the proportion of scores at the extremes, suggesting that they would differ in their capacity to measure the extent of true underlying change in the construct of balance.

Types of instruments

Direct clinical testing

Traditionally, clinicians have used a number of physical tests to assess aspects of function and disability, for example, by timing how long it took patients to complete tasks such as walking given distances, or by assessing the performance of particular tasks such as buttoning and unbuttoning. One problem with such assessments is that they may be unrepresentative of the challenges faced by the patient in the usual environment. A more fundamental problem is that such tests can be very unreliable, although by careful standardizing of instruction to patients and methods of recording observations, it is possible to obtain very good inter-rater reliability (Pincus et al., 1991). Clinical tests such as walking time can be useful but are inevitably limited in scope because of inherent difficulties of directly observing many IADLs such as shopping and use of transport.

Observer-based assessments

One of the first, and still most commonly used, of such assessments is the Index of ADL developed by Katz and colleagues (1963). Individuals are rated by observers on a three-point scale of degree of independence for each of six activities: bathing, dressing, toileting, transfer (moving in and out of bed and chairs), continence and feeding. It clearly concentrates on more basic ADLs and uses rather broad categories of assessment so that it may not be appropriate as an outcome for the majority of interventions from which only modest benefits are expected.

Probably more widely used now is the Barthel Index which assesses patients on ten dimensions: feeding, grooming, bathing, dressing, bowel and bladder care, toilet use, ambulation, transfers and stair climbing. The Barthel Index exists in a variety of forms which differ in items and methods of scoring. Studies comparing different forms of the Barthel Index with each other and with comparable measures of disability are inconclusive but generally seem to indicate that shorter and simpler measures are often as reliable valid and responsive as longer forms (Hsueh et al., 2002). Because no single measure of observer-assessed disability clearly dominates others in terms of measurement properties, there is now a growing proliferation of instruments, either modifying existing scales for generic use, or designed for specific use with particular conditions such as stroke or multiple sclerosis or particular functions such as mobility.

Standardized interviews and questionnaires

There is now increased emphasis upon instruments either in the form of standardized instruments or self completed questionnaires that focus on the individual's own perception and experience of disability. An example is the Sickness Impact Profile (SIP) (Bergner et al., 1981). It comprises 136 statements with 'yes' or 'no' responses. Items contribute to one of 12 scales: walking, body care and movement, mobility, work, sleeping and rest, eating, housework, recreation, emotion, social interaction, alertness and communication. The first three scales can be combined to produce a 'physical scale' which most closely resembles a disability assessment. Scoring of items is weighted on the basis of extensive prior rating exercises of panels to assess severity. It has been shown to be valid in a wide range of disabling conditions. Nevertheless its relatively large number of items has resulted in efforts to shorten and simplify it. Thus, van de Port and colleagues (2004) devised a shorter version of SIP with items tailored to individuals with stroke; they demonstrated validity and concluded that measurement properties were not inferior to those of the longer original SIP.

Probably more extensively used now is the SF-36 which comprises 36 items each contributing to one of eight scales: limitations in physical activities because of health problems, limitations in social activities because of physical or emotional problems, limitations in usual role activities because of physical health problems, bodily pain, general mental health (psychological distress and wellbeing), limitations in usual role activities because of emotional problems, vitality (energy and fatigue) and general health perceptions (Brazier et al., 1992). Items can also be summarized in terms of two broader scales to simplify reporting: physical and mental health summary scales. Unfortunately the success in terms of rate of uptake of the instrument has resulted in a number of varying forms of the basic instrument. As with clinician- and observer-based scales, there is also a tendency for investigators to develop disease-specific adaptations of the core instrument. For example the Multiple Sclerosis Quality of Life Health Survey is an instrument intended for use with individuals with multiple sclerosis; it comprises the SF-36 with 18 disease-specific items added on (Pittock et al., 2004). One major advantage of SF-36 is that the relative ease of use and wide-ranging applicability of its content has resulted in frequent use in general population surveys so that scores for specific groups can be compared with normative evidence (see also 'Quality of life assessment').

A wide range of disease-specific instruments have also appeared that have relevance to assessment of disability in specific populations. For example the Health Assessment Questionnaire (HAQ) (Fries, Spitz & Young, 1982) is widely used for individuals with rheumatoid arthritis and related conditions. It contains 20 items across 8 areas of function: dressing and grooming, rising, eating, walking, hygiene, reach, grip and outside activity. The HAQ is very widely used: it is, for example, a powerful predictor of future health status and use of healthcare services by those with arthritis (Ethgen et al., 2002).

Handicap and participation

Recently, efforts have been made explicitly to address broader aspects of disability emphasized by WHO models discussed earlier.

Amongst the earliest of instruments to address the WHO agenda for disability was the London Handicap Scale (Harwood *et al.*, 1994). The scale generates a profile of handicaps on six different dimensions (mobility, physical independence, occupation, social integration, orientation and economic self-sufficiency) by asking respondents to select between six levels on each item. It has been shown to be sensitive to change in an evaluation of a day hospital rehabilitation programme for stroke patients (Hershkowitz *et al.*, 2004).

Similarly Noreau and colleagues (2004) developed the LIFE-H instrument specifically to assess social participation in individuals with disability focusing on items to assess a person's performance in daily activities, social roles (life habits) leisure and community participation. It should be noted that many instruments such as SIP and SF-36 do contain items and dimensions addressing WHO-type concerns regarding handicap and social participation, but were not explicitly developed and tested against the WHO-based conceptualization of disability.

Individualized measures

An important approach to rehabilitation in disability is 'goal attainment scaling' in which patient and therapist jointly set priorities in terms of specific targets for particular functional problems. The idea of personalizing or individualizing has been adopted in the field of assessment, moving away from the idea of assessing a standard list of pre-selected items to assessing items identified by the patient. Tugwell and colleagues (1990) developed an instrument to assess disability in arthritis (the Patient Preference Disability Questionnaire) in which patients identify up to five functional problems of concern to them arising from their disease. The instrument proved sensitive to changes in a placebo controlled drug trial. A number of instruments have been developed based on the same principles of individuals selecting issues of concern to them. A systematic review assessed available evidence for such instruments (Patel and colleagues, 2003). The authors concluded that whilst some instruments had good evidence of measurement properties, they were all fairly impractical for the purposes of clinical trials and related evaluative research because of

practical difficulties arising from the need for in-depth interviews to collect data. By contrast, the principle of personalizing goals remains of fundamental importance in clinical aspects of disability.

Issues for the future

Two major developments are now needed in the field of disability assessment. The first development is that recent advances in statistical analysis of data such as scales and additive scores need to be fully applied and tested in the context of disability assessment. There are numerous scales now available to assess disability. However none is free of possible problems to do with redundancy of items, floor or ceiling effects, difficulties of assuming equivalence and additivity of items and other such statistical problems. It has been argued that recently developed statistical methods such as item response theory may overcome such problems, in particular by identifying items that address the full spectrum of phenomena such as disability with true interval or even ratio-level measurement (Lindeboom *et al.*, 2003).

The second development that is required is increased effort directly to compare the performance of measures of assessment of disability. A start has been made. A study made by Katz and colleagues (1992) found that shorter measures of disability were no less sensitive to change than were longer and more detailed instruments. Similarly Wiebe and colleagues (2003) carried out a systematic review of measures of outcome that had been used in randomized controlled trials. They concluded that generic or general-purpose measures of health status were less sensitive to important changes in patients than were more disease-specific measures. More such direct head-to-head comparison of instruments to assess disability is needed mainly to produce a stronger evidence base regarding the comparative performance of instruments, but also to reduce the volume of instruments available.

It is unlikely that major breakthroughs will now occur through development of new instruments. Instead existing methods need to be applied more clearly to identify the value and relevance of existing measures.

REFERENCES

Bergner, M., Bobbitt, R., Carter, W. & Gilson, B. (1981). The Sickness Impact Profile: development and final revision of a health status measure. *Medical Care*, **19**, 787–805.

Brazier, J., Harper, R. & Jones, N. (1992). Validating the SF-36 health survey questionnaire: new outcome measure for primary care. *British Medical Journal*, **305**, 160–4.

Centers for Disease Control, and Prevention. (2000). *Measuring healthy days*. Atlanta, GA: CDC.

Ethgen, O., Kahler, K. H., Kong, S. X., Reginster, J. Y. & Wolfe, F. (2002). The effect of health related quality of life on reported use of health care resources in

patients with osteoarthritis and rheumatoid arthritis: a longitudinal analysis. *Journal of Rheumatology*, **29**, 1147–55.

Fitzpatrick, R., Peto, V., Jenkinson, C., Greenhall, R. & Hyman, N. (1997). Health-related quality of life in Parkinson's disease: a study of out-patient clinic attenders. *Movement Disorders*, **12**, 916–22.

Fitzpatrick, R., Norquist, J. & Jenkinson, C. (2004). Distribution-based criteria for change in health-related quality of life in Parkinson's disease. *Journal of Clinical Epidemiology*, **57**, 40–4.

Fries, J., Spitz, P. & Young, D. (1982). The dimensions of health outcomes: the Health Assessment Questionnaire, disability and

pain scales. *Journal of Rheumatology*, **9**, 789–93.

Greenhalgh, J. & Meadows, K. (1999). The effectiveness of the use of patient-based measures of health in routine practice in improving the process and outcomes of patient care: a literature review. *Journal of Evaluation in Clinical Practice*, **5**, 401–16.

Harwood, R., Gompertz, P. & Ebrahim, S. (1994). Handicap one year after stroke: validity of a new scale. *Journal of Neurology, Neurosurgery and Psychiatry*, **57**, 825–9.

Hershkovitz, A., Beloosesky, Y., Brill, S. & Gottlieb, D. (2004) Is a day hospital rehabilitation programme associated with reduction of handicap in stroke patients? *Clinical Rehabilitation*, **8**, 261–6.

Hsueh, I. P., Lin, J. H., Jeng, J. S. & Hsieh, C. L. (2002). Comparison of the psychometric characteristics of the functional independence measure, 5 item Barthel index, and 10 item Barthel index in patients with stroke. *Journal of Neurology Neurosurgery and Psychiatry*, **73**, 188–90.

Katz, S., Ford, A., Moskowitz, R., Jackson, D. & Jaffer, M. (1963). Studies of illness in the aged: the Index of ADL: a standardized measure of biological and psychosocial function. *Journal of the American Medical Association*, **85**, 914–19.

Katz, J., Larson, M., Phillips, C., Fossel, A. & Liang, M. (1992). Comparative measurement sensitivity of short and longer health status instruments. *Medical Care*, **30**, 917–25.

Keysor, J., Sokka, T., Krishnan, E., Callahan, L. F. & Pincus, T. (2004). Patient questionnaires and formal education level as prospective predictors of mortality over 10 years in 97% of 1416 patients with rheumatoid arthritis from 15 United States private practices. *Journal of Rheumatology*, **31**, 229–34.

Lindeboom, R., Vermeulen, M., Holman, R. & De Haan, R. J. (2003). Activities of daily living instruments: optimizing scales for

neurologic assessments. *Neurology*, **60**, 738–42.

Mao, H. F., Hsueh, I. P., Tang, P. F., Sheu, C. F. & Hsieh, C. L. (2002). Analysis and comparison of the psychometric properties of three balance measures for stroke patients. *Stroke*, **33**, 1022–7.

Messier, S. P., Loeser, R. F., Miller, G. D. *et al.* (2004). Exercise and dietary weight loss in overweight and obese older adults with knee osteoarthritis: the Arthritis, Diet, and Activity Promotion Trial. *Arthritis and Rheumatism*, **50**, 1501–10.

Noreau, L., Desrosiers, J., Robichaud, L. *et al.* (2004). Measuring social participation: reliability of the LIFE-H in older adults with disabilities. *Disability and Rehabilitation*, **26**, 346–52.

Patel, K. K., Veenstra, D. L. & Patrick, D. L. (2003). A review of selected patient-generated outcome measures and their application in clinical trials. *Value and Health*, **6**, 595–603.

Pincus, T., Brooks, R. & Callahan, L. (1991). Reliability of grip strength, walking time and button test performed according to a standard protocol. *Journal of Rheuamtology* **18**, 997–1000.

Pittock, S. J., Mayr, W. T., McClelland, R. L. *et al.* (2004). Quality of life is favorable for most patients with multiple sclerosis:

a population-based cohort study. *Archives of Neurology*, **61**, 679–86.

Tugwell, P., Bombardier, C., Buchanan, W. *et al.* (1990). Methotrexate in rheumatoid arthritis: impact on quality of life assessed by traditional standard item and individualized patient preference health status questionnaire. *Archives of Internal Medicine*, **150**, 59–62.

Van de Port, I. G., Ketelaar, M., Schepers, V. P., Van den Bos, G. A. & Lindeman, E. (2004). Monitoring the functional health status of stroke patients: the value of the Stroke-Adapted Sickness Impact Profile-30. *Disability and Rehabilitation*, **26**, 635–40.

Wagner, A. K., Ehrenberg, B. L., Tran, T. A. *et al.* (1997). Patient-based health status measurement in clinical practice: a study of its impact on epilepsy patients' care. *Quality of Life Research*, **6**, 329–41.

Wiebe, S., Guyatt, G., Weaver, B., Matijevic, S. & Sidwell, C. (2003). Comparative responsiveness of generic and specific quality-of-life instruments. *Journal of Clinical Epidemiology*, **56**, 52–60.

World Health Organisation (2001). *International Classification of Functioning, Disability and Health*. Geneva: author.

Health cognition assessment

Brian McMillan and Mark Conner

University of Leeds

Introduction

Health cognitions are items of knowledge or beliefs about health and illness. These include evaluations of health-relevant behaviours, expectations about the consequences of these behaviours, self-representations, perceptions of social approval or disapproval resulting from engaging in these behaviours, perceptions about the behaviour of others, perceptions regarding one's own abilities and thoughts about ones personal disposition towards engaging in particular behaviours. The assessment of health cognitions is more than merely the rule-based assignment of numerals to objects or events. Assessment must assign values to entities that are theoretically meaningful, and in this respect assessment and theory

go hand in hand. Theory provides us with guidance as to what we should measure, but it is good measurement that theory depends upon.

Self-report methods for assessing health cognitions

Health cognitions are commonly assessed by self-reports measured using Guttman, Thurstone, Likert, or semantic differential scales (Kline, 2000), although only the latter two continue to receive significant attention. Likert scales are less cumbersome than Thurstone's technique without compromising on reliability and validity. Semantic differential scales consist of bipolar adjective scales where respondents are asked to rate an attitude object (e.g. 'Exercising for 30 minutes, 5 times a week would be …' Good–Bad). Unlike other techniques, semantic differential scales do not require the development and scaling of specific belief items (see Eagly & Chaiken, 1993).

Important considerations for self-report measures

Since good theory depends upon dependable measurement, it is disappointing that much published work examining health cognitions pays scant attention to reliability and validity. Theory-based measures of health cognitions should be developed by paying the same attention to reliability and validity as we expect from other areas of psychology. Issues which should be considered include face validity (does the measure appear to measure what it purports to measure?), content validity (does it match the defined content domains?), concurrent validity (does it correlate highly with similar measures of this construct?), predictive validity (does it predict a particular criterion?) and construct validity (are the constructs confirmed by factor analyses?). We should also expect health cognition measures to be reliable, internally consistent (commonly measured using coefficient alpha) and ideally there should be additional checks for reliability such as parallel forms reliability (do different versions of the measure correlate highly?). Use of multi-item measures can improve the reliability of measures, yet there are abundant studies in the literature using single item measures of unknown reliability. Since many health cognitions such as attitudes may vary with time, test–retest reliability (do scores from the same measures taken at two separate time points correlate highly?) is less relevant to health cognition measures (cf. Kline, 2000).

Many factors may affect the validity of health cognition measures, such as social desirability and the ordering of items within a questionnaire. Randomization of items within a questionnaire is one defence against order effects, whereas concerns over social desirability can be addressed by ensuring participant confidentiality and anonymity where possible. Inclusion of a social desirability measure will also allow for analyses to ascertain if it has an impact on the relationships between measured variables.

Ajzen's (1988) principle of compatibility emphasizes the importance of matching the elements of action, target, context and time. If we are concerned with predicting behaviour, then it is essential that we are as specific as possible about the nature of this behaviour. For example we could ask; 'I intend to cycle to work every weekday for the next month, unless I am on holiday'. This question contains reference to the action (cycling), the target (place of work), the context (unless they are on holiday) and the time period (every weekday for the next month). This may seem overly pedantic, but were we simply to ask participants if they intended to cycle to work, we would have no idea how often they intended to cycle, or even if they intended to do it any time in the near future. These considerations apply not only to predicting behaviour but also predicting health cognitions. If we wish to examine how well attitudes predict intention, the measures should also be matched in terms of action, target, context and time.

Theories incorporating health cognitions

Social cognition models have become popular frameworks for research aimed at furthering our ability to understand, predict and change health behaviours. Such models include Attribution Theory (AT), the Health Belief Model (HBM), the Theory of Planned Behaviour (TPB), Social Cognitive Theory (SCT), Protection Motivation Theory (PMT) and Health Locus of Control (HLC). Stage models such as the Transtheoretical Model of Change (TTM), and the Precaution Adoption Process Model (PAPM) have become increasingly popular, as have models which incorporate constructs from both these approaches, such as the Health Action Process Approach (HAPA). An in-depth description of each of these models is beyond the scope of this chapter. See Conner and Norman (2005) and chapters on 'Attributions and health', 'The health belief model', 'Theory of planned behaviour' and 'Transtheoretical model of behaviour change'.

Figure 1 shows the core cognitive constructs which have been used to predict health behaviour in the literature. There is much overlap between these theories and constructs often differ on little more than name.

Abraham and Sheeran (2000) identified five core cognitive antecedents of health behaviours: attitude, self-representations, norms, self-efficacy and intention. In order to include attributions and locus of control we have labelled the self-efficacy construct 'control perceptions', and replaced intention with 'disposition to act' as this incorporates constructs from a wider range of theories.

Measuring attitude

Attitudes are typically measured using semantic differential items such as;

My eating fruit as part of my	good	1 2 3 4 5 6 7	bad
midday meal tomorrow	harmful	1 2 3 4 5 6 7	beneficial
would be …	pleasant	1 2 3 4 5 6 7	unpleasant

The semantic differentials used in such measures should result from careful pilot work, as concerns have been raised that measures of attitude are frequently biased towards their cognitive component (Conner & Sparks, 2005). Weiner's attributional model (1985) includes an 'emotion' construct, but within the context of different attributions leading to different emotions, such as guilt or shame. Work into anticipated affective reactions approaches this issue in a different tense, and considers how anticipated feelings relate to the performance of a behaviour. O'Connor and Armitage (2003) measured anticipated affect with the use of semantic differentials; 'If I deliberately harmed myself I would feel …' – 'feeble–strong', 'tense–relaxed', 'sad–happy'. Others have focussed on more specific aspects of anticipated affect, such as anticipated regret (Conner & Sparks, 2005).

The evaluative component of attitude is typically measured in terms of 'Performing behaviour X would lead to outcome Y'.

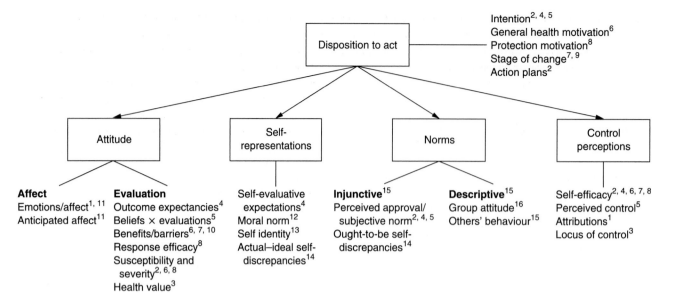

Affect
Emotions/affect[1, 11]
Anticipated affect[11]

Evaluation
Outcome expectancies[4]
Beliefs × evaluations[5]
Benefits/barriers[6, 7, 10]
Response efficacy[8]
Susceptibility and
 severity[2, 6, 8]
Health value[3]

Self-evaluative
 expectations[4]
Moral norm[12]
Self identity[13]
Actual–ideal self-
 discrepancies[14]

Injunctive[15]
Perceived approval/
 subjective norm[2, 4, 5]
Ought-to-be self-
 discrepancies[14]

Descriptive[15]
Group attitude[16]
Others' behaviour[15]

Self-efficacy[2, 4, 6, 7, 8]
Perceived control[5]
Attributions[1]
Locus of control[3]

Theories
1. Attribution Theory (e.g. Weiner, 1985, 1986)
2. Health Action Process Approach (Schwarzer et al., 2003)
3. Health Locus of Control (Wallston et al., 1978)
4. Social Cognitive Theory (Bandura, 1986, 1997)
5. Theory of Planned Behaviour (Ajzen, 1991)
6. Health Belief Model (Rosenstock et al., 1988)
7. Transtheoretical Model (Velicier et al., 1998)
8. Protection Motivation Theory (Maddux & Rogers, 1983)
9. Precaution Adoption Process Model (Weinstein, 1988)

Relevant studies
10. Sutton et al. (2005)
11. Conner & Sparks (2005)
12. O'Conner & Armitage (2003)
13. Evans & Norman (2003)
14. Higgins (1989)
15. Caldini, Kallgren & Reno (1991)
16. White, Terry & Hogg (1994)

Fig 1 Core health cognitions (adapted from Abraham & Sheeran, 2000).

Within the TPB, beliefs and evaluations are measured separately using items such as:

Eating fruit as part of my midday meal tomorrow would make me healthier	unlikely	1	2	3	4	5	6	7	likely
Being healthier would be	bad		1	2	3	4	5	6	7	good

respectively. The beliefs to be included should result from careful pilot work using open-ended questions such as 'what do you think would be the advantages/disadvantages for you of being more physically active in the next twelve months' and 'what would you like or enjoy/dislike or hate about being more physically active in the next twelve months?'.

Within the HBM and TTM, the evaluative component of attitude is measured in terms of perceived benefits or barriers of performing a behaviour. For example, Champion (1984) used items such as 'Self breast exams can help me find lumps in my breast' and 'Self breast exams are time consuming' – 'Strongly disagree–Strongly agree' to measure the pros and cons of self breast examination. In PMT, attitudes towards particular behaviours are measured in terms of response efficacy, e.g. 'Regular exercise will reduce my chances of having a heart attack'. The TPB uniquely includes separate assessments of outcome likelihood and outcome evaluation, whereas other models, such as the HAPA, HBM and PMT measure perceived susceptibility to a particular condition and perceived severity of that condition. Champion (1984) measured the HBM components of susceptibility and severity with

items such as: 'There is a good possibility that I will get breast cancer' and 'If I got breast cancer, it would be more serious than other diseases' – 'Strongly disagree–Strongly agree'. Schwarzer *et al.* (2003) recommend similar measures for the HAPA, but suggest that susceptibility should be measured in terms of absolute susceptibility – 'How do you estimate the likelihood that you will ever suffer from . . .' – 'very unlikely–very likely' and relative susceptibility 'If I compare myself to an average person of my age and sex, the risk of my suffering from . . . is . . .' – 'very unlikely–very likely' (see also 'Risk perception').

Measuring self-representations

Self-representations are an important group of health cognitions, although many popular theories fail to include them as a separate component. SCT includes self-evaluative expectations as a subset of outcome expectations. Operationalizations of SCT have measured self-evaluative expectations using items such as 'I would feel more responsible if I used a condom' (NIMH, 2001) and as such they appear very close to measures of anticipated affect. Moral norms also come under the umbrella of self-representations, and have been measured in studies applying the TPB using items such as 'It would be morally wrong for me to deliberately harm myself' and 'Deliberately harming myself goes against my principles' – 'Strongly disagree–Strongly agree' (O'Connor & Armitage, 2003). Self-identity is also an important cognitive antecedent of health behaviour and has been measured using items such as

'I like to think of myself as someone who always thinks carefully about how to cross the road' 'disagree strongly–agree strongly' (Evans & Norman, 2003). Higgins (1987) highlights the importance of perceived discrepancies between our ideal and actual self in terms of how we subsequently behave. Research into this area commonly employs the Selves Questionnaire (Higgins, 1987).

Measuring norms

Normative influences on behaviour form a part of many social cognition models, and are typically measured as perceptions of approval or disapproval of important others. In the TPB subjective norms are measured using items such as;

People who are important to me think I ...								
Should	1	2	3	4	5	6	7	Should not ... eat fruit as part of my midday meal tomorrow

and specific normative beliefs are measured using the wording of the item above but replacing 'people who are important to me' with specific referent groups identified from pilot work, such as 'my friends' or 'my partner'. In addition, the TPB includes a measure of motivation to comply for each specific referent group;

With regard to your diet, how much do you want to do what your friends think you should?	Not at all	1	2	3	4	5	6	7 Very much

Within the HAPA and SCT, normative beliefs are included in the outcome expectancies component and are measured in terms of social approval or disapproval being a pro or con of following a particular course of action, e.g. 'If I start exercising regularly, then I will receive a lot of praise form my partner'. SCT also incorporates normative beliefs as a form of outcome expectancy, e.g. 'My sex partner would get mad if I said we had to use condoms' (NIMH, 2001).

Cialdini, Reno and Kallgren (1990) noted that normative influences on behaviour should be split into two types; injunctive norms (perceived approval or disapproval) and descriptive norms (perceptions of what others think and do). Descriptive norms are typically measured in terms of perceived behaviour of others, for example 'Most of my friends/family/co-workers exercise regularly' – 'Strongly disagree–Strongly agree'. Group attitudes have been measured using items such as 'To what extent would there be agreement among the people who are important to you that to use a condom every time one had sexual intercourse is a good thing to do?' – 'to a large degree–to a small degree' (White, Terry & Hogg, 1994).

Measuring control perceptions

Self-efficacy has become a part of most major models of health behaviour (see Self-efficacy and health behaviour). It is included specifically in the HAPA, SCT, PMT and has been incorporated

into the HBM and the TTM. Self-efficacy is typically measured using items which contain the wording 'I am confident that I can [perform task X], even if [barrier Y]' (Schwarzer et al., 2003). Velicer, Prochaska, Fava, Norman, and Redding (1998) recommend measuring self-efficacy or temptation when using the TTM, and have developed a measure known as the Situational Temptation Measure. Although many researchers regard self-efficacy and perceived behavioural control as being synonymous, the items which Ajzen (1991) recommended are different from those used to measure self-efficacy. Examples of items used to measure PBC are;

How much control do you feel you have over eating fruit as part of your midday meal tomorrow?	No control	1	2	3	4	5	6	7	Complete control
For me to eat fruit as part of my midday meal tomorrow would be.	Difficult		1	2	3	4	5	6	7 Easy

Ajzen (1991) also recommended measuring the determinants of PBC with control belief measures relating to facilitators and barriers, e.g. 'When eating out there is a limited choice of fruit available' – 'strongly disagree–strongly agree', and corresponding power items, e.g. 'The limited choice of fruit when eating out makes my eating fruit as part of my midday meal tomorrow' – 'much more difficult–much easier'.

Theories which do not specifically measure self-efficacy or PBC include Weiner's (1985) attribution model, the HLC and the PAPM. Attribution theory is concerned with the underlying causes of events, and incorporates cognitions of control. Weiner proposed attributions related to stability (i.e. respondents might be asked to rate if their reasons for not giving up smoking were 'stable over time – variable over time'), locus (e.g. 'Do your reasons for not giving up smoking ... reflect an aspect of yourself – reflect an aspect of the situation') and controllability. Wallston et al.'s (1978) Health Locus of Control had split perceptions of control into three separate components a quarter of a century ago; Internal Health Locus of Control (measured with items such as 'If I get sick, it is my own behaviour which determines how soon I get well again' – 'Strongly disagree–Strongly agree'), Powerful Others Locus of Control (e.g. 'Having regular contact with my physician is the best way for me to avoid illness' – 'Strongly disagree–Strongly agree'), and Chance Locus of Control (e.g. 'No matter what I do, if I'm going to get sick, I will get sick' strongly disagree–strongly agree). Although such a measure does not take Ajzen's (1988) compatibility concerns into account, it did undergo more stringent tests for reliability and validity than many of the control measures currently in use and it came in two forms, which allowed for testing of parallel forms reliability.

Measuring disposition to act

Intention measures are employed to measure disposition to act in the HAPA, SCT and TPB and often the protection motivation component of the PMT is operationalized as intention. Conner and Sparks (2005) recommend measuring three components of intention, namely: intention (e.g. 'I intend to eat fruit as part of my midday meal tomorrow' – 'definitely do not–definitely do'), desire (e.g. 'I would like to eat fruit as part of my midday meal tomorrow' – 'definitely yes–definitely no') and expectation ('I expect to eat fruit as part of my midday meal tomorrow' – 'unlikely–likely'). They note that although multiple-item measures have a psychometric advantage, many studies continue to assess intentions using single-item measures. In the HBM model, disposition to act is termed General Health Motivation and has been measured using items such as 'I frequently do things to improve my health' – 'Strongly disagree–Strongly agree' (Champion, 1984).

Stage theories measure disposition to act in terms of what stage an individual is currently in. For example, Velicer et al. (1998) recommend using the following questions to ascertain what stage an individual is currently in: 'Are you currently a smoker' – 'yes' (Smoker), 'no, I quit within the last six months' (action stage), 'No, I quit more than 6 months ago' (maintenance stage), 'No, I have never smoked' (non-smoker). Those who reported being smokers would be asked how many times they have quit smoking in the last 24 hours, and if they are seriously thinking of quitting smoking. Those who state that they are seriously thinking of quitting smoking within the next 30 days and have had one 24 hour quit attempt in the last year are said to be in the 'preparation stage', and those who have not had a previous quit attempt are said to be in the 'contemplation stage'. Those who are thinking of quitting in the next 6 months are also said to be in the contemplation stage, and those who are not thinking of quitting are said to be in the 'precontemplation stage'. The TTM uses items which measure a combination of cognitons (i.e. intention) and behaviour, but has been criticized for numerous reasons, not least because the time periods specified within these measures seem somewhat arbitrary (Sutton, 2005; see also 'Transtheoretical model of behaviour change').

The PAPM uses more of a straightforward measure to categorize an individual into a particular stage; 'Have you ever thought about behaviour X' (those who say no are in Stage 1 – unaware of issue), 'Have you performed behaviour X' (those who say yes are in Stage 6 – acting), 'Which of the following best describes your thoughts about behaviour X' – 'I've never thought about it' (Stage 2 – unengaged), 'I'm undecided' (Stage 3 – deciding about acting), 'I've decided I don't want to ...' (Stage 4 – decided not to act), 'I've decided I do want to ...' (Stage 5 – decided to act). The HAPA similarly includes an additional stage after intention called 'action plans', which are cognitions about how and in what circumstances an intended action is to be implemented. Action plans are assessed using questions such as 'I have my own plans regarding behaviour X', 'I have already planned precisely ...': '... when I will perform behaviour X', '... where I will perform behaviour X', 'how often I will perform behaviour X', 'with whom I will perform behaviour X' – 'not at all true – exactly true' (Schwarzer et al., 2003). Measured in this way, action plans (or implementation intentions – see relevant entry in this volume) are actually very specific types of intention which take Ajzen's (1988) concerns with action, target, context and time into account.

Alternatives to self-report measures

Problems with self-report measures have led to the development of a range of alternative measures that attempt to minimize problems of socially desirable responding, either by changing the nature of the self-report measure or avoiding self-report as the basis of measurement. They also tend to have been developed in relation to the assessment of attitude (see Eagly & Chaiken, 1993). It should be noted that while, to differing degrees, these measures avoid problems of socially desirable responding, the reliability and validity of these measures is usually lower than self-report measures.

A range of behaviour measures has been used as alternatives to self-report for example in assessing attitudes. For example, in relation to assessing attitudes toward table salt one might directly assess the amount of table salt used by an individual at a meal and compare this with self-reported attitudes. Alternatively, in judging attitudes towards two different products one might allow individuals to choose one product to take away. In the consumer area, more sophisticated behavioural measures are now used through, for example, examination of supermarket checkout receipts and mapping these onto other measures (cf. Eagly & Chaiken, 1993). Whilst they represent an appealing means of avoiding socially desirable responding their validity is clearly questionable. For example, in relation to the analysis of checkout receipts it is not clear that individual purchase equates with individual use.

Similar problems surround physiological and biomarker measures. For example, both galvanic skin response and pupillary dilation have been used to assess attitudes (see Eagly & Chaiken, 1993). However, whilst strength of reaction may show some mapping onto underlying attitude strength it is not clear that this is a linear relationship and such physiological measures tell us little about the valence of such attitudes. A variety of bio-markers are also increasingly being used. For example, using expelled carbon monoxide levels to tap smoking or blood cholesterol to tap level of fat in the diet. Whilst such measures may provide good predictions of various health outcomes their relationship to behaviour may be weak. Carbon monoxide levels may only tap recent smoking and blood cholesterol is only modestly influenced by dietary changes.

There is also a range of disguised techniques such as the error choice method, estimating the plausibility of different arguments, thought listing and estimating other's responses. In each it is assumed that the individuals underlying attitude will bias their responses in a particular direction (see Eagly & Chaiken, 1993). A different technique is the bogus pipeline (Jones & Sigall, 1971). Originally this was used in relation to attitudes. The original research involved obtaining a prior measure of attitude and then using this information to convince respondents that it will be possible to detect non-accurate responding. A variant on this methodology is to inform respondents that an objective measure of behaviour will be taken and matched with self-report measures. A further set of disguised techniques are so-called projective techniques such as the Thematic Apperception Tests. Here individuals are asked to respond to ambiguous stimuli and their responses are scored in terms of what they indicated about underlying cognitions. The reliability and validity of such measures have been widely questioned, although more recent research has employed them as implicit measures of, for example, personality.

A final set of measures are the so-called implicit measures. These are in fact forms of self-report but are collected in such a way as to minimize socially desirable responding. Probably the most widely applied implicit measure is the Implicit Association Test (IAT, Greenwald, McGhee & Schwartz, 1998). The IAT is a computerized method for measuring indirectly the strength of the association between pairs of concepts via a discrimination task. It relies on the assumption that, if two concepts are highly associated (congruent), the discrimination task will be easier, and therefore quicker, when the associated concepts share the same response key than when they require a different response key (see Greenwald *et al.*, 1998). Studies have investigated the predictive power of the IAT for behaviours such as smoking (Swanson, Rudman & Greenwald, 2001). The correlations between explicit and IAT measures of attitudes tend to be low (on average in the region of 0.20 to 0.30). A range of other implicit measures have been employed including the Extrinsic Affective Simon Task Dot Probe Tasks and priming measures. Fazio and Olson (2003) provide a useful review of these measures. Whilst minimizing the effects of socially desirable responding there is continuing debate about the aspects of cognitions that these measures tap (Fazio & Olson, 2003).

Summary

The accurate assessment of health cognitions deepens our understanding of why individuals behave in ways that are detrimental to their health, or fail to behave in ways that are beneficial. The knowledge so gained can be used to develop theory-driven health education programmes and intervention strategies. Health cognitions are commonly assessed by self-reports, although there is a growing level of interest in alternate measures. There are many types of self-report measures, the most popular of which are Likert and semantic differential scales. More attention should be given to the reliability and validity of such scales, for example by the use of multi-item scales or parallel forms. Other factors that should be considered include social desirability, item ordering and the principle of compatibility (matching action, target, context and time). There are many social cognition models which incorporate health cognitions, and there is a great deal of overlap between these theories. Five core cognitive antecedents of health behaviours are: attitude, self-representations, norms, control perceptions and disposition to act.

Since good theory relies upon dependable measurement, it is important that future work in this area pays sufficient attention to the measurement issues described here. Due consideration should be given to issues relating to reliability and validity and the use of alternative techniques in conjunction with well constructed self-report measures is strongly encouraged. (See also 'Illness cognition assessment').

REFERENCES

Abraham, C. & Sheeran, P. (2000). Understanding and changing health behaviour: from health beliefs to self-regulation. In P. Norman, C. Abraham & M. Conner (Eds.). *Understanding and changing health behaviour: from health beliefs to self-regulation* (pp. 3–24). Amsterdam: Harwood Academic Publishers.

Ajzen, I. (1988). *Attitudes personality and behavior.* Milton Keynes, UK: Open University Press.

Ajzen, I. (1991). The theory of planned behavior. Special Issue: Theories of cognitive self-regulation. *Organizational Behavior and Human Decision Processes,* **50**, 179–211.

Bandura, A. (1986). *Social foundations of thought and action: a social cognitive theory.* Englewood Cliffs, NJ: Prentice Hall.

Champion, V. L. (1984) Instrument development for health belief model constructs. *Advances in Nursing Science.* **6**(3), 73–85.

Cialdini, R. B., Reno, R. R. & Kallgren, C. A. (1990). A focus theory of normative conduct: recycling the concept of norms to reduce littering in public places. *Journal of Personality and Social Psychology,* **58**, 1015–26.

Conner, M. & Sparks, P. (2005). The theory of planned behavior and health behaviors. In M. Conner & P. Norman (Eds.). *Predicting Health Behavior* (2nd edn.). (pp. 170–222). Buckingham, UK: Open University Press.

Conner, M. & Norman, P. (2005). *Predicting Health Behaviour: Research and Practise with Social Cognition Models* (2nd edn.). Buckingham, UK: Open University Press.

Eagly, A. H. & Chaiken, S. (1993). *The psychology of attitudes.* Fort Worth, Texas, US: Harcourt Brace Jovanovich College Publishers.

Evans, D. & Norman, P. (2003). Predicting adolescent pedestrians' road crossing intentions: an application and extension of the Theory of Planned Behaviour. *Health Education Research,* **18**(3), 267–77.

Fazio, R. H. & Olson, M. A. (2003). Implicit measures in social cognition research: their meaning and use. *Annual Review of Psychology,* **54**, 297–327.

Greenwald, A. G., McGhee, D. E. & Schwartz, J. L. K. (1998). Measuring individual differences in implicit cognition: the implicit association test. *Journal of Personality and Social Psychology,* **74**, 1464–80.

Higgins, E. (1987). Self-discrepancy: a theory relating self and affect. *Psychological Review,* **94**(3), 319–40.

Jones, E. E. & Sigall, H. (1971). The bogus pipeline: a new paradigm for measuring affect and attitude. *Psychological Bulletin,* **76**, 349–64.

Kline, P. (2000). *Handbook of psychological testing.* London: Routledge.

National Institute of Mental Health (NIMH) Multisite HIV Prevention Trial Group (2001). Social–cognitive theory mediators of behavior change in the National Institute of Mental Health Multisite HIV Prevention Trial. *Health Psychology,* **20**(5), 369–76.

O'Connor, R. C. & Armitage, C. J. (2003). Theory of planned behaviour and parasuicide: an exploratory study. *Current Psychology,* **22**, 196–205.

Rogers, R. W. (1983). Cognitive and physiological processes in fear appeals and attitude change: a revised theory of protection motivation. In J. T. Cacioppo & R. E. Petty (Eds.). *Social psychophysiology: a source book* (pp. 153–76). New York: Guilford Press.

Rosenstock, I. M., Strecher, V. J. & Becker, M. H. (1988). Social Learning Theory and the health belief model, *Health Education Quarterly,* **15**(2), 175–83.

Schwarzer, R., Sniehotta, F. F., Lippke, S. et al. (2003). On the assessment and analysis of variables in the Health Action Process Approach: conducting an investigation. Retrieved July 31, 2004 from http://www.fu-berlin.de/gesund/hapa_web.pdf

Sutton, S. (2005). Stage theories of health behaviour. In M. Conner & P. Norman (Eds.). *Predicting Health Behavior* (2nd edn.). (pp. 223–75). Buckingham, UK: Open University Press.

Swanson, J. E., Rudman, L. A. & Greenwald, A. G. (2001). Using the Implicit Association Test to investigate attitude–behavior consistency for stigmatized behavior. *Cognition and Emotion,* **15**, 207–30.

Velicer, W., Prochaska, J. O., Fava, J. L., Norman, G. J. & Redding, C. A. (1998). Smoking cessation and stress management: applications of the transtheoretical model of behavior change. *Homeostasis in Health and Disease.* **38**(5–6), 216–33.

Wallston, K. A., Wallston, B. S. & DeVellis, R. (1978). Development of multidimensional health locus of control (MHLC) scales. *Health Education Monographs,* **6**, 160–70.

Weiner, B. (1985). An attributional theory of achievement motivation and emotion. *Psychological Review,* **92**, 548–73.

Weinstein, W. D. (1988). The precaution adoption process. *Health Psychology,* **7**, 355–86.

White, K. M., Terry, D. J. & Hogg, M. A. (1994). Safer sex behavior: the role of attitudes, norms, and control factors. *Journal of Applied Social Psychology,* **24**(24), 2164–92.

Health status assessment

Ann Bowling

University College London

There is an increasing focus on the measurement of the health outcomes of healthcare interventions. Purchasers of health services want to know how much patients' lives will be improved by potential treatments, evidence of their effectiveness and costs and information about health gain in the broadest sense. But the conceptualization and methods of measurement of health outcomes is still controversial.

In order to measure health outcomes a measure of health status is required which needs to be based on a concept of health. Health indicators have largely been developed within the era of science based on the logical positivist paradigm. This inevitably leads to suspicion when data are presented which are based on subjective experience, rather than objective indicators. Clinicians have traditionally judged the value of an intervention mainly in terms of the five-year survival period. While obviously important in the case of life-threatening conditions, this indicator ignores the living. Many healthcare programmes and interventions will have little or no impact on mortality rates (e.g. in relation to chronic diseases). Survival needs to be interpreted more broadly in terms of the impact and consequences of treatment. And a person's 'ill health' is indicated by feelings of pain and discomfort or perceptions of change in usual functioning and feeling. Illnesses can be the result of pathological abnormality, but not necessarily so. A person can feel ill without medical science being able to detect disease. The World Health Organization's (WHO) (1947) therefore developed a multidimensional definition of health as a 'state of complete physical, mental and social wellbeing and not merely the absence of disease or infirmity'. The WHO (1984) has since added 'autonomy' to this list. Functional theory in sociology regards health broadly, and in the context of society, as the level of fitness and functioning (social, psychological or physical) which a person requires in order to fulfil expected social roles, based on his or her cultural norms. The social sciences not only focus on people's role functioning and social norms, but other perspectives emphasize people's definitions of health and illness and on individuals' subjective perceptions of their health (see Bowling, 2004 for overview). Phenomenological models hold that humans interpret and experience the world in terms of meanings and actively construct an individual social reality. These models in social science focus on the individual's unique perceptions of their circumstances (O'Boyle, 1997).

Measures of the outcome or consequences of disease, its treatment or care, which are based on patients' own perspectives ('patient-based') can be used to supplement the medical model of disease with a social model of health and ability. Their use helps to answer the question of whether the treatment leads to a life worth living from the patient's perspective. What matters is how the patient feels, rather than how others think they feel. Outcome assessment, then, needs to incorporate patient-based, subjective assessments as well as clinical indicators. In recognition of the need for a more positive focus, there has been an exponential increase in the additional use of indicators of broader health status and health related quality of life over the past two decades (Garrett *et al.*, 2002). However, most measures still take health as a starting point and measure deviations away from it (deteriorating health), rather than also encompassing gradations of healthiness. A perspective which captures the positive end of the spectrum is required to create a balance. In contrast to the emphasis on negative health, Merrell and Reed (1949) proposed a graded scale of health from positive to negative health. On such a scale people would be classified from those who are in top-notch condition with abundant energy, through to people who are well, to fairly well, down to people who are feeling rather poorly and finally to the definitely ill. The word 'health' rather than 'illness' was chosen deliberately to emphasize the positive side of this scale. Despite the existence of single item ranking scales asking people to rate their health from 'excellent' to 'very poor', the development of a broader health status scale along such a continuum is still awaited.

Broader measures of health status generally focus on individuals' subjective perceptions of their physical, psychological and social health. Many studies in medical sociology have indicated the importance of the perceptual component of illness in determining whether people feel ill or whether they seek help. Standardized items or measures of subjective, broader health status are increasingly included in population health surveys, in evaluations and clinical trials of service interventions. These are measures which ask people to rate their own health status and the impact of their health on various aspects of their lives. They are often referred to as patient-based measures. Detailed information about self-perceived health and its effects can be collected from large numbers of people using self-report questionnaires. They can be administered to the target group of interest by post, telephone, by computers, in clinic settings, or in face to face home interviews. The group of interest may be a patient or client group or a sample of the general population, depending on the aims of the study. Survey information about subjectively perceived health and illness at population level is now collected routinely by many governments worldwide.

Scales of subjective, broader-health statuses are more stable, and have better reliability and validity than single item questions and are the preferred instruments to use. The most commonly used instrument across the world is the Short Form-36 Health Survey Questionnaire (Ware *et al.*, 1993, 1997). On the other hand, some single items, despite some instability, are popularly used in general, multi-topic population surveys. A popular single-item measure consists of simply asking respondents to rate their health as 'excellent, good, fair or poor'. In order to increase the question's ability to discriminate between groups, researchers now insert a 'very good' category in between 'excellent' and 'good' (given that most respondents are affected by social desirability bias and rate their health at the 'good' end of the scale spectrum) (Ware *et al.*, 1993). This single-item measure of self-perceived health status has long been reported to be significantly and independently associated with use of health services, changes in functional status, mortality and to rates of recovery from episodes of ill health (e.g. National Heart and Lung Institute, 1976; Siegel *et al.*, 2003). The increasing emphasis on the patient's perspective has represented a paradigm shift in the approach to the operationalization and measurement of health outcomes (O'Boyle, 1997) (see also 'Quality of life assessment' and 'Disability assessment').

Self-rated health status may be contextual and vary over time with people's varying expectations. It should be cautioned that being in poor mental health can distort perceptions of health and wellbeing; being in poor physical health can lead to poor mental health and wellbeing, and vice versa. People's self-ratings of their health can also be subject to optimism, social desirability and other biases (Brissette *et al.*, 2003). Thus self-ratings of health are often criticized as subjective, although their subjectivity is their strength because they reflect personal evaluations of health.

Other health measurement formats, which are commonly used in studies of health status, are symptom checklists. These also have their limitations, but are generally considered to be useful tools if used in conjunction with scaled measurement techniques. There are numerous examples of checklists of symptoms presented to respondents in surveys. Respondents are typically asked to indicate which, if any, they currently suffer from. General symptom checklists can be found in the Rand Health Insurance Study Questionnaires (Stewart *et al.*, 1978). Disease specific quality of life questionnaires usually contain a list of symptoms relevant to the condition under study (see Bowling, 2001). However, items focusing on trivial problems are unlikely to have much discriminatory power in terms of monitoring change between groups over time. They may include response errors and diagnostic errors. Reporting of morbidity depends on symptom tolerance levels, pain thresholds; attitudes towards illness and other social and cultural factors.

The researcher also has to decide whether a general and/or specific measure of health status is required, depending on the nature of the study. There is little point in including a health status measure if it is unlikely to detect the effects of the treatment or symptoms specific to the condition. The case for using general health rather than disease-specific measures, in population surveys has been clearly argued by Kaplan (1988). For example, detailed information about specific disease categories may appear overwhelming to many respondents not suffering from them. Also the use of disease-specific measures precludes the possibility of comparing the outcomes of services that are directed at different groups suffering from different diseases. Policy analysis requires a general measure of health status, which research on clinical outcomes also requires the use of disease-specific indicators.

In sum, there are multiple influences upon patient outcome, and these require broad models of health to underpin outcome measurement. Investigators need to be clear about their definition of health status and select a measuring instrument which clearly operationalizes and measures that definition.

Acknowledgements

The information contained in this chapter is based on Bowling, A., Measuring Health, 3rd edn. Maidenhead: Open University Press, 2004 and Bowling, A., Measuring health outcomes from the patient's perspective. Chapter 18, In: A. Bowling and S. Ebrahim (Eds.). Handbook of health research methods. Maidenhead: Open University Press, Maidenhead.

REFERENCES

Bowling, A. (2001). *Measuring Disease: A Review of Disease-Specific Quality of Life Measurement Scales* (2nd edn.). Buckingham, UK: Open University Press.

Bowling, A. (2004). *Measuring Health* (3rd edn.). Maidenhead: Open University Press, 2004.

Brissette, I., Leventhal, H. & Leventhal, E. A. (2003). Observer ratings of health and sickness: can other people tell us anything about our health that we don't already know? *Health Psychology,* **22**, 471–8.

Garratt, A., Schmidt, L., Mackintosh, A. & Fitzpatrick, R. (2002). Quality of life measurement: bibliographic study of patient assessed health outcome measures. *British Medical Journal,* **324**, 1417.

Kaplan, R. M. (1988). New health promotion indicators: the general health policy model. *Health Promotion,* **3**, 35–48.

Merrell, M. & Reed, L. J. (1949). *The epidemiology of health, social medicine, its deviations and objectives.* New York: The Commonwealth Fund.

National Heart and Lung Institute (1976). Report of a task group on cardiac rehabilitation. In *Proceedings of the Heart and Lung Institute Working Conference on Health Behaviour.* Bethesda, MD: US Department of Health, Education and Welfare.

O'Boyle, C. A. (1997). Measuring the quality of later life. *Philosophy Transactions of the Royal Society of London,* **352**, 1871–9.

Siegel, M., Bradley, E. H. & Kasl, S. V. (2003). Self-rated life expectancy as a predictor of mortality: evidence from the HRS and AHEAD surveys. *Gerontology,* **49**, 265–71.

Stewart, A. L., Ware, J. E., Brook, R. H. *et al.* (1978). *Conceptualization and measurement of health for adults in the Health Insurance Study: Vol. 2. Physical health in terms of functioning.* Santa Monica, CA: Rand Corporation: R-1987/2-HEW.

Ware, J. E., Snow, K. K., Kosinski, M. & Gandek, B. (1993). *SF-36 Health Survey: manual and interpretation guide.* Boston, MA: The Health Institute, New England Medical Center.

Ware, J. E., Snow, K. K., Kosinski, M. & Gandek, B. (1997). SF-36 *Health Survey: Manual and Interpretation Guide.* (Rev. edn.). Boston, MA: The Health Institute, New England Medical Center.

World Health Organization (1947). *Constitution of the world health organization.* Geneva: WHO.

World Health Organization (1984). *Uses of epidemiology in aging: report of a scientific group, 1983.* Technical Report Series, No. 706. Geneva: WHO.

Illness cognition assessment

Ad A. Kaptein[1] and Elizabeth Broadbent[2]

[1]Leiden University Medical Center
[2]The University of Auckland

Introduction

Illness cognitions refer to 'individuals' common-sense definition of health threats' (Leventhal *et al.*, 1998, p. 719), and 'the patient's perception and understanding of the disease and treatment' (Leventhal *et al.*, 1986, p. 176). Concepts used as synonyms are illness beliefs, illness perceptions, illness representations, illness schemata and lay beliefs about illness (Scharloo & Kaptein, 1997). An elaborate and formal definition is proposed by Lacroix (1991): 'a distinct, meaningfully integrated cognitive structure that encompasses (1) a belief in the relatedness of a variety of physiological and psychological functions, which may or may not be objectively accurate; (2) a cluster of sensations, symptoms, emotions and physical limitations in keeping with that belief; (3) a naïve theory about the mechanisms that underlie the relatedness of the elements identified in (2); and (4) implicit or explicit prescriptions for corrective action' (p. 197).

Social cognitive models propose that individuals develop their own mental representation of health threats and these cognitions guide coping responses and set the criteria for appraisal of outcomes. Individuals' responses to stimuli, such as physical symptoms and signs, are partly determined by individuals' cognitions (or ideas, thoughts, views) about those stimuli. Social cognition models aim to shed light on these cognitions in order to describe, understand and change responses of individuals to these stimuli (Conner & Norman, 1996). The concept of 'lay illness models' is related to the illness cognition concept (Schober & Lacroix, 1991) (see 'Lay beliefs of health and illness'). In contrast, the concept of 'health cognition' pertains to items of knowledge or beliefs about health; it is discussed elsewhere in this Handbook (see 'Health cognition assessment'). The following sections describe the chronological development of assessment tools in illness cognition.

Interviews

A number of face to face interview techniques have been used to assess illness cognitions over the past 50 years. One of the earliest interviews was reported in a study by Bard and Dyk (1956) on the significance of beliefs of patients with various types of cancer regarding the causes of their condition. Interviews identified two categories of beliefs; self-blaming on the one hand and 'projective', i.e. blaming factors external to the patient, on the other. The authors described the relevance of causal beliefs for seeking medical care, adherence and behavioural outcomes, as well as the importance of concordance between patients and healthcare providers regarding causal beliefs.

Anthropologist and psychiatrist Kleinman used open interviews to explore illness representations in patients and healthy respondents in non-western, Asian countries. The theoretical focus was inspired by medical anthropology: to find explanations of how people make sense of health and illness in different cultures. The open interviews aimed at assessing explanatory models, 'the notions about an episode of sickness and its treatment that are employed by all those engaged in the clinical process' (Kleinman, 1980, p. 105). Observations and open interviews resulted in identifying a number of categories of illness representations that respondents used to make sense of illness and its treatment. Aetiology, onset of symptoms, pathophysiology, course of illness, treatment, were the categories observed (Kleinman *et al.*, 1978, p. 256).

These dimensions are quite similar to the ones used in illness cognition theories that were developed some 20 years later, such as the Common Sense Model of illness (Leventhal *et al.*, 1980).

Leventhal and colleagues conducted open-ended interviews with patients with chronic illness and identified four themes for how people think about illness: identity, timeline, consequences and cause (Leventhal *et al.*, 1980; Leventhal & Nerenz, 1985; Meyer *et al.*, 1985). Asking patients why they had recovered from everyday illnesses such as the flu, Lau and colleagues identified an additional cure/control theme to illness representations (Lau *et al.*, 1989; Lau & Hartman, 1983).

Some interviews have been designed for specific populations based on the themes from the Common Sense Model of illness, such as an interview for epilepsy patients (Kemp & Morley, 2001) which incorporates both open and closed questions and takes approximately 30 minutes. The Personal Models of Diabetes Interview (Hampson, Glasgow & Toobert, 1990) is also based on Leventhal's self-regulation theoretical framework and uses a combination of open and closed questions to assess 'personal models', defined as patients' cognitive representations of their disease. This research identified the dimensions: cause, symptoms (identity), treatment (cure/control) and seriousness (course and consequences). A later study (Hampson *et al.*, 1994), found similar results in a sample of patients with osteoarthritis, which lends further empirical support for the dimensions of illness representations.

One open-ended patient interview assesses the accuracy of patients' illness schemata compared with the views of their treatment specialist (Lacroix, 1991). The Schema Assessment Instrument focuses on assessing the patient's symptoms and their interpretation of these with regard to their medical condition. These are matched to medical evidence to attain an overall understanding score. Using this interview, functioning has been found to be better related to schema accuracy than to medical severity of the condition in chronic respiratory patients (Lacroix *et al.*, 1991). However, the Schema Assessment Interview is limited to assessing the objective accuracy of schemata and has received little use, as researchers more commonly assess the content of representations than their accuracy.

A review of the assessment of illness perceptions in chronic somatic patients between 1985 and 1995 found 101 studies; the most common method used to assess illness perceptions in these studies was the open-ended interview (Scharloo & Kaptein, 1997; Kaptein *et al.*, 2001). In the majority of these studies, patients' answers were recorded verbatim and then rated into categories. All interviews in the review assessed causal representations, and some interviews assessed all five dimensions of illness representation.

Many of the in-depth semi-structured interviews conducted in the early explorative phase of illness perceptions were very time-consuming and produced a large variation in the quantity and quality of response (Weinman *et al.*, 1996). Furthermore, in many cases there has been no information published on their psychometric validity. This type of assessment is most suited to the exploratory phase and instruments to assess specific attributes of representations are more useful for hypothesis testing which has led to the development of psychometrically validated questionnaires.

Questionnaires

One of the earliest questionnaires on illness cognition stemmed from the work of Osgood *et al.*, on 'The measurement of meaning', which led researchers in the public health area to use the semantic differential technique as a method to assess the meaning respondents (patients) attach to a certain stimulus or concept, relevant to health and illness (Jenkins, 1966; Osgood *et al.*, 1957). Jenkins adapted the semantic differential technique to health and illness by developing the Semantic Differential for Health (SDH). The SDH had 16 items assessing various dimensions of beliefs about different illnesses (e.g. poliomyelitis, tuberculosis, cancer, mental illness). The three original semantic differential dimensions – evaluative, potency, activity – were operationalized in a questionnaire with the 16 items that had 2 to 6 response categories, depending on the item. Factor analysis produced dimensions of beliefs about illness that were labelled personal involvement, human mastery and social acceptability (Jenkins & Zyzanski, 1968). This work is important in itself within the context of assessing illness cognitions, and it laid the foundations for work on the Health Belief Model (Becker *et al.*, 1977; see 'Health belief model').

Rating scales have been a popular way to assess illness perceptions, but in many cases studies have assessed just one or two dimensions and used separate scales for each dimension (Scharloo & Kaptein, 1997), such as the Multidimensional Health Locus of Control Scale (Wallston *et al.*, 1978) to measure control beliefs. Some measures of illness cognitions have been developed for use with specific populations, for example, the Pain Beliefs and Perceptions Inventory (Williams & Thorn, 1989), which assesses causes and timeline using a 16-item scale scored on a 4-point Likert scale, and the 24-item true–false response Survey of Pain Attitudes (Jensen *et al.*, 1987) (measuring dimensions akin to consequences and control). These scales are limited in their applicability to illness population types other than pain. Other scales have been designed with the ability to be applied to many different patient populations, and an advantage of these generic questionnaires is that they facilitate comparisons across illness populations.

Turk *et al.* (1986) set out to examine 'implicit models of illness' and to clarify differences in outcome between patients with various illnesses and complaints, chronic pain in particular. The Implicit Model of Illness Questionnaire (IMIQ) was developed as a generic instrument to assess illness cognitions. The questionnaire contains 38 items on a 9-point scale that are theoretically based, i.e. it aimed to examine whether the dimensions in Leventhal & Nerenz model (1985) could be identified. It was found via factor analytic techniques that the IMIQ items had four dimensions: seriousness, personal responsibility, controllability and changeability. In this study the respondents were not only groups of patients, but also nurses and healthy students using contrasting illnesses such as the flu, cancer and diabetes. This research has been criticized for not constructing the scale with patient samples rating their own illness (Weinman *et al.*, 1996), as well as the way the data were analysed (Lau *et al.*, 1989). Subsequent research with a rheumatic arthritis sample found a different factor structure: curability, personal responsibility, symptom variability and serious consequences (Schiaffino & Cea, 1995). These problems have resulted in little subsequent use of the questionnaire.

Other studies have also found that factor analysis of theoretically derived items from the Common Sense Model reveals different clustering of items depending on the illness. For example, in a study of chronic fatigue patients, factor analysis revealed four factors identified as manageability, seriousness, personal responsibility and external cause, while in Addison's disease patients the factors were seriousness, cause, chronicity and controllability (Heijmans & de Ridder, 1998). Some researchers argue that assessment should involve factor analysis of the items (Heijmans & de Ridder, 1998; Turk et al., 1986), but analysis usually reveals dimensions that are similar to the theoretical domains (Hagger & Orbell, 2003). Keeping the theoretical factor structure of the core domains keeps the representations true to theory derived from open-ended interviews, and allows comparisons across studies and across illnesses.

The publications by Leventhal and his associates are a major source of theoretical and empirical work in the illness cognition or illness representation field (e.g. Leventhal et al., 2003). This theoretical work led Weinman, Petrie, Moss-Morris & Horne (1996) to develop the Illness Perception Questionnaire (IPQ). The IPQ is a theoretically-derived 38-item multifactorial pencil and paper questionnaire which assesses all five cognitive components of illness representations: identity, timeline, consequences' cause and cure/control. Identity is assessed by asking respondents how frequently s/he now experiences 12 symptoms as part of their illness. The cause, timeline, consequences and control/cure dimensions are assessed with 26 5-point Likert type questions, ranging from 'strongly agree' to 'strongly disagree'. Examples of items are, 'My illness will last a short time' (timeline), 'My illness has major consequences on my life' (consequences) and 'There is a lot which I can do to control my symptoms' (control/cure) and 'Stress was a major factor in causing my illness' (cause). The IPQ timeline scale has lower than desirable internal consistency and the cure/control scale loads on two factors, self-efficacy and treatment beliefs; the IPQ was therefore revised to improve its measurement properties and to extend its scope (Moss-Morris et al., 2002). The Illness Perception Questionnaire – Revised (IPQ-R), extends the original scale by adding more items, splitting the control dimension into personal control and treatment control, incorporating a cyclical timeline dimension, an overall comprehension of illness factor and an emotional representation (Moss-Morris et al., 2002). The IPQ-R assesses identity by asking patients whether or not s/he has experienced each of 14 symptoms since their illness; then they are asked whether they believe the symptom is specifically related to their illness. Causes are assessed by asking patients whether they agree or disagree with a list of causes for their illness and the scale also includes an open-ended item asking patients to list the three most important causes for their illness. However, with all these additions, a drawback of the IPQ-R is that it has over 80 items. In some situations such a long questionnaire can be prohibitive.

The publication of the Illness Perception Questionnaire and its revised form represented a breakthrough in the area of assessing illness perceptions because the scales are theoretically derived, simple to administer, comprehensive, psychometrically validated and easily adaptable to different populations. These scales have been used in over 100 published papers and are available on the IPQ website (http://www.uib.no/ipq/).

The Brief Illness Perception Questionnaire is a newly developed 9-item scale designed to rapidly assess illness representations (Broadbent et al., 2006). It has been suggested that instruments assessing specific attributes of illness representation take one of two forms (Leventhal & Nerenz, 1985): specific scales can be used to assess factors, or single-item measures can be used to measure particular variables. As illness perceptions are now well defined, single items may be better suited to their assessment than multiple items designed to assess latent factors (Leventhal & Nerenz, 1985).

In the Brief IPQ, single-item scales from 0 to 10 are used to assess consequences, timeline, personal control, treatment control, identity, coherence, concern and emotional responses; for example, 'How long do you think your illness will continue?', answered from 0 'A very short time' to 10 'Forever' (timeline). Causes are assessed by an open-ended response item. This questionnaire is likely to be especially useful when participants are very ill or elderly, when illness perceptions are measured as only one part of a larger set of psychological constructs, in large population-based studies, when repeated measures are taken on a frequent basis and in longitudinal studies designed to demonstrate changes in illness representations as a result of coping and appraisal.

The Illness Cognition Questionnaire has been recently developed to assess adjustment cognitions, namely helplessness, acceptance and perceived benefits (Evers et al., 2001). Rather than focusing on the mental representation of illness, this questionnaire focuses on the next stage of the Common Sense Model which involves coping and appraisal. Patients are asked to rate 18 items on a 4-point agree–disagree Likert scale, for example 'My illness frequently makes me feel helpless'.

Causal attributions

Causal attribution models examine perceptions of causes of past events. Causal attributions can be assessed through open-ended questions or through participant responses to experimenter-generated causal lists, such as the list included in the IPQ-R. There is some evidence for convergent validity between open-ended and structured questionnaires for eliciting causal beliefs. The responses generated on the causal dimension for heart attacks from studies using open-ended questions have been compared to responses from studies using experimenter generated lists (French et al., 2001). The review found no evidence for different patterns of attributions when the responses were respondent-or experimenter-generated. However, there were differences in the frequency of some of the causal items endorsed when response scales were dichotomous compared to interval-rating scales. The advantage of the open-ended questions is that patients' responses are not limited to the listed items.

The Symptom Beliefs Questionnaire has been developed specifically for the assessment of causal attributions for symptoms prior to contact with a general practitioner (Salmon, Woloshynowych & Valori, 1996). Patients are asked whether they believe a list of 50 items are a cause of their symptoms with the responses 'probably has', 'don't know', or 'probably has not'. Eight dimensions emerge from factor analysis – stress, lifestyle, wearing out, environmental, internal–structural, internal–functional, weak constitution and concern.

Drawings

The assessment of illness representations has largely relied on language-based interviews and questionnaires. An alternative approach to the assessment of illness perceptions asked patients to draw what they thought had happened to their heart after a heart attack (Broadbent *et al.*, 2004). Patients tended to draw damage and/or blockages on their heart. A smaller number of patients drew emotions or the causes of their heart attack on their heart. The drawings were able to quantitatively assess damage perceptions from the percentage of the heart drawn as damaged. Greater damage perceptions predicted slower return to work and poorer perceptions of recovery at three months after the heart attack. Figure 1 shows an example of a patient's drawing of his/her heart. Drawings are able to identify idiosyncratic perceptions of illness that are not easily assessable by questionnaire. Drawings may be particularly useful for patients who cannot express themselves in language or for children. Further work needs to assess the ability of drawings to assess illness cognitions in other illnesses.

Assessment populations

The majority of studies have assessed illness cognitions in adult patient populations with chronic illness, however illness cognitions have also been assessed in other populations including: children (for example, Koopman *et al.*, 2004; Walker *et al.*, 2004); relatives of patients, for example mothers (Leiser *et al.*, 1996) and spouses (for example (Weinman *et al.*, 2000); healthcare providers (for example, Richardson *et al.*, 2001); and society (for example, Liddell *et al.*, 2005). In addition to assessing illness representations in patients with various physical disorders, illness cognitions

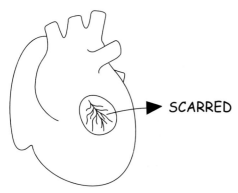

Fig 1 A patient's perception of his/her heart after a heart attack assessed through drawing.

have also been assessed in patients with psychiatric disorders (e.g. Lobban *et al.*, 2004).

Most work in assessing illness cognitions has aimed at describing the illness cognitions of various samples of respondents (e.g. patients, physicians, other healthcare providers), without paying attention to whether these cognitions are consistent with 'objective' descriptions of the illness or complaint under study. This emphasis is almost a logical consequence of the idea of illness cognitions in the first place, i.e. examining the idiosyncratic, subjective definition of symptoms and physical states. Two lines of research extend to the examining of illness representations, however, namely the work by Lacroix (1991) on concordance vs. divergence of illness perceptions with health professionals, and the work on match/mismatch between the patients' and their partners' perceptions of illness and symptoms (e.g. Figueiras & Weinman, 2003).

Examining the illness representations of not only the patient but of those around the patient, and using the degree of correspondence between the two parties is increasingly applied in health psychology research. The study by Figueiras and Weinman (2003) is a good example: patients with a myocardial infarction and their partners/spouses both completed the IPQ-R. Higher concordance (i.e. similar positive perceptions) on the dimensions of the questionnaire was associated with a more favourable outcome, expressed as better physical, psychological and sexual functioning and as less impact of the myocardial infarction on social and recreational activities.

Applications from assessing illness cognitions

Assessing illness cognitions not only allows research into how patients understand and respond to illness but also offers a theory-based intervention target to improve outcomes. Petrie *et al.*'s trial of an individually tailored psychological intervention in patients with a myocardial infarction is exemplary in this respect (Petrie *et al.*, 2002): a brief hospital-based intervention designed to alter negative cognitions resulted in quicker return to work and improved functional outcomes following myocardial infarction. In other work, negative consequence beliefs in patients with dizziness have been shown to predict sustained activity restriction and these beliefs have been shown to be modifiable by therapy (Yardley *et al.*, 2001). There has also been some promising work attempting to teach healthcare providers to recognize, challenge and change illness perceptions in their patients in order to improve illness cognitions and adherence (Theunissen *et al.*, 2003).

REFERENCES

Bard, M. & Dyk, R. B. (1956). The psychodynamic significance of beliefs regarding the cause of serious illness. *Psychoanalytic Review*, **43**, 146–62.

Becker, M. H., Haefner, D. P., Kasl, S. V. *et al.* (1977). Selected psychosocial models and correlates of individual health-related behaviors. *Medical Care*, **1977, 15**, 27–46.

Broadbent, E., Petrie, K. J., Ellis, C. J., Ying, J. & Gamble, G. (2004). A picture of health-myocardial infarction patients' drawings of their hearts and subsequent disability. A longitudinal study. *Journal of Psychosomatic Research*, **57**, 583–7.

Broadbent, E., Petrie, K. J., Main, J. & Weinman, J. (2006). The brief illness perception questionnaire. *Journal of Psychosomatic Research*, **60**, 631–37.

Conner, M. & Norman, P. (Eds.). (1996). *Predicting health behaviour*. Buckingham, UK: Open University Press.

Evers, A. W. M., Kraaimaat, F. W., van Lankveld, W. *et al.* (2001). Beyond unfavorable thinking: The Illness Cognition Questionnaire for chronic diseases. *Journal of Consulting and Clinical Psychology*, **69**, 1026–36.

Figueiras, M. J. & Weinman, J. (2003). Do similar patient and spouse perceptions of myocardial infarction predict recovery? *Psychology and Health*, **18**, 201–16.

French, D. P., Senior, V., Weinman, J. & Marteau, T. M. (2001). Causal attributions for heart disease: a systematic review. *Psychology and Health*, **16**, 77–98.

Hagger, M. S. & Orbell, S. (2003). A meta-analytic review of the common-sense model of illness representations. *Psychology and Health*, **18**, 141–84.

Hampson, S. E., Glasgow, R. E. & Toobert, D. J. (1990). Personal models of diabetes and their relations to self-care activities. *Health Psychology*, **9**, 632–46.

Hampson, S. E., Glasgow, R. E. & Zeiss, A. M. (1994). Personal models of osteoarthritis and their relation to self-management activities and quality of life. *Journal of Behavioral Medicine*, **17**, 143–58.

Heijmans, M. & de Ridder, D. (1998). Assessing illness representations of chronic illness: explorations of their disease-specific nature. *Journal of Behavioral Medicine*, **21**, 485–503.

Jenkins, C. D. (1966). The Semantic Differential for Health: a technique for measuring beliefs about diseases. *Public Health Reports*, **81**, 549–58.

Jenkins, C. D. & Zyzanski, S. J. (1968). Dimensions of belief and feeling concerning three diseases, poliomyelitis, cancer, and mental illness: a factor analytic study. *Behavioral Science*, **13**, 372–81.

Jensen, M. P., Karoly, P. & Huger, R. (1987). The development and preliminary validation of an instrument to assess patients' attitudes toward pain. *Journal of Psychosomatic Research*, **31**(3), 393–400.

Kaptein, A. A., Scharloo, M. & Weinman, J. A. (2001). Assessment of illness perceptions. In A. Vingerhoets (Ed.). *Assessment in behavioural medicine* (pp. 179–94). Hove, UK: Brunner-Routledge.

Kemp, S. & Morley, S. (2001). The development of a method to assess patients' cognitive representations of epilepsy. *Epilepsy and Behavior*, **2**, 247–71.

Kleinman, A. (1980). *Patients and healers in the context of culture*. Berkeley, CA: University of California Press.

Kleinman, A., Eisenberg, L. & Good, B. (1978). Culture, illness, and care. *Annals of Internal Medicine*, **88**, 251–8.

Koopman, H. M., Baars, R. M., Chaplin, J. & Zwinderman, K. H. (2004). Illness through the eyes of the child: the development of children's understanding of the causes of illness. *Patient Education and Counseling*, **55**, 363–70.

Lacroix, J. M. (1991). Assessing illness schemata in patient populations. In J. A. Skelton & R. T. Croyle (Eds.). *Mental representation in health and illness* (pp. 193–219). New York NY: Springer.

Lacroix, J. M., Martin, B., Avendano, M. & Goldstein, R. (1991). Symptom schemata in chronic respiratory patients. *Health Psychology*, **10**, 268–73.

Lau, R. R., Bernard, T. M. & Hartman, K. A. (1989). Further exploration of the common-sense representations of common illnesses. *Health Psychology*, **8**, 195–219.

Lau, R. R. & Hartman, K. A. (1983). Common sense representations of common illnesses. *Health Psychology*, **2**, 167–85.

Leiser, D., Doitsch, E. & Meyer, J. (1996). Mothers' lay models of the causes and treatment of fever. *Social Science and Medicine*, **43**, 379–87.

Leventhal, H., Brissette, I. & Leventhal, E. A. (2003). The common-sense model of self-regulation of health and illness. In L. D. Cameron & H. Leventhal (Eds.). *The self-regulation of health and illness behaviour* (pp. 42–65). London: Routledge.

Leventhal, H., Easterling, D. V., Coons, H. L., Luchterhand, C. M. & Love, R. R. (1986). Adaptation to chemotherapy treatments. In B. L. Andersen (Ed.). *Women with cancer – psychological perspectives* (pp. 172–203). New York: Springer.

Leventhal, H., Leventhal, E. A. & Contrada, R. J. (1998). Self-regulation, health, and behavior a perceptual–cognitive approach. *Psychology and Health*, **13**, 717–33.

Leventhal, H., Meyer, D. & Nerenz, D. R. (1980). The common sense representation of illness danger. In S. Rachman (Ed.). *Contributions to medical psychology*. Vol. 2 (pp. 7–30). New York: Pergamon.

Leventhal, H. & Nerenz, D. R. (1985). The assessment of illness cognition. In P. Karoly (Ed.). *Measurement strategies in health psychology* (pp. 517–54). New York: John Wiley & Sons.

Liddell, C., Barrett, L. & Bydawell, M. (2005). Indigenous representations of illness and AIDS in sub-Saharan Africa. *Social Science and Medicine*, **60**, 691–700.

Lobban, F., Barrowclough, C. & Jones, S. (2004). The impact of beliefs about mental health problems and coping on outcome in schizophrenia. *Psychological Medicine*, **34**, 1165–76.

Meyer, D., Leventhal, H. & Gutmann, M. (1985). Common-sense models of illness: the example of hypertension. *Health Psychology*, **4**, 115–35.

Moss-Morris, R., Weinman, J., Petrie, K. J. *et al.* (2002). The Revised Illness Perception Questionnaire (IPQ-R). *Psychology and Health*, **17**, 1–16.

Osgood, C. E., Suci, G. & Tannenbaum, P. (1957). *The measurement of meaning*. Urbana, IL: The University of Illinois Press.

Petrie, K. J., Cameron, L. D., Ellis, C. J., Buick, D. L. & Weinman, J. (2002). Changing illness perceptions following myocardial infarction: an early intervention randomized controlled trial. *Psychosomatic Medicine*, **64**, 580–6.

Richardson, R. D., Engel, C. C., McFall, M., McKnight, K., Boehnlein, J. K. & Hunt, S. C. (2001). Clinician attributions for symptoms and treatment of Gulf War-related health concerns. *Archives of Internal Medicine*, **161**, 1289–94.

Salmon, P., Woloshynowych, M. & Valori, R. (1996). The measurement of beliefs about physical symptoms in English general practice patients. *Social Science and Medicine*, **42**, 1561–7.

Scharloo, M. & Kaptein, A. A. (1997). Measurement of illness perceptions in patients with chronic somatic illness: a review. In K. J. Petrie & J. A. Weinman (Eds.). *Perceptions of health and illness*. (pp. 103–4). Amsterdam: Harwood Academic Publishers.

Schiaffino, K. M. & Cea, C. D. (1995). Assessing chronic illness representations: the implicit models of illness questionnaire. *Journal of Behavioral Medicine*, **18**, 531–48.

Schober, R. & Lacroix, J. M. (1991). Lay illness models in the Enlightenment and the 20th century: some historical lessons. In J. A. Skelton & R. T. Croyle (Eds.). *Mental representation in health and illness* (pp. 10–31). New York: Springer.

Theunissen, N. C. M., de Ridder, D. T. D., Bensing, J. M. & Rutten, G. E. H. M. (2003). Manipulation of patient–provider interaction: discussing illness representations or action plans concerning adherence. *Patient Education and Counseling*, **51**, 247–58.

Turk, D. C., Rudy, T. E. & Salovey, P. (1986). Implicit models of illness. *Journal of Behavioral Medicine*, **9**, 453–74.

Walker, C., Papadopoulos, L., Hussein, M. & Lipton, M. (2004). Paediatric eczema, illness beliefs and psychosocial morbidity: how does eczema affect children (in their own words)? *Dermatology + Psychosomatics*, **5**, 126–31.

Wallston, K. A., Wallston, B. S. & DeVellis, R. (1978). Development of the multidimensional health locus of control (MHLC) Scales. *Health Education Monographs*, **6**, 160–70.

Weinman, J., Petrie, K. J., Moss-Morris, R. & Horne, R. (1996). The Illness Perception Questionnaire: a new method for assessing the cognitive representation of illness. *Psychology and Health*, **11**, 431–46.

Weinman, J., Petrie, K. J., Sharpe, N. & Walker, S. (2000). Causal attributions in patients and spouses following first-time myocardial infarction and subsequent lifestyle changes. *British Journal of Health Psychology*, **5**, 263–3.

Williams, D. A. & Thorn, B.E. (1989). An empirical assessment of pain beliefs. *Pain*, **36**, 351–8.

Yardley, L., Beech, S. & Weinman, J. (2001). Influence of beliefs about the consequences of dizziness on handicap in people with dizziness, and the effect of therapy on beliefs. *Journal of Psychosomatic Research*, **50**, 1–6.

IQ testing

Robert J. Sternberg

Tufts University

In this chapter, we first consider what intelligence is. Then we discuss the nature of IQ and its relation to intelligence. The two main test batteries that are used to assess IQ are described. Next we discuss the history of intelligence testing that led up to these tests and some of the main psychometric theories which underlie IQ testing. Mean differences among various groups in scores on tests of IQ are defined and illustrated. Finally we draw some conclusions.

What is intelligence?

In 1921, 14 famous psychologists presented their views on the nature of intelligence in a symposium organized in the *Journal of Educational Psychology* (see 'Intelligence and its measurement: a symposium', 1921). Although their responses varied, two themes became clear: intelligence comprises (1) the ability to learn from experience and (2) the ability to adapt to the surrounding environment. These themes are important. Ability to learn from experience implies, for example, that more intelligent people learn from their mistakes. They do not keep making the same ones again and again. Adaptation to the environment means that being intelligent goes beyond getting high scores on tests. It includes how you perform in school, handle a job, get along with other people and manage your life in general.

Sixty-five years after the initial symposium, 24 different experts of a later generation were asked to give their views on the nature of intelligence (R.J. Sternberg & Detterman, 1986). They too noted the standard themes of learning from experience and adapting to the environment. However, these experts also put more emphasis on the role of 'metacognition', i.e., people's understanding and control of their own thinking processes (during problem-solving, reasoning and decision-making), than did earlier experts. Contemporary experts also more heavily emphasized the role of culture.

They pointed out that what is considered intelligent in one society may be considered stupid in another.

Some psychologists, such as Edwin Boring (1923), have been content to define intelligence as whatever it is that what sometimes are called 'IQ tests' measure. This definition, unfortunately, is circular because according to it, the nature of intelligence is what is tested, but what is tested must necessarily be determined by the nature of intelligence. Moreover, what different tests of intelligence test is not always exactly the same thing. Different tests measure somewhat different constructs (Daniel, 1997, 2000; Kaufman, 2000; Kaufman & Lichtenberger, 1998), so it is not feasible to define intelligence by what tests test, as though they all measured precisely the same thing. What they test is due, in large part, to a Frenchman of the early twentieth century named Alfred Binet.

The Intelligence Quotient (IQ)

To this day, schools usually segregate children according to their physical, or chronological, age. In the early twentieth century, Alfred Binet, a Frenchman, suggested that we might assess children's intelligence on the basis of their mental age. This age is a score indicating the chronological age of persons who typically perform at the same level of intelligence as a test taker. If, for example, someone's performance on a test is at a level comparable to that of an average 12-year-old, the person's mental age will be 12, regardless of the chronological age. Suppose, for example, that José is 10 years old, but his performance on a test of intelligence is equal to that of the average 12-year-old. His mental age would be 12. Mental age also conveniently might suggest an appropriate grade placement in school.

William Stern, a German psychologist, noted that mental age is of doubtful usefulness for comparing levels of intelligence in children who differ in chronological age. Stern (1912) suggested instead that we measure intelligence by using an intelligence quotient (IQ): a ratio of mental age (MA) divided by chronological age (CA), multiplied by 100. This ratio can be expressed mathematically as follows:

$$IQ = (MA/CA) \times 100$$

Thus, if Anita's mental age of 5 equals her chronological age of 5, then her intelligence is average, and her IQ is 100, because $(5/5)(100) = 100$. People whose mental age equals their chronological age always have IQs of 100 because the numerator of the equation equals the denominator, giving a quotient of 1. Suppose Bill's mental age of 4 is only half of his chronological age of 8. Then his IQ is 50, because the quotient is ½, and half of 100 is 50. Subsequent investigators have suggested further modifications of the IQ. As a result, Stern's particular conception of expressing intelligence in terms of a ratio of mental age to chronological age, multiplied by 100, is now termed a ratio IQ.

Unfortunately, the concept of mental age proved to be a weak link in the measurement of intelligence, even when used for calculating a ratio IQ. First, increases in measured mental age slow down at about the age of 16 years. Compare what you knew and how you thought when you were 8 years old with what you knew and how you thought when you reached 12 years old. Quite a difference! Now think about someone who is 30 years old. Do you imagine that person's knowledge and thought processes to be very different from what they will be at age 45? It makes sense to say that an 8-year-old who performs at the level of a 12-year-old has an IQ of 150. But it makes no sense at all to say that a 30-year-old who performs at the level of a 45-year-old has an IQ of 150. The reason is that the intellectual performance of a typical 45-year-old usually differs only minimally from that of a typical 30-year-old. Indeed, in older age, scores on some kinds of mental tests actually may start to decrease. When measuring across the whole life span, it seems less than effective to base the calculation of intelligence on mental age.

Intelligence tests

A number of tests of intelligence measure various kinds of cognitive skills (Daniel, 1997, 2000; Kaufman, 2000). These tests are based largely on the notion that intelligence is a function of judgments of a fairly academic kind. The two main tests derive respectively from the work of Alfred Binet and David Wechsler.

The Stanford–Binet Intelligence Scales

One major test derives from the work of Alfred Binet, mentioned above. The most recent revision, the Stanford–Binet Intelligence Scales, fifth edition (Roid, 2003), or Stanford–Binet V, as it is sometimes called, is designed for age levels ranging from two to ninety+ years and, like the original test, is administered to people individually in an untimed fashion. The ten tests in the scale together measure reasoning abilities, general knowledge, visual–spatial abilities and working memory (simultaneous storage and processing of information). The Stanford–Binet V emphasizes verbal and nonverbal abilities equally. Also, for this scale and all

other modern intelligence scales, the traditional ratio IQ has been replaced by a deviation IQ, which indicates a person's performance relative to other people of the same chronological age.

The Wechsler scales

There are three Wechsler scales. Each of the Wechsler scales currently used is designed for a different age group. The Wechsler Preschool and Primary Scale of Intelligence, Version III (WPPSI-III), is administered to children ranging in age from two and a half years to approximately seven years. Younger children are administered a different part of the scale than are older children. For younger children, the verbal part of the WPPSI-III contains tests of vocabulary and basic knowledge about the world. The performance part of the scale includes tests that require children to create pictures of common objects using jigsaw puzzle pieces and to reproduce a design using building blocks. For older children there are additional tests of verbal comprehension and perceptual classification skills. Also, both the verbal and performance parts of the WPPSI-III for older children contain additional tests which assess reasoning.

The Wechsler Intelligence Scale for Children, Version IV (WISC-IV), is administered to children ranging in age from 6 years to 16 years. The tests on the WISC-IV are similar in nature to the WPPSI-III, though they are more difficult as is appropriate for older children. The WISC-IV also includes tests of memory and reasoning that the WPPSI-III does not include.

The Wechsler Adult Intelligence Scale, Version III (WAIS-III), is administered to adults ranging in age from 16 to 89 years, and contains 14 tests. The primary difference between the WAIS-III and its companion scale for children, the WISC-IV, is the inclusion of several tests that assess working memory and more difficult items. Like Binet, Wechsler (1974) recognized that intelligence goes beyond what his own test measures. We use our intelligence in relating to people, in doing our jobs effectively and in managing our lives in general. In fact, intelligence tests predict performance in a variety of real-world pursuits, such as education (R. Mayer, 2000) and the work force (Schmidt et al., 1992; Wagner, 1997).

Where do tests such as the Stanford–Binet and the Wechsler come from? The next section explores their origins and history.

The history of IQ testing

In 1904, the Minister of Public Instruction in Paris named a commission to find a means to differentiate mentally 'defective' children from those who were unsuccessful in school for other reasons. The commission was to ensure that no child suspected of retardation be placed in a special class without first being given an examination. Alfred Binet and his collaborator, Theodore Simon, devised tests to meet this requirement. Thus, theory and research in the tradition of Binet grew out of practical educational concerns. To Binet and Simon (1916), the core of intelligence is judgement and common sense.

Binet's ideas were brought to the United States primarily by Lewis Terman. The first major revision was completed by Terman (1916), who translated and renamed the test (to the Stanford–Binet Intelligence Scales) for American use. In the United States, intelligence testing came into its own in World War I. Practical concerns regarding military recruitment and placement required tests that could be administered to several people at one time in order to meet the US Army's demands for the rapid testing of a large number of men. The shift from one-on-one testing to group testing required substantial changes to intelligence test design. These changes included (1) the presentation of brief, written items in lieu of more complicated tasks requiring detailed instructions; (2) the replacement of examiner judgement with objective, right/wrong scoring techniques; (3) the imposition of time limits for test completion; and (4) the development of test problems appropriate for adults. The familiarity of these test characteristics to most readers of this book shows how lasting these changes have proven to be.

The staying power of group intelligence tests can be attributed primarily to their tremendous efficiency relative to assessments that must be administered individually. Brief, written items with simple instructions eliminate the need for a highly trained examiner to explain the requirements of each test in the scale. In addition, objective scoring techniques are much quicker and less prone to error than are scoring techniques dependent on the subjective judgement of the examiner. Time limits for test completion have obvious implications for the efficiency of test administration. An important disadvantage of group testing, however, is that it often limits the kinds of performances which can be assessed. For example, basic motor abilities, such as finger tapping or bodily coordination, are not easily assessed when the examinee–examiner ratio is greater than 1 : 1.

The Army Alpha, created by Arthur Otis as an adaptation of the Stanford–Binet intelligence scale, was the first group intelligence test developed to meet the army's recruitment and placement needs. It assessed various reasoning skills and basic cultural knowledge. Due to high rates of illiteracy among military recruits, a companion test, the Army Beta, was designed to use nonverbal means for assessing intelligence. Instead of presenting examinees with written instructions, pictorial instructions were used and examiners pantomimed the requirements of each test. The Army Beta assessed perceptual speed, memory and reasoning with pictures. Together, the Army Alpha and Army Beta were administered to over a million men, and proved useful for making placement decisions.

A major contributor to testing in the early twentieth century was David Wechsler, the modern versions of whose tests are discussed above. Based on his experiences scoring and administering intelligence exams for the army, he developed his own series of intelligence scales, starting with the Wechsler–Bellevue Intelligence Scale (Wechsler, 1939). This individually-administered scale featured both verbal and non-verbal, or performance, tests, reflecting Wechsler's belief that intelligence is expressed in both verbal and nonverbal ways. Although Wechsler's ideas ran against the commonsense belief that nonverbal, or performance, testing was inefficient, the revised and expanded versions of his intelligence scales are probably the most widely used today.

Theories of intelligence underlying IQ tests

Underlying IQ tests is a notion of intelligence as some kind of 'map of the mind' (Sternberg, 1990). The view of intelligence as a map of the mind extends back at least to the 1800s, when phrenology was in vogue. During the first half of the twentieth century, the idea that intelligence is something to be mapped dominated theory and research. The psychologist studying intelligence was both an explorer and a cartographer, seeking to chart the innermost regions of the mind. Like other explorers, those psychologists needed tools. In the case of research on intelligence, a useful tool appeared to be factor analysis. This method of statistical analysis allows an investigator to infer distinct hypothetical constructs, elements, or structures (called factors) that underlie a phenomenon. In this case, some intelligence researchers have believed that these factors form the basis of individual differences in test performance. The actual factors derived, of course, depend on the particular questions being asked and the tasks being evaluated. This approach continues to be used actively today (see e.g. J.B. Carroll, 1993; Brody, 2000; Embretson & McCollam, 2000; Jensen, 1998).

Among the many competing theories, the main ones have been of a single general factor that dominates intelligence; of multiple, equally important abilities constituting intelligence; and of a hierarchy of abilities contributing to intelligence.

Charles Spearman: the *g* factor

Charles Spearman is usually credited with inventing factor analysis. Using factor-analytic studies, Spearman (1927) concluded that intelligence could be understood in terms of both a single general factor (called *g*). This factor pervades performance on all tests of mental ability and a set of specific factors (called *s*), each involved in performance on only a single type of mental ability test. (A specific ability might be arithmetic computation.) In Spearman's view, the specific factors are of only casual interest, due to their narrow applicability. The general factor, however, provides the key to understanding intelligence. Spearman believed that *g* derives from individual differences in mental energy. The view that there is a general factor of intelligence persists among many contemporary psychologists (e.g. Demetriou, 2002; Detterman, 2002; Gottfredson, 2002; Kyllonen, 2002; Humphreys & Stark, 2002; Jensen, 1998, 2002; Petrill, 2002), although other psychologists furiously debate this issue (Berg & Klaczynski, 2002; Grigorenko, 2002; Kray & Frensch, 2002; Lautrey, 2002; Naglieri & Das, 2002; Stankov, 2002; Sternberg, 1999, 2002; Wahlsten, 2002).

Louis Thurstone: primary mental abilities

In contrast to Spearman, Louis Thurstone (1938) concluded that the core of intelligence resides not in one single factor but in seven factors of equal importance. He referred to these factors as primary mental abilities. According to Thurstone, the primary mental abilities and typical measures of them are (1) verbal comprehension – vocabulary tests; (2) verbal fluency – tests requiring the test taker to think of as many words as possible that begin with a given letter, in a limited amount of time; (3) inductive reasoning – tests such as analogies and number-series completion tasks; (4) spatial visualization – tests requiring mental rotation of pictures of objects; (5) number – computation and simple mathematical problem-solving tests; (6) memory – picture and word-recall tests; and

(7) perceptual speed – tests that require the test taker to recognize small differences in pictures or to cross out the A's in strings of various letters.

Raymond Cattell and John Carroll: hierarchical models

A more parsimonious way of handling a number of factors is through a hierarchical model of intelligence. Two models of this sort are those of Raymond Cattell and John Carroll.

The model developed by Cattell (1971) proposes that general intelligence comprises two major subfactors: fluid intelligence and crystallized intelligence. Fluid intelligence represents the acquisition of new information, or the grasping of new relations and abstractions regarding known information. These skills are required in inductive reasoning tests such as analogies and series completions. Crystallized intelligence represents the accumulation of knowledge over the life span of the individual and is measured. This knowledge is required in tests of vocabulary, of general information and of achievement. Subsumed within these two major subfactors are more specific factors. An intelligence test based on this model is the Kaufman Adolescent and Adult Intelligence Test.

A more detailed hierarchical model, based on a reanalysis of many data sets from studies, has been proposed by Carroll (1993). At the top of the hierarchy is general ability; in the middle of the hierarchy are various broad abilities (including learning and memory processes and the effortless production of many ideas). At the bottom of the hierarchy are many narrow, specific abilities such as spelling ability and reasoning speed.

Group differences

Cultural and societal analyses of intelligence render it particularly important to consider carefully the meaning of group differences in measured IQ (Fischer et al., 1996; Loehlin, 2000; Sternberg, 1997, 2004). For example, on average, African Americans score somewhat lower than White Americans on conventional standardized tests of intelligence (Herrnstein & Murray, 1994). Italian American scores used to be considerably lower than they are now. Test scores of African Americans have been increasing over time, just as have scores for other groups. Available evidence suggests an environmental explanation for these group differences (Mackintosh, 1998; Nisbett, 1995), although opinions vary. Moreover, differences between groups in societal outcomes, such as likelihood of graduating from high school or going on welfare, cannot really be attributed simply to differences in IQ, as some people have tried to do. Removing IQ as a source of group differences, African Americans are still considerably more likely than Whites to be born out of wedlock, born into poverty and be underweight at birth (Herrnstein & Murray, 1994). Group differences may thus originate from a number of factors, many of which change over time. The result is that group differences are not immutable. A group that scores, on average, lower than another group at one given time may score, on average, lower, the same, or even higher at another time.

Sex differences

An example of a change in the nature of group differences is that males and females do about the same on cognitive ability tests, although differences have been noted on specific ability tests. Analyses of trends over time suggest that sex differences in scores on these cognitive-ability tests have been shrinking over the years (Feingold, 1988). Nevertheless, there do appear to be some differences that remain. In particular, males, on average, tend to score higher on tasks that require visual and spatial working memory, motor skills that are involved in aiming at a target, and certain aspects of mathematical performance. Females tend to score higher on tasks that require rapid access to phonological and semantic information in long-term memory, production and comprehension of complex prose, fine motor skills and perceptual speed (Halpern, 1997). These differences refer only to averages. There are many individuals of one sex who do better than individuals of the other sex, regardless of the particular skill measured by a given test. In any case, these score differences are not easily interpretable.

Steele (1997), for example, has found that when boys and girls take difficult mathematical tests, boys often do better. But when the two groups are told in advance that a particular test will show no difference, on average, scores of boys and girls converge, with girls' scores increasing and boys' scores actually decreasing.

Socially defined racial/ethnic group differences

Racial and ethnic groups are referred to here as 'socially-defined' because these constructs are culturally constructed, not biological. Different societies have different definitions of what constitute races and ethnic groups. For example, South Africa recognizes two groups of 'Coloured' and 'Black' people who would be lumped into a single category in the United States. In the United States, reference is sometimes made to 'hispanic Americans', but Puerto Rican Americans, Mexican Americans, Dominican Americans and members of many other groups are distinct in numerous ways.

A group difference which has received considerable study is between African Americans and Whites. As mentioned earlier, African Americans tend to score lower than do White Americans on conventional tests of intelligence. The available evidence is largely consistent with an environmental explanation (Nisbett, 1995). For example, in one study, offspring of American servicemen born to German women during the Allied occupation of Germany after the Second World War revealed no significant difference between IQs of children of African American and children of white servicemen (Eyferth, 1961). This result suggests that as a result of similar environments, the children of the two groups of servicemen performed equally on tests of intelligence. Another study found that children adopted by white families obtained higher IQ scores than children adopted by African American families, again suggesting environmental factors contributing to the difference between the two groups (Moore, 1986). Another way of studying group differences has been through trans-racial adoption studies. In such studies, white parents have adopted African American children (Scarr & Weinberg, 1976; Scarr et al., 1993; Weinberg et al., 1992). The results of these studies have been somewhat difficult to interpret. Both White and African American children who were adopted in the study showed decreased IQ in a 10-year follow-up on their performance.

Environmental differences

There are a number of mechanisms by which environmental factors such as poverty, undernutrition and illness might affect intelligence (Sternberg et al., 2000; Sternberg & Grigorenko, 2001). One mechanism is resources. Children who are poor often do not have the resources in the home and school which are enjoyed by children in more affluent environments. Another mechanism is attention to and concentration on the skills taught in school. Children who are under-nourished or ill may find it hard to concentrate in school. They may therefore profit less from the instruction they receive. A third mechanism is the system of rewards in the environment. Children who grow up in economically deprived environments may note that those who are most rewarded are not necessarily those who do well in school. Rather, they may be those who earn the money they need to survive, whatever these ways may be. It is unlikely that any one mechanism fully explains the effects of these various variables. It is also important to realize that whatever the mechanisms are, they can start in utero, not just after birth. For example, foetal alcohol syndrome results in reduced IQ and has its initial effects prenatally, before the child even enters the world.

Conclusions

IQ is not the entirety of intelligence but its measurement can serve a useful purpose for predicting school and work performance. The two main IQ used today are descendants of those originated by Alfred Binet, on the one hand, and David Wechsler, on the other. Groups differ in IQ scores, for reasons that are complex and not fully determined.

REFERENCES

Berg, C. A. & Klaczynski, P. A. (2002). Contextual variability in the expression and meaning of intelligence. In R. J. Sternberg & E. L. Grigorenko (Eds.). *General factor of intelligence: How general is it?* (pp. 281–98). Mahwah, NJ: Lawrence Erlbaum.

Binet, A. & Simon, T. (1916). *The development of intelligence in children.* Baltimore: Williams & Wilkins. (Originally published in 1905.)

Boring, E. G. (1923, June 6). Intelligence as the tests test it. *New Republic*, 35–7.

Brody, N. (2000). History of theories and measurements of intelligence. In R. J. Sternberg (Ed.). *Handbook of intelligence* (pp. 16–33). New York: Cambridge University Press.

Carroll, J. B. (1993). *Human cognitive abilities: a survey of factor-analytic studies.* New York: Cambridge University Press.

Cattell, R. B. (1971). *Abilities: their structure, growth and action.* Boston: Houghton Mifflin.

Daniel, M. H. (1997). Intelligence testing: status and trends. *American Psychologist*, **52**, 1038–45.

Daniel, M. H. (2000). Interpretation of intelligence test scores. In R. J. Sternberg (Ed.). *Handbook of intelligence* (pp. 477–91). New York: Cambridge University Press.

Demetriou, A. (2002). Tracing psychology's invisible g$_{iant}$ and its visible guards. In R. J. Sternberg & E. L. Grigorenko (Eds.). *The general factor of intelligence: how general is it?* (pp. 3–18). Mahwah, NJ: Lawrence Erlbaum Associates.

Detterman, D. K. (2002). General intelligence: cognitive and biological explanations. In R. J. Sternberg & E. L. Grigorenko (Eds.). *The general factor of intelligence: how general is it?* (pp. 223–43). Mahwah, NJ: Lawrence Erlbaum Associates.

Embretson, S. & McCollam, K. (2000). Psychometric approaches to the understanding and measurement of intelligence. In R. J. Sternberg (Ed.). *Handbook of intelligence* (pp. 423–44). New York: Cambridge University Press.

Eyferth, K. (1961). Leistungen verschiedener Gruppen von Besatzungskindern im Hamburg-Wechsler Intelligenztest für Kinder (HAWIK). *Archiv für die gesamte Psychologie*, **113**, 222–41.

Feingold, A. (1988). Cognitive gender differences are disappearing. *American Psychologist*, **43**, 95–103.

Fischer, C. S., Hout, M., Sanchez Janowski, M. et al. (1996). *Inequality by design: cracking the bell curve myth.* Princeton, NJ: Princeton University Press.

Gottfredson, L. S. (2002). g: Highly general and highly practical. In R. J. Sternberg & E. L. Grigorenko (Eds.). *The general factor of intelligence: how general is it?* (pp. 331–80). Mahwah, NJ: Lawrence Erlbaum Associates.

Grigorenko, E. L. (2002). Other than g: the value of persistence. In R. J. Sternberg & E. L. Grigorenko (Eds.). *The general factor of intelligence: how general is it?* (pp. 299–327). Mahwah, NJ: Lawrence Erlbaum Associates.

Halpern, D. F. (1997). Sex differences in intelligence: implications for education. *American Psychologist*, **52**, 1091–102.

Herrnstein, R. J. & Murray, C. (1994). *The bell curve.* New York: Free Press.

Humphreys, L. G. & Stark, S. (2002). General intelligence: measurement, correlates, and interpretations of the cultural-genetic construct. In R. J. Sternberg & E. L. Grigorenko (Eds.). *The general factor of intelligence: how general is it?* (pp. 87–115). Mahwah, NJ: Erlbaum.

"Intelligence and its measurement": a symposium. (1921). *Journal of Educational Psychology*, **12**, 123–47, 195–216, 271–5.

Jensen, A. R. (1998). *The g factor: the science of mental ability.* Westport, CT: Praeger/Greenwoood.

Jensen, A. R. (2002). Psychometric g: Definition and substantiation. In R. J. Sternberg & E. L. Grigorenko (Eds.). *General factor of intelligence: how general is it?* (pp. 39–54). Mahwah, NJ: Lawrence Erlbaum.

Kaufman, A. S. (2000). Tests of intelligence. In R. J. Sternberg (Ed.). *Handbook of intelligence* (pp. 445–76) New York: Cambridge University Press.

Kaufman, A. S. & Lichtenberger, E. O. (1998). Intellectual assessment. In C. R. Reynolds (Ed.). *Comprehensive clinical psychology: Vol. 4: Assessment* (pp. 203–38). Tarrytown, NY: Elsevier Science.

Kray, J. & Frensch, P. A. (2002). A view from cognitive psychology: g – (G)host in the correlation matrix? In R. J. Sternberg & E. L. Grigorenko (Eds.). *The general factor of intelligence: How general is it?* (pp. 183–220). Mahwah, NJ: Lawrence Erlbaum Associates.

Kyllonen, P. C. (2002). g: Knowledge, speed, strategies, or working-memory capacity? A systems perspective. In R. J. Sternberg & E. L. Grigorenko (Eds.). *The general factor of intelligence: how general is it?* (pp. 415–45). Mahwah, NJ: Erlbaum.

Lautrey, J. (2002). Is there a general factor of cognitive development? In R. J. Sternberg & E. L. Grigorenko (Eds.) *The general factor of intelligence: how general is it?*

(pp. 117–48). Mahwah, NJ: Lawrence Erlbaum Associates.

Loehlin, J. C. (2000). Group differences in intelligence. In R.J. Sternberg (Ed.). *Handbook of intelligence* (pp. 176–93). New York: Cambridge University Press.

Mackintosh, N. J. (1998). *IQ and human intelligence.* Oxford: Oxford University Press.

Mayer, R. E. (2000). Intelligence and education. In R.J. Sternberg (Ed.). *Handbook of intelligence* (pp. 519–33). New York: Cambridge University Press.

Moore, E. G. J. (1986). Family socialization and the IQ test performance of traditionally and transracially adopted black children. *Developmental Psychology,* **22**, 317–26.

Naglieri, J. A. & Das, J. P. (2002). Practical implications of general intelligence and PASS cognitive processes. In R. J. Sternberg & E. L. Grigorenko (Eds.). *The general factor of intelligence: how general is it?* (pp. 55–86). Mahwah, NJ: Lawrence Erlbaum Associates.

Nisbett, R. (1995). Race, IQ, and scientism. In S. Fraser (Ed.). *The bell curve wars: race, intelligence and the future of America* (pp. 36–57). New York: Basic Books.

Petrill, S. A. (2002). The case for general intelligence: a behavioral genetic perspective. In R. J. Sternberg & E. L. Grigorenko (Eds.). *The general factor of intelligence: how general is it?* (pp. 281–98). Mahwah, NJ: Lawrence Erlbaum.

Roid, G. (2003). *Stanford–Binet Intelligence Scales* (5th edn.). Itasca, IL: Riverside.

Scarr, S. & Weinberg, R. A. (1976). IQ test performance of black children adopted by white families. *American Psychologist,* **31**, 726–39.

Scarr, S., Weinberg, R. A. & Waldman, L. D. (1993). IQ correlations in transracial adoptive families. *Intelligence,* **17**, 541–5.

Schmidt, F. L., Ones, D. S. & Hunter, J. E. (1992). Personnel selection. *Annual Review of Psychology,* **43**, 627–70.

Spearman, C. (1927). *The abilities of man.* London: Macmillan.

Stankov, L. (2002). *g*: A diminutive general. In R. J. Sternberg & E. L. Grigorenko (Eds.). *The general factor of intelligence: how general is it?* (pp. 19–37). Mahwah, NJ: Lawrence Erlbaum Associates.

Steele, C. M. (1997). A threat in the air: how stereotypes shape intellectual identity and performance. *American Psychologist,* **52**(6), 613–29.

Stern, W. (1912). *Psychologische methoden der Intelligenz-Prüfung.* Leipzig, Germany: Barth.

Sternberg, R. J. (1990). *Metaphors of mind: conceptions of the nature of intelligence.* New York: Cambridge University Press.

Sternberg, R. J. (1997). *Successful intelligence.* New York: Plume.

Sternberg, R. J. (1999). The theory of successful intelligence. *Review of General Psychology,* **3**, 292–316.

Sternberg, R. J. (2002). Beyond *g*: the theory of successful intelligence. In R. J. Sternberg & E. L. Grigorenko (Eds.). *The general factor of intelligence: how general is it?* Mahwah, NJ: Lawrence Erlbaum Associates.

Sternberg, R. J. (2004). Culture and intelligence. *American Psychologist,* **59**, 325–38.

Sternberg, R. J. & Detterman, D. K. (Eds.). (1986). *What is intelligence?* Norwood, NJ.: Ablex Publishing Corporation.

Sternberg, R. J., Forsythe, G. B., Hedlund, J. *et al.* (2000). *Practical intelligence in everyday life.* New York: Cambridge University Press.

Sternberg, R. J. & Grigorenko, E. L. (Eds.). (2001). *Environmental effects on cognitive abilities.* Mahwah, NJ: Lawrence Erlbaum Associates.

Terman, L. M. (1916). *The measurement of intelligence: an explanation of and a complete guide for the use of the Stanford revision and extension of the Binet–Simon Intelligence Scale.* Boston: Houghton Mifflin.

Thurstone, L. L. (1938). *Primary mental abilities.* Chicago, IL: University of Chicago Press.

Wagner, R. K. (1997). Intelligence, training, and employment. *American Psychologist,* **52**, 1059–69.

Wahlsten, D. (2002). The theory of biological intelligence: History and a critical appraisal. In R. J. Sternberg & E. L. Grigorenko (Eds.). *The general factor of intelligence: how general is it?* (pp. 245–77). Mahwah, NJ: Lawrence Erlbaum Associates.

Wechsler, D. (1939). *The measurement of adult intelligence.* Baltimore: Williams & Wilkins.

Wechsler, D. (1974). *The measurement and appraisal of adult intelligence.* Baltimore: Williams & Wilkins.

Weinberg, R. A., Scarr, S. & Waldman, I. D. (1992). The Minnesota Transracial Adoption Study: A follow-up of IQ test performance at adolescence. *Intelligence,* **16**(1), 117–35.

Assessment of mood

Michele M. Tugade[1], Tamlin Conner[2] and Lisa Feldman Barrett[3]

[1]Vassar College
[2]University of Connecticut Health Center
[3]Boston College

Theoretical and methodological advances in psychology, physiology and medicine have led to rigorous examinations of the role of affect and emotion in health. In this chapter, we review the role of negative and positive emotions in health research and then discuss some of the most prominent measures currently used to measure mood in this research. We conclude with specific recommendations for the measurement of mood and emotion in the context of studies of physical health. Across different samples and studies in health psychology, there is little variation in mood assessment procedures. As a consequence, we focus our discussions primarily on the cardiovascular system, with a shorter discussion of relations between cancer and mood.

Negative emotions and health

Much of the research that examines the relation between mood and health addresses the impact of negative or unpleasant affect. Although the experience of negative affect is generally adaptive in preparing the body for fight-or-flight, it can have adverse consequences when the body is continually taxed. In particular, researchers have focused on how particular experiences of negative affect (e.g. anger, anxiety and depression) have emerged as important risk factors in health (see Gallo & Matthews, 2003; Kubzansky & Kawachi, 2000).

Anger

Several studies have reported on the negative health consequences of anger on cardiovascular responses (e.g. Kawachi *et al.*, 1996), particularly in relation to incidence of coronary heart disease (CHD). Hostility appeared to be a greater risk factor than smoking, high blood pressure and high cholesterol (Chaput *et al.*, 2002). Hostility is related to heightened cardiovascular stress (Davis *et al.*, 2000; see also 'Hostility, Type A behaviour and coronary heart Disease') and the speed of cardiovascular recovery from evocative situations, increasing the allostatic load or the total time that cardiovascular indices remain elevated, which itself is an important factor in the development of later hypertension and cardiovascular disease (Faber & Burns, 1996; Gerin & Pickering, 1995; Jamieson & Lavoie, 1987; Lai & Linden, 1992). There is also some evidence that inhibiting anger expression is related to heart disease (including essential hypertension and CHD; e.g. Appel *et al.*, 1983; Diamond, 1982; MacDougall *et al.*, 1985; also see Engebretson *et al.*, 1989). It is also consistent with the more general finding that emotional suppression produces increases cardiovascular reactivity (Gross & Levenson, 1993; see 'Emotional expression and health'). Almost all of the studies assessed anger-related experiences using general or summary type self-report measures (detailed below in the 'Mood assessment procedures' section; e.g. the MMPI-2 Anger Content Scale, Hathaway & McKinley, 1989, in Kawachi *et al.*, 1996; the Speilberger Anger-Out Expression scale, Speilberger, 1988, in Eng *et al.*, 2003; dispositional hostility measured by a composite index including cynicism, anger, mistrust and aggression, in Rozanski *et al.*, 1999). Taken together, this body of research suggests that respondents' reports of anger experiences in general are related to cardiovascular functioning.

Anxiety

Most prospective epidemiological studies have found an association between self-reported symptoms of anxiety and risk of developing CHD, even when other factors were considered (e.g. a family history of heart disease; Kubzansky & Kawachi, 2000). This link could exist in individuals who report anxiety symptoms because they have repeated activation of the sympathetic nervous system and suppression of immune system function (Schneiderman, 1987), because they are less likely to engage in health-promoting behaviours (Kubzansky *et al.*, 1998) or because they are more likely to engage in risky health behaviours (e.g. increased smoking, alcohol or drug consumption; Kubzansky & Arthur, 2004). Indeed, individuals who report anxiety are at increased risk of atherosclerosis (Paterniti *et al.*, 2001) and hypertension (Markovitz *et al.*, 1991). These studies assessed anxiety-related experiences using global measures of anxiety and anxiety symptoms, such as: the Framingham Tension Scale (Haynes *et al.*, 1978) in Markovitz *et al.* (1991); the Speilberger State-Trait Anxiety Inventory (Spielberger *et al.*, 1970) in Paterniti *et al.* (2001); and the Hopkins Symptoms Checklist (Derogatis *et al.*, 1973). Taken together, these studies indicate that reports of anxiety-related experiences are associated to CHD.

Depression

Studies provide convincing evidence that clinical depression contributes significantly to the onset of heart disease. Clinical depression is a mood-related disorder that can lead to a three-fold increase in risk for heart disease (see Anderson, 2003) and it is therefore especially dangerous for people with existing heart ailments. Numerous epidemiological studies consistently demonstrate a prospective relation between the occurrence of major depressive episodes and the incidence of myocardial infarction, ischemic heart disease and cardiac death (Anderson, 2003), as well as a dose–response association between the magnitude of depression and future cardiac events (cf. Rosanski *et al.*, 1999; see 'Coronary heart disease: cardiac psychology'). These studies use clinical assessments of depression (as reported in Rozanski *et al.*, 1999), such as the Centre for Epidemiological Studies-Depression Scale (CES-D; Radloff, 1977), MMPI Depression Scale (Hathaway & McKinley, 1989) and the Beck Depression Inventory (BDI; Beck, 1996). Together, these data suggest that risk for coronary artery disease associated with depression exists along a continuum, according to the magnitude of depressive symptoms.

The assessment of depression also plays an important role in the diagnosis of cancer. Although the direct pathways by which mood might influence cancer etiology remain unclear (Croyle & Rowland, 2003), evidence indicates that self-reported experiences of negative affect (e.g. depression) are related to an increased risk of developing cancer (Pennix *et al.*, 1998). One groundbreaking prospective study examined the links between depression and cancer incidence in 4825 participants. After controlling for factors such as age, sex, race, disabilities, alcohol use and smoking, the researchers found that participants who had been chronically depressed for at least six years had an 88% greater risk of developing cancer within the following four years. In this study, chronically depressed mood was defined as being present when the number of depressive symptoms exceeded 20 on the Centre for Epidemiologic Studies-Depression scale (CES-D; Radloff, 1977) during three timepoints: baseline, 3 years before baseline and 6 years before baseline. The CES-D measures depressive feelings and behaviours experienced during the past week (e.g. feelings of sadness or feelings that life had been a failure, lack of appetite, having a restless sleep, or having crying spells). Although the results of this study are compelling, the researchers cautioned that further studies are needed to determine the direction of causality in their findings. For instance, it is possible that depressed mood was a consequence of early-stage cancer that had yet to be detected (Pennix et al., 1998).

Previous to the Pennix et al. (1998) study, prospective studies used a single measurement occasion to assess depressed mood and the development of cancer. Obtaining only a single measure of depression in the absence of assessment of duration or frequency, however, may be incomplete. A single estimate may classify persons as depressed as a result of temporary stressful life circumstances or health problems present at that moment. There is also variability in the frequency of depression across the cancer disease course (Croyle & Rowland, 2003). Such variability may reflect an inconsistency among several factors, including type of assessment, timing of assessment, type of cancer, concurrent treatment and comorbidity (e.g. Croyle & Rowland, 2003). Moreover, most clinical assessments rely on patient self-report. Although symptoms of depression (e.g. fatigue, reduced appetite, sleep problems, concentration problems) are best reported by the patient, most depressed cancer patients may not be able to complete assessments or may not seek treatment for cancer-related depression at all (Croyle & Rowland, 2003).

Research also indicates that repression of negative affect (i.e. having no cognitive awareness of feelings of anger, sadness, anxiety, worry, or fear related to cancer) has been identified as the single most important predictor of cancer incidence (McKenna et al., 1999). It is also related to faster cancer progression (Jenson, 1987) and is a risk factor for early mortality in women with breast cancer (Giese-Davis et al., 2004). Examining the links between mood and cancer, therefore, can be important in understanding the course of the disease and a cancer patient's overall quality of life.

Positive emotions and health

Just as individuals with a negative affective style are at greater risk for developing health problems, individuals with a positive emotional style (including a tendency to report positive emotions such as feeling happy, pleased and relaxed) experience potential health benefits. Recent research, for instance, has demonstrated that positive emotional experiences serve as a protective factor against the common cold even after controlling for a number of risk factors (e.g. age, sex, education, race, body mass and season; Cohen et al., 2003). Physical health benefits associated with positive emotions are further established in research on optimism, a dispositional attribute associated with positive emotions. For example, optimists (compared with pessimists) are less likely to suffer from angina and myocardial infarction (Kubzansky & Kawachi, 2002) and they show better physical recovery immediately after coronary artery bypass surgery and up to six months post-surgery (Carver & Scheier, 1998). Other research corroborates this pattern, showing that the tendencies to maintain optimistic (even unrealistically optimistic) beliefs about the future act to buffer against the advancement of disease and death (Aspinwall & Taylor, 1997; Taylor & Brown, 1988; Taylor et al., 2000). Taken together, these studies suggest that the relation between physical health and positive dispositional styles (e.g. optimism) may be due in part to the chronic positive emotional states engendered by the personality style.

One of the most important functions of positive emotion is to undo the cardiovascular reactivity associated with negative emotion. Recent research indicates that positive emotional experiences may be important in accelerating cardiovascular recovery from stressful experiences. Theory and research have shown that positive and negative emotions have unique and complementary adaptive functions and physiological effects (see Fredrickson, 1998, 2001). Experiences of negative emotions are associated with autonomic nervous system activation, such as changes in heart rate, vascular resistance and blood pressure (for meta-analytic evidence, see Cacioppo et al., 2000) that prepare the body for fight or flight. Experiences of positive emotions function as efficient antidotes for the lingering cardiovascular effects of negative emotions, in a sense 'undoing' the lingering after-effects of negative emotional experiences (Fredrickson & Levenson, 1998; Fredrickson et al., 2000). Experimental evidence suggests that participants induced to experience both high activation positive emotions (i.e. joy/amusement) and low activation positive emotions (i.e. contentment/serenity) exhibited faster cardiovascular recovery after exposure to emotionally evocative films than those in a neutral control condition (Fredrickson & Levenson, 1998; Fredrickson et al., 2000). In this way, positive emotions are not only a form of psychological resilience (Tugade & Fredrickson, 2004) but may also serve as a protective factor for cardiovascular and other stress-related illnesses.

Now that we have provided a brief review of the links between mood and health, in the next section, we will highlight some of the most prominent measures currently used to measure mood in health psychology.

Mood assessment procedures in health psychology

Self-report measures

Self-report methods are popular for measuring mood. Their use is grounded in the first-person perspective that the best way to know how people feel is to ask them. This contrasts with a third-person perspective whereby feeling is inferred from instrument-based observational methods (e.g. using physiological measures, facial affect coding, etc.). Self-report procedures vary in the content of the measures (i.e. the experiences that are sampled) and the time-frame of the assessment period. Moods can be assessed as they are currently experienced, called a 'state' or 'momentary report'; over a specified time frame, called a 'retrospective report'; or in general, often called a 'trait or global report'.

Content

There are numerous self-report measures currently used in the health sciences and each assesses different aspects of mood. Some measures target a single type of mood-related experience, for example, feelings of anxiety, depression, or anger. The most widely-used measure of anxious mood is the Spielberger State–Trait Anxiety Inventory (STAI; Spielberger, 1983; Marteau & Bekker, 1992). Popular measures of depressed mood include the 20-item Centre for Epidemiologic Studies-Depression Scale (CES-D; Radloff, 1977) and variants of the Beck Depression Inventory (original, Version II and fast screen for medical patients, Beck et al., 1961, Beck et al., 1996; 2000; see also Richter et al., 1998, for a validity review). Commonly used anger-related mood measures include the

MMPI-2 Anger Content Scale (Hathaway & McKinley, 1989) and the Spielberger Anger-Out Expression Inventory (Spielberger, 1988).

Other measures include a wider range of items to sample more than one type of mood-related experience. For example, the widely-used Profile of Mood States (POMS; McNair et al., 1971/1981) is a 65-item rating scale that yields a total mood index, plus a single index of positive mood (Vigour) and five indices of negative mood (tension/anxiety; depression/dejection; anger/hostility; fatigue; and confusion/bewilderment), the latter two presumably measuring more physically-based mood states. Respondents rate the extent to which they are experiencing or have experienced 65 affect states (e.g. sad, tense, energetic, cheerful) using a 5-point scale (0 = not at all, 5 = extremely). There are also several shortened versions, which appear to show adequate internal consistency (see Guadagnoli & Mor, 1989; Shacham, 1983). Similarly, the Mood Adjective Checklist (MACL, Nowlis, 1965) is a 50-item affect rating scale that yields 12 separate mood indices – aggression, anxiety, surgency, elation, concentration, fatigue, social affection, sadness, skepticism, egotism, vigor and nonchalance. It also attempts to differentiate between physical versus emotion-based mood states, although it should be noted that some of the terms are outdated (e.g. 'clutched up' as a marker of anxiety). The 40-item Derogatis Affects Balance Scale (DABS; Derogatis, 1996) measures several positive mood dimensions (joy, contentment, vigour and affection) and several negative mood dimensions (anxiety, depression, guilt and hostility) and is often used in clinical psychology related fields. The Multiple Affect Adjective Check List Revised (MAACL-R; Zuckerman & Lubin, 1985) is a 132-item scale that assesses five dimensions of mood (anxiety, depression, hostility, positive affect and sensation-seeking), and combines these for superordinate measures of dysphoria (sum of anxiety, depression and hostility) and positivity (sum of sensation-seeking and positive affect). All of these scales have shown adequate internal consistency and reliability.

Even though these scales purport to measure distinct mood states, respondents typically have some difficulty distinguishing mood states of the same valence. Reports of negative mood experience tend to correlate so highly that measures of anxiety, sadness, fear and so on, often fail capture any unique variance (e.g. Feldman, 1993; Watson & Clark, 1984; Watson & Tellegen, 1985). Even scales that are explicitly built to measure discrete emotions tend to suffer from high correlations between like-valenced states (e.g. Boyle, 1986; Watson & Clark, 1994; Zuckerman & Lubin, 1985). Individuals also vary a great deal in the tendency with which they represent feelings as distinctive experiences (Carstensen et al., 2000; Lane et al., 1990; Lane & Schwartz, 1987; Larsen & Cutler, 1996), with some individuals making categorical distinctions between like valenced states in their reports of experience and others making fewer distinctions (Barrett, 1998, 2004; Barrett et al., 2001; Feldman, 1995b) – an individual difference termed 'emotional granularity' (Barrett, 2004).

Several strategies can address the weak discriminant validity in discrete mood reports and granularity differences across people. Single mood measures (e.g. STAI; BDI) are best used in conjunction with other mood measures to determine whether participants are feeling 'anxiety' or 'depression' per se or whether they using the scales simply to record undifferentiated feelings of negativity (Watson & Clark, 1984) or dysphoric mood (Feldman, 1993;

1995a). Measures which sample more than one type of mood-related experience should be analyzed for their psychometric properties, but at minimum can be considered valid measures of positive and negative affective states (Feldman, 1993, 1995a; Watson & Tellegen, 1985). Also, regardless of whether people are high or low in emotional granularity, their verbal reports do seem to convey something valid about the two broad dimensions of mood – their feelings of valence (pleasure–displeasure) and arousal (high activation–low activation) (Barrett & Niedenthal, 2004; Barrett et al., 2004).

Another option is to measure the broad dimensions of mood more explicitly. One popular measure is the Positive and Negative Activation Schedule (once called the Positive and Negative Affect Schedule; PANAS; Watson, Clark & Tellegen, 1988; Watson et al., 1999). The PANAS is a 20-item scale that assesses positive and negative activation (that is, high arousal positive and negative states; e.g. excited, interested, proud; ashamed, nervous, scared). Importantly, the PANAS is not a measure of both dimensions of affectivity (pleasure–displeasure; high activation–low activation) (Barrett & Russell, 1998; Carroll et al., 1999), although it is often treated as such, because it does not capture lower activation feelings of calmness, depression, sadness, or even happiness. An extended version, the PANAS-X, is available to measure more discrete feelings including some, but not all, lower level activation states (sadness, serenity, fatigue) in addition to the broader positive and negative activation states (Watson & Clark, 1994). In general, both the PANAS and PANAS-X show good validity and reliability for measuring high activation, valenced mood states in a variety of time frame formats (see Watson, 1988; Watson & Clark, 1997). Other measures have been developed to sample the affective space more completely by including items reflecting all combinations of valence and arousal. For examples, see Barrett and Russell (1998), Carroll et al. (1999), Larsen and Diener (1992), Mayer and Gaschke, 1988; Russell, Weiss and Mendelsohn, 1989; and Yik et al. (1999).

An alternative to the PANAS and other existing measures is to develop (or modify) one's own measure. In doing so, it is advisable to include a broad range of adjectives reflecting all combinations of valence (pleasant–unpleasant) and arousal levels (high activation–low activation) (see Barrett & Russell, 1998). Also, accumulating evidence strongly suggests that all self-report scales of mood should use unambiguously unipolar (rather than bipolar) scales, where respondents first judge the absence or presence of affective feeling, and only then judge the intensity of the feeling if it is present (e.g. 0 = no feeling at all, but if feeling is present, and then 1 = mild intensity to 5 = strong intensity; for a discussion of why this is so, see Russell & Carroll, 1999). Failure to do so can cause systematic artifacts in measurement that can influence, among other things, the extent to which self-reports positive and negative affect are correlated (Russell & Barrett, 1999).

The time frame of mood assessment

Time frame is another important issue in the measurement of self-reported mood. Mood can be measured in the present moment (How do you feel right now?), retrospectively over increasingly extended time intervals (How have you felt this day? week? month? past year?) and globally (How do you feel in general?). Momentary and shorter interval retrospective reports capture immediate affective states which fluctuate in response to changing events and conditions, and constitute a form of episodic or state mood. In contrast, global or longer term retrospective reports capture enduring beliefs about the types of moods we experience, and constitute a form of semantic or trait mood (for a review, see Robinson & Clore, 2002). Many existing mood measures come in state and trait forms or can be easily adapted to different time frames. Choosing the appropriate time frame in measurement is important because state and trait reports are psychologically distinct and each is suited to different types of health-related investigations.

State mood measures reflect people's transient mood states and should be used when seeking to measure mood as it occurs or how it changes in response to events or situations (e.g. laboratory or real-world stressors). The strictest state format is to ask people how they feel right now (a momentary self-report) either at a single time point (typically in the lab), or on repeated occasions (typically outside the lab) using a method called Ecological Momentary Assessment (EMA) or experience-sampling methods (ESM).[1] These intensive, longitudinal self-report procedures are designed to allow respondents to document their thoughts, feelings and behaviours on repeated occasions within the context of everyday life. Sampling is typically accomplished through the use of a device (like a Palm, a pager, or cell phone) that allows respondents to report their momentary experience multiple times a day (either in response to a random signal, a fixed signal and/or self-initiated). Momentary self-reports, like those used in EMA and ESM, are often considered the gold standard of state mood measurement because they capture mood as it happens in real life, unbiased by memory processes. For these reasons, EMA and ESM are playing increasingly vital roles in the scientific study of health. They have been used to evaluate the efficacy of clinical interventions and health treatments with presumed mood components, and to test the links between mood and important health factors including coping, cardiovascular function and salivary cortisol levels *in situ* (for examples see Steptoe *et al.*, 2000; Stone & Shiffman, 1994). For a full review of these procedures, the interested reader is referred to Barrett and Barrett (2001), Bolger, Davis and Rafaeli, (2003), Conner *et al.* (2003), Reis and Gable (2000) and Stone *et al.* (1999).

Short term retrospective reports also measure state mood and can be used when practicalities prohibit the use of EMA, or when researchers are expressly seeking to measure people's retrospections of their mood states. A short-term retrospective report may ask people how they felt over the past hour, day, or week. When people retrospect over such short time intervals, reports tend to be fairly accurate when they are compared to momentary self-reports averaged over that interval (Thomas & Diener, 1990; Hedges *et al.*, 1985; Parkinson *et al.*, 1995); however, retrospections across a span of a week appear to relate more to averaged end-of-day reports than to averaged momentary reports over the interval suggesting that weekly reports are retrospections on already aggregated memories (Parkinson *et al.*, 1995). Although generally accurate, short-term retrospective reports can reflect several systematic biases, deriving from people's attempts to recall and aggregate past experiences over time. Short-term retrospective reports are often disproportionately influenced by people's affective state at the time of recall (Singer & Salovey, 1988), by the most intense experience that is remembered ('peak effect'), and to a lesser extent by the most recent experience remembered ('end effect') (see Fredrickson, 2000). Also, as a general rule, people tend to over-estimate the intensity of their positive and negative moods in retrospect, in part, because they neglect to incorporate the duration of certain neutral experiences into memory (Barrett, 1997; Thomas & Diener, 1990). These biases should be kept in mind when using short-term retrospective self-reports as proxies for momentary mood.

Despite the biases associated with short-term retrospective reports, there may be times when researchers would want expressly to target these retrospections. Recent research suggests that people make important decisions about their future behaviours based on how they remember their experiences, not necessarily what 'objectively' happened in the moment. For example, retrospective pain, more than momentary pain, has been shown to predict people's decisions about whether to undergo follow-up colonoscopies (Redelmeier, Katz & Kahneman, 2003). The same patterns could hold for other types of decisions regarding mood and health. At the end of a long working week, it may be how people remember their mood – more than an objective average of their moment-to-moment mood – that will predict risky health related behaviours over the weekend (e.g. binge drinking, smoking etc.). Thus, retrospective reports may be the best measure and not simply a more convenient substitute for momentary reports in cases where people retrospect on their mood to make health-related decisions.

When people recollect on their mood over longer time frames (e.g. two weeks or more), they are typically very poor at accurately recalling their states. People forget the details of their original experiences and instead report their beliefs or theories about how they felt during that time (for a review, see Robinson & Clore, 2002). As evidence of this distortion, longer term retrospections of mood are often biased by theories of one's own emotionality (Barrett, 1997; Larsen, 1992), including gender stereotypes (Barrett *et al.*, 1998). For these reasons, longer term retrospections are best considered measures of trait mood and/or recollected experience and should not be used as proxies for actual state experience. While it may be tempting to use long term retrospective reports as a 'short-cut' for measuring state mood over a long time period, such decisions are not justifiable. In that circumstance, researchers would be better served by using a series of daily or weekly reports. Of course, there may be times when it is important and appropriate to measure people's longer term recollections of their mood states (i.e. to the extent that participants use their memories to inform health-related behaviours).

For other investigations, it may be important to tap people's trait beliefs about their mood-related experiences using global self-reports (e.g. How one feels in general). Trait beliefs are typically stable and shaped by a multitude of factors, including one's actual experience. As such, these reports can be strong predictors of

---

[1] The term 'experience-sampling' is used more in social and clinical psychology, whereas the term 'ecological momentary assessment' is used more in health-related fields, referring to procedures that may also incorporate the ambulatory monitoring of physical states, like blood pressure, in addition to self-report.

enduring health related risk factors. For example, people who describe themselves as generally anxious or high in hostility tend to show a higher risk for coronary heart disease and hypertension, presumably because their global self-reports are tapping something about their enduring affective reactions. But trait beliefs are also shaped by other factors beyond actual experience, including cultural norms (e.g. gender or cultural stereotypes) and personal values. Trait beliefs are also limited by how people filter and label their past experiences. As such, it is important not to use trait ratings as proxies for state mood or to assume that trait ratings will necessarily predict affective experience in a given instance.

A final consideration occurs when adapting an existing measure to alternate time frames. Some measures, like the STAI, the POMS and the PANAS and PANAS-X, already exist in various state and trait forms, which have been validated and found to be reliable. Other measures have only been validated in one form or the other. Most mood measures are robust enough to be adapted to state and trait forms simply by changing the nature of the instructions. Past research has shown that psychometric properties for trait adjective rating scales are typically preserved across time frames (e.g. mood adjectives correlate in the same fashion in both state and trait formats) (Watson & Clark, 1994). This bodes well for adaptive other measures with generally similar formats. Of course, it is crucial to run comparative psychometric analyses for any adapted measure. It is also essential to remember that state and trait forms are not interchangeable and neither is inherently 'better' than the other – they measure different types of mood-related experiences and are suited to different types of research questions.

Psychophysiological measures

William James (1884) proposed one of the most compelling ideas in the science of emotion – that emotional states have specific and unique patterns of somatovisceral changes, and the perception of these bodily events constitutes an emotion. As a result, many researchers have assumed that it is possible to measure anger, sadness, fear and other emotional states more objectively by assessing their psychophysiological correlates. According to this approach, specific emotions are comprised of unique patterns of behavioural and physiological activation and these specific patterns underlie distinct subjective experiences of emotion. Theories which propose emotion-specific physiological patterning often examine cardiovascular (e.g. heart rate, finger pulse amplitude, blood pressure), electrodermal (e.g. digital skin temperature) and facial (e.g. facial electromyography) indices. Despite rigorous research efforts, consistent evidence for emotion-specific patterning of peripheral nervous system responses remains elusive. Certainly, people have well developed beliefs about the patterns of bodily cues that distinguish discrete emotional episodes and these beliefs display great stability across individuals within a culture, as well as across cultures (e.g. see Pennebaker, 1982; Scherer et al., 1986; Wallbott & Scherer, 1986). Despite the intuitive appeal, research has not produced a strong evidentiary basis for distinctive physiological patterns that characterize anger, sadness, fear and so on. Although individual studies sometimes report distinct autonomic correlates for different emotion categories (e.g. Christie & Friedman, 2004; Ekman et al., 1983; Levenson, Ekman & Friesen, 1990), meta-analytic

summaries generally fail to find distinct patterns of peripheral nervous system responses for each basic discrete emotion (Cacioppo et al., 2000). Peripheral nervous system responses do appear to configure for conditions of threat and challenge, however (Quigley et al., 2002; Tomaka et al., 1993, Tomaka et al., 1997), and for positive versus negative affect (Cacioppo et al., 2000; Lang et al., 1993) suggesting that patterns of cardiovascular responding can be used to characterize appraisals (threat, challenge) and affect (positive, negative), but not necessarily discrete emotions per se. Facial electromyography and vocal acoustic assessments generally produce the same findings as the cardiovascular measures. Facial electromyography measurements coordinate around positive versus negative affect (Cacioppo et al., 2000) or intensity of affect (Messinger, 2002). A similar case holds for vocal acoustics, which indicate a person's arousal level (e.g. Bachorowski 1999; Bachorowski & Owren 1995; Kappas et al., 1991), but do not indicate discrete emotional states per se (for a review, see Russell et al., 2003). The fact that people can automatically and effortlessly perceive anger, sadness, fear and so on, in others suggests the hypothesis that they are imposing, rather than detecting, categorical distinctions in the facial configurations or vocal signals that they rate (Barrett, 2005).

Recommendations for measurement

Based on the evidence summarised here, it is possible to offer several recommendations when measuring affect and emotion in health-related research. First, although many scientists continue to assume that each category of discrete or 'basic' emotion, referred to by such English words as 'anger', 'sadness' and 'fear', is an inherited, reflex-like module that causes a distinct and recognizable behavioural and physiological pattern, the empirical evidence does not strongly support this view. Self-reports of experience, cardiovascular measures, facial and vocal measurements, reliably and validly seem to index something about a person's affective state, so it may make the most sense to address the role of affective functioning (e.g. affective reactivity, propensity to be threatened or challenged) in questions about health and human functioning. Second, in the face of evidence that people vary in the granularity of their emotion reports, and in general tend to use discrete emotion scales to report positive and negative affect, it is important to assess the discriminant validity in reports of anger, sadness, fear and so on. Scientific studies that include only one measure of emotion (e.g. hostility) in the absence of others (e.g. anxiety) may mistakenly assume that there is a specific emotional effect driving health effects when in fact it is something about affect more broadly defined. Finally, momentary (state) and summary (trait) reports of emotion are not synonymous, and whether a researcher uses one over the other should not be a matter of convenience, but rather should depend on whether episodic or semantic representations of experience are of interest.

Acknowledgements

Preparation of this chapter was supported by NSF grants SBR-9727896, BCS 0074688, BCS 0092224, and NIMH grant K02 MH001981 awarded to Lisa Feldman Barrett.

Anderson, N. B. (2003). *Emotional longevity.* New York: Viking.

Appel, M. A., Holroyd, K. A. & Gorkin, L. (1983). Anger and the etiology and progression of physical illness. In L. Temoshok, L. van Dyke & L. S. Zegans (Eds.). *Emotions in health and illness: theoretical and research foundations.* Orlando, FL: Grune und Stratton.

Aspinwall, L. G. & Taylor, S. E. (1997). A stitch in time: self-regulation and proactive coping. *Psychological Bulletin, 121*, 417–36.

Bachorowski, J.-A. & Owren, M. J. (1995). Vocal expression of emotion: acoustic properties of speech are associated with emotional intensity and context. *Psychological Science, 6*, 219–24.

Bachorowski, J.-A. (1999). Vocal expression and perception of emotion. *Current Directions in Psychological Science, 8*, 53–7.

Barrett, L. F. (1997). The relationships among momentary emotion experiences, personality descriptions, and retrospective ratings of emotion. *Personality and Social Psychology Bulletin, 23*, 1100–10.

Barrett, L. F. (1998). Discrete emotions or dimensions? The role of valence focus and arousal focus. *Cognition and Emotion, 12*, 579–99.

Barrett, L. F. (2004). Feelings or words? Understanding the content in self-report ratings of emotional experience. *Journal of Personality and Social Psychology, 87*, 266–81.

Barrett, L. F. (2005). Feeling is perceiving: core effect and conceptualization in the experience of emotion. In L. F. Barrett, P. Niedenthal & P. Winkielman (Eds.). *Emotions: conscious and unconscious.* (pp. 255–84). New York: Guilford.

Barrett, L. F. & Barrett, D. J. (2001). Computerized experience-sampling: how technology facilitates the study of conscious experience. *Social Science Computer Review, 19*, 175–85. (Invited contribution).

Barrett, L. F. & Niedenthal, P. M. (2004). Valence focus and the perception of facial affect. *Emotion, 4*, 266–74.

Barrett, L. F., Pietromonaco, P. R. & Eyssell, K. M. (1998). Are women the "more emotional sex?" Evidence from emotional experiences in social context. *Cognition and Emotion, 12*, 555–78.

Barrett, L. F. & Russell, J. A. (1998). Independence and bipolarity in the structure of current affect. *Journal of Personality and Social Psychology, 74*, 967–84.

Barrett, L. F., Gross, J., Conner, T. & Benvenuto, M. (2001). Emotion differentiation and regulation. *Cognition and Emotion, 15*, 713–24.

Barrett, L. F., Quigley, K., Bliss-Moreau, E. & Aronson, K. R. (2004). Arousal focus and interoceptive sensitivity. *Journal of Personality and Social Psychology, 87*, 684–97.

Beck, A. T. (1996). *Beck depression inventory.* New York: Harcourt.

Beck, A. T., Steer, R. A. & Brown, G. K. (1996). *Beck depression inventory – Second edition manual.* USA: Harcourt Assessment/The Psychological Corporation.

Beck, A. T., Steer, R. A. & Brown, G. K. (2000). *Beck depression inventory – fast screen for medical patients.* USA: Harcourt Assessment/The Psychological Corporation.

Beck, A. T., Ward, C. H., Mendelson, M., Mock, J. & Erbaugh, J. (1961). An inventory for measuring depression. *Archives of General Psychiatry 4*, 561–71.

Bolger, N., Davis, A. & Rafaeli, E. (2003). Diary methods: capturing life as it is lived. *Annual Review of Psychology, 54*, 579–616.

Boyle, G. J. (1986). Higher-order factors in the differential emotions scale (DES-III). *Personality and Individual Differences, 7*, 305–10.

Cacioppo, J. T., Bernston, G. G., Larsen, J. T., Poehlmann, K. M. & Ito, T. A. (2000). The psychophysiology of emotion. In R. Lewis & J. M. Haviland-Jones (Eds.). *The Handbook of Emotion* (2nd edn.). (pp. 173–191). New York: Guilford

Carroll, J. M., Yik, M. S. M., Russell, J. A. & Barrett, L. F. (1999). On the psychometric principles of affect. *Review of General Psychology, 3*, 14–22.

Carstensen, L. L., Pasupathi, M., Mayr, U. & Nesselroade, J. R. (2000). Emotional experience in everyday life across the adult life span. *Journal of Personality and Social Psychology, 79*(4), 644–55.

Carver, C. S. & Scheier, M. F. (1998). *On the self-regulation of behavior.* New York: Cambridge University Press.

Chaput, L. A., Adams, S. H., Simon, J. A. et al. (2002). Hostility predicts recurrent events among postmenopausal women with coronary heart disease. *American Journal of Epidemiology, 156*, 1092–99.

Christie, I. C. & Friedman, B. H. (2004). Autonomic specificity of discrete emotion and dimensions of affective space: A multivariate approach. *International Journal of Psychophysiology, 51*, 143–53.

Cohen, S., Doyle, W. J., Turner, R., Alper, C. M. & Skoner, D. P. (2003). Sociability and susceptibility to the common cold. *Psychological Science, 14*(5), 389–95.

Conner, T., Feldman Barrett, L., Bliss-Moreau, E., Lebo, K. & Kaschub, C. (2003). A practical guide to experience – sampling procedures. *Journal of Happiness Studies, 4*, 53–78.

Croyle, R. T. & Rowland, J. H. (2003). Mood disorders and cancer: a national cancer institute perspective. *Biological Psychiatry, 54*, 191–4.

Davis, M. C., Matthews, K. A. & McGrath, C. (2000). Hostile attitudes predict elevated vascular resistance to interpersonal stress in both men and women. *Psychosomatic Medicine, 62*, 17–25.

Derogatis, L. R. (1996). *Derogatis affects balance scale (DABS): Preliminary scoring, procedures & administration manual.* Baltimore, MD, Clinical Psychometric Research.

Derogatis, L. R., Lipman, R. S. & Covi, L. (1973). SCL–90, an outpatient psychiatric rating scale – preliminary report. *Psychopharmacology Bulletin, 9*, 13–28.

Diamond, E. L. (1982). The role of anger and hostility in essential hypertension and coronary heart disease. *Psychological Bulletin, 92*, 410–33.

Ekman, P., Levenson, R. W. & Friesen, W. V. (1983). Autonomic nervous system activity distinguishes among emotions, *Science, 221*, 1208–10.

Eng, P. M., Fitzmaurice, G., Kubzansky, L. D., Rimm, E. B. & Kawachi, I. (2003). Anger expression and risk for stroke and coronary heart disease among male health professionals. *Psychosomatic Medicine, 65*, 100–10.

Engebretson, T. O., Matthews, K. A. & Scheier, M. F. (1989). Relations between anger expression and cardiovascular reactivity: Reconciling inconsistent findings through a matching hypothesis. *Journal of Personality and Social Psychology, 57*, 513–21.

Faber, S. D. & Burns, J. W. (1996). Anger management style, degree of expressed anger, and gender influence cardiovascular recovery from interpersonal harassment. *Journal of Behavioral Medicine, 19*, 31–53.

Feldman, L. A. (1993). Distinguishing depression from anxiety in self-report: evidence from confirmatory factor analysis on nonclinical and clinical samples. *Journal of Consulting and Clinical Psychology, 61*, 631–8.

Feldman, L. A. (1995a). Variations in the circumplex structure of emotion. *Personality and Social Psychology Bulletin, 21*, 806–17.

Feldman, L. A. (1995b). Valence focus and arousal focus: individual differences in the structure of affective experience. *Journal of Personality and Social Psychology, 69*, 153–66.

Fredrickson, B. L. (1998). What good are positive emotions? *Review of general psychology: special issue: new directions in research on emotion*, 2, 300–19.

Fredrickson, B. L. (2000). Extracting meaning from past affective experiences: the importance of peaks, ends, and specific emotions. *Cognition and Emotion*, 14(4), 577–606.

Fredrickson, B. L. (2001). The role of positive emotions in positive psychology: the broaden-and-build theory of positive emotions. *American Psychologist: Special Issue*, 56, 218–26.

Fredrickson, B. L. & Levenson, R. W. (1998). Positive emotions speed recovery from the cardiovascular sequelae of negative emotions. *Cognition and Emotion*, 12, 191–220.

Fredrickson, B. L., Mancuso, R. A., Branigan, C. & Tugade, M. M. (2000). The undoing effect of positive emotions. *Motivation and Emotion*, 24, 237–58.

Gallo, L. C. & Matthews, K. A. (2003). Understanding the association between socioeconomic status and health: do negative emotions play a role? *Psychological Bulletin*, 129, 10–51.

Gerin, W. & Pickering, T. G. (1995). Association between delayed recovery of blood pressure after acute mental stress and parental history of hypertension. *Journal of Hypertension*, 13, 603–10.

Giese-Davis, J., Sephton, S. E., Abercrombie, H., Duran, R. E. F. & Spiegel, D. (2004). Repression and high anxiety are associated with aberrant diurnal cortisol rhythms in women with metastatic breast cancer. *Health Psychology*, 23, 645–50.

Gross, J. J. & Levenson, R. W. (1993). Emotional suppression: physiology, self-report, and expressive behavior. *Journal of Personality and Social Psychology*, 64, 970–86.

Guadagnoli, E. & Mor, V. (1989). Measuring cancer patients' affect: revision and psychometric properties of the profile of mood states (POMS). *Psychological Assessment*, 1, 150–54.

Hathaway, S. R. & McKinley, J. C. (1989). *Minnesota multiphasic personality inventory-2 (MMPI-2): manual for administration and scoring*. Minneapolis: University of Minnesota Press.

Haynes, S. G., Levine, S., Scotch, N., Feinleb, M. & Kannel, W. B. (1978). The relationship of psychological factors to coronary heart disease in the Framingham study: methods and risk factors. *American Journal of Epidemiology*, 107, 362–83.

Hedges, S., Jandorf, L. & Stone, A. (1985). Meaning of daily mood assessments.

Journal of Personality and Social Psychology, 48, 428–34.

James, W. (1884/1969). *What is an emotion?* In *William James: Collected essays and reviews* (pp. 244–80). New York: Russell and Russell.

Jamieson, J. L. & Lavoie, N. P. (1987). Type A behavior, aerobic power and cardiovascular recovery from a psychosocial stressor. *Health Psychology*, 6, 361–71.

Jenson, M. R. (1987). Psychobiological factors predicting the course of breast cancer. *Journal of Personality*, 55, 317–42.

Kappas, A., Hess, U. & Scherer, K. R. (1991). Voice and emotion. In B. Rime & R. Feldman (Eds.). *Fundamentals of nonverbal behavior* (pp. 200–38). Cambridge: Cambridge University Press.

Kawachi, I., Sparrow, D., Spiro, A., Vokonas, P. & Weiss, S. T. (1996). A prospective study of anger and coronary heart disease: the normative aging study. *Circulation*, 94(9), 2090–5.

Kubzansky, L. D. & Arthur, C. M. (2004). Anxiety, heart disease, and mortality. In N. Anderson (Ed.). *Emotional longevity* (pp. 55–59). New York: Viking.

Kubzansky, L. D. & Kawachi, I. (2000). Going to the heart of the matter: Do negative emotions cause coronary heart disease? *Journal of Psychosomatic Research*, 48, 323–37.

Kubzansky, L. D., Berkman, L. F., Glass, T. A. & Seeman, T. E. (1998). Is educational attainment associated with shared determinants of health in the elderly? Findings from the MacArthur studies of Successful aging. *Psychosomatic Medicine*, 60, 578–85.

Kubzansky, L. D. & Kawachi, I. (2002). Affective states and health. In L. F. Berkman & I. Kawachi (Eds.). *Social epidemiology* (pp. 213–41). New York: Oxford University Press.

Lai, J.Y. & Linden, W. (1992). Gender, anger expression style, and opportunity for anger release determine cardiovascular reaction to and recovery from anger provocation, *Psychosomatic Medicine*, 54, 297–310.

Lane, R. D. & Schwartz, G. E. (1987). Levels of emotional awareness: A cognitive–developmental theory and its application to psychopathology. *American Journal of Psychiatry*, 144(2), 133–43.

Lane, R. D., Quinlan, D. M., Schwartz, G. E., Walker, P. A. & Zeitlin, S. B. (1990). The Levels of emotional awareness scale: a cognitive-developmental measure of emotion. *Journal of Personality Assessment*, 55(1–2), 124–34.

Lang, P. J, Greenwald, M. K., Bradley, M. M. & Hamm, A. O. (1993). Looking at pictures:

affective, facial, visceral and behavioural reactions. *Psychophysiology*, 30, 261–73.

Larsen, R. J. (1992). Neuroticism and selective encoding and recall of symptoms: evidence from a combined concurrent–retrospective study. *Journal of Personality and Social Psychology*, 62(3), 480–8.

Larsen, R. J. & Cutler, S. E. (1996). The complexity of individual emotional lives: a within-subject analysis of affect structure. *Journal of Social and Clinical Psychology*, 15(2), 206–30.

Larsen, R. & Diener, E. (1992). Promises and problems with the circumplex model of emotion. In M. S. Clarke (Ed.). *Emotion* (pp. 25–59). Newbury Park, CA: Sage.

Levenson, R. W., Ekman, P. & Friesen, W. V. (1990). Voluntary facial action generates emotion-specific autonomic nervous system activity. *Psychophysiology*, 27, 363–84.

MacDougall, J. M., Dembroski, T. M., Dimsdale, J. E. & Hackett, T. P. (1985). Components of Type-A, hostility and anger-in: further relationships to angiographic findings. *Health Psychology*, 4, 137–52.

Markovitz, J. H., Matthews, K. A., Wing, R. R., Kuller, L. H. & Meilahn, E. N. (1991). Psychological, biological, and health behavior predictors of blood pressure change in middle-aged women. *Journal of Hypertension*, 9, 399–406.

Marteau, T. M. & Bekker, H. (1992). The development of a six-item short-form of the state scale of the spielberger state–trait anxiety inventory (STAI). *British Journal of Clinical Psychology*, 31(3), 301–6.

Mayer, J. D. & Gaschke, Y. N. (1988). The experience and meta-experience of mood. *Journal of Personality and Social Psychology*, 55(1), 102–11.

McKenna, M. C., Zevon, M. A., Corn, B. & Rounds, J. (1999). Psychosocial factors and the development of cancer: A meta-analysis, *Health Psychology*, 18, 520–1.

McNair, D., Lorr, M. & Droppleman, L. F. (1971/1981). *EITS manual for the profile of mood states*. San Diego, CA: educational and industrial testing service.

Messinger, D. S. (2002). Positive and negative: infant facial expressions and emotions. *Current Directions in Psychological Science*, 11, 1–6.

Nowlis, V. (1965). Research with the mood adjective checklist. In S. S. Tomkins & C. E. Izard (Eds.). *Affect, cognition, and personality*, (pp. 352–89). New York: Springer.

Parkinson, B., Briner, R. B., Reynolds, S. & Totterdell, P. (1995). Time frames for mood: relations between momentary and generalized ratings of affect. *Personality and Social Psychology Bulletin,* **21**(4), 331–9.

Paterniti, M., Zureik, M., Ducimetiere, P., Feve, J. M. & Alperovitch, A. (2001). Sustained anxiety and 4-year progression of carotid atherosclerosis. *Atherosclerosis, Thrombosis and Vascular Biology,* **21**, 136–41.

Pennebaker, J. W. (1982). *The psychology of physical symptoms.* New York: Springer-Verlag.

Pennix, B. W. J. H., Guralnik, J. M., Pahor, M. *et al.* (1998). Chronically depressed mood and cancer risk in older persons. *Journal of the National Cancer Institute,* **90**, 1888–93.

Quigley, K. S., Barrett, L. F. & Weinstein, S. (2002). Cardiovascular patterns associated with threat and challenge appraisals: a within-subjects analysis. *Psychophysiology,* **39**, 292–302.

Radloff, L. S. (1977). The CES-D Scale: A self-report depression scale for research in the general population. *Applied Psychological Measurement,* **1**(3), 385–401.

Redelmeier, D. A., Katz, J. & Kahneman, D. (2003). Memories of colonoscopy: a randomized trial. *Pain,* **104**(1–2), 187–94.

Reis, H. T. & Gable, S. L. (2000). Event sampling and other methods for studying daily experience. In H. T. Reis & C. M. Judd (Eds.). *Handbook of research methods in social and personality psychology* (pp. 190–222). New York: Cambridge University Press.

Richter, P., Werner, J., Heerlien, A., Kraus, A. & Sauer, H. (1998). On the validity of the beck depression inventory: a review. *Psychopathology* **31**(3), 160–8.

Robinson, M. D. & Clore, G. L. (2002). Belief and feeling: evidence for an accessibility model of emotional self-report. *Psychological Bulletin,* **128**(6), 934–60.

Rozanski, A., Blumenthal, J. A. & Kaplan, J. (1999). Impact of psychological factors on the pathogenesis of cardiovascular disease and implications for therapy. *Circulation,* **99**, 2192–217.

Russell, J. A. & Barrett, L. F. (1999). Core affect, prototypical emotional episodes, and other things called emotion: Dissecting the elephant. *Journal of Personality and Social Psychology,* **76**, 805–19.

Russell, J. A. & Carroll, J. M. (1999). On the bipolarity of positive and negative affect. *Psychological Bulletin,* **125**(1), 3–30.

Russell, J. A., Bachorowski, J. & Fernandez-Dols, J. (2003). Facial and vocal expressions of emotions. *Annual Review of Psychology,* **54**, 329–49.

Russell, J. A., Weiss, A. & Mendelsohn, G. A. (1989) Affect Grid: a single-item scale of pleasure and arousal. *Journal of Personality and Social Psychology,* **57**(3), 493–502.

Scherer, K. R., Wallbott, H. G. & Summerfield, A. B. (1986). *Experiencing emotion. A cross-cultural study.* Cambridge, UK: Cambridge University Press.

Schneiderman, N. (1987). Psychophysiologic factors in atherogenesis and coronary artery disease. *Circulation,* **76**, 141–7.

Seyfarth, R. M. & Cheney, D. L. (2003). Signalers and receivers in animal communication. *Annual Review of Psychology,* **54**, 145–73.

Shacham, S. (1983). A shortened version of the Profile of Mood States. *Journal of Personality Assessment,* **47**(3), 305–6.

Singer, J. A. & Salovey, P. (1988). Mood and memory: evaluating the network theory of affect, *Clinical Psychology Review,* **8**(2), 211–51.

Spielberger, C. (1988). *State–Trait Anger Expression Inventory, (Res. edn.). Professional Manual.* Odessa, FL: Psychological Assessment Resources.

Spielberger, C. D. (1983). *Manual for the State-trait anxiety inventory.* Palo Alto, CA: Consulting Psychologists Press.

Spielberger, C. D., Gorsuch, R. L. & Lushene, R. D. (1970). *Manual for the State–Trait Anxiety Inventory.* Palo Alto, CA: Consulting Psychologists Press.

Steptoe, A., Cropley, M. & Joekes, K. (2000). Task demands and the pressures of everyday life: associations between cardiovascular reactivity and work blood pressure and heart rate. *Health Psychology,* **19**(1), 46–54.

Stone, A. A. & Shiffman, S. (1994). Ecological momentary assessment (EMA) in behavioral medicine. *Annals of Behavioral Medicine,* **16**, 199–202.

Stone, A. A., Shiffman, S. S. & DeVries, M. W. (1999). Ecological momentary assessment. In D. Kahneman & E. Diener (Eds.). *Well-being: the foundations of hedonic psychology* (pp. 26–39). New York: Russell Sage Foundation.

Taylor, S. E. & Brown, J. D. (1988). Illusion and well-being: a social psychological perspective on mental health. *Psychological Bulletin,* **103**, 193–210.

Taylor, S. E., Kemeny, M. E., Reed, G. M., Bower, J. E. & Gruenewald, T. L. (2000). Psychological resources, positive illusions, and health. *American Psychologist,* **55**, 99–109.

Thomas, D. L. & Diener, E. (1990). Memory accuracy in the recall of emotions. *Journal of Personality and Social Psychology,* **59**(2), 291–7.

Tomaka J., Blascovich, J., Kelsey, J. & Leitten, C. (1993). Subjective, physiological, and behavioural effects of threat and challenge appraisal. *Journal of Personality and Social Psychology.* **65**, 248–60.

Tomaka, J., Blascovich, J., Kibler, J. & Ernst, J. M. (1997). Cognitive and physiological antecedents of threat and challenge appraisal. *Journal of Personality and Social Psychology,* **73**, 63–72.

Tugade, M. M. & Fredrickson, B. L. (2004). Resilient individuals use positive emotions to bounce back from negative emotional experiences. *Journal of Personality and Social Psychology,* **86**, 320–33.

Wallbott, H. G. & Scherer, K. R. (1986). Stress specificities: differential effects of coping style, gender, and type of stressor on autonomic arousal, facial expression, and subjective feeling. *Journal of Personality and Social Psychology,* **61**, 147–56.

Watson, D. & Clark, L. A. (1984). Negative affectivity: the disposition to experience aversive emotional states. *Psychological Bulletin,* **96**(3), 465–90.

Watson, D. & Clark, L. A. (1994). *The PANAS-X:* Manual for the positive and negative affect schedule – Expanded form. Cedar Rapids: University of Iowa.

Watson, D. & Clark, L. A. (1997). Measurement and mismeasurement of mood: recurrent and emergent issues. *Journal of Personality Assessment,* **68**(2), 267–96.

Watson, D. (1988). The vicissitudes of mood measurement: effects of varying descriptors, time frames, and response formats on measures of positive and negative affect. *Journal of Personality and Social Psychology,* **55**(1), 128–41.

Watson, D., Wiese, D., Vaidya, J. & Tellegen, A. (1999). The two general activation systems of affect: structural findings, evolutionary considerations, and psychobiological evidence. *Journal of Personality and Social Psychology,* **76**(5), 820–38.

Watson, D., Clark, L. & Tellegen, A. (1988). Development and validation of a brief measure of positive and negative affect: The PANAS scales. *Journal of Personality and Social Psychology,* **54**, 1063–70.

Watson, D. & Tellegen, A. (1985). Toward a consensual structure of mood. *Psychological Bulletin,* **98**, 219–35.

Yik, M. S. M., Russell, J. A. & Barrett, L. F. (1999). Integrating four structures of current mood into a circumplex: integration and beyond. *Journal of Personality and Social Psychology,* **77**, 600–19.

Zuckerman, B. & Lubin, B. (1985). *Manual of multiple affect adjective check list revised.* San Diego: edITS.

Neuropsychological assessment

Jane Powell

University of London

Organic injury to the brain can have complex and interacting psychological effects, not only at the level of intellectual impairment but also at the levels of affective and behavioural disturbance. These sequelae may be directly or indirectly caused by the brain injury, and may vary in severity from those which are gross and obvious to those which are subtle and detectable only on detailed assessment. Nevertheless, even those which are subtle can have pervasive effects on a patient's social and occupational functioning, whilst those which are gross may arise from a variety of causes with different treatment implications. In either case, neuropsychological assessment can be highly germane to clarification of the problem, to prediction of the functional consequences and to the development of appropriate interventions or environmental adaptations.

To illustrate this, consider the case of a young man who has sustained a head injury in an assault. A year after the incident he has made a good physical recovery, but is very aggressive and has lost his job as a sales manager because of hostility towards colleagues and a general lack of organization in his work. These problems might, on the one hand, arise from organic damage to regions of the brain involved in the genesis or inhibition of aggression, or, on the other, be a psychological reaction to some more subtle cognitive deficit such as a generalized reduction in the efficiency with which information is processed or a mild but specific impairment of memory. In the former case, a pharmacological treatment to control the emotional reactions might be most appropriate, whilst in the latter it would be more relevant to address the underlying cognitive deficit directly and/or help the patient adjust his lifestyle and outlook to his new limitations.

Purposes of neuropsychological assessment

The form taken by any neuropsychological assessment will depend critically on the question which is to be answered. Frequent purpose for assessment include the following:

- description and measurement of organically based cognitive deficits
- differential diagnosis (e.g. to ascertain whether memory problems arise from organic injury or mood disturbances)
- prediction of the consequences of neurosurgical excision of brain tissue (e.g. the cost–benefits likely to accrue from a temporal lobectomy)
- monitoring improvement or deterioration associated with recovery from, or exacerbation of, a neurological condition
- evaluation of the neuropsychological effects, positive or adverse, of pharmacological and non-pharmacological treatments (e.g. to determine whether a psychological intervention has improved attention, or whether an anticonvulsant might impair learning)
- guiding rehabilitation strategies
- predicting or explaining deficits in social, educational, or occupational functioning
- medico-legal evaluations (e.g. contributing to determination of compensation awards, ascertaining fitness to plead, etc.).

Dimensions and level of assessment

The extensiveness of, and methods employed within, any individual assessment will be largely determined by the specific referral question, though a wide range of other factors will also be influential. These will include characteristics of the patient which affect his or her ability or willingness to carry out certain tests, as well as resource-based considerations, such as the location in which the assessment is to take place, or the amount of time which is available.

A major element of many neuropsychological assessments is evaluation of the patient's intellectual functioning, usually tested via formal pen-and-paper or computerized test procedures. However, this is neither the only form of assessment used nor necessarily the most important. If the presenting problem is one of behavioural or emotional disturbance, assessment may concentrate on the systematic collection of information either from the patient or from others concerning factors which may influence its occurance. Thus, although neuropsychological assessment is often perceived as a special form of cognitive assessment, it is very often much broader than this. In practice, a referral to a neuropsychologist will often result in a multidimensional assessment in which the presenting problem is analyzed from a number of perspectives rather than just one. Sometimes there may be no formal testing, if the pertinent information can be gleaned from systematic behavioural observations and interviews.

At a general level, the purpose of neuropsychological assessment may be categorized into those which are primarily descriptive and those which are explanatory. The former represents an attempt to identify the type and severity of any problems, whilst the latter entails more theoretically driven procedures designed to illuminate the causes or consequences of an observed deficit. These two aspects will be differentially important depending on the nature of the initial question. So, if the purpose of the assessment is to quantify the extent of any memory deficits (e.g. for the purposes of monitoring change over time, or for medico-legal purposes), then a standardized measurement of different aspects of the patient's memory relative to their general intellectual level may suffice. By contrast, if the purpose of the assessment is to determine why the patient has difficulty in remembering information in daily life and to make therapeutic recommendations, then more detailed probing of potential causes for the memory problem become relevant. For instance, it may be that the memory deficit is secondary to poor concentration or impaired perception, or that it is related to the form in which the information is presented (e.g. verbally vs. visually). If the assessment clarifies the mechanisms underlying the patients's problems, then treatment can focus specifically on these.

Descriptive assessments will also vary in terms of their breadth, and this again is likely to reflect the referral question. In one case the requirement may be to determine whether a brain injury has resulted in any impairment, whilst in another the emphasis may be particularly on a certain aspect of the patient's functioning. The basis for focusing on one aspect more than on others may consist in observations which have already been made (e.g. that the patient appears forgetful) or on the basis of what is known about the aetiology or location of the brain injury (e.g. that there is a focal lesion to a part of the brain which is implicated in memory functions). The prediction of neuropsychological sequelae which are likely to arise from damage to specified areas of the brain has become an increasingly sophisticated exercise over the last decade with the emergence of complex information-processing models of cognitive function, a framework which is considered briefly below.

Cognitive neuropsychology

This framework guides much of contemporary neuropsychological assessment, and derives from an integration of theory and research bearing on the elements of information-processing involved in normal cognition ('cognitive psychology') with that relating organic brain injury to alterations in psychological function defined broadly to incorporate not only cognition but also mood and behaviour ('neuro-psychology').

To illustrate the clinical utility of this approach, consider acquired deficits of spelling which can follow brain injury. Anatomically, impairments of spelling and writing seem predominantly to be associated with lesions of the left posterior region of the brain (see 'Head injury' and McCarthy & Warrington, 1990, for an overview). Although this by no means implies either that all patients with left posterior lesions will have such deficits, or that the presence of such a deficit definitively indicates left posterior damage, nevertheless the observed association is important in guiding the form of the clinical assessment. Thus, if a patient is known to have sustained an injury to the left parietal or occipital lobe, the neuropsychologist may make an informed decision to include within the assessment tests which will be specifically sensitive to possible spelling or writing difficulties.

At this point, analysis of the information-processing operations entailed in spelling guides the neuropsychologist in assessing the presence of specific deficits. These can vary in their impact, from those which give rise to extensive and very obvious difficulties with spelling to those which produce much more subtle effects that may be less obvious at first glance but which may nevertheless have the effect of slowing the patient down or causing him or her to underperform in certain situations. For instance, Ellis and

Young (1988) have proposed that one route to writing down a single word after hearing it spoken out loud entails the sequential occurrence of the following operations:

- auditory analysis (extraction of individual speech sounds from the speech wave)
- representation of word as a series of individual distinctive speech sounds (phoneme level)
- mapping of sounds on to spellings (phoneme–grapheme conversion)
- representation of letters involved in the spelling (grapheme level)
- representation of the particular form in which the letters are to be written, e.g. in upper vs. lower case (allograph level)
- generation of motor programme for writing the letters (graphic motor patterns)
- writing (activation of the motor programme).

These components have been identified through a combination of theory, experimental studies with neurologically intact individuals, and evidence that brain injury can disrupt some of these processes independently of others. Other aspects of the model are yet to be confirmed, and it is in a continuing process of development.

Using the above framework, the clinical neuropsychologist may test whether the patient's difficulty in writing to dictation reflects difficulty at the level of acoustic analysis, at the level of phoneme–grapheme conversion, or at one of the other stages. The implications are quite different: if the patient has specific difficulty at the level of acoustic analysis, then in parallel with the above problem he may have considerable difficulty in understanding other people's speech but be unimpaired in copying written words or in writing down his own thoughts. By contrast, if the deficit arises at the level of phoneme–grapheme conversion, he is not likely to have a problem in comprehending normal speech but may experience some difficulty in keeping written notes, etc. It may be that a deficit of the latter type actually has very little practical impact, in that alternative routes to spelling (e.g. from vocabulary) may be undamaged; on the other hand, if these alternative routes are not spontaneously used by the patient, then the assessment may have the practical benefit of focusing rehabilitation training and practice in use of these or other functional mechanisms (see 'Neuropsychological rehabilitation').

Approaches to assessment of cognitive functions

Neuropsychological assessments are generally highly structured, one conventional approach being to administer a set of tests which between them assess the following broad cognitive domains (Benton, 1994):

- verbal capacities and aphasia (includes expression, comprehension, fluency)
- visuoperceptual capacities (e.g. object recognition, visual discrimination, processing of spatial relationships)
- audition (e.g. recognition and identification of sounds; auditory localizations; phoneme/word discrimination)
- somesthesis (e.g. identification of objects through touch; perception of sensory stimulation on the skin)

- motor skills and praxis (e.g. fine motor co-ordination and manual dexterity; manipulation of objects; ability to execute purposeful motor acts on verbal command or by imitation)
- learning, memory and orientation (see 'Neuropsychological assessment: memory')
- executive functions and abstract reasoning (the higher level cognitive capacities such as concept formation, judgement, mental flexibility, creativity, decision-making, insight and planning) (see 'Neuropsychological assessment: attention and executive function').

Other, more general, outputs of neuropsychological assessment include indices of overall 'intelligence', effectively a composite index of the effectiveness of an individual's functioning across all of the above domains and 'intellectual efficiency' which may be manifest (for instance) in the speed with which simple information is processed, or in the ability to maintain vigilance or concentration over an extended period.

These functions are inevitably inter-related, in that deficits in some areas are likely to have adverse effects on functioning in others: for example, an impairment of verbal comprehension will impede verbal learning and memory and will be associated with deficits in many linguistic reasoning tasks. Likewise, attentional deficits will limit the extent to which new information is taken in and is retrievable from memory.

Some neuropsychologists in some settings routinely adopt the approach of conducting a comprehensive descriptive assessment, systematically testing all of the main areas of cognitive function using a standardized battery of tests such as the Halstead–Reitan or Luria Nebraska. A brief description and consideration of these batteries can be found in Kolb and Whishaw's (2003) valuable reference text. In Britain the more common clinical practice is to employ a smaller battery of standardized tests to tap broad dimensions of cognitive function and screen for deficits, and to supplement these with other tests which are of particular relevance to the individual patient.

The best known and most widely used instrument is the Wechsler Adult Intelligence Scale III (WAIS-III; Wechsler, 1997), which comprises 14 subtests from which 'intelligence quotients' (IQs) can be computed. In addition to an overall IQ, separate 'Verbal' and 'Performance' IQs can be calculated from those subtests respectively tapping verbal resoning abilities/knowledge and visuospatial problem-solving; similarly, indices of other aspects of functioning such as 'working memory' and 'processing speed' can be derived from groups of subtests sensitive to these functions. IQ scores, as well as being of interest in their own right, serve as a reference point against which to evaluate a patient's performance in specific cognitive domains: thus, if a patient of superior intelligence scores only in the average range on tests of memory, this is more likely to represent a deterioration than similar memory test scores in a patient of average IQ. This example illustrates the importance of considering the profile of a patient's performance across a range of tests in order to gauge where there are anomalies. The same philosophy also holds at the finer levels of description exemplified within the cognitive neuropsychological approach: thus, the interpretation of a spelling deficit will vary depending on whether it is associated with concomitant abnormalities of comprehension, perception, etc.

Within each domain, there exist any number of tests to probe the patterning of a patient's deficits and residual abilities (see, e.g. Lezak, 2004, for a wide-ranging inventory and discussion of specific neuropsychological instruments). Of the tests used, many have been standardized so that a patient's performance can be evaluated by comparison with normative data, but there is, in addition, a significant role for more informal, unstandardized tests which may be sensitive to idiosyncratic or qualitative aspects of a patient's functioning. These may be generated ad hoc during the assessment, as the neuropsychologist formulates hypotheses about the patient's underlying impairments and tests them out in an individualized way.

For instance, if a patient performs poorly on a test of mental arithmetic, he might have a problem either with generating strategic aspects of the computation or with remembering details of the question. The neuropsychologist might decide to pit these explanations against each other, either by presenting the question in a written format (thereby reducing the memory load but keeping the complexity of the calculation constant), or by presenting a strategically 'easier' problem containing approximately the same number of to-be-remembered facts. Although these variations on the basic theme are not standardized, they permit an individualized analysis of the stage at which an observed deficit arises.

Integration with other neurological indices

Neuropsychological assessment has a distinctive role within the multiplicity of tests the patient may undergo following brain injury, and one which is an important complement to other types of information. Physiological, biochemical and neuroimaging techniques are able to identify, often with great precision, the locus of or mechanism giving rise to a brain lesion and this information is likely to be critical in informing medical treatment and often in making a general prognosis. The neuropsychological contribution is a detailed analysis of the patient's functioning based on an understanding of brain—behaviour relationships, thereby allowing the consequences of the lesion for the patient's current and future functioning to be evaluated. An integration of the physiological and the neuropsychological information is therefore critical, both at the level of development of theory and at the level of understanding, predicting and treating the consequences of a neurological event for an individual patient.

REFERENCES

Benton, A. L. (1994). Neuropsychological assessment. *Annual Review of Psychology,* **45**, 1–23.

Ellis, A. W. & Young, A. W. (1988). *Human cognitive neuropsychology.* Hove, UK: Lawrence Erlbaum Associates.

Kolb, B. & Whishaw, I. Q. (2003). *Fundamentals of Human Neuropsychology* (5th edn.). New York: Worth.

Lezak, M. D. (2004). *Neuropsychological Assessment* (4th edn.). Oxford: Oxford University Press.

McCarthy, R. A. & Warrington, E. K. (1990). *Cognitive neuropsychology: an introduction.* London: Academic Press.

Wechsler, D. (1997). *WAIS-III administration and scoring manual.* New York: The Psychological Corporation.

Neuropsychological assessment of attention and executive functioning

Melissa Lamar[1] and Amir Raz[2]

[1]King's College London
[2]Columbia University and the New York State Psychiatric Institute

This chapter describes the cognitive neuroscience and neuropsychological assessment of attention and executive functioning. Each cognitive construct is defined within a theoretical framework. Additional information highlights the neuroanatomical and neurochemical underpinnings of specific aspects of attention and executive functioning. Adequate assessment of attention and executive functioning requires at least a basic knowledge of these features in order to choose the neuropsychological test measures best suited for a particular patient or clinical population.

Attention

Attention is one of the oldest issues in cognitive neuropsychology; its role in assessment is equally as historic and remains integral to the successful evaluation of a presenting patient. Attention is the process of selecting for active processing specific aspects of the physical environment (e.g. objects) or ideas stored in memory (Raz, 2004). Originally, attention was thought of as a unitary concept akin to a filter (Broadbent, 1958) or a spotlight (Shalev & Algom, 2000). More recent theories suggest that attention is a system of disparate networks including alerting, orienting and selection (Fan et al., 2002).

Alerting involves particular changes in the internal state of an individual in preparation for perceiving a stimulus otherwise thought of as vigilance. Alerting is critical for optimal performance in tasks involving higher cognitive functions. With the use of neuroimaging technologies, alerting has been associated with the frontal and parietal regions of the right hemisphere. Lesions within these regions will reduce the ability to maintain the alert state. For example, right frontal lesion patients show an impaired ability to voluntarily sustain attention during continuous performance tests, displaying a larger number of errors over time when compared to left frontal lesion patients (Raz, 2004). It has long been established that right parietal lobe lesions, particularly those secondary to stroke, disrupt one's ability to remain alert and orient to stimuli in left hemispace, producing a profound and sometimes permanent neglect (Heilman & Van Den Abell, 1980). Alerting is thought to involve the cortical distribution of the brain's norepinephrine system arising in the locus coeruleus of the midbrain (Coull et al., 2001).

Orienting involves the selection of information from sensory input which can be triggered by the stimulus or shifted as a result of voluntary control. Thus, orienting can be reflexive as when a sudden target event directs attention to its location, or it can be more voluntary as when a person searches the visual field looking for a particular target. Even though orienting typically involves head and/or eye movements toward the target or overt orienting, it can also be covert. Orienting has been associated with areas of the parietal and frontal lobes, particularly the superior parietal lobe and frontal eye fields. Lesions within these regions will negatively impair the ability to determine a point of reference to sensory objects. Basal forebrain cholinergic systems play an important role in orienting (Beane & Marrocco, 2004).

Selection involves choosing among multiple conflicting actions or responses. Selection is critical for optimal performance in tasks involving decision making, error detection, or over-riding a habitual response. Neuroimaging data consistently reveals the anterior cingulate cortex as a central node in this attentional network (Posner & Rothbart, 1998). Additional brain areas involved in selection include the lateral prefrontal cortex and basal ganglia. Focal brain lesions to the anterior cingulate reduce and can often annihilate specific aspects of self-regulation and voluntary control making the inhibition of a pre-potent response difficult if not impossible. Selection is thought to involve the dopaminergic system given that both the anterior cingulate and lateral prefrontal cortex serve as target areas to this neurotransmitter system (Deth et al., 2004).

These largely orthogonal attentional networks interact in many practical contexts to compute different aspects of cognitive and emotional tasks; however, they also retain a certain degree of functional and anatomical independence. Variations in the operational efficiency of these various attentional networks serve as a basis for differences in such complex cognitive neuropsychological processes as self-regulation and emotional control as well as more basic mechanisms of volition and sustained effort. Thus, evaluating each aspect of attention that is, alerting, orienting and selection, is advised if one is to gain a complete picture of the attentional functioning of the presenting patient.

Assessment measures of attention

We now highlight measures of attention that assess aspects of the alerting, orienting or selection networks. Please consult the references associated with each test measure for a more in-depth discussion of administration, scoring and interpretation procedures.

- *Digit Span–Forward* (DSp-F; Wechsler, 1981) DSp-F is a measure of immediate attention and rote recall. It requires participants to listen to increasingly longer lists of digits and recite them in the exact order presented. Scores range from 0–14 and each point reflects successful completion of one trial of a particular list length.

There are visual variants of the traditional digit span task which involve learning increasingly longer lengths of 3-dimensional spatial positions as represented by raised blocks on a stimulus board (Milner, 1971) or 2-dimensional visual locations as represented by coloured circles on a visual display (Wechsler, 1945).

- *Trail Making Test – Part A* (TMT-A; Army, 1944) TMT-A is a test of speeded attention, mental tracking and visual search. Participants are required to connect a series of circles containing numbers randomly arranged in a spatial array. Both time-to-completion in seconds as well as error rate give an indication of an individual's level of attention.

- *Visual Search and Cancellation Tasks* (Diller *et al.*, 1974) Many forms of these measures exist but the underlying instructions remain the same: to 'cancel' or indicate by either crossing out or circling a particular target stimulus embedded in a larger array of distracter items. Traditional cancellations tasks include identifying the letter 'A' within a complex visual array of various letters and finding a variant of a star within a complex visual array of abstract designs. The number of items omitted is an indication of vigilance and the proportion of items omitted in each quadrant of the test page can suggest the presence of a possible neglect.

- *Stroop Colour Word Interference Test* (Stroop, 1935) In the classic Stroop task experienced readers are asked to name the ink colour of a displayed word. Responding to the ink colour of an incompatible colour word (e.g. the word 'RED' displayed in blue ink), subjects are usually slower and less accurate than identifying the ink colour of a control item (e.g. ''XXX'' or ''LOT'' inked in red). This difference in performance is called the Stroop Interference Effect (SIE).

- *Global Local Test* (Robertson *et al.*, 1988) Assesses attentional preference and the ability to reorient attention (i.e. from the global, or overall gestalt of a figure, to the local, or more detailed level of analysis). Thus, individuals are presented with a large number or letter (e.g. a 2) made up of smaller numbers or letters (e.g. strategically positioned 1's) at a rapid rate of visual presentation and asked to indicate what number or letter they perceive. Alternatively, individuals may be asked to indicate what object (e.g. number), is represented at either the global or the local level. Reaction time data indicates which level of analysis, global or local, is more taxing with slower reaction times suggesting greater difficulty. Error rates can also be informative.

- *Flanker Tasks* (Eriksen & Eriksen, 1974) Subjects respond to the direction of a central arrow when flanking arrows could either point in the same, that is congruent, or opposite, that is incongruent, direction.

- *Attention Network Test* (ANT; Fan *et al.*, 2002) The ANT, a variation of the Flanker task, requires subjects to determine whether a central arrow points rightward or leftward while the surrounding arrows may be either congruent or incongruent. Targets are arrows above or below fixation, pointing to the left or right and they are flanked on both sides by congruent or incongruent arrows. Targets are preceded by informative or uninformative spatial cues. The ANT provides three numbers that indicate the efficiency of the networks that perform the alert, orient and conflict resolution functions of attention and can be performed by adults, children, patients and even non-human animals.

- *Lateralized Attention Network Test* (LANT; Barnea *et al.*, in press) A variation of the ANT, the LANT was developed to measure the sensitivity and reliability of the three networks of attention in each hemisphere and demonstrate their validity in relation to standardized clinical measures of attention. The promise of the LANT centres on its potential to critically assess training protocols for modulating the relative attentional engagement of the two hemispheres. Furthermore, the LANT can be used, together with EEG, on self-regulation protocols to rehabilitate normal human attention.

Executive functioning

The role of executive functioning has long been to coordinate other neurocognitive systems through activities such as working memory, planning and monitoring (Stuss & Alexander, 2000). A number of authors have presented conceptual definitions of different aspects of executive functioning including models of working memory (Baddeley, 1992) and the organization of complex behaviours (Luria, 1980). Based on a review of such definitions, executive functioning appears to encompass a network of cognitive operation involving mental coordination of behaviour including planning, monitoring and mental tracking; self-regulation of behaviour including mental flexibility and the capacity to shift mental set; and complex purposive action involving self-initiated and goal-directed behaviour (Lamar *et al.*, 2002). In breaking down executive functioning into a network of cognitive operations, one is better able to determine the neuroanatomical underpinnings of this complex construct and to conduct a more complete neuropsychological evaluation.

There is a long history of non-human lesion studies as well as an increasing amount of in vivo human neuroimaging studies describing the neural substrates involved in various aspects of executive functioning (see Fuster, 1997 for review). The dorsolateral prefrontal cortex, Brodman's area (BA) 46 (Figure 1), is associated with the successful mental coordination and manipulation of information. The dopaminergic system is most affiliated with this aspect of executive functioning although other neurotransmitter systems may modulate performance on select measures of working memory and mental manipulation (Ellis & Nathan, 2001). The orbitofrontal cortex is associated with the acquisition of appropriate behaviours and the inhibition of inappropriate ones with medial orbitofrontal cortex (BA 25) associated with error detection and positive reward and lateral orbitofrontal cortex (BA 11) responsible for the inhibition of a prepotent response (see Elliott *et al.*, 2000 for review). Investigations repeatedly suggest that decreases in serotonin negatively impact various measures of orbitofrontal functioning, particularly decision making (Rogers *et al.*, 2003).

Neuroimaging studies corroborate the notion that there are separable components of executive functioning which may not reside within prefrontal cortex but are nonetheless integral to and supervised by this region. For example, specific areas within the

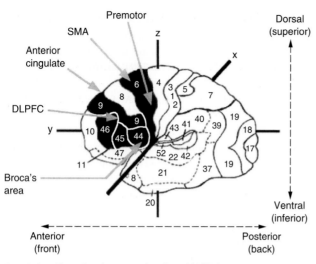

Fig 1 Brain with Brodman's areas and prefrontal highlights.

parietal lobe (BA 40; BA 7) have been associated with storage and mental coordination whose purpose is to maintain information online; while Broca's area (BA 44) appears responsible for the rehearsal of information that resides in short-term memory (see Smith & Jonides, 1998 for review). Thus, a thorough assessment of executive functioning should be a part of any neuropsychological evaluation when assessing individuals with frank frontal lobe lesions as well as individuals without obvious damage to prefrontal cortex.

Due to the complexity of the behaviours in question and the multifaceted nature of most tests of executive functioning, it is difficult to say with certainty what any particular executive function task assesses. The variability present in the literature to describe any single measure of executive functioning (Lezak, 1982) illustrates the trouble in measuring a single aspect of executive ability or developing a consensus regarding the specific abilities tapped by any particular executive function task. Therefore, it is advised to rely on several measures to gain a global picture of executive functioning.

Assessment measures of executive functioning

We now highlight measures of executive functioning that primarily assess some aspects of mental coordination, self-regulation or complex purposive action. Please consult the references affiliated with each measure for a more in-depth discussion of administration, scoring and interpretation.

- *WAIS-R Digit Span Backward* (DSp-B; Wechsler, 1981) DSp-B is a measure of mental tracking as well as brief storage and mental manipulation. It requires participants to listen to increasingly longer lists of digits presented for immediate recall in the reverse order from what was originally presented. In addition to the attentional requirements also evident in DSp-F, DSp-B requires mental manipulation for successful completion. Scores range from 0–14 and each point reflects successful completion of one trial of a particular list length. Visual variants of DSp-B are described within the section 'Assessment measures of attention' with the

caveat that these measures require recall in the reverse order from the initial visual presentation.

- *WAIS-R Similarities subtest* (Wechsler, 1981). Similarities is a measure of concept formation and reasoning which relies on continuous monitoring of output. It requires participants to find associations between word pairs of increasing complexity. Points are given based on the nature of the response and calculated using standardized procedures.

- *Trail Making Test Part B* (TMT-B; Army, 1944) The TMT-B is a test of speeded attention, mental tracking and visual search, as well as sequencing and mental flexibility. In addition to the attentional demands evident in TMT-A, TMT-B requires the additional processes of mental flexibility and set shifting as participants alternate between connecting a series of circles containing numbers and letters randomly arranged in a spatial array. Variables indicating an individual's performance include time-to-completion and errors. Some researchers subtract the scores of TMT-B from TMT-A to further isolate executive functioning from attention.

- *Alpha Span* (Asp; Craik, 1990) ASp involves short-term memory and mental tracking. It requires participants to listen to increasingly longer lists of common words presented for immediate recall in alphabetical order. Participants receive two trials of each list length, and the task is terminated after the failure of both trials. ASp scores range from 0–14, and each point reflects successful completion of one trial of a particular list length.

- *Porteus Maze Test* (Porteus, 1959) The Porteus Maze test involves the planning aspect of executive functioning. It requires participants to navigate through increasingly difficult 2-dimensional mazes. A mental age score is calculated according to standard procedures.

- *Rivermead Behavioural Memory Prospective Memory Tasks* (Wilson, Cockburn & Baddeley, 1985) Prospective memory involves planning, monitoring and purposive action. Items require participants to remember to execute different activities in the future (e.g. remembering to: ask about the next appointment when an alarm clock goes off). All tasks are introduced within 15 minutes of the beginning of the test session and interspersed throughout the course of a complete neuropsychological evaluation. Two, one, or zero points are given for each activity depending on the level of cueing needed at the time of recall. Higher scores indicate better performance.

- *Verbal Fluency* (Spreen & Benton, 1969) Although measures of verbal fluency primarily tap language functions, they also assess spontaneous flexibility through the generation of responses within a particular set of constraints and the capacity to shift mental set. Fluency tests require participants to generate as many words as possible in one minute for a given letter (F, A, S) or category (animals, fruits, vegetables), excluding proper nouns and variations of the same word. Separate scores for letter and category fluency reflect total output across all three trials (see also 'Communication assessment').

- *Wisconsin Card Sorting Test* (WCST; Grant & Berg, 1948) The WCST assesses many aspects of executive functioning including mental flexibility and concept formation. Individuals are given individual cards containing one of four forms (triangles, stars, crosses, or circles) in one of four colours (red, yellow, green or blue) presented one of four times per card. They are required to match each card to one of four target cards based on a series of rules. These rules are not explicitly stated but must be deduced based on examiner feedback. Only when 10 cards have been placed correctly under a specific rule does the rule change. Thus, sorting to colour would require 10 successful matches based on colour before the rules changed to either form or number. A total of 6 rule changes are possible and a variety of scores including the number of categories achieved and perseverative errors may be calculated.

- *The Graphical Sequence Test* (Bilder & Goldberg, 1987); *The Graphical Sequence Test – Dementia Version* (Lamar *et al.*, 1997) These measures, designed to elicit perseverative behaviour across a wide variety of clinical populations, consist of a series of consecutive verbal commands to write or draw simple geometric shapes, e.g. circles and squares, or common figures, e.g. flowers and houses. The total number of errors provides a measure of overall executive dysfunction and various error types represent increasingly lower levels of executive dysfunction.
- *The Self-Ordered Pointing Task* (SOPT; Petrides & Milner, 1982) This task assesses planning and self-monitoring through sequential selection of visual or verbal stimuli. The SOPT consists of a set number of stimuli per page with the number of pages dependent upon the number of stimuli (e.g. 12-items/12 pages). Each page contains all the same stimuli; however, the position of each stimulus on any given page varies so that no stimulus is in the same location twice. For each page, participants are instructed to select a different stimulus from those selected on previous pages in the trial. A trial is complete when all pages in the series have been presented. A total of three trials are administered. The number of items selected more than once is summed across all trial blocks with higher scores indicative of greater executive dysfunction.
- *Intra/Extra-Dimensional Shift Task* (CANTAB, Cambridge, UK). This task assesses participants' ability to attend to specific attributes of compound stimuli and to shift mental set based on feedback. Dimensions for visually presented stimuli consist of colour-filled shapes and white lines. Participants are required to choose the correct stimulus from a set of stimuli. Initial responses are to simple or unidimensional stimuli but as the task progresses, stimuli become more complex, consisting of both colour and line dimensions. Correct responses are based on criterion learned as the task progresses and become increasingly difficult to determine; that is, moving from simple, intra-dimensional shifts (e.g. colour rules only) to more difficult, extra-dimensional shifts, (i.e. colour and line rule combinations). A variety of shift scores

may be determined based on the total correct at each stage of difficulty.

Assessment batteries of executive functioning

- *Delis-Kaplan Executive Function System* (D–KEFS; Delis *et al.*, 2001) This battery consists of nine sub-tests that tap such areas of executive functioning as mental flexibility, planning, concept formation, the ability to attain and maintain mental set and self-regulation. Thus, the D-KEFS evaluates the majority of executive function aspects outlined throughout this chapter. Comprehensive normative data assists in the evaluation of all age ranges and the qualitative scoring system allows for an error analysis that may help explain subtle nuances of behaviour not addressed by more traditional measures of executive functioning.
- *The Executive Control Battery* (ECB; Goldberg *et al.*, 2000) The ECB takes an error production approach to assessing executive functioning through a series of subtests designed to elicit perseverations, inertia, stereotyped behaviour and mimicry. In addition to the Graphical Sequences Test, a version of the Go/No-Go task assesses self-regulation by either rewarding the selection of a prepotent response or the inhibition of it, respectively. Two remaining sub-tests require the repetition or mirroring of various motor programmes and sequences to evaluate more basic aspects of executive control involving the premotor cortex.

Conclusion

We have attempted to highlight the various component parts or networks that constitute attention and executive functioning. Furthermore, we have outlined the neuroanatomy and neurochemistry involved in each of these cognitive constructs and the neuropsychological test measures that may be used to investigate performance. In order to pick the most appropriate measures of attention and executive functioning for a particular evaluation, one should always consider the referral question, the presenting symptomatology and/or diagnosis of the client. Given this information, one can then attempt to predict the expected functional and/or structural areas of involvement. These predictions will make choosing the appropriate neuropsychological test measures easier. However, if little or no information exists, it is advised to select a few neuropsychological test measures that assess various aspects of attention and executive functioning to adequately cover these cognitive abilities (see also 'Neuropsychological assessment: general principles').

REFERENCES

Army Individual Test Battery (1944). *Manual of directions and scoring.* Washington, D C: Adjutant General's Office, The War Department.

Baddeley, A. (1992). Working memory. *Science*, **255**(5044), 556–9.

Barnea, A., Rassis, A., Raz, A. & Zaidel, E. (in press) Performance of adults and children on the lateralized attention network test (LANT). *Brain and Cognition.*

Beane, M. & Marrocco, R. T. (2004). Norepinephrine and acetylcholine mediation of the components of reflexive attention: implications for attention deficit disorders. *Progression in Neurobiology*, **74**(3), 167–81.

Bilder, R. M. & Goldberg, E. (1987). Motor perseverations in schizophrenia. *Archives of Clinical Neuropsychology*, **2**(3), 195–214.

Broadbent, D. E. (1958). *Perception and communication.* New York: Pergamon Press.

Coull, J. T., Nobre, A. C. & Frith, C. D. (2001). The noradrenergic alpha2 agonist clonidine modulates behavioural and neuroanatomical correlates of human attentional orienting and alerting. *Cerebral Cortex*, **11**(1), 73–84.

Craik, F. I. M. (1990). Changes in memory with normal aging: a functional view. In R. J. Wurtman (Ed.). *Alzheimer's disease (Advances in neurology) Vol. 51.* New York: Raven Press.

Delis, D. C., Kaplan, E. & Kramer, J. H. (2001). *Delis–Kaplan executive function system (D-KEFS)*. San Antonio: The Psychological Corporation.

Deth, R., Kuznetsova, A. & Waly, M. (2004). Attention-related signaling activities of the d4 dopamine receptor. In M. Posner (Ed.). *Cognitive neuroscience of attention* (pp. 269–82) New York: Guilford Press.

Diller, L., Ben-Yishay, Y., Gerstman, L. J. et al. (1974). *Studies in cognition and rehabilitation in hemiplegia*. (No. 50). New York: Behavioral Science Institute of Rehabilitation Medicine, New York University Medical Center.

Elliott, R., Dolan, R. J. & Frith, C. D. (2000). Dissociable functions in the medial and lateral orbitofrontal cortex: evidence from human neuroimaging studies. *Cerebral Cortex*, **10**(3), 308–17.

Ellis, K. A. & Nathan, P. J. (2001). The pharmacology of human working memory. *International Journal of Neuropsychopharmacology*, **4**(3), 299–313.

Eriksen, B. & Eriksen, C. (1974). Effects of noise letters upon the identification of a target letter in a nonsearch task. *Perceptual Psychophysics*, **16**, 143–9.

Fan, J., McCandliss, B. D., Sommer, T., Raz, A. & Posner, M. I. (2002). Testing the efficiency and independence of attentional networks. *Journal of Cognitive Neuroscience*, **14**(3), 340–7.

Fuster, J. M. (1997). *The Prefrontal Cortex: Anatomy, Physiology, and Neuropsychology of the Executive Lobe* (2nd edn.). New York: Lippincott-Raven Press.

Goldberg, E., Podell, K., Bilder, R. & Jaeger, J. (2000). *The executive control battery*. Melbourne: Psychology Press.

Grant, D. A. & Berg, E. A. (1948). A behavioral analysis of degree of reinforcement and ease of shifting to new responses in a weight-type card-sorting problem. *Journal of Experimental Psychology*, **38**, 404–11.

Heilman, K. M. & van den Abell, T. (1980). Right hemisphere dominance for attention: the mechanism underlying hemispheric asymmetries of inattention (neglect). *Neurology*, **30**(3), 327–30.

Lamar, M., Podell, K., Carew, T.G. et al. (1997). Perseverative behavior in Alzheimer's disease and subcortical ischemic vascular dementia. *Neuropsychology*, **11**(4), 523–34.

Lamar, M., Zonderman, A. B. & Resnick, S. (2002). Contribution of specific cognitive processes to executive functioning in an aging population. *Neuropsychology*, **16**(2), 156–62.

Lezak, M. D. (1982). The problem of assessing executive functions. *International Journal of Psychology*, **17**, 281–97.

Luria, A. R. (1980). *Higher cortical functions* (pp. 246–360). New York: Basic Books.

Milner, B. (1971). Interhemispheric differences in the localization of psychological processes in man. *British Medical Bulletin*, **27**(3), 272–7.

Petrides, M. & Milner, B. (1982). Deficits on subject-ordered tasks after frontal- and temporal-lobe lesions in man. *Neuropsychologia*, **20**, 249–62.

Porteus, S. D. (1959). *The Maze Test and clinical psychology*. Palo Alto, CA: Pacific Books.

Posner, M. I. & Rothbart, M. K. (1998). Attention, self-regulation and consciousness. *Philosophical Transactions of the Royal Society B: Biological Sciences*, **353**(1377), 1915–27.

Raz, A. (2004). Attention. In *Encyclopedia of applied psychology* (pp. 203–8). Oxford: Elsevier, Inc.

Robertson, L. C., Lamb, M. R. & Knight, R. T. (1988). Effects of lesions of temporal–parietal junction on perceptual and attentional processing in humans. *Journal of Neuroscience*, **8**(10), 3757–69.

Rogers, R. D., Tunbridge, E. M., Bhagwagar, Z., Drevets, W. C., Sahakian, B. J. & Carter, C. S. (2003). Tryptophan depletion alters the decision-making of healthy volunteers through altered processing of reward cues. *Neuropsychopharmacology*, **28**(1), 153–62.

Shalev, L. & Algom, D. (2000). Stroop and Garner effects in and out of Posner's beam: reconciling two conceptions of selective attention. *Journal of Experimental Psychology: Human Perception and Performance*, **26**(3), 997–1017.

Smith, E. E. & Jonides, J. (1998). Neuroimaging analyses of human working memory. *Proceedings of the National Academy of Sciences USA*, **95**(20), 12061–8.

Spreen, O. & Benton, A. L. (1969). *Neurosensory centre comprehensive examination for aphasia (NCCEA)*. Victoria, British Columbia:University of Victoria Neuropsychology Laboratory.

Stroop, J. (1935). Studies of interference in serial verbal reactions. *Journal of Experimental Psychology*, **18**, 643–61.

Stuss, D. T. & Alexander, M. P. (2000). Executive functions and the frontal lobes: a conceptual view. *Psychology Research*, **63**(3-4), 289–98.

Wechsler, D. (1945). A standardized memory scale for clinical use. *Journal of Psychology*, **19**, 87–95.

Wechsler, D. A. (1981). *The Wechsler adult intelligence scale–revised*. San Antonio TX: Psychology Corporation.

Wilson, B., Cockburn, J. & Baddeley, A. (2003). *The rivermead behavioral memory test (RBMT-II)*. Harcourt Assessment: Oxford, England.

Neuropsychological assessment of learning and memory

Nancy D. Chiaravalloti, Amanda O'Brien and John DeLuca

Kessler Medical Rehabilitation Research and Education Corporation

With over 100 different theorized types of memory in existence (Tulving, 2002) it is no wonder that the assessment of learning and memory can be quite complex. However, despite our current knowledge, memory is often conceptualized as a unitary concept, especially by non-psychologist health professionals. Memory is actually a multidimensional construct with dissociable sub-systems, or processes. Many of these subsystems are particularly sensitive to impairment following trauma or other acquired brain insult. Therefore, understanding how the brain represents and processes information is essential in the clinical assessment of learning and memory. Despite the major advances in the understanding of cognitive and cerebral aspects of learning and memory in the last century, clinical assessment has lagged behind the research knowledge in this area.

This chapter will present a basic overview of modern clinical assessment of learning and memory in adults. It begins with a brief historical perspective on views of memory followed by a discussion of the different approaches to the conceptual understanding of learning and memory (e.g. 'process' versus 'systems' approach). The chapter will also touch upon the key brain structures responsible for aspects of memory. We will address the role of learning, current debates in assessment, comprehensive assessment techniques and other cognitive functions that impact memory. Finally, a discussion of future directions and recommendations for improving the quality of memory assessment is presented.

The history of learning and memory assessment

There have been significant advances in the knowledge of learning and memory (and related brain structures) over the past 50 years. However, the 'formal' scientific study of learning and memory actually began in the late 1800s, with the work of Ebbinghaus, who established several cognitive principles of memory. By the early 1900s, the existence of an 'amnestic syndrome' (primarily Korsakoff's syndrome) became widely accepted and became associated with damage to diencephalic structures (i.e. thalamic nuclei and mammillary bodies). By the 1950s and 1960s, mesial temporal structures also became a primary focus of understanding the cerebral substrates of human memory. More recent conceptualizations of learning and memory have returned to the important role played by the basal forebrain and the frontal lobes.

Despite a solid body of research, the clinical assessment of memory still largely neglects the experimental study of learning and memory in psychology as well as the vast cognitive psychology and cognitive neuroscience literature. This has often resulted in an assessment which seems clinically meaningful, but is typically not well grounded theoretically. Although the original development of a memory 'test battery' was a landmark event in psychology, it was abundantly criticized due to statistical and methodological issues in its development (Prigatano, 1978). More recent memory assessments (i.e. Wechsler Memory Scale (WMS)-III; Wechsler 1997) have made major advances by including a large standardization sample, improving face validity (particularly evident in the visual memory sub-tests) and expanding the sub-tests measuring visual memory functions. However, the clinical assessment of learning and memory continues to lag behind the knowledge gained through research.

Defining learning and memory

It is necessary to understand that memory cannot be properly assessed without first addressing learning. 'Learning' can be defined as 'the process of acquiring new information', whereas the term 'memory' refers to 'the persistence of learning in a state that can be revealed at a later time' (Squire, 1987). As such, memory cannot be adequately assessed unless it is verified that the to-be-remembered information has indeed been learned.

Despite the many theories regarding types of memory and memory systems (Lezak et al., 2004) two of the most widely accepted approaches to memory are the systems approach and the process approach. Although distinctly different, these approaches can be seen as complimentary (Schacter et al., 2000). In the 'systems' approach to memory functioning, each inter-related but dissociable system is somewhat independent, in that different brain structures and resources may be utilized by each system in order to function (see Figure 1). A major distinction in this approach to human memory is the dichotomy between the procedural memory system and the declarative memory system (Tulving, 2000).

The declarative memory system consists of knowing *that* something, such as a skill or an element of information, was learned. In contrast, the procedural memory system represents knowing *how* to perform a skill, without consciously reflecting on the steps to perform the skill (Bauret et al., 1993). The declarative memory system consists of a complex interaction between mesial temporal (especially hippocampus), diencephalic (primarily anterior structures), basal forebrain and frontal lobe structures and is sensitive to acquired brain damage. In contrast, the procedural memory system is less sensitive to such damage.

One can also conceptualize learning and memory as a process, in an information processing framework (Tulving, 2000) (see Figure 2). In this model, information moves through several stages from temporary to long-term storage in the brain. An important component of this model is 'working memory'. The term 'working memory' refers to the temporary storage, maintenance and manipulation

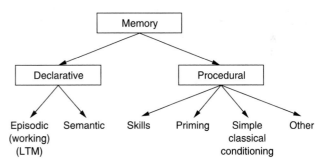

Fig 1 The structure of the memory system.

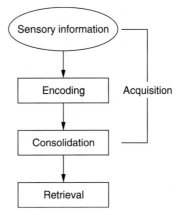

Fig 2 The memory process.

of information in the brain (Baddeley, 2000). This process is vital to the new learning and long-term memory processes.

When information is rehearsed in working memory, it is encoded due to the development of memory traces. Once information is encoded, it is transferred from this short-term temporary store to more long-term storage, a process referred to as 'consolidation', or 'elaboration' (Squire *et al.*, 1983). Numerous structures, including the hippocampus and surrounding regions, diencephalic structures, basal forebrain and the cingulate gyrus are involved in the consolidation of declarative information (see Markowitsch, 2000). The combined processes of initial encoding and subsequent consolidation of learned material in long term storage is called memory 'acquisition' (see Figure 2). 'Retrieval' is the process of tapping into previously encoded information from long-term storage for use (Squire *et al.*, 1983).

Interestingly, even the most modern imaging studies have not yet been able to definitively identify the structures responsible for the process of retrieval. As retrieval tasks often simultaneously involve re-encoding of the information retrieved, it makes identification of such structures more complex (Markowitsch, 2000). Tulving and colleagues (1994) posit a model called the Hemispheric Encoding/Retrieval Asymmetry (HERA) model. In this model, a left hemisphere prefrontal pattern of activation for the encoding of episodic memory is seen, with a right hemisphere prefrontal pattern of activation for retrieval from episodic memory. However, additional regions may be involved with distinct types of information. For example, temporo-polar regions may be involved when autobiographical memories are being retrieved (Fink *et al.*, 1996).

Comprehensive assessment of learning and memory

The clinical assessment of learning and memory is multifaceted and is not simply the administration of psychometric tests. Rather, it consists of several levels of evaluation, beginning with the referral question and including activities such as record review(s), the clinical interview and concluding with the actual psychometric testing (see Lezak *et al.*, 2004). The efficient assessment of learning and memory must begin with a specific referral question. Unfortunately, referrals are too often vague and therefore of limited use for identifying the need for an evaluation. Questions such as 'characterize strengths and weaknesses', or 'examine functional versus organic factors', offer little guidance to the evaluating clinician. The comprehensive clinical interview gathers a complete patient history including topics such as alcohol or substance use, learning disabilities, educational and work history and relevant medical history (see 'Medical interviewing'). A hypothesis testing approach to assessment gathers all of this data in order to integrate background information and draw conclusions from later testing outcomes.

Psychometric assessment

A psychometric approach to assessing learning and memory is based on quantitative measurements of samples of behaviour (e.g. learning and remembering a list of words), and a subsequent determination as to whether or not a person is 'impaired' on that sample of behaviour, compared to a normative group.

Table 1. Common neuropsychological tests of memory ability

Verbal memory	Non-verbal memory
Rey Auditory Verbal Learning Test	Rey Osterrieth
California Verbal Learning Test	Benton Visual Retention Test
Hopkins Verbal Learning Test	Brief Visuospatial Memory Test
Selective Reminding Procedure	Warrington Facial Recognition Test
	Biber Figural Learning Test
Test batteries	
Wechsler Memory Scale III	
Memory Assessment Scales	

One's 'performance' is considered to be impaired when it is below expected levels, given the patient's age, education and estimated pre-morbid intelligence. This inference is then used to determine if, and to what degree, a person has a deficit in learning and/or memory (see 'Neuropsychological assessment: general principles').

The quantitative assessment of learning and memory includes the use of test instruments or batteries that have been standardized in terms of administration, and evaluated in terms of basic psychometric properties. Some of the more popular instruments are listed in Table 1 (see Lezak *et al.*, 2004 for a thorough discussion). Interestingly, because episodic memory is the system most vulnerable to brain damage or dysfunction, virtually all tests of 'memory' that are popularly used are actually tests of episodic memory.

Memory cannot be adequately assessed without first knowing if the target information had been acquired. The importance of learning has been addressed in a series of studies by DeLuca and colleagues (1994, 1998, 2000). In one study (DeLuca *et al.*, 2000), persons with traumatic brain injury (TBI) were equated with healthy controls on the amount of information initially learned. Specifically, target material was presented repeatedly until a pre-set learning criterion was reached by both groups. Once both groups were equated on acquisition, recall and recognition was assessed and was not significantly different between the two groups. Using this design, a better understanding of the nature of impaired learning and memory (i.e. acquisition versus retrieval) was achieved. These data argue that individuals with TBI suffer from significant problems in the acquisition of new information and that recall and recognition abilities are not impaired once acquisition deficits are taken into account. Interestingly, these same results have been replicated by others (e.g. Vanderploeg *et al.*, 2001) and have also been shown in samples of individuals with multiple sclerosis (DeLuca *et al.*, 1994, 1998; Demaree *et al.*, 2000).

Unfortunately, most current clinical tools generally do not assess learning directly or comprehensively. As a result, interpretation of recall and recognition is typically confounded. (See Table 2 for common memory assessment measures and the degree to which they assess learning.)

Today, with an increased understanding of the complexity of learning and memory, a clinical assessment should be designed to determine at what point within the memory process (i.e., encoding–consolidation–retrieval) a patient is exhibiting difficulty, as this issue significantly impacts the approach to treatment. For example the treatment for difficulties in acquisition would be vastly different

Table 2. Common neuropsychological tests of memory functioning, strengths and weaknesses

Name	Form	Adequacy of assessing learning	Strengths	Weakness
California Verbal Learning Test (CVLT)–II	List Learning Test	Good	• Multiple trials • Many indices available • Good difficulty level • Good norms • 16 items are in 4 categories allowing assessment of organization	• Fixed number of learning trials
Rey Auditory Verbal Learning Test (RAVLT)	List Learning Test	Not adequate	• Multiple trials	• No formal measure of learning
Bushke Selective Reminding Test (SRT)	List Learning Test	Not adequate	• Multiple trials • Many alternate forms	• Many versions, making decision of which to use is difficult
Hopkins Verbal Learning Test – Revised	List Learning Test	Not adequate	• Multiple trials • Simple words are easier for those with lower education • Many alternate forms • 12 items are in 4 categories allowing assessment of organization	• Many higher functioning patients ceiling out • Only 3 learning trials
Rey Osterrieth Complex Figure	Figure Copy	Not adequate	• Figure is complex, allowing assessment of complex figural memory • Allows assessment of organizational ability	• No learning trials
Brief Visual Spatial Memory Test	Figural 'List' Learning	Not adequate	• Multiple trials • Nonverbal list learning task is fairly rare, but useful	• Only 3 learning trials • Stimuli can be verbalized fairly easily
Biber Figural Learning Test	Figural 'List' Learning	Not adequate	• Multiple trials • Nonverbal list learning task is fairly rare, but useful • Many learning items in each trial, making the task more difficult	• Fixed number of learning trials • Certain stimuli can be verbalized fairly easily
Wechsler Memory Scale – Revised	Battery of Sub-tests	Not adequate	• Multiple types of memory assessed, both verbal and nonverbal	• Nonverbal tasks are easily verbalized and limited in difficulty
Wechsler Memory Scale – III	Battery of Sub-tests	Not adequate, but better than the revised edition	• Multiple types of memory assessed, both verbal and nonverbal • Includes facial memory and memory for everyday scenes	• Few measures of learning for a very extensive battery • Time consuming to administer
Memory Assessment Scales	Battery of Sub-tests	Not adequate	• Multiple types of memory assessed, both verbal and nonverbal	• Few measures of learning for a very extensive battery • Sub-tests are limited in difficulty level
Warrington Recognition Memory Test	Facial memory and word memory	Not adequate	• Includes verbal and nonverbal stimuli	• Only uses a recognition format

than the treatment of a patient with difficulties in the retrieval of information from long term storage (Cicerone *et al.*, 2000).

The California Verbal Learning Test (CVLT, Delis, Kramer & Kaplan, 1987) is perhaps the best test available that allows for differentiation between learning and retrieval. The CVLT allows for the examination of the learning process through a variety of procedures, based on principles from cognitive psychology, including quantifying the rate of learning, examining recall consistency and quantifying the learning strategy employed (i.e. serial vs. semantic clustering). The CVLT also generates traditional measures of free and cued recall and recognition.

However, many clinicians continue to rely on the recall versus recognition contrast in their clinical assessments to draw conclusions regarding 'memory' with little or no regard to the learning indices available. By assuming that initial learning is intact due to the presence of adequate recognition abilities, one may make a number of erroneous assumptions. First, one is assuming that recall and recognition procedures are matched for difficulty. However, free recall is a more difficult task than recognition for both healthy and impaired individuals (Lezak *et al.*, 2004; Johnson, 1992). Second, it is often assumed that 'learning' is an all-or-none phenomenon. However, cognitive psychologists often talk about depth or quality of encoding (Brown & Craik, 2000), which refer to the strength of the memory trace. Research in learning and memory present a strong argument that a simple recall vs. recognition analysis of clinical data is insufficient to determine whether impaired performance is due to deficient acquisition or a retrieval failure.

Other considerations for comprehensive learning and memory assessment

It is important to emphasize that the clinical assessment of learning and memory is not simply the administration of tests that measure memory. There are numerous factors, both cognitive and non-cognitive, that affect the ability to acquire and subsequently recall or recognize target material. Some of these factors include working memory, information processing speed, executive abilities and 'effort'. These factors must also be assessed to provide an understanding as to why an individual may perform poorly on tests of learning and memory.

Working memory

As mentioned above, working memory is a pivotal component for many cognitive skills, such as active listening, problem-solving and planning and is often considered the first step in the encoding of information into episodic memory (Johnson, 1992; Jonides, 1995). Impairments in working memory can lead to decreased learning efficiency, which leads to impaired recall and recognition in long-term memory (Kyllonen & Christal, 1990).

The best known theory of working memory was posited by Baddeley (1992) and includes two slave systems and a central executive system. The slave systems (a phonological loop and a visuo-spatial sketchpad) maintain and rehearse information for a limited period of time. The central executive system is then responsible for processing and manipulating this stored information for use.

As working memory has a significant impact on long-term episodic memory, its proper assessment is critical within a comprehensive evaluation of long-term episodic memory ability. Despite well developed mutli-factorial theories, working memory is often conceptualized and assessed as if it is a unitary construct. There is a solid body of research, including neuroimaging studies, which support the assertion that working memory is a multifactorial construct. Unfortunately, many tests that claim to assess working memory do not do so purely. For example, the Paced Auditory Serial Addition Test (PASAT) is commonly utilized to assess working memory. However, performance on this task is confounded by attention and processing speed, making a true determination of working memory skills very difficult. There is a current need for clinical assessments to reflect the current research knowledge in order to properly assess working memory in adults.

Information processing speed

Research demonstrates that an analysis of processing speed must be part of the clinical assessment of learning and memory due to the intricate relationship between processing speed and acquisition of information. For example, in persons with multiple sclerosis, speed of processing has been found to be correlated with the number of learning trials it takes to achieve a learning criterion (DeLuca *et al.*, 1994; Gaudino *et al.*, 2001). There is also research that posits that decreased processing speed is responsible for impaired working memory and skill acquisition in older adults (e.g. Salthouse, 1996).

A challenge in assessing information-processing speed is that clinical tests of pure 'processing speed' are non-existent. Therefore, multiple instruments should be used so that related cognitive constructs can be 'factored out' in an attempt to isolate speed of processing deficits (Kalmar *et al.*, 2004). For example, if a patient's assessment results included an impaired PASAT, coupled with impairment on the WAIS-III Processing Speed Index in the presence of an intact Working Memory Index on the WAIS-III, evidence of a specific impairment in processing speed would be supported. If the same patient had an impaired verbal memory performance on the Logical Memory subtest of the WMS-III, a clinician may conclude that the impairment in verbal memory is at least partially confounded by the processing speed deficit. As this example illustrates, information processing speed can have a significant impact on learning and memory and must be integrated into an assessment in order to correctly interpret results of a learning and memory evaluation.

Executive functions and 'frontal lobe' factors

Executive functions are complex and multidimensional and include complex cognitive processes including initiating, motivating, processing, organizing and planning goal-directed behaviours and are thought to be related to frontal lobe structures (Lezak *et al.*, 2004, Fletcher & Henson, 2001). Although a number of studies point to a significant relationship between executive functions and memory, it should be recognized that not all aspects of executive functions will necessarily be associated with learning and memory, due to its multidimensional nature (e.g. Tremont and colleagues, 2000). Clinical assessment of learning and memory must account for the potential influence of executive dysfunction on tests of learning and memory. See 'Neuropsychological assessment of attention and executive function' for a more detailed discussion of this topic.

Evaluating effort

A participant's level of effort can also significantly influence performance on tests of learning and memory. This is a particularly important issue in the forensic arena where secondary gains (e.g. financial) may provide the motivation to perform below one's true abilities. In addition, the feigning of symptoms, such as cognitive deficits, can be a marker for psychiatric syndromes. The inclusion of tests designed to measure symptom validity is therefore a necessary component in a neuropsychological assessment of learning and memory.

To evaluate 'effort', a number of objective tests have been designed such that even impaired individuals are able to perform adequately (i.e. they are 'too easy to fail') (Lezak *et al.*, 2004). Examples include the Rey 15-Item Memory Task, the Portland Digit Recognition (Binder, 1993) and the TOMM (Tombaugh, 1997). Impaired performance on tasks such as these may suggest poor effort or malingering, but cannot 'prove' either. The results of effort testing must be integrated with information from other sources such as the clinical interview, records, etc. in order to form a meaningful conclusion.

Conclusions and recommendations

The fields of cognitive psychology, neuropsychology and neuroscience have greatly advanced our understanding of the learning and memory process and related brain structures over the past 50 years. However, the clinical assessment of learning and memory has not fully translated research findings into practice. With such a solid base of research as a guide, clinicians must take this information into account in the development of new assessments and in their interpretations of clinical assessment outcomes.

Several conclusions can be drawn from the information highlighted in this chapter. First, research must be translated into practice. Although determining the presence or absence of a memory problem is often the primary referral question, an assessment should also include where in the process of learning and memory (i.e. encoding, consolidation, retrieval) a patient is experiencing difficulty. Such information can be utilized to design more specific and effective treatment interventions aimed toward improving functional ability. Second, it is necessary for clinicians to demonstrate that preliminary steps in the learning and memory process (i.e. attention) are intact before they are able to conclude that a later process (i.e. retrieval) is impaired. A more appropriate conclusion may be that the integrity of the memory system is compromised, potentially secondary to impaired attention or executive functioning skills. Third, learning and memory cannot be assessed simply by the administration of tests of memory alone. Several other cognitive constructs can significantly influence whether information is adequately learned and therefore available for later retrieval from long-term storage. The clinical assessment of learning and memory must include both qualitative and quantitative assessment as well as careful interpretation of results.

Finally, new research-based approaches to the clinical assessment of learning and memory must be developed. One potentially valuable approach is criterion-based assessment. In this approach, tests would be designed to measure the ability to achieve a learning criterion (e.g. number of trials to learn a list of 12 words). However, assessments of learning and memory continue to utilize a traditional normative-based approach to understanding cognitive abilities and impairments (Anastasi, 1988). An integration of both a criterion-based approach with more traditional normative-based approach may provide a more comprehensive and complete clinical picture.

REFERENCES

Anastasi, A. (1988). *Psychological Testing* (6th edn.). New York: MacMillan.

Baddeley, A. (1992). Working memory. *Science*, **255**, 556–9.

Baddeley, A. (2000). Short-term and working memory. In E. Tulving & F. I. M. Craik (Eds.). *The Oxford handbook of memory* (pp. 77–92). New York: Oxford University Press.

Baur, R. M., Tobias, B. & Valenstien, E. (1993). Amnestic disorders. In K. M. Heilman & E. Valenstein (Eds.). *Clinical neuropsychology*. New York: Oxford University Press.

Binder, L. M. (1993). Assessment of malingering after mild head trauma with the Portland digit recognition test. *Journal of Clinical and Experimental Neuropsychology*, **15**, 170–82.

Brown, S. C. & Craik, F. I. M. (2000). Encoding and retrieval of information. In E. Tulving & F. I. M. Craik (Eds.). *The Oxford handbook of memory* (pp. 93–108). New York: Oxford University Press.

Cicerone, K. D., Dahlberg, C., Kalmar, K. et al. (2000). Evidence-based cognitive rehabilitation: recommendations for clinical practice. *Archives of Physical Medicine and Rehabilitation*, **81**, 1596–615.

Delis, D. C., Kramer, J. H., Kaplan, E. & Ober, B. A. (1987). *California verbal learning test*. San Antonio, TX: The Psychological Corporation.

DeLuca, J., Schultheis, M. T., Madigan, N. K., Christodoulou, C. & Averill, A. (2000). Acquisition versus retrieval deficits in traumatic brain injury: implications for memory rehabilitation. *Archives of Physical Medicine and Rehabilitation*, **81**(10), 1327–33.

DeLuca, J., Barbieri-Berger, S. & Johnson, S. K. (1994). The nature of memory impairments in multiple sclerosis: acquisition versus retrieval. *Journal of Clinical and Experimental Neuropsychology*, **16**, 183–9.

DeLuca, J., Gaudino, E. A., Diamond, B. J., Christodoulou, C. & Engel, R. A. (1998). Acquisition and storage deficits in multiple sclerosis. *Journal of Clinical and Experimental Neuropsychology*, **20**, 376–90.

Demaree, H. A., Gaudino, E. A., DeLuca, J. & Ricker, J. H. (2000). Learning impairment is associated with recall ability in multiple sclerosis. *Journal of Clinical and Experimental Neuropsychology*, **22**, 865–73.

Fink, G. R., Markowitsch, H. J., Reinkemeier, M., Kessler, J. & Heiss, W. D. (1996). A PET study of autobiographical memory recognition. *Journal of Neuroscience*, **16**, 4275–82.

Fletcher, P. C. & Henson, R. N. (2001). Frontal lobes and human memory: insights from functional neuroimaging. *Brain*, **124**, 849–81.

Gaudino, E. A., Chiaravalloti, N. D., DeLuca, J. & Diamond, B. J. (2001). A comparison of memory performance in relapse-remitting, primary progressive and secondary progressive multiple sclerosis. *Neuropsychiatry, Neuropsychology, and Behavioral Neurology*, **14**, 32–44.

Johnson, M. K. (1992). MEM: mechanisms of recollection. *Journal of Cognitive Neuroscience*, **4**(3), 268–80.

Jonides J. (1995). Working memory and thinking. In E. E. Smith & D. N. Osheron (Eds.). *Invitation to Cognitive Science: Thinking* (2nd edn.) (pp. 215–65). Cambridge, MA: MIT Press.

Kalmar, J., Bryant, D., Tulsky, D. & DeLuca, J. (2004). Information processing deficits in multiple sclerosis: does screening instrument make a difference? *Rehabilitation Psychology*, **49**, 213–18.

Kyllonen, P. C. & Christal, R. E. (1990). Reasoning ability is (little more than) working-memory capacity. *Intelligence*, **14**, 389–433.

Lezak, M., Howieson, D. & Loring, D. (2004). *Neuropsychological Assessment* (4th edn.). New York: Oxford University Press.

Markowitsch, H. J. (2000). Neuroanatomy of memory. In E. Tulving, & F. I. M. Craik (Eds.). *The Oxford handbook of memory* (pp. 465–84). New York: Oxford University Press.

Prigatano, G. P. (1978). Wechsler memory scale: a selective review of the literature. *Journal of Clinical Psychology*, **34**, 816–32.

Salthouse, T. A. (1996). The processing speed theory of adult age differences in cognition. *Psychological Review*, **103**, 403–28.

Schacter, D. L., Wagner, A. D. & Buckner, R. L. (2000). Memory systems of 1999. In E. Tulving & F. I. M. Craik (Eds.). *The Oxford handbook of memory* (pp. 627–43). New York: Oxford University Press.

Squire, L. R. (1987). *Memory and brain*. New York: Oxford University Press.

Squire, L. R., Cohen, N. J. & Nadel, L. (1983). The medial temporal region and memory consolidation: a new hypothesis. In H. Weingartner & E. Parker (Eds.). *Memory consolidation* (pp. 185–210). Hillsdale, NJ: Erlbaum.

Tombaugh, T. N. (1997). The test of memory malingering (TOMM): normative data from cognitively intact and cognitively impaired individuals. *Psychological Assessment*, **9**, 260–8.

Tremont, G., Halpert, S., Javorsky, D. J. & Stern, R. A. (2000). Differential impact of executive dysfunction on verbal list learning and story recall. *The Clinical Neuropsychologist*, **14**(3), 295–302.

Tulving, E. (2000). Concepts of memory. In E. Tulving & F. I. M. Craik (Eds.). *The Oxford handbook of memory* (pp. 33–44). New York: Oxford University Press.

Tulving, E., Kapur, S., Craik, F. I. M., Moscovitch, M. & Houle, S. (1994). Hemispheric encoding/retrieval asymmetry in episodic memory: positron emission tomography findings. *Proceedings of the National Academy of Sciences of the USA*, **91**, 2016–20.

Vanderploeg, R. D., Crowell, T. A. & Curtiss, G. (2001). Verbal learning and memory deficits in traumatic brain injury: encoding, consolidation and retrieval. *Journal of Clinical and Experimental Neuropsychology*, **23**, 185–95.

Wechsler, D. (1997). *Wechsler Memory Scale* (3rd edn.). San Antonio, TX: The Psychological Corporation.

Pain assessment

Sandra J. Waters, Kim E. Dixon, Lisa Caitlin Perri and Francis J. Keefe

Duke University Medical Center

Over the past four decades, approaches to the assessment of chronic pain have evolved substantially within the field of behavioural medicine. During this time, it has become apparent that what we label as 'pain' is the result of complex interactions among biological, psychological and social factors. The gate control theory of pain (Melzack & Wall, 1965) supports this paradigm in that it confirms that pain is a complex experience involving sensory–discriminative, evaluative–cognitive and affective–motivational components, thus emphasizing the role of the central nervous system in nociceptive perception and processing. Further, the gate control theory provides a foundation for the development and refinement of integrated pain assessment models, such as the biopsychosocial model of pain (Turk, 1996).

The biopsychosocial model of pain acknowledges that the experience of pain often is the result of physiological changes occurring after peripheral nociceptive stimulation (Turk, 1996). However, this model also emphasizes that the pain experience is modulated by individual differences in various cognitive, affective, behavioural and social factors. People with the same level of underlying nociceptive stimulation may differ in their pain experience depending on the importance of any factor at any given time during the course of the disease or condition (Asmundson & Wright, 2004). Thus, assessing pain necessitates the examination of relations among various factors across a variety of levels (Stoney & Lentino, 2000).

During the latter part of the twentieth century, Melzack (1999) proposed an expanded model of pain which further highlights the role of psychological processes in pain. This model, the neuromatrix model, proposes the presence of a widespread network of neurons (the neuromatrix) which is distributed throughout many areas of the brain and which integrates information from multiple sources. The neuromatrix outputs information to other brain areas and produces a neurosignature pattern that may be responsible for the development of chronic pain (Melzack & Katz, 2004). The neuromatrix theory is important because it provides a theoretical framework in which a genetically determined template of a whole body (i.e. the body–self neuromatrix) is modulated by sensory inputs, the stress system and cognitive functions of the brain (Melzack & Katz, 2004). As such, it presents a more complex, psychological model of pain that warrants a broader approach for assessing pain (see 'Pain').

Pain assessment

Just as the models of pain have evolved from simple to more complex, integrated designs, so too have the measures used in the assessment of pain. Today, clinicians and researchers utilize measures designed not only to assess pain intensity, but also the psychological and sociological factors which contribute to the pain experience. This chapter provides a brief overview of assessment tools currently used by many clinicians and researchers in the field of pain. The chapter is divided into three sections in which we describe measures that assess (1) pain experience; (2) cognitive and emotional aspects of pain; and (3) functional aspects of pain. Each section includes a brief description of each measure, presents research evidence, and clinical implications of using such measures in pain assessment. The sections conclude with evaluative comments.

Pain experience measures

The experience of pain is typically assessed using single-item or multi-item scales. Pain is very often assessed using brief, single item scales such as a Numeric Rating Scale (NRS) that measures pain using a 0–10 scale on which 0 is 'no pain' and 10 is 'pain as bad as it can be'. The patient chooses the number that best represents the current intensity of their pain. It has been suggested that a reduction of 2 points on a 0 to 10 point NRS represents a clinically important improvement in pain (Farrar et al., 2001).

A Visual Analogue Scale (VAS) is another single-item scale used to measure pain. Patients place a hash mark at the location on a 10 cm line that reflects the intensity of their pain. The scale is anchored on the lower end by '0' (no pain at all) and '10' on the upper end (worst pain ever experienced). Some researchers suggest that older adults with and without cognitive impairments may find this scale hard to use because of the abstract nature of the scaling properties (Varni et al., 1986). Despite this potential shortcoming, the VAS is frequently used to assess pain intensity in both research and medical settings (e.g. Jansen & Karoly, 2001).

Single item Verbal Descriptor Scales (VDS) are also frequently used to assess the perceived intensity and unpleasantness of pain. On a VDS, a group of verbal descriptors is presented to the patient (e.g. 'none', 'mild', 'moderate', 'severe' and 'extreme') and the patient is asked to select the word that best describes their pain. The VDS is easy to score and interpret and is sensitive to both drug and non-drug treatment changes in pain levels, making it an attractive measure for use in both research and clinical settings (Burckhardt & Jones, 2003).

A drawback of single item scales is that they measure only one part of the pain experience. In an attempt to capture multidimensional aspects of the pain experience, multi-item instruments such as the McGill Pain Questionnaire (MPQ; Melzack, 1975) were developed. The MPQ contains 20 sets of adjective pain descriptors describing the sensory qualities, affective qualities and subjective intensity of pain. Patients select words from the list to describe their current pain. Pain descriptors are given a rank value based on their position within each group of words. The rank values are used to calculate (1) a Sensory sub-scale; (2) an Affective subscale; and (3) an Evaluative sub-scale. A short form of the MPQ (MPQ-SF; Melzack, 1987) is available for occasions when time constraints negate the use of the original measure. Both forms are valid, reliable and useful measures of subjective pain in clinical and research settings (Dudgeon et al., 1993). However, research has suggested some instability in the MPQ sub-scale factors in different pain populations (e.g. Holroyd et al., 1992; Cassisi et al., 2004).

The Brief Pain Inventory (BPI; Cleeland, 1989) is another multi-item, self-report questionnaire that measures current pain as well as the least, worst and average pain in the past 24 hours. On the BPI, 0 to 10 numeric rating scales are not only used to assess pain intensity but also to assess pain interference in seven quality of life domains (i.e. general activity, walking, mood, sleep, work, relations with other persons and enjoyment of life). Although initially developed to assess cancer pain, the BPI is now widely used to assess chronic non-malignant pain (Tan et al., 2004; White et al., 2003).

Direct observation of pain behaviours can be useful in gathering information on behavioural markers of pain. Pain behaviours are the verbal (e.g. sighing) and non-verbal behaviours (e.g. grimacing, rubbing) which serve to convey to others that pain is being experienced (Fordyce, 1976). In clinical settings, pain behaviours are important because they can influence physicians' decisions about pain evaluation and treatment (e.g. deciding on whether to order an invasive test or whether or not to prescribe opioids (Turk & Okifuji, 1997). Pain behaviours can be recorded through videotaped observations of overt motor behaviours (e.g. guarded movement, rubbing of the painful area; Keefe & Block, 1982) or facial expressions (Breau et al., 2001; Prkachin et al., 2002).

Comment: Single-item measures of pain are often preferred by clinicians for the assessment of pain intensity because they tap into a key dimension of pain, are quick to administer, easy to score and can be given repeatedly over time (Glajchen, 2001). Multi-item questionnaires take somewhat longer to administer and score but provide a much more comprehensive assessment of different qualities of the pain experience (Dworkin & Sherman, 2001). Observational methods of pain are useful in situations where patient self-report is not a viable option (e.g. in very young children, or in patients with cognitive deficits) or in settings in which clinicians and researchers wish to augment self-report measures with an objective measure of pain behaviour.

Cognitive and affective measures of the pain experience

The challenges of dealing with chronic pain on an ongoing basis can alter cognitive and affective functioning. Of the various measures of cognitive adjustment to pain, catastrophizing has emerged as one of the strongest predictors of poor adjustment to chronic pain Sullivan et al. (2001). Catastrophizing, 'an exaggerated negative 'mental' set brought to bear during actual or anticipated pain experience', (Sullivan et al., 2001, p. 53) has been found to explain 7–31% of the variance in pain in studies across several pain populations (e.g. low back pain, dental pain, experimental pain) (see 'Coping with chronic pain' and 'Pain management'). Pain catastrophizing has been associated with higher levels of healthcare utilization, more frequent hospitalizations and heightened disability (Sullivan et al., 2001). One of the most reliable and widely used measures of catastrophizing is the Pain Catastrophizing Scale (PCS; Sullivan et al., 1995). The PCS is a 13-item measure with three sub-scales: 'Magnification', 'Rumination' and 'Helplessness'. Scores on the PCS have been found to explain unique variance in key indices of adjustment to pain including measures of psychological functioning, social functioning and physical disability (Sullivan et al., 1998; Severeijns et al., 2002). PCS scores also have been found to significantly predict the physical and emotional distress experienced by participants undergoing experimental pain procedures (Sullivan et al., 2001). A version of the PCS has been developed for use in children and adolescents (PCS-C; Crombez et al., 2003).

Another key cognitive aspect of pain is self-efficacy, or one's perceived ability to adapt to and respond to pain. Self-efficacy is malleable and numerous studies have found that increases in self-efficacy occurring over the course of intervention are related to short- and long-term improvements in pain outcomes (see Tait, 1999, for a review of this topic). The Chronic Pain Self-Efficacy Scale (CPSS; Anderson et al., 1995) is a useful instrument which measures chronic pain patients' perception of their self-efficacy to deal with chronic pain. This brief 22-item measure has three factors; 'Self-efficacy for pain management', 'Self-efficacy for coping with symptoms' and 'Self-efficacy for physical function'. Scores on the CPSS are correlated with pain intensity, affective distress and activity levels (see also 'Self-efficacy and health behaviour').

Emotional responses to pain can have a major impact on the pain experience (Chapman, 2004). In several recent studies, pain-related anxiety has emerged as a critical factor in understanding the pain experience and how an individual responds to the thoughts about pain or the experience of pain flares (see Keefe et al., 2004). The Pain Anxiety Symptom Scale (PASS; McCracken et al., 1992) attempts to capture several dimensions of pain-related anxiety responses. It is a 40-item self-report inventory with four sub-scales; 'Cognitive anxiety', 'Escape/avoidance', 'Fearful thoughts' and 'Physiological symptoms of anxiety'. In a study of rheumatoid arthritis patients, anxiety about pain predicted patient functioning even after controlling for self-reports of health, education, active and passive coping strategies and self-efficacy (Strahl et al., 2000).

In a similar vein, fear of pain can exacerbate the experience of pain. The Fear of Pain Questionnaire-III (FPQ-III; McNeil & Rainwater, 1998) is a 30-item instrument that describes different painful situations. Patients rate how fearful they are of pain associated with each situation using a 5-point Likert scale. Three sub-scales are derived from the ratings: 'Fear of severe pain', 'Fear of minor pain' and 'Fear of medical pain'. The short length and ease of scoring of the FPQ-III make it attractive for use in both clinical and research settings. However, different response patterns have been found for various samples of chronic pain patients (Hursey & Jacks, 1992).

The prevalence of depression (in some studies exceeding 50%; e.g. Banks & Kerns, 1996) occurring after developing chronic pain suggests an aetiological role for chronic pain in the subsequent development of depression. While it is not uncommon for chronic pain patients to develop depression, somatic symptoms presenting in patients with chronic pain may artificially inflate scores on the most commonly used self-report depression measures (Bradley & McKendree-Smith, 2001). One such instrument is the Beck Depression Inventory (BDI; Beck et al., 1961), which is a 21-item self-report inventory that assesses cognitive, affective, motivational and physiological levels of depressive symptoms. Revisions have been made to the original BDI (i.e. BDI-II; Beck et al., 1996), to better align items with the current major depression criteria from the Diagnostic and Statistical Manual, Fourth edition, Text revision (DSM-IV-TR; American Psychiatric Association, 2000). A similar self-report instrument, the Centre for Epidemiologic Studies – Depression Scale (CES-D; Radloff, 1977), has 20 items rating depressive symptoms on a 0–3 point Likert-like scale, but few items directly assess physical complaints. In either case, the predictive ability of both instruments to detect depression in chronic pain patients is acceptable, but higher cut-off scores (21 for BDI; 27 for CES-D) should be employed in this population before a diagnosis of depression is rendered (Geisser et al., 2000).

Comment: Research has shown that catastrophizing as well as pain-related anxiety and fear are concepts that are important for our understanding of how persons adjust to persistent pain (see Keefe et al., 2004). Use of the measures described in this section may give researchers and clinicians further insight into the interplay between cognition and emotions and the experience of pain (see Price, 2001, for a more comprehensive review) and the factors that contribute to the strong relationship between pain and depression.

Functional aspects of pain

The impact of persistent pain on a person's life can vary substantially. One person with persistent arthritis pain, for example, may be unable to carry out home or work responsibilities, and report being resentful because he or she has become dependent on family and friends. Another person having the same pain level, may be involved in a wide array of social and work activities, and report being satisfied with the support and encouragement received from family and friends. Psychologists have developed several instruments to assess these variations in functional aspects of pain. One of the most widely used instruments is the Multidimensional Pain Inventory (MPI; Kerns et al., 1985), a 13-item scale that assesses the impact of pain on various aspects of the patients' lives including beliefs about how significant others respond to expressions of pain and pain interference with domestic, social and recreational activities. Internal consistency of the original instrument ranges from 0.70 to 0.92 and the test–retest reliability ranges from, 0.62–0.91 (Kerns et al., 1985). Responses on the MPI are often used to classify patients into three pain sub-types (i.e. 'dysfunctional', 'adaptive coper' and 'interpersonally distressed'; Turk & Rudy, 1988). More recently, researchers have suggested that the MPI contains a fourth group, 'repressors', characterized by high pain levels, low activity and low distress (Burns et al., 2001).

Comment: Unlike acute pain, where the focus of assessment is on finding a cure, chronic pain assessment is more likely to be focused on self-management issues (Turk et al., 2004). Multidimensional inventories, such as the MPI, identify aspects of daily functioning and social interactions being impacted by, or having an impact on, pain. The information obtained from these measures may facilitate individualized treatment planning (see also 'Disability assessment' and 'Quality of life assessment').

underscore the contributions which health psychologists can make in the understanding, assessment and treatment of complex pain conditions.

Conclusion

Over the past two decades, a number of reliable and valid pain measures have been developed by psychologists. These measures are increasingly being incorporated into clinical settings. Their growing use has heightened recognition of the psychosocial impact of both chronic pain and disease-related pain conditions. It has also increased interest in psychosocial interventions designed to improve patients' abilities to manage pain. Considered overall, these measures

Acknowledgements

Preparation of this chapter was supported, in part, by the following grants from the National Institutes of Health: NIAMS AR 46305, AR047218, P01 AR50245, NIMH MH63429; Cancer Institute grants: R21-CA88049-01, CA91947-01, National Institute of Neurological Diseases and Stroke grant: NS46422 and by support from the Arthritis Foundation and Fetzer Institute.

REFERENCES

American Psychiatric Association (2000). *Diagnostic and statistical manual of mental disorders (DSM-IV-TR) – text revision.* Washington, DC: American Psychiatric Association.

Anderson, K. O., Dowds, B. N., Pelletz, R. E., Edwards, W. T. & Peeters-Asdourian, C. (1995). Development and initial validation of a scale to measure self-efficacy beliefs in patients with chronic pain. *Pain,* **63**, 77–84.

Asmundson, G. J. G. & Wright, K. D. (2004). Biopsychosocial approaches to pain. In T. Hadjistavropoulos & K. D. Craig (Eds.). *Pain: psychological perspectives* (pp. 13–34). Mahwah, NJ: Lawrence Erlbaum Associates.

Banks, S. M. & Kerns, R. D. (1996). Explaining high rates of depression in chronic pain: a diathesis–stress framework. *Psychological Bulletin,* **119**, 95–110.

Beck, A. T., Steer, R. A. & Brown, G. K. (1996). *Beck Depression Inventory Manual* (2nd edn.). San Antonio, TX: Psychological Corporation.

Beck, A. T., Ward, C. H. & Mendelson, M. (1961). An inventory for measuring depression. *Archives of General Psychiatry,* **4**, 561–71.

Bradley, L. A. & McKendree-Smith, N. L. (2001). Assessment of psychological status using interviews and self-report instruments. In D.C. Turk & R. Melzack (Eds.). *Handbook of pain assessment* (pp. 292–319). New York: Guilford Press.

Breau, L. M., McGrath, P. J., Craig, K. D. *et al.* (2001). Facial expression of children receiving immunizations: a principal components analysis of the child facial coding system. *Clinical Journal of Pain,* **17**, 178–86.

Burckhardt, C. S. & Jones, K. D. (2003). Adult measures of pain. *Arthritis and Rheumatism,* **9**, S96–S104.

Burns, J. W., Kubilus, A., Bruehl, S. & Harden, R. N. (2001). A fourth empirically derived cluster of chronic pain patients based on the

multidimensional pain inventory: evidence for repression within the dysfunctional group. *Journal of Consulting and Clinical Psychology,* **69**, 663–73.

Cassisi, J. E., Umeda, M., Deisinger, J. A. *et al.* (2004). Patterns of pain descriptor usage in African Americans and European Americans with chronic pain. *Cultural Diversity and Ethnic Minority Psychology,* **10**, 81–9.

Chapman, C. R. (2004). Pain perception, affective mechanisms, and conscious experience. In T. Hadjistavropoulos & K. D. Craig (Eds.). *Pain: psychological perspectives* (pp. 59–86). Mahwah, NJ: Lawrence Erlbaum Associates.

Cleeland, C. S. (1989). Measurement of pain by subjective report. In C.R. Chapman & J. D. Loeser (Eds.). *Advances in pain research and therapy. Issues in pain measurement* (pp. 391–403). New York: Raven Press.

Crombez, G., Bijttebier, P., Eccleston, C. *et al.* (2003). The child version of the pain catastrophizing scale (PCS-C): a preliminary validation. *Pain,* **104**, 639–46.

Dudgeon, D., Raubertas, R. F. & Rosenthal, S. N. (1993). The short-form McGill Pain Questionnaire in chronic cancer pain. *Journal of Pain and Symptom Management,* **8**, 191–5.

Dworkin, S. F. & Sherman, J. J. (2001). Relying on objective and subjective measures of chronic pain: guidelines for use and interpretation. In D. C. Turk & R. Melzack (Eds.). *Handbook of Pain Assessment* (2nd edn.). (pp. 619–38). New York: Guilford Press.

Farrar, J. T., Young, J. P., Jr., LaMoreaux, L., Werth, J. L. & Poole, R.M. (2001). Clinical importance of changes in chronic pain intensity measured on an 11-point numerical pain rating scale. *Pain,* **9**, 149–58.

Fordyce, W. E. (1976). *Behavioral methods for chronic pain and illness.* St. Louis, MO: Mosby.

Geisser, M. E., Roth, R. S., Theisen, M. E., Robinson, M. E. & Riley, J. L. (2000). Negative affect, self-report of depressive symptoms, and clinical depression: relation to the experience of chronic pain. *Clinical Journal of Pain,* **16**, 110–20.

Glajchen, M. (2001). Chronic pain: treatment barriers and strategies for clinical practice. *The Journal of the American Board of Family Practice,* **14**, 211–18.

Holroyd, K. A., Holm, J., Keefe, F. J. *et al.* (1992). A multi-center evaluation of the McGill Pain Questionnaire: results from more than 1700 chronic pain patients. *Pain,* **48**, 301–11.

Hurscy, K. G. & Jacks, S. D. (1992). Fear of pain in recurrent headache sufferers. *Headache: The Journal of Head and Face Pain,* **32**, 283–6.

Jensen, M. P. & Karoly, P. (2001). Self-report scales and procedures for assessing pain in adults. In D. C. Turk & R. Melzack (Eds.). *Handbook of pain assessment* (pp. 15–34). New York: Guilford Press.

Keefe, F. J. & Block, A. R. (1982). Development of an observation method for assessing pain behavior in chronic low back pain patients. *Behaviour Therapy,* **13**, 363–75.

Keefe, F. J., Rumble, M. E., Scipio, C. D., Giordano, L. A. & Perri, L. M. (2004). Psychological aspects of persistent pain: current state of the science. *Journal of Pain,* **5**, 195–211.

Kerns, R. D., Turk, D. C. & Rudy, T. E. (1985). The West Haven–Yale Multidimensional Pain Inventory (WHYMPI). *Pain,* **23**, 345–56.

McCracken, L. M., Zayfert, C. & Gross, R. T. (1992). The pain anxiety symptoms scale: development and validation of a scale to measure fear of pain. *Pain,* **50**, 67–73.

McNeil, D. W. & Rainwater III, A. J. (1998). Development of the fear of pain questionnaire-III. *Journal of Behavioural Medicine,* **21**, 389–410.

Melzack, R. (1999). From the gate to the neuromatrix. *Pain Supplement*, **6**, S121–S26.

Melzack, R. (1987). The short-form McGill pain questionnaire. *Pain*, **30**, 191–7.

Melzack, R. (1975). The McGill pain questionnaire: major properties and scoring methods. *Pain*, **1**, 277–99.

Melzack, R. & Katz, J. (2004). The gate control theory: reaching for the brain. In T. Hadjistravropoulos & K. D. Craig (Eds.). *Pain: psychological perspectives* (pp. 13–34). Mahwah, NJ: Lawrence Erlbaum Associates.

Melzack, R., & Wall, P. D. (1965). Pain mechanisms: a new theory. *Science*, **150**, 971–9.

Prince, D. D. (2000). Psychological and neural mechanisms of the affective dimension of pain. *Science*, **9**, 1769–72.

Prkachin, K. M., Hughes, E., Schultz, I., Joy, P. & Hunt, D. (2002). Real-time assessment of pain behavior during clinical assessment of low back pain patients. *Pain*, **95**, 23–30.

Radloff, L. S. (1977). The CES-D Scale: a self-report depression scale for research in the general population. *Applied Psychological Measurement*, **1**, 385–401.

Severijns, S., van den Hout, M., Vlaeyen, J. & Picavet, H. (2002). Pain catastrophizing and general health status in a large Dutch community sample. *Pain*, **99**, 367–76.

Stoney, C. M. & Lentino, L. M. (2000). Psychophysiological applications in clinical health psychology. In J. T. Cacioppo, L.G. Tassinary & G.G. Berntson (Eds.). *Handbook of psychophysiology* (pp. 751–71). Cambridge, UK: Cambridge University Press.

Strahl, C., Kleinknecht, R. A. & Dinnel, D. L. (2000). The role of pain anxiety, coping and pain self-efficacy in rheumatoid arthritis patient functioning. *Behaviour Research and Therapy*, **38**, 863–73.

Sullivan, M. J., Bishop, S. R. & Pivik, J. (1995). The pain catastrophizing scale: development and validation. *Psychological Assessment*, **7**, 524–32.

Sullivan, M. J., Stanish, W., Waite, H., Sullivan, M. & Tripp, D. A. (1998). Catastrophizing, pain, and disability in patients with soft-tissue injuries. *Pain*, **77**, 253–60.

Sullivan, M. J., Thorn, B., Haythornthwaite, J. *et al.* (2001). Theoretical perspectives on the relation between catastrophizing and pain. *The Clinical Journal of Pain*, **17**, 52–64.

Tait, R. (1999). Evaluation of treatment effectiveness in patients with intractable pain: measures and methods. In R.J. Gatchel & D. C. Turk (Eds.). *Psychosocial factors in pain: critical perspectives* (pp. 457–80). New York: Guilford Press.

Tan, G., Jensen, M. P., Thornby, J. I. & Shanti, B.F. (2004). Validation of the brief pain inventory for chronic nonmalignant pain. *The Journal of Pain*, **5**, 133–7.

Turk, D. C. (1996). Biopsychosocial perspective on chronic pain.

In R. J. Gatchel & D. C. Turk (Eds.). *Psychological approaches to pain management: a practitioner's handbook* (pp. 3–32). Baltimore, MD: Williams & Wilkins.

Turk, D. C., Monarch, E. S. & Williams, A. D. (2004). Assessment of chronic pain sufferers. In T. Hadjistravropoulos & K. D. Craig (Eds.). *Pain: psychological perspectives* (pp. 209–43). Mahwah, NJ: Lawrence Erlbaum Associates.

Turk, D. C. & Okifuji, A. (1997). What factors affect physicians' decisions to prescribe opioids for chronic noncancer pain patients? *Clinical Journal of Pain*, **13**, 330–6.

Turk, D. C. & Rudy, T. E. (1988). Toward an empirically derived taxonomy of chronic pain patients: Integration of psychological assessment data. *Journal of Consulting and Clinical Psychology*, **56**, 233–8.

Varni, J. W., Jay, S. M., Masek, B. J. & Thompson, K. L. (1986). Cognitive–behavioral assessment and management of pediatric pain. In A. D. Holzman & D. C. Turk (Eds.). *Pain management: a handbook of psychological treatment approaches.* New York: Pergamon, 1986.

White, W. T., Patel, N., Drass, M. & Nalamachu, S. (2003). Lidocain patch 5% with systemic analgesics such as gabapentin: a rational polypharmacy approach for the treatment of chronic pain. *Pain Medicine*, **4**, 321–30.

Patient satisfaction assessment

Susan V. Eisen

Edith Nourse Rogers Memorial Veterans Hospital

Overview

In recent years, assessment of patient satisfaction has become ubiquitous among health care providers and systems in much of the developed world. In the United States, the Joint Commission on Accreditation of Healthcare Organizations (JCAHO, the accrediting organization for hospitals) and the National Committee on Quality Assurance (NCQA, the accrediting organization for managed healthcare plans and physician organizations) have identified patient satisfaction as an important quality indicator, and have required its measurement to meet accreditation requirements (JCAHO, 1997; http://www.ncqa.org/about/timeline.htm.) Specific approaches to meeting patient satisfaction assessment requirements vary. JCAHO allows for patient satisfaction instruments to be incorporated into 'performance measurement systems'. Following submission to JCAHO of documentation regarding reliability, validity and use of specific quality indicators, JCAHO reviews and approves performance measurement systems that meet their standards. Accredited facilities can then choose from dozens of approved performance measurement systems, all of which include quality indicators that meet accreditation requirements. This system allows for potential use of different satisfaction surveys by different facilities.

In Europe, the Verona Service Satisfaction Scale (VSSS) is included in a 5-nation study to develop standardized instruments to facilitate cross-national research, specifically addressing characteristics, needs, quality of life, patterns of care, service costs and satisfaction of individuals with schizophrenia (Ruggeri *et al.*, 2000).

Globally, the World Health Organization (WHO) has developed a framework for measuring health system performance that includes 'responsiveness' as an important criterion. The 'responsiveness' construct includes domains commonly assessed in patient satisfaction instruments such as dignity, communication, access to care, etc. WHO has implemented a health and responsiveness study that includes 70 developed and developing countries across six continents (Valentine *et al.*, 2003).

These efforts and many other smaller scale projects have approached the challenge of assessing patient satisfaction in a variety of ways using varied methods, sometimes derived from different conceptualizations of satisfaction. This chapter presents an overview of current thinking about patient satisfaction, paradigms and strategies for assessing patient satisfaction, challenges for the assessment process and clinical implications.

Conceptualization of patient satisfaction

Early conceptualizations of patient satisfaction were based on a discrepancy model in which perception of services received is compared to expectations or ideals regarding those services. Satisfaction is the difference between perception of actual services vs. expectations or ideals (Campbell & Einspahr, 2001; Pascoe, 1983). Other conceptualizations view patient satisfaction as a global, unidimensional or multidimensional indicator of the quality and/or outcome of care (Attkisson & Greenfield, 1994; Cleary & McNeil, 1988; Davies & Ware, 1988; Donabedian, 1980; Marshall *et al.*, 1993). Donabedian (1980) describes a three-part approach to understanding quality of care in terms of the structure, process and outcome of care. Within this framework, patient satisfaction is seen both as an outcome distinct from health status and as a judgement about the quality of care. Within processes of care, a distinction is made between the technical; that is, the science of care; and the interpersonal, the art of care (Donabedian, 1980). Technical care is the application of medical science and technology to the management of a health problem. It includes accuracy of diagnosis; appropriateness of treatment; clinician competence and skill in performing medical and surgical procedures; and medical errors. Interpersonal care includes communication of information about diagnosis; results of tests; prognosis and treatment options; listening to patients' concerns; mutuality; treatment with courtesy; dignity and respect; and patients' active participation in treatment decisions (Donabedian, 1980). Because of concerns regarding consumers' ability to evaluate technical aspects of care, some satisfaction surveys focus exclusively on interpersonal aspects of care. However, Davies and Ware (1988) provide evidence that in addition to being excellent sources of data on the interpersonal aspects of care, consumers can distinguish between levels of technical quality care as well (see also 'Patient satisfaction').

The recent focus on patient-centred care, recovery and empowerment (particularly with regard to mental health services) has raised questions about earlier conceptualizations of satisfaction.

Campbell and Einspahr (2001) note that focus group participants suggested that 'satisfaction assessments are often guided by political agendas, that serve to support programmes and funding for providers rather than accurately assess the needs and feelings of consumers' (p. 103). They suggest elimination of the 'professional' definition of satisfaction created by providers, and implementation of consumer-oriented measures of quality, with inclusion of qualitative, rather than quantitative data. Recognizing the value of consumer involvement in determining optimal ways to assess healthcare quality and satisfaction, a number of efforts have incorporated consumer input into the development of healthcare quality indicators. The results have identified several concerns expressed by consumers that are not often included in measures of patient satisfaction, such as the threat of involuntary treatments, intolerable side effects of medications and exclusion from the treatment decision-making process (Campbell & Einspahr, 2001). As a result of the consumer movement in health care, more recent efforts to assess patient satisfaction have included consumers and family members in the process of identifying priority areas, in questionnaire development and as interviewers (Kaufmann & Phillips, 2000). For example, both the MHSIP (Mental Health Statistics Improvement Programme) consumer survey and the CAHPS® (Consumer Assessment of Health Plans Study) survey involved consumers in the development and early testing of these instruments (Center for Mental Health Services, 1996; Edgman-Levitan & Cleary, 1996; Harris-Kojetin *et al.*, 1999) (see also 'Patient-centred healthcare').

Purposes of patient satisfaction assessment

The ultimate purpose of assessing patient satisfaction is to improve the quality (including outcomes) of care. For this reason organizations with oversight responsibilities have identified patient satisfaction as an important quality indicator and required its systematic assessment for accreditation, reimbursement or other accountability reasons. Improved quality may occur in a variety of ways, including improving optimal utilization of appropriate services, enhancing patient–provider communication and increasing adherence to treatment recommendations (Cleary & McNeil, 1988; Marquis *et al.*, 1983).

At the programme or facility level, within the Continuous Quality Improvement (CQI) paradigm, results are reported at regular intervals (usually monthly or quarterly) to administrators and clinical providers who work to develop strategies to improve aspects of care identified as needing improvement. The formats and methods for reporting results vary. Eisen *et al.* (2002) discuss the use of control and comparison charts in comparing performance within a facility over time, as well as comparing a programme's performance to external benchmarks derived from multiple facilities that use the same patient satisfaction instrument. Control charts are standardized statistical tools that plot means and standard deviations over time (Lee & McGreevey, 2002a). Recommended by JCAHO, they are used to determine whether variation over time in either standard deviations or mean satisfaction ratings are within or outside expected limits. If they are outside expected limits, facilities are advised to look into possible causes for such variations. Comparison charts show a programme's satisfaction ratings compared with expected performance, based on a benchmark

(Lee & McGreevey, 2002*b*). If performance falls below the expectation, Continuous Quality Improvement teams meet to determine possible explanations for poor performance and develop strategies for improvement.

In addition to improving quality, assessment of patient satisfaction is increasingly used for marketing purposes (Cleary & McNeil, 1988). As the cost of healthcare rises and as the number of for-profit healthcare organizations increases, so does competition among providers. A survey of more than 500 patients reported that over a 5-year period, 85% either changed their physician or were thinking of doing so (Cousins, 1985). Patient satisfaction surveys have potential for increasing business for provider organizations that can show favourable results. At the health insurance plan level, employers commonly use health plan 'report cards' showing patient satisfaction results for the different health plans offered to employees. These report cards can be used by employees to choose a health plan that best meets their needs. However, such report cards are also used by oversight organizations and by states to provide information to consumers that could hurt marketing efforts of health plans whose ratings are unfavourable. NCQA posts results for accredited health plans on its web site (hprc.ncqa.org/Result.asp) for the following quality domains; access and service, qualified providers, staying healthy, getting better and living with illness.

Patient satisfaction assessment paradigms

The great majority of efforts to assess patient satisfaction use quantitative (rating scale) surveys. Across both technical and interpersonal realms, researchers in the field have used conceptual frameworks and empirical (factor analytic) methods to identify satisfaction domains. The CAHPS survey assesses specific domains as well as global ratings of doctors, care received and health insurance plans. The specific domains include access to care (getting needed care and getting care quickly); doctor–patient communication and interaction; respect, courtesy and helpfulness of office staff; and health plan service information and paperwork. Other relevant domains of care that have been identified in the literature include physical surroundings; competence of treatment staff; continuity of care; outcomes of care; and billing procedures (Steiber & Krowinski, 1990). Domains of care that are unique to hospital settings also include nursing care; hospital environment (cleanliness and condition of rooms, quality of food, etc.); admissions process; discharge process; and information provided (Meterko & Rubin, 1990; Eisen *et al.*, 2002).

Although many widely used patient satisfaction questionnaires include multiple domains, correlations among the domains tend to be high, raising questions about their differentiability (Marshall *et al.*, 1993). Despite high correlations, there may be value in assessing different domains depending on the purposes of particular satisfaction assessment efforts. For example, although correlations among domains may be high, average ratings may vary considerably among domains, thus providing important information about specific aspects of care that may need improvement.

Quantitative patient satisfaction surveys are popular because results can be easily summarized and reported. However, they have been criticized for a number of reasons. One problem is that results tend to be positively skewed, that is, respondents tend to report high levels of satisfaction with care, resulting in poor discrimination among domains of care, inadequate information for targeting quality improvement efforts and insensitivity to detection of areas of dissatisfaction (Campbell & Einspahr, 2001; Steiber & Krowinski, 1990). Positively skewed results are particularly problematic when a small number of response options are offered that are evenly distributed across the spectrum of satisfaction (e.g. 'very dissatisfied', 'somewhat dissatisfied', 'mixed, somewhat satisfied' and 'very satisfied'). This problem can be addressed in a number of ways. One is to include more response options representing the satisfied end of the spectrum. For example, an alternative to response options ranging from very dissatisfied to very satisfied, might be 'not at all satisfied', 'somewhat satisfied', 'moderately satisfied', 'very satisfied', 'extremely satisfied'. These options are more likely to spread out favorable opinions over a wider range and provide better discrimination. Ware and Hays (1988) found that 'excellent … poor' response options also resulted in greater variance and less skewness. Harris-Kojetin *et al.* (1999) suggest multiple benefits of a 0…10 rating scale in which 0 is the worst possible care and 10 is the best possible care. This rating scale produces greater distribution of responses and increased ability to distinguish among programmes or providers. In addition, the numerical rating scale is easier to translate into foreign languages and can more easily be administered by telephone than rating scales with adjectival descriptors.

Other concerns about quantitative surveys are that they do not adequately reflect consumers' concerns or priorities and that their results contradict information obtained using qualitative methods such as focus groups, open-ended questions, interviews, patient narratives and content analysis of relevant material (Campbell & Einspahr, 2001; Edgman-Levitan & Cleary, 1996; Eisen & Grob, 1982). When qualitative questions supplement quantitative items, the likelihood of identifying important areas of dissatisfaction increases. This point is illustrated by data from a hospital's ongoing assessment of patient perceptions of care which includes 18 forced-choice questions and one open-ended question asking respondents if 'there is anything else you would like to tell us about your care'. The forced-choice questions focus on communication and information received from the provider; interpersonal aspects of care; continuity and coordination of care; and global evaluation of care, with scores that can range from 0 to 100. For each of the four domains scores ranged from 77.8 to 83.0, suggesting high levels of satisfaction. However, in response to the open-ended question many respondents identified areas of dissatisfaction. Open-ended responses were coded as to subject (staff, aspects of treatment and other) and favourability (favourable or unfavourable). Regarding staff, three times as many patients reported favourable comments as unfavourable comments. However, regarding treatment, 57% of patients reported favourable comments compared with 43% of patients reporting unfavourable comments. Regarding 'other' aspects of care, favourable and unfavourable comments were almost evenly divided (51% favourable and 49% unfavourable (Eisen *et al.*, 2001). In addition, many unfavourable comments provided specific information regarding aspects of treatment or services; for example, 'There should be skills-building groups added; more groups would be beneficial'. Favourable comments tended to be more general; for example, 'It's a good hospital'. 'Thank you'. 'Staff were very helpful and caring'.

Assessment challenges

A wide range of methodological decisions must be made in the course of selecting or developing instruments, implementing surveys, analyzing data and reporting patient satisfaction results. A number of these issues are discussed below.

Standardized vs. customized instruments

A basic question to consider is whether to use an existing standardized instrument or to create a new one. Many programmes are tempted to create their own customized instruments that will capture unique features of their programme. However, customized instruments have two major limitations: their reliability and validity would need to be assessed, and they do not permit comparison with other providers, programmes or system of care. In this era of accountability, with increasing emphasis on comparison with other programmes, an instrument that is widely used across a range of programmes can be extremely valuable. Consequently, it is increasingly difficult to justify creation of customized instruments. Dozens of patient satisfaction and/or perceptions of care instruments exist. A thorough review of existing instruments should be undertaken before a decision is made to create a new one. If a programme does have unique features it may be appropriate to use both a standardized instrument with supplemental questions developed for specific programmes.

In developing a new survey or supplemental items the surveyor must select questions and response options that best meet the needs of the commissioning organization are appropriate for the target population. Principles of question and survey design including reading level, survey layout, use of screening questions to determine whether questions are applicable and methods of minimizing response bias should also be considered (Fowler, 1995).

Reports vs. ratings

Ware *et al.* (1983) distinguish between reports and ratings of care. Reports ask factual questions such as, 'Were you given information about the benefits and risks of medication you received?'. Reports may also ask for the frequency with which particular events occurred. For example, 'How often did you have to wait more than 15 minutes past your appointment time?' Response options might include 'never', 'sometimes', 'usually', or 'always'. Ratings ask respondents to evaluate an aspect of care. For example, 'How would you rate the amount of information you received about your medications?'. Response options might include 'poor', 'fair', 'good', 'very good', 'excellent'. Alternatively, one might ask 'How satisfied were you with the amount of information you received about your medications?' ('very dissatisfied', 'somewhat dissatisfied', 'mixed', 'somewhat satisfied', 'very satisfied'). Harris-Kojetin *et al.* (1999) suggest that details about healthcare received (e.g. communication with providers, waiting times, etc.) are better captured using report formats, whereas ratings are more effective in summarizing overall experiences.

Mode of administration

Several modes of survey administration are commonly used including self-administered questionnaires, telephone or personal interviews. More recently, computer-administered and Internet surveys have come into use. Both mode of administration and even setting (home vs. clinic) have been found to affect both response rates and survey results (Fowler *et al.*, 1999). By using a consistent mode of survey administration any effect of mode of administration will apply equally across patients or programmes. If mode of survey administration varies, it would be wise to document mode of administration and control for it in the analysis of results.

Sampling

Sampling is of major importance in assessing patient satisfaction because response rates can vary widely and bias results. Low response rates are unlikely to be representative of the population. Many survey efforts, particularly those done at the point of service, may not be able to compute response rates because the number of eligible respondents is not systematically tracked. Telephone surveys will not reach potential respondents who do not have telephones or stable living arrangements, problems that are more likely to occur among populations who are at greatest risk for poor quality care. Consequently, every effort should be made to obtain representative samples and to maximize response rates.

Risk adjustment

Any attempt to compare patient satisfaction across providers, programmes or healthcare systems should not be undertaken without appropriate risk adjustment. Risk adjustment is a statistical method of adjusting for differences in patient, provider and programme characteristics to allow for more appropriate comparisons of quality and outcome, so that one is not comparing apples with oranges. 'The goal of risk-adjustment is to account for pertinent patient characteristics before making inferences about the effectiveness or quality of care ...' (Iezzoni, 1997, pp. 3–4) Variables commonly used for risk adjustment include age, gender, socioeconomic status, diagnosis and comorbidity, although any data that correlate with the outcome of interest is appropriate to include in a risk adjustment model. Failure to risk adjust for patient characteristics can lead to misleading, embarrassing and even libellous conclusions. For example, the first public release of hospital mortality data by the US Healthcare Financing Administration compared actual mortality with expected mortality based on mortality rates from several hundred US hospitals. At the hospital with the most aberrant death rate, 86.7% of Medicare patients died, much higher than the expected death rate for that hospital (22.5%). However, the model did not account for the fact that the facility in question was a hospice, caring for terminally ill patients.

With regard to patient satisfaction, Medicare beneficiaries with psychiatric disorders have been found to report lower levels of satisfaction with both overall quality of care and with specific aspects of care including health information received, follow-up care and physicians' concern for their health, compared with Medicare beneficiaries without psychiatric disorders (Hermann *et al.*, 1998). Consequently, it would be important to control for presence of psychiatric illness in comparing patient satisfaction across providers or programmes.

Clinical and policy implications

To the extent that patient satisfaction assessment efforts are reliable, valid and appropriately used, their results hold promise for improving particularly, interpersonal aspects of healthcare quality. After much concern about increasing impersonalization in the current healthcare system and pressure on providers to see more patients in less time, efforts to assess patient satisfaction should, at least, serve to raise the consciousness of healthcare providers, administrators and health plan organizations about the importance of attending to patients' needs, listening to their concerns and treating them with respect and dignity. At best, efforts to assess patient perceptions of care may help to change providers' behaviour regarding appropriate treatment of patients, their involvement in treatment decisions and attention to patient preferences and concerns. Increasing emphasis on patients' rights may also be incorporated into the training of new healthcare providers.

Patient satisfaction assessment efforts have also begun to influence policy. More than 35 health plans in the United States, covering more than 30 million patients, have programmes tying doctor bonuses to performance. These 'pay for performance' programmes are likely to further increase providers' interest in meeting patients' needs in ways that will enhance satisfaction with care. Although most of these bonuses are offered for adhering to practice guidelines for preventive care and chronic conditions, extra points can be earned for high levels of patient satisfaction (Landro, 2004). The challenge to the field will be to ensure that patient satisfaction data are appropriately collected, reported and used to improve care. (See also 'Patient satisfaction references').

REFERENCES

Attkisson, C. C. & Greenfield, T. K. (1994). The client satisfaction questionnaire-8 and the service satisfaction questionnaire-30. In M. E. Maruish (Ed.). *The use of psychological testing for treatment planning and outcome assessment*. Hillsdale, NJ: Lawrence Erlbaum Associates.

Campbell, J. & Einspahr, K. (2001). Building partnerships in accountability. Consumer satisfaction. In B. Dickey & L. I. Sederer (Eds.). *Improving mental health care. Commitment to quality*. Washington, DC: American Psychiatric Publishing, Inc.

Center for Mental Health Services (1996). The MHSIP consumer-oriented mental health report card. *The final report of the mental health statistics improvement program (MHSIP) task force on a consumer-oriented mental health report card*. Washington, DC.

Cleary, P. D. & McNeil, B. J. (1988). Patient satisfaction as an indicator of quality care. *Inquiry*, **23**, 25–36.

Crofton, C., Lubalin, J. S. & Darby, C. (1999). Foreword. Consumer assessments of health plans study. (CAHPS™). *Medical Care*, **37**(33) Suppl., MS1–MS9.

Cousins, N. (1985). How patients appraise physicians. *New England Journal of Medicine*, **313**, 1422–4.

Davies, A. R. & Ware, J. E. (1988). Involving consumers in quality of care assessment. *Health Affairs*, **7**, 33–48.

Donabedian, A. (1980). *Explorations in quality assessment and monitoring: the definition of quality and approaches to its assessment*. Ann Arbor, Michigan: Health Administration Press.

Edgman-Levitan, S. & Cleary, P. D. (1996). What information do consumers want and need? *Health Affairs*, **15**, 42–56.

Eisen, S. V. & Grob, M. C. (1982). Measuring discharged patients' satisfaction with hospital care at a private psychiatric hospital. *Hospital and Community Psychiatry*, **33**, 227–8.

Eisen, S. V., Idiculla, T., Speredelozzi, A., Gebre-Medhin, P. & Egan, A. (2001). *Quality Indicators Report. McLean Hospital*. (Unpublished). Belmont, MA.

Eisen, S. V., Wilcox, M. A., Idiculla, T., Speredelozzi, A. & Dickey, B. (2002). Assessing consumer perceptions of inpatient psychiatric treatment: the perceptions of care survey. *The Joint Commission Journal on Quality Improvement*, **28**(9), 511–26.

Fowler, F. J. (1995). *Improving survey questions. Design and evaluation. Applied social research methods series. Vol. 38*. Thousand Oaks, CA: Sage Publications.

Fowler, F. J., Gallagher, P. M. & Nederend, S. (1999). Comparing telephone and mail responses to the CAHPS™ survey instrument. *Medical Care*, **37**(3) Suppl., MS41–MS49.

Harris-Kojetin, L. D., Fowler, F. J., Brown, J. A. Schnaier, J. A. & Sweeny, S. F. (1999) The use of cognitive testing to develop and evaluate CAHPS™; 1.0 core survey items. *Medical Care*, **37**(3) Suppl., MS10–MS21.

Hermann, R. C., Ettner, S. L. & Dorwart, R. A. (1998). The influence of psychiatric disorders on patients' ratings of satisfaction with health care. *Medical Care*, **36**, 720–7. http://www.ncqa.org/about/timeline.htm.

Iezzoni, L. I. (Ed.). (1997). *Risk adjustment for measuring healthcare outcomes* (2nd edn.). Chicago: Health Administration Press.

Joint Commission on Accreditation of Healthcare Organizations (1997). *Oryx outcomes: the next evolution in accreditation*. Oakbrook Terrace, IL: JCAHO.

Kaufmann, C. & Phillips, D. (2000). *Survey of state consumer surveys* (pp. 1–24). Rockville, MD: Substance Abuse and Mental Health Services Administration, US Department of Health & Human Services.

Landro, L. (September 17, 2004). Booster shot. To get doctors to do better, health plans try cash bonuses. *The Wall Street Journal*. New York.

Lee, K. & McGreevey, C. (2002a). Using control charts to assess performance measurement data. *The Joint Commission Journal on Quality Improvement*, **28**, 90–101.

Lee, K & McGreevey, C. (2002b). Using comparison charts to assess performance measurement data. *The Joint Commission Journal on Quality Improvement*, **28**, 129–38.

Marquis, M. S., Davies, A. R. & Ware, J. E. (1983). Patient satisfaction and change in medical care providers: a longitudinal study. *Medical Care*, **21**, 821–9.

Marshall, G. N., Hays, R. D., Sherbourne, C. D. & Wells, K. B. (1993). The structure of patient satisfaction with outpatient medical care. *Psychological Assessment*, **5**, 477–83.

Meterko, M. & Rubin, H. R. (1990). Patient judgments of hospital quality A taxonomy. *Medical Care*, **28**, S10–S14.

Pascoe, J. M. (1983). Patient satisfaction in primary health care. *Evaluation and Program Planning*, **6**, 185–210.

Ruggeri, M., Lasalvia, A., Dall'Agnola, R. et al. (2000). Development, internal consistency and reliability of the Verona Service Satisfaction Scale – European Version. EPSILON Study 7. European psychiatric services: inputs Linked to outcome domains and needs. *British Journal of Psychiatry*, **39**, (Suppl.) S41–8.

Steiber, S. R. & Krowinski, W. J. (1990). *Measuring and managing patient satisfaction*. Chicago, USA: American Hospital Association Company.

Valentine, N. B., De Silva, A., Kawabata, K. et al. (2003). Health system responsiveness: consepts, domains and operationalization. In C. J. L. Murrary & D. B. Evans (Eds.). *Health systems performance assessment: debates, methods and empiricism.*

(pp. 573–96). Geneva: World Health Organization.

Ware, J. E. & Hays, R. D. (1988). Methods for measuring patient satisfaction with specific medical encounters. *Medical Care*, **26**, 393–402.

Ware, J. E., Snyder, M. K., Wright, W. R. & Davies, A. R. (1983). Defining and measuring patient satisfaction with medical care. *Evaluation and Program Planning*, **6**, 247–63.

Psychoneuroimmunology assessments

Andrew Baum[1] and Angela Liegey Dougall[2]

[1]University of Pittsburgh Medical Center
[2]University of Pittsburgh

Overview

The immune system is a complex system of cells, organs and secretory agents that plays a key role in defence against pathogens, healing and communication with a large number of other systems in the body. It contains a large number of different cells, each with different functions, advantages and limitations, most of which secrete a dizzying variety of substances or cytokines that permit intercellular communication and which enhance or effect the cells' function. There are components of immunity that are primarily responsible for defence against pathogens, altered cells, or other foreign agents and there are components of the system that regulate inflammation and healing of wounds. Communication with nervous and metabolic systems is accomplished by other substances and structures. Many of these processes require coordinated collaboration among cells and substances and nearly all appear to be sensitive to internal rhythms and external events. In the rapidly growing field of psychoneuroimmunology (PNI), this complexity has added to the challenge of studying behaviour or central nervous system (CNS) interactions with the immune system (see also 'Psychoneuroimmunology').

In the face of the rapid growth of molecular biology and bioassay capabilities, PNI investigators now have access to a number of methods and measures that capture this complexity. In this chapter, we will review some of these newer approaches as well as some more traditional, widely used measures. Emphasis will be on what each measure tells us, how feasible and reliable it is and when it is appropriate.

Although there are many different emphases in the field of PNI, a great deal of research has focused on the effects of stress

and emotion on immunity. This work has generally found effects of stress on some measures, accomplished either through stress-related behaviour change (e.g. changes in diet, smoking, exercise) or by virtue of physiological changes tied to stress (e.g. changes in stress hormones, blood flow). Measures that have evolved have been aimed at aspects of the immune system that affect disease susceptibility or general 'immunocompetence'. Other measures have been used in conditioning studies, investigation of interactions with other bodily systems and studies of other phenomena use these and other measures.

Assays of cell numbers

As noted, the immune system includes a large number of cells specialized for the performance of particular functions in detecting foreign substances or altered cells or eliminating them. Measures of the number of each of these different cells can be accomplished by doing simple complete blood counts (CBCs, also known as whole blood counts, or WBCs) which provide an estimate of how many of each of a small number of immune cell types are present in a defined volume of blood. These ordinarily include numbers of lymphocytes and several other types, including eosonophils, neutrophils and monocytes. These measures are gross estimates of very general categories of cells and only reflect the number of cells in peripheral blood flow. These limit the value of these measures, but they are used extensively as rough clinical screens and are often needed to interpret more sophisticated measures of cells and cell subtypes.

Table 1. Measurable cells or functions of the immune system

Immune index	Measure
Cell number	Complete blood count with differential
	Lymphocyte subsets (e.g.)
	T-cells
	CD4$^+$ T-cells
	CD8$^+$ T-cells
	NK cells
	B-cells
Cell activity/function	Mitogen-stimulated proliferation
	Cell lysis (e.g. NK chromium release measure)
	Stimulated release of cytokines (e.g.)
	Interleukin-1
	Interleukin-2
	Interleukin-5
	Interleukin-6
	Interleukin-12
	Interferon
	Tumour Necrosis Factor
	Seroconversion/antibody response
Intrinsic function	Chemotactic response
	Adherence
	Phagocytosis
	Release of reactive oxygen species
	Delayed-type hypersensitivity

More fine-grained analysis can be accomplished by flow cytometry and cell sorting. These include measures of T- and B-cell subtypes and natural killer (NK) cell numbers (see Table 1). These technologies use monoclonal antibodies to tag cell surface receptors and these tags are then detected and measured.

In general, flow cytometry provides information about numbers of cells carrying specific proteins on their surfaces that identify them as one or another type of cell. This is done by culturing monoclonal antibodies for a particular protein marker with peripheral blood samples (Ruiz-Argüelles & Pérez-Romano, 2000). These antibodies are previously labelled with a fluorescent dye and bind to cells bearing the appropriate cell-surface proteins, 'tagging' them with the dye. Mononuclear cells from the peripheral blood are sent through a cell sorter that emits a laser which activates the dye and allows the cell to be identified. The detection systems associated with flow cytometry can measure the size and granularity of the cells as well as different intensities of fluorescence allowing evaluation of numbers of each of several subsets of lymphocytes (Table 1), measuring other proteins on cell membranes, detection of activation and amount of intracellular cytokines.

Assessment of cell numbers or of activated cells, cytokines and the like can be useful measures for PNI research, but must be interpreted cautiously. Stress and other psychosocial variables have been associated with changes in numbers of particular cells and other quantitative indices and differential changes may help to explain differences in antecedent conditions. For example, acute laboratory stressors produce increases in some cells (T, NK) but more chronic, naturalistic stressors produce decreases in these same cells in circulation. Although these changes are probably due to cell migration in and out of lymphoid storage areas (e.g. spleen), we typically do not know the specific causes or clinical impacts of these changes in numbers of cells in peripheral blood.

Cell activity and lytic capcity

In part due to these limitations on interpreting measures of cell numbers, researchers have also devised measures of cell or other structural function. These measures evaluate the capacity of cells, for example, to 'conduct their business', be it cell replication and proliferation, killing, or releasing/evoking release of cytokines and other important components of immunity.

There are several ways to organize the cells of the immune system. One of the most traditional is to separate the overall activity of the system into 'innate' and 'acquired' immunity. Innate immunity refers to elements of the immune system that are not specific to a particular pathogen. They are not antigen-dependent and mount maximal responses immediately upon activation. Because they are not antigen-specific there is no acquisition of memory; each encounter with a particular antigen occurs *de novo*. Barrier structures such as the skin or mucosa and cells such as macrophages, neutrophils, dendritic cells and natural killer (NK) cells are considered key elements of innate immunity.

Acquired immunity reflects more advanced forms of immune response, present only in vertebrate species. It includes immune responses and cells that are antigen-dependent and -specific (specific cells are only active against a particular antigen). Immunologic memory that underlies these characteristics and the strength of immune responses lags behind exposures. After an initial exposure, subsequent contact with an antigen evokes an adaptive response that strengthens over time.

There are two 'branches' of acquired immunity. The first consists of humoral responses that are focused on activity of B lymphocytes and antibodies which are produced by these cells. B cells are plentiful and continuously produced in the bone marrow. They are chiefly responsible for producing antibodies, immunoglobulins, that act to assist in killing or inactivating antigen. There are several classes of antibody corresponding to the type of immunoglobulin (Ig) involved. IgG is the most plentiful, composing nearly three-quarters of all antibodies produced in the body. IgG activates complement and NK cells and osporizes antigen, coating it to decrease its activity and attract other immune agents (e.g. phagocytes). IgM is less common and shares these functions. IgA is often found in the digestive tract (e.g. in saliva, stomach secretions) and respiratory system and is effective in helping disable antigens for removal by mucosa. IgE is important in allergic responses, shock and in disabling parasites. Antibodies also bind viruses and deactivate them.

Cell-mediated immunity is the second type of acquired immunity, focused primarily on activity by T lymphocytes. There are two main types of T cells; T helper and cytotoxic T cells. Helper cells (CD4 cells) coordinate immune responses by producing cytokines that direct larger responses. Cytotoxic T cells attack and lyse virally infected cells and other pathogens. They are directly involved in killing of pathogens.

Each of these branches of immunity have unique functions and investigators have devised a number of reliable methods of assessing the functions and killing activity accomplished by cells under varying circumstances. Some of these methods are described below.

Proliferation

One general indicator of immune system reactivity is the proliferative response of human peripheral blood mononuclear cells (PBMC) to antigen-nonspecific reagents or mitogens. Proliferation measures estimate the response by selected immune cells when stimulated to proliferate, that is to rapidly make a large number of replicates of specific cell types. The change in number of cells before and after culture with a mitogen is approximated by estimating the incorporation of [^{3}H]thymidine into the DNA of the replicating cells (James, 1994). When T- and B-cells are activated by the mitogen, they begin to replicate. During the replication process [^{3}H]thymidine is incorporated into the dividing cell's DNA. The radiation emitted from the incorporated [^{3}H]thymidine is then measured to estimate changes in cell number. The mitogen chosen determines what type of cells are stimulated. Three commonly used mitogens are phytohemagglutinin (PHA), Concanavalin A (Con A) that primarily stimulate T-cells and pokeweed mitogen which stimulates T-cell dependent activation of B-cells.

The greater the proliferative response, the 'better' the function of these cells, at least to a point and such estimates have consistently been used as an index of immunocompetence in PNI research. However, stimulated proliferation is only one way to measure cell function and it is not clear how well this index models overall efficacy of the system. Other measures model different aspects of immune system function, assessing the ability to kill infected or altered cells, phagocytize foreign material, or release cytokines.

Natural killer cell activity

A good example of one of these measures is a chromium-release assay of NK cell activity (Whiteside, 1996). NK cells are large granulocytes that attack tumours and bacteria, virally-infected cells and parasites by lysing them (drilling small holes in the membrane of the target) and injecting enzymes that kill the target. These cells are able to kill pathogens without prior experience with them. If one can isolate a known number of NK cells, culture them with cells that NK cells will attack and measure the rate at which these target cells are killed, the result would be a good estimate of NK cell activity. This is exactly what the chromium-release-assay for NK cell activity does. After tagging tumour cells with radioactive chromium which is released when the cell is lysed, they are cultured with live NK cells that attack and kill a substantial number of target cells. The amount of radioactivity released in the process can be measured and used as an estimate of lytic activity by the NK cells. Resulting measures of lysis can be combined with counts of the number of NK cells available and yield lytic units, which are reliable estimates of NK cell activity.

Cytokines

Cytokines are endocrine-like substances which are produced by various cells of the immune system (Leonard, 2003; Moldawer, 2003). These chemical compounds act as messengers and also stimulate cells to act or produce components of an immune response. They interact with immune cells, with the nervous system and with endocrines to enhance or regulate immune activity or facilitate organism activity that is restorative and facilitates healing. For example, interleukin-1 (IL-1) is produced by monocytes and stimulates body temperature to increase. It also induces 'illness behaviour' and contributes to inflammatory responses. Interleukin-2 (IL-2) is produced by T-cells and is integral in the Type 1 Helper T-cell response. It stimulates recruitment, activation and differentiation of B cells and supports local inflammation via activation of monocytes and macrophages. The Type 2 helper T-cell response is stimulated by cytokines such as IL-5 and IL-6 and assists in the activation, proliferation and differentiation of B-cells. Other interleukins (e.g. IL-6, IL-12) contribute to inflammatory responses, as does tumor necrosis factor (TNF) which is released by all cells except erthrocytes and mediates the sepsis response and cell death as well as the development of lymphoid organs. Interferon is released by almost all cells and acts on T- and NK cells to promote antiviral and antitumour responses.

A widely used assay technique, called enzyme-linked immunosorbent assay (ELISA) has become the most common and preferred method for quantifying antibodies, antigens, cytokines, or other immunologic agents. Commercially available kits with well validated procedures and standards are a strength for many measurable entities and the relative ease and safety level are also reasons for the current popularity of this method. Newer developments such as technology designed to yield estimates of panels of interrelated cytokines are more useful in some contexts but when the objective is to measure one or a few cytokines, antibodies, or antigens, ELISA remains an excellent option.

An ELISA is conducted using standard 96-well plates, but for these assays the plates are pretreated with antibody for the substance being measured. If one is interested, for example, in IL-1 the wells will have been pretreated with antibody for IL-1. serum or plasma from participants are added to the wells and incubated, allowing the target cytokine (IL-1) to bind to the antibody in the wells. The plate is then washed and a second antibody to IL-1 is added, this one linked to an enzyme. The amount of this enzyme-linked antibody that binds depends on the amount of IL-1 in the sample. Once this has been accomplished, a substrate that reacts with the enzyme is added and the intensity of the subsequent chromatic reaction is a measure of the amount of enzyme (and IL-1) that was bound. Determination of the amounts of cytokine is made by comparing the sample with standards that have known quantities of cytokine. A listing of basic ELISA protocols can be found at http://www.protocol-online.org/prot/Immunology/ELISA/index.html.

The ELISA can be used to measure the amount of cytokine in the peripheral blood, the amount produced by activated cells (e.g. cells stimulated by mitogens or mixed antigens) and/or quantities of other messengers released by cells trying to communicate with the immune system (e.g. leptin, adipocytes). Differences in study design and purpose will dictate which, if any, of these measures should be used, but once the decision is made, the only major differences in measurement are the kit target and the sample used (i.e. peripheral blood or supernatant from stimulating peripheral blood cells).

B cell activity

Similar ELISA methods can be used to assess antibody production by activated B-cells. Antibodies can be measured from bodily fluids such as blood and saliva. One common method in PNI is to assay levels of antibody titers in human blood to common viruses that people have likely been exposed to in the past, for example, *herpes simplex* virus (HSV), Epstein–Barr virus (EBV) and cytomegalovirus (CMV) (Ironson *et al.*, 2002; Jenkins & Baum, 1995). Most adults have been exposed and infected with these viruses even if they never displayed illness symptoms. After infection, the cellular immune system acts to contain the virus and keep it in latency. Therefore, some levels of antibody titer are present in most adults. However, if the immune system is compromised by factors such as medication, disease, or chronic stress, it can lose control over the virus and the virus will reactivate. Reactivation of a latent virus prompts a T-cell mediated immune response and production of more antibody titers. In studies assessing naturalistic chronic stressors, such as exam stress, marital discord and exposure to natural and man-made disasters, antibody titers in the blood are assessed as a marker of the overall integrity of cellular and humoral immunity. High levels of latent virus antibody titers suggest immunosuppression.

Another approach in PNI research is to use ELISA to assess the body's ability to mount an antibody response to a novel antigen. An in vivo immunization paradigm is used to assess change in antibody titers following inoculation with antigens such as hepatitis B, influenza, keyhole limpet hemocyanin (KLH) and attenuated rubella virus (Cohen *et al.*, 2001). In addition to the first or primary response, antibody production following a subsequent or secondary challenge can also be measured. Seroconversion, or the detection of antigen-specific antibodies in the serum, is usually used as a marker of primary response. Delays in seroconversion or failure to seroconvert are thought to indicate immunosuppression. Likewise, attenuation of antibody production in response to a secondary challenge indicates immunosuppression.

Assays of intrinsic function

Phagocytosis

Cells in the innate immune system also help provide a first-line defence against microbes, tumour cells and cellular debris by ingesting (phagocytosis) and then digesting pathogens. Phagocytic cells, primarily monocytes, macrophages, neutrophils and dendritic cells engulf and destroy pathogens such as bacteria by attaching membrane projections to the pathogen, surrounding the antigen with cytoplasm and ingesting it. Eventually enzymes are released from lysosomes in the phagocytic cell, destroying the antigen. This process is called phagocytosis and can be quantified by culturing phagocytic cells (e.g. macrophages or neutrophils) with appropriate target cells (e.g. bacteria or tumour cells) and then measuring incorporation. Phagocytic activity of macrophages is quantified by staining the bacterial target cells, culturing the bacteria with the macrophages and then counting the number of internalized bacteria in each macrophage using a fluorescence microscope (Campbell *et al.*, 1994). Assays for phagocytic activity of neutrophils are similar, except the target cells are radiolabelled with ^{14}C and counted with a liquid scintillation counter to determine the percentage of phagocytosis (Clark & Nauseef, 1996). The ability of macrophages

and neutrophils to digest or kill the target cells can be assessed by lysing the macrophages and neutrophils after phagocytosis. The remaining live bacteria are cultured and then counted to determine bactericidal activity.

Phagocytic activity can be augmented by the presence of stimulating cytokines. Macrophages can be stimulated by cytokines such as interferon gamma released from antigen-stimulated T-cells (see 'Delayed type hypersensitivity'). Macrophages, in turn, release cytokines that stimulate other immune cells such as T-cells, neutrophils and other mononuclear phagocytes. Activated macrophages release inflammatory cytokines (e.g. IL-6) and other substances that attract other cells (chemotaxis) and can serve antigen-presenting processes important in seroconversion.

Release of reactive oxygen species

During phagocytosis, macrophages and neutrophils release reactive oxygen species (ROS) such as superoxide anion (O_2^-), inorganic nitrite (NO_2^-) and hydrogen peroxide (H_2O_2) that produce cell damage and have potent antimicrobial and antitumour effects themselves. ROS are produced by other cells as well and this reflects normal function of the system. Changes in ROS that produce the potential for cell damage and mutation is referred to as oxidative stress and can be measured in several different ways (Epel *et al.*, 2004; Irie *et al.*, 2001).

Delayed-type hypersensitivity

Delayed-type hypersensitivity (DTH) is an in vivo assay of cell-mediated immunity, in which T-cells recognize an antigen, proliferate and secrete cytokines that then induce inflammation and activate macrophages that act to eliminate or resolve the foreign antigen (Abbas & Lichtman, 2005). In the classic animal model, a guinea pig or other animal is immunized with a specific antigen by injecting the antigen subcutaneously (Luo & Dorf, 1993). After 6 to 14 days of sensitization, the animal is then challenged with a new dose of the antigen and the inflammatory response is measured. The delayed-type peak inflammatory reaction occurs 24 to 48 hours after antigenic challenge. The intensity of DTH is quantified by using calipers to measure the swelling and induration (hardness) in the area of the skin at the site of injection. In humans, the challenge test of DTH is used to assess immune response to antigens to which people may have been previously exposed through infection or immunization, such as tuberculin, tetanus, diphtheria, streptococcus and *Candida albicans*.

The DTH response provides important information regarding the in vivo functioning of T cells and an overall assessment of immunocompetence. Failure to elicit a sufficient inflammatory response to a battery of common antigens suggests a defect in cellular immunity or a condition known as anergy. These individuals are more susceptible to viral, bacterial or fungal infections that are normally resisted by cell-mediated immunity. Intense DTH reactions indicate an enhanced or hypersensitive immune response that may reflect an underlying susceptibility to allergic or autoimmune disorders such as contact dermatitis and insulin-dependent diabetes mellitus.

Although DTH responses protect a host by eradicating invading micro-organisms, they also cause injury to normal host tissues. If a DTH response is elicited to a non-injurious agent only the destructive and not the protective functions occur (hypersensitivity), such as those seen in allergy and autoimmunity.

Conclusions

This discussion has been limited to immunologic measures that have been used in PNI studies, typically to assess the effects of stress or emotional expression on immunity. This is not an exhaustive review: it has focused on the most commonly used measures and a few newer assessments that have particular promise. The revolution in molecular biology during the past 25 years has revealed several previously unknown 'layers' of function and ways to assess them. This offers researchers the opportunity to answer questions that were previously not addressable due to measurement limitations. Together with biomarkers and other intermediate measures of pathogenesis, these developments will contribute greatly to successful mapping and prevention of immunologically-mediated diseases.

REFERENCES

Abbas, A. K. & Lichtman, A. H. (2005). *Cellular and Molecular Immunology* (5th edn.). Philadelphia, PA: W.B. Saunders Co.

Campbell, P. A., Canono, B. P. & Drevets, D. A. (1994). Measurement of bacterial ingestion and killing by macrophages. In J. E. Coligan, A. M. Kruisbeek, D. H. Margulies, E. M. Shevach & W. Strober (Eds.). *Current protocols in immunology*, (pp. 14.6.1–13). On-line. Avaiable at http://www.mrw.interscience.wiley.com/cp/cpim/articles/im1406/frame.html.

Clark, R. A. & Nauseef, W. M. (1996). Isolation and functional analysis of neutrophils. In J. E. Coligan, A. M. Kruisbeek, D. H. Margulies, E. M. Shevach & W. Strober (Eds.). *Current protocols in immunology*, (pp. 7.23.1–17). On-line. Avaiable at http://www.mrw.interscience.wiley.com/cp/cpim/articles/im0723/frame.html.

Cohen, S., Miller, G. E. & Rabin, B. S. (2001). Psychological stress and antibody response to immunization: a critical review of the human literature. *Psychosomatic Medicine*, **63**, 7–18.

Epel, E. S., Blackburn, E. H., Lin, J. *et al.* (2004). Accelerated telomere shortening in response to life stress. *Proceedings of the National Academy of Sciences*, **101**, 17312–15.

Irie, M., Asami, S., Nagata, S., Miyata, M. & Kasai, H. (2001). Relationships between perceived workload, stress and oxidative DNA damage. *International Archives of Occupational and Environmental Health*, **74**, 153–7.

Ironson, G., Balbin, E. & Schneiderman, N. (2002). Health psychology and infectious diseases. In T. J. Boll, S. B. Johnson, N. W., Perry Jr. & R. H. Rozensky (Eds.). *Handbook of clinical health psychology: Vol. 1. Medical disorders and behavioral applications.* (pp. 5–36). Washington, DC: American Psychological Association.

James, S. P. (1994). Measurement of proliferative responses of cultured lymphocytes. In J. E. Coligan, A. M. Kruisbeek, D. H. Margulies, E. M. Shevach & W. Strober (Eds.). *Current protocols in immunology* (pp. 7.10.1–10). On-line. Avaiable at http://www.mrw.interscience.wiley.com/cp/cpim/articles/im0710/frame.html.

Jenkins, F. J. & Baum, A. (1995). Stress and reactivation of latent herpes simplex virus: a fusion of behavioral medicine and molecular biology. *Annals of Behavioral Medicine*, **17**, 116–23.

Leonard, W. J. (2003). Type 1 cytokines and interferons and their receptors. In W. E. Paul (Ed.). *Fundamental immunology.* (pp. 701–47). Philadelphia: Lippincott, Williams & Wilkins.

Luo, Y. & Dorf, M. E. (1993). Delayed-type hypersensitivity. In J. E. Coligan, A. M. Kruisbeek, D. H. Margulies, E. M. Shevach & W. Strober (Eds.). *Current protocols in immunology* (pp. 4.5.1–5). On-line. Avaiable at http://www.mrw.interscience.wiley.com/cp/cpim/articles/im0405/frame.html.

Moldawer, L. L. (2003). The tumor necrosis factor superfamily and its receptors. In W. E. Paul (Ed.). *Fundamental immunology.* (pp. 749–73). Philadelphia: Lippincott, Williams & Wilkins.

Ruiz-Argüelles, A. & Pérez-Romano, B. (2000). Immunophenotypic analysis of peripheral blood lymphocytes. In J. P. Robinson, Z. Darzynkiewicz, P. N. Dean *et al.* (Eds.). *Current protocols in cytometry* (pp. 6.5.1–14). On-line. Available at http://www.mrw.interscience.wiley.com/cp/cpcy/articles/cy0605/frame.html.

Whiteside, T. L. (2000). Measurement of cytotoxic activity of NK/LAK cells. In J. E. Coligan, A. M. Kruisbeek, D. H. Margulies, E. M. Shevach & W. Strober (Eds.). *Current protocols in immunology* (pp. 7.18.1–13). On-line. Avaiable at http://www.mrw.interscience.wiley.com/cp/cpim/articles/im0718/frame.html.

Qualitative assessment

Felicity L. Bishop[1] and Lucy Yardley[2]

[1]Aldemoor Health Centre
[2]University of Southampton

Introduction

Qualitative assessment has long made a central contribution not only to psychological approaches to health and illness but also to traditional medical practice itself. In taking a case history a medical practitioner is engaged in a process of interviewing a patient to find out about their experiences. During this process the questioning is flexible and is influenced by the patient's previous answers. The practitioner must listen to and interpret what the patient tells them. The practitioner then uses their own explanatory framework to try to understand the patient's experience and determine an appropriate course of action. These processes of adaptable questioning and interpretation are central to qualitative assessment. In qualitative assessment, the researcher (or practitioner) begins with a question about experience or process, flexibly seeks out the information to answer that question and then uses interpretative skills to provide an explanation and understanding of the phenomena of interest. The development of explanations often highlights changes or interventions which can be implemented to enhance health care provision. Also central to traditional medicine is the use of the concept of cases, for example in everyday clinical practice and as exemplars in teaching. The study of cases in health psychology has been reinvigorated by Radley and Chamberlain (2001) and is well suited to qualitative, rather then quantitative, approaches to assessment.

A wide variety of qualitative methods has been applied to the study of health and illness. In comparison with quantitative methods, qualitative methods focus on providing in-depth analyses of individual perspectives and interpersonal processes. The value of qualitative methods lies in their ability to provide insights into the lived experience of healthcare. Qualitative methods are well suited to questions about patients' experiences of health and illness and the processes involved in health-related behaviours, including healthcare delivery. In an era of patient-centred care, qualitative techniques provide a means to assess patients' concerns and suggest ways in which care can become more patient-centred. Returning to the example of the consultation, qualitative methods can provide answers to such questions as: What do patients want from consultations?, What interpersonal processes are involved in consultations? Qualitative approaches can also improve understandings of the experiences and needs of health care professionals. For example, qualitative methods can answer questions such as: How do health care professionals cope with delivering bad news? How does the working environment constrain and/or facilitate the delivery of health care?

The aims, purposes and methods differ widely across different qualitative approaches. However, there are some typical characteristics of most (though not all) qualitative research.

1. An emphasis on the contextual nature of knowledge, and a view of knowledge as embedded in cultural systems of value and meaning. This means that whereas much quantitative work seeks to minimize the impact of extraneous variables on research, qualitative work embraces the way in which people are shaped by social and cultural situations, such as social networks (family, friends), upbringing, economic factors, the media and so on. Qualitative work acknowledges and often takes as its focus this view of individuals and their stories as contextually situated, seeking to explore this context and trying to generate understandings which do not abstract individuals from their everyday lives.

2. An emphasis on the ways in which people make sense of their experiences and their subjective meanings, rather than causal mechanisms. Because qualitative researchers are usually interested in the variety of different people's perspectives, qualitative work is not intended to establish generally applicable laws, but instead to provide an in-depth understanding of a particular situation that may have relevance to other, similar, situations.

3. An interplay between data and theory. Whereas quantitative assessment generally uses empirical data to test theory, in qualitative research data is often the inspiration for theoretical insights and developments.

4. Since the aim of much qualitative research is to understand the perspective of those who are the subject of research, a close, subjective relationship between researcher and participants is often desirable. It is therefore necessary to acknowledge and examine the influence of the researcher on the data and its interpretation.

Qualitative data

Qualitative data can include naturally occurring data and researcher-instigated data. For example, audio or videotape-recorded consultations, patients' medical records, one-on-one interviews and focus group discussions are all forms of qualitative data. Given that many qualitative approaches understand knowledge to be context dependent, naturalistic data is often highly valued, and where researcher-instigated data is used, the researcher's role in the generation of data is openly acknowledged and reflected on. Indeed, the contributions of a researcher, for example in an interview, may be analyzed as data alongside the contributions of the person being interviewed.

Qualitative interviewing

Interviewing is the most commonly used qualitative data collection technique, but is more involved than may seem at first glance (see Kvale, 1996). One-on-one interviews can provide detailed insights into individual experiences and perspectives. Most qualitative interviews are semi-structured, which means that 'open-ended' questionning is used which does not restrict participants to yes or no answers, or any other predetermined 'closed' set of responses. Some qualitative interviewers use a conversational style of interviewing, in which questions and comments from interviewees are responded to by the interviewer. While the questions asked will necessarily reflect the interests of the interviewer, questions should be worded in a neutral way to avoid leading the interviewee to frame their answer in a particular way. For example, questions such as 'how did you feel about your consultation' or 'tell me about your illness' allow participants to talk freely about whatever aspect of their experiences that they want to. While questions are devised before interviews commence, the interview content should be flexible: the order of questions can be changed and prompts can be used if necessary. Furthermore, the interviewer is able to take the lead from the interviewee and follow up issues of interest which emerge during individual interviews.

Wright *et al.* (2004) conducted an interview study to investigate patients' perceptions of doctors' communication in breast cancer. They interviewed women about the aspects of consultations they valued or disliked, using recordings of consultations as a starting point to guide the interview schedule. Using grounded theory techniques (see below), it was found that women valued the perception that doctors had formed an individual relationship with them, had relevant expertise and demonstrated respect for them as individual people. These findings highlight the need to take patients' views into account in developing training in communication skills, since the aspects of communication valued by the patients were not the same as those emphasized in current communication skills training.

Focus groups

Focus groups are group discussions around a specific topic which commonly involve between 4 and 15 participants (Morgan, 1992). Discussions are often led by the researcher, who acts as a 'moderator', to encourage involvement of all individuals and keep discussions on topic. Focus groups can provide information on the views and understandings of groups of people and it is the interaction between participants which distinguishes focus groups from group interviews (Wilkinson, 1998).

The public nature of focus groups must be considered when deciding whether and how to use them. Participants may be unwilling to 'stand out from the crowd' and voice minority opinions, thus the resulting data can demonstrate socially sanctioned normative perspectives. However, the inherently social nature of focus groups can provide valuable data which would not arise from questionnaires or one-to-one interviews. Focus groups can facilitate the discussion of sensitive issues in that where the participants have shared experiences and understandings they may be more likely

to discuss these issues with each other than alone in an interview with a researcher (Wilkinson, 1998). Participants' talk may be more natural in focus groups than in one-to-one interviews, and the interactions between participants can themselves be an interesting topic (Kitzinger, 1995).

Wilkinson and Kitzinger (2000) conducted focus groups with women with breast cancer. They used a relatively unstructured approach and the topic of the analysis, 'thinking positive', emerged as an important issue from women's general talk about their illness. Through their use of focus groups and discursive analytic techniques (see below) Wilkinson and Kitzinger were able to focus on the social functions of talk about positive thinking, and to examine the ways in which women themselves talk about positive thinking.

Participant observation

Participant observation, often known as 'ethnography', involves spending a prolonged period of time in a particular setting, such as a hospital ward, in order to provide insight into the social processes at work in that setting (Hammersley & Atkinson, 1995). Participant observation is a way to observe actual behaviour, rather than relying solely on verbal reports. By spending time in a setting the researcher can develop relationships and gain the trust of participants, thus developing understandings which are derived from the perspective of the participants themselves. Such observation can provide valuable insights into how things are achieved in real life settings and how changes could improve practice. Participant observation studies generally involve the collection of a wide range of data to supplement and complement observations. This can include informal and formal interviews with a range of participants as well as documentary or even photographic evidence.

An ethnographic study of doctor–patient communication about death was conducted by The *et al.* (2000). Observations of patients and medical staff both in and outside consultations were combined with interviews, medical notes and fieldwork diaries to provide an in-depth analysis of the processes involved in doctor–patient communication about death. The results showed that both doctors and patients colluded in a false optimism about recovery, drawing on a recovery story in which short-term possibilities are prioritized over the future. Doctors found it difficult to break bad news to patients, often mentioning the bad prognosis and then offering short-term hope through further (often palliative) treatments. Patients accepted this hope, focusing on offers of treatment and the action this entailed while not asking about or actively resisting information about long-term prognoses. The ethnographic approach enabled the researchers to develop trusting relationships with participants and to develop an in-depth analysis which incorporated both doctors and patients and the interactions between them.

Documentary evidence

Documents constitute relatively permanent records which have been created for specific purposes, and constitute a valuable resource for qualitative researchers (Prior, 2003). Documents such as medical records can be analyzed to provide insight into healthcare provision and the doctor–patient relationship. Other documents such as magazine and newspaper articles can be analyzed in terms of examining the social and cultural context of illness. Printed material is commonly used in healthcare and documents such as health promotion leaflets can be analyzed from a qualitative perspective to provide insight into the medical perspective, which can then be compared with patients' perspectives.

Lupton (1994) used discourse analysis (see below) to examine the representation of breast cancer in the Australian press. By examining articles in the public domain she was able to show that certain themes, or discourses, dominated the portrayal of breast cancer in the media. Of particular interest was the emphasis on individual responsibility which was central to many of the articles. Lupton argued that such a discourse could have a negative impact not only on women's beliefs but also on their behaviour. If breast cancer is seen as the individual's responsibility, then so is the responsibility for prevention and recovery – but in the context of breast cancer where there are no absolute right or wrong answers in relation to prevention or treatment, this puts an impossible burden on individual women to make the right lifestyle and treatment choices.

Major qualitative methods

Qualitative coding: thematic and content analyses

Coding is central to much qualitative assessment. At its most basic, coding involves the organisation of qualitative data into analytically meaningful categories. For example in a study of the experience of pain, all occurrences of talk about pain might be coded into categories such as 'talk about the causes of pain', 'the effects of pain' and 'treatments used to alleviate pain'. Coding can also be used to look at latent patterns in the data. For example, some talk about pain might be interpreted as representing talk about coping strategies, such as denial or avoidance.

Coding can be deductive, i.e. codes are established before the coding begins using categories from previous research or theory to code the new qualitative data. However, coding is often inductive, in that codes are developed from the qualitative data itself; rather than applying existing categories to the data the researcher identifies themes and patterns that emerge through analysis and may be new and unexpected. Whichever approach to coding is used, explicit detailed definitions of codes are essential.

Traditional approaches to coding involve making notes on interview transcripts or other texts, and using card index systems to record names, definitions and examples of codes. The advent of computer software designed specifically for qualitative data has somewhat eased the labour intensive management and analysis of large volumes of qualitative data (see Joffe & Yardley, 2003).

Content analysis represents a relatively quantitative approach to coding. In content analysis a qualitative data set is examined and instances of particular words, phrases or codes are counted. Statistical analyses can be carried out on the count measures that result from content analysis. Thematic analysis takes a more qualitative approach to coding. In thematic analysis either theoretically derived or inductive themes are coded in the dataset and the

meanings, context and implications of these themes are examined and described (Joffe & Yardley, 2003).

Grounded theory

Grounded theory was developed in the context of research on healthcare by Glaser and Strauss (1967). Since its inception, different versions of grounded theory have been developed (see Charmaz, 2000). Grounded theory is a complete and rigorous approach to qualitative research which provides an explicit, detailed methodological framework to guide researchers from an initial research topic through to a theory about that topic. The aim of grounded theory is to generate theory which is grounded in data. Data and theory are closely linked, and so are the processes of data collection and analysis (Charmaz, 1990).

Initial data collection is guided by 'purposive sampling', which involves gathering data from a wide range of sources relevant to the topic. Data for grounded theory studies can consist of any of the forms mentioned above, but often interviews constitute the primary source of data. A number of analytic procedures are employed in the coding of data and there is a general movement through coding from concrete, descriptive coding which stays close to the data to more abstract, analytical coding which moves towards theory and explanation. The technique of 'constant comparison' is a key feature of grounded theory, and refers to the process by which the analyst makes comparisons between examples of the same or different codes or between definitions of codes and examples of codes in the data. This technique helps to refine codes and to keep the emerging theory grounded in the data itself.

The generation of theory proceeds iteratively and initial analyses are used to guide further data collection. Inductive and deductive processes are used throughout this iterative process and as theories evolve and are refined data collection becomes driven by the theory (theoretical sampling), in an attempt to deepen and validate the emerging theory.

Yardley *et al.* (2001) developed a grounded theory model of treatment perceptions. They conducted initial interviews with chiropractic patients and analysed them inductively using techniques such as the constant comparative method, which resulted in the development of a model of the processes involved in patients' perceptions of treatment that was grounded in the analysis of interview texts but also integrated this analysis with existing literature. The emerging model was then tested by further, deductive, analysis of interviews with a sample drawn from a different treatment population (people consulting their GP for dizziness). The outcome of this study was an explication of patients' perceptions of treatment which highlighted the influence of processes occurring during treatment, in particular the relationship with the therapist and perceptions of the effects of the treatment on symptoms.

Phenomenological analysis

Phenomenological analysis is concerned with examining the subjective experiences and meanings of individuals. Non-directive in-depth interviews are an important source of data in phenomenology, although naturally occurring texts such as diaries can also be used. Interpretative Phenomenological Analysis is an example of a system of phenomenological research, in which the researcher attempts to gain an insider view point, engaging with and making sense of participants' own personal accounts and understandings (Smith, 1996). This approach requires the researcher to be open to participants' perspectives and to use their own interpretative skills to produce a co-construction (between researcher and participant) of participants' experiences. Interpretative Phenomenological Analysis is an idiographic approach in that the primary focus is on the experiences of individual participants, and it is only in the later stages of analysis that researchers look for patterns of themes across individuals.

Smith *et al.* (2002) used Interpretative Phenomenological Analysis to investigate perceptions of risk and decision-making about genetic testing in Huntington's disease. They showed that their interview participants (five women, all of whom had children), found it difficult to deal with the objective 50% risk of having the disease and that this risk was often reinterpreted and situated within considerations of the family context and the women's own beliefs about inheritance. The process of decision-making that women went through concerning whether or not to have genetic testing was removed from and in some cases inconsistent with the model of informed decision making favoured by current healthcare systems. By analyzing individual women's accounts and then making comparisons between and examining common themes across the different accounts the analysis provided insight into the complex issues which the participants were dealing with and suggested ways in which genetic testing and counselling might address patients' perspectives (see 'Screening: genetic').

Discourse analysis

Discourse analysis involves a focus on 'discourse', or language, as the way in which the social world is created and maintained. Discourse analysis is not a single unified method, but it is beyond the scope of this chapter to explore the range of forms of discourse analysis (see Willig, 2001). From a discursive perspective, psychological entities such as attitudes and beliefs have no existence beyond their expression, and in the expression of attitudes people are not reporting on an internal state but are engaged in a social act which achieves certain things (Wetherell *et al.*, 2001). Discourse analysts draw on a range of data sources, including naturally occurring dialogue, interviews, focus groups and documentary evidence. Spoken data, such as interviews, are transcribed in full, in other words features such as laughter, pauses, intakes of breath, loudness and emphasis are included in transcriptions. Analysis consists of examining texts for patterns of discourse, paying attention to the possible and actual effects of language both in the immediate context (e.g. the interview) and in the wider social context. Discourse analysis can provide valuable insights into how people talk about their experiences and the implications this has, and analysis can focus on levels ranging from one phrase to complete discourses.

Wilkinson and Kitzinger (2000) carried out a discourse analysis of cancer patients' talk, focusing on the phrase 'thinking positive'. Previous research had investigated positive thinking as a coping strategy related to adjustment to illness. By taking a discursive perspective Wilkinson and Kitzinger showed that rather than being a report of an internal cognitive state, the phrase thinking positive could be interpreted as a conversational idiom which, when used, demonstrates a speaker's awareness of the socially normative requirement of cancer patients to be optimistic and fight their cancer. Lupton (1994) demonstrated a similar theme in her analysis of media representations of breast cancer, showing how the media linked fighting spirit to cancer survival. Here discourse analysis was able to show how coping strategies are represented in the mass media, and the potential for such discourses to shape social requirements for women to adopt certain attitudes.

Evaluation

Well established criteria for judging the quality of quantitative research, such as statistical validity and reliability, are not appropriate for the evaluation of qualitative work and a number of authors have suggested alternative criteria (e.g. Mays & Pope, 2000; Yardley, 2000). The quality of qualitative assessment can be judged on the clarity, coherence and systematic nature of data collection and analysis. A number of specific individual criteria can also assist in evaluation.

1. Transparency refers to the ability of a reader to follow exactly what a researcher has done, both in the collection and analysis of their data. The provision of excerpts from interview transcripts and worked through examples of the process of analysis can help to create paper trails which enhance the transparency of qualitative work.

2. The role of the researcher in qualitative research is often acknowledged and it is important to know about any techniques used to examine, account for or minimize the impact of the researcher on the data collection and analysis. This enables readers to judge for themselves the influence of the researcher on the project.

3. Negative or deviant case analysis is a technique which involves searching a qualitative data set for instances that do not fit with emerging analytical or explanatory frameworks. This demonstrates rigour and openness to alternative explanations and can help to determine the limits of an analysis.

4. Triangulation involves the use of multiple sources of data or types of data, or multiple analytic strategies or analysts, in order to examine phenomena from a range of angles. Rather than being a technique to examine the reliability of findings, triangulation may be used to provide more complete understandings of phenomena.

5. Respondent validation can be appropriate for some forms of qualitative assessment, and involves feeding back the analysis to participants to check if the results of the analysis correspond to participants' own understandings. This can be particularly important for approaches which seek to explore participants' own subjective understandings and systems of meaning, but may be less appropriate for approaches such as discourse analysis where technical analyses are used which do not focus on participants' meanings.

6. It is important to be able to judge the transferability of qualitative findings, in other words the extent to which findings might hold true in other settings, contexts or population groups. Transparency in terms of the provision of adequate detail about settings and participants can facilitate this process.

Using qualitative and quantitative assessment

The techniques and studies discussed above demonstrate a range of applications of qualitative approaches as stand-alone systems of inquiry. However, qualitative techniques can also be successfully combined with quantitative techniques in mixed method approaches. Qualitative techniques are often used in the development of questionnaire measures, in order to ground questionnaires in participants' own language and understandings and to ensure the questionnaire covers the range of issues important to participants. Qualitative assessment can also be used to investigate in more depth findings from quantitative research. For example Williams *et al.* (1998) used a qualitative approach to explore possible reasons for high levels of patient satisfaction found in questionnaire studies. They showed that patients' evaluations of care were more complex than existing questionnaires suggested and that reports of high satisfaction often masked more negative evaluations.

Recently there has been interest in the integration of evidence from qualitative and quantitative studies. Thomas *et al.* (2004) provide an example of how qualitative research can be integrated with evidence from clinical trials and the value of such integrations: qualitative findings provide insight into patients' perspectives on interventions and can help to explain heterogeneous trial results, for example through examining the relationship between patients' outcome priorities identified in qualitative work and the measures of outcomes used in trials.

Conclusions

Qualitative assessment techniques are central to patient-centred healthcare. The inclusion of qualitative studies in the *British Medical Journal* in recent times demonstrates the recognition of the valuable insights that they can offer. Qualitative techniques provide a means to explore the subjective, personal, interpersonal and cultural aspects of health and illness. They can offer a sophisticated understanding of linguistic and social processes, as well as the variety of meanings of health and illness for different individuals. Furthermore, qualitative techniques provide a means to go beyond existing theory, to explore new areas and poorly understood phenomena and to incorporate patients' perspectives into the development of interventions and the delivery of healthcare.

REFERENCES

Charmaz, K. (2000). Grounded theory: objectivist and constructivist methods. In N.K. Denzin & Y.S. Lincoln (Eds.). *Handbook Of Qualitative Research* (2nd edn.) (pp. 509–35). Thousand Oaks, CA: Sage Publications.

Charmaz, K. (1990). 'Discovering' chronic illness: using grounded theory. *Social Science and Medicine*, **30**, 1161–72.

Glaser, B. & Strauss, A. (1967). *The discovery of grounded theory.* London: Weidenfeld and Nicolson.

Hammersley, M. & Atkinson, P. (1995). *Ethnography. Principles in practice* (2nd edn.) London: Routledge.

Joffe, H. & Yardley, L. (2003). Content and thematic analysis. In D. Marks & L. Yardley (Eds.). *Research methods in clinical and health psychology* (pp. 56–68). London: Sage Publications.

Kitzingers, J. (1995). Qualitative research: introducing focus groups. *British Medical Journal*, **311**, 299–302.

Kvale, S. (1996). Interviews. *An introduction to qualitative research interviewing.* Thousand Oaks, CA: Sage.

Lupton, D. (1994). Femininity, responsibility, and the technological imperative: discourses on breast cancer in the Australian press. *International Journal of Health Services*, **24**, 73–89.

Mays, N. & Pope, C. (2000). Assessing quality in qualitative research. *British Medical Journal*, **320**, 50–2.

Morgan, D.L. (1992). Designing focus group research. In M. Steward (Ed.). *Tools for primary care research*, *Vol.* 2 (pp. 177–93). Newbury Park, CA: Sage Publications.

Prior, L. (2003). *Using documents in social research.* London: Sage Publications.

Radley, A. & Chamberlain, K. (2001). Health psychology and the study of the case: from method to analytic concern. *Social Science and Medicine*, **53**, 321–32.

Smith, J.A. (1996). Beyond the divide between cognition and discourse: using interpretative phenomenological analysis in health psychology. *Psychology and Health*, **11**, 261–71.

Smith, J.A., Michie, S., Stephenson, M. & Quarrell, O. (2002). Risk perception and decision-making processes in candidates for genetic testing for Huntington's disease: an interpretative phenomenological analysis. *Journal of Health Psychology*, **7**, 131–44.

The, A., Hak, T., Koëter, G. & van der Wal, G. (2000). Collusion in doctor–patient communication about imminent death: an ethnographic study. *British Medical Journal*, **321**, 1376–81.

Thomas, J., Harden, A., Oakley, A. *et al.* (2004). Integrating qualitative research with trials in systematic reviews. *British Medical Journal*, **328**, 1010–12.

Wetherell, M., Taylor, S. & Yates, S. (2001). *Discourse theory and practice: a reader.* London: Sage.

Wilkinson, S. (1998). Focus groups in health research. Exploring the meanings of health and illness. *Journal of Health Psychology*, **3**, 329–48.

Wilkinson, S. & Kitzinger, C. (2000). Thinking differently about thinking positive: a discursive approach to cancer patients' talk. *Social Science and Medicine*, **50**, 797–811.

Williams, B., Coyle, J. & Healy, D. (1998). The meaning of patient satisfaction: an explanation of high reported levels. *Social Science and Medicine*, **47**, 1351–9.

Willig, C. (2001). *Introducing qualitative research in psychology.* Buckingham, UK: Open University Press.

Wright, E.B., Holcombe, C. & Salmon, P. (2004). Doctors' communication of trust, care, and respect in breast cancer: qualitative study. *British Medical Journal*, **328**, 864–8.

Yardley, L. (2000). Dilemmas in qualitative health research. *Psychology and Health*, **15**, 215–28.

Yardley, L., Sharples, K., Beech, S. & Lewith, G. (2001). Developing a dynamic model of treatment perceptions. *Journal of Health Psychology*, **6**, 269–82.

Quality of life assessment

Ann Bowling

University College London

Quality of life, and its sub-domain of health-related quality of life (the effects of health on quality of life), are increasingly popular concepts as endpoints in the evaluation of outcomes of health and social care. But the wider research community has accepted no common definition or definitive theoretical framework of quality of life or health-related quality of life. The wide range of definitions of these concepts was reviewed by Farquhar (1995), and the diverse contributions of sociology (functionalism) and psychology (subjective wellbeing) to the theoretical foundations of the concept of quality of life were described by Patrick and Erickson (1993) (See 'Quality of life').

Quality of life is a complex collection of interacting objective and subjective dimensions (Lawton, 1991). Like health, health-related quality of life (and broader quality of life), includes positive as well as negative aspects of wellbeing and life, it is multidimensional and is a dynamic concept: perspectives can change with the onset of major illness. Relevant cognitive or affective processes in individuals when faced with changing circumstances (e.g. in their health or lives) include making comparisons of one's situation with others who are better or worse off, cognitive dissonance reduction, re-ordering of goals and values and response shift whereby internal standards and values are changed – and hence the perception of one's health and life changes (Sprangers & Schwartz, 1999). People may adjust to deteriorating circumstances because they want to feel as good as possible about themselves. The roots of this process are in psychological control theory, with goals of homeostasis. Investigators need to be aware of these problems, and attempt to control for them.

The main theoretical models of quality of life include needs based approaches derived from Maslow's (1954, 1962) hierarchy of human needs (deficiency needs – hunger, thirst, loneliness, security; and growth needs – learning, mastery and self-actualization); (overlapping with) social–psychological models which emphasize autonomy and control, self-sufficiency, internal control and self-assessed technical performance, social competence (Abbey & Andrews, 1986; Fry, 2000); classic models based on subjective wellbeing, happiness, morale, life satisfaction (Andrews, 1986; Andrews & Withey, 1976; Larson, 1978); social expectations or gap models based on the discrepancy between desired and actual circumstances (Michalos, 1986); and phenomenological models of individuals' unique perceptions of their circumstances, based on the concept that quality of life is dependent on the individuals who experience it and should be measured using their own value systems (Rosenberg, 1995; O'Boyle, 1997). In relation to the latter perspective, O'Boyle and his colleagues developed the Schedule for the Evaluation of Individual Quality of Life (SEIQoL), as a generic, individualized quality of life scale (Browne *et al.*, 1997). This has been used in many clinical contexts. It is based on the rationale that it works within the value system of the individual being assessed, rather than the value systems of others. It derived its cognitive aspects from theoretical studies of perception and their extension to Social Judgement Theory, and enables individuals to nominate the areas of life they consider to be the most important to their quality of life, based on their own values.

Also in recognition of the importance of the individual's perspective, the World Health Organization included in its definition of quality of life in the context of health, individuals' perceptions of their position in life in the context of the culture and value systems in which they live and in relation to their goals. While its measure of quality of life (the WHOQoL) is subjective, it uses structured scales rather than individualized items to tap perceptions (WHOQoL Group, 1993, 1995; Skevington, 1999; Skevington *et al.*, 2001).

It could be argued that multidimensional definitions of quality of life confound the dimensionality of the concept with the multiplicity of their causal sources. Beckie and Hayduk (1997) argued that quality of life could be considered as a unidimensional concept with multiple causes, and a unidimensional QoL rating, such as 'How do you feel about your life as a whole?' could be the consequence of global assessments of a range of diverse and complex factors. Thus it would be logical for a unidimensional indicator of quality of life (e.g. a self-rating global QoL uniscale) to be the dependent variable in analyses and the predictor variables include the range of health, social and psychological variables. An appreciation of the distinction between these types of variables in needed by investigators (Zizzi *et al.*, 1998; Fayers & Hand, 2002).

In addition, the effects of personality on perceived wellbeing and quality of life are controversial, partly because of the debate about causal versus mediating variables. Extroversion and neuroticism have been reported to account for a moderate amount of the variation in subjective wellbeing (the trait of extraversion is associated with positive affect and with wellbeing; emotionality is associated with negative affect and poor wellbeing) (Spiro & Bossé, 2000). However, these personality factors are highly stable traits, while subjective wellbeing has been shown to have only moderate stability over time (Headey *et al.*, 1985) (see 'Personality and health').

Zissi et al. (1998) also argued that perceived quality of life is likely to be mediated by several inter-related variables, including self-related constructs (e.g. self-mastery) and these perceptions are likely to be influenced by cognitive mechanisms (e.g. expectations of life). There is still little empirical data to support or refute the distinction between psychological constructs as mediating or influencing variables in determining the quality of life.

Regardless of the conceptual debates and distinctions between health status, quality of life and health-related quality of life, few health researchers have defined these terms in their investigations and many have inappropriately used measures of broader health status to measure health-related quality of life or broader quality of life. This has been justified on the basis of the untested assumption that broader measurement scales of health status (e.g. the SF-36; Ware *et al.*, 1993, 1997) include the main areas in which health can affect one's life, and which are relevant for health services. These concepts may overlap (Ware *et al.*, 1993), but they are not synonymous. In addition, a plethora of disease-specific quality of life measures has been developed, with little standardization of measurement approaches between studies (Garrett *et al.*, 2002) (see also 'Health status assessment').

The investigator should define the concepts used, and select an appropriate measure, which may be generic, health-related (Bowling, 2004) or designed to relate to a specific disease (Bowling, 2001). It is important that the measure selected for use should include topics relevant to the research question and questions which are considered to be important by the target group (e.g. patients). Measures should be based on a theoretical model; incorporate the perceptions of the target population (i.e. items generated from interviews); be directly relevant to, and appropriate for, the research population; contain items related to the target population's identified needs and outcomes; be reliable, valid, precise and responsive to changes associated with treatment; have scale scores which are interpretable (i.e. associated with severity of condition with a guide to cut-off points/ranges); minimize respondent and interviewer burden and be acceptable to respondents; have alternative forms available (interviewer and self-administration versions); and have made cultural and language adaptations, in accordance with good practice on obtaining cultural equivalence.

The choice of whether to use a measure of generic quality of life, health-related or disease-specific quality of life depends on the aims of the study and the type of population or intervention studied. There is little point in including a broad generic measure if it is unlikely to detect the specific effects of treatment, although the use of disease-specific measures precludes the possibility of comparing the outcomes of services that are directed at different groups suffering from different diseases. It is not possible within the space of this chapter to review available measures of generic, health-related and disease-specific quality of life and interested readers are referred to the several existing reviews of measures of health status, generic, health-related and disease-specific quality of life (McDowell & Newell, 1996; Spilker, 1996; Bowling, 2001, 2004).

Acknowledgement

This chapter is based on material from: Bowling, A. *Measuring health*, 3rd edn., Maidenhead: Open University Press, 2004; and Bowling, A. '*Measuring health outcomes from the patient's perspective*'. In Bowling, A. and Ebrahim, S. (eds). *Handbook of Research Methods in Health*, (Chapter 18). Maidenhead: Open University Press, 2005. The material is reproduced with the kind permission of the Open University Press/McGraw-Hill Publishing Company.

REFERENCES

Abbey, A. & Andrews, F. M. (1986). Modelling the psychological determinants of life quality. In F. M. Andrews (Ed.). *Research on the quality of life*. Ann Arbor, Michigan: Survey Research Center, Institute for Social Research, University of Michigan.

Andrews, F. M. (Ed.). (1986). *Research on the quality of life*. Ann Arbor, Michigan: University of Michigan: Institute for Social Research.

Andrews, F. M. & Withey, S. B. (1976). Developing measures of perceived life quality: results from several national surveys. *Social Indicators Research*, **1**, 1–26.

Beckie, T. M. & Hayduk, L. A. (1997). Measuring quality of life. *Social Indicators Research*, **42**, 21–39.

Bowling, A. (2001). *Measuring Disease: A Review of Disease-Specific Quality of Life Measurement Scales* (2nd edn.). Buckingham, UK: Open University Press.

Bowling, A. (2004). *Measuring Health* (3rd edn.). Maidenhead, UK: Open University Press.

Browne, J. P., O'Boyle, C. A., McGee, H. M. et al. (1997). Development of a direct weighing procedure for quality of life domains. *Quality of Life Research*, **6**, 301–9.

Farquhar, M. (1995). Definitions of quality of life: a taxonomy. *Journal of Advanced Nursing*, **22**, 502–8.

Fayers, P. M. & Hand, D. J. (2002). Causal variables, indicator variables and measurement scales: an example from quality of life. *Journal of the Royal Statistical Association*, **165**, Part 2:1–21.

Fry, P. S. (2000). Whose quality of life is it anyway? Why not ask seniors to tell us about it? *International Journal of Aging and Human Development*, **50**, 361–83.

Garratt, A., Schmidt, L., Mackintosh, A. & Fitzpatrick, R. (2002). Quality of life measurement: bibliographic study of patient assessed health outcome measures. *British Medical Journal*, **324**, 1417.

Headey, B. W., Glowacki, T., Holmstrom, E. L. & Wearing, A. J. (1985). Modelling change in perceived quality of life, *Social Indicators Research*, **17**, 276–98.

Larson, R. (1978). Thirty years of research on the subjective well-being of older Americans. *Journal of Gerontology*, **33**, 109–25.

Maslow, A. H. (1954). *Motivation and personality*. Harper: New York.

Maslow, A. H. (1962). *Toward a Psychology of Being* (2nd edn.). Princeton, NJ: Van Nostrand.

McDowell, I. & Newell, C. (1996). *Measuring Health: A Guide to Rating Scales and Questionnaires* (2nd edn.). New York: Oxford University Press.

Michalos, A. C. (1986). Job satisfaction, marital satisfaction and the quality of life: a review and preview. In F. M. Andrews (Ed.). *Research on the quality of life*. Ann Arbor, Michigan: Survey Research Center, Institute for Social research, University of Michigan.

O'Boyle, C. A. (1997). Measuring the quality of later life. *Philosophy Transactions of the Royal Society of London*, **352**, 1871–9.

Patrick, D. L. & Erickson, P. (1993). Health status and health policy. *Quality of life in health care evaluation and resource allocation*. New York: Oxford University Press.

Rosenberg, R. (1995). Health-related quality of life between naturalism and hermeneutics. *Special Issue 'Quality of Life' in Social Science and Medicine*, **10**, 1411–15.

Skevington, S. M. (1999). Measuring quality of life in Britain: introducing the WHOQoL-100. *Psychomatic Research*, **47**, 449–59.

Skevington, S. M., Carse, M. S. & Williams, de C. (2001). Validation of the WHOQoL-100: pain management improves quality of life for chronic pain patients. *Clinical Journal of Pain,* **17**, 264–75.

Spilker, B. (Ed.). (1996). *Pharmacoeconomics and Quality of Life in Clinical Trials* (2nd edn.). Philadelphia: Lippincott-Raven.

Spiro, A. & Bossé, R. (2000). Relations between health-related quality of life and well-being: the gerontologist's new clothes. *International Journal of Aging and Human Development,* **50**, 297–318.

Sprangers, M. A. G. & Schwartz, C. E. (1999). Integrating response shift into health-related quality of life research:

a theoretical model. *Social Science and Medicine,* **48**, 1507–15.

Ware, J. E., Snow, K.K., Kosinski, M. & Gandek, B. (1993). *SF-36 Health Survey: manual and interpretation guide.* Boston, MA: The Health Institute, New England Medical Center.

Ware, J. E., Snow, K. K., Kosinski, M. & Gandek, B. (1997). *SF-36 Health Survey: manual and interpretation guide* (Rev. edn.). Boston, MA: The Health Institute, New England Medical Center.

WHOQoL Group (1993). Measuring quality of life: the development of the World Health Organization Quality of Life

Instrument (WHOQOL). Geneva: World Health Organization.

WHOQoL Group (1995). The World Health Organization quality of life assessment (WHOQoL): position paper from the World Health Organization. *Special Issue 'Quality of Life' in Social Science and Medicine,* **10**, 1403–9.

Zissi, A., Barry, M. M. & Cochrane, R. (1998). A mediational model of quality of life for individuals with severe mental health problems. *Psychological Medicine,* **28**, 1221–30.

Social support assessment

Brian Lakey and Jay L. Cohen

Wayne State University

In this chapter, we review different approaches to assessing social support, as well as research evidence indicating the psychological and environmental characteristics that these measures reflect. A comprehensive review of all of the major social support measures is beyond the focus of this chapter, and we refer readers to recent comprehensive reviews (e.g. Brissette *et al.*, 2000; Wills & Shinar, 2000). In this chapter, we briefly describe different types of social support measures, and review research bearing on their validity. We focus on the most widely used types of measures, although we also briefly describe under-utilized and more recently developed approaches.

Types of social support measures

There are at least three different types of social support constructs and measures; perceived support, enacted support and social integration/network characteristics (Barrera, 1986) (see 'Social support and health'). Each type is most often assessed by self-report, whereby research participants complete questionnaires about participants' perceived availability of support (perceived support), the amount of specific supportive actions received (enacted support), or the number of different types of relationships in which people participate (social integration). Measures of these different types of support are only modestly related to each other, and relate to mental health, physical health and other constructs in different ways (Barrera, 1986).

Description of types of social support measures

Measures of perceived support

Measures of perceived support (also termed 'functional support', see chapter on 'Social support and health') ask respondents to make subjective judgments about the availability of support, or for some measures, about the quality of the support typically received. Two prototypical measures of perceived support are the Interpersonal Support Evaluation List (S. Cohen & Hoberman, 1983; S. Cohen *et al.*, 1985) and the Social Provisions Scale (SPS; Cutrona & Russell, 1987). Both measures are used very widely in research. Detailed descriptions of a wide range of measures of perceived support are provided by Wills and Shinar (2000).

Measures of enacted support

Measures of enacted support (also termed 'received support') ask respondents to report the frequency by which (or simply whether or not) they have received various supportive actions over a specific period of time (e.g. 30 days). Perhaps the most widely used measure of enacted support is the Inventory of Socially Supportive Behaviours (ISSB; Barrera *et al.*, 1981). Detailed descriptions of a range of measures of enacted support can be found in Wills and Shinar (2000).

Measures of social integration and social networks

Measures of social integration and social networks typically assess the number of important relationships or roles in which respondents participate, or may assess more detailed characteristics of social networks such as the extent to which different network members know each other (i.e. network density). One prototypic measure of social integration is S. Cohen's (1991; Cohen *et al.*, 1997) Social Network Index (SNI). Detailed descriptions of a range of measures of social integration and network characteristics can be found in Brissette *et al.* (2000).

Construct validity

Readers interested in understanding the scientific basis for determining the validity of measures of psychological constructs should study Cronbach and Meehl's (1955) definitive statement on construct validity. An adequate account of construct validity cannot be provided in a short paragraph, but here is a summary of some of the key points, as applied to social support. First, there will never be a single gold standard for the assessment of social support, because social support is a human abstraction used to organize and make sense of complex psychological phenomena. Instead, different measures of social support will be more or less useful for different purposes. Second, the validity of social support measures is based solely on the measures' correlations with other constructs and variables, as determined by quantitative research methods. The label applied to the measure, or the intentions of the measure's developers do not count as evidence for construct validity. Third, validity occurs on a continuum rather than as a dichotomy. That is, measures have more or less validity, rather than are valid or invalid. Further, validity may vary depending upon the purposes for which the measure is used. A given scale might have good validity for predicting mortality, but poor validity for predicting changes in mental health. In the next section, we describe the construct validity of measures of perceived support, enacted support and social integration.

Construct validity for perceived social support

The most important fact regarding the validity of measures of perceived support is the consistent and strong finding that people who report higher levels of perceived support have better mental health and lower rates of psychopathology than do people with lower perceived support (Cohen & Wills, 1985; Sarason *et al.*, 2001). Nonetheless, measures of perceived support are not so highly correlated with mental health as to suggest that measures of perceived support reflect mental health primarily. Similar findings have been observed for a range of physical health indices, although the magnitude of the link between perceived support and physical health often is smaller than the link between perceived support and mental health (Uchino, 2004; see 'Social support and health').

From the beginning of social support research, scholars assumed that measures of perceived support primarily reflected respondents' social environments. If so, then people who perceive their relationships as supportive should perceive other aspects of their relationships positively as well. In fact, people who perceive their relationships as supportive also report high satisfaction (Kaul & Lakey, 2003), intimacy (Reis & Franks, 1994) and low levels of conflict (Okun & Lockwood, 2003) with important relationship partners, less loneliness (Joiner, 1997) and more secure adult romantic attachments (Davis *et al.*, 1998). Although people who perceive their relationships as more supportive also report receiving more enacted support, the magnitude of this correlation is not as strong as most social support models imply (Barrera, 1986). A recent meta-analysis estimated the link between perceived and enacted support at $r = 0.34$ (Haber *et al.*, 2003). Thus, perceived support is only partly a reflection of the amount of enacted support received.

Another indicator of the extent to which perceived support reflects the characteristics of personal relationships is the extent to which relationship partners agree about the supportiveness of their relationships. A number of studies have found modest agreement among friends, couples and diverse family members on perceived supportiveness, with indices of agreement ranging from $r = 0.32$ to 0.55 (Abbey *et al.*, 1995; Cutrona, 1989; McCaskill & Lakey, 2000; Vinokur *et al.*, 1987).

Although people with high levels of perceived support describe other aspects of their relationships positively, these people also describe their own personality characteristics favourably. People with high levels of perceived support report higher self-esteem, a greater sense of personal control and fewer irrational beliefs (Lakey & Cassady, 1990). With regard to personality traits, people with high levels of perceived support describe themselves as agreeable, extraverted, emotionally stable, conscientious and open to experience, (Branje *et al.*, 2004; Finch *et al.*, 1999; Colby & Emmons, 1997; but see Tonga *et al.*, 2004, for an exception). Such people also describe themselves as not sensitive to rejection, not alienated and as having high levels of interpersonal trust (Lakey *et al.*, 1994). They describe themselves as socially skilled (Cohen *et al.*, 1986) and independent observers agree to some extent (Sarason *et al.*, 1985). Thus, although people with high levels of perceived support describe other aspects of their personal relationships favourably, they also describe their own personality characteristics favourably (see 'Personality and health').

Although most research on perceived support has focused on the characteristics of support recipients, other research has focused on the characteristics of people who are seen as good support providers. Recipients see supportive providers as agreeable, similar to recipients in attitudes and values and emotionally stable (Branje *et al.*, 2004; Lakey *et al.*, 2002), although recipients vary substantially in the particular provider personality traits which they use to judge supportiveness (Lutz & Lakey, 2001).

Thus, the evidence reviewed so far provides a murky view of the extent to which measures of perceived support reflect the personal qualities of support recipients and the characteristics of the social environment. Recent research using Generalizability Theory (Cronbach *et al.*, 1972) and the Social Relations Model (Kenny, 1994) provide more precise estimates of the extent to which perceived support reflects the characteristics of support recipients (also termed perceiver or actor effects) and two different forms of social influence; the objectively supportive properties of providers (also termed target or partner effects) and the unique relationships among recipients and providers. The 'recipient' component represents individual differences in how favourably recipients see support providers, on average, regardless of the characteristics of providers. The provider component represents the extent to which recipients agree on the relative supportiveness of the same providers; that is, the extent to which supportiveness is an objective quality of providers. Here we operationalize 'objective' as inter-rater agreement. Most social support models emphasize the provider component. The 'relationship' component reflects systematic disagreement among recipients about the relative supportiveness of the same providers. This component reflects the extent to which supportiveness is a matter of personal taste and it reflects the unique matches between specific recipients and specific providers.

Our research group's current best estimate of the relative magnitude of recipient, provider and relationship effects, is derived from three studies in which recipients rated individuals who were well known to them (Studies 1 and 2 in Lakey *et al.*, 1996, and one unpublished study). We estimate that approximately 14% of perceived support reflects the personality characteristics of recipients, 6% reflects the objectively supportive properties of providers and 51% reflects the unique relationships among providers and recipients. Branje *et al.* (2002) have conducted an independent replication in Holland and reported very similar findings, although Branje obtained slightly higher estimates for recipient personality and slightly lower estimates for unique relationships. Thus, measures of perceived support reflect a blend of the personality characteristics of recipients, as well as two distinct kinds of social influence. On the whole, however, the large majority of the variance in perceived support measures reflects social influence, although not the kind emphasized by most social support models.

Construct validity for enacted social support

One of the major differences between measures of perceived and enacted support is that measures of enacted support are not consistently linked to mental and physical health (Barrera, 1986; Finch *et al.*, 1999; Uchino, 2004). When measures of enacted support are significantly related to mental health, the direction of the correlation frequently is opposite to expectations: people who receive the most enacted support have the worst mental health (Barrera, 1986). More recent evidence suggests that only enacted support involving positive social exchanges (Finch *et al.*, 1997), support that goes un-noticed by support recipients (Bolger *et al.*, 2000) and support that is desired by recipients (Reynolds & Perrin, 2004) is related to mental health.

Unlike measures of perceived support, measures of enacted support do not appear to have strong links to recipients' reports of self-esteem, irrational beliefs and personal control (Lakey & Cassady, 1990; Lakey *et al.*, 1994), although like perceived support, people who report receiving high levels of enacted support express more positive affect (Lakey *et al.*, 1994) and extroversion (Finch *et al.*, 1997) than people who express low levels.

Although measures of enacted support do not have as many documented links to other constructs as does perceived support, recipients appear to report enacted support more accurately than they report perceived support and personality (Cohen *et al.*, in press). After controlling for a variety of artifacts that inflate agreement, agreement between providers and recipients was

$r = 0.50$ for enacted support and $r = 0.29$ for perceived support. Agreement on providers' personality traits was much lower. Other investigators also report significant agreement between dyads on enacted support (Antonucci & Israel, 1986; Coriell & S. Cohen, 1995).

Construct validity for social integration and social network characteristics

Most research on social integration and social network characteristics examines links to health outcomes, as reviewed by Wills and Ainette (see 'Social support and health') and Uchino (2004). Compared with perceived support, less is known about the construct validity of social integration. In one study (Cohen *et al.*, 1987), people with more diverse social networks smoked less and exercised more, but did not drink less alcohol than people with less diverse social networks. The same study found that people with more diverse social networks were more extraverted than people with less diverse networks, but not more neurotic, conscientiousness, open to experience or agreeable. Cohen (1991) also reported that people with more diverse networks had more positive affect, stronger beliefs in their own personal control and higher self-esteem than people with less diverse networks. Similarly, people with larger social networks (all relationships not limited by type of relationship) reported more extroversion and positive affect, but not negative affect, neuroticism, perceived stress or hostility, than people with smaller networks (Pressman *et al.*, 2005). Thus, social integration appears to be related to extroversion and positive affect, as well as to some positive health practices.

Incremental validity

Incremental validity is the extent to which a given measure predicts outcomes of interest above and beyond other constructs (Sechrest, 1963). For example, do measures of social support predict health beyond other related constructs, or other risk factors? As reviewed elsewhere (Sarason *et al.*, 2001), measures of perceived support and social integration forecast changes in both mental and physical health incrementally beyond pre-existing mental and physical health. With regard to mental health, measures of perceived support show incremental validity beyond social desirability (Cohen *et al.*, 1985; Cutrona & Russell, 1987) and social competence (Cohen *et al.*, 1986). In spite of these favourable findings for measures of perceived support, additional work is needed to demonstrate that measures of social support can predict incrementally beyond other measures of personal relationships. For example, Finch *et al.* (1999) found that perceived social support was related to mental health incrementally beyond interpersonal stress. However, Kaul and Lakey (2003) failed to find incremental validity for perceived support beyond generic relationship satisfaction in predicting mental health, raising the question of the extent to which reports of social support captured social support per se, or a more general evaluation of relationships.

In addition to showing that total social support scores have incremental validity beyond other constructs, it is also important to demonstrate that various social support subscales have incremental validity beyond other subscales. Otherwise, it is difficult to argue that a given sub-scale measures a unique aspect of social support that is not shared with other sub-scales. Establishing incremental validity for sub-scales is especially important because the sub-scales typically are moderately to strongly inter-correlated and display similar patterns of correlations with other constructs (Cohen *et al.*, 1985; Cutrona & Russell, 1987). Cohen and Hoberman (1983) found that self-esteem support and appraisal support each displayed buffering effects with stressful life events in predicting depression, even when all other sub-scales of the ISEL were controlled. In a sample of married people, Cutrona (personal communication, November, 2004) found that the SPS sub-scales of attachment, guidance, social integration and reassurance of worth each were uniquely related to marital satisfaction. For enacted support, Finch *et al.* (1997) found that positive social exchange was linked to less depression but that tangible assistance and directive guidance were linked to more depression, when all other sub-scales and personality measures were controlled. Although these studies are promising, there are not enough studies of this kind to fully resolve the question of incremental validity for social support sub-scales.

Under-utilized approaches to measurement

The vast majority of studies use self-report measures that assess social support in a global sense. Although such measures are valuable, it is important to remember that they only partly reflect the objective properties of social environments (Lakey *et al.*, 1996). In addition, global measures of social support do not capture moment-by-moment social interactions. Although used infrequently, there are behavioural observation and diary measures of social support that can provide more objective and moment-by-moment assessments.

Cutrona and her colleagues (Cutrona *et al.*, 1997) developed the Social Support Behaviour Code (SSBC), a behavioural observation measure designed to assess the extent to which a provider engages in specific, observable supportive actions in a specific conversation. The SSBC has not been used extensively in research and so there is comparatively little information about its construct validity. However, preliminary findings indicate that extraverted providers give more support than do introverted providers, and providers give more support when they themselves received more support in a previous interaction (Cutrona *et al.*, 1997). Consistent with research based on questionnaires, recipients' perceptions of support are not very closely related to the receipt of support, as rated by observers (Cutrona *et al.*, 1997).

Diary measures are another form of under-utilized social support assessment. For example, Bolger and his colleagues (Bolger *et al.*, 2000) developed a diary method whereby respondents reported social support on a daily basis. In Bolger *et al.* (2000), recipients preparing to take the bar exam reported on a daily basis whether their romantic partners 'listened to and comforted' them. Partners also reported whether they provided such support. Couples agreed on whether support was provided on 61% of diary days, indicating modest agreement on support provision. However, this method revealed a fascinating effect: recipients were least depressed on days in which partners reported providing support, but

recipients did not see it. Recipients were most depressed when they reported receiving support, but providers reported not providing it. Bolger *et al.* (2000) termed this phenomenon, 'invisible support' because recipients appeared to benefit most from support that was invisible to them. Using the same method, Gleason *et al.* (2003) reported that reciprocity in the exchange of support was associated with higher levels of positive affect and lower levels of negative affect.

Summary and conclusions

Perceived support, enacted support and social integration/ network characteristics are the three major types of social support constructs and measures. Of these, the construct validity of perceived support is the best understood. Perceived support represents a blend of the personality characteristics of recipients, the objectively supportive properties of providers and the unique relationships among recipients and providers. Of these, relationships are the most important influence. Thus, most of the variance in measures of perceived support reflects the social environment, although it is not the aspect of the social environment that has been emphasized by most social support models. Recipients see supportive providers as similar to recipients in attitudes and values, as agreeable and as providing enacted support. People who report high levels of perceived support also have more favourable scores on a wide range of personal characteristics. The construct validity of measures of enacted support is less well understood than for perceived support. Although people who receive more enacted support express more extraversion and positive affect than people who receive less enacted support, enacted support is not as strongly correlated with the same wide range of favourable personal characteristics as is perceived support. Nonetheless, recipients and providers display good agreement about the enacted support that is received and therefore measures of enacted support appear to reflect the objective features of social interactions more so than do measures of perceived support. Beyond the abundant research linking social integration to health, there is relatively little research on the construct validity of such measures. What is available suggests that people with more diverse social networks express more positive affect and extroversion than do people with less diverse social networks.

In choosing social support measures for research or clinical applications it is essential to verify that the type of social support measure under consideration is relevant to the clinical problem or outcome of interest. For example, although researchers often believe that the more objective types of social support measures (e.g. social integration or enacted support) are preferred because of their apparent objectivity, the more subjective measures of perceived support are much more closely tied to mental health. In contrast, measures of social integration do quite well in predicting a variety of health outcomes, including mortality. It is important to remember that the three different types of social support measures are not closely related and reflect different psychological and social processes.

REFERENCES

Abbey, A., Andrews, F. M. & Halman, L. J. (1995). Provision and receipt of social support and disregard: what is the impact on the marital life quality of fertile and infertile couples? *Journal of Personality and Social Psychology*, **68**, 455–69.

Antonucci, T. C. & Israel, B. (1986). Veridicality of social support: a comparison of principal and network members' responses. *Journal of Consulting and Clinical Psychology*, **54**, 432–37.

Barerra, M., Jr. (1986). Distinctions between social support concepts, measures, and models. *American Journal of Community Psychology*, **14**, 413–45.

Barrera, M., Sandler, I. N. & Ramsey, T. B. (1981). Preliminary development of a scale of social support: studies on college students. *American Journal of Community Psychology*, **9**, 435–47.

Bolger, N., Zuckerman, A. & Kessler, R. C. (2000). Invisible support and adjustment to stress. *Journal of Personality and Social Psychology*, **79**, 953–61.

Branje, S. J. T., van Aken, M. A. G. & van Lieshout, C. F.M. (2002). Relational support in families with adolescents, *Journal of Family Psychology*, **16**, 351–62.

Branje, S. J. T., van Lieshout, C. F. M. & van Aken, M. A.G. (2004). Relations between big five personality characteristics and perceived support in adolescents' families, *Journal of Personality and Social Psychology*, **86**, 615–28.

Brissette, I., Cohen, S. & Seeman, T. E. (2000). Measuring social integration and social networks. In S. Cohen, L. G. Underwood & B. H. Gottlieb (Eds.). *Social support measurement and intervention* (pp. 53–85). New York: Oxford University Press.

Cohen, J. L., Lakey, B., Tiell, K. & Neely, L. C. (in press). Recipient-provider agreement on enacted support, perceived support and provider personality. *Psychological Assessment*.

Cohen, S. (1991). Social supports and physical health: symptoms, health behaviors, and infectious diseases. In A. L. Greene, E. M. Cummings & K. H. Karraker (Eds.). *Life-span developmental psychology: perspectives on stress and coping* (pp. 213–34). Hillsdale, NJ: Erlbaum.

Cohen, S., Doyle, W. J., Skoner, D. P., Rabin, B. S. & Gwaltnery, J. M. (1997). Social ties and suspectibility to the common cold. *Journal of the American Medical Association*, **277**, 1940–4.

Cohen, S. & Hoberman, H. M. (1983). Positive events and social supports as buffers of life change stress. *Journal of Applied Social Psychology*, **13**, 99–125.

Cohen, S., Mermelstein, R., Kamarck, T. & Hoberman, H. (1985). Measuring the functional components of social support. In I. G. Sarason & B. R. Sarason (Eds.). *Social support: theory research and application* (pp. 73–94). The Hague: Martinus Nijhoff.

Cohen, S., Sherrod, D. R. & Clark, M. S. (1986). Social skills and the stress-protective role of social support. *Journal of Personality and Social Psychology*, **50**, 963–73.

Cohen, S. & Wills, T. A. (1985). Stress, social support, and the buffering hypothesis. *Psychological Bulletin*, **98**, 310–57.

Colby, P. M. & Emmons, R. A. (1997). Openness to emotion as a predictor of perceived, requested, and observer reports of social support. In G. R. Pierce, B. Lakey, I. G. Sarason, & B. R. Sarason (Eds.). *Sourcebook of social support and personality* (pp. 3–18). New York: Plenum Press.

Coriell, M. & Cohen, S. (1995). Concordance in the face of a stressful event: when do members of a dyad agree that one person supported the other? *Journal of Personality and Social Psychology*, **69**, 289–99.

Cronbach, L. J., Gleser, G. C., Nanda, H. & Rajaratnam, N. (1972). The dependability of behavioral measurements: theory of generalizability of scores and profiles. New York: John Wiley.

Cronbach, L. J. & Meehl, P. E. (1955). Construct validity in psychological tests. *Psychological Bulletin*, **52**, 281–302.

Cutrona, C. E. (1989). Ratings of social support by adolescents and adult informants: degree of correspondence and prediction of depressive symptoms. *Journal of Personality and Social Psychology*, **57**, 723–30.

Cutrona, C. E., Hessling, R. M. & Suhr, J. A. (1997). The influence of husband and wife personality on marital social support interactions. *Personal Relationships*, **4**, 379–93.

Cutrona, C. E. & Russell, D. W. (1987). The provisions of social relationships and adaptation to stress. *Advances in Personal Relationships*, **1**, 37–67.

Davis, M. H., Morris, M. M. & Kraus, L. A. (1998). Relationship-specific and global perceptions of social support: associations with well-being and attachment. *Journal of Personality and Social Psychology*, **74**, 468–81.

Finch, J. F., Barrera, M. Jr., Okun, M. A. *et al.* (1997). The factor structure of received social support: dimensionality and the prediction of depression and life satisfaction. *Journal of Social and Clinical Psychology*, **16**, 323–42.

Finch, J. F., Okun, M. A., Pool, G. J. & Ruehlman, L. S. (1999). Comparison of the influence of conflictual and supportive social interactions on psychological distress. *Journal of Personality*, **67**, 581–621.

Gleason, M. E. J., Iida, M., Bolger, N. & Shrout, P. E. (2003). Daily supportive equity in close relationships. *Personality and Social Psychology Bulletin*, **29**, 1036–45.

Haber, M. G., Cohen, J. L. & Lucas, T. (February, 2003). *The relationship between support behaviors and support perceptions: a meta-analytic review*. Presented at the annual meeting of the Society for Personality and Social Psychology, Los Angeles, CA.

Joiner, T. E., Jr. (1997). Shyness and low social support as interactive diatheses, with loneliness as mediator: testing an interpersonal-personality view of vulnerability to depressive symptoms. *Journal of Abnormal Psychology*, **106**, 386–94.

Kaul, M. & Lakey, B. (2003). Where is the support in perceived support? The role of generic relationship satisfaction and enacted support in perceived support's relation to low distress. *Journal of Social and Clinical Psychology*, **22**, 59–78.

Kenny, D. A. (1994). *Interpersonal perception: a social relations analysis*. New York: Guilford.

Lakey, B., Adams, K., Neely, L. *et al.* (2002). Perceived support and low emotional distress: the role of enacted support, dyad similarity and provider personality. *Personality and Social Psychology Bulletin*, **28**, 1546–55.

Lakey, B. & Cassady, P. B. (1990). Cognitive processes in perceived social support. *Journal of Personality and Social Psychology*, **59**, 337–43.

Lakey, B., McCabe, K. M., Fisicaro, S. A. & Drew, J. B. (1996). Environmental and personal determinants of support perceptions: three generalizability studies. *Journal of Personality and Social Psychology*, **70**, 1270–80.

Lakey, B., Tardiff, T. & Drew, J. B. (1994). Interpersonal stress: assessment and relations to social support, personality and psychological distress. *Journal of Social and Clinical Psychology*, **13**, 42–62.

Lutz, C. J. & Lakey, B. (2001). How people make support judgments: individual differences in the traits used to infer supportiveness in others. *Journal of Personality and Social Psychology*, **81**, 1070–9.

McCaskill, J. & Lakey, B. (2000). Perceived support, social undermining, and emotion: idiosyncratic and shared perspectives of adolescents and their families. *Personality and Social Psychology Bulletin*, **26**, 820–32.

Okun, M. A. & Lockwood, C. M. (2003). Does level of assessment moderate the relation between social support and social negativity?: a meta-analysis. *Basic and Applied Social Psychology*, **25**, 15–35.

Pressman, S., Cohen, S., Miller, G. E. *et al.* (2005). Loneliness, social network size, and immune response to influenza vaccination in college freshmen. *Health Psychology*, **24**, 297–306.

Reis, H. T. & Franks, P. (1994). The role of intimacy and social support in health outcomes: two processes or one? *Personal Relationships*, **1**, 185–97.

Reynolds, J. S. & Perrin, N. A. (2004). Mismatches in social support and

psychosocial adjustment to breast cancer. *Health Psychology*, **23**, 425–30.

Sarason, B. R., Sarason, I. G. & Gurung, R. A. R. (2001). Close personal relationships and health outcomes: a key to the role of social support. In B.R. Sarason & S. Duck (Eds.). *Personal relationships: implications for clinical and community psychology* (pp. 15–41). Chichester, UK: Wiley.

Sarason, B. R., Sarason, I. G., Hacker, T. A. & Basham, R. B. (1985). Concomitants of social support: social skills, physical attractiveness and gender. *Journal of Personality and Social Psychology*, **49**, 469–80.

Sechrest, L. (1963). Incremental validity: a recommendation. *Educational and Psychological Measurement*, **23**, 153–8.

Tonga, E. M. W., Bishopa, G. D., Dionga, S. M. *et al.* (2004). Social support and personality among male police officers in Singapore. *Personality and Individual Differences*, **36**, 109–23.

Uchino, B. N. (2004). *Social support and physical health outcomes: understanding the health consequences of our relationships*. New Haven, CT: Yale University Press.

Vinokur, A., Schul, Y. & Caplan, R. D. (1987). Determinants of perceived social support: interpersonal transactions, personal outlook, and transient affective states. *Journal of Personality and Social Psychology*, **53**, 1137–45.

Wills, T. A. & Ainette, M. G. (2005). Social Support and Health. In S. Ayers, A. Baum, C. McManus. *et al.* (Eds.). *Cambridge Handbook of Psychology, Health, & Medicine* (2nd edn.). Cambridge, UK: Cambridge University Press.

Wills, T. A. & Shinar, O. (2000). Measuring perceived and received social support. In S. Cohen, L. G. Underwood & B. H. Gottlieb (Eds.). *Social support measurement and intervention* (pp. 86–135). New York: Oxford University Press.

Stress assessment

Andrew Baum and Angela Liegey Dougall

University of Pittsburgh

Overview

Because stress is a complex process and occurs broadly and at many levels, assessment of it has been difficult and at times controversial. The proliferation of measurement protocols, continued confusion or inconsistency among theories and operational variables and the pervasiveness and depth of stress responses themselves all contribute to these difficulties. Regardless, a useful set of measures of stress-related phenomena has emerged and although several problems remain to be worked out, the development of comprehensive, convergent assessment strategies has allowed significant advances in our knowledge of stress and its contributions to health and illness. These approaches to measuring stress reflect prognostic solutions to key conceptual controversies in the field and permit measurement across different levels of response, points in the stress process, and acute and chronic timeframes. Here, we briefly consider some issues that complicate stress assessment and review available measures.

The most significant of these issues reflects the many different definitions of stress and conceptions of the nature and duration of its effects. Different assumptions and definitions will affect the operationalization of key constructs and the measures selected or developed. As discussed by Ayers and Steptoe in the chapter on 'Stress & health', the stress process includes environmental events and intrapsychic sources of stress that are called 'stressors', cognitive interpretation of these events and of one's capacity to adapt ('appraisal'), emotional behavioural and biological changes associated with these variables ('stress responses', 'strain') and effects of these changes ('consequences'). Measurement can address any one of these levels or can include simultaneous assessments of two or more.

Within these levels of analysis, measures can vary in the way they target aspects of each or in the time frame that is adopted, and because stress is essentially a 'whole body' response, it is expressed as changes in all or nearly all bodily systems and psychological dimensions. As a result, the number of variables that can be observed is large. Even brief consideration of these issues should guide choices among potential measurement approaches. Decisions about targets for measurement ultimately rest on the nature of the questions being asked.

Assessment of stressors

Assessment of stressors and/or of appraisal of them will yield different information than will measurement of response or consequence. Measures of stressors are possible and useful because specific events or conditions often cause stress appraisals and/or responses. The frequency and duration of these events or conditions can be reliably quantified. There are clear advantages to these measures but there are major limitations on their use and value as well. To some extent the use of these measures and the choices among them are related to availability of sources of data (e.g. study participants, archival data) and to the questions under investigation.

The most common or well known measures of stressors are counts or descriptions of significant 'life events' or changes. Pioneering studies of the contributions of the frequency and distribution of major life changes used the Social Readjustment Rating Questionnaire and, more recently, the Recent Life Changes Questionnaire (Holmes & Rahe, 1967; Rahe, 1975). These instruments consist of inventories of life events or changes that occur variably in peoples' lives. Respondents indicate which have been experienced and when they were experienced and sufficient data are generated to allow estimates of the frequency and clustering/dispersal of these events over time. These variables are often correlated with physical and psychological outcomes. Some forms of these life event measures ask respondents to rate the impact of each experienced event, and others rely on consensus about the relative effects of different events.

Variability in perceived impact of stressors is one source of error in these assessments and limitations imposed by lack of reliable or standardized impact estimates are key limitations of these measures. Unless detailed records exist or are compiled for other reasons, measures of life events are self-reports and are also vulnerable to recall bias, limiting the time frame that can be reliably measured. Overlap among listed items and common responses to stress have also introduced concerns about some of these measures. However, despite these problems, studies of life events and health outcomes generally produce modest but robust correlations among events and outcomes (Sarason et al., 1975).

A different body of research has focused on studying minor, mundane stressors that occur in everyday life. Lazarus and colleagues have proposed that an accumulation of these daily stressors, or 'hassles', should prospectively predict mood, distress and physical health (Lazarus et al., 1980). Research using the Hassles and Uplifts Scale has confirmed these relationships and has suggested that daily hassles were a better predictor of psychological symptoms than were life events (DeLongis et al., 1988; Kanner et al., 1981). A concern with these measures is that they may reflect mood as much as the occurrence of an annoying event or condition. Hassles are by definition minor and may normally escape detection or recollection: they may be more memorable when one is in a 'bad' mood. As a result, reporting may be inflated and the predictive value of stressor assessments influenced by associated mood changes.

To minimize bias due to an individual's appraisal and mood in the measurement of life stressors, structured interviews have been developed such as the Life Events and Difficulties Schedule (LEDS; Brown & Harris, 1989). These interview techniques are useful for gathering specific information on the actual event and its context that can then be rated by objective reviewers. This approach has increased the magnitude of the relationships found between life stress and outcomes and has shown that life events and chronic difficulties may contribute to the risk of developing many mental and physical disorders. Training for and administration of interviews like the LEDS are both time-consuming and costly and limit the feasibility and dissemination of this approach. Additionally, these techniques provide little information about how stress works or why it has these effects, nor do they measure mediators or effectors (e.g. response) to allow examination of consequences.

Measures of stressors can also focus on specific types of stressors, as, for example, with the Traumatic Stress Schedule or the Traumatic Life Events Questionnaire (Kubany et al., 2000; Norris, 1990). These target specific types of stressors or general source differences and allow more precise predictions or hypotheses when appropriate. Whether narrowly focused or more broadly inclusive, these measures are useful in evaluating gross relationships in larger samples and in evaluating other sources of stress-related variance when one or a few specific sources are targeted.

Measuring appraisal

Measures of stress appraisal are at once disarmingly simple and deceptively complex. At some level measures of appraisal can serve as 'manipulation checks' and as such can (and often are) measured with single items or brief home-grown scales that ask whether respondents felt stressed at a particular time. These questions can take many forms and can focus on specific sources of stress (e.g. Are you stressed on the job? Do you feel crowded?) or acute responses to laboratory stressors (e.g. Did you find the task stressful?). These measures fulfill the conditions specifying appraisal and appraisal process but do not reflect how this general assessment was generated. For example, part of the appraisal of whether a situation is stressful or not depends on perceptions of one's ability to adapt. Part of this evaluation consists of appraisals of one's resources, including social support or coping style and efficacy. Simple measures of stress may not reflect this complexity and tell us little about the relative contributions of stressor characteristics and appraisals of resources and assets to these summary conclusions.

There have been efforts to develop broader measures of stress appraisal. Folkman et al. (1986) developed scales for primary appraisal (determining what is at risk in the stressful encounter) and secondary appraisal (determining coping options) based on their theoretical work on stress and coping (Lazarus & Folkman, 1984). Expanding on this seminal work, investigators have developed other scales that emphasize different aspects of appraisal such as centrality or trait–state differences and include instruments such as the Stress Appraisal Measure (Peacock & Wong, 1990), the Dimensions of Stress Scale (Vitaliano et al., 1993), the Perceived Stress Scale (Cohen et al., 1983) and the Cognitive Appraisal Scale (Skinner and Brewer, 2002). Many researchers have used these scales or a modified version of them to show that the types of appraisals people make predicted the coping strategies used and psychological adaptation.

As part of the ongoing cognitive processing of stressful events, people may experience intrusive thoughts or unwanted, unbidden and uncontrollable thoughts about the event (Creamer et al., 1992;

A. Baum and A.L. Dougall

Greenberg, 1995). A popular measure of intrusive thoughts is the Impact of Event Scale and its revision (Horowitz *et al.*, 1979; Weiss & Marmar, 1997), which also assesses the incidence of avoidance and hyper-arousal symptoms that commonly occur following extreme stressors. Intrusive thoughts may help an individual work through the situation and generally decrease in frequency as people recover from stressful events (Delahanty *et al.*, 1997). However, the unwanted and uncontrollable nature of intrusive thoughts may make them stressful in their own right possibly sensitizing individuals to other reminiscent stimuli. Stressor-related intrusions, combined with other cognitive processes and environmental stimuli, may serve to perpetuate stress by eliciting acute stress episodes and maintaining stress appraisals. Research indicates that intrusive thoughts are a strong predictor of chronic stress responding (Dougall *et al.*, 1999).

Together with the availability of a number of good measures of resource appraisal and efficacy, measures of general or summary appraisals can be used to evaluate individual variation in response to events or conditions that often induce stress (see also 'Coping assessment' and 'Social support assessment'). The essential distinction between appraisal and response measures is derived from the putative role of the variable. Appraisal theoretically initiates responses. Some variables or measures, such as intrusions and the Impact of Event Scale, may represent elements of both.

Stress responses

Stress responses occur at several different levels. Both acute and more chronic stressors are associated with emotional changes, cognitive and behavioural responses and far-reaching biological changes in nearly every system in the body. There are many measures at each of these levels, varying in the extent to which they rely on self-report, the duration and timing of responses, and the system or response that they target. Mood measures, such as the Profile of Mood States (POMS; McNair *et al.*, 1981), anxiety assessments such as the State–Trait Anxiety Inventory (STAI, Spielberger, 1983) and state/trait assessments of one or several mood states, such as the Positive and Negative Affect Schedule (PANAS, Watson *et al.*, 1988) are useful in measuring changes in mood associated with exposure to experimental stressors or naturalistic stressors (see 'Mood assessment'). Cognitive aspects of stress response, including increased use of short-cutting or heuristics in decision making under stress (Shaham *et al.*, 1992), tolerance for frustration (Glass and Singer, 1972) and concentration/problem-solving (Baum *et al.*, 1983) can also be assessed during or after experimental or ongoing naturalistic stressors. Although less common, behavioural measures can be collected through observation or by presentation of experimental conditions that evoke and allow measurement of persistent or over-generalized responses to situational demands (Baum & Valins, 1977). Finally, biological measures include many different estimates of many different bodily processes. The most common include measures of blood pressure and heart rate (particularly in studies of stress reactivity), other peripheral psychophysiological measures (e.g. skin conductance, EMG) and stress hormones (e.g. cortisol, epinephrine and norepinephrine) although recent developments in psychoneuroimmunology have increased use of immune

measures of response as well (see 'Psychoneuroimmunology assessments').

Self-report measures are typically used to assess stress-related increases in negative emotions such as depression, anxiety, anger, fear and overall symptom reporting. In addition to the mood measures mentioned above, instruments used to assess general levels of distress or symptoms such as the Symptom Checklist 90 – Revised (Derogatis, 1994) and abbreviated forms are used extensively to measure general distress. These inventories typically ask a respondent to rate either how frequently a list of symptoms occurred or to rate how much the symptoms distressed or bothered them. A referent timeframe of a week or a month is given so that respondents can provide a general rating of distress.

Stress may also be manifested as decrements in behavioural performance. People may not be able to attend well to routine, mundane tasks, like driving an automobile, balancing a checkbook, or monitoring a computer screen, while their attention is focused on dealing with a stressor (Krueger, 1989). Behavioural tasks such as the proofreading task devised by Glass and Singer (1972) or an embedded figures task (Witkin *et al.*, 1979) have been used to document acute stress effects as well as chronic stress responding in people exposed to stressors such as disasters (Baum *et al.*, 1983). People experiencing chronic stress find fewer errors in the proofreading task or solve fewer puzzles and make fewer attempts to solve puzzles on the embedded figures task. Even exposure to a brief, laboratory task can result in transient performance deficits in tasks given during the stressor or after it (Cohen, 1980). These negative after-effects have been shown to occur even after a person appears to have psychologically and physiologically adapted to an acute stressor.

An important direction for stress research is measurement of stress effects on health and wellbeing. Behavioural responses during or after stress can reflect attempts to cope with a stressor deemed harmful and represent a primary pathway by which stress affects health. Many of these coping behaviours facilitate appropriate responses to the stressful event and promote successful resolution of or adaptation to the stressor. There are several chapters dealing with coping in this Handbook and the reader is referred to these for more detailed discussion of this key construct.

Some of the coping behaviours people use may increase their risk for disease or injury regardless of whether they promote successful adaptation. For example, many people under stress smoke more cigarettes, drink more alcohol and are less likely to engage in physical activity (Alexander & Walker, 1994; Ng & Jeffery, 2003). These behaviours, in turn, can negatively impact health status (see 'Health-related behaviours'). Inventories designed to specifically measure these health behaviours should be included in addition to traditional coping checklists. The Fagerström Test for Nicotine Dependence (Heatherton *et al.*, 1991) is commonly used to assess physical dependence to nicotine and includes items that assess quantity of use as well as smoking habits. Other measures, like the Wisconsin Inventory of Smoking Dependence Motives (Piper *et al.*, 2004), are used to assess the types of motivational domains that promote nicotine use. Frequency and quantity of alcohol use are assessed with questionnaires like the Quantity/Variability/Frequency Scale of Alcohol Use (Q-V-F; Cahalan *et al.*, 1969). The four-item CAGE (Ewing, 1984) and the Michigan Alcoholism Screening Test (Selzer, 1971) are popular inventories used to screen for problem drinking. Leisure-time physical activity is another important health behaviour and can be measured by having a participant wear a small device such as an actigraph or pedometer that records bodily movement or can be approximated by having people recall their activities using instruments such as the Paffenbarger Activity Questionnaire (Paffenbarger *et al.*, 1986) and the Godin Leisure Time Exercise Questionnaire (Godin *et al.*, 1986).

In addition to psychological and behavioural changes, stress responding is manifested in many physiological systems within the body. The effects of stress on the sympathetic nervous system (SNS) and the hypothalamic–pituitary–adrenal cortical (HPA) axis were introduced and documented in the seminal work of Cannon (1914) and by Selye (1956/1984). The effects generally consisted of measures of heart rate, blood pressure and the release of epinephrine and norepinephrine by the SNS and the release of adrenocorticotropic hormone (ACTH) and glucocorticoids (i.e. cortisol in humans) from the HPA axis. Heart rate and blood pressure are among the easiest and least expensive measures and have clear implications for health status. In more complex experimental designs an ambulatory blood pressure monitor is attached to a person using electrodes and leads and can be used to record multiple readings and to reduce interference caused by motion.

Depending on the nature of the experiment and the hypotheses tested, neuroendocrine measures such as epinephrine, norepinephrine, ACTH and cortisol can be assessed in the blood, urine, or saliva (Baum & Grunberg, 1997). Acute or momentary changes in these neuroendocrine factors are typically measured in serum. Cortisol can also be measured in saliva, a technique that is less invasive than blood measurements and can be used to examine cortisol's diurnal rhythm. Aggregate measures of neuroendocrine levels over a 15- or 24-hour period of time can be assessed by collecting all urine voided during that time frame. Levels of epinephrine and norepinephrine can also be estimated for the previous seven days by measuring levels of these catecholamines absorbed by blood platelets. Biochemical assays for all of these neuroendocrine factors are readily available and can be performed at moderate expense. Catecholamines such as epinephrine and norepinephrine are typically assessed using radioenzymatic assay (REA) or high-performance liquid chromatography (HPLC). In contrast, corticosteroid and ACTH levels are often assessed by competitive immunoassay, radioimmunoassay (RIA), enzyme-linked immunosorbent assay (ELISA), or double antibody sandwich immunoradiometric assay (IRMA).

Stress-related alterations in immune system functioning have also been observed and appear to be dependent on the nature and duration of the stressor (Segerstrom & Miller, 2004). Acute stressors of limited duration (i.e. minutes) have been generally associated with activation of natural immunity (the more primitive, non-specific markers of immunity such as natural killer cells and macrophages), but with reductions in markers of specific immunity (the slower, more targeted markers of immunity such as B and T cells). In contrast, stress responding of longer duration has been generally characterized by reductions in both types of immunity and has been associated with the onset and course of many diseases such as infectious diseases, cardiovascular disease, arthritis and Type 2 diabetes (Kiecolt-Glaser *et al.*, 2002). For a more detailed description of immune system changes and measures (see 'Psychoneuroimmunology assessments').

Conclusions

The nature of stress has led to a proliferation of measures which has complicated theoretical consolidation and research on the consequences of stress. Depending on the target of a particular investigation, measures should be selected because of their proximal relationship to outcomes of interest or because they are available and collectable. Systematic consideration of the needs of a particular study, as well as the limitations on data collection and sources of data that are available, will typically yield useful measurement approaches. Combinations of measurement, particularly when convergence is possible, constitute one approach to stress assessment.

REFERENCES

Alexander, D. A. & Walker, L. G. (1994). A study of methods used by Scottish police officers to cope with work-induced stress. *Stress Medicine*, 10, 131–8.

Baum, A., Gatchel, R. J. & Schaeffer, M. A. (1983). Emotional, behavioral, and physiological effects of chronic stress at Three Mile Island. *Journal of Consulting and Clinical Psychology*, 51, 565–72.

Baum, A. & Grunberg, N. (1997). Measurement of stress hormones, In S. Cohen, R. C. Kessler & L. U. Gordon (Eds.). *Measuring stress: a guide for health and social scientists* (pp. 175–92). London: Oxford University Press.

Baum, A. & Valins, S. (1977). *Architecture and social behavior: psychological studies of social density*. Hillsdale, NJ: L. Erlbaum Associates.

Brown, G. W. & Harris, T. O. (Eds.). (1989). *Life events and illness*. New York, NY: Guilford Press.

Cahalan, D., Cisin, I. H. & Crossley, H. M. (1969). *American drinking practices: a national study of drinking behavior and attitudes*. New Haven, CT: College and University Press.

Cannon, W. B. (1914). The interrelations of emotions as suggested by recent physiological researches. *American Journal of Physiology*, 25, 256–82.

Cohen, S. (1980). Aftereffects of stress on human performance and social behavior: a review of research and theory. *Psychological Bulletin*, 88, 82–108.

Cohen, S., Kamarck, T. & Mermelstein, R. (1983). A global measure of perceived stress. *Journal of Health and Social Behavior*, 24, 385–96.

Creamer, M., Burgess, P. & Pattison, P. (1992). Reaction to trauma: a cognitive processing model. *Journal of Abnormal Psychology*, 101, 452–9.

Delahanty, D. L., Dougall, A. L., Craig, K. J., Jenkins, F. J. & Baum, A. (1997). Chronic stress and natural killer cell activity following exposure to traumatic death. *Psychosomatic Medicine*, 59, 467–76.

Delongis, A., Folkman, S. & Lazarus, R. S. (1988). The impact of daily stress on health and mood: psychological and social resources as mediators. *Journal of Personality and Social Psychology*, 54, 486–95.

Derogatis, L. R. (1994). *Symptom Checklist-90-R (SCL-90-R): Administration, Scoring, and Procedures Manual* (3rd edn.). Minneapolis, MN: National Computer Systems.

Dougall, A. L., Craig, K. J. & Baum, A. (1999). Assessment of characteristics of intrusive thoughts and their impact on distress among victims of traumatic events. *Psychosomatic Medicine*, **61**, 38–48.

Ewing, J. A. (1984). Detecting alcoholism: the CAGE questionnaire. *Journal of the American Medical Association*, **252** 1905–7.

Folkman, S., Lazarus, R. S., Dunkel-Schetter, C., DeLongis, A. & Gruen, R. J. (1986). Dynamics of a stressful encounter: cognitive appraisal, coping, and encounter outcomes. *Journal of Personality and Social Psychology*, **50**, 992–1003.

Glass, D. C. & Singer, J. E. (1972). *Urban stress: experiments on noise and social stressors*. New York: Academic Press.

Godin, G., Jobin, J. & Bouillon, J. (1986). Assessment of leisure time exercise behavior by self-report: a concurrent validity study. *Canadian Journal of Public Health*, **77**, 359–61.

Greenberg, M. A. (1995). Cognitive processing of traumas: the role of intrusive thoughts and reappraisals. *Journal of Applied Social Psychology*, **25**, 1262–96.

Heatherton, T. F., Kozlowski, L. T., Frecker, R. C. & Fagerström, K. O. (1991). The Fagerström test for nicotine dependence: a revision of the Fagerström tolerance questionnaire. *British Journal of Addiction*, **86**, 1119–27.

Holmes, T. H. & Rahe, R. H. (1967). The social readjustment rating scale. *Journal of Psychosomatic Research*, **11**, 213–18.

Horowitz, M., Wilner, N. & Alvarez, W. (1979). Impact of event scale: a measure of subjective stress. *Psychosomatic Medicine*, **41**, 209–18.

Kanner, A. D., Coyne, J. C., Schaefer, C. & Lazarus, R. S. (1981). Comparison of two modes of stress measurement: daily hassles and uplifts versus major life events. *Journal of Behavioral Medicine*, **4**, 1–39.

Kiecolt-Glaser, J. K., McGuire, L., Robles, T. F. & Glaser, R. (2002). Psychoneuroimmunology: psychological influences on immune function and health.

Journal of Consulting and Clinical Psychology, **70**, 537–47.

Krueger, G. P. (1989). Sustained work, fatigue, sleep loss and performance: a review of the issues. *Work and Stress*, **3**, 129–41.

Kubany, E. S., Haynes, S. N., Leisen, M. B. et al. (2000). Development and preliminary validation of a brief broad-spectrum measure of trauma exposure: the traumatic life events questionnaire. *Psychological Assessment*, **12**, 210–24.

Lazarus, R. S. & Folkman, S. (1984). *Stress, appraisal, and coping*. New York: Springer.

Lazarus, R. S., Kanner, A. & Folkman, S. (1980). Emotions: a cognitive–phenomenological analysis. In R. Plutchik & H. Kellerman (Eds.). *Theories of emotion* (pp. 189–217). New York: Academic Press.

McNair, P. M., Lorr, M. & Droppleman, L. F. (1981). *POMS Manual* (2nd edn.). San Diego: Educational and Industrial Testing Service.

Ng, D. M. & Jeffery, R. W. (2003). Relationships between perceived stress and health behaviors in a sample of working adults. *Health Psychology*, **22**, 638–42.

Norris, F. H. (1990). Screening for traumatic stress: a scale for use in the general population. *Journal of Applied Social Psychology*, **20**, 1704–18.

Paffenbarger, R. S., Hyde, R. T., Wing, A. L. & Hsieh, C. C. (1986). Physical activity, all-cause mortality, and longevity of college alumni. *New England Journal of Medicine*, **314**, 605–13.

Peacock, E. J. & Wong, P. T. (1990). The stress appraisal measure (SAM): a multidimensional approach to cognitive appraisal. *Stress Medicine*, **6**, 227–36.

Piper, M. E., Piasecki, T. M., Federman, E. B. et al. (2004). A multiple motives approach to tobacco dependence: the Wisconsin inventory of smoking dependence motives (WISDM-68). *Journal of Consulting and Clinical Psychology*, **72**, 139–54.

Rahe, R. H. (1975). Epidemiological studies of life change and illness. *International*

Journal of Psychiatry in Medicine, **6**, 133–46.

Sarason, I. G., de Monchaux, C. & Hunt, T. (1975). Methodological issues in the assessment of life stress. In L. Levi (Ed.). *Emotions: their parameters and measurement* (pp. 499–509). New York: Raven Press.

Segerstrom, S. C. & Miller, G. E. (2004). Psychological stress and the human immune system: a meta-analytic study of 30 years of inquiry. *Psychological Bulletin*, **130**, 601–30.

Selye, H. (1984). *The stress of life* (Rev. edn.). New York: McGraw-Hill. (Original work published in 1956.)

Selzer, M. L. (1971). The Michigan alcoholism screening test: the quest for a new diagnostic instrument. *American Journal of Psychiatry*, **127**, 1653–8.

Shaham, Y., Singer, J. E. & Schaeffer, M. H. (1992). Stability/instability of cognitive strategies across tasks determine whether stress will affect judgmental processes. *Journal of Applied Social Psychology*, **22**, 691–713.

Skinner, N. & Brewer, N. (2002). The dynamics of threat and challenge appraisals prior to stressful achievement events. *Journal of Personality and Social Psychology*, **83**, 678–92.

Spielberger, C. D. (1983). *State–trait anxiety inventory*. Palo Alto, CA: Mind Garden.

Vitaliano, P. P., Russo, J., Weber, L. & Celum, C. (1993). The dimensions of stress scale: psychometric properties. *Journal of Applied Social Psychology*, **23**, 1847–78.

Watson, D., Clark, L. A. & Tellegen, A. (1988). Development and validation of brief measures of positive and negative affect: the PANAS scales. *Journal of Personality and Social Psychology*, **54**, 1063–70.

Weiss, D. S. & Marmar, C. R. (1997). The impact of event scale – revised. In J. P. Wilson & T. M. Keane (Eds.). *Assessing psychological trauma and PTSD* (pp. 399–411). New York: Guilford Press.

Witkin, C. B., Goodenough, D. R. & Oltman, D. K. (1979). Psychological differentiation: current status. *Journal of Personality and Social Psychology*, **37**, 1127–45.

Section III

Psychological intervention

Behaviour therapy

Gerald C. Davison

University of Southern California

Behaviour therapy, sometimes also called behaviour modification, developed initially during the 1950s through the work of people like B.F. Skinner (1953) and Joseph Wolpe (1958). The attempt was to create an approach to intervention that relied on experimentally tested principles of learning. In its earliest years the emphasis in behaviour therapy was on classical and operant conditioning and throughout the 1960s and thereafter a number of therapeutic techniques were developed that purportedly rested on these experimental foundations. The word 'purportedly' is used intentionally here because an ongoing scientific controversy has surrounded the extent to which behaviour therapy techniques truly derive their effectiveness from learning principles developed primarily from infrahuman experimentation. Suffice it to say that the most innovative techniques came from practising clinicians whose thinking was guided and enriched by their awareness of certain learning principles and by their creative attempts to apply them in the complex and often chaotic domain of clinical intervention. There is considerable evidence from numerous research settings worldwide that many of these techniques are helpful for dealing with a wide range of psychological disorders (see Davison *et al.*, 2004). This chapter will provide a historical overview of the development on behaviour therapy, followed by a description of some of the techniques encompassed by this approach, and conclude with a consideration of some conceptual issues in behaviour therapy.

An early behaviour therapy effort was by Andrew Salter (1949), whose book *Condition reflex therapy* represented an attempt to rationalize assertion training in Pavlovian conditioning terms. Salter was perhaps the first to argue that many anxious and depressed individuals could be helped by encouraging them to express openly to others both their likes and dislikes. He used Pavlovian theorizing to argue that much human psychological suffering arises from an excess of cortical inhibition, a state that could be reversed by an increase in emotional expressiveness. While the theorizing is doubtful, the approach in general is widely employed and even has links with humanistic emphases on become more aware of and expressing one's basic needs (Perls, 1969; Rogers, 1951).

Also in the classical conditioning camp is Joseph Wolpe, whose book *Psychotherapy by reciprocal inhibition* has had an enormous impact on the thinking and practices of behaviourally oriented clinicians. Trained in medicine and basing his work on Mary Cover Jones's (1924) classic case study with a fearful child, Wolpe conducted experiments with cats to show that pairing the pleasure of eating with graduated exposure to conditioned aversive stimuli (harmless situations that had been paired with painful electric shock) could markedly reduce, if not altogether eliminate, acquired fear and avoidance. Extrapolating from this and related research on conditioned fear (e.g. Miller, 1948; Mowrer, 1939), Wolpe devised his technique of systematic desensitization, which entails training the patient in deep muscle relaxation, constructing with the patient a hierarchy of situations that elicit varying degrees of unwarranted and unwanted fear and presenting each situation seriatim to the imagination of the person in a relaxed, non-anxious state. The idea is to counter-condition the fear, that is, enable the patient to confront a fearsome event without experiencing the usual anxiety, thereby changing the response to the presumed conditioned stimulus from fear to neutrality or even positive interest. It would appear that the applicability of this technique is limited only by the ingenuity of the clinician in construing a patient's problems in terms that permit the construction of an anxiety hierarchy (Goldfried & Davison, 1994). Usually these imaginal exposures are supplemented, sometimes even replaced, by real-life exposures to what the person needlessly fears, cf. in vivo desensitization, especially in the treatment of agoraphobia. Recently the technological innovation of virtual reality (VR) has been introduced to present patients with very realistic representations of what they fear. Driven by high-speed computers, a device mounted on the person's head creates a lifelike depiction of a fearsome situation, enhancing the capacity to become immersed in simulated situations that are more controllable than during in vivo exposures and perhaps closer to reality than what the person could imagine.

In recent years the efficacy of extended exposure without anxiety-inhibiting responses like relaxation has been demonstrated for a variety of disorders, especially obsessive–compulsive disorder. It is now argued that gradual approaches, such as Wolpe's technique of systematic desensitization, which allow escape from anxiety-provoking situations, may impede the reduction of unwarranted anxieties (Emmelkamp, 2004). On the other hand, the more confrontive procedures involved in extended exposure can produce greater stress in patients and as a consequence, a greater tendency to drop out of treatment.

Another approach usually considered to derive its efficacy from classical conditioning is aversion therapy, which involves pairing an undesirably attractive event or stimulus with a negative emotional state such as fear or disgust. The effectiveness as well as the morality of aversive procedures have been a subject of heated debate over the past three decades, but many reports attest to its usefulness in dealing with problems such as excessive drinking of alcohol, smoking, overeating and the paraphilias (Emmelkamp, 2004).

The general approach other than classical conditioning that historically lies at the core of behaviour therapy is operant conditioning, deriving from Skinner's work on the importance of contingencies in behaviour, that is, whether a given response is followed by a positive reinforcer like food or praise, or by a negative reinforcer like pain or disapproval. Operant techniques attracted a great deal of favourable attention in the 1960s through the seminal work of Staats and Staats (1963) and others, who showed that reinforcement contingencies could favourably affect such problems as regressive crawling in children, poor academic performance, inappropriate social behaviour of various kinds and non-compliance to therapeutic instructions. The positive reinforcement of adaptive interpersonal skills is emerging as a likely active ingredient in Aaron Beck's cognitive therapy for depression (see 'Cognitive behaviour therapy'). A notable achievement of the operant approach is the token economy (Ayllon & Azrin, 1968), a system whereby tokens are awarded for desirable behaviour and sometimes also taken away for undesirable behaviour and later exchanged for goodies like sweets or access to better dining facilities for hospitalized adult patients. In a functional sense, the token economy brings to the institutionalized setting the orderliness of a market economy, whereby particular behaviours are given a certain value within the parameters of a monetary system.

A particularly significant example of the power of a token economy is provided by Paul and Lentz (1977), who studied three methods of rehabilitating severely impaired chronic mental patients. The comparison treatments were (1) milieu therapy, which essentially set expectations for the patients but without the highly structured contingencies of the token economy; and (2) a routine hospital management group, which entailed continued usage of heavy doses of neuroleptic medication. The token economy achieved better success in reducing symptomatology and shaping useful self-care and social skills. It should be mentioned that there were cognitive elements as well within the token economy condition, an issue we explore below.

While difficult to categorize as behaviour therapy, modelling is widely used by behaviour therapists as an efficient way to teach complex patterns of behaviour. The early research programme of Albert Bandura (Bandura & Walters, 1963) documented the powerful effects of observing another person perform sometimes complex patterns of behaviour. Evidence indicates that people can acquire behavioural patterns without reinforcement, but that their performance of what they have learned is indeed influenced by expected contingencies. A noteworthy application of modelling can be found in role-playing or behaviour rehearsal (Lazarus, 1971), whereby a therapist models effective behaviour and then encourages the patient to follow suit. This has become a central part of the treatment of social phobia, especially when the patient lacks the interpersonal skills which are necessary for positive social interactions. It is likely as well that anxiety is extinguished by exposure to situations like talking with others or being evaluated on one's performance. Irrational fears can also be reduced by watching a fearless model interact with the frightening stimulus (Bandura & Menlove, 1968). The fact that something important is learned by watching another person suggests that cognitive processes are important.

The foregoing summarizes briefly the techniques and approaches usually associated with the phrases 'behaviour therapy' or 'behaviour modification'. However, since the late 1960s, there has been increasing recognition of the role of cognitive processes in therapeutic behaviour change, not only in the form of the cognitive therapies described in a separate entry but within those therapies judged to rely on classical and operant conditioning. For example, Wolpe's systematic desensitization has been conceptualized as a cognitive change technique or at least a procedure that relies on the patient's cognitive abilities (Davison & Wilson, 1973). After all, patients imagine what is troubling them and these symbolic exposures lead to anxiety reduction in actual fearsome situations.

What then is behaviour therapy? It can be seen from this chapter that whether behaviour therapy should include explicit attention to cognition or be restricted to conditioning principles is dependent upon the theoretical stance one takes. For example, the Skinnerian legacy would purport that behaviour therapy should concentrate only on overt behaviours; yet the tradition of Mowrer, Miller and Wolpe would also include mediating behaviours. Ultimately answers depend upon who is responding. To this writer and many others, behaviour therapy refers most generally and most usefully to a laboratory-based, empirical approach to therapeutic change. There need not be any prior allegiance to particular theories or principles of change. Behaviour therapists strive to use rigorous standards of proof rather than to rely on untested and sometimes even untestable concepts such as the Freudian unconscious (see 'Psychodynamic psychotherapy'). In sum, behaviour therapy/behaviour modification is an attempt to change abnormal behaviour, thoughts and feelings by applying in the clinical context the epistemologies, methods and discoveries made by non-applied behavioural scientists in their study of both normal and abnormal behaviour. Viewed in this way, any consideration of behaviour therapy would be incomplete without the inclusion of cognitive concepts (see also 'Biofeedback', 'Cognitive behaviour therapy' and 'Group therapy').

REFERENCES

Ayllon, T. & Azrin, N. H. (1968). *The token ceremony: a motivational system for therapy and rehabilitation.* New York: Appleton–Century–Crofts.

Bandura, A. & Menlove, F. L. (1968). Factors determining vicarious extinction of avoidance behavior through symbolic modelling. *Journal of Personality and Social Psychology, 8,* 99–108.

Bandura, A. & Walters, R. H. (1963). *Social learning and personality development.* New York: Holt, Rinehart & Winston.

Davison, G. C., Neale, J. M. & Kring, A. M. (2004). *Abnormal Psychology* (9th edn.). New York: Wiley.

Davison, G. C. & Wilson, G. T. (1973). Processes of fear-reduction in systematic desensitization: cognitive and social reinforcement factors in humans. *Behavior Therapy, 4,* 1–21.

Emmelkamp, P. M. G. (2004). Behavior therapy with adults. In M. J. Lambert (Ed.). *Bergin and Garfield's Handbook of Psychotherapy and Behavior Change* (5th edn.) (pp. 393–446). New York: Wiley.

Goldfried, M. R. & Davison, G. C. (1994). *Clinical behavior therapy.* Expanded edition. New York: Wiley-Interscience.

Jones, M. C. (1924). A laboratory study of fear: the case of Peter. *Pedagogical Seminary, 31,* 308–15.

Lazarus, A. A. (1971). *Behavior therapy and beyond.* New York: McGraw-Hill.

Miller, N. E. (1948). Studies of fear as an acquirable drive: I. Fear as motivation and fear-reduction as reinforcement in the learning of new responses. *Journal of Experimental Psychology, 38,* 89–101.

Mowrer, O. H. (1939). A stimulus–response analysis of anxiety and its role as a reinforcing agent. *Psychological Review*, **46**, 553–65.

Paul, G. I. & Lentz, R. J. (1977). *Psychological treatment of chronic mental patients: milieu versus social learning programs.* Cambridge, MA: Harvard University Press.

Perls, F. S. (1969). *Gestalt therapy verbatim.* Moab, UT: Real People Press.

Rogers, C. R. (1951). *Client-centered therapy.* Boston: Houghton-Mifflin.

Salter, A. (1949). *Conditioned reflex therapy.* New York: Farrar, Straus.

Skinner, B. F. (1953). *Science and human behavior.* New York: Macmillan.

Staats, A. W. & Staats, C. K. (1963). *Complex human behavior.* New York: Holt, Rinehart & Winston.

Wolpe, J. (1958). *Psychotherapy by reciprocal inhibition.* Stanford, CA: Stanford University Press.

Biofeedback

Robert J. Gatchel[1], Carl Noe[2] and Raymond Gaeta[3]

[1]The University of Texas at Arlington
[2]Baylor University Medical Center
[3]Stanford University

Over the years, there have been various unusual instances of the voluntary control over physiological functions noted in the scientific literature. Luria (1958) presented a case of a mnemonist who had remarkable control of his heart rate and skin temperature to the degree that he could abruptly alter his heart rate by 50 beats per minute, and could also raise the skin temperature of one hand while simultaneously lowering the temperature of the other hand. The modification of physiological activities such as this has been the subject of anecdotal reports for a considerable period of time. Although true empirical investigation into such self-regulation through biofeedback began in the 1960s, gaining voluntary control of various physiological activities has been a goal in many different cultures for a variety of reasons. Gatchel (1999) and Gatchel *et al.* (2003*b*) have reviewed the goals that have been traditionally sought with regard to gaining control of physiological functioning:

- In order to achieve spiritual enlightenment, yogis and other mystics of the eastern tradition have demonstrated that through certain physical exercises, or by a sheer act of will, that individuals are capable of producing significant physiochemical changes in their bodies which, in turn, produce perceived pleasant states of consciousness (Bagchi, 1959; Bagchi & Wenger, 1957).
- In order to test various theories of learning, psychologists have long debated the issue of whether autonomic nervous system responses could be operantly conditioned.
- During the 1960s, biofeedback was viewed as a potential clinical treatment procedure for modifying psychological and medical disorders.

The major focus of this present chapter is on the third category of how voluntary control of physiological activity can be used as a clinical treatment modality for medically related disorders. This particular area has contributed significantly to the growing field of behavioural medicine and health psychology. Indeed, as mentioned earlier, beginning in the 1960s, clinical researchers have gained control of physiological functions which were previously considered to be outside the realm of volitional control. The biofeedback method was the most popular of these training methods, and it also afforded clinical researchers the ability to translate the research in the laboratory setting to more practical clinical applications. For example, biofeedback was used to teach individuals to lower their blood pressure to manage hypertension, or to decrease muscle tension to treat musculo-skeletal pain. Biofeedback and other techniques, such as relaxation training, were used to address clinical problems and were developed to the point that Birk (1973) eventually coined the term 'behavioural medicine' to describe the application of a behavioural treatment technique (biofeedback) that could be applied to medicine or medical problems (e.g. headache pain).

The biofeedback technique

The biofeedback technique itself is based on the fundamental learning principle that people learn to perform a particular response when they receive feedback or information about the consequences of that response, and then make the appropriate compensatory behaviour adjustments. This is how individuals have learned to perform the wide variety of skills and behaviours utilized in the activities of everyday living. The availability of feedback is also of extreme importance in learning how to control internal physiological responses. However, much of our biological behaviour is concerned with maintaining a constant internal 'homeostasis' and is not

Table 1. Summary of medical and pain disorders for which biofeedback has been applied

Medical disorder	Summary of findings
Asthma	Although clinical studies have suggested the effectiveness of EMG biofeedback for asthma reduction, there have been a number of methodological problems associated with such studies. Non-specific placebo factors may play an important role in asthma reduction.
Cardiac arrhythmias	The few cases available indicate that heart rate biofeedback seems to be effective in the treatment of cardiac arrhythmias such as sinus tachycardia, atrial fibrillation and premature ventricular contractions. However, judgement must be withheld with regard to therapeutic value of biofeedback for such disorders generally until more research is conducted.
Dermatological disorders	Although there have been some case studies suggesting the therapeutic effectiveness of biofeedback-assisted behavioural treatment techniques, there have been no well controlled studies conducted to date. Moreover, there are various forms of dermatological disorders which may be differentially responsive to such treatment.
Dyskinesias	Biofeedback techniques have been used to treat a number of different dyskinesias, including spasmatic torticollis, Parkinson's disease tardive dyskinesia and Huntington's disease. Individual and multiple case reports suggest a possible use of EMG in the treatment of these disorders. However, the role of biofeedback is unclear because controls were not used.
Epileptic seizures	At this time, the amount of control group research concerning possible therapeutic effects of EEG biofeedback for the treatment of epileptic seizures is limited and all but the most speculative conclusions are premature. Positive results have been reported that are encouraging and it would seem to justify additional research.
Essential hypertension	Research has shown some degree of success in reducing the symptoms of essential hypertension with biofeedback. Blood pressure can be effectively reduced using biofeedback. However, biofeedback is still an experimental form of treatment for hypertension, with little known about the exact physiological mechanisms involved in the process. Thus, it cannot be considered an alternative to pharmacological treatment at this time. Biofeedback is often used as one component in a more comprehensive behavioural intervention.
Gastrointestinal disorders	Research results of the biofeedback-assisted modification of gastrointestinal disorders are encouraging. Biofeedback by means of rectal or anal devices is currently the treatment of choice for many types of fecal incontinence. Moreover, it is likely to become a preferred treatment method for patients with constipation related to the inability to relax the striated pelvic floor muscles during defaecation. In addition, thermal-biofeedback, as part of a comprehensive behavioural treatment programme is a promising approach to the treatment of irritable bowel syndrome.
Insomnia	There is a great deal of evidence indicating that biofeedback and relaxation techniques, as components of a more comprehensive behavioural treatment programme, are effective in the treatment of insomnia.
Lower motor neuron dysfunctions	The case studies reporting the successful application of biofeedback in the treatment of lower motor neuron dysfunction (EEG, peripheral nerve injury, Bell's Palsy) must currently be interpreted with some caution, given the lack of control procedures.
Migraine headache	Research suggests that temperature biofeedback, combined with autogenic training, is more effective than no treatment and possibly superior to placebo treatments. Thus, such an approach is warranted for the treatment of migraine.
Muscle contraction headaches	The effects of EMG biofeedback exceed those for medication placebo, biofeedback placebo and psychotherapy procedures. In addition, although research suggests that biofeedback and relaxation produce similar levels of improvement, biofeedback may offer greater benefits to a sub-set of patients.
Postural hypotension	There is no effective treatment for this disorder, and severely affected patients must remain in the supine position. Although control group studies are not yet available, several good case studies have demonstrated that systolic blood pressure biofeedback training has enabled some patients to sit upright or to stand with crutches, whereas prior to training these actions produced fainting.
Raynaud's disease	Recent controlled research studies involving over 160 patients have shown that behavioural treatment, with biofeedback as a key modality, can be very effective, equalling the best clinical effects of many medical and surgical interventions. In the light of the limitations of current medical and surgical treatments for Raynaud's disease, behavioural interventions appear to have much to offer for these patients.
Sexual dysfunction	Although genital responses have been shown to be responsive to both instructional control and biofeedback, there is no evidence that the direct conditioning of genital responses through biofeedback has therapeutic value. However, biofeedback may have a role to play in guiding the development of erotic and non-erotic fantasy, which can, in turn, have significant therapeutic value.
Tinnitus	There have been a few case studies indicating the effectiveness of biofeedback and relaxation methods in reducing the severity of tinnitus symptoms.
Upper motor neuron dysfunctions	A number of well designed individual and multiple case studies has suggested the therapeutic effectiveness of biofeedback in the treatment of upper motor neuron disorders such as paresis, cerebral palsy and incomplete spinal cord lesion. However, an appropriate number of control group experiments is still lacking except in the biofeedback treatment of paresis, where results are negative of ambiguous.

Table 1. (*cont.*)

Pain disorder	Summary of research findings
Back pain	Low back pain is one of the most costly of the musculoskeletal disorders. Flor and Birbaumer (1994) have provided some support for EMG biofeedback being more effective than cognitive behavioural therapy or conservative medical therapy with patients suffering from chronic back pain and temporomandibular pain.
Fibromyalgia syndrome	Widespread musculo-skeletal pain, fatigue and multiple tender points characterize fibromyalgia syndrome. Many practitioners use multiple recording sites and simultaneous EMG biofeedback while patients are in multiple postures, positions and acute stressor conditions. While muscle relaxation therapies and EMG biofeedback are logical parts of the recommended multidisciplinary treatment approaches, to date there is very little research on this topic.
Headache	Studies have found successful outcomes using EMG to reduce pain in these disorders. It should be noted that individuals presenting with headaches often suffer from more than one variety, making treatment and debates regarding aetiology difficult. Research, however, suggests that temperature/thermal biofeedback is more effective than no treatment when combined with autogenic/relaxation training for migraine headache. In addition, these treatments may be superior to placebo treatments. For tension/muscle contraction headaches, EMG biofeedback effects may exceed those of medication placebo, biofeedback placebo and psychotherapy procedures. Moreover, while research suggests that biofeedback and relaxation produce similar levels of improvement for this type of headache, biofeedback may offer greater benefits for a subset of patients.
Temporomandibular Disorders (TMD)	The use of biofeedback technique to cultivate low arousal in TMD patients appears to be effective. EMG and other biofeedback techniques can be improved both to improve the comprehension of individual patient issues, as well as to improve functioning. EMG, in particular, is often used to evaluate appliances for particular individuals, re-educate the masticatory, facial, postural and potentially respiratory muscles and aid in proprioceptive deficits and psychophysiologic problems. Overall, a considerable number of studies attest to the efficacy of biofeedback training, especially when accompanied by relaxation or general stress management training.
Upper extremity disorders	Upper extremity disorders, such as carpal tunnel syndrome, are a growing problem in occupational settings. Although there have been few well controlled studies in this area, those that exist suggest that biofeedback can aid in treatment effectiveness when used in unison with a more comprehensive interdisciplinary programme.

readily accessible to conscious awareness. Indeed, individuals do not consciously experience some interoceptive awareness of internal biological activity, such as their blood pressure or muscle tension, because there is normally an adaptive advantage to not having to consciously attend or control these activities on a continuous basis. Moreover, interoceptors do not normally have the extensive afferent representation at the cortical level that is needed for a high degree of perceptual acuity or the fine discriminating characteristics of audition or vision (Gatchel, 1999).

Because individuals do not normally receive feedback of these internal events in day-to-day situations, they cannot be expected to control them. However, if they are provided biofeedback of, say, heart rate via a visual display monitor, they can become more aware of the consequences of heart rate changes and the ways adjustments can be made to modify and eventually control it. Receiving feedback serves to remove the 'blindfold', and enables individuals to voluntarily control their response. The development of sensitive physiological recording devices and digital logic technology has made it possible to detect small changes in visceral events and provide subjects with immediate feedback of these biological responses. Thus, biofeedback involves developing an individual's ability to alter a particular physiological response by providing them with feedback about the response which they are attempting to control. For example, an individual may attempt to alter muscle tension, blood flow, or surface skin temperature. Subjects are most commonly provided feedback in the form of a tone, or other auditory signals, or a visual display, such as a line that moves up or down on a computer screen. Electromyography (EMG) which involves feedback of muscle tension is one of the most common types of biofeedback. Other types of biofeedback include thermal biofeedback, which provides information on skin temperatures; electroencephalography (EEG), which provides information on brain wave activity; an electrodermal response (EDR), which provides information on sweat gland activity. Often, individuals may receive biofeedback information from more than one of these modalities (Green & Shellenberger, 1999).

Today, biofeedback is broadly and loosely, defined as a procedure for transforming some aspect of physiological behaviour into electrical signals that are made accessible to exteroception or awareness (usually vision or audition). Sometimes, the feedback signal is combined with a tangible reward, such as money or the opportunity to view attractive pictures, in an attempt to motivate the individual and strengthen the effect of the target physiological response. In other cases, the clinician provides verbal praise for success in addition to the feedback. These latter practices are also forms of biofeedback, because they too convey information to learners about their biological performance. In most instances, however, response-contingent lights or tones alone can be shown to augment voluntary control of physiological activity.

The growth in the utilization of biofeedback techniques

Borrowing heavily from operant conditioning techniques developed in psychology, the early biofeedback investigators during the 1960s and 1970s began to demonstrate some degree of operant or voluntary control in a wide variety of visceral, central nervous system and somato motor functions. Gatchel and Price (1979) provided an early review of this research that demonstrated learned control by human subjects of a wide variety of 'involuntary responses' including cardiac ventricular rate, systolic and diastolic blood pressure, peripheral vascular responses, electrodermal activity, gastric motility, skin temperature, penile tumescence and various brain wave rhythms. Encouraged by these early successes demonstrating voluntary control of normal physiological activity, medical and psychological clinicians soon began to address the issue of whether pathophysiological activity could also be controlled with the goal of restoring health or preventing illness. This stimulated a rapid growth of the scientific literature evaluating the clinical effectiveness of biofeedback. This research has been reviewed in a number of different sources (e.g. Green & Shellenberger, 1999; Hatch *et al.*, 1987; White & Tursky, 1982). A journal was also established (*Biofeedback and Self-Regulation*, which is now called *Applied Psychophysiology and Biofeedback*) and a professional society specializing in biofeedback and self-regulation (Association for Applied Psychophysiology and Biofeedback) was founded. There are also a number of useful practitioner guides which have been published (e.g. Basmajian, 1989; Schwartz & Andrasik, 2003).

To date, the clinical research literature has clearly demonstrated that some degree of self-control is possible over behaviours long assumed to be completely involuntary. It has also been shown that, with biofeedback, it is possible to extend voluntary control to pathophysiological responding in order to modify the maladaptive behaviour in the direction of health. Table 1 summarizes the various disorders for which biofeedback has been applied.

As can be seen in Table 1, in some areas, such as treatment of insomnia and headache, biofeedback has been successful. However, as reviewed elsewhere (Gatchel, 1997, 1999), many important questions still remain concerning the extent to which biofeedback and other physiological self-control techniques will be medically effective. Unfortunately, the current research evaluating therapeutic effectiveness of these procedures has been plagued by a number of problems. For example, there have been very few well controlled clinical outcome studies that have been conducted using large numbers of patients having well confirmed medical diagnoses. Moreover, the few comparative outcome studies that have been performed evaluate the relative effectiveness of biofeedback and various other behavioural techniques (e.g. simple relaxation training). It is extremely helpful to also compare biofeedback techniques with more traditional medical treatments, some of which have fairly well established success rates. Combinations of medical and behavioural techniques should also be explored and evaluated.

It should also be pointed out that, unfortunately, there have been claims for the therapeutic efficacy of biofeedback which have been grossly exaggerated and even wrong. Overall, it is justifiable to conclude that relevant and encouraging data do exist but, at the present time, the value of biofeedback still has to be questioned in some areas. Moreover, terms such as 'biofeedback therapist' and 'biofeedback clinic', which are now regularly encountered in many medical centres, are difficult to justify. They imply that a form of treatment exists that is more or less generally applicable for a variety of illnesses. Worse yet, they imply, at least in the minds of some, that biofeedback is a new alternative treatment modality. Currently, in the majority of areas in which it is applied, biofeedback should be viewed merely as an adjunctive treatment modality.

Biofeedback and pain

One area where biofeedback is being increasingly used as an adjunctive treatment modality is pain management. Pain is a complex and debilitating medical condition which affects more than 50 million people in the United States alone. Pain also accounts for approximately 80% of all physician visits (Gatchel & Turk, 1996). The number of Americans utilizing pain management programmes has increased 64% from 1998 to 2000 (Marketdata Enterprises, 2001). The complexity of pain and the absence of any one simple method to treat pain necessitates examining which treatments will have the highest likelihood of success for any given patient (Gatchel *et al.*, 2003*a*). In an early review of research on the application of biofeedback for the regulation of pain, Turk *et al.* (1979) concluded that biofeedback was no better than other less expensive and less instrument-oriented treatments such as progressive relaxation training and coping skills training. In addition, evidence for the effectiveness of biofeedback in reducing pain was marginal at best. The evidence was based mainly on case studies and poorly controlled research. Although this status has not changed much since the 1979 review, some subsequent studies have found that biofeedback is useful in reducing pain. In fact, since the earlier pessimistic view of biofeedback, training in biofeedback does appear to provide patients with information that enables them to control voluntarily some aspect of their physiology that may contribute to the pain experience. Currently, biofeedback is viewed as beneficial for patients when used as one component of an interdisciplinary pain-management programme (Gatchel, 2004; Gatchel *et al.*, 2003*b*). For example, biofeedback, in combination with cognitive behavioural therapy, provides powerful evidence of the relationship between thoughts, feelings and physiological functioning. In addition, cognitive behavioural therapy with biofeedback increases the patient's sense of self-efficacy by providing clear and unequivocal feedback about a person's ability to gain control over certain physiological responses. However, because pain is a complex behaviour and not merely a pure sensory experience, biofeedback is most beneficial for patients when used as one adjunctive component of an interdisciplinary pain management programme (Gatchel *et al.*, 2003*b*). In this context, a true biopsychosocial approach to the patient can be undertaken, and an interdisciplinary team can address the 'whole person', rather than just the pathophysiology. Moreover, biofeedback is then performed not only within the larger context of the interdisciplinary pain clinic, but also in the context of cognitive behavioural therapy. A summary of specific pain disorders in which biofeedback has been effectively utilized appears in Table 1. It should be noted that most of these pain conditions were treated from a biopsychosocial perspective in an interdisciplinary setting.

Biofeedback and the placebo effect

When considering the use of biofeedback as a treatment modality, it should be clearly kept in mind that research has demonstrated the important impact that the placebo effect has in biofeedback and other physiological self-control techniques directed at eliminating emotional distress. The placebo effect itself was originally shown to be an important factor in medical research when it was found that inert chemical drugs, which had no direct effects on physical events underlying various medical disorders, were often found to produce symptom reduction. An extensive scientific literature on the placebo effect in medicine unequivocally demonstrated that a patient's belief that a prescribed medication is active, even if it was in fact chemically inert, often led to significant symptom reduction (e.g. Honigfeld, 1964; Shapiro, 1971). Indeed, Shapiro (1959, p. 303) noted that 'The history of medical treatment until relatively recently is the history of the placebo effect'. Even response to a chemically active drug to some degree depends on a belief in the drug's actions and faith in the doctor prescribing it (see 'Placebos').

As Gatchel (2004) has recently noted, the placebo effect has been shown to be involved in the reduction of pain. In a number of painful conditions, up to one-third of individuals experiencing pain can obtain significant relief following the administration of a placebo (in the form of either a non-active drug or a strong suggestion that increases a patient's expectancy of therapeutic improvement). The mechanisms involved in this placebo analgesia effect are still not totally understood, although factors affecting endogenous opioid activity appear important (Baum *et al.*, 1997). Moreover, recent imaging studies of the brain are beginning to isolate other biological bases of the placebo effect (e.g. Mayberg *et al.*, 2002). Despite this, it is clear that a clinician can help decrease pain in a certain percentage of patients by simply providing a placebo or a strong expectation of therapeutic improvement. Enthusiastic management of patients' ability to manage their pain by controlling physiological activity through biofeedback goes a long way in maximizing the efficacy of the biofeedback technique itself.

Conclusions

Physiological self-regulation techniques such as biofeedback have an important place in the rapidly growing field of health psychology. To date, there is a great deal of research demonstrating the efficacy of biofeedback as an adjunctive treatment modality in helping to manage a wide variety of medically related disorders. It should be emphasized, however, that more controlled research is still required to unequivocally document its effectiveness for many of the disorders. In addition, biofeedback should be viewed merely as an important adjunctive treatment modality to use as part of a more comprehensive treatment programme. Many disorders are complex, biopsychosocial illnesses which will not be totally responsive to a single treatment modality. Finally, the therapeutic effects of biofeedback are not due solely to the direct link to physiological activity, but also to the psychological process of perceived control which is often associated with the placebo effect. Further investigation of the complex biopsychosocial mechanisms underlying the therapeutic efficacy of biofeedback should lead to a greater refinement of training methods and a resultant more effective overall treatment strategy.

REFERENCES

Ader, R. (2000). The placebo effect: if it's all in your head, does that mean you only think you feel better? *Advances In Mind-Body Medicine*, **16**(1), 7–11.

Annent, J. (1969). *Feedback and human behavior*. Baltimore: Penguin Books.

Bagchi, B. K. (1959). Mysticism and mist in India. *Journal of the Denver Society of Psychosomatic Dentistry and Medicine*, **16**, 1–32.

Bagchi, B. K. & Wenger, M. A. (1957). Electro-physiological correlates of some yogi exercises. *Electroencephalography and Clinical Neurophysiology* (Supp. 7), 132–49.

Basmajian, J. V. (Ed.). (1989). *Biofeedback: principles and practice for clinicians*. Baltimore: Williams & Wilkins.

Baum, A., Gatchel, R. J. & Krantz, D. S. (Eds.). (1997). *An Introduction To Health Psychology* (3rd edn.) New York: McGraw-Hill.

Birk, L. (1973). *Biofeedback: behavioral medicine*. New York: Grune & Stratton.

Flor, H. & Birbaumer, N. (1994). Psychophysiological methods in the assessment and treatment of chronic musculoskeletal pain. In J. G. Carlson, A. R. Seifert & N. Birbaumer (Eds.). *Clinical applied psychophysiology*. New York: Plenum.

Gatchel, R. J. (1997). Biofeedback. In A. Baum, C. McManus, S. Newman, J. Weinman & R. West (Eds.). *Cambridge Handbook of Psychology, Health and Medicine*. London: Cambridge University Press.

Gatchel, R. J. (1999). Biofeedback and self-regulation of physiological activity: a major adjunctive treatment modality in health psychology. In A. Baum, T. Revensen & J. E. Singer (Eds.). *Handbook Of Health Psychology*. Hillsdale, NJ: Erlbaum.

Gatchel, R. J. (2004). *Clinical essentials of pain management*. Washington, DC: American Psychological Association.

Gatchel, R. J., Polatin, P. B., Noe, C. E. *et al.* (2003*a*). Treatment and cost-effectiveness of early intervention for acute low back pain patients: a one-year prospective study. *Journal of Occupational Rehabilitation*, **13**, 1–9.

Gatchel, R. J. & Price, K. P. (1979). Biofeedback: an introduction and historical overview. In R. J. Gatchel & K. P. Price (Eds.). *Clinical applications of biofeedback: appraisal and status*. Elmsford: Pergamon.

Gatchel, R. J., Robinson, R. C., Pulliam, C. & Maddrey, A. M. (2003*b*). Biofeedback with pain patients: evidence for its effectiveness. *Seminars In Pain Management*, **1**, 55–66.

Gatchel, R. J. & Turk, D. C. (1996). *Psychological approaches to pain management: a practitioner's handbook*. New York: Guilford Publications, Inc.

Green, J. A. & Shellenberger, R. (1999). Biofeedback therapy. In W. B. Jonas & J. S. Levin (Eds.). *Essentials of complementary and alternative medicine*, (pp. 410–25). Baltimore, MD: Lippincott Williams & Wilkins.

Hatch, J. P., Fisher, J. G. & Rugh, J. D. (Eds.). (1987). *Biofeedback: studies in clinical efficacy*. New York: Plenum.

Honigfeld, G. (1964). Non-Specific factors in treatment. I. Review of placebo reactions and placebo reactors. *Diseases of the Nervous Systems*, **25**, 145–56.

Lang, P. J. (1970). Autonomic control or learning to play the internal organs. *Psychology* (October), 19–33.

Lindsley, D. B. & Sassaman, W. H. (1938). Autonomic activity and brain potentials associated with voluntary control of pilomotors. *Journal Of Neurophysiology*, **1**, 342–9.

Luria, A. R. (1958). *The mind of a mnemonist* (L. Solotaroff, Trans.). New York: Basic Books.

Marketdata Enterprises. (2001). Chronic pain management clinics. A market analysis. Tampa, FL: Author.

Mayberg, H. S., Silva, J. A., Brannan, S. K. *et al.* (2002). The functional neuroanatomy of the placebo effect. *American Journal of Psychiatry*, **159**, 728–37.

McClure, C. M. (1959). Cardiac arrest through volition. *California Medicine*, **90**, 440–8.

Ogden, E. & Shock, N. W. (1939). Voluntary hypercirculation. *American Journal of the Medical Sciences*, **198**, 329–42.

Schwartz, M. S. & Andrasik, F. (Eds.). (2003). *Biofeedback: A Practitioner's Guide* (3rd edn.). New York: Guilford Publications.

Shapiro, A. K. (1959). The placebo effect in the history of medical treatment – implications for psychiatry. *American Journal of Psychiatry*, **116**, 298–304.

Shapiro, A. K. (1971). Placebo effects in medicine, psychotherapy, and psychoanalysis. In A. E. Bergen & S. L. Garfield (Eds.). *Handbook of psychotherapy and behavior change.* New York: Wiley.

Turk, D. C., Meichenbaum, D. H. & Berman, W. H. (1979). Application of biofeedback for the regulation of pain: a critical review. *Psychological Bulletin*, **86**, 1322–38.

White, L. & Tursky, B. (Eds.). (1982). *Clinical biofeedback: efficacy and mechanisms.* New York: Guilford Press.

Cognitive behaviour therapy

Andrew Eagle[1] and Michael Worrell[2]

[1]CNWL NHS Mental Health Trust
[2]Royal Holloway, University of London

Introduction

Cognitive behavioural therapy (CBT) may be defined as a set of empirically grounded clinical interventions implemented by therapists who understand themselves to be operating as scientist-practitioners (Salkovskis, 2002). These interventions, however, must be understood as being far more than the mere application of ready to hand techniques or 'tools' but rather as direct expressions of an explicit, sophisticated and continually developing, theoretical model(s) of the nature of psychopathology and the processes of human change.

Despite its being a relatively young psychotherapy, CBT has clearly come of age over the past decade and is widely recognized as the 'treatment of choice' for an ever expanding range of clinical presentations. For example, evidence for the effectiveness of CBT has been gained in the treatment of depression (Young *et al.*, 2001), panic disorder (Clark *et al.*, 1994) and eating disorders (Wilson & Fairburn, 1998). The approach has also gained supporting evidence in the area of more severe presentations including personality disorders (Beck & Freeman, 1990) and schizophrenia (Fowler *et al.*, 1995). In addition to its growing empirical support and popularity, the approach has also attracted its fair share of challenges and criticisms. While the field of psychotherapy often continues to be characterized by a competitive 'all or nothing' stance in which only one model may emerge victorious, an important and developing movement in the field is the interest in integrative approaches which emphasize a more respectful dialogue and openness between different styles of approach. CBT has in many respects always been an integrative approach and continues to have much to offer to the development of empirically grounded integrative therapeutic interventions (Beck, 1991).

In this brief article we have set ourselves the following objectives:

1. To attempt to define the 'essence' of CBT and its theoretical underpinnings.
2. To briefly consider the application of CBT to physical health problems.
3. To describe what we regard as some of the most interesting contemporary developments and controversies in the field.

Defining CBT

As is the case with other well known 'branded' therapies such as psychodynamic psychotherapy (see 'Psychodynamic psychotherapy') or systemic therapy, it would be misleading to assert that there is a singular unitary entity called CBT. As early as 1978, Mahoney and Arnkoff noted the existence of a range of therapeutic procedures which are subsumed under the heading of CBT. These included Cognitive Therapy, Rational Emotive Therapy (now known as Rational Emotive Behaviour Therapy), Problem Solving Therapy, Coping Skills Therapy, Stress Inoculation Training, etc. The contemporary scene is even richer with the addition of therapies such as Functional Analytic Therapy (Kohlenberg & Tsai, 1991), Dialectical Behaviour Therapy (Linehan, 1993), Acceptance and Commitment Therapy (Hayes *et al.*, 1999) and Schema Focused Therapy (Young *et al.*, 2003). Each of these may be described as belonging to the family of cognitive behavioural psychotherapies.

In many respects, however, it is Aaron Beck's cognitive behaviour therapy that has come to be taken as the foundational model for what CBT is in its essence (Beck, 1976, Beck *et al.*, 1979). In what follows we outline the defining theoretical and practice based features of this 'Beckian' approach.

The theoretical foundations of CBT

The primacy of cognition

From a CBT perspective, all acts of perception, learning and knowing are the products of an active information processing system which selectively attends to the environment, filters and then interprets the information impinging upon the organism. Such 'processing' of information is seen as evolutionarily adaptive. In psychopathological conditions, particular aspects of the information processing system are seen as having become 'distorted', biased or maladaptive, leading to experiences of emotional, behavioural and relational distress. The role of the CBT therapist is seen as that of assisting individuals to clarify their current patterns of information processing and to modify this through a range of strategies which encourage individuals to take on a more 'scientific' stance towards their own experiences and their experience of their interpersonal world. Within CBT, a clear therapeutic priority is placed on cognition. Achieving change in cognitive content, processes and structures is seen as the most effective means of achieving clinically significant change. In a stance of 'technical eclecticism' a wide range of strategies, including experiential, behavioural or relational strategies may be employed to achieve this end.

CBT is a mediational theory

A central tenet of CBT is that cognitive content, processes and structures directly influence both emotional experience and behaviour (Clark, 1995; Dobson & Block, 1988). It is vital to stress that the CBT model does not assert that cognition is *causal* in relation to any of these other factors. Nevertheless there has been considerable debate between cognitive and emotion theorists as to whether or not cognition always or usually precedes emotional experience (see Lazarus, 1984; Zajonc, 1984).

CBT is an empirical approach

One of the strengths of CBT is that it is an empirically based approach where theoretical concepts are operationally defined, measured and subject to research. Consistent with this approach, CBT has emphasized that the relevant cognitive content, processes and structures can be accessed, clarified and measured. No reliance is made on notions of an unconscious to which the client has no direct access but which the therapist may be in a position to interpret. This does not mean however that all cognitive activity is consciously experienced, subject to control or deliberate. An important strand of cognitive research is upon the relatively automatic, involuntary and preconscious processes that may be implicated in a range of psychopathological conditions such as anxiety and depression (see Mathews & McLeod, 1987).

CBT is a 'here and now' therapy

Consistent with its behavioural heritage, CBT asserts that it is current cognitive factors which are central in the maintenance of psychopathological difficulties. Hence, therapeutic attention is focused on the present situation rather than historical or childhood fact These are not neglected entirely however, and are seen as particularly relevant in more serious conditions such as personality disorders. Even here however, information concerning development origins is sought primarily to more adequately formulate currently relevant cognitive factors.

Defining procedural features of CBT

CBT is a short-term structured therapy. A typical course of CBT lasts from 12–24 sessions in addition to follow-up sessions to ensure the maintenance of gains. The CBT therapist approaches each session in a structured fashion. There is a shared plan or agenda for each session that the therapist encourages the client to take an active part in co-constructing. Goals are clearly defined in measurable and operationalized terms. Progress is continually monitored and evaluated and feedback is sought from the client during each therapy session.

CBT is based on the principle of 'collaborative empiricism'. Rather than the therapist being seen as the expert on the clients experience, therapist and client work together to resolve the clients problems. The client is seen as the expert on their own problems and experience. In the words of Beck *et al:*

'The cognitive therapist implies that there is a team approach to the solution of a patient's problem: that is, a therapeutic alliance where the patient supplies the raw data (reports on thoughts and behaviour…) while the therapist provides structure and expertize on how to solve problems. The emphasis is on working on problems rather correcting deficits or changing personality'. (Beck et al., 1985, p. 175).

An explicit goal of the CBT therapist is to teach clients the model of CBT and to assist them in becoming their own therapist. Rather than direct instruction, the therapist adopts a Socratic stance which involves the use of questioning to assist clients in clarifying and challenging their own thoughts and beliefs.

CBT interventions are based on a comprehensive formulation of the client's presenting problems (Needleman, 1999). The CBT formulation is a working hypothesis which attempts to explain the genesis and maintenance of a client's difficulties according to current CBT theory and the data gathered from assessment. The formulation is explicitly shared with the client and modified by his or her feedback. The formulation provides a blueprint or touchstone for the rest of the therapy.

CBT involves the co-construction of therapeutic tasks or homework which the client carries out between sessions. In certain respects what happens between sessions in the client's normal environment is seen as more important than what happens during sessions themselves. While earlier versions of behavioural therapy may have stressed homework tasks in terms of behavioural rehearsal or exposure to feared situations, in CBT, homework tasks are understood primarily in terms of the particular cognitive variables which they are designed to clarify or challenge (Bennett-Levy et al., 2004).

CBT is based on a positive, collaborative therapeutic relationship. In their seminal text Beck *et al.* (1979) clarified that the therapeutic relationship is crucial in the successful practice of CBT. However while 'Rogerian' conditions of empathy, warmth and positive regard and other relational factors are seen as necessary for the application of cognitive change strategies, they are not regarded as sufficient in themselves to produce the required cognitive changes.

Applications of CBT to physical health problems

While the principles of CBT were established in the treatment of psychiatric problems, there are good reasons why CBT is also proving effective in the treatment of physical health problems. Chronic medical conditions are frequently associated with psychological problems such as anxiety and depression, for which CBT is an effective treatment. There is no reason to anticipate that CBT should be less effective in treating psychological conditions co-morbid with physical illness. Furthermore effective treatment of psychological dysfunction is often an important step in enabling patients to cope better with physical illness.

The central role of 'illness perception' or 'cognitive representations of illness' in adjustment to physical illness is a well established theme in the health psychology literature (Weinman & Petrie, 1997). The way people think about their physical health problems has been explored using a range of social cognition models (Connor & Norman, 1995). The influential Self-regulation Model (SRM) (Leventhal *et al.*, 1984) has focused on five dimensions of health belief (identity, consequences, causes, timeline and control, or cure) which are seen as being key to guiding individual responses to physical illness. The model emphasizes that the coping strategies which people select for coping with health problems are influenced by their perceptions of their illness (see 'Lay beliefs about health and illness').

CBT with its emphasis on the central role of cognition and appraisals in mediating patients' experience of physical illness shares a consistent theoretical rationale with these approaches. The cognitive processes that are targeted by CBT in psychiatric conditions are equally amenable to treatment in physical illness.

Salkovskis (1989) summarizes the cognitive processes relevant to treatment of most physical problems. These include patients' beliefs about bodily functioning and the causation of physical problems; misinterpretations of bodily symptoms and signs; evaluations of the threat to self and future wellbeing associated with illness; and changes in behaviour and mood following perceived impairment which may increase emotional distress and the degree of handicap. CBT is particularly interested in modifying thoughts and behaviours, which may function to maintain physical problems, even when these originally had a physical cause (see, for example, 'Pain management').

Space does not permit any in-depth review of the application of CBT to specific physical disorders. It is sufficient to say that CBT is demonstrating effectiveness in treatment of a wide range of chronic illnesses and disabilities. For example, there is promising evidence for the use of CBT in treating chronic fatigue syndrome (Deale *et al.*, 1997); rheumatoid arthritis, (Sharpe *et al.*, 2003) and chronic pain (Morley *et al.*, 1999). There is also evidence to support the use of CBT to treat somatisation (Kroenke & Swindle, 2000) and hypochondriasis (Barsky & Ahern, 2004; Warwick *et al.*, 1996) (see 'Psychosomatics'). It should be noted that a recurring methodological limitation of certain outcome studies is that they do not adequately measure treatment fidelity and thus cannot reliably determine whether the effectiveness of CBT reflects the training and experience of the therapist or the efficacy of the intervention (Raine *et al.*, 2002).

Moorey (1996) has discussed the use of Cognitive Therapy in situations where people face objectively adverse life circumstances such as cancer or other potentially terminal illnesses. In these situations the negative thoughts verbalized by patients may reflect an accurate view of their circumstances and are not 'distortions' of external reality. Moorey suggests that in situations where a process of adjustment to life-threatening illness is ongoing, formal cognitive therapy may be inappropriate and a more flexible supportive approach may be preferable. Notwithstanding this, he also argues that maladaptive beliefs such as over-generalization of the consequences of illness, can hinder the normal process of adjustment.

Controversies and developments

As CBT has been applied to an ever widening range of clinical problems, various authors have proposed revisions and adaptations of Beck's original model of CBT. Many of these may be seen as welcome developments that may greatly increase the flexibility and therapeutic power of CBT. Other authors such as Clark (1995), however, have suggested that some of these developments are sufficiently dissimilar to the original model that they could be seen as alternative or competing models.

One of the most significant developments in CBT over the past decade has been the increasing significance given to the role of the therapeutic relationship in CBT. Safran and his colleagues (Safran & Segal, 1990; Safran & Muran, 2000) have strongly argued for the integration of an interpersonal perspective into CBT. These authors have proposed novel understandings of the varieties of 'ruptures' which can occur in the working relationship between therapist and client and how these may be most fruitfully addressed to improve therapeutic outcome. In a review of the available research literature, Waddington (2002) concluded that there is robust evidence for the impact of the therapeutic relationship in determining therapeutic outcome in CBT. Increasing attention is likely to be paid to the complexities of the therapeutic relationship in CBT as the approach continues to be applied to more challenging clinical presentations. The work of Leahy (2001), for example, has provided an interesting analysis of how the phenomena of transference and counter-transference (concepts originating from within psychoanalysis) can be understood and worked with from within a CBT perspective.

A related development has been the influence of what has come to be known as 'social constructivism' in CBT (Mahoney, 2003). Social constructivism emphasizes how human beings 'construct' narratives or 'personal realities' in order for them to be able to make sense of relational experience and maintain a sense of their own continuity through time. Social constructivists have challenged what they have understood to be the overly 'rationalistic' tendencies in standard CBT and have proposed a version of 'post-rationalist CBT' which does not rely on any notion of 'distorted' or 'irrational' thinking (Guidano, 1991). Social constructivist versions of CBT tend to be less structured, pay a great deal of attention to the therapeutic relationship, are more exploratory rather than focused on specific problem solving and tend to take more account of early developmental issues.

A significant development within standard CBT has been that of Schema Focused Therapy (Young *et al.*, 2003) which has been developed specifically to help individuals presenting with varieties of personality disorders. Schema therapy tends to be longer-term, to focus on the therapeutic relationship as a vehicle for achieving change and to emphasize the concept of 'early maladaptive schemas' – deep cognitive structures which have their origin in toxic relationships with care givers when the individual was a child. This new emphasis on 'deep' cognitive structures and early developmental issues has not been uncontroversial however, and a number of authors have suggested caution in using these methods as standard practice and have emphasized the need to submit these models to further empirical testing (James, 2001).

Hayes (2004) has argued that the history of the behavioural and cognitive psychotherapies can be described as having taken place in three 'waves'. The first wave of Behaviour Therapy was characterized by the development of strategies arising from the models of classical and operant conditioning (see 'Behaviour therapy'). The second wave, according to these authors, was characterized by cognitivism and is most clearly expressed in the model of CBT developed by Beck. 'Third Wave CBT' is argued to be a very recent phenomenon. Hayes *et al.* (in press) suggest that recent developments including Dialectical Behaviour Therapy (Linehan, 1993), Acceptance and Commitment Therapy (Hayes *et al.*, 1999)

and Mindfulness Based Cognitive Therapy (Segal *et al.*, 2002) have moved CBT into areas traditionally seen as less empirical and therefore requiring novel philosophical, conceptual and theoretical development and debate. An example of an important concept from Acceptance and Commitment Therapy is that of 'acceptance'. Acceptance strategies are significantly different from standard CBT strategies which attempt to modify the content of cognitive structures. Acceptance strategies encourage the client to distance themselves from their cognitive processes but not attempt to change them. This is held to result in a weakening of the link between cognition and behaviour and to aid the individual in overcoming varieties of 'experiential avoidance' which are seen as intrinsic to psychopathology.

Conclusion

The field of the Cognitive and Behavioural Psychotherapies is a rich, complex and developing one. The model has gained a good deal of empirical evidence for its usefulness and has become the treatment of choice for many forms of psychological disorder. There is a growing body of evidence to support its application to *physical* health problems. CBT continues to grow in novel directions and to develop new understandings of the nature of psychological problems and new treatment strategies for their alleviation.

REFERENCES

Barsky, A.J. & Ahern, D.K. (2004). Cognitive behaviour therapy for hypochondriasis: a randomised controlled trial. *Journal of American Medical Association*, **291**, 1464–70.

Beck, A.T. (1976). *Cognitive therapy of the emotional disorders.* New York: New American Library.

Beck, A.T. (1991). Cognitive therapy as the integrative therapy. *Journal of Psychotherapy Integration*, **1**, 191–8.

Beck, A.T., Rush, A.J., Shaw, B.F. & Emery, G. (1979). *Cognitive therapy of depression.* New York: The Guilford Press.

Beck, A.T., Emery, G. & Greenberg, R.L. (1985). *Anxiety disorders and phobias: a cognitive perspective.* New York: Basic Books.

Beck, A.T., Freeman, A. & Associates. (1990). *Cognitive therapy of personality disorders.* New York: Guilford Press.

Bennett-Levy, J.B., Butler, G., Fennell, M. *et al.* (2004). *Oxford guide to behavioural experiments in cognitive therapy.* Oxford: Oxford University Press.

Clark, D.A. (1995). Perceived limitations of standard cognitive therapy: a consideration of efforts to revise Beck's theory and therapy. *Journal of Cognitive Psychotherapy: An International Quarterly*, **9**(3), 153–72.

Clark, D.M., Salkovskis, P.M., Hackmann, A. *et al.* (1994). A comparison of cognitive therapy, applied relaxation and imipramine in the treatment of panic disorder. *British Journal of Psychiatry*, **164**, 759–69.

Connor, M. & Norman, P. (1995). The role of social cognition in health behaviour. In M. Connor & P. Norman (Eds.). *Predicting health behaviour* (pp. 1–22). Buckingham, UK: Open University Press.

Deal, A., Chalder, T., Marks, I. & Wessely, S. (1997). Cognitive behaviour therapy for chronic fatigue syndrome: a randomised controlled trial. *American Journal of Psychiatry*, **154**(3), 408–14.

Dobson, K.S. & Block, L. (1988). Historical and philosophical bases of the cognitive behavioural therapies. In K.S. Dobson (Ed.). *Handbook of cognitive–behavioural therapies* (pp. 3–38). New York: Guildford Press.

Fowler, D., Garety, P. & Kuioers, E. (1995). *Cognitive behaviour therapy for psychosis.* West Sussex: Wiley.

Guidano, V.F. (1991). *The self in process: towards a post-rationalist cognitive therapy.* New York: Guilford Press.

Hayes, S.C. (2004). Acceptance and commitment therapy and the new behavior therapies. Mindfulness, acceptance, and relationship. In S.C. Hayes, V.M. Follette & M.M. Linehan (Eds.). *Mindfulness and*

acceptance. Expanding the cognitive behavioral tradition. New York: Guilford Press.

Hayes, S.C., Masuda, A. & De May, H. (in press). Acceptance and commitment therapy and the third wave of behaviour therapy. *Gedragstherapie* (Dutch Journal of Behaviour Therapy).

Hayes, S.C., Strosahl, K.D. & Wilson, N.G. (1999). *Acceptance and commitment therapy: an experimental approach to behaviour change.* New York: Guilford.

James, I. (2001). Schema therapy: the next generation, but should it carry a health warning? *Behavioural and Cognitive Psychotherapy*, **29**(4), 401–7.

Kohlenberg, R.J. & Tsai, M. (1991). *Functional analytic psychotherapy: creating intense and curative therapeutic relationships.* New York: Plennum.

Kroenke, K. & Swindle, R. (2000). Cognitive–behavioural therapy for somatization and symptom syndromes: a critical review of controlled clinical trials. *Psychotherapy and Psychomatics*, **69**, 205–15.

Lazarus, R.S. (1984). On the primacy of cognition. *American Psychologist*, **39**, 124–9.

Leahy, R.L. (2001). *Overcoming resistance in cognitive therapy.* New York: Guilford Press.

Leventhal, H., Nerenzu, D. R. & Steele, D. F. (1984). Illness representations and coping with health threats. In A. Baum & J. Singer (Eds.). *A handbook of psychology and health* (pp. 229–52). Hillsdale, NJ: Earlbaum.

Linehan, M. M. (1993). *Cognitive–behavioural treatment of borderline personality disorders.* New York: The Guilford press.

Mahoney, M. (2003). *Constructive psychotherapy: a practical guide.* New York: Guilford Press.

Mahoney, M. & Arnkoff, D. (1978). Cognitive and self-control therapies. In S. Garfield & A. Bergin (Eds.). *Handbook of psychotherapy and behaviour change.* New York: Wiley.

Mathews, A. & McLeod, C. (1987). An information-processing approach to anxiety. *Journal of Cognitive Psychotherapy: An International Quarterly,* **1**, 105–15.

Moorey, S. (1996). When bad things happen to rational people: cognitive therapy in adverse life circumstances. In P. Salkovskis (Ed.). *Frontiers of cognitive therapy* (pp. 450–69). New York: Guildford Press.

Morley, S., Greer, S., Bliss, J. & Law, M. (1999). Systematic review and meta analysis of randomised controlled trials of cognitive behaviour therapy and behaviour therapy for chronic pain in adults, excluding headaches. *Pain,* **80**, 1–13.

Needleman, L. D. (1999). *Cognitive case conceptualisation: a guidebook for practitioners.* London: Lawrence Erlbaum.

Raine, R., Haines, A., Sensky, T. *et al.* (2002). Systematic review of mental health interventions for patients with common somatic symptoms: can research from secondary car be extrapolated to primary care? *British Medical Journal,* **325**, 1082.

Safran, J. D. & Segal, Z. V. (1990). *Interpersonal process in cognitive therapy.* New York: Basic Books.

Safran, J. D. & Muran, J. C. (2000). *Negotiating the therapeutic alliance: a relational treatment guide.* New York: Guilford Press.

Salkovskis, P. M. (1989). Somatic Problems. In K. Hawton, P. M. Salkovskis, J. Kirk & D. M. Clark (Eds.). *Cognitive behaviour therapy for psychiatric problems: a practical guide* (pp. 235–76). New York: Oxford University Press.

Salkovskis, P. M. (2002). Empirically grounded clinical interventions: cognitive–behavioural therapy progresses through a multi-dimensional approach to clinical science. *Behavioural and Cognitive Psychotherapy,* **30**(1), 3–11.

Segal, Z. V., Williams, J. M. G. & Teasdale, J. D. (2002). *Mindfulness-based cognitive therapy for depression: a new approach for preventing relapse.* New York: Guilford Press.

Sharpe, L., Sensky, T., Timberlake, N., Ryan, B. & Allard, S. (2003). Long-term efficacy of a cognitive behavioural treatment from a randomised controlled trial for patients recently diagnosed with rheumatoid arthritis. *Rheumatology,* **42**(3), 435–41.

Waddington, L. (2002). The therapy relationship in cognitive therapy: a review. *Behavioural and Cognitive Psychotherapy,* **30**, 2, 179–92.

Warwick, H. M. C., Clark, D. M., Cobb, A. M. & Salkovskis, P. M. (1996). A controlled trial of cognitive–behavioural treatment of hypochondriasis. *British Journal of Psychiatry,* **169**, 189–95.

Weinman, J. & Petrie, K. J. (1997). Introduction to the perceptions of health and illness. In J. Weinman & K. J. Petrie (Eds.). *Perceptions of health and illness* (pp. 1–19). Amsterdam: Harwood Academic.

Wilson, G. T. & Fairburn, C. G. (1998). Treatment of eating disorders. In P. E. Nathan & J. M. Gorman (Eds.). *Treatments that Work* (pp. 501–30). New York: Oxford University Press.

Young, J. E., Klosko, J. S. & Weishaar, M. E. (2003). *Schema therapy: a practitioners guide.* New York: Guilford Press.

Young, J. E., Weinberger, A. D. & Beck, A. T. (2001). Cognitive Therapy for Depression. In D. Barlow (Ed.). *Clinical handbook of psychological disorders* (pp. 264–308). London: Guilford Press.

Zajonc, R. B. (1984). On the primacy of affect. *American Psychologist,* **37**, 117–23.

Community-based interventions

Deborah E. Polk[1], Christie M. King[2] and Kenneth Heller[3]

[1]University of Pittsburgh
[2]F. Spellacy & Associates
[3]Indiana University

Public health practitioners who design community-based, health interventions base their work on evidence that social and environmental processes impact upon health and wellbeing, and contribute to health decline, morbidity and mortality. Furthermore, rather than assuming that negative environmental conditions are fixed and immutable aspects of industrial society, designers of community-based interventions believe that with sufficient encouragement, education and skills, citizens can become more active in modifying and overcoming unhealthy social conditions. The goals of community health interventions, then, are to help set in place social structures that support and reinforce individual and group efforts at improving health and the quality of life.

The emphasis on facilitative social structures is not intended to minimize the efforts that individuals can take to improve their own health. Indeed, much can be accomplished by encouraging patients to change unhealthful practices which contribute to increased risk for disease. For example, convincing patients to adopt a healthy diet, decrease smoking, drug and alcohol intake and engage in moderate exercise have been prime ingredients in the reduction of cardiovascular risk that has taken place within the last two decades. However, there is a limit to what individuals can do on their own when confronted with adverse environmental conditions. The barriers to continued improvements in community health are not only in the individual citizen's knowledge of proper health practices, but also in economic factors and social customs that maintain risk-producing conditions. Since there is now a substantial body of research indicating that rates of morbidity and mortality are linked to social conditions such as poverty, community disintegration, poor education and social isolation (Adler *et al.*, 1994; Williams *et al.*, 1992), the dilemma for modern community health practice is how to help individuals come together to deal with these negative social conditions.

While the correction of adverse social conditions can be difficult to accomplish, we believe that health practitioners need not wait for some golden age of social enlightenment before acting to improve community health. There are many examples of local projects in which citizens have developed effective action plans in collaboration with health professionals. The key ingredients in these efforts involve a mobilized and informed community group in which social structures have been developed that encourage concerted action. The idea is to find ways to encourage the development of community groups that can provide the structure for citizens to become proactive in health maintenance, and that then become institutionalized as an ongoing part of community life.

The purpose of this chapter is to review key ingredients of successful community-based interventions, discuss impediments to their implementation and how these might be overcome, and outline the possible roles of the healthcare provider in a community-based intervention. Our goal is that by the end of the chapter, the reader will understand the role of community-based interventions in the toolkit of techniques used to address health and disease, be introduced to key ideas and know how to obtain additional information.

Key ingredients in successful community-based interventions

Citizen ownership

Project adoption and retention is enhanced when citizens are seen as equal partners in an intervention project (Wagenaar *et al.*, 1999). Although interventions are sometimes initiated by concerned persons outside the community of interest, the greatest and most lasting changes occur when community members themselves take part in identifying a need and designing an intervention to meet that need. A major weakness of many externally funded health projects is that they do not survive once project demonstration funds are used up because not enough effort was given to ensuring community ownership.

An example of how community members might become involved in a planned intervention is the establishment of a community advisory board to help fashion the content of the programme, publicize it and recruit participants. Choosing an advisory board requires some knowledge of the leadership structure of the community because community leaders can serve a vital 'gatekeeper'

role. Their views of the project can either facilitate or retard acceptance. For example, in a study targeting child malnutrition and pregnant and lactating women in Mexico, a community assembly served a gatekeeper function by approving the list of low-income households who were to receive the intervention (Rivera *et al.*, 2004).

Essential to the success of a community intervention is that the content of the intervention and its manner of implementation be acceptable to the community. So for example, in a study of the efficacy of permethrin-treated bed nets to prevent malaria among children in Western Kenya, open community meetings were held in each of 33 communities to discuss the project and allow villagers to ask questions. At the end of these meetings, participants themselves provided authorization for the trial to be conducted in their communities (Phillips-Howard *et al.*, 2003).

Building trust

Efforts to promote community change are maximized when intervention recipients trust and respect the people promoting the new behaviours. The heart of organizing is careful building of interpersonal relations, often one at a time (Wagenaar *et al.*, 1999). However, this essential process of relationship building can take time. In a study examining mammography adherence in the United States, prior to participant recruitment, 10 months were spent in building community support through group breakfasts for pastors and follow-up involving meetings with the pastor and church governing body (Derose *et al.*, 2000). This extended period of relationship building through community-based activities was a key to the project's ultimate success.

To maximize trust, careful selection of community members to deliver the intervention can be a key element in its ultimate success. Research has shown that intervention specialists are most effective when they are already known to the intervention recipient; have equal or slightly higher status than the recipient; and are credible and empathic. Community workers need to know and understand the people they are working with – their values, perspectives, needs and strengths (Wagenaar *et al.*, 1999). For example, in a study designed to increase the utilization of cervical smear tests among Vietnamese-American women, utilization was greater among women receiving both a media education campaign and outreach visits by a lay health worker than among women receiving the media education campaign only (Lam *et al.*, 2003).

Of course, lay intervention agents must be well trained and must be provided with effective support (Nation *et al.*, 2003). In a study in Pakistan to prevent infant diarrhoea through family handwashing, lay field workers were most effective and were more satisfied with their jobs when they were extensively trained. Their training included discussions of interviewing techniques, how to encourage handwashing by mothers, data recording and measuring and weighing children (Luby *et al.*, 2004).

Changing social norms

Changing social customs and practices is perhaps the most powerful way of instituting changes in health practices that are likely to endure. Psychological research shows that humans are usually motivated to belong to social groups (Baumeister & Leary, 1995).

Furthermore, if they believe that adhering to the social norm of the group requires them to change their behaviour, they will probably be motivated to do so. Thus social norms and recipients' understandings of these norms are crucial in instituting behaviour change.

For example, in a 15-community randomized trial to change policies and practices with regard to the sale of alcohol to minors, the target of the intervention was the entire community rather than individual young people (Wagenaar *et al.*, 1999; Wagenaar *et al.*, 2000). Over a two-and-a-half-year period, contact was made with merchants, hotels, bars, law enforcement personnel, religious organizations and parents, with events and training sessions designed for each group. As a result there was a reduced propensity for merchants to sell alcohol to minors, and a reduction in the tendency for older teens to provide alcohol to younger teens.

Another example is the need for many HIV/AIDS prevention programmes to be aware of social norms associated with men and women's sexual practices. One such programme in rural Uganda used television-based plays and video programmes to raise awareness of risky behaviours and offer culturally acceptable solutions (Kinsman *et al.*, 2002). For example, one video illustrated the problem of extra-marital sex by men working away from home, and how this can lead to HIV contracted by the men and subsequently their spouses. In another play, a wife finds a condom that her husband had hidden in anticipation of introducing it to her. A friend resolves their argument, explaining to her the benefits of condoms as well as how to use and store them (Kinsman *et al.*, 2002).

The influence of social norms and individual beliefs also can be seen in a large scale HIV/AIDS prevention programme developed within the school system for high school students in South Africa. The researchers noted that high-risk behaviours appeared to increase over the evaluation year despite increases in knowledge related to the disease and protective behaviours (Visser & Schoeman, 2004). Focus group discussions with the student participants revealed that possible underlying factors which may have maintained high-risk sexual behaviours despite the change in knowledge were based on social norms. For example, sexual experience was perceived as normative for that peer group, was a status symbol, particularly for boys, and was much more important than engaging in HIV-protective behaviours. In addition, the social norms surrounding girls saying 'no' to sex were unclear, leaving girls confused about what was acceptable and whether they might lose the relationship if they did not comply.

Multiple intervention points

There are several reasons why multiple components in an intervention are important to its success (Nation *et al.*, 2003). Studies have demonstrated that providing information alone is not sufficient to change behaviour (Botvin & Griffin, 2002; Botvin & Tortu, 1988). The research literature is rife with examples of trials that failed because they tried to change behaviour only by providing information. Also, research shows that different people learn in different ways, so having multiple components increases the chances that an intervention will have a broader appeal (Bloom, 1976; Wagenaar *et al.*, 1999). Research also demonstrates the power of repetition in learning. Seeing the same material presented in different ways reinforces the message. For example, in the study designed to prevent infant diarrhoea described above (Luby *et al.*, 2004), field workers conducted neighbourhood meetings at which information about handwashing was presented in slide shows, videotapes, and pamphlets. Additionally, they made weekly visits to households to describe specifics of the handwashing protocol. Similarly, in a study designed to increase the consumption of fruits and vegetables among rural African American church members in North Carolina (Campbell *et al.*, 1999), church members were encouraged to plant victory gardens and fruit trees and were encouraged to serve fruits and vegetables at church functions. Pastors received a newsletter and were encouraged to promote the project from the pulpit, and church members received personalized, tailored messages based on their responses to survey questions on fruit and vegetable consumption, their health beliefs, readiness to change and support from others for changes in diet. Intervention counties formed coalitions that included representatives from the churches, local agencies, grocers and farmers. Finally a cookbook based on church members' own recipes, modified to meet the dietary guidelines, was created and distributed to all intervention recipients

In sum, for an intervention to succeed, it is important to collaborate with community members as equal partners in the intervention process. Community members can serve as 'gatekeepers' to the community; they understand the concerns and culturally appropriate responses in their community, and can help to ensure that the content of the intervention is designed in such a way as to be consistent with the community's culture and norms. Additionally, interventions drawing on the knowledge and strengths of both healthcare providers and community members should strive to disseminate their messages through as many different means as possible.

Impediments to community-based health programmes

Professional attitudes

There continues to be an ongoing debate in medical education about the extent to which public health and prevention concepts should be taught in the medical school curriculum (Altman, 1990; Colwill, 2004). Despite the value of community-based prevention programmes, the reward structure in medicine, particularly in the USA, has not been on public health, but on the treatment of complex disorders whose occurrence in the general population may be relatively infrequent. Unfortunately, the model in clinical medicine of treating individuals in isolation from their social milieu has had limited effectiveness in dealing with the health problems of the vast majority of citizens (Ewart, 1991). This is because social factors play a large role in facilitating or inhibiting the adoption of effective health practices. Dealing with these social factors, then, becomes a key ingredient in community health programmes.

Lack of knowledge, distrust and discouragement

Decisions to adopt positive health behaviours are influenced by diverse social and psychological motives. These can include concerns about personal appearance, maintaining perceived respect of one's peers, the desire to avoid social rejection, the need for

material and financial security as well as actual knowledge of effective health practices. These factors either facilitate or impede the adoption of new behaviour, and should be anticipated in the design of health programmes.

Research has demonstrated that those most at risk are usually those who are most reluctant to volunteer for community programmes. For example, Fink and Shapiro (1990) found that mortality rates from all causes were highest among women who refused to participate in a voluntary breast cancer screening programme conducted by their health insurance plan. Reaching these reluctant participants required personal contact and intensive outreach as demonstrated by Lacey et al. (1989). In their cancer screening project, public health outreach workers, culturally sensitive to the target population, visited places frequented by women (such as beauty shops, grocery stores, housing projects and currency exchanges) to bring word of the programme and allay fears which only surfaced after personal contact had been established.

Addressing difficulties in recruiting and engaging at-risk participants improves the ability of the intervention to reach its target participants. Lindenberg and her colleagues (2001) recognized that even traditional health education programme approaches using schools, health centres, and churches were not accessible to many of the young, Hispanic women they were targeting in their intervention designed to reduce substance use and risky sexual behaviour. For these young women, commitments to work, studying, childcare and household activities precluded regular attendance at programme classes. These researchers found that mailing health education materials which were personalized, in Spanish, and at a 10–12-year-old reading level was a successful strategy for reaching many woman who many not have participated otherwise. In addition, bilingual telephone consultation was also a useful strategy in contacting participants, especially since the telephone afforded the privacy essential given the nature of the intervention.

Inadequate resources

Despite the advancement of prevention as a science and the success of many community intervention programmes, many communities have been unable to implement effective programming due to limitations in funding, resources, technical and organization capacities and community readiness (Goodman, 2000; Wandersman & Florin, 2003).

The research on preschool education programmes provides a useful illustration. Demonstration projects that serve as models for broader implementation generally show both immediate and long-term benefits. However, the evidence for the efficacy of Head Start programmes which have been implemented community-wide with the model programmes as a guide, show less consistent effects (Haskins, 1989). The reasons for the less successful dissemination of model programmes are not clear, but one reason that widespread

implementation might be less successful is that resources to administer programmes never match what is available to the demonstration projects. Real programmes are usually inadequately funded and are required to service more children with fewer resources than is true for model research programmes.

The lesson is that any large-scale community health programme must be aware of both predictable and unpredictable costs that may occur, and must make plans to deal with inadequate resources. For example, distribution of HIV/AIDS leaflets in a Ugandan community fell significantly for an extended period of time when technical problems with a photocopier arose (Kinsman et al., 2002). However, it is possible to build on community support for the programme in order to restrain costs. In a study of mammography screening in Los Angeles, church-member volunteers were an integral part of developing a cost-effective programme (Stockdale et al., 2000). This strategy could only have been adopted with a sufficient amount of community support for the programme. In addition to saving money, the use of community volunteers reinforced both the importance and acceptability of mammography for the participants.

Conclusion

The strategies for community intervention outlined in this chapter may seem daunting to an individual healthcare practitioner. Although the current medical model focuses more on the treatment of illness in individuals than on the prevention of health problems in a population, healthcare providers can integrate aspects of community-based intervention into their practice. Healthcare providers can assess the important social influences in a patient's life (e.g. spouse, family, friends, other caregivers, co-workers, religious affiliations, employment, social clubs, etc.) and how those persons or structures may facilitate or impede prescribed health behaviour changes. For example, it may be useful to know about the smoking patterns of a patient's co-workers and whether the employer offers on-site cessation clinics. Health care providers frequently hear first-hand from patients (i.e. community members) about community health concerns such as those described in this chapter. For example, patients may tell their physician about common community sexual practices that might put them at risk. Although physicians (nurses, etc.) may not have the resources themselves to initiate a community intervention, s/he may use her standing in the community and expertize to inspire others (e.g. university researcher, public health officials, advocacy groups) or consult with others (e.g. other healthcare providers, community leaders, school officials) who may be able to address the problem. After all, a health professional cannot expect to achieve success by working alone without the involvement of significant others in the community. Working at the community level is worthwhile because even small changes in health care practices on a community level can significantly reduce mortality and morbidity over time. (See also 'Health promotion'.)

REFERENCES

Adler, N. E., Boyce, T., Chesney, M. A. et al. (1994). Socioeconomic status and health: the challenge of the gradient. *American Psychologist*, **49**, 15–24.

Altman, L. K. (1990). A profession divided is finding it hard to teach prevention.

New York Times, (Medical Science Section) August 14, C3.

Baumeister, R. F. & Leary, M. R. (1995). The need to belong: desire for interpersonal attachments as a fundamental human

motivation. *Psychological Bulletin*, **117**, 497–529.

Bloom, B. S. (1976). Learning for mastery. In D. T. Gow (Ed.). *Design and development of curriculum materials Vol. 2. Instruction design* articles. Pittsburgh, PA: University of Pittsburgh.

Botvin, G. J. & Griffin, K. W. (2002). Life skills training as a primary prevention approach for adolescent drug abuse and other problem behaviors. *International Journal of Emergency Mental Health*, **4**, 41–8.

Botvin, G. J. & Tortu, S. (1988). Preventing adolescent substance abuse through life skills training. In R. H. Price, E. L. Cowen, R. P. Lorion & J. Ramos McKay (Eds.). *Fourteen ounces of prevention: a casebook for practitioners* (p. 110). Washington, DC: American Psychological Association.

Campbell, M. K., Demark-Wahnefried, W., Symons, M. *et al.* (1999). Fruit and vegetable consumption and prevention of cancer: the black churches united for better health project. *American Journal of Public Health*, **89**, 1390–6.

Colwill, J. M. (2004). Primary care medicine and the education of generalist physicians. In S. L. Isaacs & J. R. Knickman (Eds.). *Generalist medicine and the U. S. health system* (pp. 5–47). San Francisco, CA: Jossey-Bass.

Derose, K. P., Hawes-Dawson, J., Fox, S. A. *et al.* (2000). Dealing with diversity: recruiting churches and women for a randomized trial of mammography promotion. *Health Education and Behavior*, **27**, 632–48.

Ewart, C. K. (1991). Social action theory for a public health psychology. *American Psychologist*, **46**, 931–46.

Fink, R. & Shapiro, S. (1990). Significance of increased efforts to gain participation in screening for breast cancer. *American Journal of Preventive Medicine*, **6**, 34–41.

Goodman, R. M. (2000). Bridging the gap in effective program implementation: from concept to application. *Journal of Community Psychology*, **28**, 309–21.

Haskins, R. (1989). Beyond metaphor: the efficacy of early childhood education. *American Psychologist*, **44**, 274–82.

Kinsman, J., Kamali, A., Kanyesigye, E. *et al.* (2002). Quantitative process evaluation of a community-based HIV/AIDS behavioral intervention in rural Uganda. *Health Education Research*, **17**, 253–65.

Lacey, L. P., Phillips, C. W., Ansell, D. *et al.* (1989). An urban community-based cancer prevention screening and health eduction intervention in Chicago. *Public Health Reports*, **104**, 526–41.

Lam, T. K., McPhee, S. J., Mock, J. *et al.* (2003). Encouraging Vietnamese-American women to obtain Pap tests through lay health worker outreach and media education. *Journal of General Internal Medicine*, **18**, 516–24.

Lindenberg, C. S., Solorzano, R. M., Vilaro, F. M. & Westbrook, L. O. (2001). Challenges and strategies for conducting intervention research with culturally diverse populations. *Journal of Transcultural Nursing*, **12**, 132–9.

Luby, S. P., Agboatwalla, M., Painter, J. *et al.* (2004). Effect of intensive handwashing promotion on childhood diarrhea in high-risk communities in Pakistan: a randomized controlled trial. *JAMA*, **291**, 2547–54.

Nation, M., Crusto, C., Wandersman, A. *et al.* (2003). What works in prevention: principles of effective prevention programs. *American Psychologist*, **58**, 449–56.

Phillips-Howard, P. A., Nahlen, B. L., Alaii, J. A. *et al.* (2003). The efficacy of permethrin-treated bed nets on child mortality and morbidity in Western Kenya.

I. Development of infrastructure and description of study site. *The American Journal of Tropical Medicine and Hygiene*, **68**, 3–9.

Rivera, J. A., Sotres-Alvarez, D., Habicht, J. P., Shamah, T. & Villalpando, S. (2004). Impact of the Mexican program for education, health, and nutrition (Progresa) on rates of growth and anemia in infants and young children. *JAMA*, **291**, 2563–70.

Stockdale, S. E., Keeler, E., Duan, N., Derose, K. P. & Fox, S. A. (2000). Costs and cost-effectiveness of a church-based intervention to promote mammography screening. *Health Sciences Research*, **35**, 1037–57.

Visser, M. J. & Schoeman, J. B. (2004). Implementing a community intervention to reduce young people's risks for getting HIV: unraveling the complexities. *Journal of Community Psychology*, **32**, 145–65.

Wagenaar, A. C., Gehan, J. P., Jones-Webb, R., Toomey, T. L. & Forster, J. L. (1999). Communities mobilizing for change on alcohol: lessons and results from a 15-community randomized trial. *Journal of Community Psychology*, **27**, 315–26.

Wagenaar, A. C., Murray, D. M. & Gehan, J. P. (2000). Communities mobilizing for change on alcohol: outcomes from a randomized community trial. *Journal of Studies on Alcohol*, **61**, 85–94.

Wandersman, A. & Florin, P. (2003). Community interventions and effective prevention. *American Psychologist*, **58**, 441–8.

Williams, R. B., Barefoot, J. C., Califf, R. M. *et al.* (1992). Prognostic importance of social and economic resources among medically treated patients with angiographically documented coronary artery disease. *JAMA*, **267**, 520–4.

Counselling

Robert Bor and John Allen

Royal Free Hospital

Introduction

It has been estimated that as many as one-third of all patients who consult a doctor do so because they have a 'personal problem', or real physical symptoms, causing them distress and reflecting an underlying psycho-social problem (Pereira Gray, 1988). Often patients first present with such 'life-problems' or psychosomatic symptoms during a medical consultation lasting a matter of minutes. If the doctor has no psychological training, the 'life-problem', or psychosomatic symptoms may well be medicalized, i.e. treated solely or principally as an organic complaint. Treatment then tends to take the form of psychotropic drugs. The consequence may well be that the condition becomes chronic, or fails to improve, resulting in yet more frequent consultations and further prescriptions. Many observers have commented on the enormous amount of personal distress that this scenario causes to patients and the huge resulting costs to healthcare providers (Maguire & Pitceathly, 2002).

Counselling, among other forms of psychological help, may well be beneficial for patients presenting with such problems. The counsellor working with people in medical settings can provide time in which patients may express feelings about loss of abilities, roles and self-esteem and assist them in coming to terms and/or coping with these and other changes. In addition to the psychological benefits of counselling, there are at least some indications that the presence of a counsellor in the primary healthcare team leads to a reduction in patients' psychosomatic symptoms, a consequent reduction in drug prescription rates and a reduction in the demand for the time of medical staff. Other claimed benefits include a better shared understanding of the role of counselling in the work of the therapeutic team; fewer inappropriate referrals and investigations; and fewer hospital admissions. Moreover, it appears that the division of workload leads to increased satisfaction for GPs and greater mutual respect within the primary healthcare team.

The nature of counselling

If counselling is to have these beneficial effects, it is imperative that the appropriate conditions should be provided for its effective practice. There needs to be a clear appreciation within each medical team of the nature of counselling and the ways in which it differs from other forms of helping. The definition of counselling has always been problematic but one which is espoused by the British Association for Counselling and Psychotherapy (BACP) states: 'people become engaged in counselling when a person, occupying regularly or temporarily the role of counsellor offers or agrees explicitly to offer time attention and respect to another person or persons temporarily in the role of client' (BACP, 1985). The Code for Counsellors published by the BACP also states:

the overall aim of counselling is to provide an opportunity for a client to work towards living in a more satisfying and resourceful way ... Counselling may be concerned with developmental issues, addressing and resolving specific problems, making decisions, coping with crisis, developing personal insight and knowledge, working through feelings of inner conflict or improving relationships with others. The counsellor's role is to facilitate the client's work in ways which respect the client's values, personal resources and capacity for self-determination. (BACP, 1992)

One of the clear implications of the stress on self-determination is that in counselling, the patient, or client, is involved in an active and to a large extent autonomous, process of exploration, clarification and problem-solving. (This autonomy is often explicitly recognized by the use of the preferred title of 'client' rather than patient in the counselling context.) The emphasis on enabling or facilitating the client's decision-making in 'client-centred' approaches to counselling can be sharply contrasted with the traditional 'doctor-centred', or biomedical model, of patient care. In counselling, the 'expert' role

is abandoned in favour of a consultative style which values client responsibility and freedom. This may well involve the sharing of specialist knowledge, particularly about medical issues but the use of such information is seen ultimately as the client's responsibility. The biopsychosocial model (Engel, 1977) encourages patients, healthcare providers and counsellors to adopt an holistic and integrative approach to health problems. Narratives and experiences of illness and related problems have more relevance than linear or reductionistic explanations within this counselling approach (Bor et al., 2007).

The impact of counselling on medical practice

Interestingly in recent years the 'client-centred' approach has had a significant impact on medical practice especially among those practitioners who have become dissatisfied with the older 'doctor-centred' model of patient care (see 'Patient-centred healthcare'). Both in primary care and in postgraduate training, psychological and social approaches to the understanding of health and illness have led to alternative ways of working with patients. There has, for example, been increasing acceptance by medical practitioners that an understanding of the patient's view is vital to the process of consultation and that medical treatment should be based on shared involvement in decision-making. To facilitate this in practice, many of the skills developed in the counselling context such as active listening, empathic responding and reflection have been adopted by medical practitioners. Davis and Fallowfield (1991) argue that the use of counselling skills within a 'patient-centred' approach to medical care results in many benefits for patients and health professionals. These include increased patient and professional satisfaction, greater diagnostic adequacy and improved adherence to treatment. Where they occur, these benefits are thought to be largely due to improved communication between patients and health professionals. (See 'Compliance among patients', 'Healthcare professional–patient communication', 'Medical interviewing' and 'Patient satisfaction')

Counselling in the medical context

The origins of professional counselling for medical problems lie in efforts to improve patients' knowledge in order to help them to make informed decisions about treatment and care (such as with counselling for treatment for infertility, HIV antibody test counselling and termination of pregnancy counselling among others). More recently, this has extended to psychological support counselling. Counselling in medical settings is frequently associated with the following issues or problems: post-traumatic stress, coping and adjustment, pain management, pre- and postoperative stress, HIV disease, adjustment to coronary heart disease, substance misuse, renal disease, treatment non-compliance, infertility, anxiety, helping sick children and their families cope, among many others. There is rapid growth in the area of counselling in primary healthcare settings. Not only is this a context in which counsellors can work with patients at the first point of diagnosis, treatment and care, but it also provides an opportunity for focused health education and preventative counselling (Bor & McCann, 1999).

R. Bor and J. Allen

Many of the interactions between healthcare professionals and patients may not involve counselling as defined above but they may involve the use of counselling skills. The distinction between the use of counselling skills and counselling as a discrete activity is an important one but one which is often not made explicit. Bond (1993) has pointed out that counselling skills may be seen as a group of interpersonal, or communication, skills which share the common purpose of assisting the self-expression and autonomy of the recipient. Thus the purpose or values they serve are similar, if not identical, to those of counselling; namely empowerment and the encouragement of self-determination.

Counselling skills can, therefore, be regarded as providing ways of helping patients make informed choices from a range of health options. In this way counselling skills may be distinguished from the use of other communication skills such as those employed to advise, influence and persuade. Bond (1993) also points out that counselling and the use of counselling skills may be distinguished from each other, at least in part, by noting whether the contracting between the parties concerned is explicit or not. The BACP definition of counselling given earlier expressly addresses this issue by noting the need for clear understanding of the roles of counsellor and client. Confusion of roles has often arisen, particularly in healthcare and medical contexts because counselling has been practised by those who occupy dual roles such as counsellor and doctor, nurse or health visitor. Where dual relationships apply, it is especially important to make the boundaries between roles clear and appropriately manage overlap between professional roles. The pitfalls of dual relationships in the context of general practice have been examined with insight by Kelleher (1989) and it seems that, in the context of health counselling, such problems can best be avoided by ensuring that where possible the role of counsellor is separate from the provision of other services.

It is possible to envisage the relationship between counselling skills as a continuum as described in Table 1 (although for a contrary view on the relationship between counselling and counselling skills see Pratt, 1990). Here counselling skills and counselling are seen as overlapping activities which play more or less prominent roles in different kinds of health-related consultations.

Evaluation of counselling

In a climate in which competition for resources is acute, it is essential that the effectiveness of counselling be demonstrated in order to justify its continued support. There is now a well recognized need to determine the efficacy of counselling in medical settings (Tolley & Rowlands, 1995). Some studies have attempted to do this by asking whether counselling is cost-effective. Maguire *et al.* (1982), for example, reported considerable savings to the British National Health Service through the early recognition and treatment of psychiatric problems in counselled mastectomy patients, as compared with a control group. Other studies have examined changes in patients' use of medical services or reductions in the number of drugs prescribed following counselling. Whilst the results of these studies have generally been favourable, it is necessary to interpret these outcomes with caution. In many of these studies there have been serious methodical flaws such as the absence of control groups; sample attenuation; non-independent evaluation; and lack of appropriate statistical comparison (Brown & Abel Smith, 1985).

Table 1. Levels of psychological counselling

Counselling skills – the provision of factual information and advice about medical conditions, assessment, laboratory tests, treatment, drug trials, disease prevention and health promotion.

Counselling skills/Implications counselling – discussion with the patient and others which addresses the meaning of the information for the patient, personal relationships and taking into account the patient's unique circumstances.

Support counselling – in which the emotional consequences of implications can be expressed and acknowledged in a caring environment.

Therapeutic counselling – which focuses on healing, psychological adjustment, coping and problem resolutions.

(Adapted from The King's Fund Report, 1991)

Most evaluation studies have concentrated on psychological outcomes such as the alleviation of distress, psychological adjustment and the amelioration of psychiatric conditions. Here again methodological difficulties abound. As with the psychotherapies, efficacy depends on the goals of the counsellor, the conceptual framework used and the methodologies which are employed. The research literature contains many examples of evaluation studies where researchers have used outcome measures of doubtful validity and reliability, research designs have been oversimplified and data has been over-interpreted. Moreover, the situation is not eased by the determination among some researchers to apply criteria for conducting evaluation studies of counselling which are almost identical to those used in clinical drugs trials (Andrews, 1993). However, some recent studies have addressed many of the flaws which bedevilled earlier attempts to establish the psychological efficacy of counselling in the medical context. For example, Milne and Souter (1988) studied the effects of counselling on assessed levels of stress in a study which used patients as their own controls by incorporating a waiting list before counselling began. Significant increases in the use of coping skills and decreases in the levels of strain where found. Moreover, these results were not the results of normal crisis resolution because those with the most chronic problems developed more adequate coping skills whilst showing increased stressor scores. Patients who improved showed significant reductions in treatment cost in terms of hospitalization, visits by primary care physicians and drug prescription rates.

Other studies have examined the efficacy of counselling as an adjunct to medical treatment of cardiovascular problems and cancer. Maes (1992) has pointed out that psychosocial interventions, including counselling, may affect cardiac rehabilitation in two ways. First, such interventions may facilitate psychosocial recovery and thus aid return to everyday activities. Secondly, they may play an important role in secondary prevention, by improving compliance with medical advice concerning medication and lifestyle changes. Many of the studies of counselling and cardiac rehabilitation have been reviewed by Maes (1992) and Davis and Fallowfield (1991), who conclude that there is now considerable evidence that counselling, and related forms of intervention, can have beneficial effects on reported stress levels, professional reintegration, necessary lifestyle changes and even perhaps morbidity and mortality. Davis and Fallowfield (1991) also provide a review of studies in which counselling has been employed as an adjunct to physical treatment for many other medical conditions ranging from diabetes mellitus to spinal cord injury.

Although gross measures may indicate the effectiveness of counselling, we still know little about the psychological processes underlying such changes. We also need to know more about which kinds of counselling interventions are particularly beneficial for which patients and at what stage of their illness. This requires detailed consideration of patient characteristics, the nature and time course of the presenting problems, patients' previous coping strategies and the impact of family and other supports. Research into counsellor characteristics and their impact on counselling is also much needed.

Training issues

To date, there has been enormous variability in the experience and qualifications of those employed as counsellors in medical settings. The situation has been unsatisfactory partly because until recently in the UK, there were no statutory regulations governing the qualifications of counsellors. However, helpful recommendations have been drawn up by the BACP, which also operates a voluntary counsellor accreditation procedure. The Counselling in Primary Health Care Trust has also been active in promoting courses at postgraduate level for counsellors working in general practice and other settings. Chartered Counselling Psychologists in the UK are governed by statutory regulations through a route to qualification regulated by the British Psychological Society. With more courses emerging in counselling and counselling psychology at masters and postmasters level, it can be hoped that the qualifications of those working as counsellors will improve and higher levels of professional practice will be provided.

Emerging issues

An increasing number of counsellors working in medical settings provide brief, evidence-based counselling sessions focusing on symptom control or alleviation and helping to enhance patient autonomy and coping (Bor *et al.*, 2004). Extending counselling to carers and other family members is an important new trend which requires specialist training beyond traditional one-to-one therapeutic skills. Counsellors also have an important contribution to make to team resource management and patient safety programmes. Lessons taken from team management programmes in the airline industry are being applied to help improve team performance in healthcare settings, reduce error and prevent the risk of litigation. Counselling and communication skills are central to this initiative in healthcare settings.

REFERENCES

Andrews, G. (1993). The essential psychotherapies. *British Journal of Psychiatry*, **162**, 447–51.

Bond, T. (1993). *Standards and ethics for counselling in action*. London: Sage.

Bor, R. & McCann, D. (Eds.). (1999). *The practice of counselling in primary care*. London: Sage.

Bor, R., Gill, S., Miller, R. & Parrott, C. (2004). *Doing therapy briefly*. Basingtoke: Palgrave Macmillan.

Bor, R., Miller, R., Gill, S. & Evans, A. (2007). *Counselling in health care settings*. Basingtoke: Palgrave Macmillan.

Brown, P. & Abel Smith, A. (1985). Counselling in medical settings. *British Journal of Guidance and Counselling*, **13**, 75–88.

British Association for Counselling (1985). *Counselling definitions of terms in use with expansion and rationale*. Rugby: British Association for Counselling.

British Association of Counselling. (1992). *Code for counsellors*. Rugby: British Association for Counselling.

Davis, H. & Fallowfield, I. (1991). *Counselling and communication in health care*. Chichester: John Wiley.

Engel, G. (1977). The need for a new medical model: a challenge to modern medicine. *Science*, **196**, 129–36.

Kelleher, D. (1989). The GP a counsellor: an examination of counselling in general practice. *Counselling Psychology Section Review*, **4**, 7–13.

King's Fund Report. (1991). *Counselling for regulated infertility treatments*. London: The King's Fund.

Maes, S. (1992). Psychosocial aspects of cardiac rehabilitation in Europe. *British Journal of Clinical Psychology*, **1**, 473–83.

Maguire, P., Oentol, A., Allen, D. *et al.* (1982). Cost of counselling women who undergo mastectomy. *British Medical Journal*, **284**, 1933–5.

Maguire, P & Pitceathly, C. (2002). Key communication skills and how to acquire them. *British Medical Journal*, **325**, 697–700.

Milne, D. & Souter, K. (1988). A re-evaluation of the clinical psychologist in general practice. *Journal of the Royal College of General Practitioners*, **38**, 457–60.

Pereira Gray, D. (1988). Counselling in general practice. *Journal of the Royal College of General Practitioners*, **38**, 50–1.

Pratt, J. W. (1990). The meaning of counselling skills. *Counselling*, **1**, 21–2.

Tolley, K. & Rowlands, N. (1995). *Evaluating the cost-effectiveness of counselling in health care*. London: Routledge.

Group therapy

Peter Hajek

University of London

This chapter will (1) outline the main approaches to using groups to help people deal with psychological problems, (2) examine briefly the relevant outcome research and (3) describe the main applications of group therapy, with particular focus on groups in a medical setting.

Models of group therapy

There is an obvious intuitive and experiential validity in the notion that cohesive groups can provide considerable support and psychological help to their members. Throughout our lives the features of our membership in various groups such as the primary and secondary family, school class, work groups and networks of friends are of great importance. Social interactions within such structures are one of the major sources of human happiness and fulfilment, as well as of human misery.

Various religious and secular groups have always helped to alleviate their members' psychological distress. However, the idea of creating groups for an explicitly therapeutic purpose is relatively new. The first account of such groups was published in 1907. Rather surprisingly, this pioneering report is from a general medical rather than psychiatric setting. An American internist, Joseph Pratt, organized group meetings to provide support and encouragement to patients with tuberculosis, and to demonstrate the benefits of compliance with the therapeutic regimen of the day. In recent years, support groups for people with physical or externally-based problems are becoming popular again. Throughout the intervening period however, group therapy has been practised primarily in psychiatric settings, and the most influential approaches were informed predominantly by the work with neurotic populations.

Groups are a complex and multivariate tool and there exists a large number of styles of group work. Well over 100 'group therapies' have been described in the literature. Most of them, however, derive from four basic approaches, and could be in broad terms allocated to one of them, or to their combinations. These four major strands can be labelled 'analytical', 'interpersonal', 'experiential' and 'didactic'. They correspond to the main work styles a group can adopt, i.e. to analyze motives for group members' behaviour; to provide an opportunity for social learning; to generate emotional experience; and to impart information and teach new skills.

In practice, group therapists working with similar types of clients often converge on a similar integrated package of interventions and skills, spanning across these different approaches. For an observer it would often be impossible to say which particular 'school' the therapist subscribes to. Throughout this chapter, this amalgam which characterizes the practice of many experienced group therapists is labelled 'mainstream practice'. Even the principal proponents of the four alternative forms of group treatment include at least some elements of the other approaches in their work.

The analytical approach

(See 'Psychodynamic psychotherapy'.) This has a historical primacy as the first to apply a theory of psychological functioning and disorders to group treatment. Its influence is waning, but some of its marks remain visible on the eclectic mainstream practice of group therapy. In broad terms, the goal of treatment is to uncover and resolve hypothetical unconscious conflicts. This is expected to lead to the patient's recovery. The mainstream practice has adopted elements of two particular hallmarks of group analytical treatments, i.e. attention to hidden motivation behind group members' interactions, and attention to the relationship of group members to the group leader (transference).

The interpersonal approach

The interpersonal approach emphasizes the opportunity for social learning which groups can provide. Its origin is in the 'laboratory' groups initiated by Kurt Lewin in 1947 and intended as an in vitro social environment in which group members can learn about how groups function and how participants behave in them. Treatment applications of a combination of this and other approaches are associated primarily with the work of Irvin Yalom (1995). The mainstream practice has adopted the concept of social feedback (i.e. allowing group members to learn how their behaviour affects others), and an empirically derived outline of typical developmental processes and stages in an unstructured group. 'Training groups' also provide a model for training group therapists in awareness of group processes.

The experiential approach

The experiential approach to groups is characterized by working primarily with the client's current awareness of their experience. The most important source for this approach were 'encounter groups' inspired by Carl Rogers and aimed primarily at experiences of closeness and acceptance. Jacob Moreno's psychodrama and other developments such as gestalt therapy by Fritz Perls represent other important influences. The contribution of this approach to mainstream practice is primarily in encouraging group therapists to use techniques aimed at stimulating desirable group experiences. (The label 'experiential' is used here for convenience. It often appears in various other contexts as well.)

Didactic approaches

Didactic approaches are connected primarily with behavioural and cognitive treatments administered in groups, but are also widely practised in various health promotion/education contexts. The therapist usually has a set agenda for each session, group members are given concrete tasks and group interaction and group processes are not the main focus of attention. Behaviour and cognitive therapists and health education workers usually lack a background in group dynamics and tend to automatically adopt the simplest group model we are all familiar with, i.e. that of a classroom with a teacher and pupils. Behaviour approaches have developed in opposition to the older models, and there has been little cross-fertilization so far.

Further details of different approaches to group treatment, and descriptions of group processes and of practical skills involved in running groups can be found in Yalom and Leszcz (2005) and Aveline and Dryden (1988).

Therapeutic factors in group therapy

There are a number of hypothetical processes through which groups are supposed to exercise their therapeutic effects. Different applications of group treatment concentrate on different therapeutic factors. A description of group treatment in terms of therapeutic factors expected to foster specific treatment goals is a useful practical alternative to describing a groupwork style only in terms of the therapist's theoretical orientation. This 'transtheoretical' approach to group treatment is also amenable to empirical research.

Several categorizations of therapeutic factors have been proposed. Table 1 provides one of them, based on a list by Bloch and Crouch (1985) with the last item, Group Pressure, added by the present author. The pressure to conform to group norms seems to go against the individualistic self-actualization philosophy endorsed in most writings on groups and therapy. However, where the goal of the group includes e.g. modification of health behaviours, drug use, or antisocial behaviour and where the group manages to establish norms conducive to desirable behaviour change, group pressure can be a major therapeutic influence. Different factors become prominent in different types of groups. For example, a group aiming at uncovering hidden motives behind self-defeating neurotic behaviours would focus on self-understanding more than on guidance; an Alcoholics Anonymous group would rely on instillation of hope more than on catharsis; and a support group for patients diagnosed with cancer would emphasize universality and altruism more than insight.

Efficacy of group therapy

The main and obvious argument in favour of group treatments is that, assuming there is little difference in efficacy between individual and group approaches, treating people in groups is much more cost-effective. Running a group with ten patients for the same length of time that individual treatment would take means that group therapy achieves the same effect as individual therapy ten times faster; or to put the identical argument differently, in the same time period,

Table 1. Therapeutic factors in group therapy

1. *Acceptance* – patients feel a sense of belonging and being valued (cohesiveness).
2. *Universality* – patients discover that they are not unique with their problems.
3. *Altruism* – patients learn with satisfaction that they can be helpful to others in the group.
4. *Instillation of hope* – patients gain a sense of optimism about their potential to benefit from treatment.
5. *Guidance* – patients receive useful information in the form of advice, suggestions, explanation and instruction.
6. *Vicarious learning* – patients benefit (e.g. by learning about themselves) by observing the therapeutic experience of fellow group members.
7. *Self-understanding* – patients learn something important about themselves (insight).
8. *Learning from interpersonal action* – patients learn from thier attempts to relate constructively and adaptively within the group (interpersonal learning).
9. *Self-disclosure* – patients reveal highly personal information to the group and thus 'get it off their chest'.
10. *Catharsis* – patients release intense feelings which bring them a sense of relief.
11. *Group pressure* – patients alter undesirable behaviours/attitudes to gain or to retain group approval.

group therapy helps ten times as many people as the individual approach.

A more involved issue concerns the specificity of any group treatment effects. In most contexts, group treatments have been shown to be effective compared with no treatment, and direct and meta-analytical comparisons have not found much difference between individual and group approaches (Burlingame *et al.*, 2004). Apart from this broad brush conclusion, it is the basic assumption of all types of group therapy that the processes generated in group setting (which are not available in an individual setting) are conducive to patients' recovery. To empirically demonstrate this hypothetical active ingredient of group treatment is not easy. The question of specific efficacy of a treatment which can be applied in different forms with different conditions may appear too unfocused. However, to consider any treatment approach valid and deserving of further study, some proof is needed of the existence of the presumed effect in whatever form and context.

Research in efficacy of psychological treatments is generally difficult and plagued with methodological problems (Kendall *et al.*, 2004). Research in the efficacy of group treatments has the additional handicap of extra demands on sample size because the units of observation are groups rather than individual patients, and it may be even more difficult to find a suitable control condition for group treatments than it is for individual treatments. Comparisons of groups with no treatment or with individual treatments cannot demonstrate the specific effects of groups. More promising are mutual comparisons of group treatments which only differ in group-specific variables. One area uniquely suited to this type of research are smoking cessation groups. This is because there is an almost unlimited supply of patients, treatment is brief and outcome (i.e. tobacco abstinence) is clearly defined and can be objectively verified. In this population there are suggestions that variations in group format can affect outcome, and that individual's chances of success can be influenced by group membership (group effect) (Hajek *et al.*, 1985). At least in this particular area, processes generated by groups seem to have specific effects on therapeutic outcome.

Research in efficacy of group treatments has some way to go. A telling sign is the fact that, as in psychotherapy literature generally, books advising readers on minutiae of treatment still outnumber studies examining whether such manipulations actually have the promised effect. However, over the last few years, good quality randomized trials, particularly of groups in medical settings, are increasingly appearing in respected medical journals. The most recent review of group therapy outcome studies can be found in Burlingame *et al.*, 2004.

Applications of group therapy

Table 2 lists some of the standard uses of group therapy. The remainder of this chapter concentrates on groups for medically ill people.

Medical patients can derive a number of benefits from participating in support groups. The largest available experimental literature concerns groups for cancer patients. There is good evidence that in this patient category, group treatment leads to improvements in coping skills and quality of life and decrease in emotional distress, anxiety and depression (Burlingame *et al.*, 2004). Medical care traditionally focuses on medical illness, and patients' concerns tend to remain unexplored. Yet it is obvious that learning that one has a terminal or debilitating illness has a profound psychological impact, which deeply affects patient's psychological wellbeing, and can possibly affect the course of the illness itself. It appears that group support can ameliorate some of these effects.

The goals of groups with physically ill members differ from the focus of traditional group therapy. Most 'medical' groups concentrate primarily on providing general support to group members, although some would also aim at influencing their health behaviours (e.g. cardiac rehabilitation groups). The group camaraderie and 'common bond in common disease' have already been described by Yalom and Leszcz (2005). In the current revival of medical groups, the emphasis on sharing mutual concerns and feeling understood and accepted remains central. Other elements include relinquishing the unhealthy 'silent sufferer' role often adopted to protect others; the opportunity to learn from other group members about ways of coping with illness; sharing relevant information and resources; maintaining social interest and involvement; etc. Groups are often also an ideal forum for health professionals to impart and discuss medical advice affecting patients' lifestyle.

Table 2. Common uses of group therapy

Groups for normals – assisting personal development in individuals who are not experiencing specific problems. Examples: staff groups, parents' groups, women's groups, etc.

Group counselling for externally-based problems. Examples: groups for rape victims, disaster victims, relatives of mentally or terminally ill, etc.

Group support for physically ill patients. Examples: cardiac rehabilitation, pain management, groups for cancer patients, etc. (see text).

Group treatment for antisocial and addictive behaviours. Examples: groups for delinquents and inmates, Alcoholics Anonymous, group clinics for smokers, etc.

Group therapy for people with neurotic problems and personality disorders. Traditional area of group therapy, usually psychiatric out-patients.

Groups for people with severe mental disorders. Psychiatric in-patients and out-patients (rehabilitation, occupational therapy, 'living skills', etc.).

Groups with patients are usually dependent on health professionals in both their organization and content. Within the health service, group leaders come from diverse professional backgrounds, including psychology, medicine, social work, psychiatry, nursing and rehabilitation.

Examples of 'disease management' groups include groups for chronic pain sufferers (in addition to general support, cognitive–behavioural principles are usually included), coronary artery disease patients (cardiac rehabilitation programmes are possibly the largest application of disease management groups and typically include exercise, stress management, smoking cessation and health education in addition to group support), cancer patients, diabetics, patients with HIV, etc. Even in didactically oriented groups, elements of group support tend to have bigger impact than other components (e.g. Rahe *et al.*, 1979).

An important branch of this work consists of groups with relatives of patients who have chronic debilitating conditions. These groups often have a self-help format. If health professionals are involved at all, it may be only in the initiation stage, or possibly in an ongoing consulting capacity. Support groups for patients' families have been described for parents of newborn children who died, family members of cancer patients, of patients with Alzheimer's disease, etc. Particulars of some of the developments in groups for physically ill and their families can be found in Roback, 1984.

Group counselling for patients with serious medical conditions and for their families is by no means commonplace. However, the merits of this approach are increasingly recognized and various approaches are being formally evaluated. The idea of using group support to alleviate the psychological distress accompanying certain diseases and to improve disease management has taken root, and is likely to continue to develop.

REFERENCES

Aveline, M. & Dryden, W. (Eds.). (1988). *Group therapy in Britain*. Milton Keynes, UK: Open University Press.

Bloch, S. & Crouch, E. (1985). *Therapeutic factors in group psychotherapy*. Oxford: Oxford Medical Publications.

Burlingame, G., MacKenzie, K. & Strauss, B. (2004). Small-group treatment: evidence for effectiveness and mechanisms of change. In M. Lambert (Ed.). *Bergin and Garfield's handbook of psychotherapy and behaviour change*. New York: Wiley.

Hajek, P., Belcher, M. & Stapleton, J. (1985). Enhancing the impact of groups: an evaluation of two group formats for smokers. *British Journal of Clinical Psychology*, **24**, 289–94.

Kendall, P., Holmbeck, G. & Verduin, T. (2004). Methodology, design, and evaluation in psychotherapy research. In M. Lambert (Ed.). *Bergin and Garfield's handbook of psychotherapy and behaviour change.* New York: Wiley.

Rahe, R., Ward, H. & Hayes, V. (1979). Brief group therapy in myocardial

infarction rehabilitation: three-to four-year follow-up of a controlled trial. *Psychosomatic Medicine*, **41**, 229–42.

Roback, H. (Ed.). (1984). Helping patients and their families cope with medical problems. San Francisco: Jossey-Bass.

Yalom, I. & Leszcz, M. (2005). The Theory and Practice of Group Psychotherapy (5th edn.). New York: Basic Books.

Health promotion

Gerjo Kok

University of Maastricht

Health promotion, health education and prevention

Health promotion is any planned combination of educational, political, regulatory and organizational supports for actions and conditions of living conducive to the health of individuals, groups, or communities (Green & Kreuter, 2004). Involving the target individuals, groups, or communities in the development of programmes, is a prerequisite for effective health promotion. Three types of prevention are the goals of health promotion: (i) primary prevention; (ii) early detection and treatment; and (iii) patient care and support. Health education is one type of health promotion intervention. Health education is a planned activity, stimulating learning through communication, to promote health behaviour. Other health promotion instruments are resources and regulation. Health education is based on voluntary change, while regulation is based on forced compliance and will only be effective in combination with control and sanctions. In general, interventions that are directed at several levels and which use more means, will be more effective.

An example of this last statement is the prevention of drunk driving. There is regulation: most countries have laws against driving under the influence of alcohol. Often there is control: drivers are stopped by the police and may be tested, although countries differ in their commitment to these control activities. There are resources: public transport is available and, especially in the weekends and during the night, cheap taxis for adolescents. There is education: information is provided about the rules and possible sanctions, about resources and about drunk driving itself, i.e. the consequences of drunken driving, but also on ways to prevent getting into that situation. The combination of control, resources and education is more effective than any one of these elements alone.

Health promotion as an intervention for patient care, and support is usually called patient education instead of health promotion. Sometimes patient education supports patients who recover, for instance, after surgery. Sometimes the focus is on chronic patients, such as patients with asthma or diabetes. Patient education also includes support for people who are dying, for instance in the case of terminal cancer. Patient education is not only directed at the patient but also at the patient's family, at health professionals and at other environmental factors. Health workers such as physicians and nurses are the primary providers of patient education. Frequently, many different health workers are involved in the treatment of the same patient. Patient education by each of these professionals is not always attuned to the needs of the patient. This calls for the development of patient education programmes that co-ordinate the educational activities of the different health professionals involved, for example, by developing protocols for continuity of care (Mesters *et al.*, 2002).

The planning of health promotion

Health promotion is a planned activity. The best known and most often used planning model in health promotion is Green's PRECEDE-PROCEED model (Green & Kreuter, 2005); see Figure 1.

In short, Green starts with the social assessment: what is the quality of life of a certain group, community or country, and the epidemiological assessment; is health relevant for the quality of life and if it is, what are the most serious health problems? With the epidemiological assessment, the causes of health in terms of behaviour/ lifestyle, genetics and environment can be analyzed. With the educational and ecological assessment analysis can be made of the determinants of the relevant behaviours, in terms of predisposing, reinforcing and enabling factors, and selection can be made of the variables that are desired to be influenced. With the intervention alignment and administrative and policy assessment the possible usefulness of health education and other potential interventions, of resources and regulations can be analyzed. Health promotion interventions are developed and then implemented. Finally, evaluation is made of the process, impact and outcome of these interventions, resulting in feedback and improvement of the interventions.

For example, in most western countries, the quality of life in general is high. People value health as one of the most important aspects

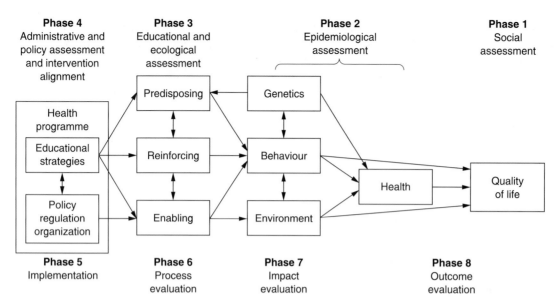

Fig 1 The PRECEDE–PROCEED model for health programme planning (Green & Kreuter, 2005).

of their quality of life. What are the most important health problems? In terms of mortality cardiovascular disease (CVD) and cancer fulfil this role. What are the causes of CVD and cancer? In terms of environment these are, for instance, industrialization and unhealthy working environments. In terms of behaviour and lifestyle, smoking and unhealthy diet are major causes. Let us select smoking and, in particular, the prevention of the onset of smoking, as a relevant behaviour that we might want to influence. Why do adolescents start smoking? Not because they like it and not because they don't know about the dangers. One reason they start smoking is social pressure, mostly from peers, family or mass media. In terms of predisposing factors: adolescents often do not know how to resist social pressure. In terms of reinforcing factors, belonging to a peer group is very important for adolescents. In terms of enabling factors, cigarettes are easy to obtain and sanctions against smoking are weak. What can we do? In terms of health education, we might want to improve adolescents' self-efficacy in resisting social pressure. There are a number of techniques that help adolescents to learn how to resist pressure to smoke, for instance, through positive role modelling (see Bartholomew *et al.*, 2006). In terms of resources and regulation we want to develop anti-smoking policies, for instance, in schools, or through community action against vendors who sell cigarettes to adolescents under legal age. The implementation of such a health promotion programme is organized in co-operation with schools, parents and students. Finally, the effectiveness of the programme is measured. In terms of process evaluation the central question is: was the programme implemented as planned and was the supposed self-efficacy improvement actually realized? In terms of impact evaluation: did fewer students in our programme group start smoking that in a comparison group? It may be clear that an improvement in terms of outcomes, reduction of CVD and cancer and quality of life, cannot be expected for several years.

Quality of the planning

The process of planning health promotion programmes is a cumulative and iterative process. On the one hand, we need answers on earlier planning questions to decide about later phases. On the other hand, the process is not rigid but flexible and we go back and forth through the model. During the planning process we make use of existing knowledge that is systematized in theories, and which is available as empirical data. Why does it have to be so complex? Certainly not because health promoters admire complicated models, but because careful planning is essential if we strive for effect. A very important study in this respect is a meta-analysis by Mullen *et al.* (1985) on 70 patient education studies that were methodologically sound and which included knowledge and compliance as effect variables. Several diseases and several types of interventions were represented. Mullen *et al.* estimated the quality of the interventions using six criteria that they derived from the literature and that can also be seen as guidelines for intervention development:

1. Consonance: the degree of fit between the programme and the programme objectives.
2. Relevance: the tailoring of the programme to knowledge, beliefs, circumstances and prior experiences of the learner, as assessed by pilot-testing or other means.
3. Individualization: the provision of opportunities for learners to have personal questions answered or instructions paced according to their individual progress.
4. Feedback: information given to the learner regarding the extent of which learning is being accomplished (e.g. blood pressure reading).
5. Reinforcement: any component of the intervention that is designed to reward the behaviour (other than feedback) after the behaviour has been enacted (e.g. social support).
6. Facilitation: the provision of means for the learner to take action and/or means to reduce barriers to action (e.g. subsidies).

Mullen *et al.* show that the best predictor of success was the rating score for the quality of the educational intervention. The choice for a specific educational technique was not related to effectiveness, again demonstrating that there is no such thing as a 'magic bullet'. Thus, the effectiveness of a health promotion intervention is determined by the quality of the planning process.

In the six criteria that Mullen *et al.* used, we recognize different concepts from Green's planning model: the choice of relevant behavioural objectives, tailoring to determinants of behaviour, learning (health education), reinforcement, support and facilitation (health promotion). There are also some additional concepts that have not been described in the PRECEDE-PROCEED model, but which are selected from behavioural science theories.

Using theories in health promotion: determinants

At different phases in the planning process different theories will be most relevant (Glanz *et al.*, 2002). The first phases rely on epidemiological theories; the later phases, when the intervention is developed, rely on theories from the behavioural sciences, especially social psychology. In this and the next two paragraphs we will describe theories that can be applied in the three phases: determinants, intervention and implementation.

In the phase of looking at determinants we try to understand why people behave as they do. Current social psychological models indicate three types of determinants of behaviour (Ajzen, 1988; Bandura, 1997):

1. Attitude: beliefs about advantages and disadvantages of behaviour resulting in an attitude about the behaviour, also described as outcome expectations.
2. Social influence: beliefs about social norms, behaviour of others (modelling).
3. Self-efficacy: beliefs about perceived control, self-efficacy expectations.

Models about determinants of behaviour do not imply a one-directional influence; attitudes, social influence, self-efficacy and habits can be antecedents as well as consequences of behaviour (see 'Health Belief Model'). In interventions we try to change determinants in order to change behaviour, but we also use techniques that influence behaviour rather directly, such as reinforcement and having people publicly commit themselves to the desired behaviour. Positive experiences with behaviour, in turn, may change psychosocial determinants of behaviour, thus creating reciprocal determinism (Bandura, 1997). Recently, there has been greater focus on habitual or automated behaviour (Aarts & Dijksterhuis, 2000); interventions to change this kind of behaviour first have to break through the habitual nature of the behaviour.

Using theories in health promotion: interventions

Current general social and health psychological models on behaviour change distinguish steps, phases or stages of change. Within those steps, a number of different specific theories can be applied. One general framework for theories on behaviour change is provided by McGuire's (1985) persuasion–communication model. He describes different steps that people take, from the initial response to the message to, hopefully, a continuous change of behaviour in the desired direction. Simplified, the first steps indicate successful communication, the next steps involve changes of determinants and behaviour and the last step is concerned with maintenance of that behaviour change. Going through these steps, McGuire argues that the educational interventions should change with each step. The choices that have to be made about the message, the target group, the channel and the source, will be different, or may even by conflicting, depending on the particular step that is addressed: for example, mass media may reach many people but are not adequate for self-efficacy improvement.

Prochaska & DiClemente's (1984) Transtheoretical or Stages of Change model distinguishes stages of change within the person: precontemplation; contemplation; preparing for action; action; and maintenance or relapse (see 'Transtheoretical model of behaviour change'). An important contribution of the stage model is the specific tailoring of health promotion efforts to groups of people in different stages. Interventions based on the model normally have completely different methods or strategies for each stage. A frequently used application of the theory is the so-called Motivational Interviewing counselling method (Miller & Rollnick, 2002). Recently, computer-based tailoring programmes based on the stages of change model have been shown to be effective in changing people's behaviour (Kreuter *et al.*, 2000).

Within these general frameworks, a number of other theories can be applied (Glanz *et al.*, 2002). To get people motivated for change, we apply theories on risk perception (Weinstein, 1987); to help people change, goal-setting theory (Strecher *et al.*, 1995); to maintain behavioural change, relapse prevention theories (Marlatt & Gordon, 1985). Although these theories often cover only steps, or even only parts of steps, they can be helpful in developing interventions that focus on particular aspects of change.

Theories can suggest techniques, but the actual application of these techniques in the intervention requires practical experience, creativity and thorough pilot testing.

Using theory in health promotion: implementation

Development of an educational intervention includes making plans for programme implementation. The adoption of innovations is a systematic process, following the pattern of diffusion (Rogers, 2003). A number of characteristics of the intervention are related to faster adoption: compatibility; relative advantage; flexibility; observability; 'trialability' (can the innovation be tried before making a decision?); low risk; reversibility; and low complexity.

Currently, diffusion researchers stress the importance of carefully developing the linkage between the change agent system and the target group system (Oldenburg & Parcel, 2002). In the example of smoking prevention in schools, it is important to involve teachers and students in the development of the programme, as well as principals and parents. In the example of co-operation among different health professionals to achieve continuity of care, it is important to involve all those groups in the development of the protocol.

Intervention mapping

Recently, a protocol was published that describes a process for developing theory-based and evidence-based health promotion programmes, i.e. Intervention Mapping (Bartholomew *et al.*, 2006).

Intervention Mapping describes the process of health promotion programme development in six steps: (1) the needs assessment based on the PRECEDE-PROCEED (2) the definition of performance and change objectives based upon scientific analyses of health problems and problem causing factors; (3) the selection of theory-based intervention methods and practical strategies to change (determinants of) health-related behaviour; (4) the production of programme components, design and production; (5) the anticipation of programme adoption, implementation and sustainability; and (6) the anticipation of process and effect evaluation.

An example of Intervention Mapping is the Long Live Love HIV-prevention programme for Dutch adolescents (Bartholomew *et al.*, 2006, Chapter 10):

1. *Needs assessment*: HIV is a serious health problem and young people today face increased risk of infection. In addition health promotion programmes are most effective when the population has not yet formed risky behaviour pattern and habits.

2. One *change objective* for an HIV-prevention programme in schools would be: 'adolescents (target population) express their confidence (determinant) in successfully negotiating with the partner about condom use (performance objective)'. Performance objectives are the specific behaviours that we want the target group (or the environmental agents) to 'do', as a result of the programme. For example, in the case of HIV prevention; buy condoms; have them with you; negotiate with your partner; use them correctly; and keep using them.

3. The *theoretical method* is the technique derived from theory and research to realize the proximal programme objective; the *strategy* is the practical application of that method. For instance, the method for self-efficacy improvement (for negotiating) could be modelling, and the strategy could be peer modelling by video. An important task in this step is to identify the conditions or parameters that limit the effectiveness of theoretical models, such as identification, observability and reinforcement as necessary conditions for the effectiveness of learning by modelling.

4. The actual designing of the *programme* involves organizing the strategies into a deliverable programme and producing and pre-testing the materials. In the example of HIV-prevention in

schools, the programme comprised five lessons, an interactive video, a brochure for students and a workbook for teachers.

5. The first activity to *anticipate implementation*, actually at the start of intervention development, is the development of a linkage system, linking programme developers with programme users. Then, an intervention is developed to promote adoption and implementation of the programme by the intended programme users.

6. Finally, Intervention Mapping step 6 *anticipates process and effects evaluation*. Again, this is relevant from the start. For instance, 'adolescents express their confidence in successfully negotiating with the partner about condom use' is an objective, but is also a measure of that objective, that can be asked in pre- and post-interviews with experimental and control group subjects.

Although Intervention Mapping is presented as a series of steps, Bartholomew *et al.* (2006) see the planning process as iterative rather than linear. Programme planners move back and forth between tasks and steps. The process is also cumulative: each step is based on previous steps, and inattention to a particular step may lead to mistakes and inadequate decisions.

Epilogue: planned health promotion

Health promotion is a planned activity, stimulating learning through communication in order to promote health behaviour. Health promotion planning involves a series of phases where quality of life, health problems, health behaviour, determinants of behaviour and possible interventions are successively analyzed, followed by the development and implementation of the intervention and evaluation of the process, impact and outcome. Careful planning is important, since quality of planning has been shown to determine effectiveness of the intervention.

A wide range of theories from the behavioural sciences may contribute fruitfully to the analysis of determinants and to the development and implementation of health promotion interventions. Intervention Mapping provides a helpful protocol for theory-based and evidence-based health promotion planning.

REFERENCES

Aarts, H. & Dijksterhuis, A. (2000). Habits as knowledge structures: automaticity in goal-directed behavior. *Journal of Personality and Social Psychology*, **78**, 53–63.

Ajzen, I. (1988). *Attitudes, personality, and behavior*. Milton Keynes, UK: Open University Press.

Bandura, A. (1997). *Self-efficacy: the exercise of control*. New York: Freeman.

Bartholomew, L. K., Parcel, G. S., Kok, G. & Gottlieb, N. H. (2006). *Planning Health Promotion Programs; An Intervention Mapping Approach* (2nd edn.). San Francisco: Jossey-Bass.

Glanz, K., Lewis, F. M. & Rimer, B. (2002). *Health Behavior and Health Education* (3rd edn.). San Francisco: Jossey-Bass.

Green, L. W. & Kreuter, M. W. (2005). *Health Program Planning: An Educational and Ecological Approach* (4th edn.). St. Louis: McGraw-Hill.

Kreuter, M., Farrell, D., Olevitch, L. & Brennan, L. (2000). *Tailoring health messages: customizing communication with computer technology*. Mahwah, NJ: Lawrence Erlbaum.

Marlatt, G. A. & Gordon, J. R. (1985). *Relapse prevention; maintenance strategies in the*

treatment of addictive behaviors. New York: Guilford.

McGuire, W. J. (1985). Attitudes and attitude change. In G. Lindsay & E. Aronson (Eds.). *The handbook of social psychology, Vol. 2* (pp. 233–346). New York: Random House.

Mesters, I., Greer, Th. & Gerards, F. (2002). Self-management and respiratory disorders; guiding patients from health counselling and self-management perspectives. In: A. Kaptein & Th. Creer (Eds.). *Respiratory disorders and behavioural medicine*. London: Martin Dunitz Ltd.

G. Kok

Miller, W. R. & Rollnick, S. (2002). *Motivational Interviewing; Preparing People for Change* (2nd edn.). New York: Guilford.

Mullen, P. D., Green, L. W. & Persinger, G. (1985). Clinical trials for patient education for chronic conditions; a comparative meta-analysis of intervention types. *Preventive Medicine*, **14**, 753–81.

Oldenburg, B. & Parcel, G. S. (2002). Diffusion of innovations. In K. Glanz, F. M. Lewis & B. K. Rimmer (Eds.). *Health Behavior and Health Education: Theory, Research and Practice* (2nd edn.). San Francisco, CA: Jossey-Bass.

Prochaska, J. O. & DiClemente, C. C. (1984). *The transtheoretical approach: crossing traditional boundaries of therapy*. Illinois: Dow Jones–Irwin Homewood.

Rogers, E. M. (2003). *Diffusion of Innovations* (5th edn.). New York: The Free Press.

Strecher, V. J., Seijts, G. H., Kok, G. *et al.* (1995). Goal setting as a strategy for health behaviour change. *Health Education Quarterly*, **22**, 190–200.

Weinstein, N. D. (1987). *Taking care; understanding and encouraging self-protective behavior*. Cambridge University Press.

Hypnosis

Michael Heap

Wathwood Hospital RSU

The nature of hypnosis

Hypnosis is a complex psychological phenomenon. It is an interaction between two people, one of whom is identified as the 'hypnotist', the other as the 'hypnotic subject' (or there may be a group of subjects). In practice it involves a variety of psychological processes and phenomena: selective attention, usually (though not necessarily) relaxation, imagination, expectation, role-playing, compliance and attribution. The significance of each of these ingredients varies according to the situation. There are, however, two additional phenomena related to the above which are central to a discussion of hypnosis, namely suggestion and trance.

Suggestion

Suggestions are communications conveyed verbally by the hypnotist that direct the subject's imagination in such a way as to elicit intended alterations in the way he or she is behaving, thinking, perceiving or feeling. The word 'intended' is meant to convey a key defining property, which is that these changes approximate those that would occur were the imagined events to be taking place in reality. (The reader may also find that the term 'suggestion' is often used to denote the process of responding by the subject to the communication.)

A corollary of the above is that the subjective experience of responding to suggestion has an automatic or involuntary quality. For example, the hypnotist may ask the subject to concentrate on his or her arm; suggestions are then conveyed that the arm is becoming very light and beginning to rise in the air. Associated imagery may be provided – for instance a helium-filled balloon tugging at the wrist. The arm may indeed lift up, but the subjective impression must be that the arm is lifting unaided (or largely so) by conscious effort; the intended response is not that the subject compliantly lifts the arm to placate the hypnotist.

Suggestions which elicit changes in motor behaviour are described as 'ideomotor'. Inhibition of a movement may also be suggested, such as arm immobility or eye catalepsy, in which case the term 'challenge suggestions' is often used. 'Cognitive suggestions' involve changes in perception or cognitive function, including somatosensory changes (anaesthesia, analgesia, warmth, etc.); visual, auditory, olfactory and gustatory 'hallucinations'; and memory inhibition (amnesia). Suggestions may be intended either to take effect immediately or some time after the session of hypnosis. The latter type, termed 'post-hypnotic suggestions' are widely used in therapy. Two examples which illustrate their characteristic form are 'Each and every time you put a cigarette to your lips, you will immediately experience this terrible taste in you mouth' and 'Between now and your next session you will have a dream at night which will help you understand your problem and how to overcome it'.

Trance and the induction of hypnosis

The concept of 'trance' as an altered state of consciousness is more contentious than that of suggestion but it is a very useful one, at least from the standpoint of the clinical applications of hypnosis. Trance is here defined as a waking state in which the subject's attention is detached from his or her immediate environment and is absorbed by inner experiences such as feelings, cognitions and imagery.

It is useful for therapeutic purposes to distinguish between 'inner experiences' that are consciously driven (that is, effortful, verbal, reality-based, etc.) and those that are less so (not goal-directed, not concerned with immediate realities, creative, involving spontaneous imagery, etc.), the latter type being more associated with therapeutic trance experience.

The state of mind here identified as 'trance' is traditionally achieved by the process of 'hypnotic induction' administered by the hypnotist. Typically the induction of hypnosis consists of a series of suggestions that direct the subjects to relax and to become absorbed in inner processes, as described above, and to let immediate realities and concerns become part of the background of their experience. Common methods of induction are progressive muscular relaxation and guided imagery. Many therapists include a procedure such as arm levitation, which allows the patient to experience automatic responding. The later stages of this manoeuvre are termed 'deepening'. Note that during this process the hypnotist does not 'become part of the background'; subjects must attend to the hypnotist and allow him or her to guide and orchestrate the content of their subjective inner world. However, during self-hypnosis, subjects go through the process under their own direction.

Further properties of trance, as defined above, have been determined by empirical research and include the following which, though not guaranteed, may be said to have an increased probability of occurrence due to trance:

i) with regular practice, alleviation of the effects of stress (Benson, 1975);

ii) alteration in the experience of the passage of time, usually leading to under-estimation (Naish, 2003);

iii) some amnesia for events which clearly registered because the subject responded overtly to them;

iv) attenuation of the experience of and increased tolerance of ongoing discomfort and pain.

v) with physical relaxation, an enhanced predisposition to go to sleep (Anderson et al., 1979).

This description of trance includes everyday daydreaming or meditative states and the aforementioned properties may all be exploited formally or informally for beneficial purposes. Such is obviously the case with property (i); the regular practice of self-hypnosis is a common component of hypnotherapy. Properties (ii) and (iv) are useful in treatments for pain management, either where the pain results from some physical condition or where the patient is undergoing some uncomfortable medical intervention. The possibility of selective amnesia (property (iii)) is occasionally exploited in analytical applications of hypnosis which will be discussed later. Finally, the obvious application of property (v) is in the area of insomnia.

Another, rather more contentious claim is that trance facilitates access to unconscious material – memories, feelings, fantasies and so on – which are normally below the level of conscious awareness but which may nevertheless exert an influence on the patient's behaviour, thoughts and feelings. Evidence for this tends to come from single case illustrations rather than empirical research.

There is in fact a tradition in hypnotherapy of perceiving the unconscious in two ways, firstly in the psychoanalytic manner as a repository of anxiety- and guilt-provoking memories, impulses, conflicts and so on, and secondly as a store of

untapped or under-used strengths and resources which the patient may be assisted in bringing to bear on his or her problem. The latter idea is associated with the late American psychiatrist, Milton Erickson. Other features of this approach are, as in this chapter, a broad definition of trance, and the use of story and metaphor as therapeutic communications by the hypnotist. The latter methods are now popular in the use of hypnosis with children.

A final claim is that during the trance the subject is hyper-suggestible, i.e. is more responsive to the hypnotist's suggestions. This is plausible on the basis that in order to respond to a suggestion, for example that their hand is feeling cold and numb or that they are reliving events of childhood, subjects must focus awareness away from the immediate external surroundings and concerns and concentrate on the suggested ideas and images. Hence, a major purpose of the hypnotic induction in therapy may be to enhance the patient's response to the therapist's suggestions that are to follow. However, laboratory research has now established that the increment in suggestibility observed following hypnotic induction and deepening may be due to enhanced motivation, commitment and expectancy on the subject's part, and any set of instructions that has this effect will suffice to enhance responsiveness to suggestion, even those that call for increased alertness and activity.

Theories of hypnosis

Modern theories of hypnosis have tended to emphasize the importance of one or more psychological processes at the expense of others. One of the major distinctions, however, has been the significance attached to the traditional concept of trance or altered state of consciousness. This controversy has in fact been present since the time of Mesmer, but it was around the middle of the last century that psychologists began to provide detailed accounts of hypnosis, later known as 'sociocognitive theories', which were constructed from concepts provided by mainstream psychology, such as imagination, role enactment compliance, strategic enactment and response expectancy and did not require the assumption that hypnotic subjects were placed in a special psychological state (see 'Expectations and health').

An example of a modern 'state' theory is the dissociated control theory of Woody & Bowers (1994). This hypothesizes that during hypnosis there is a disengagement of the frontal lobe executive control system so that responding becomes more automatic and determined by the suggestions of the hypnotist. An earlier theory that also made dissociation a central mechanism was the neo-dissociation theory of Ernest Hilgard (1986), which has greatly influenced practitioners of clinical hypnosis. Nowadays there is much greater overlap in the accounts of hypnosis given by prominent theorists and a willingness to acknowledge that multiple processes are involved. A good example of a recent integrative model of hypnosis is that provided by Brown & Oakley (2004).

The clinical application of hypnosis

The above description of hypnosis in terms of trance and suggestion contains most of the ingredients we need in order to develop therapeutic strategies for a wide range of problems. A traditional hypnotherapeutic intervention consists of the following overlapping stages.

i) a pre-hypnotic stage of rapport-building, information-gathering, allaying of misconceptions and so on;

ii) hypnotic induction and deepening which, as was stated earlier, usually consist of suggestions and imagery conducive to relaxation, an internal focus of attention and perhaps the experience of automatic responding;

iii) the treatment phase, which consists of various kinds of suggestions and imagery, either intended to promote the desired changes in experience and responding or to facilitate access to unconscious processes which may have a bearing on the patient's problem;

iv) a consolidation phase incorporating post-hypnotic suggestions aimed at reinforcing the therapeutic strategies adopted: this stage often includes a series of positive suggestions of a general nature, intended to encourage a sense of self-confidence and optimism, and termed 'ego-strengthening';

v) the alerting of the patient and the post-hypnosis phase of enquiry, clarification of the therapeutic work done, recapitulation of instructions for homework assignments and so on.

We may also include as an additional stage the practice of self-hypnosis by the patient between appointments. The purpose of this for patients may simply be to learn to control and alleviate anxiety and tension but they may also be instructed to rehearse suggestions and imagery specific to their problem. For example, migraine sufferers may imagine hand-warming, or smokers or slimmers may repeat self-statements (affirmations) concerning the reasons for their not smoking or over-eating. The self-hypnosis routine may be practised with the aid of an audiotaped recording.

Specific clinical applications of hypnosis

The above format lends itself well to the treatment of a wide range of medical and psychological disorders and there is virtually no problem for which one can confidently assert that hypnosis has no conceivable role. There exist however certain distinctions and constraints which regulate the useful application of hypnotherapeutic procedures.

Firstly, we may draw a distinction between hypnosis intended for direct symptom alleviation as opposed to hypnosis for resolving memories, feelings, conflicts and so on which may underlie the presenting problem. Examples of the former approach, which is often termed 'suggestive', are provided by the use of suggestion and post-hypnotic suggestion, ego-strengthening and self-hypnosis, for problems such as smoking, obesity, social anxiety, medical complaints which may be aggravated by psychological factors (e.g. irritable bowel syndrome, skin disorders and migraine) and painful conditions. We may include here the use of hypnosis to help patients undergo painful or stressful medical or surgical interventions (such as chemotherapy for cancer) and, for the anxious patient, dental treatment and childbirth.

The second approach of hypnosis is termed 'hypnoanalysis' and is based on a rather simplistic dichotomy of the conscious and unconscious mind. This model has generated a variety of ingenious therapeutic manoeuvres. Examples are the 'uncovering' of material by asking the patient to imagine a theatre stage or cinema screen as a metaphor for 'the unconscious mind' (which, it may be argued, is itself a metaphor), dream suggestion and interpretation, age regression and the use of ideomotor finger signals to denote the responses 'Yes', 'No', 'Don't know', etc. to questions posed by the therapist concerning the possible origins of the patient's problem. Hypnoanalysis may be used for many of the previously mentioned problems, but it tends to be favoured for those in which there is evidence of previous trauma.

A second distinction was made over 20 years ago by Wadden and Anderton (1982) in an influential review of outcome studies using the suggestive approach. These authors contrasted certain problems such as over-eating, smoking and alcoholism with others such as warts, asthma and clinical pain, referring to the former as 'self-initiated' and the latter as 'non-voluntary'. They concluded that the effects of suggestive hypnotherapy for the former were probably largely non-specific and placebo-based (see 'Placebos'). There was, however, good evidence for the specific effects of hypnosis in the treatment of 'non-voluntary' disorders.

We are probably justified in extending the category 'non-voluntary' to a wider range of problems which have a predominantly somatic component and for which we find support in the research literature for the effectiveness of suggestive hypnotherapy (see Heap & Aravind, 2002). Amongst these are certain gastrointestinal disorders such as irritable bowel syndrome and peptic ulceration and eczema. Relaxation and stress control are a substantial component of therapy, but suggestions also target the affected organ or body part. Examples are imagining the warm, healing rays of the sun on the skin in the case of eczema and the release of colonic spasm and the smooth passage of stool in the case of irritable bowel syndrome (see 'Relaxation training'). Whorwell, who has, with his colleagues, undertaken a major study of hypnosis for irritable bowel syndrome (see Gonsalkorale et al., 2003) insists that in the treatment of this disorder, suggestions must focus on bowel activity itself (hence the term 'gut-directed hypnotherapy'): suggestions of general relaxation on their own are insufficient. This claim raises the question of how specifically one can target an autonomic or physiological function by hypnotic suggestion.

Next we may note that it is most appropriate to think of hypnosis not so much as a therapy itself but as a procedure (or a set of procedures) which may be used to augment a broader course of treatment. In fact there is a spectrum of treatments ranging from those where the entire therapy consists of just one or a small number of sessions based on the format outlined earlier, to those where hypnotherapy constitutes a small component of a much more extensive treatment programme. Typifying the former is the single session treatment of warts (induction, deepening, post-hypnotic suggestions of symptom removal, ego-strengthening and de-hypnotising); similarly a single session treatment for smoking cessation. At the other end of the spectrum we see the judicious use of manoeuvres such as age regression and dream suggestion in a course of long-term analytical psychotherapy and the augmentation of a programme of cognitive therapy by hypnotic suggestions and imagery calculated to reinforce the restructuring of maladaptive beliefs and cognitions (Alladin & Heap, 1991; Ellis, 1993).

Contraindications and precautions

It is not easy to define succinctly those occasions when hypnosis should be proscribed. It is generally inadvisable to use it with psychotic patients, although its application here has occasionally been reported. Some caveats concerning hypnosis are applicable to psychological therapies generally, such as the importance of a thorough medical examination, the recognition and treatment of clinical depression and the inclusion of the patient's spouse and family in treatment when they are implicated in the presenting problem. There is concern nowadays about the authenticity of traumatic memories elicited by the indiscreet use of regressive methods, particularly where sexual abuse is claimed. However, probably the most common consequence of misapplying hypnosis is simply time-wasting if a preferred treatment exists, such as in vivo exposure in the case of a phobia or response prevention in the case of obsessive–compulsive disorder (see 'Behaviour therapy' and 'Cognitive behaviour therapy').

Conclusions

In practice, hypnosis is a relatively benign procedure. In the past, its clinical application has suffered through its being uninformed by a rigorous body of academic knowledge and by the unwillingness or incapacity of many practitioners, and indeed authors on the subject, to commit themselves to a proper scientific understanding. There is evidence that this is changing as laboratory evidence on the nature of hypnosis and hypnotic susceptibility accumulates and theory becomes more grounded in mainstream psychology and related disciplines. Reviews of clinical outcome studies for a wide range of disorders have been presented by Heap et al. (2001), and Heap and Aravind (2002) as well as for specific purposes such as pain management (Montgomery et al., 2000), weight reduction (Kirsch et al., 1995) and for smoking cessation (Green & Lynn, 2000). This literature confirms that hypnosis provides therapeutic techniques that are simple and of proven efficacy and which can be unreservedly recommended for inclusion in the clinical practitioner's range of therapeutic skills.

REFERENCES

Alladin, A. & Heap, M. (1991). Hypnosis and depression. In M. Heap & W. Dryden (Eds.). *Hypnotherapy: a handbook* (pp. 49–67). Buckingham, UK: Open University Press.

Anderson, J. A. D., Dalton, E. R. & Basker, M. A. (1979). Insomnia and hypnotherapy. *Journal of the Royal Society of Medicine*, 72, 734–39.

Benson, H. (1975). *The relaxation response.* New York: William Morrow & Co.

Brown, R. J. & Oakley, D. A. (2004). An integrative cognitive theory of hypnosis and high hypnotizability. In M. Heap, R. J. Brown & D. A. Oakley (Eds.). *The highly hypnotizable person: theoretical experimental and clinical issues* (pp. 152–86). London: Brunner-Routledge.

Ellis, A. (1993). Hypnosis and rational emotive therapy. In J. W. Rhue, S. J. Lynn & I. Kirsch (Eds.). *Handbook of clinical hypnosis* (pp. 173–86). Washington, DC: American Psychological Association.

Gonsalkorale W. M., Miller V., Afzal A. & Whorwell P. J. (2003). Long term benefits of hypnotherapy for irritable bowel syndrome. *Gut*, 52, 1623–9.

Green, J. P. & Lynn, S. J. (2000). Hypnosis and suggestion-based approaches to smoking cessation: an examination of the evidence. *International Journal of Clinical and Experimental Hypnosis*, 48, 195–224.

Heap, M., Alden, P., Brown, R. J. et al. (2001). *The nature of hypnosis: report prepared by a working party at the request of the professional affairs board of the British psychological society.* Leicester: British Psychological Society.

Heap, M. & Aravind, K. K. (2002). *Hartland's Medical and Dental Hypnosis* (4th edn.). London: Churchill Livingston/Harcourt Health Sciences.

Hilgard, E. R. (1986). *Divided consciousness: multiple controls in human thought and action:* Expanded edn. New York: Wiley.

Kirsch, I., Montgomery, G. H. & Sapirstein, G. (1995). Hypnosis as an adjunct to cognitive–behavioral psychotherapy: a meta-analysis. *Journal of Consulting and Clinical Psychology*, 63, 214–20.

Montgomery, G. H., DuHamel, K. N. & Redd, W. H. (2000). A meta-analysis of hypnotically induced analgesia: how effective is hypnosis? *International Journal of Clinical and Experimental Hypnosis*, 48, 138–53.

Naish, P. L. N. (2003). The problem of time distortion: determining the necessary conditions. *Contemporary Hypnosis*, 20, 3–15.

Wadden, T. A. & Anderton, C. H. (1982). The clinical use of hypnosis. *Psychological Bulletin*, 91, 215–43.

Woody, E. Z. & Bowers, K. S. (1994). A frontal assault on dissociated control. In S. J. Lynn & J. W. Rhue (Eds.). *Dissociation: clinical and theoretical perspectives* (pp. 52–79). New York: Guilford Press.

Motivational interviewing

Janet Treasure[1] and Esther Maissi[2]

[1]Guy's Campus
[2]King's College London

Motivational Interviewing (MI) is a directive, patient-centred counselling style that aims to help patients explore and resolve their ambivalence about behaviour change. It combines elements of style, such as warmth and empathy, with technique, for instance, focused reflective listening and the skilful development of discrepancy. A core tenet of the technique is that a patient's motivation to change is enhanced if there is a gentle process of negotiation in which the patient, rather than the practitioner, articulates the benefits and costs involved. A strong principle of this approach is that conflict is unhelpful and that a collaborative relationship between therapist and patient in which they tackle the problem together is essential. The four central principles of MI are shown in Box 1.

Reflective listening is a core skill whereby the therapist encourages patients to explore their thoughts and beliefs by using short summarizing statements which attempt to encapsulate (a) the overt content of the patient's utterance (simple reflection) or (b) the underlying and possibly covert emotional content (complex reflection). Rollnick and Miller (1995) were able to define specific and trainable therapist behaviours that they felt led to a better therapeutic alliance and better outcome. These skills are summarized in Box 2.

The first four items in Box 2 explore the factors that sustain the behaviour and aim to help the patient shift the decisional balance of pros and cons into the direction of change. The last two items cover the interpersonal aspects of the relationship. The therapist provides warmth and optimism, and takes a subordinate, non-powerful position, which emphasises the patient's autonomy and right to choose whether to avail him/herself of the therapist's knowledge and skills.

Motivational therapists need to suppress any propensity they might have to show the 'righting reflex', that is to help solve problems and set things right by giving advice. They need to be flexible

---

> **Box 2.** The skills of a good motivational therapist
>
> 1. Understand the patient's frame of reference
> 2. Filter the patient's thoughts so that statements conducive of change are amplified and statements that reflect the status quo are dampened down
> 3. Elicit statements encouraging change from the patient, such as expressions of problem recognition, concern, desire, intention to change and ability to change
> 4. Ensure that patient is not forced to make premature statements about his or her commitment to change
> 5. Express acceptance and affirmation
> 6. Affirm the patient's freedom of choice and self-direction

and have an appropriate balance between acceptance and drive for change towards the desired direction.

Within MI there are special techniques of working with resistance. These are variations on reflective listening, such as 'amplified' reflection, in which the patient's resistance and position is overstated. This works on the assumption that the oppositional tendency of the patient will lead to a withdrawal back to the middle ground. Another approach is to use a 'double-sided' reflection, which highlights the patient's ambivalence. The emphasis is on the individual's autonomy in the matter of change coupled with the therapist holding an appropriate investment in change.

MI helps change behavioural patterns that have become habitual. It works in small doses to produce a large effect. It seems to work by reducing behaviours that interfere with therapy. Patient attributes considered as markers of a poor prognosis, for instance anger and low motivation, are less serious obstacles with MI.

Mode of delivery

Normally MI is a brief intervention lasting for one or two sessions. In various contexts it has also been used as an initial motivational warm-up before other types of treatment, which do not explicitly focus on motivation. Researchers have further adapted MI to suit more specific behaviours and/or research contexts. Motivational Enhancement Therapy (MET) is such an adaptation to MI, which was developed into a manualized four-session therapeutic intervention for alcohol problems (Miller et al., 1992). Similarly, MET has been developed for bulimia nervosa (Schmidt & Treasure, 1997).

> **Box 1.** The four central principles of Motivational Interviewing
>
> 1. Express empathy by using reflective listening to convey understanding of the patient's point of view and his/her underlying drives
> 2. Develop a discrepancy between the patient's most deeply held values and his/her current behaviour
> 3. Sidestep resistance to change by responding with empathy and understanding rather than confrontation
> 4. Support self-efficacy by building the patient's confidence that change is possible

MET incorporated, in the context of the Matching Alchoholism Treatments to Client Heterogeneity (MATCH) study, a 'check-up' form of feedback (Project MATCH, 1997). Most recently, motivational techniques have been integrated with cognitive behaviour therapy and used as a combined behavioural intervention.

Theoretical framework for Motivational Interviewing

MI initially started from a basis of clinical empiricism. Empathy, its central principle, and the various forms of reflective listening, are based on Rogers's (1951) client-centred therapy. Through his work with patients with alcohol problems Miller gradually described more accurately the techniques used in MI. The approach has been fine-tuned from the first manual (Miller & Rollnick, 1991) into a second rewritten edition (Miller & Rollnick, 2002). Several theories have been borrowed to provide MI with a research framework, either with regard to its implementation in the clinical context or to its core components.

A theory that has been linked to one of the core elements of MI is cognitive dissonance theory (Festinger, 1957). This is relevant to therapists' encouragement of patients to resolve their ambivalence about behaviour change. Patients are urged to become aware of their dissonant beliefs, feelings and behaviours and are encouraged to reduce the psychological discomfort associated with such a dissonance by changing their behaviours. Bem's self-perception theory (1967) complements aspects of this process by suggesting that once patients start articulating their own beliefs and pro-change arguments, their commitment towards change strengthens as well as their self-efficacy beliefs, i.e. their feeling of being capable of achieving change.

Self-efficacy beliefs and the process of change

The basic principle that underpins most health behaviour models (e.g. Bandura, 1997) is that people hold a range of beliefs about their self, their behaviours, their illness and symptoms. Thus people can be stoical or in denial and neglect themselves and their symptoms. At the other extreme they may display maladaptive illness behaviour and readily adopt the sick role. Most models of health behaviour change include the idea that there are at least two components to readiness to change. These are perceived importance/conviction and confidence/self-efficacy (Keller & Kemp-White, 1997; Rollnick et al., 1999), being encapsulated in the adage 'ready, willing and able' (see 'Self-efficacy and health behaviour'). Importance relates to why change is needed. This concept includes the personal values and expectations that will accrue from change. Confidence relates to a person's belief that they have the ability to master behaviour change. Motivational Interviewing works on both of these dimensions by helping the client to articulate why it is important for them to change and by increasing self-efficacy so that they have confidence to change.

The Transtheoretical Model (TTM) of change is the model most frequently associated with MI. The TTM was developed by Prochaska and co-workers (Prochaska & Velicer, 1997; Prochaska & Norcross, 1994) and it suggests that a person changes by going through a specific sequence of the following five distinct stages: (1) precontemplation ('I am not thinking of changing my behaviour in the next six months'); (2) contemplation ('I intend to change my behaviour in the next six months'); (3) preparation ('I plan to change within the next month'); (4) action ('I have managed to achieve change from one day up to six months'); and (5) maintenance ('I have not relapsed back to my old behaviour for at least six months') (Prochaska et al., 2002). MI and TTM developed as ideas separately but synchronously. TTM suggested that treatment matched to the stage that a patient is in will be more successful than generic treatments. Two of the core concepts of the TTM are self-efficacy and the cost–benefit analysis pertaining change. One hypothesis drawing from this was that MI might be more useful to those patients who place themselves in the pre-contemplation stage and are hence more resistant to change. Findings, so far, have not supported this hypothesis (Project MATCH, (1997) Treasure et al., 1999; Wilson & Schlam, 2004).

The overall validity of the TTM and, hence its assumed clinical importance, have been criticized by various researchers in the field of behavioural change. With regard to the TTM's relation to MI and MET, there are problems with the stage definition and measurement, their hypothesized distinctness and ability to predict behaviour change following stage-matching according to readiness to change assessments (Sutton, 2001; Weinstein et al., 1998; Wilson & Schlam, 2004; Bandura, 1997). There seems to be no inherent correspondence between TTM and MI or MET (see 'Transtheoretical model of behaviour change').

Resistance to behaviour change

There are two forms of resistance which can impede behaviour change. The first relates to the 'problem' that is being considered and the second to the therapeutic relationship. There may be a conflict between an individual's conceptualization of his or her behaviour and that of family members or society. Thus individuals with drug and alcohol abuse may not see any need to change their behaviour and will have been coerced into treatment by family/ friends or statutory agencies. The other source of resistance often relates to unusual representations of helping/parental/authoritarian relationships or to values about individual rights. Individuals posses an inherent intolerance to a perceived lack of choice and can become motivated to do the opposite of what is requested, the so-called 'reactance'. The propensity to this response lies on a dimension with the poles ranging from oppositional to compliant behaviours. Patients who are prone to resistance are those with high levels of anger, aggressiveness and impulsivity and those with a need for control and with high levels of avoidance.

The effect of resistance in therapy has been reviewed in several studies (Beutler et al., 2002). Resistance, which is marked by anger or defensiveness in therapy, is associated with a poor outcome to therapy. MI has an explicit focus on resistance in therapy.

Evidence on the effectiveness of MI

MI and its adaptations have been evaluated in the contexts of various problematic behaviours and study designs. The diversity of these applications and the research quality make it difficult to combine findings meta-analytically and assess the mechanisms through which MI brings about change.

MI has been found to be effective for different forms of health behaviour change (Dunn *et al.*, 2001). Adaptations of MI have been found to be more effective than no treatment or placebo and as effective as other active treatments for people with problems related to alcohol, drug abuse, diet and exercise, diabetes, hypertension and bulimia. Mixed results have been found for its efficacy in smoking and HIV-related risk behaviours (Burke *et al.*, 2003).

In the most recently published meta-analysis of 72 clinical trials (Hettama *et al.*, 2005) where MI and its adaptations were tested across a range of contexts and behaviours, MI was found to have a good effect early (average between-group effect size was equal to 0.77) but the effect diminished at 12-months follow-up (average effect size was about 0.30). In studies where MI was added to a standard/specified treatment, the effect size was either stable or it increased over time, being on average about 0.60.

Exploring the predictors of MI outcome

The process of change within MI interventions has been studied in order to highlight its key and necessary strategies. It has been demonstrated that the style of the therapist's interaction is a critical component in facilitating change (Miller, 1995).

Therapists differ in their adherence to the principles of MI. Within Project MATCH, in which there was intensive training and monitoring to ensure equitable delivery between therapists, therapist effects on outcome persisted even after controlling for the effects of other variables.

Empathy, demonstrated as accurate reflective listening, is a strong predictor of therapist efficacy. Other elements, which are more difficult to measure, include a stance that communicates belief in the patient's innate abilities and judgement. Thus the role of the therapist is to respect the patient and to hold an optimistic concept of the patient's potential for 'goodness' (i.e. high self-esteem and self-efficacy) and to help the patient work within this framework. The therapist needs to be able to be able to flexibly shift between acceptance and change. Therapist expectancies for patient change have been found to influence patient adherence and outcomes.

A low level of resistance within the session seems to predict behaviour change also (Miller *et al.*, 1993). Resistance often arises in the presence of confrontation. When therapists behave in a way that minimizes resistance, change is more likely to ensue. An increase in the rate of change of 'self-motivational statements', i.e. utterances by the patient that express interest and/or intent to change, is associated with behaviour change. Motivational feedback using the 'drinker's check-up' instrument was compared with a standard approach based on confrontation. The outcome, in terms of drinking one year later, was worse in the group of patients who were given confrontational feedback (Miller *et al.*, 1993). In a further study it was found that if the motivational feedback of the drinker's check-up was given as an initial intervention prior to entry into an in-patient clinic, it led to an improvement in outcome (abstinence rates doubled 57% vs. 29% 3 months after discharge). The therapists (unaware of group assignment) reported that patients given this intervention had participated more fully in treatment and appeared to be more motivated (Brown & Miller, 1993;

Bien *et al.*, 1993). A dose-effect via the delivery of MI-based adaptations, rather than 'pure' MI, and the effectiveness of MI when used as a therapy prelude seem to result in better study outcomes. This, however, is an area that needs more carefully designed future research.

One randomized trial of manual-guided one-session MI for drug abusers failed to replicate the positive results found in the pilot study (Miller *et al.*, 2003). The explanation for this was found when the transcripts of the MI session were analyzed (Amrhein *et al.*, 2003). The need to complete the process of commitment to change within one session interfered with the development of the patient's motivation and some therapists, despite patient resistance, were moving ahead of their patients in an attempt to adhere to the study protocol and the manual.

Training in Motivational Interviewing

Training courses in MI are often relatively short (two to three days). Miller and Mount (2001) evaluated the effectiveness of a two-day training workshop in MI by studying samples of practice before and after the training. They found statistically significant changes in counsellor's behaviours consistent with the principles of MI, but these changes were not large enough to make a difference for patients. Patients did not change either in their resistance levels or in the frequency of expressing commitment to change. Thus, continued practice, regular supervision and monitoring are needed in addition to two to three-day training workshops to attain and maintain standards. Instruments to measure therapist adherence to MI principles are being developed. Two of these are currently available: The Motivational Interviewing Skill Code (MISC) and the Motivational Interviewing Treatment Integrity code (MITI) (http://casaa.umn.edu/tandc.html).

Conclusion

Motivational Interviewing (MI) is a style of therapy that has many applications within general medicine. It is particularly helpful for use in settings where patients show resistance to change. The principles are simple but practice is less easy, and stringent quality control is needed to ensure that therapists adhere to the spirit of the therapeutic process. However, once the overall skill is integrated, honed and maintained it can be adapted to many situations. Practitioners can be flexible in their use of MI-based interventions; they can use this style particularly with patients who are ambivalent about change and later shift to a style of therapy informed more by cognitive and behavioural techniques when the person is committed to change. This is where the art and judgement of therapy come into play. People do not simply switch into a stable motivational state. A sensitive and empathic therapist will know when to move from a skills-based approach into a more motivational stance. Unfortunately, time-limited and/or manualized therapy does not lend itself to such an approach. There always needs to be room for flexibility to adjust for individual differences in the readiness to change, as this is a psychological state that fluctuates within and between therapy sessions.

Existing theories about behavioural change, and specifically the Transtheoretical Model of behavioural change, do not provide a solid framework for MI. Some components of MI have been associated with the cognitive dissonance theory and the social perception theory. Variability exists in the efficacy of MI and its adaptations across studies (even in the same behavioural problem domain) and across therapists. Future research should be directed towards conducting well designed and clinically-based randomized controlled trials. This will shed more light on the effectiveness of MI in various contexts, and help us understand what its 'active ingredients' and the exact predictors of outcome are.

Acknowledgements

JT acknowledges the support of the Nina Jackson Eating Disorders Research Charity.

REFERENCES

Amrhein, P. C., Miller, W. R., Yahne, C. E., Palmer, M. & Fulcher, L. (2003). Client commitment language during motivational interviewing predicts drug use outcomes. *Journal of Consulting and Clinical Psychology*, **71**, 862–78.

Bandura, A. (1997). *Self-efficacy: the exercise of control*. San Francisco: Freeman.

Bem, D. J. (1967). Self-perception: an alternative interpretation of cognitive dissonance phenomena. *Psychological Review*, **74**, 183–200.

Beutler, L. E., Moleiro, C. & Talebi, H. (2002). Resistance in psychotherapy: what conclusions are supported by research. *Journal of Clinical Psychology*, **58**, 207–17.

Bien, T. H., Miller, W. R. & Tonigan, J. S. (1993). Brief interventions for alcohol problems: a review. *Addiction*, **88**, 315–35.

Brown, K. L. & Miller, W. R. (1993). Impact of motivational interviewing on participation and outcome in residential alcoholism treatment. *Psychology of Addictive Behaviors*, **7**, 238–45.

Burke, B. L., Arkowitz, H. & Menchola, M. (2003). The efficacy of motivational interviewing: a meta-analysis of controlled clinical trials. *Journal of Consulting and Clinical Psychology*, **71**(5), 843–61.

Dunn, C., Deroo, L. & Rivara, F. P. (2001). The use of brief interventions adapted from motivational interviewing across behavioral domains: a systematic review. *Addiction*, **96**, 1725–42.

Festinger, L. (1957). *A theory of cognitive dissonance*. Evanston, IL: Row, Peterson.

Hettama, J., Steele, J. & Miller, W. R. (2005). Motivational interviewing. *Annual Review of Clinical Psychology*, **1**, 91–111.

Keller, V. F. & Kemp-White, M. (1997). Choices and changes: a new model for influencing patient health behaviour. *Journal of Clinical Outcomes Management*, **4**, 33–6.

Miller, W. (1995). Increasing motivation for change. In R. K. Hester & W. R. Miller (Eds.). *Handbook of alcoholism treatment approaches: effective alternatives*. Boston, MA: Allyn and Bacon.

Miller, W. R. & Rollnick, S. (1991). *Motivational interviewing: preparing people to change addictive behavior*. New York: Guilford Press.

Miller, W. R. & Rollnick, S. (2002). *Motivational Interviewing: Preparing People for Change* (2nd edn.). New York: Guilford Press.

Miller, W. R., Benefield, R. G. & Tonigan, J. S. (1993). Enhancing motivation for change in problem drinking: a controlled comparison of two therapist styles. *Journal of Consulting and Clinical Psychology*, **61**, 455–61.

Miller, W. R. & Mount, K. A. (2001). A small study of training in motivational interviewing: does one workshop change clinician and client behavior? *Behavioural and Cognitive Psychotherapy*, **29**, 457–71.

Miller, W. R., Yahne, C. E. & Tonigan, J. S. (2003). Motivational interviewing in drug abuse services: a randomized trial. *Journal of Consulting and Clinical Psychology*, **71**, 754–63.

Miller, W. R., Zweben, A., DiClemente, C. C. & Rychtarik, R. (1992). *Motivational enhancement manual: a clinical research guide for therapists treating individuals with alcohol abuse and dependence*. Project MATCH Monograph Series, Vol. 2. Rockville, MD, National Institute of Alcohol Abuse and Alcoholism.

Prochaska, J. O. & Norcross, J. (1994). *Systems of psychotherapy: a transtheoretical analysis*. Pacific Grove California: Brooks/Cole Publishing Company.

Prochaska, J. O., Redding, C. A. & Evers, K. E. (2002). The transtheoretical model of change and stages of change. In K. Glanz, B. K. Rimer & F. M. Lewis (Eds.), *Health behaviour and health education: theory, research and practice*. San Fransisco: Jossey-Bass.

Prochaska, J. O. & Velicer, W. F. (1997). The transtheoretical model of health behavior change. *American Journal of Health Promotion*, **12**, 38–48.

Project MATCH Research Group (1997). Matching alcoholism treatments to client heterogeneity: project MATCH posttreatment drinking outcomes. *Journal of Studies on Alcohol*, **58**, 7–29.

Rogers, C. R. (1951). *Client-centered therapy*. Boston: Houghton-Mifflin.

Rollnick, S., Mason, P. & Butler, C. (1999). *Health Behaviour Change*. Edinburgh: Churchill Livingstone.

Rollnick, S. & Miller, W. R. (1995). What is motivational interviewing? *Behavioural and Cognitive Psychotherapy*, **23**, 325–34.

Schmidt, U. & Treasure, J. (1997). *A clinicians guide to management of bulimia nervosa (Motivational Enhancement Therapy for Bulimia Nervosa)*. Psychology Press Hove, UK: Psychology Press.

Sutton, S. (2001). Back to the drawing board? A review of applications of the transtheoretical model to substance use. *Addiction*, **96**, 175–86.

Treasure, J. L., Katzman, M., Schmidt, U., Troop, N., Todd, G. & de Silva, P. (1999). Engagement and outcome in the treatment of bulimia nervosa: first phase of a sequential design comparing motivation enhancement therapy and cognitive behaviour therapy. *Behavioral Research and Therapy*, **37**, 405–18.

Weinstein, N. D., Rothman, A. J. & Sutton, S. R. (1998). Stage theories of health behaviour: conceptual and methodological issues. *Health Psychology*, **17**, 290–9.

Wilson, G. T. & Schlam, T. R. (2004). The transtheoretical model and motivational interviewing in the treatment of eating and weight disorders. *Clinical Psychology Review*, **24**, 361–78.

Neuropsychological rehabilitation

Barbara A. Wilson

MRC Cognition and Brain Sciences Unit

Introduction

Neuropsychological rehabilitation is concerned with the assessment, treatment and recovery of brain-injured people and aims to reduce the impact of disability and handicapping conditions and, indirectly, to improve the quality of life of patients.

For the most part, neuropsychological rehabilitation concentrates on cognitive and emotional deficits following brain injury, although physical, social and behavioural disorders are also addressed. It can therefore be distinguished from cognitive rehabilitation in that it encompasses a wider range of deficits.

Modern rehabilitation of brain-injured people probably began in Germany during World War I as a result of improvements in survival rates of head-injured soldiers (Goldstein, 1942). Goldstein stressed the importance of cognitive and personality deficits following brain injury, and described principles which are almost identical to those used in current neuropsychological rehabilitation. A further impetus to neuropsychological rehabilitation came during World War II, with developments in Germany, the UK, the Soviet Union and the USA (Boake, 1989, Prigatano, 1986). An important paper by Zangwill (1947) discussed principles of re-education and referred to three main approaches – compensation, substitution and direct retraining.

At the same time, Luria and his colleagues were treating head-injured soldiers in the Soviet Union, and describing their activities (Luria, 1979). These early papers by Zangwill and Luria still provide a rich source of ideas for contemporary neuropsychologists interested in rehabilitation.

Recent developments in neuropsychological rehabilitation

There have been a number of changes in the practice of neuropsychological rehabilitation over the past 15 or so years. There are five changes that would appear to have been particularly influential: (1) rehabilitation is now seen as a partnership between patients, families and healthcare staff; (2) goal setting is now well established as a means of planning rehabilitation programmes; (3) there is general recognition that cognition, emotion, social functioning and behaviour are interlinked and should all be addressed in the rehabilitation process; (4) there has been an increase in the use of technology to help people compensate for their difficulties; and (5) there is a greater acknowledgement that rehabilitation requires a broad theoretical base; no one theory, model or framework is sufficient to address all the problems faced by people with neuropsychological deficits.

Rehabilitation as a partnership

Over the past 10–15 years, patients and families have become increasingly involved in making decisions about rehabilitation. Gone are the days, in most brain injury rehabilitation centres, when doctors, psychologists, therapists and nurses decided what patients would do, achieve or work on during rehabilitation. Instead, patients together with their families and healthcare staff discuss the aims and goals of rehabilitation and negotiate these. This partnership is reflected in McLellan's (1991) definition of rehabilitation as a two-way interactive process between the disabled person and others to achieve their optimum physical, psychological, social and vocational wellbeing.

Goal setting as a means of planning rehabilitation programmes

Goal planning has been used in rehabilitation for a number of years with various diagnostic groups including people with cerebral palsy, spinal injuries, developmental learning difficulties and acquired brain injury (McMillan & Sparkes, 1999). Because goal planning is simple, focuses on practical everyday problems, is tailored to individual needs and avoids the artificial distinction between many outcome measures and real life functioning, it is used increasingly in rehabilitation programmes.

Houts and Scott (1975) and McMillan and Sparkes (1999) put forward several principles of the goal planning approach. First, the patient should be involved in setting his or her goals. Second, The goals set should be reasonable ones and client centred. Third, they should describe the patient's behaviour when a goal is reached. Fourth, they should spell out the method to be used in achieving the goals in such a manner that anyone reading the plan would know what to do. In addition, goals should be specific and measurable and have a definite time deadline. In most rehabilitation centres, long-term goals are those which the patient or client is expected to achieve by the time of discharge from the programme while short-term goals are the steps set each week or fortnight to achieve the long-term goals.

Cognition, emotion, social functioning and behaviour are interlinked (the holistic approach)

Although cognitive problems are among the most handicapping for brain-injured people, they are not generally seen in isolation. Emotional and behavioural problems are common, and may indeed worsen over time. Depression, anxiety, irritability and aggression may all occur. Social isolation is often reported by brain-injured people and their families. Different personality characteristics and pre-morbid lifestyles may exacerbate or diminish the relevance of current problems for everyday functioning, and may influence the effectiveness of rehabilitation.

Such a multitude of sequelae following brain injury has led to the development of holistic approaches whereby rehabilitation programmes attempt to deal with the 'whole person'. The original holistic neuropsychological rehabilitation regime for brain-injured people appears to be that of Ben Yishay and his colleagues in Israel in 1974 (Prigatano, 1986), with a few others following Ben Yishay's model elsewhere in the USA and in Europe.

Major themes of these programmes include the development of increased awareness, acceptance and understanding, cognitive retraining, development of compensatory skills and vocational counselling. Evidence is provided of increased self-esteem among patients, reduction in anxiety and depression and greater social interaction (Ben Yishay & Prigatano, 1990).

Increasing use of technology in neuro-rehabilitation

In the early part of the 1980s there was considerable excitement concerning the use of computers, which were expected to revolutionize cognitive rehabilitation. It was thought they would assist neuropsychologists with assessment, monitoring treatment effectiveness and retraining. Numerous software programmes appeared, despite the fact that they were not subjected to controlled investigation at that time. Robertson (1990) published a review of computerized rehabilitation and focused on programmes for language, memory, attention, visuoperceptual and visuospatial disorders. His concern was with adults with non-progressive, acquired brain damage, so he excluded computer programmes used for assessment, recreation, teaching aids, or prosthetic devices. He found no evidence that computerized memory, visuoperceptual or visuospatial training produced significant changes in cognitive functioning. Language training programmes fared a little better, although there was no published evidence for general effectiveness of computerized language training. Only in attention training were there some positive results, although even here the evidence was contradictory. Since Robertson's (1990) review, further studies of computerized attentional training programmes appear to support the tentative evidence from the 1980s that they can be effective.

Already useful as prosthetic devices for people with language or physical impairments, computers are likely to play more important roles in other areas of cognitive disability. For example, they could be used as aids in activities of daily living by providing series of cues to guide patients through the steps needed to perform practical tasks such as cooking, janitorial activities or money management. Kapur et al. (2004) point out that computers have great power for storing and producing on demand all kinds of information relevant to an individual's functioning in everyday life.

Another area of current interest is in the use of computers as memory aids. Much of the work in memory rehabilitation involves teaching people to compensate for their impairments by employing aids such as diaries, tape recorders and electronic organizers. Work in this area of rehabilitation is difficult, however, because remembering to use an aid is in itself a memory task that

brain-injured people may forget to employ. Additionally, memory-impaired people will probably experience great difficulty in learning to programme an electronic or computerized aid or they may use them in unsystematic and inefficient ways. Kapur (1995) discusses a number of external memory aids and suggests ways of teaching their use. Wilson et al. (2001) report on one particular computerized memory aid, NeuroPage®, developed by a neuropsychologist, Neil Hersh and Larry Treadgold, the engineer father of a head-injured son. NeuroPage® is a simple and portable paging system with a screen that can be attached to a waist belt. The system uses an arrangement of microcomputers linked to a conventional computer memory and, by telephone, to a paging company. The scheduling of reminders or cues for each individual is entered into a computer and from then on no further human interfacing is required. On the appropriate date and time, the reminder is transmitted to the individual, and all that person has to learn is to press one fairly large and obvious button on receipt of the signal. A randomized control trial of the system in which people were randomly allocated to a pager first or to a waiting list first, showed that the pager significantly reduced the everyday failures of memory and planning in people with brain injury. More than 80% of those who completed the trial were significantly more successful in carrying out activities such as self-care, self-medication and keeping appointments when using the pager compared with the baseline period.

Neuropsychological rehabilitation requires a broad theoretical base

People surviving brain injury are likely to have several cognitive problems including attention, memory and planning problems and they are likely to have additional non-cognitive problems such as anxiety, depression and social skills deficits. Consequently, it is unlikely that any one model, theory or framework can address all of these difficulties and neuropsychological rehabilitation requires a broad theoretical base (or several theoretical bases). A theoretical model can be regarded as a representation that may help to explain and increase our understanding of related phenomena. They vary in complexity and detail, ranging from highly complex computer-based structures such as connectionist models of brain damage through to simple analogues that assist in the explanation of relatively complex situations like comparing memory storage to various library systems (Baddeley, 1992).

In rehabilitation, models are useful for facilitating thinking about assessment and treatment, for explaining deficits to therapists and relatives and for enabling us to conceptualize outcomes. No one model can answer all our questions, deal with all the complexities of treatment and management or address all the needs of patients and families. Wilson (2002) attempted to integrate many of the existing models that are useful for neuropsychological rehabilitation into a comprehensive model of rehabilitation. This synthesis of models that have influenced rehabilitation including models of cognitive functioning, emotion, learning, personality, recovery and others. In order to understand which parts of the synthesized model were most used by practising psychologists engaged in neuropsychological rehabilitation, a questionnaire was designed and sent to psychologists working in brain injury rehabilitation. Psychologists were asked to confirm all the components of the model that they assessed in their practice, e.g. personality, cognitive functioning, emotion, behaviour and to provide further comments. Approaches to treatment were also surveyed.

Forty-five people responded. Some of the main results are summarized. One hundred per cent of the respondents said they tried to find out about patients' likes and dislikes and the same percentage said that they employed a goal-setting approach. All but two said they assessed pre-morbid personality and all but three said they assessed present personality. The most frequently used treatment approaches derived from models of cognitive behaviour therapy, (67%) cognitive neuropsychological theory (37%) and behavioural models (24%) (see 'Behaviour therapy' and 'Cognitive behaviour therapy'). Psychodynamic models were only used by 3% of respondents (see 'Psychodynamic psychotherapy'). Most practitioners tried to reduce disabilities and handicaps rather than impairments. They made use of several strategies to do this, with the most frequent being compensatory techniques, making use of residual skills and restructuring the environment (between 90 and 100% using these) Restorative approaches and attempts at anatomical reorganization were rarely used.

Practising psychologists in rehabilitation use a range of theoretical models and approaches in their clinical work, confirming the view that we need a broad theoretical base when dealing with the complex problems faced by people with brain injury.

Conclusions

Neuropsychological rehabilitation has reached an exciting stage of development with a worldwide growing interest in the subject as reflected in numerous conferences, debates, books and papers in journals relevant to the field. This interest has been stimulated by scientific research, on the one hand, and by improved and more sophisticated clinical practice, on the other. A wide range of methodologies is available to practitioners of neuropsychological rehabilitation, including those from cognitive neuropsychology, learning theory, developmental psychology, linguistics and, more recently, connectionist modelling. It is to be hoped that a recent comprehensive model of neuropsychological rehabilitation will inform psychologists and therapists working in the field and lead to even more improvements. (See also 'Neuropsychological assessment' and 'Head injury').

REFERENCES

Baddeley, A. D. (1992). Memory theory and memory therapy. In B. A. Wilson & N. Moffat (Eds.). *Clinical management of memory problems* (pp. 1–31). London: Chapman & Hall.

Ben-Yishay, Y. & Prigatano, G. (1990). Cognitive remediation. In E. Griffith, M. Rosenthal, M. R. Bond & J. D. Miller (Eds.). *Rehabilitation of the adult and child with traumatic brain injury* (pp. 393–409). Philadelphia: F. A. Davis.

Boake, C. (1989). A history of cognitive rehabilitation of head-injured patients, 1915 to 1980. *Journal of Head Trauma Rehabilitation*, **4**, 1–8.

Goldstein, K. (1942). *Aftereffects of brain injury in war.* New York: Grune and Stratton.

Houts, P. S. & Scott, R. A. (1975). *Goal planning with developmentally disabled persons: procedures for developing an individualized client plan.* Hershey, PA: Department of Behavioral Science, Pennsylvania State University College of Medicine.

Kapur, N. (1995). Memory aids in the rehabilitation of memory disordered patients. In A. D. Baddeley, B. A. Wilson & F. N. Watts (Eds.). *Handbook of memory disorders* (pp. 533–56). Chichester: John Wiley.

Kapur, N., Glisky, E. L. & Wilson, B. A. (2004). External memory aids and computers in memory rehabilitation. In A. D. Baddeley, M. D. Kopelman & B. A. Wilson (Eds.). *The essential handbook of memory disorders for clinicians* (pp. 301–27). Chichester: John Wiley.

Luria, A. R. (1979). *The making of mind: a personal account of Soviet psychology* M. Cole & S. Cole (Eds.). Cambridge, MA: Harvard University Press.

McLellan, D. L. (1991). Functional recovery and the principles of disability medicine. In M. Swash & J. Oxbury (Eds.). *Clinical neurology* (pp. 768–90). Edinburgh: Churchill Livingstone.

McMillan, T. & Sparkes, C. (1999). Goal planning and neurorehabilitation: the Wolfson neurorehabilitation centre

approach. *Neuropsychological Rehabilitation*, **9**, 241–51.

Prigatano, G. P. (1986). Personality and psychosocial consequences of brain injury. In G. P. Prigatano, D. J. Fordyce, H. K. Zeiner *et al.* (Eds.). *Neuropsychological rehabilitation after brain injury* (pp. 29–50). Baltimore; London: The Johns Hopkins University Press.

Robertson, I. H. (1990). Does computerised cognitive rehabilitation work? A review. *Aphasiology*, **4**, 381–405.

Wilson, B. A. (2002). Towards a comprehensive model of cognitive rehabilitation. *Neuropsychological Rehabilitation*, **12**, 97–110.

Wilson, B. A., Emslie, H. C., Quirk, K. & Evans, J. J. (2001). Reducing everyday memory and planning problems by means of a paging system: a randomised control crossover study. *Journal of Neurology, Neurosurgery and Psychiatry*, **70**, 477–82.

Zangwill, O. L. (1947). Psychological aspects of rehabilitation in cases of brain injury. *British Journal of Psychology*, **37**, 60–9.

Pain management

Stephen Morley

University of Leeds

The term pain management applies mainly to chronic pain rather than acute pain. In its broadest sense it includes a range of physical (e.g. spinal cord stimulation) and pharmacological (e.g. opioid drugs, intrathecal pumps, facet joint injections) as well as psychological interventions. Although the purpose of physical interventions is to reduce the intensity, frequency and duration with which pain is experienced, the overall aim of pain management is to ameliorate the experience of pain in its broadest sense rather than to eradicate it. Acute pain, such as postoperative pain, is expected to have a self-limiting time course and treatments are primarily directed at preventing its occurrence or reducing the magnitude of experienced pain during this period of time. This approach has been transferred to many medical treatments of chronic pain (such as those listed above) but while the elimination of pain is a worthy goal for chronic pain sufferers it is generally not possible with our present understanding of the neurobiology of chronic pain. By definition chronic pain is longstanding, usually defined as greater than six months but often many years. Most sufferers will have received a wide range of pharmacological treatments without experiencing complete relief. When pain persists over a period of time its impact becomes widespread, it needs to be considered as a multifaceted construct and its treatment is necessarily more complex. This chapter is therefore concerned primarily with psychological approaches to this problem.

Chronic pain as a construct

In order to understand psychological approaches to pain management, it is necessary to examine the contemporary psychological analysis of pain. This analysis conceptualizes pain as a meta-construct: a set of inter-related components none of which uniquely defines pain. Moreover, each component is itself a complex construct and the subject of scientific and clinical investigation. The experimental analysis of these components has developed considerably in recent years but many problems remain. As a result of this, psychological treatments are only partly based on a fully rational analysis of the problem.

The main biological elements underpinning the experience of pain are nociception, transmission and modification of nociceptive inputs and the central representation of pain in the brain. Pharmacological and physiological therapies (neurostimulation) are all directed at these elements. Although many biological pain processes are not directly addressed by psychological treatments, treatments such as relaxation training and biofeedback are directed at some physiological responses to painful stimuli e.g. increased muscle tension and sympathetically mediated responses (see 'Relaxation training' and 'Biofeedback').

For acute somatic pain there is good evidence that the immediate experience of pain is correlated with basic neurophysiological parameters (Price, 1999). Current thinking considers the primary experience of pain to comprize two inter-related dimensions; a sensory–intensity dimension characterized by the sensory quality of the pain (reflected by descriptors such as 'throbbing' and 'shooting') and a primary affective dimension (reflected by descriptors such as 'unpleasant' and 'agonizing'). The relationship between neurophysiological parameters and immediate pain experience in chronic pain is not well established but the same sensory–intensity and affective experiences are present. However the persistence of pain leads to a more complex range of emotional experiences as would be expected when a person is forced to re-evaluate him- or herself in the face of an adverse experience. The main emotional states observed in chronic pain patients are frustration, anxiety and depression. Understanding what shapes individuals' emotional responses to persistent pain is an important topic of contemporary research, with relevance for the development of treatments (Asmundson et al., 2004; Banks & Kerns, 1996).

Chronic pain is also associated with marked cognitive changes. The phrase 'cognitive' is used broadly to refer to a wide range of psychological phenomena, including a person's attitudes and beliefs about pain as well as more fundamental appraizal mechanisms which incorporate attention, perception and memory processes. It also refers to the mental activity in which people engage while experiencing pain. Current research indicates that certain types of activity, such as thinking about catastrophic outcomes (catastrophizing) intensify the experience of pain and distress (Sullivan et al., 2001). Not surprisingly catastrophizing is a major target for intervention in therapy.

Acute pain is often associated with distinct behavioural acts; the sudden reflex withdrawal from the pain stimulus, para-vocalizations and changes to facial expression. When pain persists the behavioural consequences become greatly elaborated and may include persistent verbal complaints and expressions of pain, postural changes, use of mobility and support aids, reduction in the general activity level, increased medication consumption and a range of other placatory behaviour. Psychological theorizing has applied the concepts of classical and operant conditioning in the analysis to behaviour associated with pain. It is important to note that behavioural activity is a public event and it is therefore subject to modification by social reinforcement contingencies. This process has been invoked to explain variation in pain behaviour between individuals and is also applied therapeutically. The major behavioural treatment is concerned with analysis of the contingent relationship between pain and behaviour and the subsequent modification of the contingencies (Fordyce, 1976; Sanders, 2002).

Finally, we must consider the social context in which pain occurs. Factors known to influence several aspects of pain include the age and gender of the person, family characteristics, culture and the behaviour of professionals and carers. These may all be important when considering treatment options (Morris, 1998). In addition to these features there are influences from work and employment status and, in some cases, the legal status of the person, i.e. whether compensation claims are pending.

Implications

This brief résumé indicates the breadth of factors considered by psychological approaches to pain. It may be useful to simplify the complexity surrounding chronic pain if we construe it as comprising three major components; interruption, interference and identity. A primary feature of pain is to interrupt ongoing behaviour and cognitive activity on a moment by moment basis. The extent of the interruption is related to the intensity, novelty and threat value of the pain. Patients with chronic pain have constantly to manage this interruption and to incorporate it into their daily functioning. Interruption can also lead to interference with behaviour that has a visible impact on the pain sufferer. Patients with chronic pain frequently report high levels of frustration attributable to their incapacity to complete normal behavioural routines or to complete them in an acceptable timescale. For example, even dressing can be a major source of frustration. The degree of interference with life is reflected in the extent of disability reported by patients. Finally when interference occurs in many behavioural activities, or in particularly important ones, then pain has the capacity to impact on a person's identity i.e. his or her sense of who s/he are and perhaps more importantly who s/he might become (Morley & Eccleston, 2004). It is at this level that we can understand the suffering caused by chronic pain (Chapman & Gavrin, 1999).

Not all treatments embrace all the factors. Medical treatments are primarily targeted at reducing the interruptive impact of pain by moderating the sensory–intensity and primary affective responses to pain. Psychological treatments may also target interruption e.g. attention management. They more frequently attempt to modify the extent of interference by increasing meaningful behavioural activity and coping strategies. More recent work on acceptance is clearly targeting identity as a significant focus for treatment (McCracken *et al.*, 2004).

Psychological treatments in pain management

Psychological approaches to pain management are multimodal, presenting the patient with a series of interventions throughout treatment. Meta-analytic reviews of the psychological management of pain (Morley *et al.*, 1999) and of multidisciplinary approaches incorporating substantial psychological components (Flor *et al.*, 1992), testify to the effectiveness of psychological approaches to pain management.

Psychological management is characterized by several features which are common to treatment programmes despite variations in their content. Psychological treatments require the active engagement of the patient. Rather than being a passive recipient of a treatment delivered by a professional the patient is explicitly assigned personal responsibility for the planning and implementation of treatment. The initial assessment phase provides the therapist with information about the patient's understanding of his or her pain and an assessment of his or her attitudes, beliefs and cognitive state. The assessment also provides the therapist with an educational opportunity to both give information about chronic pain and begin to help patients to elaborate alternative ways of construing their experiences. Emphasis is placed on the co-variation between psychological states and the experience of pain. For example, patients are frequently required to keep pain diaries to help them discover the reciprocal influences between events, their mood, behaviour and pain. Psychological management also requires patients to set specific goals for treatment and specify ways in which they may be achieved. In the case of chronic pain, goal setting often requires the patient to shift from unrealistic outcome expectations of 'no-pain' to expectations that they will be able to manage their pain, so that its impact on their life is reduced. The aim of assessment is to elaborate the patient's view of pain and in doing so help them generate a range of treatment options which they will be able to apply outside the clinic. Psychological management therefore explicitly considers how treatments may be generalized and maintained out of the clinic and over a prolonged period of time.

Education

Education always forms a part of multidisciplinary pain treatment programmes and good practice incorporates this element during the assessment phase. The educational process is active and requires patients to reflect on their own understanding of pain. The educational component of treatment is an integral part of contemporary psychological management (Turk, 2002) and serves to engage the patient as an active collaborator in the process of treatment.

Relaxation and biofeedback

There are two broad classes of treatments; biofeedback and relaxation, which are aimed at modifying a biological aspect of pain. In biofeedback physiological signals (e.g. Electromyography (EMG), skin temperature) are processed and displayed as auditory or visual information to the patient. The patient is instructed to attempt to change a feature of the display in a direction corresponding to the required change in physiological functioning. For example, the pitch of an auditory signal might correlate with EMG activity, so that reduction in EMG will be reflected by a lowering of pitch. Biofeedback has been extensively investigated as a standalone treatment over 30 years (Arena & Blanchard, 2002). There is substantial evidence that it can be effective in the treatment of a variety of painful disorders, e.g. headache. Recent reconsideration of biofeedback as a treatment has been stimulated by experimental analysis of chronic pain problems which has identified specific peripheral dysfunctions hypothesized to be responsible for nociceptive input. For example (Flor & Birbaumer, 1993) treated patients with low back pain and temporomandibular pain with EMG biofeedback derived from the appropriate paraspinal or facial muscles. Their data indicated that biofeedback training was more effective than a relatively brief cognitive–behavioural programme and standard, conservative, medical treatment.

Biofeedback may also be used non-specifically to help induce a general state of relaxation. Relaxation is a widely used component of psychological treatment packages. The primary purpose of relaxation is to reduce the psychophysiological arousal frequently associated with pain. It is also frequently taught as a coping resource which patients can use at times of heightened pain and distress. Biofeedback procedures are not generally necessary as there is a range of relaxation procedures (active progressive relaxation, autogenic training and varieties of breathing exercises) which are relatively easily applied within a clinical setting (see 'Relaxation training' and 'Biofeedback').

Attention management

Methods designed to modify attentional focus are frequently incorporated into cognitive–behavioural pain management programmes and presented as part of a relaxation strategy. The rationale for this approach is a widely held view that the content of conscious awareness is determined by a limited capacity channel with attentional mechanisms controlling which aspects of a person's external and internal environment enter into consciousness (Cioffi, 1991). Pain may be considered as a stimulus which vies for finite attentional resources. The purpose of treatment is therefore to teach patients to switch attention to other sources of stimulation or to change the interpretation placed on the current focus of awareness. For example, a patient may be taught to construct a vivid mental image which includes features from a number of sensory dimensions, e.g. cutting a lemon and squeezing a drop of the juice onto the tongue. The elaborated sensory features of this image compete with the painful stimulus and reduce its impact. Alternatively, the patient may be encouraged to alter the focus of their attention to the pain without switching attention away from the pain. In this instance, the subject may be asked to focus on the sensory quality of the pain and transform it to a less threatening quality (Morley et al., 2004). While these procedures are undoubtedly popular, empirical evidence for their effectiveness is difficult to obtain (Eccleston, 1995). On balance, it would appear that attention switching/distraction strategies do have a role to play in the management of pain although it is probable that they are most effective at low to medium levels of pain intensity (Jensen & Karoly, 1991). Hypnotic methods may also be employed to modify the subjective experience of pain (Syrajala & Abrams, 2002).

Cognitive–behavioural strategies

Cognitive–behavioural strategies are predicated on the hypothesis that it is a person's interpretation of events rather than the events themselves which determines the subjective experience and behavioural response to the event. In the context of pain the critical determinants of individuals' emotional and behavioural adaptations to the pain are their thoughts (appraisals, expectations and beliefs about the origin and consequences of the pain), rather than the nociceptive and biological events per se. Cognitive–behavioural methods seek to modify a person's thinking about pain, and in doing so to change their pattern of adaptation to it. The central technique of cognitive–behavioural strategies is the identification of the sequence of thoughts and actions exhibited during painful episodes. A common content of patient's mental activity is 'catastrophizing', the expectation of worst-state outcomes (Sullivan et al., 2001). These and other dysfunctional methods of thinking about pain can be modified by a set of techniques which include cognitive challenges to the belief, provision of alternative ways of construing events (reattribution) and self-instructional behavioural experimentation with alternative adaptive coping responses. Treatment is through guided rehearsal under the supervision of a therapist with subsequent monitoring and modification as patients introduce the methods into their daily lives (Hanson & Gerber, 1990; Keefe et al., 2002; Turk, 2002) (see 'Cognitive behavioural therapy').

Behavioural

Behavioural approaches to pain are directed at modifying pain behaviour rather than the subjective experience of pain. Pain behaviour includes maladaptive postural changes, excessive resting and dysfunctional rest–activity cycles. The application of principles of operant behaviour modification has been paramount in the development of behavioural treatments (Fordyce, 1976; Sanders, 2002). Frequent targets for intervention are patients' activity levels (physical fitness), medication intake and social interactions with family members. Behavioural assessment identifies the events which precede (discriminative stimuli) the target pain behaviour and the consequences of the behaviour (the reinforcers). Treatment consists of manipulating the contingencies between these events in order to decrease non-functional responses and increase positive adaptive ways of behaving. Features of behavioural treatments include graded programmes to increase exercise and alter the contingent relationship between exercise and pain; modification of social reinforcement given by solicitous spouses and family members; and modification of the contingencies between pain and medication intake. Behavioural treatments have been frequently delivered as inpatient programmes as this allows the treatment environment to be carefully controlled. A behavioural approach to pain also implies that it is necessary for family members to change their behaviour towards the patient. The typical pattern of behaviour between spouses is described as 'solicitous'; the patient's partner is unduly attentive and responsive to signs of pain thereby positively reinforcing patterns of rest and non-participation in family and household activity. Family members are therefore, frequently involved in treatment programmes (Kerns et al., 2002) (see 'Behaviour therapy').

Evidence of effectiveness

There is good evidence for the effectiveness of psychologically based treatment for chronic pain problems. Morley et al. (1999) reported a systematic review and meta-analysis of the extant published randomized controlled trials. The trials were characterized by marked heterogeneity in a number of respects: (1) the clinical diagnoses of patients included low back pain, osteo- and rheumatoid arthritis, fibromyalgia, upper limb pain and several trials with patient groups with mixed diagnoses; (2) nearly all trials used multiple outcome measures; (3) many trials used more than a simple comparison between a treatment and control group; (4) the trials reported using a wide range of treatment components, while one or two trials used a single treatment such as biofeedback, most used treatments comprising a number of the components described earlier.

Morley *et al.* (1999) dealt with the problem of heterogeneity in the data in several ways. First, they grouped the outcome measures into domains of measurement; these included many of the concepts described earlier in the chapter, e.g. pain experience, mood and affect. Secondly, they carried out two sets of analyses; in the first they compared active psychological treatments, i.e. those treatments that included one or more of the treatment components described earlier (with the exception of education when delivered alone) with waiting list control groups. In the second analysis they compared active psychological treatments with active control groups such as patients receiving treatment as usual or patients on an active educational programme. A summary of these analyses is shown graphically in Figure 1. These figures display the average effect sizes and their 95% confidence intervals for the two sets of comparisons for each of the measurement domains. The upper panel clearly shows that when considered as a class of treatments (CBT-) cognitive behaviour therapy-based treatments are effective compared with a waiting list control treatment. The lower panel indicates that, on average, CBT-based treatments are at least as effective as other active treatments across the range of measures. In no case was CBT significantly worse than the controls and for several measurement domains it was slightly better.

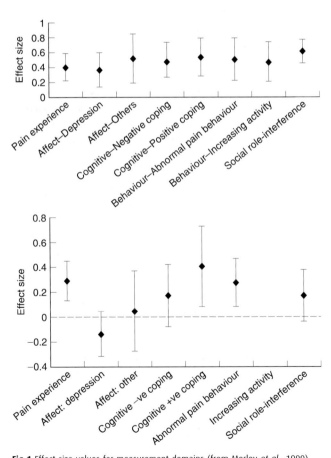

Fig 1 Effect size values for measurement domains (from Morley *et al.,* 1999). The upper shows the effect size values when active CBT is compared with waiting list controls; the lower panel the effect size values when CBT is compared with other active treatments.

Future developments and conclusions

Several additional randomized controlled trials (RCT) of CBT-based treatments for chronic pain have been published since Morley *et al.*'s (1999) review and these generally provide support for the effectiveness of CBT-based treatments for chronic pain management. However the complex multi-component treatment and its multiple outcomes means that it is difficult to discern if different aspects of therapy are responsible for different outcomes and it is not clear whether current treatment is optimal for all patients with chronic pain. In part, this is attributable to the rather general and imprecise way in which the problem of chronic pain has been construed (Morley & Williams, 2002).

Several strands of current research are tackling this problem. One approach has been to identify groups of patients who appear to be psychologically similar and to customize treatment for particular profiles. This line of research has been stimulated by Turk *et al.* (Turk, 2005) who have consistently identified three groups; 'adaptive copers', 'dysfunctional' and 'interpersonally distressed'. These groups have been replicated across research groups in North America, Europe and Oceania and they are found independently of medical diagnoses. There is a small amount of evidence that they respond differently to a standard pain management programme but as yet there is no compelling evidence for a specific treatment by group interaction.

A second approach has been to develop a more precise model of chronic pain with an explicit intervention targeted at particular sub-group of patients. Vlaeyen and Linton (2000) have described a fear-avoidance model which applies to a section of the chronic pain population. These patients are excessively fearful of activity because they believe that movement will result in some catastrophic outcome e.g. a broken back. Vlaeyen and his colleagues have obtained experimental evidence for the elements of this model and preliminary case series have demonstrated a treatment called graded exposure based on well validated fear reduction principles is effective (Vlaeyen *et al.*, 2001). A randomized controlled trial is now being performed.

The fear-avoidance model does not apply to all chronic pain patients and other models may be developed to account for different aspect of pain. Recently, Vlaeyen and Morley (2004) have considered how to account for the development of pain in people who appear to persist rather than avoid when faced with pain. They have suggested an approach based on the phenomenon of stop-rules. This approach also incorporates the fear-avoidance model and appears to account for some observed anomalies in the fear-avoidance model. Other researchers have begun to apply general models in clinical health psychology in an attempt to optimize treatment outcome. A number of researchers have applied the transtheoretical model of behaviour change (see 'Transtheoretical model of behaviour change') (Dijkstra, 2005) while others have developed motivational interviewing protocols to preparing patients for pain management programmes (Jensen, 2002; Jensen *et al.*, 2003). Finally, considerable effort has been invested in trying to identify those at risk for the development of chronic pain (Linton, 2002) and to devise interventions that might prevent chronic pain.

See also 'Coping with Chronic Pain', 'Pain', 'Pain Assessment', 'Amputation and Phantom Limb Pain', 'Back Pain', 'Noncardiac Chest Pain' and 'Pelvic Pain'.

REFERENCES

Arena, J. G. & Blanchard, E. B. (2002). Biofeedback training for chronic pain disorders. In D. C. Turk & R. J. Gatchel (Eds.). *Psychological Approaches to Pain Management: A Practitioner's (Handbook)* (2nd edn.). (pp. 138–58). New York: Guilford.

Asmundson, G. J. G., Vlaeyen, J. W. S. & Crombez, G. (Eds.). (2004). *Understanding and treating fear of pain.* Oxford: Oxford University Press.

Banks, S. M. & Kerns, R. D. (1996). Explaining high rates of depression in chronic pain: A diathesis–stress framework. *Psychological Bulletin,* **119**(1), 95–110.

Chapman, C. R. & Gavrin, J. (1999). Suffering: the contributions of persistent pain. *The Lancet,* **353**(9171), 2233–7.

Cioffi, D. (1991). Beyond attentional strategies: a cognitive–perceptual model of somatic interpretation. *Psychological Bulletin,* **109**(1), 25–41.

Dijkstra, A. (2005). The validity of the Stages of Change model in the adoption of the self-management approach in chronic pain. *Clinical Journal of Pain,* **21**(1), 27–37.

Eccleston, C. (1995). The attentional control of pain: methodological and theoretical concerns. *Pain,* **63**(1), 3–10.

Flor, H. & Birbaumer, N. (1993). Comparison of the efficacy of electromyographic biofeedback, cognitive–behavioral therapy, and conservative medical interventions in the treatment of chronic musculoskeletal pain. *Journal of Consulting and Clinical Psychology,* **61**(4), 653–8.

Flor, H., Fydrich, T. & Turk, D. C. (1992). Efficacy of multidisciplinary pain treatment centers: a meta-analytic review. *Pain,* **49**(2), 221–30.

Fordyce, W. E. (1976). *Behavioral methods for chronic pain and illness.* St Louis: Mosby.

Hanson, R. W. & Gerber, K. E. (1990). *Coping with chronic pain.* New York: Guilford Press.

Jensen, M. P. (2002). Enhancing motivation to change in pain treatment. In D. C. Turk & R. J. Gatchel (Eds.). *Psychological Approaches to Pain Management: A Practitioner's Handbook* (2nd edn.). (pp. 71–93). New York: Guilford.

Jensen, M. P. & Karoly, P. (1991). Control beliefs, coping efforts, and adjustment to chronic pain. *Journal of Consulting and Clinical Psychology,* **59**(3), 431–8.

Jensen, M. P., Nielson, W. R. & Kerns, R. D. (2003). Toward the development of a motivational model of pain self-management. *Journal of Pain,* **4**(9), 477–92.

Keefe, F. J., Beaupré, P. M., Gil, K. M., Rumble, M. E. & Aspnes, A. K. (2002). Group therapy with patients with chronic pain. In D. C. Turk & R. J. Gatchel (Eds.). *Psychological Approaches to Pain Management: A Practitioner's Handbook* (2nd edn.). (pp. 234–55). New York: Guilford Press.

Kerns, R. D., Otis, J. D. & Wise, E. A. (2002). Treating families of chronic pain patients: application of a cognitive–behavioral model. In R. J. Gatchel & D. C. Turk (Eds.). *Psychosocial Factors in Pain* (2nd edn.). (pp. 256–75). New York: Guilford Press.

Linton, S. J. (Ed.). (2002). *New avenues for the prevention of chronic musculoskeletal pain and disability Vol. 12.* Amsterdam: Elsevier.

McCracken, L. M., Carson, J. W., Eccleston, C. & Keefe, F. J. (2004). Acceptance and change in the context of chronic pain. *Pain,* **109**(1–2), 4–7.

Morley, S. & Eccleston, C. (2004). The object of fear in pain. In G. J. Asmundson, J. Vlaeyen & G. Crombez (Eds.). *Understanding and treating fear of pain* (pp. 163–88). Oxford: Oxford University Press.

Morley, S., Eccleston, C. & Williams, A. (1999). Systematic review and meta-analysis of randomized controlled trials of cognitive behaviour therapy and behaviour therapy for chronic pain in adults, excluding headache. *Pain,* **80**(1–2), 1–13.

Morley, S., Shapiro, D. A. & Biggs, J. (2004). Developing a treatment manual for attention management in chronic pain. *Cognitive Behaviour Therapy,* **33**(1), 1–11.

Morley, S. & Williams, A. C. de C. (2002). Conducting and evaluating treatment outcome studies. In R. J. Gatchel & D. C. Turk (Eds.). *Psychosocial Factors in Pain* (2nd edn.). (pp. 52–68). New York: Guilford.

Morris, D. B. (1998). *Illness and culture in a postmodern age.* Berkeley: University of California Press.

Price, D. D. (1999). *Psychological mechanisms of pain and analgesia.* Seattle: IASP Press.

Sanders, S. H. (2002). Operant conditioning with chronic pain: back to basics. In D. C. Turk & R. J. Gatchel (Eds.). *Psychological Approaches to Pain Management: A Practitioner's Handbook* (2nd edn.). (pp. 128–37). New York: Guilford Press.

Sullivan, M. J. L., Thorn, B. E., Haythornthwaite, J. A. *et al.* (2001). Theoretical perspectives on the relationship between catastrophizing and pain. *The Clinical Journal of Pain,* **17**, 52–64.

Syrajala, K. L. & Abrams, J. R. (2002). Hypnosis and imagery in the treatment of pain. In D. C. Turk & R. J. Gatchel (Eds.). *Psychological Approaches to Pain Management: A Practitioner's Handbook* (2nd edn.). (pp. 187–209). New York: Guilford Press.

Turk, D. C. (2002). A cognitive–behavioral perspective on treatment of chronic pain patients. In R. J. Gatchel & D. C. Turk (Eds.). *Psychosocial Factors in Pain* (2nd edn.). (pp. 138–58). New York: Guilford.

Turk, D. C. (2005). The potential of treatment matching for subgroups of chronic pain patients: Lumping vs. splitting. *Clinical Journal of Pain,* **21**(1), 44–55.

Vlaeyen, J. W., de Jong, J., Geilen, M., Heuts, P. H. & van Breukelen, G. (2001). Graded exposure in vivo in the treatment of pain-related fear: a replicated single-case experimental design in four patients with chronic low back pain. *Behaviour Research and Therapy,* **39**(2), 151–66.

Vlaeyen, J. W. & Linton, S. J. (2000). Fear-avoidance and its consequences in chronic musculoskeletal pain: a state of the art. *Pain,* **85**(3), 317–32.

Vlaeyen, J. W. S. & Morley, S. (2004). Active despite pain: the putative role of stop-rules and current mood. *Pain,* **110**(3), 512–16.

Physical activity interventions

Michael Ussher

St. George's, University of London

Introduction

Sedentary lifestyles are a global public health problem (World Health Organization (WHO), 2004). Those who are physically inactive have an increased risk of premature death and of developing major chronic diseases; including coronary heart disease, cancers and diabetes (Baumann, 2004). Physical activity (PA) refers to any bodily movement resulting in energy expenditure (Caspersen, 1989) and includes routine activities such as walking and housework, as well as structured exercise, sport and occupational activity. For general health benefits, it is recommended that adults accumulate a total of at least 30 minutes a day of at least moderate intensity PA on five or more days a week (Department of Health (DOH), 2004). Children are advised to accumulate at least 60 minutes of at least moderate intensity activity every day (DOH, 2004). Over the last 20 to 30 years PA levels have declined, largely due to a reduction in PA at work, in the home and as a means of transport (DOH, 2004). It is estimated that 60% to 85% of adults are insufficiently active to benefit their health and promoting PA is a priority for health policy in most developed nations (WHO, 2004).

This chapter provides an overview of the application of psychological theory in PA interventions. Discussion is mostly restricted to adult populations as very few studies have examined the effect of psychologically-based interventions on PA levels in children (Lewis et al., 2002). Exercise has been shown to provide psychological benefits, most notably in the management of depression and anxiety; therefore, evidence for the role of exercise in mental health is also summarized.

Physical activity and mental health

There is some evidence to suggest that regular PA can benefit the mental health of both adolescents and adults. There is little research on the psychological benefits of exercise for younger children. Cross-sectional, longitudinal and intervention studies have shown benefits of PA among adolescents for reducing anxiety, stress and depression and for fostering self-esteem and emotional wellbeing (e.g. Calfas & Taylor, 1994; Field et al., 2001; Steptoe & Butler, 1996; Motl et al., 2004). However, many of these studies have methodological limitations including the use of psychological measures which may not be appropriate for adolescents; not controlling for potential confounders, such as smoking status and body mass index; and not considering selection bias, whereby those not completing the study questionnaire due to truancy, sickness or drop-out were more likely to have emotional difficulties. In the cross-sectional studies it is not clear whether those with poorer mental health have difficulty maintaining PA, or whether taking regular PA results in improved mental health.

Among adults, a number of adequately designed studies have shown that a sedentary lifestyle is associated with an increased risk of developing clinically defined depression (e.g. Camacho et al., 1991; Farmer et al., 1988), although the optimal dose of PA necessary to prevent depression is not known (Dunn et al., 2002). Meta-analyses have established that both aerobic and resistance-type exercise programmes are effective for treating mild to severe depression and that exercise is at least as effective as psychotherapy and medication (Craft & Landers, 1998; Lawlor & Hopkin, 2001). However, many of these studies have flaws (Lawlor & Hopkin, 2001); including, exclusion of drop-outs from the analyses, assessment of outcome not being blinded and use of symptom ratings rather than clinical diagnosis as the outcome.

Those with mental illness have higher levels of mortality and morbidity than the general population (Davidson et al., 2001); therefore the general health benefits of exercise may be particularly important for this population. Exercise may be especially attractive to patients not responding to conventional treatments or those who want to reduce medications. There is some evidence to suggest that where exercise is offered routinely as part of the psychiatric service adherence is likely to be comparable to that of the general population (Martinsen, 1993), although further studies are needed of exercise adherence among those with psychiatric illness.

Exercise has been shown to have some modest benefits for reducing generalized anxiety disorder, panic attacks and stress disorders and for improving psychological health among those with schizophrenia, although insufficient studies have been conducted with these populations to draw firm conclusions (O'Connor et al., 2000; Faulkner & Biddle, 1999). A few studies have shown that PA is beneficial as an aid for achieving smoking cessation and during alcohol and drug rehabilitation, although there are too few well designed studies to evaluate the role of PA in these areas (Donaghy & Ussher, 2005; Ussher, 2005).

In the general population there is some evidence to suggest that regular PA can have beneficial effects on depression, anxiety, emotional wellbeing, self-esteem, perceived stress and sleep disturbance (Biddle & Mutrie, 2001; Department of Health, 2004). However, many of the studies have limitations which are similar to those found in studies with clinical populations; therefore definitive recommendations for exercise and mental health cannot be made at this time. Moreover, the mechanisms underlying any beneficial effects of PA on mental health have yet to be determined (Buckworth & Dishman, 2002).

Psychological theory and physical activity interventions

Psychological theory has been used to generate hypotheses concerning the psychosocial mediators of changes in PA and to provide a rationale for incorporating psychological strategies in PA interventions. This section presents an overview of the main psychological theories which have been applied to PA behaviour and summarizes the evidence for the effectiveness of PA interventions based on these theories.

Behaviour modification and learning theories

(See 'Behaviour therapy').

Behaviour modification and learning theories propose that PA is more likely to occur when environmental and situational stimuli encourage it and when it leads to rewards or avoidance of punishment (Skinner, 1953). For example, signs promoting the health benefits of stair use have been shown to increase stair use (Andersen et al., 1998) and offering incentives, such as attendance lotteries, gifts and behavioural contracts has been shown to increase PA levels by up to 75% (King et al., 1992). Providing rewards is likely to be most important during the early phases of a PA programme when the punishing side of PA (e.g. fatigue, stiffness) is often more apparent than the rewards (e.g. feeling fitter and healthier). Reward-based interventions have been shown to be effective in the short-term, but less so in the long-term (Glanz & Rimmer, 1995; King et al., 1992). In the long-term, intrinsic rewards (e.g. enjoyment) are likely to be more important (Sher, 1998) and enjoyment is a reliable predictor of adherence to PA (Lewis et al., 2002).

Relapse prevention model (RPM)

Fifty per cent of those starting an organized PA programme are likely to drop out within six months (Dishman, 1994) and the relapse prevention model (RPM), (Marlatt & Gordon, 1985) postulates that relapse begins with high-risk barriers (e.g. 'It's raining too heavily to jog') at which point, it is argued, a lapse (e.g. 'I will not jog today') leads to reduced self-efficacy (confidence towards PA), whereas, appropriate coping (e.g. 'I will work out to an exercise video today') leads to enhanced self-efficacy and a reduced chance of further lapses. There is some evidence to suggest that preparing for high-risk situations and setbacks and setting realistic goals leads to increased PA adherence (e.g. Baum et al., 1991; King & Fredricksen, 1984), but other studies have found that such strategies do not aid adherence (e.g. Marcus & Stanton, 1993). Further work is needed to test the RPM for PA and to identify the most critical PA barriers and lapses at different stages of PA adoption and with different populations.

Health belief model

(See 'Health belief model').

The health belief model (HBM), (Becker et al., 1977) proposes that becoming physically active is largely dependent upon a sedentary lifestyle being perceived as a threat to health. Prospective and retrospective studies, of both healthy and ill populations, have consistently shown either no relationship between perceived threat and PA levels (Biddle & Mutrie, 2001) or have found that a greater perceived threat of illness is associated with less PA (e.g. Lindsay-Reid & Osborn, 1980). This may be because PA is associated with being well and people may be cautious about being physically active when they are unwell. The HBM fails to take account of motives for PA which are unrelated to illness, such as appearance, enjoyment and social contact and has limited applicability to PA behaviour.

Theory of planned behaviour

(See 'Theory of planned behaviour').

The theory of planned behaviour (TPB), (Ajzen, 1988) argues that the main determinant of changes in PA behaviour is intention to be physically active. This intention is said to be influenced by (i) attitudes or evaluative beliefs towards physical activity (e.g. 'Exercise helps with managing my weight, but I find it boring'), (ii) subjective norms (e.g. 'Most of my friends have joined exercise classes') and (iii) perceived behavioural control (perception of resources and barriers for PA). In this theory perceived behavioural control is also considered to be a direct influence on PA behaviour. The constructs in the TPB have consistently been shown to be valid for modelling PA behaviour (e.g. Blanchard et al., 2003; Hausenblas et al., 1997; Okun et al., 2003) and this model is important in that it highlights social influences and barriers as mediators of PA behaviour. Most studies have tested elements of the TPB rather than the whole model and the definition and measurement of constructs (e.g. perceived behavioural control) varies greatly, which makes comparison of studies difficult.

Transtheoretical model

(See 'Transtheoretical model of behaviour change').

The transtheoretical model (TTM), or stages of change model, defines an individual's intention to change towards a more active lifestyle by five main stages: (i) precontemplation – inactive and not intending to become more active in the next six months; (ii) contemplation – inactive but intending to become more active in the next six months; (iii) preparation – active but at less than recommended levels and may or may not intend to become more active; (iv) action – active at the recommended level but for less than six months; and (v) maintenance – active at the recommended level for at least six months (Marcus et al., 1992). The TTM hypothesizes that PA behaviour is influenced by self-efficacy, decisional balance and processes of change (e.g. cognitive processes: increasing knowledge, being aware of risks for lapse; and behavioural processes: enlisting social support, rewarding oneself) which vary in importance according to the stage of change.

The TTM integrates concepts from other models. For instance, self-efficacy is central to Bandura's (1986) social cognitive theory and is similar to perceived behavioural control in the TPB. Decisional balance is derived from decision-making theory (Janis & Mann, 1977) and proposes that we are more likely to be physically active if we perceive that the benefits of PA (e.g. improved mood) outweigh the costs (e.g. time taken for PA). Through considering the environmental influences on PA (e.g. safe areas for walking), the TTM acknowledges ecological models (McLeroy *et al.*, 1988). The TTM is similar to the TPB in as much as stage of change is partly distinguished by intention. However, stage of change is also distinguished by actual PA behaviours and the algorithm for defining which behaviours are associated with which stage varies greatly between studies, making interpretation of findings difficult.

There is mixed evidence to suggest that interventions which are tailored to an individual's stage and processes of change are effective for increasing PA (e.g. Bock *et al.*, 2001; Calfas *et al.*, 1997; Pinto *et al.*, 2001). Where such interventions have been effective it is not always clear whether this is due to changes in theoretical constructs. There is evidence for some of the constructs in the transtheoretical model predicting changes in PA. For example, increases in PA have been associated with greater self-efficacy and with the behavioural processes of change, but there is little evidence to support the value of the other constructs in the TTM (Lewis *et al.*, 2002).

Multi-component exercise interventions

In practice, psychological strategies for promoting PA are most often employed in combination and as part of an individual or group consultation, whether in primary care, in the community or in the workplace (Marcus & Forsyth, 2003). Different strategies tend to be emphasized at different phases of the PA programme, although there is limited evidence to show the benefits of this approach (Bock *et al.*, 2001) and studies need to compare mediators and interventions at different stages of exercise adoption and maintenance.

Decision-making for PA can be assessed using decision balance sheets and scaling questions can be used to assess self-efficacy, barriers to PA and social support. As part of a relapse prevention plan, strategies can be identified to help the client overcome barriers and lapses. Self-monitoring encourages adherence to the PA regimen and assists health professionals in monitoring their clients' PA levels (Martin *et al.*, 1984; Oldridge & Jones, 1983). Self-monitoring is usually in the form of a brief daily record, for instance, stating the mode and duration of PA (e.g. brisk walking for 20 minutes). Self-monitoring requiring a high level of attention to the process of PA (e.g. using pedometers) has been used in practice but no adequately controlled studies have assessed the impact of such devices on exercise adherence (Croteau, 2004).

As a relapse prevention and motivational strategy, it is recommended that clients set realistic goals and that these goals are revised during future consultations. Realistic goals ensure a gradual progression in levels of PA and foster self-efficacy for PA. Ideally, goals are specific to the mode, intensity, duration and frequency of PA (e.g. 'To walk briskly so that I am breathing heavier than normal for 30 minutes on five days a week'). The client can be asked to sign a contract outlining PA goals and specifying rewards or penalties relating to the achievement of these goals (e.g. 'If I attend the exercise class twice a week for two months I will receive a free tea-shirt, pedometer and certificate').

Discussion and future directions

Interventions which target multiple psychosocial variables are more likely to lead to maintenance of regular PA (Sallis *et al.*, 1998) and multi-component interventions are often used in research studies; however, in these studies it is not clear which elements of the intervention are effective. More studies are required which examine the effectiveness of specific psychological strategies for promoting PA, which compare different strategies within the same study and which control for the effects of reinforcement and social support. These strategies are most often employed in face-to-face consultations, which are costly and have limited dissemination. Therefore, further research is needed to investigate interventions delivered via telephone, internet contact or leaflet (Marcus *et al.*, 2000; Sciamanna *et al.*, 2002).

Many of the interventions discussed in this chapter have focused on short-term increases in PA levels and further work is needed to understand the processes involved in the maintenance of regular PA for 12 months or longer. Increasing use of personal computers and video games presents a barrier to regular PA and novel theories of PA behaviour are required which address both motivations towards PA and motivations towards sedentary activities. Interventions which target changes in multiple health behaviours; such as exercise, diet and smoking behaviours, are now common (e.g. Avenell *et al.*, 2004; Ussher, 2005); therefore, theories also need to be extended to accommodate changes in multiple health behaviours (King *et al.*, 1996).

In some of the studies described in this chapter the direction of the relationship between the psychosocial mediator and PA behaviour is not clear; for example, research is needed to establish whether individuals become more active as they overcome barriers to PA or whether people perceive fewer barriers following success at raising PA levels. At this time, it is not possible to make definitive conclusions about the importance of psychosocial mediators in the application of PA interventions. Nor is it possible to define the intensity of PA intervention necessary to produce sustained changes in these psychosocial mediators.

REFERENCES

Ajzen, I. (1988) *Attitudes, personality and behavior.* Chicago: Dorsey Press.

Andersen, R. E., Franckowiak, S. C., Snyder, J., Bartlett, S. J. & Fontaine, K. R. (1998). Can inexpensive signs encourage the use of stairs? Results from a community intervention. *Annals of Internal Medicine,* **129**, 363–9.

Avenell, A., Brown, T. J., McGee, M. A. et al. (2004). What interventions should we add to weight reducing diets in adults with obesity? A systematic review of randomized controlled trials of adding drug therapy, exercise, behaviour therapy or combinations of these interventions. *Journal of* Human Nutrition and Dietetics, **17**, 293–316.

Bandura, A. (1986). *Social foundations of thought and action: a social cognitive theory.* New Jersey: Prentice-Hall.

Baum, J. G., Clark, H. B. & Sandler, J. (1991). Preventing relapse obesity through post-treatment maintenance system: comparing the relative efficacy of two levels of therapist support. *Journal of Behavioral Medicine*, **14**, 287–302.

Bauman, A. E. (2004). Updating the evidence that physical activity is good for health: an epidemiological review 2000–2003. *Journal of Science and Medicine in Sport*, **7**(Suppl.), 6–19.

Becker, M. H., Haefner, D. P., Kasl, S. V. *et al.* (1977). Selected psychosocial models and correlates of individual health-related behaviors. *Medical Care*, **15**(Suppl.), 27–46.

Biddle, S. J. H. & Mutrie, N. (2001). *Psychology of physical activity: determinants, well-being and interventions.* London: Routledge.

Blanchard, C. M., Courneya, K. S., Rodgers, W. M. *et al.* (2003). Is the theory of planned behavior a useful framework for understanding exercise adherence during phase II cardiac rehabilitation? *Journal of Cardiopulmonary Rehabilitation*, **23**, 29–39.

Bock, B. C., Marcus, B. H., Pinto, B. M. & Forsyth, L. H. (2001). Maintenance of physical activity following an individualized motivationally tailored intervention. *Annals of Behavioral Medicine*, **23**, 79–87.

Buckworth, J. & Dishman, R. K. (2002). *Exercise psychology.* Champaign, IL: Human Kinetics.

Calfas, K. J., Sallis, J. F., Oldenburg, B. & Ffrench, M. (1997). Mediators of change in physical activity following an intervention in primary care: PACE. *Preventive Medicine*, **26**, 297–304.

Calfas, K. J. & Taylor, W. C. (1994). Effects of physical activity on psychological variables in adolescents. *Pediatric Exercise Science*, **6**, 406–23.

Camacho, T. C., Roberts, R. E., Lazarus, N. B., Kaplan, G. A. & Cohen, R. D. (1991). Physical activity and depression: evidence from the Alameda County Study. *American Journal of Epidemiology*, **134**, 220–31.

Caspersen, C. J. (1989). Physical activity epidemiology: concepts, methods, and applications to exercise science. *Exercise and Sport Sciences Reviews*, **17**, 423–73.

Craft, L. L. & Landers, D. M. (1998). The effect of exercise on clinical depression and depression resulting from mental illness: a meta-analysis. *Journal of Sport and Exercise Psychology*, **20**, 339–57.

Croteau, K. A. (2004). A preliminary study on the impact of a pedometer-based intervention on daily steps. *American Journal of Health Promotion*, **18**, 217–20.

Davidson, S., Judd, F., Jolley, D. *et al.* (2001). Cardiovascular risk factors for people with mental illness. *Australian and New Zealand Journal of Psychiatry*, **35**, 196–202.

Department of Health (2004). *At least five a week: evidence on the impact of physical activity and its relationship to health, a report from the Chief Medical Officer.* London: Department of Health.

Dishman, R. K. (1994). The measurement conundrum in exercise adherence research. *Medicine and Science in Sports and Exercise*, **26**, 1382–90.

Donaghy, M. & Ussher, M. (2005). Exercise interventions in drug and alcohol rehabilitation. In G. E. J. Faulkner & A. H. Taylor (Eds.). *Exercise, health and mental health: emerging relationships.* (pp. 48–69). Routledge: London.

Dunn, A. L., Trivedi, M. H. & O'Neal, H. A. (2002). Physical activity dose–response effects on outcomes of depression and anxiety. *Controlled Clinical Trials*, **23**, 584–603.

Farmer, M. E., Locke, B. Z., Moscicki, E. K. *et al.* (1988). Physical activity and depressive symptoms: the NHANES I epidemiologic follow-up study. *American Journal of Epidemiology*, **128**, 1340–51.

Faulkner, G. & Biddle, S. (1999). Exercise as an adjunct treatment for schizophrenia: a review of the literature. *Journal of Mental Health*, **8**, 441–57.

Field, T., Diego, M. & Sanders, C. (2001). Adolescent depression and risk factors. *Adolescence*, **36**, 491–8.

Glanz, K. & Rimer, B. K. (1995). *Theory at a glance: a guide for health promotion practice.* Bethesda, MD: US Department of Health and Human Services.

Hausenblas, H., Carron, A. V. & Mack, D. E. (1997). Application of the theories of reasoned action and planned behavior to exercise behavior: a meta-analysis. *Journal of Sport and Exercise Psychology*, **19**, 36–51.

Janis, I. L. & Mann, L. (1977). *Decision making: a psychological analysis of conflict, choice, and commitment.* New York: Collier Macmillan.

King, A. C., Blair, S. N., Bild, D. E. *et al.* (1992). Determinants of physical activity and interventions in adults. *Medicine and Science in Sports and Exercise*, **24**(Suppl.), 221–36.

King, A. C. & Fredericksen, L. W. (1984). Low-cost strategies for increasing exercise behavior: relapse preparation training and support. *Behavior Modification*, **8**, 3–21.

King, T. K., Marcus, B. H., Pinto, B. M., Emmons, K. M. & Abrams, D. B. (1996). Cognitive–behavioral mediators of changing multiple behaviors: smoking and a sedentary lifestyle. *Preventive Medicine*, **25**, 684–91.

Lawlor, D. A. & Hopker, S. W. (2001). The effectiveness of exercise as an intervention

in the management of depression: systematic review and meta-regression analysis of randomised controlled trials. *British Medical Journal*, **322**, 763–7.

Lewis, B. A., Marcus, B. H., Pate, R. R. & Dunn, A. L. (2002). Psychosocial mediators of physical activity behavior among adults and children. *American Journal of Preventive Medicine*, **23**(Suppl.), 26–35.

Lindsay-Reid, E. & Osborn, R. W. (1980). Readiness for exercise adoption. *Social Science and Medicine*, **14A**, 139–46.

Marcus, B. H. & Forsyth, L. H. (2003). *Motivating people to be physically active.* Champaign, IL: Human Kinetics.

Marcus, B. H., Nigg, C. R., Riebe, D. & Forsyth, L. H. (2000). Interactive communication strategies: implications for population-based physical-activity promotion. *American Journal of Preventive Medicine*, **19**, 121–6.

Marcus, B. H., Selby, V. C., Niaura, R. S. & Rossi, J. S. (1992). Self-efficacy and the stages of exercise behavior change. *Research Quarterly for Exercise and Sport*, **63**, 60–6.

Marcus, B. H. & Stanton, A. L. (1993). Evaluation of relapse prevention and reinforcement interventions to promote exercise adherence in sedentary females. *Research Quarterly for Exercise and Sport*, **64**, 447–52.

Marlatt, G. A. & Gordon, J. R. (1985). *Relapse prevention: maintenance strategies in addictive behavior change.* New York: Guilford Press.

Martin, J. E., Dubbert, P. M., Katell, A. D. *et al.* (1984). Behavioural control of exercise in sedentary adults: Studies 1 through 6. *Journal of Consulting and Clinical Psychology*, **52**, 795–811.

Martinsen, E. W. (1993). Therapeutic implications of exercise for clinically anxious and depressed patients. *International Journal of Sport Psychology*, **24**, 185–99.

McLeroy, K. R., Bibeau, D., Steckler, A. & Glanz, K. (1988). An ecological perspective on health promotion programs. *Health Education Quarterly*, **15**, 351–77.

Motl, R. W., Birnbaum, A. S., Kubik, M. Y. & Dishman, R. K. (2004). Naturally occurring changes in physical activity are inversely related to depressive symptoms during early adolescence. *Psychosomatic Medicine*, **66**, 336–42.

Nies, M. A. & Kershaw, T. C. (2002). Psychosocial and environmental influences on physical activity and health outcomes in sedentary women. *Journal of Nursing Scholarship*, **34**, 243–9.

O'Connor, P. J., Raglin, J. S. & Martinsen, E. W. (2000). Physical activity, anxiety and anxiety disorders. *International Journal of Sport Psychology*, **31**, 136–55.

Okun, M. A., Ruehlman, L., Karoly, P., Lutz, R., Fairholme, C. & Schaub, R. (2003). Social support and social norms: do both contribute to predicting leisure-time exercise? *American Journal of Health Behavior*, **27**, 493–507.

Oldridge, N. B. & Jones, N. L. (1983). Improving patient compliance in cardiac rehabilitation: effects of written agreement and self-monitoring. *Journal of Cardiopulmonary Rehabilitation*, **3**, 257–62.

Pinto, B. M., Lynn, H., Marcus, B. H., DePue, J. & Goldstein, M. G. (2001). Physician-based activity counseling: intervention effects on mediators of motivational readiness for physical activity. *Annals of Behavioral Medicine*, **23**, 2–10.

Sallis, J. F., Bauman, A. & Pratt, M. (1998). Environmental and policy interventions to promote physical activity. *American Journal of Preventive Medicine*, **15**, 379–97.

Sciamanna, C. N., Lewis, B., Tate, D. *et al.* (2002). User attitudes toward a physical activity promotion website. *Preventive Medicine*, **35**, 612–15.

Sher, L. (1998). The endogenous euphoric reward system that reinforces physical training: a mechanism for mankind's survival. *Medical Hypotheses*, **51**, 449–50.

Skinner, B. F. (1953). *Science and human behaviour*. New York: Free Press.

Steptoe, A. & Butler, N. (1996). Sports participation and emotional wellbeing in adolescents. *Lancet*, **347**, 1789–92.

Ussher, M. (2005). *Exercise interventions in smoking cessation*. Tobacco addiction module of the cochrane database of systematic reviews. Oxford: The Cochrane Collaboration, Update Software.

World Health Organization (2004). *Sedentary lifestyle: a global public health problem*. www.who.int/hpr/physactiv/sedentary.lifestyle1.shtml, accessed March 30, 2005.

Psychodynamic psychotherapy

Jo-anne Carlyle

Tavistock Clinic

Overview

What sets the psychodynamic psychotherapies apart from other traditions of psychological therapy is centrality of a dynamic unconscious. It is not only taken as fact that there are large parts of our psychological life of which we are unaware but also that there is a level of dynamic activity in these unconscious processes which contributes to our emotional and behavioural life (Laplanche & Pontalis, 1973). This idea takes us beyond a notion of a static unconscious where previous thoughts or experiences are 'laid down' in a way that is isolated from relationships with other experiences. It refers to processes whereby aspects of emotional life, particularly conflicts between different instincts, feelings and thoughts, actively impinge on one another. The product or evidence of this activity may be in dreams or symptoms. Shakespeare, who so often anticipates our understanding of the mind, puts it eloquently thus:

And since you know you cannot see yourself, so well as by reflection,
I, your glass, will modestly discover to yourself,
that of yourself which you yet know not of.
(William Shakespeare, Julius Caesar, Act 1, Scene II)

Although Freud is recognized as the modern founder of psychoanalysis (on which the psychodynamic therapies are based), the principles and foundations of psychodynamic theory are revealed in many of the compelling and elemental stories which have endured throughout history, from religious texts to the role of myths, as universal means of describing the experience of society and the individual. These stories speak of key experiences of love and hate, of envy and rivalry, of grievance and forgiveness. Perhaps most importantly, they tell how human beings act beyond their conscious logic and rationality and are affected by their experiences and by one another in profound ways.

There are many strands of psychodynamic theory that derive from the different psychoanalytic traditions as they have developed both in the UK and in other parts of the world. The differences in these are, for the purposes of this chapter, less important than their common features, which will be described below. In addition it should be noted that the theoretical and clinical developments within the psychodynamic traditions have been applied in a variety of modalities, including individual therapy, group therapy, couples work, as well as a particular form of family therapy (see 'Group therapy'). They have also been very influential in the areas of experiential learning, consultancy work for organizations, as well as in some forms of executive coaching, particularly through the area of group relations.

Early experience and the internal world

A key feature of the theoretical models that underpin psychodynamic psychotherapy sets out the importance of early experience. There continue to be debates about how much an individual brings constitutionally (genetically) and prenatally to their situation and also about the effects that such resiliences and vulnerabilities bring to bear on subsequent experience. However, it is generally acknowledged and evidenced that early caregiver experience is crucial for determining later development. (Enns *et al.*, 2002; Fonagy *et al.*, 2002). The theoretical model of Attachment Theory is often used to help understand the importance of early development. Attachment Theory emphasizes the behaviour and responsivity of the primary caregiver(s) as well as the need for a secure base, the problematic effects of poor attachments, of separation and of loss. It is in some ways a more rational and behavioural approach to key aspects of such early relationships than the more psychoanalytic models, for example, Object Relations Theory. The work of Winnicott, Fairbairn, Klein and Bion takes the Attachment Theory understanding a stage further for psychodynamic psychotherapy, by taking as a key point of focus the 'intra-psychic' experience and the unconscious activity which contributes to or hinders development (see 'Child abuse and neglect').

Being sensitive to the processes and experiences of deprivation and also of intrusion is clearly an important part of the caregiving role to a young child. However, we also play more appropriate games with young infants that introduce them to these processes and through which we begin to help them develop an internal understanding of the boundaries which are fundamental both in external relationships and also in internal object relationships. Peek-a-boo games, hide-and-seek and games of tickling all use processes of withdrawal and separation and also of pain in normal development. These games involve hiding a face or hiding a loved transitional object like a teddy bear to a point where excitation and a level of anxiety is provoked, but is managed and contained. There is a transaction between infant and carer as to what is manageable and exciting and what induces fear or loss. Tickling (an important activity with babies and young children and later incorporated into sexual activity) borders the boundary between pain and pleasure and is a sensitive area in which the carer can interpret the state of mind of the baby and respond. These relational skills are essential to developing both an experience of separateness as well as dependency.

The processes of 'introjection' and 'projection' that make up the relationship between infant and carer are, in Kleinian theory, seen to provide the mechanism for the development of the ego from the very primitive ego with which the child is born. This is the cornerstone of object relations theory, but it does depart from the more stage-dependent model that was originally set out by Freud.

These relational aspects of psychodynamic understanding can be seen in relation to the developments made by Freud. His Topographical Theory, perhaps best set out in '*The interpretation of dreams*' (Freud, 1900) and developed in the late 1880s and early 1900s, comprises of three levels of awareness: the 'Conscious' – what we are aware of and cognisant of; the 'pre-conscious' – sense impressions, things that can be brought to conscious awareness without much effort; and the 'unconscious' – primitive emotions and impulses, drives, phantasies, repressed memories and feelings. These ideas are important in that they state explicitly that there are things of which not only are we unaware, but of which we cannot gain awareness by our own activity.

In 1923, Freud published '*The ego and the id*' (Freud, 1923) which introduces what is known as the Structural Theory. It sets out the concepts of the 'id', 'ego' and 'super-ego' which now form part of our ordinary language. The id refers to the basic and instinctual impulses or parts of the personality; the ego employs our conscious mind to think about the consequences of our actions and the demands of living in the real world; whereas the super-ego can be understood as a part of the ego in which moral judgement, or perhaps conscience, are located. The super-ego is often thought to embody the authority figures in our lives and to convey censure or approval for our actions.

The structural model conceptually includes the ideas of the dynamic relationship between impulses and fantasies (derived from the id), of which we are not aware, being mediated by other aspects of our experience which are derived from our own capacities (via the ego) and also includes the experiences which we internalize from key figures, parents, carers, teachers, etc. (super-ego). In addition it allows for the experience of unconscious conflict, for example between id and super-ego. The role of the ego as a kind of mediator is relaxed during sleep (which allows for dreaming) and also when we are affected by other factors such as alcohol or drugs and stress.

The therapeutic frame

The theories set out above – attachment theory, object relations theory and also Freud's structural theory – are useful in that, as well as setting out processes of normal development, they also provide an understanding of abnormal development. Where early caregiver containment is inadequate or lacking, or where there are other significant stresses on development, for example through trauma, illness, separation, etc., then these theories set out how problems including difficulties coping with the pressures of life, struggles in relationships and difficulties with dependency or autonomy are more likely to emerge. The nature and particularities of such difficulties are likely to be related to the nature of the developmental failure or impediment. These are not pathological or stigmatizing realities; they are part of the human condition and to a greater or lesser extent are relevant to all of our experiences.

Psychodynamic psychotherapy provides a context where such early deprivations or injuries can be thought about and understood. More importantly it provides a setting based on consistency, regularity, predictability, firm boundaries of time and setting and a protective function. In this way such early difficulties can re-emerge within the therapeutic relationship (transference) and the therapeutic situation can symbolically function in the way that a 'good enough' carer might have done for the young infant.

These often physical manifestations of the containment function of the setting are clearly very important and need to be rigorously applied to be effective. However, as described above, this is not a simple process of ensuring that they take place; it demands an active attention and listening on the part of the therapist. The very fact of consistency in setting means that the therapist can be attentive to the patient's response to the setting or frame, and work with him or her to understand attempts to breach it, or attempts to pretend that it produces no effect or sense of deprivation on the individual.

This begins to bring us to the process of the analytic attitude that constitutes the internal frame which guides the therapist's stance and attitude to the patient. Psychodynamic therapists are sometimes caricatured for being rigid in these attitudes, however the employment of them goes beyond whether the therapist smiles, or says good morning, or whether she shakes hands (all of which are important). It refers to a process of attuned listening and to the fact that the analyst sets aside his or her other preoccupations and emotions and develops a capacity to focus and concentrate on the patient's communication. This process requires a capacity for neutrality, the ability not to be pulled into personal feelings. It is a process of dual listening – both to the actual content of what the patient says and also to the deeper meanings which are revealed beneath the surface or deeper than the apparent overt content.

As a patient enters the room, the therapist is interested not only in the content of his or her story, that is, the description of difficulties, social situation, experiences etc., but also in the form that the description takes and the ways in which it relates to the therapist. The therapist is watching for particular patterns of coping with difficult experiences or relationships and of constructing the patient's own experience of him- or herself. Psychodynamic theory and experience expects that the way in which the patient sees and relates to the therapist is central (transference in the broadest of terms). There is also the expectation that the way in which the patient describes his or her ideas and the way in which movement is made between ideas will illustrate something of the his or her unconscious processes, the ways of thinking, relating, understanding, behaving etc., which are not available to the conscious awareness of the patient. The focus of sessions is often not particularly on past traumas or disappointments per se, so much as on the current experiences and consequences of those happenings or emotions, i.e. what it is in the person's current conflicts that gets in the way of coming to terms with those painful past events.

Means of protecting the self – defences

One way in which the therapist might begin to understand patients' unconscious processes is to identify the ways in which patients try to protect themselves by keeping uncomfortable or painful thoughts out of conscious awareness. These 'defences' provide clues about the kind of damage that might have happened to the patients' developmental processes. One of the main functions of defences is to keep such thoughts or knowledge out of conscious awareness.

Defences are one of the features of psychoanalytic theory that have been absorbed into our everyday understandings of behaviour and also into our language. 'You are so defensive' is a familiar accusation, as are: 'you are so repressed (or anal)'; 'he is in denial'; 'she projects all the time'; and so on. The fact that they are part of our discourse is partly because they make sense of our experience of ourselves and of those around us, of the people we live with, look after, work with and love.

A crucial point to be made here is that, as with most psychoanalytic phenomena, defences are universal. We all use them, we can observe them in our own behaviour as well as that of those around us – in our families, our social circle, amongst our work colleagues and so on. Thus, although there is some implication that they are 'pathological' or maladaptive, in fact the situation is not as simple as this. In situations of extreme danger, it is quite appropriate to repress previous experiences of being afraid or deny certain aspects of the situation that faces us. These are adaptive strategies which allow us to focus our attention on the more pressing concerns that arise in the situation.

Vaillant (1971) suggested four groups of defences, characterized in hierarchical terms for levels of maturity: psychotic; immature; neurotic; and mature. He tested these on various samples in some longitudinal studies and found that mature defences were associated with adult adjustment (work, marriage, etc.) and that there were negative correlations between immature defences and adjustment. In this hierarchy, mature defences included humour, anticipation, suppression, altruism and sublimation, whereas immature defences included fantasy; hypochondriasis; acting out and passive aggression. More recently, Perry (1989) developed rating scales for 28 different defences, again arranged in hierarchical order. This provided an empirical tool for looking at the relationship of defence mechanisms with particular diagnoses and also with outcomes in psychotherapy (Høglend & Perry, 1998).

Social and cultural relevance

It has been argued that psychodynamic therapies and theories are outdated and are drawn from a Western Judaeo-Christian model of the world that is not sufficiently universally applicable to be relevant in a multicultural society. It is not within the scope of this chapter to address the theoretical arguments that support these views other than to acknowledge that they are equally applicable to most other psychological and medical interventions.

What is possible within the psychodynamic model however is the scope to specifically look directly at the interpersonal and intra-psychic (as opposed to societal and economic) impact of features of difference and to understand something of the process of prejudice from this position. The concept of discrimination is an interesting one to look at here. For example, it can be held to mean the capacity to discern the difference between one thing and another, i.e. to distinguish. Sometimes this requires real skill and a balanced understanding of the nature of differences between two things. However 'discrimination' also carries a related but almost opposing meaning – to discriminate is to notice the differences between two aspects of things (for example, gender; ethnicity; religion; disability) and to make judgements based, not on balanced reflections, but on prejudice (born of instinctual wishes or of anxiety). Both definitions of discrimination are served by underlying defences but they operate at different hierarchical levels. For example, attempts to work against inequity are often driven by the more mature defences such as altruism, sublimation. However, the means of justifying discrimination and prejudice are serviced by what we have described as the immature defences (for example, altruison and sublimation). Whereas prejudice is serviced by what we have described as the immature defence (for example, projective identification; omnipotence and grandiosity; and acting out). The intensity and directness of a psychodynamic treatment allows the honest and direct exploration of feelings such as these as they are revealed within the transference and as they represent key internal conflicts and insecurities.

Research evidence

As the Roth and Fonagy (2004) review of the evidence for the psychotherapies indicates, psychodynamic psychotherapy is not marked by evidence against its effectiveness as by a lack of evidence.

It is commonly accepted in most western healthcare systems that strong evidence supporting the effectiveness of treatments must take the form of the randomized controlled trial (RCT), a research design useful for developing and testing drugs. The fact is that insufficient research of this sort has been conducted to look at effectiveness of all the psychotherapies and in particular the psychodynamic therapies. Psychodynamic treatments are practised widely in the Western world for a range of mental health problems and in a range of settings from primary care (e.g. counsellors) to secondary care and dedicated specialist inpatient and outpatient services. Despite this, it is notoriously difficult to get funding for RCTs of psychoanalytic psychotherapy in the UK, where the National Health Service (NHS) has limited funds and where the small proportion of funding designated for mental health research is usually allocated to psychiatric drug trials which are more familiar to funding bodies. Lack of funding breeds further difficulties as there are few publicly funded centres where researcher-clinicians can locate themselves to take up an apprenticeship in good quality programmatic research, whereas those practitioners practising privately do not have the infrastructure or numbers to set up the good quality research trials required. In this context it is interesting to note how much evidence there is, but it also clear that most of it comes from other parts of Europe and North America.

Although psychodynamic treatment is often seen as more costly to deliver (because of longer training and also longer interventions) this should be placed in context. Some studies show that the more complex psychodynamic interventions actually keep working after the end of treatment, with maintained or continued improvement after termination (Svartberg & Stiles, 1999) or that reductions in service utilization after treatment means that they are very cost-effective (Guthrie et al., 1999). Finally the fact that Cognitive Behavioural Therapy interventions for more complex cases are now being set up to include interventions at a greater frequency than once a week (DeRubeis et al., 2005) and over longer periods of time (for example with boosters extending treatment to up to a year, (Hollon et al., 2005) supports the need for longer and more complex interventions (see 'Cognitive behavioural therapy').

There are a number of publications reviewing the evidence for the psychodynamic psychotherapies (Fonagy, 2002; Leuzinger-Bohleber & Target, 2003; Richardson et al., 2004; Wallerstein, 1986) and these are supplemented by a developing literature in counselling (e.g. McLeod, 2001; Rowland & Goss, 2000) much of which is derived from a more psychodynamic model.

It can also be argued that the huge demand for this type of talking therapy by referrers and by clients themselves also provides a kind of evidence for its relevance. In 1998, 40% of primary care practices in the UK employed a counsellor psychotherapist and this number is growing (Counselling in Primary Care, 1998, Report by National Medical Advisory Committee). The lack of an evidence-base means that recommendations made for clinical practice are largely, though not exclusively, derived from clinical settings.

Clinical implications and conclusions

The delivery of psychodynamic treatments varies from short-term, very focussed interventions (as assessments or consultations, usually better for crises or as a way of finding out if the method is one that is found helpful by the client) to time-limited groups; open-ended groups (often called 'slow open'); once-weekly treatment, extending over longer periods of time or being open-ended; and finally to more intensive treatments that take place at a frequency of greater than one session a week. Although all of these options can be found in the NHS, the longer and more intensive ones are more common in the private sector.

In previous decades there had been a suggestion that people being considered for psychodynamic treatments should display certain features (psychological mindedness, average to high intelligence, etc.). It is now recognized that this is not the case. Psychodynamic psychotherapy is used with people with learning difficulties (Sinason, 1992), autism (Alvares & Reid, 1999), severe mental health problems, including personality disorder, (Bateman & Fonagy, 1999) and psychotic illnesses (Martindale et al., 2000).

It is important that patients considering this treatment have some idea of what to expect and recognize that it is not an advice-giving approach and can sometimes seem tough in its attention to the features that maintain difficulties rather than sympathizing with the symptoms. In fact, many people find considerable relief in the consistency of the treatment and the non-judgemental preparedness to face painful and uncomfortable realities.

REFERENCES

Alvarez, A. & Reid, S. (Eds.). (1999). *Autism and personality: findings from the Tavistock Clinic workshop.* London: Routledge.

Bateman, A. & Fonagy, P. (1999). The effectiveness of partial hospitalisation in the treatment of borderline personality disorder – a randomised controlled trial. *American Journal of Psychiatry,* **156,** 1563–9.

DeRubeis, R., Hollon, S., Amsterdam, J. *et al.* (2005). Cognitive therapy vs medications in the treatment of moderate to severe depression. *Archives of General Psychiatry,* **62**(4), 409–16.

Enns, M., Cox, B. & Clara, I. (2002). Parental bonding and adult psychopathology: results from the US National Comorbidity Survey. *Psychological Medicine,* **32,** 997–1008.

Fonagy, P. (Ed.). (2002). *An open door review of outcome studies in psychoanalysis* (2nd edn.). London: International Psychoanalytic Association.

Fonagy, P., Gergely, G., Jurist, E. & Target, M. (2002). *Affect regulation, mentalisation and the development of the self.* New York: The Other Press.

Freud, S. (1900). The Interpretation of Dreams. In, J. Strachey (Ed.). *The standard edition of the complete psychological work of sigmund freud, Vol. 4–5.* London: Hogarth Press.

Freud, S. (1923). The Ego and the Id. In, J. Strachey (Ed.). *The standard edition of the complete psychological works of sigmund freud, Vol. 19.* London: Hogarth Press.

Guthrie, E., Moorey, J., Margison, F. *et al.* (1999). Cost effectiveness of brief psychodynamic–interpersonal therapy in high utilizers of psychiatric services. *Archives of General Psychiatry,* **56,** 519–26.

Hollon, S., DeRubeis, R., Shelton, R. *et al.* (2005). Prevention of relapse following cognitive therapy vs medications in moderate to severe depression. *Archives of General Psychiatry,* **62**(4), 417–22.

Høglend, P. & Perry, J. C. (1998). Defensive functioning predicts improvement in major depressive episodes. *Journal of Nervous and Mental Disease*, **186**, 238–43.

Laplanche, J. & Pontalis, J. B. (1988, (1973)). *The language of psychoanalysis*. London: Karnac.

Leuzinger-Bohleber, M. & Target, M. (2003). *Outcomes of Psychoanalytic Treatment*. Brunner-Routledge.

McLeod, J. (2001). *Qualitative research in counselling and psychotherapy*. London: Sage.

Martindale, B., Bateman, A., Crowe, M. & Margison, F. (Eds.). (2000). *Psychosis: psychological approaches and their effectiveness*. London: Gaskell.

National Medical Advisory Committee. (1998). *Counselling in primary care*. The Scottish Office, Department of Health.

Perry, J. C. (1989). *Defence Mechanism Rating Scales* (5th edn.). Cambridge MA: Cambridge Hospital.

Richardson, P., Kaechele, H. & Renlund, C. (Eds.). (2004). *Research on psychoanalytic psychotherapy with adults*. EFPP Monograph. London: Karnac Books.

Roth, A. & Fonagy, P. (2004). *What work for whom? A Critical Review of Psychotherapy Research* (2nd edn.). New York: Guilford.

Rowland, N. & Goss, S. (Eds.). (2000). *Evidence-based counselling and psychological therapies*. London: Routledge.

Sinason, V. (1992). *Mental handicap and the human condition*. Oxford: Free Association Books.

Svartberg, M. & Stiles, T. (1999). *The Trondheim Psychotherapy Study: a randomised trial of short term dynamic therapy versus cognitive therapy for cluster C personality disorder*. Paper presented to the 30th International Conference, Society for Psychotherapy Research. Braga, Portugal, June.

Vaillant, G. (1971). Theoretical hierarchy of adaptive ego mechanisms. *Archives of General Psychiatry*, **24**, 107–18.

Wallerstein, R. (1986). *Forty-two lives: A study of psychoanalysis and psychotherapy*. New York: The Other Press.

Psychosocial care of the elderly

Jennifer Q. Morse and Charles F. Reynolds, III

Western Psychiatric Institute and Clinic

Mood disorders are among the most significant and often overlooked disorders in later life (Consensus Development Panel of the Depression and Bipolar Support Alliance, 2003). Because there is relatively little research on late-life bipolar disorder, this chapter will focus on depression. Depression is the most frequently diagnosed psychiatric disorder in late life (Verhey & Honig, 1997), particularly among the chronically or acutely medically ill, those in residential facilities, or community dwellers who have recently been bereaved or assumed caregiving roles (Koenig et al., 1997). The prevalence of major depression in community samples ranges from 1% to 5% (Pahkala et al., 1995) but clinically significant depressive symptoms occur more frequently (Verhey & Honig, 1997).

Barriers to effective treatment

One of the biggest barriers to effective treatment of late-life depression may be under-recognition by older adults, their families and their physicians. Late-life depression is significantly under-diagnosed (Mulsant & Ganguli, 1999), particularly in primary care settings (Harman et al., 2001), the healthcare setting used most often by older adults (Unutzer et al., 1999). Many older adults and their physicians assume that low energy, loss of interest and somatic symptoms are part of being old or physically ill, rather than symptoms of depression (Karel & Hinrichsen, 2000) (see 'Ageing and health behaviour'). Sleep disturbance, failure to care for oneself, withdrawal from social activities, unexplained somatic complaints and hopelessness may be important clinical clues for depression (Gallo et al., 1997). In addition to under-recognition, under-treatment of late-life depression is common (Hirshfield et al., 1997), despite available and effective pharmacological treatments and psychosocial interventions: the latter will be reviewed in this chapter.

Under-recognition and under-treatment of late-life depression are critical issues because depression is associated with a number of costly consequences: emotional suffering, caregiver burden, excess disability, increased use of health services, risk of hospitalization, decreased quality of life and mortality from comorbid medical conditions or suicide (Ganguli et al., 2002; Unutzer et al., 2000). In fact, depression is likely to be a leading cause of death and disability by 2020 (Murray & Lopez, 1996). On the other hand, mental health treatment may lead to reductions in subsequent medical costs (Mumford et al., 1984), but this remains a controversial point. In this chapter we review the evidence-based psychosocial interventions for late-life depression, considering first a rationale for their use and then what is known about the efficacy of each and the putative mechanism of action (change).

Psychosocial treatments

Rationale

Psychosocial interventions generally address psychosocial risk factors for depression, with the rationale that targeting *modifiable* factors may decrease depression and reduce the risk of later depression (Bruce, 2002), particularly if medications are not likely to address these vulnerabilities (Niederehe, 1994). The modifiable risk factors for developing late-life depression include stressful life events, low social support, physical illness and disability; more importantly, change in these factors is associated with recovery (Kennedy, 1995). Psychotherapy can also help older adults to cope with psychosocial risk factors that cannot be easily modified, including caregiver strain, bereavement and role transitions (Bruce, 2002) (see 'Disability', 'Social support and health' and 'Stress and health').

Psychotherapy is infrequently prescribed by primary care physicians (PCPs) (Alvidrez & Arean, 2002), but older adults not only consider psychotherapy a viable option, but prefer it over medication (Landreville et al., 2001). In early studies, older adults had better compliance with psychotherapy protocols, lower drop-out rates and more positive responses than younger adults (Brink, 1979; Sparacino, 1978–79). Later work confirmed that the ability to benefit from psychotherapy does not diminish with age (Knight, 1988). Psychotherapy may also be the only viable treatment option for depressed older adults who cannot tolerate antidepressant medications because of dangerous side-effects (like gait instability or falls), comorbid medical illnesses, or drug interactions with medications for comorbid medical illnesses.

Evidence base

There have been several meta-analyses which suggest that psychotherapy in general is a well established treatment for late-life depression (see Arean & Cook, 2002; Niederehe, 1994). Across depression severity levels, depressed older adults receiving psychotherapy showed less post-treatment depression than no-treatment or placebo controls. The average effect size in these meta-analyses is 0.78 or greater – patients in psychotherapy do more than $\frac{3}{4}$ standard deviation better on outcome measures than patients in no-treatment or placebo-control conditions. Most meta-analyses indicate that the immediate effects of treatment are greater than the long-term effects and that improvement on clinician-rated scales of depression is often greater than improvement on self-rated depression scales. In general, the efficacy of acute treatment for late-life depression is not different from that with mid-life adults, with about 60% recovered after six months. We now turn to empirically validated psychosocial interventions for late-life depression.

Specific interventions – classification

The psychosocial interventions that have been empirically validated for treating late-life depression fall into two general classes – behavioural therapies and interpersonal or psychodynamic-rooted therapies – each of which will be described specifically, along with empirical evidence supporting its use. Behaviour therapies include classic behaviour therapy (BT), cognitive or cognitive–behavioural therapy (CT or CBT), dialectical behaviour therapy (DBT) and problem-solving therapy (PST). These interventions largely rest on the assumption that human behaviour, including influencing one's environment, regulating one's mood and managing one's thoughts, is learned. Thus, behaviour therapies focus on skill-building. More interpersonal or psychoanalytically rooted therapies focus on interpersonal relationships and are based on the finding that

depression is associated with long-term and short-term disruption of interpersonal relationships (Coryell et al., 1993), or the absence of social resources like family support or confidants (Barnett & Gotlib, 1988). The interpersonal or psychodynamic interventions include brief dynamic therapy (BDT), interpersonal psychotherapy (IPT) and reminiscence therapy (RT). We will briefly describe each specific intervention along with the rationale for treatment, the purported mechanism for change and empirical support for the intervention in acute treatment, follow-up or maintenance and in combination with medication, as available.

Behaviour therapies

Behaviour therapy (BT) asserts that changes in information processing are attained by experiencing more positive events through new behaviour (Lewinsohn et al., 1984). The mechanism of change is behavioural activation and changing the reinforcement schedule by behaviour. BT is often used as a comparison treatment for CBT interventions. In Arean and Miranda's review (1996), there were no differences between BT, CBT and social PST and each was at least as effective as placebo, usual care and medication in acute treatment. Treatment gains made in BT are generally maintained following treatment (Gallagher & Thompson, 1983) (see 'Behaviour therapy').

According to cognitive–behavioural therapy (CBT), errors in thinking about oneself, one's experience and one's future maintain a depressed patient's negative or depressed mood (Beck, 1983). The central mechanism for change in CBT is 'stepping back', labelling cognitive errors, examining the evidence for specific thoughts and rejecting those that are likely to be false or of low probability and responding to negative thoughts or emotions as transitory events rather than self-defining ones. For depressed older adults, CBT is a superior treatment to usual care (Campbell, 1992), waiting list control (Rokke et al., 2000), pill placebo (Jarvik et al., 1982) and no treatment (Viney et al., 1989). There is evidence that treatment gains are maintained up to two years after treatment (Rokke et al., 2000). Finally, CBT combined with medication has been demonstrated to be more efficacious that medication alone (Thompson et al., 2001) (see 'Cognitive behaviour therapy').

Rather than focusing on affect and cognitive regulation skills, social problem-solving therapy (PST) focuses on problem-solving skills. The mechanism of change in social PST includes behavioural activation, increased exposure to positive events, and increased interpersonal skills, including increased sensitivity to interpersonal cues and improved communication (Nezu et al., 1989). Social PST is superior to waiting list control and reminiscence therapy and equivalent, to or better than, medication (Alexopoulos et al., 2003; Mynors-Wallis, 1996). Treatment gains are maintained three months after treatment (Arean et al., 1993). Social PST may be particularly effective for depressed older adults with cognitive (executive functional) impairment. For these populations, PST has been more effective than supportive therapy (Alexopoulos et al., 2003).

A treatment initially formulated for suicidal and self-injuring women, dialectical behaviour therapy (DBT), has also been adapted for depressed older adults (Lynch, 2000). DBT focuses on skills deficits in several key areas – mindfulness or attention control; interpersonal skills; crisis management skills; and emotion regulation. The mechanism of change in DBT is skill acquisition which improves emotion regulation. Though not yet studied as a stand-alone treatment, group DBT plus antidepressant had a better remission rate than antidepressant plus clinical management in acute treatment, with gains maintained six months later (Lynch et al., 2003).

Interpersonal therapies

Moving from behavioural interventions to interpersonal or psycho-dynamic ones, brief dynamic therapy (BDT) views psychopathology, including depression, as rooted in developmental difficulties that promote ineffective coping. Treatment focuses on insight, achieved through the relationship with the therapist, as the mechanism of change. Adaptations of BDT for older adults focus on ineffective coping with losses or stresses in late life. BDT has been as effective as CBT at reducing symptoms (Gallagher & Thompson, 1982), but other therapies may show greater reduction in symptoms (Arean et al., 1993). One problem with the existing literature on BDT is that it has not been directly compared with antidepressants (Arean & Cook, 2002) and while there is some evidence of problem resolution, there is no evidence of increased insight, the purported mechanism of change (Karel & Hinrichsen, 2000) (see 'Psychodynamic psychotherapy').

IPT is a research-oriented operationalization of psychodynamic treatment for depressed patients with foci that are particularly relevant for older adults. It uses exploration, clarification of affect and some change techniques to target four areas: unresolved grief; role transitions; interpersonal role conflict; and interpersonal deficit. The mechanism of change in IPT is resolving the interpersonal context in which depression arose. IPT has been as effective as antidepressant pharmacotherapy in acute treatment and had a lower dropout rate than medication (Schneider et al., 1986). In addition, the combination of IPT plus medication is the most efficacious treatment for depressed older adults (Reynolds et al., 1999a) and bereavement-related episodes (Reynolds et al., 1999b). IPT also receives significant attention as a maintenance treatment. Following stable remission, IPT plus medication produces the best recurrence prevention rates among depressed older adults (Reynolds et al., 1999a). However IPT has rarely been studied as a stand-alone treatment: IPT plus placebo cannot be interpreted as being the same thing as IPT alone because of patient expectations about being treated with a medication or not (Arean & Cook, 2002).

Reminiscence therapy (RT) is also called life review therapy. It bears mention because of its specificity to elderly people. RT argues that reminiscence is a normal experience to resolve Erikson's (1963) final developmental stage, sense of integrity or despair. Techniques to operationalize RT have varied greatly and its treatment manuals are not as well developed than other interventions. RT has been studied predominantly in non-clinical samples seeking personal growth or in cognitively impaired nursing home residents. In these settings it is generally reported to be effective at decreasing mild depressive symptoms (Dhooper et al., 1993) or increasing life satisfaction (Haight, 1988). While RT seems useful for mild to moderate depression, some are concerned about the viability of life review for more severely depressed patients whose characteristics or life histories make a positive review unlikely (Niederehe, 1994).

Comment

A number of adaptations must be made in order to offer older adults effective treatments. More initial education about the nature of depression and the process of psychotherapy, indicating for example that participating in psychotherapy is not a sign that the patient is weak or crazy, is essential. Gaining insight or learning new skills must take into account changes associated with ageing (cognitive changes, memory changes, cohort biases, disability and greater experiences and learning history) by slowing the pace of therapy, emphasizing repetition and using multiple modes of presentation (Karel & Hinrichsen, 2000). Therapist flexibility in delivering care and willingness to communicate with, or involve, family members or other healthcare professionals is also essential. An example of modifications that did not help older adults was an abbreviated version of PST designed for primary care (PST-PC) (Mynors-Wallis, 1996). The modifications included brief sessions, fewer sessions and only one presentation of model, which has been suggested as inappropriate for older adults (Arean & Cook, 2002). These were not responsive to the needs of older adults, but PST in its traditional presentation is effective for treating late-life depression.

Special populations in late life

Now that general treatments have been reviewed, several special populations of older adults deserve attention: depressed medically ill older adults, depression treatment in primary care, depressed caregivers, depressed older adults with cognitive impairment, suicidal older adults, older adults experiencing subclinical depression and populations for whom more research is needed. Exhaustive examination of these 'special populations' is beyond the scope of this chapter: these descriptions are intended to alert the reader and to suggest further reading.

Depression in medically ill older adults

Depression often accompanies chronic illness (see 'Coping with chronic illness'). For example, about 20% of people with coronary artery disease have depression, especially following myocardial infarction (MI) (Frasure-Smith et al., 1993). Recognizing and treating post-MI depression is critical because depression is associated with an increased mortality rate after MI (Frasure-Smith et al., 1993) and with cardiac complications (Roose et al., 1991) (see 'Coronary heart disease: cardiac psychology'). Similarly, depression is the most common psychiatric disorder in post-stroke patients (Robinson & Starkstein, 1990) and has a negative impact on recovery of activities of daily living (ADLs) and the outcome of rehabilitation (Verhey & Honig, 1997). Depression is also common following organ transplant (Dew et al., 1997) and may impact treatment adherence following transplant. Depression is common following hip fracture and negatively impacts recovery and disability (Lenze et al., 2004). Depression is also prevalent among patients with Parkinson's disease, but it is difficult to disentangle the psychiatric, neuropsychological and neurological deficits and symptoms. The bottom line is that recognizing and treating depression among medically ill older adults is essential because of the negative impact of depression has on recovery and treatment adherence.

Depression in primary care

Most older adults receive their healthcare in primary care practices (Unutzer *et al.*, 1999), thus it will be essential to extend empirically validated interventions for depression to this setting. Depressed older adults in primary care are reported to respond well to CBT (Arean & Miranda, 1996) and IPC (a modification of IPT) (Mossey *et al.*, 1996), but not to PST (Williams *et al.*, 2000). A recent innovation was for depression researchers to place a depression care manager in primary care practices in an attempt to increase the recognition of depression, improve its treatment and enhance functional outcomes for comorbid medical illnesses (Williams *et al.*, 2004). A similar strategy was used to reduce late-life suicide (Reynolds *et al.*, 2001). More approaches like these successful integrations of primary care and on site mental health services are needed to meet the needs of depressed older adults and to provide care where it is most accessible to them.

Depression in caregivers

Depression in response to chronic situational stress such as caring for a physically or mentally disabled family member is common, with prevalence rates as high as 50% in some studies of caregivers of dementia patients (Gallagher *et al.*, 1989), even after placement or death of the patient receiving caregiving (Schulz *et al.*, 2004). While studies of caregiver support groups often do not often meet criteria for inclusion in scientific reviews or meta-analyses of depression treatment studies (Niederehe, 1994), there are two points to mention. First, more benefit for caregivers may be derived from psychoeducational groups that specifically target managing depressive symptoms rather than general support groups (Lovett & Gallagher, 1988). And second, the amount of time spent in caregiving may also be critical in treatment recommendations. In a study comparing CBT and BDT, there were no differences between the groups in aggregate. However, for caregivers who had been caring for a family member for more that 44 weeks, CBT was more effective (Gallagher-Thompson & Steffen, 1994). The authors concluded that 'old' dementia caregivers need more structured problem-solving while 'young' caregivers need to cope with processing the affect around the diagnosis of dementia.

Depression in Alzheimer's disease

Approximately 10–30% of Alzheimer's disease (AD) patients will meet criteria for depression (Verhey & Honig, 1997). Reversible depression-induced dementia ('true pseudodementia') is rare. In terms of treating depression among AD patients, BT produced improvements in depressive symptoms for both AD patients and their caregivers (Teri *et al.*, 1997). Reminiscence therapy delivered in nursing homes to AD patients showed greater reduction in depressive symptoms than supportive therapy and no treatment (Goldwasser *et al.*, 1987). As noted previously, PST has been effective in treating depression in older adults with executive dysfunction (Alexopoulos *et al.*, 2003). Many efficacy studies exclude older adults with cognitive impairment, but more research is needed to improve treatment of depression with mild cognitive impairment or dementia.

Reducing the risk of suicide

Suicide rates increase with age, with the highest suicide rates among older white males. Suicide in late life is more directly related to underlying depression than in other age groups, particularly among completed suicides (Conwell & Caine, 1991). Thus this group requires particular clinical attention and suicidality should be directly assessed in depressed older adult patients. The use of depression care managers was found to effectively reduce suicidal ideation more than usual care in PCP practices (Bruce *et al.*, 2004). Additional research efforts to intervene effectively with this high-risk group are needed (see 'Suicide').

Subsyndromal depression

Seemingly opposite to suicidal older adults, those who experience minor or subclinical depression also warrant particular attention. While major depression may decline with age, other depressive syndromes and depressive symptoms that do not meet criteria for major depressive episode increase (Verhey & Honig, 1997). There is evidence that subclinical depression may be more consequential in older adults because of its association with disability, medical burden and vulnerability to further psychiatric disorder or chronic course (Lyness *et al.*, 2002). And while some conclude that psychosocial interventions are equally effective for clinical and subclinical depression (Scogin & Mcelreath, 1994), others point out that the literature is limited and that more research needs to be done (Arean & Cook, 2002).

Minority, homebound or rural and the oldest old

Additional research is also needed to address the treatment needs for other groups of older adults, including minority, homebound or rural elders and the oldest old. Few of the empirically validated interventions have been examined with sufficient minority samples to draw conclusions about which interventions are effective for this group. A single non-randomized trial has found CBT to be effective in treating depressed minority older adults (Arean & Miranda, 1996). Clearly more research with minority older adults is needed. Similarly, there is little research focusing on rural or homebound older adults. Researchers focused on this group have found that bibliotherapy plus check-ups by phone or in person is superior to usual care (Landreville & Bissonnette, 1997). These innovations may help to reach this difficult group. Although research studies are beginning to include older participants, a particular focus still needs to be placed on the needs of the oldest old; earlier work often did not include these participants and it is difficult to know if findings with young old will generalize to the oldest old. Data from our group (Gildengers *et al.*, 2002), suggest that the oldest old can and do respond well to treatment for depression.

Conclusions

In conclusion both behavioural and interpersonal interventions are effective in treating late-life depression in ambulatory older adults. Clinical practice should include therapy plus medication for serious depression and may include psychotherapy alone for those with mild to moderate depression who are unwilling or unable to tolerate medications (Karel & Hinrichsen, 2000). Intervention research needs to focus on long-term and functional outcomes and the goal of getting well and staying well (Reynolds *et al.*, 1999*a*). There are still gaps between the efficacy of treatments demonstrated in controlled clinical trials and the effectiveness of treatments in real-world settings (Consensus Development Panel of the Depression and Bipolar Support Alliance, 2003). Thus researchers need to recruit medically ill and/or cognitively impaired patients. In addition, more trials are needed for BDT, IPT alone and for combinations of medication plus CBT, PST and BDT. Empirically validated interventions for late-life depression need to be examined in rural or homebound older adults, minority older adults and subclinically depressed older adults. Perhaps most importantly, because most studies found non-significant differences between psychosocial treatments, other variables may predict differences in therapy outcomes (Niederehe, 1994). Currently, there are no known factors to help patients, families or care providers choose between psychosocial inventions. Such examinations would be helpful.

Acknowledgement

Manuscript preparation by Dr. Morse was supported by NIMH training grants (T32 MH 18269, PI: Paul Pilkonis, PhD, T32 MH19986-08, PI: Charles Reynolds, MD, and P30 MH52247, PI: Charles Reynolds, MD). We would like to thank Valerie Anderson at the Western Psychiatric Institute and Clinic's Intervention Research Centre for Late Life Mood Disorders for help with the case vignette.

REFERENCES

Alexopoulos, G. S., Raue, P. & Arean, P. (2003). Problem-solving therapy versus supportive therapy in geriatric major depression with executive dysfunction. *American Journal of Geriatric Psychiatry*, **11**, 46–52.

Alvidrez, J. & Arean, P. (2002). Physician willingness to refer older depressed patients for psychotherapy. *International Journal of Psychiatry in Medicine*, **32**, 21–35.

Arean, P. A. & Cook, B. L. (2002). Psychotherapy and combined psychotherapy/pharmacotherapy for late life depression. *Biological Psychiatry*, **52**, 293–303.

Arean, P. A. & Miranda, J. (1996). The treatment of depression in elderly primary care patients: a naturalistic study. *Journal of Clinical Geropsychology*, **2**, 153–60.

Arean, P. A., Perri, M. G., Nezu, A. M. *et al.* (1993). Comparative effectiveness of social problem-solving therapy and reminiscence therapy as treatments for depression in older adults. *Journal of Consulting and Clinical Psychology*, **61**, 1003–10.

Barnett, P. A. & Gotlib, I. H. (1988). Psychosocial functioning and depression: distinguishing among antecedents, concomitants, and consequences. *Psychological Bulletin*, **104**, 97–126.

Beck, A. T. (1983). Cognitive therapy of depression: new perspectives. In P. J. Clayton & J. E. Barrett (Eds.). *Treatment of depression: old controversies and new approaches*. New York: Raven Press.

Brink, T. L. (1979). *Geriatric psychotherapy*. New York: Human Sciences Press.

Bruce, M. L. (2002). Psychosocial risk factors for depressive disorders in late life. *Biological Psychiatry*, **52**, 175–84.

Bruce, M. L., Ten Have, T. R., Reynolds III, C. F. *et al.* (2004). Reducing suicidal ideation and depressive symptoms in depressed older primary care patients: a randomized controlled trial. *Journal of the American Medical Association*, **291**, 1081–91.

Campbell, J. M. (1992). Treating depression in well older adults: use of diaries in cognitive therapy. *Issues in Mental Health Nursing*, **13**, 19–29.

Consensus Development Panel of the Depression and Bipolar Support Alliance (2003). Depression and bipolar support alliance consensus statement on the unmet needs in diagnosis and treatment of mood disorders in late life. *Archives of General Psychiatry*, **60**, 664–72.

Conwell, Y. & Caine, E. D. (1991). Rational suicide and the right to die: reality and myth. *New England Journal of Medicine*, **325**, 1100–3.

Coryell, W., Scheftner, W., Keller, M. *et al.* (1993). The enduring psychosocial consequences of mania and depression. *American Journal of Psychiatry*, **150**, 720–7.

Dew, M. A., Switzer, G. E., Goycoolea, J. M. *et al.* (1997). Does transplantation produce quality of life benefits? A quantitative review of the literature. *Transplantation*, **64**, 1261–73.

Dhooper, S. S., Green, S. M., Huff, M. B. & Austin-Murphy, J. (1993). Efficacy of a group approach to reducing depression in nursing home elderly residents. *Journal of Gerontological Social Work*, **20**, 87–100.

Erikson, E. (1963). *Childhood and society*. New York: W. W. Norton.

Frasure-Smith, N., Lesperance, F. & Talajic, M. (1993). Depression following myocardial infarction: Impact on 6-month survival. *Journal of the American Medical Association*, **270**, 1819–25.

Gallagher-Thompson, D. & Steffen, A. M. (1994). Comparative effects of cognitive–behavioral and brief psychodynamic psychotherapies for depressed family caregivers. *Journal of Consulting and Clinical Psychology*, **62**, 543–9.

Gallagher, D. E. & Thompson, L. W. (1982). Treatment of major depressive disorder in older adult outpatients with brief psychotherapies. *Psychotherapy: Theory, Research and Practice*, **19**, 482–90.

Gallagher, D. E. & Thompson, L. W. (1983). Effectiveness of psychotherapy for both endogenous and nonendogenous depression in older adult outpatients. *Journal of Gerontology*, **38**, 707–12.

Gallagher, D., Rose, J. & Rivera, P. (1989). Prevalence of depression in family caregivers. *Gerontologist*, **29**, 449–56.

Gallo, J. J., Rabins, P. V. & Iliffe, S. (1997). The "research magnificent" in late life: psychiatric epidemiology and the primary health care of older adults. *International Journal of Psychiatry in Medicine*, **27**, 185–204.

Ganguli, M., Dodge, H. H. & Mulsant, B. H. (2002). Rates and predictors of mortality in an aging, rural, community-based cohort: the role of depression. *Archives of General Psychiatry*, **59**, 1046–52.

Gildengers, A. G., Houck, P. R., Mulsant, B. H. *et al.* (2002). Course and rate of antidepressant response in the very old. *Journal of Affective Disorders*, **69**, 177–84.

Goldwasser, A. N., Auerbach, S. M. & Harkins, S. W. (1987). Cognitive, affective, and behavioral effects of reminiscence group therapy on demented elderly.

International Journal of Aging and Human Development, **25**, 209–22.

Haight, B. K. (1988). The therapeutic role of a structured life review process in homebound elderly subjects. *Journals of Gerontology Series B Psychological Sciences and Social Sciences*, **43**, P40–4.

Harman, J. S., Schulberg, H. C., Mulsant, B. H. & Reynolds III, C. F. (2001). The effect of patient and visit characteristics on diagnosis of depression in primary care. *Journal of Family Practice*, **50**, 1068.

Hirshfield, R. M. A., Keller, M. B., Panico, S. et al. (1997). The national depressive and manic-depressive association consensus statement on the undertreatment of depression. *Journal of the American Medical Association*, **277**(4), 333–40.

Jarvik, L. F., Mintz, J., Steuer, J. L. & Gerner, R. (1982). Treating geriatric depression: a 26-week interim analysis. *Journal of the American Geriatrics Society*, **30**, 713–17.

Karel, M. J. & Hinrichsen, G. (2000). Treatment of depression in late life: psychotherapeutic interventions. *Clinical Psychology Review*, **20**, 707–29.

Kennedy, G. J. (1995). The geriatric syndrome of late-life depression. *Psychiatric Services*, **46**, 43–8.

Knight, B. (1988). Factors influencing therapist-rated change in older adults. *Journal of Gerontology*, **43**, 111–12.

Koenig, H. G., George, L. K., Peterson, B. L. & Pieper, C. F. (1997). Depression in medically ill hospitalized older adults: prevalence, characteristics, and course of symptoms according to six diagnostic schemes. *American Journal of Psychiatry*, **154**, 1376–83.

Landreville, P. & Bissonnette, L. (1997). Effects of cognitive bibliotherapy for depressed older adults with a disability. *Clinical Gerontologist*, **17**, 35–55.

Landreville, P., Landry, J., Baillargeon, L., Guerette, A. & Matteau, E. (2001). Older adults' acceptance of psychological and pharmacological treatments for depression. *Journals of Gerontology Series B-Psychological Sciences and Social Sciences*, **56B**, P285–91.

Lenze, E. J., Munin, M. C., Dew, M. A. et al. (2004). Adverse effects of depression and cognitive impairment on rehabilitation participation and recovery from hip fracture. *International Journal of Geriatric Psychiatry*, **19**, 472–8.

Lewinsohn, P. M., Antonuccio, D. O., Steinmetz, J. L. & Teri, L. (1984). *The coping with depression course: a psychoeducational intervention for unipolar depression*. Eugene, OR: Castalia.

Lovett, S. & Gallagher, D. E. (1988). Psychoeducational interventions for family caregivers: preliminary efficacy data. *Behavior Therapy*, **19**, 321–30.

Lynch, T. R. (2000). Treatment of elderly depression with personality disorder comorbidity using dialectical behavior therapy. *Cognitive and Behavioral Practice*, **7**, 468–77.

Lynch, T. R., Morse, J. Q., Mendelson, T. & Robins, C. J. (2003). Dialectical behavior therapy for depressed older adults: a randomized pilot study. *American Journal of Geriatric Psychiatry*, **11**, 33–45.

Lyness, J. M., Caine, E. D., King, D. A. et al. (2002). Depressive disorders and symptoms in older primary care patients: one-year outcomes. *American Journal of Geriatric Psychiatry*, **10**, 275–82.

Mossey, J. M., Knott, K. A., Higgins, M. & Talerico, K. (1996). Effectiveness of a psychosocial intervention, interpersonal counseling, for subdysthymic depression in medically ill elderly. *Journals of Gerontology Series A Biological Sciences and Medical Sciences*, **51**, M172–8.

Mulsant, B. H. & Ganguli, M. (1999). Epidemiology and diagnosis of depression in late life. *Journal of Clinical Psychiatry*, **20**, 9–15.

Mumford, E., Schlesinger, H. J., Glass, G. V., Patrick, C. & Cuerdon, T. (1984). A new look at evidence about the reduced cost of medical utilization following mental health treatment. *American Journal of Psychiatry*, **141**, 1145–58.

Murray, C. J. L. & Lopez, A. D. (1996). *The global burden of disease: a comprehensive assessment of mortality and disability from diseases, injuries, and risk factors in 1990 and projected to 2020*. Cambridge, MA: Harvard University Press.

Mynors-Wallis, L. (1996). Problem-solving treatment: evidence for effectiveness and feasibility in primary care. *International Journal of Psychiatry in Medicine*, **26**, 249–62.

Nezu, A. M., Nezu, C. M. & Perri, M. G. (1989). *Problem-solving therapy for depression: theory, research, and clinical guidelines*. Oxford, UK: John Wiley & Sons.

Niederehe, G. T. (1994). Psychosocial therapies with depressed older adults. In L. S. Schneider, C. F. Reynolds, III, B. D. Lebowitz & A. J. Friedhoff (Eds.). *Diagnosis and treatment of depression in late life: results of the NIH Consensus Development Conference*. Washington, DC: American Psychiatric Association.

Pahkala, K., Kesti, E., Kongas-Saviaro, P., Laippala, P. & Kivela, S. L. (1995). Prevalence of depression in an aged population in Finland. *Social Psychiatry and Psychiatric Epidemiology*, **30**, 99–106.

Reynolds III, C. F., Degenholtz, H., Parker, L. S. et al. (2001). Treatment as usual (TAU) control practices in the PROSPECT Study: managing the interaction and tension between research design and ethics. *International Journal of Geriatric Psychiatry*, **16**, 602–8.

Reynolds III, C. F., Frank, E., Perel, J. M. et al. (1999a). Nortriptyline and interpersonal psychotherapy as maintenance therapies for recurrent major depression: a randomized controlled trial in patients older than 59 years. *Journal of the American Medical Association*, **218**, 39–45.

Reynolds III, C. F., Miller, M. D., Pasternak, R. E. et al. (1999b). Treatment of bereavement-related major depressive episodes in later life: a controlled study of acute and continuation treatment with nortriptyline and interpersonal psychotherapy. *American Journal of Psychiatry*, **156**, 202–8.

Robinson, R. G. & Starkstein, S. E. (1990). Current research in affective disorders following stroke. *Journal of Neuropsychiatry and Clinical Neurosciences*, **2**, 1–14.

Rokke, P. D., Tomhave, J. A. & Jocic, Z. (2000). Self-managment therapy and educational group therapy for depressed elders. *Cognitive Therapy and Research*, **24**, 99–119.

Roose, S. P., Dalack, G. W. & Woordring, S. (1991). Death, depression and heart disease. *Journal of Clinical Psychiatry*, **52**, 34–9.

Schneider, L. S., Sloane, R. B., Staples, F. R. & Bender, M. (1986). Pretreatment orthostatic hypotension as a predictor of response to nortriptyline in geriatric depression. *Journal of Clinical Psychopharmacology*, **6**, 172–6.

Schulz, R., Belle, S. H., Czaja, S. J. et al. (2004). Long-term care placement of dementia patients and caregiver health and well-being. *Journal of the American Medical Association*, **292**, 961–7.

Scogin, F. & McElreath, L. (1994). Efficacy of psychosocial treatments for geriatric depression: a quantitative review. *Journal of Consulting and Clinical Psychology*, **62**, 69–73.

Sparacino, J. (1978–79). Individual psychotherapy with the aged: a selective review. *International Journal of Aging and Human Development*, **9**, 197–220.

Teri, L., Logsdon, R. G., Uomoto, J. & McCurry, S. M. (1997). Behavioral treatment of depression in dementia patients: a controlled clinical trial. *Journals of Gerontology Series B Psychological Sciences and Social Sciences*, **52**, 159–66.

Thompson, L. W., Coon, D. W., Gallagher-Thompson, D., Sommer, B. R. & Koin, D. (2001). Comparison of desipramine and cognitive/behavioral therapy in the treatment of elderly outpatients with mild-to-moderate depression. *American Journal of Geriatric Psychiatry*, **9**, 225–40.

Unutzer, J., Katon, W., Russo, J. *et al.* (1999). Patterns of care for depressed older adults in a large-staff model HMO. *American Journal of Geriatric Psychiatry*, **7**, 235–43.

Unutzer, J., Patrick, D. L., Diehr, P. *et al.* (2000). Quality adjusted life years in older adults with depressive symptoms and

chronic medical disorders. *International Psychogeriatrics*, **12**, 15–33.

Verhey, F. R. J. & Honig, A. (1997). Depression in the elderly. In A. Honig & H. M. Van Praag (Eds.). *Depression: neurobiological, psychopathological and therapeutic advances.* (Wiley series on clinical and neurobiological advances in psychiatry). New York: John Wiley & Sons, Inc.

Viney, L. L., Benjamin, Y. N. & Preston, C. A. (1989). An evaluation of personal construct therapy for the elderly. *British Journal of Medical Psychology*, **62**, 35–41.

Williams Jr., J. W., Barrett, J., Oxman, T. *et al.* (2000). Treatment of dysthymia and minor depression in primary care: a randomized controlled trial in older adults. *Journal of the American Medical Association*, **284**, 1519–26.

Williams Jr. J. W., Katon, W., Lin, E. H. *et al.* (2004). The effectiveness of depression care management on diabetes-related outcomes in older patients. *Annals of Internal Medicine*, **140**, 1015–24.

Relaxation training

Michael H. Bruch

University College London

Introduction

Procedures for the relaxation of body and mind have been known for thousands of years. In some cultures relaxation methods have even become an integral part of philosophical, religious value systems. In view of this it is perhaps surprising that relaxation techniques have gained clinical interest only fairly recently. Early pioneers include J.H. Schultz (autogenic training; e.g. Schultz & Luthe, 1959) and Edmund Jacobsen (progressive muscle relaxation; Jacobson, 1929). Davidson and Schwartz (1976) found it surprising that the subject had been absent from psychological examination for so long, despite obvious links between psychological and physiological arousal and emotional disorders.

Furthermore, perhaps as a result of its varied nature and ideographic meaning for different individuals, there were no generally agreed definitions of the concept. Jacobson attempted to define relaxation by describing its effects thus: 'respiration loses the slight irregularities, the pulse rate may decline to normal, the knee jerk diminishes or disappears along with the pharyngeal and flexion reflexes and nervous start, the esophagus … relaxes in all its parts, while mental and emotional activity dwindle or disappear for brief periods' (Davidson & Schwartz, 1976, p. 400).

In modern clinical psychotherapy and behavioural medicine the focus for relaxation is on emotional and health problems which are perceived to be associated with increased levels of tension. In such clinical contexts therapists make frequent use of stress reduction or relaxation techniques. The aim for the patient is to learn to recognize, control and modify somatic and cognitive responses in such a way that they become incompatible with subjective anxiety, pain or tension. Typical targets are reduction of anxiety-provoking thought processes, muscular tension, hyperventilation, tachycardia and

gastrointestinal responses. Other techniques may involve vasodilatation to reduce blood pressure, regular breathing, positive thinking to achieve feelings of relaxation.

Methods

To this day a vast array of methods and respective variations, as well as combinations thereof, has been reported. Comprehensive discussions of this can be found in Lehrer and Woolfolk (1993) or more recently in publications by Smith (2001, 2002).

Methods include progressive relaxation, autogenic training, breathing, meditational techniques (as developed from Hindu philosophy (i.e. yoga) and Zen Buddhism, hypnosis, biofeedback, cognitive approaches, music therapy, aerobic exercises and pharmacological methods. These are the most commonly used techniques which have also been evaluated by research to varying degrees. The wide range of procedures seems to suggest individual differences both in the modes of arousal and in the responsiveness to intervention methods. In addition one may speculate as to what extent respective methods might have generic or more limited specific effects. We shall address these questions later on when discussing theoretical issues and clinical applications.

Brief descriptions of the most commonly used methods are given below, however, for more detailed accounts of these approaches and their variations readers are referred to the above-mentioned sources.

Progressive relaxation

This technique was originally developed by Edmund Jacobson (1929). He regarded it as a therapeutic method to achieve muscular quiescence to effect cognitive and somatic relaxation. The patient is trained to recognize and to control decreasingly intense levels of muscular tension. As Woolfolk and Lehrer (1984) point out: 'The primary aim is to make the individual able to recognize and eliminate even the most minute levels of tension, to remain as tension free as possible at all times, and to eliminate unnecessary tension continuously during everyday activities.' (p. 5). The method was originally designed as an independent psychotherapy to achieve deep relaxation. The emphasis was for the patient to discover minute changes in tension for him- or herself. The therapist would not make suggestions regarding the expected effects but encourage proprioceptive experience to facilitate learning.

In later use the method was abbreviated for flexible and integrated use with other therapeutic approaches. According to Woolfolk and Lehrer (1984) this was also accompanied by a shift from awareness training to maximum relaxation effect. Such applications are more directive and suggestive with the aim of achieving deep relaxation as quickly as possible. Typical examples can be found within the fields of behavioural and cognitive therapies as described by Hawton *et al.* (1989). These deal mainly with anxiety states and phobic disorders. Such an approach was first pioneered by Wolpe (1958) and labelled 'systematic desensitization'. Here, relaxation is used as a stimulus for counter conditioning. A more recent development is applied relaxation, a comprehensive step by step guide building on progressive relaxation but also utilizing additional methods. (Öst, 1987).

Autogenic training

This method was originally developed by Schultz in the early part of this century (English version by Schultz & Luthe, 1959) on the basis of his experience with hypnosis. Autogenic training (AT) can be described as a form of autosuggestion to influence physiological processes. Similar as in biofeedback facilitation of self-regulation processes is intended. The goal is to reduce excessive autonomic arousal and the patient is asked to concentrate on his bodily sensations in a passive, accepting style. As Linden (1993) has noted, it is especially the principle of passive concentration that distinguishes AT from progressive muscle relaxation and biofeedback, where emphasis is on active concentration. The method is supported by an impressive body of research (Linden, 1990) and, although it had fallen slightly out of fashion, there appears to be growing interest currently.

Meditational techniques

Meditational procedures can be found in many cultures, including western societies. Traditionally meditation was associated with philosophical and religious contexts. As discussed by Patel (1993) it was only recently that such methods were considered to be useful for the reduction of stress induced tension and anxiety. She describes the nature of meditation as follows:

...meditation practice involves taking a comfortable position ... it then involves being in a quiet environment, regulating the breath, adopting a physically relaxed and mentally passive attitude, and dwelling single-mindedly upon an object ... the ultimate idea is to learn the discipline of concentrating on one

thing and only one thing at a time, to the exclusion of everything else ... giving voluntary concentration to a subject not only enables a person to see and think about that subject with greater clarity, but also brings into consciousness all the different ideas and memories associated with the subject. A practical result is an increased ability to find a solution to any problem. (p. 127)

More recently, Smith (2002) has suggested eight types of meditation which are described as follows:

- meditation on a relaxing body sensation
- meditation on movement or posture
- breath meditation
- mantra meditation
- meditation on an internal visual image
- meditation on an external visual stimulus
- meditation on a simple sound
- mindfulness meditation.

Such a comprehensive list clearly indicates that meditation is attempting to address somatic as well as cognitive systems.

Biofeedback

(See also 'Biofeedback').

Biofeedback is a fairly recent method which came into clinical use in the late 1960s. It may be simply defined as any technique which increases the ability of a person to control voluntary physiological activities by providing information about those activities: biofeedback is information about the state of biological processes. The technique of biofeedback is the most technical of the major established relaxation methods, as it requires sophisticated electronic equipment. The main intention is to teach the individual self-control over processes which are normally subject to autonomic functioning. Or, as Woolfolk and Lehrer (1993) describe it '...biofeedback is a method for representing somatic activity as information available to cognition' (p. 7). The procedure is highly specific and focuses on one autonomic response system at a time. Rimm and Masters (1979) have compiled a comprehensive list of clinical applications which can involve heart rate, blood pressure, skin temperature, skin conductivity, electroencephalogram (EEG), electromyogram (EMG) and other responses. According to Stoyva and Budzyenski (1993) also pioneers in the field,

the object of such training is to achieve control over biological systems that previously have been operating in a maladaptive fashion and have been beyond conscious control ... biofeedback training essentially involves three stages. The first stage is acquiring awareness of the maladaptive response ... next, guided by the biofeedback signal, he or she learns to control the response. Finally, the client learns to transfer the control into everyday life. (p. 263)

Although it is not entirely clear how feedback control is mediated and, despite mixed results, the method has been firmly established in the behavioural treatment of some psychological and physical disorders.

Cognitive techniques

The relationship between maladaptive thinking and anxiety/stress is well documented (e.g. Beck *et al.*, 1985) and has inspired the development of cognitive behaviour therapy. It is assumed that negative, irrational thought patterns distort perception and evaluation of threatening stimuli and thus prevent adaptive and coping oriented behaviours. Cognitive approaches to effect relaxation would thus seek to modify negative and dysfunctional thought patterns which are seen to promote tension and anxiety in the first place. The causal role of cognitive appraisal in the genesis of pathological emotionality is emphasized. Typical treatments involve identification and re-interpretation of internal events such as thoughts, images, bodily sensations. Cognitive techniques are employed to raise awareness for negative thoughts, cognitive distortions and dysfunctional schemas which may serve as an underlying condition.

Finally, Woolfolk and Lehrer (1993) list a number of additional relaxation techniques which are increasingly used by clinicians of various persuasions but have not yet been subject to scientific enquiry. These include the Alexander technique which focuses on posture and movement of the body; tai chi, an ancient Chinese technique which focuses on '...balance, muscular relaxation, deep breathing and mental concentration during a complex series of slow, dance-like movements' (p. 4); also, the Japanese method of *Akaido*, which is based on Zen Buddhism, is becoming increasingly popular in the West.

Theoretical issues

Despite recent rigorous development in clinical psychology and behavioural medicine, there have been few attempts to develop general theories of relaxation. To date, only three general frameworks can be identified; the relaxation response theory by Benson (1975), the multiprocess theory by Davidson and Schwartz (1976) and attentional behavioural cognitive (ABC) relaxation theory by Smith (1999).

The relaxation response theory postulates that all applied relaxation techniques produce a similar relaxation response which leads to reduction of sympathetic arousal. The antithesis to this is the multiprocess model which suggest specific effects of the various techniques. More recently Smith (Smith, 2001) has proposed an embracing of both aspects and has offered a somewhat compromise conceptualization which he labels 'Attentional Behavioural Cognitive (ABC) Relaxation Training'. It is claimed, on the basis of reported research evidence, that six basic approaches (largely the ones discussed above – progressive muscle relaxation, autogenic training, breathing exercises, yoga, imagery and visualization, meditation) to relaxation will have quite different effects on different people and different types of problems. More specifically, ABC relaxation theory proposes that all methods work when they evoke one or more 'relaxation states'. Smith has identified 15 of those which he has labelled 'R-states' and described as follows:

- Sleepiness
- feeling disengaged
- feeling physically relaxed
- feeling rested and refreshed
- feeling energized
- feeling at ease/peaceful
- feeling joyful and happy
- feeling mentally quiet

- feeling innocent and childlike
- feeling thankful and loving
- feeling the great mystery of things beyond one's understanding
- feeling awe and wonder
- feeling prayerful
- feeling timeless/boundless/infinite
- feeling aware.

Although Smith acknowledges the existence of a non-specific relaxation response (Benson, 1975), R-states are proposed as outcomes of different methods and should be regarded as targets in a relaxation programme according to individual requirements. Consequently, Smith proposes that clients should become competent in all basic relaxation procedures to enable access to all identified R-states. In a further development, Smith (2004*a*) has added 'relaxation access skills' and 'initial specific effects' to the model. These two components are designed as a link between the relaxation technique and the relaxation response as well as R-states. This is done to enable an improved matching of individual skills to desired outcomes.

Perhaps it is timely to favour such a compromise position as clinical evidence points to some generalized relaxation effect with most established techniques (Woolfolk & Lehrer, 1993). Smith's model may be regarded as a first attempt towards a unifying framework in trying to explain the effects of various techniques, as well as respective interactions with individual responding and presenting problems.

Another concern is the gap between theoretical understanding and clinical application. For example, when the theorist-researcher attempts to clarify the efficacy of different techniques, the clinician may simply use intuition regarding selection or combination of several methods. Typically, clinicians tend to apply their favourite method and use it to maximum effect. It is not always clear to what extent non-specific aspects, such as the therapeutic relationship come into play, especially when similar results are achieved across different patients and disorders.

Clinical application

Relaxation techniques have been applied as an independent therapeutic approach to relieve problems related to chronically elevated level of arousal. Examples include insomnia, nervousness, headaches, hypertension etc. The goal is to achieve a reduction of a chronically high level of arousal by sustained practice, initially under the supervision of a therapist.

Also, relaxation may be designed as an integral part of a comprehensive treatment programme. Stress inoculation training (Meichenbaum, 1993), anxiety management training (Suinn, 1990) or stess management (Smith, 2002) may serve as the typical examples. In this way relaxation training is employed as a more active and flexible tool. Typically one starts with deep relaxation and once the patient is able to relax, a shortened and individualized version is directly applied to stress- or anxiety-inducing situations. This approach is designed to facilitate coping behaviours and prevent avoidances.

Applied relaxation (Öst, 1987) can serve as a typical example for a well documented and successful relaxation programme in the cognitive–behavioural framework. Such programmes typically last between 8–12 sessions and consists of the following steps:

- training in recognizing early signs of anxiety
- progressive relaxation
- tension release training
- cue-controlled relaxation
- differential relaxation
- rapid relaxation
- application training
- maintenance.

The main objectives are to provide a rationale and motivate the patient to enable short, effective techniques which can be applied in realistic anxiety situations as opposed to the consulting room. Emphasis is on intensive training and self-control.

Furthermore, the question arises as to whether relaxation techniques should be differentially applied, depending on the nature of problems as well as individual response mechanisms. In clinical work it is useful to seek guidance by the tripartite response system analysis as originally put forward by ŠPeter Lang (1969) who has proposed behavioural responses as three Š behavioural - motoric which have been demonstrated to be highly interactive. This conceptualization allows us to examine the nature of subjective anxiety or stress. For example, one may be able to identify a dominant response mode (e.g. cognitive or physiological) which has causal impact on the other systems. In other cases there may be an enhancing interaction between cognitive and autonomic variables, as is typical for the anticipatory anxiety syndrome.

Such investigations are expected to provide vital clues for relaxation procedures. For example, an anxiety response which is predominantly cognitively manifested would obviously require a different therapeutic focus (e.g. cognitive restructuring) as compared with a strong autonomic reaction (e.g. biofeedback).

Tripartite analysis would thus suggest that tailor-made techniques may be suitable for individual circumstances. Woolfolk and Lehrer (1993) have reviewed this issue by comparing techniques across problems as well as within problems with different individuals. They conclude the following:

We find that each of the various techniques has specific effects, in addition to a global, undifferentiated relaxation effect. There are few kinds of problems for which one technique is clearly superior to another, but, for the most part, the effects of the various techniques are similar. Combinations of techniques often produce better results than single techniques do. Also, there is some evidence that particular individuals may be differentially motivated by and attracted to specific techniques. (p. 11)

However, most studies need cautious evaluation as techniques may have lost their clinical significance through abbreviation and standardization procedures, or non-clinical samples were used. Similar points were made by Smith (2004b); in the context of the

evaluation of mindfulness training, this author urges caution regarding the number of possible factors involved.

Lehrer and Woolfolk (1993) also emphasize the importance of motivation and compliance, especially in consideration of the enormous dropout rate. It seems important that clients understand the rationale of relaxation principles and are prepared to practice on a daily basis. Clients show individual preferences and some data suggest that compliance is best, with meditation followed by progressive relaxation, autogenic training and biofeedback. Subjects who feel more in control of themselves tend to do better with all techniques except for biofeedback.

Summary and conclusion

In reviewing various relaxation approaches one can confirm the prevailing clinical view that the various techniques work differently with different individuals in different problem situations. In more detail, it appears that best results are obtained when modalities of individual responses are matched with corresponding treatments.

In addition, Lehrer and Woolfolk (1993) and Smith (2001) conclude that most methods are likely to achieve also some general relaxation effect. Also, combinations of techniques tend to be more effective than singular treatments. Most experts in the field have developed such treatment packages to enhance relaxation effects (examples were given above). Clinicians tend to use relaxation techniques and combinations on a trial-and-error basis, which makes it difficult to assess the outcome of specific techniques in applied settings. Some clinicians have claimed synergistic effects when using a variety of modalities.

To facilitate relaxation it thus seems crucial to conduct a comprehensive cognitive–behavioural assessment of relevant target complaints in order to identify individual response modalities. Further, non-specific factors such as motivation; the therapeutic relationship; the level of self-regulation ability; and expectations according to personal preferences need to be assessed. Linden (1993) has suggested that it may be useful to present model options and their rationale to the patient in order to encourage a choice. It is assumed that what is understood well, credible and self-chosen may work best for the individual patient. The ultimate goal is to generalize relaxation skills so that they can be applied actively to all relevant settings reported by the sufferer.

Finally, relaxation techniques have been demonstrated to be highly successful in the fields of emotional disorders and behavioural medicine. With emotional disorders, the emphasis appears to be more 'cognitive' as one intends to adjust the perception and evaluation of stress and tension, whereas in behavioural medicine techniques tend to focus predominantly on the modification of somatic states, such as pain, hypertension, or other physical conditions.

REFERENCES

Beck, A. T., Emery, G. & Greenberg, R. L. (1985). *Anxiety disorders and phobias.* New York: Basic Books.

Benson, H. (1975). *The relaxation response.* New York: Morrow.

Davidson, R. J. & Schwartz, G. E. (1976). Psychobiology of relaxation and related stress: a multiprocess theory. In D. Mostofsky (Ed.). *Behaviour modification and control of*

physiological activity. Englewood Cliffs: Prentice-Hall.

Hawton, K., Salkovskis, P. M., Kirk, J. & Clark, D. M. (1989). *Cognitive behaviour therapy for psychiatric* *problems*. Oxford: Oxford Medical Publications.

Jacobson, E. (1929). *Progressive relaxation*. Chicago: University of Chicago Press.

Lang, P. J. (1969). The mechanics of desensitisation and the laboratory study of human fear. In C. Franks (Ed.). *Behaviour therapy: appraisal and status*. New York: McGraw-Hill.

Lehrer, P. M. & Woolfolk, R. L. (1993). Principles and Practice of Stress Management (2nd edn.). New York: Guilford Press.

Linden, W. (1990). *Autogenic training: a clinical guide*. New York: Guilford Press.

Linden, W. (1993). The autogenic training method of J. H. Schultz. In P. M. Lehrer & R. L. Woolfolk (Eds.). *Principles and Practice of Stress Management* (2nd edn.). New York: Guilford Press.

Meichenbaum, D. (1993). Stress inoculation training: a 20 year update. In R. L. Woolfolk & P. M. Lehrer (Eds.). *Principles and practice of stress management*. New York: Guilford Press.

Miller, N. E. (1978). Biofeedback and visceral learning. *Annual Review of Psychology*, **29**, 373–404.

Öst, L. G. (1987). Applied relaxation: description of a coping technique and review of controlled studies. *Behaviour Research and Therapy*, **25**, 397–410.

Patel, C. (1993). Yoga-based therapy. In R. L. Woolfolk & P. M. Lehrer (Eds.). *Principles and practice of stress management*. New York: Guilford Press.

Rimm, D. C. & Masters, J. C. (1979). *Behaviour Therapy* (2nd edn.). New York: Academic Press.

Schultz, J. H. & Luthe, W. (1959). *Autogenic training: a psychophysiological approach to psychotherapy*. New York: Grune and Stratton.

Smith, J. C. (1999). *ABC relaxation theory*. New York: Springer.

Smith, J. C. (2001). *Advances in ABC relaxation. Applications and inventories*. New York: Springer Publishing Company.

Smith, J. C. (2002). *Stress management. A comprehensive handbook of techniques and strategies*. New York: Springer Publishing Company.

Smith, J. C. (2004*a*). Revised ABC relaxation theory. Personal communication.

Smith, J. C. (2004*b*). Alterations in brain and immune function produced by mindfulness meditation: three caveats. *Journal of Psychosomatic Medicine*, **66**(1), 148–9.

Stoyva, J. M. & Budzyenski, T. H. (1993). Biofeedback methods in the treatment of anxiety and stress disorders. In P. M. Lehrer & R. L. Woolfolk (Eds.). *Principles and Practice of Stress Management* (2nd edn.). New York: Guilford Press.

Suinn, R. M. (1990). *Anxiety management training*. New York: Plenum.

Wolpe, J. (1958). *Psychotherapy by reciprocal inhibition*. Stanford: Stanford University Press.

Woolfolk, R. L. & Lehrer, P. M. (1984). *Principles and practice of stress management*. New York: Guilford Press.

Woolfolk, R. L. & Lehrer, P. M. (1993). The Context of Stress Management. In P. M. Lehrer & R. L. Woolfolk (Eds.). *Principles and Practice of Stress Management* (2nd edn.). New York: Guilford Press.

Self-management interventions

Kathleen Mulligan and Stanton Newman

University College London

Background

Living with a chronic illness places many demands on the patient. These may include self-monitoring of symptoms or physiological measures, such as blood sugar in diabetes, taking medication and making lifestyle changes. Healthcare professionals provide advice about what action to take, but the responsibility for integrating these actions into their daily lives rests with the patients who also have to cope with changes in life roles and the emotional demands a chronic illness can bring (see 'Coping with chronic illness'). The patients' role in their care is referred to as 'self-management', which has been defined as 'the individual's ability to manage the symptoms, treatment, physical and psychosocial consequences and life style changes inherent in living with a chronic condition' (Barlow *et al.*, 2002). It can, however, be difficult for people to self-manage all of these aspects of their illness effectively, resulting in poor health outcomes and impaired quality of life.

Theoretical influences

While 'self-management' refers to what individuals do to deal with their illnesses, it is also the term that is increasingly used to describe interventions that have been developed to help patients self-manage more effectively. A traditional approach to addressing self-management is for healthcare professionals to provide patients with more information about their illness and its treatment in the expectation that increased knowledge will lead to enhanced self-management. This approach tends to pay little attention to patients' beliefs about their illness and its treatment or the difficulties they may have in incorporating medical recommendations into their daily lives. A consistent finding from the literature is that interventions that provide information alone are not usually successful in improving outcomes for people with chronic illness (Coates & Boore, 1996; Gibson *et al.*, 2002; Taal *et al.*, 1997).

As a result of these findings, many self-management interventions now incorporate concepts developed within psychological theories. These theories provide a framework for considering the complex nature of health behaviour change and have drawn attention to the importance of people's beliefs about themselves, their illness and its treatments and how these affect self-management. One of the key concepts to emerge has been that of self-efficacy, which Bandura (1997) described as the level of confidence individuals have in their ability to perform a given behaviour. A number of studies have found that enhancing self-efficacy makes performance of a given health-related behaviour more likely. Self-efficacy can be enhanced through a variety of routes, including modelling, social persuasion and mastery over the skills required. Modelling may involve teaching self-management skills and also learning from others in a group setting. In group based interventions, performance of a behaviour by some participants can act as social persuasion, encouraging others to take part. Skills mastery can be facilitated by setting goals and learning problem-solving skills. Breaking down what is perhaps a complex behaviour into smaller, more manageable, specific goals increases the likelihood of success and each success helps to build self-efficacy and so encourage the maintenance of a behaviour (see 'Self-efficacy and health behaviour').

Other theories which have influenced the development of self-management interventions include the Stress–Coping Model (Lazarus, 1992), the Transtheoretical Model of readiness to change (Prochaska & Velicer, 1997) and the Self-regulatory Model (Leventhal *et al.*, 1984). The Stress–Coping Model focuses on the strategies people use to cope with a stressor such as a chronic illness. The use of passive or avoidant strategies has generally been found to have a detrimental effect on health outcomes and psychological wellbeing, while active coping strategies are more helpful. Interventions based on this model frequently use cognitive–behavioural techniques to encourage the use of more effective coping strategies (see 'Cognitive behavioural therapy' and 'Stress and health'). The Transtheoretical Model highlights the importance of a person's readiness to make behaviour changes. The model incorporates five stages, from 'precontemplation', in which change is not being considered to 'maintenance' in which the self-management behaviour has been performed for some time. Self-management interventions based on this model incorporate strategies such as Motivational Interviewing which focus on increasing participants' readiness to change (see Motivational interviewing and 'The transactional model of behaviour change'). Interventions based on the Self-regulatory Model focus upon altering individuals' views about their illness and its treatments which are seen as the drivers of both coping and health-related behaviours (Hirani & Newman, in press; Petrie *et al.*, 2002) (see 'Lay beliefs about health and illness').

It is apparent that the theories applied in self-management interventions vary in their emphasis, with some focusing primarily on behaviour change and others addressing the more cognitive and emotional aspects of coping with a chronic illness.

Although many of the interventions have roots in a particular theoretical approach, in practice many draw on concepts from more than one theory.

Content of self-management interventions

Over the past two to three decades a large number of self-management interventions have been developed for a range of different illnesses. Three conditions which have placed particular emphasis on self-management are arthritis, asthma and diabetes (Lorig *et al.*, 1987; Norris *et al.*, 2001; Sudre *et al.*, 1999). Self-management approaches have been introduced in several other chronic illnesses, including hypertension, chronic obstructive pulmonary disease, headache and back pain (Barlow, Wright, Sheasby *et al.*, 2002) and a generic chronic disease self-management programme has also been developed (Lorig *et al.*, 1999, 2001). There is considerable variety in the content of these interventions, partly due to the diversity of the routes through which they developed but also due to differences between the illnesses that they have been designed to address (Newman *et al.*, 2004).

Most interventions include some form of general education about the illness and its treatment and discussion amongst participants or with a healthcare professional. Other commonly used components include monitoring features of the illness (symptoms or a physiological measure) and taking appropriate action, management of symptoms (e.g. pain or fatigue) or disability and, as living with a chronic illness involves considerable contact with healthcare professionals, many teach communication skills to enable people to make the most of these encounters. Because most adaptation to a chronic illness involves making and maintaining lifestyle changes, the incorporation of strategies to facilitate behaviour change such as setting goals and learning problem-solving skills, features in many interventions.

Variation in self-management interventions arising from the differing demands of the illnesses can be seen in a comparison of arthritis, asthma and diabetes (Newman *et al.*, 2004). Coping with the emotional consequences and changed life roles, as well as some changes in health behaviours, is required in all three illnesses. However, in arthritis, the major concerns are to manage symptoms, particularly pain and to optimize physical functioning, while asthma self-management has been concerned mainly with minimizing the risk of acute exacerbation of symptoms. Diabetes requires lifestyle changes in order to stabilize blood glucose levels and prevent long-term complications. As a consequence, adherence to medication is an important part of asthma self-management interventions but is not a major issue in osteoarthritis. Pain management is an important part of arthritis self-management but this is not the case for diabetes and asthma. Self-monitoring, of symptoms in the case of asthma and blood glucose in the case of diabetes, is an important aspect of self-management in these illnesses but such detailed self-monitoring is not usually a component of arthritis self-management. Anxiety about and/or during an asthma exacerbation may require quite specific anxiety management techniques that are not necessarily relevant in diabetes and arthritis. In general, however, the asthma interventions have been narrowly focused in comparison to the other two conditions and have not addressed broader psychological issues.

Disease-specific and generic approaches

Traditionally, self-management interventions have been disease-specific but a significant recent development has been the introduction of a generic programme, the Chronic Disease Self-Management Programme (CDSMP), developed at Stanford University Patient Education Research Centre (Lorig et al., 1999, 2001). The approach of the CDSMP is to focus on problems and strategies which are common across illnesses. It consists of community-based group sessions which combine participants with different chronic illnesses. Strategies such as problem-solving techniques, goal-setting and behavioural modelling are included as they are considered to be helpful in all chronic illnesses (see 'Behaviour therapy' and 'Cognitive behaviour therapy'). There is no disease-specific advice but participants are taught to manage their illness through correct medication use; relaxation; diet; exercise; managing sleep and fatigue; and effective communication with health professionals.

Delivery of self-management interventions

The review by Newman et al. (2004) found that two-thirds of interventions in arthritis and about half in asthma and diabetes were delivered in group settings. Comparison of the relative benefits of group versus individual delivery is rare but one study that compared them in diabetes found that the group programme resulted in a greater improvement in blood glucose. Group programmes have the advantage of the opportunity for group learning and support as well as reducing costs. In contrast individual programmes can be tailored to each person's needs and can be designed to be more easily incorporated into standard care (Clark & Hampson, 2001). Although it is also likely that some individuals will be less willing to take part in group programmes, there is no research on this issue (see 'Group therapy').

The duration of self-management interventions varies a great deal from brief, single sessions to several sessions over many months. The type of illness has influenced the objectives of self-management interventions and hence their length. For example in asthma, self-management interventions have tended to be brief and focused on symptom monitoring and medication adherence. In diabetes and arthritis, self-management interventions often address a range of health behaviours and strategies for managing many aspects of living with the illnesses and as a consequence involve multiple sessions. There has been little systematic examination of the optimum duration of these interventions in different conditions. In one study, Lorig et al. compared their standard 6-week Arthritis Self-Management Programme with a reduced 3-week version and found that the original obtained better results (Lorig et al., 1998). Decisions about duration are affected not only by breadth of intervention content but also by cost implications and the greater time demand that several sessions places on patients, with the consequent risk of lower participation and higher dropout rates.

Self-management interventions have been delivered by a variety of healthcare professionals, including dieticians, nurses, occupational therapists, physicians, physiotherapists, psychologists and social workers. Although many self-management interventions are multidisciplinary, nursing is the professional group which tends to dominate, perhaps because of nurses' greater numbers and availability, but also because of their ability to provide detailed illness-related information. There is also a trend, as evidenced in the Arthritis Self-Management Programme (Lorig, 1986), the Chronic Disease Self-Management Programme (Lorig et al., 1999, 2001) and the Expert Patient Programme in the UK (Wright et al., 2003), for trained lay people, most of whom themselves have a chronic illness, to deliver self-management interventions.

Regardless of who delivers the intervention, effective delivery requires appropriate training and experience in facilitation skills and behaviour change strategies. Leaders need to be trained to deal with emotional issues that may arise. These skills are not taught routinely to most healthcare professionals and this raises the issue of what training is needed for both professional and lay leaders. This issue is frequently neglected and inappropriate assumptions are made regarding the ability, of both professionals and lay individuals, to easily take on the role of facilitating self-management interventions.

Uptake and attrition

Many self-management interventions require a considerable commitment by participants in terms of both time and emotional investment. One measure of the acceptability of a self-management intervention is provided by the percentage of people approached who decide to take part. This information is often not reported, but in studies recruiting from a circumscribed population the suggestion is that self-management interventions are not attractive to a proportion of individuals. If the numbers who choose not to participate are large it limits the generalizability of the findings from these studies. The reasons for non-participation are likely to be many and include convenience, scepticism of the process and likely benefits, amongst others. There is a need to assess reasons for lack of participation to understand these processes well.

Another indicator of acceptability is the number of people who begin but do not complete the intervention. Study attrition rates vary widely; the reasons are not clear but there is some indication that longer interventions have higher attrition rates (Newman et al., 2004). The method of delivery of the self-management intervention could also affect uptake and attrition rates. Although most interventions are delivered face-to-face, some with telephone follow-up, they could also be delivered either partially or fully via a self-administered manual or using the internet. These methods have had limited application to date but are likely to grow in use and may prove popular to individuals who find travelling to the clinic and the time of the interventions too burdensome.

Efficacy

Research studies evaluating the efficacy of self-management interventions typically assess several outcomes such as physiological measures, symptoms, physical functioning, psychological wellbeing, performance of health behaviours, quality of life and use of healthcare resources. In assessing self-management interventions it is important to be clear about what a self-management approach can reasonably be expected to influence and to target the assessment of efficacy accordingly. For example, better self-management of diet in diabetes would be expected to affect a measure of blood glucose (HbA1c), but in rheumatoid arthritis, better self-management of symptoms and physical functioning is unlikely to affect erythrocyte sedimentation rate (ESR), a physiological marker of disease activity. Many studies measure mood state and this is important because depressed mood will affect many other factors, but it is nevertheless unrealistic to expect to see a reduction in depression scores if the study population was not depressed at the outset (see 'Mood assessment'). An understanding of other variables that may influence the effectiveness of a self-management intervention, commonly known as 'process' variables, such as self-efficacy, illness beliefs and coping strategies, is also important.

One approach to assessing the efficacy of self-management interventions has been to combine studies in a meta-analysis, which provides a statistical analysis of their combined effect. A problem with this approach is that it does not take into account the diversity of the interventions and is only suitable where data are homogeneous (Eysenck, 1995). A more descriptive approach to the different interventions and study outcomes is likely to be more informative regarding what interventions, or components of interventions, are efficacious.

Several reviews of the efficacy of self-management interventions have been conducted in individual illnesses (Gibson *et al.*, 2002; Norris *et al.*, 2001; Riemsma *et al.*, 2002) and a small number have compared across illnesses, using arthritis, asthma and diabetes as examples (Barlow *et al.*, 2002; Bodenheimer *et al.*, 2002; Newman *et al.*, 2004; Warsi *et al.*, 2004). These reviews have shown that some self-management interventions have resulted in beneficial outcomes in the performance of self-management behaviours, clinical outcomes, symptoms, physical functioning and emotional wellbeing. There is, nevertheless, considerable variation both between and within illnesses in the level and duration of effects.

In reviews of specific illnesses, it has generally been found that self-management interventions can be effective in improving HbA1c in diabetes (Norris *et al.*, 2001), small effects have been found on pain and disability in arthritis (Astin *et al.*, 2002; Riemsma *et al.*, 2002; Taal *et al.*, 1997) and reductions in health care utilization for acute exacerbation have been achieved in asthma (Gibson *et al.*, 2002). Self-management interventions have also been quite successful in achieving change in behaviours such as diet, exercise, medication adherence and cognitive coping strategies (Newman *et al.*, 2004).

Further development in the field of self-management requires a better understanding of which component or groups of components of these complex interventions are most important and for which outcomes. Studies that compare two or more self-management interventions, varying a single component, are necessary. This type of design is becoming more common in diabetes but remains relatively rare in other chronic illnesses.

Interventions that can extend the duration of effects are also required. Most evaluations of self-management interventions have not examined their efficacy beyond a few months but where longer-term studies have been conducted, effects tend not to be maintained. Booster sessions at intervals may provide one way of maintaining the benefits of self-management interventions but given that the illnesses, by definition, will last for the patient's lifetime, further research is necessary to examine how frequently and for how long, booster sessions would need to be provided.

REFERENCES

Astin, J. A., Beckner, W., Soeken, K., Hochberg, M. C. & Berman, B. (2002). Psychological interventions for rheumatoid arthritis: a meta-analysis of randomized controlled trials. *Arthritis and Rheumatism*, **47**, 291–302.

Bandura, A. (1997). *Self-efficacy: the exercise of control*. New York: Freeman & Co.

Barlow, J. H., Hearnshaw, H. & Sturt, J. (2002). Self-management interventions for people with chronic conditions in primary care: examples from arthritis, asthma and diabetes. *Health Education Journal*, **61**, 365–78.

Barlow, J., Wright, C., Sheasby, J., Turner, A. & Hainsworth, J. (2002). Self-management approaches for people with chronic conditions: a review. *Patient Education and Counseling*, **48**, 177–87.

Bodenheimer, T., Lorig, K., Holman, H. & Grumbach, K. (2002). Patient self-management of chronic disease in primary care. *JAMA*, **288**, 2469–75.

Clark, M. & Hampson, S. E. (2001). Implementing a psychological intervention to improve lifestyle self-management in patients with Type 2 diabetes. *Patient Education and Counselling.*, **42**, 247–56.

Coates, V. E. & Boore, J. R. (1996). Knowledge and diabetes self-management. *Patient Education and Counselling.*, **29**, 99–108.

Eysenck, H. J. (1995). Problems with meta-analysis. In I. Chalmers & D. G. Altman (Eds.). *Systematic reviews*, (pp. 64–74). London: BMJ Publishing Group.

Gibson, P. G., Powell, H., Coughlan, J. *et al.* (2002). Self-management education and regular practitioner review for adults with asthma. *The cochrane database of systematic reviews 2002*, Issue 3. Art. No.: CD001117.

Hirani, S. & Newman, S. (2005). Patients' beliefs about their cardiovascular disease. *Heart*, **91**, 1235-9.

Lazarus, R. S. (1992). Coping with the stress of illness. *WHO Regional Publications. European Series*, **44**, 11–31.

Leventhal, H., Nerenz, D. R. & Steele, D. J. (1984). Illness representations and coping with health threats. In A. Baum, S. E. Taylor & J. E. Singer (Eds.). *Social psychological aspects of health* (pp. 219–52). Erlbaum, New Jersey.

Lorig, K. (1986). Development and dissemination of an arthritis patient education course. *Family and Community Health*, **9**, 23–32.

Lorig, K., Gonzalez, V. M., Laurent, D. D., Morgan, L. & Laris, B. A. (1998). Arthritis self-management program variations: three studies. *Arthritis Care and Research*, **11**, 448–54.

Lorig, K., Konkol, L. & Gonzalez, V. (1987). Arthritis patient education: a review of the literature. *Patient Education and Counselling.*, **10**, 207–52.

Lorig, K. R., Ritter, P., Stewart, A. L. *et al.* (2001). Chronic disease self-management program: 2-year health status and health care utilization outcomes. *Medical Care*, **39**, 1217–23.

Lorig, K. R., Sobel, D. S., Stewart, A. L. *et al.* (1999). Evidence suggesting that a chronic disease self-management program can improve health status while reducing hospitalization: a randomized trial. *Medical Care*, **37**, 5–14.

Newman, S., Steed, L. & Mulligan, K. (2004). Self-management interventions for chronic illness. *The Lancet*, **364**, 1523–37.

Norris, S. L., Engelgau, M. M. & Narayan, K. M. (2001). Effectiveness of self-management training in type 2 diabetes: a systematic review of randomized controlled trials. *Diabetes Care*, **24**, 561–87.

Petrie, K. J., Cameron, L. D., Ellis, C. J., Buick, D. & Weinman, J. (2002). Changing illness perceptions after myocardial infarction: an early intervention randomized controlled trial. *Psychosomatic Medicine*, **6**(4), 580–6.

Prochaska, J. O. & Velicer, W. F. (1997). The transtheoretical model of health behavior change. *American Journal of Health Promotion*, **12**, 38–48.

Riemsma, R. P., Taal, E., Kirwan, J. R. & Rasker, J. J. (2002). Patient education

programmes for adults with rheumatoid arthritis. *British Medical Journal*, **325**, 559.

Sudre, P., Jacquemet, S., Uldry, C. & Perneger, T. V. (1999). Objectives, methods and content of patient education programmes for adults with asthma: systematic review of studies published between 1979 and 1998. *Thorax*, **54**, 681–7.

Taal, E., Rasker, J. J. & Wiegman, O. (1997). Group education for rheumatoid arthritis patients. *Seminars in Arthritis and Rheumatism*, **26**, 805–16.

Warsi, A., Wang, P. S., LaValley, M. P., Avorn, J. & Solomon, D. H. (2004).

Self-management education programs in chronic disease: a systematic review and methodological critique of the literature. *Archives of Internal Medicine*, **164**, 1641–9.

Wright, C. C., Barlow, J. H., Turner, A. P. & Bancroft, G. V. (2003). Self-management training for people with chronic disease: an exploratory study. *British Journal of Health Psychology*, **8**, 465–76.

Social support interventions

Benjamin Gottlieb

University of Guelph

Introduction

If we knew that our social relationships had the power to shield us from adversity and to prevent us from succumbing to stress-induced anguish and disability, then we would do everything possible to ensure that people are equipped with these protective social resources. However, since some of these people will not have the skills, motivation, or coping propensities to engage in support-relevant interactions with others, we will need to invest effort in determining how to select the best candidates for such interventions and how to design them in a way that has broad appeal. For those practitioners who wish to capitalize on social support's protective potential, all of these activities constitute a challenging agenda for planning and implementing such interventions in the health field.

This chapter begins by setting out the rationale for the development of support interventions, and then distinguishes between interventions in the natural network and interventions that introduce one or more new social ties. In the health field, the latter strategies predominate. Hence, the chapter consists of two main sections, the first concentrating on the design and effectiveness of support groups and the second focusing on ways of marshalling individual supportive allies. Several critical issues and uncertainties about the optimal design of these initiatives are considered, including the importance of properly matching them to certain characteristics of the intended beneficiaries. Questions that need to be

addressed in the next generation of support studies are sprinkled throughout the chapter.

Rationale for support interventions

There are three main justifications for planned programmes designed to augment, specialize, intensify, or prolong social support. First, epidemiological research amply testifies to the proposition that both absolute and relative social isolation are risk factors for numerous adverse health developments (Berkman & Syme, 1979; House *et al.*, 1982 (see 'Social support and health'). Second, there is much empirical evidence showing that people who believe that they can gain support from their social network experience lower levels of stress and its adverse health-related sequelae than those who do not harbour such beliefs (Cohen & Wills, 1985). A third rationale for planned support interventions is based on evidence of the fallibility of natural support. Several studies have documented the ways in which well-intentioned support from network members can miscarry and either aggravate the problems or increase the distress experienced by the would-be recipient (Coyne & Smith, 1994; Dakof & Taylor, 1990; Lehman & Hemphill, 1990). It follows that interventions which remediate the helping skills of natural network members or interventions which replace them with more relevant and effective supporters are needed.

In fact, the two main social support strategies involve either intervening in natural social networks in order to improve their responsiveness to the needs of an associate (Cutrona & Cole, 2000) or introducing the individual to one or more new social ties who presumably can provide more relevant and less flawed support than the natural network (Gottlieb, 1988). Furthermore, both of these strategies offer opportunities to intervene at the dyadic or the group level. Whereas early intervention studies focused on improving natural support (see Cutrona & Cole, 2000 for a review), they have given way to a plethora of grafted tie interventions, of which the most popular in the health field are support groups and individual supportive allies. Hence, this chapter concentrates on recent developments concerning the latter two types of interventions.

Support groups

Support groups usually consist of 6–12 people who share a similar life stressor, transition, affliction, disability, diagnosis, or noxious habit and meet in this face-to-face small group to engage in mutual aid and receive expert information and/or training. Support groups differ from mutual aid self-help (MASH) groups and peer discussion groups by virtue of the fact that they have a professional or quasi-professional leader who usually is responsible for the group's composition, and injects expert knowledge while guiding the group process.

To prepare this chapter, a search was conducted of the PsycInfo database from 1985 onward, specifying that the term 'support group' must appear in the journal article's title. The search yielded 262 English language citations, the vast majority of the studies describing the groups' formats, composition, themes and subjectively rated satisfaction of members. However, compared to a review conducted almost 20 years ago (Gottlieb, 1988), several new developments have occurred in that literature. They include: (1) more studies that adopt the strict procedures of a randomized controlled trial; (2) more studies comparing the effects of support groups with other intervention strategies rather than with a treatment as usual or untreated control group; (3) a new cluster of studies which report on the reasons why prospective support group candidates decline participation, or the factors that distinguish participants from non-participants; (4) a new set of studies which aims to identify the characteristics of those who benefit most and least from support groups; and (5) several reports of on-line support groups. All five of these trends reflect the growth of intelligence about the candidates and the conditions which are most conducive to the beneficial effects of support groups.

Who attends and benefits from support groups?

One indication of the maturation of research on support interventions is the acknowledgement that support groups are not universally attractive or effective vehicles for promoting health and wellbeing. For example, Winefield et al. (2003) asked 93 women who had been diagnosed with breast cancer an average of 7.4 months earlier whether they were interested in joining a support group. Almost 60% of the women stated that they would not attend such a group, whereas 22% did enrol in one. These figures are almost identical to those reported for 218 women who tested positive for the gene mutation associated with breast and ovarian cancer (Hamann et al. 2000). Four to seven months after receiving their test results only about 25% of the women expressed interest in participating in a hypothetical support group for women with this gene mutation.

What detracts from support groups? More precisely, what are the characteristics of those who find support groups appealing and those who do not? Although we have some clues, the answers to these questions are largely unknown because so few studies report the characteristics of those who decline participation and those who drop out. We know that some people shy away from support groups because they anticipate hearing frightening stories or meeting people whose disease has progressed further than their own and therefore is interpreted as a preview of their own decline. Others may simply be afraid of the unknown, worried that they will be coerced to disclose too much, or that they will be confronted with a group of strangers with whom they share nothing but a common misfortune. There are also people who cannot commit the time or funds to attend a group and others who are content with the support they already receive from their social network. In fact, a recent study showed that support groups are not only of little measurable benefit to those who have access to natural support, but also can backfire by communicating to participants that their natural supporters are not doing as much as they could to render support (Helgeson et al., 2000). Moreover, such communication need not be direct but can result from private social comparisons.

Empirical data about the people who are attracted to support groups suggest that they are relatively well-educated, white, female, middle-class individuals who are high service users and who report more problems or worse mental health (Taylor et al., 1986; Winefield et al., 2003). Since these are largely demographic variables, the quest should be expanded to other situational and individual differences variables that may affect initial entry and later attrition. For example, McGovern et al. (2002) found that men who joined a prostate cancer support group engaged in a coping style that reflected low helplessness and hopelessness and high fighting spirit. Edgar et al. (2001) also found that many breast and colon cancer patients who were randomized to support groups did not attend all five of the group sessions because they did not enjoy this format. The authors suggest experimenting with randomized control trials (RCTs) that allow for a preference arm so that the effect of treatment preference can be discerned.

Moreover, the factors that distinguish attenders from non-attenders may also distinguish between participants who benefit most and least from their group experience. Both Andersen (1992) and Helgeson et al. (2000) suggest that people who have less support or troubled relationships with their family and friends might benefit most from the compensatory group support, unless the reason for deficient network support stems from poor social skills which make the individual less supportable by co-participants. Perhaps other personal liabilities may limit the gains which individuals derive from support groups. For example, future studies may find that gains are limited by such pre-existing interpersonal vulnerabilities as an insecure attachment history or excessive reassurance seeking (Potthoff et al., 1995), or by individuals' preferences for employing a 'blunting' style of coping that runs counter to the 'monitoring' style of the group (Miller, 1995). In addition, although more educated, middle-class people tend to join support groups, when less educated people can be recruited, they tend to experience the greatest benefit (e.g. Lepore *et al.*, 2003). Less education may reflect less knowledge about health matters and services, which is another example of the selective benefits of support groups that accrue to those in greatest need.

The effectiveness of support groups

In a *New England Journal of Medicine* editorial, Spiegel (2001) summarized the findings of 10 published RCTs that examined the effects of support groups for cancer patients on both psychological and survival outcomes. He reported that, whereas virtually every study showed improvements in quality of life indicators (e.g. Classen *et al.*, 2001), only half the studies obtained evidence of moderately prolonged survival (e.g. Cunningham *et al.*, 1998). Among these studies is Spiegel's own trial that initiated this line of investigation by documenting an 18-month survival advantage for breast cancer patients who attended a long-term 'supportive-expressive' group (Spiegel *et al.*, 1989). However, it has been suggested that Spiegel's impressive results are attributable to the fact that breast cancer was a hidden disease in the late 1970s, hence the absence of public awareness of breast cancer and the dearth of informational and service resources for its victims (Nekhlyudov & Yaker, 2002). The introduction of a group that openly discussed the disease, promoted emotional expressiveness, and addressed existential issues seemed to mitigate the emotional and social isolation characterizing the lives of women with breast cancer at that time.

Along with other investigators, Spiegel (2001) suggests investing more efforts in screening and identifying people who, still today, are most likely to need and respond to emotional support. Participants who are more distressed (Antoni *et al.*, 2001; Goodwin *et al.*, 2001) and who report inadequate natural support at the outset (Helgeson *et al.*, 2000) would meet these criteria as long as they also have the social skills and adopt a coping style that suits the group's interpersonal processes. An alternative option is to design support groups in ways that suit the varied skills and styles of the prospective participants. For example, the 'blunters' might be more attracted to a group that is highly structured, focuses on overt or cognitive–behavioural training and in which a leader guides the group's interactions rather than fostering unfettered experience-swapping among participants. Indeed, it would be instructive to design several support groups that differ in their organization and social process, create videotaped sample sessions for 'the prospective participants' and then ask them to self-select into the group that appears most comfortable for them. Although this strategy violates the strictures of random assignment, it would yield valuable knowledge about the bases on which people choose supportive milieux and about the effects of people exercising control over the means of coping.

Intervention trials comparing the effects of groups that are strictly educational in nature, groups that are strictly peer discussion and groups that combine the two elements have yielded mixed results. For example, Helgeson *et al.* (1999, 2000) found that pure education had an edge over peer discussion immediately, 6 months and 3 years after the 8-week trial ended. Specifically, the women in the education-only group experienced significant gains in self-esteem and reductions in intrusive thoughts about their illness. But several caveats are in order, including the facts that the sample was composed of highly educated, middle-income women, the short-term nature of the intervention, which may have limited the extent of mutual aid that arose in the peer discussion groups, and the exclusion from the 3-year analysis of women who experienced breast cancer recurrence. Moreover, questions arise about the distinctiveness of the three conditions; can peer discussion occur without any elements of education about the disease, and can educational sessions that are followed by a question and answer period eliminate any opportunities for peer support, including the indirect support that occurs through social comparisons? In contrast, Lepore *et al.* (2003) found that, compared with a control condition, 6-week groups focusing only on education and groups combining education and peer discussion had equivalent superior effects on the knowledge, physical functioning and health behaviour of men with prostate cancer. In addition, they found that the men in the education plus peer discussion group had significantly more stable employment and felt significantly less bothered by sexual difficulties than those in the other two conditions. The authors speculate that the peer discussion helped to normalize and validate the men's treatment-induced poorer sexual functioning and thereby moderated their distress about it.

Surprisingly, investigators rarely inquire about what prospective support group members want from their group experience, much less whether they prefer a group or a one-to-one supportive ally. Nor do investigators ask whether the outcome measures they plan to adopt coincide with participants' goals or needs. Related to this, several investigators have reported that group members' scores on the outcomes of interest were so high at baseline that it was impossible to detect any significant improvement over time due to this ceiling effect (Demers & Lavoie, 1996; Haley *et al.*, 1987). Investigators also need to more carefully consider the appropriate duration of support groups. The modal duration has been 6–8 weeks or sessions, regardless of the participants' requests and needs for more extensive support. Especially when facing the changing demands associated with the chronic stress of caring for individuals affected by multiple sclerosis, cancer, dementia and intellectual impairments, longer-term support is called for (Helgeson & Gottlieb, 2000) (see 'Coping with chronic illness'). In this regard, Edmonds *et al.* (1999) maintain that, for cancer patients, longer interventions have different effects from short-term interventions because they demand more commitment from the participants, expose them to the harsh realities of the disease and give way to the work of coping after the initial honeymoon period that is marked by enthusiasm and hope.

Research on support groups for the family caregivers of persons affected by dementia shows growing evidence that groups which provide behavioural or cognitive training in addition to peer discussion have effects that are superior to groups which only emphasize education and peer discussion (Bourgeois *et al.*, 1996). Because it has been consistently found that the behavioural management challenges contribute most to the prediction of caregiver burden, it stands to reason that groups delivering problem-solving skills (Lovett & Gallagher, 1988) and anger management (Gallagher-Thompson & DeVries, 1994) should have a value-added positive impact on the caregiver (See 'Cognitive behaviour therapy and group therapy').

Finally, in the future, complete description of the intervention, ideally in the form of a manual, and evidence that actual or perceived support increased prior to the measurement of the intended outcomes, should become standard components of any assessment protocol. However, increased support is only one possible mechanism through which the intervention may affect its endpoints; other potential mediators include changes in coping and health behaviours, and changes in physiological functioning. In this regard, Andersen et al. (2004) implemented an exemplary assessment protocol, measuring not only emotional distress, but also its precursors, including perceived support, health behaviours, adherence to chemotherapy and immune system functioning. This RCT resulted in significant reductions in anxiety, increases in perceived support from network members, improved health behaviours involving diet and smoking, and selective improvements in immune system functioning among women who had been surgically treated for breast cancer. The intervention was more intensive than most, involving 27 hours of weekly small group sessions over a 4-month period. An in-depth review of cancer support group designs and effects appears in Gottlieb and Wachala (in press).

Individual supportive allies

Although far more limited in number, there have been trials of the effects of providing supplemental one-to-one support to people experiencing various stressful health events and conditions. Dyadic support strategies lack the influence derived from the consensual validation and social comparisons that occur in support groups, but they have the advantage that they can be deployed in a more flexible manner. This augmentation and specialization of support can derive from either a peer who is a 'veteran sufferer', and therefore possesses the experiential knowledge necessary to be useful to the recipient, or from someone who has full or semi-professional qualifications and therefore can offer expert knowledge in addition to emotional support. Obviously, from the recipient's standpoint, these two types of support providers will be viewed quite differently, the peer perceived to be capable of communicating an insider's perspective from having 'walked in the same shoes' and the professional perceived as more authoritative. In principle, the peer supporter's influence also derives from being a target of social comparison, as well as a model of healthy adjustment, whereas the professional's influence derives from his or her perceived knowledge of what is best for the patient.

One important implication is that more care needs to be taken in selecting the peer supporter than the professional supporter because the peer must be viewed by the patient as a relevant and similar other. For example, a 50-year-old employed Hispanic man who has opted for a radical prostatectomy would not tend to view a retired Caucasian 70-year-old man who has had radiation treatment for his prostate cancer as a similar peer. In fact, one study has illustrated the extent to which being 'in the same boat' matters to support recipients. Thoits et al. (2000) designed a trial in which men undergoing bypass surgery received either routine hospital care or the support of a man who had undergone the same surgery previously and who had been trained to provide simple supportive behaviours. Although they found null effects of the extra support, meaning that the trial was a failure, they discovered that virtually all the study participants had talked with one or more fellow patients while they were in the hospital, before and/or after their surgery.

Moreover, frequent conversations with fellow patients were associated with better perceived health 1 month after surgery, greater health satisfaction 1 and 6 months after surgery fewer activity limitations 12 months after surgery and lower symptoms of depression and distress at all 3 time points after surgery.

The authors argue that the support of other patients was more 'natural' than the introduction of a formal volunteer supporter. In addition, it is very likely that the study participants perceived their hospital mates as more similar to themselves than the volunteer helpers because the former men were in exactly the same stressful circumstances, namely awaiting or recovering from heart surgery, whereas the volunteers had already resumed their daily lives. Not only were hospital mates more relevant targets of social comparison, but they also may have offered less conspicuous expressions of support and accepted whatever support was extended by their mates. The effect was to make the support process more reciprocal, and therefore more acceptable than the more one-sided interactions with the volunteer supporters.

In the most commonly implemented one-to-one support initiatives a professional, paraprofessional, or trained staff member periodically renders face-to-face or phone support. For example, Mishel et al. (2002) implemented an 8-week telephone intervention in which nurses were trained to provide information and to enhance the self-efficacy of men recently treated for prostate cancer. The nurses' ethnicity was matched to that of the patients and their emphasis was on helping the patients to reframe their situation as manageable and on improving their problem-solving skills. The results showed improvement in the latter two mediators, and significantly improved bladder control 4 months after the intervention ended. A similar dyadic telephone support strategy was implemented by Dennis et al. (2002), except that in this case the support was provided by a peer for the purpose of extending the duration of breastfeeding among primaparous mothers. The support providers were women with breastfeeding experience who were matched to the new mothers on age, cultural background and SES. They were trained to provide optimal telephone support and referral skills. Contact was made with the new mothers within 48 hours of their discharge from hospital, and as frequently thereafter as the new mother wanted. The actual average amount of contact proved to be 5.4 calls over the 3-month study period, the benefit being that significantly more of these mothers continued to breastfeed at 3 months postpartum compared with mothers who had been randomly assigned to the conventional care condition.

Yet a third variation of this method of marshalling support involves more costly and time-consuming home visitation. In a widely cited study, Olds and his colleagues assigned nurses to make home visits to unmarried, low-income teenaged mothers, half the mothers receiving the home visits only during pregnancy and half until the child's second birthday (Olds et al., 1986). The nurses were trained to provide health education, emotional and practical support, parenting skills and links to community services. Both short-term and long-term (15 years) outcomes have shown that the more extensive home visitation resulted in fewer pre-term deliveries, fewer child maltreatment reports, fewer emergency hospital visits for injuries and ingestions up to the child's fourth year and both fewer subsequent pregnancies and a longer interval between those that did occur. In subsequent studies, Olds and his colleagues have experimented with different types of home visitors and concluded that nurses are the visitors of choice. As Olds *et al.* (1998) observe: 'We have chosen nurses because of their formal training regarding women's and children's health and because of their competence in managing the types of complex clinical situations often presented by at-risk families' (p. 99). Furthermore, the programme planners maintain that registered nurses are in the best position to address mothers' concerns about complications in pregnancy, the biological changes entailed in pregnancy, labour and delivery, as well as the physical health and cognitive and emotional development of the infant. In addition, nurses have been found to have more credibility with low-income, high-risk mothers and can teach them how to use the healthcare system most effectively.

Disappointing and even disquieting evidence about the effects of dyadic support comes from other experimental trials. Frasure-Smith *et al.* (1997) conducted an RCT assessing the effects of dual support interventions on depression, anxiety and survival of 1376 male and female post-myocardial infarction (MI) patients. Specifically, they hypothesized '... that patients who participated, after leaving hospital, in a 1-year programme of monthly telephone monitoring of psychological distress symptoms, combined with home-nursing visits in response to high levels of distress, would be less likely to die from cardiac causes during the first post-MI year than patients receiving usual care' (p. 473). This hypothesis was informed by evidence revealing not only that life events hasten the death of post-MI patients via the mediating role of depressive affect, but also that post-MI men who had received the same support protocol in a prior pilot study were about half as likely to die of cardiac causes as men receiving usual care. Hence, this was a replication of the earlier study, but with a much larger sample that included women patients. The results of this enlarged trial differed vastly from those of the pilot study: after one year, patients in the experimental condition had no overall survival advantage and the women in this condition evidenced higher cardiac and all-cause mortality. At one year, there was a negligible impact of the intervention on the survivors' reports of depressive affect and anxiety, the hypothesized mediating mechanisms.

The study investigators' intriguing interpretation of these disconcerting results serves as a caution regarding the potential adverse effects of support programmes. They argue that the monthly telephone screening for possible distress, combined with an average of 5–6 home-nursing visits paid to 75% of the patients in the intervention condition, may have inadvertently compounded the patients' distress, especially among the women. This is because the supporters' intense interest in the mental health of the patients may have reminded them of their serious conditions, disrupting their efforts to cope by denying problems, and by uncovering family strains and raising expectations that long-standing problems could be resolved. It is also possible that the psychological symptom threshold for triggering the extra nurse home visits was too low, and alarmed the women who received them.

Whatever the reasons why this intervention backfired, the message it leaves is that the delivery of support must be carefully planned with respect to its source, timing, content and amount. In addition, attention should be paid to the inferences which support recipients draw about themselves and their wellbeing when they are selected or invited to participate in support programmes but have not solicited the support themselves. The social–psychological dynamics affecting the recipient of support deserve as much attention as those which concern the provider and the structure of the larger intervention (Heller *et al.*, 1991; Rook, 1991; Vaux, 1991).

Conclusion

Much thoughtful planning and careful evaluation efforts are yielding valuable knowledge about the combinations of conditions and candidates that make these grafted support interventions most attractive and effective. We know that groups that provide specific cognitive or behavioural skills in addition to support tend to be more effective than those offering only support. We also know that candidates who lack sufficient natural support and who are motivated to compare their own experiences with similar peers tend to benefit most from their group experience. Yet how far the benefits reach and for how long is uncertain: there is no conclusive evidence that support groups alone can affect length of survival from serious disease, even though they exercise a significant improvement in mental health and quality of life. Similarly, few firm conclusions can be drawn about the impact of supplemental support from a peer or professional who is dedicated to this role. More research is needed in order to identify the social–psychological conditions and the interpersonal transactions which are most favourable for relationship development and for the relationship's influence on the intended health outcomes. However, given the substantial progress that has been made in the past 20 years, there is good reason to believe that we are on the threshold of discovering how to mobilize support in ways that are acceptable and health-protective.

REFERENCES

Andersen, B. L. (1992). Psychological interventions for cancer patients to enhance the quality of life. *Journal of Consulting and Clinical Psychology*, **60**, 552–68.

Andersen, B., Farrar, W., Golden-Kreutz, D. *et al.* (2004). Psychological, behavioral, and immune changes after a psychological intervention: a clinical trial. *Journal of Clinical Oncology*, **22**(17), 3570–80.

Antoni, M. H., Lehman, J. M., Kilbourn, K. M. *et al.* (2001). Cognitive–behavioral stress management interventiondecreases the

prevalence of depression and enhances benefit-finding among women under treatment for early-stage breast cancer. *Health Psychology*, **20**, 20–32.

Berkman, L. F. & Syme, L. (1979). Social networks, host resistance, and mortality: a nine-year follow-up study of Alameda County residents. *American Journal of Epidemiology*, **109**, 186–204.

Bourgeois, M. S., Schulz, R. & Burgio, L. (1996). Interventions for caregivers of patients with Alzheimer's Disease: a review

and analysis of content, process, and outcomes. *International Journal of Aging and Human Development*, **43**(1), 35–92.

Classen, C., Butler, L. D., Koopman, C. *et al.* (2001). Supportive-expressive group therapy and distress in patients with metastatic breast cancer: a randomized clinical intervention trial. *Archives of General Psychiatry*, **58**, 494–501.

Cohen, S. & Wills, T. (1985). Stress, social support, and the buffering hypothesis. *Psychological Bulletin*, **98**, 310–57.

Coyne, J. & Smith, D. (1994). Couples coping with myocardial infarction: contextual perspective on patient's self-efficacy. *Journal of Family Psychology*, **8**, 43–54.

Cunningham, A. J., Edmonds, C. V. I. & Jenkins, G. (1998). A randomized controlled trial of the effects of group psychological therapy on survival in woman with metastatic breast cancer. *Psychooncology*, **7**, 508–17.

Cutrona, C. & Cole, V. (2000). Optimizing support in the natural network. In S. Cohen, L. Underwood & B. H. Gottlieb (Eds.). *Social support measurement and intervention* (pp. 278–308). New York: Oxford University Press.

Dakoff & Taylor, S. E. (1990). Victims' perceptions of social support: what is helpful from whom? *Journal of Personality and Social Psychology*, **58**, 80–9.

Demers, A. & Lavoie, J. P. (1996). Effect of support groups on family caregivers to the frail elderly. *Canadian Journal on Aging*, **15**(1), 129–44.

Dennis, C.-L., Hodnett, E., Gallop, R. & Chalmers, B. (2002). The effect of peer support on breast-feeding duration among primaparous women: a randomized controlled trial. *Canadian Medical Association Journal*, **166**(1), 21–8.

Edgar, L., Collet, J.-P. & Rosberger, Z. (2001). Lessons learned: outcomes and methodology of a coping skills intervention trial comparing individual and group formats for patients with cancer. *International Journal of Psychiatry in Medicine*, **31**(3), 305–20.

Edmonds, C. V. I., Lockwood, G. A. & Cunningham, A. J. (1999). Psychological response to long term group therapy: a randomized trial with metastatic breast cancer patients. *Psychooncology*, **8**, 74–91.

Frasure-Smith, N., Lesperance, F., Prince, R. et al. (1997). Randomised trial of home-based psychosocial nursing intervention for patients recovering from myocardial infarction. *The Lancet*, **350**, 473–9.

Gallagher-Thompson, D. & DeVries, H. (1994). 'Coping with Frustration' classes: development and preliminary outcomes with women who care for relatives with dementia. *The Gerontologist*, **34**, 548–52.

Goodwin, P. J., Leszez, M., Ennis, M. et al. (2001). The effect of group psychosocial support on survival in metastatic breast cancer. *New England Journal of Medicine*, **345**(24), 1719–26.

Gottlieb, B. H. (1988). Support interventions: a typology and agenda for research. In S. W. Duck (Ed.). *Handbook of personal relationships* (pp. 519–41). New York: Wiley.

Gottlieb, B. H. & Wachala, E. D. (in press). Cancer support group: a critical review of empirical studies. *Psychoncology*.

Haley, W., Brown, S. L. & Levine, E. G. (1987). Experimental evaluation of the effectiveness of group intervention for dementia caregivers. *The Gerontologist*, **27**(3), 376–82.

Hamann, H. A., Croyle, R. T., Smith, K. R. et al. (2000). Interest in a support group among individuals tested for a BRCA1 gene mutation. *Journal of Psychosocial Oncology*, **18**(4), 15–37.

Helgeson, V., Cohen, S., Schulz, R. & Yasko, J. (1999). Education and peer discussion group interventions and adjustment to breast cancer. *Archives of General Psychiatry*, **56**, 340–7.

Helgeson, V., Cohen, S., Schulz, R. & Yasko, J. (2000). Group support interventions for women with breast cancer: who benefits from what? *Health Psychology*, **19**(2), 107–14.

Helgeson, V. & Gottlieb, B. H. (2000). Support groups. In S. Cohen, L. Underwood & B. H. Gottlieb (Eds.). *Social support measurement and intervention* (pp. 221–45). New York: Oxford University Press.

Heller, K., Thompson, M., Trueba, P., Hogg, J. & Vlachos-Weber, I. (1991). Peer support telephone dyads for elderly women: was this the wrong intervention? *American Journal of Community Psychology*, **19**, 53–74.

House, J., Robbins, C. & Metzner, H. (1982). The association of social relationships and activities with mortality: prospective evidence from the Tecumseh Community Health Study. *American Journal of Epidemiology*, **116**, 123–40.

Lehman, D. & Hemphill, K. (1990). Recipients' perceptions of support attempts and attributions for support attempts that fail. *Journal of Social and Personal Relationships*, **7**, 563–74.

Lepore, S., Helgeson, V., Eton, D. & Schulz, R. (2003). Improving quality of life in men with prostate cancer: a randomized controlled trial of group education interventions. *Health Psychology*, **22**(5), 443–52.

Lovett, S. & Gallagher, D. (1988). Psychoeducational interventions for family caregivers: preliminary efficacy data. *Behavior Therapy*, **19**, 321–30.

McGovern, R. J., Heyman, E. N. & Resnick, M. I. (2002). An examination of coping style and quality of life of cancer patients who attend a prostate support group. *Journal of Psychosocial Oncology*, **20**(3), 57–68.

Miller, S. M. (1995). Monitoring versus blunting styles of coping with cancer influence the information patients want and need about their disease. *Cancer*, **76**, 167–77.

Mishel, M., Belyea, M., Germino, B. et al. (2002). Helping patients with localized prostate carcinoma manage uncertainty and treatment side effects. *Cancer*, **94**(6), 1854–66.

Nekhlyudov, L. & Yaker, A. (2002). Group psychosocial support in metastatic breast cancer. *New England Journal of Medicine*, **346**(16), 1247–8.

Olds, D., Eckenrode, J., Henderson, C. et al. (1998). Long-term effects of home visitation on maternal life course and child abuse and neglect: 15-year follow-up of a randomized trial. *Journal of the American Medical Association*, **278**, 637–43.

Olds, D., Henderson, C., Chamberlin, R. & Tatelbaum, R. (1986). Preventing child abuse and neglect: a randomized trial of nurse home visitation. *Pediatrics*, **78**, 65–78.

Potthoff, J. G., Holahan, C. J. & Joiner Jr., T. E. (1995). Reassurance seeking, stress generation, and depressive symptoms: an integrative model. *Journal of Personality and Social Psychology*, **68**(4), 664–70.

Rook, K. (1991). Facilitating friendship formation in late life: puzzles and challenges. *American Journal of Community Psychology*, **19**, 103–10.

Schulz, R., O'Brian, A., Czaja, S. et al. (2002). Dementia caregiver intervention research: in search of clinical significance. *The Gerontologist*, **42**(5), 589–602.

Spiegel, D. (2001). Mind matters – group therapy and survival in breast cancer. *New England Journal of Medicine*, **345**(24), 1767–8.

Spiegel, D., Bloom, J. R., Kraemer, H. C. & Gottheil, E. (1989). Effect of psychosocial treatment on survival of patients with metastatic breast cancer. *Lancet*, **2**, 888–91.

Taylor, S. E., Falke, R. L., Shoptaw, S. J. & Lichtman, R. R. (1986). Social support, support groups, and the cancer patient. *Journal of Consulting and Clinical Psychology*, **54**(5), 608–15.

Thoits, P., Hohmann, A., Harvey, M. & Fletcher, B. (2000). Similar-other support for men undergoing coronary artery bypass surgery. *Health Psychology*, **19**(3), 264–73.

Vaux, A. (1991). Let's hang up and try again: lessons learned from a social support intervention. *American Journal of Community Psychology*, **19**, 85–90.

Winefield, H. R., Coventry, B. J., Lewis, M. & Harvey, E. J. (2003). Attitudes of patients with breast cancer toward support groups. *Journal of Psychosocial Oncology*, **21**(2), 39–54.

Stress management

Dianna T. Kenny

University of Sydney

Overview

What is stress management?

Stress management interventions arose in the 1960s with the growth of the community mental health and crisis intervention movements, disenchantment with medical model approaches to mental health and dissatisfaction with traditional psychiatry, the development of behavioural and cognitive–behavioural therapies, the growing acceptance of psychological problems within the community and the surgence of self-help approaches to psychological wellbeing (Auerbach, 1986).

There have been literally thousands of articles written about stress management. A search of the PsychInfo datatbase shows 3433 articles published between 1958 and 2004 on various applications of stress management, such as stress management in health care, occupational settings, educational settings, community programmes and critical incident stress management.

It is difficult to find an adequate definition of stress management that is sufficiently inclusive to incorporate all the stress management strategies and interventions which currently occur in the literature under this nomenclature and to be sufficiently exclusive so as to differentiate these interventions from other types of psychological treatments. In its broadest definition, stress management interventions are designed to assist people to cope with stressors and with the negative emotions, physiological arousal and/or health consequences that arise from these stressors by changing their cognitive and emotional responses to the trigger events. To distinguish stress management from many psychological interventions, a number of caveats must be invoked. Firstly, stress management is generally applied to adequately functioning individuals who may be facing difficult circumstances in their occupational or social settings. Secondly, the focus of stress management is primarily educational rather than psychotherapeutic. Programmes are generally derived from the principles of learning theory; cognitive theory; and stress and coping theory and aim to change some aspect of behaviour or thinking related to a particular environment or circumstance. Thirdly, the duration is shorter rather than longer, usually with a fixed number of sessions. Fourthly, the service is more often delivered to groups than to individuals. Fifthly, the deliverers of stress management interventions do not generally form a therapeutic relationship with participants. Rather, they act as facilitators/educators, encouraging group members to establish their own goals, and to self-administer and self-monitor progress. There is rarely any long-term follow-up once the programme has been completed (Auerbach & Gramling, 1998).

Stress management interventions vary widely in content and duration and may include progressive muscle relaxation, meditation, guided imagery, autogenics training, biofeedback, cognitive restructuring, problem-solving skills, anger management, social skills training and assertiveness training, as well as educative components related to general health, diet, exercise and wellbeing.

This chapter will review the three main areas in which stress management approaches are applied:

1. Stress management in occupational settings
2. Stress management in healthcare settings
3. Critical incident stress management (psychological debriefing).

The review will conclude with a brief discussion of recent new directions in stress management research.

Stress management in occupational settings

Occupational stress arises in the complex interaction between organizational and work demands and individual and interpersonal characteristics. Candidate occupational stressors include job tasks (e.g. monotonous); the organization of work (e.g. fast-paced, low control, shift work); the physical work environment (e.g. noise, temperature, chemical fumes, ventilation); the fit between the worker and the work (e.g. overload, underload); role in the organization (e.g. lack of status, lack of prospects for promotion, lack of a career path, job insecurity) and the social work environment (e.g. lack of support, exposure to interpersonal conflict, discrimination, bullying); and home and work interface (e.g. conflict between domestic and work roles, lack of spousal support for remaining in the workforce).

Occupational stress has been held responsible for almost every category of ill health, both physical and psychological by both researchers in the area and lay people (see 'Stress and health'). The effects of occupational stress may be direct, as in the case of workers on a fast-paced production line showing chronic increased blood pressure and muscular tension, or indirect, as may occur when work-related stressors trigger pathogenic health-related behaviours, such as increased alcohol or drug consumption. The empirically established connections between occupational stressors and health outcomes are more robust for some conditions than others and some types of occupational stressors appear more closely related to health outcomes than others. For example, high psychological demand, low control, low social support and lack of reward for high effort increase the risk of cardiovascular morbidity and mortality. The evidence is much less conclusive with regard to stroke and cancer. Occupational stress, in the form of job dissatisfaction and interpersonal distress may also mediate injury, compensation claims and poor return to work outcomes following injury (Kenny & McIntyre, 2005).

There is a vast and truly daunting literature on occupational stress, one that can at times generates more heat than light. A number of recent editions of journals have been devoted to the topic of occupational stress and its management (see, for example, Kenny & Cooper, 2003). There have been many conflicting views of the nature and cause of occupational stress, ranging from a problem that resides within individuals (i.e. personality, cognitions (cognitive appraisals) and coping behaviours) to one that has its roots in the organization of work, organizational climate and the structure of power and authority in the workplace (Kenny & McIntyre, 2005). Context, interactional and multilevel factors may each contribute to the overall stress quotient. That is, occupational stress may be rooted in the job itself, in the way the job is perceived, in the way employees are managed as a group and in the overall organizational climate and leadership of the workplace. For each putative cause, methods of occupational stress management have been developed. Just as root causes have been identified at the level of the individual, the level of interaction between individual and organizations and at the organizational (climate/managerial) level, so too do interventions occur on these three levels:

- individual (relaxation, meditation, cognitive behaviour therapy, exercise, time management, employee assistance programmes)
- individual/organizational (co-worker support groups, role clarification, person–environment fit and participation and autonomy programmes)
- organizational (selection and placement, training and education, interpersonal skill development in managers, work environment changes and job redesign and restructuring) (Giga et al., 2003; Kenny & McIntyre, 2005; Morrison & Payne, 2003).

The critical question is whether any of these interventions has a significant positive impact on measurable outcomes such as absenteeism, sick leave, claims for workers' compensation and productivity. The converging consensus is that individual person-directed stress management programmes – those that attempt to empower workers to deal with demanding situations by developing their own coping skills and abilities – are unlikely to maintain employee health and wellbeing in the long term without procedures in place within organizations to reduce or prevent environmental stressors. Individual level approaches which focus on skill development and job control appear to fare better, but organizational strategies in the form of management/supervisor training and organizational climate yield the best results (Morrison & Payne, 2003). There is some evidence to show that individual distress and morale have different determinants, with personality factors accounting mostly for distress and organizational factors for morale. Low morale is more likely than distress to lead to work withdrawal. Cotton and Hart (2003) argue that workplaces can address organizational factors impacting on morale through provision of a supportive organizational climate and appropriate leadership behaviours.

Stress management in healthcare settings

Since stress has been strongly associated with morbidity and mortality in a number of chronic and life threatening medical illnesses (see 'Stress and health'), it is not difficult to argue that offering stress management programmes to these individuals with these conditions is likely to have a positive impact on the course and outcome of their illnesses. There are direct and indirect pathways through which psychosocial stressors are thought to contribute to disease onset and exacerbation. In the direct pathway, psychosocial stressors promote pathophysiological processes such as altered immune functioning, atherosclerosis and vascular dysfunction. In the indirect pathway, psychosocial stressors contribute to unhealthy lifestyle choices such poor diet, smoking, alcohol abuse, risky behaviours and low physical activity that are the direct causes of the pathophysiological processes which lead to illnesses such as coronary heart disease (CHD) and cancer.

The evidence for the effectiveness of stress management in reducing morbidity and mortality from CHD is not strong. Although some programmes that included a cognitive restructuring component reported a decrease in behaviours (collectively called Type A behaviours) known to be associated with myocardial infarction (Friedman et al., 1986), and others have achieved reductions in depression (ENRICHD, 2000), neither programme was associated with decreased morbidity or mortality at 12-month and 2-year follow-up respectively, although the Friedman study found small decreases in mortality at 4.5 years and decreased cardiac recurrence in the stress management group. Trials using short duration stress management programmes (Frasure-Smith et al., 1997) reported neither improved psychological functioning, nor heart disease outcomes. However, Blumenthal et al. (1997) found decreased incidence of myocardial ischemia and reduced myocardial infarction at 5-year follow-up in stress management participants compared with a standard care control group.

The findings for the effect of stress management on cancer parallel to some extent the findings for CHD. While early studies reported significant improvements in life expectancy of women with breast cancer (Spiegel et al., 1989) and malignant melanoma (Fawzy et al., 1990) as a result of participation in stress management programmes, more recent studies have been unable to replicate these positive findings and concluded that they were due to methodological problems in the early studies (Claar & Blumenthal, 2003). Current studies about the use of stress management programmes in cancer treatment support the conclusion that while such programmes may have a significant positive influence on depression, anxiety and perceived pain in women with breast cancer, there is little evidence for reductions in morbidity or mortality (Goodwin et al., 2001).

Headache (both chronic tension type and migraine) has also been of interest to researchers in stress management. Recent randomized controlled trials have indicated that a combined treatment of antidepressant medication and stress management programmes produces larger reductions in tension-type headaches (64% of participants) than either drug (38%) or stress management (35%) alone. Interestingly, placebo fared only marginally worse (29%) than these active monotherapies (Holroyd et al., 2001). Another study on migraine reported similar improvements in self-reported outcomes such as pain frequency and intensity but no change in medication use or work status compared with the control group (Lemstra et al., 2002).

Critical incident stress management (CISM)

There are many conceptual and classification issues in the psychology of trauma and its attendant psychological manifestations as post-traumatic stress disorder (PTSD), acute stress disorder (ASD) and expectable distress reactions in response, either directly or indirectly, to traumatic events (see 'Post-traumatic stress disorder'). The lack of clear definitional boundaries for psychological conditions leads to problems in identifying suitable and effective treatments and in evaluating those treatments. An additional complication in PTSD is that diagnosis may change, depending on how long after the traumatic event a person is assessed. Many studies indicate that people are resilient in the face of catastrophe and the majority recover spontaneously, including those with symptoms of PTSD immediately after the event (DeLisi *et al.*, 2003; Kessler *et al.*, 1995). Thus, timing of the intervention is also important, as those who are treated early may have recovered without treatment.

The terms Critical Incident Stress Management (CISM), Critical Incident Stress Debriefing (CISD) and Psychological Debriefing (PD) have been used interchangeably in the literature to describe a form of secondary prevention delivered as soon after exposure to trauma as possible to reduce symptoms and prevent PTSD. PD originated on the battlefields of World War I for use with both combat and peace keeping forces (Litz *et al.*, 2002). Mitchell (1983) applied the principles of PD employed in the armed services to emergency services personnel (firefighters, police, ambulance). Originally intended for the so-called secondary victims of trauma (i.e. those persons assisting the primary victims), Mitchell's model of CISD was applied widely to both primary and secondary victims in diverse settings. CISD is delivered to a group of individuals all of whom have been exposed to, or have assisted a victim of, trauma. It typically occurs immediately or soon after the critical incident, and involves a standard procedure in which a facilitator explains the procedure and ground rules (e.g. confidentiality of the group, suspension of rank, voluntary participation) and invites all members to present their account of the incident and their reactions, thoughts and feelings at the time. The session concludes with an educational component in which participants are advised about the nature of normal stress reactions, what they might expect to experience in the next few days and some stress management strategies that they might employ to alleviate symptoms. The group often ends with an informal, social component (see Mitchell & Bray, 1990). Some countries have made the offer of CISD compulsory to avoid possible negligence claims from employees in the event that they develop PTSD (Rose *et al.*, 2001).

Recently, the terms PD, CISD and CISM have become more differentiated. CISM is the generic term now used for a number of strategies employed in critical incidents. Everly and Mitchell (1999) have described six distinct components as follows: pre-incident preparedness training; individual crisis support; demobilization (provision of food, rest and information about coping to emergency staff as they complete their shifts); defusing (small group meetings along the lines of the CISD model discussed above); family support; and referral. However, Devilly and Cotton (2003) reported continuing difficulty in distinguishing between CISM and CISD and prefer the use of the term PD to describe any immediate intervention following trauma in contrast to structured CISM and CISD programmes, as described by Mitchell (1983).

Despite its intuitive appeal and ubiquitous presence globally, a heated debate is being waged in the academic literature as to whether CISM in its various manifestations is effective in preventing the onset of PTSD (McNally *et al.*, 2003). In order to resolve the question, researchers should consider only those studies which meet the gold standard for treatment outcome studies. Foa and Meadows (1997) itemize the factors needed to meet this yardstick. They include clearly defined target symptoms, specifying a threshold of symptom severity;

exclusion of subjects with comorbid diagnoses; the use of reliable and valid measures; the use of blind evaluators; standardized training of assessors and those delivering the treatment; manualized, replicable, specific treatment programmes; unbiased assignment to treatment; and adherence to treatment. Interestingly, most of the studies cited in support of the efficacy of CISM in reducing stress and the onset of PTSD do not meet some or all of the benchmarks for treatment outcome studies and hence are either difficult to interpret or produce findings in which one can have little confidence (Campfield & Hills, 2001; Deahl *et al.*, 2000; Nurmi, 1999; Yule, 1992).

There is a larger body of better designed studies which is converging on the conclusion that CISD either has no effect (Conlon *et al.*, 1999; Rose *et al.*, 1999) or indeed has a deleterious effect (Bisson *et al.*, 1997; Hobbs *et al.*, 1996; Kenardy *et al.*, 1996; Mayou *et al.*, 2000) on victims of trauma. Ironically, even in studies where debriefed participants fared worse than those who were not debriefed in terms of the number and severity of PTSD symptoms, the majority of those undertaking debriefing reported the experience to be helpful and positive (Carlier *et al.*, 1998; Raphael *et al.*, 1995; Small *et al.*, 2000).

The controversy is not resolved because there are many differences within and between groups of supportive and non-supportive studies; for example, the type of trauma (victims of crime, victims of natural disasters); the type of participants (primary or secondary victims of trauma); the type of service delivery (group vs. individual); the timing of service delivery (immediately after trauma or later); the outcome measures used to assess efficacy of CISD (symptoms of PTSD, depression, adaptive function, return to work, sick leave); and variations in the actual protocol (Everly & Mitchell, 1999; Mitchell, 2002). The assumption underpinning CISM, that it is helpful to express thoughts and feelings about the trauma immediately after the incident, is currently being re-examined in the light of this body of evidence. The emerging view is that the focus should shift from CISD to screening and provision of early intervention for those at risk or actually suffering from adverse reactions as a result of trauma (Devilly & Cotton, 2003).

New directions in stress management

Changing views of the nature of stress

In recent years, there has been a gradual shift in the way that stress itself has been understood, and this, in time, will affect the way in which stress management programmes are developed and delivered. Current models of stress emphasize the role of cognitive appraisal (e.g. perceiving the event as a threat or a challenge, as controllable or uncontrollable) in determining stress responses, and that social factors such as social isolation or position in a dominance hierarchy all play a role in the intensity of the physiological response (Kemeny, 2003). These are all factors that will need to be considered in the development of the next generation of stress management programmes.

New approaches to stress management

Mindfulness

Western medicine has been complemented in recent years by the practices of the East. Chinese herbal medicine, homeopathy, acupuncture, various forms of massage therapy, meditation and Tai Chi have gained increasing acceptance over the past 20 years. A newer form of stress management, called Mindfulness Based Stress Reduction (MBSR) '. . . is a clinical program originally developed to facilitate adaptation to medical illness that provides systematic training in mindfulness meditation as a self-regulation approach to stress reduction and emotion management' (Bishop, 2002, p. 71). The primary goal is '. . . to provide patients with training in meditation techniques to foster the quality of mindfulness, broadly conceptualized as a state in which one is highly award and focused on the reality of the present moment, accepting and acknowledging it, without getting caught up in thoughts that are about the situation or in emotional reactions to the situation' (Bishop, 2002).

The enthusiasm with which this form of stress management has been embraced is not matched by evidence to support its effectiveness from quality controlled studies. However, although such studies are urgently needed, the approach does appear promising and certainly warrants further large-scale investigation.

Service delivery via the Internet

There has been a growing interest in the use of the Internet as a means of delivering psychological interventions (King & Moreggi, 1998). There are some clear advantages to this form of delivery including reduced costs, easy access, particularly for those with agoraphobia or mobility problems, participant control over therapy and anonymity for those who feel uncomfortable with face-to-face contact with psychologists and counsellors. However, obtaining accurate assessment and diagnosis via the Internet may cause difficulty because therapists have no cues on which to form an opinion about their clients other than the completed self-assessments provided electronically. Attrition has also been identified as an issue, but this problem is universal to all forms of therapy. Early indications point to potential benefits of online (i.e. Internet-based), self-help stress management interventions (Zetterqvist et al., 2003) although further research is needed to confirm its effectiveness.

REFERENCES

Auerbach, S. M. (1986). Assumptions of crisis theory and a temporal model of crisis intervention. In S. M. Auerbach & A. L. Stolberg (Eds.). *Crisis intervention with children and families.* Washington, DC: Hemisphere.

Auerbach, S. M. & Gramling, S. E. (1998). *Stress management: psychological foundations.* England Cliffs, NJ: Prentice Hall.

Bishop, S. R. (2002). What do we really know about mindfulness-based stress reduction? *Psychosomatic Medicine,* **64,** 71–84.

Bisson, J., Jenkins, P. L., Alexander, J. & Bannister, C. (1997). Randomised controlled trial of psychological debriefing for victims of acute burn trauma. *British Journal of Psychiatry,* **171,** 78–81.

Blumenthal, J. A., Jiang, W., Babyak, M. et al. (1997). Stress management and exercise training in cardiac patients with myo-cardial ischemia: effects on prognosis and evaluation of mechanisms. *Archives of Internal Medicine,* **157,** 2213–23.

Bryant, R. A. & Harvey, A. G. (2000). *Acute stress disorder: a handbook of theory, assessment and treatment.* Washington, DC: American Psychological Association.

Campfield, K. M. & Hills, A. M. (2001). Effect of timing of critical incident stress debriefing (CISD) on posttraumatic symptoms. *Journal of Traumatic Stress,* **14,** 327–40.

Carlier, I. V. E., Lamberts, R. D., van Uchelen, A. J. & Gersons, B. P. R. (1998). Disaster-related post-traumatic stress in police officers: a field study of the impact of debriefing. *Stress Medicine,* **14,** 143–8.

Claar, R. L. & Blumenthal, J. A. (2003). The value of stress-management interventions in life-threatening medical conditions. *Current Directions in Psychological Science,* **17,** 133–7.

Conlon, L., Fahy, T. J. & Conroy, R. (1999). PTSD in ambulant RTA victims: a randomized controlled trial of debriefing. *Journal of Psychosomatic Research,* **46,** 37–44.

Cotton, P. & Hart, P. M. (2003). Occupational wellbeing and performance: a review of organisational health research, *Australian Psychologist,* **38**(1), 118–27.

Deahl, M., Srinivasan, M., Jones, N. et al. (2000). Preventing psychological trauma in soldiers: the role of operational stress training and psychological debriefing. *British Journal of Medical Psychology,* **73,** 77–85.

DeLisi, L. E., Maurizio, A., Yost, M. et al. (2003). A survey of New Yorkers after the Sept. 11, 2001, terrorist attacks. *American Journal of Psychiatry,* **160,** 780–3.

Devilly, G. J. & Cotton, P. (2003). Psychological debriefing and the workplace: defining a concept, controversies and guidelines for intervention. *Australian Psychologist,* **38**(2), 144–50.

DSM-III. (1980). *Diagnostic and Statistical Manual of Mental Disorders* (3rd edn.). Washington, DC: American Psychiatric Association.

DSM-IV. (1994). *Diagnostic and Statistical Manual of Mental Disorders* (4th edn.). Washington, DC: American Psychiatric Association.

ENRICHD. (2000). *Enhancing recovery in coronary heart disease.* Retrieved from: http://www.bios.unc.edu/units/cscc/ENRI/index.html.

Everly Jr., G. S. & Mitchell, J. T. (1999). *Critical Incident Stress Management (CISM): A New Era and Standard of Care in Crisis Intervention* (2nd edn.). Ellicott City, MD: Chevron.

Fawzy, F. I., Cousins, N., Fawzy, N. W. et al. (1990). A structured psychiatric intervention for cancer patients: I. Changes over time in methods of coping and affective disturbance. *Archives of General Psychiatry,* **50,** 681–9.

Foa, E. B. & Meadows, E. A. (1997). Psychosocial treatments for posttraumatic stress disorder: a critical review. *Annual Review of Psychology,* **48,** 449–80.

Frasure-Smith, N., Lesperance, F., Prince, R. H. et al. (1997). Randomised trial of home-based psychosocial intervention and breast cancer survival. *Psycho-Oncology,* **7,** 361–70.

Friedman, M., Thoresen, C. E., Gill, J. J. et al. (1986). Alteration of Type A behavior and its effect on cardiac recurrences in post myocardial infarction patients: summary results of the recurrent coronary prevention project. *American Heart Journal,* **112,** 653–65.

Giga, S. I., Cooper, C. L. & Faragher, B. (2003). The development of a framework for a comprehensive approach to stress management interventions at work. *International Journal of Stress Management,* **10,** 280–96.

Goodwin, P. J., Leszcz, M., Ennis, M. et al. (2001). The effect of group psychosocial support on survival in metastatic breast cancer. *New England Journal of Medicine,* **345,** 1517–21.

Hobbs, M., Mayou, R., Harrison, B. & Worlock, P. (1996). A randomised controlled trial of psychological debriefing for victims of road traffic accidents. *British Medical Journal,* **313**, 1438–9.

Holroyd, K. A., O'Donnell, F. J., Stensland, M. et al. (2001). Management of chronic tension-type headache with tricyclic antidepressant medication, stress management therapy and their combination: a randomized controlled trial. *Journal of the American Medical Association,* **285**, 2208–15.

Kemeny, M. E. (2003). The psychology of stress, *Current Directions in Psychological Science,* **12**, 124–9.

Kenardy, J. A., Webster, R. A., Lewin, T. J. et al. (1996). Stress debriefing and patterns of recovery following a natural disaster. *Journal of Traumatic Stress,* **9**, 37–49.

Kenny, D. T. & Cooper, C. L. (2003). Introduction to the Special Issue on occupational stress and its management. *International Journal of Stress Management,* **10**, 275–9.

Kenny, D. T. & McIntyre, D. (2005). Constructions of occupational stress: nuance or novelty? In A.-S. Antoniou & C. Cooper (Eds.). *Research companion to organizational health psychology.* Cheltenham, UK: Edward Elgar Publishing.

Kessler, R. C., Sonnega, A., Bromet, E., Hughes, M. & Nelson, C. B. (1995). Posttraumatic stress disorder in the National Comorbidity Survey. *Archives of General Psychiatry,* **52**, 1048–60.

King, S. A. & Moreggi, D. (1998). Internet therapy and self-help groups – the pros and cons, In J. Gackenbach (Ed.). *Psychology and the internet: intrapersonal, interpersonal and transpersonal implications* (pp. 77–109). San Diego, CA: Academic Press.

Lemstra, M., Stewart, B. & Olszynski, W. P. (2002). Effectiveness of multidisciplinary intervention in the treatment of migraine: a randomized clinical trial. *Headache,* **42**, 845–54.

Litz, B. T., Gray, M. J., Bryant, R. A. & Adler, A. B. (2002). Early intervention for trauma: current status and future directions. *Clinical Psychology: Science and Practice,* **9**, 112–34.

Mayou, R. A., Ehlers, A. & Hobbs, M. (2000). Psychological debriefing for road traffic accidents: three-year follow-up of a randomised controlled trial. *British Journal of Psychiatry,* **176**, 589–93.

McDonald Jr., J. J. (2003). Posttraumatic stress dishonesty. *Employee Relations Law Journal,* **28**, 93–111.

McNally, R. J., Bryant, R. A. & Ehlers, A. (2003). Does early psychological intervention promote recovery from posttraumatic stress? *Psychological Science in the Public Interest,* **4**, 45–79.

Mitchell, J. T. (1983). When disaster strikes . . . the Critical Incident Stress Debriefing process. *Journal of Emergency Medical Sciences,* **8**, 36–9.

Mitchell, J. T. (2002). *CISM research summary.* Retrieved from: http://www.icisf.org/articles/cism_research_summary.pdf

Mitchell, J. T. & Bray, G. (1990). *Emergency Services stress: guidelines for preserving the health and careers of Emergency Services personnel.* Englewood Cliffs, NJ: Prentice Hall.

Morrison, D. L. & Payne, R. L. (2003). Multilevel approaches to stress management. *Australian Psychologist,* **38**, 128–37.

Nurmi, L. A. (1999). The sinking of the *"Estonia"*: the effects of critical incident stress debriefing (CISD) on rescuers. *International Journal of Emergency Mental Health,* **1**, 23–31.

Raphael, B., Meldrum, L. & McFarlane, A. (1995). Does debriefing after psychological trauma work? *British Medical Journal,* **310**, 1479–80.

Rose, S., Bisson, J., Churchill, R., Wessely, S. (2006). *Psychological debriefing for preventing post traumatic stress disorder (PTSD).* [Systematic Review] Cochrane Depression, Anxiety and Neurosis Group cochrane Database of Systematic Reviews. **4**.

Rose, S., Brewin, C. R., Andrews, B. & Kirk, M. (1999). A randomized controlled trial of individual psychological debriefing for victims of violent crime. *Psychological Medicine,* **29**, 793–9.

Small, R., Lumley, J., Donohue, L., Potter, A. & Waldenstrom, U. (2000). Randomised controlled trial of midwife lead debriefing to reduce maternal depression after operative childbirth. *British Medical Journal,* **321**, 1043–7.

Spiegel, D., Bloom, J. R., Kraemer, H. C. & Gottheil, E. (1989). Effect of psychosocial treatment on survival of patients with coronary artery disease: a meta-analysis. *Archives of Internal Medicine,* **156**, 745–52.

Yule, W. (1992). Post-traumatic stress disorder in child survivors of shipping disasters: the sinking of the "Jupiter". *Psychotherapy and Psychosomatics,* **57**, 200–5.

Zetterqvist, K., Maanmies, J., Ström, L. & Andersson, G. (2003). Randomized controlled trial of internet-based stress management. *Cognitive Behaviour Therapy,* **32**, 151–60.

Worksite interventions

Paul A. Estabrooks and Russell E. Glasgow

Kaiser Permanente-Colorado

Overview

There are numerous theoretical and practical reasons for delivering health promotion programmes in work places. First, the worksite is an environment in which many adults spend a large percentage of their waking hours. Secondly, interventions conducted in a person's relevant physical and social environment – rather than in clinical settings that are not frequented by most individuals – have fewer problems with generalization. Thirdly, worksites offer the opportunity to combine policy, organizational and individual behaviour change strategies: conceptually the combination of such strategies should be more powerful than any one in isolation (Glasgow *et al.*, 1990; Sorensen *et al.*, 2000). Fourthly, the common and consistent interactions among employees within worksites offers the potential for various social support intervention components such as group rewards, participatory employee steering committees, co-worker support and incentive programmes. Fifthly, worksite programmes can increase the reach of health promotion by getting many persons to take advantage of health promotion offerings who may not otherwise participate (Glasgow *et al.*, 1993). Finally, there are also good reasons for employers to offer such programmes. Worksite interventions can potentially increase employee recruitment and retention, reduce health care costs and absenteeism and enhance employee morale and productivity (Pelletier, 2001; Riedel *et al.*, 2001).

There are also complexities and potential downsides to worksite interventions. Some employees may feel that such programmes are coercive, especially in cases in which there are workplace exposures or safety hazards that are not concurrently addressed. Secondly, even if there is strong top management support, which has been documented as essential (Sorensen *et al.*, 1996*b*), front line supervisors may not be as supportive or allow workers to use company time to participate. Finally, there are also logistical challenges such as competing demands, availability of appropriate meeting rooms and facilities, difficulties of reaching part-time and night shift employees.

Definition and scope

We define worksite health promotion (WHP) as the delivery of educational or behavioural change materials or activities to maintain or improve employee fitness, health or wellbeing and changes in organizational practices and policies conducive to health promotion. The variability in the types of WHP programmes has increased over the past decade. Because of the large amount of literature on this topic, for this review we have restricted our focus to WHP programmes that target one or more of the following factors: physical activity, eating patterns and smoking cessation behaviours. We included programmes that addressed both employee behaviour change and environmental or policy change. We did not include worksite-based employee assistance or mental health interventions, or programmes that focused exclusively on occupational safety or workplace hazards. We also excluded worksite interventions that focused solely on cancer screening or assessment of health risks (that did not provide risk reduction activities) although those are also active areas. Finally, given the increased attention on translation of research findings to practice (Glasgow *et al.*, 1999), we have emphasized studies that have implications for dissemination, generalizability of findings and sustainable interventions.

Research evidence

Given that smoking, poor nutrition and physical inactivity are leading behavioural causes of death (Mokdad *et al.*, 2004) there has been a strong emphasis in developing WHP initiatives with the potential to have a broad public health impact (Bull *et al.*, 2003) (see 'Diet and

health', 'Physical activity and health' and 'Tobacco use'). Unfortunately, although WHP strategies have great potential to have a broad reach into the adult population, there is evidence that this potential is not being realized (Bull *et al.*, 2003). This evidence highlights the paucity of literature that reports on essential WHP programme characteristics related to generalization (or robustness) across different types of employees and worksites.

To evaluate the potential public health impact of WHP programmes, we used the RE-AIM evaluation framework to structure our review of the research evidence (Glasgow *et al.*, 1999). The RE-AIM framework was designed to place balanced emphasis on internal and external validity by addressing five issues that combine to determine the overall public health impact of an intervention (www.re-aim.org). These issues are: (1) Reach, or the percentage and representativeness of employees who are willing to participate in a given programme; (2) Effectiveness, or the impact of a WHP programme on important outcomes, including potential negative effects, quality of life and economic outcomes; (3) Adoption, or the percentage and representativeness of settings where personnel are willing to conduct a WHP programme; (4) Implementation, or how consistently various elements of a programme are delivered as intended and by different types of staff and modalities; and (5) Maintenance, or the extent to which a programme or policy becomes institutionalized or part of the routine worksite practices and policies. Maintenance also refers to the ability of employees to sustain healthy behaviour changes for six months (or longer) following the most recent intervention contact.

Recently, our research team completed a review of 24 WHP studies that were published in prominent health promotion and behaviour change journals between 1995–2000 (Bull *et al.*, 2003). Inclusion criteria for this review included a controlled (but not necessarily a randomized control trial) intervention study published in one of the 11 journals identified. In that review we documented the state of the literature related to reporting on the dimensions of the RE-AIM framework. A summary of our findings across RE-AIM dimensions is given below.

Reach

Employee participation rate was reported in 87.5% of the 24 studies (Bull *et al.*, 2003). Rates varied across studies; from 8–97%, with a median of 61%. An earlier comprehensive review demonstrated that WHPs, on average, recruited approximately 39% of overweight employees and that recruitment rates were better for programmes in which less time and effort was required for participation (Hennrikus & Jeffery, 1996). Further, incentives-based programmes have doubled recruitment to worksite health programmes (Hennrikus *et al.*, 2002). Finally, participation rates could be increased by offering free programmes and allowing participants some choice in programme components (Hennrikus & Jeffery, 1996).

It should be noted that the 'denominator' for estimating reach in many studies was based on volunteers who completed a survey, a risk assessment or who sought information, rather than all employees in the worksite, while other studies included all potentially eligible participants as the denominator. The lack of clarity on the population denominator limits the potential of a study to examine the representativeness of the participants to the entire worksite population. For example, WHP programmes often include time and resource costs that result in only a sub-set of employees volunteering to participate. As such, a high participation rate like 90% suggests that the sample is likely to be representative of the larger population, but by basing this rate on a denominator of volunteers, or by excluding certain types of employees (e.g. part-time or night shift workers, blue collar employees) the conclusion of representativeness would be erroneous.

Unfortunately, few studies compare the representativeness of the study sample to a sample of non-participants or all eligible workers (Bull *et al.*, 2003). Those that have included these analyses found that participants were more frequently older, retired, better educated and White (Kristal *et al.*, 2000; Marcus *et al.*, 1998). They also found that participants ate more fruits and vegetables and less fat at baseline, suggesting that the participants may have been more motivated to change behaviours than the general worksite population. The limited reporting of recruitment protocols (i.e. volunteer or passive vs. active, or how many participants were excluded a priori) and lack of comparisons between those who enrolled and those who did not reduces our ability to discern how representative study participants were of the general workforce.

The Next Step Trial (Kristal *et al.*, 2000) provides a template for other worksite interventions for the documentation of the reach of an intervention. The protocol included the reporting of recruitment method used, participation rates and representativeness of participants. Kristal *et al.* indicate the voluntary nature of recruitment: 'both active and retired employees were offered all activities (p.118).' They note the total number of eligible employees, total number of employees taking part in each of the intervention activities and overall intervention participation rates by different employee groups (e.g. active vs. retired). Additionally, this study compared characteristics of all eligible employees and the sample of individuals who chose to participate.

Effectiveness

The utility of WHP programmes is typically judged on data that demonstrate if it worked or if it did not in changing employee behaviour(s). This context exemplifies the effectiveness dimension of the RE-AIM framework – with the caveat that it is one of five equally important dimensions. Nonetheless the documentation of effectiveness (or efficacy – dependent on the type of trial) is the most consistently reported RE-AIM dimension. Research on the effectiveness of WHP interventions has been summarized in a number of review articles (Hennrikus & Jeffery, 1996; McTigue *et al.*, 2003). Each of these reviews highlighted both promise and disappointment with the current state of the literature. The reviews demonstrated that published reports on WHP programmes typically have been adaptations of clinic-based approaches (e.g. education classes). Behaviour modification and incentives were also used regularly, while competitions and capitalizing on the worksite organizational characteristics were used less frequently. A recent study which suggested that high intensity interventions (i.e. person-to-person contact more frequently than once a month) were most likely to be successful for behaviour change and weight loss at 12 months following the initiation of intervention (McTigue *et al.*, 2003). The effectiveness of incentives to improve behavioural outcomes has been equivocal. For example, participants who were given incentives for increased walking during a WHP programme, completed more sessions than

those that were not (Jeffery *et al.*, 1998). Furthermore, although the study was not designed to detect a significant interaction, there was a trend that participants who received both incentives and personal coach support completed more walking sessions than those who received only the incentives or the coach in isolation (Jeffery *et al.*, 1998). In contrast, the use of incentives based on weight loss did not significantly improve the effectiveness of standard behavioural therapy and participants in both conditions suffered similar weight re-gain following the completion of the intervention (Jeffery & Wing, 1995). When contrasted with the findings on strategies to improve reach (e.g. incentives, low-intensity programmes) these studies suggest that programme characteristics which will attract a higher proportion of employees may be different from programme characteristics which lead to successful weight loss.

More recent literature has highlighted specific strategies and delivery methods for WHP programmes that show promise for future research. For example, friendly competition seems to promote healthy eating, physical activity and worksite cessation rates, without increasing unintended consequences of rapid weight loss or increasing physical activity at an unsafe rate (Klesges *et al.*, 1986; Patterson *et al.*, 1997). Similarly, utilizing interactive computer technologies such as telephone counselling, web-based education, personalized email support and tailored print strategies to provide behavioural therapy may be as effective as time intensive and costly individual face-to-face sessions (Harvey-Berino *et al.*, 2004). Unfortunately, the optimal content and method of delivery for WHPs is still unknown. For example, Internet education alone does not seem to be very effective; however when offered in conjunction with behaviour therapy which included weekly email contact and individualized feedback, weight loss was significantly enhanced (Tate *et al.*, 2001). Similarly, tailored magazines combined with trained employee volunteers were successful in changing F&V (fruit and vegetables) and fat intake in female blue collar workers (Campbell *et al.*, 2002).

Utilizing more participatory methods in programme development and delivery is also an emerging area of potential promise. Studies that have utilized employee steering committees or advisory boards demonstrated improved delivery of health programmes on site and programmes that are appealing to the employees (Hunt *et al.*, 2000). Interactive technologies, participatory research methods and the use of employee volunteers are all promising, but understudied, avenues for future WHP initiatives.

The effectiveness dimension of the RE-AIM framework is also defined by the assessment of quality of life outcomes in addition to unintended negative consequences – which include programme drop out rate. In our review of the recent literature none of the 24 studies that we reviewed reported on quality of life issues for participants; and none of the papers reported measuring potential negative effects that may have been produced (Bull *et al.*, 2003). Approximately half the 24 studies reported attrition rates, with a median rate of 28%. To compound the issue of attrition only 1 of the 24 studies used an intention-to-treat analysis, opting instead to only examine outcomes based on those present at follow-up, thereby potentially overestimating the effect of the programme.

Adoption

All 24 studies in our review reported the number of worksites, and some characteristics of worksites that participated in the research

(Bull *et al.*, 2003). A quarter of the studies reported on the proportion of worksites that participated compared to those which were eligible and the median adoption participation rate among those studies was 56.5%. Only two studies identified exclusion criteria and the number of worksites that were excluded from the research. Number of employees, high employee turnover and non-English speaking employees were the common exclusion criteria. No study reported on the representativeness of the participating worksites on issues of resources, type of business, or median salaries of the employees when compared to the population of eligible worksites. Adding to concerns about the generalization of findings across settings, only 25% of the studies reported any information on characteristics of or participation among staff or persons who conducted the WHP. The interventions were primarily delivered by research staff rather than by regular employees or the in-house departments who would ultimately deliver the programme if it were taken to scale or sustained.

The Well Works Project (Sorensen *et al.*, 1996*a*) provides a good example of reporting on organizational adoption of a research intervention. In that study, the investigators reported the protocol for eligible worksite identification (i.e. they used the Dun and Bradstreet Direct Access Database to identify worksites meeting the eligibility criteria), indicated total number of eligible worksites and the proportion of those approached who agreed to participate. The only aspect of adoption not recounted in Well Works articles was a comparison of the characteristics of adopting vs. non-adopting organizations.

Implementation

Given the strong focus on internal validity within the research community and the relationship between internal validity and treatment fidelity, we were surprised to find that only 3 of the 24 studies we reviewed documented the extent to which the WHP programme was delivered as intended; indicating the degree to which the programme was appropriately implemented (Bull *et al.*, 2003). Each of these studies provided a detailed description of the proportion of process objectives related to the intervention that were achieved, for example, the number of class hours that were taught compared with the number that were prescribed.

In searching for a strong example of the need to document implementation activities, we selected a school-based rather than a worksite-based study. Baranowski and colleagues (Baranowski *et al.*, 2000) provide a good example of rigorously documenting implementation rates of the 'Gimme 5 Fruit, Juice and Vegetables for Fun and Health Trial.' In their study, the intervention curriculum included components to be delivered at the school and newsletters with family activities and instructions for intervention at home. Researchers documented the delivery of the curriculum as intended through classroom observations and teacher self-reports of the completion of the curriculum activities. All teachers were observed at least once during the 6-week intervention. The observations revealed that only about half of the curriculum activities were completed. In addition, the components of the intervention that were not delivered were those which were most likely to lead to behaviour changes. In contrast, teacher self-reported delivery was 90%. Baranowski *et al.* (2000) also documented the delivery of 6 newsletters to parents through follow-up telephone calls to a randomly

selected number of households participating in the study. They found that only 1 in 5 parents recalled receiving all 6 newsletters, while half reported receiving between 3 and 5 newsletters. One caveat to these findings, which raises questions regarding the reliability of participant estimates, is that a small proportion of parents reported receiving more than six newsletters (18%), which was not possible. There is a clear and important need for future WHP studies to document consistency in intervention delivery, provide data on the characteristics of intervention staff who best implement programmes and evaluate how programmes are implemented or adapted. Similarly, there is an area of assessment ripe for research which relate to how evidence-based programmes might be adapted rather than implemented in their entirety and the influence adaptation may have on effectiveness (potentially positive or negative).

Maintenance

Because the majority of WHP studies in our review concentrated on reporting early findings related to their interventions, it is not surprising that only 2 of the 24 (8%) discussed long-term follow-up of study participants or programme sustainability (Bull *et al.*, 2003). One study reported on how well intervention effects were sustained at the individual level two years following the first evaluation; the authors of this study did not indicate whether the programme itself was still in place. One other study did return to worksites two years after the research was complete and reported that the intervention was still in place. Nutrition activities in the Working Well intervention worksites declined over time, but that overall many nutrition activities remained viable. The authors point out, however, that this viability was related to the overall support the institution had for nutrition activities from the start of the study and not necessarily to a change in attitude towards nutrition activities during the intervention (Patterson *et al.*, 1997).

Evidence summary

Our brief review of literature demonstrates that, to date, researchers have focused primarily on an individual rather than on an organizational level of evaluation. Specifically, WHP programmes are associated with some encouraging results related to the effectiveness of different intervention strategies to change health behaviours. However, data on characteristics of participants vs. non-participants and participating settings vs. non-participating settings are limited and this reduces the conclusions that can be made related to the generalizability of these findings. Similarly, indices of the extent to which interventions were delivered as intended (or can be successfully delivered by different types of staff, or regular worksite vs. paid research staff) were rarely reported. Finally, there were few WHP studies that reported on either individual and setting level maintenance effects.

Using research evidence and theory to aid WHP practice

In the face of the current state of WHP research, one emerging area is the use of theory as the basis for intervention development.

Historically WHP studies that have capitalized on theoretical models which attempt to predict behaviour from an individual perspective. A number of notable and effective WHP strategies have been developed based exclusively on individually targeted strategies (Kristal *et al.*, 2000). However, recent research suggests that policy and environmental approaches may also be effective for worksite health promotion programmes. Policy and environmental strategies reflect a social-ecological and public health approach to reducing disparities among employees since such policy changes influence all employees, regardless of demographic and worker characteristics. (French *et al.*, 2001) provided an excellent description of the environmental influences on eating and physical activity. They identified a number of environmental change strategies that could be utilized in worksite settings. Unfortunately, such attempts to exploit the worksite environment, communication systems and social context are rare (Sorensen *et al.*, 2004).

Because initial WHP strategies typically focused on a myriad of activities that targeted individuals to change their behaviour or worksites to change their environment, it is hard to identify which components were responsible for effectiveness. As a result of this lack of detailed understanding, a number of authors have posited that any health behaviour intervention should be based on a sound theory. In a review of physical activity interventions, Baranowski and colleagues (Baranowski *et al.*, 1998) found that interventions based on theoretical models were more effective than those that were not. Using a theoretical basis for intervention has two key benefits. First, a sound theory will provide a blue print for strategies that target theoretical variables thought to lead to behaviour change. In the case of WHP interventions, we agree with the work of Sorensen and colleagues which suggests a sound theory should be operationalized as one that identifies the need to develop strategies

to target both environmental (i.e. organizational) and individual strategies for behaviour change (Sorensen *et al.*, 2004). Second, theory provides a description of mediators of intervention effectiveness (or ineffectiveness) that can be measured and tested to determine why an intervention works or not (for examples of theoretical frameworks see 'Health belief model', 'Health promotion', 'theory of planned behaviour' and 'The transtheoretical model of behaviour change').

The Working Well Trial provides a good example of using theory as the basis for intervention development and assessment of potential mediators of health behaviour change. The intervention model was based in social ecology (Krasnik & Rasmussen, 2002) and highlighted the need to understand the interaction between an individual and her/his environment. Based on the findings from the Working Well Trial, a review of current theories of behaviour change and practical experience developing and testing WHP strategies, Sorensen *et al.* (Sorensen *et al.*, 1996*b*; Sorensen *et al.*, 2004) refined a social ecological framework for WHP which provides an excellent theoretical schematic for intervention development. The model provides the detail necessary to develop interventions and to explicitly test the hypothesis that adding environmental intervention components (i.e. setting and organizational level strategies) will enhance the effectiveness of individually targeted intervention strategies.

The Sorensen *et al.* model describes the importance of social contextual factors that may modify intervention effects, i.e. the social demographic characteristics associated with those factors, and potential social context/setting level and individual level mediating factors. Figure 1 below is a schematic adapted from Sorensen's work and includes example variables for consideration in a WHP. The solid lines in Figure 1 represent hypothesized relationships

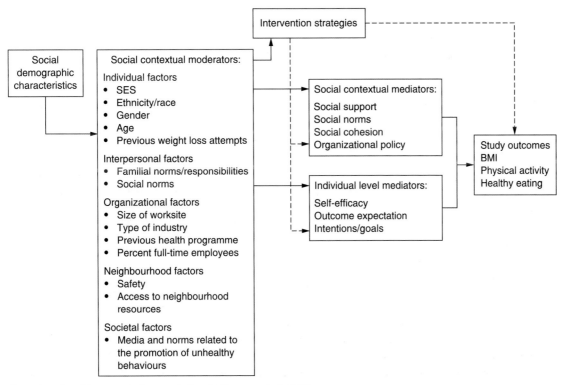

Fig 1 Adaptation of Sorensen *et al*'s conceptual model (Sorensen *et al.*, 2004).

between variables or sets of variables and dashed lines represent intervention effects. The implication of this model is that comprehensive intervention strategies should be developed to change proposed environmental level and individual level mediators, which in turn are hypothesized to have a direct relationship with changes of health behaviour outcomes. There is also the potential that there are additional mediating variables which may not be accounted for in this model and as such it is hypothesized that the intervention may also have direct effects on the outcomes in addition to the indirect effects through the proposed mediating variables.

Summary and future directions

There has been considerable progress in WHP research over the past decade. In particular, many investigations are now evaluating how well WHP reach all employees and also designing interventions for the types of blue-collar, small worksites that were often left out of earlier investigations. One innovative line of research is that of Linnan et al. (Linnan et al., 2002), who have studied beauty parlours as settings for WHPs that also target customers.

Led by a number of investigators from the Working Well and subsequent trials, there has also been a recent increased emphasis on understanding theoretical mechanisms underlying both participation (Linnan et al., 2002a, 2002b; Linnan & Marcus, 2001) and

outcomes (Glanz, 1997; Sorensen et al., 1996b) of WHP. Equally important, the methodological sophistication of WHP research has increased over the past decade, with most studies now including multi-level analyses.

Several challenges remain, however. Few studies have designed interventions for, or evaluated their sustainability after, the time that research funding is removed (i.e. the end of a study). Attrition also remains a challenge in WHP and innovative theoretically based approaches to enhance retention are needed. Greater study of the robustness and generality of WHP effects across key variables such as race and ethnicity; risk level; health literacy; part- vs. full-time status; and of organizational characteristics that may moderate outcomes are needed. Given the social–ecological conceptual model in Figure 1, we predict that the greatest future advances will be made by interventions that address environmental, physical and social as well as individual factors. We predict that such multi-level interventions should be especially effective in producing superior long-term results, but this hypothesis needs to be empirically tested. Although there have been reports of cost-effectiveness (Pelletier, 2001), more such studies, using standard economic methods of determining costs and conducting sensitivity analyses are needed (Gold et al., 2003). Finally, future studies should include both quality of life measures and outcomes important to employers (e.g. presenteeism, impact on recruitment and employee retention).

REFERENCES

Baranowski, T., Anderson, C. & Carmack, C. (1998). Mediating variable framework in physical activity intervention: How are we doing? How might we do better? *American Journal of Preventive Medicine*, **15**, 266–97.

Baranowski, T., Davis, M., Resnicow, K. et al. (2000). Gimme 5 fruit, juice, and vegetables for fun and health: outcome evaluation. *Health Education and Behavior*, **27**, 96–111.

Bull, S. S., Gillette, C., Glasgow, R. E. & Estabrooks, P. (2003). Worksite health promotion research: to what extent can we generalize the results and what is needed to translate research to practice? *Health Education and Behavior*, **30**, 537–49.

Campbell, M. K., Tessaro, I., DeVellis, B. et al. (2002). Effects of a tailored health promotion program for female blue-collar workers: Health Works for Women. *Preventive Medicine*, **34**, 313–23.

French, S. A., Story, M. & Jeffery, R. W. (2001). Environmental influences on eating and physical activity. *Annual Review of Public*, **22**, 309–35.

Glanz, K. (1997). Behavioral research contributions and needs in cancer prevention and control: dietary change. *Preventive Medicine*, **26**, S43–S55.

Glasgow, R. E., Hollis, J. F., Ary, D. V. & Lando, H. A. (1990). Employee and

organizational factors associated with participation in an incentive-based worksite smoking cessation program. *Journal of Behavioral Medicine*, **13**, 403–18.

Glasgow, R. E., McCaul, K. D. & Fisher, K. J. (1993). Participation in worksite health promotion: a critique of the literature and recommendations for future practice. *Health Education Quarterly*, **20**, 291–408.

Glasgow, R. E., Vogt, T. M. & Boles, S. M. (1999). Evaluating the public health impact of health promotion interventions: the RE-AIM framework. *American Journal of Public Health*, **89**, 1322–7.

Gold, M. R., Siegel, J. E., Russell, L. B. & Wenstein, M. C. (2003). *Cost effectiveness in health and medicine.* New York, NY: Oxford University Press.

Harvey-Berino, J., Pintauro, S., Buzzell, P. & Gold, E. C. (2004). Effect of Internet support on the long-term maintenance of weight loss. *Obesity Research*, **12**, 320–9.

Hennrikus, D. & Jeffery, R. W. (1996). Worksite intervention for weight control: a review of the literature. *The Science of Health Promotion*, **10**, 471–98.

Hennrikus, D., Jeffery, R. W., Lando, H. et al. (2002). The SUCCESS Project: the effect of program format and incentives on participation and cessation in worksite smoking cessation programs.

American Journal of Public Health, **92**, 274–9.

Hunt, M. K., Lederman, R., Potter, S., Stoddard, A. & Sorensen, G. (2000). Results of employee involvement in planning and implementing the Treatwell 5-a-day work-site study. *Health Education and Behavior*, **27**, 223–31.

Jeffery, R. W., Thorson, C., Wing, R. R. & Burton, L. R. (1998). Use of personal trainers and financial incentives to increase exercise in a behavioral weight-loss program. *Journal of Consulting and Clinical Psychology*, **66**, 777–83.

Jeffery, R. W. & Wing, R. R. (1995). Long-term effects of interventions for weight loss using food provision and monetary incentives. *Journal of Consulting and Clinical Psychology*, **63**, 793–6.

Klesges, R. C., Vasey, M. M. & Glasgow, R. E. (1986). A worksite smoking modification competition: potential for public health impact. *American Journal of Public Health*, **76**, 198–200.

Krasnik, A. & Rasmussen, N. K. (2002). Reducing social inequalities in health: evidence, policy, and practice. *Scandinavian Journal of Public Health*, **30**(Suppl. 59), 1–5.

Kristal, A. R., Glanz, K., Tilley, B. C. & Li, S. (2000). Mediating factors in dietary change: understanding the impact of a worksite nutrition intervention. *Health Education and Behavior*, **27**, 112–25.

Linnan, L. A., Emmons, K. & Abrams, D. B. (2002*a*). Beauty and the Beast: results of the Rhode Island Smokefree Shop Initiative. *American Journal of Public Health*, **92**, 27–8.

Linnan, L. A., Emmons, K. M., Klar, N. *et al.* (2002*b*). Challenges to improving the impact of worksite cancer prevention programs: comparing reach, enrollment, and attrition using active versus passive recruitment strategies. *Annals of Behavioral Medicine*, **24**, 157–66.

Linnan, L. A. & Marcus, B. (2001). Worksite-based physical activity programs and older adults: current status and priorities for the future. *Journal of Aging and Physical Activity*, **9**, S59–S70.

Marcus, B. H., Emmons, K. M., Simkin-Silverman, L. R. *et al.* (1998). Evaluation of a motivationally tailored vs. standard self-help physical activity interventions at the workplace. *American Journal of Health Promotion*, **12**, 246–53.

McTigue, K. M., Harris, R., Hemphill, B., Lux, L. & Sutton, S. (2003). Screening and interventions for obesity in adults: summary of the evidence for the U. S. preventive services task force. *Annals of Internal Medicine*, **139**, 933–49.

Mokdad, A. H., Marks, J. F., Stroup, D. F. & Gerdes, D. A. (2004). Actual causes of death in the United States, 2000. *Journal of American Medical Association*, **291**, 1238–45.

Patterson, R. E., Kristal, A. R., Glanz, K. *et al.* (1997). Components of the Working Well trial intervention associated with adoption of healthful diets. *American Journal of Preventive Medicine*, **13**, 271–6.

Pelletier, K. R. (2001). A review and analysis of the clinical- and cost-effectiveness studies of comprehensive health promotion and disease management programs at the worksite: 1998–2000 update. *The Science of Health Promotion*, **16**, 107–16.

Riedel, J. E., Lynch, W., Baase, C., Hymel, P. & Peterson, K. W. (2001). The effect of disease prevention and health promotion on workplace productivity: a literature review. *American Journal of Health Behavior*, **15**, 167–91.

Sorensen, G., Barbeau, E., Hunt, M. K. & Emmons, K. (2004). Reducing social disparities in tobacco use: a social–contextual model for reducing tobacco use among blue-collar workers. *American Journal of Public Health*, **94**, 230–9.

Sorensen, G., Stoddard, A., LaMontagne, A. D. *et al.* (2000). A comprehensive worksite cancer prevention intervention: behavior change results from a randomized controlled trial (United States). *Journal of Public Health Policy*, **24**, 5–25.

Sorensen, G., Stoddard, A., Ockene, J. K., Hunt, M. K. & Youngstrom, R. (1996*a*). Worker participation in an integrated health promotion/health protection program: results from the WellWorks project. *Health Education Quarterly*, **23**, 191–203.

Sorensen, G., Thompson, B., Glanz, K. *et al.* (1996*b*). Work site-based cancer prevention: primary results from the Working Well Trial. *American Journal of Public Health*, **86**, 939–47.

Tate, D. F., Wing, R. R. & Winett, R. A. (2001). Using Internet technology to deliver a behavioral weight loss program. *Journal of American Medical Association*, **285**, 1172–7.

Healthcare practice

Adherence to treatment

Rob Horne

University of London

Introduction

Non-adherence is perceived to be a significant problem in all aspects of healthcare from taking medication to attending counselling sessions. Thousands of research papers have been published on the topic in the last few decades yet non-adherence remains a key challenge in modern healthcare. The main focus of research and reviews has been on adherence to medication prescribed for long-term medical conditions. This is hardly surprising. In affluent countries, most healthcare resources are devoted to the management of chronic diseases such as coronary heart disease, diabetes and asthma. Here, good outcomes depend as much on self-management by the patient as on good medical care and, for most of these conditions, self-management hinges on the appropriate use of medicines. However many patients fail to achieve this. Estimates of the incidence of non-adherence to medication range widely from 2–98%, partly because of differences in the way adherence is defined and measured across studies. Most reviews estimates that 30–50% of medication prescribed for chronic illness is not taken as directed (Meichenbaum & Turk, 1987; Myers & Midence, 1998; World Health Organization, 2003). If the prescription was appropriate, then this level of non-adherence is a concern for those providing, receiving or funding healthcare because it not only entails a waste of resources but also a missed opportunity for therapeutic benefit (DiMatteo et al., 2002). Unfortunately, effective interventions remain elusive (Haynes et al., 2002).

This chapter will focus on medication adherence. It will begin by summarizing our current understanding of the causes of non-adherence and from this explain why interventions have so far met with such disappointing results will then go on to suggest how we might rectify the problem. Although a full review of adherence to all health-related behaviour is beyond the scope of this chapter, many of the insights from research into medication adherence might be applied to other behaviours such as diet, exercise and smoking cessation.

The causes of non-adherence

Dispelling common myths

Non-adherence is not significantly related to the type or severity of disease with rates of between 25–30% noted across 17 disease conditions (DiMatteo, 2004b). Furthermore, providing clear information, although essential, is not enough to guarantee adherence (Weinman, 1990). Likewise, a plethora of studies have failed to identify clear and consistent relations between adherence and sociodemographic variables such as gender and age in adults (DiMatteo, 2004a;

Horne, 1998). Adherence is positively correlated with income when the patient is paying for treatment (Piette et al., 2004) but not with general socioeconomic status (DiMatteo, 2004a). Non-adherence is often lower for more complex regimens, but reducing the frequency of dosage administrations does not always solve the problem (Claxton et al., 2001). There is little evidence that adherence behaviours can be explained in terms of trait personality characteristics. Even if stable associations existed between sociodemographic or trait characteristics, they would serve to identify certain 'at risk' groups so that interventions could be targeted but could do little to inform the type or content of these interventions. This is not to say that sociodemographic or dispositional characteristics are irrelevant. Rather, the associations with adherence appear to be indirect and are best explained by the influence of sociodemographic and dispositional characteristics on other relevant parameters. For example, correlations between adherence and educational status or race may simply be a reflection of income and ability to afford prescription costs.

The notion of the 'non-adherent patient' is a myth: most of us are non-adherent some of the time. Stable characteristics such as the nature of the disease and treatment, or sociodemographic variables, influence the adherence behaviour of some patients more than others. Non-adherence is therefore best seen as a variable behaviour.

Non-adherence as a variable behaviour with intentional and unintentional causes

There are many causes of non-adherence but they fall into two overlapping categories – intentional and unintentional. Unintentional non-adherence occurs when the patient's intentions to take the medication are thwarted by barriers such as poor recall or comprehension of instructions, difficulties in administering the treatment or simply forgetting. Deliberate or intentional non-compliance arises when the patient decides not to follow the treatment recommendations. It follows that we need to consider two issues – resources and motivation. Unintentional non-compliance is linked to problems of resources. To understand intentional non-adherence we need to consider the processes influencing motivation to start and continue with treatment. Clearly, there is a degree of overlap between these behaviours: motivation may overcome resource barriers and resource barriers may reduce motivation. However, this simple model is useful because it helps us to understand why previous attempts have met with only limited success.

Why adherence interventions have had limited effect

Literature searches using established search terms (Haynes et al., 2002) suggest that over 120 articles reporting unconfounded

R. Horne

randomized controlled trials of adherence interventions have been published since 1972. This literature has been subjected to a range of systematic reviews (Haynes *et al.*, 1996; Peterson *et al.*, 2003; Roter *et al.*, 1998) including a recent Cochrane systematic review (Haynes *et al.*, 2002). The overall conclusion of these systematic reviews is that, 'complex strategies for improving adherence with long-term medication prescriptions are not very effective despite the amount of effort and resources they consume' (Haynes *et al.*, 2002, p. 9). Even successful interventions have modest or short-lived effects.

The main problem relates to the design of the interventions themselves. Few interventions have targeted proven determinants of non-adherence. Instead they typically use ad hoc approaches that are not well described or standardized. Most interventions are not sufficiently comprehensive. The majority have addressed unintentional non-adherence with an implicit assumption that adherence can be improved through more effective communication of instructions; by better patient education; or by addressing non-volitional barriers such as forgetting or poor recall of instructions (by issuing reminders), or by addressing failure to make plans when attempting to adhere to a complex regimen (see, for example, 'Healthcare professional–patient communication' and 'Neuropsychological rehabilitation'). Although this approach may be helpful for many patients, its efficacy is likely to be limited because it fails to address the causes of intentional non-adherence.

A further problem is that it is difficult to judge why some interventions work and others do not. Interventions that are complex, addressing both intentional and unintentional non-adherence tend to be more effective than single component interventions. Few papers describe the content of the interventions in sufficient detail. Most studies assessing complex interventions did not evaluate the separate components ('black box' approach) or assess process variables, so that we remain uncertain about what was effective or whether all elements of the intervention were required.

Potential solutions

The need for theory-based interventions

A core recommendation of the UK Medical Research Council's (2000) framework for the development of complex interventions to improve health is that the intervention should be based on a sound theoretical model. This is germane to adherence where few interventions have used psychological theories to identify the salient factors influencing motivation to start and persist with medication.

Several theoretical models have been developed to explain how people initiate and maintain actions to preserve or improve health status. These models share the common assumption that the motivation to engage in and maintain health-related behaviours arises from beliefs that influence the interpretation of information and experiences and which guide behaviour (Conner & Norman, 1996; Horne & Weinman, 1998). The capacity of theoretical models to explain variance in adherence and other behaviours is of course determined by the validity of the model and whether it contains the right 'constructs'. It is also influenced by the way in which the constructs are operationalized. In social cognition models, the antecedents of behaviour are specified at the 'process'

level (e.g. attitudes inform intentions and behaviour) (see 'Theory of planned behaviour').

When theoretical models are used to develop interventions then they are likely to be more effective if they also specify content (e.g. the beliefs that contribute to the positive or negative evaluations which constitute the attitude towards the behaviour). This is recognized within the Common-Sense Model of self-regulation (CSM) where the content as well as the process of illness representations is specified (Leventhal *et al.*, 1998) (see 'Lay beliefs about health and illness'). However, theoretical models of health behaviour are likely to be more explanatory as their contents become more specific to the behaviour in question (Fishbein & Ajzen, 1975). Although representations of coping procedures are implicit within the CSM a more explicit consideration of perceptions of treatment may be useful when the model is applied to adherence(Horne, 2003). A better understanding of how people perceive treatments will improve our ability to operationalize theories of social cognition and self-regulation and enhance their power to explain variations in adherence (see also 'Health cognition assessment' and 'Illness cognition assessment').

Operationalizing the salient beliefs influencing treatment adherence: the example of general and specific beliefs about medication

The first step in identifying salient beliefs about treatment (i.e. those beliefs influencing behaviour) is to conduct interview-based studies to examine beliefs about the behaviour, their expectancies and the value they place on the expected outcome (Ajzen & Fishbein, 1980). In the case of medication, qualitative studies have suggested that many people seem to hold prototypic beliefs about pharmaceuticals as a class of treatment and their capacity to produce harm as well as benefit and beliefs about the appropriateness of doctors' prescribing of medicines (Horne, 1997). Moreover, many people seem to be have a fairly negative orientation to pharmaceuticals perceiving them to be fundamentally harmful, addictive substance that should not be taken for long periods of time but that tend to be over-prescribed by doctors (Horne *et al.*, 1999). These 'social representations' of medicines are linked to wider concerns about scientific medicine, lack of trust in doctors and an increasing interest in alternative or complementary healthcare (Calnan *et al.*, 2005). These general beliefs influence the way in which people evaluate specific medication prescribed for a particular medical condition. They frame initial expectations of the outcome of taking the prescribed medication (Cooper *et al.*, 2004), as well as how subsequent events are interpreted – for example whether symptoms are attributed to the illness or the treatment (Siegel *et al.*, 1999) (see 'Symptom perception'). They may even influence outcome directly through the placebo/nocebo effect (see Di Blasi *et al.*, (2001) for a review of non-specific treatment effects) (see also 'Placebos').

Making decisions about adherence: judging perceived necessity and concerns

One method for operationalizing people's initial and subsequent evaluation of medicines prescribed for specific conditions ('specific medication beliefs') that has been quite widely applied in adherence research is the necessity–concerns framework (Horne *et al.*, 1999).

This suggests that the motivation to start and persist with prescribed treatment regimens is influenced by the way in which the individual judges their personal need for the treatment relative to their concerns about potential adverse effects of taking it as recommended. Studies involving patients from a wide range of illness groups including asthma (Horne & Weinman, 2002), renal disease (Horne *et al.*, 2001), diabetes, cancer and coronary heart disease (Horne & Weinman, 1999), hypertension (Ross *et al.*, 2004), HIV/AIDS (Horne *et al.*, 2004), haemophilia (Llewellyn *et al.*, 2003) and depression (Aikens *et al.*, 2005) have consistently found that low rates of adherence are related to doubts about personal need for medication and concerns about potential adverse effects.

It is worth noting that perceived necessity is not a form of efficacy belief. Although views about medication efficacy are likely to contribute to perceived need, the constructs are not synonymous. We might believe that a treatment will be effective but yet not perceive a personal need for it. Conversely, we might perceive a strong need for a treatment that we believe to be only moderately effective, because we know that it is the only treatment that is available. Necessity beliefs are influenced by perceptions of the condition being treated (Horne & Weinman, 2002) as well as by symptom expectations and experiences (Cooper, 2004).

There is a striking similarity in the type of concerns that patients report about prescription medicines. One obvious source of concern is the experience of symptoms as medication 'side-effects' and the disruptive effects of medication on daily living; but this is not the whole picture. Many patients receiving regular medication who have not experienced adverse effects are still worried about possible problems in the future. These often arise from the belief that regular use can lead to dependence, or that the medication will accumulate within the body and lead to long-term effects and these problems are related to the social representations of medicines as being harmful and over-used as discussed above (Horne *et al.*, 1999). Other concerns are specific to the particular class of medicine (Horne & Weinman, 2002). For example, worries that corticosteroid inhalers prescribed for asthma will result in weight gain (Hand & Bradley, 1996) or that regular use of analgesic medication now will make it less effective in the future (Gill & Williams, 2001).

Evidence to date is consistent with the notion that medication adherence is influenced by a cost–benefit analysis in which patients' beliefs about the necessity of their medication are weighed against concerns about the potential adverse effects of taking it. The 'cost–benefit analysis' may be implicit rather than explicit. For example, in some situations, non-adherence could be the result of a deliberate strategy to minimize harm by taking less medication. Alternatively, it might simply be a reflection of the fact that patients who do not perceive their medication to be important are more likely to forget to take it. The impact of perceptions of treatment on adherence will also influenced by beliefs about adherence, such as the importance of strict adherence to achieve the desired outcome (Siegel *et al.*, 2000).

Prior to treatment, necessity beliefs and concerns may be thought of as higher order outcome expectancies which are influenced by beliefs about the illness and treatment as well as more general 'social representations' of, and preferences for, classes of treatments. Once treatment has commenced they are influenced by appraisal processes (Horne, 2003).

Preliminary evidence suggests that the framework can be used to operationalize 'treatment representations' within Leventhal's CSM and adds to the variance in reported adherence than can be explained by illness representations alone (Horne & Weinman, 2002; Ross *et al.*, 2004). Recent research suggests that the necessity–concerns framework may also be applied to other treatment-related behaviours such as attendance at cardiac rehabilitation classes (Cooper *et al.*, in press). However, futher research is needed to establish the utility of the framework in prospective studies and in interventions studies.

Other factors and challenges

Several other important issues need to be addressed in operationalizing social cognition and self-regulatory theories as a basis for adherence interventions. The effects of emotion and mood are likely to be important. A meta-analysis of 25 high quality studies investigating the relationship between depression (12 studies) and anxiety (13 studies) found that the relationship between depression and non-adherence to medication prescribed for chronic illnesses (other than depression) was substantial. Anxiety had little effect (DiMatteo *et al.*, 2000). A further aspect that needs attention is how we enable patients to overcome the resource and capacity limitations that act as barriers to the implementation of intentions to adhere to treatment. An example of promising work in this area utilizes the concept of 'implementation intentions' or action plans (Gollwitzer, 1999) to tie specific behaviours to environmental cues by prompting the planning of when and how the behaviour can be carried out (Sheeran & Orbell, 1999) (see 'Theory of planned behaviour').

A further area for future research is the effect of social support. Social support appears to have broadly positive effects on adherence but we know little about the mechanism or the type of support that works best in what situations (DiMatteo, 2004). A further challenge to adherence research includes the issue of measurement and how to reduce self-presentational bias so that adherence behaviour can be reliably and accurately assessed.

Developing complex intervention to facilitate adherence

The main priority for research is to develop effective, equitable and efficient interventions to facilitate informed adherence where adherence matters most. Previous interventions have had limited effects partly because they have not been comprehensive enough. Many have focused on single causal factors whereas adherence is best seen as unintentional and intentional behaviours with internal and external determinants. The 'internal' factors influencing motivation and capacity may be moderated by 'external' variables, such as the quality of communication between the patient and healthcare provider and by the wider societal contexts such as access to resources and societal policy and practice. Future interventions may be more effective if they address both the perceptual factors influencing motivation to initiate and persist with the recommended behaviour, as well as facilitating the implantation of intentions to adhere, for example by addressing the capacity and resource limitations that act as barriers.

REFERENCES

Aikens, J. E., Nease, D. E., Jr., Nau, D. P., Klinkman, M. S. & Schwenk, T. L. (2005). Adherence to maintenance-phrase antidepressant medication as a function of patient beliefs about medication. *Annals of Family Medicine*, **3**(1), 23–30.

Ajzen, I. & Fishbein, M. (1980). *Understanding attitudes and predicting social behaviour*. Englewood Cliffs, NJ: Prentice-Hall.

Calnan, M., Montaner, D. & Horne, R. (2005). How acceptable are innovative health-care technologies? A survey of public beliefs and attitudes in England and Wales. *Social Science and Medicine*, **60**(9), 1937–48.

Claxton, A.J., Cramer, J. & Pierce, C. (2001). A systematic review of the associations between dose regimens and medication compliance 1. *Clinical Therapeutics*, **23**(8), 1296–310.

Conner, M. & Norman, P. (1996). The role of social cognition in health behaviours. In P. Norman (Ed.). *Predicting health behaviour: research and practice with social cognition models* (pp. 1–22). Buckingham, UK: Open University Press.

Cooper, A.F., Jackson, G., Weinman, J. & Horne, R. (in press). A qualitative study investigating patients beliefs about cardiac rehabilitation. *Journal of Clinical Rehabilitation*.

Cooper, V. (2004). Explaining adherence to Highly Active Anti-Retroviral Therapy (HAART): the utility of an extended self-regulatory model. Unpublished PhD thesis. Brighton, UK: University of Brighton.

Cooper, V., Gelliatry, G. & Horne, R. (2004). Treatment perceptions and self-regulation in adherence to HAART. *International Journal of Behavioral Medicine*, **11**(Suppl.), 81.

Di Blasi, Z., Harkness, E., Ernst, E., Georgiou, A. & Kleijnen, J. (2001). Influence of context effects on health outcomes: a systematic review. *Lancet*, **357**, 757–62.

DiMatteo, M.R. (2004a). Social support and patient adherence to medical treatment: a meta-analysis 1. *Health Psychology*, **23**(2), 207–18.

DiMatteo, M.R. (2004b). Variations in patients' adherence to medical recommendations: a quantitative review of 50 years of research. *Medical Care*, **42**(3), 200–9.

DiMatteo, M.R., Giordani, P.J., Lepper, H.S. & Croghan, T.W. (2002). Patient adherence and medical treatment outcomes: a meta-analysis. *Medical Care*, **40**(9), 794–811.

DiMatteo, M.R., Lepper, H.S. & Croghan, T.W. (2000). Depression is a risk factor for noncompliance with medical treatment: meta-analysis of the effects of anxiety and depression on patient adherence. *Archives of Internal Medicine*, **160**(14), 2101–7.

Fishbein, M. & Ajzen, I. (1975). *Belief, attitude, intention, and behavior: an introduction to theory and research*. Reading, MA; London: Addison-Wesley.

Gill, A. & Williams, A.C. (2001). Preliminary study of chronic pain patients' concerns about cannabinoids as analgesics. *Clinical Journal of Pain*, **17**(3), 245–8.

Gollwitzer, P.M. (1999). Implementation intentions – strong effects of simple plans. *American Psychologist*, **54**(7), 493–503.

Gollwitzer, P.M. & Brandstatter, V. (1997). Implementation intentions and effective goal pursuit. *Journal of Personality and Social Psychology*, **73**(1), 186–99.

Hand, C.H. & Bradley, C. (1996). Health beliefs of adults with asthma: toward an understanding of the difference between symptomatic and preventive use of inhaler treatment. *Journal of Asthma*, **33**(5), 331–8.

Haynes, R.B., McDonald, H., Garg, A.X. & Montague, P. (2002). Interventions for helping patients to follow prescriptions for medications. Cochrane Database of Systematic Reviews, *Issue 2*. Art. No.: CD000011.DOI: 10.1002/14651858.

Haynes, R.B., McKibbon, K.A. & Kanani, R. (1996). Systematic review of randomised clinical trials of interventions to assist patients to follow prescriptions for medications. *Lancet*, **348**, 383–86.

Horne, R. (1997). Representations of medication and treatment: advances in theory and measurement. In K.J. Petrie & J.A. Weinman (Eds.). *Perceptions of health and illness: current research and applications* (pp. 155–88). London: Harwood Academic Press.

Horne, R. (1998). Adherence to medication: a review of existing research. In L. Myers & K. Midence (Eds.). *Adherence to treatment in medical conditions* (pp. 285–310). London: Harwood Academic Press.

Horne, R. (2003). Treatment perceptions and self regulation. In L.D. Cameron & H. Leventhal (Eds.). *The self-regulation of health and illness behaviour* (pp. 138–53). London: Routledge.

Horne, R., Buick, D., Fisher, M. *et al.* (2004). Doubts about necessity and concerns about adverse effects: identifying the types of beliefs that are associated with non-adherence to HAART. *International Journal of STD and AIDS*, (**15**), 38–44.

Horne, R., Sumner, S., Jubraj, B., Weinman, J. & Frost, S. (2001). Haemodialysis patients' beliefs about treatment: implications for adherence to medication and fluid-diet restrictions. *International Journal of Pharmacy Practice*, **9**, 169–75.

Horne, R. & Weinman, J. (1998). Predicting treatment adherence: an overview of theoretical models. In L. Myers & K. Midence (Eds.). *Adherence to treatment in medical conditions* (pp. 25–50). London: Harwood Academic Press.

Horne, R. & Weinman, J. (1999). Patients' beliefs about prescribed medicines and their role in adherence to treatment in chronic physical illness. *Journal of Psychosomatic Research*, **47**(6), 555–67.

Horne, R. & Weinman, J. (2002). Self-regulation and self-management in asthma: exploring the role of illness perceptions and treatment beliefs in explaining non-adherence to preventer medication. *Psychology and Health*, **17**(1), 17–32.

Horne, R., Weinman, J. & Hankins, M. (1999). The beliefs about medicines questionnaire: the development and evaluation of a new method for assessing the cognitive representation of medication. *Psychology and Health*, **14**, 1–24.

Leventhal, H., Leventhal, E.A. & Contrada, R.J. (1998). Self-regulation, health and behavior: a perceptual–cognitive approach. *Psychology and Health*, **13**, 717–33.

Llewellyn, C., Miners, A., Lee, C., Harrington, C. & Weinman, J. (2003). The illness perceptions and treatment beliefs of individuals with severe haemophilia and their role in adherence to home treatment. *Health Psychology*, **18**(2), 185–200.

Medical Research Council (2000). *A framework for development and evaluation of RCTs for complex interventions to improve health*. Oxford: MRC.

Meichenbaum, D. & Turk, D.C. (1987). *Facilitating treatment adherence: a practitioner's handbook*. New York: Plenum Press.

Myers, L.B. & Midence, K. (1998). Methodological and conceptual issues in adherence. In L.B. Myers & K. Midence (Eds.). *Adherence to treatment in medical conditions*. Amsterdam: Harwood Academic Publishers.

Peterson, A.M., Takiya, L. & Finley, R. (2003). Meta-analysis of interventions to improve drug adherence in patients with hyperlipidemia. *Pharmacotherapy*, **23**(1), 80–7.

Piette, J.D., Heisler, M. & Wagner, T.H. (2004). Cost-related medication underuse: an analysis of tough choices by chronically ill patients. *American Journal of Public Health*.

Ross, S., Walker, A. & MacLeod, M.J. (2004). Patient compliance in hypertension: role of illness perceptions and treatment beliefs.

Journal of Human Hypertension, **18**(9), 607–13.

Roter, D.L., Hall, J.A., Merisca, R. *et al.* (1998). Effectiveness of interventions to improve patient compliance: a meta-analysis. *Medical Care*, **36**(8), 1138–61.

Sheeran, P. & Orbell, S. (1999). Implementation intentions and repeated behaviour: augmenting the predictive validity of the Theory of Planned Behaviour. *European Journal of Social Psychology*, **29**(2/3), 349–70.

Siegel, K., Dean, L. & Schrimshaw, E. (1999). Symptom ambiguity among late middle aged and older adults with HIV. *Research on Aging*, **21**(4), 595–618.

Siegel, K., Schrimshaw, E.W. & Raveis, V.H. (2000). Accounts for non-adherence to antiviral combination therapies among older HIV-infected adults. *Psychology, Health and Medicine*, **5**(1), 29–42.

Weinman, J. (1990). Providing written information for patients: psychological considerations. *Journal of the Royal Society of Medicine*, **83**, 303–5.

World Health Organization (2003). *Adherence to long-term therapies: evidence for action.* Geneva: World Health Organization.

Attitudes of health professionals

Hannah M. McGee

Royal College of Surgeons in Ireland

Introduction

Research on attitudes of health professionals has been a relatively marginal activity until recently. This has been because of what Marteau and Johnston (1990) describe as the implicit model of health professional attitudes and beliefs, i.e. that they are knowledge-based and invariant. Health professionals have been seen as having an empirically derived set of shared beliefs. However, a developing literature demonstrates wide variability in health professional attitudes. The importance of this variability is illustrated here in a range of studies which depict the presentation of treatment options for healthcare users, the professional choices made about access to services and the overall outcome of healthcare for patients and professionals. Many of the studies to date have been atheoretical, focusing instead on a description of attitudes themselves or on their associates. Attitudes of health professionals are often inferred rather than being directly assessed. For instance, previous experience is often assessed in relation to current behaviour with attitudes then inferred, as in the finding that patterns of greater hospital referral for childhood gastroenteritis by general practitioners was associated with prior specialist training in infectious diseases settings (McGee & Fitzgerald, 1991). Divergent current behaviour, e.g. higher levels of referral to cardiac surgery for male than female patients (King *et al.*, 1992) are also documented and attitudinal influences inferred (in this case a range of attitudes including those relating to the severity of symptoms as presented by men and women). Some cognitive and social psychological constructs have been incorporated in research studies of health professional attitudes, and these are illustrated alongside methodological strategies in the next sections.

Attitudes of health professionals to varying characteristics of healthcare users

Health professionals attribute a range of treatment-relevant characteristics to service users based on information available to them. Thus patients who are reported to practice lifestyle habits associated with the disorder which has been diagnosed, e.g. smoking with lung cancer, are believed to be less concerned about their health and less adherent to medical recommendations (Marteau & Riordan, 1992). Recall of details regarding individuals is greater when it fits with the expected stereotypes of health professionals. For instance, when specific characteristics (e.g. 'promiscuous') were paired with particular background details (e.g. 'homosexual'), they were recalled more readily by counsellors (Casas *et al.*, 1983). Professional attributions may also differ in relation to patient gender. Cardiac staff have been shown to attribute psychological difficulties following coronary artery bypass surgery to 'emotional problems' in women and to 'organic problems' in men (King *et al.*, 1992) (see 'Gender issues and women's health'). Attitudes also vary in relation to the particular type of health professional involved and in relation to the type of health problem under consideration. In general, health professionals are less willing to work with patients with more chronic disorders and with those individuals having a poorer prognosis. Margolies *et al.* (1983) demonstrated that medical students want more professional distance from psychiatric than from cancer patients and from cancer than myocardial infarction patients. Similarly, they want more distance from male than female patients and from those with a poor rather than good prognosis. With regard to differences associated with the type of health professional training undertaken, occupational therapists and physiotherapists have been found to rate the likely benefit of health care to disabled individuals as being higher than do nurses (Johnston *et al.*, 1987).

Professional choices about access to health services

It is difficult to directly document how professional attitudes per se influence choices about treatment for particular patients. A classic experimental study by McNeil and colleagues (1982) demonstrated that the format in which information is presented can influence healthcare choices for patients, students and physicians. The research task involved choosing between surgical and medical management of cancer given various facts about short- and long-term risks and framing the information in either a positive (survival statistics) or a negative (mortality statistics) manner. For all groups, information presented in a positive framework led to higher levels of adoption of the treatment alternative than did the same statistics presented negatively (i.e. as mortality data). Service availability may be influenced by implicit beliefs about appropriate behaviour by different groups, e.g. women and men. One illustration in the cardiac setting showed that physicians were perceived as providing stronger recommendations to attend cardiac rehabilitation programmes to male than to female patients (Ades *et al.*, 1992). In a study of prescribing of antibiotics by primary care physicians, Walker *et al.* (2001) showed that professional attitudes influenced intention to prescribe. This study used a theoretical model to consider the relationship of factors such as social norm and attitudes in determining professional behaviour (see 'Theory of planned behaviour'). More generally, a theoretically based approach to changing health professional, as distinct from patient, behaviour has recently been described. The PRIME project includes assessment of professional attitudes, alongside other factors in a variety of professional settings (Walker *et al.*, 2003). This work explicitly uses social cognition models (in particular the Theory of Planned Behaviour) to assess health professional attitudes. The work focuses on variation in adoption of evidence-based recommendation, rather than just prescribing behaviour.

Outcome of health services for users and professionals

The attitudes and behaviour of health professionals are often influenced by expectations regarding individuals or health problems. Thus, a review of studies which have documented the under-diagnosis of mental health problems in patients with physical disorders and vice versa (Lopez, 1989) suggests a dualist understanding of physical and psychological health problems and illustrates that those with both types of problem may be under-served by the current approach of health professionals. More generally, the literature on the placebo effect demonstrates how the attitudes of professionals to health service users and their health problems may be a powerful influence in accelerating or retarding recovery (Di Blasi *et al.*, 2001) (see 'Placebos').

Health services may be withheld because of a range of attitudes and beliefs of health professionals; thus advice on smoking cessation may be withheld because professionals either believe that patients are not receptive to advice or because they believe that they themselves are not capable of providing the appropriate advice (Braun *et al.*, 2004) with differences across professionals, e.g. nurses less

willing to provide advice than physicians. The attitude of the health professional may be expressed in his or her interactions and may thus influence the health outcome. In an early study, Milmoe *et al.* (1967) demonstrated that the degree of hostility expressed in a physician's voice tone while talking about alcoholic patients was positively associated with physician failure in getting patients into treatment for alcohol problems.

Future directions

The developing literature on attitudes of health professionals is complemented by a more rapidly expanding research focus on cognitive aspects of decision-making in health settings. From the work of Tversky and Kahneman (1981), a large literature on clinical decision-making has evolved (see 'Medical decision-making'). There is overlap between these two approaches, i.e. one approach which focuses on cognitive processes which are seen to be universal influences on health professional decision-making and another which documents attitudes (affective processes) seen to be exhibited by particular individuals or groups of professionals. Attention to this overlap may lead to a greater understanding of the nature of health professional behaviour and to more effective methods of educating health professionals as active evaluators of their own influence on the practice of, and outcome from, their interventions. An illustration of research at this level is the evolution of work on adherence to health professional recommendations. Here, rather than searching for the 'non-compliant personality' of the 'patient', recent research has focused on the interaction between health professional and service user and on how characteristics of the health professional and the context influence levels of adherence to health recommendations. Another example of the likely application of a joint approach is the area of professional preferences where, for instance, professionals and service users are both influenced in their choice of treatment by a positive framing (survival rather than mortality data) of information (McNeil *et al.*, 1982). Here, the evaluation of affective influences on choice for individual professionals, e.g. the influence of exposure to the disorder in one's own family or the influence of a poor outcome for a previous case in one's care, could complement the documentation of these general cognitive processes as displayed in decision-making.

Further study of the attitudes of health professionals may counterbalance previous attention which was restricted to the attitudes of service users only. If included in a wider research agenda as suggested here, the findings should positively influence the individual professional's understanding and management of his or her role and thereby improve the delivery of health services in the future.

REFERENCES

Ades, P.A., Wildmann, M.L., Polk, D.M. & Coflesky, J.T. (1992). Referral patterns and exercise response in the rehabilitation of female coronary patients aged >62 years. *American Journal of Cardiology*, **69**, 1422–5.

Braun, B.L., Fowles, J.B., Solberg, L.I. *et al.* (2004). Smoking-related attitudes and clinical practices of medical personnel

in Minnesota. *American Journal of Preventive Medicine*, **27**, 316–22.

Casas, J.M., Brady, S. & Ponterotto, J.G. (1983). Sexual preference biases in counselling: an information processing approach. *Journal of Counselling Psychology*, **30**, 139–45.

Di Blasi, Z., Harkness, E., Ernst, E., Georgiou, A. & Kleijnen, J. (2001).

Influence of context effects on health outcomes: a systematic review. *Lancet*, **357**, 757–62.

Johnston, M., Bromley, I., Boothroyd-Brooks, M. *et al.* (1987). Behavioural assessments of physically disabled patients: agreement between rehabilitation therapists and nurses.

International Journal of Research in Rehabilitation, **10**, 205–3.

King, K.B., Dark, P.C. & Hich, G.L. Jr. (1992). Patterns of referral and recovery in men and women undergoing coronary artery bypass grafting. *American Journal of Cardiology,* **69**, 179–82.

Lopez, S.R. (1989). Patient variable biases in clinical judgment: conceptual overview and methodological considerations. *Psychological Bulletin,* **106**, 184–203.

Margolies, R., Wachtel, A.B., Sutherland, K.R. & Blum, R.H. (1983). Medical students' attitudes towards cancer: concepts of professional distance. *Journal of Psychosocial Oncology,* **1**, 35–49.

Marteau, T.M. & Johnston, M. (1990). Health professionals: a source of variance in patient outcomes. *Psychology and Health,* **5**, 47–58.

Marteau, T.M. & Riordan, D.C. (1992). Staff attitudes towards patients: the influence of causal attributions for illness. *British Journal of Clinical Psychology,* **31**, 107–10.

McGee, H.M. & Fitzgerald, M. (1991). The impact of hospital experiences during training on GP referral rates. *Irish Journal of Psychological Medicine,* **7**, 22–3.

McNeil, B., Pauker, S., Sox, H. & Tversky, A. (1982). On the elicitation of preferences: for alternative therapies. *The New England Journal of Medicine,* **306**, 1259–62.

Milmoe, S., Rosenthal, R., Blane, H.T., Chafetz, M.L. & Wolf, I. (1967). The doctor's voice: postdictor of successful referral of alcoholic patients. *Journal of Abnormal Psychology,* **72**, 78–84.

Tversky, A. & Kahneman, D. (1981). The framing of decisions and the psychology of choice. *Science,* **211**, 453–8.

Walker, A., Grimshaw, J.M. & Armstrong, E.M. (2001). Salient beliefs and intentions to prescribe antibiotics for patients with a sore throat. *British Journal of Health Psychology,* **6**, 347–60.

Walker, A.E., Grimshaw, J.M., Johnston, M. et al. (2003). PRIME: process modelling in implementation research: selecting a theoretical basis for interventions to change clinical practice. *BMC Health Services Research,* **3**, 22. http://www.biomedcentral.com/1472–6963/3/22.

Breaking bad news

Katherine Joekes

Leiden University

What constitutes 'bad news'

Many healthcare professionals will find themselves in a situation where they have to break bad or difficult news to patients and/or their relatives. A broad definition of what constitutes bad news includes situations where there is a threat to a person's mental or physical wellbeing, a risk of upsetting an established lifestyle, or where a message is given which conveys to an individual fewer choices in his or her life (Ptacek & Eberhardt, 1996). This indicates that bad news contains an element of loss or anticipated loss and will, to a certain extent, be subjective. Generally, news of death, terminal illness or deformity constitute the more extreme situations, and will generally be accepted as 'bad news' for the recipient. However, news of chronic illnesses or the need for medical intervention, which at first glance would appear less disastrous, could for the recipient have far-reaching or negative implications for their personal or working life, or their hopes for the future.

The breaking of bad news is stressful for both the messenger and the recipient. Because the manner in which bad news is given will impact the recipient and the decisions he or she needs to make (e.g. Roberts *et al.,* 1994), there has been increased emphasis over the last decades on teaching appropriate communications skills to healthcare professionals. Factors that may create barriers to breaking bad news appropriately are outlined in this chapter, followed by general guidelines on how to break bad news. A review of the literature on how patients perceive bad news gives further insight into the relevance of these guidelines. Furthermore, issues related to communication skills training will be discussed.

Barriers to breaking bad news

Healthcare professionals are faced with a difficult task when having to impart bad or sad news (Buckman, 1984) and several obstacles to delivering bad news appropriately may arise. Factors such as age, gender, social status and race can generally create barriers in communication. Further to this, there are factors related to chaotic hospital settings (including lack of private spaces, time restraints and lack of support from team members) which can hinder the process of communication. The physician's lack of training, fears or sense of powerlessness can result in inadequate or incomplete information giving, and in particular may affect the way in which the clinician deals with the patient's emotions. These emotions (e.g. guilt or fear) can also cause the patient to behave in a manner that hampers the process. Furthermore, differences between what is perceived as bad news by the patient and by the clinician (Dosanjh *et al.,* 2001) can create misunderstanding and confusion. On the other hand, physicians and patients will often collude to limit the communication (The *et al.,* 2000; Dias *et al.,* 2003).

Guidelines and recommendations

It is now generally accepted that breaking bad news appropriately rarely comes naturally to healthcare professionals. Different 'models' for breaking bad news can be identified in the literature. One model distinguished between non-disclosure, full disclosure

423

and individualized disclosure (Girgis & Sanson-Fisher, 1995), whilst Brewin (1991) differentiates the 'unfeeling way' from the 'kind and caring way' and from the 'understanding and positive way' of breaking bad news. Such descriptive models may be too abstract to create useful guidelines for clinicians, but will have aided in the generation of more detailed recommendations on how best to break bad news. Several guidelines or protocols for the delivery of bad news have been drawn up in the past decade (e.g. Baile *et al.*, 2000; Buckman, 1992; Dias *et al.*, 2003; Girgis & Sanson-Fisher, 1995; SCOPE, 1999). Although such guidelines have primarily been generated from a consensus process rather than based on empirical findings, there is an increasing emphasis in the literature on assessment of the relevance and efficacy of these guidelines.

The six-step approach

A six-step approach to breaking bad news has been suggested (Buckman, 1992; SPIKES by Baile *et al.*, 2000), which shows considerable overlap with the principles suggested by other authors. The six steps are outlined below.

Setting up

Setting up the interview starts with the clinician preparing thoroughly and ensuring that he/she has all relevant information to hand. A private setting without disruption, where both clinician and patient or relatives can sit and feel comfortable, helps all parties to focus on the conversation and respond more freely. The clinician should allow enough time to impart the information and deal with the recipient's response. Patients may prefer to have a significant other present. If the situation allows this, the clinician could check with the patient whether he/she would wish for a relative or friend to attend the interview.

Assessment of patient's perception

It is important to assess the patient's perception of the medical situation by using open questions (e.g. 'What have you been told about the tests that have been carried out?'). This gives the clinician insight into what the patient knows and understands and allows him/her to tailor the bad news appropriately. It can also give the clinician an indication of the recipient's expectations of the interview.

Agreement about amount of information

Obtaining a patient's invitation about the amount of information he/she desires to receive about diagnosis, prognosis and treatment allows the clinician to match the amount of detail given to the patient's wishes. In a situation where medical tests are ordered, the clinician can ascertain in advance how much the patient may wish to know about the test results. Patients will have different coping styles (Miller, 1995), and the clinician should allow for this.

Imparting knowledge and information

The consultation centres on giving knowledge and information to a patient or relative. A verbal warning that bad news is coming can help prepare the recipient and may lessen the shock (Maynard, 1996). Following this, the use of clear and unambiguous

(but not blunt) language avoids misunderstanding or confusion. Information should be given in small chunks and may need to be repeated. This, and checking that the patient or relative has understood, will help him/her to take in as much of the information as possible.

Emotional responses

When addressing patient's emotions, it is important to keep in mind that a wide array of emotions can be experienced (e.g. shock, disbelief, anger, fear), and that clinicians should respond with empathic statements, exploratory questions and validating responses. Responding appropriately to a patient's emotions is perceived to be one of the most difficult aspects of breaking bad news (Ptacek & Eberhardt, 1996), but also one of the most important elements of the bad news consultation. The clinician needs to identify the emotional response, check this with the patient and indicate that he/she understands the reason for this emotion (e.g. when a patient responds with disbelief and shock to news, the clinician may respond with 'I realize that this is not what you expected to hear. I understand this must be a shock for you'.). Non-verbal behaviour should match the verbal messages, i.e. facial expression and touch (where deemed appropriate).

Summarizing and future strategy

Before ending the interview, the clinician needs to summarize and consider a strategy for the future. This should match the patient's readiness to move on. In cases of chronic or terminal illness, a discussion of continuous, curative or palliative treatment can provide the patient with a sense of certainty and a clear plan for the future. This could include future appointments and/or lines of communication. At this stage additional sources of support can usefully be identified.

Evaluation of guidelines

The six-step approach and similar guidelines make intuitive sense, and certain aspects of the guidelines find resonance in research on patient's experience of hearing bad news, as described in the following section of this chapter. More systematic research on the validity, efficacy and practicality of these guidelines is necessary (Baile *et al.*, 2000; Fallowfield & Jenkins, 2004). There is an indication that the presence of a protocol specifying how to proceed following disclosure of bad news may reduce stress for health care professionals (Simpson & Bor, 2001). Therefore, implementation and evaluation of these guidelines in medical education, both at undergraduate and postgraduate level, should continue to be developed.

The patient's perspective

The general view is that the manner in which bad news is conveyed can have an impact on factors such as patient satisfaction (Fallowfield & Jenkins, 2004), comprehension of information (Maynard, 1996), coping and psychological adjustment (Roberts *et al.*, 1994) and levels of hopefulness (The *et al.*, 2000) (see 'Coping with chronic illness' and 'Patient satisfaction'). In the last decade there has been increasing emphasis on research to further investigate these preferences in delivery of bad news. Reviews of this research (Fallowfield & Jenkins, 2004; Ptacek et al., 2001) identify three main areas of research, i.e. in cancer care, in acute trauma situations and in obstetrics and paediatrics settings. The issues in these three areas will be quite different. Cancer patients receive news about diagnosis or recurrence of terminal or serious illness, which will be followed by information and discussion about curative or palliative treatment. In instances of acute trauma, family members are likely to be confronted with unexpected bad news (e.g. of death after a road traffic accident) delivered by a person they have never met before. In obstetrics and paedicatrics departments parents or prospective parents can be confronted with news of a child's death or disability. Although the news and settings vary widely, the research generates three themes. Firstly, recipients of bad news tend to value the informant being kind, confident, sensitive and caring. They appreciate the informant showing concern and distress, rather than a cool or detached attitude. This underlines the necessity for showing empathy and having an understanding of the impact that the news will have on the patient and the family. Secondly, there is a strong desire for information to be imparted in a clear and unambiguous manner using simple terms, whilst blunt or abrupt communication is perceived as distressing. Patients appreciate being given time to talk and to ask questions. For cancer patients there is an important balance to be struck between the physician being truthful and not being too negative. There appear to be large personal differences between patients regarding the amount of detail they wish to know, for example about prognosis (Salander, 2002; Dias et al., 2003). Such findings underline the guideline of matching information given to the patient's desire for such information. The third main theme is the setting in which a patient receives the bad news, with privacy being of importance. These themes, also identified in other studies (Parker et al., 2001; McCulloch, 2004), give credence to the guidelines set out above.

There has been less emphasis in research on the potential consequences of the bad news consultation on longer-term psychological adjustment, and results are equivocal. Barnett (2002) reported no difference on psychological distress between cancer patients who had negative perceptions of the interaction with the physician (i.e. displaying brusque, unsympathetic or impatient behaviour) and those who had a positive perception of the interaction. Mager and Andrykowski (2002), however, found a weak correlation between a negative consultation experience and increased levels of distress in cancer patients. Furthermore, a study by Schofield and colleagues (2003) provides preliminary evidence that communications strategies recommended in the literature are associated with reduced anxiety and depression in patients with newly diagnosed melanoma.

Teaching skills for delivering bad news

Medical education in developed countries increasingly incorporates relevant communications skills training (see 'Teaching communications skills' and 'Medical interviewing'). One aspect of this training should deal with appropriate communication skills for breaking bad news. Although a detailed discussion of such training lies beyond the scope of this chapter, a brief overview is given. The literature identifies that adequate education of communication skills requires evidence-based rationale for the training (Maguire & Pitceathly, 2002), multiple sessions and opportunities for demonstration, reflection, discussion, practice and feedback (Fallowfield, 1996; Rosenbaum et al., 2004). Postgraduate workshops may also benefit physicians (Ladouceur et al., 2003). Whilst training sessions on breaking bad news emphasize acquisition of skills, they should simultaneously pay attention to the clinician's own emotions. Many clinicians report that breaking bad news remains a difficult task throughout their career, which can be accompanied by negative emotions, in particular feelings of guilt. It is important for them to understand that the manner in which the news is imparted can support the patient and their family and make a positive contribution in such difficult times. This knowledge may give the clinician a sense of purpose and hope and can assist effective and compassionate communication.

Evaluation of training and workshops is vital in order to establish both short-term and long-term efficacy. Rather than assessing clinician satisfaction and confidence, evaluation procedures should include observation of actual behaviour (Rosenbaum et al., 2004).

Other issues

Cultural diversity

The medical profession in the western world will increasingly be treating patients from a culturally diverse background, which has repercussions for the patient's response to medical issues. This will be reflected in communication of bad news and end-of-life decisions (Searight & Gafford, 2005). Although it may be too much to expect practitioners to be fully conversant with all subtleties of cultural diversity, it is important that they are sensitive to the needs of the specific ethnic minority groups that they mostly encounter in daily practice (see 'Cultural and ethnic factors in health').

Breaking bad news to children

When children are seriously ill or lose a parent, the bad news will be all the harder to impart appropriately. The child's developmental stage and understanding of death and illness needs to be taken into consideration. Clinicians need to work closely with parents or other relatives whose response may greatly influence the child's perceptions (Forrest, 1989) (see 'Children's perceptions of illness and death' and 'Coping with death and dying').

Summary

In summary, research has shown that the manner in which bad or sad news is broken influences patient satisfaction and possibly their future psychological adjustment. Guidelines have been generated primarily from a consensus process: however, these can aid the healthcare professional. The available literature shows that guidelines are relevant, in particular with regard to the settings, language used and the manner in which the clinician responds to the patient. Future research would benefit from audiotapes, videotapes or direct observation of bad news consultation, although there are ethical issues to consider. The patient's and family's wellbeing will always be a priority: asking consent to take part in a research project could be perceived as difficult or indeed inappropriate. Medical education increasingly focuses on teaching and evaluating communications skills, including those skills relevant for breaking bad news.

See also 'Healthcare professional–patient communication', 'Medical interviewing' and 'Teaching communication skills'.

REFERENCES

Baile, W.F., Buckman, R., Lenzi, R. *et al.* (2000). SPIKES – a six-step protocol for delivering bad news: application to the patient with cancer. *The Oncologist*, **5**, 302–11.

Barnett, M.M. (2002). Effect of breaking bad news on patients' perceptions of doctors. *Journal of the Royal Society of Medicine*, **95**, 343–7.

Brewin, T.B. (1991). Three ways of giving bad news. *Lancet*, **337**, 1207–9.

Buckman, R. (1984). Breaking bad news: why is it so difficult? *British Medical Journal*, **288**, 1597–9.

Buckman, R. (1992). *How to break bad news*. UK: Papermac.

Dias, L., Chabner, B.A., Lynch, T.J. & Penson, R.T. (2003). Breaking bad news: patient's perspective. *The Oncologist*, **8**, 587–96.

Dosanjh, S., Barnes, J. & Bhandari, M. (2001). Barriers to breaking bad news among medical and surgical residents. *Medical Education*, **35**, 197–205.

Fallowfield, L.J. (1996). Things to consider when teaching doctors how to deliver good, bad and sad news. *Medical Teaching*, **18**, 27–30.

Fallowfield, L.J. & Jenkins, V. (2004). Communicating bad, sad, and difficult news in medicine. *Lancet*, **363**, 312–19.

Forrest, G. (1989). Breaking bad news to children in paediatric care. In J. Couriel (Ed.). *Breaking bad news* (pp. 10–16). London: Duphar Medical Relations.

Girgis, A. & Sanson-Fisher, R.W. (1995). Breaking bad news: consensus guidelines for medical practitioner. *Journal of Clinical Oncology*, **13**, 2449–56.

Ladouceur, R., Goulet, F., Gagnon, R. *et al.* (2003). Breaking bad news: impact of a continuing medical education workshop. *Journal of Palliative Care*, **19**, 238–45.

Mager, W.M. & Andrykowski, M.A. (2002). Communication in the cancer "bad news" consultation: patient perceptions and psychological adjustment. *Psycho-Oncology*, **11**, 35–46.

Maguire, P. & Pitceathly, C. (2002). Key communications skills and how to acquire them. *British Medical Journal*, **325**, 697–700.

Maynard, D.W. (1996). On "realization" in everyday life: the forecasting of bad news as a social relation. *American Sociological Review*, **61**, 109–31.

Miller, S.M. (1995). Monitoring versus blunting styles of coping with cancer influence the information patients want and need about their disease. Implications for cancer screening and management. *Cancer*, **76**, 167–77.

McCulloch, P. (2004). The patient experience of receiving bad news from a health professional. *Professional Nurse*, **19**, 276–80.

Parker, P.A., Baile, W.F., de Moor, C. *et al.* (2001). Breaking bad news about cancer: patients' preferences for communication. *Journal of Clinical Oncology*, **19**, 2049–56.

Ptacek, J.T. & Eberhardt, T.L. (1996). Breaking bad news. A review of the literature. *JAMA*, **276**, 496–502.

Ptacek, J.T., Ptacek, J.J. & Ellison, N.M. (2001). "I'm sorry to tell you . . ." Physicians' reports of breaking bad news. *Journal of Behavioral Medicine*, **24**, 205–17.

Roberts, C.S., Cox, C.E., Reintgen, D.S., Baile, W.F. & Gibertini, M. (1994). Influence of physician communication on newly diagnosed breast patients' psychologic adjustment and decision making. *Cancer*, **74**, 336–41.

Rosenbaum, M.E., Ferguson, K.J. & Lobas, J.G. (2004). Teaching medical students and residents skills for delivering bad news: a review of strategies. *Academic Medicine*, **79**, 107–17.

Salander, P. (2002). Bad news from the patient's perspective: an analysis of the written narratives of the newly diagnosed cancer patients. *Social Science and Medicine*, **55**, 721–32.

Schofield, P.E., Butow, P.N., Thompson, J.F. *et al.* (2003). Psychological responses of patients receiving a diagnosis of cancer. *Annals of Oncology*, **14**, 48–56.

SCOPE (1999). *Right from the start. Looking at diagnosis and disclosure*. London: SCOPE Campaigns and Parliamentary Affairs Department.

Searight, H.R. & Gafford, J. (2005). Cultural diversity at the end of life: issues and guidelines for family physicians. *American Family Physician*, **71**, 515–22.

Simpson, R. & Bor, R. (2001). 'I'm not picking up a heart-beat. Experience of sonographers giving bad news to women during ultrasound. *British Journal of Medical Psychology*, **74**, 255–72.

The, A.M., Hak, T., Koëter, G. & van der Wal, G. (2000). Collusion in doctor–patients communication about imminent death: an ethnographic study. *British Medical Journal*, **321**, 1376–81.

Burnout in health professionals

Christina Maslach

University of California, Berkeley

Burnout in health professionals

Burnout is a psychological syndrome that involves a prolonged response to chronic emotional and interpersonal stressors on the job (Maslach, 1982; Maslach *et al.*, 2001). As such, it has been an issue of particular concern for human services occupations where: (a) the relationship between providers and recipients is central to the work, and (b) the provision of service, care, treatment or education can be a highly emotional experience. Within such occupations, the norms are clear, if not always stated explicitly: to be selfless and put others' needs first; to work long hours and do whatever it takes to help a client or patient or student; to go the extra mile and to give one's all. When such norms are combined with work settings that are high in demands and low in resources, then the risk for burnout is high (Maslach & Goldberg, 1998). All of these criteria certainly apply to health professions, which have long been recognized as stressful occupations (Cartwright, 1979). Indeed, much of the earliest research on burnout was conducted in the area of healthcare (Maslach & Jackson, 1982), and this focus has continued up to the present (Maslach & Ozer, 1995; Leiter & Maslach, 2000).

The multidimensional model of burnout

Burnout has been conceptualized as an individual stress experience that is embedded in a context of social relationships and thus involves the person's conception of both self and others (Maslach, 1998). The three key dimensions of this experience are exhaustion; feelings of cynicism and detachment from the job; and a sense of ineffectiveness and lack of accomplishment. Exhaustion is the individual stress dimension of burnout, and it refers to feelings of being physically over-extended and depleted of one's emotional resources (it has also been described as wearing out, loss of energy, depletion, debilitation and fatigue). Cynicism (or depersonalization) refers to a negative, callous or excessively detached response to other people, who are usually the recipients of one's service or care (it has also been described as negative or inappropriate attitudes towards patients, loss of idealism and irritability). Inefficacy refers to a decline in one's feelings of competence and successful achievement in one's work (it has also been described as reduced productivity or capability, low morale, withdrawal and an inability to cope).

These three dimensions of burnout can be illustrated by the experiences of healthcare professionals. Clearly, there are significant emotional experiences linked to the caregiving relationship between health worker and patient. Some of these experiences are enormously rewarding and uplifting, as when patients recover because of the worker's efforts. However, other experiences are emotionally stressful for the health practitioner, such as working with difficult or unpleasant patients, having to give 'bad news' to patients or their families, dealing with patient deaths or having conflicts with co-workers or supervisors. These emotional strains are sometimes overwhelming and lead to exhaustion.

To protect themselves against such disruptive feelings, health professionals may moderate their compassion for patients by distancing themselves psychologically, avoiding over-involvement and maintaining a more detached objectivity (a process known as 'detached concern'; Lief & Fox, 1963). For example, if a patient has a condition that is upsetting to see or otherwise difficult to work with, it is easier for the practitioner to provide the necessary care if he or she thinks of the patient as a particular 'case' or 'symptom' rather than as a human being who is suffering. However, the blend of compassion and emotional distance is difficult to achieve in actual practice, and too often the balance shifts toward a negative and depersonalized perception of patients. A derogatory and demeaning view of patients is likely to be matched by a decline in the quality of the care that is provided to them.

Many health professionals have not had sufficient preparation for the emotional reality of their work and its subsequent impact on their personal functioning. Thus, the experience of emotional turmoil on the job is likely to be interpreted as a failure to 'be professional' (i.e. to be non-emotional, cool and objective). Consequently, these health workers begin to question their own ability to work in a health career and to feel that their personal accomplishments are falling short of their expectations. These failures may be as much a function of the work setting as of any personal shortcomings: providing good healthcare may be difficult to accomplish in the context of staff shortages, poor training or inadequate resources. Nevertheless, health workers may begin to develop a negative self-evaluation, which can impair their job performance or even lead them to quit the job altogether.

Consequences of burnout

Burnout has been associated with various forms of negative responses to the job, including job dissatisfaction, low organizational commitment, absenteeism, intention to leave the job and rapid turnover (see Schaufeli & Enzmann, 1998, for a review). People who are experiencing burnout can have a negative impact on their colleagues, both by causing greater personal conflict and by disrupting job tasks. Thus, burnout can be 'contagious' and perpetuate itself through informal interactions on the job. When burnout reaches the high cynicism stage, it can result in higher absenteeism and increased turnover. Furthermore, burnout is linked to poorer quality of work, as people shift to doing the bare minimum, rather than performing at their best. They make more errors, become less thorough and have less creativity for solving problems. For example, one study found that nurses experiencing higher levels of burnout were judged by their patients to be providing a lower level of patient care (Leiter *et al.*, 1998), while another study found that the risk of patient mortality was higher when nurses had a higher patient workload and were experiencing greater burnout (Aiken *et al.*, 2002).

Because burnout is a prolonged response to chronic interpersonal stressors on the job, it tends to be fairly stable over time. Unlike depression, which is considered to be context-free and pervasive across all situations, burnout is regarded as job-related and situation-specific. Burnout symptoms tend to manifest themselves in normal persons who do not suffer from prior psychopathology or an identifiable organic illness. As such, burnout seems to fit the diagnostic criteria for job-related neurasthenia (Schaufeli *et al.*, 2001).

As one would expect from the research on stress and health, the exhaustion dimension of burnout has been correlated with various physical symptoms of stress: headaches, gastrointestinal disorders, muscle tension, hypertension, cold/flu episodes and sleep disturbances (see Leiter & Maslach, 2000*a*, for a review). Although there has been less research on how burnout affects one's home life, studies have found a fairly consistent negative 'spillover' effect. For example, nurses who experienced burnout reported that their job had a negative impact on their family and that their marriage was unsatisfactory (Burke & Greenglass, 2001). (See also 'Psychosomatics' and 'stress and health').

Job engagement

Burnout is one end of a continuum in the relationship people establish with their jobs, standing in contrast to the positive state of engagement with work. Recently, the multidimensional model of burnout has been expanded to this other end of the continuum (Leiter & Maslach, 1998). Job engagement is defined in terms of the same three dimensions as burnout, but at the positive end of those dimensions rather than the negative. Thus, engagement consists of a state of high energy (rather than exhaustion), strong involvement (rather than cynicism) and a sense of efficacy (rather than inefficacy).

The concept of a burnout-to-engagement continuum enhances the understanding of how the organizational context of work can affect workers' wellbeing. It recognizes the variety of reactions that people can have to the organizational environment, ranging from the intense involvement and satisfaction of engagement, through indifference to the exhausted, distant and discouraged state of burnout. One important implication of the burnout–engagement continuum is that strategies to promote engagement may be just as important for burnout prevention as strategies to reduce the risk of burnout. A work setting designed to support the positive development of the three core qualities of energy, involvement and effectiveness should be successful in promoting the wellbeing and productivity of its employees.

Key risk factors for burnout

Although there is some evidence for individual risk factors for burnout, there is far more research evidence for the importance of situational variables. Over two decades of research on burnout have identified a plethora of organizational risk factors across many occupations in various countries (see Maslach *et al.*, 2001; Schaufeli & Enzmann, 1998). Building on earlier models of job–person fit, in which better fit was assumed to predict better adjustment and less stress, Maslach and Leiter (1997) formulated a burnout model that focuses on the degree of match, or mismatch, between the individual and key aspects of his or her organizational environment. The greater the gap, or mismatch, between the person and the job, the greater the likelihood of burnout; conversely, the greater the match (or fit), the greater the likelihood of engagement with work. In analyzing the research literature, Maslach and Leiter (1997, 1999) identified six key areas of worklife in which a job–person mismatch is predictive of burnout: workload, control, reward, community, fairness and values.

Work overload

A commonly discussed source of burnout is overload: job demands exceeding human limits. People feel that they have too much to do, not enough time to perform required tasks and not enough resources to do the work well. There clearly is an imbalance, or mismatch, between the demands of the job and the individual's capacity to meet those demands. Not surprisingly, work overload is the single best predictor of the exhaustion dimension of burnout.

Patient workload has consistently been found to predict burnout in healthcare professionals. Both the quantity and quality of the contact between health professional and patient are important risk factors. The strain of working with patients can be multiplied by the need to deal with the patients' families as well, and by the challenges of working with colleagues.

Lack of control

Burnout is consistently linked to job factors in the healthcare setting that entail greater ambiguity and less control. Health professionals must often work closely and interdependently with each other, but may differ in status and power (as in the case of physicians and nurses). Consequently, some people have little control over the decisions that determine their daily activities and may receive little feedback about the results of their efforts. They may feel they are being held accountable, and yet they don't have the ability to control what it is they are being held accountable for. In other cases, people will feel a lack of control because working life has become more chaotic and ambiguous as a result of economic downturns. Many health professionals find themselves worrying about mergers, downsizing, layoffs and changes in management. In some cases, health workers have no influence on institutional policies that govern the hours and conditions of their work, and few opportunities for creativity and autonomy in carrying out their job tasks.

Insufficient rewards

Another type of job–person mismatch occurs when health professionals believe they are not getting rewarded appropriately for their performance. The standard rewards that most people think of are salary or benefits or special 'perks'. However, in many cases the more important rewards involve recognition. Lack of recognition from patients, colleagues, managers and external stakeholders devalues both the work and the workers, and is closely associated with feelings of inefficacy. It matters a great deal to people that somebody else notices what they do and that somebody cares about the quality of their work. When employees are working hard and feel that they are doing their best, they want to get some feedback on their efforts. The value of such concepts as 'walk-around' management lies in its power to reward: there is explicit interest in what people are doing, and the direct acknowledgement and appreciation of their accomplishments. Employee morale is heavily dependent on rewards and recognition.

Breakdown in community

Community is the overall quality of social interaction at work, including issues of conflict, mutual support, closeness and the capacity to work as a team. Work relationships include the full range of people that health professionals deal with on a regular basis, such as their patients, their co-workers, their boss, the people they supervise or people in the larger community (such as the patients' families). When these relationships are characterized by a lack of support and trust and by unresolved conflict, then there is a breakdown in the sense of community. If work-related relationships are working well, then there is a great deal of social support, and people have effective means of working out disagreements. But when there is a breakdown in community and there is not much support, there is real hostility and competition, which makes conflicts difficult to resolve. Under such conditions, stress and burnout are high and work becomes difficult (see also 'Social support and health').

Absence of fairness

The fifth area, an absence of fairness in the workplace, seems to be quite important for burnout, although it is a relatively new area of burnout research. The perception that the workplace is unfair and inequitable is probably the best predictor of the cynicism dimension of burnout. Anger and hostility are likely to arise when people feel they are not being treated with the respect that comes from being treated fairly. Even incidents that appear to be insignificant or trivial can, if they signal unfair treatment, generate intense emotions and have great psychological significance.

When people are experiencing the imbalance of inequity, they will take various actions to try to restore equity. Some actions might involve standard organizational procedures (e.g. for resolving grievances), but if employees do not believe there is any hope of a fair resolution, they may take other actions in areas that they can control. For instance, if employees think they are not being paid as well as they deserve, they may leave work early or take company supplies home with them, because 'they owe it to me'. It is possible that, in some extreme instances, employees might take action against the person (or persons) whom they may consider responsible for the inequity.

Value conflicts

Although there has not been a lot of research on the impact of values, current work suggests that it may play a key role in predicting levels of burnout (Leiter & Maslach, 2004). Values are the ideals and goals that originally attracted people to their job and thus they are the motivating connection between the worker and the workplace (beyond the utilitarian exchange of time and labour for salary). Value conflicts arise when people are working in a situation where there is a conflict between personal and organizational values. Under these conditions, people may have to grapple with the conflict between what they want to do and what they have to do. For example, people whose personal values dictate that it is wrong to tell a lie may find themselves in a job where it is necessary to lie or to shade the truth (e.g. to get the necessary authorization, or to avoid upsetting the patient). People who experience such a value conflict will give the following kinds of comments: 'This job is eroding my soul', or 'I cannot look at myself in the mirror any more knowing what I'm doing. I can't live with myself. I don't like this'. If workers are experiencing this kind of mismatch in values on a chronic basis, then burnout is likely to arise.

Implications for intervention

What can be done to alleviate burnout? One approach is to focus on the individual who is experiencing stress and help him or her to either reduce it or cope with it. Another approach is to focus on the workplace, rather than just the worker, and change the conditions that are causing the stress. A focus on the workplace is the clear implication of the organizational research on burnout, which posits that the six key areas of work-life affect people's experience of burnout or engagement, which, in turn, affect attitudes and behaviour at work. Thus, an effective approach to intervention would be to change workplace policies and practices that shape these six areas. The challenge for organizations is to identify which of the areas are most problematic, and then designing interventions that target those particular areas (see 'Worksite interventions').

Assessment of these six areas, as well as assessment of burnout, is a key element in the organizational checkup survey (Leiter & Maslach, 2000b), which has proved to be a useful tool for mobilizing both individual and organizational self-reflection and change. This organizational approach, which utilizes the six-area framework, makes a major contribution to making burnout a problem that can be solved in better ways than having employees either endure the chronic stress or quit their jobs. For the individual employees, the organizations for which they work, and the clients whom they serve, the preferred solution is to build a work environment that supports the ideals to which people wish to devote their efforts. This is a formidable challenge, but one that becomes more possible with the development of effective measures and a conceptual framework to guide intervention.

The practice of medicine has long been regarded as one of the noblest of occupations. To cure illness, repair injury, promote health and even forestall death are skills that are highly esteemed in all societies. Although the personal rewards and satisfactions of a health career are many, it is not without its hazards, including that of burnout. However, recent research has improved our understanding of the workplace dynamics of this syndrome and provides new insights into possible solutions to this important problem.

REFERENCES

Aiken, L.H., Clarke, S.P., Sloane, D.M., Sochalski, J. & Silber, J.H. (2002). Hospital nurse staffing and patient mortality, nurse burnout, and job dissatisfaction. *Journal of the American Medical Association*, **288**(16), 1987–93.

Burke, R.J. & Greenglass, E.R. (2001). Hospital restructuring, work–family conflict and psychological burnout among nursing staff. *Psychology and Health*, **16**, 83–94.

Cartwright, L.K. (1979). Sources and effects of stress in health careers. In G.C. Stone, F. Cohen & N.E. Adler (Eds.). *Health psychology* (pp. 419–45). San Francisco: Jossey-Bass.

Leiter, M.P., Harvie, P. & Frizzell, C. (1998). The correspondence of patient satisfaction and nurse burnout. *Social Science and Medicine*, **47**, 1611–17.

Leiter, M.P. & Maslach, C. (1998). Burnout. In H. Friedman (Ed.). *Encyclopedia of mental health* (pp. 347–57). San Diego, CA: Academic Press.

Leiter, M.P. & Maslach, C. (2000a). Burnout and health. In A. Baum, T. Revenson & J. Singer (Eds.). *Handbook of health psychology* (pp. 415–26). Hillsdale, NJ: Lawrence Erlbaum.

Leiter, M.P. & Maslach, C. (2000b). *Preventing burnout and building engagement: a complete program for organizational renewal*. San Francisco: Jossey-Bass.

Leiter, M.P. & Maslach, C. (2004). Areas of worklife: a structured approach to organizational predictors of job burnout. In P.L. Perrewe & D.C. Ganster (Eds.). *Research in occupational stress and well-being Vol. 3* (pp. 91–134). Oxford: Elsevier.

Lief, H.I. & Fox, R.C. (1963). Training for "detached concern" in medical students. In H.I. Lief, V.F. Lief & N.R. Lief (Eds.). *The psychological basis of medical practice*. New York: Harper & Row.

Maslach, C. (1982). *Burnout: the cost of caring*. Englewood Cliffs, NJ: Prentice-Hall. Reprinted in 2003. Cambridge, MA: Malor Books.

Maslach, C. (1998). A multidimensional theory of burnout. In C.L. Cooper (Ed.). *Theories of organizational stress* (pp. 68–85). Oxford, UK: Oxford University Press.

Maslach, C. & Goldberg, J. (1998). Prevention of burnout: new perspectives. *Applied and Preventive Psychology*, **7**, 63–74.

Maslach, C. & Jackson, S.E. (1982). Burnout in health professions: a social psychological analysis. In G. Sanders & J. Suls (Eds.). *Social psychology of health and illness*. Hillsdale, NJ: Erlbaum.

Maslach, C. & Leiter, M.P. (1997). *The truth about burnout*. San Francisco, CA: Jossey-Bass.

Maslach, C. & Ozer, E. (1995). Theoretical issues related to burnout in health workers. In L. Bennett, D. Miller & M. Ross (Eds.). *Health workers and AIDS: research, intervention and current issues in burnout and response* (pp. 1–14). London: Harwood Academic.

Maslach, C., Schaufeli, W.B. & Leiter, M.P. (2001). Job burnout. In S.T. Fiske, D.L. Schacter & C. Zahn-Waxler (Eds.). *Annual review of psychology. Vol. 52* (pp. 397–422).

Schaufeli, W.B., Bakker, A.B., Hoogduin, K., Schaap, C. & Kladler, A. (2001). The clinical validity of the Maslach Burnout Inventory and the Burnout Measure. *Psychology and Health*, **16**, 565–82.

Schaufeli, W.B. & Enzmann, D. (1998). *The burnout companion to study and practice: a critical analysis*. London: Taylor & Francis.

Communicating risk

David P. French[1] and Theresa M. Marteau[2]

[1]University of Birmingham
[2]King's College London

Introduction

There is an increasing move towards communicating risk information to both patients and the wider public, fuelled by increasingly
precise epidemiological estimates, technological developments
allowing the use of biomarkers of risk as communication tools and
the rise of interest in informed choice (see, for example, 'Screening in
healthcare'). As a consequence, concern about how best to communicate risk information and evaluate the impact of different methods
of communicating risk has risen correspondingly. Communicating
risk information should not be seen as an end in itself, but rather as
a means to achieving one or more ultimate aims. Principally, these
include communicating risk information to (a) facilitate informed
choices; (b) motivate behaviour change to reduce identified risks
and (c) provide reassurance while avoiding false reassurance.
This chapter discusses why the current focus on communicating
probabilistic information is insufficient for achieving these outcomes
and describes other approaches which have shown more promise.

Risk communication as presenting probabilities

Much recent discussion of risk communication has centred on how
numerical probability information should be presented (Calman &
Royston, 1997; Edwards et al., 2001, 2002, 2003; Paling, 2003). At face
value, presenting risk information in a probabilistic form is entirely
reasonable: the information derives from epidemiological studies,
which yield information about disease risks in terms of probabilities.
However, there are reliable and systematic differences between
estimates of actual risks, as calculated from mortality statistics
and the public's perception of these (Lichtenstein et al., 1978)
(see 'Risk perception'). These include a tendency to under-estimate
the frequency of large risks and over-estimate small risks, with
over-estimation being more likely when the risks were dramatic, e.g. murder, than when they were less so, e.g. diabetes
(see Schwarz & Vaughn, 2002). An understandable response to this
has been to try to reduce this gap by providing people with the
epidemiological risks, presented in terms of the probability of an
adverse outcome, such as disease or death. However, providing
probabilities to people has made little impact on informing choices,
providing reassurance or altering risk-related behaviour.

Why does providing probabilistic risk information have little impact?

It is now well established that providing information about the
probability of health risks alone has, at best, only a small influence
on how people think about those risks and on their risk-related
behaviour. One review concluded: 'it would appear that people
cannot reliably understand and interpret numerical probability
statistics' (Rothman & Kiviniemi, 1999, p. 46). Similarly, meta-
analyses of studies investigating the effects of fear-rousing communications show that perceptions of vulnerability have on average a
small effect on intentions to change behaviour and on concurrent
and subsequent behaviour (Floyd et al., 2000; Milne et al., 2000;
Witte & Allen, 2000). We now consider three of the reasons
why providing probabilistic risk information has minimal effects
on how people think and behave: (a) people have difficulty understanding and remembering probabilities, (b) people find it difficult
to evaluate probabilities without supplementary information and (c)
even if probabilistic information is understood, perception of risk
comprises more than perception of probability.

Understanding and remembering probabilities

Both health professionals and patients have difficulties in understanding probabilities (Rothman & Kiviniemi, 1999). Several studies
have shown that many people are unable to handle even simple
numerical operations, such as converting a percentage into a proportion (e.g. Lipkus et al., 2001; Schwartz et al., 1997). Many people,
including physicians, are unable to correctly calculate the likelihood
that a person being screened has a particular condition, when
provided with information in the form of percentages about the
base rate, sensitivity and false-positive rate of the screening test
(Hoffrage et al., 2000). Even when probabilistic information is
understood, people still tend to remember it in terms of a
small number of discrete categories (Axworthy et al., 1996;
Lippman-Hand & Fraser, 1979). For example, while over 90% of
those testing negative for being a cystic fibrosis carrier understood
at the time of testing that they had a residual risk of being a carrier
(about 1:130), three years later, fewer than 50% had retained this
information, with many believing they were at no risk (Axworthy
et al., 1996). Thus, even when numerical probabilities appear to
be understood, what is often remembered is only the 'gist' of the
communication (Reyna & Brainerd, 1991).

Evaluating probabilistic information through comparisons

People do not generally carry around accurate numerical estimates
of probabilities of harm in their heads, only vague senses of
'riskiness'. For this reason, when they receive a new piece of probabilistic risk information, it can be difficult to evaluate this, if they

have nothing against which to compare it. At a minimum, people need additional information to clarify the implications of absolute risk information. This includes the risk that others similar to them have, or their own risk if they were to adhere to recommended medical advice. Thus, when asked what information they want in order to understand a health risk, people typically ask for comparative information about the probability of other risks (Roth *et al.*, 1990). In keeping with the evaluative function of relative risk information, presenting information about relative risks generally has more impact on perceptions of likelihood, emotion and decision-making, than information about absolute risks (Edwards *et al.*, 2001; Klein, 1997; Nexoe *et al.*, 2002).

Beyond probability

One fundamental problem with viewing risk as probability is that it fails to take into account the value that people attach to different outcomes. Thus, although two people may have identical beliefs about the probability of the same adverse outcome, such as having a child with Down's syndrome, their decision about whether to have a screening test depends critically upon their evaluation of that outcome (Lawson, 2001). Equally, people vary widely in their perception of how severe they view even common conditions such as diabetes (Farmer *et al.*, 1999). Reviews of experimental studies which have provided people with information about both the severity and the likelihood of health threats have shown that perceptions of severity have as much impact as perceptions of likelihood on motivation to take protective action against the threat and on behaviour itself (Milne *et al.*, 2000; Witte & Allen, 2000). The impact of likelihood information may even be reduced in the presence of information about severity (Hendrickx *et al.*, 1989).

Towards effective risk communication

The aims of communicating risk information are often implicit. However, to be able to judge the effectiveness or otherwise of risk communication, explicit criteria are needed. These criteria will vary with the aims of the communication. The aim of communicating risk information should affect both the content and framing of the information provided. This is described below in considering effective ways of achieving three of the more common aims of communicating risk information: informing choices; facilitating risk reducing behaviour; and providing appropriate reassurance.

Informing choices

Changes both within and outside of healthcare have resulted in an increasing emphasis upon providing services in ways to facilitate patients making informed choices (see 'Patient-centred healthcare'). Core elements of definitions of informed choice are an understanding of the different options and their likelihoods (Bekker *et al.*, 1999; Marteau *et al.*, 2001*a*). Despite understanding being a central outcome to risk communication, there have been few attempts to define what it means to understand a risk (Weinstein,

1999). In addition to likelihood of harm, other important dimensions include an appreciation of the nature of the potential harm, the risk in comparison with other hazards, the factors that lead to this risk, the excess risk due to these factors and the difficulty of avoiding the harmful consequences of these factors, once exposed (Weinstein, 1999). Although people may have a good appreciation of some of these dimensions, e.g. that smoking is bad for one's health, appreciation of other elements of understanding, e.g. the nature and severity of the health consequences of smoking, can still be lacking (Weinstein *et al.*, 2004). Thus, the first choice in communicating risk information to facilitate informed choices concerns selecting the appropriate information to communicate.

A general framework for selecting the appropriate strategy for communicating risk information and supporting decisions has been developed (O'Connor *et al.*, 2003). According to this framework, the most appropriate risk communication strategies depend upon whether patients are faced with decisions concerning either 'effective' health services, where the benefits are large compared with harms, or 'preference-sensitive' health services, where it is unclear how much benefit is provided relative to harms, or where the ratio of benefits to harms is dependent on patient values. Where clinicians are discussing 'effective' health services with patients, consultations surrounding risk may be more directive and may concern motivations and barriers to change. On the other hand, where clinicians are discussing 'preference-sensitive' health services, counselling is non-directive, where more discussion of potential benefits and harms, probabilities and options is suitable.

Where probabilistic information is to be communicated, understanding and manipulation of that information is facilitated when it is presented using natural frequencies (Hoffrage *et al.*, 2000). Natural frequency information is given when all the information provided relates to an overall sample, e.g. of 1000 people, 40 people are infected, of whom 30 test positive and 10 test negative (see Hoffrage *et al.*, 2002). More generally, there is now an evidence base for how to communicate other written information to maximize the likelihood that people will understand it and be able to extract the information in which they are particularly interested (Wright, 1999).

As noted above, over time people tend to remember risk information in terms of simpler discrete categories: they extract the 'gist' of the message (Reyna & Brainerd, 1991). How this 'gist' is recalled depends critically upon the prior understanding of the health threat. Such information is better recalled if it is congruent with how people already think about that disease (Bishop, 1991). The important point is that people are not blank slates onto which risk communications can be written: people already have an understanding of health and disease, albeit often simplistic and discrepant from current medical understanding (Bostrom *et al.*, 1992; Leventhal *et al.*, 1997).

There are many areas where disease-related communications may not fit with pre-existing understandings of disease. For example, many women appear to lack a plausible explanation for how smoking increases the risk of cervical abnormalities (Marteau *et al.*, 2002). Consequently, informing women with cervical abnormalities that quitting smoking would help them will not make sense to them and they are therefore unlikely to do so (McBride *et al.*, 1999). Providing such women with a coherent model of the nature of the risk is more effective at promoting understanding and recall of likelihood of cervical abnormalities, than probabilistic information which will soon be forgotten (Hall *et al.*, 2004).

Facilitating risk-reducing behaviour

It has been known for some time now that communicating risk information on its own is rarely sufficient to bring about changes in behaviour to reduce risk, and under some circumstances may even be counter-productive (Leventhal, 1970). Behaviour change is more likely when information about likelihood and severity are presented alongside information about the action needed to reduce this threat (Witte & Allen, 2000). Experimental manipulations of information about the effectiveness of behaviour change in reducing health threats have been consistently shown to have as much of an impact on behaviour as do manipulations of likelihood and severity combined (Milne *et al.*, 2000). Thus, although most smokers have some awareness of the high likelihood that their smoking will lead to severe disease (Weinstein, 1998), whether they even attempt to stop smoking is highly dependent on whether they believe that quitting will substantially reduce their chances of avoiding disease (Christensen *et al.*, 1999), as well as whether they think they can stop (Dijkstra & deVries, 2000). These beliefs depend critically upon how people understand the process by which the risk leads to disease, and how avoidance of the risk can reduce chances of disease.

Health communications aimed at achieving behaviour change should therefore aim to provide a clear and simple explanation of these factors, rather than just a bald statement of likelihood. They also need to be accompanied by an explicit plan concerning exactly when and where the recommended risk-reducing behaviour will be performed (Sheeran, 2002). However, even when all these recommendations are followed, risk communications will not provide a 'magic bullet' to alter behaviour. They need to be seen as part of a broader strategy to reduce population risks of common conditions (Crawford, 2002) (see 'Health promotion').

Providing appropriate reassurance

The majority of health risk assessments and many diagnostic test procedures yield 'negative' or 'normal' results. Such results indicate that there is a low chance, but do not indicate that there is absolutely no chance, of developing or having the tested condition. An important aim when communicating negative results, therefore, is to present these results to provide appropriate reassurance. That is, to communicate that the result is 'good news' and hence anxiety about the residual risk is unwarranted, whilst avoiding false reassurance, i.e. the belief that low risk means no risk.

A major concern in much risk communication to date has been to avoid generating high levels of distress. Information on test sensitivity, i.e. the proportion of cases that it can detect, and by implication, the number of cases it can not, is often not provided. For example, one analysis found that information on the proportion of breast cancers detected by screening was mentioned in just 15 of 58 patient information leaflets (Slaytor & Ward, 1998).

This lack of provision of information on test sensitivity may lead to a number of unfortunate consequences due to false reassurance, i.e. erroneously believing that negative or normal test results indicate an absence of residual risk. These include reinforcement of unhealthy lifestyles (Tymstra & Bieleman, 1987), poorer adjustment following the birth of a child with a disability (Hall *et al.*, 2000) and delay in seeking help when symptoms of disease arise, as well as delay in health professionals responding to such symptoms, along with associated litigation (Petticrew *et al.*, 2000). There is evidence that using the term 'normal' to describe test results encourages false reassurance with as many as 50% believing their results indicate no residual risk (Axworthy *et al.*, 1996; Marteau *et al.*, 2001*b*).

Communicating residual risks using numbers rather than words has been found to have a small beneficial effect of increasing awareness of residual risks without raising anxiety (Marteau *et al.*, 2000). Further, whilst only 52% of women who were informed that their smear test result was 'normal' understood that cervical smear tests entail a residual risk, 70% of women given an additional sentence explaining the meaning of a normal smear result using a verbal probability of absolute risk, appreciated that there was a residual risk (Marteau *et al.*, 2001*b*). To date, however, few studies have been conducted on how to reduce rates of false reassurance and there is a particular need to understand the emotional and cognitive processes that affect longer-term recall.

Conclusions

To help people understand risk information, they should be presented not only with the likelihood of harm, but also with a clear description of the nature of the harm to which they are exposed. To help people make informed decisions, any information about risk communicated should take into account their likely prior understanding and what are the features of the risk information in which people will already have an interest. To help people change their behaviour to reduce risk, they should be given explicit information about how altering their behaviour might result in a reduction in risk and helped to develop a clear plan of action to alter their behaviour. To provide reassurance but avoid false reassurance, information on test sensitivity and in particular on residual risk with 'normal' test results should be presented. In all these cases, these recommendations are tentative: there is insufficient reliable data on the long-term effects of different approaches to communicating risk information to be more conclusive.

It is important to appreciate that these different aims of risk communication may sometimes conflict: although presenting information on the sensitivity and specificity of screening programmes should promote informed choice, it may lead to lower programme uptake and possibly reduce their public health impact (Marteau & Kinmonth, 2002). However, a clear idea of why risk information is being communicated will undoubtedly be helpful in optimizing risk communication and in evaluating whether the goals of such communications have been met (see also 'Risk perception').

REFERENCES

Axworthy, D., Brock, D.J., Bobrow, M. & Marteau, T.M. (1996). Psychological impact of population-based carrier testing for cystic fibrosis: 3-year follow-up. *Lancet*, **347**, 1443–6.

Bekker, H., Thornton, J.G., Airey, C.M. *et al.* (1999). Informed decision making: an annotated bibliography and systematic review. *Health Technology Assessment*, **3**(1).

Bishop, G.D. (1991). Understanding the understanding of illness. In J.A. Skelton & R.T. Croyle (Eds.). *Mental representation in health and illness* (pp. 32–59). New York: Springer-Verlag.

Bostrom, A., Fischhoff, B. & Morgan, M.G. (1992). Characterizing mental models of hazardous processes: a methodology and an application to radon. *Journal of Social Issues*, **48**, 85–100.

Calman, K. & Royston, G. (1997). Risk language and dialects. *British Medical Journal*, **315**, 939–42.

Christensen, A.J., Moran, P.J., Ehlers, S.L. *et al.* (1999). Smoking and drinking behavior in patients with head and neck cancer: effects of behavioral self-blame and perceived control. *Journal of Behavioral Medicine*, **22**, 407–18.

Crawford, D. (2002). Population strategies to prevent obesity. *British Medical Journal*, **325**, 728–9.

Dijkstra, A. & deVries, H. (2000). Self-efficacy expectations with regard to different tasks in smoking cessation. *Psychology and Health*, **15**, 501–11.

Edwards, A.G.K., Elwyn, G.J., Mathews, E. & Pill, R. (2001). Presenting risk information – a review of the effects of "framing" and other manipulations on patient outcomes. *Journal of Health Communication*, **6**, 61–2.

Edwards, A., Elwyn, G. & Mulley, A. (2002). Explaining risks: turning numerical data into meaningful pictures. *British Medical Journal*, **324**, 827–30.

Edwards, A., Unigwe, S., Elwyn, G. & Hood, K. (2003). Effects of communicating individual risks in screening programmes: Cochrane systematic review. *British Medical Journal*, **327**, 703–9.

Farmer, A., Levy, J.C. & Turner, R.C. (1999). Knowledge of risk of developing diabetes mellitus among siblings of Type 2 diabetic patients. *Diabetic Medicine*, **16**, 233–7.

Floyd, D.L., Prentice-Dunn, S. & Rogers, R.W. (2000). A meta-analysis of research on protection motivation theory. *Journal of Applied Social Psychology*, **30**, 407–29.

Hall, S., Bobrow, M. & Marteau, T.M. (2000). Psychological consequences for parents of false negative results on prenatal screening for Down's syndrome: retrospective interview study. *British Medical Journal*, **320**, 407–12.

Hall, S., Weinman, J. & Marteau, T.M. (2004). The motivating impact of informing women smokers of a link between smoking and cervical cancer: the role of coherence. *Health Psychology*, **23**, 419–24.

Hendrickx, L., Vlek, C. & Oppewal, H. (1989). Relative importance of scenario information and frequency information in the judgment of risk. *Acta Psychologica*, **72**, 41–63.

Hoffrage, U., Gigerenzer, G., Krauss, S. & Martignon, L. (2002). Representation facilitates reasoning: what natural frequencies are and what they are not. *Cognition*, **84**, 343–52.

Hoffrage, U., Lindsey, S., Hertwig, R. & Gigerenzer, G. (2000). Communicating statistical information. *Science*, **290**, 2261–2.

Klein, W.M. (1997). Objective standards are not enough: affective, self-evaluative, and behavioral responses to social cognition information. *Journal of Personality and Social Psychology*, **72**, 763–74.

Lawson, K.L. (2001). Contemplating selective reproduction: the subjective appraisal of parenting a child with a disability. *Journal of Reproductive and Infant Psychology*, **19**, 73–82.

Leventhal, H. (1970). Findings and theory in the study of fear communications. *Advances in Experimental Social Psychology*, **5**, 119–86.

Leventhal, H., Benyamini, Y., Brownlee, S. *et al.* (1997). Illness representations: theoretical foundations. In K.J. Petrie & J.A. Weinman (Eds.). *Perceptions of health and illness: current research and applications* (pp. 19–45). Amsterdam: Harwood Academic.

Lichtenstein, S., Slovic, P., Fischhoff, B., Layman, M. & Combs, B. (1978). Judged frequency of lethal events. *Journal of Experimental Psychology: Human Learning and Memory*, **4**, 551–78.

Lipkus, I.M., Samsa, G. & Rimer, B.K. (2001). General performance on a numeracy scale among highly education samples. *Medical Decision Making*, **21**, 37–44.

Lippman-Hand, A. & Fraser, F.C. (1979). Genetic counseling: provision and reception of information. *American Journal of Medical Genetics*, **3**, 113–27.

Marteau, T.M., Dormandy, E. & Michie, S. (2001*a*). A measure of informed choice. *Health Expectations*, **4**, 99–108.

Marteau, T.M. & Kinmonth, A.L. (2002). Screening for cardiovascular risk: public health imperative or matter for individual informed choice? *British Medical Journal*, **325**, 78–80.

Marteau, T.M., Rana, S. & Kubba, A. (2002). Smoking and cervical cancer: a qualitative study of the explanatory models of smokers with cervical abnormalities. *Psychology, Health and Medicine*, **7**, 107–9.

Marteau, T.M., Saidi, G., Goodburn, S. *et al.* (2000). Numbers or words? A randomised controlled trial of presenting screen negative results to pregnant women. *Prenatal Diagnosis*, **20**, 714–18.

Marteau, T.M., Senior, V. & Sasieni, P. (2001*b*). Women's understanding of a "normal smear test result": experimental questionnaire based study. *British Medical Journal*, **322**, 526–8.

McBride, C.M., Scholes, D., Grothaus, L.C. *et al.* (1999). Evaluation of a minimal self-help smoking cessation intervention following cervical cancer screening. *Preventive Medicine*, **20**, 133–8.

Milne, S., Sheeran, P. & Orbell, S. (2000). Prediction and intervention in health-related behavior: a meta-analytic review of protection motivation theory. *Journal of Applied Social Psychology*, **30**, 106–43.

Nexoe, J., Gyrd-Hansen, D., Kragstrup, J., Kristiansen, I.S. & Nielsen, J.B. (2002). Danish GPs' perception of disease risk and benefit of prevention. *Family Practice*, **19**, 3–6.

O'Connor, A.M., Legare, F. & Stacey, D. (2003). Risk communication in practice: the contribution of decision aids. *British Medical Journal*, **327**, 736–40.

Paling, J. (2003). Strategies to help patients understand risks. *British Medical Journal*, **327**, 745–8.

Petticrew, M.P., Sowden, A.J., Lister-Sharp, D. & Wright, K. (2000). False-negative results in screening programmes: systematic review of impact and implications. *Health Technology Assessment*, **4**(5).

Reyna, V.F. & Brainerd, C.J. (1991). Fuzzy-trace theory and framing effects in choice: gist extraction, truncation, and conversion. *Journal of Behavioral Decision Making*, **4**, 249–62.

Roth, E., Morgan, M.G., Fischhoff, B., Lave, L. & Bostrom, A. (1990). What do we know about making risk comparisons? *Risk Analysis*, **10**, 375–80.

Rothman, A.J. & Kiviniemi, M.T. (1999). Treating people with information: an analysis and review of approaches to communicating health risk information. *Journal of the National Cancer Institute Monographs*, **25**, 44–51.

Schwartz, L.M., Woloshin, S., Black, W.C. & Welch, G.H. (1997). The role of numeracy in understanding the benefit of screening mammography. *Annals of Internal Medicine*, **127**, 966–71.

Schwarz, N. & Vaughn, L.A. (2002). The availability heuristic revisited: ease of recall and content of recall as distinct sources of information. In T. Gilovich, D. Griffin & D. Kahneman (Eds.). *Heuristics and biases: the psychology of intuitive judgment* (pp. 103–19). Cambridge: Cambridge University Press.

Sheeran, P. (2002). Intention–behaviour relations: a conceptual and empirical review. *European Review of Social Psychology*, **12**, 1–36.

Slaytor, E.K. & Ward, J.E. (1998). How risks of breast cancer and benefits of screening are communicated to women: analysis of 58 pamphlets. *British Medical Journal*, **317**, 263–4.

Tymstra, T. & Bieleman, B. (1987). The psychosocial impact of mass-screening for cardiovascular risk-factors. *Family Practice*, **4**, 287–90.

Weinstein, N.D. (1998). Accuracy of smokers' risk perceptions. *Annals of Behavioral Medicine*, **20**, 135–40.

Weinstein, N.D. (1999). What does it mean to understand a risk? Evaluating risk communication. *Journal of the National Cancer Institute Monographs*, **25**, 15–20.

Weinstein, N.D., Slovic, P., Waters, E. & Gibson, G. (2004). Public understanding of the illnesses caused by cigarette smoking. *Nicotine and Tobacco Research*, **6**, 349–55.

Witte, K. & Allen, M. (2000). A meta-analysis of fear appeals: implications for effective public health campaigns. *Health Education and Behavior*, **27**, 591–615.

Wright, P. (1999). Designing healthcare advice for the public. In F.T. Durso, R.S. Nickerson, *et al.* (Eds.). *Handbook of applied cognition* (pp. 695–723). New York: John Wiley & Sons.

Healthcare professional–patient communication

John Weinman

King's College London

Effective healthcare professional–patient communication is necessary to ensure not only that the patients' problems and concerns are understood by the healthcare professional (HCP) but also that relevant information, advice and treatment is received and acted upon by the patient. HCP–patient communication has been the object of considerable research, which has attempted not only to describe the interaction processes involved but also to show how these affect a range of patient outcomes. Early research revealed quite high levels of patient dissatisfaction which were often associated with insufficient information, poor understanding of the medical advice and subsequent reluctance or inability to follow recommended treatment or advice (Korsch & Negrete, 1972). The development of relatively unobtrusive audio- and video-recording techniques allowed researchers to obtain an 'inside view' of the consultation and many studies have analyzed the process of the consultation and attempted to relate process variables or characteristics to outcome. However, these studies, while identifying important themes, have not always been successful in making clear links between process and outcome (Stiles, 1989). One reason for this is that patients vary in their expectations and preferences. As a result, many current frameworks for understanding HCP–patient communication (e.g. Friedrikson, 1993) are based on the relations between inputs (i.e. the attitudes, beliefs, expectations, etc., which patient and HCP bring to the consultation), process (the nature of the encounter) and outcome (the short and longer-term effects on the patient).

Input factors in communication

Patients cope with health threats in diverse ways and show consistent differences in the extent to which they want to be involved in the healthcare process (Krantz *et al.*, 1980) as well as in the amount of information which they would like to receive about their health problems. Similarly, a distinction has been made by Miller (1995) between 'monitors' and 'blunters', with the former being more inclined to need and seek out information about their problem and treatment, whereas the latter group prefer consultations in which relatively limited information is provided. Miller and colleagues have shown how these two different styles of coping with health threats can influence how patients respond to communication in many areas of healthcare, including cancer screening and treatment.

Patients have differing expectations for specific consultations. Contrary to medical opinion, patients do not always want or expect diagnosis or treatment since they may be looking to the consultation to gain more understanding of their health problem or may be hoping for support or understanding from their HCP (Barry *et al.*, 2000). These prior expectations can be important in determining outcomes since consultations in which patient expectations are met result in greater satisfaction and an increased willingness to follow advice or treatment (Williams *et al.*, 1995). Thus an important starting point for any consultation is to identify the patients' own expectations, as well as their own preferences and beliefs.

Healthcare professionals can also vary considerably in the attitudes and beliefs, which they have not only about their own and the patient's role, but also about the function and conduct of the consultation. For example, doctors have been categorized in various ways according to their role perceptions and the extent to which they concentrate on the technical or more psychosocial aspects of patient care, as well as their beliefs about whether patients should be actively involved in the consultation and in decision-making about the management of the clinical problem (e.g. Grol *et al.*, 1990). Inevitably these broad attitudinal differences are reflected in differences in the way in which the consultation is conducted (see 'Attitudes of health professionals').

The consultation process

There is a range of methods and frameworks for analyzing and describing the process of the consultation. One of the broadest distinctions made has been between consultations which are described as patient-centred and those which are doctor-centred, reflecting the extent to which the doctor or patient determines what is discussed (see 'Patient-centred healthcare'). Doctor-centred consultations are ones in which closed questions are used more often and the direction is determined by the doctor atypically with a primary focus on medical problems. In contrast, patient-centred encounters involve more open-ended questions with greater scope for patients to raise their own concerns and agendas. Related to this are consistent differences in the extent to which the doctor responds to the emotional agendas and the non-verbal cues of the patient. Although there has been a tendency to consider the more patient-centred/emotion-focused approach as preferable, the evidence of the effects on health outcomes is equivocal (Kinmonth *et al.*, 1998; Michie *et al.*, 2003). What may be more important is for HCP and patient to be in agreement over the nature of the problem and the best course of action (Starfield *et al.*, 1981).

A number of specific methods have been developed for carrying detailed analyses of the social interaction between HCP and patient based on audio or videotapes or transcripts of the consultations. Good overviews of these different approaches are available elsewhere (e.g. Roter & Hall, 1989) and attempts have been made to define a number of more general ways of classifying doctor–patient interactions. For example, one can distinguish between verbal and non-verbal information and within the verbal domain, six broad categories can be defined (information-giving; information-seeking; social conversation; positive talk; negative talk; partnership building). From a meta-analysis of these broad categories (Roter, 1989) it has been found that for the doctor, information-giving occurs most frequently (approximately 35% of the doctor's communication) followed by information-seeking (approximately 22%), positive talk (15%), partnership building (10%), social conversation (6%) and negative talk (1%). In contrast, the main type of patient communication consists of information giving (approximately 50%) with less than 10% involving question-asking. Using cluster analysis of these different categories of communication, Roter and colleagues (Roter *et al.*, 1997) identified five broad patterns of relationship in primary care consultations: narrowly biomedical; biomedical (in transition); biopsychosocial; psychosocial; and consumerist. They also showed

that doctors show a fair degree of consistency in their style of communication.

A more specific approach to process analysis is found in the studies of Ley and colleagues (Ley, 1988), who concentrated on the informational content of the consultation and the quality of information provided by the HCP. In particular, they analyzed the content in terms of its level of complexity, comprehensibility and the extent to which the information was organized. They and others have found that medical information may be too detailed or too complex with the result that important information may not be understood or retained by the patient. There is even evidence that patients and HCPs may interpret the same information in different ways: this communication gap can occur around anatomical information or other technical terms which are used to describe illness or treatment.

These various ways of conceptualizing and analyzing the consultation process have given rise to a large number of indices or categories which have been related to outcome, often in quite a limited fashion. Outcomes, such as patient satisfaction or adherence to treatment are likely to be determined by a range of factors, reflecting a complex interaction of input, process and situational variables. Hence it is not surprising that attempts to derive simple process–outcome models have been disappointing in their predictive value (Stiles, 1989). Moreover, there are various ways of defining outcomes and it is very likely that different process variables will affect different outcome indicators.

Outcomes of the consultation

One of the most common outcomes which has been used in studies of healthcare communication is patient satisfaction. This has been investigated as an endpoint in its own right as well as a possible mediator of more distal outcomes including treatment adherence and health. Fitzpatrick (this volume) maintains that the concept of patient satisfaction is important because it focuses on the need to understand how patients respond to healthcare. As a result, it is increasingly being assessed in surveys of healthcare settings, as a marker of quality of care, along with such other dimensions of quality as access, relevance to need, effectiveness, equity and efficiency. Patient satisfaction is a multidimensional concept since patients have been found to have differing views about different aspects of their healthcare, such as the HCP's behaviour towards them, the information provided and their technical skills. Nevertheless there is evidence that the HCP's behaviour during the consultation is the critical determinant and one which can significantly influence satisfaction ratings of all the other aspects of healthcare. Although patient satisfaction can provide a useful general indicator of the patient's experience, there are some associated problems with its use, since many measures appear to be insensitive to variations in patient satisfaction and often do not distinguish between different categories of satisfaction (see 'Patient satisfaction').

In their studies of the quality of information transmission, Ley and colleagues have used patient knowledge and recall as outcome measures and these do show a clearer relation with process variables, such as the complexity and level of organization of the information presented (Ley, 1988). Moreover, their interventions to improve the clarity or comprehensibility of the information consistently resulted in better recall and understanding (see below). Despite this, there is still abundant evidence that patients often emerge from consultations with insufficient information or understanding of their problems. As a result, they forget a great deal of what they have been told. Consultation skills which facilitate the effective communication of information include using language that is readily understood, presenting information in a way that takes account of the patient's beliefs and checking understanding of any information that has been given (Ley, 1988). Videorecordings of consultations show that these skills are frequently absent in routine consultations (Braddock et al., 1997; Campion et al., 2002). Thus, for example, recording of consultations conducted by primary care physicians in the United States revealed that in just 2% were direct questions asked of the patient to check understanding (Braddock et al., 1997). Similarly in an analysis of videotaped consultations selected by candidates as part of a qualifying examination for membership of the Royal College of General Practitioners, checking patient understanding was evident in just 20% of the consultations (Campion et al., 2002).

Patient satisfaction, understanding and beliefs can play a major role in influencing another important and widely studied outcome variable, namely compliance or adherence with treatment or advice. This is discussed in detail elsewhere in this volume (see 'Adherence to treatment') and is obviously an important outcome in situations where non-adherence results in adverse health consequences. There is evidence of high levels of non-adherence and this can clearly affect other outcomes including health and wellbeing. The latter have not often been studied as communication outcomes but there are a few studies which demonstrate positive effects on patients' health and wellbeing arising from positive experiences in medical consultations (Stewart, 1995).

Improving healthcare professional–patient communication

In the undergraduate and postgraduate medical curriculum, communication skills training is now regarded as a fundamental component, but this varies considerably in terms of the amount and type of teaching and the stage at which it is taught. Typically, students are provided with an overview of the basic skills of 'active' listening, which facilitate patient communication. At a basic level these include the importance of developing good rapport and the use of open-ended questions early in the consultation, appropriate eye contact and other facilitatory responses to help the patient talk, together with the ability to summarize and arrive at a shared understanding of the patients' problem. These skills can be taught in a number of ways, but the successful courses inevitably involve active learning, using role-plays with simulated patients as well as real patient interviews. Feedback is important to identify problem areas and directions for improvement and increasing use is made of videotape for this purpose. There is now consistent evidence that this type of training can result in clear improvements in basic communication skills which are maintained for a number of years. In addition to these basic packages, it is also necessary for students to learn how to communicate about sensitive or difficult areas of medical practice, including dealing with distressed patients or relatives and giving 'bad news'. Given the intrinsic difficulties in

many of these areas, training packages have made good use of role-play often involving the use of actors, for developing these skills (see 'Teaching communication skills').

A recent Cochrane review of training interventions to increase patient-centredness in consultations showed that these are generally successful in modifying styles of communication and increasing rates of patient satisfaction (Lewin et al., 2004). However the evidence was much less convincing as to whether these interventions result in improvements in either adherence to treatment or advice or in more positive health outcomes. Moreover, some studies (e.g. Kinmonth et al., 1998) have shown negative effects and this has led to a more critical approach to this area (Michie et al., 2003) and the proposal that facilitating patient adherence and/or behaviour change needs to involve the use of motivational strategies as well as patient-centred communication skills.

A number of studies have also evaluated training packages for patients prior to medical consultations with the aim of helping patients to be clear about their needs and to maximize the chances of achieving these. While early studies provided some encouraging findings, particularly for health outcomes (e.g. Greenfield et al., 1985), the results have been equivocal. Just as with training interventions for doctors, the evidence indicates that while specific behaviours (e.g. question-asking) can be modified, the impact on adherence and health outcomes is less clear (Harrington et al., 2004) and there is considerable scope for further research on this.

Finally, mention should be made of two specific patient-based approaches which have been very successful. The first by Ley and colleagues (see Ley, 1988) involved hospital patients and an additional short visit, which allowed them to ask for any information to be clarified. Compared with control groups these patients had a much higher level of satisfaction with communication, indicating that effective interventions need not be complex or time-consuming. In the more difficult area of the 'bad news' consultation, Hogbin and Fallowfield (1989) describe a simple yet effective intervention which consisted of tape-recording the consultation and allowing patients to keep the tape. Since this type of consultation is often very distressing, patients may often find it very difficult to take in all the information. Thus it was found patients welcomed the use of these tapes as something which they could go back to, and which other could also listen to. A review of consultation audio-taping studies in cancer care showed that this provision of a tape-recording holds promise as an effective adjunct to communication in this setting (McClement & Hack, 1999).

Communicating with different groups

There are ethnic and social inequalities in healthcare and health outcomes and there is some evidence to show that the quality of healthcare professionals' communication with these groups may contribute to these inequalities (Cooper & Roter, 2003). Ethnic minority patients report less involvement in consultations and lower levels of satisfaction with care, and patients from lower socioeconomic groups are given less information in consultations. Cooper and Roter (2003) recommend that communication skills training programmes need to be more broadly based to train healthcare practitioners to communicate in a culturally more sensitive way, and that strategies are needed to empower patients across ethnic and social groups to participate more in their care. Communicating effectively with those with low levels of literacy and those from minority ethnic groups requires some different considerations to those that govern communication with those who are literate and those from dominant ethnic groups.

With patients from different backgrounds, HCPs also need to be aware of possible differences in their beliefs about illness and treatment. Since these beliefs are very likely to play a major role in patients' evaluation of and use of treatment, effective communication will need to incorporate the elicitation and acknowledgement of patients' beliefs as a fundamental part of the consultation.

The benefits of good communication

One of the most widely reported effects of good medical communication is a higher level of patient satisfaction which also brings other benefits, such as increasing adherence to advice or treatment, for a number of reasons (Ley, 1988). First, effective communication should result in increased patient understanding recall of the information given in the consultation. Second, if the patient feels that the HCP understands their concerns and is empathic towards them, they may have more confidence in the advice which is offered. Furthermore, empathic communication may result in reduced levels of patient anxiety, which may not only facilitate recall of information but also promote better coping with the problem. With chronic conditions, improved self-management resulting from a greater involvement in the consultation has also been shown to lead to improved health outcome (Stewart, 1995).

Effective medical communication may be crucial in the many situations where patients are required to make important decisions relating to their own or another's health. For example, in genetic counselling, individuals may be required to process quite complex risk information, which is often couched in terms of probabilities and may be difficult to take in (see 'Communicating risk'). However, since the information may relate to the individual's long-term health prospects or may influence reproductive decisions, it is clearly vital not only that communication is clear but also that it takes account of the beliefs, expectations and needs of the individual in order that these major decisions can be taken in an informed way and that any recommended behavioural changes can be achieved more effectively (Marteau & Lerman, 2001).

A final example of a situation in which effective communication can be beneficial is prior to stressful medical procedures or investigations. There is now considerable evidence that the provision of clear sensory and procedural information about an impending medical procedure can be extremely beneficial in helping patients to cope with the procedure as well as promoting better recovery (Johnston & Vogele, 1993) (see 'Coping with stressful medical procedures').

In view of the many problems which have been identified in HCP–patient communication and the documented benefits arising from effective communication, it is not surprising that communication teaching is now regarded as a critical component of medical training. The evidence from the detailed studies of input, process and outcome components of communication can provide an excellent basis for this training and for improving the quality of patient care.

(See also 'Medical interviewing' and 'Written communication'.)

REFERENCES

Barry, C., Bradley, C., Britten, N., Stevenson, F.A. & Barber, N. (2000). Patients' unvoiced agendas in general practice consultations. *British Medical Journal*, **320**, 1246–50.

Braddock, III, C.H., Fihn, S.D., Levinson, W., Jonsen, A.R. & Pearlman, R.A. (1997). How doctors and patients discuss routine clinical decisions: informed decision making in the outpatient setting. *Journal of General Internal Medicine*, **12**, 339–45.

Campion, P., Foulkes, J., Neighbour, R. & Tate, P. (2002). Patient-centredness in the MRCGP videoexamination: analysis of large cohort. *British Medical Journal*, **325**, 691–2.

Cooper, L.A. & Roter, D.L. (2003). Patient–Provider communication: the effect of race and ethnicity on process and outcomes of health care. In B.D. Smedley, A.Y. Stith & A.R. Nelson, (Eds.). *Unequal treatment: confronting racial and ethnic disparities in health care* (pp. 552–93). Committee on Understanding and Eliminating Racial and Ethnic Disparities in Health Care. Washington, DC: National Academics Press.

Friedrikson, L.G. (1993). Development of an integrative model for the medical consultation. *Health Communication*, **5**, 225–37.

Greenfield, S., Kaplan, S. & Ware, J.E. (1985). Expanding patient involvement in care: effects on patient outcomes. *Annals of Internal Medicine*, **102**, 520–8.

Grol, R., de Maeseneer, J., Whitfield, M. & Mokkink, H. (1990). Disease-centred versus patient-centred attitudes: comparison of general practitioners in Belgium, Britain and the Netherlands. *Family Practice*, **7**, 100–4.

Harrington, J., Noble, L. & Newman, S.P. (2004). Improving patients' communication with doctors: a systematic review of intervention studies. *Patient Education and Counselling*, **52**, 7–16.

Hogbin, B. & Fallowfield, L.J. (1989). Getting it taped: the bad news consultation with cancer patients. *British Journal of Hospital Medicine*, **41**, 330–3.

Johnston, M. & Vogele, C. (1993). Benefits of psychological preparation for surgery: a meta-analysis. *Annals of Behavioural Medicine*, **15**, 245–56.

Kinmonth, A.L., Woodcock, A., Griffin, S., Spiegal, N., Campbell, M. & Diabetes Care from Diagnosis Team (1998). Randomised controlled trial of patient centred care of diabetes in general practice: impact on current well-being and future risk. *British Medical Journal*, **317**, 1202–8.

Korsch, B.M. & Negrete, V.F. (1972). Doctor–patient communication. *Scientific American*, **227**, 66–74.

Krantz, D., Baum, A. & Wideman, M. (1980). Assessment of preferences for self treatment and information in health care. *Journal of Personality and Social Psychology*, **39**, 977–90.

Lewin, S., Skea, Z., Entwhistle, V., Zwarenstein, M. & Dick, J. (2004). Intervention for providers to promote a patient centred approach in clinical consultations. *The Cochrane Library, Issue 1*. Chichester: John Wiley & Sons.

Ley, P. (1988). *Communicating with patients*. London: Croom Helm.

Marteau, T.M. & Lerman, C. (2001). Genetic risk and behavioural change. *British Medical Journal*, **22**, 1056–9.

McClement, S.E. & Hack, T.F. (1999).
Audio-taping the oncology treatment
consultation: a literature review.
Patient Education and Counselling,
36(3), 229–38.

Michie, S., Miles, J. & Weinman, J. (2003).
Patient-centredness in chronic illness:
what is it and does it matter? *Patient
Education and Counselling,* **51**, 197–206.

Miller, S.M. (1995). Monitoring versus
blunting styles of coping with cancer
influence the information patients
want and need about their disease.
Implications for cancer screening and
management. *Cancer,* **76**(2), 167–77.

Roter, D. (1989). Which facets of
communications have strong effects on

outcome: a meta-analysis. In M. Stewart &
D. Roter (Eds.). *Communicating with
medical patients* (pp. 283–96). Newbury
Park: Sage.

Roter, D. & Hall, J.A. (1989). Studies of
doctor–patient interactions. *Annual Review
of Public Health,* **10**, 163–80.

Roter, D.L., Stewart, M., Putnam, S.M.
et al. (1997). Communication patterns
of primary care physicians. *Journal of the
American Medical Association,* **277**, 350–6.

Starfield, B., Wray, C., Hess, K. *et al.* (1981).
The influence of patient–practitioner
agreement on outcome of care. *American
Journal of Public Health,* **71**, 127–31.

Stewart, M.A. (1995). Effective
physician–patient communication

and health outcomes: a review.
Canadian Medical Association Journal,
152, 1423–33.

Stiles, W.B. (1989). Evaluating medical
interview process, components:
null correlations with outcomes
may be misleading. *Medical Care,* **27**,
212–20.

Williams, S., Weinman, J., Dale, J. &
Newman, S. (1995). Patient expectations:
what do primary care patients want
from the GP and how far does
meeting patient expectations affect
patient satisfaction? *Family Practice,*
12, 193–201.

Healthcare work environments

Rudolf H. Moos, Jeanne A. Schaefer and Bernice S. Moos

Center for Health Care Evaluation, Veterans Affairs Health Care System and Stanford University

Introduction

Over the past 80 years, organization theorists have formulated three main conceptual frameworks to examine the relationship between employees and their work environment. An emphasis on employee productivity in the 1920s led to Taylorism and the scientific school of management, which focused on how to maximize task efficiency and production. Scientific management sees the work environment as a set of conditions for ensuring task performance and controlling employees: there is little regard for interpersonal issues or individual differences.

The human relations approach was shaped by concern about employee alienation and the conviction that a narrow focus on productivity could lead to poorer job performance. This approach emphasizes the value of individual and small group relationships and focuses special attention on organizational development and the quality of work life. Most recently, proponents of the socio-technical school have encompassed the technological or task attributes of a job as well as the interpersonal and organizational context in which it is performed.

These three approaches provide a gradually evolving perspective on the work environment and its connections to personal characteristics and work outcomes. We use these ideas here by describing a systems perspective that considers job-related and personal factors, the salient aspects of healthcare work environments and their impact on healthcare staff and how staff morale and performance can affect the quality of patient care and treatment outcome.

An integrated systems framework

The model shown in Figure 1 depicts the healthcare system (Panel I) as composed of organizational structure and policies; staffing and task factors; and work climate. The personal system (Panel II) encompasses staff members' characteristics, including their job position and work role; level of experience; demographic factors; and personal resources such as knowledge and self-confidence.

The model posits that the link between healthcare system factors (Panel I) and work morale and performance (Panel V) is affected by the personal system (Panel II), as well as by specific work stressors (Panel III) and staff members' coping responses (Panel IV). Work stressors (Panel III) and the organizational and personal factors (Panels I and II) that contribute to them can shape coping responses (Panel IV) and staff morale and performance (Panel V). For example, organizational factors, such as the adequacy of staffing and resources, the level of staff autonomy and control and an emphasis on good interpersonal relationships, affect staff outcomes. In turn, these staff outcomes ultimately affect the quality of care and patient outcomes (Panel VI). As the bi-directional paths in the model indicate, these processes are transactional: feedback can occur at each stage.

The healthcare system

Within the healthcare system, the work climate is linked to specific work stressors that affect employees directly. The work climate and

439

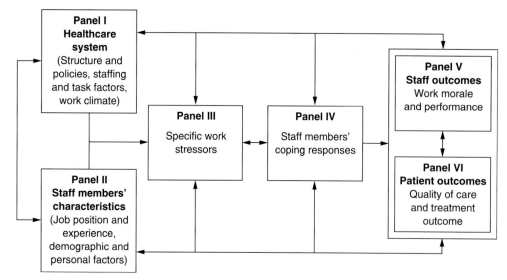

Fig 1 Conceptual model of healthcare system, staff members' personal characteristics and staff and patient outcomes.

work stressors transmit and alter the influence of other sets of healthcare system factors on staff and patient outcomes.

Work climate and work stressors

The underlying facets of work climates and specific work stressors can be organized into relationship, task and system maintenance dimensions (Moos, 1994). Relationship dimensions measure the extent to which employees and supervisors are involved with and supportive of one another. Relationship stressors arise from inter-actions with co-workers, supervisors and other healthcare staff and typically include communication problems, lack of teamwork and interpersonal conflicts among employees.

Task dimensions cover the goals and responsibilities in the work setting, such as the level of autonomy, task orientation and work pressure. Task-related stressors stem from the duties staff members perform in their job and how well prepared they are to handle them. Some salient task stressors are caring for dying, chronically ill or uncooperative patients; facing distraught and angry family members; and learning how to use increasingly complex equipment.

System maintenance dimensions assess the amount of structure, clarity and openness to change in the workplace. System stressors stem from problems in how the work unit or facility is managed and the lack of resources available to staff. Staff members frequently cite heavy workload and understaffing as major stressors. Other system stressors arise from scheduling problems; scarcity of equipment and supplies; and adverse aspects of the physical environment, such as too little space and too much noise.

Work-related stressors have increased exponentially in the last decade. Healthcare staff members are confronted with increasingly heavy responsibilities; more acutely ill patients and higher caseloads; a shortfall of resources; lack of management concern and support; and continual restructuring of the workplace. Extensive cross-cultural research highlights these special problems. Compared with employees in other types of work settings, health-care employees report less job involvement, co-worker cohesion and supervisor support. Moreover, they see healthcare settings as lacking in autonomy and clarity, characterized by high work demands and managerial control and short on physical ame-nities that make for a pleasant workplace (Aiken *et al.*, 2002*a*; Moos, 1994).

As the model indicates, these aspects of the work climate elicit specific work stressors. A difficult work climate typically is asso-ciated with more relationship and task stressors. For example, when the workplace has high work pressure and managerial control and lacks support, autonomy and clarity, staff members are likely to experience conflicts with co-workers and supervisors and problems associated with patient care tasks, such as incongruence between multiple job demands and distress resulting from patients' suffering and death (Hemingway & Smith, 1999) (see 'Burnout in health professionals').

Determinants of work climates and work stressors

Healthcare work settings vary widely in the quality of interpersonal relationships, the level of task stressors and work demands and the adequacy of clarity and management support. Organizational struc-ture and policies, and staffing and related patient care tasks account for these differences.

Organizational structure and policies

The guiding policies of a healthcare organization can affect the workplace. Compared with healthcare facilities that follow a professional model, those with a bureaucratic model are likely to have more centralized decision-making and formalized jobs, which are associated with a lack of support and autonomy, ambiguous work-related practices and high work demands and managerial control. In contrast, participative leadership helps to foster a clearer, more task-focused and innovative work climate.

The organization of nursing services also influences the work environment. In primary nursing, each nurse is responsible for the care of specific patients; in team and functional nursing, however, the head nurse retains overall responsibility for patient care and each nurse performs specific limited tasks for a group of patients. Nurses in Primary Nursing Units tend to report more involvement, support and autonomy and less management control than their team and functional nursing counterparts. Similarly, Nursing Development Units, which provide nursing staff with opportunities for decision-making and career development, tend to create supportive and stimulating work climates that emphasize autonomy and innovation (Avallone & Gibbon, 1998; Thomas, 1992).

Some work settings, such as magnet hospitals that attract and retain nurses and specialized units for the care of patients with Acquired Immune Deficiency Syndrome (AIDS), are designed to provide nurses with more autonomy and status and to enable them to widen their scope of practice. In these settings, nursing services tend to be organized in a flat structure with few supervisory personnel: decision making is decentralized, giving nurses more authority; management supports nurses' patient care decisions; and there is good communication between nurses and physicians. Nurses in these settings tend to report more job satisfaction and less emotional distress; patients in these settings are more satisfied with their care (Aolen *et al.*, 1999).

Staffing and task factors

The primary task performed by healthcare personnel can influence the workplace. Compared with staff members not involved in patient care, such as dietitians and laundry workers, staff involved in patient care, such as nurses and nurses' aides, tend to report less support, autonomy and clarity and experience their work as more demanding. Staffing and the amount of patient contact are related to work climate also. Compared with healthcare personnel in well staffed units, personnel in poorly staffed areas typically see their workplace as less cohesive and supportive, less independent and clear and more demanding. Employees who spend more time in direct contact with patients tend to rate their workplace as less innovative and higher on managerial control: they also report more alienation from their patients (Moos, 1994).

Lack of adequate staffing and resulting work overload are key factors that contribute to poorer quality care. For example, after adjusting for nurse and hospital characteristics, each additional patient per nurse may contribute to a 15–20% increase in the odds of emotional distress and job dissatisfaction among nurses. Moreover, each additional patient per nurse has been associated with a 7% increase in patient mortality within 30 days of hospital admission and a 7% increase in the odds of failure-to-rescue (deaths within 30 days of hospital admission among patients who experience complications). Nurses monitor and intervene when patients' conditions deteriorate; more patients per nurse contribute to a more harried work milieu and distress and make this job more difficult (Aiken *et al.*, 2002*b*).

Consistent with the socio-technical perspective, both patient care tasks and social systems factors, such as authority patterns and the division of labour, affect nurses' work-related attitudes and distress. Thus, the specialized nature of the tasks in intensive care units (ICUs) may create a particular work climate. For example, ICU nurses reported more involvement, support and task orientation than did nurses working in general medical-surgical units (Hipwell *et al.*, 1989) (see 'Intensive care unit'). These findings imply that

social systems factors, such as a supportive work milieu, can reduce the perception of high work demands and that, in a task-focused workplace in which there is a strong sense of involvement, high demands may contribute to team spirit and a sense of accomplishment.

The impact of work climates and work stressors

Healthcare work climates and work stressors are predictably linked to staff morale and job performance. In turn, as indicated by the conceptual model (Figure 1), characteristics of the workplace and staff members' reactions to it can influence the quality of patient care and patient outcomes.

Staff outcomes: work morale and performance

Staff members in more positive work climates typically have higher morale and are more likely to intend to stay in their job. Staff members who experience high job autonomy, empowerment, task focus and innovation tend to have more positive mood and a stronger sense of personal accomplishment and to be more satisfied with their work. In contrast, staff members who lack support and job clarity and have little influence on decision making are likely to experience emotional distress related to their work and detachment from their patients (Aiken *et al.*, 2002*a*; Laschinger *et al.*, 2004; Moos, 1994; Vahey *et al.*, 2004).

Work stressors are also predictably associated with staff members' satisfaction and job-related mood. In general, staff members who experience more work stressors, especially with regard to relationships with fellow employees and supervisors and workload and scheduling problems, report less satisfaction and more job-related distress and depression. However, staff members who are challenged by patient care tasks and successfully manage them may put more effort into their work and, in turn, be given more autonomy and responsibility (Schaefer & Moos, 1996).

Lack of organizational support and inadequate staffing are also associated with more risk of injuries to staff. Compared with nurses on units with adequate resources and staffing, nurses on units with scarce resources, poorer staffing, heavy workloads, less administrative support and innovation and more emotional distress are more likely to experience needlestick injuries. Nurses on these units also report more injuries due to staff careless-ness and inexperience, lack of patient cooperation and inadequate knowledge or supplies. The mechanisms underlying these effects likely involve the impact of the organizational climate on safety-related resources, as well as a direct influence of staffing levels and working conditions on how well nurses carry out risky procedures (Clarke *et al.*, 2002*a*; 2002*b*; Hemingway & Smith, 1999).

Patient outcomes: satisfaction, involvement in care and improvement

As the model indicates, the healthcare work environment affects staff members' morale and performance and, in turn, influences patients' satisfaction and other outcomes of care. Patients on units where nurses had a high sense of accomplishment and less emotional distress were more than twice as likely to be satisfied with their nursing care as were patients on units where nurses lacked a sense of professional efficacy and experienced more emotional distress. When nurses find their work meaningful and fulfilling, patients are more satisfied with their care and the outcomes of care (Leiter *et al.*, 1998; Vahey *et al.*, 2004) (see 'Patient satisfaction').

High morale may be especially important in enhancing staff members' relationships with patients who have mental health and behavioural problems. Staff members who take pride in their work accomplishments and are resilient to emotional distress may be better able to support patients and provide high quality mental health care. Consistent with these ideas, patients treated by staff members who experienced more professional self-efficacy and less distress were more satisfied with their treatment and preparation for independence. When the therapeutic relationship is a key aspect of service provision, problems that interfere with a staff member's ability to develop a strong alliance with patients are likely to diminish patients' satisfaction with their care (Garman *et al.*, 2002).

The work environment may also be associated with staff members' attitudes toward patients and, in turn, patients' reactions toward staff. For example, mental health staff members who perceive less autonomy and task orientation and more managerial control in the workplace are likely to be more authoritarian and restrictive; that is, to believe that persons with mental illness are threatening and require coercive management. These work-related and staff characteristics may be associated with less job satisfaction and, in turn, with more anger and violence directed from patients to staff (Morrison, 1998) (see 'Attitudes of health professionals').

Most broadly, there is a connection between the work environment and staff members' beliefs about treatment, the quality of the treatment environment, patients' involvement in treatment and self-help activities and patients' improvement during treatment. For example, staff members in substance abuse treatment programmes with supportive and goal-directed work environments were more likely to develop supportive and goal-directed treatment environments. Patients in these treatment environments participated in more treatment services, were more involved in self-help groups, were more satisfied with the programme, improved more during treatment and were more likely to participate in outpatient mental health care after discharge (Moos & Moos, 1998). Taken together, these findings confirm that the healthcare workplace is a key component of the overall healthcare treatment system.

The interplay of relationship, task and management factors

It is important to consider the connections between relationship, task and management factors when examining the impact of healthcare work settings. Work groups characterized by independence and task orientation tend to enhance morale and performance. In contrast, the combination of high job demands and lack of autonomy has a detrimental influence on employee health and satisfaction. However, challenging work can compensate somewhat for an unfavourable organizational climate.

Good management can promote task orientation and job performance. Clear job tasks and policies, adequate performance feedback and moderate structure all contribute to satisfaction and effectiveness. In the relative absence of these factors, staff members

experience low morale and distress. However, personal relationships in the workplace can alter these associations. In general, cohesive co-worker and supervisor relationships can amplify the influence of autonomy and task orientation and moderate the problematic consequences of demanding and constrained work settings.

Improving healthcare work settings

The framework we have described can be useful to healthcare managers and staff who wish to improve the quality of their work settings. In this respect, Shinn *et al.* (1993) proposed a tripartite model of coping with work stressors. There are coping strategies used by individuals (setting limits on one's activities, focusing on the positive aspects of work), strategies undertaken by groups of individuals to aid one another (mutual support groups) and strategies initiated by agencies themselves (changing job designs, providing recreational facilities). Many of the stressors which staff members confront stem from the organization of the healthcare system and are beyond the control of individual employees. Thus, management interventions to improve group and agency coping are required.

Team building and collaborative change

One type of intervention is to provide supervisors and staff with feedback about the work climate and work stressors and use it to increase communication among them. In one mental health centre, for example, staff members appraised the workplace as below average in co-worker cohesion, supervisor support, clarity and innovation, and they wanted more emphasis in each of these areas. This information was used in a teambuilding workshop to address these issues, set new goals and strengthen staff team functioning. At follow-up six months later, cohesion and support increased, but work pressure rose, perhaps because staff focused primarily on the need to complete work-related tasks (Davidson & Elliot, 1997).

Staff mutual support groups also can use feedback about the workplace to identify major problems such as lack of staff communication and confusion about work procedures and guide staff problem-solving efforts. In one example, information about the work climate enabled a staff support group to increase clarity and organization closer to the levels staff members preferred (Tommasini, 1992). This process can be taken one step further by developing a collaborative design process in which staff and management work with patients to improve the healthcare work climate and quality of care. In one chronic care hospital, the design process resulted in staff and patients identifying workplace problems, feeling more empowered to voice their concerns and enhancing their understanding of the impact of the social context and management style (Belicki & Woolcott, 1996).

Process consultation and continuous quality improvement

Over the last decade, there has been a shift away from quality assurance to process consultation and continuous quality improvement (CQI), and to a 'bottom-up' approach with ongoing feedback about the quality of care from line staff and sometimes also from patients. CQI procedures embody the principles that quality management should be a systematic and integral part of everyday healthcare work, be focused on patient-centred practice and encompass information about ongoing care and outcomes.

In one controlled trial, nurse managers were paired with nurse consultants in problem-solving leadership development meetings. On units in which nurse managers participated more fully in the intervention, staff reported greater increases in co-worker cohesion and clarity and less alienation from work than did staff on units in which nurse managers participated less (Weir et al., 1997).

In another relevant project, a CQI process was used to evaluate clinical supervision and its effect on the quality of care. CQI was implemented on five medical wards with team supervision supported by ongoing self-appraisal of work and systematic feedback from patients. After the intervention, staff monitored their work more carefully and the quality of care and patient satisfaction improved (Hyrkas & Lehti, 2003). Overall, studies in this area show that staff involvement in decision-making and team problem-solving can improve the work climate, reduce job stressors and promote better individual and organizational outcomes.

Future directions

Work stressors are likely to continue to intensify as healthcare staff encounter more acutely ill patients; cost containment efforts and competition; new medical technologies and associated ethical dilemmas; and performance monitoring and quality improvement programmes that demand ever greater accountability and perfection. To cope with these changes, healthcare staff members need to be empowered; that is, to be involved in the development of responsive organizations in which they can participate actively in improving the workplace and healthcare services. Such an approach can enhance the work climate and contribute to better staff performance and patient outcomes.

Acknowledgements

Preparation of this manuscript was supported by the Department of Veterans Affairs Health Services Research and Development Service research funds and by NIAAA Grant AA12718. The views expressed here are the authors' and do not necessarily represent the views of the Department of Veterans Affairs.

REFERENCES

Aiken, L.H., Clarke, S.P. & Sloane, D.M. (2002a). Hospital staffing, organization, and quality of care: cross-national findings. *International Journal for Quality in Health Care*, **14**, 5–13.

Aiken, L.H., Clarke, S.P., Sloane, D.M., Sochalski, J. & Silber, J.H. (2002b). Hospital nurse staffing and patient mortality, nurse burnout, and job dissatisfaction. *Journal of the American Medical Association*, **288**, 1987–93.

Aolen, L.H., Sloane, D.M., Lake, E.T., Sochalski, J. & Weber, A.L. (1999). Organization and outcomes of inpatient AIDS care. *Medical Care*, **37**, 760–72.

Avallone, A. & Gibbon, B. (1998). Nurses' perceptions of their work environment in a Nursing Development Unit. *Journal of Advanced Nursing*, **27**, 1193–201.

Belicki, K. & Woolcot, R. (1996). Employee and patient-designed study of burnout and job satisfaction in a chronic care hospital. *Employee Assistance Quarterly*, **12**, 37–45.

Clarke, S.P., Rockett, J.L., Sloane, D.M. & Aiken, L.H. (2002a). Organizational climate, staffing, and safety equipment as predictors of needlestick injuries and near-misses in hospital nurses. *American Journal of Infection Control*, **30**, 207–16.

Clarke, S.P., Sloane, D.M. & Aiken, L.H. (2002b). Effects of hospital staffing and organizational climate on needlestick injuries to nurses. *American Journal of Public Health*, **92**, 1115–19.

Davidson, G. & Elliot, B.V. (1997). Teambuilding in a rural mental health center: a case study. *Organization Development Journal*, **15**, 27–33.

Garman, A.N., Corrigan, P.W. & Morris, S. (2002). Staff burnout and patient satisfaction: evidence of relationships at the care unit level. *Journal of Occupational Health Psychology*, **7**, 235–41.

Hemingway, M.A. & Smith, C.S. (1999). Organizational climate and occupational stressors as predictors of withdrawal behaviours and injuries in nurses. *Journal of Occupational and Organizational Psychology*, **72**, 285–99.

Hipwell, A.A., Tyler, P.A. & Wilson, C.M. (1989). Sources of stress and dissatisfaction among nurses in four hospital environments. *British Journal of Medical Psychology*, **62**, 71–9.

Hyrkas, K. & Lehti, K. (2003). Continuous quality improvement through team supervision supported by continuous self-monitoring of work and systematic patient feedback. *Journal of Nursing Management*, **11**, 177–88.

Laschinger, H.K.S., Finegan, J., Shamian, J. & Wilk, P. (2004). A longitudinal analysis of the impact of workplace empowerment on work satisfaction. *Journal of Organizational Behavior*, **25**, 527–45.

Leiter, M.P., Harvie, P. & Frizzell, C. (1998). The correspondence of patient satisfaction and nurse burnout. *Social Science and Medicine*, **47**, 1611–17.

Moos, R. (1994). *Work environment scale manual*. Palo Alto, CA: Consulting Psychologists Press.

Moos, R. & Moos, B. (1998). The staff workplace and the quality and outcome of substance abuse treatment. *Journal of Studies on Alcohol*, **59**, 43–51.

Morrison, E.F. (1998). The culture of caregiving and aggression in psychiatric settings. *Archives of Psychiatric Nursing*, **12**, 21–31.

Schaefer, J. & Moos, R. (1996). Effects of work stressors and work climate on long-term care staff's job morale and functioning. *Research in Nursing and Health*, **19**, 63–73.

Shinn, M., Morch, H., Robinson, P.E. & Neuner, R.A. (1993). Individual, group, and agency strategies for coping with job stressors in residential child care programs. *Journal of Community and Applied Social Psychology*, **3**, 313–24.

Thomas, L.H. (1992). Qualified nurse and nursing auxiliary perceptions of their work environment in primary, team, and functional nursing wards. *Journal of Advanced Nursing*, **17**, 373–82.

Tommasini, N.R. (1992). The impact of a staff support group on the work environment of a specialty unit. *Archives of Psychiatric Nursing*, **6**, 40–7.

Vahey, D.C., Aiken, L.H., Sloane, D.M., Clarke, S.P. & Vargas, D. (2004). Nurse burnout and patient satisfaction. *Medical Care*, **42**, (Suppl.), II-57–66.

Weir, R., Stewart, L., Browne, G. *et al.* (1997). The efficacy and effectiveness of

process consultation in improving staff morale and absenteeism. *Medical Care*, **35**, 334–53.

Informed consent

Robin N. Fiore

Florida Atlantic University

Introduction

"Respect for persons requires that … to the degree that they are capable, [they] be given the opportunity to choose what shall or shall not happen to them. This opportunity is provided when adequate standards for informed consent are satisfied." (Belmont Report, 1979)

The doctrine of informed consent is the cornerstone of contemporary ethical practice in clinical medicine and psychology, and in research involving human subjects or human tissue. For the last quarter of a century, the principal framework for understanding informed consent in ethics and at law has been its role in promoting personal autonomy. The central ethical idea is that self-determination – here with regard to medical care/participation in research – is desirable in and of itself; it is through consent or refusal that we make our lives consistent with our values. Valid informed consent is the practical means by which the fundamental moral value of autonomy, in the sense of self-determination, is realized in healthcare decision-making.

Additionally, the practice of informed consent is thought to facilitate other factors integral to healthcare relationships. In both clinical and research encounters, patients and subjects are vulnerable parties in virtue of their lack of knowledge and in many cases, their ill health. Information and shared decision-making are thought to be potentially empowering. First, the information deficit is repaired. Secondly, since patients personally bear the burden of healthcare decisions, assisting them to make the best possible choices for themselves also realizes the professional goals of healthcare providers. Lastly, transparency encourages healthcare professionals to act responsibly in their interactions with patients and subjects.

Development of doctrine of informed consent

The association of informed consent with the facilitation of autonomous choices by patients and research subjects is relatively recent.

Indeed, modern-day elements of informed consent date only to the second half of the twentieth century (Faden & Beauchamp, 1986). For centuries, physicians followed the Hippocratic instruction to 'reveal nothing of the patient's future or present' in order to keep them from harm, deciding what information, if any, to tell patients and families and making treatment decisions on their behalf. Any responsibility to inform and obtain consent was derived from the principle of beneficence, the overarching obligation to benefit the patient: what the patient was told was largely a matter of therapeutic judgement and professional custom.

The legal history of informed consent is grounded in common law protections of bodily integrity. Physicians who did not obtain the consent of competent adult patients to medical interventions committed bodily trespass, or the intentional tort of battery. Later developments linked consent to disclosure, with the idea that consent to treatment based on inadequate or defective information was invalid, a violation of the person. Today, most jurisdictions now consider a failure to disclose as a matter of negligence rather than medical battery, that is a failure on the part of physicians with respect to regulatory standards of care.

Advance directives and 'living wills' are now recognized as part of the apparatus of informed consent. Typically, healthcare providers who abide by advance directives are protected from civil or criminal liability. In the event of provider conscientious objection, immunity and ethical practice requires that the patient be referred to someone willing to implement the advance directive or living will. Some jurisdictions expressly permit legal actions for non-compliance with valid advance directives or living wills. Institutions and physicians have been sued for medical battery and/or wrongful life (intentional or negligent interference with an individual's right to refuse medical treatment) for example, resuscitating someone who didn't want to be resuscitated or, continuing dialysis for patients with final stage renal disease who have declined dialysis (http://www.painlaw.org/).

Following revelations of experiments by the Nazis on concentration camp prisoners, the emerging doctrine of informed consent underwent specification for the special circumstances of non-therapeutic research and the promulgation of voluntary informed consent as an essential ethical prerequisite in the following international conventions for the protection of human subjects of research: *Nuremberg code on medical intervention and experimentation* (1945/1964); *Declaration of Helsinki: ethical principles for medical research involving human subjects* (World Medical Association, 1964/2004); and later *Belmont Report: ethical principles and guidelines for the protection of human subjects of research* (National Commission for the Protection of Human Subjects of Biomedical and Behavioral Research, 1979*)*. More detail is given below in the section on clinical research.

Elements of informed consent

According to the most widely referenced conceptual analysis of informed consent, five elements distinguish valid consent: competence; disclosure; understanding; voluntariness; and authorization (Faden & Beauchamp, 1986). The translation of ethical principles into practical guidelines for healthcare providers has been largely a function of court decisions and, to a lesser extent, legislation. Thus, legal requirements of disclosure and valid consent vary by jurisdiction. The discussion that follows offers general guidance with respect to ethical considerations: appropriate authorities must be consulted for specific legal rules and institutional policies.

As with all bureaucratic institutions, healthcare is replete with policies and protocols, as well as procedures for documenting compliance. Informed consent discussions usually conclude with the execution of a consent document. The signature attests to the authorization (or refusal) but does not add to the effective force of the authorization, which is only effective in virtue of the ethical elements having been satisfied.

Competence

Valid consent can only be obtained from a competent individual, or a designated proxy or surrogate on behalf of an incompetent individual. Adults are presumed competent, subject to medical and legal protocols for rebuttal. At a minimum, individuals must be able to communicate, to evidence a preference; thus unconscious or completely paralyzed persons are paradigmatically incompetent.

Competence is best understood as a contextual rather than a global concept; the capacity required for a determination that an individual is competent should be adjusted to the issues in question and their consequences. One might not be competent to stand trial yet still have the capacity to make certain medical decisions, or have the capacity to assent but not to refuse. Physical and mental status, as well as external factors (e.g. medication) and situational issues (e.g. language competency) must be taken into account.

Certain individuals, such as minors, may be incompetent by statute, though empowered in some jurisdictions to authorize specific kinds of medical care, such as reproductive healthcare.

Disclosure

The two most common standards for determining the adequacy of disclosure, and thus the validity of consent, are 'the professional standard' and the 'prudent or reasonable patient standard'. The professional standard, adopted in a British case in 1767, requires that patients be given information that physicians similarly situated (possessing the same skills and practicing in a similar community) would disclose (*Slater v. Baker & Stapleton*, 95 Eng. 860, 2 Wils. KB 359 1767). The more common standard obtaining in the United States requires that physicians disclose information that a hypothetical 'reasonable patient' in similar circumstances would regard as material to decision-making (*Canterbury v. Spence*, 464 F.2d 772, D.C. Cir. 1972). Courts in England, Canada and Australia have been moving recently towards the latter lay standard (Mazur, 2003).

There is general agreement that satisfactory disclosure includes: purpose of seeking consent (treatment authorization, research participation); nature of proposed treatment or research (therapeutic or non-therapeutic, invasive or diagnostic, investigational status); alternatives (including no treatment/non-participation); associated risks and benefits of alternatives (including likelihood and degree); and professional recommendation. There is less agreement about whether provider-specific information – such as HIV status, financial interests, success rates, experience level – should be disclosed routinely.

Understanding

Valid consent requires that the individual or surrogate must be able to comprehend general information regarding condition and prognosis, possible treatments, risks and benefits and so forth. Moreover, the patient's or subject's understanding must encompass the relevance of the information to the decision being undertaken. The patient or subject must be able to make use of the information in forming preferences, that is, must be able to weigh alternatives and to appreciate the implications of information for the individual's own situation, given that individual's particular goals, values and other preferences. Depression, anxiety, pain, etc. may interfere with the evaluation of information. However, the decision-maker's capacity may be enhanced by addressing the sources of incapacity, providing assistance, moderating external influences, etc.

Voluntariness

In order to be valid, consent or refusal must not only be un-coerced, it must be free of excessive or inappropriate influence by healthcare providers or researchers, caregivers, family members and friends. Desperate prognosis, financial distress and fear of abandonment may also invalidate consent. What counts as excessive or inappropriate influence is a normative judgement that must take particular facts about particular cases into account. However, autonomous decision-making is consistent with the idea that various moral actors and relationships may strongly influence beliefs, value commitments and judgements concerning personal wellbeing. For example, cultural traditions of family decision-making do not necessarily compromise autonomy if the individual is genuinely committed to those values. This is explored further in the section on cultural pluralism below.

Authorization (consent or refusal)

The requirement that healthcare providers/researchers obtain valid consent before initiating treatment or research protocols protects persons' interests in preventing unwanted treatment. The philosopher John Harris has characterized consents and refusals as 'the Janus faces of autonomous capacity to choose' (Harris, 2003). Competent adults may refuse care or cure, including life-saving treatment (exceptions noted below); they may consent and subsequently revoke consent. In some jurisdictions, surrogates may refuse on behalf of incompetent individuals, although the refusal of life-saving treatment on behalf of others, especially minors, usually becomes a matter for the courts. There are several standards variously available for proxy decision-making, depending on jurisdiction: 'substituted judgement', 'best interests' and 'reasonable person' standards. Under substituted judgement, the proxy does not choose but rather attempts to give the best account of the patient's hypothetical choice based on available information, including the patient's written directives and reliable oral declarations. Where no such directives or declarations are available, less subjective standards may be implemented by courts or authorized persons. Since these are not based on patient specific understandings, such standards are often controversial.

Exceptions to informed consent

Exceptions to some elements of informed consent requirements may be justified when complying would be impossible or pose a detriment to the patient's welfare.

Emergency

In an emergency situation, time and/or the patient's condition may not permit full disclosure or valid consent. If a surrogate decision maker is unavailable, procedures necessary to stabilize the patient are authorized unless the patient has a valid advance directive refusing such procedures, e.g. a 'Do Not Resuscitate Order' (DNR).

Therapeutic privilege

Under certain circumstances, a physician's ethical obligation to avoid harm may conflict with legal obligations with regard to disclosure. Physicians have historically claimed a 'therapeutic privilege' of non-disclosure (from omission of information to outright falsehood) in cases where the standard of disclosure is a threat to the wellbeing of patients, deemed likely to produce extremely adverse reactions, or expected to make rational participation in medical decisions impossible. Court decisions have constrained the circumstances in which therapeutic privilege may operate and have specifically rejected non-disclosure which has as its object pre-empting refusals of potentially beneficial treatment. Studies indicate that physicians tend to underestimate the degree to which patients would like to be informed (Appelbaum & Grisso, 1995) and that patients desired more involvement in their treatment as they acquired more information about their condition (Meisel *et al.*, 1977).

Waiver

Patients are empowered by determining what information they desire as well as their desired level of participation in medical decision-making. Thus, under certain conditions, a competent patient may voluntarily relinquish the right to make decisions and/or to receive certain disclosures. In order for such a waiver to be valid, it must be 'informed, reasoned and voluntary' (Beauchamp & Childress, 2001). Moreover, the waiver may be partial: that is, pertaining to decision-making but not information, or concerning certain types of information, e.g. decline prognosis, but not risk information. However, competent patients who have waived information that is highly relevant to decision-making cannot be regarded as having full capacity. In the case of waiver, the healthcare practitioner may not assume surrogate decision-making authority and should make every effort to obtain valid consent from an appropriate third party, as well as assent from the patient.

Compulsory treatment

Certain kinds of treatment may be legally mandated and, strictly speaking, do not require the individual's consent. Depending on the jurisdiction, compulsory treatment for infectious diseases, vaccinations for military personnel, involuntary commitment, AIDS screening for newborns, etc. may be justified by society's overriding interest in protecting public health and welfare. Nevertheless, despite the absence of choice, it is appropriate to disclose information and obtain assent wherever possible.

Incompetence

Strictly speaking, incompetence does not provide an exception to the requirements of informed consent. Disclosure and consent are properly obtained from designated healthcare surrogates, court-appointed guardians, or the courts themselves.

Special contexts

A number of special contexts pose compliance and other concerns in connection with informed consent. Two briefly addressed here are psychotherapy and clinical research.

Psychotherapy

Material risk disclosure in psychotherapeutic contexts may require more attention to the limits of confidentiality, especially legally mandated reporting requirements and the degree of patient–professional privilege accorded to different classifications of practitioners. Specific consent must be obtained from patients as well as research participants prior to recording their voices or images. In discussing alternative treatments, opinion divides on whether treatment modalities not within the expertise of the therapist should be presented. Finally, consent may need to be updated or revised in the light of information or direction developed as the therapeutic relationship proceeds.

Clinical research

While all healthcare decisions are subject to informed consent, decisions to participate in research are recognized as a special case since the beneficiaries of research are not necessarily the individuals who are assuming the burdens of participating in research (Siminoff *et al.*, 2004). Moreover, research subjects and participants confuse scientific experiments with treatment, known as the 'therapeutic misconception', often over-estimating the benefits of participating in clinical trials (Appelbaum *et al.*, 1982). In the Belmont report (United States) the 'reasonable patient standard' is replaced with a 'reasonable *volunteer*' standard of disclosure to ensure that the risks of harm and the likelihood of personal benefit (as distinguished from benefit to others or to the knowledge building enterprise) are properly distinguished.

Current debates

Rapid changes in clinical healthcare and scientific research will continue to challenge the sufficiency of consensus and codes governing informed consent.

Third party information

Medical treatment of individuals often involves personal information that implicates third parties: genetic information, family history, information about exposure to infectious disease, community information about behaviour, criminal actions, etc. The information is disclosed or collected without the knowledge or informed consent of family members and social contacts, both living and departed. Research on human tissues and genetic materials may likewise reveal information about past, present and future family members; about one's ethnic group or tribe; about one's residential community or fellow employees, without their having agreed to the risks such information poses – employment and insurance discrimination; paternity disclosure; unwanted information about future health; diminished property values, etc. While it is impractical and probably impossible to obtain the informed consent of all who are/will be adversely affected by information disclosed during clinical care or collected for research, protection against harmful or unnecessary revelation of information must be a priority.

Genetics

Informed consent applies equally to decisions about predictive genetic testing (see 'Screening: genetic'). In addition to standard disclosure elements, the consequences of having such information on the individual's record, confidentiality issues and information about the accuracy of tests and the limits of their predictive capacity should be thoroughly understood. In situations where testing for more than one condition is combined in a single testing session, commentators disagree on whether consent ought to be obtained separately for each test in the panel, or whether the requirements of disclosure and consent are satisfied by addressing 'common denominator issues' (New York State Task Force, 2004). Where tests may reveal unsolicited and perhaps unwanted information about conditions other than those for which testing is proposed, the disclosure should cover all conditions not just the intended use of the test.

Computing

The Internet has become a research site in which the health behaviours of users are observed or analyzed, and through which subsequent public health outreach may take place. Typical disclosure and consent protocols are likely to change the behaviour of those being observed and to render research less useful (Goodman, 2003). Goodman argues that health data is regularly collected and studied without giving citizens the ability to opt out – e.g. disease registries, death records – and that citizens permit this because of presumed offsetting public health benefits. However, we have yet to reach consensus on how 'public' Internet chats and blogs are and what expectations of privacy ought to prevail in this area.

Conflicts of interest

In both clinical care and clinical research, healthcare providers and investigators may have interests – financial incentives or non-financial but self-serving interests – that conflict with their primary professional duty to advocate for patients and avoid harm. In clinical care, providers may be under contract to healthcare delivery systems that provide disincentives for certain types of care, or providers may be in a position to recommend and to channel services to facilities in which he or she has a proprietary interest is held (self-referral). Disclosure of financial interests that a patient would be unlikely to know about, or be able to judge the significance of, ought to be disclosed and properly framed in terms of community standards, alternatives in which the provider does not have a conflicting interest, and available research regarding the health implications of such conflicting interest.

In research contexts, the dominant conflict of interest concern relates to equity interests in pharmaceuticals and devices under study (Fiore, 2003). Few research institutions currently require investigators to disclose 'significant financial interests' to Institutional Review Boards (IRB's) and/or subjects/participants (McCrary *et al.*, 2000). Critics argue that the failure to disclose financial conflicts of interest violates the ethical obligation to provide subjects and potential participants with information that is relevant to the choice to participate. Further, some argue that failure to disclose is fundamentally deceptive and that without complete information about the risks of participation, including the possibility that financial arrangements of the investigator might influence their judgement, consent is invalid. Others have argued that disclosure merely confuses or disturbs subjects/participants and does nothing to fundamentally eliminate or reduce conflicts of interest (Shimm & Spence, 1996). It is worth noting that the World Medical Association's 2000 revision of the *Declaration of Helsinki* now lists 'sources of funding' as information that should be provided to subjects.

Cultural diversity

The doctrine of informed consent, grounded in ideals of individual rights and self-determination, assumes a view of persons as moral agents, of physician–patient interactions and of personal relationships that is peculiarly Western. How is the autonomous decision-making model to be reconciled with divergent cultural values and customs? The argument from human rights asserts that local custom is not sufficiently weighty to override fundamental rights, specifically, the right of self-determination on which informed consent is based (Angell, 1988). Advocates of cultural sensitivity respond that the emphasis on patient autonomy arose in reaction to physician paternalism, not with the intention of alienating patients from family influences or indoctrinating liberal values. On this view, a patient's right to full participation in medical care decisions is consistent with an important role for family members. Thus the healthcare provider's obligation to disclose information and obtain voluntary consent may need to be 'relativized' to permit fuller participation by families than the standard autonomous decision-making model anticipates (Macklin, 1999) (see also 'Medical decision-making').

Conclusion

The prospect of momentous scientific advances in medicine, information and biotechnology and associated social and cultural changes suggests that informed consent and other bioethical norms will be subject to continuing reflection, debate and adaptation. The ethical doctrine of informed consent can provide a 'moral counterweight' to practical necessity.

REFERENCES

Angell, M. (1988). Ethical imperialism? Ethics in international collaborative clinical research. *New England Journal of Medicine*, **319**, 1081–3.

Appelbaum, P., Roth, L. *et al.* (1982). The therapeutic misconception: informed consent in psychiatric research. *International Journal of Law and Psychiatry*, **5**, 319–25.

Appelbaum, P.S. & Grisso, T. (1995). The MacArthur treatment competence study I: mental illness and competence to consent to treatment. *Law and Human Behavior*, **19**, 105–26.

Beauchamp, T. & Childress, J. (2001). *Principles of biomedical ethics*. New York: Oxford University Press.

Faden, R.R. & Beauchamp, T.L. (1986). *A history and theory of informed consent*. New York: Oxford University Press.

Fiore, R.N. (2003). *Conflicts of Interest in Research Involving Human Subjects*. Miami, FL: Collaborative IRB Training Initiative (CITI) Course in The Protection of Human Research Subjects. http://www.citiprogram.org

Goodman, K.W. (2003). *Ethics and evidence-based medicine: fallibility and responsibility in clinical science*. Cambridge University Press.

Harris, J. (2003). Consent and end of life decisions. *Journal of Medical Ethics*, **29**, 10–15.

Macklin, R. (1999). *Against relativism: cultural diversity and the search for ethical universals in medicine*. New York: Oxford University Press.

Mazur, D.J. (2003). Influence of the law on risk and informed consent. *British Medical Journal*, **327**, 731–4.

McCrary, S.V., Anderson, C.B. *et al.* (2000). A national survey of policies on disclosure of conflicts of interest in biomedical research. *New England Journal of Medicine*, **343**, 1621–6.

Meisel, A., Roth, L. *et al.* (1977). Toward a model of the legal doctrine of informed consent. *American Journal of Psychiatry*, **134**, 285–9.

New York State Task Force on Life and the Law (2004). *Genetic testing and screening in the age of genomic medicine*. http://www.health.state.ny.us/nysdoh/taskfce/

Shimm, D.S. & Spence, R.D. (1996). An introduction to conflicts of interest in clinical research. In J. Roy, G. Spence, D.S. Shimm & A.E. Buchanan (Eds.). *Conflicts of interest in clinical practice and research* (pp. 361–76). New York: Oxford University Press.

Siminoff, L.A., Caputo, M. *et al.* (2004). The promise of empirical research in the study of informed consent theory and practice. *HEC Forum*, **16**, 53–71.

Interprofessional education in essence

Hugh Barr

University of Westminster

Interprofessional education is taking root in increasing numbers of countries and fields of practice. Encouraging though that is, its essence becomes correspondingly harder to capture. Different health and social care policies, priorities and practices carry different implications for objectives, content and learning methods compounded by lack of a unifying rationale, a fragmented (some may say fragile) evidence base and a seemingly perverse insistence on employing terminology in bewildering disarray.

Much, however, is being done to establish interprofessional education as a coherent and cohesive movement worldwide as this chapter explains. Terminology is being clarified. Principles are being enunciated. Types of interprofessional education are being distinguished. Theoretical perspectives are being compared. Evidence is being assembled. Communications channels are being opened and mutual support networks established.

Setting the agenda

Credit for promoting interprofessional education globally goes to a World Health Organization Working Group meeting in Geneva (World Health Organization, 1988), which advocated shared learning to complement profession-specific programmes. Students, said its members, should learn together during certain periods of their education, to acquire the skills necessary to solve the priority problems of individuals and communities known to be particularly amenable to teamwork. Emphasis should be put on learning how to interact with one another, on community orientation to ensure relevance to the health needs of people and team competence.

The WHO Group was influenced by a previous WHO European Regional Working Group which had met in Copenhagen. At that meeting delegates had argued that students from health professions with complementary roles in teams should share learning in order to discover the value of working together as they defined and solved problems within a common frame of reference. Such learning should employ participatory learning methods to modify reciprocal attitudes, foster team spirit and identify and value respective roles, while effecting change in both practice and the professions. This approach would support the development of integrated health care, based on common values, knowledge and skills (d'Ivernois & Vadoratski, 1988).

With hindsight, the lead given by the WHO can be seen to have had more impact in developing countries than so-called developed countries with the exception of some smaller European states. Developments in, for example, the United States, and for the most part the United Kingdom, responded to local and national, not international, 'drivers'.

Blazing the trail

Interprofessional education had, however, already been pioneered in many countries during the preceding twenty years (Meads *et al.*, 2005) providing a fund of experience and examples on which both WHO groups drew.

The advent of interprofessional education in some countries was associated with a shift of emphasis from hospital-based to community-based healthcare as long-stay hospitals closed and community mental health and learning disabilities services developed. Charged with responsibility for long institutionalized and highly dependent ex-patients, members of multidisciplinary teams joined forces to respond flexibly to growing demands. Primary care was also developing, bringing together hitherto separate services and taking over responsibilities from hospitals. Here too multidisciplinary teams were being convened.

To attribute the rise of interprofessional education solely to the development of community-based services would, however, be less than the whole truth. In the United States much of the pioneering work was in hospitals, notably those of the Veterans' Administration. In community or hospital, the unifying factor was the need to respond to complex conditions which exceeded the capacity of any one profession acting alone. Mental illness and learning disabilities were two of these; others were physical disabilities and chronic or terminal illnesses for all age groups, but especially older people.

Emphasis on adults and older people was, however, soon redressed in countries such as the UK, where abuse of children, often leading to their death, was attributed time and again by Official Inquiries to failures in communication, collaboration and trust between professions and their respective agencies. Collaborative mechanisms were reinforced. The emphasis was further redressed as collaboration was strengthened in special needs education and juvenile justice.

Nor was collaboration limited to casework with individuals and families. It also included moves to combine energy and expertise across professions to promote health education and, in developing countries especially, public health strategies.

As the fields of collaboration multiplied so too did the number of professions participating. Different fields involved different configurations reaching beyond the health and care professions as commonly understood to include, for example, clergy, police officers, probation officers, psychologists and schoolteachers.

If most put education, health or social care at the centre, others focused, for example, on community development or the built environment.

Collaboration, which had long characterized good practice in these and other fields, was now required by policy-makers and service managers, enshrined in guidelines, included in performance appraisal and, not least, valued by practitioners themselves, but it could not be taken for granted. Miscommunication, misunderstanding and sometimes rivalry and territorial disputes too easily frustrated best laid plans, reinforcing the case for interprofessional education to cultivate collaboration in general and teamwork in particular.

Finding the focus

Given the stress put in the literature on teamwork, readers might reasonably expect it to feature strongly in objectives and content for interprofessional education. Many of the early interprofessional 'initiatives' were indeed team-based. Most, however, went unrecorded, still less evaluated, to be lost in the mists of time, although the early literature includes reports of initiatives where members of different teams were released to attend workshops where they could compare perspectives as they planned collaborative projects to implement in their teams (Spratley, 1990*a*; 1990*b*).

The notion of the learning team was, however, taking root and has since gained ground. Ways were being found to mobilize the resources of the team to respond to the learning needs of its members individually and collectively within and across professional and non-professional groupings (see, for example, Bateman *et al.*, 2003).

But teaching teamwork in pre-qualifying interprofessional education in college, at least in the UK, remained the exception (Miller *et al.*, 1999). Early examples reported of such education focused on modifying reciprocal attitudes or perceptions (e.g. Carpenter, 1995). Recent commentaries on interprofessional education put more emphasis on the reinforcement of competence (e.g. Barr, 1996; Whittington, 2004) for collaborative practice, although this has yet to be reported in evaluations of programmes (Barr *et al.*, 2005).

Furthermore, many policy-makers and service managers now look to interprofessional education to generate a multi-skilled and flexible workforce within which professions have the ability to substitute for each other and the opportunity to progress from one occupation to another without beginning their specialist professional education again from scratch. Only then, the argument runs, can the professionals be deployed optimally in the spirit of the modernization agenda set for health and social care by governments around the world and become agents of change (e.g. Meads *et al.*, 2005).

The implications for interprofessional education are far-reaching. Collaboration may still head the agenda, but it is an agenda which is growing longer and now includes items with quite different implications for objectives, content and learning methods.

Defining terms

The more diverse the fields of practice and the more varied the expectations, the greater the need for clarity of definition.

In response, the UK Centre for the Advancement of Interprofessional Education (CAIPE, 1997) defined interprofessional education as: 'Occasions when two or more professions learn from and about each other to improve collaboration and the quality of care'. It saw interprofessional education as a subset of multiprofessional education, which it defined as: 'Occasions when two or more professions learn side by side for whatever reason'.

Distinguished thus, interprofessional education is multiprofessional education with value added resulting from the methods that it employs and the ends for which it strives.

Enunciating principles

CAIPE (1996) has also published a set of principles for interprofessional education from which we select two in this context.

Alive to the dangers that interprofessional education can threaten the identity, integrity and territory of professions, CAIPE emphasized mutual respect, but went further. It asserted the need to enhance satisfaction for each of the participant professions in its own right and as a means to improve quality of care for individuals, families and communities.

In addition CAIPE asserted that effective interprofessional education will not only focus on the needs of service users and carers, but also engage them actively in planning, teaching and mentoring and as co-participants. This is easily said but less easily and less often done.

Building models

Numerous models can be devised to establish the organizational relationship between uniprofessional and interprofessional education. Each has its strengths and weaknesses. The following list is not exhaustive. Nor are the types mutually exclusive.

The marginal model

Early interprofessional education 'initiatives' were often freestanding, i.e. outside the mainstream of uniprofessional education associated with practice learning or part of continuing professional development. Either way, teachers were free to innovate unfettered by the need to win the support of profession-specific teachers for each of the professions involved or to jump through regulatory 'hoops'. Students or workers were, however, left to relate such learning as best they might to their uniprofessional education. Impact on mainstream uniprofessional education was minimal and initiatives vulnerable and short-lived when 'funny money' ran out or the champion of the cause moved on.

An early example of the marginal model organized lunchtime debates and case discussions for students concurrently on placement in Thamesmead during the 1980s (Jaques, 1986), whilst a more recent one in Vancouver organized extra-curricular team-building sessions on Saturday mornings (Gilbert *et al.*, 2000).

The block model

Early moves in Linkoping in Sweden to integrate interprofessional education into the mainstream took the form of a ten-week block before students embarked upon their uniprofessional courses. Albeit positively evaluated by its champion (Areskog, 1995), lasting benefits were harder to establish and depended on continuing opportunities for students to learn together during the remainder of their pre-qualifying studies which Linkoping subsequently added.

The cross-bar model

A more familiar model in the UK and other countries where interprofessional is being 'mainstreamed' is the cross-bar model, where specified subjects, e.g. ethics and communication studies, are ceded from two or more uniprofessional programmes to be taught across them. Such studies are, however, no more than multiprofessional unless and until their objectives and learning methods are modified to become interprofessional. This model sets limits on the degree of intrusion on profession-specific curricula, but again leaves students to integrate inter- and uniprofessional studies as best they may.

The composite model

The nature and extent of integration is often governed by 'the art of the possible'; planners looking for a number of opportunity to introduce interprofessional education. King's College London, for example, provides combined (cross-bar) studies in communications and ethics in college during the first year, complemented later by patient mapping exercises for students concurrently on placement and learning at any time on the web about a virtual extended family with multiple health and social needs (Norman, 2004).

The comprehensive model

A more radical model exemplified by the New Generation Project in Southampton and Portsmouth (http://www.mhbs.soton.ac.uk/newgeneration) devises an overall multiprofessional curriculum from the outset within which uniprofessional and interprofessional sequences of study are embedded. Logistical constraints have, however, precluded initial plans for the different professions to share their multiprofessional education at the same time and place, which prompts questions about how similar the learning will be even though the outcomes prescribed are the same.

Each of these models has advantages and disadvantages at different stages in evolution of interprofessional education, depending on the resources available and the degree of support forthcoming from teachers, colleges, employers and regulatory bodies.

Comparing theoretical perspectives

Interprofessional education applies and augments principles of adult learning (Barr, 2002). It capitalizes on the widespread application of those principles in uniprofessional education, but goes further. To take two examples, building on Knowles' (1990) argument that adult learners are intrinsically motivated by the problems they identify and seek to resolve for themselves, interprofessional learning engages participants from different professions collectively in problem-solving. Building on Lave Wenger's (1991) argument that adult learners enter into communities of practice where learning is participative, embedded and situated, interprofessional educators agrees with Strauss and Corbin (1990) that such learning involves shared commitments, shared resources, shared ideologies and shared meaning.

None of this is enough to change reciprocal attitudes for the better without also ensuring that conditions enshrined in contact theory are met, according to its exponents in interprofessional education (see, for example, Carpenter, 1995; McMichael & Gilloran, 1984). According to Allport (1979), who originated the theory, three conditions had to be met before such prejudice could be reduced: equality of status between the groups; group members working towards common goals; and cooperation during the contact. For Hewstone and Brown (1986), there were three more: positive expectations by participants; successful experience of joint working; and a focus on understanding differences as well as similarities between themselves.

Helpful though contact theory can be in formulating and testing favourable conditions necessary to effect attitudinal change during interprofessional education, it does not hypothesize conditions necessary to change behaviour.

Changing attitudes and behaviour are indeed required, but also action to improve services needs to be instigated if interprofessional education is to measure up to all the expectations now demanded. At this point it calls upon organizational learning theory (Argyris and Schon, 1978) whereby individuals work and learn collectively to improve the quality of their environment and the products or services they deliver. This theoretical perspective ties in with the notion of the learning organization which fosters a culture of questioning and enquiry, reframing information as learning and adopting a cyclical process of change given practical expression in work-based interprofessional education by the application of continuous quality improvement (Wilcock et al., 2003).

Numerous other theoretical perspectives have been introduced (see Barr et al., 2005) of which systems theory (Von Bertalanffy, 1971) is perhaps the most pertinent, applying as it does expressly to interprofessional learning and working as an antidote to the limitations of specialist disciplines in addressing complex problems, seeing wholes as more than the sum of their parts, interactions between parties as purposeful, boundaries between them as permeable and cause and effect as interdependent not linear. It is associated in interprofessional learning and working with the biopsychosocial model to counter the perceived limitations of a narrowly medical model (Engel, 1977).

Systems theory has multiple applications in interprofessional education and practice. It offers a unifying and dynamic framework within which all the participant professions can relate – person, family, community and environment – one or more of which may be points of intervention interacting with the whole. It can also be used to understand relationships within and between professions, between service agencies, between education and practice and between stakeholders planning and managing programmes.

The development of a systems theory in interprofessional education and practice which has the most potential may be activity theory (Engestrom, 1999). This offers a systemic approach to the understanding of, and intervention in, relations at micro- and macro-levels to effect change in interpersonal, interprofessional and inter-agency relations. However, much remains to be done to express its analytical model in operational terms and language with which practitioners and their managers can readily engage.

Like all education, interprofessional education is grounded in an admixture of theories. It calls on academic disciplines which contribute to the uniprofessional education systems to which it relates. It would therefore be neither appropriate nor helpful to discriminate in favour of theories from one discipline or school of thought, or to press prematurely for a unifying theoretical frame of reference, to the exclusion of the many new and creative perspectives being brought to bear.

Assembling evidence

The World Health Organization stressed that claims that interprofessional education could improve collaboration, to which it subscribed, should be subject to critical evaluation (WHO, 1976, 1978, 1988).

That argument grew stronger as evidence-based practice gained ground in the healthcare sector during the 1990s. The case for the evaluation of interprofessional education became more compelling as it became more widespread. Furthermore, investment in small group interactive learning, to which many teachers were committed on the basis of their experience, was open to challenge in cost conscious times in the absence of evidence that it was needed.

Against this backdrop a Cochrane Review was undertaken (Zwarenstein et al., 2000).[1] Criteria for inclusion were one of three experimental designs for evaluation (randomized controlled trials, controlled before and after studies and interrupted time series studies) *and* one or both of two outcomes (organizational changes and benefit to patients). Searches were carried out in Medline (1966–98) and CINAHL (1982–98) and the grey literature, but no studies met both methodological and outcome criteria (Zwarenstein et al., 2000).

That review would be repeated. Meanwhile, some members of the team saw merit in conducting a review applying less constrained criteria (Barr et al., 2005). The team therefore re-formed to become the Interprofessional Education Joint Evaluation Team (JET). Two members left and one joined at this stage.[2]

No longer simply concerned with whether interprofessional education 'worked', the research question was re-framed as follows: 'In what ways can interprofessional education contribute to improvements in collaboration between health and social care professions and in what circumstances?'

The team agreed to include a wider range of research methodologies – qualitative and quantitative – and the following continuum of outcomes adapted from the work of Kirkpatrick (1967):

- Learners' reactions
- Modification of attitudes or perceptions
- Acquisition of knowledge/skills
- Behavioural change

- Organizational change
- Benefit to patients

Medline (1966–2003) and CINAHL (1982–2001) were searched afresh plus the British Education Index (1964–2001) and the Allied Social Sciences Index and Abstracts (1990–2003).

Over 10 000 abstracts were scanned from which some 800 papers were selected for critical appraisal. Of these, 353 qualified for inclusion in the review, but power, rigour and presentation were uneven prompting a further selection of 107 higher quality studies to be made (Barr et al., 2005).

Seventy-six (71%) of the reports had been published since 1996 and the number was continuing to increase year on year. Fifty-eight (54%) originated in the United States and 35 (33%) in the United Kingdom with the remainder spread thinly. Only one was from a developing country. The most commonly involved professions were nurses followed by doctors, allied health professionals and social workers. The most common research design was before and after measurement found in 58 (55%) of the sample, but only 12 (11%) of these included controls. Five (5%) were randomized controlled trials.

Outcomes reported were overwhelmingly positive, almost certainly reflecting bias in the publishing process. Employing multiple coding to the modified Kirkpatrick classification, positive responses most frequently reported were students' satisfaction with their interprofessional learning experience (45, 42%) followed by the acquisition of knowledge and skills relating to interprofessional working (38, 36%) and changes in organizational practice (37, 35%). The other three outcomes were similar: changing attitudes or perceptions (21, 20%), changing individual behaviour (21, 20%) and benefiting patients (20, 19%).

Further analyses indicated that reporting student satisfaction, acquiring knowledge and skills and modifying attitudes were more often associated with college-led interprofessional education and changing behaviour, changing organizational practice and benefiting patients with work-led interprofessional education. In other words, the college-led initiatives can meet intermediate objectives that may be taken further by work-led ones at a later stage. Much remains to be done to formulate the continuum of interprofessional education led by college and agency over time.

Opening channels for communication

Interprofessional education is reported more and more often in journals, books and conference proceedings and on websites. The *Journal of Interprofessional Care* (see www.caipe.org.uk) is wholly dedicated to the exchange of experience about collaboration in education, practice and research throughout health and social care worldwide. Books on matters interprofessional, including two derived from the work of JET (Barr et al., 2005 and Freeth et al., 2005) in a new series by Blackwell, are growing in number, while relevant websites multiply (e.g. www.caipe.org.uk, www.hea.health.ac.uk, www.commonlearning.net and www.nipnet.org).

---

[1] The Cochrane Team comprised Jo Atkins, Hugh Barr, Marilyn Hammick, Ivan Koppel, Scott Reeves and Merrick Zwarenstein.
[2] JET comprised Hugh Barr, Marilyn Hammick, Della Freeth, Ivan Koppel and Scott Reeves.

Building mutual support

International conferences, wholly or partly dedicated to matters interprofessional, inform, challenge, stimulate and extend mutual support as partnerships are forged between nations. They are backed up by national and regional networks such as CAIPE, the Nordic Interprofessional Network (NIPNET) and, the International Association for Interprofessional Education as Collaborative Practice (Inter Ed).

Building on the basics

Much remains to be done in interprofessional education to:

- encourage consistent use of concepts and terminology
- refine, apply and test principles
- discriminate between learning methods and test their efficacy
- develop a coherent but multifaceted rationale
- weave college-led and work-led uni- multi- and interprofessional education into a mutually reinforcing and progressive continuum of learning
- raise the general standard of evaluation to that of the best
- improve update and elaborate the evidence base
- strengthen channels for communication and mutual support

Gone are the days, however, when interprofessional education could be dismissed as a passing whim, comprising assorted, ephemeral and marginal activities. More complex and perhaps more confusing and more controversial than it once seemed, interprofessional education is responding to the agenda set internationally by the World Health Organization and nationally by reformist governments (Meads *et al.*, 2005) to become a force for change in education, health and social care policies. It remains, however, in essence a collective response by practitioners from increasing numbers of professions to the complexity of the human condition.

REFERENCES

Agyris, C. & Schon, D. (1978). *Organizational learning: a theory of action perspective.* New York: McGraw Hill.

Allport, G. (1979). *The Nature of Prejudice* (25th edn.). Cambridge, MA: Perseus Books Publishing.

Areskog, N. (1995). Multiprofessional education at the undergraduate level. In K. Soothill, L. Mackay & C. Webb (Eds.). *Interprofessional relations in health care* (pp. 125–39). London: Edward Arnold.

Barr, H. (1996). Ends and means in interprofessional education: towards a typology. *Education for Health*, **9**, 341–52.

Barr, H. (2002). *Interprofessional education: today, yesterday and tomorrow.* Occasional Paper 1. London: The Learning and Teaching Support Network for Health Sciences and Practice.

Barr, H., Koppel, I., Reeves, S., Freeth, D.S. & Hammick, M. (2005). *Effective interprofessional education: argument, assumption and evidence.* Oxford: Blackwell.

Bateman, H., Bailey, P. & MacLellan, H. (2003). Of rocks and safe channels: learning to navigate. *Journal of Interprofessional Care*, **17**, 141–50.

Bertalanffy, L. von (1971). *General systems theory.* London: Allen Lane.

CAIPE (1996). *Principles of interprofessional education.* London: CAIPE.

CAIPE (1997). Interprofessional education: a definition. *CAIPE Bulletin*, **13**, 19.

Carpenter, J. (1995). Doctors and nurses: stereotype and stereotype change in interprofessional education. *Journal of Interprofessional Care*, **9**, 151–62.

d'Ivernois, J.-F. & Vadoratski, V. (1988). *Multiprofessional education of health personnel in then European region.* Copenhagen: WHO.

Engel, G. (1977). The need for a new medical model: a challenge for biomedical. *Science*, **196**(4286), 129–36.

Engestrom, I. (1999). Expansive visibilization of work: an activity–theoretical reconceptualization. Kluwer Academic Publishing, the Netherlands. *Computer Supported Cooperative Work*, **8**, 63–93.

Freeth, D.S., Hammick, H., Reeves, S., Koppel, I. & Barr, H. (2005). *Effective interprofessional education: development, delivery and evaluation.* Oxford: Blackwell.

Gilbert, J., Camp, R., Cole, C. *et al.* (2000). Preparing students for interprofessional teamwork in health care. *Journal of Interprofessional Care*, **14**, 223–36.

Hewstone, M. & Brown, R. (1986). Contact is not enough: an intergroup perspective on the contact hypothesis. In M. Hewstone & R. Brown (Eds.). *Contact and conflict in intergroup encounters.* Oxford: Blackwell.

Jaques, D. (1986). *Training for teamwork: the report of the Thamesmead Interdisciplinary Project.* Oxford: Educational Methods Unit, Oxford Polytechnic.

Kirkpatrick, D.L. (1967). Evaluation of training. In R. Craig & L. Bittel (Eds.). *Training and development handbook.* New York: McGraw Hill.

Knowles, M. (1990). *The Adult Learner: a Neglected Species* (4th edn.). Houston, TX: Gulf.

Lave, J. & Wenger, E. (1991). *Situated learning: legitimate peripheral participation.* Cambridge: Cambridge University Press.

McMichael, P. & Gilloran, A. (1984). *Exchanging views: courses in collaboration.* Edinburgh: Moray House College of Education.

Meads, G., Ashcroft, J., Barr, H., Scott, R. & Wild, A. (2005). *The case for interprofessional collaboration.* Oxford: Blackwell Science.

Miller, C., Ross, N. & Freeman, M. (1999). *Shared learning and clinical teamwork: new directions in education for multiprofessional practice.* London: English National Board for Nursing, Midwifery and Health Visiting.

Norman, I. (2003). *Inter-professional education for undergraduates in south east London: a progress report.* Conference presentation at London South Bank University, 21st November 2003.

Spratley, J. (1990a). *Disease prevention and health promotion in primary health.* London: Health Education Authority.

Spratley, J. (1990b). *Joint planning for the development and management of disease prevention and health promotion strategies in primary health care.* London: Health Education Authority.

Strauss, A. & Corbin, J. (1990). *Basics of qualitative research: grounded theory procedures and techniques.* London: Sage.

Whittington, C. (2004). A model for collaboration. In J. Weinstein, C. Whittington & T. Leiba (Eds.).

Collaboration in social work practice. London: Jessica Kingsley Publisher.

World Health Organization (1976). Health manpower development. Doc./A29/15 (unpublished). Presented at the 29th World Health Assembly.

World Health Organization (1978). *Report of the international conference on primary*

healthcare: the Alma Ata Declaration. Geneva: WHO.

World Health Organization (1988). *Learning together to work together for health.* Geneva: WHO.

Wilcock, P., Campion-Smith, C. & Elston, S. (2003). *Practice professional development planning: a guide for*

primary care. Oxford: Radcliffe Medical Press.

Zwarenstein, M., Reeves, S., Barr, H. *et al.* (2000). *Interprofessional education: effects on professional practice and health.* Oxford: The Cochrane Library.

Medical decision-making

Clare Harries[1] and Peter Ayton[2]

[1]University College London
[2]City University, London

Introduction

Doctors constantly make decisions that affect the health and lives of other people. They gather evidence by interpreting the signs and symptoms of the patient, conducting examinations and determining appropriate tests. All of these actions imply the use of judgement and decision-making. Using such evidence they may form a diagnosis and conclude what, if anything, is to be done. In the current healthcare climate, patients are also encouraged to participate in decision-making, either by sharing in it, or by making their own informed decisions, on the basis of the evidence presented to them by doctors (Charles *et al.*, 1997). Many of these decisions will be based on clear evidence from the patient and tried and tested methods drawn from the doctor's medical knowledge and may seem quite straightforward. However, very often, simple medical principles and rules will not be available. From the perspective of formal Decision Analysis, in order to make an optimal decision, a doctor and patient must identify all the options available, work out their potential outcomes and the probability that these outcomes will occur. They also need to assess how good or bad that outcome occurring would be. Such a process is often difficult for several reasons. Firstly, it is difficult to identify the options and outcomes and their associated probabilities. As the evidence base of medicine develops this may become easier, but where clear evidence about options, or actuarial statistics about their outcomes, are not available doctors have to rely on their judgement. Secondly, people find it difficult to understand and clearly communicate probabilities. Thirdly, we find it difficult to assess the utility, or the potential good or bad, of outcomes. Beyond these three aspects of decision-making, the combination of this information is hampered by the fact that the number of components in even relatively straightforward decisions soon expands beyond human information processing capacities (estimated at $7+/-2$ pieces of information, or 4 chunks; Simon, 1979). This capacity may be reduced given the unpleasant emotions and stress associated with considerations of potentially negative outcomes. In this chapter we shall review the evidence that these aspects of decision-making are difficult, discuss the psychological processes underlying them and briefly review the techniques that have emerged which seem to make good medical decision-making easier.

Clinical judgement

Although identification of the options and outcomes and their associated probabilities is partly the role of evidence-based medicine, the evidence may be uncertain: signs and symptoms can be ambiguous and tests results are rarely 100% accurate. Tests and treatments can involve adverse side effects or a risk of permanent damage or even death. In the absence of a clear rule for such situations doctors will be obliged to apply their own judgement.

Research investigating the topic of medical judgement has a fairly short, but intense, history. The first significant development was Meehl's (1954) book which evaluated clinical judgement. Meehl compared the intuitive clinical judgements made by experts (e.g. 'is this patient schizophrenic?') with those that could be made by a statistical formula using the same information. The statistical decisions were based on a 'linear model'. A linear model summarizes the relationship between a set of predictor variables and some criterion value – the outcome to be predicted. For example, if predicting the chances of survival from major surgery, relevant predictor variables may be the age, weight and general fitness of the patient. The linear model is constructed in such a way as to maximize the statistical relationship between the predictor variables and the criterion to be predicted. The value of each of the predictor variables is differentially weighted according to the strength of its diagnostic relationship to the criterion and then all the variables are summed.

In approximately 20 studies which compared clinical decisions with statistical decisions, Meehl found that the statistical model provided more accurate predictions or the two models were equally accurate. Over the years since there have been many more studies comparing clinical and statistical judgement in an enormous range of areas of judgement. The superiority of the statistical method over clinical judgement has been replicated in all of these studies. Meehl (1986) commented: 'There is no controversy in social science which shows such a large body of qualitatively diverse studies coming out so uniformly in the same direction as this one'.

Despite this claim, the effect of the research on the practice of clinical judgement has been limited; according to Dawes (1988) it is 'almost zilch'. Dawes argues that this is because the findings are a challenge to the self-perceptions of experts. It is difficult for highly trained clinicians to accept that they cannot outperform a procedure which simply adds up the cues in favour of each judgement and picks the one with the highest score. This resistance may well be stiffened by the knowledge that the statistical method will not be perfect. There is evidence that resistance to the use of simple decision rules, which (given present knowledge) cannot be outperformed, increases with expertise and the importance of the decision. Doctors may find it unacceptable to settle for the given number of errors implied by the statistical approach when they feel that their judgement might do better. Moreover, when the statistical decision conflicts with the doctor's decision, the statistical decision may be seen as risky while their own judgement is seen as safe, quite opposite to the conclusion drawn from research.

So why is statistical judgement superior? Of course the statistical approach relies on all the relevant evidence being coded in a quantitative fashion, something which may itself require considerable clinical skill but which would not ordinarily be performed in clinical situations. The statistical model will, moreover, utilize this evidence in an entirely consistent fashion. The statistical model will not be influenced by fatigue and boredom or distracted by spurious factors as human judgement is. A large number of studies have discovered inconsistency in medical judgements. Studies reviewed by Schwartz and Griffin (1986) have shown that doctors will show substantial disagreement with each other when interpreting chest X-rays, electrocardiograms and electroencephalograms, as well as more global quantities such as severity of depression. They will also sometimes disagree with their own previous judgements. One study that asked pathologists to examine the same tissue sample on two different occasions found that the conclusions (malign or benign) differed 28% of the time.

The statistical modelling approach of Meehl and others makes no claims to investigate how medical judgements are actually made. However, other studies of medical judgement have sought to examine the extent to which descriptive theories of human judgement, developed in the psychological laboratory, apply in medical contexts. One theoretical approach to judgement assumes that, because human information processing capacity is limited, people do not judge under uncertainty using systematic strategies. Instead they use mental heuristics (rules of thumb) to judge uncertainties (Kahneman et al., 1982). One such heuristic is representativeness. This heuristic determines how likely it is that an event is a member of a category according to how similar or typical the event is to the category. In a medical situation this may seem a reasonable strategy: a doctor might judge how likely a person is to have a disease on the basis of the similarity between their symptoms and those typical of the disease. For example, if a person walks in with all the symptoms of a cold it seems reasonable to judge it highly probable that they

have a cold. However, this strategy neglects consideration of the relative prevalence of cold symptoms in the presence or absence of a cold: such judgements need to be made on the basis of diagnostic, rather than typical information. When base-rates of different categories vary, judgements may be correspondingly biased.

Another heuristic used for probabilistic judgement is availability. This heuristic is invoked when people estimate likelihood or relative frequency by the ease with which instances can be brought to mind. Instances of frequent events are typically easier to recall than instances of less frequent events so availability will often be a valid cue for estimates of likelihood. However, availability is affected by factors other than likelihood. For example, recent events and emotionally salient events are more easy to recollect. Dawson and Arkes (1987) report the following anecdote to illustrate this point. An older practising physician had non-specific abdominal discomfort and had not been feeling well for several days. Chronic appendicitis was diagnosed and treated surgically. After having this experience he began diagnosing 'chronic appendicitis' in many of his older patients who presented with new-onset, non-specific abdominal discomfort and referred them for surgery.

Christensen-Szalanski et al. (1983) discovered an availability bias in physicians' estimates of the risk (mortality rate) of various diseases. They studied physicians and students and found that both groups over-estimated the risks. In general, physicians were more accurate than the students but the estimates of both groups were found to be biased by actual encounters with people with the disease. Judgements made on the basis of availability then are vulnerable to bias (see also 'Risk perception').

The literature reporting investigations of expert medical judgements provides several instances of poor judgement attributable to heuristic processing, some of which may have serious potential consequences. Eddy (1982) set a sample of physicians the task of estimating the likelihood that a patient had cancer given that, prior to the X-ray, their examination of the patient indicated a 99% probability that the lesion was benign but that the X-ray test was positive and had indicated it was malignant. They were told that research into the accuracy of the test showed that 79.2% of malignant lesions were correctly diagnosed and 90.4% of benign lesions were correctly diagnosed by the test. Applying a probability rule known as Bayes' theorem to this evidence allows us to consider the diagnosis as a statistical inference and calculate that the probability of cancer, in the light of the positive test, is nearly 8%.

However, most of the physicians misinterpreted the information about the reliability of the test and estimated the likelihood of cancer to be about 75%. When asked about their reasoning the physicians report that they assumed that the probability of cancer given a positive test result [p(cancer/positive)] is equal to the probability of a positive test result in a patient with cancer [p(positive/cancer)]. They seem to have used a representativeness heuristic in that they judged the likelihood of cancer in patients with a positive test in terms of how typical (or representative) they were of patients with cancer. They failed to properly consider the impact on the outcome of the very low incidence of the disease together with the tendency of the test to (falsely) show positive test results.

Confirmation that, in fact, real decisions are taken on the basis of such misunderstandings is provided by Dawes (1988). He cites a case of a doctor performing mastectomy operations on women judged to have high risk of breast cancer. The surgery was justified on the basis of the supposition that 'one in two or three DY (highest-risk) women will develop breast cancer between the ages of 40 and 59'. However, it turns out that this conclusion was based on the probability that a woman with cancer will have DY breasts [p(DY/cancer)], not on the relevant probability that a woman with DY breasts will develop cancer [p(cancer/DY)]. The relevant probability, that a woman with DY breasts will develop cancer [p(cancer/DY)], is approximately one in eight.

In order to make a clinical diagnosis the doctor must make an inference that involves assessing the probability that a patient has the disease given some pattern of symptoms [p(disease/symptoms)]. However, according to Eddy and Clanton (1982), medical knowledge is not organized to assist this process. Most medical texts discuss the probability that patients will present a certain pattern of symptoms given that they have the disease [p(symptoms/disease)]. This information is not sufficient for making a diagnosis and the focus on it may well encourage the false notion that p(disease/symptoms) is the same as p(symptoms/disease). The confusion between the two probabilities may be further engendered by the type of instruction that trainee physicians receive. On ward rounds patients with certain diseases are examined and the co-occurrence of symptoms is noted. However, people with the same symptoms but without the disease (healthy people not in hospital and patients with similar symptoms and different diseases) will not be subject to the same scrutiny. As a result the diagnostic significance of a given set of symptoms may be over-estimated.

Communication and understanding of probabilities

We have already seen an indication that physicians' judgements may be influenced by their use of rules of thumb. But there are several other notable features of the judgement and perception of probability. When people communicate about risk, they may be communicating one of several different things (Gigerenzer, 2003). Gigerenzer illustrates the potential for confusion in risk communications with an anecdote from a physician colleague whose patients were interpreting his advice that they had a 30–50% chance of a developing a sexual problem from taking a particular antidepressant as indicative of the fact that they had a propensity to have sexual problems – on 30–50% of all occasions. In fact such problems occured for only 30–50% of people.

Whilst risk communication in medicine is often in verbal terms, these do not map clearly onto numerical terms, their mapping is context–specific and verbal terms contain additional directional information. For example, an event with a probability of 0.3 of occurring may be 'doubtful', or 'possible'. Doctors communicating in numerical terms are trusted more, and seen as less likely to distort the probability. But such numerical terms are subject to classical psychophysical phenomena (Lloyd, 2001). They are perceived categorically (e.g. no risk, low risk, medium risk, high risk). Their meaning is context specific. And perception of changes in risk will depend upon the risk levels involved. For example, we find it hard to distinguish between small probabilities (such as 1 in 20 000 and 1 in 200 000), and we tend to perceive situations as dangerous or safe, rather than integrating different risks. Such effects can be exacerbated when information is presented in terms of relative risk.

A treatment that reduces fatalities by 50% (a relative risk statement) sounds better than one that reduces fatalities by 5%, nonetheless the latter treatment might be more valuable than the former; reducing a tiny risk by 50% might be trivial relative to reducing a large risk by 5%. For example, media reports on the association between the contraceptive pill and thrombosis in 1995 were followed by a 16% increase in abortions in the first quarter of 1996. Arguably, the reports of the doubling of the risk of thrombosis with the pill led to its reclassification by the public as dangerous even though the risk that was doubled was still very small (Lloyd, 2001).

Even numerical probabilities are understood context-specifically: for example the difference between a 0% chance of dying and a 10% chance of dying is more salient than a 90% chance of survival and a 100% chance of survival. Such framing effects are largest when relative risk rather than absolute risk is presented. The strong effect of context is also seen in the contrast between people's perception of risk to themselves, and to other people, known as 'unrealistic optimism'. A striking example of this is seen in a study, cited in Lloyd (2001), in which 80% of cancer patients told there was no chance of cure, thought that there was some chance.

Two methods are currently being promoted to improve risk communications. Firstly, there is evidence to suggest that numerical probabilities can be communicated more clearly in terms of frequencies than probabilities, percentages etc. For example, when test information is presented as frequencies, the majority of physicians and other people reason correctly about conditional probability. Gigerenzer (1994) reviews a number of studies that show a dramatic improvement in reasoning with probabilities if they are converted into frequencies. For instance, we can change the mammography example above as follows:

Imagine 100 people (think of a 10 x 10 grid). We expect that one woman has cancer and a positive mammography. Also we expect that there are 10 more women with positive mammographies but no cancer. Thus we expect 11 people with positive mammographies. How many women with positive mammographies will actually have breast cancer?

With frequencies you immediately 'see' that only about 1 out of 11 women who test positive will have cancer. Although Harvard medical school staff have difficulties with the probability version (the majority give wrong answers) most undergraduates readily provide the correct answer to similar problems constructed with frequencies. Gigerenzer's physician colleague could also more clearly explain the risks involved with the antidepressant by talking in terms of the number of people taking the medication who would experience sexual problems.

A second method adopted to improve communication of risk is to present the information pictorially. A range of pictorial types can be used: bar charts, pie charts, sets of happy and sad faces, or different coloured human figures. Relatively little research has been carried out on the impact of such pictures though it is clear that they influence risk perceptions. Whilst one study found that the improvements with frequency formats were amplified when pictorial information was also available (Cosmides & Tooby, 1996), other studies have found that graphical information leads to greater risk aversion compared with numerical information. Presenting mortality risks in icons is associated with higher perceived risk and results in a lower number of participants choosing what may be the optimal choice (Timmermans *et al.*, 2004). Risks represented as pictorial figures are perceived as riskier than risks presented as numbers (Stone *et al.*, 1997). This reiterates the findings of a review which suggests that providing more information which is understandable is associated with improved patient knowledge but greater wariness to take treatments or participate in trials (Edwards *et al.*, 2001) (see 'Communicating risk').

Ascertaining utilities

The third component of decision-making is the identification of the utility of potential outcomes. A distinction can be made between experienced utilities, or the pleasure and pain experienced during a particular moment; and decision utilities, the underlying valuation of outcomes that drive decision-making. Such utilities are often inferred from people's preferences and used to explain people's preferences. Psychologists have long realized that such valuations are not simply waiting to be uncovered, but rather are constructed by decision-makers (patients and physicians) as they consider the options and outcomes available. What is preferred depends upon what's on offer, how it's evaluated or assessed, how it's presented and when it's offered.

The effect of what's on offer can be seen both in patients' and in physicians' preferences. For example, preferences can be affected by whether options are evaluated one at a time, or side by side. In a study by Zikmund-Fisher *et al.* (2004), participants rated two eye surgeons. The two surgeons available were similar but one was Harvard-educated and had completed 80 successful operations; the other was Iowa educated and had completed 300 successful operations. Evaluated independently, the Harvard-educated surgeon was given a higher rating. However, when both surgeons were evaluated side-by-side, the Iowa surgeon was given the higer rating. The psychological explanation for this effect focuses on the evaluability of certain criteria. In this example, 80 successful operations indicates a reasonable performance, until a participant realizes that there are surgeons out there with 300 successful operations under their belt. Such contrast effects can be reduced by providing patients with reference points such as the minimum, maximum or average performance, when evaluating just one option.

But the ability to evaluate is not the only phenomenon underlying changes in preference with changes in options. In a study by Redelmeier and Shafir (1995), physicians were asked to prioritize for surgery someone from a choice of either a 52-year-old woman or a 72-year-old man; or prioritize someone from a choice of these two plus a 55-year-old woman. With a choice of two people most physicians prioritized the woman. With the choice of three, most prioritized the older man. This behaviour can be understood as an example of the effects of reason-based choice: decision-making is driven by identifiable reasons or arguments. But in choice the reasons that are used are affected by contrasts between the options available. Since any reason that led to a priority of the 52-year-old woman over the 72-year-old man also applied to the 55-year-old woman, they were not useful as a basis for decision-making. Those that become useful are those which prioritized the 72-year-old man. Plainly, the reasons that are salient and influential depend on the alternatives confronting the decision-maker.

Preferences are also affected by the method we use to make them. For example we could judge how much one would have to adjust an attribute of one option to make it as good as another, or we could simply choose between them. In a study by Sumner and Nease (2001), participants choosing between living for 30 years with migraines for 10 days per month, and living for 20 years with migraines for 4 days per month, tended to prefer to live for longer. But participants who were asked to state how many days of migraine during 30 years would make that option equivalent to living for 20 with migraine for 4 days per month gave a figure indicating that had they had the choice, they would prefer to live for a shorter period. There are several explanations of this pattern of results. It may be that asking for a judgement of one attribute led to an increase in salience (and therefore influence) of the attribute being judged (in this case days of migraine) or any attribute on a similar dimension. This effect has been labelled 'scale compatibility'. But there are also arguments that, in changing from judgement to choice, people change the way they process information. In judgement, the attributes or outcomes of an option must be traded off or compensate for each other, but in a choice people might just refer to prominent attributes (such as years of life) to resolve the dilemma.

In addition there is clear evidence that choosing an option encourages decision-makers to focus on positive attributes, while rejecting an option encourages a focus on negative attributes. The resulting inconsistency in attention to features can result in people both preferring *and* rejecting the same option depending on whether they are asked which option they want or which option they don't want (Shafir, 1993).

The effects of framing of information can be seen when preferences change depending on whether the probability of outcomes in surgery are presented as death or survival. But outcomes can also be framed as resulting from your action, or from inaction. People are reluctant to make choices in which harm is the result of their action. For example, most people will not accept a risk of 9 in 10 000 of death from a vaccine that eliminates a 10 in 10 000 probability of fatal flu, even though the result would be a reduction in risk (Ritov & Baron, 1990). However, what is seen as an action, or seen as leading to potential regret, depends upon what is seen as the status quo, or the norm in that situation.

Finally, people's preferences, and therefore their apparent utilities, change depending upon how soon the outcome will occur. In a study by Christensen-Szalanski (1984), one month before labour women expressed a preference to avoid anaesthesia during labour. During labour most chose to have anaesthesia, but one month later they again preferred the idea of avoiding anaesthesia during labour. Arguably, such preference differences result from our inability to predict how we will feel in a different emotional state (an intrapersonal empathy gap). We are over-influenced by our current emotional state in decision-making, and are particularly poor at making predictions across 'hot–cold' gaps. Which decision is the optimal one in the labour situation might be a matter of debate, but the attractiveness of vices over virtues (immediately fun but ultimately health-depreciating activities over steady health-promoting activities) has been explained in terms of these temporal and emotional effects (Loewenstein *et al.*, 2003).

Assisting medical decision-making

The prescriptive approach to decision-making seeks to identify the ideal method by which decisions should be made. We have already suggested that choice of actions should reflect both probabilities and utilities. Expected Utility theory, the major theory defining rational decisions, also prescribes evaluation of different courses of action in order to choose the best. Each option is evaluated in terms of the probabilities of achieving all of the possible outcomes that may ensue from it and their relative value. For each option these two quantities are multiplied together to determine the expected utility. Accordingly, the option which has the highest expected utility is chosen. At an individual decision-making level, Decision Analysis (the term given to the application of Expected Utility theory) encourages the expression of values that reflect individual patient's utilities for the outcomes. The method can thereby be used as a means for involving patients in decisions about their own treatment (important when informed consent is required) and it has been developed as a counselling technique to help pregnant women make decisions about risky tests for foetal abnormalities. The approach can also accommodate problems of allocation of limited resources and decisions about administering tests given that costs and risks are involved.

The strategy of Decision Analysis is to decompose what may be very complex decisions involving many considerations into basic components. Using a decision tree the components are then evaluated so that the attractiveness of each option can be determined. The appeal of the procedure is that it represents a systematic attempt to analyze all relevant considerations and give them their appropriate weight. Studies of decision analysis used in real clinical settings indicate that the procedure results in different decisions being made from those that would have been made intuitively; doctors are sometimes surprised by the recommendations of the analysis (Sonnenberg & Pauker, 1986) which is one reason why they may be reluctant to accept the result. To this extent then the procedure is clearly not redundant, but does it produce *better* decisions? Many patient decision aids aim to help reduce decision conflict, and to encourage decisions that are consistent with patients' values (in other words help patients work out how they value different attributes or goals and how to trade these off against each other), but there is evidence that decision aids without an explicit utility assessment procedure facilitate decision-making. The decomposition rationale (break the decision down and consider each element separately) suggests that it prevents information overload and permits consideration of more factors than unaided intuition would allow.

Elstein *et al.* (1986) studied decisions regarding oestrogen replacement therapy, a treatment for osteoporosis which entails an increased risk of cancer, for a sample of women with varying levels of cancer risk, fracture risk and symptom severity. They compared intuitive decisions made by the doctors with those made by decision analysis where the same doctors provided their own estimates of all the relevant probabilities and utilities for all the possible outcomes. The decision analysis recommended the treatment far more often than the clinicians' intuitions. Intuitively the clinicians appeared to give far too much weight to the risk of cancer. Calculations indicated that as very poor outcomes are so rare the increased risk was heavily outweighed by the powerful benefits of the therapy. The idea that the doctors' component probabilities and utilities were somehow in error was rejected. In general the component estimates of likelihood were accurate and sensitivity analysis on the values used showed that any reasonable set of values entered in the decision analysis recommended treatment. Decisions therefore appeared to hinge on the sub-optimal way different bits of information were combined, not on (un)awareness of specific risks and benefits.

Conclusion

Traditionally, medical training has been largely concerned with the biomedical sciences. Increasingly however, competence in the decision sciences is being seen as vital to good medical practice. The methods for making a decision become crucial when the physician is uncertain through incomplete or ambiguous information, when risks are involved, and when the patient is participating in the decision. The growing mass of psychological research investigating medical decision-making presents a strong argument for the view that these decisions may not always be ideal and that, with the application of developing methods, they can be improved.

REFERENCES

Charles, C., Gafni, A. & Whelan, T. (1997). Shared decision-making in the medical encounter: what does it mean? (or it takes at least two to tango). *Social Science and Medicine*, **44**, 681–92.

Christensen-Szalanski, J.J.J. (1984). Discount functions and the measurement of patients' values: womens' decisions during childbirth. *Medical Decision Making*, **4**, 47–58.

Christensen-Szalanski, J.J.J., Beck, D.E., Christensen-Szalanski, C.M. & Koepsell, T.D. (1983). Effects of expertise and experience on risk judgements. *Journal of Applied Psychology*, **68**, 278–84.

Cosmides, L. & Tooby, J. (1996). Are humans good intuitive statisticians after all? Rethinking some conclusions from the literature on judgement under uncertainty. *Cognition*, **58**, 1–73.

Dawes, R.M. (1988). *Rational choice in an uncertain world*. Orlando, FL: Harcourt.

Dawson, N.V. & Arkes, H.R. (1987). Systematic errors in medical decision making: judgement limitations. *Journal of General Internal Medicine*, **2**, 183–7.

Eddy, D.M. (1982). Probabilistic reasoning in clinical medicine: Problems and opportunities. In D. Kahneman, P. Slovic & A. Tversky (Eds.). *Judgement under uncertainty: heuristics and biases.* Cambridge University Press.

Eddy, D.M. & Clanton, C.H. (1982). The art of clinical diagnosis: solving the clinicopathological exercise. *The New England Journal of Medicine*, **306**, 1263–8.

Edwards, A., Elwyn, G., Covey, J., Matthews, E. & Pill, R. (2001). Presenting risk information – a review of the effects of "framing" and other manipulations on patient outcomes. *Journal of Health Communication*, **6**, 61–82.

Elstein, A.S., Holzman, G.B., Ravitch, M.M. *et al.* (1986). Comparisons of physicians' decisions regarding estrogen replacement therapy for menopausal women and decisons derived from a decision analytic model. *American Journal of Medicine*, **80**, 246–58.

Gigerenzer, G. (1994). Why the distinction between single event probabilities and frequencies is important for psychology (and vice-versa). In G. Wright & P. Ayton (Eds.). *Subjective probability* (pp. 129–61). Chichester, UK: Wiley.

Gigerenzer, G. (2003). *Reckoning with risk.* London: Penguin Books Ltd.

Kahneman, D., Slovic, P. & Tversky, A. (1982). *Judgement under uncertainty: heuristics and biases.* Cambridge University Press.

Lloyd, A.J. (2001). The extent of patients' understanding of the risk of treatments. *Quality in Health Care*, **10**, 114–18.

Loewenstein, G., Read, D. & Baumeister, D.F. (2003). *Time and decision: economic and psychological perspectives on intertemporal choice.* Russell Sage Foundation.

McNeil, B.J., Pauker, S.G., Sox, H.E. & Tversky, A. (1982). On the elicitation of preferences for alternative therapies. *New England Journal of Medicine*, **306**, 1259–62.

Meehl, P.E. (1954). *Clinical versus statistical prediction: a theoretical analysis and a review of the evidence.* Minneapolis: University of Minnesota Press.

Meehl, P.E. (1986). Causes and effects of my disturbing little book. *Journal of Personality Assessment*, **50**, 370–5.

Redelmeier, D.A. & Shafir, E. (1995). Medical decision making in situations that offer multiple alternatives. *Journal of the American Medical Association*, **273**, 302–5.

Ritov, I. & Baron, J. (1990). Reluctance to vaccinate: omission bias and ambiguity. *Journal of Behavioral Decision-making*, **3**, 263–77.

Schwartz, S. & Griffin, T. (1986). *Medical thinking: the psychology of medical judgement and decision making.* New York: Springer Verlag.

Shafir, E. (1993). Choosing versus rejecting: why some options are both better and worse than others. *Memory and Cognition*, **21**, 546–56.

Simon, H. (1979). How big is a chunk? In H.A. Simon (Ed.). *Models of thought.* New Haven: Yale University Press.

Sonnenberg, F.A. & Pauker, S.G. (1986). Elecive pericardiectomy for tuberculous pericarditis: should the snappers be snipped? *Medical Decision-making*, **6**, 110–23.

Stone, E.R., Yates, J.F. & Parker, A.M. (1997). Effects of numerical and graphical displays on professed risk-taking behavior. *Journal of Experimental Psychology: Applied*, **3**, 243–56.

Sumner, W. & Nease, R.F. (2001). Choice-matching preference reversals in health outcome assessments. *Medical Decision Making*, **21**, 208–18.

Timmermans, D., Molewijk, B., Stiggelbout, A. & Kievit, J. (2004). Different formats for communicating surgical risks to patients and the effect on choice of treatment. *Patient Education and Counseling*, **54**, 255–63.

Tversky, A. & Kahneman, D. (1981). The framing of decisions and the psychology of choice. *Science*, **211**, 453–8.

Zikmund-Fisher, B.J., Fagerlin, A. & Ubel, P.A. (2004). "Is 28% good or bad?": evaluability and preference reversals. *Medical Decision Making*, **24**, 142–8.

Medical interviewing

Jonathan Silverman

School of Clinical Medicine, University of Cambridge

Introduction

The medical interview is central to clinical practice. It is the essential unit of medical time, a critical few minutes for the doctor to help the patient with his or her problems. To achieve an effective interview, doctors need to be able to integrate four aspects of their work which together determine their overall clinical competence:

- knowledge
- communication skills
- problem solving
- physical examination

These four essential components of clinical competence are inextricably linked: outstanding expertise in any one alone is not sufficient.

Strangely then, traditionally the medical interview has been described only in terms of its output, the information that needs to be gathered from the patient in order to make a diagnosis. Until recently, very little attention has been paid to how to go about the process of such information gathering, or to what skills or techniques would aid the retrieval of the data required by the doctor.

Of course, data gathering is only one of the goals of medical interviewing. Even less attention has been traditionally paid to how to build a relationship with the patient, how to organize and structure an interview, how to explain and make plans with the patient or indeed to how the patient feels about the process.

There is also a strong argument to be made that the traditional data set required by doctors has been too restrictive, focusing only on the symptoms and signs of disease that help the clinician to make a diagnosis, at the expense of gathering information about the patient's perspective of the illness and in particular his or her ideas, concerns, expectations and feelings.

This chapter looks at the medical interview more widely and attempts to bring together two different approaches to the medical interview; traditional history taking and the study of communication process skills, so that they form a seamless whole, indeed a 'comprehensive clinical method'.

Historical perspective

Generations of doctors have learnt a system of medical interviewing known as the traditional medical history which lists the data required by the clinician from the patient that could then be applied to solving the diagnostic puzzle. These are shown in Fig. 1.

This traditional method of history-taking is so firmly established in medical practice that it is easy to assume that it is the correct approach. Yet often in medicine we make such assumptions without considering the origins of what we do and their relevance to modern-day practice (McWhinney, 1989).

It was at the beginning of the nineteenth century that a new method of clinical medicine emerged. Prior to this, medicine had lacked any scientific basis: patients' symptoms had been the focus of doctors' attention and there had been little understanding of underlying disease processes. Innovations such as the stethoscope now revealed a whole new range of clinical information. At the same time, physicians began to correlate physical signs in life with post mortem findings in death. From this time onwards, the physical expression of the patient's illness became central to the profession's approach: it became the aim of the diagnostician to interpret the patient's symptoms in terms of specific diseases and to provide a scientific explanation.

By 1880, a fully defined clinical method had become established. This is apparent from hospital clinical records where the structured method of recording the history and examination that we are all so familiar with today had taken root (Tait, 1979; Roter, 2000). The history of present complaint, history of past illness, medication and allergy history, family history, personal and social history and functional enquiry provided a standard method of recording clinical enquiries and forged an ordered approach to history taking (see Fig. 1).

This method is still in use today, almost unchanged. Its greatest strength is that it provides physicians with a clear method of taking and recording the clinical history, supplying a carefully structured template with which to arrive at a diagnosis or to exclude physical disease. It simplified and unified a very complex process

and enabled the data extracted from the patient to appear in a standard form.

A new approach

So what is missing from the traditional clinical method? First we will look at what vital elements of content are not represented in the framework of the traditional clinical interview. Then our attention is turned to the process of the interview.

Content

Content is what healthcare professionals communicate; the substance of their questions, the information they gather and give, the treatments they discuss. Content is the information that clinicians obtain when taking a clinical history, that they consider when formulating a diagnosis and that they discuss with their patients. It is *what* is written down in clinical records and discussed with other health professionals and with patients and relatives.

The patient's perspective

The strength of the traditional clinical method is also its weakness. As the profession embraced the objectivity required to diagnose disease in terms of underlying pathology, it increasingly concentrated on the individual parts of the body that are malfunctioning and honed this process down to a cellular or molecular level. Yet this very detached objectivity so easily misses the patient as a whole: as Cassell says 'the patient's individual concerns are brushed aside to support the function of their organs' (Cassell, 1985).

The scientific approach does not aim to understand the meaning of the illness for the patient or place it in the context of his life and family. Subjective matters such as beliefs, anxieties and concerns are not the remit of the traditional approach: science deals with the objective, that which can be measured, whereas the patient's feelings, thoughts and concerns are unquantifiable and subjective and therefore are deemed less worthy of consideration.

The traditional medical history concentrates on pathological disease at the expense of understanding the highly individual needs and perspectives of each patient. As a consequence, much of the information required to understand and deal with patients' problems is never elicited. Studies of patient satisfaction, adherence, recall and physiological outcome validate the need for a broader view of history-taking that encompasses patients' life world as well as doctors' more limited biological prospective (The Headache Study Group of The University of Western Ontario, 1986; Roter *et al.*, 1995; Stevenson *et al.*, 2000; Joos *et al.*, 1993; Bell *et al.*, 2002; Dowell *et al.*, 2002; Little *et al.*, 1997; Abdel-Tawab & Roter, 2002; Tuckett *et al.*, 1985). We need to move the concept of history-taking as diagnostic problem-solving to a much wider view of patient care in the real world. For this to be effective, doctors need not only to be good diagnosticians but also to care for their patients, understand their needs and negotiate effective plans.

McWhinney and his colleagues at the University of Western Ontario (McWhinney, 1989) therefore proposed a new approach

---

TRADITIONAL MEDICAL HISTORY

- Chief complaint
- History of the present complaint
- Past medical history
- Family history
- Personal and social history
- Drug and allergy history
- Functional enquiry/systems review

Fig 1 Traditional medical history.

'patient-centred clinical interviewing' which encouraged doctors to consider *both* the doctor's and patient's perspectives in each interview (Mishler, 1984; Campion *et al.*, 1992; Epstein, 2000; Stewart *et al.*, 2003). The disease–illness model (Fig. 2) attempts to provide a practical way of using these ideas in everyday clinical practice:

The beauty of this analysis of gathering information is the clarity with which it demonstrates how we need to explore both 'disease' and 'illness' to fulfil our unique role as medical practitioners. 'Disease' is the biomedical cause of sickness in terms of pathophysiology. Clearly it is the doctor's role to search for symptoms and signs of underlying disease. Discovering a diagnosis for the patient's disease is the doctor's traditional and central agenda. 'Illness', in contrast, is the individual patient's unique experience of sickness, how each patient perceives, experiences and copes with their illness. The patient's perspective is not as narrow as the doctor's and includes the feelings, thoughts, concerns and effect on life that any episode of sickness induces. It represents the patient's response to events around him, his understanding of what is happening to him and his expectations of help.

The disease–illness model does not in any way negate the scientific disease approach but adds a patient-centred arm as well. Doctors are not counsellors whose sole aim is to help patients to become aware of how their thoughts and feelings are influencing their lives and their illness: they have the extra responsibility and burden of diagnosing and treating disease. But if doctors consider their role as purely that of discovering disease, they will not fully help their patients' very individual needs. The patient-centred approach enlarges the doctor's agenda to take account of both disease and illness.

Other changes to the content of the medical interview

As well as the patient's perspective, there are other omissions of content in the traditional medical history:

(a) *A list of the problems that the patient wishes to address* The traditional medical history starts with a chief complaint and the history of that complaint. Yet we know from research that patients present with more than one symptom or problem and that the serial order in which they are presented is not related to their clinical importance: the first concern presented is no more likely than the second or third to be the most important as judged by either the patient or the doctor (Starfield *et al.*, 1981; Beckman & Frankel, 1984; Barry *et al.*, 2000; Greenfield *et al.*, 1985). A list of problems rather than a single complaint helps prevent a biased and blinkered approach to history taking.

(b) *Progression of events* Discovering a temporal sequence of events is essential to effective clinical reasoning, yet is not explicitly requested in the traditional clinical method.

(c) *A record of what the patient has been told* Increasingly modern medicine is conducted in teams with shift work and hand-overs becoming more and more important. Yet nowhere in the clinical method is a record of the information provided to the patient.

(d) *Plan of action that has been negotiated* Similarly no record is made of the plan of action negotiated despite modern approaches towards a collaborative shared decision-making model of practice.

An alternative template for the content of the medical interview

The disease–illness model provides the foundation for an alternative template for the content of information gathering which retains all the elements of the traditional medical history but in addition includes the 'new' content of the patient's perspective (Kurtz *et al.*, 2003). This template forms the backbone of how physicians can record information in the medical records and present their findings to others.

This template, as shown in Fig. 3, explicitly demonstrates how the discrete elements of the traditional medical history and the components of the disease–illness model can seamlessly work together in clinical practice.

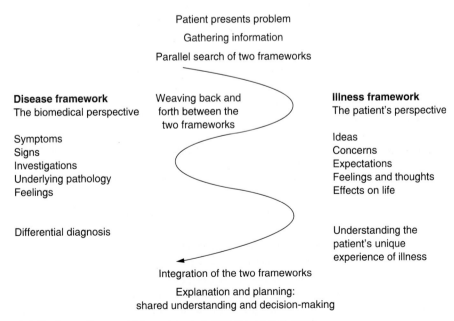

Fig 2 The disease–illness model (Levenstein *et al.*, 1998, Stewart *et al.*, 2003).

```
┌─────────────────────────────────────────────────┐
│ REVISED CONTENT OF THE MEDICAL INTERVIEW          │
│                                                   │
│ PATIENT'S PROBLEM LIST:                           │
│                                                   │
│      1.                                           │
│      2.                                           │
│      3.                                           │
│      4.                                           │
│      5.                                           │
│                                                   │
│ BIOMEDICAL PERSPECTIVE:      (DISEASE)            │
│ sequence of events                                │
│                                                   │
│ symptom analysis                                  │
│                                                   │
│ relevant systems review                           │
│                                                   │
│ PATIENT'S PERSPECTIVE:       (ILLNESS)            │
│ ideas                                             │
│ concerns                                          │
│ expectations                                      │
│ effects on life                                   │
│ feelings                                          │
│                                                   │
│ BACKGROUND INFORMATION–CONTEXT                    │
│ past medical history                              │
│                                                   │
│ drug and allergy                                  │
│                                                   │
│ family history                                    │
│                                                   │
│ personal and social history                       │
│                                                   │
│ review of systems                                 │
│                                                   │
│ PHYSICAL EXAMINATION                              │
│                                                   │
│ DIFFERENTIAL DIAGNOSIS–HYPOTHESES                 │
│ including both disease and illness issues         │
│                                                   │
│ PHYSICIAN'S PLAN OF MANAGEMENT                    │
│ investigations; treatment alternatives            │
│                                                   │
│ EXPLANATION AND PLANNING                          │
│ what the patient has been told;                   │
│ plan of action negotiated                         │
│                                                   │
└─────────────────────────────────────────────────┘
```

Fig 3 Revised content of the medical history.

This new template fits with what happens in real life clinical practice: clinicians can readily see how the new and traditional content fit together. It is important that this template makes intuitive sense to both practising physicians and teachers in communication courses (see 'Teaching communication skills'). Both these groups need to be able to embrace the same template with enthusiasm so that students, whether in the formal communication course or on the wards, can receive a consistent message about the content of the medical interview.

Process

There is a further even more fundamental problem with the classical method of history-taking. Students often erroneously perceive that the format in which they present their findings or record information in the case records is that in which they should obtain the information. They mistake the *content* of the traditional medical history for the *process* of medical interviewing. The way that doctors

have been taught about the symptoms that we need to explore in order to make a diagnosis suggests that if we ask the 15 questions we have learned about the functioning of a particular organ system, we will gather all the information that we need. But this closed approach to questioning actually encourages an inefficient and inaccurate method of history-taking (Evans *et al.*, 1991). In fact, it is the premature search for scientific facts that stops us from listening, that prevents us from both taking an accurate history and picking up the cues to our patient's problems and concerns (see 'Healthcare professional–patient communication' and 'Patient-centred healthcare').

Above we have described the changes required to the recording of the content of the medical history. Now we need to turn our attention to the process of the medical interview, how we go about communicating with our patients so that we obtain the above information and achieve so much more. Paying attention to the process of communication within the medical interview is essential if we are to make the most of our time with patients and enable both doctors and patients to achieve their goals.

But what exactly are the specific process skills of doctor–patient communication? How can we define the individual skills that together make up the medical interview?

Here we describe the Calgary–Cambridge Guides, an example of a process guide to the medical interview (Kurtz & Silverman, 1996; Kurtz *et al.*, 2003, 2005; Silverman *et al.*, 2005). Although numerous guides and checklists have been available in the past (Stillman *et al.*, 1976; Cassata, 1978; Carroll & Monroe, 1979; Riccardi & Kurtz, 1983; Tuckett *et al.*, 1985; Maguire *et al.*, 1986; Cohen-Cole, 1991; Sanson-Fisher R.W. *et al.*, 1991; van Thiel *et al.*, 1991; Novack *et al.*, 1992; van Thiel & van Dalen, 1995; Towle & Godolphin, 1999; Edwards & Elwyn, 2001) the Calgary–Cambridge Guides make significant advances by:

- providing a comprehensive repertoire of skills that is validated by research and theoretical evidence
- referencing the skills to current evidence
- taking into account the move to a more patient-centred and collaborative style
- increasing the emphasis on the highly important area of explanation and planning (see Carroll & Monroe, 1979; Tuckett *et al.*, 1985; Maguire *et al.*, 1986; Sanson-Fisher R.W. *et al.*, 1991; Towle & Godolphin, 1999; Edwards & Elwyn, 2001)

Firstly, the guides provide a set of three diagrams which outline the framework of the process of the medical interview and place it in the context of a comprehensive clinical method. The three diagrams depict this framework graphically in increasing detail and provide a logical organizational schema for both doctor–patient interactions and communication skills education. Secondly, the guides provide a comprehensive list of communication process skills that fit explicitly into this framework.

Three diagrams: the framework of the enhanced Calgary–Cambridge Guides

The three diagrams depicting the Calgary–Cambridge Guides make it easier to conceptualize firstly what is happening in a medical interview and secondly how the skills of communication and physical examination work together in an integrated way.

The basic framework

Figure 4a is a diagrammatic representation of the medical interview. This 'bare bones' map introduces five key tasks that physicians tend to carry out in temporal sequence during a full medical interview (initiating the session, gathering information, physical examination, explanation and planning and closing the session) and two that occur as continuous threads throughout the interview, building the relationship and structuring the interview. These tasks made intuitive sense and provided a logical organizational schema for both physician–patient interactions and communication skill education. This structure was first proposed by Riccardi and Kurtz (Riccardi & Kurtz, 1983) and is similar to that adopted by Cohen-Cole (Cohen-Cole, 1991).

The expanded framework

Figure 4b expands the basic framework by identifying the key objectives to be achieved within each of its six communication tasks.

An example of the inter-relationship between content and process

Figure 5 takes one task, i.e. gathering information, as an example and shows an expanded view of how content and process specifically inter-relate in the medical interview.

Together the diagrams in Figures 4a, 4b and 5 form a framework for conceptualizing the tasks of a physician–patient encounter and the way they flow in real time. This framework helps us to visualize the relationships between the discrete elements of communication content and process.

Calgary–Cambridge Guides: communication process skills

More detail is then needed to move from merely thinking about the objectives of physician–patient interaction to actually identifying the communication process skills involved in the medical interview. The more complex Calgary–Cambridge process guide, as shown in Table 1, spells out the specific, evidence-based skills needed to accomplish each objective in the expanded framework of Fig. 4b.

Conclusion

This chapter makes the case that traditional ways of describing clinical interviewing have favoured the biomedical approach, limited doctors' understanding of the patient as a person and over-emphasized content over process issues in medical interviewing. Here we have described how both content and process need equal attention and how marrying process and content into a comprehensive clinical method carries considerable benefits. Doctors need to understand that *how* they approach the patient, and *what* information they are gathering and explaining, are inextricably linked and that they need to very deliberately focus on both.

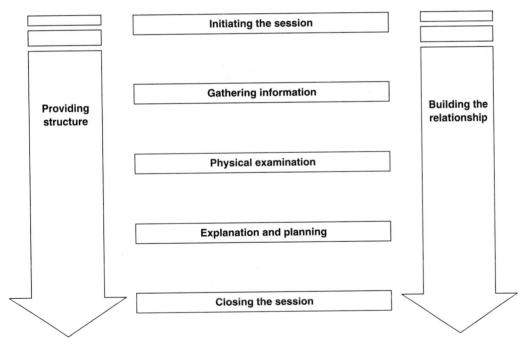

Fig 4a Basic framework of the Calgary–Cambridge guides.

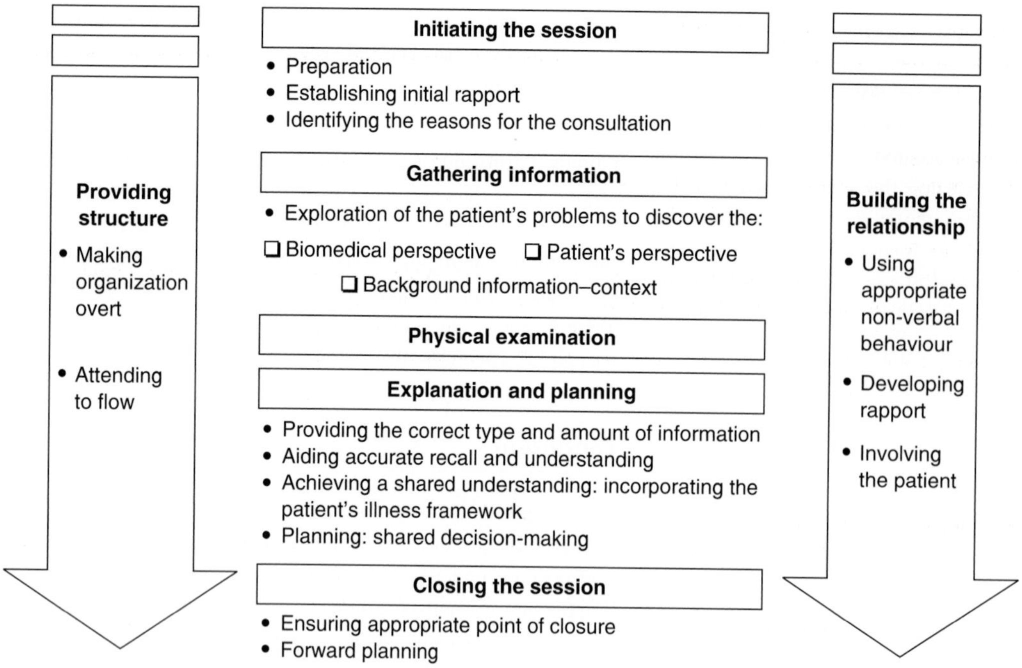

Initiating the session

- Preparation
- Establishing initial rapport
- Identifying the reasons for the consultation

Gathering information

- Exploration of the patient's problems to discover the:

  ☐ Biomedical perspective   ☐ Patient's perspective

  ☐ Background information–context

Physical examination

Explanation and planning

- Providing the correct type and amount of information
- Aiding accurate recall and understanding
- Achieving a shared understanding: incorporating the patient's illness framework
- Planning: shared decision-making

Closing the session

- Ensuring appropriate point of closure
- Forward planning

Providing structure

- Making organization overt
- Attending to flow

Building the relationship

- Using appropriate non-verbal behaviour
- Developing rapport
- Involving the patient

Fig 4b Expanded framework of the Calgary–Cambridge guides.

Gathering information

Process skills for exploration of the patient's problems
- Patient's narrative
- Question style: open to closed cone
- Attentive listening
- Facilitative response
- Picking up cues
- Clarification
- Time-framing
- Internal summary
- Appropriate use of language
- Additional skills for understanding patient's perspective

Content to be discovered

The biomedical perspective (disease)
Sequence of events
Symptom analysis
Relevant systems review

The patient's perspective (illness)
Ideas and beliefs
Concerns
Expectations
Effects on life
Feelings

Background information–context
Past medical history
Drug and allergy history
Family history
Personal and social history
Review of systems

Fig 5 An example of the interrelationship between content and process.

Table 1. Calgary–Cambridge Guides: communcation process skills

INITIATING THE SESSION

Establishing initial rapport

1. **Greets** patient and obtains patient's name
2. **Introduces** self, role and nature of interview; obtains consent if necessary
3. **Demonstrates respect** and interest, attends to patient's physical comfort

Identifying the reason(s) for the consultation

4. **Identifies** the **patient's problems** or the issues that the patient wishes to address with appropriate **opening question** (e.g. 'What problems brought you to the hospital?' or 'What would you like to discuss today?' or 'What questions did you hope to get answered today?')
5. **Listens** attentively to the patient's opening statement, without interrupting or directing patient's response
6. **Confirms list and screens** for further problems (e.g. 'So that's headaches and tiredness, anything else?')
7. **Negotiates agenda** taking both patient's and physician's needs into account

GATHERING INFORMATION

Exploration of patient's problems

8. **Encourages patient to tell the story** of the problem(s) from when first started to the present in own words (clarifying reason for presenting now)
9. **Uses open and closed questioning techniques**, appropriately moving from open to closed
10. **Listens** attentively, allowing patient to complete statements without interruption and leaving space for patient to think before answering or go on after pausing
11. **Facilitates** patient's responses verbally and non-verbally e.g. use of encouragement, silence, repetition, paraphrasing, interpretation
12. **Picks up** verbal and non-verbal **cues** (body language, speech, facial expression, affect); **checks out and acknowledges** as appropriate
13. **Clarifies** patient's statements that are unclear or need amplification (e.g. 'Could you explain what you mean by light headed')
14. Periodically **summarizes** to verify own understanding of what the patient has said; invites patient to correct interpretation or provide further information.
15. **Uses** concise, **easily understood questions and comments**, avoids or adequately explains jargon
16. **Establishes dates and sequence** of events

Additional skills for understanding the patient's perspective

17. **Actively determines and appropriately explores:**
    - patient's **ideas** (i.e. beliefs re cause)
    - patient's **concerns** (i.e. worries) regarding each problem
    - patient's **expectations:** (i.e. goals, what help the patient had expected for each problem)
    - **effects:** how each problem affects the patient's life
18. **Encourages patient to express feelings**

PROVIDING STRUCTURE TO THE CONSULTATION

Making organization overt

19. **Summarizes** at the end of a specific line of inquiry to confirm understanding before moving on to the next section
20. Progresses from one section to another using **signposting, transitional statements**; includes rationale for next section

Attending to flow

21. Structures interview in logical **sequence**
22. Attends to **timing** and keeping interview on task

BUILDING RELATIONSHIP

Using appropriate non-verbal behaviour

23. **Demonstrates appropriate non-verbal behaviour**
    - eye contact, facial expression
    - posture, position and movement
    - vocal cues, e.g. rate, volume, intonation
24. If reads, writes notes or uses computer, does so in a **manner that does not interfere with dialogue or rapport**
25. **Demonstrates** appropriate **confidence**

Developing rapport

26. **Accepts legitimacy** of patient's views and feelings; is **not judgmental**
27. **Uses empathy** to communicate understanding and appreciation of the patient's feelings or predicament, overtly **acknowledges patient's views and feelings**
28. **Provides support**: expresses concern, understanding, willingness to help; acknowledges coping efforts and appropriate self-care; offers partnership
29. **Deals sensitively** with embarrassing and disturbing topics and physical pain, including when associated with physical examination

Involving the patient

30. **Shares thinking** with patient to encourage patient's involvement (e.g. 'What I'm thinking now is ......')
31. **Explains rationale** for questions or parts of physical examination that could appear to be non sequiturs
32. During **physical examination**, explains process, asks permission

Table 1. (*cont.*)

EXPLANATION AND PLANNING

Providing the correct amount and type of information

Aims: to give comprehensive and appropriate information
to assess each individual patient's information needs
to neither restrict or overload

33. **Chunks and checks**: gives information in easily assimilated chunks, checks for understanding, uses patient's response as a guide to how to proceed
34. **Assesses patient's starting point**: asks for patient's prior knowledge early on when giving information, discovers extent of patient's wish for information
35. **Asks patients what other information would be helpful** e.g. aetiology, prognosis
36. **Gives explanation at appropriate times**: avoids giving advice, information or reassurance prematurely

Aiding accurate recall and understanding

Aims: to make information easier for the patient to remember and understand

37. **Organizes explanation**: divides into discrete sections, develops a logical sequence
38. **Uses explicit categorization or signposting** (e.g. 'There are three important things that I would like to discuss. 1st …' 'Now, shall we move on to…')
39. **Uses repetition and summarizing** to reinforce information
40. **Uses concise, easily understood language**, avoids or explains jargon
41. **Uses visual methods of conveying information**: diagrams, models, written information and instructions
42. **Checks patient's understanding** of information given (or plans made): e.g. by asking patient to restate in own words; clarifies as necessary

Achieving a shared understanding: incorporating the patient's perspective

Aims: to provide explanations and plans that relate to the patient's perspective
to discover the patient's thoughts and feelings about information given
to encourage an interaction rather than one-way transmission

43. **Relates explanations to patient's perspective**: to previously elicited ideas, concerns and expectations
44. **Provides opportunities and encourages patient to contribute**: to ask questions, seek clarification or express doubts; responds appropriately
45. **Picks up and responds to verbal and non-verbal cues** e.g. patient's need to contribute information or ask questions, information overload, distress
46. **Elicits patient's beliefs, reactions and feelings** re information given, terms used; acknowledges and addresses where necessary

Planning: shared decision making

Aims: to allow patients to understand the decision-making process
to involve patients in decision-making to the level they wish
in order to increase patients' commitment to plans made

47. **Shares own thinking as appropriate**: ideas, thought processes and dilemmas
48. **Involves patient:**
    – offers suggestions and choices rather than directives
    – encourages patient to contribute their own ideas, suggestions
49. **Explores management options**
50. **Ascertains level of involvement patient wishes in making the decision at hand**
51. **Negotiates a mutually acceptable plan**
    – signposts own position of equipoise or preference regarding available options
    – determines patient's preferences
52. **Checks with patient**
    – if accepts plans
    – if concerns have been addressed

CLOSING THE SESSION

Forward planning

53. **Contracts** with patient re next steps for patient and physician
54. **Safety nets**, explaining possible unexpected outcomes, what to do if plan is not working, when and how to seek help

Ensuring appropriate point of closure

55. **Summarizes** session briefly and clarifies plan of care
56. **Final check** that patient agrees and is comfortable with plan and asks if any corrections, questions or other issues

REFERENCES

Abdel-Tawab, N. & Roter, D. (2002). *Social Science and Medicine*, **54**, 1357–68.

Barry, C.A., Bradley, C.P., Britten, N., Stevenson, F.A. & Barber, N. (2000). *British Medical Journal*, **320**, 1246–50.

Beckman, H.B. & Frankel, R.M. (1984). *Annals of Internal Medicine*, **101**, 692–6.

Bell, R.A., Kravitz, R.L., Thom, D., Krupat, E. & Azari, R. (2002). *J Gen Intern Med*, **17**, 817–24.

Campion, P.D., Butler, N.M. & Cox, A.D. (1992). *Family Practice*, **9**, 181–90.

Carroll, J.G. & Monroe, J. (1979). *Journal of Medical Education*, **54**, 498–500.

Cassata, D.M. (1978). In B.D. Ruben (Ed.). *Communication Yearbook* New Brunswick, NJ: Transaction Books.

Cassell, E.J. (1985). *Talking with patients. Volume 2: clinical technique.* Cambridge MA: MIT Press.

Cohen-Cole, S.A. (1991). *The medical interview: a three function approach.* St. Louis: Mosby Year Book.

Dowell, J., Jones, A. & Snadden, D. (2002). *British Journal of General Practice*, **52**, 24–32.

Edwards, A. & Elwyn, G. (2001). *Evidence based patient choice: inevitable or impossible?* Oxford: Oxford University Press.

Epstein, R.M. (2000). *J Fam Pract*, **49**, 805–7.

Evans, B.J., Stanley, R.O., Mestrovic, R. & Rose, L. (1991). *Medical Education*, **25**, 517–26.

Greenfield, S., Kaplan, S.H. & Ware, J.E. (1985). *Annals of Internal Medicine*, **102**, 520–8.

Joos, S.K., Hickam, D.H. & Borders, L.M. (1993). In *Public Health Reports, Vol. 108*, (pp. 751–9).

Kurtz, S., Silverman, J., Benson, J. & Draper, J. (2003). *Academic Medicine*, **78**, 802–9.

Kurtz, S., Silverman, J. & Draper, J. (2005). *Teaching and Learning Communication Skills in Medicine* (2nd edn.). Oxford: Radcliffe Publishing.

Kurtz, S.M. & Silverman, J.D. (1996). *Medical Education*, **30**, 83–9.

Levenstein, J.H., Belle Brown, J., Weston, W.W. *et al.* (1989). In M. Stewart & D. Roter (Eds.). *Communicating with medical patients.* Newbury Park, CA: Sage Publications Inc.

Little, P., Williamson, I., Warner, G. *et al.* (1997). *British Medical Journal*, **314**, 722–7.

Maguire, P., Fairbairn, S. & Fletcher, C. (1986). *British Medical Journal*, **292**, 1576–8.

McWhinney, I. (1989). In M. Stewart & D. Roter (Eds.). *Communicating with medical patients.* Newbury Park, CA: Sage Publications Inc.

Mishler, E.G. (1984). *The discourse of medicine: dialectics of medical interviews.* Norwood, NJ: Ablex.

Novack, D.H., Dube, C. & Goldstein, M.G. (1992). *Archieves of Internal Medicine*, **152**, 1814–20.

Riccardi, V.M. & Kurtz, S.M. (1983). *Communication and counselling in health care.* Springfield, IL: Charles C Thomas.

Roter, D. (2000). *Patient Education and Counseling*, **39**, 5–15.

Roter, D.L., Hall, J.A., Kern, D.E. *et al.* (1995). *Archieves of Internal Medicine*, **155**, 1877–84.

Sanson-Fisher, R.W., Redman, S., Walsh, R. *et al.* (1991). *Medical Education*, **25**, 322–33.

Silverman, J., Kurtz, S. & Draper, J. (2005). *Skills for Communicating with Patients* (2nd edn.). Oxford: Radcliffe Publishing.

Starfield, B., Wray, C., Hess, K. *et al.* (1981). *American Journal of Public Health*, **71**, 127–31.

Stevenson, F.A., Barry, C.A., Britten, N., Barber, N. & Bradley, C.P. (2000). *Social Science and Medicine*, **50**, 829–40.

Stewart, M.A., Brown, J.B., Weston, W.W. *et al.* (2003). *Patient-centered medicine: transforming the clinical method.* Oxford: Radcliffe Medical Press.

Stillman, P.L., Sabars, D.L. & Redfield, D.L. (1976). *Pediatrics*, **57**, 769–74.

Tait, I. (1979). *The history and function of clinical records.* Cambridge: University of Cambridge.

The Headache Study Group of The University of Western Ontario (1986). *Headache Journal*, **26**, 285–94.

Towle, A. & Godolphin, W. (1999). *British Medical Journal*, **319**, 766–71.

Tuckett, D., Boulton, M., Olson, C. & Williams, A. (1985). *Meetings between experts: an approach to sharing ideas in medical consultations.* London: Tavistock.

Van Thiel, J., Kraan, H.F. & Van Der Vleuten, C.P. (1991). *Med Educ*, **25**, 224–9.

Van Thiel, J. & van Dalen, J. (1995). *MAAS-Globaal criterialijst, versie voor de vaardigheidstoets Medisch Basiscurriculum.* Maastricht, Netherlands: Universiteit Maastricht.

Patient-centred healthcare

Peter Bower and Nicki Mead

University of Manchester

Introduction

The delivery of healthcare is increasingly influenced by two funda-mental philosophies. The first is evidence-based healthcare, which is defined as the 'the conscientious, explicit, and judicious use of current best evidence in making decisions about the care of individ-ual patients' (Kleijnen et al., 1997; Sackett et al., 1996). However, in the past 30 years, an extensive body of literature has emerged advo-cating another key philosophy, which is described as patient-centred healthcare. This notion is commonly discussed in both the professional and health policy literature. This chapter will con-sider the nature of patient-centred healthcare, and review current research of relevance to this complex concept.

The definition of patient-centred healthcare

Despite the increasing popularity of the concept of patient-centred healthcare in the literature, there is little consensus as to its exact meaning. In fact, patient-centred healthcare has been most commonly understood in terms of its opposition to the philo-sophy of evidence-based healthcare (Bensing, 2000; Stewart, 2001). Evidence-based healthcare is generally based on rigorous outcomes research, characterized by the randomized controlled trial, which is itself concerned with the response of the 'average' patient receiving defined, conventional treatment for distinct, biomedical disorders. Evidence-based healthcare has a focus on treatments and technol-ogies, often provided in specialist hospital settings. The style of healthcare practice engendered by this philosophy has been described as 'doctor-centred'[1]. This means that evidence derived from controlled outcomes research on populations is to be inter-preted and applied by the professional to the care of individual patients. This in turn means that healthcare consultations are driven by the agenda of the professional; the professional's need to know (i.e. to make an accurate diagnosis) and to control (i.e. to ensure that the prescribed treatments are delivered and adhered to by the patient, in line with the research evidence) (Byrne & Long, 1976). Patient-centred health care is often viewed as simply the antithesis of this style of practice.

Fortunately, more specific definitions have also been proposed. Patient-centred healthcare has been described as 'understanding the patient as a unique human being' (Balint, 1969) (p. 269) or as an approach whereby 'the physician tries to enter the patient's world, to see the illness through the patient's eyes' (McWhinney, 1985) (p. 35)

Other authors have highlighted sharing information and decision-making (Grol et al., 1990; Verhaak, 1988; Winefield et al., 1996) and providing care which is 'closely congruent with, and responsive to patients' wants, needs and preferences' (Laine & Davidoff, 1996). It is increasingly accepted that patient-centred healthcare is a multi-dimensional construct, and more comprehensive descriptions have identified a number of interconnecting components from a theoret-ical perspective (Mead & Bower, 2000b; Stewart et al., 1995):

1. *The biopsychosocial perspective*: patient-centred healthcare involves exploring both the disease and the illness experience. This means that the professional needs to respond to any bio-medical disorder, *and* to the patient's understanding of, and reaction to the problem they have brought to the consultation (Engel, 1977, 1980).

2. *The patient as person*: as noted above, evidence-based healthcare is concerned with the application of clinical data derived from groups of patients to the individual, whereas patient-centred healthcare is concerned with understanding the individual patient in his or her unique context (Bower, 1998).

3. *Sharing power and responsibility*: patient-centred healthcare involves a shift in the traditional dynamic of the doctor–patient relationship. The traditional dynamic has been described as the 'co-operation–guidance' model (analogous to a parent–adolescent relationship), whereas in patient-centred healthcare, the dynamic is one of 'mutual participation' (analogous to a rela-tionship between adults), where power and responsibility are shared with the patient (Szasz & Hollender, 1956).

4. *The therapeutic alliance*: in patient-centred healthcare, the pro-fessional is expected to attend to the therapeutic nature of the professional–patient relationship (Browne & Freeling, 1976). This was described as 'the doctor as drug' (Balint, 1964), and relates to what is described as the 'therapeutic alliance' in the psychological therapy literature (Horvath et al., 1993; Roth & Fonagy, 1996).

5. *The doctor as person*: this involves taking account of the subjec-tivity of the doctor as an influence on, or possible aid to diagnosis and treatment (Balint, 1964; Balint et al., 1993). This is in contrast to evidence-based healthcare, where the subjectivity of the doctor is seen largely as a source of bias.

Although developed from within medicine, the concept of patient-centred healthcare has many roots in the psychological therapy research literature, and one of the first uses of the term related it to work conducted by psychoanalytic practitioners working with

---

[1] The term 'doctor-centred' is that commonly found in the literature, but here the term 'doctor' should be understood as referring to the broader notion of the healthcare professional

general practitioners in the United Kingdom (Balint, 1964; Balint, 1969). For example, understanding the perspective of clients in psychotherapy has been traditionally highlighted in discussions of empathy within client-centred therapy (Rogers, 1967), and it has long been suggested that the therapeutic alliance is a fundamental driver of change in psychological therapy (Roth & Fonagy, 1996).

However, the development of patient-centred healthcare also has its roots in the evolution of particular disciplines within healthcare. Many of the attributes of patient-centred healthcare have been championed by general practitioners as part of their professional differentiation from specialist, hospital-based medicine. Sensitivity to the ongoing doctor–patient relationship, respect for the patient as an individual and a belief in the intrinsic therapeutic potential of the consultation are all core themes in the academic literature of general practice. Lacking the complex diagnostic technologies of hospital medicine, general practice has instead defined for itself a model of care focused on the 'whole person' in his or her wider psychological and social context (May & Mead, 1999).

Patient-centred healthcare in the consultation

Given its origins within the disciplines of psychological therapy and general practice, it is no surprise that much of the development of the concept of patient-centred healthcare has been in relation to the individual consultation between professional and patient, and the content and quality of the actual process of care between doctor and patient. That is, patient-centred healthcare is conceptualized as a clinical method. This perspective is best exemplified by the literature concerning the role and function of patient-centred healthcare in the clinical setting, and the training and educational issues associated with it (Stewart et al., 1995). Table 1 details examples of types of doctor behaviours indicative of the different dimensions of patient-centred healthcare described above.

It should be noted that the concept of patient-centred healthcare can also be applied at another level, that of health policy, where it concerns the organization of healthcare systems at a local, national or international level. For example, the blueprint for the National Health Service in the United Kingdom, the NHS Plan, states that 'The NHS must be redesigned to be patient-centred – to offer a personalised service' (Secretary of State for Health, 2000), (p. 20).

When used in this fashion, the concept is less concerned with the specific behaviours of health professionals, and more with broader values such as empowerment of patients and the need to design health services to fit in with their preferences and needs, as opposed to the convenience of professionals.

Research on patient-centred healthcare

Just as some critics have questioned the degree to which evidence-based medicine is patient-centred, it is possible to ask the degree to which the provision of patient-centred medicine is supported by the available evidence (Bensing, 2000). One of the first issues concerning research on patient-centred healthcare regards its measurement. Given the complex definition of patient-centred healthcare described above, it is clear that this is a significant challenge.

A plethora of different measurements of patient-centred healthcare have been used in the research and training literature (Mead & Bower, 2000b). These can involve measurements of the attitudes of professionals, global ratings of the quality of consultations, or microanalyses of actual behaviours demonstrated in the consultation which are hypothesized to correspond to patient-centred healthcare (Table 1) (see also 'Healthcare professional–patient communication').

However, attempts to measure this complex construct have highlighted significant problems. For example, there is some evidence that measurement tools which are ostensibly measuring the same concept are not always in agreement (Mead & Bower, 2000a). Furthermore, there is also evidence that measures of professional behaviour which are theoretically related to patient-centred healthcare are not in close agreement with ratings of the same consultations made by patients (Cape, 1996; McKinstry et al., 2004; Mead et al., 2002; Stewart et al., 2000). This might suggest that professional and patient concepts of quality in healthcare consultations differ significantly (Burkitt Wright et al., 2004). Alternatively, this may reflect the fact that a concept such as patient-centred healthcare is difficult to quantify. Patients judgements as to what appears to them to be 'patient-centred' may be highly idiosyncratic and variable: indeed, such variability may be highly appropriate, given the nature of the patient-centred philosophy and its focus on the subjectivity of the patient.

Table 1. Examples of patient-centred behaviours

Dimension of patient-centred healthcare	Examples of patient-centred healthcare
The biopsychosocial perspective	Discussion of psychosocial/lifestyle issues (Ford et al., 1996), counselling about prevention (Roter et al., 1987)
The patient-as-person	Eliciting patient's assumptions about diagnosis and treatment (Langewitz et al., 1998), responding to patient's 'offers' of thoughts, feelings, symptoms, expectations or prompts (Henbest & Stewart, 1989)
Sharing power and responsibility	Giving information (Ford et al., 1996; Roter et al., 1987; Wissow et al., 1998), assisting patients to participate in decision-making about diagnosis and therapy (Verhaak, 1988); soliciting and encouraging patient questions, opinions and suggestions (Stewart, 1984; Street, 1992)
The therapeutic alliance	Responding to patients with empathy and assurance (Ockene et al., 1988); partnership-building statements (Ford et al., 1996; Wissow et al., 1998); statements of reassurance, support, empathy and inter-personal sensitivity (Street, 1992); talking about non-medical matters (Butow et al., 1995)
The doctor-as-person	Self-awareness of limitations and personal response to stress; acceptance of risk of exposing own weakness and vulnerability; understanding of transference/counter-transference (Stewart et al., 1995)

Notwithstanding difficulties in measurement, it is probably true that the 'gold standard' test of the utility of patient-centred healthcare is whether it has an impact on outcomes: that is, does practising in a patient-centred manner make any difference to the end result of the consultation? A number of studies have examined this issue, and a systematic overview of their results is beyond the scope of the current discussion. However, some relevant reviews will be discussed in detail.

The first examined the relationship between doctor behaviours within the consultation and patient outcomes such as satisfaction with healthcare, adherence with medical advice and health status. In this review, 16 out of 21 studies reported improvement in various outcomes, including distress, functioning, physiological measures (e.g. blood pressure) and health service utilization (Stewart, 1995). However, the reviewed studies covered a wide variety of clinical settings and patient populations and, importantly, none measured aspects of doctor–patient communication explicitly defined as 'patient-centred' by the respective investigators (Graugaard & Finset, 2004). A second review was restricted to primary care settings, and used a more clearly specified definition of patient-centred healthcare. Although there were some positive relationships, generally the pattern of results was much more inconsistent (Mead & Bower, 2002). There are a number of possible reasons for the differences in the results of these reviews, such as the types of professionals and patients included, and the study designs deemed eligible. However, the somewhat inconsistent results do suggest that an uncritical acceptance of the benefits of patient-centred healthcare may be inappropriate. A recent review of the effect of patient-centred healthcare in chronic illness has thrown some light on this inconsistency, suggesting that taking the patient's perspective (i.e. the patient as person) may have a different pattern of effect on outcomes than 'activating' the patient (i.e. sharing power and responsibility) (Michie et al., 2003). Even then, there is also some evidence from diabetes research that improving patient outcomes through self-care may be more easily achieved by intervening directly with patients, rather than attempting to modify patients by teaching patient-centred skills to clinicians (van Dam et al., 2003).

A related question concerns whether patient-centred skills can be taught, or whether they reflect more fundamental personality attributes that may not be amenable to change. At least one author has suggested that some aspects of patient-centred healthcare require 'a limited though considerable change in personality' (Balint, 1964) (p. 121)

However, others suggest that patient-centred skills can be learned without such profound psychological change (Gask & McGrath, 1989). A systematic review published in the Cochrane Library has examined the effects of interventions for health professionals who aim to promote patient-centred approaches in consultations (Lewin et al., 2001). All the interventions involved training of professionals, but some included other interventions, such as materials for patients. Generally, interventions were successful in increasing the patient-centred nature of consultations in terms of the process of those consultations, and there was some support for the hypothesis that the interventions improved patient satisfaction with care. However, there was generally less evidence that the interventions impacted on patient health behaviours such as adherence to treatment, or on health outcomes. Again, this suggests that the benefits of patient-centred healthcare cannot be assumed.

Discussion

The question 'is patient-centred medicine evidence-based?' is difficult to answer definitively. Although it might seem self-evident that the behaviours described in Table 1 would lead to more satisfied patients and improvement in other health outcomes, current evidence is far from unequivocal. This last section will discuss some reasons for this, and consider implications for the future development of patient-centred healthcare.

It is a legitimate question whether patient-centred healthcare should be evaluated using the same standards of evidence-based healthcare that are applied to treatments and technologies. Firstly, the available measurement methodologies may be insufficiently sensitive to the complex nature of the concept. For example, in the psychological therapy literature, it has been suggested that research examining the relationship between certain behaviours (such as empathy) and patient outcomes are unwittingly applying what is called the 'drug metaphor' (Stiles et al., 1995; Stiles & Shapiro, 1989), whereby the content of the consultation can be seen as analogous to drug ingredients and analyzable in terms of 'strength' and 'dosage'. Thus there may be an expectation that greater amounts of 'sharing of information' will be associated with greater patient satisfaction, irrespective of the appropriateness of the behaviour, the particular requirements of individual patients or the responsiveness of the professional to the patient and to the context of the consultation. This argument would suggest the need for more complex and sensitive research methodologies involving in-depth qualitative and quantitative research.

Issues of appropriateness and responsiveness relate to the question of whether patients actually want 'patient-centred healthcare', as currently defined. There are aspects of patient-centred healthcare that are generally considered relevant for all patients (e.g. developing a positive therapeutic alliance, understanding the patient experience), but patients may differ in their preferences for other aspects. For example, in terms of the issue of sharing power and control, it is possible some patients will prefer the doctor to make decisions, and have no great interest or desire to become more actively involved in the process of their medical care and clinical decision-making. Therefore, studies that attempt to increase involvement with all patients may actually worsen outcomes for some patients (Roter, 1977; Savage & Armstrong, 1990). Indeed, it is increasingly recognized that one of the key aspects of patient-centred healthcare is the ability of the professional to recognise or negotiate with the patient as to their preferred level of involvement in decision-making, so as to overcome this problem (Guadagnoli & Ward, 1998; Winefield et al., 1996).

On a more fundamental level, patient-centred healthcare reflects value judgements concerning the way patients should be treated within healthcare (Laine & Davidoff, 1996; McWhinney, 1989), as well as being a way of encouraging 'instrumental' benefits such as improvements in health behaviours and outcomes (Lewin et al., 2001). Even if there is no direct evidence that sharing control improves patient outcomes, there is an argument that such an approach is morally and ethically appropriate in the context of providing healthcare in societies which increasingly value individual rights.

Finally, it is important to consider the potential tension between the philosophies of evidence-based and patient-centred healthcare. Although in principle it should be possible to provide both, and that is still seen as the gold standard for healthcare delivery, it is equally possible that there are trade-offs to be made in terms of the benefits of the two different approaches. This was neatly demonstrated by a randomized controlled trial of the delivery of patient-centred diabetes advice in primary care (Kinmonth *et al.*, 1998). Practice teams received training in the provision of patient-centred healthcare, and the study found that increased patient-centred healthcare (as reported by patients) was associated with a reduction in quality of care as defined by objective biomedical indicators.

Summary

Patient-centred healthcare is a complex construct that defines a number of important processes in healthcare provision, focussing on the subjectivity of individual patients and their particular perspectives, needs and preferences. There is a growing literature on the methods by which this approach can be demonstrated in consultations between patient and professionals, and suggestive evidence that providing healthcare that is patient-centred improves outcomes, especially patient satisfaction. However, there are also emerging controversies concerning patient-centred healthcare that have important implications for research, clinical practice and health policy.

REFERENCES

Balint, E. (1969). The possibilities of patient-centred medicine. *Journal of the Royal College of General Practitioners*, **17**, 269–76.

Balint, E., Courtenay, M., Elder, A., Hull, S. & Julian, P. (1993). *The doctor, the patient and the group: Balint revisited*. London: Routledge.

Balint, M. (1964). *The doctor, his patient and the illness*. London: Pitman Medical.

Bensing, J. (2000). Bridging the gap: the separate worlds of evidence-based medicine and patient-centered medicine. *Patient Education and Counseling*, **39**, 17–25.

Bower, P. (1998). Understanding patients: implicit personality theory and the general practitioner. *British Journal of Medical Psychology*, **71**, 153–63.

Browne, K. & Freeling, P. (1976). *The doctor–patient relationship*. London: Churchill Livingstone.

Burkitt Wright, E., Holcombe, C. & Salmon, P. (2004). Doctors' communication of trust, care, and respect in breast cancer: qualitative study. *British Medical Journal*, **328**, 864–8.

Butow, P., Dunn, S., Tattersall, M. & Jones, R. (1995). Computer-based interaction analysis of the cancer consultation. *British Journal of Cancer*, **71**, 1115–21.

Byrne, P. & Long, B. (1976). *Doctors talking to patients*. London: HMSO.

Cape, J. (1996). Psychological treatment of emotional problems by general practitioners. *British Journal of Medical Psychology*, **69**, 85–99.

Engel, G. (1977). The need for a new medical model: a challenge for biomedicine. *Science*, **196**, 129–35.

Engel, G. (1980). The clinical application of the biopsychosocial model. *American Journal of Psychiatry*, **137:5**, 535–43.

Ford, S., Fallowfield, L. & Lewis, S. (1996). Doctor–patient interactions in oncology. *Social Science and Medicine*, **42**, 1511–19.

Gask, L. & McGrath, G. (1989). Psychotherapy and general practice. *British Journal of Psychiatry*, **154**, 445–53.

Graugaard, P. & Finset, A. (2004). Trait anxiety and reactions to patient-centered and doctor-centered styles of communication: an experimental study. *Psychosomatic Medicine*, **62**, 33–9.

Grol, R., de Maeseneer, J., Whitfield, M. & Mokkink, H. (1990). Disease-centred versus patient-centred attitudes: comparison of general practitioners in Belgium, Britain and the Netherlands. *Family Practice*, **7**(2), 100–4.

Guadagnoli, E. & Ward, P. (1998). Patient participation in decision-making. *Social Science and Medicine*, **47**, 329–39.

Henbest, R. & Stewart, M. (1989). Patient-centredness in the consultation. 1: A method for measurement. *Family Practice*, **6**, 249–54.

Horvath, A., Gaston, L. & Luborsky, L. (1993). The therapeutic alliance and its measures. In N. Miller *et al.* (Eds.). *Psychodymaic treatment research: a handbook for clinical practice* (pp. 247–73). New York: Basic Books.

Kinmonth, A., Woodcock, A., Griffin, S., Spiegal, N., Campbell, M. & Diabetes Care from Diagnosis Team (1998). Randomised controlled trial of patient centred care of diabetes in general practice: impact on current wellbeing and future disease risk. *British Medical Journal*, **317**, 1202–8.

Kleijnen, J., Gotzsche, P., Kunz, R., Oxman, A. & Chalmers, I. (1997). So what's so special about randomisation? In A. Maynard & I. Chalmers (Eds.). *Non-random reflections on health services research* (pp. 93–106). London: BMJ Publishing Group.

Laine, C. & Davidoff, F. (1996). Patient-centered medicine: a professional evolution. *Journal of the American Medical Association*, **275**, 152–6.

Langewitz, W., Phillipp, E., Kiss, A. & Wossmer, B. (1998). Improving communication skills: a randomized controlled behaviorally-oriented intervention study for residents in internal medicine. *Psychosomatic Medicine*, **60**, 268–76.

Lewin, S., Skea, Z., Entwistle, V., Zwarenstein, M. & Dick, J. (2001). Interventions for providers to promote a patient-centred approach in clinical consultations. Cochrane database of systematic reviews, *Issue 4*, Art. No. CD003267. DOI: 10.1002/14651858. CD003267.

May, C. & Mead, N. (1999). Patient-centredness: a history. In C. Dowrick & L. Frith (Eds.). *General practice and ethics: uncertainty and responsibility* (pp. 76–90). London: Routledge.

McKinstry, B., Walker, J., Blaney, D., Heaney, D. & Begg, D. (2004). Do patients and expert doctors agree on the assessment of consultation skills? A comparison of two patient consultation scales with the video component of the MRCGP. *Family Practice*, **21**, 75–80.

McWhinney, I. (1985). Patient-centred and doctor-centred models of clinical decision making. In M. Sheldon *et al.* (Eds.). *Decision making in general practice* (pp. 31–46). London: Stockton.

McWhinney, I. (1989). The need for a transformed clinical method. In M. Stewart & D. Roter (Eds.). *Communicating with medical patients* (pp. 25–40). London: Sage.

Mead, N. & Bower, P. (2000*a*). Measuring patient-centredness: a comparison of three observation-based instruments. *Patient Education and Counseling*, **39**, 71–80.

Mead, N. & Bower, P. (2000*b*). Patient-centredness: a conceptual framework and review of the empirical literature. *Social Science and Medicine*, **51**, 1087–110.

Mead, N. & Bower, P. (2002). Patient-centred consultations and outcomes in primary care: a review of the literature. *Patient Education and Counseling*, **48**, 51–61.

Mead, N., Bower, P. & Hann, M. (2002). The impact of general practioners' patient-centredness on patients' post-consultation satisfaction and enablement. *Social Science and Medicine*, **55**, 283–99.

Michie, S., Miles, J. & Weinman, J. (2003). Patient-centredness in chronic illness: what is it and does it matter? *Patient Education and Counseling*, **51**, 197–206.

Ockene, J., Quirk, M., Goldberg, R. *et al.* (1988). A residents' training program for the development of smoking intervention skills. *Archives of Internal Medicine*, **148**, 1039–45.

Rogers, C. (1967). *On becoming a person: a therapist's view of psychotherapy.* London: Constable.

Roter, D. (1977). Patient participation in patient–provider interactions: the effects of patient question asking on the quality of interaction, satisfaction, and compliance. *Health Education Monographs*, **5**, 281–315.

Roter, D., Hall, J. & Katz, N. (1987). Relations between physicians' behaviors and analogue patients' satisfaction, recall and impressions. *Medical Care*, **25**, 437–51.

Roth, A. & Fonagy, P. (1996). *What works for whom? A critical review of psychotherapy research.* London: Guildford.

Sackett, D., Rosenberg, W., Gray, J., Haynes, B. & Richardson, W. (1996). Evidence-based medicine: what it is and what it is not. *British Medical Journal*, **312**, 71–2.

Savage, R. & Armstrong, D. (1990). Effect of a general practitioners' consulting style on patients' satisfaction: a controlled study. *British Medical Journal*, **301**, 968–70.

Secretary of State for Health (2000). *The NHS Plan.* London: HMSO.

Stewart, M. (1984). What is a succesful doctor–patient interview? a study of interactions and outcomes. *Social Science and Medicine*, **19**, 167–75.

Stewart, M. (1995). Effective physician–patient communication and health outcomes: a review. *Canadian Medical Association Journal*, **152**, 1423–33.

Stewart, M. (2001). Towards a global definition of patient centred care. *British Medical Journal*, **322**, 444–5.

Stewart, M., Brown, J., Donner, A. *et al.* (2000). The impact of patient-centred care on outcomes. *Journal of Family Practice*, **49**, 796–804.

Stewart, M., Brown, J., Weston, W. *et al.* (1995). *Patient-centred medicine: transforming the clinical method.* London: Sage.

Stiles, W. & Shapiro, D. (1989). Abuse of the drug metaphor in psychotherapy process–outcome research. *Clinical Psychology Review*, **9**, 521–43.

Stiles, W., Shapiro, D., Harper, H. & Morrison, L. (1995). Therapist contributions to psychotherapeutic assimiliation: an alternative to the drug metaphor. *British Journal of Medical Psychology*, **68**, 1–13.

Street, R. (1992). Analyzing communication in medical consultations: do behavioral measures correspond to patients' perceptions? *Medical Care*, **30**, 976–88.

Szasz, T. & Hollender, M. (1956). A contribution to the philosophy of medicine: the basic models of the doctor–patient relationship. *Archives of Internal Medicine*, **97**, 585–92.

van Dam, H., van der Horst, F., van der Borne, B., Ryckman, R. & Crebolder, H. (2003). Provider–patient interaction in diabetes care: effects on patient self-care and outcomes. A systematic review. *Patient Education and Counseling*, **51**, 17–28.

Verhaak, P. (1988). Detection of psychologic complaints by general practitioners. *Medical Care*, **26**, 1009–20.

Winefield, H., Murrel, T., Clifford, J. & Farmer, E. (1996). The search for reliable and valid measures of patient-centredness. *Psychology and Health*, **11**, 811–24.

Wissow, L., Roter, D., Bauman, L. *et al.* (1998). Patient–provider communication during the emergency department care of children with asthma. *Medical Care*, **36**, 1439–50.

Patient safety and iatrogenesis

Maria Woloshynowych and Charles Vincent

Imperial College School of Medicine

Treatment for disease or ill-health is not without its risks. These risks may be inherent to the treatment, such as known side effects of medication, or due to the actions or omissions of healthcare professionals, such as accidentally cutting an adjacent organ during surgery or failing to give the patient prophylactic antibiotics to prevent post-operative infection. Terms used to describe treatment complications and injury to patients include the following: iatrogenic injury or iatrogenic disease; medical accidents; medical mishaps; adverse events; negligence; adverse events; medical mistakes; medical error and critical incidents. Some of these terms have specific definitions while others are general terms that are often used interchangeably. The definition, use and development of these terms are described below. This is followed by an outline of methods used to help our understanding of medical harm, the impact on patients, families and staff, and concludes with a section on how harm to patients can be prevented.

Iatrogenic disease and patient harm

The term 'iatrogenic' comes from the Greek word for physician 'iatros' and from 'genesis', meaning origin; iatrogenic disease therefore is illness which is induced, in some way, by a physician. With the advances of medical science in the mid-twentieth century, particularly the development of penicillin and other antibiotics, the term iatrogenic disease broadened in scope. By the mid-1950s some doctors were beginning to realize that there were potential hazards associated with the enormous increase in drug use and availability (Sharpe & Faden, 1998).

In the 1960s Schimmel (1964) instituted one of the first systematic studies of harm that resulted from 'acceptable diagnostic or therapeutic measures deliberately instituted in the hospital'. Reactions due to error or from previous treatment, and situations that were only potentially harmful were excluded. Even without errors more than 20% of patients experienced one or more episodes of harm and 16 fatalities resulted partly from diagnosis and treatment. In 1981, Steel and colleagues set out to reassess Schimmel's findings, noting that since his time the number and complexity of diagnostic procedures and the number of drugs used had increased and the patient population had aged. Of 815 patients surveyed, 36% suffered a iatrogenic illness, with 9% being major in that they threatened life or produced a major disability. Exposure to drugs was the main factor leading to adverse effects, with nitrates, digoxin, lidocaine, aminophylline and heparin being the most dangerous. Cardiac catheterization, urinary catheterization and intravenous therapy were the principal procedures leading to problems. Falls were also a serious issue.

Steel *et al.* (1981) were willing to admit that some of these episodes might have been preventable, but did not discuss error and were at pains to point out that there was no suggestion of culpability. Gradually however, there has been a greater willingness to examine the problem of patient harm and to speak explicitly of medical error; in the last 10 years the numbers of studies of medical error have increased dramatically. A particular terminology has also developed:

- *adverse events* refer to injury or complication caused by healthcare management (and not due to the disease process) which have resulted in extended hospital stay or disability at the time of discharge from hospital. These events may or may not be preventable
- *critical incidents* generally include harm due to treatment which have *not* resulted in extended stay or disability
- *near misses* refer to errors or circumstances, which if not averted might have resulted in an adverse event or critical incident
- *negligence* is a legal term, which refers to care clearly below the accepted standard of care and resulting in definite harm. In practice events that might be termed negligent are a sub-set of adverse events and critical incidents.

As well as a change in the terms used to describe harm to patients, there has also been a change in emphasis in the phrase used to describe the attempts to reduce harm to patients. Risk management is sometimes, for instance in the United States, oriented more towards resolving legal problems and protecting the organization. In Britain however, the term clinical risk management included attempts to make care safer and prevent harm. Increasingly the reduction of error and harm are encapsulated in the more positive term 'patient safety'. Patient safety activities and initiatives are described in the next two sections.

The nature and frequency of adverse events and critical incidents

In the last 20 years a number of factors combined to bring medical error and the associated harm to the attention of both patients and professionals. These factors include rising rates of litigation, the emergence of risk management, the influence of safety theories and practices from high-risk industries, high profile cases, major government reports and increasing research activity. Perhaps the most powerful driver of all however has been epidemiological studies of harm to patients, defined as adverse events.

The definition for adverse events originated from a study in the United States, the Harvard Medical Practice Study (Brennan *et al.*, 1991), carried out in New York in the mid-1980s, sought to examine the scale of harm to patients in hospital. The researchers needed a measurable definition of adverse events and chose extended stay and disability at the time of discharge as these could be identified with retrospective record review of medical records. The initial findings were substantiated in further retrospective studies in the United States (Thomas *et al.*, 1999), Australia (Wilson *et al.*, 1995), the UK (Vincent *et al.*, 2000), New Zealand (Davis *et al.*, 2001), Denmark (Schiolar *et al.*, 2001), France (Michel *et al.*, 2004) and Canada (Baker *et al.*, 2004).

The incidence of adverse events in these studies vary, with rates ranging from 2.9% in the USA to 16.6% in Australia. However, subsequent analysis has revealed that this can be explained to some extent by differences in definitions, exclusion/inclusion criteria and purpose of the studies (Thomas *et al.*, 2000; Runciman *et al.*, 2000). Studies which have focused on quality of care have reported that 37–60% of adverse events were judged to be preventable (Wilson *et al.*, 1995; Vincent *et al.*, 2000; Davis *et al.*, 2003; Michel *et al.*, 2004; Baker *et al.*, 2004) and have attempted to identify the underlying causes for the adverse events and how to address these. For example, the Australian study recommended better implementation of policies and protocols, better formal quality monitoring, better education and training and more consultation (Wilson *et al.*, 1995); and subsequent US studies have shown how information and decision support systems can reduce medication events (Bates *et al.*, 1993).

Michel *et al.* (2004) have shown that prospective record review is comparable to retrospective record review and in fact identified more preventable adverse events. Prospective review studies are also being carried out in the UK (Chapman *et al.*, 2003). These review studies differ from the earlier, traditional adverse event studies in that they have widened the definition of adverse events to include critical incidents and potential harm. Preliminary results show that on six medical and surgical units 15% of patients experienced an adverse event and a further 14% experienced a critical incident. 72% of adverse events, and 90% of critical incidents, were judged to be preventable. Most adverse events caused little harm but had a negative impact on hospital resources (S. Olsen & G. Neale, personal communication).

Examination of cases identified in the preliminary feasibility study suggested that a significant proportion of critical incidents may be specific to a particular hospital, ward or unit (Chapman *et al.*, 2003). As such it is amenable to local action and this is a good starting point for strategies to improve patient safety. This could be included as part of the ongoing process of clinical risk management or quality improvement. For example, contributory factors may be difficult to assess in retrospective reviews, but prospective methods would enable the staff to further explore causes for particular types of adverse events or critical incidents.

Table 1. Framework of factors influencing clinical practice

Factor types	Influencing Contributory factors	Examples
Institutional Context	Economic and regulatory context; National Health Service Executive; Clinical negligence scheme for NHS trusts	Inconsistent policies; funding problems
Organizational and management factors	Financial resources & constraints; Organizational structure; Policy standards and goals; Safety culture and priorities	Lack of senior management procedure for risk reduction
Work environment factors	Staffing levels and skills mix; Workload and shift patterns; Design, availability and maintenance of equipment; Administrative and managerial support	High workload, inadequate staffing or limited access to essential equipment
Team factors	Verbal communication; Written communication; Supervision and seeking help; Team structure (consistency, leadership, etc.)	Poor supervision of junior staff, poor communication between staff
Individual (staff) factors	Knowledge and skills; Competence; Physical and mental health	Lack of knowledge or experience of specific staff
Task factors	Task design and clarity of structure; Availability and use of protocols; Availability and accuracy of test results	Non-availablity of test results or protocols
Patient factors	Condition (complexity & seriousness); Language and communication; Personality and social factors	Distressed patient or language problem

Understanding adverse events

When the first edition of this book was published, very few studies focused directly on the causes of harm to patients. Confidential enquiries into maternal and postoperative deaths had revealed problems with supervision of junior staff and a higher mortality from surgeons operating outside their own speciality. Critical incident studies, which analyze potentially dangerous incidents reported by staff, have identified other common themes. Cooper *et al.* (1984) examined anaesthetic incidents such as breathing circuit disconnections, drug-syringe swaps and losses of gas supply. Failure to check equipment, unfamiliarity with the equipment, inattention and haste were frequently implicated. Closed claims analyses had also been instructive. For instance Ennis and Vincent (1990) summarized the findings of expert obstetricians in claims involving a stillbirth, perinatal or neonatal death, severe handicap or maternal death. Three major areas of concern were identified: inadequate fetal monitoring; mismanagement of forceps; and lack of involvement of senior staff – inexperienced doctors were left alone for long periods and could not get help when difficulties arose.

The complexity and nature of the factors that combine to cause harm to patients has been illuminated by studies of single cases and case series. In most high-risk industries learning from accidents and near misses is a long-established practice and a cornerstone of safety analysis and improvement. Aviation accidents for instance are exhaustively investigated and the lessons learnt disseminated widely, with important changes made mandatory by the regulatory authorities. In contrast learning within healthcare, with some notable exceptions, has generally been fragmentary and uncertain. Studies of accidents in industry, transport and military spheres have led to a much broader understanding of accident causation, with less focus on the individual who makes the error and more on pre-existing organizational factors.

There are a number of methods of investigation and analysis available in healthcare, though these tend to be under-developed compared with methods available in industry. In the USA the most familiar is the root cause analysis approach of the Joint Commission, an intensive process with its origins in Total Quality Management approaches to healthcare improvement (Spath, 2000). The Veterans Hospital Administration has developed a highly structured system of triage questions which is being disseminated throughout their system (see the National Center for Patient Safety (NCPS) website). In Britain we have developed a method based on Reason's model and on the framework of contributory factors developed by Vincent *et al.* (Vincent *et al.*, 2000b; see Clinical Safety Research Unit website). Reason's essential insights are as follows: incidents and accidents are usually preceded by some kind of unsafe act, in which a person makes an error or mistake. However to understand how this occurred it is necessary to look further back to the 'error producing conditions' which led to the unsafe act and also to 'latent failures', decisions taken by management and others which may have had a bearing on the outcome. Reason's model has been extended and adapted for use in healthcare by developing a broad framework of 'contributory factors' which can impact on clinical practice (Vincent *et al.*, 1998; Table 1).

Information is gleaned from a variety of sources. Case records, statements and any other relevant documentation are reviewed. Structured interviews with key members of staff are undertaken to establish the chronology of events, the main care management problems and their respective contributory factors. The key questions are: 'What happened?' (the outcome and chronology); 'How did it happen?' (the care management problems); and 'Why did it happen?' (the contributory factors).

Analyses using this method have been conducted in hospitals, primary care settings and mental health units. The protocol may be used in a variety of formats, by individual clinicians, researchers, risk managers or clinical teams. For serious incidents a team of individuals with different skills and backgrounds may be assembled for a major incident. A clinical team may use the method to guide and structure reflection on an incident, to ensure that the analysis is full and comprehensive. The group approach is also useful for teaching, both as an aid to understanding the protocol itself and as a vehicle for introducing systems thinking.

The contributory factors that reflect more general problems in a unit are the targets for change and systems improvement. When obvious problems are identified, action may be taken after a single incident, but when more substantial changes are being considered other incident analyses and sources of data (routine audits and outcome data) should also be taken into account. Recommendations may be made in a formal report but it is essential to follow these up with monitoring of action and outcome and to specify who is responsible for implementation.

After the event: the impact on patients, families and staff

Patients are often in a vulnerable psychological state, even when diagnosis is clear and treatment goes according to plan. Even routine procedures and normal childbirth may produce post-traumatic symptoms (Clarke *et al.*, 1997; Czarnocka & Slade, 2000). When patients experience harm or misadventure therefore, their reaction is likely to be particularly severe. Patients and relatives may suffer in two distinct ways after an adverse outcome, firstly from the incident itself and secondly from the manner in which the incident is handled. Many people harmed by their treatment suffer further trauma through the incident being insensitively and inadequately handled. Conversely when staff come forward, acknowledge the damage and take the necessary action, the overall impact can be greatly reduced.

The impact of a medical injury differs from most other accidents in two important respects. Firstly, patients have been harmed, unintentionally, by people in whom they placed considerable trust, so their reaction may be especially powerful and complex. Secondly, they are often cared for by the same professions, and perhaps the same people, as those involved in the original injury. They may have been very frightened by what happened to them and have a range of conflicting feelings about those involved. This can be very difficult, even when staff are sympathetic and supportive (Vincent *et al.*, 1993; Vincent, 2001).

The initial reaction to a medical injury is likely to be one of fear, loss of trust and feelings of isolation. Traumatic and life-threatening events produce a variety of symptoms, over and above any physical injury. Anxiety, intrusive memories, emotional numbing and flashbacks are all common sequelae and are important components of post-traumatic stress disorder (Brewin *et al.*, 1996) (see 'Post-traumatic stress disorder'). The full impact of most incidents only becomes apparent in the longer term. A perforated bowel, for example, may require a series of further operations and time in hospital. The long-term consequences may include chronic pain, disability and depression, with a deleterious effect on family relationships and ability to work. When a patient dies the trauma is obviously severe, especially after a potentially avoidable death (Lundin, 1984), when relatives may face an unusually traumatic and prolonged bereavement (see 'Coping with bereavement').

The aftermath of an adverse event can also have profound consequences for the staff involved, particularly if an individual is perceived as primarily responsible for the outcome. Staff may experience shame, guilt and depression after making a mistake, with litigation and complaints imposing an additional burden. In some cases doctors or nurses may become very nervous of clinical medicine, seek out a specialty with less direct patient contact or abandon medicine entirely. The reaction of the patient and their family may be especially hard to bear, especially when the outcome is severe and if there has been a close involvement over a long period. The reaction of colleagues, whether supportive or defensive and critical, may be equally powerful. Guidelines and practical advice on caring for injured patients and supporting staff can be found elsewhere (Vincent, 2001).

Preventing harm to patients

With the proliferation of studies on medical error and patient harm, it is becoming clear that making healthcare safer is a massive and extremely difficult task. There are clear examples of rapid and obvious safety improvements, such as taking Potassium Chloride and other dangerous drugs off wards to avoid erroneous use. However, while incident reports and basic risk management programmes provide a starting point, fundamental changes are required to many healthcare processes and systems.

Compared with other hazardous enterprises like aviation and nuclear power, healthcare is extraordinarily diverse in nature and highly reliant on human beings, rather than technology, to ensure safety. Solutions required to ensure high reliability in, for instance, blood transfusion services, will obviously differ from those aimed at reducing suicides in mental health. Some factors, perhaps leadership and attitudes to safety, will be important in all environments. Improving safety is likely to require some generic, crossorganizational action, coupled with specialty and process specific changes. The way in which the specific and generic might combine (or interfere) has not yet been established. In this chapter we can only highlight some areas which are held to be of particular importance.

Culture and leadership

Almost everyone involved in patient safety is agreed that progress will depend to some extent on a change in attitudes to error, with more reflection and analysis and less blame and disciplinary action. The development of a 'safety culture' is often held up as the foundation of all approaches to improving patient safety. This term is not well defined, but tends to include an open and fair response to error, a more general awareness of the potential for error and harm, and a willingness to report and discuss error. Crucially, a strong organizational and management commitment is implied. Safety is taken seriously at every level of the organization: the cleaner on the wards is conscious of infection risks, the nurse is alert for potential equipment problems and drug hazards, and managers are monitoring incident reports. The hospital's chief executive should be setting the pace with clear and committed leadership that gives the safety of patients and staff a priority.

Reporting and learning systems

At the heart of most programmes are methods for early identification of adverse events, using staff reports or a systematic screening of records. Similar systems are already in operation in respect of the safety of medicines and medical devices. The reports are used to create a database to identify common patterns and prevent future incidents. The development of clinical risk management in the United Kingdom and elsewhere led to the establishment of local incident reporting systems in hospitals, usually run centrally. Typically there is a standard incident form, asking for basic clinical details and a brief narrative describing the incident. Sometimes staff are asked to report any incident which concerns them or might endanger a patient; in more sophisticated systems, where staff within a unit may be trying to routinely monitor and address specific problems, there may be a designated list of incidents, although staff are free to report other issues that do not fall into these categories. Local systems are ideally used as part of an overall quality improvement strategy but in practice are often dominated by managing claims and complaints. The NHS has a well developed clinical incidents reporting system and this system should be seen as a tool by which patient safety issues can be identified and addressed to reduce the occurrence of clinical incidents and to improve both patient and staff experience. However, there still exist a number of barriers to reporting, such as fear of reprisals or poor understanding of the process of investigation of an incident.

Training, supervision and working conditions

Many senior doctors, and probably hospital management, may be unaware of the extent to which junior doctors are called upon to act beyond their competence. Poor communication between professions is another source of errors and lost information. Linked to the need for better training and supervision is the question of error-producing working conditions, particularly the excessive hours or long shifts that junior staff are required to work in Britain and many other countries. It is a curious paradox that it is illegal to drive a coachload of healthy passengers without regular rest, yet until August 2004, with the introduction of European directives on doctors' working hours, it was considered acceptable to care for a ward of desperately sick patients when close to exhaustion (Vincent et al., 1993). There is still however, in all healthcare systems, serious concern about the impact of workload and fatigue on liability to error (Gaba & Howard, 2002).

Information technology

Bates and Gawande (2003) identify a number of ways in which information technology can reduce error: improving communication; making knowledge more readily accessible; prompting for key information (such as the dose of a drug); assisting with calculations, monitoring and checking in real time; and providing decision support. The use of information technology is accompanied by some degree of standardization and reduction in the variability of provision provided by human beings. Such standardization, when in the form of guidelines and protocols, can be criticized as being overly prescriptive and not taking a patient's particular constellation of symptoms into account. Computers however, when provided with the appropriate information, can completely tailor their guidance or output to the individual patient. Thus technology potentially provides a marriage between the need for standardization and less reliance on human memory and decision-making, with the clinician's necessary insistence that treatment is tailored to the individual patient. Bates et al. (1998) have shown that the introduction of a computerized order entry system resulted in a 55% reduction in medication errors. With the addition of higher levels of decision support, in the form of more comprehensive checking for allergies and drug interactions, there was an overall reduction of 83% in medication errors.

Patient empowerment

A further initiative which is becoming more widespread is to involve the patient in reducing risks and promoting safety. Patients are usually thought of as passive receivers of treatment once they are admitted to hospital, but there is considerable scope for them to contribute to their own safety without placing an too much of a burden of responsibility on them (Vincent & Coulter, 2002). Some patients and relatives already do this, particularly when they suffer from a chronic condition and often may understand their treatment requirements better than a junior doctor. The ways in which patients can be involved in promoting safety are by helping to reach an accurate diagnosis; deciding on appropriate treatment or management strategy; choosing a suitably experienced and safe provider; ensuring that treatment is appropriately administered, monitored and adhered to; and identifying side effects or adverse events quickly and taking appropriate action (Vincent & Coulter, 2002).

In summary, we have shown that a growing awareness of iatrogenic injury led to the development of clinical risk management and then patient safety. Patient safety initiatives were driven and influenced by rising rates of litigation, the emergence of risk management, safety theories and practices from high-risk industries, high profile cases, major government reports and research activity, including epidemiological studies of harm to patients. Earlier initiatives such as confidential enquiries, critical incident studies, analyses of closed claims and case analyses also created a climate in which the systematic study of harm to patients became possible. We have described subsequent impact of critical incidents or adverse events, and stressed the importance of how incidents are handled, both for patients and staff. Improving safety for patients is likely to require some general as well as specific interventions and will include exploration of the following areas: culture and leadership; reporting and learning systems; training, supervision and working conditions; information technology and patient empowerment.

REFERENCES

Baker, G. R., Norton, P. G., Flintoft, V. et al. (2004). The Canadian adverse events study: the incidence of adverse events among hospital patients in Canada. Canadian Medical Association Journal, 170, 1678–86.

Bates, D. W., Leape, L. L. & Petrycki, S. (1993). Incidence and preventability of adverse drug events in hospitalised adults. Journal of General Internal Medicine, 8, 289–94.

Bates, D. W. & Gawande, A. A. (2003). Improving safety with information technology. New England Journal of Medicine, 348(25), 2526–34.

Bates, D. W., Leape, L. L., Cullen, D. J. et al. (1998). Effect of computerised physician order entry and a team intervention on prevention of serious medication errors. Journal of the American Medical Association, 80, 1311–16.

Brennan, T. A., Leape, L. L., Laird, N. M. *et al.* (1991). Incidence of adverse events and negligence in hospitalised patients. Results of the Harvard medical practice study I. *New England Journal of Medicine*, 324, 370–6.

Brewin, C. R., Dalgleish, T. & Joseph, S. (1996). A dual representation theory of posttraumatic stress disorder. *Psychology Review*, 103, 670–86.

Chapman, E. J., Hewish, M., Logan, S. *et al.* (2003). Detection of critical incidents in hospital practice: a preliminary feasibility study. *Clinical Governance Bulletin*, 4, 8–9.

Clarke, D. M., Russell, T. A., Proglase, A. L. & McKenzie, D. P. (1997). Psychiatric disturbance and acute stress response in surgical patients. *Australian and New Zealand Journal of Surgery*, 67,115–18.

Clinical Safety Research Unit website, 2004. http://www.csru.org.uk

Cooper, J. B., Newbower, R. S. & Kitz, R. J. (1984). An analysis of major errors and equipment failures in anaesthesia management: considerations for prevention and detection. *Anaesthesiology*, 60, 34–42.

Czarnocka, J. & Slade, P. (2000). Prevalence and predictors of post-traumatic stress symptoms following childbirth. *British Journal of Clinical Psychology*, 39, 35–51.

Davis, P., Lay-Yee, R., Briant, R. *et al.* (2003). Preventable in-hospital medical injury under the "no fault" system in New Zealand. *Quality and Safety in Health Care*, 12, 251–6.

Davis, P., Lay-Yee, R., Schug, S. *et al.* (2001). Adverse events regional feasibility study: indicative findings. *New Zealand Medical Journal*, 114, 203–5.

Ennis, M. & Vincent, C. A. (1990). Obstetric accidents: a review of 64 cases. *British Medical Journal*, 300, 1365–7.

Gaba, D. M. & Howard, S. K. (2002). Fatigue among clinicians and the safety of patients. *New England Journal of Medicine*, 347, 1249–55.

Lundin, T. (1984). Morbidity following sudden and unexpected bereavement. *British Journal of Psychiatry*, 144, 84–8.

Michel, P., Quenon, J. L., de Sarasqueta, A. M. *et al.* (2004). Comparison of three methods for estimating rates of adverse events and rates of preventable adverse events in acute care hospitals. *British Medical Journal*, 328, 199–202.

The National Center for Patient Safety (NCPS) website. http://www.patientsafety.gov

Runciman, W. B., Webb, R. K., Helps, S. C. *et al.* (2000). A comparison of iatrogenic injury studies in Australia and the USA. II: Reviewer behaviour and quality of care. *International Journal of Quality in Health Care*, 12, 379–88.

Schimmel, B. M. (1964). The hazards of hospitalization. *Annals of Internal Medicine*, 60, 100–10.

Schiolar, T., Lipczak, H., Pedersen, B. L. *et al.* (2001). Forekomsten af utilsigtede haendesler pa sygehuse. En retrospektiv gennemgang af journaler. *Ugeskrift for Laeger*, 163, 5370–8.

Sharpe, V. A. & Faden, A. I. (1998). *Medical harm. Historical, conceptual and ethical dimensions of iatrogenic illness.* Cambridge: Cambridge University Press.

Spath, P. L. (Ed.). (2000). *Error reduction in health care: a systems approach to improving patient safety.* Washington, DC: AHA Press.

Steel, K., Gertman, P. M., Crescenzi, C. & Anderson, J. (1981). Iatrogenic illness on a general medical service at a university hospital. *New England Journal of Medicine*, 304(11), 638–42.

Thomas, E. J., Studdart, D. M., Burstin, H. R. *et al.* (1999). Incidence and types of adverse events and negligent care in Utah and Colorado. *Medical Care*, 38, 261–71.

Thomas, E. J., Studdert, D. M., Runciman, W. B. *et al.* (2000). A comparison of iatrogenic injury studies in Australia and the USA. I: Context, methods, casemix, population, patient and hospital characteristics. *International Journal of Quality in Health Care*, 12, 371–8.

Vincent, C. A. (2001). Caring for patients harmed by treatment. In C. A. Vincent (Ed.). *Clinical Risk Management. Enhancing Patient Safety* (2nd edn.). London: BMJ Publications.

Vincent, C. A. & Coulter, A. (2002). Patient safety: what about the patient? *Quality and Safety in Health Care*, 11, 76–80.

Vincent, C. A., Ennis, M. & Audley, R. J. (Eds.). (1993). *Medical accidents.* Oxford: Oxford University Press.

Vincent, C., Neale, G. & Woloshynowych, M. (2000a). Adverse events in British hospitalised patients: preliminary retrospective record review. *British Medical Journal*, 322, 517–19.

Vincent, C. A., Pincus, T. & Scurr, J. H. (1993). Patient's experience of surgical accidents. *Quality in Health Care*, 2, 77–82.

Vincent, C., Taylor-Adams, S., Chapman, E. J. *et al.* (2000b). How to investigate and analyse clinical incidents: clinical risk unit and association of litigation and risk management protocol. *British Medical Journal*, 320, 777–81.

Vincent, C. A., Taylor-Adams, S. & Stanhope, N. (1998). A framework for the analysis of risk and safety in medicine. *British Medical Journal*, 316, 1154–7.

Wilson, R. M., Runciman, W. B., Gibberd, R. W. *et al.* (1995). The quality in Australian health care study. *Medical Journal of Australia*, 163, 458–71.

Patient satisfaction

Raymond Fitzpatrick

University of Oxford

The concept of satisfaction

There are three distinct reasons why we are interested in patient satisfaction. Firstly, the concept of patient satisfaction enables us to view healthcare services from the patient's point of view. Secondly, patient satisfaction provides a practical means of identifying problems in the processes of care, that is, how care is provided, so that such problems can be addressed and services improved. In this applied use of the term, patient satisfaction is normally listed alongside five other dimensions whereby quality of health services should be assessed: access; relevance to need; effectiveness; equity; and efficiency. A third purpose, related to the second, is to contribute to the formal evaluation of health services (Sitzia & Wood, 1997). Although the theoretical and conceptual clarity of the term 'satisfaction' is generally agreed to be poor, the general emphasis of approaches is upon some form of discrepancy between the patient's expectations and actual experience. The concept of patient satisfaction reflects increasing emphasis upon the patient as 'customer', concerned to judge the value of a service. However it can be argued that the idea of patient as customer has some limitations: patients often do not feel like customers when seeking solutions to problems concerning their own bodies and wellbeing, being rather more intimately concerned in the product than the metaphor of customer implies (Hudak et al., 2003).

There is a tension in the vast array of evidence regarding patient satisfaction. Many studies have focused upon patients' evaluations of their care, ultimately focusing on whether they were 'satisfied' or some related subjective appraisal. By contrast a distinct body of evidence prefers to focus upon patients' reported experiences; whether they have experienced particular problems or shortcomings of health services. Advocates of the former approach argue that the key issue is how patients feel about their healthcare. Advocates for the latter approach are less worried about whether patients accept or tolerate shortcomings; the value of the patient is in reporting experiences that in principle are capable of remedy. The two approaches can provide different assessments of the quality of a service. Patients frequently report themselves as satisfied with a service despite identifying one or more important problems (Jenkinson et al., 2002). The two approaches are probably complementary rather than in contradiction. Inviting patients to say whether they have experienced any of a list of specific problems is a way of identifying specific components of services that we can remedy. Identifying which specific problems are most related to patients' judgements of satisfaction helps us to target and prioritize amongst perceived problems (Fitzpatrick, 2002).

Despite being of importance to our understanding of the behaviour of patients, it is remarkable how neglected patient satisfaction is in terms of theoretical discussion in psychology. A number of models have been proposed to explain available evidence regarding patient satisfaction. Thus satisfaction may be seen as the product of the discrepancies between patients' expectations of care and their perceptions of actual care received (see 'Expectations and health'). Other approaches emphasize the anxiety and uncertainty that attends illness, and argue that satisfaction is determined by the extent of emotional support and reassurance that patients receive. However, to date, no model or theory has emerged that fully encompasses the range of available evidence and more effort has gone into refining measures of satisfaction and applying them in the context of pragmatic evaluations of the quality of care (Fitzpatrick, 1993). It is useful to consider patient satisfaction as an evaluation by the patient of a received service, where the evaluation contains both cognitive and emotional reactions.

A multidimensional construct

Patient satisfaction is best considered as a multidimensional construct. Patients may hold quite distinct views in relation to different aspects of their healthcare. Cleary and McNeil (1988) distinguish nine different dimensions of health care on which patients' views can be obtained: 'the art of care' (i.e. health professionals' interpersonal skills); technical quality; accessibility; convenience; finance; physical environment; availability; continuity; and outcome. As will be evidenced below, the first category of influences, 'the art of care', contains elements of healthcare, such as health professionals' communication skills and sensitivity to patients' concerns, that have a particularly strong influence on patient satisfaction. Some evidence suggests that, so influential are such factors, patients are unable to distinguish between interpersonal skills on the one hand and technical competence on the other hand (Ware & Snyder, 1975). It may be argued that such 'halo effects' reduce the value of patient satisfaction surveys, at least in assessing the quality of healthcare. However, there is sufficient evidence that, in response to well designed questionnaires, patients are capable of distinguishing between technical and interpersonal aspects of the care that they receive (Fitzpatrick, 1993). It remains true that patients place great value on health professionals' empathic and communication skills and value them as least as highly as technical proficiency. Moreover, patients are best convinced that the health professional's technical skills have been appropriately applied when they feel that effort has been made by the doctor personally to understand the patient.

Relationship to other outcomes

As well as being of primary importance as an objective of health care, patient satisfaction is also of importance because its relationship to other outcomes of healthcare. In the first place it has been related to whether patients comply with their treatment regimen. In a study of a paediatric clinic in Los Angeles, mothers were interviewed by researchers immediately after their consultation and then visited at home a fortnight later (Korsch et al., 1968). Three-quarters of mothers had been satisfied with the consultation, the rest were dissatisfied. The satisfied group were three times more likely eventually to have complied with the paediatrician's advice. The observation of a relationship between satisfaction and compliance has been noted in several other studies; for example, in a longitudinal study of patients attending a variety of neurological clinics in South-east England, dissatisfaction with consultations was found to be a significant predictor of non-compliance with drug regimes one year later (Fitzpatrick & Hopkins, 1981) (see 'Adherence to treatment').

A number of studies have also noted that satisfied patients are more likely to continue with their current healthcare provider. Thus, Baker and Whitfield (1992) sent two patient satisfaction questionnaires to the patients of two primary care practices and also to patients who had recently changed surgeries without changing their home addresses. The two instruments assessed satisfaction with different aspects of the general practice and with consultations. Patients who had changed their doctor produced poorer satisfaction scores on all dimensions of the two satisfaction instruments. A number of other studies have shown similar relationships to related variables such as re-attendance at a given healthcare facility, change to alternative provider or health plan, or resort to unorthodox medicine (Fitzpatrick, 1993).

Patient satisfaction and health status

The most intriguing evidence is of a relationship between patient satisfaction and health status: more positively satisfied patients report better health. Thus Cleary and colleagues (1991) carried out a telephone interview survey of 6455 adult patients recently discharged from medical or surgical services of 62 hospitals around the United States. Patients who reported their health as poor reported twice as many problems with regard to satisfaction with care as did those who rated their health as excellent. The same pattern was found when other indicators of health were used such as number of days in bed with ill-health. This relationship between satisfaction and poorer health status and dissatisfaction has now been reported for a wide range of inpatient, outpatient and primary care settings (Fitzpatrick, 1993). A number of quite different explanations are possible. Patients may express greater dissatisfaction because of their failure to make progress in response to treatment. Both satisfaction and health outcomes could be produced by higher quality care. Dissatisfied patients may comply less with treatment regimens, as a result of which they make less progress in terms of health. General psychological wellbeing could influence responses to both health status and satisfaction questionnaires. In addition, there are a number of intervening non-specific or psychosomatic mechanisms that make it plausible that dissatisfaction may directly lead to poorer health. Longitudinal research designs are more likely to throw light on such processes. One such study examined the relationship between immediate satisfaction with consultations with a neurologist for headache and symptomatic change one year later (Fitzpatrick *et al.*, 1983). Patients who had expressed satisfaction with the neurological consultation were significantly more likely to report improvements in headaches one year later. Possible confounding variables such as severity of initial symptoms did not explain the relationship; nor were relationships due to intervening processes such as compliance. At present, it is not clear why relationships are consistently observed between satisfaction and health status. It is clear that satisfaction is positively related to a wide range of other desirable outcomes of healthcare.

Factors that influence patient satisfaction

A number of aspects of healthcare have been shown to influence patient satisfaction. Research evidence for such influences is most convincing when patient satisfaction has been measured by means of some standardized quantifiable instrument and measures have been obtained of the relevant component of healthcare independently of patients' reports. Roter (1989) carried out a meta-analysis of 41 such studies reporting aspects of doctor's behaviour and patient satisfaction. By far the most consistent influence upon patient satisfaction was found to be the doctor's information-giving. This overview confirms what is commonly assumed to be the case, that patients particularly appreciate receiving more information about their health problems and treatment. The importance of information-giving for patient satisfaction is

confirmed by experimental as well as observational studies. Information needs to be appropriate and comprehensible to be fully appreciated by patients (see 'Healthcare professional–patient communication').

Evidence from surveys of patients' experiences suggests poor communication is an organizational feature of hospital care across healthcare systems. Large independent surveys of patients discharged from hospitals in the USA, the UK and Canada all found similar problems of communication. Patients were not told what to expect in terms of daily hospital routines, were not told about side effects of medicines and received no information and advice about resuming normal activities after hospital discharge to their homes (Coulter & Fitzpatrick, 2000).

Effective communication between health professionals and patients is bidirectional; doctors need to be able to obtain medical histories and identify patients' main concerns as well as to give information. Aspects of how doctors obtain information can also influence patient satisfaction. Thus Stiles *et al.* (1979) recorded the consultations of 19 doctors providing general medical care, and then interviewed their patients subsequently to assess satisfaction with consultations. The consultations were analyzed by investigators rating the supposed intention of either the patient or doctor. Patients' satisfaction with the doctor was highest amongst those patients who had experienced consultations in which the doctor used a style of asking questions which invited patients to tell their stories in their own terms, what is often termed a 'patient-centred' rather than 'doctor-centred' form of history-taking (see 'Patient-centred healthcare'). Patients were more likely to feel, in response to this form of questioning, that the doctor had listened to them and understood their problem. In the meta-analysis of studies referred to above (Roter, 1989), a broad category of 'partnership building' processes had the biggest effect on patient satisfaction after information-giving. Roter includes in this category a wide range of behaviours by the doctor, including asking the patient's opinion, facilitating the patient's response or reflecting on statements by the patient. These may all be considered aspects of patient-centred communication and it is clear that such approaches have positive relationships with patient satisfaction. However, such effects are rarely large and not consistently found. Thus Henbest and Stewart (1990) studied the consultations of a sample of patients with six experienced family practitioners in Ontario. Consultations were recorded and rated in patients' views obtained by a follow-up questionnaire and interview. Some positive relationships were obtained in the predicted direction. Patient-centred consultations were more likely to result in the patient feeling that the doctor knew why they had consulted him or her. However, no significant effect could be found upon satisfaction scores. It may be that patient-centred forms of communication are only appropriate to certain presenting problems or patient's concerns and beneficial effects of this approach are less visible where all consultations are included in the analysis. Above all, it is of importance that patients and professionals may value different skills when rating consultations between doctors and patients. There were no correlations when professional examiners' ratings of communication skills of doctors in training were assessed in relation to patients' ratings of the same consultations via a satisfaction questionnaire (McKinstry *et al.*, 2004). The authors suggest that practices such as exploring the patient's reason for consulting or challenging patients' requests for a prescription may be considered up-to-date practice in professional opinion but be considered invasive or unfriendly by the patients.

A number of other factors measured independently of patients' opinions have been shown to influence patient satisfaction. Thus, DiMatteo and colleagues (1980) assessed 71 doctors in a New York hospital for their sensitivity to human emotions by rating their performance in interpreting non-verbal emotions expressed in films and also by their own ability to demonstrate a range of emotions in experimental tasks. Patients consulting at the hospital were asked to assess the doctors via a patient satisfaction questionnaire. Patients' ratings of the doctors' interpersonal skills, but not of their technical skills, were found to correlate with the independently derived measures of doctors' interpersonal sensitivity. Such results are consistent with a wide range of evidence that patients are particularly aware of health professionals' interpersonal skills (Fitzpatrick, 1993). The study is also an example of how patient satisfaction questionnaires can be tested for discriminant validity. Other factors that have been independently measured and shown to influence patient satisfaction include length of time of consultations, continuity in the doctor–patient relationship and accessibility and availability of doctors (Baker & Whitfield, 1992; Fitzpatrick, 1993).

Several studies have shown that one of the main consequences of patient dissatisfaction with the consultation is a reduction of trust. In a study of patients attending primary care services in several cities in the United States, the more that patients experienced problems of communication with the doctor in consultations, the greater the likelihood that they reported themselves not trusting the doctor and also considering changing healthcare provider (Keating et al., 2002). Similarly in a large survey of patients discharged from 51 hospitals in Massachusetts, trust and confidence in hospital staff was strongly associated with willingness to recommend the hospital to others (Joffe et al., 2003).

Patients' views are of enormous value in evaluating the impact of organizational and delivery aspects of the health service and in the highly diverse and constantly changing pattern of services found in the United States especially, patient satisfaction surveys are used to assess such changes. Thus Landon and colleagues (2004) surveyed nearly half a million Medicare patients receiving care under different organizational arrangements. Patients receiving traditional fee-for-service care were more generally satisfied with their care than were patients under managed care. Managed care, by contrast appeared to be better in delivering preventative services. Another study experimented with different primary care providers in the managed care environment (Roblin et al., 2004). Overall, patients receiving primary care from a physician assistant or nurse practitioner were as satisfied as those who received care from traditional medical practitioners. These examples illustrate the central role of patients' views and experiences to evaluate innovation in how healthcare is provided.

The measurement of patient satisfaction

There remain a number of measurement problems in the field of patient satisfaction. One difficulty is that several sociodemographic variables appear to exert consistent influence on patterns of response. In a meta-analysis of published patient satisfaction surveys Hall and Dornan (1990) found that the largest and most consistent variable to influence results was age, with older patients reporting more positive satisfaction. A weaker but significant influence was that of education with less well-educated respondents expressing more favourable responses. Other sociodemographic variables were less consistent in effects. It is not clear why such influences occur, although it seems more likely that age effects are due to normative influences than to real differences in the quality of healthcare received. Other influences already cited, such as health status and psychological wellbeing, are more difficult to interpret. It is at least clear that studies that fail to control for sociodemographic and other known influences should be interpreted with great caution. In particular, variations in satisfaction levels between different healthcare providers may be due to other factors than the quality of care.

Results from satisfaction surveys tend to be positively skewed, with small minorities expressing dissatisfaction. Hall and Dornan (1988) carried out a meta-analysis of 68 published studies and found a median of 84% satisfied across surveys (range 43%–99%). It is not clear to what extent such skewness is due to methodological problems arising either from normative influences, which inhibit patients from expressing criticism of healthcare providers and services, or from limitations inherent in structured questionnaires. It is clear that the modest variability in satisfaction levels in some surveys makes identifying explanatory factors from modelling of results implausible (Hall & Dornan, 1988).

Considerable effort has been put into improving measurement properties of some satisfaction instruments. Increasingly, views are assessed via scales rather than single items in order to improve reliability. Ware and Hays (1988) review a number of scales from patient satisfaction instruments that have internal reliability coefficients which exceed 0.90. Test–retest reliability of instruments is less commonly examined, but results are often very satisfactory (Fitzpatrick, 1993). Ware and Hays (1988) report a study to examine effects of alternative wording of questionnaires. Patients attending outpatient clinics were randomly assigned to receive satisfaction questionnaires after their visit that either involved six point ('very satisfied' to 'very dissatisfied') or five point response options ('excellent' to 'poor'). The five-point format consistently produced more variability and greater construct validity in that answers were more strongly related to other variables such as readiness to comply with medical regimen and whether respondents would recommend the doctor just visited to a friend.

Because there is enormous diversity of healthcare settings and issues may be specific to particular settings, few questionnaires have become 'standard' in the sense of being widely and regularly used. Nevertheless there are a few instruments that have been quite widely applied and found to be of particular use. Thus, the consultation satisfaction questionnaire, comprising 18 items, is a well validated and extensively applied instrument assessing three key aspects of patients' experiences of primary care: the professional aspects of the consultation, the depth of the patient's relationship with the doctor, and the perceived length of the consultation (Baker, 1996). Similarly, the Picker Patient Experience Questionnaire is a 40-item instrument addressing seven core issues: information and education; coordination of care; physical comfort; emotional support; respect for patient preferences; involvement of family/friends; and continuity of care (Jenkinson et al., 2003).

It has been widely employed to assess patients' views of hospital care.

Alternatives to the standardized questionnaire

Investigators remain concerned however that fixed-choice format questionnaires may not elicit patients' concerns fully or may not supply healthcare providers with the kinds of feedback from patients that lead to improvements in services. An increasingly wide range of alternative forms of obtaining patients' views about their healthcare is available (Fitzpatrick & Hopkins, 1993). On the one hand, a number of standardized instruments which have reasonably well-established psychometric properties are available. On the other hand, a variety of more in-depth methodologies have also been developed. Critical incident analysis requires trained interviewers to obtain detailed narratives of their healthcare encounters from which incidents which attract respondents' positive or negative reactions are abstracted for (largely) qualitative analysis.

In a similar vein, non-schedule standardized interviews have been used to obtain detailed qualitatively rich accounts of medical encounters on which conventional quantitative analysis can be performed. Finally, focus groups are increasingly used as a technique for eliciting patients' concerns and views in a way that is least contaminated by investigators' preconceptions. Examples of systematic approaches to these different methods exist but, to date, studies in which comparative advantages are directly compared are lacking (Fitzpatrick & Hopkins, 1993).

Ultimately, a large part of the purpose in assessing patient satisfaction is to provide evidence to healthcare providers of the scope for improvement revealed by patients' views. It is not yet clear that the increasing sophistication observed in measurement systems is matched by practical arrangements within healthcare organizations to respond constructively to evidence obtained from surveys. Increasingly, it will be necessary to examine the practical utility of alternative approaches to the assessment of patient satisfaction.

REFERENCES

Baker, R. (1996) Characteristics of practices, general practitioners and patients related to levels of patients' satisfaction with consultations. *British Journal of General Practice*, **46**, 601–5.

Baker, R. & Whitfield, M. (1992). Measuring patient satisfaction: a test of construct validity. *Quality in Health Care*, **1**, 104–9.

Cleary, P. & McNeill, B. (1988). Patient satisfaction as indicator of quality of care. *Inquiry*, **25**, 25–36.

Cleary, P., Edgman-Levitan, S., Roberts, M. et al. (1991). Patients evaluate their hospital care: a national survey. *Health Affairs*, **10**, 254–67.

Coulter, A. & Fitzpatrick, R. (2000). The patient's perspective regarding appropriate health care. In G. Albrecht, R. Fitzpatrick & C. Scrimshaw (Eds.). *The handbook of social studies in health and medicine* (pp. 454–64). London: Sage Publications.

DiMatteo, M., Taranta, A., Friedman, H. & Prince, L. (1980). Predicting patient satisfaction from physicians' non verbal communication skills. *Medical Care*, **18**, 376–87.

Fitzpatrick, R. (1993). Scope and measurement of patient satisfaction. In R. Fitzpatrick & A. Hopkins (Eds.). *Measurement of patients' satisfaction with their care* (pp. 1–17). London: Royal College of Physicians of London.

Fitzpatrick, R. (2002). Capturing what matters to patients when they evaluate their hospital care. *Quality and Safety in Health Care*, **11**, 306–7.

Fitzpatrick, R. & Hopkins, A. (1981). Patients' satisfaction with communication in neurological outpatient clinics. *Journal of Psychosomatic Research*, **25**, 329–34.

Fitzpatrick, R. & Hopkins, A. (Eds.). (1993). *Measurement of patients' satisfaction with their care*. London: Royal College of Physicians of London.

Fitzpatrick, R., Hopkins, A. & Harvard-Watts, O. (1983). Social dimensions of healing: a longitudinal study of outcomes of medical management of headache. *Social Science Medicine*, **17**, 501–10.

Hall, J. & Dornan, M. (1988). Meta-analysis of satisfaction with medical care: description of research domain and analysis of overall satisfaction levels. *Social Science Medicine*, **27**, 637–44.

Hall, J. & Dornan, M. (1990). Patient sociodemographic characteristics as predictors of satisfaction with medical care: a meta-analysis. *Social Science Medicine*, **7**, 811–18.

Henbest, R. & Stewart, M. (1990). Patient-centredness in the consultation. 2: Does it really make a difference? *Family Practice*, **7**, 28–33.

Hudak, P., McKeever, P. & Wright, J. (2003). The metaphor of patients as customers: implications for measuring satisfaction. *Journal of Clinical Epidemiology*, **56**, 103–8.

Jenkinson, C., Coulter, A., Bruster, S., Richards, N. & Chandola, T. (2002). Patients' experiences and satisfaction with health care: results from a questionnaire study of specific aspects of care. *Quality and Safety in Health Care*, **11**, 335–9.

Jenkinson, C., Coulter, A., Reeves, R., Bruster, S. & Richards, N. (2003). Properties of the picker patient experience questionnaire in a randomized controlled trial of long versus short form survey instruments. *Journal of Public Health Medicine*, **25**, 197–201.

Joffe, S., Manocchia, M., Weeks, J. & Cleary, P. (2003). What do patients value in their hospital care? An empirical perspective on autnomy centred bioethics. *Journal of Medical Ethics*, **29**, 103–8.

Keating, N., Green, D., Kao, A. et al. (2002). How are patients' specific ambulatory care experiences related to trust, satisfaction, and considering changing physicians. *Journal of General Internal Medicine*, **17**, 29–39.

Korsch, B., Gozzi, E. & Francis, V. (1968). Gaps in doctor–patient communications. I: Doctor–patient interaction and patient satisfaction. *Paediatrics*, **42**, 855–71.

Landon, B., Zaslavsky, A. M., Bernard, S., Cioffi, M. J. & Cleary, P. (2004). Comparison of performance of traditional Medicare vs Medicare managed care. *Journal of the American Medical Association*, **291**, 1744–52.

McKinstry, B., Walker, J., Blaney, D., Heaney, D. & Begg, D. (2004). Do patients and expert doctors agree on the assessment of consultation skills? *Family Practice*, **21**, 75–80.

Roblin, D., Becker, E., Adams, E., Howard, D. & Roberts, M. (2004). Patient satisfaction with primary care: does type of practitioner matter? *Medical Care*, **42**, 579–90.

Roter, D. (1989). Which facets of communication have strong effects on outcome – a meta analysis. In M. Stewart & D. Roter (Eds.). *Communicating with medical patients* (pp. 183–96). Newbury Park, CA: Sage Publications.

Sitzia, J. & Wood, N. (1997). Patient satisfaction: a review of issues and concepts. *Social Science and Medicine*, **45**, 1829–43.

Stiles, W., Putnam, S., Wolf, M. & James, S. (1979). Interaction exchange structure and patient satisfaction with medical interviews. *Medical Care*, **17**, 667–79.

Ware, J. & Snyder, M. (1975). Dimensions of patients' attitudes regarding doctors and medical care services. *Medical Care*, **13**, 669–79.

Ware, J. & Hays, R. (1988). Methods for measuring patient satisfaction with specific medical encounters. *Medical Care*, **26**, 393–402.

Psychological support for healthcare professionals

Valerie Sutherland

Sutherland Bradley Associates

The importance of psychological support in the health and wellbeing of patients and clients is well documented and acknowledged by healthcare professionals. However, it is suggested that healthcare systems and the professionals employed as carers do not optimize the benefits associated with psychological support as a stress reduction strategy. This article explores the concept and impact of psychological support as a mediator and moderator of the stress response and suggests ways in which social support systems for healthcare professionals might be improved.

Empirical evidence continues to highlight the negative impact and high costs associated with mismanaged stress in the workplace. It remains a significant problem associated with poor performance, high levels of sickness absence and increasing violence in the healthcare work environment. Jobs in human services share many of the sources of stress present in other occupations in addition to the potential strains associated with intense involvement in the lives of others. This requires a caring commitment and the ability to respond with empathy usually in high demand situations where staff shortages are a common feature of the healthcare environment. A negative spiral of stress can develop when staff shortages, caused by recruitment and retention problems, create high levels of job demand and work stress, leading to yet more strain, sickness absence, or withdrawal from the job because the employee cannot face further pressure. Verhaeghe *et al.* (2003) observed higher levels of 'job-demand' and lower levels of 'decision latitude' among Flemish healthcare workers (aged 35–59 years) compared with a control group. A clear association between high job demand, lack of social support and absenteeism was observed for this group of healthcare workers working under 'job strain' conditions (see also 'Healthcare work environments' and 'Patient safety and iatrogenisis').

Such conditions are optimal for psychological burnout and this has serious, deleterious consequences for both health professionals and patients. In addition, individuals working in healthcare occupations continually have their competence on trial in a highly visible way and in an environment where mistakes can be very costly. It is evident that the job of the healthcare professional is inherently stressful and the recruitment and retention of healthcare professionals remains a key concern in several countries. It has been suggested (Sutherland & Cooper, 1990, 2000, 2003) that healthcare professionals will perform more effectively and suffer less negative effect or personal harm if they understand the role of stress and social support in their own lives and the impact that it could have on patients, clients, colleagues and staff.

A conceptual framework for social support

Dunkel-Schetter and Bennett (1990) provide a framework to guide our understanding of the concept of social support based on the following assumptions.

1. Social support is defined in functional terms as an interpersonal transaction. Therefore, a distinction is made between the existence of social relationships (social integration), the structure of social relationships (social networks) and the function of social interactions/relationships (see 'Social support and health'). Although some authors believe that the term 'social support' should be reserved for this latter interpretation, research evidence indicates the importance of social integration, i.e. the existence of social relationships. For example, Knox *et al.* (1985) found that the actual number of contacts and acquaintances was one of the significant factors inversely related to elevated blood pressure among young, male hypertensives. However, a six-month, longitudinal study of 350 nurses in the northwest of England concluded that perceived organizational support was also related to nurses' health and job satisfaction. This means that interventions designed to increase support, which typically operate at individual or group level, may be limited in their effectiveness unless nurses' perceptions of organizational support are taken into account (Bradley & Cartwright, 2002).

2. It is also necessary to differentiate between the availability of social support and the activation of it. The interactive model of stress defines a state of stress as an imbalance

between perceived demand and perceived ability to meet that demand (see 'Stress and health'). The processes that follow are the coping process and the consequences of the coping strategy applied. This means that stress is a subjective experience contingent upon the perception of a situation. Likewise, it is the belief about social support available, if needed, rather than the actual support available, which influences one's cognitive appraisal of the situation and is the determinant of effective coping and crucial to health protection. It is this assumption that provides a rationale for the interchangeable usage of the terms 'social support' and 'psychological support'.

3. Individual differences in terms of needs, desires and social support seeking behaviour will have an impact on the activation of, receipt of, and perceived satisfaction with social support. Chay (1993) suggests that personality dispositions interact to influence the appraisal of a situation and supportive relationships; affect one's readiness to seek help from others; influence the need for sociable and intimate interaction; and influence one's response to feedback from others. Chay (1993) found that higher levels of perceived availability of support were associated with a combination of trait extraversion, internal locus of control and a high need for achievement among self-employed individuals and small business owners, suggesting that individual differences played a role in the utilization of support services (see also 'Personality and health').

Since the term 'healthcare professional' embraces a very wide range of employee groups working under quite different contractual arrangements, including both self-employed and employed status, it is important to include these factors in any operational model of social support for this occupational group. For example, in a survey of 882 consultants, Graham et al. (2001) observed that just 2% reported obtaining formal psychological support and only 12% coped with stress by formally talking to colleagues in a regular support group. However, the informal use of social support was a coping strategy used by more than two-thirds of this cohort. Consultants stated that talking to a partner, family or friends, or informally with colleagues helped as a stress-coping strategy. However, junior house doctors cite difficult relationships with senior doctors as a key source of stress (Firth-Cozens, 1993), indicating a lack of available social support from a boss or significant others at work. Powerful evidence indicates that a lack of psychological support from one's boss is associated with perceived job strain, job dissatisfaction and poor physical and psychological health.

Types of social support

It is also necessary to acknowledge that different types of social support exist which will have a variable impact on strains and pressures. These have been described in various ways, although it would seem that the four classifications proposed by House (1981) tend to include recent citations:

Emotional support

Emotional Support which involves providing love, caring, empathy and trust, is regarded by House as the most crucial because individuals tend to think of 'being supportive' in terms of emotional support. Research evidence suggests that dentists tend to experience high levels of stress at work because of the nature of the job. However, it is the routine problems in dentistry associated with time pressures, high caseload and falling behind with schedules that cause most concern. These pressures are probably exacerbated because dentists tend to work in isolation from their peers and interact with clients who would, perhaps, rather not attend the surgery. The provision of effective emotional support would thus seem to be important for this occupational group. All branches of the nursing profession are subjected to high levels of stress and burnout and forensic nursing has been perceived as an area of high risk despite the paucity of research evidence. An in-depth study of 51 forensic psychiatric nurses (Happell et al., 2003) found that relatively few suffered from 'high levels of burnout' and the least reported stressor appeared to be the lack of staff support for nursing activities. This work suggests that this form of emotional support may have accounted for the lower than expected levels of stress and burnout (see 'Burnout in health professionals').

Instrumental support

This involves actual assistance through an intervention. It refers to behaviour that directly helps the person in need. For example, to physically take over some aspect of a task for someone is instrumental support. It can also be described as 'material or tangible aid'. Many healthcare professionals have described work overload conditions and time pressures as the most stressful aspects of their job (Sutherland & Cooper, 1991, 1993; Tyler & Cushway, 1992). Having someone to physically provide help would alleviate these pressures but financial constraints do not permit this simple solution to a stressful situation. Usually the individual is required to cope with the strain and pressure of such overload conditions.

Informational support

This means providing a person with information that can be used in the coping process. The information itself is not viewed as instrumental support because it is usually aimed at helping the individual to help him- or herself. Tutoring or coaching a person to help that individual to reach a desired goal is an example of informational support. Beehr et al. (1990) found evidence for the supportive value of informational and emotional support from supervisors among occupational, registered nurses. Both positive job-related and non-job-related communications (versus negative job-related communications) were associated with the perception of the supervisor as supportive, and this had a positive, main effect on individual job strain. Evidence for a buffering effect (i.e. the interaction between social support and job stressors to reduce the strength of the stressor–strain relationship) was also found for non-job-related communication as a form of social support.

Appraisal support

This involves the transmission of self-evaluation information. Feedback from the environment, i.e. social comparison, is derived from information supplied directly and indirectly by the people around us. For example, we gauge our own work performance either from being told by significant others, or by interpreting what we see. At exam time, medical students all face the same challenge and potential threat. Knowing that everyone is in the same circumstance has an impact on the way in which that situation is perceived. An increased understanding of the role of social support will enable an organization to maximize support networks in the workplace, especially during the times when strains and pressures are greatest (for example, threats to jobs, restructuring and during examinations etc.). Research evidence also suggests that there are psychological and physical health benefits, in terms of better immune function and blood pressure, associated with self-disclosure, including the sharing of personal secrets and disclosure of traumatic events (Kennedy *et al.*, 1990). Therefore, reciprocity in the transmission of appraisal and informational support would seem to be the most beneficial support strategy. However, many healthcare professionals tend to feel that they do not have other people around them to provide this form of support. Although general practitioners and dentists rarely operate in single-practice surgeries and tend to work as part of a multidisciplinary team with other autonomous professionals, the working structure and climate does not facilitate the supportive environment which is beneficial to the health and wellbeing of these carers.

Some authorities are attempting to overcome such problems by providing counselling services and/or employee assistance programmes for healthcare professionals. Nevertheless, there is also scope for improvement in the levels of social support within a group practice or team of health professionals, and the quality of interpersonal relationships at work is an area which would typically be addressed by a stress management intervention. Toloczko (1989) reports on the effectiveness of social support training on burnout and improving working relationships among nurses. Measures taken following a six week training programme (one two-and-a-half hour session per week) showed significant reductions in emotional exhaustion and depersonalization, compared with a no-training control group of nurses, even though measures of total life experiences remained consistent for both groups.

The importance of appraisal on stress-coping style was demonstrated in an evaluation study reported by Hirokawa *et al.* (2002). A 14-week stress management programme was provided for trainee social workers. They attended sessions on progressive muscle training, cognitive–behavioural skills training and assertion training. Pre- and post-measures of life events, stress symptoms and stress-coping skills (i.e. active and passive coping) were obtained. Compared with a control group, passive coping strategies had decreased and active coping skills had improved among the trainee social workers following the programme. An ability to identify a potentially stressful or negative situation, and actively seek social support would appear to be a crucial coping skill for healthcare workers (see 'Stress management').

Sources of social support

In addition to the existence of different types of social support it must also be acknowledged that sources of social support have a varying effect on outcomes, i.e. a specific source of support (e.g. a nurse manager) may buffer the effects of a specific source of stress (e.g. work overload) on a job-related strain (e.g. job dissatisfaction) and/or mental or physical health outcomes for a student nurse. Investigating these relationships is complex. For example, Tyler and Cushway (1992) found that having a friend, a partner,

or a member of the family to whom nurses could talk about problems at work had a small but beneficial effect on mental wellbeing. However, levels of anxiety and insomnia were higher in single/ unpartnered people if they could talk to a partner, but higher in married/partnered people if they could not. This highlights the need to consider:

1. Perceptions held about the skill of the support givers (i.e. a partner may be there to help but is unable to engage in any clinically oriented discussion about a stressful experience at work, or understand the situation).
2. Stress experiences may be more acute when expectations of support are too high and therefore, are not realized. Support providers may feel unable to help or to meet the continual demands made which might elicit emotional reactions such as fear, embarrassment, discomfort or helplessness (Dunkel-Schetter & Bennett, 1990). Indeed, it is suggested that informal support providers may experience the same burnout and emotional exhaustion that occurs when professional care providers are over-extended. The outcome tends to be physical and/or psychological withdrawal, i.e. avoidance and detachment.

These results highlight the importance of having supportive work colleagues (or perceiving them to be supportive), because they share similar experiences and can help each other in a reciprocal manner. A formal way to maximize this form of social support is the introduction of co-counselling in the workplace. However, it is likely that much of this is already available informally. For example, Fletcher *et al.* (1991) found that 87% of health visitors screened ($N = 124$) believed that support and encouragement from work colleagues made the job easier most or all of the time. Performance feedback from colleagues and the ability to talk to colleagues during breaks were perceived as supportive in the work environment, and were ranked higher than support from the spouse and family. Nevertheless, for individuals who work in isolation from other healthcare workers, social support from a spouse/partner, or family or friends is clearly desirable. In a prospective study of case managers hired to work with seriously and persistently mentally ill clients, Koeske *et al.* (1993) found control coping strategies (which included talking to spouse, family and friends about the problems) facilitated the workers' ability to deal with a difficult and challenging work obligation. Workers who relied on avoidance coping strategies showed significantly poorer outcomes three months after starting the job (e.g. this included, 'keeping my feelings to myself', 'avoided being with people in general', 'drinking more' etc). Also, the study reported by Graham *et al.* (2001) indicates that a high percentage of consultants report talking to colleagues and family as a stress-coping strategy. However, we still need research evidence to evaluate the efficacy of informal versus formal sources of psychological support as a stress-coping strategy.

Developing psychological support systems

Social support as a stress management strategy could be developed for healthcare professionals in the following ways:

• Emphasize the importance of supportive relationships and networks during the selection, recruitment and training of healthcare professionals in order to promote a supportive work climate and culture. As workload pressures among healthcare professionals continue to create strains and pressures, the importance of coping style is an important variable in the stress management process. In a large scale study of consultants, Graham *et al.* (2001) observed consultants who reported using alcohol or non-prescriptive drugs in response to stress were more than twice as likely to experience psychiatric morbidity as those who maintained a balanced, healthy lifestyle while experiencing stress at work. For example, out of a sample of 882 consultants, 70% coped by talking to a partner, family or friends and 67% coped by talking informally to a colleague. However, only 12% coped by talking formally to colleagues in a regular support group, suggesting that the role of social support among these healthcare professionals is acknowledged but not formalized.

- Social support from the boss appears to be very important. Lack of support is associated with perceived job strain, job dissatisfaction and poor wellbeing. Bennett *et al.* (2001) examined the relationship between stress within work and managerial support available, the strategies used to cope with work stress and levels of anxiety, depression and work satisfaction among one hundred and six ward-based nurses. Consistent relationships between work stress and each of these outcomes were observed. They also found that lack of managerial support was associated both with negative mood states and low levels of work satisfaction. The key predictors of negative affect were lack of management support, job overspill, having to make decisions under time pressure and lack of recognition by the organization.

Therefore it is necessary that healthcare professionals as managers of other people are trained to understand the role and importance of managerial support and reflect this in their style of leadership and supervision.

The support derived from a mentoring relationship can also provide a strong psychological support structure for the healthcare professional. Some Health Care Trusts in the UK have introduced mentoring as a professional development technique and this type of mentoring relationship can be found outside of the normal chain of reporting. In fact, there may be greater benefit in having a significant other as a mentor rather than one's manager (Young & Perrewe, 2000; Vance & Olsen, 2002).

- Coherent teamwork is crucial for the delivery of good quality patient care both directly in terms of efficient and effective services and indirectly via the impact on stress reduction (Firth-Cozens, 1998). Teamworking provides opportunity for support especially among multiprofessional clinical teams. Self-managed work teams and action groups help to develop support networks and provide opportunity for strong bonding. This is useful for healthcare professionals who spend much of their day working in relative isolation. For example, community nurses and doctors in the practice surgery lack opportunity to meet and socialize with peers and colleagues for much of the working day.
- Develop and provide psychological support services, such as employee assistance programmes, occupational health and counselling services for healthcare professionals. The need to ensure that a culture and climate exists that actively and overtly encourages the use of such services cannot be over-estimated. Staff will not seek help if they fear blame, or perceive that their

actions might jeopardize future employment or career opportunities.

- Each practice, ward, surgery or department should be encouraged to develop social networks, both at work and socially. Self-help groups such as health circles also provide a psychological support structure and forum (Kuhn, cited ILO, 1993).
- Education about the beneficial effects of social support between work-and home-life is necessary so that healthcare professionals and their significant others can build strong support networks as a buffer against the stress that is an inevitable part of working and living in the healthcare service.

Effects of social support

Much of the literature on the effectiveness of social support has focused on two sorts of health effects; main effects and buffer effects. The way in which social support works has generated considerable disagreement, but many of the differences in the findings appear to arise from the variation in the conceptual definition of the concept, the way in which it is operationalized, and the reliance on cross-sectional research designs (Thoits, 1986). However, evidence exists to support the various hypotheses proposed, but the findings may be affected by the actual source and type of support studied, and the stressor(s), outcome measure(s) and the person variables measured (e.g. gender, age and socioeconomic status). For example, Sutherland and Cooper (1993) found that reported use of social support, as a stress-coping strategy, was a significant predictor of job satisfaction among general practitioners. Low use of social support was a predictor of depression among this occupational group, and female general practitioners were significantly more likely to use this as a coping strategy than the males, who also evidenced a poorer level of psychological wellbeing than their female counterparts.

It is suggested that social support works in the following ways. Perceived social support can have a main effect on perceived job stress, job-related strain and/or mental and physical health. It can lessen the effect of perceived job stress on job-related strain, moderates job stress on mental and physical health, and it can ameliorate the effects of job-related strain on mental and physical health. Some authors have suggested that a 'coping' hypothesis best explains their findings, believing that social support is a coping mechanism that individuals use under stressful conditions. Thoits (1986) described similarities between social support and coping with stress:

1. Instrumental support was identified with problem focused coping strategies. This implies direct action on the environment or self to remove or alter the circumstances perceived of as a threat.
2. Emotional support was identified with emotion focused coping in that cognitive appraisal is used to control the undesirable feelings that result from a stressful situation.
3. Informational support is identified with perception-focused coping, which consists of cognitive attempts to alter the meaning of a situation so it is perceived as less threatening.

Therefore, both support and coping act to change the situation, the emotional reaction to the situation and/or the meaning of the situation. Indeed, it has been suggested that knowing help is available, but coping with one's problems without using outside assistance leads to the best outcomes in terms of confidence in one's own capabilities (i.e. self-confidence, a sense of mastery and high self-esteem) (see 'Self-efficacy and health').

Conclusion

The individual who chooses to become a healthcare professional seeks a satisfying and challenging occupation. By definition it involves close contact and responsibility for the good health and life of another person. Mastery of sometimes difficult and demanding situations can provide stimulation and tremendous job satisfaction and it is likely that this protects healthcare professionals from some of the negative and stressful aspects of the job. However, there are greater perceived burdens that exist outside of the actual role of caring. Change seems to be a constant theme in health practice and this is a potent source of stress. It includes changes to systems and practice as medical research advances, changes brought by legislation and government that bring new roles for health carers, and the changes in society that alter demands and the structure of support networks in our environment. The presence of psychological support can buffer against the negative impact of strain and job demand and an increased understanding of the role of psychological support as a stress coping strategy will help healthcare professionals to adapt to inevitable change. It is essential if they are to remain in the job, stay fit, healthy and happy, and deliver a quality service to patients and clients. Organizations who endorse the maxim, 'healthy workforce – healthy business' will achieve these objectives by the provision of systems and structures for the development and maintenance of psychological support for healthcare professionals.

(See also 'Stress management', 'Social support and health', 'Social support assessment' and 'social support interventions'.)

REFERENCES

Bechr, T. A., King, L. A. & King, D. W. (1990). Social support and occupational stress: talking to supervisors. *Journal of Vocational Behaviour*, **36**, 61–81.

Bennett, P., Lowe, R., Matthews, V., Dourali, M. & Tattersall, A. (2001). Stress in nurses: coping, managerial support and work demand. *Stress & Health*, **17**, 55–63.

Bradley, J. R. & Cartwright, S. (2002). Social support, job stress, health and job satisfaction among nurses in the United Kingdom. *International Journal of Stress Management*, **9**, 163–82.

Chay, Yue Wah (1993). Social support, individual differences and well-being. A study of small business entrepreneurs and employees. *Journal of Occupational and Organizational Psychology*, **66**, 285–302.

Dunkel-Schetter, C. & Bennett, T. L. (1990). Differentiating the cognitive and behavioural aspects of social support. In B. R. Sarason, I. G. Sarason & G. R. Pierce (Eds.). *Social support: an international view*. New York: John Wiley.

Firth-Cozens, J. (1993). Stress, psychological problems and clinical performance. In C. Vincent, A. Ennis & R. M. J. Audley (Eds.). *Medical accidents*. Oxford: Oxford University Press.

Firth-Cozens, J. (1998). Hours, sleep, teamwork and stress. *British Medical Journal*, **317**, 1335–6.

Fletcher, B. C., Jones, F. & McGregor-Cheers, J. (1991). The stressors and strains of health visiting: demands, supports, constraints and psychological health. *Journal of Advanced Nursing*, **16**, 1078–89.

Graham, J., Albery, I. P., Ramirez, A. J. & Richards, M. A. (2001). How hospital consultants cope with stress at work: implications for their mental health. *Stress and Health*, **17**, 85–98.

Happell, B., Pinikahana, J. & Martin, T. (2003). Stress and burnout in forensic psychiatric nursing. *Stress and Health*, **19**, 63–8.

Hirokawa, K., Yagi, A. & Miyata, Y. (2002). An examination of the effects of stress management training for Japanese college students of social work. *International Journal of Stress Management*, **9**, 113–23.

House, J. S. (1981). *Work stress and social support*. Reading, MA: Addison-Wesley.

International Labour Office (1993). Safety and related issues pertaining to work on offshore petroleum installations. Tripartite Meeting Report. Geneva: International Labour Office.

Kennedy, S., Kiecolt-Glaser, J. K. & Glaser, R. (1990). Social support, stress, and the immune system. In B. R. Sarason, I. G. Sarason & G. R. Pierce (Eds.). *Social support: an international view*. New York: John Wiley.

Koeske, G. F., Kirk, S. A. & Koeske, R. D. (1993). Coping with job stress: Which strategies work best? *Journal of Occupational and Organisational Psychology*, **66**, 319–35.

Knox, S. S., Theorell, T., Svensson, J. & Walker, D. (1985). The relation of social support and working environment to medical variables associated with elevated blood pressure in young males: a structural model. *Social Science and Medicine*, **21**, 525–31.

Sutherland, V. J. & Cooper, C. L. (1991). *Understanding stress: a psychological perspective for health professionals*. London: Chapman and Hall.

Sutherland, V. J. & Cooper, C. L. (1993). Identifying distress among general practitioners: predictors of psychological ill health and job dissatisfaction. *Social Science and Medicine*, **37**, 575–81.

Sutherland, V. J. & Cooper, C. L. (2000). *Strategic stress management: an organizational approach* (p. 145). Basingstoke, UK: Macmillan Business.

Sutherland, V. & Cooper, C. L. (2003). *De-stressing doctors: a self-management guide* (p. 161–2). China: Butterworth Heinemann.

Thoits, P. A. (1986). Social support as coping assistance. *Journal of Consulting and Clinical Psychology*, **54**, 416–23.

Toloczko, A. M. (1989). The effects of social support training and stress inoculation training on burnout in nurses. Ph.D. Thesis, Lehigh University, Bethlehem, Pennsylvannia, USA.

Tyler, P. & Cushway, D. (1992). Stress, coping and mental well-being in hospital nurses. *Stress Medicine*, **8**, 91–8.

Vance, C. & Olsen, R. K. (2002). *The mentor connection in nursing*. New York: Springer Publishing Company.

Verhaeghe, R., Mak, R., Van Maele, G. Kornitzer, M. & De Backer, G. (2003). Job stress among middle-aged health care workers and its relation to sickness absence. *Stress and Health*, **19**, 265–74.

Young, A. M. & Perrewe, P. L. (2000). What did you expect? An examination of career-related support and social support among mentors and protégés. *Journal of Management*, **26**, 1–17.

Reassurance

Patricia Loft, Geraldine Meechan and Keith J. Petrie

The University of Auckland

What is reassurance?

Patients with physical symptoms attend medical consultations expecting a clear and valid explanation for their health complaints. Patient reassurance is a central component of the medical consultation and is the most commonly occurring and important aspect of patient care. After being reassured by their doctor, many patients are unconvinced that their symptoms do not relate to physical disease and continue to experience ongoing health-related distress. Whether in primary care or following a diagnostic test, effective patient reassurance is essential to promote wellbeing and prevent future unnecessary medical visits and investigations.

In most cases reassurance is offered following the history taking and physical examination, although often the process may occur after further diagnostic or laboratory testing. Reassurance can be defined as communication between doctor and patient that is intended to allay the patient's health related fears and anxieties. Typically, the process involves the doctor providing an explanation of the patient's symptoms and confirmation that the patient has no serious illness. To be effective reassurance needs to adequately address the patient's worries about the health threat.

Reassurance following investigative tests

Patient reassurance has received only minimal attention in current empirical research, with much of this research focusing on the effectiveness of reassurance following diagnostic medical tests. Evidence shows that many patients are not reassured following a negative test result and in some patients diagnostic tests may cause more harm than good by increasing patient perceptions of disease vulnerability. For example, women undergoing diagnostic laparoscopy for chronic pelvic pain experienced more pain and disturbed daily activities following the procedure even though no pathology was found, compared with a comparison group who underwent solely psychological and physiotherapy treatment (Peters et al., 1991).

Ambiguous test results can elevate health concerns, particularly in patients who already have high health anxiety (Howard & Wessely, 1996; Verrilli & Welch, 1996). Lucock et al. (1997) found patients who reported high health anxiety prior to a gastroscopic investigation reported a decline in feelings of reassurance 24 hours later and continued to be concerned about their health when followed up a year after the test (Lucock et al., 1997).

The process of diagnostic testing can in itself, make feelings of vulnerability to illness more salient and reinforce the patient's belief that there is something wrong with their health. Several studies have found evidence that cardiac investigations may not always be useful in reassuring patients, but rather they may cause harm by creating anxiety and encouraging the patient's illness beliefs (Howard & Wessely, 1996; Mayou et al., 1999). The process of cardiac investigation typically involves a hospital visit, patient consent for a procedure that is not without risk and the investigation itself, all of which may also encourage focusing on symptoms and reinforce the belief that the complaints are serious.

Research suggests that the more invasive the investigation, the more likely it is that illness concerns are activated. For example, more serious and frequent pain symptoms were reported by patients six weeks after receiving a negative test result following angiography, compared with patients who underwent a non-invasive assessment for chest pain symptoms. In addition, these individuals continued to use anti-anginal medication and had more hospital emergency admissions compared with those undergoing non-invasive assessment (Mayou et al., 1999). A similar pattern of failed reassurance was reported in patients with normal coronary arteries as confirmed by angiography, with patients reporting continuing incapacity, distressing symptoms and ongoing medical visits two years following the procedure (Potts & Bass, 1993).

Why does reassurance fail?

Both doctor and patient factors contribute to successful reassurance and influence misunderstandings during doctor–patient communication. The doctor may assume the patient clearly understands that there is no physical pathology following a negative investigative result. However, the patient may come to the medical consultation with specific illness beliefs and ideas which significantly affect the interpretation of the reassurance offered by the doctor. Poor medical knowledge and previous experience of medical misdiagnosis can all undermine successful reassurance. For example, minimal reassurance was found in patients undergoing echocardiography for chest pain symptoms or a benign heart murmur even though heart disease was ruled out by a normal test result (McDonald et al., 1996). Later interviews with the patients revealed that many lacked the important understanding that a murmur or symptoms could continue even though there was no heart pathology, whilst patients with a better understanding had reduced anxiety about their symptoms.

Individual differences also play a role in reducing reassurance. Some individuals have a high focus on their internal bodily state, making them sensitive to symptom detection and leading to misinterpretation of symptoms and subsequent failure of reassurance by a medical professional (Barsky & Borus, 1995) (see 'Symptom perception'). Other patients may be prone to catastrophic thinking following symptom discovery (Howard & Wessely, 1996). In such cases, the doctor may be unaware of the extent of the 'worst case scenario' thinking which the patient has engaged in and the level of reassurance offered by the doctor may not be enough to overcome the patient's level of concern. Alternatively, the level of emotional distress developed from the patient's fear of a life-threatening condition may interfere with effective reception of the information provided by the doctor.

Even though reassurance may appear successful during the medical consultation, once the patient leaves the medical environment they may be influenced by a number of social factors that present obstacles to reassurance (McDonald *et al.*, 1996). For example, a patient may watch a graphic portrayal of death from heart disease on television, or a family member may develop cancer despite an earlier negative diagnostic scan, both of these being scenarios that may encourage fear and undermine reassurance. Stories concerning health threats have become commonplace in all areas of the media. This has the effect of undermining individuals' perception of their own health, heightening vigilance for symptoms and increasing the likelihood that symptoms will be interpreted negatively (Barsky & Borus, 1995).

Ambiguous behaviour on the part of the doctor may also impede patient reassurance. For example, many negative cardiac investigations fail to reassure patients simply because the doctor continues to prescribe anti-anginal or other cardiac medication. This communicates an ambiguous message to the patient regarding cardiac health (Mayou *et al.*, 2000). Additionally, a long delay before the diagnostic test is undertaken allows more time for negative illness beliefs to become established. This may include lifestyle changes geared to a different illness outcome, such as a reduction in work hours or leisure activities, which will make subsequent reassurance considerably more difficult (Nijher *et al.*, 2001).

Psychological morbidity

Patients who frequently attend medical clinics seeking reassurance for benign symptoms often suffer psychological morbidity and research suggests that these patients are more difficult to reassure. A study of women undergoing bone screening for osteoporosis found that women with high health anxiety were only temporarily reassured following a high bone density result. Long-term follow-up showed a return to baseline levels of worry and perceived likelihood of developing osteoporosis (Rimes & Salkovskis, 2002). Similarly, patients with high levels of both anxiety and depression continued to experience chest pain symptoms after a negative exercise test ruled out cardiac problems, compared with those low in psychological morbidity who became pain-free following a negative result (Channer *et al.*, 1987). Again, individuals with severe headaches who also suffered from anxiety and depression did not feel reassured following a neurological consultation (Fitzpatrick & Hopkins, 1981).

High trait anxiety has been found to be associated with an increased focus on internal bodily states, which leads to more symptoms being detected and reported (Watson & Pennebaker, 1989). A heightened sensitivity to the frequency and intensity of physical symptoms can make anxious or depressed patients extremely resistant to medical reassurance. Many patients who do not have significant medical illness but consistently seek medical care for reassurance about their symptoms tend to be high in trait anxiety

(Banks *et al.*, 1975) and tend to be less likely to make normalizing attributions for common somatic symptoms than other people are (Sensky *et al.*, 1996) (see 'Psychosomatics').

Patients with medically unexplained symptoms are a common occurrence in medical practice and much time and effort is devoted to patients where no medical diagnosis can account for persistent and disabling symptoms. Often these patients have multiple symptoms, experience considerable distress and are high users of medical resources. A number of syndromes have evolved from clusters of unexplained physical symptoms, such as irritable bowel syndrome and chronic fatigue syndrome. Reassurance is often extremely challenging with these patients as there is uncertainty as to why symptoms persist even though serious illness has been ruled out. Also, patient support groups may provide information that inadvertently validates symptoms, encourages further investigations and undermines reassurance provided during the medical consultation (Page & Wessely, 2003).

Improving reassurance

Poor communication is frequently the most significant cause of unsuccessful reassurance and both verbal and non-verbal cues contribute to this problem. Reassurance is improved when the provision of information is clear and unambiguous. If a clinician offers reassurance in an unsure manner this may encourage the patient's resolve that the condition is incurable or life threatening. Similarly, the patient may be left with ambiguities if vague words are used, such as 'probably' – a word that embodies some doubt and may encourage catastrophic thoughts and speculation (Coia & Morley, 1998). A recent study of patients with minor to severe arthritis found that although patients were given reassurance that the condition was 'low' in seriousness, at an 'early stage' or the prognosis was 'mild', many patients misinterpreted this information to mean that their condition would change in the future and would eventually progress to more intense pain and disability (Donovan & Blake, 2000).

Building rapport with the patient and adopting a patient-centred communication style is a useful method for alleviating illness concerns and increasing reassurance (Kessel, 1979). This can be achieved by ensuring that the patient's thoughts and fears have been adequately addressed, thereby conveying to the patient that they have been heard and understood. Patient-centred consultation styles significantly increased patient reassurance in a study of Ontario family doctors, where patients who were encouraged to express their thoughts and feelings felt significantly more reassured following the consultation (Henbest & Stewart, 1990) (see 'Patient-centred healthcare' and 'healthcare professional–patient communication').

Reassurance following invasive diagnostic tests can also be improved if medical professionals prepare patients for the possibility of normal findings. Additionally, structured interventions that address patient's maladaptive cognitions following a negative investigative result may also enhance patient reassurance. Klimes *et al.* (1990) employed a psychological intervention to enhance reassurance in patients who continued to experience chest pain symptoms following negative cardiac investigation. The cognitive behavioural therapy challenged incapacitating beliefs and behaviours and provided patients with training in relaxation, distraction and breathing. Significant reductions in chest pain were reported by patients as well as better mood and less disruption in daily life compared with a control group, suggesting that this type of programme may be very effective in patients where initial reassurance has failed (Klimes *et al.*, 1990). Moreover, in order to prevent the development of negative illness cognitions in patients waiting for medical investigations, shorter waiting times prior to the diagnostic test may also improve patient reassurance (Nijher *et al.*, 2001).

The challenges involved in reassuring patients with medically unexplained symptoms, have led to the development of a number of interventions to improve the management and treatment of these patients. A meta-analysis of studies utilizing cognitive behavioural therapy for patients with somatoform disorders has revealed significant success for this type of treatment option (Looper & Kirmayer, 2002). These interventions typically include methods such as exploring the patient's illness beliefs and behaviours, developing normalizing cognitive strategies, reducing body scanning for symptoms and enhancing physical activity (Rief & Nanke, 2004) (see 'Cognitive behaviour therapy').

Recent research has also found that training primary care physicians to effectively manage frequent medical attenders was helpful in reducing subsequent medical visits (Rief *et al.*, 2006).

The general practitioners received training in patient communication, in managing the patient's organic health beliefs and avoidance of physical activity, beginning and stopping medical examinations and patient reassurance. Subsequent patient visits to the trained doctors declined, whereas patient visits to the untrained doctors did not, which suggests that this type of training programme is a useful and effective tool in assisting doctors to manage these patients.

Conclusions

Reassurance is at the heart of many medical consultations. To provide effective reassurance the clinician needs to provide an explanation for symptoms that fits into the patient's knowledge of the condition and addresses the patient's concerns about the health threat. Patients with high health anxiety and fixed negative health cognitions provide a particular challenge for clinicians. More research needs to be completed to identify effective strategies for clinicians working with such patients to improve levels of reassurance and resist pressure for inappropriate investigations. Cognitive behavioural approaches have the potential to reduce illness concerns in patients following failed reassurance but need to be based on a more detailed theoretical understanding of the reassurance process.

REFERENCES

Banks, M. H., Beresford, S. A., Morrell, D. C., Waller, J. J. & Watkins, C. J. (1975). Factors influencing demand for primary medical care in women aged 20–44 years: a preliminary report. *International Journal of Epidemiology*, **4**(3), 189–95.

Barsky, A. J. & Borus, J. F. (1995). Somatization and medicalization in the era of managed care. *Journal of American Medical Association*, **274**, 1931–4.

Channer, K. S., James, M. A., Papouchado, M. & Rees, J. R. (1987). Failure of a negative exercise test to reassure patients with chest pain. *Quarterly Journal of Medicine*, **63**(240), 315–22.

Coia, P. & Morley, S. (1998). Medical reassurance and patients' responses. *Journal of Psychosomatic Research*, **45**(5), 377–86.

Donovan, J. L. & Blake, D. R. (2000). Qualitative study of interpretation of reassurance among patients attending rheumatology clinics: "just a touch of arthritis, doctor?" *British Medical Journal*, **320**, 541–4.

Fitzpatrick, R. & Hopkins, A. (1981). Referrals to neurologists for headaches not due to structural disease. *Journal of Neurology, Neurosurgery & Psychiatry*, **44**(12), 1061–7.

Henbest, R. & Stewart, M. (1990). Patient-centredness in the consultation. Does it really make a difference? *Family Practice*, **7**, 28–33.

Howard, L. & Wessely, S. (1996). Reappraising reassurance: the role of investigations. *Journal of Psychosomatic Research*, **41**(4), 307–11.

Kessel, N. (1979). Reassurance. *Lancet*, **1**(8126), 1128–33.

Klimes, I., Mayou, R. A., Pearce, M. J., Coles, L. & Fagg, J. R. (1990). Psychological treatment for atypical non-cardiac chest pain: a controlled evaluation. *Psychological Medicine*, **20**, 605–11.

Looper, K. J. & Kirmayer, L. J. (2002). Behavioral medicine approaches to somatoform disorders. *Journal of Consulting and Clinical Psychology*, **70**(3), 810–27.

Lucock, M. P., Morley, S., White, C. & Peake, M. D. (1997). Responses of consecutive patients to reassurance after gastroscopy: results of self administered questionnaire survey. *British Medical Journal*, **315**, 572–5.

Mayou, R. A., Bass, C. M. & Bryant, B. M. (1999). Management of non-cardiac chest pain: from research to clinical practice. *Heart*, **81**(4), 387–92.

Mayou, R. A., Bass, C., Hart, G., Tyndel, S. & Bryant, B. (2000). Can clinical assessment of chest pain be made more therapeutic? *Quarterly Journal of Medicine*, **93**, 805–11.

McDonald, I. G., Daly, J., Jelinek, V. M., Panetta, F. & Gutman, J. M. (1996). Opening Pandora's box: the unpredictability of reassurance by a normal test result. *British Medical Journal*, **313**, 329–32.

Nijher, G., Weinman, J., Bass, C. & Chambers, J. (2001). Chest pain in people with normal coronary anatomy. *British Medical Journal*, **323**, 1319–20.

Page, L. A. & Wessely, S. (2003). Medically unexplained symptoms: exacerbating factors in the doctor–patient encounter. *Journal of the Royal Society of Medicine*, **96**(5), 223–7.

Peters, A. A., van Dorst, E., Jellis, B. *et al.* (1991). A randomised clinical trial to compare two different approaches in women with chronic pelvic pain. *Obstetrics & Gynaecology*, **77**(5), 740–4.

Potts, S. G. & Bass, C. M. (1993). Psychosocial outcome and use of medical resources in patients with chest pain and normal or near-normal coronary arteries: a long term follow-up study. *Quarterly Journal of Medicine*, **86**, 583–93.

Rief, W. & Nanke, A. (2004). Somatoform disorders in primary care and inpatient settings. *Advances in Psychosomatic Medicine*, **26**, 144–58.

Rief, W., Nanke, A., Rauh, E., Zech, T. & Bender, A. (2006). Evaluation of a general practitioners' training: "how to manage patients with unexplained physical symptoms". *Psychological Medicine*, **47**, 304–11.

Rimes, K. A. & Salkovskis, P. M.
(2002). Prediction of psychological
reactions to bone density screening
for osteoporosis using a
cognitive–behavioral model of health
anxiety. *Behaviour Research and Therapy*,
40(4), 359–81.

Sensky, T., MacLeod, A. K. &
Rigby, M. F. (1996). Causal attributions

about common somatic sensations
among frequent general practice
attenders. *Psychological Medicine*, **26**(3),
641–6.

Verrilli, D. & Welch, H. G. (1996).
The impact of diagnostic testing on
therapeutic interventions. *Journal of
American Medical Association*, **275**(15),
1189–91.

Watson, D. & Pennebaker, J. W. (1989).
Health complaints, stress, and distress:
exploring the central role of negative
activity. *Psychological Review*, **96**(2),
234–54.

Screening in healthcare: general issues

Anne Miles

University College London

People are offered screening tests throughout their lifetime, from birth through to old age. But although screening for certain diseases/disorders is widely accepted, screening for other types remains controversial. The aim of this chapter is to provide a general outline of the current debates and developments within screening, and it draws principally on examples from the field of cancer screening. More detailed discussion of the issues surrounding cardiac, genetic and antenatal screening and further discussion of cancer screening, can be found in other chapters in this book (see 'Screening: antenatal', 'Screening: cancer', 'Screening: cardiac' and 'Screening: genetic').

The aims of screening

The term 'screening' is usually reserved to describe the testing of all people within a specific sector of the population (e.g. people within a particular age range) who have no symptoms, and who appear to be at 'average risk' of getting the target disease. Although, in the case of neonates, screening might be used to enhance the medical management of the future date (i.e. once the child has been born) or to give parents the opportunity to terminate a pregnancy if they do not wish to have a child who has a particular disability or condition, the main purpose of screening is often to reduce disease-related morbidity and mortality by detecting disease at an early stage, when treatment is more likely to be successful.

Early detection can lead to fewer disease-related complications, because simpler, less toxic treatment is required. It can also dramatically enhance a person's chance of survival. For example, five-year survival rates for colorectal cancer are 90% if the disease is detected whilst still localized, but drop to 10% if the disease is detected after it has spread to vital organs, such as the liver. Screening for colorectal cancer can reduce mortality from the disease by as much as 33%, but the benefits of screening can be even greater if the pre-disease stage is identified. Most colorectal cancers develop from pre-malignant adenomatous polyps. If polyps are removed, this type of cancer can be prevented altogether, sparing people both the trauma of a cancer diagnosis and obviating the need for major interventions such as surgery and chemotherapy.

Many types of screening aim to detect signs of disease; as a result, screening is usually classified as a type of secondary prevention. Increasingly, though, tests have become available that identify individuals at 'enhanced susceptibility' to developing a disease at some point in the future, which means that screening has begun to play a role in primary prevention.

Identifying people who are susceptible to developing future disease, or who have pre-disease states, is clearly preferable to finding active disease because it can lead to a reduction in disease incidence as well as mortality. However, this is not always possible. In the case of cancer, whilst some types of the disease, such as cervical cancer and colorectal cancer, have an identifiable 'pre-malignant' stage, other types do not. So whether a particular screening test aims to detect enhanced susceptibility towards developing a disease, pre-disease states, or early-stage disease, depends on what is known about how a particular disease progresses and whether an appropriate test is available.

Although screening is widespread, it provokes a number of debates. How should screening be offered? Should it be tightly controlled or should people be free to choose which screening tests they have? How can people be encouraged to have screening and how do motivational efforts square with the move towards greater informed choice? What are the psychological and behavioural consequences of screening and how can these be minimized?

Offering screening

There is little doubt that screening can help to prevent or cure a number of diseases, but it does not always lead to an improvement in health outcomes. Detecting a disease at an earlier stage may fail to improve a person's prognosis, it may only increase the length of time that they are aware they have the disease. For example, there is no evidence at the moment that screening for cancers of the prostate and lung increases survival, although research into the efficacy of screening for these types of cancer is continuing (Prorok *et al.*, 2000). In addition, screening tests, and the treatment of any screen-detected abnormalities, may have adverse consequences that offset any health gains. So how do people decide which types of screening should be encouraged and which should not?

The guidelines issued by the World Health Organization specify that screening should only be offered if the disease is common; has high levels of associated morbidity or mortality; effective treatment is available that can reduce morbidity and mortality; and screening and treatment for the disease are acceptable, safe and relatively inexpensive (Wilson, 1968). In short, screening should do more good than harm at reasonable cost.

The benefits, harms and costs of screening can all be established through Health Technology Assessment (HTA). Randomized controlled trials can demonstrate whether screening is effective in reducing disease morbidity/mortality and what the harmful effects of screening might be. However, although such studies may show how effective screening is in theory, in practice things may turn out rather differently. High levels of population coverage, good quality screening and the effective follow-up and treatment of any screen-detected abnormalities are all needed if screening is to be effective in reducing disease incidence/mortality. Simply offering screening is not enough. In Mexico, cervical screening has been available since 1974, but mortality rates have failed to decline, because of low uptake rates and poor quality screening (Lazcano-Ponce *et al.*, 1999).

Screening is more likely to be effective in reducing disease morbidity and mortality if it is offered as part of an organized programme. This is because targets for screening uptake, quality and follow-up, are set and monitored within organized settings as part of a coordinated system of care; and if standards are not met, coordinated efforts are made to attain them. In contrast, where screening is 'opportunistic' there are fewer opportunities for recording screening uptake and monitoring the effectiveness of treatment and follow-up (Lurie & Welch, 1999) and hence failings in the screening service may remain undetected.

The greater potential for organized programmes to reduce disease related morbidity/mortality is reflected in the WHO guidelines, which state that screening should be offered as part of an organized system. Despite this recommendation, countries differ in their screening provision. Such inter-country differences are determined partly by financial resources. Certain types of screening can be expensive to set up and co-ordinate, for example mammography screening for breast cancer, and they may be too costly for poorer countries to provide. In countries with similar wealth status, the price of introducing organized screening will depend on how much of the necessary infrastructure is already in place. In countries where opportunistic screening is already widespread, many of the required services, e.g. trained staff and equipment, will already exist, making the introduction of an organized programme less expensive. But the way screening is offered is also determined by the political values which underlie healthcare provision. Countries that value equality of access are likely to offer centralized, publicly-funded

healthcare where screening is offered as part of an organized programme. In contrast, those countries that value individual choice will promote the use of private healthcare services, and screening will tend to be more opportunistic, with individuals deciding when to be screened and what to be screened for.

Decisions about how to offer screening have important consequences for the individual. Organized programmes focus on benefits, harms and costs at a population level. As a result, the individual may not be offered maximum protection from a particular disease: rare disorders may not be screened for, screening may be less frequent than optimal, and those most at risk of getting the disease may not be screened due to insufficient gain in terms of life-years saved. Whilst screening done in less regulated settings may afford greater protection to the individual, people are less likely to be protected from the harms of screening: they are more likely to be over-screened, have poor quality screening and have access to screening of unproven benefit.

Because screening in opportunistic settings is not as tightly regulated, there is less attention to Health Technology Assessment (HTA). This can result in screening activity which conflicts with the available evidence. For example, in the United States, prostate screening is more common than colorectal cancer screening, despite the fact that the efficacy data for the latter is much stronger (Sirovich *et al.*, 2003). However, a plus-side to this more flexible attitude towards HTA is that new screening technologies will be available to the general population more quickly and, if beneficial, may mean much earlier adoption of a successful screening test. This can be seen in colorectal cancer screening which has been offered in the USA for the last 10 years, but is only now becoming available in the UK through the introduction of a nationwide screening programme (see Miles *et al.* (2004) for a more detailed comparison of organized and opportunistic screening).

Adherence to screening

Screening uptake

In order to reduce disease prevalence or mortality, a high proportion of the population needs to be screened so that enough cases can be detected and treated for prevalence/mortality rates to drop. Achieving high population coverage is therefore an essential part of delivering an effective screening service.

The particular strategies used by healthcare providers depend to some extent on how screening is offered. In places where invitations are issued to all those within the target population, methods to increase uptake may focus on the content and source of invitation letters, and the number of reminders that are sent. For example, research has shown that adherence is increased if the invitation letter comes from a primary care provider (King *et al.*, 1992) and a timed, dated appointment is offered rather than an open invitation (Stead *et al.*, 1998). Where there is no call–recall service, healthcare providers may themselves need reminders to ensure that they offer screening tests to those eligible (Zapka & Lemon, 2004).

Despite the success of such approaches, a substantial proportion of the population still under-use screening services. In particular, there is evidence across countries and screening modalities that socioeconomically deprived and ethnic minority groups are less likely to receive screening than more affluent groups and members of the ethnic majority (Streetly *et al.*, 1994; Kim *et al.*, 2004). This is the case even in countries where screening is heavily reimbursed or offered for free, and so cannot be attributed simply to lack of access to screening.

A number of theories have been forwarded to understand why people use screening services and hence how they might be persuaded to adhere. One of the most widely used is the Health Belief Model (HBM). This model was initially developed to understand why people took up the offer of X-ray screening for tuberculosis. It proposes that six factors determine whether someone will accept an offer of screening. Two relate to 'threat perception': (i) the likelihood of experiencing the health problem, and (ii) the perceived severity of the health problem were it to develop; and another two relate to 'behavioural evaluation': (iii) the benefits of doing something to prevent the health problem from occurring, and (iv) the costs (or barriers) to taking preventive action. A fifth factor, 'cues to action' (e.g. noticing a symptom or seeing a health education campaign), promotes health behaviour if the appropriate positive beliefs about the particular behaviour are held. A further factor, added to the model at a later date, is 'health motivation' or 'readiness to be concerned' about a particular health issue (see 'Health belief model').

Consistent with this model, threat evaluation and behavioural evaluation variables have been found to significantly predict adherence to screening. Believing oneself to be at risk from the disease has been associated with higher participation at screening (Vernon, 1999) and a variety of barriers to screening have predicted lower screening adherence, including concerns about the procedure, such as anticipated embarrassment or discomfort, refusal to believe the test can help decrease cancer morbidity or mortality, and fear of a cancer diagnosis (Wender, 2002; UK CRC Screening Pilot Evaluation Team, 2003). Conversely, screening rates are consistently higher among those who have a preventive orientation and participate in other preventive activities (Sutton *et al.*, 1994). Cues to action, such as the presence of symptoms, have also been associated with screening, but the role of health motivation has rarely been examined.

Other theories of behaviour have also been used to predict participation in screening, such as the Theory of Planned Behaviour (TPB) and Protection Motivation Theory (PMT). Like the Health Belief Model, PMT proposes that perceived susceptibility and disease severity will predict adherence to screening. Where it differs from the HBM is in its claim that efficacy beliefs also play a role. According to PMT, beliefs that one can perform the recommended behaviour (self-efficacy) and beliefs in the effectiveness of the recommended behaviour in reducing the health threat (response-efficacy) are considered important. Perceived control is also identified as a predictor of behaviour by the TPB, along with perceived social norms, attitudes and behavioural intentions, and there is evidence of the predictive value of both PMT and TPB in understanding screening uptake (see Connor & Norman, (1995) for an overview of these theories and Weinstein, (1993) for a discussion of the conceptual overlap between them) (see also 'Theory of planned behaviour').

Strategies to target people's beliefs and thereby enhance adherence to screening have included sending leaflets aimed at reducing perceived barriers to screening, informing people of the benefits, modifying threat and efficacy beliefs and enhancing perceived social norms. However, some of the erroneous and negative beliefs about screening appear to be attributable to low levels of 'health literacy', either due to illiteracy or a failure to understand commonly used medical terms (Lindau *et al.*, 2002). Hence, non-written methods of persuasion may be required to reach this group (see Meissner *et al.* (2004) for a review of methods to promote adherence).

In addition to ensuring adherence to screening, people also need to be persuaded to attend for any treatment or make any lifestyle changes recommended as a result of their screening test. For example, individuals identified as susceptible to future disease may need to adopt one of a number of different primary prevention strategies to prevent pathological changes from developing. These strategies may involve the use of drugs or dietary change to reduce risk factors such as raised cholesterol levels, or more invasive methods, such as the removal of tissue that may develop cancer in the future (e.g. prophylactic surgery to remove ovaries/breasts following the detection of genes such as BrCa1 and BrCa2). If such interventions are not adhered to, then screening will fail to reduce incidence/mortality rates.

Informed consent, and informed and shared decision making

Previously, where screening was endorsed by the government/healthcare provider, the main aim was to achieve high population coverage. As a result, people were encouraged to go for screening, and were often poorly informed of its limitations and potential to cause harm. However this is no longer the case. Now, the main goal is to ensure that individuals are fully informed of the benefits and harms of screening, and people are encouraged to make a decision about whether or not to be screened based on their own values.

This move towards informed consent, and informed and shared decision-making, has been attributed to concerns among healthcare bodies about litigation; pressure from patient advocacy organizations; and the increased availability of health information, notably via the World Wide Web (Wilson, 2000; Rimer *et al.*, 2004). Litigation is particularly likely following false negative results whereby a screening test fails to detect a disease, leading to delay in diagnosis and treatment (Brenner, 2004). Unfortunately, such outcomes are an inevitable part of screening, because many screening tests are not 100% sensitive (Wilson, 2000). The hope is that, by raising awareness of the inherent limitations of screening, litigation surrounding missed disease might reduce.

Whilst the move towards informed consent is to be welcomed, it has its disadvantages. The additional burden it places on staff time is one (Laing & McIntosh, 2004). Informed consent may also raise anxiety by drawing attention to the limitations of screening, for example, that it offers no guarantee of prevention or cure, although relatively little work has examined this possibility (see Goldberger *et al.*, 1997). A further problem is the impact that informed consent might have on the perceived benefits of screening. Fully informing people of the benefits and harms of screening has the potential to put people off. At the very least, it conflicts with strategies that have been successful in promoting uptake, such as payment incentives to primary care providers. At present, though, little research has examined the impact of informed consent and decision-aids on screening uptake. The limited research done in the area of cancer screening has shown informed decision-making leads to small changes in uptake with decreases in prostate screening and increases in breast and cervical screening. Hence the observed shifts have been in line with screening recommendations, where there is stronger evidence to support the efficacy of breast and cervical screening than prostate (see Rimer *et al.* (2004) for a review).

It has been suggested that, where the evidence clearly points to the benefits of screening, efforts should be made to fully inform people of associated harms, but minimal physician time should be expended on discussing the pros and cons. Rather, an explicit recommendation to be screened should be issued (Rimer *et al.*, 2004). This view is in agreement with the general proposal that informed consent should be used where there is only one sensible course of action, whilst shared decision-making (where the patient is involved in the decision process) should be reserved for situations that involve at least two sensible alternative routes to medical care which the patient must decide between (Whitney *et al.*, 2004). However, this approach conflicts with the idea that the patient's values, rather than scientific evidence, should guide screening decisions.

Advocates of informed consent often propose that individual-level benefits should be made explicit (Marshall & Adab, 2003) and that this should be done using absolute risk information rather than relative risk information because the former is easier to understand (Gigerenzer & Edwards, 2003). However, people may attend screening out of a sense of social obligation, that is, people may value actions that benefit society. This suggests that people should be informed about both the population-level and individual-level benefits that screening confers (see also 'Communicating risk', 'Informed consent' and 'Risk perception').

Psychological and behavioural consequences of screening

Screening involves testing asymptomatic 'healthy' people for a disease they are unlikely to have. There is therefore understandable concern that any adverse effects are kept to a minimum. One of four outcomes can arise as a result of screening: true positives, where disease is correctly identified; false positives, where people have a suspicious result which, on further investigation, turns out to be normal; true negatives, where disease is correctly judged to be absent; and false negative, where disease is missed. All have the potential to cause adverse effects.

Very little research has examined the impact of false negative results, and the work that has been done is almost exclusively in the realm of antenatal screening (Petticrew *et al.*, 2000). This is because it is easier to identify false negatives in tests for antenatal disorders, as they often become apparent with the birth of the baby. In adult diseases, however, false negative results are harder to establish. They may only become evident if there is further screening (which correctly identifies the disease) or the disease becomes symptomatic. However, it is hard to determine whether the disease was missed by the previous screening or developed subsequently. Some diseases may remain asymptomatic and never be diagnosed.

Based on the limited evidence available it appears that, in the field of antenatal screening, a false negative result may lead to poorer acceptance of a child with chromosomal abnormalities (Down's Syndrome) than if no screening had taken place (Hall *et al.*, 2000). And one of few studies on the impact of false negatives in cancer screening showed that such error led to reduced confidence in the screening programme, but did not alter people's intention to be screened in the future (Houston *et al.*, 2001).

Research into the psychological impact of false positive results is more extensive. False positives usually involve further medical investigations and a period of waiting before a 'normal' result is verified. In breast cancer screening there is strong evidence that the psychological distress arising from false positives is relatively short-lived (Rimer & Bluman, 1997). Although anxiety is raised when people are recalled for further investigation of suspicious findings, this returns to baseline levels once people have been informed their result is normal (Lampic *et al.*, 2001). However a number of studies have shown that cancer-specific worries may persist for months and even years after screening, e.g. Aro *et al.* (2000).

True positive results may also lead to further investigations or treatment, for example cervical screening can detect pre-cancerous cells which may require minor surgery to be removed. As with false positives, there is anxiety related to the duration of medical surveillance and treatment, and evidence that cancer-specific worry, though not anxiety, may persist for months afterwards (Wardle *et al.*, 1995). Evidence for the adverse effects of 'susceptibility' testing, though is mixed. Some research into the impact of familial hypercholesterolaemia in children has shown little effect on anxiety and quality of life but heightened disease-specific concerns (de Jongh *et al.*, 2003). Behavioural problems in children identified as at high risk for hyperlipidemia in routine screening have also been observed (Rosenberg *et al.*, 1997), but other studies, albeit on adults, have shown no such effects. For example, no indication of adverse effects on psychological wellbeing and absenteeism from work has been observed among a community sample of people attending blood cholesterol screening (Havas *et al.*, 1991). However, the way in which information about enhanced susceptibility is communicated is a key factor in determining its impact. For example, men identified as being at increased risk of cardiovascular disease were less likely to view this information as threatening if they were provided with individually-tailored and supportive information about risk factors for cardiovascular disease (Troein *et al.*, 2002).

Although true positive results are the main aim of screening, screening can detect disease states or abnormalities that the individual may never have become aware of. The increased detection of so-called 'pseudo-disease' is a problem for many types of screening, but relatively little research has been conducted into the psychological consequences of over-diagnosis. This is mainly because it is currently impossible to identify those individuals who have pseudo- rather than true disease.

The majority of people screened will receive a clear (or true negative) screening result. Whilst this might be seen as the best outcome of screening, concerns have been raised that clear results may promote complacency about health. People may believe that any poor health habits to date, such as smoking, have had no ill effects and may be continued (Hoff *et al.*, 2001). Equally, a clear result may lead people to conclude that they do not need to look out for symptoms or attend for screening in the future, a phenomenon known as 'false reassurance'. Relatively little research has been done in this area although some work has shown that screening results may stimulate positive changes in health behaviours (Bankhead *et al.*, 2003).

A number of strategies may reduce the impact of screening. Anxiety tends to be raised until testing and investigations are complete, and waiting is often seen as an unpleasant aspect of screening. Speeding up the investigation of screen-detected abnormalities will therefore help to reduce any unnecessary anxiety. Further issues, such as false reassurance, complacency about health and the adverse effects of false positives can potentially be attenuated through careful provision of information. For example, informing women undergoing breast cancer screening of the possibility of further investigations, and the fact that such investigations rarely lead to a diagnosis of cancer, has successfully reduced anxiety associated with recall for the follow-up of suspicious findings (Austoker & Ong, 1994).

Conclusion

Screening technologies are proliferating. Efficacy trials for prostate, ovarian and lung cancer screening are taking place; the search for genes that place people at above average risk of developing diseases, such as coronary heart disease and cancer, is continuing; and a variety of tests for antenatal, neonatal and adult testing are currently being considered for introduction into routine care. All these factors mean an increasing proportion of the population will find themselves eligible for one form of screening or another. The ethical, social and psychological implications of this increase in health surveillance need to be carefully monitored. It is important to ensure, for example, that such information is not used to discriminate unfairly against people.

These concerns notwithstanding, more specific issues surrounding screening will require attention. The emphasis on screening methods which aim to prevent disease is likely to increase. As a result, the use of tests that label people as 'at risk' of developing future disease will rise. Consequently, a key challenge concerns how to convey complex and probabilistic information to achieve the desired level of informed consent.

In addition, this increased focus on prevention means new sectors of the population will find themselves eligible for screening. Adolescents and young adults are likely to be at the forefront of efforts to prevent chronic disease, because the earlier the intervention the greater the potential benefits. This will set new challenges for health professionals because a new group will need to be persuaded of the benefits of prevention and early detection at an age when the long-term consequences of behaviours are unlikely to be salient.

Finally, and perhaps of prime importance, is the impact screening may have on socioeconomic gradients in health. There is strong evidence that deprived groups are 'late adopters' of primary prevention advice and screening. For example, acceptance of a new screening test of prevent the development of colorectal showed a strong socioeconomic status (SES) gradient, with lower update among more deprived member of the community (MacCaffery *et al*). The introduction of new types of screening is therefore likely to benefit higher socioeconomic groups the most, and the pre-existing difference in premature mortality rates between low and high SES will therefore become more pronounced if lower SES group consistently fail to engage in efforts to prevent and treat chronic disease. Ethnic differences in uptake of screening have also been observed. Efforts are therefore urgently needed to engage more deprived and ethnic minority groups in the screening effort so that all sectors of the community can benefit from the health gains that screening can offer.

REFERENCES

Aro, A. R., Pilvikki Absetz, S., van Elderen, T. M. *et al.* (2000). False-positive findings in mammography screening induces short-term distress – breast cancer-specific concern prevails longer. *European Journal of Cancer*, **36**, 1089–97.

Austoker, J. & Ong, G. (1994). Written information needs of women who are recalled for further investigation of breast screening: results of a multicentre study. *Journal of Medical Screening*, **1**, 238–44.

Bankhead, C. R., Brett, J., Bukach, C. *et al.* (2003). The impact of screening on future health-promoting behaviours and health beliefs: a systematic review. *Health Technology Assessment*, **7**, 1–92.

Brenner, R. J. (2004). Breast cancer evaluation: medical legal issues. *The Breast Journal*, **10**, 6–9.

Connor, M. & Norman, P. (Eds.). (1995). *Predicting health behaviour*. Buckingham, UK: Open University Press.

de Jongh, S., Kerckhoffs, M. C., Grootenhuis, M. A. *et al.* (2003). Quality of life, anxiety and concerns among statin-treated children with familial hypercholesterolaemia and their parents. *Acta Paediatrica*, **92**, 1096–101.

Gigerenzer, G. & Edwards, A. (2003). Simple tools for understanding risks: from innumeracy to insight. *British Medical Journal*, **327**, 741–4.

Goldberger, J. J., Kruse, J., Parker, M. A. & Kadish, A. H. (1997). Effect of informed consent on anxiety in patients undergoing diagnostic electrophysiology studies. *American Heart Journal*, **134**, 119–26.

Green, J. M., Hewison, J., Bekker, H. L., Bryant, L. D. & Cuckle, H. S. (2004). Psychosocial aspects of genetic screening of pregnant women and newborns: a systematic review. *Health Technology Assessment*, **8**, 1–109.

Hall, S., Bobrow, M. & Marteau, T. M. (2000). Psychological consequences for parents of false negative results on prenatal screening for Down's syndrome: retrospective interview study. *British Medical Journal*, **320**, 407–12.

Havas, S., Reisman, J., Hsu, L. & Koumjian, L. (1991). Does cholesterol screening result in negative labeling effects? Results of the Massachusetts model systems for blood cholesterol screening project. *Archives of Internal Medicine*, **151**, 113–19.

Hoff, G., Thiis-Evensen, E., Grotmol, T. *et al.* (2001). Do undesirable effects of screening affect all-cause mortality in flexible sigmoidoscopy programmes? Experience from the Telemark polyp study 1983–1996. *European Journal of Cancer Prevention*, **10**, 131–7.

Houston, D. M., Lloyd, K., Drysdale, S. & Farmer, M. (2001). The benefits of uncertainty: changes in women's perceptions of the cervical screening programme as a consequence of screening errors by Kent and Canterbury NHS Trust. *Psychology, Health and Medicine*, **6**, 107–13.

Kim, L. G., Thompson, S. G., Marteau, T. M. & Scott, R. A. (2004). Screening for abdominal aortic aneurysms: the effects of age and social deprivation on screening uptake, prevalence and attendance at follow-up in the MASS trial. *Journal of Medical Screening*, **11**, 50–3.

King, J., Fairbrother, G., Thompson, C. & Morris, D. L. (1992) Colorectal cancer screening: optimal compliance with postal faecal occult blood test. *Australian and New Zealand Journal of Surgery*, **62**, 714–19.

Laing, I. A. & McIntosh, N. (2004). Practicalities of consent. *Lancet*, **364**, 659.

Lampic, C., Thurfjell, E., Bergh, J. & Sjoden, P. O. (2001). Short- and long-term anxiety and depression in women recalled after breast cancer screening. *European Journal of Cancer*, **37**, 463–9.

Lazcano-Ponce, E. C., Moss, S., Alonso, D. R., Salmeron, C. J. & Hernandez, A. M. (1999). Cervical cancer screening in developing countries: why is it ineffective? The case of Mexico. *Archives of Medical Research*, **30**, 240–50.

Lindau, S. T., Tomori, C., Lyons, T. et al. (2002). The association of health literacy with cervical cancer prevention knowledge and health behaviors in a multiethnic cohort of women. *American Journal of Obstetrics and Gynecology*, **186**, 938–43.

Lurie, J. & Welch, H. (1999). Diagnostic testing following fecal occult blood screening in the elderly. *Journal of the National Cancer Institute*, **91**, 1616.

Marshall, T. & Adab, P. (2003). Informed consent for breast screening: what should we tell women? *Journal of Medical Screening*, **10**, 22–6.

McCaffery, K., Wardle, J., Nadel, M. & Atkin, W. (2002). Socioeconomic variation in participation in colorectal cancer screening. *Journal of Medical Screening*, **9**, 104–8.

Meissner, H. I., Smith, R. A., Rimer, B. K. et al. (2004). Promoting cancer screening: learning from experience. *Cancer*, **101**, 1107–17.

Miles, A., Cockburn, J., Smith, R. A. & Wardle, J. (2004). A perspective from countries using organized screening programs. *Cancer*, **101**, 1201–13.

Petticrew, M. P., Sowden, A. J., Lister-Sharp, D. & Wright, K. (2000).

False-negative results in screening programmes: systematic review of impact and implications. *Health Technology Assessment*, **4**, 1–120.

Prorok, P. C., Andriole, G. L., Bresalier, R. S. et al. (2000). Design of the Prostate, Lung, Colorectal and Ovarian (PLCO) Cancer Screening Trial. *Controlled Clinical Trials*, **21**, 273S–309S.

Rimer, B. K. & Bluman, L. G. (1997). The psychosocial consequences of mammography. *Journal of the National Cancer Institute Monographs*, 131–8.

Rimer, B. K., Briss, P. A., Zeller, P. K., Chan, E. C. & Woolf, S. H. (2004). Informed decision making: what is its role in cancer screening? *Cancer*, **101**, 1214–28.

Rosenberg, E., Lamping, D. L., Joseph, L., Pless, I. B. & Franco, E. D. (1997). Cholesterol screening of children at high risk: behavioural and psychological effects. *Canadian Medical Association Journal*, **156**, 489–96.

Sirovich, B. E., Schwartz, L. M. & Woloshin, S. (2003). Screening men for prostate and colorectal cancer in the United States: does practice reflect the evidence? *Journal of the American Medical Association*, **289**, 1414–20.

Stead, M. J., Wallis, M. G. & Wheaton, M. E. (1998). Improving uptake in non-attenders of breast screening: selective use of second appointment. *Journal of Medical Screening*, **5**, 69–72.

Streetly, A., Grant, C., Bickler, G. et al. (1994). Variation in coverage by ethnic group of neonatal (Guthrie) screening programme in south London. *British Medical Journal*, **309**, 372–4.

Sutton, S., Bickler, G., Sancho-Aldridge, J. & Saidi, G. (1994). Prospective study of predictors of attendance for breast screening in inner London. *Journal of Epidemiology and Community Health*, **48**, 65–73.

Troein, M., Rastam, L. & Selander, S. (2002). Changes in health beliefs after labelling with hypercholesterolaemia. *Scandinavian Journal of Public Health*, **30**, 76–9.

UK CRC Screening Pilot Evaluation Team. (2003). Evaluation of the UK Colorectal Cancer Screening Pilot. Available from URL: http://www.cancerscreening.nhs.uk/colorectal/finalreport.pdf.

Vernon, S. W. (1999). Risk perception and risk communication for cancer screening behaviours: a review. *Journal of the National Cancer Institute Monographs*, **25**, 101–19.

Wardle, J., Pernet, A. & Stephens, D. (1995). Psychological consequences of positive results in cervical cancer screening. *Psychology and Health*, **10**, 185–94.

Weinstein, N. D. (1993). Testing four competing theories of health-protective behavior. *Health Psychology*, **12**, 324–33.

Wender, R. C. (2002). Barriers to screening for colorectal cancer. *Gastrointestinal Endoscopy Clinics of North America*, **12**, 145–70.

Whitney, S. N., McGuire, A. L. & McCullough, L. B. (2004). A typology of shared decision making, informed consent, and simple consent. *Annals of Internal Medicine*, **140**, 54–9.

Wilson, J. M. (1968). *Principles and Practice of Screening for Diseases.* Geneva, World Health Organization.

Wilson, R. M. (2000). Screening for breast and cervical cancer as a common cause for litigation. A false negative result may be one of an irreducible minimum of errors. *British Medical Journal*, **320**, 1352–3.

Zapka, J. G. & Lemon, S. C. (2004). Interventions for patients, providers, and health care organizations. *Cancer*, **101**, 1165–87.

Shiftwork and health

Katharine R. Parkes

University of Oxford

Current trends in shiftwork

Industrial and commercial activities that operate outside normal work hours have become widespread in recent years; services such as banking, communications, transport, catering and retailing are routinely available during evening hours, and often round-the-clock. Consequently, the work patterns of a substantial proportion of the population now extend beyond regular daytime working hours; variable schedules (often including evening or night work) and rotating shifts are both widespread. In a recent European survey, 28% of the workforce had variable work patterns, 10% had evening or night schedules, while 17% worked two-shift or three-shift rotating schedules (Boisard et al., 2003). Further analyses showed that the proportion of shift workers remained relatively constant up to age 45 years, but fell sharply at higher ages, particularly over 55 years (European Foundation for the Improvement of Living and Working Conditions, 2003), reflecting older workers' difficulties in adjusting to shiftwork.

Similarly, analyses of US survey data showed that, in 1997, 27.6% of the workforce had flexible work schedules, while 16.8% of full-time employees had 'alternative' schedules involving work outside normal daytime hours (06.00–18.00 hrs), 6.4% of whom worked night or rotating shifts (Beers, 2000). These proportions varied by occupation; rotating shifts were particularly common in security services (16.3%), mining (12.5%) and catering (8.7%), but infrequent among professionals and managers (1.7%). Night work was prevalent in healthcare, manufacturing and manual occupations. Global trends towards a '24-hour society' suggest that these proportions are likely to rise; thus, the implications of shiftwork for physical and mental health are not only a matter of current concern but are also likely to become increasingly important in the future (Costa, 2001; Rajaratnam & Arendt, 2001).

Mechanisms underlying the health effects of shiftwork

Shiftwork has been empirically linked to a variety of diseases although evidence does not suggest an effect on all-cause mortality (Knutsson, 2003). Three pathways have been implicated in associations between shiftwork and disease (Boggild & Knutsson, 1999; Knutsson, 1989; Knutsson & Boggild, 2000): disruption of circadian rhythms (leading to sleep/wake disturbances, desynchronisation of internal processes, and increased susceptibility to disease); disturbed socio-temporal patterns (resulting from atypical work hours leading to family problems, reduced social support and stress); and unfavourable changes in health behaviours (increased smoking, poor diet and irregular meals). Moreover, there is evidence that biomarkers, such as cholesterol and other lipids, plasminogen, blood pressure and cardiac activity show changes related to shiftwork, and may act as mediators of disease processes (Boggild & Knutsson, 1999).

The general pattern of findings is that shift workers, as compared with day workers, exhibit less favourable profiles of lifestyle, behavioural and biological risk factors (e.g. Lac & Chamoux, 2004; Morikawa et al., 1999; Parkes, 2002). Psychosocial factors are also relevant; for instance, Smith et al. (1999) found that chronic fatigue and ineffective coping behaviour acted to mediate the process by which sleep loss and social disruption led to disease endpoints. Shiftwork may also interact with individual and environmental factors (e.g. age, personality, poor physical work conditions) to increase the risk of health problems (Smith et al., 2003).

Shiftwork in relation to particular health outcomes

Findings relating shiftwork to particular health problems and diseases are summarized in the sections below. In interpreting the findings reviewed, several methodological problems of shiftwork research should be noted. Specifically, shiftworkers tend to differ from day workers in factors such as age, socioeconomic status, job demands and physical/psychosocial work environment characteristics, all of which may contribute to disease outcomes. Moreover, those who are selected (either by self or employer) into, and survive in, shiftwork may differ from day workers in age, personality and initial health status. Comparisons of shiftworkers and day workers may therefore be confounded by pre-existing differences between the groups and by environmental factors. Whilst statistical methods potentially allow control of these effects, stronger evidence of the causal role of shiftwork in relation to disease risk can be derived from prospective studies which assess baseline data prior to exposure (e.g. van Amelsvoort et al., 2004).

Sleep, fatigue and mental health

Disturbed sleep is an almost inevitable outcome of the disruption to normal circadian rhythms associated with shiftwork, particularly night work. The fundamental problem is the mismatch between the need for wakefulness and work activity during night hours when circadian rhythms are conducive to sleep, and for sleep during daylight hours, normally the time of wakefulness and activity (Akerstedt, 1998; 2003; Smith et al., 1999). This reversal of the usual diurnal pattern underlies many of the sleep problems experienced by shiftworkers; environmental conditions (e.g. domestic and traffic noise, presence of children and normal social activities) may also disturb shiftworkers' daytime sleep.

Consistent with the empirical evidence (e.g. Harma *et al.*, 2002; Ohayon *et al.*, 2002), delayed onset of sleep, reduced sleep duration and sleepiness and fatigue during working hours are seen as characteristic sleep disturbances among night shiftworkers (Akerstedt, 1990). Adaptation to a new sleep/wake pattern occurs at a rate of ~1 hr per day (Akerstedt, 2003). Thus, for rotating schedules, adaptation to one shift may not be complete before a further shift change occurs; sleep disturbances and fatigue may also continue into rest days. The nature and magnitude of shiftwork effects depend on the type of schedule, particularly the direction and speed of rotation (Akerstedt, 2003). These factors combine to influence sleep, fatigue and performance differently during morning, afternoon and night shifts, but productivity tends to be most adversely affected during night work (Folkard & Tucker, 2003) (see 'Sleep and health')

The combination of chronic fatigue resulting from sleep disturbances and the disruption of family life and leisure activities associated with shiftwork, may give rise to social stress and work–family conflict, and to psychological distress, particularly anxiety and depression (e.g. Gordon *et al.*, 1986; Jamal, 2004; Jansen *et al.*, 2004; Parkes, 1999; Pisarski *et al.*, 2002). Impairment of psychological health often leads shift workers to change to day-work jobs; Costa (1996) estimates that 20% of workers leave shiftwork after a relatively short time because of its adverse effects, that only 10% do not complain about shiftwork, and that the remaining 70% withstand shiftwork with varying degrees of tolerance.

Gastrointestinal disorders

Gastrointestinal complaints are among the most frequently reported health problems of shift workers; these problems are estimated to be two to five times more common among night-shift workers as compared with those not working nights (Costa, 1996). Circadian disturbance affecting the intake, digestion and absorption of food are thought to play a major aetiological role, but sleep loss, fatigue and the social stress of shiftwork may also be implicated. Typically, shiftworkers have higher levels of gastric symptoms (e.g. indigestion, heartburn, constipation, loss of appetite and nausea) than dayworkers, even with control for demographic, job and lifestyle variables (e.g. Caruso *et al.*, 2004; Costa *et al.*, 2001; Parkes, 1999). Evidence also links shiftwork to peptic ulcers (Knutsson, 2003). In particular, in a study based on endoscopic examination of suspected cases, the prevalence of gastric ulcers among Japanese workers was 2.38% among current shiftworkers, 1.52% among past shiftworkers, and 1.03% in day-workers (Segawa *et al.*, 1987). Duodenal ulcers also showed higher prevalence among shiftworkers in this study.

Cardiovascular disease

Evidence accumulated over the past two decades suggests that shiftwork is a significant risk factor for cardiovascular disease. Thus, a recent review by Knutsson (2003) concluded 'there is rather strong evidence in favour of an association between shiftwork and coronary heart disease' (p. 105). Findings from a meta-analysis of 17 studies of cardiovascular disease in relation to shiftwork (Boggild & Knutsson, 1999) support this view. Overall, shift workers were found to have a 40% excess risk for cardiovascular disease relative to day-workers, although there was wide variation across studies.

Findings of two major studies included in this analysis are outlined below.

In a six-year prospective study of cardiovascular (CHD) risk, Tenkanen *et al.* (1997) followed up 1806 industrial workers, assessing lifestyle factors, blood pressure and serum lipid levels, and identifying CHD cases from official health records. Overall, the relative risk of CHD among shiftworkers as compared with day-workers was 1.5 (CI 1.1–2.1), decreasing to 1.4 (CI 1.0–1.9) with control for physiological and lifestyle variables. Among blue-collar employees, day-workers, 2-shift and 3-shift workers had relative risks of 1.3 (CI 0.8–2.0), 1.9 (CI 1.1–3.4) and 1.7 (CI 1.1–2.7) respectively. Shiftwork was also found to interact with smoking and obesity to increase CHD risk (Tenkanen *et al.*, 1998).

Kawachi *et al.* (1995) examined the incidence of CHD over a four-year period among 79 109 female nurses in relation to the total years of rotating night shiftwork. The age-adjusted relative risk was 1.38 (95% CI, 1.08–1.76) in women who reported ever doing shiftwork compared with those who had never done so. This excess risk remained significant after adjustment for cigarette smoking and other cardiovascular risk factors. The analyses also demonstrated a dose–response relationship between CHD risk and duration of shiftwork (greater risk being associated with longer durations), consistent with earlier findings (Knutsson *et al.*, 1986).

Cancer

Empirical studies demonstrate associations between night work and elevated risk of breast cancer (e.g. Hansen, 2001; Tynes *et al.*, 1996). In each of these studies, shiftwork was associated with an overall risk ratio for breast cancer of 1.5, but the risk increased with age and length of exposure to night work. Similarly, in a prospective study of nurses, positive associations were found between breast cancer and extended periods (>30 years) of intermittent night work (Schernhammer *et al.*, 2001); among postmenopausal women, the risk ratio also increased for 1–14 years and 15–29 years of rotating night work. One mechanism by which shiftwork may lead to breast cancer is that the normal production of melatonin during hours of darkness is disrupted by working at night; suppression of melatonin is thought to lead to an increase in reproductive hormones (particularly oestrogen), acting to increase hormone-sensitive cells in the breast (Schernhammer & Schulmeister, 2004). However, other pathways may also exist; for instance, Bovbjerg (2003) suggests that alterations in immune function associated with circadian disruption may be implicated.

Evidence linking night work and cancer is largely specific to breast cancer; little is known about other types of cancer in this context, or about the possible mechanisms involved. Although Taylor and Pocock (1972) reported an increased incidence of cancer among shiftworkers, Tynes *et al.* (1996) found that cancer incidence among female shiftworkers was not different from that of the general female population. However, increased risk of colorectal cancer among female nurses working rotating night shifts for >15 years has recently been reported (Schernhammer *et al.*, 2003).

Pregnancy and reproductive disorders

Two review articles (Costa, 1996; Scott, 2000) summarize evidence linking shiftwork to adverse pregnancy outcomes (e.g. premature births, miscarriages and low birth weight). For instance, a meta-analysis of 29 studies identified shiftwork as a significant risk factor (OR 1.24) for pre-term birth (Mozurkewich *et al.*, 2000). In the light of the evidence, Knutsson (2003) recommended that women should avoid shiftwork during pregnancy. Recent studies (using data from the Danish National Birth Cohort) also indicate that shiftwork, especially fixed night work, is associated with adverse pregnancy outcomes (e.g. Zhu *et al.*, 2004).

Other aspects of reproductive dysfunction (e.g. irregular menstruation) have also been linked to shiftwork (e.g. Hatch *et al.*, 1999; Labyak *et al.*, 2002). Disruption of circadian rhythms, and the resulting desyncronization of cyclic physiological functions (including hormonal activity), is thought to be the most likely cause of menstrual problems among shiftworkers (Costa, 1996; Smith *et al.*, 2003).

Accidents and injuries

Sleep loss and fatigue associated with circadian disruption impairs cognitive performance, particularly in tasks requiring vigilance, concentration and decision-making (e.g. Meijman *et al.*, 1993); this impairment potentially increases the risk of accident and injury incidents. However, in many work situations, the number of personnel exposed, the nature of the work done, the level of supervision and the likelihood of an accident being reported, differ across the 24-hour workday; thus, incident rates cannot be directly compared across shifts (Folkard & Tucker, 2003). Nonetheless, a few studies in which confounding factors are adequately controlled do allow such comparisons.

Thus, Smith *et al.* (1994) found that, relative to the morning shift, the overall risk of an injury incident during the night shift was 1.23 (CI 1.14–1.31), with a higher risk for self-paced work at night, 1.82 (CI 1.30–2.34). Folkard & Tucker (2003), combining five data sets, found that risk increased approximately linearly across the three shifts. Relative to the morning shift, the increase was 18.3% for afternoon shifts, and 30.4% for night shifts. More generally, Smith *et al.* (2003) note that the disasters of Three Mile Island, Chernobyl and the Challenger space shuttle all occurred during the night.

Use of statistical methods to estimate risk from large-scale exposure data provides an alternative (although less precise) method of studying accidents in relation to shift patterns. For instance, Williamson and Feyer (1995) analyzed a total of 1020 work-related fatalities occurring over a two-year period in Australia. To estimate exposure rates, they used national survey data to determine the proportion of the employed population engaged in night work as compared with day work. Taking into account the difference in exposure rates between night hours and day hours, the risk of fatality was found to be more than twice as high for night work (19.00–07.00 hours) as compared with day work (07.00–19.00 hours). However, Laundry and Lees (1991) found no evidence of elevated rates of minor accidents during night work, although they did find a circadian pattern of accident frequency with morning (0800–1000 hrs) and afternoon (1400–1600 hrs) peak periods. Using more complex statistical methods, Hanecke *et al.* (1998) found that, beyond the eighth or ninth hour of work, there was a marked increase in relative risk particularly for afternoon and night shifts.

Tolerance to shiftwork and intervention strategies

Shiftwork tolerance

Individual variation in the ability to adjust to shiftwork has been widely noted (e.g. Costa, 2003; Smith *et al.*, 2003). Age is a particularly important factor. Individuals older than 45 years experience increasing difficulty in adjusting to altered sleep–wake cycles; reduced fitness, decreased restorative powers of sleep and greater proneness to internal desynchronization of circadian rhythms, all contribute to decreased shiftwork tolerance. However, other individual factors, including circadian type ('morningness' versus 'eveningness'), and personality traits (e.g. extraversion) also affect shiftwork adaptation. These traits are related to circadian cycle characteristics that influence preferences for morning or evening activities (Tankova *et al.*, 1994); however, in the absence of validation data, Smith *et al.* (2003) caution against the use of such measures for selection purposes.

Interventions to facilitate shiftwork adaptation

Several types of interventions can be effective in facilitating shiftwork adaptation (for reviews, see Knauth & Hornberger, 2003; Smith *et al.*, 2003). At the organizational level, shift schedule design is particularly important; although there are no ideal shift patterns, factors such as shift duration, direction of rotation, changeover times and work/rest sequences all affect adaptation. Other recommended strategies include worker participation in the design and implementation of shift schedules and attention to work conditions (e.g. staffing levels, workload, rest breaks and the physical environment, especially lighting levels) that may accentuate or mitigate the effects of shiftwork.

At the individual level, recommendations for favourable adaptation include 'sleep hygiene' (e.g. regular sleep routine, quiet bedroom, curtains or blinds to eliminate sunlight during sleep hours, avoidance of caffeine or alcohol prior to sleep); healthy diet and fixed meal times; active coping; and ensuring a balance between sleep and family time (Knauth & Hornberger, 2003). Exposure to bright light during specific circadian phases has also been found to speed adaptation (e.g. Bjorvatn *et al.*, 1999), but use of melatonin as a sleep medication to aid adjustment to shift changes, whilst potentially effective, is subject to some safety concerns (Smith *et al.*, 2003).

Conclusions

The material reviewed in this chapter suggests that shiftwork significantly increases risks of cardiovascular disease, cancer and several other major illnesses: shiftwork is also implicated in psychosomatic problems, particularly sleep disturbance and fatigue, in psychological distress and in the occurrence of accidents. However, the mechanisms by which shiftwork impacts on physical and psychological health are still not fully understood. Whilst evidence suggests that each of the three pathways identified earlier in this chapter (circadian disruption, behavioural change and disturbed socio-temporal patterns) are involved, it is likely that their relative importance varies across different health outcomes, and in relation to individual and environmental characteristics, including the particular shift hours and rotation patterns worked. Nonetheless, the desynchronization of normal psychophysiological functions associated with circadian disruption (particularly during night work) is generally thought to play a key role (Costa, 2003; Knutsson & Boggild, 2000). It is therefore unlikely that the health impact of shiftwork can be entirely eliminated, although identifying individuals with greater tolerance to shift changes, and implementing organizational and individual strategies to facilitate adaptation, can help to alleviate some adverse outcomes.

REFERENCES

Akerstedt, T. (1990). Psychological and psychophysiological effects of shift work. *Scandinavian Journal of Work, Environment and Health,* **16**(Suppl. 1), 67–73.

Akerstedt, T. (1998). Shift work and disturbed sleep/wakefulness. *Sleep Medicine Reviews,* **2**, 117–28.

Akerstedt, T. (2003). Shift work and disturbed sleep/wakefulness. *Occupational Medicine,* **53**, 89–94.

Beers, T. M. (2000). Flexible schedules and shift work: replacing the '9–5' workday. *Monthly Labor Review,* June, 33–40.

Bjorvatn, B., Kecklund, G. & Akerstedt, T. (1999). Bright light treatment used for adaptation to night work and re-adaptation back to day life. A field study at an oil platform in the North Sea. *Journal of Sleep Research,* **8**, 105–12.

Boggild, H. & Knutsson, A. (1999). Shift work, risk factors and cardiovascular disease. *Scandinavian Journal of Work, Environment & Health,* **25**, 85–99.

Boisard, P., Cartron, D., Gollac, M. & Valeyre, A. (2003). *Time and work: duration of work.* Dublin, Ireland: European Foundation for the Improvement of Living and Working Conditions.

Bovbjerg, D. H. (2003). Circadian disruption and cancer: sleep and immune regulation. *Brain, Behavior, and Immunity,* **17**(Suppl. 1), S48–50.

Caruso, C. C., Lusk, S. L. & Gillespie, B. W. (2004). Relationship of work schedules to gastrointestinal diagnoses, symptoms, and medication use in auto factory workers. *American Journal of Industrial Medicine,* **46**, 586–98.

Costa, G. (1996). The impact of shift and night work on health. *Applied Ergonomics,* **27**, 9–16.

Costa, G. (2001). The 24-hour society: between myth and reality. *Journal of Human Ergology,* **30**, 15–20.

Costa, G. (2003). Shift work and occupational medicine: an overview. *Occupational Medicine,* **53**, 83–8.

Costa, G., Sartori, S., Facco, P. & Apostoli, P. (2001). Health conditions of bus drivers in a 6 year follow up study. *Journal of Human Ergology,* **30**, 405–10.

European Foundation for the Improvement of Living and Working Conditions (2003). *Age and working conditions in the European Union.* Dublin, Ireland: Author.

Folkard, S. & Tucker, P. (2003). Shift work, safety and productivity. *Occupational Medicine,* **53**, 95–101.

Gordon, N. P., Cleary, P. D., Parker, C. E. & Czeisler, C. A. (1986). The prevalence and health impact of shiftwork. *American Journal of Public Health,* **76**, 1225–8.

Hanecke, K., Tiedemann, S., Nachreiner, F. & Grzech-Sukalo, H. (1998). Accident risk as a function of hour at work and time of day as determined from accident data and exposure models for the German working population. *Scandinavian Journal of Work, Environment & Health,* **24**(Suppl. 3), 43–8.

Hansen, J. (2001). Increased breast cancer risk among women who work predominantly at night. *Epidemiology,* **12**, 74–7.

Harma, M., Sallinen, M., Ranta, R., Mutanen, P. & Muller, K. (2002). The effect of an irregular shift system on sleepiness at work in train drivers and railway traffic controllers. *Journal of Sleep Research,* **11**, 141–51.

Hatch, M. C., Figa Talamanca, I. & Salerno, S. (1999). Work stress and menstrual patterns among American and Italian nurses. *Scandinavian Journal of Work, Environment and Health,* **25**, 144–50.

Jamal, M. (2004). Burnout, stress and health of employees on non-standard work schedules: a study of Canadian workers. *Stress and Health,* **20**, 113–19.

Jansen, N. W., Kant, I., Nijhuis, F. J., Swaen, G. M. & Kristensen, T. S. (2004). Impact of worktime arrangements on work-home interference among Dutch employees. *Scandinavian Journal of Work, Environment and Health,* **30**, 139–48.

Kawachi, I., Colditz, G. A., Stampfer, M. J. et al. (1995). Prospective study of shift work and risk of coronary heart disease in women. *Circulation,* **92**, 3178–82.

Knauth, P. & Hornberger, S. (2003). Preventive and compensatory measures for shift workers. *Occupational Medicine,* **53**, 109–16.

Knutsson, A. (1989). Shift work and coronary heart disease. *Scandinavian Journal of Social Medicine. Supplementum,* **44**, 1–36.

Knutsson, A. (2003). Health disorders of shift workers. *Occupational Medicine,* **53**, 103–8.

Knutsson, A., Akerstedt, T., Jonsson, B. G. & Orth Gomer, K. (1986). Increased risk of ischaemic heart disease in shift workers. *Lancet,* **2**, 89–92.

Knutsson, A. & Boggild, H. (2000). Shiftwork and cardiovascular disease: review of disease mechanisms. *Reviews on Environmental Health,* **15**, 359–72.

Labyak, S., Lava, S., Turek, F. & Zee, P. (2002). Effects of shiftwork on sleep and menstrual function in nurses. *Health Care for Women International,* **23**, 703–14.

Lac, G. & Chamoux, A. (2004). Biological and psychological responses to two rapid shiftwork schedules. *Ergonomics,* **47**, 1339–49.

Laundry, B. R. & Lees, R. E. (1991). Industrial accident experience of one company on 8- and 12-hour shift systems. *Journal of Occupational Medicine,* **33**, 903–6.

Meijman, T., Van-Der-Meer, O. & Van-Dormolen, M. (1993). The after-effects of night work on short-term memory performance. *Ergonomics,* **36**, 37–42.

Morikawa, Y., Nakagawa, H., Miura, K. et al. (1999). Relationship between shift work and onset of hypertension in a cohort of manual workers. *Scandinavian Journal of Work, Environment & Health,* **25**, 100–4.

Mozurkewich, E. L., Luke, B., Avni, M. & Wolf, F. M. (2000). Working conditions and adverse pregnancy outcome: a meta-analysis. *Obstetrics and Gynecology,* **95**, 623–35.

Ohayon, M. M., Lemoine, P., Arnaud Briant, V. & Dreyfus, M. (2002). Prevalence and consequences of sleep disorders in a shift worker population. *Journal of Psychosomatic Research,* **53**, 577–83.

Parkes, K. R. (1999). Shiftwork, job type, and the work environment as joint predictors of health outcomes. *Journal of Occupational Health Psychology,* **4**, 256–68.

Parkes, K. R. (2002). Shift work and age as interactive predictors of body mass index among offshore workers. *Scandinavian Journal of Work, Environment & Health*, **28**, 64–71.

Pisarski, A., Bohle, P. & Callan, V. J. (2002). Extended shifts in ambulance work: influences on health. *Stress and Health*, **18**, 119–26.

Rajaratnam, S. M. & Arendt, J. (2001). Health in a 24-h society. *Lancet*, **358**, 999–1005.

Schernhammer, E. S., Laden, F., Speizer, F. E. *et al.* (2001). Rotating night shifts and risk of breast cancer in women participating in the nurses' health study. *Journal of the National Cancer Institute*, **93**, 1563–8.

Schernhammer, E. S., Laden, F., Speizer, F. E. *et al.* (2003). Night-shift work and risk of colorectal cancer in the nurses' health study. *Journal of the National Cancer Institute*, **95**, 825–8.

Schernhammer, E. S. & Schulmeister, K. (2004). Melatonin and cancer risk: does light at night compromise physiologic cancer protection by lowering serum melatonin levels? *British Journal of Cancer*, **90**, 941–3.

Scott, A. J. (2000). Shift work and health. *Primary Care*, **27**, 1057–70.

Segawa, K., Nakazawa, S., Tsukamoto, Y. *et al.* (1987). Peptic ulcer is prevalent among shift workers. *Digestive Diseases and Sciences*, **32**, 449–53.

Smith, C. S., Folkard, S. & Fuller, J. A. (2003). Shiftwork and working hours. In J. C. Quick (Ed.). *Handbook of occupational health psychology*. Washington, DC: American Psychological Association.

Smith, C. S., Robie, C., Folkard, S. *et al.* (1999). A process model of shiftwork and health. *Journal of Occupational Health Psychology*, **4**, 207–18.

Smith, L., Folkard, S. & Poole, C. J. (1994). Increased injuries on night shift. *Lancet*, **344**, 1137–9.

Tankova, I., Adan, A. & Buela-Casal, G. (1994). Circadian typology and individual differences: a review. *Personality and Individual Differences*, **16**, 671–84.

Taylor, P. J. & Pocock, S. J. (1972). Mortality of shift and day workers, 1956–68. *British Journal of Industrial Medicine*, **29**, 201–7.

Tenkanen, L., Sjoblom, T. & Harma, M. (1998). Joint effect of shift work and adverse life-style factors on the risk of coronary heart disease. *Scandinavian Journal of Work, Environment and Health*, **24**, 351–7.

Tenkanen, L., Sjoblom, T., Kalimo, R., Alikoski, T. & Harma, M. (1997). Shift work, occupation and coronary heart disease over 6 years of follow-up in the Helsinki Heart Study. *Scandinavian Journal of Work, Environment and Health*, **23**, 257–65.

Tynes, T., Hannevik, M., Andersen, A., Vistnes, A. I. & Haldorsen, T. (1996). Incidence of breast cancer in Norwegian female radio and telegraph operators. *Cancer Causes and Control*, **7**, 197–204.

Van Amelsvoort, L. G., Schouten, E. G. & Kok, F. J. (2004). Impact of one year of shift work on cardiovascular disease risk factors. *Journal of Occupational and Environmental Medicine*, **46**, 699–706.

Williamson, A. M. & Feyer, A.-M. (1995). Causes of accidents and time of day. *Work and Stress*, **9**, 158–64.

Zhu, J. L., Hjollund, N. H. & Olsen, J. (2004). Shift work, duration of pregnancy, and birth weight: the National Birth Cohort in Denmark. *American Journal of Obstetrics and Gynecology*, **191**, 285–91.

Stress in health professionals

Chris McManus

University College London

Stress and burnout are inevitable problems for the highly committed, highly involved individuals who work in healthcare services, as they deal with the physical and emotional problems of seriously ill and sometimes emotionally disturbed patients, while also having to cope with running effective teams, dealing with complex management structures and conflicting demands at all hours of the day and night. Anyone working in such conditions will inevitably become stressed if enough such pressures are placed upon them. Having said that, not everyone in practice does become stressed, and that raises a host of questions about who becomes stressed, why people become stressed, what are the precipitating and protective factors and what are the causal processes underlying the separate but related conditions of stress and burnout. A brief review such as this can inevitably only present a personal view of a large research area. Several recent edited volumes are recommended as good starting places for studying the field further (Dollard *et al.*, 2003; Cooper, 2005).

Defining and measuring stress and burnout

Stress

As p. 1 of Cox (1978) pointed out long ago, 'the concept of stress is elusive... It is a concept which familiar to both layman and professional alike; it is understood by all when used in a general context but by very few when a more precise account is required...'. Stress suffers from the conceptual confusion of both referring to the external event and to the internal response (just as in engineering, a stress is a force upon an object such as an aircraft wing, and the damage that results from that force, as in metal fatigue). It also suffers from the problems that beset technical terms within psychology which are also used in everyday language, so that hardly a person nowadays describes their work as anything other than 'stressful', or describes themselves as anything other than 'stressed out'. Amongst the various definitions of stress and stress responses, perhaps a common denominator is a failure of normal, effective functioning, which can manifest in disordered, ineffective behaviour, of which perhaps the symptoms of anxiety-related and depressive disorders are the first and commonest signs (see 'Stress and health').

For research purposes, many empirical studies have resorted to defining stress in terms of conventional measuring instruments, typically questionnaires, of which the General Health Questionnaire (GHQ) has become the most popular, not least because of its conceptual and research links to the diagnosis of anxiety and depressive disorder. The GHQ was originally introduced by Goldberg (1972), as an instrument to be used in general medical practice for detecting undiagnosed psychiatric disorders in general medical and surgical patients. The original 140-item scale was also presented as a more popular 60-item scale (GHQ-60) which had several sub-scales. Subsequently, shorter versions of the instrument have been used, including the 28-item scale (GHQ-28), and the very popular 12-item questionnaire (GHQ-12), which conventionally is regarded as having only a single scale, but probably assesses two correlated factors, i.e. anxiety/depression and social dysfunction (Kalliath *et al.*, 2004). An important feature of the original GHQ was that a scoring method was devised which was validated against independent, psychiatric assessments of the individuals using standardized clinical interviews. A score of four or more on the GHQ-12 has been shown, in its proper context, to have about an 80% sensitivity and 80% specificity for detecting psychiatric illness, with good comparability even when used cross-culturally in a range of countries, and after translation into ten different languages (Goldberg *et al.*, 1997), and a positive predictive value of about 65% (Schmitz *et al.*, 1999).

Because of its success as a screening instrument for detecting psychiatric illness ('caseness'), the GHQ began to be seen as a useful instrument for assessing psychiatric morbidity which could then be used as a proxy for stress and stress-related illnesses. There are many such studies in the literature, and a recent review summarized the result in these terms: "Although stress is common in most professions, the figures for doctors suggest that 28–30% of them suffer above the threshold level of stress as measured by the General Health Questionnaire" (Maxwell & Squire, 2000). Such studies typically do not include a population control, but where such data are available, as in the Health and Lifestyle Survey in the UK, the rate of caseness was about 14% (McManus *et al.*, 1999), seeming to support the idea that doctors and health professionals may indeed be particularly stressed.

An important problem in using the GHQ for assessing stress is that it is typically not used in the context for which it was originally devised. The rubric for the GHQ very carefully does not make any mention of stress (and indeed the term is not even found in the index to Goldberg's 1972 monograph). Instead it asks, 'how your health has been in general, over the past few weeks'. However many of the studies, which have used versions of the GHQ for estimating stress rates in health professionals, present the questionnaire in an explicit context of stress, often with a covering letter with a title such as, 'Stress in doctors'. Such phraseology potentially primes respondents to answer in particular ways if they feel that they are indeed 'stressed' in the everyday sense of the term, but the risk is that the validity of the instrument is threatened. Almost no studies using the GHQ to assess stress in health professionals have cross-validated GHQ-detected cases against formal psychiatric diagnosis; it is just assumed implicitly that the measure is as valid as in its original context. An important exception used the GHQ-12 to identify cases in a population of healthcare professionals and hospital staff in a hospital setting in the north of England. The proportion of cases was 27% (Weinberg & Creed, 1999). However formal psychiatric assessment found that only 52% met the criteria for a psychiatric diagnosis (Weinberg & Creed, 1999). It seems likely, therefore, that a proportion of GHQ-based studies of the absolute rate of stress in health professionals over-estimate rates of stress, a risk that will of course be exacerbated if there is response bias, with the most stressed seeing an opportunity to express their discontent. Great care should therefore be taken in interpreting such surveys, particularly when they form the basis for headlines used by medical politicians. A study in which GHQ-assessed stress rates in doctors could be assessed properly was a stratified, representatively sampled study of attitudes of 1013 UK doctors to the General Medical Council's Performance Procedures, in which we included the GHQ-12 amongst a range of questions unrelated to stress, and with its proper rubric which does not mention stress. The overall rate of caseness was 16.9%, which was similar to rates of 14.1% and 17.8% in large-scale population studies (McManus *et al.*, 1999). Interestingly there was evidence of a relationship of stress to age, doctors in mid-career showing the highest rates of stress.

In summary, the measurement of stress is not straightforward, and absolute rates should be treated with care when assessed by instruments such as the GHQ. Whether doctors and other health professionals are more stressed than the public as a whole is at best controversial. What is clear however, is that *some* doctors are more stressed than others, and it seems likely that those with high stress, as assessed by the GHQ, are neither happy nor effective doctors, often wanting to leave medicine for other careers.

Burnout

The concept of 'burnout' is less conceptually confused than that of stress, not least because of a clear articulation of the different components, and their ready measurement in a single, well-accepted measuring instrument, the Maslach Burnout Inventory (MBI) (Maslach & Jackson, 1986). Maslach has defined burnout as, "a psychological syndrome in response to chronic interpersonal stressors on the job" (Maslach *et al.*, 2001). The three separate components, measured by the MBI are:

- Emotional Exhaustion (EE; a sense of being emotionally over-extended and exhausted by one's work)
- Depersonalization (DP: an unfeeling, impersonal response towards patients; cynicism)
- Personal Accomplishment (PA: a feeling of achievement and competence in working with patients; efficacy)

These are differentiated by EE and DP being positively correlated with each other and with burnout overall, whereas PA is negatively correlated with burnout overall and with EE and DP. In more recent work Maslach has extended the conceptualization and in particular has emphasized 'engagement', the positive antithesis of burnout, which is the starting point from which 'What started out as important, meaningful and challenging work becomes unpleasant, unfulfilling and meaningless. Energy turns into exhaustion, involvement turns into cynicism, and efficacy turns into ineffectiveness' (Maslach *et al.*, 2001) (see 'Burnout in health professionals').

An important and often misunderstood feature of the MBI is that there is no absolute scoring, and unlike the GHQ there is no validation against formal psychiatric assessment. The manual (Maslach & Jackson, 1986) does describe high, medium and low scores, but these in effect are simple tertiles, dividing the original normative groups into top, middle and bottom thirds. The claim, as is sometimes seen, that in a survey, 'a third of the subjects showed high levels of burnout', is not saying that there are high levels of burnout but that there are normal levels of burnout.

An important conceptual aspect of the definition of burnout is the clear distinction between burnout and depression. Although the two conditions can co-occur, Maslach emphasizes that while burnout is job-related and situation-specific, depression in contrast is a condition which pervades every aspects of a person's life. Of course depression may cause burnout and burnout may cause depression, but their clear aetiological and diagnostic distinction must be maintained.

A similar conceptual distinction can also be made between stress and burnout, perhaps most clearly seen in the work of Pine, whose existential model clearly differentiates burnout from stress and strain (Pines & Keinan, 2005). In the existential perspective, people need their lives to be meaningful, and a sense of meaning is in part achieved by having jobs which are useful, important and of perceived significance. Burnout is the absence of such a sense of meaningfulness, and correlates principally with a lack of perceived job significance, whereas strain correlates particularly with work stressors such as workload. Pine also emphasises that the lack of significance is specific and situational, rather than generalized, so that individuals can, for instance, be burned out in one part of their life, such as at work but not in another part, such as their marriage.

The causal relationship between stress and burnout

Many studies measure levels of stress and burnout in health professionals, and the consistent finding is that doctors with higher stress levels also report more emotional exhaustion, more depersonalization and less personal accomplishment. The correlations are undisputed: much more problematic is the causal relationships between the measures, and these are much less studied. Particularly problematic is that the inference of causation from cross-sectional data is not straightforward, where stress is correlated with lowered personal accomplishment and increased depersonalization (Graham *et al.*, 2002). Proper longitudinal studies are rare, but in one study path modelling was used to interpret the relationships between stress and burnout measures in doctors assessed after a three-year interval (McManus *et al.*, 2002a). Figure 1 shows that the engine which drives the relation between stress and burnout is the causal cycle from stress to emotional exhaustion and from emotional exhaustion to stress. However the other effects are less intuitive. Longitudinally, personal accomplishment acts not to protect against stress but to increase it, whereas depersonalization acts to reduce subsequent stress. A metaphor may perhaps help in understanding the relationships; the oxygen of high personal accomplishment may initially help to ignite the fire of engagement, but just as a fire runs out of fuel, so burnout results when mental resources are consumed. To burnout one has firstly to have burned brightly and high personal accomplishment both makes the fire burn and also burn out (McManus, 2002).

Stress, personality and working conditions

A frequent assumption in the stress literature is that working conditions, and in particular in the case of doctors, a heavy workload and long working hours, including work at night and sleeplessness, are the major cause of stress (see 'Healthcare work environments' and 'Shiftwork and health'). Certainly it is the case that if one interviews doctors who are highly stressed then they will attribute their stress to working conditions. The problem, however, is that non-stressed doctors also describe similar working conditions. Systematic surveys of working conditions find a very poor, almost non-existent correlation, between working hours, patient load and

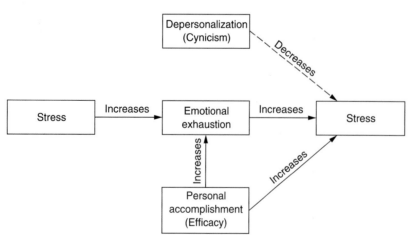

Fig 1 Causal relations between stress and burnout (for further details see text and McManus *et al.* (2002a)).

other variables describing working conditions, with stress levels (McManus *et al.*, 2002*b*; Bovier & Perneger, 2003) or with burnout (Pines, 2000). Two possibilities are therefore raised: one, is that, it is not workload per se which is stressful (and after all, many people find activation, exhilaration and excitement from working hard at a job they enjoy doing), but the imbalance between effort and reward (Tsutsumi & Kawakami, 2004): hard work for little reward, financial, psychological, social or professional, is stressful and results in burn-out. The other possibility is that stress is as much a characteristic of the doctor or health professional as it is of the work environment.

Most studies are incapable methodologically of separating effects of the individual from effects of the environment, since they assess a single health professional in a single job, the person and the situation being completely confounded. A study which shows the separation of the two looked at a large group of British doctors in their pre-registration house officer (PRHO) posts, the first year after qualification (McManus *et al.*, 2002*b*). The study was large enough to mean that many doctors had worked in the same post (i.e. for the same consultant firm, in the same hospital, which was a part of the same trust, which was supervized by the same postgraduate deanery). Such data can be analyzed by multi-level modelling, which allocates variance to different levels of the hierarchy. The analysis showed that many measures, such as reported working hours, number of patients, perceived quality of the job, etc. did indeed involve variance at the level of the consultant firm, or the hospital or trust. However, the most striking result was that stress and burnout *only* showed variance at the level of the individual doctor. In other words, two doctors working in precisely the same post showed no greater sim-ilarity of their stress levels than did two doctors working for different consultants, in different hospitals under different trusts and aca-demic deaneries (McManus *et al.*, 2002*b*). The strong implication is that stress is, to a large extent, an individual response of the health professional, rather than being directly driven by working conditions.

The clinical literature has long reported that the personality dimension of neuroticism is related to anxiety disorders (Matthews *et al.*, 2003; Tyssen & Vaglum, 2002) and an obvious personality correlate for stress and burnout in health professionals is neuroticism (see 'Personality and health'). Although personality is rarely measured in studies of stress, when it is there are clear correla-tions of neuroticism with stress levels (Deary *et al.*, 1996*a*, *b*; Tyssen *et al.*, 2002). Larger scale studies have found that other personality variables are also important in predicting stress, doctors with higher stress levels not only being more neurotic, but also being more intro-vert, and having lower levels of conscientiousness and agreeableness (McManus *et al.*, 2003, 2004). Intriguingly these are precisely the same personality variables which in meta-analyses predict low levels of job satisfaction, life satisfaction and marital satisfaction (Heller *et al.*, 2004). Particularly important is that in longitudinal studies, neuroticism measured at one time, when doctors are in a particular job, is predictive of stress and burnout levels five years later, when doctors are in an entirely different work environment (McManus *et al.*, 2004). The effects of stress on the working environ-ment are manifold, particularly when interacting with personality and study habits and learning styles, causing a surface-disorganized approach (Kirby *et al.*, 2003) and a high sense of workload, but also a less supportive–receptive working environment, and less indepen-dence of choice in work (McManus *et al.*, 2004) (see Fig. 2).

The management of stress and burnout

Whatsoever the disputes about the causes of stress in health profes-sionals, there is little doubt that many health professionals are stressed and burned out and interventions to reduce that stress would be beneficial to the professionals themselves and probably also to their patients and their colleagues. Several broad sets of intervention can be distinguished.

Stress-reduction techniques

Stress-reduction techniques for the workplace have been classified into six broad groups: relaxation; physical fitness; cognitive

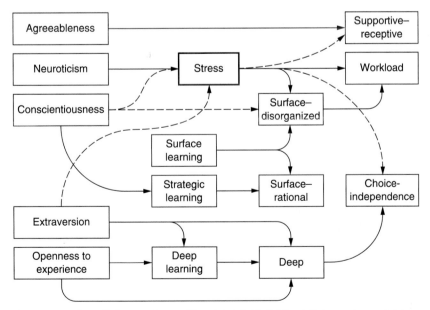

Fig 2 Summary of causal influences of personality and study habits (left-hand side) upon stress and of stress upon working styles and work environment (right-hand side). Solid lines indicate positive relationship, and dashed lines indicate negative relationships. For technical details see McManus *et al.* (2004).

restructuring; mediation; assertiveness training; and stress inoculation (Bellarosa & Chen, 1997) (see 'Cognitive behaviour therapy', 'Relaxation training' and 'Stress management'). Experts in such techniques were most familiar with relaxation, rated it as the most practical and cheapest of the methods and along with physical activity, the most effective of the methods although its effects were seen to be short-lived, with cognitive restructuring having the most long-lasting effects. Properly conducted empirical trials of the effectiveness of stress-reduction techniques are rare, one review of such interventions for mental health professionals finding only three well-evaluated studies, which found that stress reduced after attendance at workshops linked to sustained consultation, after participation in an intensive programme and after interdisciplinary education (Edwards et al., 2002). A meta-analysis of stress-reduction methods, found that the most effective techniques are cognitive–behavioural (Cohen's $d = 0.68$; 95% confidence interval CI = 0.54 to 0.82), with relaxation techniques less effective ($d = 0.35$; 95% CI = 0.22 to 0.48), and organizational interventions without any significant effect ($d = 0.08$; 95% CI = −0.03 to 0.19) (van der Klink et al., 2001); the overall effects were described as 'small but significant' (van der Klink et al., 2001). Large-scale randomized trials are unusual, not least because they are expensive, but an important exception is a study in which healthcare professionals in oncology received 105 hours of training on attitudes and communication skills, with significant reductions in stress being found three and six months later (Delvaux et al., 2004).

Lifestyle

Healthcare professionals are not only healthcare professionals, but also have lives outside of hospitals and other workplace institutions. In some cases it is events in those outside lives which have an impact on stress and burnout. In one study, many cases of stress identified by the GHQ-12 had problems outside work, including substantial health difficulties in close relatives, a past psychiatric history, marital difficulty and the lack of a confidant. These were more predictive of stress than were work problems (Weinberg et al., 1999). Family life can be a source of stress to doctors, particularly female doctors and those with children, with the problems of combining work and family being a common problem, which can result in continual compromises (Töyry et al., 2004). Although having children was a source of stress for doctors, interestingly doctors with children reported lower levels of depersonalization and higher levels of personal accomplishment than those without children (Töyry et al., 2004). GHQ scores were systematically lower in doctors who responded to stress at work by maintaining a balanced, healthy life-style (Graham et al., 2005).

Selection for hardiness

A recurrent suggestion, particularly from selectors for medical school, is that since neuroticism and other personality factors predict stress and burnout, then a sensible strategy is to select the hardiest of students, who will be the stable, conscientious extraverts. Although superficially attractive, such an approach has several problems. Firstly, it assumes that the selection ratio is sufficiently high to allow selection on multiple factors, but with only about two applicants for every medical school place, that is unlikely to be the case (McManus & Vincent, 1993). Secondly, the approach assumes that neuroticism, introversion and low conscientiousness have only negative correlates. However, that is unlikely to be the case. In the dangerous world in which early humans evolved, with the ever-likely possibility of predation and indeed in the dangerous modern technological world which modern humans have subsequently created, the risk of death or injury is always present. To have no anxiety about such possibilities is to run the risk of being eaten or run over. However, to be excessively anxious is also to run the risk of being paralyzed into inactivity. Moderate levels of neuroticism are therefore beneficial (and it is always worth remembering that, by definition, we are all the descendants of individuals who were sufficiently anxious as to make sure that they were not eaten by sabre-toothed tigers before they had reproduced). It is likely also that moderate, or even high, levels of neuroticism have their benefits in medicine: we want doctors and nurses who do sometimes go home and worry that they may have made a diagnosis wrongly, may have carried out an operation less well than they might have, or did not communicate properly with a patient or their relative. If we need such reflective individuals who worry about their jobs (and it seems likely we do) then we also need counselling and other career support systems which help them to continue coping at doing the thing at which they are good, and for which they have been so expensively trained, which is practising as health professionals.

REFERENCES

Bellarosa, C. & Chen, P. Y. (1997). The effectiveness and practicality of occupational stress management interventions: a survey of subject matter expert opinions. Journal of Occupational Health Psychology, 2, 247–62.

Bovier, P. A. & Perneger, T. V. (2003). Predictors of work satisfaction among physicians. European Journal of Public Health, 13, 299–305.

Cooper, C. L. (2005). Handbook of Stress Medicine and Health (2nd edn.). Boca Raton, FL: CRC Press.

Cox, T. (1978). Stress. Basingstoke, UK: Macmillan.

Deary, I. J., Blenkin, H., Agius, R. M. et al. (1996a). Models of job-related stress and personal achievement among consultant doctors. British Journal of Psychology, 87, 3–29.

Deary, I. J., Agius, R. M. & Sadler, A. (1996b). Personality and stress in consultant psychiatrists. International Journal of Social Psychiatry, 42, 112–23.

Delvaux, N., Razavi, D., Marchal, S. et al. (2004). Effects of a 105 hours psychological training program on attitudes, communication skills and occupational stress in oncology: a randomised study. British Journal of Cancer, 90, 106–14.

Dollard, M. F., Winefield, A. H. & Winefield, H. R. (2003). Occupational stress in the service professions. London: Taylor and Francis.

Edwards, D., Haningan, B., Fothergill, A. & Burnard, P. (2002). Stress management for mental health professionals: a review of effective techniques. Stress and Health, 18, 203–15.

Goldberg, D. P. (1972). The detection of psychiatric illness by questionnaire. London: Oxford University Press.

Goldberg, D. P., Gater, R., Sartorius, N. et al. (1997). The validity of two versions of the GHQ in the WHO study of mental illness in general health care. *Psychological Medicine*, **27**, 191–7.

Graham, J., Albery, I. P., Ramirez, A. J. & Richards, M. A. (2005). How hospital consultants cope with stress at work: implications for their mental health. *Stress and Health*, **17**, 85–9.

Graham, J., Potts, H. W. W. & Ramirez, A. J. (2002). Stress and burnout in doctors. *Lancet*, **360**, 1975–6.

Heller, D., Watson, D. & Ilies, R. (2004). The role of person versus situation in life satisfaction: a critical examination. *Psychological Bulletin*, **130**, 574–600.

Kalliath, T. J., O'Driscoll, M. P. & Brough, P. (2004). A confirmatory factor analysis of the general health questionnaire-12. *Stress and Health*, **20**, 11–20.

Kirby, J. R., Delva, M. D., Knapper, C. K. & Birtwhistle, R. V. (2003). Development of the approaches to work and workplace climate questionnaires for physicians. *Evaluation and the Health Professions*, **26**, 104–21.

Maslach, C. & Jackson, S. E. (1986). *Maslach burnout inventory*. Palo Alto, CA: Consulting Psychologists Press.

Maslach, C., Schaufeli, W. B. & Leiter, M. P. (2001). Job burnout. *Annual Review of Psychology*, **52**, 397–422.

Matthews, G., Deary, I. J. & Whiteman, M. C. (2003). *Personality Traits* (2nd edn.). Cambridge: Cambridge University Press.

Maxwell, H. & Squire, B. (2000). Feelings and counterfeelings in doctors an medical students. In H. Maxwell (Ed.). *Clinical psychotherapy for health professionals* (pp. 191–9). London: Whurr.

McManus, I. C. (2002). Stress and burnout in doctors. *Lancet*, **360**, 1976.

McManus, I. C., Keeling, A. & Paice, E. (2004). Stress, burnout and doctors' attitudes to work are determined by personality and learning style: a twelve year longitudinal study of UK medical graduates. *BMC Medicine*, **2**, 29.

McManus, I. C., Smithers, E., Partridge, P., Keeling, A. & Fleming, P. R. (2003). A levels and intelligence as predictors of medical careers in UK doctors: 20 year prospective study. *British Medical Journal*, **327**, 139–42.

McManus, I. C. & Vincent, C. A. (1993). Selecting and educating safer doctors. In C. A. Vincent, M. Ennis & R. J. Audley (Eds.). *Medical accidents* (pp. 80–105). Oxford: Oxford University Press.

McManus, I. C., Winder, B. C. & Gordon, D. (1999). Are UK doctors particularly stressed? *Lancet*, **354**, 1358–9.

McManus, I. C., Winder, B. C. & Gordon, D. (2002a). The causal links between stress and burnout in a longitudinal study of UK doctors. *Lancet*, **359**, 2089–90.

McManus, I. C., Winder, B. C. & Paice, E. (2002b). How consultants, hospitals, trusts and deaneries affect pre-registration house officer posts: a multilevel model. *Medical Education*, **36**, 35–44.

Pines, A. M. (2000). Nurses' burnout: an existential psychodynamic perspective. *Journal of Psychosocial Nursing*, **38**, 1–9.

Pines, A. M. & Keinan, G. (2005). Stress and burnout: the significant difference. *Personality and Individual Differences*, **39**, 625–35.

Schmitz, N., Kruse, J., Heckrath, C., Alberti, L. & Tress, W. (1999). Diagnosing mental disorders in primary care: the general health questionnaire (GHQ) and the symptom check list (SCL-90-R) as screening instruments. *Social Psychiatry and Psychiatric Epidemiology*, **34**, 360–6.

Töyry, S., Kalimo, R., Äärimaa, M. *et al.* (2004). Children and work-related stress among physicians. *Stress and Health*, **20**, 213–21.

Tsutsumi, A. & Kawakami, N. (2004). A review of empirical studies on the model of effort–reward imbalance at work: reducing occupational stress by implementing a new theory. *Social Science and Medicine*, **59**, 2335–539.

Tyssen, R. & Vaglum, P. (2002). Mental health problems among young doctors: an updated review of prospective studies. *Harvard Review of Psychiatry*, **10**, 154–65.

van der Klink, J. J. L., Blonk, R. W. B., Schene, A. H. & van Dijk, F. J. H. (2001). The benefits of interventions for work-related stress. *American Journal of Public Health*, **91**, 270–6.

Weinberg, A. & Creed, F. (1999). Stress and psychiatric disorder in healthcare professionals and hospital staff. *Lancet*, **355**, 533–7.

Surgery

Claus Vögele

Roehampton University

Introduction into the healthcare system and hospitalization can be a stressful experience on its own. Among the aspects of hospitalization considered to be most stressful Koenig *et al.* (1995) identified the following in a sample of elderly medical inpatients: communication problems with healthcare professionals; diagnostic and therapeutic procedures; the hospital environment (noise, rigid routines etc.); worries about the home situation and the separation from home; insufficient information about diagnosis and prognosis; and fear of dependency, loss of autonomy and control.

In addition to uncertainties about their illnesses (because of unclear communication) and the unfamiliar surroundings of a hospital ward, therefore, patients encounter additional stress because they must undergo medical procedures and examinations (see 'Hospitalization in adults'). Even some outpatient procedures such as dental treatments or blood donation can be stressful. Normally patients would report increases in anxiety in anticipation of procedures such as surgery, endoscopy, cardiac catheterization, cancer screening or chemotherapy. In addition to the anticipatory anxiety associated with the procedure itself, diagnostic procedures such as cancer screening are characterized by a prolonged period of anxiety between screening and receiving the result (Marteau *et al.*, 1993). The same is true for procedures such as HIV testing although the development of rapid testing procedures with the provision of same-day results and counselling has reduced the negative psychological consequences associated with a long wait (Kassler *et al.*, 1997) (see 'Coping with stressful medical procedures').

Of all medical procedures, surgery is perhaps the most threatening event as it contains many unpredictable and uncontrollable features such as losing consciousness due to the administration of a general anaesthetic, the anticipation of post-operative pain and the surgical trauma related to the incision. This chapter will concentrate on surgical procedures and describe the stressful characteristics associated with being hospitalized for surgery. The literature on psychological and physiological responses to the experience of surgery will be reviewed and findings from studies investigating psychological preparation for surgery will be summarized.

Stressful characteristics of the surgical situation

There are obvious potential threats for the surgical patient: anaesthesia; pain; physical restriction; life-threatening procedures; being away from home. Evidence suggests that the lack of predictability and control are significant contributors to the stressful experience of surgical patients (Slangen *et al.*, 1993). It is usually the case that we need to be able to predict an event in order to be able to control it. But the reverse does not follow: being able to predict an event does not necessarily mean we can control it. Such is the case for elective surgery, which accounts for the vast majority of surgical interventions.

This evidence confirms that there are common characteristics of the surgical situation which are identified by most patients as stressful. However, it seems likely that different types of surgical procedures produce different types of stress. Weinman and Johnston (1988) suggest that a useful way of distinguishing between the various procedures would be by considering the function of the procedure (diagnostic, treatment or both) and the timeline and nature of stress associated with the procedure. Weinman and Johnston (1988) further distinguish between procedural stress (i.e. the stress associated with the negative aspects of the actual procedure itself) and outcome stress (i.e. longer term fears and concerns related to the the results of the treatment or procedure'). To illustrate the latter point, some operations, for example, may have more positive characteristics in terms of their expected outcome than others, e.g. restoration (hip replacement) versus removal of physical function (leg amputation).

Responses of surgical patients at emotional, cognitive and physiological levels

Emotional responses

Most studies investigating emotional responses to surgery have shown elevated levels of anxiety both before and after surgery. In some groups of patients postoperative anxiety levels may be even higher than those measured preoperatively and this may reflect different sources of worry (procedural versus outcome). Vögele and Steptoe (1986) and Vögele (1992) found moderate levels of anxiety on the day before the operation and a significant increase on the days immediately following surgery in patients undergoing total hip replacement. As this particular type of surgery involved the patients to get out of bed on the second or third day after the operation it seems likely that the observed postoperative increase in anxiety was due to the anticipatory anxiety about the outcome of the operation. Interestingly, a similar pattern of responses could be observed in another patient group undergoing a much more minor orthopaedic surgical procedure (knee arthroscopy; Vögele & Steptoe, 1986).

Although anxiety has been the most frequently assessed emotional response for obvious reasons, it has been shown that surgical patients may also experience high levels of nervousness, depression, anger and boredom (Vögele, 1992).

These results indicate that emotional responses to the surgical situation may vary as a function of the type of operation, and therefore, outcome concerns. They also point to the possibility of effective interventions not only before but also after surgery.

Cognitive responses

Several studies have examined surgical patients' worries and it has been suggested that patients' main worries are more related to the outcome of the operation rather than the operation itself (Weinman & Johnston, 1988). Patients also worry significantly about normal everyday matters such as family and home, perhaps exacerbated by hospitalization and the impending surgery. As in the treatment of depression, the cognitive elements of surgical patients' stress response may be critical in indicating the most promising intervention approach to alleviate distress.

Physiological responses

The most thorough research on physiological responses to surgery has been carried out on indices of sympathetic-adrenomedullary activity. The most consistent finding is that of a reduction in palmar sweat gland activity prior to surgery followed by recovery to normal levels postoperatively (e.g. Vögele & Steptoe, 1986). Palmar sweat gland activity closely follows the pattern of subjective distress and pain, indicating that sweat gland activity is reduced by the stress of surgery. Some authors, however, have argued that the palmar sweating pattern of surgical patients is related to the effort rather than the distress aspect of stress, i.e. changes in palmar sweating are due to changes in activity levels. Indices of cardiovascular activity may be even more complicated to interpret. Goldstein *et al.* (1982) suggested that the cardiovascular responses to the stress of surgery have multiple determinants and may not be mediated by sympathetic influences. They found preoperative increases in heart rate, systolic blood pressure and cardiac output, but these persisted when noradrenaline responses were eliminated by diazepam sedation. In studies by Vögele & Steptoe (1986) and Vögele (1992), elevated heart rates before and after the operation that could not be accounted for by blood loss were consistently found.

A more recent line of research has investigated neuroendocrine and immune changes in response to surgery (Kiecolt-Glaser *et al.*, 1998) and wound healing (Ebrecht *et al.*, 2004). Post-operative elevations in plasma levels of adrenaline, cortisol and beta-endorphin reflect sympathetic nervous system and hypothalamic–pituitary–adrenal axis activation (Salomaki *et al.*, 1993). Evidence for immune suppression during surgery comes from studies showing suppression of natural killer cell activity (Pollock *et al.*, 1991), lymphocyte proliferative responses to mitogens and changes in lymphocyte populations (Tonnessen *et al.*, 1987).

In order to interpret these physiological responses to surgery as psychophysiological phenomena (including the experience of pain), it is necessary to disentangle the effects that are due to the experience of stress from those that are caused by the surgical trauma and other medical interventions (e.g. anaesthesia). Surgery represents in most cases a major trauma with a relatively stereotyped physiological response pattern (Salmon & Hall, 1997). This response pattern involves physiological changes reminiscent of Selye's 'General Adaptation Syndrome' (GAS) (Selye, 1980), and includes the release of catecholamines, glucocorticoids, growth hormone and glucagon, the suppression of insulin secretion and changes in other endocrine systems. These hormonal responses are assumed to trigger a cascade of metabolic adjustments leading to catabolism (a metabolic state of breakdown of the body's own protein) and substrate mobilization in the postoperative period.

This pattern of responses is sometimes described in the medical literature under the term 'La maladie post-opératoire' or 'Post aggression syndrome' (Moore, 1976). The implication of a unifying concept of postoperative physiological changes as suggested by this term has, however, been criticized in favour of a more differentiated view (Anand, 1986; Moore, 1976) taking into account the site and extent of the surgical trauma. In the simple uninfected elective surgical trauma, which usually forms the basis for psychological research reported in this chapter, there is little to note other than the mild tissue injury, with prompt healing, transient starvation and trivial fluid volume reduction. It could be argued, therefore, that any differences between patients in physiological responses to surgery may be attributable to psychological and behavioural factors, and this (despite all caveats) makes physiological indices of stress an attractive paradigm for the study of the impact of the surgical situation on postoperative recovery. As we will see in the following section such differences in physiological responses (including immunological and neuroendocrine changes) may have an effect on indices of postoperative recovery such as speed of wound healing.

Surgical stress and postoperative recovery

Despite a strong effect of physical factors such as extent of tissue damage caused by the surgical trauma on postoperative recovery, there is variability across patients who have undergone the same procedure. It is unclear what accounts for this variability, and this has led to the suggestion that psychological factors such as anxiety and depression may play some part in determining the duration or quality of postoperative recovery.

There is considerable theoretical and empirical support for the relevance of psychosocial factors to postoperative recovery. These include demographic variables such as age, gender and socioeconomic status, and also personality variables such as anxiety, neuroticism, coping style and social support. Most of the available literature today suggests a linear association between preoperative anxiety and success of recovery, in that the more anxious the patient before the operation the less favourable the postoperative recovery. There is even evidence that preoperative anxiety is related to intra-operative adjustment (Abbott & Abbott, 1995; de Bruin *et al.*, 2001), however with equivocal results: while in the former study highly anxious patients required more anaesthetic, the latter reports an inverse relationship: the higher the preoperative anxiety levels, the less anaesthetic was required during the operation.

In a review of studies relating anxiety and postoperative recovery, Munafò & Stevenson (2001) conclude that there is consistency across studies in finding a linear relationship between preoperative state anxiety and postoperative mood. A somewhat smaller degree of consistency is reported for the association between preoperative anxiety and other recovery variables. The authors use this finding to highlight methodological problems of these studies that prevent any firm conclusions to be drawn as yet.

Although the number of studies employing physiological recovery indices is relatively small, there is some compelling evidence for a positive relationship between preoperative self-report measures and postoperative immune function. Linn *et al.* (1988) assessed the relevance of differences in preoperative pain tolerance and stress to postoperative immune function. Physiological responses to a cold pressor test were measured the day before surgery in 24 men undergoing hernia repair. After controlling for preoperative immunological values (as well as age and social support) lymphocytes from men who reported more recent stressful life events had lower proliferative responses to an antigen (Phytohemagglutinin, PHA). In addition, high responders to the cold pressor test (i.e. a lower pain threshold) had significantly lower proliferative responses to a pokeweed mitogen after surgery (i.e. impaired immune function). They also required more pain medication and had more complications.

Across a number of studies, greater self-reported anxiety is typically related to more severe postoperative pain. In addition to direct effects on endocrine and immune function, the greater pain sensitivity of more anxious patients can have further consequences for recovery through altered behaviour. Breathing exercises, for example, can reduce the risk of pneumonia, and ambulation decreases the risk of phlebitis and may improve wound healing (Kehlet, 1997). Highly anxious patients may be more reluctant to follow recommendations for coughing, deep breathing or walking.

Personality variables may moderate post-surgical outcomes via their influence on stress, mood and coping (Mathews & Ridgeway, 1981). For example neuroticism as assessed by the Eysenck scales, has been shown in many studies to be associated with poorer surgical outcomes, such as increased postoperative pain and medical complications. Scheier *et al.* (1989) assessed the effect of dispositional optimism on recovery from coronary artery bypass surgery. After controlling for a number of confounds (extensiveness of surgery, severity of disease, smoking, hypertension, high cholesterol) the authors found that compared with pessimistic men, optimistic men fared better on perioperative physiological variables; they also began walking faster after surgery, and rehabilitation staff rated them as showing a more favourable physical recovery.

In summary, there is increasing evidence from psychoneuroimmunological work that stress and pain have a negative effect on endocrine and immune function and may thereby lead to delays in wound healing and other clinical complications. Although wound healing is only one postoperative outcome among a whole range, it is certainly a central parameter for short-term outcome in recovery from surgery. Kiecolt-Glaser *et al.* (1998) offer a biobehavioural model suggesting a number of routes through which psychological and behavioural responses can influence surgery and postoperative recovery (See 'Psychoneuroimmunology').

Psychological preparation for surgery

Most patients cope with preparations for stressful and potentially painful medical procedures as well as they can. However, the evidence reported in the previous sections of this chapter suggests that this coping ability might be compromised by a range of factors such as preceding life events, personality characteristics, demographic variables such as age and gender and previous unfavourable experiences with such procedures.

Efforts to design interventions to help surgical patients with their coping can be traced back more than four decades. Studies have investigated a diverse range of intervention techniques on equally diverse outcome measures.

Types of pre-surgical interventions

The provision of information of some kind concerning the surgical experience has perhaps been the most frequently employed. There are two types of information provision that can be distinguished; procedural information and sensory information. While the former describes the procedure and sequence of events in more detail, the latter places the emphasis on informing the patient about the sensations which they are likely to experience, e.g. nature, site and duration of pain after surgery etc. Another related intervention gives patients instructions on the behaviours they should engage in order to promote recovery (e.g. breathing, coughing, walking, eating etc.). This group of interventions is usually referred to as behavioural instructions. Although both information provision interventions are thought to act through the same mechanism of anxiety reduction, there is evidence that sensory information may be more effective by creating a 'cognitive map' within which to locate subjective (pain) experiences. It is difficult, however, to prove these claims in the context of preparation for surgery as many researchers in this area have designed interventions that contain mixtures of these three treatments.

Other, less frequently used interventions include cognitive techniques to help the patient re-appraise the surgical situation in a more positive (adaptive) way, relaxation techniques (progressive muscle relaxation, breathing techniques), hypnosis and emotion focused/psychotherapeutic interventions.

There is not only heterogeneity in interventions used but also in the way they have been delivered. Some studies use a group format, whereas others rely on low cost alternatives such as booklets, manuals, audiotapes and videotapes (e.g. Doering *et al.*, 2000). It may be worth noting, at this point, that most interventions are remarkably brief: the majority of studies employ a single session with an average duration of 30 minutes (Devine, 1992).

While being critical of the methodology of some of the studies included, several major literature reviews (e.g. Mathews & Ridgeway, 1984) and meta-analyses (e.g. Mumford *et al.*, 1982; Johnston & Vögele, 1993) are in broad agreement that prepared patients have better postoperative outcomes. In most cases 'better outcome' would relate to statistically significant differences between the group of patients receiving the preparation and an unprepared control group. Contrada *et al.* (1994), however, argue on the basis of several meta-analyses that these differences are not only statistically but also clinically meaningful. Depending on the meta-analysis, 60–75% of prepared patients had better outcomes than untreated controls, and the size of the improvement was in the order of 20–28%.

As to the question how psychological preparation for surgery promotes recovery two classes of explanations can be distinguished. The first set of assumptions stipulates that the physiological changes accompanying stress reduction resulting from psychological preparation (e.g. reduction in sympathetic arousal) improve patients' immunological responses (Kiecolt-Glaser *et al.*, 1998). There is evidence that interventions that alter appraisal, coping and/or mood may modulate immune and endocrine function (Kiecolt-Glaser & Glaser, 1992; Manyande *et al.*, 1995). An alternative explanation suggests that preparations exert their effects by reducing the frequency and extent of maladaptive behaviours that an unprepared patient might engage in (Mathews & Ridgeway, 1984). These two explanations are not mutually exclusive and can be subsumed under the biobehavioural model described by Kiecolt-Glaser *et al.* (1998).

Individual differences and psychological preparation for surgery

As discussed in the previous section, personality variables have been shown to moderate postoperative recovery via their influence on stress, mood and coping. Such individual differences may also be important in moderating the effects of psychological preparation for surgery, in particular in the area of preferred styles of coping with threat. For example, patients with a vigilant coping style (monitors) scan for threat-relevant cues, whereas those with a more avoidant coping style (blunters) try to distract themselves from threat cues. The two types of patients appear to show better adjustment in clinical settings when interventions are tailored to their coping style (Miller, 1992). Monitors fare better with voluminous sensory and procedural information, whereas the opposite is true for blunters (Prokop *et al.*, 1991).

Outcomes

In view of the heterogeneity of interventions, intervention formats, surgical procedures and the potential of individual differences to interact with treatment outcomes, the results achieved by psychological preparation for surgery are surprising and speak for the robustness of the effect.

The question remains, however: effective in gaining which benefits? It would also seem important to establish if all forms of preparation are equally effective. There are different reasons for an outcome to be valued. In a meta-analysis of the literature on preparing adult patients for surgery (Johnston & Vögele, 1993) the authors examined which benefits were sought, whether they were achieved and whether all benefits were equally likely to be gained by psychological preparation. They grouped outcomes in eight categories: negative affect; pain; pain medication; length of stay; behavioural and clinical indices of recovery; physiological indices; and satisfaction. The most important conclusion to be drawn from this analysis is that prepared patients show significant improvements in all outcomes analyzed. Given the heterogeneity in the data analyzed, the consistency of these results seems impressive. They are certainly sufficient to offer useful guidance to the medical or nursing staff or managers of a surgical unit attempting to improve outcomes for patients having routine, elective surgery under general anaesthesia.

In relation to interventions used, procedural information and behavioural instructions were found to be clearly effective in improving all eight outcomes. Relaxation is also highly effective, showing benefit on all outcomes except behavioural recovery, although this has been investigated in a number of studies. The results for cognitive interventions suggest that this type of preparation may have a specific effect on negative affect, pain, pain medication and clinical recovery, but not on length of stay in hospital, behavioural recovery, or physiological indices (see 'Cognitive behaviour therapy'). It is plausible to assume that these interventions affect a negative affect/symptom complaint dimension, but do not affect physiological or behavioural measures. Finally, it was found that sensory information, hypnotic and emotion-focused approaches to be rather less effective in improving outcome. However, these interventions have been explored in fewer studies and the procedures may be less well developed. In a more recent study comparing the effects of structured attention, self-hypnotic relaxation and standard care in a group of patients undergoing percutaneous vascular and renal procedures (angiographies) hypnosis had more pronounced effects on pain and anxiety reduction (Lang et al., 2000) (see 'Hypnosis').

Implications for research and practice in the future

As a consequence of technical advances in medicine and surgery, many operations are less invasive than in the past. They are, therefore, increasingly performed on an outpatient basis, or with a greatly reduced hospital stay. Kehlet and Wilmore (2002) estimate that in the future most elective surgical procedures will become day surgical procedures or require only one to two days of postoperative hospitalization. In addition to this development, the introduction of managed care in the healthcare systems of many countries has led to a further shortening of length of hospitalization. With any extended convalescence at home, family members or carers play a more important role. The additional demands that are placed on carers of surgical patients recovering at home should not be overlooked. Future developments should address these issues in research and in the design of flexible interventions that take into account the psychosocial context in which they take place.

REFERENCES

Abbott, J. & Abbott, P. (1995). Psychological and cardiovascular predictors of anaesthesia induction, operative and postoperative complications in minor gynecological surgery. *British Journal of Clinical Psychology*, **34**, 613–25.

Anand, K. J. (1986). The stress-response to surgical trauma: from physiological basis to therapeutic implications. *Progress in Food and Nutritional Science*, **10**, 67–132.

Contrada, R. J., Leventhal, E. A. & Anderson, J. R. (1994). Psychological preparation for surgery: marshalling individual and social resources to optimize self-regulation. In S. Maes, H. Leventhal & M. Johnston (Eds.). *International review of health psychology Vol. 3* (pp. 219–66). New York: Wiley.

De Bruin, J. T., Schaefer, M. K., Krohne, H. W. & Dreyer, A. (2001). Preoperative anxiety, coping, and intraoperative adjustment: are there mediating effects of stress-induced analgesia? *Psychology & Health*, **16**, 253–71.

Devine, E. C. (1992). Effects of psychoeducational care for adult surgical patients: a meta-analysis of 191 studies. *Patient Education and Counseling*, **19**, 129–42.

Doering, S., Katzlberger, F., Rumpold, G. et al. (2000). Videotape preparation of patients before hip replacement surgery reduces stress. *Psychosomatic Medicine*, **62**, 365–73.

Ebrecht, M., Hextall, J., Kirtley, L.-G. et al. (2004). Perceived stress and cortisol levels predict speed of wound healing in healthy male adults. *Psychoneuroendocinology*, **29**, 798–809.

Goldstein, D. S., Dionne, R., Sweet, J. et al. (1982). Circulatory, plasma catecholamine, cortisol, lipid, and psychosocial responses to a real-life stress (third molar extractions): effects of diazepam sedation and of inclusion of epinephrine with the local anaesthetic. *Psychosomatic Medicine*, **44**, 259–72.

Johnston, M. & Vögele, C. (1993). Benefits of psychological preparation for surgery: a meta-analysis. *Annals of Behavioral Medicine*, **15**, 245–56.

Kassler, W. J., Dillon, B. A., Haley, C., Jones, W. K. & Goldman, A. (1997). On-site, rapid HIV testing with same-day results and counselling. *AIDS*, **11**, 1045–51.

Kehlet, H. (1997). Multimodal approach to control postoperative pathophysiology and rehabilitation. *British Journal of Anaesthesia*, **78**, 606–17.

Kehlet, H. & Wilmore, D. W. (2002). Multimodal strategies to improve surgical outcome. *American Journal of Surgery*, **183**, 630–41.

Kiecolt-Glaser, J. K. & Glaser, R. (1992). Psychoneuroimmunology: can psychological interventions modulate immunity? *Journal of Consulting and Clinical Psychology*, **60**, 569–75.

Kiecolt-Glaser, J. K., Page, G. G., Marucha, P. T., MacCallum, R. C. & Glaser, R. (1998). Psychological influences on surgical recovery. Perspectives from psychoneuroimmunology. *American Psychologist*, **53**, 1209–18.

Koenig, H. G., George, L. K., Stangl, D. & Tweed, D. L. (1995). Hospital stressors experienced by elderly medical inpatients: developing a Hospital Stress Index. *International Journal of Psychiatry in Medicine*, **25**, 103–22.

Lang, E. V., Benotsch, E. G., Fick, L. J. et al. (2000). Adjunctive non-pharmacological analgesia for invasive medical procedures: a randomised trial. *Lancet*, **355**, 1486–90.

Linn, B. S., Linn, M. W. & Klimas, N. G. (1988). Effects of psycho-physical stress on surgical outcome. *Psychosomatic Medicine*, **50**, 230–44.

Manyande, A., Simon, B., Gettins, D. et al. (1995). Preoperative rehearsal of active coping imagery influences subjective and hormonal responses to abdominal surgery. *Psychosomatic Medicine*, **57**, 177–82.

Marteau, T. M., Kidd, J., Michie, S. *et al.* (1993). Anxiety, knowledge and satisfaction in women receiving false positive results on routine prenatal screening: a randomized controlled trial. *Journal of Psychosomatic Obstetrics and Gynaecology*, **14**, 185–96.

Mathews, A. & Ridgeway, V. (1981). Personality and surgical recovery: a review. *British Journal of Clinical Psychology*, **20**, 243–60.

Mathews, A. & Ridgeway, V. (1984). Psychological preparation for surgery. In A. Steptoe & A. Mathews (Eds.). *Health care and human behaviour* (pp. 231–59). London: Academic Press.

Miller, S. (1992). Monitoring and blunting in the face of threat: implications for adaptation and health. In L. Montada, S. Filipp & M. J. Lerner (Eds.). *Life crises and experiences of loss in adulthood* (pp. 255–73). Hillsdale, NJ: Erlbaum.

Moore, F. D. (1976). La maladie post-opératoire: is there order in variety? *Surgical Clinics of North America*, **56**, 803–15.

Mumford, E., Schlesinger, H. J. & Glass, G. V. (1982). The effects of psychological intervention on recovery from surgery and heart attacks. An analysis of the literature. *American Journal of Public Health*, **72**, 141–51.

Munafò, M. R. & Stevenson, J. (2001). Anxiety and surgical recovery. Reinterpreting the literature. *Journal of Psychosomatic Research*, **51**, 589–96.

Prokop, C. K., Bradley, L. A., Burish, T. G., Anderson, K. O. & Fox, J. E. (1991). Psychological preparation for stressful medical and dental procedures. In C. K. Prokop & L. A. Bradley (Eds.). *Health psychology: clinical methods and research* (pp. 159–96). New York: Macmillan.

Pollock, R. E., Lotzova, E. & Stanford, S. D. (1991). Mechanism of surgical stress impairment of human perioperative natural killer cell cytotoxicity. *Archives of Surgery*, **126**, 338–42.

Salmon, P. & Hall, G. M. (1997). A theory of postoperative fatigue: an interaction of biological, psychological, and social processes. *Pharmacology, Biochemistry and Behavior*, **56**, 623–8.

Salomaki, T. E., Leppaluoto, J., Laitinen, J. O., Vuolteenaho, O. & Nuutinen, L. S. (1993). Epidural versus intravenous fentanyl for reducing hormonal, metabolic, and physiologic responses after thoracotomy. *Anesthesiology*, **79**, 672–9.

Scheier, M. F., Matthews, K. A., Owens, J. F. *et al.* (1989). Dispositional optimism and recovery from coronary artery bypass surgery: the beneficial effects on physical and psychological well-being. *Journal of Personality and Social Psychology*, **57**, 1024–40.

Selye, H. (Ed.). (1980). *Guide to stress research*. New York: Van Nostrand.

Slangen, K., Krohne, H. W., Stellrecht, S. & Kleemann, P. P. (1993). Dimensionen perioperativer Belastung und ihre Auswirkungen auf intra- und postoperative Anpassung von Chirurgiepatienten. *Zeitschrift für Gesundheitspsychologie*, **1**, 123–42.

Tonnessen, E., Brinklov, M. M., Christensen, N. J., Olesen, A. S. & Madsen, T. (1987). Natural killer cell activity and lymphocyte function during and after coronary artery bypass grafting in relation to the endocrine stress response. *Anesthesiology*, **67**, 526–33.

Vögele, C. (1992). Perioperative stress. In L. R. Schmidt (Ed.). *Jahrbuch der Medizinischen Psychologie Vol. 7* (pp. 74–95). Berlin: Springer.

Vögele, C. & Steptoe, A. (1986). Physiological and subjective stress responses in surgical patients. *Journal of Psychosomatic Research*, **30**, 205–15.

Weinman, J. & Johnston, M. (1988). Stressful medical procedures: an analysis of the effects of psychological interventions and of the stressfulness of the procedures. In S. Maes, P. Defares, I. G. Sarason & C. D. Spielberger (Eds.). *Topics in health psychology* (pp. 205–17). Chichester, UK: Wiley.

Teaching communication skills

Angela Hall[1] and Jane Kidd[2]

[1]University of London
[2]University of Warwick

Background

The prevailing view in medicine that communication skills improve with practice and experience was challenged by the seminal studies published by Maguire and colleagues between 1976 and 1986. The traditional apprenticeship model of learning how to elicit information from patients was shown to have serious deficiencies. Few students managed to discover the patient's main problem or clarify its exact nature, let alone explore ambiguous statements, respond to cues or cover personal topics. Students who then underwent a training programme reported almost three times as much accurate and relevant information as the control group. A sub-sample of these students was followed up five years later to see whether their skills had persisted: both control and trained groups had improved, but the superiority in the skills associated with accurate diagnosis in the group given feedback was maintained. Both groups were poor at giving information, although this was something that these doctors were doing on a daily basis. Skills associated with information-giving had not in fact been taught to these doctors while they were undergraduates.

During the same period of time evidence was accumulating for the importance of effective communication, not only for participants in the consultation but also for the health service (see 'Healthcare professional–patient communication'). For patients, effective communication was associated with enhanced satisfaction (see 'Patient satisfaction'), enhanced adherence (see 'Adherence to treatment'), and improved health outcomes. For doctors, effective communication was associated with reduced burnout, enhanced functioning and fewer complaints and litigation. Finally, for the health service, effective communication was associated with shorter stays in hospital and less waste of drugs.

In acknowledgement of these sorts of finding, the General Medical Council in the UK has encouraged all medical schools to include the teaching of clinical communication in undergraduate curricula (1993; 2002). With the impact of modernizing medical careers and the development of new roles for junior doctors with competency-based assessment, communication skills teaching and learning continues in the postgraduate years as well (www.mmc.nhs.uk; Department of Health, 2004).

A literature review conducted by Aspergren (1999) confirmed that communication skills in medicine can be both taught and learned. Eighty-one of 180 studies fulfilled the criteria for having a high or medium methodological standard; only one study failed to show positive changes in skill following a teaching intervention. Not only did these studies demonstrate that communication skills can be learned, they also illuminate our understanding about appropriate learning methods. Learners require a framework that explicitly identifies what areas should be covered and what skills they should use. Effective learning also requires opportunities for students to be given systematic feedback on how effectively they communicate with their patients. Evans *et al.* (1989) demonstrated that didactic methods alone are not sufficient to bring about change in learners' skills. There is a place for didactic or cognitive methods, in particular, introducing conceptual frameworks through which to view the medical interview and to stimulate interest and expand the understanding of learners. There is overwhelming evidence however, that it is experiential methods of teaching that bring about lasting behavioural changes in the clinical setting. These include direct observation of the learners interviewing each other, simulated or real patients, the provision of appropriate and constructive feedback, and the facilitation of practice and rehearsal in a safe and supportive environment.

Introduction

Effective doctor–patient communication contains three categories of skills (Silverman *et al.*, 2005): those that reflect the content of a consultation (what to ask and what to provide information about), those that reflect the process (how to do it); and those that reflect the perceptual skills (awareness of the impact of certain skills and how they affect self and patient). All three sets of skills are essential in enabling a consultation to be effective for both the doctor and the patient (see 'Medical interviewing'). This chapter is going to focus primarily on the teaching and learning of the process skills.

We will start by identifying challenges for tutors as students enter medical school, looking at the effect of their prior learning. The chapter will continue by exploring the needs of undergraduate and postgraduate learners and then consider curriculum development with these needs in mind. Some models of the doctor–patient consultation will be identified as well as teaching approaches that have been shown to be effective. The chapter will close with an overview of assessment and draw some conclusions.

Challenges

There are particular challenges for students starting medical school which need to be recognized and understood by tutors. There can be few medical schools that do not consider students' ability to communicate as a key element of the selection procedure. Students are aware of this, yet when they arrive, they are required to reflect and analyse how they communicate. What is more, they are being asked to do this in what for most is a completely new context, i.e. medicine. Importantly, they are required to communicate in a professional manner which may be rather different to the way in which they normally interact with people. Even something as basic as explaining to a patient the reason why they wish to carry out a clinical interview is potentially fraught. 'A quick chat' is something that students may have with their friends, but employed in a clinical setting as an explanation, hardly conveys the purpose of the interview. It is small wonder that students may feel awkward and uncomfortable during sessions early on in the curriculum and need explicit acknowledgement of the expertise they already possess and the context in which that expertise is valued, in order not to feel de-skilled.

Needs of undergraduate and postgraduate learners

Students enter medical school with certain ideas and perceptions of themselves that may need to be reviewed in terms of effective doctor–patient communication. People who are learning skills can be working at one of four levels which are shown in Box 1.

Whether in the undergraduate or postgraduate arena, it is important not to make assumptions about the level at which a learner is

---

Box 1. Competence Learning Model

Unconscious incompetence	The person is not aware of the existence or relevance of the skill area. The person does not know what s/he does not know. The learner is in a state of 'blissful ignorance'. Confidence exceeds ability.
Conscious incompetence	The person becomes aware of the existence and relevance of the skills and also aware of their deficiency in this area. Confidence reduces with the realization that ability is limited. Practice is essential to learning.
Conscious competence	The person achieves 'conscious competence' in a skill when they can perform it reliably at will. The person needs to concentrate and think, in order to perform the skills.
Unconscious competence	The person can perform the skills but does not necessarily know how s/he does it – it becomes second nature.

www.businessballs.com/consciouscompetencelearningmodel.htm

functioning. These stages are not age-dependent and not all qualified doctors are working at the level of unconscious competence. There is a wide variation in knowledge and competence across the spectrum from initial entry to medical school through to consultant. The learning styles of learners need to be taken into account as well as where they sit on the spectrum between pedagogy (where learners are perceived to be dependent) and andragogy (where learners are perceived to be self-directed) (Knowles, 1990; Grow, 1996). For both undergraduates and postgraduates, it is necessary on occasion to revisit basic skills in order to identify that these are still in place and then to allow the learner to move forward by building on these in a helical type of model.

We need to ensure that for all learners there is a clear link to application: for junior medical students who spend most of their time in medical school, this is often more difficult to achieve than for more senior students and practising doctors. However postgraduate learners who are attempting to gain technical competence in dealing with disease, to develop their professional identity and to learn how to heal, can also at times find this difficult.

Undergraduate and postgraduate learners may differ in terms of having experienced different models of feedback and having experienced a wider range of consultations with patients. Initially a more prescriptive type of feedback may be beneficial to the learner, using guidelines such as those developed by Pendleton et al. (1984). With more experience of patients and particularly of challenges faced on a daily basis, postgraduate learners are often more able to identify where their own strengths and difficulties lie in terms of effective doctor–patient communication. They are thus more able to state what it is they would like feedback on and work with the more appropriate agenda-led outcome-based analysis (ALOBA) model of feedback described by Silverman et al. (1996).

Curriculum development

Many medical schools have now adopted a helical approach to the learning of communication skills referred to earlier and first described by Dance (1967). The helix conceptualized an important theoretical principle underpinning how we communicate, namely that effective communication depends on interaction between sender and receiver and, crucially, depends on both the giving and receiving of feedback about the impact of the message. Communication gradually evolves in a spiral fashion and demands both reiteration and repetition to become effective. The concept of the helix has been widely used by medical educators, as well as those working in the field of communication. Simply put, the communication curriculum should allow learners to 'review, refine and build on existing skills while at the same time adding in new skills and increasing complexity' (Kurtz et al., 2005). The model emphasizes that people learn in a spiral rather than a linear form. The curriculum should be delivered not as a series of isolated sessions or modules, but as opportunities for learning, review and challenge as learners move to higher levels on the helix.

Educators themselves face considerable challenges when developing a communication curriculum. In a thoughtful editorial, Cushing (1996) makes the point that the relationship between the components of the curriculum, and when and how they are taught, is crucial. The worst message that can be given to students is that communication skills are a soft add-on to the 'real' curriculum. To avoid this, teaching needs to be integrated into the curriculum as a whole and made relevant to what students are learning elsewhere in their course.

There are many creative ways in which integrated teaching and learning can be achieved. With the change in many schools from traditional, didactic, lecture-based courses towards problem-based learning, the clinical content of communication sessions can be determined by the paper problem of the week or the system being learned. Communication issues can be flagged up for discussion in tutor notes. Content can also be determined by what is expected of students on their general practice, community and hospital placements. Thus, some sessions can specifically prepare students for visits or for clinical attachments. Explicit integration with other specialisms, such as medical statistics, helps students appreciate the relevance of aspects of their curriculum to clinical practice (Sedgewick & Hall, 2003). Finally, the active involvement of practising doctors in the teaching of process skills gives a powerful message to students about the importance of communication and how it fits into medical practice.

There are other aspects of effective communication that need to be included in the medical curriculum. Written communication is one of the principal ways in which healthcare professionals communicate with each other and at the very least students need to know how to write notes, discharge summaries and referral letters (Nestel & Kidd, 2004) (see 'Written communication'). They also need to know how to present their patients to senior colleagues with a clear, succinct and relevant summary. The value of integrating teaching communication and clinical skills is also beginning to be addressed (Kidd et al., 2005).

Models of the medical interview

In teaching and learning about communication, two types of model are important. There are models (or frameworks) for the consultation and there are role models, the current practitioners of doctor–patient communication.

Models of the consultation are important as they provide a structure that can help the learner to understand that the medical interview has an internal logic with a beginning, a middle and an end. Different phases or stages of the interview have different functions and there is a range of skills that can be utilized to achieve these functions. Many models of the consultation have been proposed over the past 30 years (Stewart & Jones, 1991; Stott & Davis, 1979; Byrne & Long, 1976; Heron, 1975; Helman's 'Folk Model', 1981).

Since 1984, models have been developed that describe specific stages, functions or tasks in a consultation. Each of the models listed in Box 2 divides the consultation into stages, tasks, or areas to be explored. They identify objectives for each stage and the skills that can help the doctor to meet those objectives.

Even a quick glance at these models shows the reader that there is a lot of similarity in terms of the stages and functions identified as elements of an effective consultation. When the authors begin to describe the skills associated with effective communication for each stage or task, there is again a high degree of consistency between models.

Box 2. Models of the Medical Interview

Pendleton et al. (1984)

1. Define the reason for the patient's attendance
2. Consider other problems
3. With the patient, choose an appropriate action for each problem
4. Achieve a shared understanding of the problems with the patient
5. Involve the patient in the management and encourage him or her to accept appropriate responsibility
6. Use time and resources appropriately
7. Establish and maintain a relationship with the patient which helps to achieve other tasks

Neighbour (1987)

1. Connect – establish rapport with the patient
2. Summarize – discover why the pt has attended and summarize back
3. Hand over – agree agenda for consultation
4. Safety net – explore options for each item on agenda
5. Housekeep – Check on 'self' before seeing next patient

Disease–Illness Model (McWhinney, 1989)

This model concentrates on the task of gathering information and suggests that doctors need to explore two parallel frameworks: the disease framework of the doctor and the illness framework of the patient. In this way this model introduces new content to information-gathering from the patient's perspective

The Three-Function approach to the medical interview (Cole & Bird, 2000)

1. Develop rapport
2. Gather data
3. Educate and motivate

The Calgary–Cambridge Approach to Communication Skills Teaching (Kurtz et al., 2005)

This model identifies five sequential tasks to a consultation:

1. Initiating the session
2. Gathering information
3. Physical examination
4. Explanation and planning
5. Closing the session

and two continuous tasks:

1. Providing structure to the consultation
2. Building the relationship

However, it is perhaps the models who the learners see in action, i.e. the current practitioners, who have the most influence on the skills that the learners perceive to be important and put effort into learning. This modelling works at three levels. First, learners observe their more senior colleagues communicating with their patients and can pick up on the skills that they see being used. At the second level, they are also learning what their role models consider

important, through the topics that are chosen for discussion related to the consultation. Is the discussion always on the content of the history, physical examination and problem solving or are the process skills and the patient's perspective included in the discussion? At the third level medical students learn from observing how their role models interact with all the people around them and how they themselves are treated. If learners feel valued, they are far more able to reflect that in their relationship with patients (see also 'Medical interviewing').

Teaching methods/approaches

An effective communicator needs at the very least to have a body of knowledge, a set of skills and an appropriate attitude. To be an effective communication skills tutor one needs a parallel set of knowledge, skills and attitudes related to education, coupled with a set of tools to move learners from the level of unconscious incompetent practitioner to that of unconscious competent practitioner. Good tutors are genuinely facilitative and behave towards their students as they would in turn wish the students to behave towards their patients. There are many parallels in the relationship between teachers and learners and between doctors and patients. Characteristics of competent trainers are listed in Box 3.

Moving learners from the stage of unconscious incompetence to conscious incompetence requires introduction to cognitive material in terms of a framework, identification of skills (naming skills) and evidence of effectiveness on which learners can reflect. Such material can be delivered effectively in interactive lectures or during

Box 3. Characteristics of a competent trainer

Knowledge

Understands basic teaching methods
Understands effective communication skills (why they work, what impact they have)

Skills: ability to

use a range of teaching tools
use effective communication skills
observe keenly
analyze effectively
provide constructive feedback
foster reflection in the trainee

Attitudes

Has respect for the trainee
Has an interest in the trainee
Gives latitude to the trainee
Is available for consultation
Flexibility
Enthusiasm
Self-insight
(Amended from Boendermakers *et al.*, 2000)

group work. However, as identified earlier in the chapter, the evidence points to the need to work with experiential learning methods to enhance the skills of learners. Most communication skills learning takes place in small groups or on a one-to-one basis, which greatly enhances a feeling of safety for learners when they are in the hands of a competent trainer. Hutchinson (2003) has written an excellent and sympathetic chapter on creating an optimal context or climate for learning.

Kolb's learning cycle (Kolb, 1984) describes one way of conceptualizing how people learn skills. It has four main components: concrete experience, followed by reflective observation, abstract conceptualization and finally active experimentation. Learners carry out an interview (the concrete experience) before having the opportunity to comment on it (reflective observation) prior to considering what it might mean for them and their patient (abstract conceptualization) and deciding what it is they might do differently the next time (active experimentation).

The theory of reflective practice developed by Schon (1983) throws useful light on the reflective process in learning and its relationship to the acquisition of competence. He identifies 'reflection *in* action' as the ability to learn and develop by applying past experience to unfamiliar events as they are occurring. Observing reflection in action is one of the most rewarding experiences for tutors, as students actively demonstrate what they have learned. 'Reflection *on* action' takes place after the event and corresponds to Kolb's 'reflective observation'. Building in the opportunity to reflect is a crucial part of becoming an effective communicator, in particular because it encourages reflection on both the attitudes and the feelings of the learner.

How can we reflect the learning cycle in terms of education about effective communication? What tools do we have to work with and what are their benefits and drawbacks? There are three main experiential approaches: role-play with colleagues; working with simulated patients; and working with patients. We describe each briefly.

Role-play between peers

This process may well be one of the most misused approaches in health professional education. There is an assumption that learners can take on a role with minimal or no preparation and learn from it but this is far from the case. For such an experience to be successful with inexperienced learners, detailed attention has to be given to the questions in Box 4.

With this level of preparation learners are less likely to have difficulty in getting into role because they know their 'patient' too well and all they can do is giggle or feel so embarrassed that their performance is inhibited.

Role-play with simulated patients

Simulated (standardized) patients have been used successfully in learning and assessment settings since the early 1960s (Barrows & Abrahamson, 1964). Simulated patients are a valuable resource in the teaching of communication skills. They work with the facilitator and the learner or learning group, playing live simulations of both a clinical problem and communication challenges appropriate and

---

Box 4. Questions about using role-play in teaching sessions

How role-play fits into a teaching session

- which learning outcome is it designed to meet?
- what is the objective of the interview?
- what is the precise role of the interviewer? (is s/he playing him/herself, or a different role?)
- what is the precise role of the 'patient' (both in terms of the presenting problem and the character of the patient)?
- how much time is allocated to the exercise?
- how is that time divided between role play and feedback?
- how will the learner be given feedback on his/her performance (verbal, written, checklist, global)?
- will the learners work in trios so that there is an observer for every interview?
- will every learner have the opportunity to play the interviewer, the patient and the observer in turn? (if learning about receiving and proving feedback is a session outcome then designing a session with an observer is essential)
- will the learners work with the same role for each interview or will new roles be provided?

---

relevant to learners' needs. Simulated patients are members of the public who have an interest in medical education. They may come from different backgrounds: many are professional actors but some are members of the local community who are able to portray roles that do not reflect their own real-life experience.

Much has been written about the benefits of working with simulated patients (e.g. Kaufman *et al.*, 2000; Madan *et al.*, 1998; Stillman *et al.*, 1990). One of the major benefits for learners is that it does not matter if they make mistakes, as there are no adverse consequences for the patient. Working with simulated patients allows the learner to rehearse skills time and time again, to try new skills and approaches, to receive constructive feedback, to explore feelings associated with the behaviour of the simulator and its impact on the learners and vice versa. At the same time the simulated patient can improvise (be learner-centred) to the level of the challenge that the learners want, which may be in terms of skills they wish to practise (e.g. empathy, reflection, picking up cues), a difficult situation (e.g. breaking bad news, working with an interpreter) or the type of character they would like to practise interviewing (e.g. angry, distressed, talkative).

For simulated patients to be of maximum benefit to the teaching of clinical communication, a selection and training programme needs to be in place. Not everyone who wants to participate in sessions as a simulated patient has the necessary qualities: the ability to play a role, reflect on it while it is happening in order to identify why they are reacting to the 'doctor' in the way that they are, and then phrase that feedback constructively to the learner. It is essential that during feedback, the simulated patient reinforces the tutor's teaching messages. Some learners have difficulty with simulated patients in that they perceive them as 'not real' or that they are 'being set up'. With appropriate introduction and honesty between trainer and trainee these perceptions can be minimized and overcome. Guidelines for introducing and setting up a simulated patient role-play are given in Box 5.

Box 5. Introducing simulated patient role-play

- Discuss the scenario and interviewer task with the group
- Brainstorm any clinical information that might be needed
- Ask for a volunteer (or more than one and share the interview)
- Discuss objectives – ask the learner what they want to achieve
- Any challenges? Any strategies? (these can be discussed with the group)
- Ask the learner to decide on a few things they would like feedback on
- Allocate specific feedback to each group member – ask them to write comments down and be able to give verbatim quotes
- Flag up to the learner that they can stop at any time during the scenario and take time out to discuss what they would like to do next
- Negotiate how long the interview will be (make it clear that they should only get as far as they can in the time, not necessarily get to the end)
- Flag up that at the end of the interview, the learner comments first on how it went

Working with patients

There are several ways in which to gain access to this rich resource. Learners at both under- and postgraduate level can videotape their interviews with patients on the wards or in outpatient clinics, to review later with their tutor. They may also carry out the same exercise in general practice and video an entire surgery from which to select material for review. From the learner's perspective, the great advantage of working with a patient is that they are real. From the educator's perspective, the advantage is that learners can be observed at the performance level of Miller's 'pyramid of assessment' hierarchy (Miller, 1990).

Medical schools involve real patients through volunteer programmes and community programmes. These are patients who are willing to come into the medical school and be available for students to elicit their history, in full or in part. Patients can be selected for given sessions on the basis of having a particular condition or experience. Increasingly schools are setting up programmes to support and train patients to give feedback to learners, which enhances the experience for both sides. Patients can also help students' learning by allowing filming of their consultation with an experienced doctor, so that students can subsequently observe and give feedback about both the content and process skills of the interviewer. Capturing appropriate material can be time-consuming but is worthwhile, because students respond so positively to the real thing.

It is very important to pay attention to how patients have been invited to participate in teaching: taking care to elicit properly informed consent is crucial. Patients need to be very clear about the purpose of the exercise and not be constrained by power imbalance. Their concerns should be addressed about whether refusal might have an impact on their treatment and care. Tutors need to be aware of the possibility of patients feeling coerced and this also applies to opportunistic approaches for bedside or outpatient teaching.

Without training, patients are not usually in a position to give constructive feedback nor is it usually possible to rehearse skills or ask the patient 'could I try that again?'. However, the benefits of working with real, carefully selected patients, usually far outweigh these constraints.

Videotaping

All three of the above experiential learning opportunities can be enhanced if it is possible to video-record the consultations. Videotape is a powerful tool for self-observation and enables learners to make detailed and accurate assessments of themselves. Learners do not have to rely on reflection alone but can observe and hear themselves in action and identify their own strengths and weaknesses. Recordings can be looked at over time to review learning goals and track progress.

Some learners have difficulty with the idea of being video-recorded, and as with the use of role-play, this may be related to a previous poorly structured learning experience. In such cases the tutor needs to work with the individual to determine their barriers to working in this way. It can be helpful to discuss the benefits that such an experience can bring, identifying that feedback will be constructive (not humiliating), re-emphasizing the formative nature of the experience and who will see the video-recording.

As we have seen, reflection on performance is a key aspect of learning how to be an effective communicator in the clinical context. It is particularly useful to be able to revisit exact points in an interview and discuss them without disagreement about whether recall about what happened was accurate. Although more complicated to set up and manage, videotape is superior to audiotape because it provides an unparalleled opportunity to observe non-verbal communication.

Assessment

Care and thought should be given to the assessment of skills. Measurement of knowledge, skills and competencies has always been an essential part of medical education. However, both reliability and validity were frequently compromised in traditional long and short cases; to measure skills reliably, performance of candidates has to be sampled across a range of problems. The Objective Structured Clinical Examination (OSCE) was introduced more than 30 years ago as a flexible format to administer assessment (Harden, 1979) and is based on a circuit around which all candidates rotate. In this way all students can be tested on a number of patient-based problems and all carry out the same tests. This assessment format is now used by many healthcare professionals at both under- and postgraduate level. For those who wish to know more about the OSCE, including its limitations, Smee (2003) has written a succinct introduction. From this chapter's perspective of teaching communication skills, it is essential that OSCE stations assess skills that have been taught to all students, reflected in the learning objectives for the curriculum.

Conclusion

There is much evidence that skills for effective communication in clinical practice can be taught, learned and will persist, given the opportunity for practice, reflection and feedback. Understanding what the skills are and appreciating their effectiveness smoothes the path for learners as they make the transition to competent practitioner. The skills are the building blocks or tools. Students need to learn not only the skills themselves but also how to select those appropriate to the individual and for the task in front of them. In the same way that patients always bring the psychosocial dimension of their illness to the medical interview, so learners bring their own attitudes, values, feelings and personal history, which play out in their behaviour. Attitudes influence skills and skills acquisition can lead to changes in attitude. Paying attention to both increases understanding, insight and job satisfaction for both learners and their teachers.

(See also 'Breaking bad news', 'Healthcare professional–patient communication', 'Medical interviewing' and 'Written communication'.)

REFERENCES

Aspergren, K. (1999). Teaching and learning communication skills in medicine: a review with quality grading of articles. *Medical Teacher*, **21**(6), 563–70.

Boendermaker, P., Schuling, J., Meyboom-de Jong, B., Zwierstra, R. P. & Metz, J. (2000). What are the characteristics of the competent general practitioner trainer? *Family Practice*, **17**, 547–53.

Barrows, H. & Abrahamson, S. (1964). The programmed patient: a technique for appraising clinical performance in clinical neurology. *Journal of Medical Education*, **39**, 802–5.

Byrne, P. & Long, B. (1976). *Doctors talking to patients*. London: HMSO.

Cole, S. & Bird, J. (2000). *The Medical Interview: The Three-Function Approach* (2nd edn.). St. Louis: Mosby.

Cushing, A. (1996). Editorial: communication skills. *Medical Education*, **30**, 316–8.

Dance, F. (1967). Toward a theory of human communication. In F. Dance (Ed.). *Human communication theory: original essays*, New York: Holt, Reinhart and Winston.

Department of Health. (2004). *The next steps – the future shape of foundation, specialist and general practice training programmes*. London: DoH.

Evans, B., Stanley, R., Burrows, G. & Sweet, B. (1989). Lecture and skills workshops as teaching formats in a history-taking skills course for medical students. *Medical Education*, **23**, 364–70.

General Medical Council (1993). *Tomorrow's doctors: recommendations on undergraduate medical education*. London: General Medical Council.

General Medical Council (2002). *Tomorrow's Doctors: Recommendations on Undergraduate Medical Education* (2nd edn.). London: General Medical Council.

Grow, G. (1996). Teaching learners to be self-directed. *Adult Education Quarterly*, **41**(3), 125–49.

Harden, R. & Gleeson, F. (1979). Assessment of clinical competence using an objective structured clinical examination (OSCE). *Medical Education*, **13**, 41–54.

Helman, C. (1981). Disease versus illness in general practice. *Journal Royal College of General Practitioners*, **31**, 548–62.

Heron, J. (1975). *A six category intervention analysis: human potential research project*. Guildford, UK: University of Surrey.

Hutchinson, L. (2003). Educational environment. In P. Cantillon, L. Hutchinson & D. Wood (Eds.). *ABC of learning and teaching in medicine* (pp. 39–41). London: BMJ Books.

Kaufman, D., Laidlaw, T. & MacLeod, H. (2000). Communication skills in Medical school: exposure, confidence and performance. *Academic Medicine*, **75**(Suppl.), s90–2.

Kidd, J., Patel, V., Peile, E. & Carter, Y. (2005). Clinical and communication skills. *British Medical Journal*, **330**, 374–5.

Knowles, M. S. (1990). *The Adult Learner: A Neglected Species* (4th edn.). Houston: Gulf Publishing.

Kolb, D. (1984). *Experiential learning: experience as the source of learning and development*. Englewood Cliffs, NJ: Prentice-Hall.

Kurtz, S., Silverman, J. & Draper, J. (2005). *Teaching and Learning Communication Skills in Medicine* (2nd edn.). Oxford: Radcliffe Medical Press.

Madan, A., Caruso, B., Lopes, J. & Gracely, E. (1998). Comparison of simulated patients and didactic methods of teaching HIV risk assessment to medical residents. *American Journal of Preventative Medicine*, **15**, 114–19.

Maguire, P. & Rutter, D. (1976). History taking for medical students. 1. Deficiencies in performance. *Lancet*, **2**, 556–8.

Maguire, P., Roe, P., Goldberg, D. *et al.* (1978). The value of feedback in teaching interviewing skills to medical students. *Psychological Medicine*, **8**, 695–704.

Maguire, P., Fairbairn, S. & Fletcher, C. (1986). Consultation skills of young doctors: I – Benefits of feedback training in interviewing as students persists. *British Medical Journal*, **292**, 1573–6.

Mc Whinney, I. (1989). The need for a transformed clinical method. In M. Stewart and D. Roter (Eds.). *Communicating with Patients* (2nd edn.). Newbury Park, CA: Sage Publications.

Miller, G. (1990). The assessment of clinical skills/competence/performance. *Academic Medicine*, **65**(Suppl.), S63–7.

Neighbour, R. (1987). The inner consultation: how to develop an effective and intuitive consulting style. Lancaster: MTP Press Ltd.

Nestel, D. & Kidd, J. (2004). Teaching and learning about written communications in a United Kingdom medical school. *Education for Health*, **17**, 27–34.

Pendelton, D., Schofield, T., Tate, P. & Havelock, P. (1984). *The consultation: an approach to learning and teaching*. Oxford: Oxford University Press.

Sedgewick, P. & Hall, A. (2003). Editorial: teaching medical students and doctors how to communicate risk. *British Medical Journal*, **7417**, 694.

Schon, D. (1983). *The reflective practitioner: how professionals think in action*. New York: Basic Books.

Silverman, J., Kurtz & Draper, J. (1996). The Calgary–Cambridge approach to communication skills teaching. 1. Agenda-led, outcome-based analysis of the consultation. *Education in General Practice*, **7**, 288–9.

Silverman, J., Kurtz, S. & Draper, J (2005). *Skills For Communicating with Patients* (2nd edn.). Oxford: Radcliffe Medical Press.

Stewart, I. & Jones, V. (1991). TA Today: *a new introduction to transactional analysis*. Reyworth, Leicestershire: Lifespace Publishing.

Stillman, P., Regan, M., Philbin, M. & Haley, H. (1990). Results of a survey on the use of standardised patients to teach and evaluate skills. *Academic Medicine*, **65**, 288–92.

Stott, N. & Davis, R. (1979). The exceptional potential in each primary care consultation. *Journal of the Royal College of General Practitioners*, **29**, 201–5.

Smee, S. (2003). Skilled based assessment. In P. Cantillon, L. Hutchinson & D. Wood (Eds.). (pp. 32–5). *ABC of learning and teaching in medicine*. London: BMJ Books.

www.businessballs.com/ consciouscompetencelearningmodel.htm

www.mmc.nhs.uk/pages/assessment

Written communication

Lorraine M. Noble

University College London

This chapter considers two domains of written communication in health care: (1) written information *for* patients, and (2) written information *about* patients.

Written information for patients

What is it for?

Written materials are used:

1. to provide information, for example, about investigations, screening, health promotion, diagnosis, prognosis, treatment and aftercare (e.g. discharge planning)
2. to aid decision-making, for example, about investigations, treatments or screening, or as part of a process to obtain a record of informed consent to treatment or a clinical trial
3. to encourage uptake of healthcare (e.g. investigations, screening, or treatment)
4. to train patients to communicate more effectively in consultations with healthcare professionals.

When is it needed?

Studies have consistently found that the majority of patients want to be kept informed about their condition and treatment, and that they want more information than they are typically provided (Audit Commission, 1993; Benbassat *et al.*, 1998). In addition, many studies have shown that patients have gaps in understanding and recall following face-to-face consultations (Ley, 1988). Investigators have concluded that written information plays an important role in routine care, either to provide a reminder of what has been discussed or more detailed information.

Supplementary written information is also useful when there are problems which create barriers to the effectiveness of face-to-face communication, for example:

i. when there are high levels of emotion (such as fear) or 'high stakes' consultations (e.g. serious illness)
ii. due to the complexity or quantity of information (e.g. presenting statistical information about treatment options, or lists of medication side effects)
iii. when communication is affected by patient factors (e.g. age, disability, cognitive impairments, language or cultural issues).

Research has indicated that patients are more passive in consultations than they intend to be, and that improving patient participation leads to improved outcomes (Harrington *et al.*, 2004). The evidence suggests that interventions to facilitate patients' communication with professionals could be beneficial in routine care. This complements current practice in the training of health professionals, who receive skills-based teaching on all aspects of their communication with patients (see 'Medical interviewing' and 'Teaching communication skills').

What form does it take?

Information is usually given in the form of leaflets (either prepared locally or by organizations such as charities, government departments or companies), notes written by the health professional for the patient, or copies of letters or reports. Interventions have included booklets, prompt sheets and guidance for patients to make their own notes either before or during a consultation.

Increasingly, information is available online. Recent developments such as interactive healthcare applications have made use of technological advances by providing electronic fora for peer information-exchange and decision-support (Eng *et al.*, 1999).

Do written materials address patients' needs?

Problems with the quality of information provided for patients has been noted for written materials and online resources (Audit Commission, 1993; Eysenbach *et al.*, 2002). Patient focus groups have reported a number of problems with written information, such as omission of topics of importance to them, over-optimism, avoidance of uncertainty and lack of detail (Coulter *et al.*, 1999). Feedback from patients is not commonly sought when written materials are being prepared, despite the use of techniques such as lists of 'frequently asked questions'.

The literature on patient leaflets was examined by Dixon-Woods (2001), who identified two discourses: a 'patient education' theme, where patients are perceived as passive recipients of information and healthcare in general; and a 'patient empowerment' theme, which takes into account patients' priorities and promotes active participation in decision-making. Dixon-Woods argued that the majority of patient leaflets serve a biomedical agenda, by aiming to save time in the consultation, reduce staff boredom and promote behaviour changes desired by professionals (such as compliance and a reduction in consulting rates). Other investigators have concluded that written materials may serve professional or commercial agendas, such as encouraging an uncritical approach to treatment (e.g. Kenny *et al.*, 1998).

The use of written materials in line with a biomedical approach tends to assume that the provision of information acts as an 'endpoint' in communication. For example, it is assumed that after reading the information given in a medication leaflet, the patient then proceeds to take the medication. In practice, written information forms part of a more dynamic process. For example, patients may seek out written information as a means of enabling them to prepare questions to ask healthcare providers (e.g. Ehrenberger, 2001).

Coulter *et al.* (1999) made a series of recommendations for the preparation of written materials, which included involving patients throughout the process, being honest about uncertainty and risks, and educating clinicians about techniques to promote shared decision-making.

Is written information effective?

Ley (1988) noted that, in order to be effective, written materials must be noticed, read, understood, believed and remembered. Much research has focused on determining whether materials are understandable and whether they aid recall. A number of tests have been developed to assess the understandability of leaflets, such as readability indices (e.g. the Flesch Reading Ease formula or the SMOG Index), word familiarity indices and tests of comprehension (such as the Cloze technique) (e.g. Beaver & Luker, 1997). In addition, controlled trials have considered the effectiveness of different formats and presentation styles (for example, verbal compared with pictorial or graphical presentation).

The unanimous conclusion from these studies has been that written materials for patients are not understandable by the majority of the population. Furthermore, there are concerns more generally about the level of functional health literacy, defined as the ability of people to read, understand and act on health information (Andrus & Roth, 2002). It has been noted that people with 'low functional health literacy' also have difficulty with oral communication, and are therefore doubly vulnerable to not getting the information they need from healthcare providers (Schillinger *et al.*, 2004).

The focus on readability, comprehension and recall has been criticized as a simplistic approach to assessing the quality and utility of written communications, as it implies that problems with effectiveness are due to 'patient incompetence' (e.g. low literacy and forgetfulness), rather than the appropriateness of the information for the individual (Dixon-Woods, 2001). Conclusions from surveys of written materials inevitably recommend that information is kept short and simple, but this contradicts the consistent finding that patients want more detailed information (e.g. Coulter *et al.*, 1999).

Indices of effectiveness have varied, depending on researchers' conceptions of the purpose of written materials. Investigators have examined the effects of written information on outcomes including knowledge and recall; uptake of screening; anxiety; satisfaction; intensity of pain; appropriate prescription of medication; compliance with treatment plans; and promotion of an active role in decision-making (e.g. Johnson *et al.*, 2003; Miaskowski *et al.*, 2004; Davison *et al.*, 1999). The consistent finding from this literature is that written information in addition to normal care is superior to normal care. In addition, in studies where no positive effect on observable outcomes was reported (e.g. on knowledge or recall), investigators have noted that patients still appreciated being given written information.

Written materials used to facilitate patients' communication with professionals have mainly been used to encourage patients to identify and verbalize their requests, problems and concerns. Whilst benefits in outcomes, such as patient question-asking, have been reported, generally the evidence indicates that written interventions are not as effective as interventions based on face-to-face coaching (Harrington *et al.*, 2004). This concurs with findings suggesting that other media can be equally or more effective in providing information. For example, studies have indicated that giving patients an audiotape of their consultation improves recall and decreases the need for repetition of information in subsequent consultations (e.g. Bruera *et al.*, 1999).

Do patients want written communication?

The consensus from the literature is that patients do want written information, but that they prefer information to be given by a person (e.g. Maly *et al.*, 2003; Wald *et al.*, 2003). Written information is perceived as a helpful addition to, but not as a substitute for, a face-to-face consultation with a health professional. This is partly explainable from the point of view of information flow: consultations are interactive, thus increasing the likelihood that information can be tailored to patients' needs. However, a consultation provides not only information, but a whole package of care, including a sense of reassurance and trust in a professional–patient relationship. That said, a recent initiative in Sweden giving free access to online consultations with a doctor was also found to be popular, with patients valuing the convenience and anonymity afforded (Umefjord *et al.*, 2003).

Individual differences have been noted in whether people actively seek written information (for example, on the Internet) or only access sources when specifically directed by health professionals. Overall, the literature suggests that there is no 'one-size-fits-all' model, i.e. that it is naïve to assume that a leaflet can be designed which meets the needs of all patients in a target population. Rather, written information should be given as part of a package which is tailored to the individual. Ideally, the health professional should go through written materials with the patient (Kenny *et al.*, 1998). Note that this approach does not assume that the aim of providing written information is to save time.

Is written communication based on psychological theories?

Much research has focussed on developing pamphlets, which are not theoretically driven, but rather created in response to a perceived clinical need to provide information and improve compliance. Although an underlying approach to the professional–patient relationship (e.g. biomedical, biopsychosocial, patient-centred) may be inferred from their content, these materials tend not to be tested for effectiveness using a psychological model.

However, some investigators have produced written materials (which include computer- and Web-based materials), specifically based on theories such as the Health Belief Model, the Transtheoretical Model, or message-framing (such as the use of 'threat appeals') (e.g. McKay *et al.*, 2004). Written materials which form part of an intervention package, such as self-management programmes, are more likely to be theoretically-driven, as such interventions have been routinely based on models such as

Social Cognitive Theory or Self-Regulation Theory (see 'Self-management' and 'Self-efficacy and health behaviour').

Written information about patients

What form does it take?

Letters, reports, medical notes, medication charts, as well as informal notes (known as 'scraps') which do not form a part of the patient's record, all have a significant role in the communication of information and delivery of care.

Is it good enough?

Problems with written communications result from:

a. poor quality of information, for example, incomplete or inaccurate information
b. systems failures in the transmission of information
c. differences of opinion among professional groups about what is important to include in the communication
d. alternative channels of communication being used.

Quality of care is affected by problems with written communication. Considerable attention has focused on medication errors (e.g. Benjamin, 2003), probably due to the salience of the written record in this aspect of care and ease of comparison with prescribing standards. However, close examination of any situation involving written communication can reveal deficiencies with implications for quality of care. For example, one study found that surgeons misunderstood pathologists' reports 30% of the time (Powsner et al., 2000).

Increasingly, written communication skills are being taught and assessed in undergraduate and postgraduate medicine. However, this component of training curricula is relatively new and needs to include information about systems issues and multi-disciplinary communication in addition to training in medical record-keeping.

Do health professionals want written communication?

Whilst written communication is required in many aspects of service delivery, in practice it may be superseded by other forms of communication, or may play a smaller role than intended. Many studies have shown that professionals prefer oral communication (either face-to-face or by telephone), supplemented by written communication (e.g. Forrest et al., 2000; Blankenship et al., 1999). Furthermore, there is evidence that oral inter-professional communication can be more effective in achieving a result (Martin et al., 2003).

As perceptions of the nature of the doctor–patient relationship have changed, there has been a corresponding attitudinal shift regarding medical record-keeping. Until relatively recently, there was an accepted stereotype of a 'heartsink' patient, who typically had a 'fat file' or who brought a list of questions. It is now more accepted for patients to keep a diary or record of symptoms to bring to a consultation, although there remains a variable response to patients who bring written information to discuss or a list of questions.

How much are patients involved?

The increasing involvement of patients in their own care has been supported by a number of government initiatives regarding written communication, particularly changes to the law regarding patients' access to their own medical records. The right of access of persons to data about themselves has been established in the UK in the Access to Health Records Act 1990 and Data Protection Act 1998. Furthermore, the recent National Health Service Plan (Department of Health, 2000) directed that from April 2004, patients should routinely be offered copies of letters about themselves. However, professional reservations regarding patients' access to their own records have been repeated in the more recent debate about access to letters (White, 2004).

There have been many trials of patient-held records, particularly in services for cancer, antenatal and mental health care. However, it is likely that technological advances will supersede these initiatives. Current developments in electronic patient records (EPR) are expected in time to allow patients to access information held about themselves by all healthcare providers. This technology may include patient-held 'smart cards'.

Patients have the right, protected by law, to decide whether or not to have any given medical intervention, which includes investigations, treatment, screening or research. A written record of informed consent is expected in certain situations, for example, when the intervention is complex, involves significant risks, or is part of a research programme (Department of Health, 2002) (see 'Informed consent'). The 'consent form' documents the discussion with the patient. Professional guidelines note that obtaining consent is not an isolated event, but involves a continuing dialogue, and that a signed consent form is not sufficient evidence that a patient has given informed consent. However, problems with the process of obtaining informed consent have been reported. For example, studies have found that a third of patients do not understand the purpose of the consent form, and that the majority of patients sign the form without reading it (Lavelle-Jones et al., 1993; Olver et al., 1995).

A further area in which patients have been involved in preparing written documentation is advanced care planning. This takes place when a patient is expected at some future point to become incapacitated to the extent of being unable to express their wishes regarding treatment. In preparation for this, a patient's wishes may be documented in an advance directive (also known as a 'living will'). However, as with informed consent, there is a common misconception that the purpose of advanced care planning is to make a written document. In addition, differences of opinion between professionals and patients about the purpose of advanced care planning have been identified. Investigators have found that patients view it as more of a social process, involving their relatives, and with a wider remit than choosing among treatment options (e.g. preparing for death) (Singer et al., 1998). Often patients regard the completion of a written document as unnecessary. Furthermore, there is evidence that increasing documentation of advance directives has not resulted in an increase in care which is consistent with patients' preferences (Covinsky et al., 2000).

A specific aspect of advanced care planning which has caused much controversy is the documentation of 'do not resuscitate' (DNR) orders. A DNR order is written into the patient's medical notes to record the decision that interventions to attempt to sustain life should not be conducted (e.g. cardio-pulmonary resuscitation, CPR, in the event of heart failure). Traditionally, there has been considerable variability in whether DNR orders have been discussed with patients at all, and there remains considerable debate about the involvement of patients in this process (Biegler, 2003; Cantor et al., 2003).

Conclusions

Written communication plays an important role in many aspects of health care, but it is best viewed as one part of a dynamic process involving other channels of information flow. The future of written information is electronic (e.g. online resources, electronic patient records) which should enable easier access to information and is intended to improve patients' involvement in their own care. However, it is important to remember that both patients and professionals prefer information to be given by a person.

REFERENCES

Access to Health Records Act (1990). London: HMSO.

Andrus, M. R. & Roth, M. T. (2002). Health literacy: a review. *Pharmacotherapy*, **22**, 282–302.

Audit Commission (1993). *What seems to be the matter: communication between hospitals and patients*. London: HMSO.

Beaver, K. & Luker, K. (1997). Readability of patient information booklets for women with breast cancer. *Patient Education and Counseling*, **31**, 95–102.

Benbassat, J., Pilpel, D. & Tidhar, M. (1998). Patients' preferences for participation in clinical decision making: a review of published surveys. *Behavioral Medicine*, **24**, 81–8.

Benjamin, D. M. (2003). Reducing medication errors and increasing patient safety: case studies in clinical pharmacology. *Journal of Clinical Pharmacology*, **43**, 768–83.

Biegler, P. (2003). Should patient consent be required to write a do not resuscitate order? *Journal of Medical Ethics*, **29**, 359–63.

Blankenship, J. C., Menapace, F. J., Fox, L. S. & Frey, C. M. (1999). Telephone reporting of the results of cardiac procedures: feasibility and primary care physician preferences. *American Journal of Medicine*, **106**, 521–6.

Bruera, E., Pituskin, E., Calder, K., Neumann, C. M. & Hanson, J. (1999). The addition of an audiocassette recording of a consultation to written recommendations for patients with advanced cancer: a randomized, controlled trial. *Cancer*, **86**, 2420–5.

Cantor, M. D., Braddock, C. H. III, Derse, A. R. *et al.* (2003). Do not resuscitate orders and medical futility. *Archieves of Internal Medicine*, **163**, 2689–94.

Coulter, A., Entwhistle, V. & Gilbert, D. (1999). Sharing decisions with patients: is the information good enough? *British Medical Journal*, **318**, 318–22.

Covinsky, K. E., Fuller, J. D., Yaffe, K. *et al.* (2000). Communication and decision-making in seriously ill patients: findings of the SUPPORT project. The study to understand prognoses and preferences for outcomes and risks of treatments. *Journal of the American Geriatrics Society*, **48**(Suppl. 5), S187–93.

Data Protection Act (1998). London: The Stationery Office.

Davison, B. J., Kirk, P., Degner, L. F. & Hassard, T. H. (1999). Information and patient participation in screening for prostate cancer. *Patient Education and Counseling*, **37**, 255–63.

Department of Health (2000). *The NHS Plan*. London: The Stationery Office.

Department of Health (2002). *Good practice in consent implementation guide: consent to examination or treatment*. London: Department of Health.

Dixon-Woods, M. (2001). Writing wrongs? An analysis of published discourses about the use of patient information leaflets. *Social Science and Medicine*, **52**, 1417–32.

Ehrenberger, H. E. (2001). Cancer clinical trial patients in the information age: a pilot study. *Cancer Practice*, **9**, 191–7.

Eng, T. R., Gustafson, D. H., Henderson, J., Jimison, H. & Patrick, K. (1999). Introduction to evaluation of interactive health communication applications. Science Panel on interactive communication and health. *American Journal of Preventative Medicine*, **16**, 10–15.

Eysenbach, G., Powell, J., Kuss, O. & Sa, E. R. (2002). Empirical studies assessing the quality of health information for consumers on the world wide web: a systematic review. *Journal of the American Medical Association*, **287**, 2691–700.

Forrest, C. B., Glade, G. B., Baker, A. E. *et al.* (2000). Coordination of specialty referrals and physician satisfaction with referral care. *Archives of Pediatrics and Adolescent Medicine*, **154**, 499–506.

Harrington, J., Noble, L. M. & Newman, S. P. (2004). Improving patients' communication with doctors: a systematic review of intervention studies. *Patient Education and Counseling*, **52**, 7–16.

Johnson, A., Sandford, J. & Tyndall, J. (2003). Written and verbal information versus verbal information only for patients being discharged from acute hospital settings to home. *Cochrane Database of Systematic Reviews*, Issue 4, Art. no. CD003716.

Kenny, T., Wilson, R. G., Purves, I. N. *et al.* (1998). A PIL for every ill? Patient information leaflets (PILs): a review of past, present and future use. *Family Practice*, **15**, 471–9.

Lavelle-Jones, C., Byrne, D. J., Rice, P. & Cuschieri, A. (1993). Factors affecting quality of informed consent. *British Medical Journal*, **306**, 885–90.

Ley, P. (1988). *Communicating with patients*. London: Chapman & Hall.

Maly, R. C., Leake, B. & Silliman, R. A. (2003). Health care disparities in older patients with breast carcinoma: informational support from physicians. *Cancer*, **97**, 1517–27.

Martin, K., Carter, L., Balciunas, D. *et al.* (2003). The impact of verbal communication on physician prescribing patterns in hospitalized patients with diabetes. *Diabetes Educator*, **29**, 827–36.

McKay, D. L., Berkowitz, J. M., Blumberg, J. B. & Goldberg, J. P. (2004). Communicating cardiovascular disease risk due to elevated homocysteine levels: using the EPPM to develop print materials. *Health Education and Behavior*, **31**, 355–71.

Miaskowski, C., Dodd, M., West, C. *et al.* (2004). Randomized clinical trial of the effectiveness of a self-care intervention to improve cancer pain management. *Journal of Clinical Oncology*, **22**, 1713–20.

Olver, I. N., Turrell, S. J., Olszewski, N. A. & Willson, K. J. (1995). Impact of an information and consent form on patients having chemotherapy. *Medical Journal of Australia*, **162**, 82–3.

Powsner, S. M., Costa, J. & Homer, R. J. (2000). Clinicians are from Mars and pathologists are from Venus. *Archives of Pathology and Laboratory Medicine*, **124**, 1040–6.

Schillinger, D., Bindman, A., Wang, F., Stewart, A. & Piette, J. (2004). Functional health literacy and the quality of physician–patient communication among diabetes patients. *Patient Education and Counseling*, **52**, 315–23.

Singer, P. A., Martin, D. K., Lavery, J. V. *et al.* (1998). Reconceptualizing advance care planning from the patient's perspective. *Archives of Internal Medicine*, **158**, 879–84.

Umefjord, G., Petersson, G. & Hamberg, K. (2003). Reasons for consulting a doctor on the Internet: web survey of users of an ask the doctor service. *Journal of Medical Internet Research*, **5**, Article e26.

Wald, C., Fahy, M., Walker, Z. & Livingstone, G. (2003). What to tell dimensia caregivers: the rule of threes. *International Journal of Geriatric Psychiatry*, **18**, 313–17.

White, P. (2004) Copying referral letters to patients: prepare for change. *Patient Education and Counseling*, **54**, 159–61.

Part II

Medical topics

Abortion

Pauline Slade

University of Sheffield

Abortion

Although induced and spontaneous abortion both involve the death of a fetus there are important differences in these experiences. In the former, pregnancy ends through an individual's choice while the latter is not because of, but often in spite of, the woman's and professionals' best efforts to save the baby. Women who have miscarried are often distressed by staff usage of the term 'spontaneous' abortion as this carries an unpleasant connotation and so this will be referred to as 'miscarriage' in this chapter.

Miscarriage

Up to 20% of recognized pregnancies end in miscarriage, defined as a pregnancy loss up to 24 weeks of gestation. Studies suggest that anxiety symptoms may be elevated for many months afterwards and a proportion of women may show depressive symptoms (Geller et al., 2004). Miscarriage has been compared to bereavement but the process of coping may be complicated by the abstract nature of the loss and the absence of memories of an individual. The loss is often hidden as many women will not have shared the news of their pregnancy at such an early stage and the support that unpleasant events often generates, may be absent. Our society lacks ritual acknowledgement of miscarriage and the prevailing view is often exemplified by the phrase 'it was for the best'. A further aspect that is increasingly recognized is that miscarriage can be considered as a potentially traumatic experience. It clearly involves loss of life, and often fear, pain and loss of blood (Lee & Slade, 1996). Many women do report elements of involuntary reliving of aspects of the experience and attempts to avoid reminders. The woman may also subsequently have fears about her future fertility and there is evidence that anxiety symptoms are elevated in subsequent pregnancies even though the risk of miscarriage is not itself increased (Geller et al., 2004). The impact on the relationship between the expectant parents is increasingly recognized (Swanson et al., 2003). The evidence is generally that impact on the male partner is less significant than for the woman although this is disputed by Conway and Russell (2000). There is a need, however to consider the partner's loss in its own right. Earlier work has tended to consider only the potential support he could provide to the woman.

Whilst demographic factors or aspects of the event have been suggested as being linked to the impact of miscarriage it is recognized that it is the personal meaning to the individual that is primarily important. Viewing this in a stress and coping framework (Lazarus & Folkman, 1994) is probably most useful. In this context, emotional responses are influenced by the appraisal of the event in terms of its meaning, which is potentially balanced by the appraisal of coping in terms of factors such as individual resources and social support from others (see 'Stress and health').

Coping is also likely to be influenced by the quality of care provided. For medical and nursing staff, miscarriage can be viewed as a routine and/or trivial event. Such a mismatch of perceptions between the staff and patients can lead to care being experienced as insensitive (Evans et al., 2002). One aspect of care that seems to be particularly important is that women should be given the news about viability or non-viability of their pregnancy as soon as this is available, that is at the scan, rather than after a protracted wait. They should be given the news in circumstances of privacy, in a sensitive manner and also provided with an opportunity to talk with appropriately trained staff about their feelings and concerns (see 'Breaking bad news'). In addition, women express a need for information about potential physical and emotional consequences together with an opportunity to discuss these issues at a follow-up appointment two to three weeks after the event. There is evidence that psychological counselling in combination with medical follow-up is potentially beneficial: the value of such services is now established (Nickevic, 2003) although unfortunately not routinely available.

It is also important to recognize that miscarriage should not just be considered as 'a pathway to pathology'. Qualitative studies have identified positive growth experiences in terms of impact on the couple's relationship, and revaluation of life values and goals that may facilitate wellbeing (Maker & Ogden, 2003).

Whilst there is no evidence to suggest that low mood contributes to the occurrence of first miscarriage (Nelson et al., 2003), there are tentative suggestions that this may increase risk in those with recurrent abortion (Sugiura-Ogasawara et al., 2002). High emotional distress in the 1% of women who may experience three or more miscarriages has been linked to cognitive processes such as degree of investment in the parenting role and low levels of non-child-related positive thoughts (McGee et al., 2003). These factors lead to the potential for cognition-focused interventions should the impact be severe, although few intervention studies are available.

Induced abortions

Countries differ in the legal limit for induced abortion. The legal situation in Britain is now governed by the 1990 amendment of the 1967 Abortion Act. This provides an upper time limit of 24 weeks gestation for most abortions, but there is no time limit if there is a risk to the life of the mother, risk of grave permanent injury or serious fetal handicap. Termination takes place within an evolving socio-political context. The rate of termination of pregnancy in the UK has been rising and there is particular concern about the number of women undergoing repeat terminations. There is also debate about the capacities of the fetus, its ability to feel pain and consequent unease about the paradox of babies born within the window for termination surviving through technological developments in neonatal intensive care. Alongside these factors within the UK there is evidence that social attitudes towards abortion in general have become more liberal between 1990 and 2000, possibly as its use has become more commonplace (Scott, 1998). The social acceptability and indeed the legality of abortion varies considerably within different societies. It is likely that the emotional consequences of the process may be significantly influenced by cultural values.

In terms of the processes involved, pregnancies of less than 13 weeks (the first trimester of pregnancy) may be terminated via surgical or medical means. The former typically involves a general anaesthetic and evacuation of the contents of the womb by suction. The latter involves the administration of prostaglandins to trigger contractions of the uterus. In medical abortion, the woman is conscious throughout, may see the fetus and the process may be protracted.

At later stages of pregnancy the woman is also likely to involve a hormonally induced labour. Many of the later induced abortions occur because of detection of abnormality in the fetus through the use of blood tests and amniocentesis. As the motivation is different this may be an important sub-group in terms of psychological issues raised.

The literature suggests that the emotional consequences of induced abortion in the first trimester in general are unremarkable, with many women, at least initially, showing a sense of relief. Bradshaw and Slade (2003) in a review of the area suggest that after recognition of the pregnancy and prior to the termination, distress, particularly in the form of anxiety, is high. However, there is a dramatic reduction of distress post termination and this seems to be maintained in the longer term. It is perhaps important to note that follow-ups beyond a year are rare and participation rates rather poor. Whilst follow-ups of cohorts have not indicated evidence of emotional distress, there have been criticisms that the more distressed may absent themselves from studies, thereby biasing findings. It appears to be important that the woman should feel that she has made the decision herself and that she has not been coerced by partner or parent. Although it has been hypothesized that medical terminations may be experienced as more traumatic because of conscious awareness, the level of exposure to blood and pain and the longer duration of the process, there is little evidence to support this notion (Slade *et al.*, 1998). It does seem that there may be a sub-sample of women who react to the experience of termination of pregnancy with more adverse consequences and there is an indication that the rate of psychiatric admission which is recognized to be high in the postnatal period is much higher post termination. (Reardon *et al.*, 2003)

As with miscarriage, there are issues about the quality of care for women undergoing induced abortions. Censorious attitudes or insensitive care from staff may enhance guilt and may negatively affect emotional outcome. It is important that staff involved in such care provision examine their own attitudes and values and are aware of their own potential for influencing adjustment in a positive or negative way (Slade *et al.*, 2001). As with the miscarriage literature, the body of published work has been criticized for being negative in focus and failing to investigate potential benefits (Boyle, 1997).

In summary, whilst the physical processes of miscarriage and induced abortion have some similarities, the psychological experience and implications may be very different. Other commonalities concern the need to consider not just the implications for the woman but also her partner, the key role of staff attitudes in promoting positive adjustment and possible impact in future pregnancy. Finally, such experiences should not just be considered as pathways to pathology and the potential for positive effect has perhaps received less attention than required.

(See also 'Screening: antenatal, pregnancy and childbirth', and 'Foetal wellbeing'.)

REFERENCES

Boyle, M. (1997). *Rethinking abortion*. London, UK: Routledge.

Bradshaw, Z. & Slade, P. (2003). The impact of termination of pregnancy on emotions and relationships. *Clinical Psychology Review*, **23**, 929–58.

Conway, K. & Russell, G. (2000). Couples' grief experience and support in the aftermath of miscarriage. *British Journal of Medical Psychology*, **73**, 531–45.

Evans, L., Lloyd, D., Considine, R. & Hancock, L. (2002). Contrasting views of staff and patients regarding psychosocial care for Australian women who miscarry: a hospital study. *Australian and New Zealand Journal of Obstetrics and Gynaecology*, **42**, 155–60.

Geller, P. A., Kerns, D. & Klier, C. M. (2004). Anxiety following miscarriage and the subsequent future pregnancy: a review of literature and future directions. *Journal of Psychosomatic Research*, **56**, 35–45.

Lazarus, R. & Folkman, S. (1994). *Stress appraisal and coping*. New York: Springer.

Lee, C. & Slade, P. (1996). Miscarriage as a traumatic event – a review of the literature and new implications for treatment. *Journal Psychosomatic Research*, **40**, 235–44.

Magee, P. C., MacLeod, A. K., Tata, P. & Regan, L. (2003). Psychological distress in recurrent miscarriage: the role of prospective thinking and role and goal investment. *Journal of Reproductive and Infant Psychology*, **21**, 35–47.

Maker, C. & Ogden, J. (2003). The miscarriage experience: more than just a trigger to psychological morbidity? *Psychology and Health*, **18**, 403–15.

Nelson, D. B., McMahon, K., Joffe, M. & Brensinger, C. (2003). The effect of depressive symptoms and optimism on the risk of spontaneous abortion. *Journal of Women's Health and Gender Based Medicine*, **12**, 569–76.

Nikcevic, A. V. (2003). Development and evaluation of a miscarriage follow up clinic. *Journal of Reproductive and Infant Psychology*, **21**, 207–17.

Reardon, D. C., Couge, J. R., Rue, V. M. et al. (2003). Psychiatric admission of low income women following abortion and childbirth. *Canadian Medical Association Journal*, **168**, 1253–6.

Scott, J. (1998). Generation changes in attitudes to abortion: a cross-national comparison. *European Sociological Review*, **14**, 177–90.

Slade, P., Heke, S., Fletcher, J. & Stewart, P. (1998). A comparison of medical and surgical termination of pregnancy: choice, emotional impact and satisfaction with care. *British Journal of Obstetrics and Gynaecology*, **105**, 1288–95.

Slade, P., Heke, S., Fletcher, J. & Stewart, P. (2001). Termination of pregnancy; patients' perceptions of care. *British Journal of*

Family Planning and Reproductive Health Care, **27**, 72–7.

Surgiara-Ogasawara, M., Furukawa, T., Nakanu, Y. *et al.* (2002). Depression as potential causal factor subsequent to

miscarriage in recurrent spontaneous abortion. *Human Reproduction*, **17**, 2580–4.

Swanson, K. M., Karmali, Z. A., Powell, S. H. & Pulvemaker, F. (2003). Miscarriage effects on couples' interpersonal and

sexual relationships during the first year after loss: women's perceptions. *Psychosomatic Medicine*, **65**, 902–10.

Accidents and unintentional injuries

Robert G. Frank and Andrea M. Lee

University of Florida

Injury is a leading cause of death and disability for America's young adults and children. It is the leading cause of death for those from ages 1 to 44 (Mokdad *et al.*, 2004) and is the fifth leading cause of death for all Americans (Centers for Disease Control and Prevention, 2001). Injuries are associated with higher treatment costs than the other three leading causes of death. Traffic accidents are the leading cause of severe brain injury, as well as most paraplegic and quadraplegic cases (Spielberger & Frank, 1992).

For many years, injuries were viewed as 'accidents' that were inevitable and not responsive to prevention efforts. Injury events tended to be attributed to human error or misaction; individuals died or were injured due to driving while intoxicated or a leg was broken when someone failed to watch their step. This psychological model of injury was related to the emergence of the concept of 'accident-proneness' during the 1930s and 1940s. In this approach, accidents occurred to individuals as a function of unconscious wishes or desires (Waller, 1994).

Injury events were also attributed to human error or misaction because they often involved relatively rare events that were perceived as unpredictable. Many data systems tended to record only 'single' causes of injury, negating the idea that a crash may occur both because the driver is impaired by alcohol and because the roadway geometry at the crash location is inadequate (Waller, 1994). Rarely did anyone examine the overall frequency of injuries to determine if higher risk existed under certain circumstances. For example, lacking statistics, the crash risk at a particular bend in a roadway may go unrecognized. Only when examined will the 1 per 250 000 vehicle risk achievable with improved roadway design, compared with the existing crash risk of 1 per 50 000, be recognized (Waller, 1994).

Models of injury control

In 1959, James J. Gibson, an experimental psychologist, recognized that injury was caused by energy interchange which occurred at the moment of, and subsequent to, the incident. Gibson suggested the most effective method of classifying sources of energy is the form of the physical energy involved (Rosenberg & Fenley, 1992). Gibson's observation became the lifework of Dr William Haddon, Jr, an

engineer and public health physician. Haddon narrowed the potential agents to five forms of physical energy: kinetic, chemical, thermo, electrical and radiation. Haddon also recognized 'negative agents' for injuries produced by the absence of critical elements such as oxygen or heat. Haddon labelled these agents as vectors and the vehicles as energy forms. He divided injuries into three phases: (i) a preinjury; (ii) a very brief injury phase; and (iii) a postinjury phase.

During the preinjury phase, the control of the energy source is lost. The preinjury phase includes everything that determines whether a crash will occur (e.g. driver ability, vehicle functioning, seat belt usage). The injury phase typically lasts less than a second and transfers energy to the individual, thereby causing damage. The postinjury phase determines whether the injuries and consequences could be reduced with subsequent prevention of further disability (e.g. speed, inefficiency of first responders). During the postinjury phase, attempts are made to retain physiological homeostasis and repair damage. Haddon also observed that injuries can often be prevented by attending to the vector (Rosenberg & Fenley, 1992; Waller, 1994).

Using this model, Haddon developed an innovative plan to intervene upon injury events by: (i) preventing or limiting energy build-up; (ii) controlling the circumstances of energy to prevent unlimited release; (iii) modifying the energy in transfer phase to limit damage; and (iv) improving emergency, acute and rehabilitative care to affect recovery (Waller, 1994).

Haddon's model led to the development of the Haddon Matrix. Haddon's 'phase-factor matrix' is actually a series of matrices developed for different purposes. The Haddon Matrix emphasizes the preventive value of the epidemiological approach to injury control. In the matrix, the host, agent (vector) and environment are seen as factors that interact over time to cause injury.

Haddon's work led to the recognition that, during each of the three phases, preinjury, injury and postinjury, injury likelihood can be reduced by changes in the driver (in the case of vehicular injury), the agent (or vehicle), or the environment. Previous models of injury prevention have emphasized psychological factors, thereby allowing only one intervention point. In contrast, the Haddon Matrix creates nine cells, each of which offers an opportunity for intervention. While behaviour is undeniably an important factor in injury causation, the Haddon Matrix demonstrates that it is only one of several areas where intervention may be effective. In determining the appropriate intervention, it is important to recognize that injury prevention is not necessarily based upon the most obvious cause of contributing factors. Interventions may occur at a number of points in the chain of events that can lead to injury (Williams & Lund, 1992). Adoption of an energy control strategy to injury prevention led to discarding the term 'accident'. The connotation of chance, fate and unexpectedness has been replaced by descriptions of injuries and physical and chemical injuries involved (Williams & Lund, 1992).

Psychological factors and injury control

Human behaviour remains an important factor in injury control. This view has been reinforced in recent years as psychologists and others have begun to contribute to our understanding of the behavioural and social causes. Within the field of injury prevention, a dialectic has developed between proponents of individually directed interventions and those who support public health models (Frank et al., 1992). These approaches to prevention have been characterized as active versus passive or individual versus population. Active individual injury prevention requires action by the individual to reduce risk (e.g. wearing a seat belt, using a motorcycle helmet, exercising or maintaining proper diet). Active or individual approaches reflect the legacy of health psychology, with its emphasis upon individuals assuming responsibility for their own behaviour (Frank et al., 1992).

The passive intervention model, derived from public health approaches, emphasizes altering health behaviours at the population level (Frank et al., 1992). In this approach, intervention is designed to automatically affect all individuals. Passive intervention models are viewed as most effective because they avoid difficulties associated with individuals making consecutive decisions regarding health and safety behaviours. Examples of the passive or population approach include automatic seat belts, mandatory air bags, locking systems to prevent drunken driving and air safety restraints.

Most often, active and passive approaches have been viewed as mutually exclusive. Others have suggested that active and passive approaches to injury reflect a continuum (Frank et al., 1992). Models of health psychology have included a broader emphasis upon the health of communities (Winett et al., 1989). Roberts (1987) has suggested that a multilevel approach is the most effective approach to injury control. In this approach, the active individual model congruent with health psychology is viewed as one end of a continuum, while the passive approach that matches public health models anchors the other end of the continuum.

Recently, a health promotion approach has been recognized as useful to injury prevention (Sleet et al., 2004). Health promotion, by definition, involves targeting behaviours, environments and policies in the prevention of injury (see 'Health promotion'). The immediate goals of health promotion strategies with regard to injury prevention are to reduce individual risk factors, minimize exposure to hazards in the environment and remove unsafe products. These goals are achieved by individual and community efforts through education, social and organizational change, and public policy, legislation and enforcement (Sleet et al., 2004).

In the area of health education, the PRECEDE model (Predisposing, Reinforcing, and Enabling Causes in Educational Diagnosis and Evaluation) was developed for planning education programmes (Fee et al., 2000). In this model, prevention strategies are dictated by three sets of factors: predisposing factors (individual characteristics), enabling factors (aspects of the environment) and reinforcing factors (rewards or punishment of behaviour). Once prevention strategies are implemented, evaluation of the prescribed programme is an integral part of the PRECEDE model (Fee et al., 2000).

Although many opportunities exist for psychologists to be involved in the community approach to prevention of injury, the traditional niche occupied by health psychologists with its emphasis upon the individual has most often been the focus of the profession. Because injury most often affects individuals under the age of 24, a disproportionate emphasis has been placed upon injury prevention among children and adolescents.

The prevention of childhood injuries continues to be a major research area (Peterson & Roberts, 1992). It is now clear that the parents whose children are most at risk (poor, under-educated, disturbed, or from single parent families) are least likely to utilize safety precautions. Children most at risk are preschoolers older than 2.5 years and children who display difficult behaviours are at higher risk than other children (Dal Santo et al., 2004). Many parents do not appreciate, or are indifferent to, factors that may contribute to injury. Often, even middle-class parents lack a strong sense of risk factors for their children. Children are rarely taught safety behaviours (Peterson & Roberts, 1992). Too often, injury prevention is based upon single presentations of safety material in classrooms. Peterson and Roberts (1992) observed that educators would never consider teaching maths by working arithmetic problems before children for one hour, or teaching spelling by having the teacher discuss spelling. These methods often serve as a safety curriculum in schools. Parents greatly over-estimate their children's safety knowledge, and when asked where the child acquired these presumed skills, parents most frequently cite visits of police or fire officials to the class (Peterson & Roberts, 1992).

Injury prevention in children includes a wide variety of interventions. Injury prevention methods have been classified according to level: national and state level, community level, family level, caregiver and child level initiatives (Damashek & Peterson, 2002). As has been the case with adult and adolescent populations, the two predominant methods have been legislation and education. Legislative changes have often been directed at product manufacturers. In contrast, educational efforts are most often directed at children's caregivers and may be direct, utilizing weak contingencies (such as suggestion that a low probability negative event may be prevented) or immediate rewards (such as a lottery ticket or prize to a child). In general, the stronger the contingency, the more effective the intervention (Peterson & Roberts, 1992).

The most frequently cited legislative success, aimed directly at the injury vector, was a 1973 mandate requiring child-resistant packaging and limiting the amount of a drug contained in any one package (Peterson & Roberts, 1992). Although legislation can be very successful, the large number of products known to cause injury to children are inadequately controlled for a variety of reasons. Many known hazards to children, such as guns, have political connotations making legislation problematic in some countries. In other cases, items directly marketed to children are hazardous, but have not been prohibited. For example, as many as 42% of accidental injuries to children under one year of age may be due to 'baby walkers' (Peterson & Roberts, 1992) which offer no developmental advantage to children. Similarly, under-inflated or uninflated balloons also pose a high risk to small children. Failure to regulate these items may stem from the perception that injury is as much a function of poor parental supervision as it is of the product alone. Thus, regulation may not be sufficient.

Persuasion to behave differently through mass media campaigns, enhanced product availability and social sanctions may rival legislative change. For example, the first child restraint law in Tennessee was accompanied by extensive publicity and media coverage. The eventual success of this legislation may reflect the publicity as much as the legislation (Peterson & Roberts, 1992).

Efforts to use education to prevent injury have yielded an uneven history. Most successful have been recent programmes that target caregivers with simple interventions requiring minimal consumer effort. When safety products are freely available, or available at a reduced cost in exchange for safety behaviour, education is effective. For example, smoke detectors, lightweight rails to guard windows, or programmes providing individualized attention rewards for decreasing hazards have all been shown to be highly effective (Peterson & Roberts, 1992). How mass media tends to influence children's safety has rarely been evaluated. Programmes aimed directly at children have had some success (Peterson, 1989). Young children can successfully learn a variety of skills ranging from bicycle safety, management of small emergencies like house fires and serious cuts, to the preparation of safe snacks, if provided with intensive modelling, rehearsal and explanation of clear, positive consequences (Peterson, 1989).

Because adolescence is a time of particular risk for injury, as well as the period when many patterns of behaviour are established, it has been a developmental epoch that has been the target of many intervention efforts (see 'Adolescent lifestyle'). Although it is a critical developmental period for the consolidation of cognitions, behaviour and learning, many common adolescent beliefs make intervention particularly problematic. Teens have strong beliefs of personal immortality and invulnerability. Adolescence is a period of increased testing of autonomy and growing identification with peers. Risky behaviours are common, and peer pressure may increase risk-taking activities. Even when the risk of injury is understood, avoiding danger may be less important than obtaining peer approval. Attempts by adults to minimize this behaviour may simply increase peer pressure to engage in such activities (Frank *et al.*, 1992).

The highest rate of fatalities and injuries in traffic crashes is among young men from ages 15 to 24 years (Centers for Disease Control and Prevention, 2001). Because young drivers are involved in the disproportionate number of traffic injuries and fatalities, many prevention programmes have focused on altering the behaviour of the driver. The most common example of these are driver education programmes which have been implemented throughout high schools in the United States. Unfortunately, these educational programmes, at best, have had limited success. There is no evidence that driver education programmes result in a reduction of the number of crashes (Robertson, 1986).

An alternative approach designed to increase safe behaviours among adolescents utilizes behavioural and/or mass media approaches to increase the use of seat belts. Behaviour approaches

have been criticized by authors such as Robertson (1986), who note that while contingencies are in effect, there is an increase in seat belt behaviour use. However, when rewards are withdrawn, seat belt use declines. What has often been ignored is that decline typically does not return to baseline, but nets a gain in overall belt usage. Similar improvements have been reported in other behavioural interventions to reduce injury risk, such as high noise environments and child restraint programmes (Frank *et al.*, 1992).

The high personal and emotional costs of catastrophic injuries, such as head and spinal cord injuries, have resulted in the proliferation of programmes designed to change behaviours associated with injury risk (see 'Head injuries' and 'Spinal cord injury'). Many hospitals have viewed these prevention programmes as an attractive way to provide a public service while marketing their name. Schools are particularly eager to endorse such programmes (Frank *et al.*, 1992). These programmes often utilize a 'shotgun' approach which includes education, modelling and persuasion. Evaluation of the efficacy of these programmes has been problematic for a number of reasons. First, the injuries the programmes are designed to prevent are low frequency events. The number of injuries occurring in any area covered by a prevention programme is likely to be small, thus complicating statistical inferences. Secondly, the proliferation of prevention programmes combined with public media efforts has resulted in a barrage of prevention type interventions. Adolescents are often exposed to a variety of such messages, making it virtually impossible to find an unexposed sample of teenagers.

As was discussed with regard to child injury prevention efforts, adolescent injury prevention programmes are often provided in a single presentation. There is little reason to believe that, regardless of the emotional or educational content of the programme, a single presentation will be sufficient to alter the complex and diverse behavioural factors involved in injury in adolescents. In general, evaluation of injury prevention programmes is demonstrated by increased knowledge and improved attitudes regarding safe behaviours in students who are exposed to the programme. Students exposed to prevention programmes show long-term maintenance of improved knowledge, better attitudes and more safe behaviours than children not exposed to programmes. However, specific analysis after exposure to a prevention programme does not demonstrate improved driving habits or increased perceived vulnerability to injury either immediately after exposure to the prevention programme or at a one-month follow-up (Bouman, 1992). Taken together, it appears that prevention programmes influence attitudes and knowledge, but may have little effect upon behavioural change. Again, expectations of behavioural changes after exposure to a single programme are naive.

In addition to modifying behaviours as a prevention strategy, it has been suggested that personalized interventions, such as mentoring programmes, would be effective in reducing injury risk (Sleet & Mercy, 2003). Furthermore, family therapy and the quality of parental involvement have been shown to reduce adolescent risk-taking behaviours (Sleet & Mercy, 2003).

In general, altering of adolescent injury risk is more complex than most studies have recognized. Evaluation of the multiple determinants, the gradual nature of behavioural change, assessment of the individual's current behaviour, beliefs, social support and alternative responses, as well as the maintenance of behaviour, are all essential steps (Frank *et al.*, 1992). Most injury prevention programmes have addressed only one or two of these issues. Successful implementation of safe behaviours will require cognizance of the individual, the community and national health priorities. Interventions must recognize an altered perceived vulnerability to injury, as well as social support factors.

Conclusions

Injury is the leading cause of death in Americans under age 44. Narrow prevention interventions designed to assess or alter injury, based on unidimensional concepts, whether psychological, behavioural, or environmental have been shown to rarely succeed. Successful prevention of injury is more likely to occur when injury is viewed from an epidemiological perspective with multiple causations. Recognition of the interaction between these causal factors and development of multiple interventions is critical to successful prevention of injury. Psychological factors comprise one element of the matrix leading to injury. Psychologists and other researchers interested in preventing injury have been most successful when they designed interventions targeting the individual, the community and state and national policy.

REFERENCES

Bouman, D. E. (1992). Examination of a traumatic injury prevention program: Adolescent's reactions and program efficiency. Unpublished doctoral dissertation. University of Missouri-Columbia.

Centers for Disease Control and Prevention. (2001). Retrieved September 16, 2004, from http://www.cdc.gov/nchs/hus.htm

Dal Santo, J. A., Goodman, R. M., Glik, D. & Jackson, K. (2004). Childhood unintentional injuries: factors predicting injury risk among preschoolers. *Journal of Pediatric Psychology*, **29**(4), 273–83.

Damashek, A. & Peterson, L. (2002). Unintentional injury prevention efforts for young children: levels, methods, types, and targets. *Journal of Developmental and Behavioral Pediatrics*, **23**(6), 443–55.

Fee, F. A., Bouman, D. E. & Corbin, P. A. (2000). Injury prevention. In R. G. Frank & T. R. Elliot (Eds.). *Handbook of rehabilitation psychology* (pp. 519–35). Washington, DC: American Psychological Association.

Frank, R. G., Bouman, D. E., Cain, K. & Watts, C. (1992). Primary prevention of injury. *American Psychologist*, **47**, 1045–9.

Mokdad, A. H., Marks, J. S., Stroup, D. F. & Gerberding, J. L. (2004). Actual causes of death in the United States, 2000. *Journal of the American Medical Association*, **291**(10), 1238–45.

Peterson, L. (1989). Latchkey children's preparation for self-care; overestimated, underdeveloped and unsafe. *Journal of Clinical Child Psychology*, **18**, 36–43.

Peterson, L. & Roberts, M. C. (1992). Complacency, misdirection and effective prevention of children's injuries. *American Psychologist*, **47**, 1040–4.

Roberts, M. C. (1987). Public health and health psychology: two cats of Kilkenny? *Professional Psychology Research and Practice*, **18**, 145–9.

Robertson, L. S. (1986). Injury. In B. A. Edelstein & L. Michelson (Eds.). *Handbook on prevention* (pp. 343–60). New York: Plenum Press.

Rosenberg, M. L. & Fenley, M. A. (1992). The federal role in injury control. *American Psychologist*, **47**, 1031–5.

Sleet, D. A., Hammond, W. R., Jones, R. T., Thomas, N. & Whitt, B. (2004). Using psychology for injury and violence prevention in the community.

In R. H. Rozensky, G. J. Norine, C. D. Goodheart & W. R. Hammond (Eds.). *Psychology builds a healthy world* (pp. 185–216). Washington, DC: American Psychological Association.

Sleet, D. A. & Mercy, J. A. (2003). Promotion of safety, security, and well-being. In M. H. Bornstein, L. Davidson, C. L. M. Keyes & K. A. Moore (Eds.). *Well-being: positive development across the life course* (pp. 81–97). Mahwah, NJ: Lawrence Erlbaum Associates.

Spielberger, C. D. & Frank, R. G. (1992). Injury control: a promising field for psychologists. *American Psychologist*, **47**, 1029–30.

Waller, J. A. (1994). Reflections on a half century of injury control. *American Journal of Public Health*, **84**, 664–70.

Williams, A. F. & Lund, A. K. (1992). Injury control: what psychologists can contribute. *American Psychologist*, **47**, 1036–9.

Winett, R. A., King, A. C. & Altman, D. G. (1989). *Health psychology and public health: an integrative approach.* New York: Pergamon Press.

Acne

Stephen Kellett

Barnsley Primary Care NHS Trust

Introduction

Of all the skin diseases, acne is the most common with approximately 85% of people affected to some degree at some time in their lives (Rapp *et al.*, 2004). In males, acne typically presents in early adolescence, with the greatest disturbance to skin being observed between the years of 16 to 19 (Hurwitz, 1993). In females, acne tends to present at an earlier age and then subsequently lasts longer than in males (Fallon, 1992). Acne therefore unfortunately tends to occur during adolescence, precisely at a time of simultaneous and significant psychological, physical and social changes (Yazici *et al.*, 2004).

The biological model of acne points to the increased metabolism of androgens in the dermis, in combination with sebaceous gland sensitivity to androgens creating varying degrees of comedones, papules and pustules ('spots')(Cunliffe & Simpson, 1998). The most common form of acne is that of *acne vulgaris*. In about 20% of such cases, the disease necessitates contact with health services (Munro-Ashman, 1963). There are a number of less common variants of acne termed nodular and cystic acne, which have a far more serious prognosis for ongoing and distal physical appearance; *acne conglobata, acne fulminans* and Gram-negative folliculitis (Cunliffe & Simpson, 1998). The raison d'être of physical intervention with regard to treating all variants of acne, is the prevention of physical scarring, by limiting the number of skin lesions and thereby minimizing the potential psychological implications of the disease (Healy & Simpson, 1994). In psychological terms, it is possible to equate and locate the psychological effects of the skin disease of acne within an internal scarring metaphor (Layton *et al.*, 1997).

In recent years within dermatological research, biological models have been supplanted with more expansive and inclusive biopsychosocial approaches (Rapp *et al.*, 1998). Biopsychosocial disease models tend to emphasize the multifactorial nature of the aetiology of skin disease by highlighting the interaction of factors such as biological, environmental, psychoemotional and interpersonal factors. Kellett & Gilbert (2001) presented a biopsychosocial model of acne, which integrated previous psychological and biological models. This model emphasized the role of shame as a stressor that functioned to maintain the skin disease of acne, via increased arousal and associated lowered immune system functioning (Teshima *et al.*, 1982), which subsequently and reciprocally reinforced shame reactions and responses through the continuation of the skin disease.

Skin diseases such as acne tend to be unfortunately and short-sightedly dismissed as inconsequential, trivial and trifling in some medical quarters, when compared with diseases of other organ systems, simply because skin diseases do not directly cause death (Mallon *et al.*, 1999). Some evidence exists that 'skin failure' exerts such a degree of psycho-emotional strain on some sufferers, that acne indirectly causes death due to those sufferers eventually progressing to commit suicide (Cotterill & Cunliffe, 1997). The fact that acne is primarily active on the face (Cunliffe & Simpson, 1998) and hence the skin pathology is observable and visible at all times during social interactions, has been hypothesized as the key reason why acne is potentially psychologically potent and pathogenic (Kellett, 2002).

Research indicates the number of people suffering from acne in the adult years is on the increase (Cunliffe & Simpson, 1998) and has been attributed to a combination of an increase in environmental pathogens and the stress–diathesis model (Kellett & Gilbert, 2001). Cunliffe and Gould (1997) illustrated that 25% of patients attending a skin clinic suffering from acne had a mean age of 34 years. Individuals who develop acne in the adult years may be equated with burns victims in that the acne, as the burn, is unwanted and unexpected and therefore difficult to integrate into already well established self-perceptions regarding body image (Couglan & Clarke, 2002). Although acne may obviously take longer to develop than a burn, the end result is identical in that the skin surface is radically altered in comparison to previous appearance. Psychologically, such events can be linked by the theme of loss. The acne sufferers 'lose' their previous clear skin and therefore are presented with a body image at odds with previous body precepts. The burns victim may also earn the sympathy of others, a sympathy which may not be extended to acne suffers, due to the presence of various 'acne myths' (Alderman, 1989). Such 'myths' regarding the aetiology of acne, include excessive masturbation, lack of hygiene and poor dietary control (Alderman, 1989). Such myths essentially represent the dual stigma of acne; the stigma of having the skin disease in the first place and the secondary stigma of the myths regarding acne causation. Unfortunately, community research regarding sufferer's knowledge concerning acne tends to mirror such acne myths, in that sufferers tend to primarily believe that a lack of general cleanliness represents the main cause of their acne (Smithard *et al.*, 2001).

The effects of dermatological difference

Once skin disease causes disruption to the presentation of the skin, three typical responses (Thompson & Kent, 2001) have been demonstrated; (a) stigma (b) psychological consequences and (c) the individual variability of such psychological responses. These issues will now be considered in relation to acne.

In terms of stigma, individuals with acne consistently report instances of discrimination, which has tended to be termed 'enacted stigma' (Scambler & Hopkins, 1986). Krowchuk *et al.* (1991) have shown that acne sufferers tend to believe that they are seen and treated by others as socially unattractive, repugnant beings. Such discrimination tends to be reported in terms of social rejections, with experimental studies illustrating that such rejections are a tangible reality, rather than a figment of the sufferer's imagination. Rumsey *et al.* (1982) illustrated that when actors are made up to appear dermatologically different from that of a control condition, then the public tended to try to ignore the presence of that person, found gaze difficult and tended to stand further apart. Marshall (1941) illustrated that, in relation to acne, prospective employers made consistent negative attributions concerning acne sufferers, regarding the degree to which potential customers would be 'repelled' by the person and hence tended not to employ acne sufferers. Interestingly, experimental evidence indicates that being dermatologically different, can also negatively influence and slant the sufferer's perceptions of social interaction. Strenta & Kleck (1985) illustrated that actors who believed that they were being made to appear dermatologically different, but then actually had any such differences removed, tended to report stronger reactions from the public in comparison with a control group. The everyday reality of coping with acne, probably represents an uncomfortable interaction of both of the aforementioned processes (see also 'Stigma').

In terms of psychological consequences of acne (point b), there is evidence that acne can exert significant negative effects upon wellbeing. Many studies have indicated that, as a group, people with acne tend to experience and report lower levels of self-esteem (Gupta & Gupta, 1998), increased depression (Cotterill & Cunliffe, 1997), heightened anxiety (Wu *et al.*, 1988) and generalized problems with socializing and social contact (Koo, 1995).

Thirdly, there is considerable individual variation between sufferers in terms of the manner in which they react and adapt to being dermatologically different. There does not appear to be a manifest relationship between the severity of presenting acne and the degree of associated psychological distress. A collection of fairly minor blemishes can result in marked mental health problems in one person, whereas another can cope relatively well with more severe disruptions to the appearance of their skin (MacGregor, 1990). Interestingly, there is also a schism between the manner in which dermatology patients and dermatologists assess symptom severity and associated quality of life (Jemec, 1996).

The measurement of psychological distress in acne

Researchers have set out in the attempt to provide an objective index of the distress associated with acne, primarily through the development and usage of self-report questionnaires (Salek *et al.*, 1996). Although there are quantitative measures of psychodermatological quality of life and associated distress (Klassen *et al.*, 2000), such measures tend to tap broadbrush and generic psychodermatological issues. Acne-specific scales, as they are disease-specific scales, are more sensitive (Morgan *et al.*, 1997) and more responsive to change (Newton *et al.*, 1997), than the generic measures available.

The aim of the following section is to review the commonly used acne-specific measures in terms of their overall purpose, psychometric foundations and to inform measure selection in the clinical and research forums. Methods of measuring acne-related distress are necessary and important due to increasing the scope and range of assessment possible in the skin clinic, the psychological assessment of new physical management techniques in clinical research (Salek *et al.*, 1996) and the evaluation of innovative psychological interventions in dermatological settings (Fortune *et al.*, 2004). The measures developed to assess 'acne handicap' (Salek *et al.*, 1996) have tended to fall into two camps: (1) the assessment of quality of life issues in acne and (2) psychosocial issues in acne. The following sections structured accordingly.

Quality of life measures

Acne-QoL

The Acne-QoL scale (Martin *et al.*, 2001) was developed to assess quality of life issues specific to facial acne samples. The 19 item Acne-QoL purports to measure four aspects of quality of life: self-perception, role-social, role-emotional and acne symptoms. In terms of reliability, the Acne-QoL has acceptable internal consistency on individual scales, sufficient stability over time and displays sensitivity to intervention effects. In terms of validity, the Acne-QoL displays adequate convergent and discriminant validity (Martin *et al.*, 2001) (see also 'Quality of life' and 'Quality of life assessment').

Psychosocial measures

Acne disability index (ADI)

The ADI (Motley & Finley, 1989) is a 48-item questionnaire, which is completed using linear analogue procedures. The ADI is purported to measure eight categories: psychological (14 items), recreation (3 items), employment (3 items), self-awareness (3 items), social reaction (14 items), skin care (3 items) and financial (4 items). The internal consistency of the total scale is high, with sound test-retest reliabilities for the whole and sub-scales. The total scale score also displays satisfactory convergent and discriminant validities (Salek *et al.*, 1996). However, the lack of clarification regarding the construct validity of the ADI represents a major psychometric concern.

Cardiff acne disability index (CADI)

The CADI (Motley & Finley, 1992) is a shortened version of the ADI, consisting of 5 questions presented in a Likert format. The CADI is scored and treated as a unidimensional construct. The measure has been illustrated to have sound internal and test-retest reliabilities and demonstrated to be a valid measure with which to assess the degree of handicap and disability experienced by a patient in relation to their acne (Salek *et al.*, 1996). The CADI has been piloted in a New Zealand sample (Oakley, 1996) and found to be useful in identifying the functional disability caused by acne.

Conclusions

This chapter has illustrated that acne is likely to exert a considerable amount of psychosocial strain upon sufferers. The measures for assessing such acne disability have been reviewed. Although there is a growing body of literature regarding the psychological implications of acne, there are a number of concerns regarding the of evidence base: (a) the lack of psychological theory regarding the impact of acne guiding resultant research; (b) the lack of testing of biopsychosocial models; (c) the lack of qualitative evidence; (d) the lack of triangulated evidence; (e) the lack of evidence regarding how sufferers cope effectively with acne; and (f) broader investigations of psychological interventions for acne. Methodologies that attempt to address the aforementioned issues would provide a far greater understanding of the psychosocial impact of acne and provide further opportunities to increase the breadth of care offered to acne patients.

(See also 'Eczema and skin disorders'.)

Acknowledgement

With thanks to Nicky Ridgway for literature searches.

REFERENCES

Alderman, C. (1989). Not just skin deep. *Nursing Standard*, **37**(3), 22–4.

Coughlan, G. & Clarke, A. (2002). Shame and burns. In P. Gilbert & J. Miles (Eds.). *Body shame: conceptualisation, research and treatment*. Hove: Brunner-Routledge.

Cotterill, J. A. & Cunliffe, W. J. (1997). Suicide in dermatology patients. *British Journal of Dermatology*, **137**, 246–50.

Cunliffe, W. J. & Gould, D. J. (1979). Prevalence of facial acne vulgaris in late

adolescence and in adults. *British Medical Journal*, **138**, 1109–10.

Cunliffe, W. J. & Simpson, N. B. (1998). Disorders of the sebaceous gland. In R. H. Champion, J. L. Burton, D. A. Burns & S. M. Breathnach (Eds.). *Textbook of* *dermatology* Vol. 2 (pp. 1927–84). Oxford: Blackwell Scientific.

Fallon, J. D. (1992). Acne. In S. M. Olbricht, M. E. Bigby & K. A. Arndt (Eds.). *Manual of clinical problems in dermatology*. Boston: Little-Brown.

Fortune, D. G., Richards, H. L. C., Griffiths, E. M. G. & Main, C. J. (2004). Targetting CBT to patients' implicit models of psoriasis: results from a patient preference controlled trial. *British Journal of Clinical Psychology*, **43**, 65–82.

Gupta, M. A & Gupta, A. K. (1998). Depression and suicidal ideation in dermatology patients with acne, alopecia areata, attopic dermatitis and psoriasis. *British Journal of Dermatology*, **139**, 846–50.

Healy, E. & Simpson, N. (1994). Acne vulgaris. *British Medical Journal*, **308**, 831–3.

Hurwitz, S. (1993). Disorders of the sebaceous and sweat glands. In S. Hurwitz (Ed.). *Clinical Paediatric Dermatology* (2nd edn.). Philadelphia: W. B. Saunders.

Jemec, G. B. E. (1996). Patient–physician consensus on quality of life in dermatology. *Clinical & Experimental Dermatology*, **21**, 177–9.

Kellett, S. & Gilbert, P. (2001). Acne; a biopsychosocial and evolutionary perspective with a focus on shame. *British Journal of Health Psychology*, **6**, 1–24.

Kellett, S. (2002). Shame-fused acne: a biopsychosocial conceptualisation and treatment rationale. In P. Gilbert & J. Miles (Eds.). *Body shame: conceptualisation, research and treatment*. Hove: Brunner-Routledge.

Klassen, A. F., Newton, J. N. & Mallon, E. (2000). Measuring quality of life in people referred for specialist care of acne: comparing generic and disease-specific measures. *Archives of the Academy of Dermatology*, **43**, 229–33.

Koo, J. (1995). The psychosocial impact of acne: patients' perceptions. *Journal of the American Academy of Dermatology*, **32**, 526–30.

Krowchuk, D. P., Stancin, T., Keskinen, R. *et al.* (1991). The psychological effect of acne on adolescents. *Paediatric Dermatology*, **8**, 332–8.

Layton, A. M., Seukeran, D. & Cunliffe, W. J. (1997). Scarred for life? *Dermatology*, **195**, 15–21.

MacGregor, F. (1990). Facial disfigurement: problems and management of social interactions and implications for mental health. *Aesthetic Plastic Surgery*, **14**, 249–57.

Mallon, E., Newton, J. N. & Klassen, A. (1999). The quality of life in acne: a comparison with general medical conditions using generic questionnaires. *British Journal of Dermatology*, **140**, 672–6.

Marshall, W. (1941). The psychology of the general public with regard to acne vulgaris. *Canadian Medical Association Journal*, **44**, 599–603.

Martin, A. R., Lookingbill, D. P., Botek, A. *et al.* (2001). Health-related quality of life among patients with facial acne – assessment of a new acne-specific questionnaire. *Clinical and Experimental Dermatology*, **26**, 380–5.

Morgan, M., McCreedy, R., Simpson, J. & Hay, R. J. (1997). Dermatology quality of life scales – a measure of the impact of skin diseases. *British Journal of Dermatology*, **136**, 202–6.

Motley, R. J. & Finlay, A. Y. (1989). How much disability is caused by acne? *Clinical and Experimental Dermatology*, **14**, 194–8.

Motley, R. J. & Finlay, A. Y. (1992). Practical use of a disability index in the routine management of acne. *Clinical and Experimental Dermatology*, **17**, 1–3.

Munroe-Ashman, D. (1963). Acne vulgaris in a public school. *Transcripts of St John's Hospital Dermatological Society*, **49**, 144–8.

Newton, J. N., Mallon, E. & Klassen, A. (1997). The effectiveness of acne treatment: an assessment by patients of the outcome of therapy. *British Journal of Dermatology*, **137**, 563–7.

Oakley, A. M. M. (1996). The Acne Disability Index: usefulness confirmed. *Australian Journal of Dermatology*, **37**, 37–9.

Rapp, S. R., Feldman, S. R. & Fleischer, A. B. (1998). Health-related quality of life in psoriasis: a biopsychosocial model and measures. In R. Rajagopalan, E. Sherritz & R. Anderson (Eds.). *Care management of skin diseases: life quality and economic impact*. New York: Marcel Dekker, Inc.

Rapp, D. A., Brenes, G. A., Feldman, S. R. *et al.* (2004). Anger and acne: implications for quality of life, patient satisfaction and clinical care. *British Journal of Dermatology*, **151**, 183–9.

Rumsey, N., Bull, R. & Gahagen, D. (1982). The effect of facial disfigurement on the proxemic behaviour of the general public. *Journal of Applied Social Psychology*, **12**, 137–50.

Salek, M. S., Khan, G. K. & Finlay, A. Y. (1996). Questionnaire techniques in assessing acne handicap: reliability and validity issues. *Quality of Life Research*, **5**, 131–8.

Scambler, G. & Hopkins, A. (1986). Being epileptic: coming to terms with stigma. *Sociology of Health and Illness*, **8**, 26–43.

Smithard, A., Glazebrook, C. & Williams, H. C. (2001). Acne prevalence, knowledge about acne and psychological morbidity in mid-adolescence; a community-based study. *British Journal of Dermatology*, **145**, 274–9.

Strenta, F. & Kleck, R. (1985). Physical disability and the attribution dilemma: perceiving the causes of social behaviour. *Journal of Social and Clinical Psychology*, **3**, 129–42.

Teshima, H., Kubo, C., Kohara, H. *et al.* (1982). Psychosomatic aspects of skin disease from the standpoint of immunology. *Psychotherapy and Psychosomatics*, **37**(3), 165–75.

Thompson, A. R. & Kent, G. (2001). Adjusting to disfigurement; processes involved in dealing with being visibly different. *Clinical Psychology Review*, **21**, 663–82.

Wu, S. F., Kinder, B. N., Trunnell, T. N. & Fulton, J. E. (1988). Role of anxiety and anger in acne patients: a relationship with the severity of the disorder. *Journal of American Academy of Dermatology*, **18**, 325–32.

Yazici, K., Baz, K., Yazici, A. *et al.* (2004). Disease-specific quality of life is associated with anxiety and depression in patients with acne. *Journal of the European Academy of Dermatology & Venereology*, **18**, 435–9.

Alcohol abuse

Michael A. Sayette

University of Pittsburgh

Alcohol has been consumed by people in all parts of the world for thousands of years. Most people who routinely consume alcohol generally do not develop drinking problems. Nevertheless, the millions of people who do develop problems associated with alcohol create enormous social, economic and medical costs to society. Complications resulting from chronic alcohol problems include liver damage, strokes and memory loss, as well as a host of negative life events. Although the term 'alcoholism' is used widely in both the lay and professional communities, its lack of specificity and moralistic overtones have led to use of alternative terms such as 'alcohol abuse' and 'alcohol dependence' in recent diagnostic formulations.

In the most recent edition of the *Diagnostic and Statistical Manual of the Mental Disorders (DSM-IV-text revision*: American Psychiatric Association, 2000), 'alcohol dependence' includes biological, psychological and social components. Most importantly, alcohol dependence involves difficulty controlling alcohol consumption and continued drinking despite aversive consequences. Edwards (1986) notes an increase in the salience of drinking, with alcohol taking on an increasingly dominant role in a drinker's life, as an important element in the alcohol dependence syndrome. Although none of the following is required for diagnosis, alcohol dependence symptoms include: tolerance (a diminished effect of alcohol, usually accompanied by increased consumption); withdrawal symptoms following reduced consumption; consumption of larger amounts or for a longer time period than was intended; persistent desire or unsuccessful efforts to cut down or control drinking; excessive time spent obtaining, consuming, or recovering from the effects of alcohol; reduction of important activities due to drinking; and continued drinking despite knowledge that it is causing or exacerbating a physical or psychological problem.

'Alcohol abuse' is conceptualized by DSM-IV-TR as a maladaptive drinking pattern (i.e. continued drinking despite knowledge that it is causing or exacerbating a problem). Individuals diagnosed with alcohol abuse must not meet the criteria for alcohol dependence and manifest at least one of the following: recurrent drinking despite its interference with the execution of major role obligations; continued drinking despite legal, social, or interpersonal problems related to its use; and recurrent drinking in situations where intoxication is dangerous. Data from the Epidemiological Catchment Area study (Robins & Reiger, 1991) indicated a lifetime prevalence rate for either alcohol abuse or dependence of 13.8%, with men being significantly more likely than women to develop drinking problems.

For heuristic purposes, this chapter will use the term 'alcoholism' to denote alcohol abuse or dependence. Alcoholism is a heterogenous disorder that is multiply determined by both genetic and psychological factors. Support for a genetic aetiology for alcoholism is derived from adoption, twin and family studies, as well as from animal studies in which rodents are bred for sensitivity to alcohol's effects and alcohol-seeking behaviour. Both twin studies and research identifying cultural and occupational differences in alcoholism rates reveal that environmental and psychological factors also contribute to the development of alcoholism. (See McGue (1999) for review of both genetic and environmental influences.) From a psychological perspective, alcoholism can be considered to be a disorder of behavioural excess, a maladaptive habit that has developed through powerful reinforcement contingencies, rather than a biomedical disease (Marlatt & Gordon, 1985).

A number of psychological theories have been developed to understand alcohol use and alcoholism (Leonard & Blane, 1999). Generally these theories state that people drink alcohol to increase pleasant feelings (positive reinforcement) or to decrease unpleasant feelings (negative reinforcement). Often these theories lead to predictions about which people will be most sensitive to these reinforcing effects, and thus will be at greatest risk for developing alcoholism.

Many people, including both those who treat and those who suffer from alcoholism, believe that alcohol is consumed because it reduces anxiety. This tension reduction hypothesis has spawned more than 50 years of experimental research. Although the data have been mixed, it appears that under certain conditions, alcohol does provide anxiolytic effects and that anxiety symptoms can sometimes precipitate drinking or relapse. Recent models have attempted to explore the mechanisms underlying these anxiolytic effects. These include models positing direct pharmacological effects of alcohol on the nervous system and the notion that anxiolytic effects are mediated by alcohol's effects on information processing (Sayette, 1999). This latter position is represented in a number of recent social–cognitive models.

Hull (1987) has proposed that alcohol's anxiolytic properties are cognitively mediated. By impairing the encoding of information in terms of self-relevance, intoxication decreases self-awareness. The inhibition of encoding processes reduces performance-based self-evaluation which, in situations where such evaluation is unpleasant, increases the probability of drinking. Alternatively, intoxication may interfere with self-evaluation rather than self-awareness of one's vulnerabilities. That is, we may know that we were judged unfavourably by another, but this information does not adversely affect the way that we view ourselves. Other cognitive mechanisms proposed to account for alcohol's anxiolytic effects include effects on attentional capacity, and initial appraisal of stressful information. (See Sayette (1999) for a review of the preceding theories.)

Although alcohol's effects on anxiety have received the most scrutiny, other negatively reinforcing effects have also been investigated. For example, alcohol has been consumed to cope with a variety of life events or situations. From this social learning perspective, alcoholism may result when one becomes overwhelmed by the demands of a situation (Maisto *et al.*, 1999). In addition to these negative reinforcing effects, alcohol often is consumed in order to produce positive effects such as enhanced arousal and positive mood. For instance, alcohol can enhance feelings of power. The euphoric effects of alcohol generally appear while blood alcohol concentrations are rising and are thought to be important in decisions concerning drinking, as people's beliefs about drinking will be most affected by the most immediate consequences of alcohol consumption (Marlatt, 1987).

Vulnerability to alcoholism

Children of alcoholics are at heightened risk to develop alcoholism compared with children without this background (Sher, 1991). Considerable research is underway to explore the genetic and environmental moderators and mediators of this relationship. Individuals at risk for alcoholism due to a family history of the disorder tend to show stronger effects of alcohol during the ascending limb of the blood alcohol curve yet weaker effects on the descending limb than those without familial risk (Newlin & Thomson, 1990). Although the evidence is mixed, some investigators have observed that alcohol's anxiolytic effects are enhanced among children of alcoholics (Sher, 1991). Research also has documented relationships between certain personality traits such as impulsivity and habituation to stimuli and the development of alcoholism. Because alcoholism is recognized to be a heterogenous disorder, current personality theories of alcoholism have shifted away from identifying a unitary alcoholic personality and instead focus on specific personality dimensions, such as behavioural undercontrol or negative emotionality, that may place an individual at increased risk (Sher, Trull, Barthalow, & Vieth, 1999).

Psychological contributions to the treatment of alcoholism

Approaches to alcoholism treatment are becoming increasingly integrated with attempts to address biological, psychological and social aspects of the disorder. A number of pharmacological treatments continue to be developed to treat alcoholism (Fuller & Hiller-Sturmhöfel, 1999). Disulfiram (Antabuse) has long been used to deter persons from drinking. When alcohol is consumed, disulphiram produces an accumulation of the toxic metabolite acetaldehyde, causing nausea and hypotension. If disulphiram is reliably used, these extremely unpleasant sensations often can deter an individual from drinking. Other drugs, such as Acamprosite and Naltrexone, have been posited to reduce alcohol craving and drinking. In addition to these pharmacological agents, a number of psychosocial interventions have been developed, which are summarized below.

Relapse prevention

Because the majority of people with alcoholism who quit drinking relapse, a trend in alcoholism treatment has been on maintaining treatment gains rather than focusing entirely on initial cessation. Marlatt and his colleagues (e.g. Marlatt & Gordon, 1985; Witkiewitz & Marlatt, 2004) have developed a model of relapse prevention that focuses on factors that can promote relapse. This model posits that particular situations, and not just personality traits, can precipitate a return to drinking. Marlatt argues that initial drinking following attempted abstinence (a lapse) leads to full blown relapse due to the shame involved in violating abstinence. This abstinence violation effect is treated psychologically by helping patients recognize the situational precipitants of the lapse, rather than interpreting the lapse as indisputable evidence that they are treatment failures. Thus, treatment focuses on anticipating high-risk situations that might jeopardize abstinence and identifying coping strategies. Should a lapse occur, however, relapse prevention seeks to prevent it from developing into a full-blown relapse. In this case, treatment involves exploring the events and experiences that triggered the lapse. Interest in understanding the variables that can precipitate relapse has led to a number of psychological strategies that are used in treatment programmes.

Skills training

The ability to cope effectively with high risk situations is related to effective treatment and is believed to prevent relapse. Certain situations appear to pose a high risk for relapse, including interpersonal anger and frustration, social pressure, negative emotional states and stimulus-elicited craving (Marlatt & Gordon, 1985). Communication difficulties also have been implicated as a problem for many who battle alcoholism. Deficient areas that often are targeted in coping skills interventions include assertiveness, initiating conversations, listening skills, giving and receiving compliments and criticism and enhancing close relationships. Particular attention is paid to developing skills specific to drinking situations. For instance, drink refusal training permits modelling and practising of skills needed to cope with offers to drink by peers. In addition, receiving criticism about drinking and enhancing non-alcoholic support networks are targeted in skills treatment. These coping-skills training programmes have reduced alcohol consumption and increased work days after treatment (Rohsenow *et al.*, 2001).

Cue exposure

Both clinical observations and experimental research suggest that exposure to alcohol cues can precipitate relapse. For example, being in the vicinity of alcohol at a party may lead to a return to drinking. Individuals in this situation may become physiologically aroused, experience a craving for alcohol and ultimately act on their urge and drink. Treatments have been developed in which patients are repeatedly exposed to alcohol cues (e.g. sniffing their favourite drink) but are not permitted to drink the beverage. Initially, patients experience heightened reactions such as intense cravings for the drink, increased physiological arousal and increased salivation. With repeated exposure to the drink over several sessions, however, patients' responses to the cues diminish. In conditioning terms, cue exposure attempts to extinguish or attenuate the strength of association between alcohol cues and drinking behaviour. From a social learning perspective, cue exposure permits modification of one's beliefs concerning both the reinforcing aspects of drinking (positive outcome expectancies) and the perceived ability to cope with, or resist, the urge to drink (self-efficacy judgments). Regardless of its underlying mechanisms, cue exposure treatment has shown promising results in conjunction with skills training in improving treatment success (e.g. Rohsenow *et al.*, 2001). Treatments that provide a richer presentation of the complex array of cues associated with relapse may enhance the efficacy of these interventions (Conklin & Tiffany, 2002).

Couples therapy/family therapy

The emphasis on determining triggers for drinking has led to increased focus on the patient's spouse or family members in understanding and treating alcoholism. Although family and relationship issues are generally not the primary cause of alcoholism, they often contribute to the maintenance of alcohol problems. Thus, among individuals with alcoholism, marital and family conflict can precipitate drinking. Further, the non-alcoholic spouse and family members may reinforce problem drinking by providing financial and emotional support during times of heavy consumption. These factors have led to the use of couples and family therapy as an adjunct to individual treatment (McCrady, 2001). Specifically, treatment has effectively improved (a) patients' initial motivation to quit; (b) treatment gains during the year following initiation of therapy; and (c) maintenance of treatment gains during long-term recovery (O' Farrell, 1992).

Alcohol expectancies

An individual's alcohol expectancies (i.e. beliefs about the effects of alcohol on affect, behaviour and cognition) predict drinking behaviour over time as well as treatment outcome (Goldman, 1994). Furthermore, it appears that individuals at increased risk for alcoholism, due to a personality marked by behavioural undercontrol or negative affectivity, or a family history of alcoholism, show differential patterns of alcohol expectancies relative to individuals who are not considered to be at risk. These expectancies may in turn predict drinking (Goldman, 1994; Sher, 1991). Expectancies about alcohol's effects may provide a common pathway that permits other factors such as personality variables or reactivity to alcohol's effects to influence the initiation and maintenance of alcohol use and alcoholism. Developments in the alcohol expectancy domain hold promise for providing a theoretical foundation for conceptualizing advances in the prevention of alcohol problems.

Motivation enhancement

Alcoholism treatment failure often has been attributed to poor motivation to recover on the part of individuals with alcoholism. Consequently, the ability to enhance one's motivation to quit has become a therapeutic goal (Miller, 1992). Simple interventions designed to improve motivation have produced significant changes in an individual's willingness to accept treatment. Data from a major multi-site study in the United States suggest that Motivational Enhancement Therapy may be an especially cost effective intervention (Project MATCH, 1998)

Self-help groups

Many individuals with alcoholism have derived benefit from self-help groups such as Alcoholics Anonymous (AA) or Rational Recovery. Self-help group meetings involve discussion by members of their experiences abstaining from alcohol. These groups can serve a number of important functions. Members gain a non-drinking support network, discuss their fears and concerns about relapse, and perhaps most importantly, realize that their struggle with alcohol is shared by others. More than one million people throughout the world attend AA meetings annually. AA relies on a 12-step treatment approach that emphasizes a belief in a higher power to combat what is viewed as an incurable but arrestable illness. Despite its widespread appeal, there have been few systematic evaluations of AA's effectiveness (Fuller & Hiller-Sturmhöfel, 1999). Rational Recovery offers a non-spiritual treatment alternative that appeals to those who are uncomfortable with AA.

Patient/treatment matching

Traditionally, patients being treated for alcoholism would receive the particular treatment package implemented by that agency. The degree of individualization of treatment often has been minimal (Miller, 1992). The 'Project Match' randomized clinical trial compared responses to a 12-step, a cognitive–behavioural and a motivational enhancement approach to treatment. Results generally did not, however, identify which type of treatment works best for particular types of individuals (matching patients to treatments using characteristics such as social support and degree of dependence). Currently a major study is underway (Project COMBINE) which examines combinations of varying intensities of psychological treatment along with pharmacological interventions (placebo, Naltrexone, Acamprosite). Clients in this ambitious study will be treated for 4 months and then followed for a year, and the findings should prove valuable.

Alcoholism: contextual issues

Understanding the aetiology of alcoholism requires an appreciation for a host of other psychological disturbances that may face the patient. Two such issues are comorbid psychiatric disorders and polydrug use. Mood, anxiety and personality disorders are examples of psychiatric conditions often comorbid with alcoholism. Exploring the nature of these relationships is important for understanding risk factors as well as for developing effective treatment strategies for these individuals.

Polydrug use among those with alcoholism is increasingly becoming the rule rather than the exception. Because many alcohol treatment facilities and research projects have excluded polydrug users, important information regarding these subjects has until recently been lacking. Generally, polydrug patients present with more severe problems than those whose problems are exclusive to alcohol. The nature of these differences has just begun to be explored. Research is needed to determine whether cessation is indicated for all drugs simultaneously or, if not, what the sequence of cessation ought to be. This concern typifies the current view of alcoholism that recognizes the importance of understanding the disorder within a broader biopsychosocial context.

(See also Drug Dependency.)

REFERENCES

American Psychiatric Association. (2000). *Diagnostic and Statistical Manual of Mental Disorders (4th edn.-text revision).* Washington, DC: Author.

Conklin, C. A. & Tiffany, S. T. (2002). Applying extinction research and theory to cue-exposure addiction treatments. *Addiction,* **97,** 155–67.

Edwards, G. (1986). The alcohol dependence syndrome: the concept as stimulus to inquiry. *British Journal of Addiction,* **81,** 71–84.

Fuller, R. K. & Hiller-Sturmhöfel, S. (1999). Alcoholism treatment in the United States: an overview. *Alcohol Research and Health,* **23,** 69–77.

Goldman, M. S. (1994). The alcohol expectancy concept: applications to assessment, prevention, and treatment of alcohol abuse. *Applied and Preventive Psychology,* **3,** 131–44.

Hull, J. G. (1987). Self-awareness model. In H. T. Blane & K. E. Leonard (Eds.). *Psychological theories of drinking and alcoholism* (pp. 272–304). New York: Guilford Press.

Leonard, K. E. & Blane, H. T. (Eds.). (1999). *Psychological Theories of Drinking and Alcoholism* (2nd edn.). New York: Guilford Press.

Maisto, S. A., Carey, K. B. & Bradizza, C. M. (1999). In K. E. Leonard & H. T. Blane (Eds.). *Psychological Theories of Drinking and Alcoholism* (2nd edn.). (pp. 106–63). New York: Guilford Press.

Marlatt, G. A. (1987). Alcohol, the magic elixir: stress, expectancy, and the transformation of emotional states. In E. Gottheil, K. Druley, S. Pasko & S. Weinstein (Eds.). *Stress and addiction* (pp. 302–22). New York: Brunner/Mazel.

Marlatt, G. A. & Gordon, J. R. (Eds.). (1985). *Relapse prevention.* New York: Guilford Press.

McCrady, B. S. (2001). Alcohol use disorders. In D. H. Barlow (Ed.). *Clinical Handbook of Psychological Disorders* (3rd edn.). (pp. 376–433). New York: Guilford Press.

McGue, M. (1999). Behavioral genetic models of alcoholism and drinking. In K. E. Leonard & H. T. Blane (Eds.). (1999). *Psychological Theories of Drinking and Alcoholism* (2nd edn.). (pp. 372–421). New York: Guilford Press.

Miller, W. R. (1992). Client/treatment matching in addictive behaviors. *The Behavior Therapist,* **15,** 7–8.

Newlin, D. B. & Thompson, J. B. (1990). Alcohol challenge in sons of alcoholics: a critical review and analysis. *Psychological Bulletin,* **108,** 383–402.

O'Farrell, T. J. (1992). Families and alcohol problems: an overview of treatment research. *Journal of Family Psychology,* **5,** 339–59.

Project MATCH Research Group. (1998). Matching alcoholism treatments to client heterogeneity: treatment main effects and matching effects on drinking during treatment. *Journal of Studies on Alcohol,* **59,** 631–9.

Rohsenow, D. J., Monti, P. M., Rubonis, A. V. *et al.* (2001). Cue exposure with coping skills training and communication skills training for alcohol dependence: 6- and 12-month outcomes. *Addiction,* **96,** 1161–74.

Robins, L. & Reiger, D. (Eds.). (1991). *Psychiatric disorders in America: the epidemiological catchment area study.* New York: MacMillan.

Sayette, M. A. (1999). Cognitive theory and research. In K. E. Leonard & H. T. Blane (Eds.). (1999). *Psychological Theories of Drinking and Alcoholism* (2nd edn.). (pp. 247–91). New York: Guilford Press.

Sher, K. J. (1991). *Children of alcoholics: a critical appraisal of theory and research.* Chicago: University of Chicago Press.

Sher, K., Trull, T., Bartholow, B. D. & Vieth, A. (1999). Personality and alcoholism: Issues, methods, and etiological processes. In K. E. Leonard & H. T. Blane (Eds.), *Psychological theories of drinking and alcoholism* (pp. 54–105). New York: Guilford Press.

Witkiewitz, K. & Marlatt, G. A. (2004). Relapse prevention for alcohol and drug problems: that was Zen, this is Tao. *American Psychologist,* **59,** 224–35.

Allergies to drugs

Mary Gregerson

Family Therapy Institute of Alexandria

Features

As a well-accepted medical/scientific iatrogenic problem, allergies to drugs have high human and medical costs. Human costs include discomfort, dysfunction and, sometimes, death. Medical costs concern emergency care to reverse acute hypersensitivity effects, expensive and semi-reliable diagnostic tests and the health risks of re-administration to definitively confirm the drug allergy.

These sensitivities are often termed 'side-effects' since they are epiphenomenal to the drug's intended effect. This minimization in the terminology does not reflect the medical reality either in terms of intensity or impact. These adverse reactions to drugs are real, and can be life-threatening. The phrase 'concurrent effects' better describes these effects.

Three different types of drug allergies have been detailed (Pichler, 1993): (1) classic drug allergies are immune over-reactions to the medication itself; (2) an immune reaction occurs but is not mediated by other immune substances; (3) an autoimmune reaction can occur when the drug invokes an immune reaction to autologous structures.

The physical sequelae of an allergy to drugs can vary widely. Symptoms may be as benign as simple mild skin rashes, or as threatening as potentially fatal anaphylactic reactions. Anaphylaxis, a constriction of smooth muscles, results in a reddening and swelling of affected areas. If the breathing passages are swollen, suffocation can occur. Death from drug allergies emanates from anaphylactic shock is unabated by medical counter measures.

Particular aspects of antibiotics termed beta-lactams often cause allergic reactions. Allergy to penicillin is quite common, and the most extensively researched of the known drug allergies. For example, research before 1970 identified contaminants in penicillin mixtures which were responsible for a large portion, but not all, of the adverse reactions to this drug (Knudsen et al., 1970). Subsequent penicillin compounds no longer contain these contaminant allergens.

Additionally, determination of which individuals experience drug allergies is influenced by a range of individual differences in genetics, metabolism and health. Major histocompatibility complex (MHC) class II pathways process drug allergens (Pieters, 1997). If a person has slow acetylation, which is genetically determined, metabolism of the pharmaceutical agent transforms toward reactivity (Clark, 1985; Rieder et al., 1991). The inflammation of infectious states sometimes amplifies reactivity to produce an allergic response (Moseley & Sullivan, 1991; Uetrecht, 1999). A curious medical finding is that although atopy does not mean a higher probability of a positive penicillin skin test (Adkinson, 1984), atopy is a major risk factor for penicillin anaphylaxis that is severe and even fatal (Idsoe et al., 1968).

Environmental factors also influence drug allergy reactions. Environmentally some trace antibiotics found in dairy and milk products will cross-react with a drug (Birnbaum & Vervloet, 1991), although current US regulations monitor carefully these trace elements. So, it is highly unlikely, but not impossible, for a sensitizing predisposition to evoke an allergic drug reaction (Division of Medical Science, 1980; Dewdney, 1984). Moreover, social engineering like the abolition of topical cream forms of penicillin avoid potential atopic dermatitis reactions sometimes resulting from these creams (Helton & Storrs, 1991; Holdiness, 2001).

Diagnosis

Diagnosis is challenging for drug allergies (Sabbah & Caradec, 1992). The natural history of most drug allergic reactions is complicated. First of all, the polypharmacopeia usual in hospitalization (usually more than 8 medications at any time) and outpatient management of many chronic diseases confound easy identification of the drug culprit producing the allergic reaction.

A scant number of definitive and universally accepted tests exist. Therefore, consultation for these multi-medication cases require six steps:

1) Assemble clinical data . . .; 2) Narrow candidate list of drug allergen (by time frame of drug administration and symptom onset as well as the surge and abatement of symptoms) . . .; 3) Consider pharmacoepidemiology of candidate list . . .; 4) Stop and/or substitute all drug candidates known as allergens . . .; 5) Consider skin testing . . .; and 6) Readminister incriminated drugs as clinically indicated . . . (Adkinson, 2001, p.1686)

Skin tests and lymphoblast transformation tests may imitate the drug-invoked allergic reaction or merely indicate sensitivity. A prevalent test to determine allergy to drugs is the leukocyte migration inhibition test. A simplification of this test proved 66% effective (Tarasov et al., 1991). Another common test assesses basophil degranulation against the exposition. Some evidence exists that this latter test, although more risky, is quicker, simpler, more useful and has more specificity (Rangel et al., 1991). The most definitive and highest risk test is a re-administration provocation test showing the drug's elicitation of the allergic reaction.

Pseudoallergic reactions, though, can confound successful diagnosis and treatment (Adkinson, 2001). For instance, often after the administration of anesthetic, e.g. in dentistry, vasovagal syncope can masquerade as anaphylaxis. In vasovagal syncope IgE mediation is not involved. Furthermore, a pseudoallergy and idiosyncratic allergy to drugs share the same biologic function, but cross-reactivity of the drug allergen with other drugs demonstrates a common biologic structure (Adkinson, 2001). Pseudoallergic responses must be separated from true allergic reactions since stark differences exist in prognosis, counselling and treatment/management.

T-cell mediation is implicated in the most common drug allergy which is a late onset rash (Yawalkar & Pichler, 2001). This rash symptom associated with aminopenicillin appears related to class II MHC (Romano et al., 1998). Thus, patch tests and delayed cutaneous intradermal tests appear reliably to predict responsiveness to readministration (Romano et al., 1999), and may have usefulness for other drug allergies as well a clinical sequelae for treatment.

Medical treatment

Acute and long-term treatment protocols have been developed. The three step acute protocol includes: (1) identify and cease administration of drug allergen; (2) administer counteractive, supportive, or suppressive agents and; (3) determine whether and how substitution may be made for the drug allergen. Antihistamines, in particular, may attenuate an acute reaction.

For long-term care, at least a two- to four-week waiting period after the anaphylactic event is necessary to evade the refractory period. Of course, use of the drug causing the allergic reaction is contraindicated. Other related drugs in that same class may also need to be avoided. For instance, discontinuance of histamine-releasing drugs is usually advised, although some question exists concerning this practice (Moss, 1993).

Long-term treatment focuses upon prophylaxis. Prevention includes the avoidance of identified allergen and all cross-reactive drugs. A number of different ways, such as the wearing of ID jewelry to identify those with drug allergies have been suggested to alert emergency and other medical personnel who might administer treatment to an unconscious person with a drug allergy. Consultation may also be sought on which of the three recommended alternatives would best suit a particular patient. These three approaches are: (1) using an unrelated alternative medication; (2) use of a non-identical but potentially cross-reactive drug; and (3) desensitization to the drug allergen. Each alternative has benefits and drawbacks (Adkinson, 2001).

Additional concern, based on clinical evidence, exists for indirect exposure from secondary trace sources, as mentioned earlier under environmental factors. Although injection is the most potent dosage method, oral ingestion can produce reactivity, especially if the allergen is undiluted. For instance, though, for trace form in antibiotically treated animals' meat, researchers continue to examine the potential of the ingestion to contaminate further up the food chain. Investigations have scrutinized allergic reactions to residues in foods such as dairy products and meats (for a review see Dewdney et al., 1991). Although no conclusion can be drawn at this point,

caution is warranted regarding ingestion or inhalation of the allergen or its derivatives in trace amounts. Those with a prior allergic history especially need to carefully monitor for traces of antibiotic residuals.

Of great interest to health psychologists is that presenting symptoms may seem psychological, at first glance, and treatment issues such as drug allergies can interfere with treatment adherence. At first, when no foreknowledge of medication use is available, allergic reactions may appear as a panic attack (Jasnoski et al., 1994). Psychological sequelae may include hyper-arousal, hyperactivity, feelings of impending doom, scattered cognitions, uncontrollability and 'unreasonable' fear. Adverse reactions to medications need to be ruled out before diagnosing panic attack as the primary symptom rather than as a secondary response to an allergic reaction. Finally, when adherence becomes problematic, drug allergies should be ruled out before more psychological adherence facilitation can appropriately be implemented.

(See also 'Allergies to food', 'Allergies: general' and 'Patient safety and iatrogenesis'.)

REFERENCES

Adkinson, N. F., Jr. (1984). Risk factors for drug allergy. *Journal of Allergy and Clinical Immunology*, **74**, 567.

Adkinson, N. F., Jr. (2001). Con: Immunotherapy is not clinically indicate in the management of allergic asthma. *American Journal of Respiratory and Critical Care Medicine*, **15: 164**(12), 2140–1; discussion 2141–2.

Birnbaum, J. & Vervloet, D. (1991). Allergy to muscle relaxants. *Clinical Review of Allergy*, **9**, 866–77.

Clark, D. W. (1985). Genetically determined variability in acetylation and oxidation. Therapeutic implications. *Drugs*, **29**(4), 342–75.

Dewdney, J. M. & Edwards, R. G. (1984). Penicillin hypersensitivity: is milk a significant hazard? A review. *Journal of Research in Social Medicine*, **77**, 866.

Dewdney, J. M., Maes, L., Raynaud, J. P. et al. (1991). Risk assessment of antibiotic residues of beta-lactams and macrolides in food products with regard to their immuno-allergic potential. *Food and Chemical Toxicology*, **29**(7), 477–83.

Division of Medical Sciences. (1980). *Assembly of Life Sciences*. The effects on human health of subtherapeutic use of antimicrobials in animal feeds. Washington, DC: National Research Council, National Academy of Sciences.

Helton, J. & Stross, F. J. (1991). Pilocarpine allergic contact and photocontact dermatitis. *Contact Dermatitis*, **25**(2), 133–4.

Holdiness, M. R. (2001). Contact dermatitis to topical drugs for glaucoma. *American Journal of Contact Dermatitis*, **12**, 217–19.

Idsoe, O., Guthe, T., Willcox, R. R. & De Weck, A. L. (1968). Nature and extent of penicillin side-reactions, with particular reference to fatalities from anaphylactic shock. *Bulletin of the World Health Organization*, **38**, 159–88.

Jasnoski, M. B. L., Bell, I. R. & Peterson, R. (1994). What associations exist between shyness, hay fever, anxiety, anxiety sensitivity, and panic disorder? *Anxiety, Stress, and Coping*, **7**, 1–15.

Knudsen, E. T., Dewdney, J. M. & Trafford, J. A. (1970). Reduction in incidence of ampicillin rash by purification of ampicillin. *British Medical Journal*, **169**, 469–71.

Moseley, E. K. & Sullivan, T. J. (1991). Allergic reactions to antimicrobial drugs in patients with a history of prior drug allergy. *Journal of Allergy and Immunology*, **87**, 226.

Moss, J. (1993). Are histamine-releasing drugs really contraindicated in patients with a known allergy to drugs? *Anesthesiology*, **79**(3), 623–4.

Patella, V., Casolaro, V. & Marone, G. (1990). A bacterial Ig-binding protein that activates human basophils and mast cells. *Journal of Immunology*, **145**, 3054–61.

Pichler, W. J. (1993). Diagnostic possibilities in drug allergies. *Schweizerische Medizinische Wochenschrift, Journal Suisse de Medecine*, **123**(23), 1183–92.

Pieters, J. (1997). MHC class II restricted antigen presentation. *Current Opinions in Immunology*, **9**, 89–96.

Rangel, H., Montero, P., Espinosa, F. & Castillo, F. J. (1991). Leukocyte migration inhibitory factor and basophil

degranulation in drug reactions. *Revista Alergia Mexico*, **38**(4), 105–9.

Rieder, M. J., Shear, N. H., Kanee, A., Tang, B. V. & Spielber, S. P. (1991). Prominence of slow acetylator phenotype among paitents with sulfonamide hypersensitivity reactions. *Clinical Pharmacology Therapies*, **49**, 13–17.

Romano, A., De Santis, A., Romito, A. et al. (1998). Delayed hypersensitivity to aminopenicillins is related to major hisotcompatibilty complex genes. *Annals of Allergy and Asthma Immunology*, **80**, 433.

Romano, A., Quaratino, D., Di Fonso, M., Papa, G., Venuti, A. & Gasbarrini, G. (1999). A diagnostic protocol for evaluating nonimmmediate reactions to aminopenicillins. *Journal of Allergy and Clinical Immunology*, **103**, 1186–90.

Sabbah, A. & Caradec, J. (1992). Measurement of mediators in drug allergies. Preliminary study. *Allergie et Immunologie (Paris)*, **24**(8), 289–92.

Tarasov, A. V., Zherdev, A. V. & Shuvalov, L. P. (1991). A modification of the leukocyte migration inhibition test in vivo. *Laboratornoe Delo (Moskva)*, **12**, 38–40.

Uetrecht, J. (1999). New concepts in immunology relevant to idiosyncratic drug reactions: The "danger hypothesis" and innate immune system. *Chemical Research Toxicology*, **12**, 387–95.

Yawalkar, N. & Pichler, W. J. (2001). Immunohistology of drug-induced exanthema: clues to pathogenesis. *Current Opinions in Allergy and Clinical Immunology*, **14**, 299–303.

Allergies to food

Mary Gregerson

Family Therapy Institute of Alexandria

Features

Food allergies are immunologic hyper-reactions to ingested substances considered non-pharmacologic, for the most part. Either the failure to develop or a breakdown in oral tolerance may be at fault in Immunoglobulin E (IgE) mediated allergy while inflammatory mediators are implicated in non-IgE cell mediated food allergies. Some food allergies have a mix of IgE and non-IgE mediation (Sampson, 2003). Generally, food allergies engage multiple classic immune mechanisms found in allergies (see 'Allergies: general').

Irrespective of aetiology, food allergies are the number one cause of generalized anaphylaxis treated in hospital accident and emergency (A&E) departments, and cover one-third of the total emergency room/A&E visits in the USA and the UK (respectively, Yocum & Kahn, 1994; Pumphrey & Stanworth, 1996). Anaphylaxis is when the smooth muscles vasodilate and constrict causing vasculature collapse because there is no blood pressure. Unknown, though, is why different individuals respond with different symptoms to different foods.

Food allergies can produce a range of discomfort and disease. Allergic immune dysfunction may create gastrointestinal, respiratory, or dermatologic symptoms like migraine, gluten enteropathy, Crohn's disease, eczema, wheeze, urticaria, irritable bowel syndrome or abdominal pain, and, in extreme cases, systemic anaphylactic shock (Del Rio Navarro & Sienra-Monge, 1993) (see 'Inflammatory bowel disease' and 'Irritable bowel syndrome'). Besides producing discomfort and disease, these allergies can be fatal, and need serious consideration.

Food allergies are different from food intolerance and food aversions (Ferguson, 1992). Allergy requires an immune overreaction, typically with elevated immunoglobulin E (IgE). On the other hand, food intolerance simply cannot absorb food by catabolism, resulting in sensitivity, and food aversion is a taste preference without physical problems. Allergy is certainly the most serious of these three food syndromes.

The morbidity of food allergic reactions depends upon the nature and amount of substance ingested as well as the patient's age (Esteban, 1992). Food allergens, or sensitizing substances, have been reported to various fruits, nuts, vegetables, dairy products, fish, grains and meats (Gluck, 1992). Fruit allergy usually centralizes in throat and mouth reactions like lip- or tongue-swelling, hoarseness and uncontrollable throat clearing. Nuts and vegetables, though, produce a more systemic acute attack with symptoms like laryngeal oedema, asthma, urticaria and even anaphylactic shock. Meat or fish reactions often result in asthma. Age is one component of incidence rate.

Incidence

Prevalence rate varies with age. Food allergy prevalence can only be considered estimates since no conceptual agreement and diagnostic procedures are consensually accepted (Esteban, 1992). Approximately 2% of adults may evidence food allergies while 8% of children under 3 years of age do (Bock, 1987). Between the 1970s and 1990s some allergies like peanut appeared to be increasing (Sampson, 1996).

Children (8%; Bock, 1987) compared with adults (2%; Novembre et al., 1988), though, have a greater incidence, which diminishes with age. For children under 3, 8% have food allergies, which dissipate after reaching 1 to 3 years of age (Bock, 1987). Tolerance appears to grow with age and exposure, yet food allergies can also appear initially in adulthood.

Most recent epidemiological work has found similarities in incidence across countries. For instance, the incidence of peanut allergy in children seems similar in the United States (Sicherer et al., 1999) and the United Kingdom (Tariq et al., 1996). In the United States (Sampson, 1996) from the 1980s to the 1990s and on the Isle of Wight (Grundy et al., 1994) from 1994 to 1996, children referred for atopic dermatitis had twice the incidence of peanut reactivity. Epidemiology studies have shown ~2% incidence rate of allergies in adults in the UK (Young et al., 1994) and in the Netherlands (Niestijl Jansen et al., 1994). Researchers can only extrapolate a similar incidence rate in the US since no large scale epidemiological work on food allergies has yet been conducted in that country.

Diagnosis

Allergies to food gained better clinical acceptance when diagnostic techniques improved in scientific rigour (Finn, 1992). Clinical skill, history taking and elimination diets have been the basis for many past diagnoses of food allergies. Tests for cutaneous (standardized skin pricks for immediate hypersensitivity) and for specific IgE antibodies (RAST, ELISA), for histamine (BHR, IMCHR), for intragastric provocation under endoscopy (IPEC), and for intestinal biopsy (after allergen elimination and subsequent feeding challenge) have proved useful.

A careful diagnostic evaluation would include medical history, a dietary diary, a physical examination and various in vitro and in vivo tests (Burks & Sampson, 1992). Standardized skin-prick tests and radioallergosorbent (RIA) assays may be used for screening, but their high rate of false positives require further confirmation with the 'gold standard', a double-blind, placebo-controlled food challenge (DBPCFC; May, 1976). Single-blind challenges, though, can be used to narrow down the scope of potential allergens before confirming with the more expensive, labour- and time-intensive DBPCFC. This rigorous approach eliminates psychological confounds that continue to influence patients' dietary practices when they think they have food allergies (Wisocki & King, 1992). Differential diagnosis needs to consider gastrointestinal disorder, contaminants and additives, pharmacologic agents and psychological reactions.

A number of diseases are considered food hypersensitivity disorders. General categories are IgE-mediated, cell-mediated, Mixed IgE- and cell-mediated and unclassified (Sampson, 2003). IgE mediated disorders include cutaneous (morbilliform rashes and flushing, angioedema, and urticaria), gastrointestinal (gastrointestinal anaphylaxis and oral allergy syndrome), respiratory (bronchospasm or wheezing and acute rhinoconjunctivitis) and generalized (systemic anaphylaxis without or with shock). Mainly cell-mediated disorders span cutaneous (dermatitis herpetiformis and contact dermatitis), gastrointestinal (coeliac disease, food protein-induced enterocolitis, food protein-induced enteropathy syndromes and food protein-induced proctocolitis) and respiratory (food-induced pulmonary hemosiderosis or Heiner's syndrome). Mixed IgE and cell-mediated food allergies-related diseases include cutaneous (atopic dermatitis), gastrointestinal (allergic eosinophilic gastroenteritis and allergic eosinophilic esophagitis) and respiratory (asthma). Finally, the unclassified category includes migraine, arthritis and cow's milk-induced anaemia. Both IgE antigen–antibody complexes and cell-mediated mechanisms are implicated, at least partially, in these pathological conditions.

Treatment

Prevention controversy has existed since almost seventy years ago when exclusive breastfeeding of infants was first identified as prophylactic (Grulee & Sanford, 1936). Results have been mixed in terms of maternal and infant avoidance of suspect allergens, with success with cow's milk allergy but neither peanut nor egg allergy (Zeiger & Heller, 1995). Animal (Hanson, 1981) and human (Fergusson et al., 1990) studies confirm that a varied diet early in life predicts later a higher likelihood of food sensitivities and atopic dermatitis, respectively, especially in high-risk infants (Kajosaari & Saarinen, 1983). High-risk children are those with a first order relative with atopy or food allergies. US allergists (Sampson, 2003) and the Department of Health (1998) in the United Kingdom advise avoidance or delay of introduction for suspect allergens, especially for high-risk children:

- children under 6 months of age should avoid solids
- children up to 12 months of age should avoid cow's milk
- children up to 18–24 months of age should avoid eggs and egg products
- children up to 3 years of age should avoid peanuts, tree nuts, shellfish and fish.
- mothers during pregnancy and lactation, should avoid peanuts.

Most young children acquire immune tolerance of their food (except peanuts, tree nuts and seafood) allergies by 3 years of age (Bock, 1982; Hill et al., 1989; Host, 1994). Yet for 1-year-olds with milk hypersensitivity, 35% by 3 years of age (Host & Halken, 1990)

and 25% by 20 years of age (Host et al., 1997) evidence additional food allergies to other allergens. No formal studies have examined non-IgE-mediated skin and respiratory allergies.

For treatment of existing food allergies, subcutaneous injections have been ineffective (Evans, 1992). The primary standard treatment programme consists of elimination diets as well as challenge tests (Ferguson, 1992). Elimination simply requires systematic abstinence from the suspected allergen. Then, if signs and symptoms disappear, the allergen is re-introduced and confirmed in the most rigorous fashion with a double-blind placebo-controlled provocation test. If and when symptoms re-appear determines the subsequent treatment plan. Strict elimination of the allergen is the only proven treatment for food allergies. One third of children and adults lose reactivity after complete elimination (Sampson & Scanlon, 1989; Pastorello & Stocchi, 1989; Businco et al., 1989; Hill et al., 1986). However, those with peanut, tree nut, fish, or shellfish allergies rarely lose their sensitivity.

Although their scientific validation has only started quite recently, some alternative approaches have treated food allergies (Kay & Lessof, 1992). Treatments that have been used with clinical success are clinical ecology, acupuncture, homeopathy, hypnosis and herbalism. Again, even though case studies have verified effectiveness, the mechanisms of and limits to these treatments are little known. Caution is warranted since many of the evaluative findings are not currently available (see 'Complementary medicine').

Behavioural and psychological aspects

Psychologists need to concern themselves most with the proper diagnosis of a food allergy and subsequent adherence to a diet regime. Those reporting food allergies which objective physiological tests do not confirm have a hypochondriacal and hysteric profile compared with those with tests that do confirm food allergies (Parker et al., 1991). Whether undiagnosed food allergies cause these problems or the reported 'allergies' stem from a psychological disturbance is unclear. Yet the unqualified acceptance of a double-blind procedure to definitively determine food allergies underlines the very potency of psychological aspects not only in the initial experience of food allergic symptoms but also in their maintenance into a disorder.

Furthermore, food allergies produce physical symptoms like migraine headaches which are perhaps misdiagnosed as psychological. Food allergies also need checking in psychological syndromes like attention deficit disorder (Burks & Sampson, 1992). Moreover, attention to other physical symptoms indicating allergies should assist in proper diagnosis. Biofeedback has actually been used to determine food-sensitive persons (Laird, 1986).

Adjunctive psychological interventions pertain to control, if not prevention, of food allergies. The psychological management skills from education focuses upon label reading, menu planning and food abstinence. Success of prevention and recovery efforts involving the strict avoidance of allergy-producing foods centrally concerns adherence, a medical challenge that is inherently psychological (Burks & Sampson, 1992). The final galvanizing news for the field of health psychology is that elimination diets work for about one-third of those with food allergies. Why?

So much is known about morbidity. Now is the time to pursue prevention, recovery and, ideally, cure. Certainly the thrust of inquiry now needs to determine aetiology ('how much is genetics?') and individual differences ('why don't all those at risk succumb?'). What will facilitate adherence to an allergen elimination diet? What else besides elimination might be used for control and cure?

To conclude, the health psychology field of food allergies is only just beginning to coalesce in scientific acceptance of its existence. So, the next step is a rigorous application of the scientific method for diagnosis of risk and manifestation and motivation for prevention as well as for recovery and cure. The elimination diet is really not the final solution, but rather just a 'way station' or temporary stop-off point that delays the tough challenge of cure.

(See also 'Allergies to drugs', 'Allergies: general' and 'Diet and health'.)

REFERENCES

Bock, S. A. (1987). Prospective appraisal of complaints of adverse reactions to foods in children during the first 3 years of life. *Pediatrics*, **79**, 633–8.

Bock, S. A. (1982). The natural history of food sensitivity. *Journal of Allergy and Clinical Immunology*, **69**, 173–7.

Burks, A. H. & Sampson, H. A. (1992). Diagnostic approaches to the patient with suspected food allergies. *The Journal of Pediatrics*, **121**(5, Pt. 1, Suppl.), S64–S71.

Businco, L., Benincori, N., Cantani, A. et al. (1989). Chronic diarrhea due to cow's milk allergy: A 4- to 10-year follow-up study. *Annals of Allergy*, **55**, 844–7.

Del Rio Navarro, B. E. & Sienra, Monge, J. J. (1993). Food allergy. *Boliva Medical Hospital Infant Mexico*, **50**(6), 422–9.

Department of Health (1998). *Peanut allergy*. London: HMSO

Esteban, M. M. (1992). Adverse food reactions in infancy and childhood. *The Journal of Pediatrics*, **121**(5, Pt. 2, Suppl.).

Evans, R. III (1992). Environmental control and immunotherapy for allergic disease. *Journal of Allergy and Clinical Immunology*, **90**(3, Pt. 2), 462–8.

Fergusson, D. M., Horwood, L. J. & Shannon, F. T. (1990). Early solid feeding and recurrent eczea: a 10-year longitudinal study. *Pediatrics*, **86**, 541–6.

Ferguson, A. (1992). Definitions and diagnosis of food intolerance and food allergy: consensus and controversy. *Journal of Pediatrics*, **121**(5, Pt. 2), S7–11.

Finn, R. (1992). Food allergy – fact or fiction: a review. *Journal of the Royal Society of Medicine*, **85**(9), 560–4.

Gluck, U. (1992). Neglected allergens. *Therapeutische Umschau*, **49**(10), 669–73.

Grulee, C. G. & Sanford, H. N. (1936). The influence of breast feeding and artificial feeding in infantile eczema. *Journal of Pediatrics*, **9**, 223–5.

Grundy, J., Matthews, S., Bateman, B. J. et al. (1994). Rising prevalence of allergy to peanut in children: data from 2 sequential cohorts. *Journal of Allergy and Clinical Immunology*, **110**, 784–9.

Hanson, D. G. (1981). Ontogeny of orally induced tolerance to soluble proteins in mice: priming and tolerance in newborn. *Journal of Immunology*, **127**, 1518–24.

Hill, D. J., Firer, M. A., Shelton, M. J. & Hosking, C. S. (1986). Manifestations of milk allergy in infancy: clinical and immunological findings. *Journal of Pediatrics*, **109**, 270–6.

Hill, D. J., Firer, M. A., Ball, G. & Hosking, C. S. (1989). Recovery from milk allergy in early childhood: antibody study. *Journal of Pediatrics*, **114**(5), 761–6.

Host, A. (1994). Cow's milk protein allergy and intolerance in infancy. *Pediatric Allergy Immunology*, **5**(Suppl. 5), 5–36.

Host, A. & Halken, S. (1990). A prospective study of cow milk allergy in Danish infants during the first 3 years of life. *Allergy*, **45**, 587–96.

Host, A., Halken, S., Jacobsen, H. P. et al. (1997). The natural course of cow's milk protein allergy/intolerance. *Journal of Allergy and Clinical Immunology*, **99**, S490 (abstract).

Kajosaari, M. & Saarinen, U. M. (1983). Prophylaxis of atopic disease by six months; total solid food elimination. *Archives of Paediatrics Scandinavia*, **72**, 411–14.

Kay, A. B. & Lessof, M. H. (1992). Allergy. Conventional and alternative concepts. A report of the Royal College of Physicians Committee on Clinical Immunology and Allergy. *Clinical and Experimental Allergy*, **22**(Suppl. 3), 1–44.

Laird, D. (1986). Using biofeedback to uncover food sensitive persons. *Journal of Orthomolecular Medicine*, **1**(2), 78–83.

May, C. D. (1976). Objective clinical and laboratory studies of immediate hypersensitivity reactions to food in asthmatic children. *Journal of Allergy and Clinical Immunology*, **58**(4), 500–15.

Niestijl Jansen, J. J., Kardinaal, A. F., Huijbers, G. H. et al. (1994). Prevalence of food allergy and intolerance in the adult Dutch population. *Journal of Allergy and Clinical Immunology*, **93**, 446–56.

Novembre, E., de Martino, M. & Vierucci, A. (1988). Foods and respiratory allergy. *Journal of Allergy and Clinical Immunology*, **81**, 1059–65.

Parker, S. L., Garner, D. M., Leznoff, A. et al. (1991). Psychological characteristics of patients with reported adverse reactions to foods. *International Journal of Eating Disorders*, **10**(4), 433–9.

Pastorello, E., Stocchi, L., Pravetonni, V. et al. (1989). Role of the food elimination diet in adults with food allergy. *Journal of Allergy and Clinical Immunology*, **84**, 475–83.

Pumphrey, R. S. & Stanworth, S. J. (1996). The clinical spectrum of anaphylaxis in north-west England. *Clinical Experimental Allergy*, **26**, 1364–70.

Sampson, H. A. (1996). Managing peanut allergy. *British Medical Journal*, **312**, 1050–1.

Sampson, H. A. (2003). Adverse reactions to foods. In J. W. Yunginger, W. W. Busse, B. S. Bochner et al. (Eds.). (2003). *Middleton's Allergy Principles and Practice. Vol. 2*. (6th edn.). (pp. 1619–1643), St. Louis, IL: CV Mosby Publishers.

Sampson, H. A. & Scanlon, S. M. (1989). Natural history of food hypersensitivity in children with atopic dermatitis. *Journal of Pediatrics*, **115**, 23–7.

Sicherer, S. H., Munoz-Furlong, A., Burks, A. W. & Sampson, H. A. (1999). Prevalence of peanut and tree nut allergy in the United States of America. *Journal of Allergy and Clinical Immunology*, **103**, 559–62.

Tariq, S. M., Steens, M., Matthews, S. et al. (1996). Cohort study of peanut and tree nut sensitization by age of 4 years. *British Medical Journal*, **313**, 514–17.

Wisocki, P. A. & King, D. S. (1992). *The construction of a food-behavior inventory to measure beliefs about the behavioral effects of food*. Paper presented at the annual conference of the American Psychological Association, San Francisco, CA.

Yocum, M. W. & Khan, D. A. (1994). Assessment of patients who have experienced anaphylaxis: a

3-year study. *Mayo Clinic Proceedings*, **69**, 16–23.

Young, E., Patel, S., Stoneham, M. D. *et al.* (1987). The prevalence of reactions to food additives in a survey population. *Journal of Research for College Physicians in London*, **21**, 241–71.

Young, E., Stoneham, M. D., Petruckevitch, A. *et al.* (1994). A population study of food intolerance. *Lancet*, **343**, 1127–30.

Zeiger, R. & Heller, S. (1995). The development and prediction of atopy in high-risk children: follow-up at seven years

in a prospective randomized study of combined maternal and infant food allergen avoidance. *Journal of Immunology*, **127**, 1518–24.

Allergies: general

Mary Gregerson

Family Therapy Institute of Alexandria

Features

Allergies are a T lymphocyte cell-mediated immunity (CMI) gone awry (Zweiman, 1999). Normal CMI development usually results in a synchronous, efficacious T-helper cell (Th1) mediated protection of the human from internal disruptions or against the invasion of disease provoking foreign agents. In allergies, an over-abundance of another specific type of T-helper cell named Th2 is the abnormality (Broide, 2001). After extensive research, whether the relationship between allergies and CMI is inverse remains an experimental question. For allergies, though, the elevated presence of Th2 results in an immediate hypersensitivity called Type I.

The genetic basis of allergies is commonly accepted. Even with similar genetic risk, some persons either never get allergic symptoms or theirs disappear while others continually experience allergies. Family transmission of allergy has been acknowledged since 1920. If two parents have Type I Hypersensitivity, offspring have a 50% chance to manifest atopy, and with one parent, almost a 30% chance. These individual differences in responsivity and the interruption of Mendelian genetic transmission make psychological and behavioural treatment factors important considerations in allergies.

The immune substrate of allergies is determined both by genetics (hardware) within the Type I major histocompatibilty complex (MCI) and by learning (software), for example, histamine tissue priming (Peeke *et al.*, 1987). Both hardware and software regulate the individual's allergic immune responsivity. The Th2 pattern is related to elevated emission of a cascade of other sequela, specifically, Immunoglobulin E (IgE), interleukins (4, 13 and 10) as well as eosinophil-laden inflammation. These immunological changes manifest in numerous clinical symptoms and distinct disease states.

Clinical symptoms of atopy

These biological sequela result in distinct clinical features for a myriad of diseases such as asthma, eczema, rhinitis (perennial and seasonal, which is commonly called hay fever) and urticaria. The umbrella term for these symptoms is atopy. The atopic disease allergy results from an immune over-reaction to a specific agent called an allergen or antigen. The former is from an outside source; the latter from an inner source.

Allergies cause physical and psychological discomfort, and, sometimes, death. In hay fever the mucous membranes in the nasal passages swell; in eczema the skin inflames with wheals and flares; in asthma the bronchial passages constrict severely; and in anaphylaxis the smooth muscles vasodilate and constrict causing vasculature collapse because there is no blood pressure (see 'Asthma' and 'Eczema'). Also, allergies are associated with a number of psychological symptoms (see Bell *et al.*, 1991; Jasnoski *et al.*, 1994). Specifically, depression, shyness, panic and anxiety have been connected to allergies. Recently in a large cross-sectional Norweigan twin study, allergies had a small inverse correlation with subjective wellbeing (Roysamb *et al.*, 2003). Concomitant allergies have been observed frequently in other diseases, e.g., eating disorders such as bulimia, schizophrenia and systemic lupus erythematosus.

Mechanisms

People with allergy usually, but not always, evidence higher levels of circulating IgE (up to 12 mg/ml) compared to normals (approximately 0.3 mg/ml). IgE's heat sensitivity could explain why rapid temperature or humidity changes and drafts often increase allergic nasal obstruction. IgE further degranulates histamine which produces positive immediate wheal and flare skin reactions. Sometimes independent of IgE elevation, inflammatory tissue priming itself can produce the clinical features of allergy (Peeke *et al.*, 1987).

After the activation of mast cells releasing vasoactive mediators, often a late phase reaction (LPR) follows within hours. At the LPR site, Th2 lymphocytes cause aggregation and activation of eosinophils and perhaps basophils. These Th2 are mainly memory T-lymphocytes and are often activated 6–8 hours after the allergen challenge. At the challenge site, among the cascade of biologic responses, eosinophils release possible noxious cationic proteins, basophils activate histamine release, and chemokines aggregate and/or activate inflammatory cells.

In an example of classical conditioning, sometimes histamine itself can produce allergic reactions without the involvement of IgE. Total IgE levels are elevated in only 30% to 40% of those with allergic rhinitis. A residual histamine priming could, even in the absence of IgE elevaion, conceivably result in an allergic response, thus accounting for those with allergic symptoms that do not evidence higher IgE levels. An important study (Rietveld *et al.*, 1997) demonstrated that the subjective reports of severity in children with asthma as well as their subsequent breathlessness were influenced by false feedback of high levels of wheezing after exercise.

In allergies, suggestion may be an important psychological consideration. Similar to the asthma study just cited (Rietveld *et al.*, 1997), in some instances, a 'placebo' allergic reaction has been evoked when the patient thought the allergen was present and it was not (see 'Placebos'). For instance, pictures of hayfields or misrepresented 'placebo' liquids have actually caused a full allergic attack (see Jemmott & Locke, 1984, for review). These psychological considerations figure into a real physiological picture of psychosomatic disease and distress.

In terms of physiology, some speculation exists that a depressed CMI (anergy) allows the allergic cellular substrate and subsequent symptomatology to develop. In essence, the CMI fails to activate in order to protect the individual. Whether absence of normal T cell function or the over-abundance of certain T cells with suppressive power underlies anergy is under study now. Perhaps both mechanisms play a role, interdependently or independently.

Also under scrutiny is whether anergy results in or results from particular diseases. Physical vulnerabilities like age, disease and pregnancy have been associated with immune vulnerability when stressed (Kiecolt-Glaser *et al.*, 2002; Segerstrom & Miller, 2004). For cancer patients, some in vitro evidence exists that stress interferes with normal anti-inflammatory responses to cease atopic symptoms (Miller *et al.*, 2002). Conceptually, the immune, neural and psychological systems are thought to be systemically interrelated (Lekander, 2002). In asthma, psychophysiological mediation is commonly accepted (Lehrer *et al.*, 2002).

Diagnosis

Double-blind, placebo-controlled provocation tests often discount IgE mediation for as many as 60% of those with a history of allergies (Jarvis, 1993). The question arises, though, as to what causes an allergic response to trigger histamine priming or other provocations of the allergic response. In the absence of physiological answers, psychological and behavioural factors are implicated. Even the methods to determine the existence of allergies implicate psychological factors.

Interestingly, one research study (for review see Jemmott & Locke, 1984) distinguished between clinical symptoms and cellular changes. A 'placebo' non-allergic mixture falsely represented as the allergic substance elicited symptoms and cellular changes, while the allergic mixture misrepresented as non-allergic also elicited cellular changes, but not symptoms. In other words if allergic participants thought the substance was non-allergic, although their underlying physiology changed, they did not show symptoms. Other work has shown a conditioned allergic response elicited by the color of the vial and not the substance in the vial. This growing body of evidence heavily implicates psychological factors in allergic clinical manifestations.

Skin tests, radioallergosorbent tests (RASTs) and relevant provocation tests have been effective in diagnosing allergies. Skin-prick tests and the enzyme allergosorbent test usually screen for allergy specificity. Then the 'gold standard' DTH provocation test confirms the allergy (Rosenstreich, 1993).

Five major criteria need to be met for a successful DTH skin test (Zweiman, 2003, p. 974):

1. The use of stable, standardized and non-irritating antigens;
2. A precise intradermal antigen injection;
3. Well-defined area of induration (not just erythema), with reproducible measurements by experienced observers;
4. A sufficient sensitivity so that a negative reaction is strong evidence against prior sensitization; and
5. A reproducible degree of reactivity in repeat testing.

A small percentage of disagreement may exist between these tests. Both false positives and negatives are possible.

Furthermore, one study (Rietveld *et al.*, 1997) has shown that children reported more symptoms when simply misled by hearing sounds of excessive wheezing. Such sensitization has been identified as anxiety sensitivity (Jasnoski *et al.*, 1994). Psychological considerations like this may be important in the diagnosis of severity which, in turn, determines treatment.

Treatment

Treatments can be drugs or psychotherapy. Besides allergen avoidance, immunotherapy is the main pharmacological treatment available. This treatment desensitizes the person with allergies by creating a tolerance. A number of well-designed studies have corroborated immunotherapy's effectiveness to reduce symptoms for allergies like hay fever and allergic asthma (Nicassio *et al.*, 2004).

Antihistamines can be used to curtail the intensity of allergic symptoms. This treatment interferes with the late phase following the immediate allergic response. Often this late phase correlates with severity. This approach, though, controls symptoms without decreasing the basic hypersensitivity.

With time and with change, allergies can disappear without pharmacological treatment. A relevant, well-accepted aspect of allergies is their responsiveness to adaptive patterns and changes in life situations. Although the mechanism has not yet been found (Stone *et al.*, 2000), one experimental study (Smyth *et al.*, 1999) found that journal writing about stressful events actually improved symptoms in those with the atopic diseases of rheumatoid arthritis and asthma (see 'Emotional expression and health'). Therefore, psychological and behavioural treatments are sensible adjunctives to medical treatment for those experiencing allergic symptoms. Recommendations include a close dovetailing of research, treatments and public policy for a consummate health psychology approach (Nicassio *et al.*, 2004).

Psychological and behavioural treatments

Research on the efficacy of psychological and behavioural treatments now needs increased conceptual and methodological rigour. For instance, individual differences such as absorption ability can spuriously confound results if not appropriately controlled (Gregerson, 2000, 2003). Of the different types of health psychology interventions available, the strongest evidence for allergy management exists for hypnosis and conditioning treatments, with equivocal support for disclosure and stress management and no support for relaxation (Miller & Cohen, 2001) (see 'Hypnosis' and 'Behaviour therapy'). All allergy research and treatment with psychosocial variables aims at morbidity and mortality but not etiology.

For allergies per se, emotional treatment and behavioural medical approaches (Schmidt-Traub & Bamler, 1992) have proved effective in diminishing outbreaks. Other alternative approaches have included hypnosis (for review see Jemmott & Locke, 1984) and nutrition (Van Flandern, 1985). The ubiquitous issue of adherence/compliance with allergy treatments has responded to behavioural intervention (Finney et al., 1990).

Allergies also have a strong body of research addressing the effects of the mother–child relationship and family environment upon symptom severity. For example, one study identified parent dyadic patterns which predicted allergy risk level in children (Faleide et al., 1988). Other work found that higher support, independence and organization, as well as lower religiosity, predicted lesser atopic dermatitis symptom severity in children (Gil et al., 1987). Significant relief of asthmatic symptoms has resulted from family therapy compared with conventional medical treatment (Gustafsson et al., 1986). One study pinpointed open extended discussion of conflict as the distinguishing characteristic of families without a member with asthma compared with those in which asthma was present (Northey et al., 1998), although the direction of causality was neither established nor addressed.

More definitive research needs to identify, assess and treat family patterns, among other psychsocial variables, related to allergic symptoms. In additional to familial support, a review (Uchino et al., 1996) has emphasized that emotional support appears as important as social support for its important psychoimmune influence (see 'Psychoneuroimmunology' and 'Social support and health'). Moreover, health-related behaviours appear superfluous to such psychoimmune associations like those found in allergies. Finally, stress buffering might be possible.

Conclusion

So, an array of psychological and behavioural factors appears to be implicated, at least, in allergy management. Personality characteristics such as absorption ability and anxiety sensitivity need consideration in research into and treatment of allergies. Furthermore, familial and other social support, emotional support and stress management appear worthwhile to pursue as morbidity and mortality factors. Again, no studies appear to definitively address the behavioural, psychological and social effects of allergy aetiology.

(See also 'Allergies to drugs' and 'Allergies to food'.)

REFERENCES

Bell, I. R., Jasnoski, M. L., Kagan, J. & King, D. S. (1991). Depression and allergies: survey of a nonclinical population. *Psychotherapy and Psychosomatics*, **55**(1), 24–31.

Broide, D. H. (2001). Molecular and cellular mechanisms of allergic disease. *Journal of Allergy and Clinical Immunology*, **108**, S65–S71.

Faleide, A. O., Galtung, V. K., Unger, S. & Watten, R. G. (1988). Children at risk of allergic development: the parents' dyadic relationship. *Psychotherapy and Psychosomatics*, **49**(3-4), 223–9.

Finney, J. W., Lemanek, K. L., Brohy, C. J. & Cataldo, M. F. (1990). Pediatric appointment keeping: improving adherence in a primary care allergy clinic. Special Issue: Adherence with pediatric regimens. *Journal of Pediatric Psychology*, **15**(4), 571–9.

Gil, K. M., Keefe, F. J., Sampson, H. A. *et al.* (1987). The relation of stress and family environment to atopic dermatitis symptoms in children. *Journal of Psychosomatic Research*, **31**(6), 673–84.

Gregerson (Jasnoski), M. B. (2000). The curious 2,000 year case of asthma. *Psychosomatic Medicine*, **62**(6), 816–27.

Gregerson (Jasnoski), M.B. (2003). Asthma as a psychosomatic Illness: An historical perspective. In E. S. Brown (Ed.). *Asthma: social and psychological factors and psychosomatic syndromes. advances in psychosomatic medicine* (pp. 16–41). Basel: Karger.

Gustafsson, P. A., Kjellman, N.-I. M. & Cederblad, M. (1986). Family therapy in the treatment of severe childhood asthma. *Journal of Psychosomatic Research*, **30**(3), 369–74.

Jarvis, W. T. (1993). Allergy related quackery. *New York State Journal of Medicine*, **93**(2), 100–4.

Jasnoski, M. B. L., Bell, I. R. & Peterson, R. (1994). What associations exist between shyness, hay fever, anxiety, anxiety sensitivity, and panic disorder? *Anxiety, Stress, and Coping*, **7**, 1–15.

Jemmott, J. B. III. & Locke, S. E. (1984). Psychosocial factors, immunologic mediation, and human susceptibility to infectious diseases: how much do we know? *Psychological Bulletin*, **95**(1), 78–105.

Kiecolt-Glaser, J. K., McGuire, L., Robles, T. F. & Glaser, R. (2002). Psychoneuroimmunology: psychological influences on immune function and health. *Journal of Consulting & Clinical Psychology*, **70**(3), 537–47.

Lehrer, P., Feldman, J., Giardino, N., Song, H. & Schmaling, K. (2002). Psychological aspects of asthma. *Journal of Consulting & Clinical Psychology*, **70**(3), 691–711.

Lekander, M. (2002). Ecological immunology: the role of the immune system in psychology and neuroscience. *European Psychologist*, **7**(2), 98–115.

Miller, G. E. & Cohen, S. (2001). Psychological interventions and the immune system: a meta-analytic review and critique. *Health Psychology*, **20**(1), 47–63.

Miller, G. E., Cohen, S. & Ritchey, A. K. (2002). Chronic psychological stress and the regulation of pro-inflammatory cytokines: A glucocorticoid-resistance model. *Health Psychology*, **21**(6), 531–41.

Nicassio, P. M., Meyerowitz, B. E., Kerns, R. D. (2004). The future of health psychology interventions. *Health Psychology*. **23**(2), 132–7.

Northey, S., Griffin, W. A. & Krainz, S. (1998). A partial test of the psychosomatic family model: marital interaction patterns in asthma and nonasthma families. *Journal of Family Psychology*, **12**(2), 220–33.

Peeke, H. V. S., Ellman, G., Dark, K., Salfi, M. & Reus, V. I. (1987). Cortisol and behaviorally conditioned histamine release. *Annals of the New York Academy of Science,* **496**, 583–7.

Rietveld, S., Kolk, A. M., Prins, P. J. M. & Colland, V. T. (1997). The influence of respiratory sounds on breathlessness in children with asthma: a symptom-perception approach. *Health Psychology,* **16**(6), Nov 1997, 547–53.

Rosenstreich, D. L. (1993). Evaluation of delayed hypersensitivity: from PPD to poison ivy, *Allergy Proceedings,* **14**, 395–400

Roysamb, E., Tambs, K., Reichborn-Kjennerud, T., Neale, M. C. & Harris, J. R. (2003). Happiness and health: environmental and genetic contributions to the relationship between subjective well-being, perceived health, and somatic illness. *Journal of Personality and Social Psychology,* **85**(6), 1136–46.

Schmidt-Traub, S. & Bamler, K. J. (1992). The psychoimmunological relationship among allergies, panic disorder, and agoraphobia. *Zeitschrift fur Klinische Psychologie, Psychopathologie und Psychotherapie,* **40**(4), 325–45.

Segerstrom, S. C. & Miller, G. E. (2004). Psychological stress and the human immune system: a meta-analytic study of 30 years of inquiry. *Psychological Bulletin,* **130**(4), 601–30.

Smyth, J., Stone, A., Hurewitz, A. & Kaell, A. (1999). Effects of writing about stressful experiences on symptom reduction in patients with asthma or rheumatoid arthritis: a randomized trial. *Journal of the American Medical Association,* **281**, 1304–9.

Stone, A. A., Smyth, J. M., Kaell, A. & Hurewitz, A. (2000). Structured writing about stressful events: Exploring potential psychological mediators of positive health effects. *Health Psychology,* **19**(6), 619–24.

Uchino, B. N., Cacioppo, J. T. & Kiecolt-Glaser, J. K. (1996). The relationship between social support and physiological processes: a review with emphasis on underlying mechanisms and implications for health. *Psychological Bulletin,* **119**(3), 488–531.

Van Flandern, B. A. (1985). Last chance. *Journal of Orthomolecular Psychiatry,* **14**(4), 251–6.

Zweiman, B. (1999). Inflammatory responses in late phase allergic reactions in the skin. *Canadian Journal of Allergy and Clinical Immunology,* **4**, 366.

Zweiman, B. (2003). Cell mediated immunity in health and disease. In Adkinson, N. F., Jr., Yunginer, J. W., Busse, W. W., Bochner, B. S., Holgate, S. T. & Simons, F. E. R. (Eds.). *Middleton's Allergy Principles and Practice* (6th edn.). (pp. 973–95). St. Louis, IL: CV Mosby Publishers.

Amnesia

Barbara A. Wilson[1] and Narinder Kapur[2]

[1]MRC Cognition and Brain Sciences Unit
[2]Addenbrooke's Hospital

Amnesia and organic memory impairment are commonly seen after many types of brain injury including degenerative disorders, head injury, anoxia and infections of the brain. If severe, amnesia is often more handicapping in everyday life than severe physical problems.

People with the classic amnesic syndrome show an anterograde amnesia (AA), i.e. they have great difficulty learning and remembering most kinds of new information. Immediate memory, however, is normal when this is assessed by forward digit span or the recency effect in free recall. There is usually a period of retrograde amnesia (RA), that is a loss of information acquired before the onset of the amnesia. This gap or period of RA is very variable in length and may range from a few minutes to decades. Previously acquired semantic knowledge about the world and implicit memory (remembering without awareness or conscious recollection) are typically intact in amnesic subjects. As the majority of patients with severe memory disorders present with additional cognitive problems such as attention deficits, word finding problems or slowed information processing, those with a classic amnesic syndrome are relatively rare.

Nevertheless, people with a 'pure' amnesic syndrome and people with more widespread cognitive deficits tend to share certain characteristics. In both cases, immediate memory is reasonably normal; there is difficulty in remembering after a delay or distraction; new learning is difficult and there is a tendency to remember things that happened a long time before the accident or illness better than things that happened a short time before.

A number of conceptual frameworks have been proposed to help explain the pattern of memory loss that is seen in memory-impaired patients. The reader is referred to the *Oxford handbook of memory* (Craik & Tulving, 2000) for a detailed exposition of memory models and theoretical expositions that are available for helping to consider memory loss in neurological populations. There is a broad consensus that memory is best considered as a number of dissociable systems, rather than as a unitary system (Schacter & Tulving, 1994), though it is likely that there is considerable overlap in the brain mechanisms underlying some of these systems (Rajah & McIntosh, 2005).

The commonly agreed memory systems are:

- *Episodic memory,* which refers to the retention of personally-experienced events that can be related to specific spatial and temporal contexts (e.g. remembering a recent holiday).
- *Semantic memory,* which refers to the organized knowledge about words, concepts and culturally/educationally-acquired facts (e.g. knowing what certain words mean).

- *Working memory* (sometimes called short-term memory), which refers to processes for holding and manipulating material in a temporary store, usually for seconds or a few minutes (e.g. remembering a telephone number shortly after hearing it).
- *Procedural memory*, which usually refers to the ability to acquire new skills, or use previously acquired skills, be they motor or linguistic (e.g. learning to ride a bicycle).
- *Perceptual memory*, which usually refers to the ability to retain the perceptual features of a stimulus, and is thought to underlie learning that leads to the perceptual identification of stimuli (e.g. seeing a new model of a car and being able to identify it better the second time round).

In the case of memory processes, while it is generally accepted that encoding, consolidation and retrieval represent important stages of memory processing, there are divergent views as to the specific mechanisms that underlie such stages (Meeter & Murre, 2004). The 'standard consolidation' model (Squire *et al.*, 2004) takes the view that while the medial temporal lobe plays a part in the laying down of new memories, their stored representation is eventually subserved by cortical mechanisms, especially those in the neocortex. By contrast, the multiple-trace model (Nadel *et al.*, 2000) regards the medial temporal lobe as being critical for the retention and recollection of all episodic memories, no matter how long ago they have been stored.

Although precise figures are not available, there are considerable numbers of memory impaired people in society. Some 10% of people over 65 years of age have dementia and some 36% of people with severe head injury will have permanent memory impairments (see 'Dementias' and 'Head injury'). Add to these figures those whose memory deficits result from Korsakoff's syndrome, encephalitis, anoxia, AIDS and so forth, and one can begin to appreciate the enormity of the problem.

Assessment of memory should include both neuropsychological and behavioural measures as it is important to identify cognitive strengths and weaknesses and to identify the everyday problems arising from memory impairment. Neuropsychological tests should include general intellectual functioning, language, perception and executive functioning as well as detailed memory assessments. Immediate and delayed memory, nonverbal and verbal memory, recall and recognition, semantic and episodic memory,

implicit memory (remembering without awareness) and new learning will all need to be assessed (see Wilson, 2004 for further discussion). More functional and behavioural measures will identify everyday problems causing concern and distress. These measures include observations in real life settings, interviewing patients, their relatives and care staff and the collection of information from such self report measures as diaries, checklists, questionnaires and rating scales (see 'Neuropsychological assessment').

Restoration of memory functioning or retraining of memory following brain damage appear to be unachievable goals although some recovery may occur for a period of years (Kapur & Graham, 2002; Wilson, 2003). Consequently, rehabilitation for memory-impaired people focuses on environmental adaptations, compensatory strategies, improving learning and helping them to make better use of their residual skills. For those who are very severely intellectually impaired, structuring the environment, to reduce the need to remember, is probably the most effective method. Examples include labelling doors, cupboards and drawers, drawing coloured lines from one place to another and positioning material so it cannot be missed. External memory aids are probably the most beneficial of all therapeutic approaches, although many memory-impaired people find it difficult to use these aids efficiently and it requires considerable ingenuity to teach their use (Sohlberg & Mateer, 1989). Kapur *et al.* (2004) cover aspects of external and compensatory aids in some detail. One of the recent developments for improving learning in amnesic subjects is the errorless learning approach (Baddeley & Wilson, 1994; Wilson *et al.*, 1994) whereby it was shown that preventing errors during the learning process led to improved learning by amnesic subjects. Helping people to make better use of their residual, albeit damaged, memory skills can be achieved through the use of mnemonics and study or rehearsal strategies (see 'Neuropsychological rehabilitation').

Finally, many memory-impaired people are anxious and isolated; so too are their families. Rehabilitation should address these anxieties through anxiety management programmes, information and counselling and perhaps through groups for patients and/or their relatives. Tate (2004) addresses these issues and other aspects of rehabilitation for people with amnesia.

REFERENCES

Baddeley, A. D. & Wilson, B. A. (1994). When implicit learning fails: amnesia and the problem of error elimination. *Neuropsychologia*, **32**, 53–68.

Craik, F. I. M. & Tulving, E. (2000). *Oxford handbook of memory.* Oxford: Oxford University Press.

Kapur, N., Glisky, E. L. & Wilson, B. A. (2004). External memory aids and computers in memory rehabilitation. In A. D. Baddeley, M. D. Kopelman & B. A. Wilson. *The essential handbook of memory disorders for clinicians* (pp. 301–27). Chichester: John Wiley.

Kapur, N. & Graham, K. S. (2002). Recovery of memory function in neurological disease. In A. D.

Baddeley, M. Kopelman & B. A. Wilson (Eds.). *Handbook of memory disorders* (pp. 233–48). Chichester: John Wiley.

Meeter, M. & Murre, J. M. (2004). Consolidation of long-term memory: evidence and alternatives. *Psychological Bulletin*, **130**, 843–57.

Nadel, L., Samsonovich, A., Ryan, L. & Moscovitch, M. (2000). Multiple trace theory of human memory: computational, neuroimaging and neuropsychological results. *Hippocampus*, **10**, 352–68.

Rajah, M. N. & McIntosh, A. R. (2005). Overlap in the functional neural systems involved in semantic and episodic memory

retrieval. *Journal of Cognitive Neuroscience*, **17**, 470–82.

Schacter, D. L. & Tulving, E. (1994). *Memory Systems 1994.* Cambridge: MIT Press.

Sohlberg, M. M. & Mateer, C. (1989). Training use of compensatory memory books: a three-stage behavioural approach. *Journal of Clinical and Experimental Neuropsychology*, **11**, 871–91.

Squire, L. R., Stark, C. E. & Clark, R. E. (2004). The medial temporal lobe. *Annual Review of Neuroscience*, **27**, 279–306.

Tate, R. (2004). Emotional and social consequences of memory disorders. In A. D. Baddeley, M. D. Kopelman & B. A. Wilson (Eds.). *The essential handbook* *of memory disorders for clinicians* (pp. 329–52). Chichester: John Wiley.

Wilson, B. A. (2003). Treatment and recovery from brain damage. In L. Nadel (Ed.). *Encyclopedia of Cognitive Science*, (*Vol. 1*). (pp. 410–16). London: Nature Publishing Group.

Wilson, B. A. (2004). Assessment of memory disorders. In A. D. Baddeley, M. D. Kopelman & B. A. Wilson (Eds.). *The essential handbook of memory disorders for clinicians* (pp. 159–178). Chichester: John Wiley.

Wilson, B. A., Baddeley, A. D., Evans, J. J. & Shiel, A. (1994). Errorless learning in the rehabilitation of memory impaired people. *Neuropsychological Rehabilitation*, **4**, 307–26.

Amputation and phantom limb pain

Ronald Melzack[1] and Joel Katz[2]

[1]McGill University
[2]York University

Phantom limbs occur in 95–100% of amputees who lose an arm or leg. The phantom limb is usually described as having a tingling feeling and a definite shape that resembles the somatosensory experience of the real limb before amputation. It is reported to move through space in much the same way as the normal limb would move when the person walks, sits down, or stretches out on a bed. At first, the phantom limb feels perfectly normal in size and shape, so much so that the amputee may reach out for objects with the phantom hand, or try to step on to the floor with the phantom leg. As time passes, however, the phantom limb begins to change shape. The arm or leg becomes less distinct and may fade away altogether, so that the phantom hand or foot seems to be hanging in mid-air. Sometimes, the limb is slowly 'telescoped' into the stump until only the hand or foot remain at the stump tip (Solonen, 1962). However, the neural basis of the phantom does not disappear. Injury of the stump years or decades after fading or telescoping may suddenly produce a phantom as vivid and full-sized as that felt immediately after amputation (Cohen, 1944).

Amputation is not essential for the occurrence of a phantom. After avulsion of the brachial plexus of the arm, without injury to the arm itself, most patients report a phantom arm (the 'third arm') which is usually extremely painful (Wynn-Parry, 1980). Even nerve destruction is not necessary. About 95% of patients who receive an anaesthetic block of the brachial plexus for surgery of the arm report a vivid phantom, usually at the side or over the chest, which is unrelated to the position of the real arm when the eyes are closed but 'jumps' into it when the patient looks at the arm (Melzack & Bromage, 1973). Similarly, a spinal anaesthetic block of the lower body produces reports of phantom legs in most patients (Bromage & Melzack, 1974), and a total section of the spinal cord at thoracic levels leads to reports of a phantom body including genitalia and many other body parts in virtually all patients (Bors, 1951; Conomy, 1973; Melzack & Loeser, 1978).

Phantom limb phenomena

The most astonishing feature of the phantom limb is its incredible reality to the amputee (Simmel, 1956), which is enhanced by wearing an artificial arm or leg; the prosthesis feels real, 'fleshed out'. Amputees in whom the phantom leg has begun to 'telescope' into the stump, so that the foot is felt to be above floor level, report that the phantom fills the artificial leg when it is strapped on and the phantom foot now occupies the space of the artificial foot in its shoe (Riddoch, 1941). Patients who have undergone a cleavage of the forearm stump muscles, to permit them to hold objects, report that the phantom hand also has a cleavage and lies appropriately in the stump (Kallio, 1950).

The remarkable reality of the phantom is reinforced by the experience of details of the limb before amputation (Katz & Melzack, 1990, 2003). For example, the person may feel a painful bunion that had been on the foot or even a tight ring on a phantom finger. Still more astonishing is the fact that some amputees who receive drugs that produce the tremor of tardive dyskinesia report a tremor in the phantom (Jankovic & Glass, 1985).

Phantoms of other body parts feel just as real as limbs do. Heusner (1950) describes two men who underwent amputation of the penis. One of them, during a 4-year period, was intermittently aware of a painless but always erect phantom penis. The other man had severe pain of the phantom penis. Phantom bladders and rectums have the same quality of reality (Bors, 1951; Dorpat, 1971). The bladder may feel so real that patients, after a bladder removal, sometimes complain of a full bladder and even report that they are urinating. Patients with a phantom rectum may actually feel that they are passing gas or faeces. Menstrual cramps may continue to be felt after a hysterectomy. A painless phantom breast, in which the nipple is the most vivid part, is reported by about 25% of women after a mastectomy and 13% feel pain in the phantom (Kroner *et al.*, 1989).

The reality of the phantom body is evident in paraplegics who suffer a complete break of the spinal cord. Even though they have no somatic sensation or voluntary movement below the level of the break, they often report that they still feel their legs and lower body (Bors, 1951; Burke & Woodward, 1976). The phantom appears to inhabit the body when the person's eyes are open and usually moves co-ordinately with visually perceived movements of the body. Initially, the patient may realize the dissociation between the two when he sees his legs stretched out on the road after an accident yet feels them to be over his chest or head. Later, the phantom becomes coordinate with the body, and dissociation is rare.

Descriptions given by amputees and paraplegics indicate the range of the qualities of experience of phantom body parts (Bors, 1951; Katz & Melzack, 2003, 1990). Touch, pressure, warmth, cold and many kinds of pain are common. There are also feelings of itch, tickle, wetness, sweatiness and tactile texture. Even the experience of fatigue due to movement of the phantom limb is reported (Conomy, 1973). Furthermore, male paraplegics with total spinal sections report feeling erections and paraplegic women describe sexual sensations in the perineal area. Both describe feelings of pleasure, including orgasms (Bors, 1951; Money, 1964; Verkuyl, 1969).

One of the most striking features of the phantom limb or any other body part, including half of the body in many paraplegics, is that it is perceived as an integral part of one's self. Even when a phantom foot dangles 'in mid-air' (without a connecting leg) a few inches below the stump, it still moves appropriately with the other limbs and is unmistakable felt to be part of one's body-self. So, too, the multiple phantoms sometimes felt after an amputation are all part of the self (Lacroix et al., 1992). The fact that the experience of 'self' is subserved by specific brain mechanisms is demonstrated by the converse of a phantom limb, the denial that a part of one's body belongs to one's self. Typically, the person, after a lesion of the right parietal lobe or any of several other brain areas (Mesulam, 1981) denies that a side of the body is part of him by or herself and even ignores the space on that side (Denny-Brown et al., 1952). From these cases it is evident that the brain processes which underlie the experience of our bodies must impart a special signal that provides the basis for experience of the self. When these brain areas are lost, the person denies that a part of the body belongs to the self. Even when a hand, for example, is pinched hard so that the patient winces or cries out, s/he still denies that the hand is hers/his.

There is convincing evidence that a substantial number of people who are born without all or part of a limb (congenital limb deficiency) feel a vivid phantom pain of the missing part. These phantoms are reported by children (Poeck, 1964; Weinstein et al., 1964; Melzack et al., 1997) as well as by adults (Saadah & Melzack, 1994; Brugger & Regard, 1997), and possess all the properties of phantoms described by amputees. Furthermore, the phantom may sometimes not appear until maturity, usually after a minor injury or surgery of the deficient limb (Saadah & Melzack, 1994).

The innate neural substrate implied by these data does not mean that learning experience is irrelevant. Learning obviously underlies the fact that people's phantoms assume the shape of the prosthesis, and people with a deformed leg or a painful corn often report, after amputation, that the phantom is deformed or has a corn. That is, sensory inputs play an important role in the experience of the phantom limb. Heredity and environment clearly act together to produce the phenomena of phantom limbs.

These observations can be summarized in the form of four propositions (Melzack, 1989) which derive from the data:

1. The experience of a phantom limb has the quality of reality because it is produced by the same brain processes that underlie the experience of the body when it is intact.
2. Neural networks in the brain generate all the qualities of experience that are felt to originate in the body; inputs from the body may trigger or modulate the output of the networks but are not essential for any of the qualities of experience.
3. The experience of the body has a unitary, integrated quality which includes the quality of the 'self', that the body is uniquely one's own and not that of any other individual.
4. The neural network that underlies the experience of the body-self is genetically determined but can be modified by sensory experience.

A hypothesis for phantom limbs: the neuromatrix

The anatomical substrate of the body-self, Melzack (1989) proposes, is a network of neurons that extends throughout widespread areas of the brain (which has been demonstrated in imaging studies by Ingvar & Hsieh, 1999). He has labelled the network, whose spatial distribution and synaptic links are initially determined genetically, and are later sculpted by sensory inputs, as a 'neuromatrix'. Thalamocortical and limbic loops that comprise the neuromatrix diverge to permit parallel processing in different components of the neuromatrix and converge repeatedly to permit interactions between the output products of processing. The repeated cyclical processing and synthesis of nerve impulses in the neuromatrix imparts a characteristic pattern or 'neurosignature'.

The neurosignature of the neuromatrix is imparted on all nerve impulse patterns that flow through it; the neurosignature is produced by the patterns of synaptic connections, which are initially innate and then modified by experience, in the entire neuromatrix. All inputs from the body undergo cyclical processing and synthesis so that characteristic patterns are impressed on them in the neuromatrix. Portions of the neuromatrix are assumed to be specialized to process information related to major sensory events (such as injury) and may be labelled as neuromodules which impress subsignatures on the larger neurosignature.

Phantom limb pain

About 70% of amputees suffer burning, cramping and other qualities of pain in the first few weeks after amputation. Even seven years after amputation, 50% still continue to suffer phantom limb pain (Krebs et al., 1985; Jensen & Nikolajsen, 1999). Why is there so much pain in phantom limbs? Melzack (1989) proposes that the active neuromatrix, when deprived of modulating inputs from the limbs or body, produces an abnormal signature pattern that subserves the psychological qualities of hot or burning, the most common qualities of phantom limb pain. Cramping pain, however, may be due to messages from the neuromatrix to produce movement. In the absence of the limbs, the messages to move the muscles may become more frequent and 'stronger' in the attempt to move a part of the limb. The end result of the output message may be felt as cramping muscle pain. Shooting pains may have a similar origin, in which the neuro-matrix attempts to move the whole limb and sends out abnormal patterns that are felt as pain shooting down from the groin to the foot. The origins of these pains, then, lie in the brain. Sensory inputs, however, clearly contribute to the phantom: stimulation of the stump or other body sites often produces sensations referred to the phantom limb (Katz & Melzack, 2003).

Surgical removal of the somatosensory areas of the cortex or thalamus generally fails to relieve phantom limb pain (White & Sweet, 1969). However, the new theory conceives of a neuromatrix that extends throughout selective areas of the whole brain, including the somatic, visual and limbic systems. Thus, to destroy the neuromatrix for the body-self which generates the neurosignature pattern for pain is impossible. However, if the pattern for pain is generated by cyclical processing and synthesis, then it should be possible to block it by injection of a local anesthetic into appropriate discrete areas that are hypothesized to comprise the widespread neuromatrix. Data obtained in rats have shown that localized injections of lidocaine into diverse areas, such as the lateral hypothalamus and the dentate gyrus (McKenna & Melzack, 1992) produce striking decreases in experimentally produced pain, including the pain in an animal model of phantom limb pain (Vaccarino & Melzack, 1991).

(See also 'Pain', 'Pain assessment' and 'Pain management'.)

REFERENCES

Bors, E. (1951). Phantom limbs of patients with spinal cord injury. *Archives of Neurology and Psychiatry*, **66**, 610–31.

Bromage, P. R. & Melzack, R. (1974). Phantom limbs and the body schema. *Canadian Anesthetists' Society Journal*, **21**, 267–74.

Brugger, P. & Regard, T. (1997). Illusory reduplication of one's own body: phenomenology and classification of autoscopic phenomena. *Cognitive Neuropsychiatry*, **2**, 19–38.

Burke, D. C. & Woodward, J. M. (1976). Pain and phantom sensation in spinal paralysis. *Handbook of Clinical Neurology*, **26**, 489–99.

Cohen, H. (1944). The mechanism of visceral pain. *Transactions of the Medical Society of London*, **64**, 65–99.

Conomy, J. P. (1973). Disorders of body image after spinal cord injury. *Neurology*, **23**, 842–50.

Denny-Brown, D., Meyer, J. S. & Horenstein, S. (1952). The significance of perceptual rivalry resulting from parietal lesion. *Brain*, **75**, 433–71.

Dorpat, T. L. (1971). Phantom sensations of internal organs. *Comprehensive Psychiatry*, **12**, 27–35.

Heusner, A. P. (1950). Phantom genitalia. *Transactions of the American Neurological Association*, **75**, 128–31.

Ingvar, M. & Hsieh, J. C. (1999). The image of pain. In: P. D. Wall & R. Melzack (Eds.). *Textbook of Pain* (4th edn.) (pp. 215–33). Edinburgh: Churchill Livingstone.

Jankovic, J. & Glass, J. P. (1985). Metoclopramide-induced phantom dyskinesia. *Neurology*, **35**, 432–5.

Jensen, T. S. & Nikolajsen, L. (1999). Phantom pain and other phenomena after amputation. In P. D. Wall and R. Melzack (Eds.). *Textbook of Pain* (4th edn.). (pp. 799–814). Edinburgh: Churchill Livingstone.

Kallio, K. E. (1950). Phantom limb of forearm stump cleft by kineplastic surgery. *Acta Chirurgica Scandinavica*, **99**, 121–32.

Katz, J. & Melzack, R. (1990). Pain 'memories' in phantom limbs: review and clinical observations. *Pain*, **43**, 319–26.

Katz, J. & Melzack, R. (2003). Phantom limb pain. In: J. Grafman & I. H. Robertson (Eds.). *Handbook of neuropsychology* (pp. 205–30). Amsterdam: Elsevier.

Krebs, B., Jensen, T. S., Kroner, K., Nielsen, J. & Jorgensen, H. S. (1985). Phantom limb phenomena in amputees seven years after limb amputation. In H. L. Fields, R. Dubner & F. Cervero (Eds.). *Advances in pain research and therapy*, (Vol. 9) (pp. 425–9). New York: Raven Press.

Kroner, K., Krebs, B., Skov, J. & Jorgensen, H. S. (1989). Immediate and long-term phantom breast syndrome after mastectomy: incidence, clinical characteristics and relationship to pre-mastectomy breast pain. *Pain*, **36**, 327–34.

Lacroix, R., Melzack, R., Smith, D. & Mitchell, N. (1992). Multiple phantom limbs in a child. *Cortex*, **28**, 503–7.

McKenna, J. E. & Melzack, R. (1992). Analgesia produced by lidocaine microinjection into the dentate gyrus. *Pain*, **49**, 105–12.

Melzack, R. (1989). Phantom limbs, the self and the brain. *Canadian Psychology*, **30**, 1–16.

Melzack, R. & Bromage, P. R. (1973). Experimental phantom limbs. *Experimental Neurology*, **39**, 261–9.

Melzack, R., Israel, R., Lacroix, R. & Schultz, G. (1997). Phantom limb in people with congenital limb deficiency or amputation in early childhood. *Brain*, **120**, 1603–20.

Melzack, R. & Loeser, J. D. (1978). Phantom body pain in paraplegics: evidence for a central 'pattern generating mechanism'. *Pain*, **4**, 195–210.

Mesulam, M. M. (1981). A cortical network for directed attention and unilateral neglect. *Annals of Neurology*, **19**, 309–15.

Money, J. (1964). Phantom orgasm in the dreams of paraplegic men and women. *Archives of General Psychiatry*, **3**, 373–82.

Poeck, K. (1964). Phantoms following amputation in early childhood and in congenital absence of limbs. *Cortex*, **1**, 269–75.

Riddoch, G. (1941). Phantom limbs and body shape. *Brain*, **64**, 197–222.

Saadah, E. S. M. & Melzack, R. (1994). Phantom limb experiences in congenital limb-deficient adults. *Cortex*, **30**, 479–85.

Simmel, M. (1956). On phantom limbs. *Archives of Neurology and Psychiatry*, **75**, 69–78.

Solonen, K. A. (1962). The phantom phenomenon in amputated Finnish war veterans. *Acta Orthopaedica Scandinavica*, **54** (Suppl.), 7–37.

Tasker, R. A. R., Choinière, M., Libman, S. M. & Melzack, R. (1987). Analgesia produced by injection of lidocaine into the lateral hypothalamus. *Pain*, **31**, 239–48.

Vaccarino, A. L. & Melzack, R. (1989). Analgesia produced by injection of lidocaine into the anterior cingulum bundle of the rat. *Pain*, **39**, 213–19.

Vaccarino, A. L. & Melzack, R. (1991). The role of the cingulum bundle in self-mutilation following peripheral neurectomy in the rat. *Experimental Neurology*, **111**, 131–4.

Verkuyl, A. (1969). Sexual function in paraplegia and tetraplegia. *Handbook of Clinical Neurology*, **4**, 437–65.

Weinstein, S., Sersen, E. A. & Vetter, R. T. (1964). Phantoms and somatic sensation in cases of congenital aplasia. *Cortex*, **I**, 276–90.

White, J. C. & Sweet, W. H. (1969). *Pain and the neurosurgeon*. Springfield, IL: C. C. Thomas.

Wynn-Parry, C. B. (1980). Pain in avulsion lesions of the brachial plexus. *Pain*, **9**, 41–53.

Anaesthesia and psychology

Keith Millar

University of Glasgow

The introduction of anaesthesia using ether and chloroform in the mid-nineteenth century meant that patients were largely spared the horror of surgery whilst conscious or merely sedated. Oblivion and survival were not assured, however, when those volatile agents were administered by less skilled practitioners. Now, in the twenty-first century, anaesthesia is reassuringly safe. Although estimates show that some 0.1% of patients die during anaesthesia, mortality during this period is confounded with both the effects of surgery and the patient's state of health which may compromise survival during a procedure. Deaths caused by the anaesthetic are therefore very rare. Where deaths can be attributed to the anaesthetic, they may arise from equipment malfunction or human error, rather than the anaesthetic itself (Arnstein, 1997).

Concern does attach, however, to the effects of anaesthesia upon cognitive function. The increasing trend towards day-case surgery means that patients are admitted to hospital, anaesthetized and subjected to a surgical procedure or investigation and then discharged a few hours later. The critical issue is whether patients' cognitive functioning has recovered sufficiently at the time of discharge for them to be regarded as 'street-fit'. As many patients do not heed advice to be cautious in their post-anaesthetic activities, there is clearly a practical imperative to establish the degree and duration of impairment after anaesthesia.

The typical methodology of studies of recovery

Most clinical studies estimate the 'average' recovery profile of an anaesthetic agent (in other words, the group mean response to the anaesthetic) rather than whether an individual patient has recovered their normal level of functioning. Studies commonly use test batteries to assess the main domains of cognitive functioning, many tests being derived from research into factors known to affect arousal including sleep deprivation and alcohol sedation. Others have been adapted from neuropsychological assessments (see 'Neuropsychological assessment').

Prior to anaesthesia, patients practice the tasks in order to provide a baseline with which to compare post-anaesthetic performance. In a busy day-case unit, the conditions are rarely optimal, and patients are distracted by the impending procedure, so that the baseline assessment is not a stable measure. When well enough after recovering consciousness, patients repeat the tests at intervals until time for discharge. In the immediate recovery period, performance shows highly significant impairment relative to the preoperative baseline. Over a period of a few hours, however, performance will typically recover to the level seen at baseline.

Potential shortcomings in methodologies

The problem of group mean performance

The recovery profile described above is typical of studies where performance is averaged across a group of patients. The conclusion is that the recovery profile represents the duration of impairment for the 'average' patient. In the case of modern intravenous anaesthetics, such profiles often favour a conclusion that recovery is complete after some three to four hours. However, the standard deviation of the mean reveals that many patients do not enjoy 'average' recovery and that a significant proportion must remain impaired at discharge. The 'masking' of individual impairment is long recognized (Hickey et al., 1991), and statistical solutions are readily available, but the issue continues to be neglected.

Practice effects and the omission of control groups

Few performance tasks are free of practice effects and, as noted above, day-case conditions rarely permit sufficient practice. Inclusion of a control group that does not undergo anaesthesia, but follows the same test schedule as the anaesthetized group, allows practice effects to be estimated. Regrettably, few studies employ control groups.

Insensitive assessments

Decades of human performance research have established key factors that determine whether a task will be sensitive to cognitive impairment. However, many of these factors are neglected in recovery research.

Task duration and short-term effort

Studies of sleep deprivation have shown that adverse effects on cognition are often detected only when tasks last for 20 minutes or more because, in the short-term, people can motivate themselves to perform well, even when fatigued. Similarly, even when still sedated after anaesthesia, patients can pull themselves together to perform effectively for a few minutes on a short task to give the misleading impression of normal functioning (Dijkstra et al., 1999). Many post-anaesthetic assessments employ durations of 60 seconds or less, and hence bear no resemblance to conditions encountered when discharged. As the hospital environment constrains performance assessment, a pragmatic approach might concentrate upon the extended performance of one task. Pollard et al. (1994) have confirmed the benefits to detecting residual impairment where task duration is sufficient for performance to be examined as a function of time on task.

Task complexity

Just as brief tasks may be insensitive, so, too, are those which are simple and undemanding. Tasks which require sustained attention may provide a solution because they give no opportunity for respite. They may also permit the use of relatively shorter performance periods without loss of sensitivity to impairment: for example, a stimulus-matching task employing a very fast rate of information has been shown effective even at very short task durations.

Sampling and exclusions

Patients are often excluded from anaesthetic recovery studies if they suffer conditions including cardiovascular disease, cancer, hepatic and renal disease, diabetes and affective disorder. Whilst such exclusions still permit relatively homogeneous samples, they are not representative of the population at large. Older patients will often have one or more of the above conditions, any one of which will also affect cognition, so that to exclude them is to favour a benign outcome. Where the study is conducted to evaluate a new anaesthetic agent, the outcome may give a misleading impression of the true degree and duration of impairment. Given the power of statistical modelling to account for variables such as those above, there must be an argument for recovery studies to be broad ranging in their sampling in order to derive a reliable estimate of impairment.

Effect sizes, sample size and power

In the immediate recovery period, virtually all patients show very marked performance impairment relative to their preoperative performance. The effect size of the anaesthetic at this stage is very large and, consequently, only small samples are required to demonstrate highly significant impairment. As recovery continues, impairment reduces and differences from baseline become statistically non-significant. Whilst the conclusion is then that impairment has resolved, many studies simply do not have the power to detect subtle residual impairment. Sample sizes for such studies should be estimated from the much smaller effect sizes likely to be observed later in the recovery period where a relatively smaller proportion of patients continue to suffer residual impairment. The detection of residual impairment in such vulnerable patients is of critical clinical and applied importance.

Defining impairment and the issue of pre-existing deficits

Impairment

'Impairment' is often implicitly defined as a statistically significant difference between baseline and postoperative performance: the corollary is then that impairment has resolved when such differences are not significant. However, for reasons discussed above, such a definition of impairment is inadequate. Other definitions of impairment are arbitrary; for example, that performance is impaired when it differs from baseline performance by more than one standard deviation of the baseline mean. Collie et al. (2002) have reviewed alternatives to detecting cognitive change which include the familiar reliability-change index and its modifications, and simple and multiple regression procedures.

Tasks which have extensive age- and gender-based performance norms permit estimation of whether a given patient is impaired relative to the norm (Ancelin et al., 2001). Many of the well-developed computerized test batteries provide such norms, as do the more traditional neuropsychological assessments. Such norms also afford the possibility of establishing whether a patient's performance is relatively impaired before anaesthesia.

Post-anaesthetic impairment can also be defined by comparing the effects of anaesthesia with the well-established effects of a sedative drug such as alcohol. Alcohol is a useful comparator because a specific blood-alcohol content (BAC) has been legally defined as the limit for driving safely. Given the importance that patients are 'street-fit' when discharged after anaesthesia, it has been shown that there is utility in defining their state according to the level of performance associated with the legal limit for alcohol (Grant et al., 2000; Thapar et al., 1995).

Pre-existing deficits

Pre-existing impairment is known to be a significant predictor of postoperative decline in patients having cardiac bypass surgery (Millar et al., 2001; Rankin et al., 2003). However, the role of pre-existing impairment in patients having non-cardiac procedures is little known. Ancelin et al. (2001) have, however, shown that pre-existing impairment, greater age, low educational exposure and depressive symptoms are predictive of greater postoperative impairment in patients aged over sixty-four years.

Vulnerable groups

Older adults

The vulnerability of older adults to post-anaesthetic impairment is of growing practical importance as the proportion of such patients in the population increases (see 'Ageing and health behaviour'). Moreover, advances in anaesthetic and surgical techniques mean that many more older patients can now be subjected safely to such procedures: more than half of those currently aged over 65 years will undergo anaesthesia and surgery in the years remaining to them.

A multi-centre study of 1218 patients aged greater than 60 years and having major non-cardiac surgery, reported 25.8% post-operative cognitive impairment at 1 week after surgery, and 9.9% at 3 months, in comparison with 3.4% and 2.8% respectively in a control group (Moller et al., 1998). A 10% incidence of impairment is cause enough for concern, but is probably an under-estimate because the authors acknowledge that theirs was a relatively fit sample, and that attrition was more likely in those with cognitive impairment. Re-analysis of other recovery studies confirms that substantially more patients suffer cognitive deficits than first supposed (Kneebone et al., 1998): indeed, a remarkable 56% of older patients may suffer persistent impairment at 3 months after anaesthesia (Anclein et al., op. cit.).

It is beyond the scope of this chapter to consider in detail the supposed mechanisms of post-anaesthetic cognitive impairment which are so well exemplified in older patients. Dodds and Allison (1998) provide an extensive review of physiological, neurological, biochemical and genetic factors that may explain postoperative decline.

Children

Some 60% of children exhibit behavioural disturbance immediately after anaesthesia and 30% continue to show symptoms one month later (Kotiniemi *et al.*, 1996). Children who have pre-existing behavioural problems, and younger children, are at greater risk. Little is known of the effects of anaesthesia on children's cognition, probably because of the practical difficulties in assessing them peri-operatively. Anaesthetics have different pharmacokinetics and dynamics in children so that one cannot draw implications from the cognitive effects seen in adults. There is, however, evidence that reaction time, memory and psychomotor co-ordination may be impaired for up to three hours after day-case anaesthesia, and may not have resolved at the time of discharge (Millar *et al.*, 2006; Schröter *et al.*, 1996).

Patients who are 'aware' during anaesthesia

On awakening from general anaesthesia, some 0.2–0.7% of patients report awareness and memories, sometimes traumatic, of pain and intra-operative events. The use of muscle-relaxant drugs to aid surgery prevents them from signalling their awareness at the time. Whilst some of these 'explicit' memories are explained by inadvertent or deliberate 'light' anaesthesia (for example in obstetric cases), enterprizing research has employed sensitive tests of 'implicit memory' to provide variable evidence that patients can retain implicit (unconscious) memories for verbal stimuli presented whilst they are ostensibly adequately anaesthetised. The methodology has been employed in conjunction with electrophysiological measures of brain activity and other physical indicators of awareness in an attempt to establish the precise anaesthetic conditions under which explicit and implicit memories occur.

Concern also attaches to the potential emotional consequences of such memories which may, in turn, have legal consequences when patients seek compensation for suffering such a traumatic experience. There is evidence for emotional disturbance after episodes of frank awareness, and that in some circumstances psychological disorder also follows periods of wakefulness for which no explicit memory is retained (Wang, 2001). Comprehensive coverage of this enigmatic and highly significant research is found in the text by Ghoneim (2001).

(See also 'Surgery'.)

REFERENCES

Ancelin, M.-L., De Roquefeuil, G., Ledésert, B. *et al.* (2001). Exposure to anaesthetic agents, cognitive functioning and depressive symptomatology in the elderly. *British Journal of Psychiatry*, **178**, 360–6.

Arnstein, F. (1997). Catalogue of human error. *British Journal of Anaesthesia*, **79**, 645–56.

Caldas, J. C. S., Pais-Rebeiro, J. L. & Carneiro, R. (2004). General anesthesis, surgery and hospitalisation in children and their effects upon cognitive, academic, emotional and sociobehavioral development. *Pediatric Anesthesia*, **14**, 910–15.

Collie, A., Darby, D.G., Falleti, M.G., Silbert, B.S. & Maruff, P. (2002). Determining the extent of cognitive change after coronary surgery: a review of statistical procedures. *Annals of Thoracic Surgery*, **73**, 2005–11.

Dijkstra, J.B., Houx, P.J. & Jolles, J. (1999). Cognition after major surgery in the elderly: test performance and complaints. *British Journal of Anaesthesia*, **82**, 867–74.

Dodds, C. & Allison, J. (1998). Post-operative cognitive deficit in the elderly surgical patient. *British Journal of Anaesthesia*, **81**, 449–62.

Ghoneim, M.M. (Ed.). (2001). *Awareness during anaesthesia*. Oxford: Butterworth-Heinemann.

Grant, S.A., Murdoch, J., Millar, K. & Kenny, G.N.C. (2000). Blood propofol concentration and psychomotor effects on skills associated with driving. *British Journal of Anaesthesia* 2000, **85**, 396–400.

Hickey, S., Asbury, A.J. & Millar, K. (1991). Psychomotor recovery after outpatient anaesthesia: individual impairment may be masked by group analysis. *British Journal of Anaesthesia*, **66**, 345–52.

Kotiniemi, L.H., Ryhänen, P.T. & Moilanen I.K. (1996). Behavioural changes following routine ENT operations in two-to-ten-year-old children. *Paediatric Anaesthesia*, **6**, 45–9.

Kneebone, A.C., Andrew, M.J., Baker, R.A. & Knight, J.L. (1998). Neuropsychologic changes after coronary artery bypass grafting: use of reliable change indices. *Annals of Thoracic Surgery*, **65**, 1320–5.

Millar, K., Asbury, A.J., Bowman, A.T., Hosey, M.T., Musiello, T. & Wellbury, R.R. (2006). Effects of brief sevoflurane-nitrous oxide anaesthesia upon children's postoperative cognition and behaviour. *Anaesthesia*, **61**, 541–7.

Millar, K., Asbury, A.J. & Murray, G.D. (2001). Pre-existing cognitive impairment as a factor influencing outcome after cardiac surgery and anaesthesia. *British Journal of Anaesthesia*, **86**, 63–7.

Moller, J.T., Cluitmans, P., Rasmussen, L.S. *et al.* (1998). Long-term postoperative cognitive dysfunction in the elderly: ISPOCD1 study. *Lancet*, **351**, 857–61.

Pollard, B.J., Bryan, A., Bennet, D. *et al.* (1994). Recovery after oral surgery with halothane, enflurane, isoflurane or propofol anaethesia. *British Journal of Anaesthesia*, **72**, 559–66.

Rankin, K.P., Kochamba, G.S., Boone, K.B., Petitti, D.B. & Buckwalter, J.G. (2003). Presurgical cognitive deficits in patients receiving coronary artery bypass graft surgery. *Journal of the International Neuropsychological Society*, **9**, 913–24.

Schröter, J., Motsch, J., Hufnagel, A.R., Bach, A. & Martin, E. (1996). Recovery of psychomotor function following general anaesthesia in children: a comparison of propofol and thiopentone/halothane. *Paediatric Anaesthesia*, **6**, 317–24.

Thapar, P., Zacny J.P., Choi, M. & Apfelbaum, J.L. (1995). Objective and subjective impairment of often-used sedative/analgesic combinations in ambulatory surgery, using alcohol as a benchmark. *Anesthesia and Analgesia*, **80**, 1092–8.

Wang, M. (2001). The psychological consequences of explicit and implicit memories of events during surgery. In M.M. Ghoneim (Ed.). *Awareness during anaesthesia* (pp. 145–53). Oxford: Butterworth-Heinemann.

Antenatal care

Kirstie McKenzie-McHarg and Rachel Rowe
University of Oxford

The provision and type of antenatal care varies across countries and continents, but its general aim is always to ensure that women and their unborn babies remain healthy during pregnancy and that any difficulties are diagnosed early and treated appropriately. Typical antenatal interventions include ultrasound screening, regular blood and urine tests, maternal weight checks, fetal heart monitoring and discussions relating to lifestyle changes such as diet and smoking. In addition, women are generally offered antenatal screening for chromosomal or structural fetal abnormalities and diagnostic testing if necessary (see 'Screening: antenatal'). Most women and their partners are given the opportunity to attend antenatal classes, aimed at providing information relating to labour and delivery, and some have access to parentcraft classes, aimed at teaching prospective parents about care of a newborn baby. There is also a wealth of educational material available, and women may access this via the Internet, directly from their care providers, in books or through friends and family.

In 1997, Clement et al. examined a range of methods of providing antenatal care, with the express aim of meeting women's psychological needs. They identified three strands of maternal antenatal psychological need, information and support and reassurance. They argue that the professional emphasis of routine antenatal appointments is often on medical issues, whereas women need time to ask questions, be reassured about symptoms and think through concerns. They propose a system of individualized care, where each pregnant woman and her healthcare providers work together to devise a mutually acceptable programme of antenatal care, including discussions relating to timing of antenatal visits, type and level of interventions and access to educational materials and groups. This group of researchers also recognized the need for flexibility within the antenatal system, suggesting an enhanced provision of care which could incorporate drop-in clinics, telephone counselling and targeted advice where necessary.

In the same year, the first edition of this title was published, and Hewison noted in this chapter (pp. 366–7) that the UK picture of antenatal care was changing (Hewison, 1997). At that time, the UK government's stated policy (*Changing Childbirth*, 1993) was to see maternity services become more woman-centred, giving more control of care and involvement in decision-making into each woman's hands. This sentiment has been mirrored in many parts of the world and there has been a significant increase in the level of research interested in ascertaining women's views and experiences of antenatal care generally and in relation to specific interventions. For example, Nigenda et al. (2003) undertook a study of women's opinions of antenatal care in four developing countries, while Ladfors et al. (2001) examined Swedish women's opinions of antenatal, delivery and postpartum care. In the UK, changes made as a direct result of the government's new policy were evaluated by Spurgeon et al. (2001) and the DIPEx group has been formed, aimed at qualitatively evaluating individual experiences of healthcare (www.dipex.org.uk).

Research such as this clarifies that women experience the varying types of intervention differently and that each woman will have an individual response. Inevitably, this means that the process of ensuring that all women receive personally satisfactory and appropriate antenatal care is a complex one. For example, Hildingsson et al. (2002) assessed women's preferences in terms of the number of antenatal visits, finding that around one-third of women wanted more or fewer than the standard number, highlighting the need for flexibility within the system. They also found that women who had previously experienced a stillbirth, miscarriage or negative birth experience were in need of 'special attention', emphasizing the importance of considering women's individual circumstances, personal resources and psychological responses within the antenatal care system. Even when a majority of women are positive about a specific intervention, there may be unforeseen repercussions. For example, Garcia et al. (2002) conducted a systematic review of women's views of pregnancy ultrasound, and found that although women were generally positive about having ultrasound offered and performed, there was a lack of clarity relating to the purpose of these scans, and women were often unprepared for adverse findings. A qualitative study examining women's experiences of screening and perceptions of risk of group B streptococcus, found that this intervention remained poorly understood despite the majority of women agreeing to undergo the test (Darbyshire et al., 2003). Unnecessarily high levels of psychological distress may result if there is an initial lack of understanding or preparedness for an unwanted test outcome (see 'Screening: antenatal' and 'Screening: general issues').

The importance of psychological wellbeing during pregnancy is paramount. Antenatal psychological distress has been linked to postnatal psychological distress (Green, 1990) and antenatal depression and antenatal anxiety are both significant predictors of postnatal depression (e.g. O'Hara et al., 1991; Ritter et al., 2000). Women who have low self-confidence and poor support antenatally appear to be at increased risk of a range of postnatal psychological problems including depression and post-traumatic stress disorder (Czarnocka & Slade, 2000; Keogh et al., 2002) and there is evidence that good antenatal psychosocial support may even have an impact on physical outcomes such as birthweight and fetal growth (Feldman et al., 2000; Rini et al., 1999). Many antenatal interventions can themselves create anxiety in women; Baillie et al. (2000) found that two-thirds of women identified via ultrasound screening as being 'high risk' continued to experience residual anxiety about their pregnancy even after being reassured by a negative diagnostic test, with potential implications for secure attachment. Women experiencing antenatal psychological difficulties such as anxiety or depression are likely to have increased need in terms of support, information and reassurance.

Psychological difficulties can be compounded when associated with social disadvantage (see 'Socioeconomic status and health'). Brown and Harris (1978) studied pregnant women and women caring for children at home in the 1970s and found that working class women experienced a higher frequency of life events than more affluent women. Irrespective of severe life events, women in lower social classes are more likely to suffer from anxiety, depression and phobias than higher social class women (Goldberg, 1999). While social support may have a protective effect in terms of mental health, acting as a 'buffer' against stress and anxiety (see 'Social support and health'), the effects of poverty and area deprivation may combine so that disadvantaged women may have reduced access to a range of potential sources of advice and social support such as shops, health facilities, parks and friends.

A significant UK development since the first edition of this title is the recent publication of the *Antenatal care guideline* (National Collaborating Centre for Women's and Chilren's Health, 2003). This guideline sets out the standards of antenatal care expected for the healthy pregnant woman, and includes advice relating to woman-centred care, informed decision-making, lifestyle considerations, management of pregnancy symptoms, clinical examination, screening, fetal growth and wellbeing and management of specific clinical conditions. The publication of the guideline has implications for the psychological wellbeing of pregnant women: standards of care are now described based on the best quality evidence available and services are expected to move towards delivering the standards described. One challenge faced by care providers is to meet these standards of care while remaining flexible and responsive to the needs of women from different social and ethnic backgrounds in the context of substantial and persistent social inequalities in the outcome of pregnancy. The move towards having more first trimester antenatal appointments is a good example here. The aim is to provide women with increased support and information at a time when the demands on them, in terms of learning about pregnancy and making decisions about antenatal care, are greatest. Women experiencing psychological difficulties or from particularly socially disadvantaged backgrounds may have increased needs at this time, but may also be least able to access these services in a timely way. Antenatal care providers need to consider how best to reach out to and engage those women so that they are able to take advantage of best quality care and make informed choices. It is at this point in time that services are faced with the challenge of providing best quality care, together with the range of flexibility needed to ensure that women and their families can have the level and type of care provision that is most appropriate for them medically and psychologically.

In summary, research that examines women's satisfaction with antenatal care, and their experiences of specific interventions, shows that most women do wish to be actively involved in making decisions about their own care. It also shows that there may be confusion about the purpose of interventions such as screening, and that more may need to be done to prepare women for the potentially negative findings of the tests, which can lead to psychological distress at a higher level than would be expected if women were better prepared. All women need to be given the opportunity to ask questions within an environment conducive to understanding. It is not enough to ask women to acquiesce in suggested care; the research suggests that while many women will agree to suggested interventions, additional explanation is required in order to achieve an appropriate level of understanding. Psychological distress can occur both antenatally and postnatally, but as antenatal distress is a significant risk factor for postnatal difficulties, appropriate antenatal care and support is of paramount importance.

REFERENCES

Baillie, C., Smith, J., Hewison, J. & Mason, G. (2000). Ultrasound screening for chromosomal abnormality: women's reactions to false positive results. *British Journal of Health Psychology*, **5**, 377–94.

Brown, G.W. & Harris, T. (1978). *Social origins of depression: a study of psychiatric disorder in women.* London: Tavistock.

Clement, S., Sikorski, J., Wilson, J. & Das, S. (1997). Planning antenatal services to meet women's psychological needs. *British Journal of Midwifery*, **5**, 298–305.

Czarnocka, J. & Slade, P. (2000). Prevalence and predictors of post-traumatic stress symptoms following childbirth. *British Journal of Clinical Psychology*, **39**, 35–51.

Darbyshire, P., Collins, C., McDonald, H.M. & Hiller, J.E. (2003). Taking antenatal group B streptococcus seriously: women's experiences of screening and perceptions of risk. *Birth*, **30**, 116–23.

Database of Individual Patient Experiences (DIPEx). (2004). Antenatal screening module. www.dipex.org.uk

Department of Health. (1993). *Changing Childbirth. Part 1. Report of the Expert Maternity Group* (Cumberlege report). London: HMSO.

Feldman, P.J., Dunkel-Schetter, C., Sandman, C.A. & Wadhwa, P.D. (2000). Maternal social support predicts birth weight and fetal growth in human pregnancy. *Psychosomatic Medicine*, **62**, 715–25.

Garcia, J., Bricker, L., Henderson, J. *et al.* (2002). Women's views of pregnancy ultrasound: a systematic review. *Birth*, **29**, 225–50.

Goldberg, D. (1999). Mental health. In: D. Gordon, M. Shaw, D. Dorling & G. Davey Smith (Eds.). *Inequalities in health. The evidence presented to the Independent Inquiry into Inequalities in Health, chaired by Sir Donald Acheson* (pp. 207–12). Bristol: The Policy Press.

Green, J.M. (1990). 'Who is unhappy after childbirth?': antenatal and intrapartum correlates from a prospective study. *Journal of Reproductive and Infant Psychology*, **8**, 175–83.

Hewison, J. (1997). Antenatal care. In A. Bawn, S. Newman, J. Weinman, R. West & C. McManus (Eds.). *Cambridge handbook of phycology, health and medicine* (pp. 366–7). Cambridge: Cambridge University Press.

Hildingsson, I., Waldeström, U. & Rådestad, I. (2002). Women's expectations on antenatal care as assessed in early pregnancy: number of visits, continuity of caregiver and general content. *Acta Obstetriciaet Gynecologica Scandinavica*, **81**, 118–25.

Keogh, E., Ayers, S. & Francis, H. (2002). Does anxiety sensitivity predict post-traumatic stress symptoms following childbirth?: a preliminary report. *Cognitive Behaviour Therapy*, **31**, 145–55.

Ladfors, L., Eriksson, M., Mattsson, L.-A. *et al.* (2001). A population based study of Swedish women's opinions about antenatal, delivery and postpartum care. *Acta Obstetriciaet Gynecologica Scandinavica*, **80**, 130–6.

National Collaborating Centre for Women's and Children's Health. (2003). *Antenatal care: routine care for the healthy pregnant woman.* London: National Institute for Clinical Excellence.

Nigenda, G., Langer, A., Kuchaisit, C. *et al.* (2003). Women's opinions on antenatal care in developing countries: results of a study in Cuba, Thailand, Saudi Arabia and Argentina. *BMC Public Health*, **3**, 17–28.

O'Hara, M.W., Schlechte, J.A. & Lewis, D.A. & Varner, M.W. (1991). Controlled prospective study of postpartum mood disorders: psychological, environmental, and hormonal variables. *Journal of Abnormal Psychology*, **100**, 63–73.

Rini, C.K., Dunkel-Schetter, C. & Wadhwa, P.D. (1999). Psychological adaptation and birth outcomes: the role of personal resources, stress, and sociocultural context in pregnancy. *Health Psychology*, **18**, 333–45.

Ritter, C., Hobfoll, S.E., Cameron, R.P., Lavin, J. & Hulsizer, M.R. (2000). Stress, psychosocial resources, and depressive symptomatology during pregnancy in low-income, inner-city women. *Health Psychology*, **19**, 576–85.

Spurgeon, P., Hicks, C. & Barwell, F. (2001). Antenatal, delivery and postnatal comparisons of maternal satisfaction with two pilot *Changing Childbirth* schemes compared with a traditional model of care. *Midwifery*, **17**, 123–32.

Aphasia recovery, treatment and psychosocial adjustment

Chris Code

University of Exeter

'Aphasia' is the generic term used to describe the common range of language impairments that can follow mainly left hemisphere brain damage. Neurological damage can also cause a range of communication problems that do not directly affect such 'straight' linguistic aspects of language, such as right hemisphere language impairments, impairments to the planning component of speech production (apraxias of speech) and dysarthria (i.e. articulation impairment). To distinguish aphasia from other language impairments accompanying brain damage, aphasia can be described in terms of disorders of the core components of a linguistic model; features like lexical semantics, syntax, morphology and phonology. This chapter will outline what we know about the recovery from, psychosocial adjustment to and therapy for, aphasia.

Recovery

Most research into recovery from aphasia has been without reference to any theoretical model. Group studies have shown that most aphasic people make some recovery, yet most studies have used operational definitions, based on a group's improved performance on a test battery (Basso, 1992; Code, 2001) (see 'Neuropsychological assessment').

Such operational definitions, e.g. change in an overall score or aphasia quotient on a psychometric battery, are used widely but do not help to improve understanding of the cognitive processes underlying recovery. One hypothesis (e.g. Le Vere, 1980) is that recovery is best seen as neural sparing and distinguishes between 'losses' which simply cannot be recovered, and behavioural deficits which are the result of attempts to shift control to undamaged neural systems. Real recovery requires the sparing of the underlying neural tissue. Behavioural deficits, the characteristics or symptoms of aphasia for instance, are compensatory. Recovery for an individual therefore may occur through a combination of restitution of lost cognitive functions or compensation for lost functions.

There have been three basic approaches to predicting recovery. A range of prognostic factors has been identified and significant relationships are often found between demographic variables and outcome (e.g. de Riesthal & Wertz, 2004) but reviews complain (Code, 2001; Basso, 1992) that on many of them there is disagreement. Such factors as severity, aphasia type, site and extent of lesion, presence of dysarthria and bilateral damage, are clearly inter-related and probably interdependent (Code, 1987). There is considerable controversy as to whether some are useful theoretical constructs (e.g. type of aphasia). For several, such as age, sex and handedness there is considerable disagreement between studies regarding their prognostic value (de Riesthal & Wertz, 2004; Basso, 1992).

A second approach involves classification into aphasia type. If type is known then some prognosis can be made. However, between 30–70% of aphasic speakers are not classifiable; many change type with recovery and many do not recover in predictable ways. Fundamentally, milder types ('Conduction', 'Transcortical', 'Anomia') have the best prognosis and severe types ('Global', 'Broca's', 'Wernicke's') have the least hopeful. However, 'type' correlates highly with severity.

Thirdly, Porch *et al.* (1980) developed a statistical approach to predict a likely recovery entailing detailed analysis of scores on the *Porch Index of Communicative Abilities* (the PICA) (Porch, 1967), a standardized aphasia test. Using multiple regression, they demonstrated that PICA scores at 1 month post-onset could predict an overall PICA score at 3, 6 and 12 months post-onset with correlations ranging from 0.74 to 0.94. Code *et al.* (1994) have examined the application of neural networks to predicting recovery. Initial results suggest that this method is superior to standard statistical approaches and offers the possibility of comparing a range of possible models of aphasia through 'lesioning'.

Clinicians and aphasic people are not just interested in 'psychometric' recovery, but mainly in ability to cope and function and adjust, which is what really matters to the aphasic person and family. Recovery of these aspects of communication disability has hardly been researched at all.

Therapy

Treatment for aphasia is generally targeted at language impairments and/or communication disabilities, on how the impairments impact on using communication in the aphasic person's everyday community interactions with people. Treatment aims either for restoration (or restitution or re-establishment) of lost functions or compensation (or substitution) for lost functions (Code, 2001). Therapists may employ specific re-organizational methods to achieve restoration or compensation. Aphasia therapy utilizes aspects of education, learning theory, counselling, linguistics, neuro- and cognitive psychology. Following Howard and Hatfield (1987), we can classify most approaches into several main methodologies, although in practice many clinicians adopt a fairly eclectic approach. Didactic methods aim to re-teach language utilizing traditional and intuitive educational methods from child and foreign-language teaching. Overlapping didactic methods are essentially atheoretical behavioural methods like repetition, imitation, modelling, prompting and cuing (see 'Behaviour therapy'). They are utilized in some hierarchically organized therapy approaches for apraxia of speech and contemporary computer based methods use systematic behavioural methods. (See chapters in Code and Muller, 1989, 1995 and Helm-Estabrooks and Albert, 1991).

Language stimulation is also universally used. Here functions are seen to be inaccessible, rather than lost. Language performance is impaired but language competence has survived. Therapy involves facilitating and stimulating language use. If improvement occurs it is because the aphasic speaker does not re-learn lost vocabulary or syntactic forms, but facilitates and integrates what he or she already knows. Intense auditory stimulation, maximum response from the speaker and repetition, facilitation and various types of cuing are general features.

Luria's (1970) neuropsychological model forms the basis for an approach to the re-organization of function. Intact functional sub-systems can substitute for impaired sub-systems. For instance, 'articulograms', which are drawings of the lips producing particular combinations of speech sounds, have been developed for severe apraxia of speech. Here the speaker makes use of an intact visual route into the speech production system. A range of other approaches has been developed for the teatment of the apraxia of speech, which is common in non-fluent aphasia (McNeil *et al.*, 1997; Duffy, 2005).

Approaches exist based on surviving right hemisphere processing, which are mostly reorganizational and aim to compensate for lost functions (Code, 1987, 1994). Melodic Intonation Therapy (Helm-Estabrooks & Albert, 1991), for instance, tries to re-establish some speech in speakers with apraxic problems by reorganization of the speech production process using intoned speech.

There is a range of treatment studies using gesture and drawing (Helm-Estabrooks & Albert, 1991). Group therapy is often considered relevant for development of everyday functional communication (See chapters in Chapey, 1987, 1994; Code & Muller, 1989, 1994).

The progress of cognitive neuropsychology has strongly influenced development of an hypothesis-driven single case assessment process based on an information processing model. The contention is that standardized assessment can provide only inadequate information on the specific deficits underlying individual impairment. Hypotheses concerning impairments must be tested using psycholinguistically controlled tests, and such resources have been developed (Kay *et al.*, 1992). The alternative view is that standardized and reliable tests should provide a baseline against which to measure change (Shallice, 1979). Batteries may be best seen as standardized and reliable screens providing a basic profile and to pinpoint areas for detailed investigation. Contemporary approaches based on social models are developing as therapists begin to acknowledge more the psychosocial implications of aphasia. The aim is to attempt to improve the aphasic person's quality of communicative experience by adjusting the communicative and social environment of the aphasic person by educating and 'training' those who come into contact more with aphasic people (family, shop attendants, health professionals).

Howard and Patterson (1990) outline three strategies for impairment-based therapy inspired by the cognitive neuropsychological model: (1) re-teaching of the missing information, missing rules or procedures based on detailed testing; (2) teaching a different way to do the same task; (3) facilitating the use of impaired access routes. Research suggests that person- and deficit-specific treatment can improve performance in speakers that can not be accounted for in terms of spontaneous recovery or non-specific effects (Howard & Hatfield, 1987) (see 'Neuropsychological Rehabilitation').

Psychosocial and emotional adjustment

Research has shown that recovery and response to rehabilitation in aphasia are probably significantly influenced by emotional and psychosocial factors (Hemsley & Code, 1996; Code & Herrmann, 2003).

There are three broad factors to consider concerning the emotional and psychosocial effects of brain damage on the individual with aphasia. The direct effects of neurological damage on the neurophysical and neurochemical substrate of emotional processing; the indirect effects which we should see as natural reactions to catastrophic personal circumstances; and the pre-existing psychological balance, constitution and the ways of coping that the individual can harness. While our knowledge of the significance of the first two factors is improving, little is known about the interaction of the third factor.

'Psychosocial' refers to the social context of emotional experience. Most emotions are closely associated with our interactions with others and this is what produces most of our happiness, sadness, anxiety, etc. Psychosocial adjustment to aphasia entails coming to terms with a unique constellation of life events. Because the aphasia effects others too, it has implications for the individual's whole social network, especially the immediate family (Code & Muller, 1992; Code & Herrmann, 2003; Duchan & Byng, 2004). The disability as experienced by the aphasic person, rather than the impairment itself, is of particular importance. Studies investigating how psycho-social adjustment to aphasia is perceived have concluded that aphasic people and their families suffer from considerable stressful changes resulting from professional, social and familial role changes, reductions in social contact, depression, loneliness, frustration and aggression. The value dimensions of psychosocial factors in our lives, like health, sexuality, career, creativity, marriage, intelligence, money, family, etc. are markedly affected for aphasic peoples and their relatives (Herrmann & Wallesch, 1989).

There has been increased attention to direct emotional disorders recently as interest in the cerebral representation of emotion and its relationship to language impairment has grown (see Code, 1987; Starkstein & Robinson, 1988, for reviews of issues). Post-stroke depression correlates highly with anterior lesions but does not appear to correlate with aphasia type (see also 'Stroke'). However, research also shows that as time elapses since onset there is an increase in the interaction between extent of cognitive and physical impairment and depression (Robinson *et al.*, 1986).

But there has been little research that has sought to identify reactive emotional states following brain damage and to separate them from direct effects. Herrmann *et al.* (1993) found no differences in overall depression between acute and chronic aphasic groups, but acute speakers showed significantly higher ratings for physical signs of depression and disturbances of cyclic functions (e.g. sleep), generally considered direct effects, and an association between severity of depression and anterior lesions close to the frontal pole. Further, aphasic peoples with major depression (all acute) shared a common subcortical lesion. This suggests that the symptoms of depression in acute aphasi speakers may be caused more by the direct effects of the damage. At later times post-onset it is a more reactive depression which emerges.

One approach has been to view the depression accompanying aphasia within the grief model (Tanner & Gerstenberger, 1988) where individuals grieving for the loss of the ability to communicate move through stages of denial, anger, bargaining, depression and acceptance. The extent to which aphasic people work through the stages of the model has not been investigated. The psychological processing of denial, bargaining, acceptance, are less amenable to more objective forms of measurement but have been investigated in aphasic persons through interpretive assessments, such as personal construct therapy techniques (PCT), by Brumfitt (1985, p. 93) who argues that the impact of becoming aphasic is seen as an event of such magnitude as to affect core-role construing and that the grief the aphasic individual feels concerns loss of the essential element of oneself as a speaker.

Studies of depression following brain damage have used factors considered symptomatic of depression, like diminished sleep and eating, restlessness and crying. These are the factors included in depression questionnaires, although these symptoms may be caused by physical illness and hospitalization directly unrelated to mood state (Starkstein & Robinson, 1988) (see 'Hospitalization in adults'). While the most reliable method of gaining information on the emotional state of people seems to be to ask them, language plays a special role in the problem of identifying and measuring mood for aphasic individuals. The intersection of language is further problematic because mood manifests itself externally through facial expression, voice quality, rate and amount of speech, gesture and posture, as well as linguistic expression and comprehension, all of which can be affected in impaired mood and all of which can be affected by neurological damage.

Relatives and friends can assist to verify accuracy but determining mood in an individual with aphasia presents many problems. One approach to tapping inner feelings is to use the nonverbal *Visual Analogue Mood Scale* (VAMS). Despite its simplicity the VAMS has been shown to be reliable and valid (Folstein & Luria, 1973). The VAMS can be made more meaningful to severely aphasic speakers by substituting schematic faces for words (Stern & Bachman, 1991). Facial expression is the most direct method of communicating emotion and an ability that should be preserved in most aphasic individuals.

With an improved understanding of the social context of communication and its importance to the reintegration of an aphasic person to the community, approaches have developed that concentrate on the communication, rather than the aphasic impairments, and other speakers in the communicative exchange, like relatives, healthcare professionals, shop keepers, policemen and publicans. Research indicates that targeting these 'conversational partners' who have intact resources, rather than the aphasic person with reduced resources, can make a significant contribution to improved communication (Kagan *et al.*, 2001; Togher *et al.*, 2004).

(See also 'Communication assessment', 'Neuropsychological assessment' and 'Neuropsychological rehabilitation'.)

REFERENCES

Alexopoulos, M.P., Abrams, R.C., Young, R.C. & Shamoian, C.A. (1988). Cornell scale for depression in dementia. *Biological Psychiatry*, **23**, 271–84.

Basso, A. (1992). Prognostic factors in aphasia. *Aphasiology*, **6**, 337–48.

Brumfitt, S. (1985). The use of repertory grids with aphasic people. In N. Beail (Ed.). *Repertory grid techniques and personal constructs*. London: Croom Helm.

Carlomagno, S. (1994). *Pragmatic and communication therapy in aphasia*. London: Whurr.

Chapey, R. (Ed.). (1987). *Language Intervention Strategies in Adult Aphasia* (2nd edn.). Baltimore: Williams & Wilkins.

Chapey, R. (Ed.). (1994). *Language Intervention Strategies in Adult Aphasia* (3rd edn.). Baltimore: Williams & Wilkins.

Code, C. (1987). *Language aphasia and the right hemisphere*. Chichester: Wiley.

Code, C. (1994). The role of the right hemisphere in the treatment of aphasia. In R. Chapey (Ed.). *Language Intervention Strategies in Adult Aphasia* (3rd edn.) (pp.380–386). Baltimore: Williams & Wilkins.

Code, C. (2001). Multifactorial processes in recovery from aphasia: developing the foundations for a multilevelled framework. *Brain & Language*, **77**, 25–44.

Code, C. (2003). The quantity of life for people with chronic aphasia.

Neuropsychological Rehabilitation, **13**, 365–78.

Code, C. & Herrmann, M. (2003). The Relevance of emotional and psychosocial factors in aphasia to rehabilitation. *Neuropsychological Rehabilitation*, **13**, 109–32.

Code, C. & Muller, D.J. (Eds.). (1989). *Aphasia Therapy*. London: Whurr.

Code, C. & Muller, D.J. (1992). *The Code–Muller Protocols: assessing perceptions of psychosocial adjustment to aphasia and related disorders.* London: Whurr.

Code, C. & Muller, D.J. (Eds.). (1995). *The treatment of aphasia: from theory to practice.* London: Whurr.

Code, C., Rowley, D.T. & Kertesz, A. (1994). Predicting recovery from aphasia with connectionist networks: preliminary comparisons with multiple regression. *Cortex*, **30**, 527–32.

de Riesthal, M. & Wertz, R.T. (2004). Prognosis for aphasia: relationship between selected biographical and behavioural variables and outcome and improvement. *Aphasiology*, **18**, 899–915.

Duchan, J.F. & Byng, S. (Eds.). (2004). *Challenging aphasia therapies: broadening the discourse and extending the boundaries.* Hove, UK: Psychology Press.

Duffy, J.R. (2005). *Motor speech disorders.* 2nd edn. St Louis, IL: Elsevier Mosby.

Folstein, M.F. & Luria, R. (1973). Reliability, validity, and clinical application of the visual analogue mood scale. *Psychological Medicine*, **3**, 479–86.

Helm-Estabrooks, N. & Albert, M.L. (1991). *Manual of aphasia therapy.* Austin, TX: Pro-Ed.

Hemsley, G. & Code, C. (1996). Interactions between recovery in aphasia, emotional and psychosocial factors in subjects with aphasia, their significant others and speech pathologists. *Disability & Rehabilitation*, **18**, 567–84.

Herrmann, M. & Wallesch, C.-W. (1989). Psychosocial changes and adjustment with chronic and severe nonfluent aphasia. *Aphasiology*, **3**, 513–26.

Herrmann, M., Bartells, C. & Wallesch, C.-W. (1993). Depression in acute and chronic aphasia: symptoms, pathoanatomical–clinical correlations and functional implications. *Journal of Neurology, Neurosurgery, and Psychiatry*, **56**, 672–8.

Howard, D. & Hatfield, F.M. (1987). *Aphasia therapy: historical and contemporary issues.* London: Lawrence Erlbaum Associates.

Howard, D. & Patterson, K. (1990). Methodological issues in neuropsychological therapy. In X. Seron & G. Deloche (Eds.). *Cognitive approaches in neuropsychological rehabilitation.* London: Lawrence Erlbaum Associates.

Kagan, A., Black, S., Duchan, J., Simmons Mackie, N. & Square, P. (2001). Training volunteers as conversational partners using 'Supported conversation with adults with aphasia' (SCA): a controlled trial. *Journal of Speech, Language, and Hearing Research*, **44**, 624–38.

Kay, J., Lesser, R. & Coltheart, M. (1992). *psycholinguistic assessments of language processing in aphasia.* Hove, UK: Lawrence Erlbaum Associates.

Le Vere, T.E. (1980). Recovery of function after brain damage: a theory of the behavioural deficit. *Physiological Psychology*, **8**, 297–308.

Luria, A.R. (1970). *Traumatic aphasia.* The Hague, Netherlands: Mouton.

McNeil, M.R., Robin, D.A. & Schmidt, R.A. (1997). Apraxia of speech: definition, differentiation and treatment. In. M.R. McNeil (Ed.). *Clinical management of sensorimotor speech disorders.* New York: Thieme.

Porch, B.E. (1967). *The Porch Index of Communicative Ability.* Palo Alto, CA: Consulting Psychologists Press.

Porch, B.E., Collins, M., Wertz, R.T. & Friden, T.P. (1980). Statistical prediction of change in aphasia. *Journal of Speech & Hearing Research*, **23**, 312–21.

Robinson, R. G., Bolla-Wilson, K., Kaplan, E., Lipsay, J. R., & Price, T. R. (1986). Depression influences intellectual impairment in stroke patients. *British Journal of Psychiatry*, **148**, 541–7.

Shallice, T. (1979). Case study approach in neuropsychological research. *Journal of Clinical Neuropsychology*, **1**, 183–211.

Starkstein, S.E. & Robinson, R.G. (1988). Aphasia and depression. *Aphasiology*, **2**, 1–20.

Stern, R.A. & Bachman, D.L. (1991). Depressive symptoms following stroke. *American Journal of Psychiatry*, **148**, 351–6.

Tanner, D.C. & Gerstenberger, D.L. (1988). The grief response in neuropathologies of speech and language. *Aphasiology*, **2**, 79–84.

Togher, L., MacDonald, S., Code, C. & Grant, S. (2004). Training communication partners of people with TBI: a randomised controlled trial. *Aphasiology*, **18**, 313–35.

Asthma

Ad A. Kaptein and Klaus F. Rabe

Leiden University Medical Centre

The English word 'asthma' comes from the Greek 'asthma', which means 'panting with sound, wheezing'. Patients who suffer an asthmatic episode are short of breath, wheeze, cough and experience chest tightness. Given the still incomplete understanding of the mechanisms involved in asthma, 'defining asthma is like defining love – we all know what it is, but who would trust anybody else's definition?' (Gross, 1980, p. 203). Recent guidelines give the following definition of asthma: '. . . a chronic inflammatory disorder of the airways . . . the chronic inflammation causes an associated increase in airway hyperresponsiveness that leads to recurrent episodes of wheezing, breathlessness, chest tightness and coughing. These episodes are usually associated with widespread but variable airflow obstruction that is often reversible either spontaneously or with treatment' (GINA, 2001, p. 2;

www.ginasthma.com). The reversibility of the airflow obstruction, 'spontaneously or with treatment', is the hallmark of asthma, distinguishing it from the other two major chronic respiratory disorders, chronic bronchitis and emphysema (COPD – chronic obstructive pulmonary disease) which are largely irreversible (see 'Chronic obstructive pulmonary disease').

Asthma is a highly prevalent disorder. Estimates range between virtually 0% to some 60%, illustrating the wide variations in the genetic predisposition for developing asthma in different parts of the world population, and in the environmental factors eliciting asthmatic responses. In Inuit populations in North Canada the asthma prevalence is virtually zero; on the island of Tristan da Cunha it is about 57% (Zamel et al., 1996). In industrialized countries, the asthma prevalence is on average 10% (Shafazand & Colice, 2004). In children, percentages of physician-diagnosed asthma range from 4% in Germany to 30% in Australia; in adults, these percentages range from 3% in Greece to 12% in the UK (GINA, 2001, p. 14, 16).

Asthma has become more prevalent worldwide over the past decades, although this increase may have come to a halt recently (Shafazand & Colice, 2004). There has also been an increased recognition of asthma by health professionals, and a greater willingness of asthma patients to acknowledge symptoms and seek medical care. These factors have contributed to a greater reporting and documenting of asthma cases. Recently, the so-called 'hygiene hypothesis' was put forward as another possible cause for the rise in asthma prevalence. This hypothesis posits that exposure to viruses and bacteria, in particular in the prenatal period or early childhood, protects against developing asthma. If true, this would imply that rather than aiming at a perfectly clean and allergen-free environment, living conditions that expose young children to infections and allergic stimuli would protect against developing asthma. The debate on this subject is still undecided (Strachan, 2000).

Contrary to popular belief, asthma can lead to death. Statistics indicate that in about 2 per 1 000 000 asthma patients, the respiratory disorder is the cause of death. In all likelihood, asthma medication is not a direct cause of mortality. Rather, inadequate management of asthma (by healthcare providers, patients and their social environment) is the most likely culprit. Black underprivileged women in the US, for example, constitute a high-risk group for death because of asthma, illustrating the importance of socioeconomic and psychosocial factors in asthma mortality (Beasley et al., 1998) (see 'Socioeconomic status and health').

Psychology and asthma

The contribution of behavioural scientists to asthma research has clearly increased over the past decades, broadening the number and scope of asthma-related topics about which important empirical studies have been published (Kaptein, 2002).

Four theoretical and related empirical lines of work can be discerned:

• psychosomatic views
• learning theory techniques
• self-management approaches
• illness representation approaches

Psychosomatic views

Asthma was one of 'the holy seven', a set of disorders where psychological factors were supposed to play a major role in their causation. It was believed that a constitutional or acquired organ vulnerability; a characteristic emotional conflict pattern; and a precipitating life event that led to a breakdown of the patient's psychological defences, were the three conditions that had to be fulfilled in order for the organic disorder to come about. In asthma, these conflict patterns between the mother and her child were thought to be centred on autonomy vs. dependence. Empirical studies failed to find any support for psychosomatic views on asthma. However, traces to these outdated, unscientific and damaging views can still be found. In a recent study on the views of general practitioners on asthma, one practitioner is reported to have claimed '... the main reasons for asthma are psychological factors ... as children these people very often have overprotective mothers ... when they've become adults they often live in circumstances where they don't want to share the air with other people' (Wahlström et al., 2001, p. 510). Explaining to mothers who hold such views that these views are unfounded and baseless is undoubtedly beneficial in helping them to aid their child to properly manage his or her asthma. Adults with asthma who harbour any worries about psychological factors being responsible for their asthma will also find benefit from clear and unequivocal statements from their doctor about these dubious views that go back to about half a century ago (Creer, 1979).

Learning theory techniques

In the nineteen sixties, the rapid and relatively successful involvement of (clinical) psychologists in the care for 'clients' or 'patients' with psychological problems encouraged them to extend their involvement to patients with somatic disorders (Kaptein, 2004). The 1970s and 1980s saw a series of empirical studies on learning theory applications to asthma (see 'Behaviour therapy'). Three major techniques, systematic desensitization, relaxation therapy, and biofeedback were examined closely.

In all three approaches, clinical wisdom from patients and health care providers formed the reason for examining the effects of various types of relaxation on pulmonary function and other outcome measures such as morbidity and quality of life. Patients report that they try to relax as much as possible during episodes of shortness of breath in order to control dyspnea. Healthcare providers reinforce these behaviours in patients who are short of breath. At the same time, the biological basis of breathing would dictate that relaxation would increase dyspnea rather than reduce it (Klinnert, 2003; Wright et al., 1998).

Systematic desensitization has lost its place altogether as a form of behavioural treatment of asthma. The most recent review on systematic desensitization dates back to 1986: neither pulmonary function nor behavioural outcomes were shown to be affected positively by this behavioural intervention (Cluss, 1986). Functional relaxation, progressive relaxation, yoga and autogenic training are the most frequently applied techniques in studies on relaxation in asthma. Symptoms, medication and healthcare use are the dependent variables studied most often. In a rigorous review on controlled studies on this subject, no significant positive effects were observed on any of the outcome measures (Ritz, 2001). Similar conclusions were reached in another, unrelated review (Huntley *et al.*, 2002).

Biofeedback shares a similar fate (see 'Biofeedback'). In five studies, direct biofeedback was examined (i.e. feedback on pulmonary function); seven other studies examined indirect biofeedback (e.g. feedback on facial muscle electrocardiogram (EMG), heart rate). They all raised doubts about the positive effects of biofeedback on asthma patients. A recent systematic review found that important dependent variables such as healthcare use, pulmonary function and mood, were not affected by either type of biofeedback (Ritz *et al.*, 2004).

Physiotherapy (or chiropractic care) is usually highly appreciated by patients with asthma due to the perceived reductions in dyspnea it produces, and this therapeutic approach is sometimes part of the learning theory interventions discussed above. Systematic reviews on the effects of chiropractic care in asthma patients 'showed benefit in subjective measures; however, the differences were not statistically significant between controls and treated groups' (Balon & Mior, 2004, p. S55).

Self-management approaches

Descriptive studies on perceived symptoms of asthma have been instrumental in developing self-management programmes in asthma (see 'Self-management'). Patients were asked to describe in their own words what it felt like to be breathless (Skevington *et al.*, 1997). Their responses were categorized into four dimensions: physical; affective/evaluative; energy; and hyperventilation/speechlessness. In patients with acute severe asthma, it was observed that patients reported breathlessness, described by patients as 'work' and 'breathing effort', long after their pulmonary function returning to normal (Moy *et al.*, 1998). The authors point out that in addition to objective characteristics such as pulmonary function, the subjective description of dyspnea in asthma patients should also be taken into account. These views reflect the increased recognition of 'subjective' aspects of asthma in the clinical encounter between pulmonologists and patients with asthma.

Some twenty years earlier, psychologists of the Denver-group published an impressive series of papers on the subjective symptomatology of asthma, and its relationships with various aspects of medical outcome. Personality traits (anxiety), state characteristics (anxiety, panic) and attitudes (stigma, pessimism) were found to predict length of hospitalization, rates of re-hospitalization and severity of medication at discharge. Objective asthma characteristics played a minor role in these relationships. The concept of 'psychomaintenance' was coined to point at the clinical implications of the results of this research, emphasizing the role psychological factors play in maintaining asthma symptoms and its consequences (Kinsman *et al.*, 1982).

Other research groups took up this challenge, and developed self-management programmes for children and adults with asthma, incorporating elements from the studies described above. Components of self-management programmes are transformation of information, self-monitoring of pulmonary function, regular review of asthma status by a physician and a written action plan informing patients about how to act during exacerbations.

The effects of the programmes must be characterized as positive. In adults with asthma, hospitalizations, visits to accident and emergency departments (A&E) (emergency rooms) for acute severe asthma, unscheduled doctor visits, days lost from work and episodes of nocturnal asthma, are all significantly reduced (Gibson *et al.*, 2000). In children with asthma similar results are found: school absence; days of restricted activity; and number of A&E/emergency room visits were reduced; self-efficacy increased (Wolf *et al.*, 2003). Self-management research in asthma is at a quite developed stage nowadays, as is demonstrated in the two major Cochrane reviews in this area (Gibson *et al.*, 2000; Wolf *et al.*, 2003) Guidelines on the management of asthma explicitly state that self-management must be incorporated into regular medical management, and that physicians should adhere to stimulating patients to use self-management techniques (GINA, 2001). But not all is well. The goals set in international guidelines are not met, particularly with regard to patients accepting restrictions in their daily activities and in respect of healthcare professionals' usage of available knowledge on proper medication policy to control asthma symptoms (Rabe *et al.*, 2004). A recent *Lancet* editorial is critical of physicians for not adhering to these guidelines: 'many factors contribute to the marketing success of baseless treatments and cures for asthma and allergies, not just patients' naivety' (Schaub & von Mutius, 2004, p. 1390).

Illness representation approaches

The most recent addition to the area of behavioural research on asthma pertains to symptom perception, illness perceptions and emotional expression (see 'Symptom perception', 'Lay beliefs about health and illness' and 'Emotional expression and health').

Correctly perceiving symptoms of bronchoconstriction is a conditio sine qua non for the performing of adequate self-management skills. Correlations between objective measures of airways obstruction and perception of breathlessness are far from perfect. Clinically this translates into patients seeking help (too) late, which increases the risk of morbidity and even mortality. Teaching patients to perceive asthma symptoms earlier and better seems beneficial (Rietveld, 1998). Interventions here often use the combination of having patients assess their pulmonary function together with observing their perceived breathlessness, which supposedly teaches them to refine their sensitivity to perceive the severity of bronchoconstriction more accurately (Klein *et al.*, 2004).

Research on illness perceptions in patients with asthma is a new area of psychological study (see Kaptein *et al.*, 2003, for a review on illness perceptions and asthma). In a recent study, the importance of illness representations and medication representations was illustrated: illness perceptions of adult asthma patients were found to be associated with use of healthcare services; medication representations predicted the use of preventer medication (Horne & Weinman, 2002). Intervention studies on the effects of intervening in illness representations and medication beliefs are underway (see Petrie *et al.*'s 2002 study on patients with cardiovascular disease).

A quite spectacular intervention study involved an emotional expression experiment in adult patients with asthma (Smyth *et al.*, 1999). In a randomized controlled design study adult asthma patients in the experimental condition were asked 'to write for 20 minutes on three consecutive days a week about the most stressful experience that they had ever undergone' (p. 1305). Patients in the control condition were asked to describe their plans for the day. Statistically and clinically significant improvements in pulmonary function were observed in the patients in the experimental condition. Future research in this line of work should encompass behavioural outcomes as well.

Although somewhat speculative, a psychoneuroimmunological model in which emotions and cognitions about asthma are combined with self-management skills and with medical and behavioural outcomes might be useful in explaining the findings from the emotional expression study by Smyth *et al.* Further research will be helpful in clarifying these issues.

Asthma is a disorder where a biopsychosocial approach appears to benefit the afflicted patients. Psychosomatic views have been followed by learning theory approaches and by self-management and illness perception models. Continued collaboration between medical and psychological researchers and clinicians, and with patients and their relatives, will be instrumental in improving the quality of life of patients with asthma.

REFERENCES

Balon, J.W. & Mior, S.A. (2004). Chiropractic care in asthma and allergy. *Annals of Allergy, Asthma, and Immunology*, 93, S55–S60.

Beasley, C.R.W., Pearce, N.E. & Crane, J. (1998). Worldwide trends in asthma mortality during the twentieth century. In A.L. Sheffer (Ed.). *Fatal asthma* (pp. 13–29). New York: Marcel Dekker.

Cluss, P.A. (1986). Behavioral interventions as adjunctive treatments for chronic asthma. *Progress in Behavior Modification*, 20, 123–60.

Creer, T.L. (1979). *Asthma therapy: a behavioral health care system for respiratory disorders.* New York: Springer.

Gibson, P.G., Coughlan, J., Wilson, A.J. *et al.* (2000). Self-management education and regular practitioner review for adults with asthma (Cochrane review). In *The Cochrane Library*, Issue 4. Oxford: Update Software.

GINA: Global Initiative for Asthma. (2001). *Global strategy for asthma management and prevention.* Bethesda, MD: NIH NHLBI.

Gross, N.J. (1980). What is this thing called love? – Or, defining asthma. *American Review of Respiratory Disease*, 121, 203–4.

Horne, R. & Weinman, J. (2002). Self-regulation and self-management in asthma: exploring the role of illness perceptions and treatment beliefs in explaining non-adherence to preventer medication. *Psychology & Health*, 17, 17–32.

Huntley, A., White, A.R. & Ernst, E. (2002). Relaxation therapies for asthma: a systematic review. *Thorax*, 57, 127–31.

Kaptein, A.A. (2002). Respiratory disorders and behavioral research. In A.A. Kaptein & T.L. Creer (Eds.). *Respiratory disorders and behavioral medicine* (pp. 1–17). London: Martin Dunitz Publishers.

Kaptein, A.A. (2004). Health psychology: some introductory remarks. In A. Kaptein & J. Weinman (Eds.). *Health psychology* (pp. 3–18). Oxford: Blackwell & British Psychological Society.

Kaptein, A.A., Scharloo, M., Helder, D.I. *et al.* (2003). Representations of chronic illnesses. In L.D. Cameron & H. Leventhal (Eds.). *The self-regulation of health and illness behaviour* (pp. 97–118). London: Routledge.

Kinsman, R.A., Dirks, J.F. & Jones, N.F. (1982). Psychomaintenance of chronic physical illness. In T. Millon, C. Green & R. Meagher (Eds.). *Handbook of clinical health psychology* (pp. 435–66). New York: Plenum Press.

Klein, R.B., Walders, N., McQuaid, E.L. *et al.* (2004). The Asthma Risk Grid: clinical interpretation of symptom perception. *Allergy and Asthma Proceedings*, 25, 1–6.

Klinnert, M.D. (2003). Evaluating the effects of stress on asthma: a paradoxical challenge. *European Respiratory Journal*, 22, 574–5.

Moy, M.L., Lantin, M.L., Harver, A. & Schwartzstein, R.M. (1998). Language of dyspnea in assessment of patients with acute asthma treated with nebulized Albuterol. *American Journal of Respiratory and Critical Care Medicine*, 158, 749–53.

Petrie, K.P., Cameron, L.D., Ellis, C.J., Buick, D.L. & Weinman, J. (2002). Changing illness perceptions following myocardial infarction: an early intervention randomized controlled trial. *Psychosomatic Medicine*, 64, 580–6.

Rabe, K.F., Adachi, M., Lai, C.K.W. *et al.* (2004). Worldwide severity and control of asthma in children and adults: the global Asthma Insights and Reality surveys. *Journal of Allergy and Clinical Immunology*, 114, 40–7.

Rietveld, S. (1998). Symptom perception in asthma: a multidisciplinary review. *Journal of Asthma*, 35, 137–46.

Ritz, T. (2001). Relaxation therapy in adult asthma. *Behavior Modification*, 25, 640–66.

Ritz, T., Dahme, B. & Roth, W. (2004). Behavioral interventions in asthma. Biofeedback techniques. *Journal of Psychosomatic Research*, 56, 711–20.

Schaub, B. & von Mutius, E. (2004). The marketing of asthma and allergies. *The Lancet*, 364, 1389–90.

Shafazand, S. & Colice, G. (2004). Asthma. The epidemic has ended, or has it? *Chest*, 125, 1969–70.

Skevington, S.M., Pilaar, M., Routh, D. & Macleod, R.D. (1997). On the language of breathlessness. *Psychology & Health*, 12, 677–89.

Smyth, J.M., Stone, A.A., Hurewitz, A. & Kaell, A. (1999). Effects of writing about stressful experiences on symptom reduction in patients with asthma or rheumatoid arthritis. *JAMA*, 281, 1304–9.

Strachan, D.P. (2000). Family size, infection and atopy: the first decade of the "hygiene hypothesis". *Thorax*, 55, S2–S10.

Wahlström, R., Lagerløv, P., Lundborg, C.S. *et al.* (2001). Variations in general practitioners' views of asthma management in four European countries. *Social Science & Medicine*, 53, 507–18.

Wolf, F.M., Guevera, J.P., Grum, C.M., Clark, N.M. & Cates, C.J. (2003). Educational interventions for asthma in children (Cochrane Review). In *The Cochrane Library*, Issue 2. Oxford: Update Software.

Wright, R.J., Rodriguez, M. & Cohen, S. (1998). Review of psychosocial stress and asthma: an integrated biopsychosocial approach. *Thorax*, 53, 1066–74.

Zamel, N., McClean, P.A., Sandell, P.R., Siminovitch, K.A. & Slutsky, A.S. (1996). Asthma on Tristan da Cunha: looking for the genetic link. *American Journal of Respiratory and Critical Care Medicine*, 153, 1902–6.

Back pain

Amanda C. de C. Williams

University College London

Back pain is so common its impact is often under-estimated. Chronic back pain is a seriously disabling condition, which causes much distress (Smith *et al.*, 2001; Sprangers *et al.*, 2000). A survey of Scottish adults (Smith *et al.*, 2001) showed that 14% reported continuous or intermittent pain for at least 3 months, for which they had taken analgesics and sought treatment. Nearly half of these people reported severe functional limitations in direct proportion to the severity of their pain. Chronic pain, of which back pain usually constitutes the largest category, was also associated with poorer physical and mental health.

Much back pain is dealt with in the United Kingdom in primary care and often involves physiotherapeutic intervention. If the back pain does not resolve or the individual does not adapt, referrals are often made to orthopaedics, rheumatology, or in some cases to neurosurgery. Optimal treatment consists of explanation and reassurance, with minimal rest, and encouragement to return to activities despite continuing pain. This contrasts with traditional advice, which tends towards prolonged rest and a cautious approach to physical activity. Any delay in referral for investigation and expert diagnosis tends to leave the patient in limbo with neither reassurance nor advice, thereby contributing to disability.

There are many possible causes and mechanisms of low back pain (Waddell, 2004). Some symptoms or physical signs indicate urgent and often operable conditions, such as tumours. These symptoms and physical signs are labelled 'red flag' indicators and suggest referral onto specialist services is appropriate. However, the majority of cases of back pain present with few physical signs. In addition, the presence of physical signs is poorly related to the severity of pain or extent of disability. In fact, psychosocial factors are far stronger predictors of disability and the likelihood that back pain will become chronic than medical or physical variables (Pincus *et al.*, 2001; Linton, 1999). Psychosocial variables that have been shown to be important are depression, pain-related fear and associated behaviour (Vlaeyen & Linton, 2000), and catastrophizing (over-vigilance to symptoms, their negative interpretation and the lack of confidence in capacity to cope with them: Sullivan *et al.*, 2001). The presence of any of these factors constitute 'yellow flag' indicators which, taken in conjunction with the influence of the wider environment (workplace, home and healthcare and welfare systems), suggest psychological assessment is appropriate (see Pincus *et al.*, 2002).

Despite the importance of psychosocial factors in chronic pain and the recognition of 'yellow flag' indicators, the treatment of back pain typifies an area where there is continuing difficulty in embracing a genuinely biopsychosocial model of pain (see 'Pain').

Pain and pain responses

Pain is defined as 'an unpleasant sensory and emotional experience associated with actual or potential tissue damage or described in terms of such damage' (International Association for the Study of Pain, 1979). Chronic or persistent pain is defined variously as pain which has continued beyond six months, or beyond an expected time for healing. In practice, there may also be the implication that the pain is somehow 'excessive' in relation to the physical findings (most often healed damage or long term changes related to age and use) and the apparent gap is plugged using unsatisfactory psychosomatic explanations or assumptions of moral weakness or malingering. But there is no 'right' amount of pain for a particular lesion or pathology: the processes that result in the experience of pain are complex and inherently psychological as well as physical. Further, these explanations draw on moral and political values, rather than on psychological insights, and focus inappropriately on judging the authenticity of the patient's experience. It may be that this tendency is an example of social policing of anyone who complains of illness and claims the advantages due (Mechanic, 1978; Williams, 2002), since pain has no visible confirming signs.

Humans, like (arguably) all animals, are hard-wired so that pain will grab and dominate attention. This is associated with efforts to identify the threat, to escape and to attempt to mitigate the pain. This is accompanied by rapid learning of cues for future avoidance and conservation of resources during healing. However, some pains do not represent actual or threatened damage (e.g. muscle cramp, colic and almost all headache pains). In these instances the repeated interruption of ongoing mental and physical activity by pain leads, in the longer term, to counterproductive attempts to avoid all pain on movement or to recover through rest. The immediate meaning of the pain to the individual is crucial, making the difference between being able to dismiss a familiar pain and return to task, and becoming preoccupied by the pain, by its continuation and its possible short- and long-term implications (Eccleston & Crombez, 1999).

While the contribution of descending messages from the brain on pain transmission and processing was clearly stated in the gate control model (Melzack & Wall, 1965; Wall, 1999), it was not until the era of imaging brain activation that it became possible to start to describe it (Ren & Dubner, 2002; Petrovic & Ingvar, 2002). Acute pain, particularly if it is severe and prolonged, engenders changes in excitation and inhibition at a spinal level; descending influences representing the cortical and affective state of the organism interact at spinal synapses with afferent messages.

A.C. de C. Williams

Serial and parallel processing of incoming pain information produces both immediate affective valence and response, and secondary affective and evaluative activity which further informs response priorities (Price, 2000). Early work with amputees, and subsequently on chronic back pain (Flor *et al.*, 1997), demonstrated extensive cortical reorganization in response to the pain experience and there is now a proliferation of imaging studies on such processes as catastrophizing (Gracely *et al.*, 2004; Petrovic & Ingvar, 2002) (see also 'Pain' and 'Pain assessment').

Treatment of back pain

Patients with back pain seek explanation and advice from their primary care physician rather than treatment and referral (Ring *et al.*, 2004; Salmon *et al.*, 2004; Saunders *et al.*, 1999). With good explanation and advice they are more likely to return to activity and avoid persistent pain (Burton *et al.*, 1999; Pincus *et al.*, 2001). However, it is more common for doctors to recommend or prescribe analgesics, to refer patients for physiotherapy or to other specialists in secondary care. At the same time, patients take action according to their own beliefs about what is wrong and the risks this implies, and may well be consulting alternative medical practitioners and receiving a variety of causal explanations and treatment (much of which is of unproven efficacy) (see 'Lay beliefs about health and illness' and 'Complementary medicine'). By the time it emerges that there is no remediable lesion or pathology and that the patient can 'safely' return to a normal life, s/he may have a bewildering set of pathological models of pain, entrenched habits of avoidance and secondary problems due to inactivity and attempts to minimize the pain, such as guarded movement. Over the longer term, losses of role and of valued activities can impact adversely on the person's personal identity, social and work life and contribute to depressed mood (Banks & Kerns, 1996; Pincus & Williams, 1999).

The few studies of the beliefs of healthcare professionals in relation to pain show a tendency to use an acute pain model long after resolution of any initial injury. This acute pain model includes a cautious approach to return to activity and a focus on abolition of pain as the only solution (Linton *et al.*, 2002). Patients themselves tend to hold damage-based models, which do not distinguish between acute and persistent pain (Rogers & Allison, 2004). Such confusions of models and disappointments in attempts to find treatment render many people with back pain sceptical and wary about further promises of treatment, and referral for rehabilitative treatment may be made with a sense of there being nothing else to offer, rather than of being the appropriate treatment which could have been instituted earlier.

Various reviews and large trials have demonstrated the benefits of physical reactivation, most through physiotherapy exercise programmes or behaviourally-oriented training with education (Pincus *et al.*, 2002; Hayden *et al.*, 2005) (see 'Physical activity interventions' and 'Behaviour therapy'). Yet these studies should not be interpreted as demonstrating that physical exercise alone changes patients' behaviour. Many of these studies and reviews focus on clinical measures of outcome. More recent studies that look at multiple outcomes are still heavily dependent on self-rated disability as a measure of outcome, which is problematic (see 'Disability assessment'). If individuals with persistent pain remain fearful of most normal activity, exercises performed in a physiotherapy clinic are unlikely to challenge or resolve these fears, as elegantly demonstrated by Vlaeyen *et al.* (2001).

In reality, the treatment of back pain differs widely according to dominant models of treatment and availability. For example, in the USA stepped care is the dominant approach (Von Korff & Moore, 2001). In the UK, physicians are encouraged to match patients to provision, although neither evidence nor availability permits this. Provision varies from virtual placebo self-help groups to intensive multi-component programmes of behavioural and cognitive therapy delivered by a multidisciplinary team (see 'Cognitive behaviour therapy'). This kind of psychological rehabilitation is described in more detail in the chapter on 'Pain management'. These interventions are costly but effective and can lead to reductions in disability, a return to normal activities and to a better psychological state. However, trials of the addition of a psychological component largely use weak approximations and assume an additive model of psychological and physical treatment, which is not appropriate (Morley & Williams, 2002). More sophisticated models of multicomponent treatment are at an early stage of resolving questions about cause and effect (Burns *et al.*, 2003).

Conclusions

Psychologists have made a very significant contribution to the understanding of back pain and to its treatment. However, the over-used term of the 'biopsychosocial' model is not yet widely realized in the treatment of back pain. The psychological is mostly too abstract to be mapped on to the biological, and social aspects are largely neglected or formulated entirely in operant terms. Developing an integrated understanding is the task for the next decade.

REFERENCES

Banks, S.M. & Kerns, R.D. (1996). Explaining high rates of depression in chronic pain: a diathesis-stress framework. *Psychological Bulletin*, **199**, 95–110.

Burns, J.W., Kubilus, A., Bruehl, S., Harden, R.N. & Lofland, K. (2003). Do changes in cognitive factors influence outcome following multidisciplinary treatment for chronic pain? A cross-lagged panel analysis. *Journal of Consulting and Clinical Psychology*, **71**, 81–91.

Burton, K., Waddell, G., Tillotson, M. & Summerton, N. (1999). Information and advice to patients with back pain can have a positive effect. A randomized trial of a novel education booklet in primary care, *Spine*, **24**, 2484–91.

Eccleston, C. & Crombez, G. (1999). Pain demands attention: a cognitive–affective model of the interruptive function of pain. *Psychological Bulletin*, **125**, 356–66.

Flor, H., Braun, C., Elbert, T. & Birbaumer, N. (1997). Extensive reorganization of primary somatosensory cortex in chronic back pain patients. *Neuroscience Letters*, **224**, 5–8.

Gracely, R.H., Geisser, M.E., Giesecke, T. et al. (2004). Pain catastrophizing and neural responses to pain among persons with fibromyalgia. *Brain*, **127**, 835–43.

Hayden, J.A., van Tulder, M.W., Malmivaara, A.V. & Koes, B.W. (2005). Meta-analysis: exercise therapy for nonspecific low back pain. *Annals of Internal Medicine*, **142**, 765–75.

International Association for the Study of Pain. (1979). Pain terms: a list with definitions and notes on usage. *Pain*, **6**, 249–52.

Linton, S.J. (1999). Prevention with special reference to chronic musculoskeletal disorders. In R.J. Gatchel & D.C. Turk (Eds.). *Psychosocial factors in pain: critical perspectives* (pp. 374–89). New York: The Guilford Press.

Linton, S.J., Vlaeyen, J. & Ostelo, R. (2002). The back pain beliefs of health care providers: are we fear-avoidant? *Journal of Occupational Rehabilitation*, **12**, 223–32.

Mechanic, D. (1978). *Medical Sociology* (2nd edn.). New York: Free Press.

Melzack, R. & Wall, P. (1965). Pain mechanisms: a new theory. *Science*, **150**, 971–9.

Morley, S. & Williams, A.C. de C. (2002). Conducting and evaluating treatment outcome studies. In D.C. Turk & R. Gatchel (Eds.). *Psychological Approaches to Pain Management: A Practitioners Handbook* (2nd edn.). (pp. 52–68). New York: Guilford Press.

Petrovic, P. & Ingvar, M. (2002). Imaging cognitive modulation of pain processing. *Pain*, **95**, 1–5.

Pincus, T., Burton, A.K., Vogel, S. & Field, A.P. (2001). A systematic review of psychological factors as predictors of disability in prospective cohorts of low back pain. *Spine*, **27**, 109–20.

Pincus, T., Vlaeyen, J.W.S., Kendall, N.A.S. *et al.* (2002). Cognitive–behavioral therapy and psychosocial factors: directions for the future. *Spine*, **27**, E133–8.

Pincus, T. & Williams, A. (1999). Models and measurements of depression in chronic pain. *Journal of Psychosomatic Research*, **47**, 211–19.

Price, D.D. (2000). Psychological and neural mechanisms of the affective dimension of pain. *Science*, **288**, 1769–72.

Ren, K. & Dubner, R. (2002). Descending modulation in persistent pain: an update. *Pain*, **100**, 1–6.

Ring, A., Dowrick, C., Humphris, G. & Salmon, P. (2004). Do patients with unexplained physical symptoms pressurise general practitioners for somatic treatment? A qualitative study. *British Medical Journal*, **328**, 1057–61.

Rogers, A. & Allison, T. (2004). What if my back breaks? Making sense of musculoskeletal pain among South Asian and African–Caribbean people in the North West of England. *Journal of Psychosomatic Research*, **57**, 79–87.

Salmon, P., Dowrick, C.F., Ring, A. & Humphris, G.M. (2004). Voiced but unheard agendas. *British Journal of Genetic Practice*, **54**, 171–6.

Saunders, K.W., Von Korff, M., Pruitt, S.D. & Moore, J.E. (1999). Prediction of physician visits and prescription medicine use for back pain. *Pain*, **83**, 369–77.

Sharpe, M. & Mayou, R. (2004). Somatoform disorders: a help or hindrance to good patient care? *British Journal of Psychiatry*, **184**, 465–7.

Smith, B.H., Elliott, A.M., Chambers, W.A. *et al.* (2001). The impact of chronic pain in the community. *Family Practice*, **17**, 292–9.

Sprangers, M.A., de Regt, E.B., Andries, F. *et al.* (2000). Which chronic conditions are associated with better or poorer quality of life? *Journal of Clinical Epidemiology*, **53**, 895–907.

Sullivan, M.J.L., Thorn, B.E., Haythornthwaite, J.A. *et al.* (2001). Theoretical perspectives on the relationship between catastrophizing and pain. *The Clinical Journal of Pain*, **17**, 52–64.

Vlaeyen, J.W.S., de Jong, J., Geilen, M., Heuts, P.H. & van Breukelen, G. (2001). Graded exposure in vivo in the treatment of pain-related fear: a replicated single-case experimental design in four patients with chronic low back pain. *Behavioral Research and Therapy*, **39**, 151–66.

Vlaeyen, J.W. & Linton, S.J. (2000). Fear-avoidance and its consequences in chronic musculoskeletal pain: a state of the art. *Pain*, **85**, 317–32.

Von Korff, M. & Moore, J. (2001). Stepped care for back pain: acitvating approaches for primary care. *Annals of Internal Medicine 134 (suppl.)*, **9**, 911–17.

Waddell, G. (2004). *The Back Pain Revolution* (2nd edn.). London: Churchill Livingstone.

Wall, P.D. (1999). *Pain: the science of suffering*. London: Weidenfeld & Nicolson.

Williams, A.C. de C. (2002). Facial expression of pain: an evolutionary account. *The Behavioral and Brain Sciences*, **25**, 439–88.

Blindness and visual disability

Linda Pring

University of London

According to the Royal National Institute for the Blind (1991) there are about 20 000 children and about 1 million adults who are blind or partially sighted in the UK. Rahi *et al.* (2003) reported on the incidence and causes of severe visual impairment and blindness in children in the UK suggesting that 4 of every 10 000 children born in the UK will be diagnosed as severely visually impaired or blind by their first birthday increasing to nearly 6 per 10 000 by 16 years of age. The causes of blindness are varied and complex but at least 75% of these children have disorders that are neither preventable nor treatable, in stark contrast to the situation found in underdeveloped countries. The age at which individuals with visual impairment experience sight loss, and the length of time over which their eyesight deteriorates, are both important factors in the ability to adjust. The over-75-year-old age-group make up 65% of the population who are blind. For adults, cataracts, glaucoma, general ill-health and diabetes can be singled out as commonly reported causes of eye problems, for children born blind retinopathy of prematurity, colomboma and optic nerve hypoplasia are amongst the most common (see also 'Diabetes').

From a psychological perspective, the important questions have been related to the consequences of loss of vision for general development (Lewis, 2003); the role of vision in our understanding of space; and the related question of how far our senses provide independent, unitary or complementary information (Schiff & Foulke, 1982). These perspectives have meant that relatively little research has concentrated on the psychological correlates of visual impairment for those who go blind after childhood (see also 'Vision disorders').

In terms of early development, we find that total blindness from birth causes the greatest problems for the young infant; some of these can be significantly diminished if the total loss of sight is delayed even by just a few months. There is conflicting evidence concerning the repertoire of facial expressions in blind infants and possible reductions in expressiveness during early development connected to the failure of reinforcement (e.g. Galati *et al.*, 2001; Dyck *et al.*, 2004). Social smiling occurs at the same time as that expected for children who are sighted but the responses of caregivers to similar behaviours in infants who are blind and those who are sighted differ. This may be caused, in part, by the anomalous communication pattern seen in the mother/child interactions, where the infant may show less initiation of communication, fewer vocalizations and fewer positive responses to the mother. Infants who are blind may for example 'freeze' to listen more attentively to new experiences while the reverse, increased motor activity, occurs for infants without sight problems. Thus, the loss of sight in this regard has effects on the consistency and therefore predictability of pattern of non-verbal communication between the infant and mother.

Like children and young people with autism, children with severe or profound visual impairment seldom engage in symbolic play (such as pretending that a box is a bath for a doll, or a car capable of making loud engine sounds!). They may be socially withdrawn, self-absorbed and mute. Speech, if present, is often echolalic and repetitive. Infants may lack exploratory, functional or imaginative play and resort to repetitive behaviour stereotypes like rocking and eye-poking. There is increasing interest in the connections between autism and blindness (see Pring, 2004) because of the similarities between the behavioural and developmental picture observed. A substantial minority of infants with severe visual impairment are at risk of a developmental setback or regression occurring at about 18–24 months. This has long-term consequences but is not well understood.

In terms of motor development, there is likely to be a delay of most milestones but these appear to be affected both by a lack of experience with the world as well as by the failure to 'see' the world. It is interesting to note that, regardless of sighted status, infants will reach out, in the dark, towards a sound source at the same point in development, while for those who are blind reaching for an object, crawling and walking may be substantially delayed. 'Blindism' is a label for the movements displayed by children who are blind with no obvious communication role, e.g. arm flapping or pressing the eyes: these are suppressed in adults. Mobility and the use of navigational codes may be problematic for individuals with a visual impairment. The fact that vision is specialized for picking up information about the relation between external objects and planes means that forms of coding which depend on this information will

be more difficult to acquire by the visually impaired, but should not be impossible provided the information is communicated by some other means (Millar, 1990). People with visual impairment do use spatial imagery since vision is not the only sense that can supply spatial information. However, certainly those who are blind tend to use fewer external reference cues in some forms of spatial imagery than do the sighted, but the differences tend to reflect differences in strategy rather than imagery.

Some aspects of language may be delayed in those who are blind, but most are not. If the child can make up for experiences lost through impaired sight by the use of other channels then early delays in language and social communication may be alleviated through compensatory processes. This may explain why there are few accounts of genuinely deviant or divergent psychological processes or behaviours in adulthood among people with visually impairment. Nevertheless, the influence of an early impoverishment to the understanding of some concepts and word meanings may be difficult to completely correct. This can lead to flaws in communication and has, at times, been blamed for the failure of standardized tests to measure accurately, due to a misunderstanding of the instructions followed. Finally, a word needs to be said about 'verbalisms' a term used to describe a blind child's tendency to use words for which s/he does not have first-hand sensory experience, such as colour terms. This does not seem very unusual when considering how often everyone tries to use terms for which they have had little or no direct experience, but in addition, such terms can be used consistently and meaningfully. For example (Landau & Gleitman, 1985) a young blind child used the term 'see' to mean things with which she could feel with her hands.

Educational issues connected to visual impairment including a concern with reading, drawing and memory have been the focus of a great deal of research (Tobin, 1979; Millar, 1975; Pring, 1992; Kennedy, 1982). Certainly advantages in short- and long-term memory for certain kinds of materials, including verbal information and musical pitch, are commonly reported. Interestingly, children with little or no residual sight can draw human figures that can be said to be indistinguishable from the drawings of some sighted children. However, the figure a child who is blind draws is often lying down or at an angle to the vertical. This indicates that the vertical and horizontal anchors play a less natural role for them.

Psychological issues within the area of visual impairment have tended to look for cognitive inabilities caused by the loss of vision. As I have reported already, these do exist but have surprisingly little impact, especially where residual sight can provide a spatial framework in which to place touch/haptic experience. For O'Connor and Hermelin (1978), an important consequence of visual impairment was an emphasis on a cognitive style characterized as 'sequential' rather than 'parallel or gestalt-like' caused by the dominance of language and tactual perception. However, while the style of processing may explain some behaviours in children and adults who are blind, equally of interest are the brain mechanisms. The neural activations in the brain have recently come under increased scrutiny with technological innovations in this field of scientific enquiry. For those congenitally deprived of visual input there is evidence of adaptive compensatory cortical reorganization. Functional magnetic resonance imaging (fMRI) and electro-encephalography (EEG) are types of technique for determining which parts of the brain different types of physical sensation or activity, such as listening to words or feeling tactile displays, activate. These brain imaging techniques have shown that for those with early blindness cross-modal sensory re-organization occurs such that tactual sensory input and also tactual imagery activate cortical areas traditionally associated with visual processing. Furthermore, studies have reported a higher activation level in the occipital brain areas of people who are blind with a variety of auditory tasks (e.g. Röder *et al.*, 2000). Their research shows that in some auditory tasks people who are blind outperform those who are sighted and this is linked with a neurological explanation. The pruning of over-produced neural connections as well as the process of myelination in the sensory cortical areas may be *incomplete* for the visually deprived and help explain the increased activations.

The consequences of blindness for adults are often social isolation and an increase in depression and anxiety, though the reports show higher levels of mental health problems in those with a hearing impairment than those with visual impairment. Some research suggests that help with social cognition in young children may also have positive outcomes. Society has often failed to recognize the real needs of those adults and children with visual impairment. Rehabilitation, in terms of occupational and mobility training, plays a crucial role in the lives and psychological health of those who go blind after school age. Within the field of computing, the advent of the graphical user interface, for example Microsoft Windows, has meant that problems for the blind user were very significantly increased. However, technological solutions mean that the Internet can be available for the user whatever their sight status and has provided an up-to-date environment (including the imaginative use of blue tooth, wireless technology) to begin to meet the needs of people with visual problems. Additionally, the Disability Discrimination Act, 1995 has helped to make a positive contribution, but lack of sufficient resources have limited the environmental adaptations that could impact on the quality of life and occupational choices for those living in the UK.

REFERENCES

Dyck, M.J., Farrugia, C., Shochet, I.M. & Holmes-Brown, M. (2004). Emotion recognition/understanding ability in hearing or vision-impaired children: do sounds, sights, or words make the difference? *Journal of Child Psychology and Psychiatry*, **45**, 789–800.

Gilbert, C.E. & Foster, A. (2001). Childhood blindness in the context of VISION 2020: the right to sight. *Bulletin of the World Health Organisation*, **79**, 227–32.

Galati, D., Miceli, R. & Sini, B. (2001). Judging and coding facial expression of emotions in congenitally blind children. *International Journal of Behavioural Development*, **25**, 268–78.

Kennedy, J.M. (1982). Haptic pictures. In W. Schiff & E. Foulke. (Eds.). *Tactual perception: a source book.* (pp.305–34). Cambridge: Cambridge University Press.

Landau, B. & Gleitman, L. R. (1985). *Language and experience: evidence from the blind child.* Cambridge, MA: Harvard University Press.

Lewis, V. (2003). *Development and disability.* Oxford: Blackwell Publishing.

Millar, S. (1975). Visual experience or translation rules? Drawing the human figure by blind and sighted children. *Perception*, **4**, 363–71.

Millar, S. (1990). *Imagery and blindness.* In P.J. Hampson, D.F. Marks & J.T.E. Richardson (Eds.). *Imagery: current developments* (p.179). London: Routledge.

O'Connor, N. & Hermelin, B. (1978). *Hearing and seeing and space and time.* New York: Lawrence Erlbaum and Associates.

Pring, L. (1992). More than meets the eye. In R. Campbell (Ed.). *Mental lives* (pp.1–9). Oxford: Blackwell.

Pring, L. (Ed.). (2004). *Autism and Blindness.* London and Philadelphia: Whurr.

Rahi, J.S., Cable, N. & British Childhood Visual Impairment Study Group. (2003). Severe visual impairment and blindness in children in the UK. *The Lancet*, **362**(9393), 1359–65.

Röder, B., Rösler, F. & Neville, H. J. (2000). Event-related potentials during auditory language processing in congenitally blind and sighted people. *Neuropsychologia*, **38**, 1482–502.

Royal National Institute for the Blind. (1991). *Blind and partially sighted adults in Britain: the RNIB survey.* London: HMSO.

Schiff, W. & Foulke, E. (1982). *Tactual perception: a source book.* Cambridge: Cambridge University Press.

Tobin, M.J. (1979). *A longitudinal study of blind and partially sighted children in special schools in England and Wales.* Birmingham: University of Birmingham School of Education: Research Centre for the Education of Visually Handicapped children.

Blood donation

Sarah A. Afuwape

Institute of Psychiatry

Blood donation – an overview

The donation of human blood, blood components and organs is an integral and indispensable part of modern medical care around the world with some countries having more success at the recruitment of donors than others (Ferriman, 2005). Across all blood centres, the demand for blood and blood products is steadily increasing as the population ages and innovative medical and surgical techniques are introduced. The demands for blood have begun to exceed supply, and the increase in complexity of donation has had a knock-on effect on recruitment of blood donors. Compared with two decades ago, the donation process has become increasingly regulated as attempts are made to acquire quality blood that is safe and free from disease and infection. The results of this increased regulation are increased donor loss through deferral, disqualification (Davey, 2004) and an apathy towards volunteering (Putnam, 2000). In the United States and the United Kingdom, blood stocks have been further impacted in recent years by the implementation of strict deferral guidelines for the prevention and transmission of variant Creutzfeldt-Jakob disease (vCJD) (US Department of Health and Human Services Food and Drug Administration & Centre for Biologics Evaluation and Research, 2003; United Kingdom Blood Transfusion Services, 2002; US Department of Health and Human Services & Food and Drug Administration Centre for Biologics Evaluation and Research, 2002). In the attempt to increase rates of new and returning donors, research has historically focused on investigating socio-demographic characteristics, and the attitudes and motivations of donors and non-donors (Oswalt, 1977; Piliavin, 1990).

Who are the blood donors?

Unlike in the United States, no attempt had been made in the UK prior to 1970 to fund systematic data collection of socio-demographic characteristics of blood donors. Still today, many blood centres around the world fail to routinely collect demographic data and rely upon anecdotal evidence (Wu et al., 2001). However, results from one large-scale UK study into donor motivations and characteristics showed that of a sample of 3,813 donors, over half were men, 90% were aged 18–55, and most were from the higher social economic classes (Titmuss, 1970). Findings from the United States also identified the typical blood donor at the time to be male, White and better educated than the general population (Ownby et al., 1999; Thomson et al., 1998; Titmuss, 1970). Although this is still largely the case in many European countries (Mikkelsen, 2004), more recent findings from the USA show that the social demography of the blood donor is shifting, along with its changing population. There is now a slow, but steady, increase of first-time donors from minority ethnic groups, Hispanic groups in particular (Wu et al., 2001). For other minority ethnic groups in the United States, such as those from Black and Southeast Asian groups, rates of single-time and repeat donation have increased at a much slower pace (Boulware et al., 2002; Glynn et al., 2002).

Why donate? Incentives and barriers to donation

A great deal of research has been conducted into the motivations underlying and predicting blood donation. Much of the literature has identified altruism as the primary reason for offering blood (Glynn et al., 2002), with certain minority ethnic groups showing preference towards donating to members of their own ethnic/racial group if they were to have a choice about the recipient (Amponsah-Afuwape et al., 2002). In first-time donors, other motivations have included awareness of the need for blood, a desire to be tested for infection, feeling a sense of duty and social pressure from friends and family (Fernandez-Montoya et al., 1998; Oswalt & Gordon, 1993; Piliavin & Callero, 1991). Although the desires for special recognition, or to receive an award have featured less often as reasons to donate, and have even been thought to negatively affect the intrinsic motivations of the blood donor (Glynn et al., 2002), other non-tangible incentives such as the offer of medical testing, have been suggested to be possible methods of recruiting the first-time donor (Sanchez et al., 2001). In contrast, reasons given for non-donation have included a lack of awareness of the need to donate blood, fear of contracting HIV or other diseases, fear of needles and pain, laziness and medical reasons (e.g. anaemia, being underweight) (Boulware et al., 2002; Moore, 1991; Oswalt & Gordon, 1993; Thompson, 1993).

Increasing the donor pool

In 1995, approximately 70% of the US supply of blood was donated by established donors (Schreiber et al., 2003). Whilst the potential donor pool is 60%, only 5% are blood donors and up to 50% of first-time donors often never return for subsequent donations. Although appeals for blood are still commonplace during shortages; with constant repetition, they become less effective in the recruitment of new donors and merely mobilize existing, regular donors (Davey, 2004). Others have highlighted the substantial increases in blood and blood product donation that often occur during national disasters, but have concluded that whilst increases are usually substantial during such crises (Glynn et al., 2003a; Schmidt & Bayer, 1985), the effects are often short-lived and rates return to pre-crisis level fairly rapidly afterwards (Glynn et al., 2003a). The decline in individuals' willingness to donate blood has been correlated with declining national levels of civic engagement. It has been proposed that membership of national associations and organizations, and an interest in politics and the environment brought with it a greater sense of belonging and a responsibility to respond to the civic duty to provide an adequate supply of blood to the community (Kolins & Herron, 2003). Putnam (2000) therefore calls for a greater understanding of the new values and interests of the younger generation in order to seek ways of making blood donation more convenient and meaningful. Others have suggested making a number of changes to the method by which donors are engaged, retained and qualified in an attempt to increase the donor pool and prevent 'burnout' of existing donors. Some of these include revising the donor history questionnaire and modifying the deferral criteria to exclude screening questions and tests of doubtful value; adjusting the haemoglobin cut-off levels according to age, sex and race to ensure haemoglobin levels are more physiologically sound and introducing iron supplements for women; lowering the minimum age of donation to age 16 and the use of non-monetary donor incentive (Newman, 2004). Work conducted by Glynn (2003b) and Piliavin (1990) suggest that prizes, raffles and other incentives do little to encourage donation, rather, the use of altruistic appeals with minimal social pressure as well as ensuring that first- and second-time donors are re-contacted promptly, are effective methods of recruitment and retention (Glynn et al., 2003b). Research from Denmark has shown that absolute trust in the safety of the products and the reputation of the centre, a belief in the sufficiency of the supply of blood, and a feeling that a valuable contribution is being made to the national blood supply, are all essential components (Mikkelsen, 2004). Finally, Simon (2003)

questions past research which suggests that paid donors are a less safe source of blood for transfusion, and enquires whether the time has now arrived to begin investigating the effects of monetary incentives (Simon, 2003).

REFERENCES

Amponsah-Afuwape, S.A., Myers, L.B. & Newman, S.P. (2002). Cognitive predictors of ethnic minorities' blood donation intention. *Psychology Health and Medicine*, **7**, 357–61.

Boulware, L.E., Ratner, L.E., Ness, P.M. *et al.* (2002). The contribution of sociodemographic, medical, and attitudinal factors to blood donation among the general public. *Transfusion*, **42**, 669–78.

Davey, R.J. (2004). Recruiting blood donors: challenges and opportunities. *Transfusion*, **44**(4), 597–600.

Fernandez-Montoya, A., Lopez-Berrio, A. & Luna del Castillo, J.D. (1998). How some attitudes, beliefs and motivations of Spanish blood donors evolve over time. *Vox Sanguinis*, **74**, 140–7.

Ferriman, A. (2005). Spain tops the table for organ donation. *British Medical Journal*, **321**, 1098.

Glynn, S.A., Busch, M.P., Schreiber, G.B. *et al.* (2003a). Effect of a national disaster on blood supply and safety: the September 11 experience. *Journal of the American Medical Association*, **289**(17), 2246–53.

Glynn, S.A., Kleinman, S.H., Schreiber, G.B. *et al.* (2002). Motivations to donate blood: demographic comparisons. *Transfusion*, **42**, 216–25.

Glynn, S.A., Williams, A.E., Nass, C.C. *et al.* (2003b). Attitudes toward blood donation incentives in the United States: implications for donor recruitment. *Transfusion*, **43**, 7–16.

Kolins, J. & Herron, R. (2003). On bowling alone and donor recruitment: lessons to be learned. *Transfusion*, **43**, 1634–8.

Mikkelsen, N. (2004). Who are the donors in 2003. *Transfusion Clinique et Biologique*, **11**, 47–52.

Moore, R.J. (1991). Promoting blood donation: a study of the social profile, attitudes, motivation and experience of donors. *Transfusion Medicine*, **1**, 201–7.

Newman, B.H. (2004). Adjusting our management of female blood donors: the key to an adequate blood supply. *Transfusion*, **44**, 591–6.

Oswalt, R.M. (1977). A review of blood donor motivation and recruitment. *Transfusion*, **17**, 123–35.

Oswalt, R. & Gordon, J. (1993). Blood donor motivation: a survey of minority college students. *Psychological Reports*, **72**, 785–6.

Ownby, H.E., Kong, F., Watanabe, K., Tu, Y. & Nass, C.C. (1999). Analysis of donor return behavior. Retrovirus Epidemiology Donor Study. *Transfusion*, **39**, 1128–35.

Piliavin, J.A. (1990). Why do they give the gift of life? A review of research on blood donors since 1977. *Transfusion*, **30**, 444–59.

Piliavin, J.A. & Callero, P.L. (1991). *Giving blood: the development of an altruistic identity.* Baltimore and London: The Johns Hopkins University Press.

Putnam, R.D. (2000). *Bowling alone.* New York: Simon & Schuster.

Sanchez, A.M., Ameti, D.I., Schreiber, G.B. *et al.* (2001). The potential impact of incentives on future blood donation behavior. *Transfusion*, **41**, 172–8.

Schmidt, P.J. & Bayer, W.L. (1985). Transfusion support in a community disaster. In P.C. Das, S. Smit & M.R. Halie (Eds.). *Supportive Therapy in Haematology* (pp. 371–7). Boston, MA: Martinus Nijhoff.

Schreiber, G.B., Sanchez, A.M., Glynn, S.A. & Wright, D.J. (2003). Increasing blood availability by changing donation patterns. *Transfusion*, **43**, 591–7.

Simon, T.L. (2003). Where have all the donors gone? A personal reflection on the crisis in America's volunteer blood program. *Transfusion*, **43**, 273–9.

The United Kingdom Blood Transfusion Services. (2005). *Guidelines for the Blood Transfusion Services in the United Kingdom* (7th edn.). London: The Stationery Office. Available online at http://www.transfusionguidelines.org.uk. Accessed June 2005.

Thompson, W.W. (1993). Blood donation behavior of Hispanics in the lower Rio Grande Valley. *Transfusion*, **33**, 333–5.

Thomson, R.A., Bethel, J., Lo, A.Y. *et al.* (1998). Retention of "safe" blood donors. The Retrovirus Epidemiology Donor Study. *Transfusion*, **38**, 359–67.

Titmuss, R.M. (1970). *The gift relationship.* London: Allen and Unwin.

US Dept of Health and Human Services/FDA Centre for Biologics Evaluation and Research (CBER). *Guidance for industry: an acceptable circular of information for the use of human blood and blood components.* Available online at http://www.fda.gov/cber/gd/ns/circbld.htm. Accessed 3 April 2005.

US Food and Drug Administration (FDA). Revised preventative measures to reduce the possible risk of transmission of Creutzfeldt–Jakob disease (CJD) and variant Creutzfeldt–Jakob disease (VCJD) by blood and blood products. US Dept of Health and Human Services/FDA Centre of Biologics Evaluation and Research (CBER). January 2002. Available online at http://www.fda.gov/cber/guidelines.htm. Accessed 3 April 2005.

Wu, Y., Glynn, S.A., Schreiber, G.B. *et al.* (2001). First-time blood donors: demographic trends. *Transfusion*, **41**, 360–4.

Breastfeeding

Antony S.R. Manstead

Cardiff University

Research on the psychological aspects of breastfeeding has tended to focus on one of two issues: (i) the factors that determine parental choice of infant feeding method, or (ii) the consequences of breastfeeding for the child's psychological development. This chapter will summarize the conclusions that can be drawn from research on these two issues.

Parental attitudes to and social and professional support for breastfeeding

Although the last two decades of the twentieth century witnessed an increase in the number of mothers who initiated breastfeeding, as compared with the steady decline seen during the earlier decades of the century, most mothers wean before the recommended age of six months postpartum because of perceived difficulties in breastfeeding (see Dennis, 2002). An illustrative example comes from research by Heath *et al.* (2002): although 88% of a self-selected sample of New Zealand mothers participating in this study initiated breastfeeding, only 42% were exclusively breastfeeding at three months.

In industrialized countries there are clear demographic differences between women who do and who do not breastfeed (see Dennis, 2002). Women least likely to breastfeed tend to be younger, to have lower incomes, to be from an ethnic minority, to receive less support for breastfeeding, to be employed full-time and to have more negative attitudes to breastfeeding and less confidence in their ability to breastfeed. Two sets of findings are especially noteworthy. First, there is an abundance of evidence that parental attitudes to and beliefs about breastfeeding are strongly associated with a woman's decision to breastfeed or with the duration of breastfeeding. Secondly, the degree of support a woman receives from professionals and laypersons has an impact on her breastfeeding decisions and behaviours.

With regard to the relation between attitudes and decision to breastfeed, Manstead *et al.* (1983) found that attitudes as measured in the last trimester of pregnancy were strongly predictive of whether mothers chose to feed by breast or by bottle during the first six weeks of the baby's life. Mothers who breastfed during these six weeks were significantly more likely than bottlefeeding mothers to believe that breastfeeding provides better nourishment for the baby, is good for the mother's figure, protects the baby against infection, and establishes a close bond between mother and baby. Mothers who bottlefed during the first six weeks were significantly more likely than breastfeeding mothers to believe that bottlefeeding is convenient, is trouble-free and makes it possible for the baby's father to be involved in feeding. Because these beliefs

and attitudes were assessed antenatally in a large sample of primiparous women, and were related to postnatal behaviours, it is reasonable to interpret the observed associations as reflecting the causal impact of beliefs on behaviours. Recent research by Shaker *et al.* (2004) confirmed the importance of maternal beliefs and attitudes but also showed that the father's attitudes and beliefs were associated with the decision to breastfeed or bottlefeed (for relevant theory on the role of attitudes in behaviour see 'Theory of planned behaviour').

With regard to the relation between attitudes and duration of breastfeeding, Jones (1986) interviewed 1525 mothers in hospital, shortly after delivery; those mothers who chose to breastfeed their babies ($n = 649$) were interviewed again 12 months later. The majority of these mothers reported that they had received sufficient advice about breastfeeding, that they had found it enjoyable or satisfying, that they would breastfeed their next child, and that they would encourage their friends to breastfeed. Among those who did not find breastfeeding enjoyable or satisfying, the majority reported having experienced physical problems such as sore or cracked nipples, and there was a tendency for women having their first baby to report more of these problems. Unsurprisingly, the more of these problems a woman experienced, the less satisfied she was with breastfeeding; and the less satisfied she was, the shorter was the duration of breastfeeding, with 50% of those not finding it satisfying stopping within two weeks. There was also a consistently negative relation between enjoyment and satisfaction, on the one hand, and embarrassment experienced when breastfeeding in front of other persons, on the other, and how embarrassed a mother reported feeling was negatively associated with how long she continued to breastfeed. However, physical problems were cited more often than embarrassment as a reason for not wanting to breastfeed a next child.

There is an abundance of evidence that support for breastfeeding received from professionals and laypersons plays an important role. In a meta-analytic review of the literature on support for breastfeeding mothers, Sikorski *et al.* (2003) found that any support (professional or lay) increased the duration of breastfeeding once initiated. Dennis's (2002) review also points to the importance of support from the mother's partner or other non-professional, but adds that professionals can be a negative source of support if they give inaccurate or inconsistent advice. Finally, it is worth noting that in most non-Western societies a new mother is supported by a *doula* (often the mother's own mother) who provides emotional support and also practical advice and support (Hall, 1978). The decline of the extended family in industrialized societies means that partner support is likely to play a key role in such societies (see James *et al.*, 1994), making it all the more important to take fathers' attitudes and beliefs into account.

Breastfeeding and child development

There is compelling evidence concerning the physical health benefits of breastfeeding. These benefits include reducing the incidence of infant deaths due to respiratory infection or to diarrhoea (see, for example, Arifeen et al., 2001). There is also evidence that breastfeeding is associated with reduced risk of overweight among non-Hispanic white children (Grummer-Strawn & Mei, 2004). However, there is one health consequence of breastfeeding that is undoubtedly negative, for it is clear that breastfeeding is responsible for at least a proportion of the increasing prevalence of paediatric human immunodeficiency virus. In developing countries it is estimated that breastfeeding accounts for 12–14% increased risk of HIV infection, leading to the recommendation that in areas of the world where adequate sanitary replacement for breastfeeding is available, HIV-infected women should be advised not to breastfeed (Weinberg, 2000) (see also 'HIV and AIDS').

Turning now to psychological functioning, there is fairly good evidence of a relationship between breastfeeding and cognitive development. For example, Morrow-Tlucak et al. (1988) compared (a) children who had been bottlefed, (b) those who had been breastfed for four months or less, and (c) those who had been breastfed for longer than four months. A large number of potentially confounding variables were taken into consideration and, where appropriate, statistically controlled for in the main analyses. The primary measure was the Mental Development Index (MDI) of the Bayley scales. Children were assessed at 1, 12 and 24 months. At each age, the mean MDI scores of the three groups of children fell in the same order: breastfed for longer than four months, followed by breastfed for four months or less, followed by bottlefed.

Another study using different measures of cognitive development was conducted by Niemela and Jarvenpaa (1996). They compared 363 children who had been breastfed for less than five months with 363 children (matched pairwise for sex of child and maternal education) who had been breastfed for five months or more. The children were assessed when they were around five years old. Significant differences between the two groups of children were found on measures of general cognitive capacity and of visuomotor integration.

Horwood and Fergusson (1998) report the results of a study of the association between duration of breastfeeding and childhood cognitive ability and academic achievement over a period from 8 to 18 years. The research was conducted in the context of a longitudinal study of a birth cohort of 1265 children born in 1977 in Christchurch, New Zealand. Longer duration of breastfeeding was associated with IQ assessed at 8 and at 9 years, a variety of scholastic ability measures taken between 10 and 13 years, teacher ratings of reading and mathematics ability at 8 and 12 years; and level of attainment in school leaving examinations. After adjustment for possible confounding factors, children who were breastfed for 8 months or longer had mean test scores that were between 0.11 and 0.30 SD units higher than those who were not breastfed.

Such findings can be interpreted as evidence that breastfeeding has directly beneficial effects on cognitive development, although the causal mechanisms underpinning such effects remain unclear. It has been argued that known differences between formula and breast milk with respect to long chain polyunsaturated fatty acid levels and DHA (docosahexaenoic acid) levels could account for the observed associations (see Horwood & Fergusson, 1998). Another possibility is that breastfeeding has beneficial effects on psychological development by fostering a more intense relationship between mother and child. However, in the absence of hard evidence concerning the underlying mechanism, it remains possible that the observed psychological differences between breastfed and bottlefed children stem from genetic or environmental factors that are confounded with the decision to breastfeed or bottlefeed, rather than from the infant feeding method per se.

REFERENCES

Arifeen, S., Black, R.E., Antelman, G. et al. (2001). Exclusive breastfeeding reduces acute respiratory infection and diarrhea deaths among infants in Dhaka slums. Pediatrics, **108**, E67.

Dennis, C.-L. (2002). Breastfeeding initiation and duration: a 1990–2000 literature review. Journal of Obstetric, Gynecologic and Neonatal Nursing, **31**, 12–32.

Grummer-Strawn, L.M. & Mei, Z. (2004). Does breastfeeding protect against pediatric overweight? Analysis of longitudinal data from the Centers for Disease Control and Prevention Pediatric Nutrition Surveillance System. Pediatrics, **113**, 81–6.

Hall, J.M. (1978). Influencing breastfeeding success. Journal of Obstetric, Gynecologic and Neonatal Nursing, **7**, 28–32.

Heath, A.L.M., Tuttle, C.R., Simons, M.S.L., Cleghorn, C.L. & Parnell, W.R. (2002). A longitudinal study of breastfeeding and weaning practices during the first year of life in Dunedin, New Zealand. Journal of the American Dietetic Association, **102**, 937–43.

Horwood, L.J. & Fergusson, D.M. (1998). Breastfeeding and later cognitive and academic outcomes. Pediatrics, **101**, E9.

James, D.C., Jackson, R.T. & Probart, C.K. (1994). Factors associated with breastfeeding prevalence and duration amongst international students. Journal of the American Dietetic Association, **94**, 194–6.

Jones, D.A. (1986). Attitudes of breast-feeding mothers: a survey of 649 mothers. Social Science and Medicine, **23**, 1151–6.

Manstead, A.S.R., Proffitt, C. & Smart, J.L. (1983). Predicting and understanding mothers' infant feeding intentions and behavior: testing the theory of reasoned action. Journal of Personality and Social Psychology, **44**, 657–71.

Morrow-Tlucak, M., Haude, R.H. & Ernhart, C.B. (1988). Breastfeeding and cognitive development in the first 2 years of life. Social Science and Medicine, **26**, 635–9.

Niemela, A. & Jarvenpaa, A.L. (1996). Is breastfeeding beneficial and maternal smoking harmful to the cognitivev development of children? *Acta Paediatrica*, **85**, 1202–6.

Shaker, I., Scott, J.A. & Reid, M. (2004). Infant feeding attitudes of expectant parents: breastfeeding and formula

feeding. *Journal of Advanced Nursing*, **45**, 260–8.

Sikorski, J., Renfrew, M.J., Pindoria, S. & Wade, A. (2003). Support for breastfeeding mothers: a systematic review. *Paediatric and Perinatal Epidemiology*, **17**, 407–17.

Weinberg, G.A. (2000). The dilemma of postnatal mother-to-child transmission of HIV: to breastfeed or not? *Birth-Issues in Perinatal Care*, **27**, 199–205.

Burn injuries: psychological and social aspects

Claire Phillips

University of the West of England

Background

Approximately 175 000 people per year attend Accident and Emergency departments in the UK with burn injuries, 13 000 requiring admission to hospital (British Burn Association, 2001). Recent medical advances mean those with more extensive burn injuries now survive, but a larger burn injury potentially brings more visible and physical impairment. Relative to other forms of traumatic injury (e.g. fractures), burns have a greater propensity to cause widespread disfiguring injury and dysfunction. Furthermore, the time taken to recover and rehabilitate after burn injury is often much longer than the recipient anticipates.

Psychosocial sequelae of burn injury

Burns occur in a sudden event, giving no time for individuals to gather coping resources. The potential for psychosocial sequelae after burn injury comes from not only what was experienced or witnessed during the accident, but painful hospital treatment, resulting altered appearance, physical impairment and potential social anxiety. The experience of burn injury has been described not as a single event but as a 'continuous traumatic stress' (Gilboa et al., 1994).

It has been observed for many years that burn injury brings with it the propensity for psychological disturbance (e.g. Woodward, 1959). Psychosocial sequelae researched includes depression and anxiety (e.g. Williams et al., 1991), post traumatic stress disorder (PTSD) (e.g. Fauerbach et al., 2000), body image disturbance and social anxiety (e.g. Lawrence et al., 2004), and factors associated with these adjustment difficulties.

Depression and anxiety

The painful experience of hospital treatment and subsequent helplessness are widely thought to contribute to depressed mood. The experience of burn injury also often brings with it a sense of loss and grief, not just for material items lost, but a loss of physical integrity. A sudden change in appearance, for example, is not in line with the gradual adaptation in body image that usually occurs across the lifespan. An adult with a disfiguring burn injury may mourn their lost looks (Partridge, 1990), experience depression or become anxious in social situations. For a parent whose child has been burned, a visible difference may represent the loss of their 'perfect child' or their loss of self image as a 'good' parent and may precipitate depression (Martin, 1970) and bring feelings of guilt.

Depression and anxiety are the most commonly reported psychosocial consequences of burn injury (Patterson et al., 1993). Depression has been reported both within the hospital setting, 2–3 months after burn injury, and in the longer term. The prevalence of depression in burned adults has reportedly ranged from 13–23% post-burn with feelings of anxiety often co-existing (Van Loey et al., 2003).

Post-traumatic stress disorder

More than 50% of burned adults experience some aspect of PTSD while in hospital (Ehde et al., 2000). Prevalence of either full or partial PTSD is reportedly around 29% during hospitalization (Patterson et al., 1990) and between 13–45% overall (Van Loey & Van Son, 2003). PTSD has also been identified in mothers of children with burn injuries (Fukunishi, 1998). To a certain extent, the post-traumatic stress response observed in burns is part of the normal adjustment process, perhaps part of survival – a reminder that what happened to threaten our survival must not be repeated. However, if symptoms persist and remain unchecked, there can be deleterious affects on rehabilitation both physically and mentally (see 'Post-traumatic stress disorder').

Body image dissatisfaction and social anxiety

An adult receiving an appearance-altering burn injury is also receiving a potential insult to their self-image. Adults are likely to have a mature sense of self and body image (their feelings or thoughts about their physical appearance) and a sudden, rapid change in their physical appearance will require an adjustment. Likewise, in older children who are just developing a more stable sense of self, an altered appearance will potentially impact on their developing body image. Modern society places an incredible amount of importance on physical appearance. Subsequently, individuals with severe burn injury may tend to avoid public places, a kind of 'social disability' (MacGregor, 1979). Notably after burn injury, a person's scars will continue to change in appearance for 1–2 years after the injury as the healing process continues and the scar matures (Schwanholt et al., 1994). Conceivably, body image (i.e. how we feel about our physical appearance) updating will be difficult within this period. It has been reported that up to 30% of people with burns report a life of social withdrawal and isolation 1–2 years after injury (Taal & Faber, 1998) as a consequence of their appearance.

However, not everybody with an altered appearance after burns develops a negative body image and associated social anxiety. This is where the personal and social meaning of scarring from burns becomes so important. It appears that perceived severity is important to post-burn adjustment (Kleve and Robinson, 1999).

Behavioural problems

With children, often it will be behaviour that acts as an indicator of psychological wellbeing after burn injury. Reported behavioural disturbances in children range from externalizing signs of aggression (Andersson et al., 2003) to internalizing signs such as withdrawal, and sleep disturbances (Rose et al., 2001). Blakeney et al. (1990, 1993) have demonstrated that even massive burn injuries in children need not necessarily cause psychosocial maladjustment. Several of this research group's studies highlight that most children are well adjusted and socially competent, even after severe burn injury. However, it should be borne in mind that in the USA, children with burn injuries receive more psychological input as part of their care than currently in the UK. Other researchers report more maladaptive behaviours in children with burns, compared with a normative sample (e.g. Meyer et al., 1995). Sleep disturbances after burn injury have also been noted (Kravitz et al., 1993).

Vulnerability factors, protective factors and psychosocial impact of burn injury

Having described the nature of psychological sequelae after burn injury, we have to consider why some people appear to be more vulnerable to negative outcomes. After all, not everybody who experiences burns is poorly adjusted, the majority of people appear to do quite well and many have a quality of life comparable to that of people without burns in the longer term (Altier et al., 2002).

Individual differences

One might expect that previous vulnerability to psychological distress may play a part in post-burn adjustment. Indeed, possibly one of the most robust predictors of emotional distress or depression after burn injury is a history of mental health problems (e.g.

Patterson et al., 2003; Van Loey & Van Son, 2003). Furthermore, it is also argued that the very existence of pre-burn mental health disorder predisposes an individual to burn injury. This appears to hold for both adults (Cobb et al., 1991) and parents of children with burns (Kendall-Grove et al., 1998).

Personality may also play a role in how a person adjusts after suffering a burn injury. Research has robustly demonstrated that the personality trait of neuroticism is associated with greater PTSD symptomology, whereas extraversion acts as a protective factor against PTSD (Fauerbach et al., 2000). Kildal et al. (2004) related the trait of neuroticism to poorer psychosocial outcome, affect, interpersonal relationships, and physical outcomes after burn injury. However, one point to bear in mind when thinking about personality and outcome of burns is the point at which personality was assessed. Studies can only ever achieve retrospective assessments of personality and it is not clear how the experience of trauma and, in the longer term, the experience of an altered appearance and the public's reaction may affect someone's responses on a personality checklist.

An interesting piece of research recently examined the role of coping patterns in adjustment following burn injury. Previously, research examining successful coping had noted that avoidant coping (e.g. suppressing thoughts, distraction) was associated with poorer psychosocial outcome (e.g. Browne et al., 1985) and was also linked to maladaptive personality traits such as neuroticism (Willebrand, et al., 2002). Examining coping patterns after burn injury revealed that swinging between coping styles such as suppression (e.g. mental distancing) and extensive processing (e.g. venting) predicts depression and PTSD at 2 months post-burn (Fauerbach, Richter et al., 2002). This is of interest because generally within the coping literature, having a range of coping strategies is seen as adaptive, whereas here, flitting between the two styles renders these processes useless in ameliorating the negative psychological effects of burn injury. The early use of disengagement as a coping strategy was also associated with a more negative social impact of disfigurement at 2 months (Fauerbach, Heinberg et al., 2002), whereas the early use of acceptance and positive outlook as a coping strategy was protective against PTSD, anxiety and depression (Tedstone et al., 1998).

Gender and age also appear to play a role in post-burn adjustment. It appears that females are more vulnerable to adverse psychosocial affects, being more likely to experience PTSD (e.g. Maes et al., 2001) and more likely, for example, to experience depression after facial burn injury (Van Loey & Van Son, 2003). Younger age at injury appears to play a protective role in body image of children with burns (Jessee et al., 1992). Receiving the burn before a stable body image is formed may allow an easier assimilation of the scar into the child's developing body image, whereas in adults receiving burns, relative youth was associated with more PTSD symptomology (El Hamaoui et al., 2002).

One area of psychological import, regarding trauma, is the attribution of blame made by both adults and parents. In adults who have been burned, self-blame for the accident is a protective factor against PTSD symptomology (Lambert et al., 2004), whereas in parents, self-blame is associated with poorer adaptation after their child has been burned (Ragiel, 1989). This can be understood in terms of blaming oneself as an adult means taking responsibility and gives a sense of control over the environment (Lambert et al.,

2004), whereas for parents blaming oneself adds to the sense of guilt, potentially perpetuating depression.

Social factors

In terms of social variables, it appears that socially disadvantaged families have a greater disposition to burn injury, a chaotic home life potentially creating vulnerability to injury (Kendall-Grove, 1998). This is often a cause for concern as one of the more stable protective factors for children after burns is the family environment. In particular, a cohesive, expressive family with good family relations fosters positive adjustment and body image (e.g. Blakeney et al., 1990; Landolt et al., 2002). Furthermore, a family that encourages autonomy and self-mastery over the environment seems to aid children in their post-burn adjustment (e.g. Blakeney et al., 1990), and also adults (Gilboa, 2001).

The most robust social variable associated with post-burn adjustment for children and adults is that of perceived social support from family and friends (e.g. Davidson et al., 1981). In adolescents, when peer acceptance becomes of central importance, it is the support of friends that buffers self esteem and body image, and ameliorates depression (Orr et al., 1989). The majority of evidence in this area therefore endorses the buffering hypothesis of social support on life stress, postulated by Cobb (1976).

In younger children, the mother's adjustment and coping strategies may protect the child from negative psychosocial sequelae (Browne et al., 1985), with maternal emotional distress linked to poorer adjustment in the child with burns (Sawyer et al., 1982). Family variables also play a role in PTSD symptomology in adults with burns, with family instability noted as a vulnerability factor (Kulka et al., 1990).

Positive self-regard has been suggested as a successful coping strategy for burned children. In a study by LeDoux et al. (1996), burned children actually had positive self-concepts on a standard measure. The children had re-evaluated their strengths and diminished the importance of athletic competence, physical appearance and social acceptance, compared with a non-burned group. Using a qualitative approach alongside the standard measure, such as an interview, would also have revealed how the children felt about this shift in their value system, giving a more in-depth understanding of how this re-evaluation had impacted on their daily life.

Physical factors

Research has highlighted the existence of certain factors that put an individual at more risk of experiencing negative psychosocial effects of burn injury. Contrary to lay belief, how big the burn is (i.e. total area of body surface burned), does not predict levels of psychosocial adjustment post-burn in adults (e.g. Tedstone et al., 1998), children (e.g. Orr et al., 1989), or in mothers of burned children (Kent et al., 2000).

The level of physical impairment, however, seems to relate in part to levels of depression and social withdrawal in the longer term after burn injury (Pallua et al., 2003).

Considering physical location, the literature is conflicting in terms of whether a visible burn has more negative psychosocial consequences than a hidden burn. Some report that hidden burns create more social anxiety due to concern about situations where the scar might be revealed (e.g. Doctor, 1992) and that this may hinder involvement in social situations and delay body image updating (Pruzinsky & Doctor, 1994). Others suggest that people with visible burns have less interaction with people outside of the family and withdraw from activities that draw attention to appearance (e.g. Browne et al., 1985). There are also reports that those with visible burns were no more adversely affected than those with non-visible burns, the explanation being that if a burn is visible you have no choice but to deal with the reactions of others (Landolt et al., 2000). Visibility of the burn is also said to be related to PTSD symptomology (Van Loey & Van Son, 2003). Perhaps the more visible a burn scar, the more attention it will draw from the public and so reminders or intrusive thoughts about the accident and its consequences prevail. Furthermore, self-rated visibility of the burn associates with more perceived hostility from others, and more startled responses from others (Lawrence et al., 2004).

This seems to highlight the need to understand the meaning and importance of the burn to the individual and what it will mean in their life. The physical location will have social consequences and perhaps alter the personal meaning of the burn in terms of importance to the individual, based on their everyday experiences. For a comprehensive discussion of issues and interventions with disfigurement, see Rumsey & Harcourt (2004).

Methodological issues

In the literature there is often conflicting evidence regarding the prevalence and occurrence of psychosocial maladjustment. There are several possible explanations for this. Methodological differences may play their part in that studies use a variety methods to assess psychosocial maladjustment with measures that cannot be directly compared, samples used may be small or skewed, time of follow up may vary from months to years, and in some studies there has been a lack of comparison with a non-burned or control group (see Eyles et al., 1984). Furthermore, many of the studies conducted in this area have mainly used standardized measures or checklists with the consequence that the knowledge gained is limited to the scope of the checklist. The use of mixed-methodologies incorporating both semi-structured interviews and checklists will provide a deeper understanding of the individual's perception of events by enabling their understanding and explanation of experiences to be more fully expressed. For example, Landolt et al. (2000) report that the children have no social impairment because of the burn injury, according to a child behaviour checklist completed by parents ('child' age range: 5–17 years). However, it would have been useful to ask those children themselves whether they had changed their social life, where they go, who they go with, when they go, and what they do when they are there. This level of understanding is not always possible using a fixed measure.

The future: positive psychology versus a 'pathologizing' culture

An interesting current debate regarding psychosocial outcome after burn injury concerns the 'pathologizing' approach to research in this field, as opposed to using a more positive psychology.

An old concept that is now being re-visited is that of resilience and the nature of resilience (Williams *et al.*, 2003). Is it a personality trait? Can it be fostered in individuals to increase hardiness towards the deleterious effects of burn injury? The term resilience has been around since the 1970s, following research where it became apparent that some children at high risk of developing psychopathology actually did well. These children were termed 'stress resistant' or 'resilient' (Caffo *et al.*, 2003). From recent debates, it seems that it would now be useful to further investigate 'resilience' as a psychological construct to assess its role within burns.

Camps for children with burns are now being established all over the UK, adopting an approach used in America with the notion that the chance to take part in confidence-building exercises in a place where they are perceived as and feel 'normal' will be a reparative step for self-esteem after burn injury (Williams *et al.*, 2004). Future researchers will hopefully work with these organizations to evaluate and identify aspects which are positive and foster these aspects in other areas of the children's lives.

Conclusion

There is considerable variability in psychosocial adjustment following burn injury. Difficulties reportedly lie in the areas of depression, PTSD, social anxiety and body image dissatisfaction. Regarding visible burns, attention must be paid to the personal and social meaning of the scar in order to understand why, for example, some people with visible scarring cope very well and others experience social withdrawal or social anxiety.

Individual and social factors seem to be more predictive than physical factors such as size of burn. Thus, a model incorporating physical (e.g. location, hand injury), social (e.g. perceived support) and psychological (e.g. personality, coping pattern) factors may best explain the variance observed in psychosocial adjustment after burn injury (Patterson *et al.*, 2000).

The future of research in this field appears to be in moving towards a more positive psychology, shedding light on how to foster protective factors in individuals with burn injuries.

REFERENCES

Altier, N., Malenfant, A., Forget, R. & Choiniere, M. (2002). Long term adjustment in burn victims: a matched control study. *Psychological Medicine*, **32**(4), 677–85.

Andersson, G., Sandberg, S., Rydell, A. & Gerdin, B. (2003). Social competence and behaviour problems in burned children. *Journal of Burn Care and Rehabilitation*, **29**, 25–30.

Blakeney, P., Portman, S. & Rutan, R. (1990). Familial values as factors influencing long-term psychological adjustment of children after severe burn injury. *Journal of Burn Care and Rehabilitation*, **11**, 472–5.

Blakeney, P., Meyer, W., Moore, P. *et al.* (1993). Social competence and behavioral problems of pediatric survivors of burns. *Journal of Burn Care and Rehabilitation*, **14**(1), 65–72.

British Burn Association. (2001). *National Burn Care Review Committee Report*. UK: BBA Publications.

Browne, G., Byrne, C., Brown, B. *et al.* (1985). Psychosocial adjustment of burn survivors. *Burns*, **12**, 28–35.

Caffo, E. & Belouse, C. (2003). Psychological aspects of traumatic injury in children and adolescents. *Child and Adolescent Clinics of North America*, **12**(3), 493–535.

Cobb, N., Maxwell, G. & Silverstein, P. (1991). The relationship of patient stress to burn injury. *Journal of Burn Care and Rehabilitation*, **12**(4), 334–8.

Cobb, S. (1976). Social support as a moderator of lifestyles. *Psychosomatic Medicine*, **38**, 300–12.

Davidson, T., Bowden, M., Tholen, D., James, M. & Feller, I. (1981). Social support and post-burn adjustment. *Archives of Physical Medicine and Rehabilitation*, **62**, 274–8.

Doctor, M.E. (1992). Helping the burned child to adapt. *Clinics in Plastic Surgery*, **19**(3), 607–14.

Ehde, D.M., Patterson, D.R., Wiechman, S.A. & Wilson, L.G. (2000). Post-traumatic stress symptoms and distress 1 year after burn injury. *Journal of Burn Care Rehabilitation*, **21**, 105–11.

El Hamaoui, Y., Yaalaoui, S., Chihabeddine, K., Boukind, E. & Moussaoui, D. (2002). Post-traumatic stress disorder in burned patients. *Burns*, **28**, 647–50.

Eyles, P., Browne, G., Byrne, C., Brown, B. & Pennock, M. (1984). Methodological problems in studies of burn survivors and their psychological prognosis. *Burns*, **10**, 427–33.

Fauerbach, J.A., Heinberg, L.J., Lawrence, J.W. *et al.* (2000). Effect of early body image dissatisfaction on subsequent psychological and physical adjustment after burn injury. *Psychosomatic Medicine*, **62**(4), 576–82.

Fauerbach, J.A., Heinberg, L.J., Lawrence, J.W. *et al.* (2002). Coping with body image changes following a disfiguring burn injury. *Health Psychology*, **21**(2), 115–21.

Fauerbach, J.A., Richter, L. & Lawrence, J.W. (2002). Regulating acute post-trauma distress. *Journal of Burn Care and Rehabilitation*, **23**(4), 249–57.

Fukunishi, I. (1998). Posttraumatic stress symptoms and depression in mothers of children with severe burn injuries. *Psychological Reports*, **83**(1), 331–5.

Gilboa, D. (2001). Long term psychological adjustment after burn injury. *Burns*, **27**, 335–41.

Gilboa, D., Friedman, M. & Tsur, H. (1994). The burn as a continuous traumatic stress: implications for emotional treatment during hospitalisation. *Journal of Burn Care and Rehabilitation*, **15**, 86–94.

Jessee, P.D., Strickland, M.P., Leeper, J.D. & Wales, P. (1992). Perception of body image in children with burns 5 years after burn injury. *Journal of Burn Care and Rehabilitation*, **13**, 33–8.

Kendall-Grove, K.J., Ehde, D.M., Patterson, D.R. & Johnson, V. (1998). Dysfunction in parents of pediatric patients with burns. *Journal of Burn Care and Rehabilitation*, **19**, 312–16.

Kent, G. (2000). Understanding the experiences of people with disfigurements: an integration of four models of social and psychological functioning. *Psychology, Health and Medicine*, **5**(2), 117–29.

Kildal, M., Willebrand, M., Andersson, G., Gerdin, B. & Ekselius, L. (2004). Personality characteristics and perceived health problems after burn injury. *Journal of Burn Care and Rehabilitation*, **25**(3), 228–35.

Kleve, L. & Robinson, E. (1999). A survey of psychological need amongst adult burn-injured patients. *Burns*, **25**, 575–9.

Kravitz, M., McCoy, B.J., Tompkins, D.M. *et al.* (1993). Sleep disorders in children after burn injury. *Journal of Burn Care and Rehabilitation*, **14**(1), 83–90.

Kulka, R.A., Schlenger, W.E., Fairbank, J.A. *et al.* (1990). *Trauma and the Viet Nam generation*. New York: Brunner/Mazel.

Lambert, J., Difede, J. & Contrada, R. (2004). The relationship of attribution of responsibility to acute stress disorder among hospitalised patients. *Journal of Nervous and Mental Disease*, **192**(4), 304–12.

Landolt, M.A., Grubenmann, S. & Meuli, M. (2000). Psychological long term adjustment in children with head burns. *Journal of Trauma, Infection, and Critical Care*, **49**(6), 1040–4.

Landolt, M.A., Grubenmann, S. & Meuli, M. (2002). Family impact greatest: predictors of quality of life and psychological adjustment in pediatric burn survivors. *Journal of Trauma, Injury, Infection, and Critical Care*, **53**(6), 1146–51.

Lawrence, J.W., Fauerbach, J.A., Heinberg, L. & Doctor, M. (2004). Visible vs hidden scars and their relation to body esteem. *Journal of Burn Care and Rehabilitation*, **25**, 25–32.

LeDoux, J.M., Meyer, W.J., Blakeney, P. & Herndon, D. (1996). Psychosocial forum: positive self regard as a coping mechanism for pediatric burns survivors. *Journal of Burn Care and Rehabilitation*, **17**, 472–6.

MacGregor, F. (1979). *After plastic surgery: adaptation and adjustment*. New York: Praeger.

Martin, H. (1970). Parents' and children's reactions to burns and scalds in children. *British Journal of Medicine and Psychology*, **43**, 183–91.

Maes, M., Delmeire, L., Mylle, J. & Altamura, C. (2001). Risk and preventive factors of post-traumatic stress disorder (PTSD): Alcohol consumption and intoxication prior to a traumatic event diminishes the relative risk to develop PTSD in response to that trauma. *Journal of Affective Disorders*, **63**(1), 113–21.

Meyer, W., Blakeney, P., LeDoux, J. & Herndon, D.N. (1995). Diminished adaptive behaviors among pediatric survivors of burns. *Journal of Burn Care and Rehabilitation*, **16**(5), 511–17.

Orr, D., Reznikoff, M. & Smith, G. (1989). Body image, self-esteem and depression in burn-injured adolescents and young adults. *Journal of Burn Care and Rehabilitation*, **10**(5), 454–61.

Pallua, N., Künsebeck, H.W. & Noah, E.M. (2003). Psychosocial adjustments 5 years after burn injury. *Burns*, **29**, 143–52.

Partridge, J. (1990). *Changing faces: the challenge of facial disfigurement*. London: Penguin Books.

Patterson, D.R., Carrrigan, L., Robinson, R. & Questad, K.A. (1990). Post traumatic stress disorder in hospitalised patients with burn injury. *Journal of Burn Care and Rehabilitation*, **11**, 181–4.

Patterson, D., Everett, J., Bombardier, C. *et al.* (1993). Psychological effects of severe burn injuries. *Psychological Bulletin*, **113**(2), 362–78.

Patterson, D.R., Finch, C.P., Wiechman, S.A. *et al.* (2003). Premorbid mental health status of adult burn patients: comparison with a normative sample. *Journal of Burn Care and Rehabilitation*, **24**(5), 347–50.

Patterson, D.R., Ptacek, J.T., Cromes, F., Fauerbach, J. A. & Engrav, L. (2000). Describing and predicting distress and satisfaction with life for burn survivors. *Journal of Burn Care and Rehabilitation*, **21**, 490–8.

Pruzinsky, T. & Doctor, M. (1994). Body image changes and pediatric burn injury. In K.J. Tarnowski (Ed.). *Behavioural aspects of pediatric burns* (pp. 169–91). New York: Plenum Press.

Ragiel, C.R. (1989). *The relationship between selected family characteristics, perceptions of trauma impact and post-trauma adaptability in families of thermally injured children*. Dissertation Abstract: University of Cincinnati.

Rose, M., Sanford, A., Thomas, C. & Opp, M.R. (2001). Factors altering the sleep of burned children. *Sleep*, **24**(1), 45–51.

Rumsey, N. & Harcourt, D. (2004). Body image and disfigurement: issues and interventions. *Body Image*, **1**, 83–97.

Sawyer, M.G., Minde, K. & Zuker, R. (1982). The burned child – scarred for life? *Burns*, **9**, 205–13.

Schwanholt, C.A., Ridgway, C.L. *et al.* (1994). A prospective study of scar maturation in pediatrics – does age matter? *Journal of Burn Care and Rehabilitation*, **15**, 416–20.

Taal, L. & Faber, A.W. (1998). Post-traumatic stress and maladjustment among adult burn survivors 1–2 years post burn. Part II: The interview data. *Burns*, **24**, 399–405.

Tedstone, J., Tarrier, N. & Faragher, E. (1998). An investigation of the factors associated with an increased risk of psychological morbidity in burn injured patients. *Burns*, **24**, 407–15.

Van Loey, N.E.E. & Van Son, M.J.M. (2003). Psychopathology and psychological problems in patients with burn scars. *American Journal of Clinical Dermatology*, **4**(4), 245–72.

Willebrand, M., Kildal, M., Andersson, G. & Ekselius, L. (2002). Long term assessment of personality after burn injury in adults. *Journal of Nervous and Mental Disease*, **190**, 53–6.

Williams, E. & Griffiths, T. (1991). Psychological consequences of burn injury. *Burns*, **17**(6), 478–80.

Williams, N.R., Davey, M. & Klock-Powell, K. (2003). Rising from the ashes: stories of recovery, adaptation, and resilience in burn survivors. *Social Work in Health Care*, **36**(4), 53–77.

Williams, N.R., Reeves, P.M., Cox, E.R. & Call, S.B. (2004). Creating a social work link to the burn community: a research team goes to burn camp. *Social Work in Health Care*, **38**(3), 81–103.

Woodward, J. (1959). Emotional disturbance of burned children. *British Medical Journal*, **1**, 1009–13.

C. Phillips

Cancer: breast

Alice Simon and Kathryn Robb

University College London

Prevalence and risk factors

Breast cancer is the most commonly diagnosed cancer in women in both the UK and the US (Cancer Research UK, 2005; American Cancer Society, 2005). In the UK, around 41 000 women develop breast cancer and around 13 000 die from the illness each year. In the US, approximately 210 000 women are diagnosed and 40 000 die from breast cancer every year. It is possible for men to develop breast cancer but it is rare, with annually fewer than 300 cases in the UK and 1700 in the US.

International comparisons (Parkin & Muir, 1992) and studies of migrants (Kolonel, 1980) have provided evidence for the importance of environment in causing the disease. These observations are significant because they suggest that some breast cancers are caused by lifestyle and therefore could be prevented. The major risk factors for breast cancer include (see Colditz *et al.*, 2000): older age, being overweight after the menopause, having a family history of breast cancer, taking the oral contraceptive pill or hormone replacement therapy, starting menstruation early or having a late menopause, starting to have children at an older age, having fewer children, not breastfeeding and regularly drinking large amounts of alcohol. Fewer than 5% of breast cancers arise from inherited gene mutations such as BRCA1 and BRCA2 (Hodgson & Maher, 1999).

Early detection

Screening

Screening mammography has been found to reduce breast cancer mortality in women aged between 50–74 years (Kerlikowske *et al.*, 1995), while the benefits of screening women aged 40–49 years are not so clear (Moss, 2004). Participation in mammography screening does not appear to be associated with age, ethnicity, marital status, or level of education (Jepson *et al.*, 2000). However, having attended a previous mammogram, intending to participate and receiving a general practitioner's recommendation, have all been found to relate to increased attendance (Jepson *et al.*, 2000).

Any medical intervention aimed at a 'healthy' population needs to consider not only the benefits but also the potential harms. The psychological impact of screening is one such potential harm. A recent systematic review reported that mammography screening does not raise anxiety among women given the 'all-clear' (Brett *et al.*, 2005). Indeed, there is some evidence that levels of anxiety following an 'all-clear' mammogram were lower than in the population, suggesting that the procedure may be having a positive emotional impact (Scaf-Klomp *et al.*, 1997). Some population sub-groups (younger age, lower education, living in an urban area, manual occupation, one or no children) are more likely to experience an adverse psychological impact of screening (Brett *et al.*, 2005).

A significant minority of women (5% in the UK) are recalled for further investigation (Smith-Bindman *et al.*, 2003), and among this group there is evidence of significant anxiety, at least in the short-term. Women who are required to have further investigations but are then given the 'all-clear' have been found to show a 'relief' effect, whereby they report lower levels of depression at 3 and 12 months relative to women initially given a clear result (Lampic *et al.*, 2001).

There is some concern that an 'all-clear' mammography result could cause complacency (Stewart-Brown & Farmer, 1997) and cause women to ignore future symptoms (Fowler & Austoker, 1996; Petticrew *et al.*, 2000). However, a review of the area found insufficient evidence for reassurance delaying subsequent symptom presentation (Ramirez *et al.*, 1999) (see also 'Screening: cancer' and 'Screening: general issues').

Symptoms and delay

Encouraging breast self-examination according to a regular schedule does not appear to reduce mortality from breast cancer (Thomas *et al.*, 2002); however women are encouraged to be 'breast aware' and to know what is normal for them. Symptoms of breast cancer include: a new lump or thickening in the breast or armpit; changes in the size, shape or feel; any puckering, dimpling or redness of the skin; changes in the position of the nipple, a rash or nipple discharge; and unusual pain or discomfort (see 'Self-examination').

Delay in the presentation of symptoms is associated with increased breast cancer mortality (Richards *et al.*, 1999). Older age has been identified as a strong predictor of patient delay, while fewer years of education, non-white ethnic origin, not disclosing breast symptoms to another and not attributing symptoms to breast cancer have been found to be moderate predictors of patient-related delay (Ramirez *et al.*, 1999). Younger age and the presentation of a symptom other than a breast lump have been associated with increased delay in diagnosis by health care providers (Ramirez *et al.*, 1999).

Impact of diagnosis

Treatments for breast cancer and their psychological consequences

For many women the primary treatment for breast cancer is surgery, often combined with radiotherapy. Early-stage, localized cancers are frequently treated by the removal of the lump only rather than the entire breast. Breast-conserving therapy appears to have some advantages in terms of improved body image and sexual functioning and improving psychosocial outcomes over the longer term (Engel *et al.*, 2004). Radiation following surgery is used to eliminate any remaining cancer cells and is related to increased fatigue resulting in worse quality of life (Jereczek-Fossa *et al.*, 2002) (see 'Radiotherapy'). Chemotherapy and hormone therapy are also used as adjuvants in the treatment of localized disease as well as for the control of metastatic tumours. Apart from the obvious side effects, such as hair-loss and vomiting, chemotherapy is also associated with longer term cognitive dysfunction (Ahles & Saykin, 2002) (see 'Chemotherapy'). Up to 70% of all breast cancers are hormone-sensitive and there are a number of hormonal therapies for both pre- and post-menopausal women with early or advanced disease. Hormonal treatments can have adverse side effects such as vaginal dryness and hot flushes. But there is some evidence to suggest that patients prefer hormonal treatments over chemotherapy when there is a choice to be made (Fallowfield *et al.*, 2004). Women cite the avoidance of hair-loss, the convenience of the treatment (i.e. less disruption to everyday life) and an overall perception of fewer side effects as the reasons for preference of hormonal therapy (Fallowfield *et al.*, 2004). This illustrates the value placed on quality of life during treatment (see 'Quality of life').

Treatments commonly cause symptoms such as fatigue, pain and sickness. These symptoms are often debilitating and cause psychological distress (Bennett *et al.*, 2004). Some cancer treatments are also associated with increased levels of distress as a direct side effect of treatment, e.g. immunotherapeutic agents, such as interferon-alpha and interleukin induce depressed mood (Capuron *et al.*, 2001; Musselman *et al.*, 2001). Patients currently undergoing treatment tend to have increased distress compared with those who have completed treatment.

There are also other studies which conclude that type of treatment is not associated with distress. Younger age, past history of depression or anxiety and lack of social support, could be more important risk factors for depression and anxiety than cancer-related variables (Burgess *et al.*, 2005). These variables are risk factors for depression in general population samples.

Recovery

Survival, recurrence and long term psychological consequences

A number of issues continue to affect breast cancer 'survivors' despite their disease-free status. There are long-term side effects of treatments including, for example, restricted arm movement and early menopause (Hoda *et al.*, 2003; Ernst *et al.*, 2002) which can affect quality of life. Up to 70% of breast cancer patients express fears about recurrence (Mast, 1998). Some survivors attend outpatient clinics many years after the doctor recommends discharge in order to receive reassurance about their disease-free status (Thomas *et al.*, 1997). Women fear recurrence because of its association with advancing disease, initiating new treatments and possible association with death (Johnson Vickberg, 2001). Unsurprisingly, a

recurrence of breast cancer is associated with increased levels of anxiety and depression (Burgess *et al.*, 2005).

Having had a cancer diagnosis can also seriously affect a person's social identity and role through loss of employment or change in status within the family (Zebrack, 2000). This change in a person's expected life trajectory leads to a process of long-term reorganization and a search for meaning in the experience (Utley, 1999).

Recognizing and treating distress

Prevalence of distress in breast cancer patients

Newly diagnosed breast cancer patients face a number of psychological threats. Not only does the diagnosis often have a significant impact on life expectancy but women are also faced with challenges related to their sexuality, femininity and fertility. The illness can also have knock-on effects throughout women's social life in terms of employment or ability to work and social and family life (Kunkel & Chen, 2003).

Estimates of the prevalence of psychological distress in breast cancer patients vary greatly. At the lower end, one study of a breast cancer clinic waiting-room sample found approximately 9% had major depression, 7% had minor depression, and 6% had generalized anxiety disorder (Coyne *et al.*, 2004). At the higher end, Burgess *et al.* (2005) found 50% of a sample of breast cancer patients to have depression or anxiety in the first year after diagnosis. They also report that this level declines to 25% in the second year and 15% thereafter, showing that estimates of prevalence will vary according to the timing of the assessment. Other factors also contribute to this variation. Higher estimates may reflect use of symptom reporting recorded with self-report questionnaires rather than diagnostic interviews (Hotopf *et al.*, 2002). Higher frequencies may also be seen in inpatients who have more severe symptoms or advanced stages of disease (Lynch, 1995).

Assessing distress in breast cancer patients

Some of the challenges in recognizing clinical levels of distress in breast cancer patients stem from the overlap between symptoms of cancer and the side effects of its treatment, and the defining symptoms of psychiatric disorders such as depression (e.g. fatigue, loss of appetite, cognitive impairment). Symptoms that best distinguish between distressed and non-distressed persons in the general population may not provide the best discrimination among breast cancer patients (Trask, 2004). Attention must be paid to the effects of inclusive versus exclusive evaluations of energy loss, appetite and sleep disturbance, as well as the use of substituting cognitive symptoms for these physical symptoms in making diagnoses (Endicott, 1984; Uchitomi *et al.*, 2001).

The natural course of distress in breast cancer patients is also unclear. A proportion of depression cases in breast cancer patients will be recurrent or ongoing, rather than new, instances. A past history of depression or anxiety is important for predicting which cancer patients will become distressed (Maunsell *et al.*, 1992; Harrison & Maguire, 1994; McDaniel *et al.*, 1997). These patients may already have been prescribed anti-depressant medication or other psychological treatments currently or in the past.

Treatments for psychological distress in breast cancer patients

Psychological distress in breast cancer patients has been treated in similar ways to distress in other population groups i.e. by psychotropic drugs or psychosocial intervention or some combination of both.

Prescribing of antidepressants or anti-anxiolytics to breast cancer patients can be high and sometimes inappropriately so. Coyne *et al.* (2004) reported that 48% of breast cancer patients without a psychiatric disorder had been prescribed antidepressants inappropriately. There is also evidence that many people are not being prescribed an appropriate therapeutic dose (Sharpe *et al.*, 2004b). Effective use of psychotropic drugs in appropriately identified individuals is obviously key to the efficacy of these treatments.

Psychological interventions to treat depression and anxiety in cancer patients are moderately effective (Sheard & Maguire, 1999). Targeted interventions directed at those who are suffering psychological distress have stronger clinical effects than non-targeted interventions. Studies which target all cancer patients have weak results and probably lead to under-estimates of the potential effectiveness of psychological therapies. Group therapy seems to be as effective as individual therapy (Sheard & Maguire, 1999) (see 'Group therapy'). Similarly, telephone counselling can be as effective as face-to-face therapy (Badger *et al.*, 2004, 2005). Recent studies looking at incorporating psychological therapies into the repertoire of oncology professionals, such as cancer nurses, can be effective (Greenberg, 2004; Strong *et al.*, 2004). Psychosocial interventions that reduce distress can save resources by reducing service use (e.g. number of visits to primary care physicians and specialists) (Carlson & Bultz, 2004). Unfortunately, a problem is that a high proportion of patients reject psychological intervention (Shimizu *et al.*, 2005; Sharpe *et al.*, 2004a). Referral for symptom management interventions could be a more acceptable format (McLachlan *et al.*, 2001) and could lead to a reduction in depression (Given *et al.*, 2004). Exercise interventions may also have the potential to improve psychological as well as physiological wellbeing (Oldervoll *et al.*, 2004) (see 'Physical activity interventions').

In sum, there are effective treatments for psychological distress in breast cancer patients. These include the use of antidepressants at effective doses and psychological interventions that focus on lifting depression or improving symptom management. Identifying the women who would benefit from these treatments is difficult, leading to problems estimating the need for clinical services.

(See also 'Cancer: general', 'Coping with chronic illness', 'Coping with death and dying', and 'Self-examination'.)

REFERENCES

Ahles, T.A. & Saykin, A.J. (2002). Breast cancer chemotherapy-related cognitive dysfunction. *Clinical Breast Cancer*, **3**, (Suppl. 3), S84–S90.

American Cancer Society. (2005). *Cancer facts & figures.*

Badger, T., Segrin, C., Meek, P., Lopez, A.M. & Bonham, E. (2004). A case study of telephone interpersonal counseling for women with breast cancer and their partners. *Oncology Nursing Forum*, **31**, 997–1003.

Badger, T., Segrin, C., Meek, P. *et al.* (2005). Telephone interpersonal counseling with women with breast cancer: symptom management and quality of life. *Oncology Nursing Forum*, **32**, 273–9.

Bennett, B., Goldstein, D., Lloyd, A., Davenport, T. & Hickie, I. (2004). Fatigue and psychological distress – exploring the relationship in women treated for breast cancer. *European Journal of Cancer*, **40**, 1689–95.

Brett, J., Bankhead, C., Henderson, B., Watson, E. & Austoker, J. (2005). The psychological impact of mammographic screening. A systematic review. *Psycho-oncology*, **14**, 917–38.

Burgess, C., Cornelius, V., Love, S. *et al.* (2005). Depression and anxiety in women with early breast cancer: five year observational cohort study. *British Medical Journal*, **330**, 702.

Cancer Research UK. (2005). Specific cancers: breast cancer. http://www.cancerresearchuk.org/aboutcancer/specificcancers/breastcancer?version=2 Online.

Capuron, L., Ravaud, A., Gualde, N. *et al.* (2001). Association between immune activation and early depressive symptoms in cancer patients treated with interleukin-2-based therapy. *Psychoneuroendocrinology*, **26**, 797–808.

Carlson, L.E. & Bultz, B.D. (2004). Efficacy and medical cost offset of psychosocial interventions in cancer care: making the case for economic analyses. *Psycho-oncology*, **13**, 837–49.

Colditz, G.A., Atwood, K.A., Emmons, K., *et al.* (2000). Harvard report on cancer prevention, Volume 4: Harvard Cancer Risk Index. Risk Index Working Group, Harvard Center for Cancer Prevention. *Cancer Causes Control*, **11**, 477–88.

Coyne, J.C., Palmer, S.C., Shapiro, P.J., Thompson, R. & DeMichele, A. (2004). Distress, psychiatric morbidity, and prescriptions for psychotropic medication in a breast cancer waiting room sample. *General Hospital Psychiatry*, **26**, 121–8.

Endicott, J. (1984). Measurement of depression in patients with cancer. *Cancer*, **53**, 2243–9.

Engel, J., Kerr, J., Schlesinger-Raab, A., Sauer, H. & Holzel, D. (2004). Quality of life following breast-conserving therapy or mastectomy: results of a 5-year prospective study. *The Breast Journal*, **10**, 223–31.

Ernst, M.F., Voogd, A.C., Balder, W., Klinkenbijl, J.H. & Roukema, J.A. (2002). Early and late morbidity associated with axillary levels I-III dissection in breast cancer. *Journal of Surgical Oncology*, **79**, 151–5.

Fallowfield, L., McGurk, R. & Dixon, M. (2004). Same gain, less pain: potential patient preferences for adjuvant treatment in premenopausal women with early breast cancer. *European Journal of Cancer*, **40**, 2403–10.

Fowler, G. & Austoker, J. (1996). Screening. In R. Detels, W.W. Holland, J. McEwan & G.S. Omenn (Eds.). *Oxford Textbook of Public Health* (3rd edn.). (pp. 1583–99). Oxford: Oxford Medical Publications.

Given, C., Given, B., Rahbar, M. *et al.* (2004). Does a symptom management intervention affect depression among cancer patients: results from a clinical trial. *Psycho-oncology*, **13**, 818–30.

Greenberg, D.B. (2004). Barriers to the treatment of depression in cancer patients. *Journal of the National Cancer Institute Monographs*, **32**, 127–35.

Harrison, J. & Maguire, P. (1994). Predictors of psychiatric morbidity in cancer patients. *The British Journal of Psychiatry*, **165**, 593–8.

Hoda, D., Perez, D.G. & Loprinzi, C.L. (2003). Hot flashes in breast cancer survivors. *The Breast Journal*, **9**, 431–8.

Hodgson, S. & Maher, E. (1999). *A Practical Guide to Human Cancer Genetics* (2nd edn.). Cambridge, UK: Cambridge University Press.

Hotopf, M., Chidgey, J., Addington-Hall, J. & Ly, K.L. (2002). Depression in advanced disease: a systematic review. Part 1. Prevalence and case finding. *Palliative Medicine*, **16**, 81–97.

Jepson, R., Clegg, A., Forbes, C. *et al.* (2000). The determinants of screening uptake and interventions for increasing uptake: a systematic review. *Health Technology Assessment*, **4**, 1–133.

Jereczek-Fossa, B.A., Marsiglia, H.R. & Orecchia, R. (2002). Radiotherapy-related fatigue. *Critical Reviews in Oncology Hematology*, **41**, 317–25.

Johnson Vickberg, S.M. (2001). Fears about breast cancer recurrence. *Cancer Practice*, **9**, 237–43.

Kerlikowske, K., Grady, D., Rubin, S.M., Sandrock, C. & Ernster, V.L. (1995). Efficacy of screening mammography. A meta-analysis. *Journal of American Medical Association*, **273**, 149–54.

Kolonel, L.N. (1980). Cancer patterns of four ethnic groups in Hawaii. *Journal of the National Cancer Institute*, **65**, 1127–39.

Kunkel, E.J. & Chen, E.I. (2003). Psychiatric aspects of women with breast cancer. *The Psychiatric Clinics of North America*, **26**, 713–24.

Lampic, C., Thurfjell, E., Bergh, J. & Sjoden, P.O. (2001). Short- and long-term anxiety and depression in women recalled after breast cancer screening. *European Journal of Cancer*, **37**, 463–9.

Lynch, M.E. (1995). The assessment and prevalence of affective disorders in advanced cancer. *Journal of Palliative Care*, **11**, 10–18.

Mast, M.E. (1998). Survivors of breast cancer: illness uncertainty, positive reappraisal, and emotional distress. *Oncology Nursing Forum*, **25**, 555–62.

Maunsell, E., Brisson, J. & Deschenes, L. (1992). Psychological distress after initial treatment of breast cancer. Assessment of potential risk factors. *Cancer*, **70**, 120–5.

McDaniel, J.S., Musselman, D.L. & Nemeroff, C.B. (1997). Cancer and depression: theory and treatment. *Psychiatric Annals*, **27**, 360–4.

McLachlan, S.A., Allenby, A., Matthews, J. *et al.* (2001). Randomized trial of coordinated psychosocial interventions based on patient self-assessments versus standard care to improve the psychosocial functioning of patients with cancer. *Journal of Clinical Oncology*, **19**, 4117–25.

Moss, S. (2004). Should women under 50 be screened for breast cancer? *Br. J. Cancer*, **91**, 413–17.

Musselman, D.L., Lawson, D.H., Gumnick, J.F. *et al.* (2001). Paroxetine for the prevention of depression induced by high-dose interferon alfa. *The New England Journal of Medicine*, **344**, 961–6.

Oldervoll, L.M., Kaasa, S., Hjermstad, M.J., Lund, J.A. & Loge, J.H. (2004). Physical exercise results in the improved subjective well-being of a few or is effective rehabilitation for all cancer patients? *European Journal of Cancer*, **40**, 951–62.

Parkin, D.M. & Muir, C.S. (1992). Cancer incidence in five continents. Comparability and quality of data. *IARC Scientific Publications*, **120** 45–173.

Petticrew, M.P., Sowden, A.J., Lister-Sharp, D. & Wright, K. (2000). False-negative results in screening programmes: systematic review of impact and implications. *Health Technology Assessment*, **4**.

Ramirez, A.J., Westcombe, A.M., Burgess, C.C. *et al.* (1999). Factors predicting delayed presentation of symptomatic breast cancer: a systematic review. *Lancet*, **353**, 1127–31.

Richards, M.A., Westcombe, A.M., Love, S.B., Littlejohns, P. & Ramirez, A.J. (1999). Influence of delay on survival in patients with breast cancer: a systematic review. *Lancet*, **353**, 1119–26.

Scaf-Klomp, W., Sanderman, R., van de Wiel, H.B., Otter, R. & van den Heuvel, W.J. (1997). Distressed or relieved? Psychological side effects of breast cancer screening in The Netherlands. *Journal of Epidemiology and Community Health*, **51**, 705–10.

Sharpe, M., Strong, V., Allen, K. *et al.* (2004*a*). Management of major depression in outpatients attending a cancer centre: a preliminary evaluation of a multicomponent cancer nurse-delivered intervention. *British Journal of Cancer*, **90**, 310–13.

Sharpe, M., Strong, V., Allen, K. *et al.* (2004*b*). Major depression in outpatients attending a regional cancer centre: screening and unmet treatment needs. *British Journal of Cancer*, **90**, 314–20.

Sheard, T. & Maguire, P. (1999). The effect of psychological interventions on anxiety and depression in cancer patients: results of two meta-analyses. *British Journal of Cancer*, **80**, 1770–80.

Shimizu, K., Akechi, T., Okamura, M. *et al.* (2005). Usefulness of the nurse-assisted screening and psychiatric referral program. *Cancer*, **103**, 1949–56.

Smith-Bindman, R., Chu, P.W., Miglioretti, D.L. *et al.* (2003). Comparison of screening mammography in the United States and the United kingdom. *Journal of American Medical Association*, **290**, 2129–37.

Stewart-Brown, S. & Farmer, A. (1997). Screening could seriously damage your health. *British Medical Journal*, **314**, 533–4.

Strong, V., Sharpe, M., Cull, A. *et al.* (2004). Can oncology nurses treat depression? A pilot project. *Journal of Advanced Nursing*, **46**, 542–8.

Thomas, D.B., Gao, D.L., Ray, R.M. *et al.* (2002). Randomized trial of breast self-examination in Shanghai: final results. *Journal of the National Cancer Institute*, **94**, 1445–57.

Thomas, S., Glynne-Jones, R. & Chait, I. (1997). Is it worth the wait? A survey of patients' satisfaction with an oncology outpatient clinic. *European Journal of Cancer Care (Engl.)*, **6**, 50–8.

Trask, P.C. (2004). Assessment of depression in cancer patients. *Journal of the National Cancer Institute Monograph*, **32**, 80–92.

Uchitomi, Y., Kugaya, A., Akechi, T. *et al.* (2001). Three sets of diagnostic criteria for major depression and correlations with serotonin-induced platelet calcium mobilization in cancer patients. *Psychopharmacology (Berl)*, **153**, 244–8.

Utley, R. (1999). The evolving meaning of cancer for long-term survivors of breast cancer. *Oncology Nursing Forum*, **26**, 1519–23.

Zebrack, B. (2000). Cancer survivors and quality of life: a critical review of the literature. *Oncology Nursing Forum*, **27**, 1395–401.

Cancers of the digestive tract

Sharon Manne

Fox Chase Cancer Center

Cancers of the digestive tract, which include cancer of the colon, rectum, pancreas, stomach and esophagus, are among the most common and deadly types of cancer. Colorectal cancer (cancer of the colon or rectum) is the second leading cause of cancer-related deaths in the United States. The disease surpasses both breast and prostate cancer in mortality and is second only to lung cancer in numbers of cancer deaths. Approximately 146 940 new cases of colorectal cancer were diagnosed in the United States 2004 and 56 730 people died from the disease. Although relatively uncommon, oesophageal, stomach and pancreatic cancer are among the most deadly cancers, as they are typically diagnosed at more advanced stages. For example, cancer of the pancreas is the fourth leading cause of cancer death in the United States. The tendency of these cancers to be either asymptomatic at early stages or to present with vague symptoms at more advanced stages, as well as the lack of screening procedures for these cancers, contributes to diagnosis at a more advanced stage. This chapter will discuss the psychological impact of cancers of the digestive tract according to upper digestive tract (oesophagus and stomach) and lower digestive tract (colon, rectum, pancreas).

Cancer of the upper digestive tract

Many individuals diagnosed with cancers of the oesophagus or stomach have a poor prognosis because the cancer may have metastasized prior to diagnosis. For individuals diagnosed with gastric (stomach) cancer, studies have shown only a 2.5% (distant metastatic disease) to 23% (all stages) 5-year survival rate (American Cancer Society, 2004). For individuals diagnosed with stage I oesophageal cancer, the 5-year survival rate is 29% (American Cancer Society, 2004). Survival rate for later stages of oesophageal cancer is poor (2–13%). Treatment for oesophageal cancer usually involves partial removal of the oesophagus and often part of the upper stomach. This is a difficult surgery with a long period of recovery. Difficulty swallowing food and pain are common disease-related symptoms. Treatment for gastric cancer is usually total removal of the stomach. This surgery results in weight loss, malnourishment due to malabsorption, difficulty swallowing food, acid reflux. Post-prandial discomfort, such as bloating and urgent diarrhoea, are common symptoms (Vickery *et al.*, 2001). Unfortunately, curative surgery is not an option for many patients with gastric cancer. These patients are offered palliative care to manage pain and surgical intervention to manage perforation or obstruction.

Given the poor prognosis and many difficult disease-related symptoms, patients diagnosed with either gastric or oesophageal cancer may be understandably anxious and depressed at the time of initial diagnosis and suffer from a greatly reduced quality of life. Indeed, the few studies of individuals with gastric cancer have suggested that this is the case. Svedlund and colleagues (1996) conducted a cross-sectional study evaluating quality of life among newly diagnosed, early stage gastric cancer patients one week prior to surgery. Compared with a healthy reference population, gastric cancer patients had lower health-related quality of life, with significant differences noted in eating, sleep/rest, work and home management. Psychological functioning was similar to the healthy reference population.

There have been two longitudinal studies of quality of life among gastric cancer patients. A prospective randomized clinical trial evaluating the impact of different types of gastrectomy on quality of life was conducted by Svedlund *et al.* (1997). The sample evidenced functional limitations, particularly with regard to digestive symptoms at the 3-month follow-up. Compared with the baseline assessment, patients who had total gastrectomy and those who had a total gastrectomy with a gastric substitute reported significantly lower quality of life compared with their pre-surgery functioning. Patients who had a subtotal gastrectomy did not report changes from their pre-surgery quality of life. One year after surgery, physical symptoms decreased more among patients who had a subtotal gastrectomy. These results suggest that there may be some health-related quality of life benefits of subtotal gastrectomy.

Relatively few studies have evaluated quality of life among patients with oesophageal cancer. Because swallowing food is a significant problem, alimentary comfort is generally considered the most prominent quality of life indicator (Sugimachi *et al.*, 1986). The majority of studies evaluating quality of life have investigated the effects of surgical/laser interventions to improve swallowing ability in both early stage patients whose surgery is curative, and among late stage patients, whose surgery is palliative. Sugimachi and colleagues (1986) evaluated the quality of life among early stage patients undergoing oesophageal replacement surgery one year after surgery. They reported better food tolerance, less dysphagia and less time needed to eat compared with pre-surgery functioning. Collard and colleagues (1992) evaluated quality of life among 17 patients who were disease free three years after oesophageal surgery. Patients reported that their comfort when eating was not as satisfactory as before the initial oesophageal symptoms began. However, body weight increased in three-quarters of the patients, and patients reported they were able to eat satisfactorily. The most common troubling symptoms were early fullness when eating, dysphagia and diarrhoea. Other aspects of quality of life, including mental health and social functioning, were not assessed.

van Knippenberg and colleagues (1992) assessed both physical and psychological aspects of quality of life three to four months after oesophageal surgery. In terms of physical symptoms, pain when swallowing, loss of appetite, tiredness, shortness of breath and diarrhoea all decreased significantly after surgery. However, 18% reported that swallowing problems worsened. Psychological symptoms, including degree of worry, desperation about the future and anxiety, declined significantly. About 48% of patients reported depressive symptoms at the post-surgical time point and about 37% reported anxiety. However, because a standardized scale was not used, exact distress levels were not reported, nor were comparisons with a normative sample. Modest associations were found between swallowing problems and quality of life ($r = 0.26$), suggesting that swallowing problems play a relatively small role in evaluations of quality of life. The authors suggest that patients may tolerate physical symptoms, such as difficulty swallowing, in exchange for a chance at a longer life. Two studies have evaluated the effect of two different endoscopic palliative treatments to control malignant dysphagia on quality of life of patients with advanced stages of cancer. Loizou and colleagues (1992) evaluated quality of life in a small sample of oesophageal cancer patients ($n = 43$). Results indicated that all patients followed until death reported improvements in ability to swallow with laser treatment and intubation. Treatment resulted in an initial improvement in quality of life, which was reduced over time with disease progression. The last post-treatment scores, which were taken within five weeks of death, were significantly lower than pre-treatment scores, despite continued successful palliation of dysphagia. The authors interpret these results as suggesting that dysphagia is a less important determinant of quality of life as disease progresses, because patients in terminal stages become anorexic and do not eat.

Cancer of the lower digestive tract

Only 4.4% of patients with pancreatic cancer survive beyond five years, and patients universally experience pain and associated suffering. Obviously, receiving a diagnosis of this disease can be catastrophic. An association between depression and pancreatic cancer was first reported in the 1930s when symptoms of anxiety and depression in patients diagnosed with pancreatic cancer were described (Yaskin, 1931). Indeed, a number of studies have suggested that depression is a presenting symptom at diagnosis (Joffee et al., 1986), with studies suggesting that between 50% (Joffee et al., 1986) and 76% (Fras et al., 1967) of patients either meet criterion for depression or report depressive symptoms at diagnosis. In one study, patients with pancreatic tumours had psychological symptoms 43 months before physical symptoms (Fras et al., 1967). Because depression is a presenting symptom at diagnosis, there has been more attention paid to assessing psychological distress in pancreatic cancer after diagnosis than other types of cancer. Holland and colleagues (1986) compared distress scores in patients with pancreatic cancer who were beginning chemotherapy with patients with gastric cancer. They found that distress scores were significantly higher among patients with pancreatic cancer. The prevalence of pain and depression in newly diagnosed patients with pancreatic cancer were evaluated in a cross-sectional study by Kelsen et al. (1995). Approximately 38% of patients had depression scores in the moderate to severe range on a standardized inventory (Beck Depression Inventory). Patients beginning chemotherapy had significantly higher depression scores than patients about to undergo surgery. The anxiety inventory scores did not indicate high levels of anxiety. There was a significant correlation between pain intensity and depression and anxiety scores. Zabora and colleagues (2001) examined distress in nearly 5000 cancer patients of whom 112 had pancreatic cancer. Comparisons between tumour sites indicated that pancreatic cancer patients endorsed the highest mean scores for anxiety and depression. Whether an association between depression and pancreatic cancer is due to the cancer itself, or whether depression causes pancreatic cancer, is an issue that has been raised in the literature (Carney et al., 2003).

For individuals with colorectal cancer, the only curative treatment is surgery. The type of surgery is dependent on the localization of the tumour relative to the anal verge. If the tumour is near the anal verge or if the patient presents with recurrent colorectal cancer, then the surgery performed includes the rectum and sphincter function is not preserved. With this procedure, patients must have a permanent ostomy. This is an intrusive surgery that can interfere with daily life. Patients must cope with an ostomy bag and its care along with frequent or irregular bowel movements.

Much of the literature on quality of life among individuals with colorectal cancer has focused on the impact of ostomy surgery, and the most common aspect of quality of life assessed has been depression. Several studies have reported that the prevalence of depression is higher among ostomates than non-ostomates (e.g. Wirtsching et al., 1975; Williams & Johnston, 1983). Prevalence of depression has ranged from 7% to 50% (Fresco et al., 1988). Approximately 25% of patients report anxiety (Cardoen et al., 1982), but comparisons of patients who have an ostomy with patients who do not have an ostomy do not suggest a difference in rates of anxiety (MacDonald & Andersen, 1984). Twenty-three per cent of patients report a worsening of anxiety or depression compared with pre-surgery levels of functioning (Thomas et al., 1984; White & Unwin, 1998). Risk factors for higher levels of distress include younger age, female gender, lower education level and lower levels of social support (Baider et al., 1989; Vernon et al., 1997). Among patients with ostomies, poorer adaptation has been associated with a higher level of ostomy self-care, less perceived support from family and friends and less psychosocial support to assist in accepting permanent changes in body image related to ostomy surgery (Piwonka & Merino, 1999).

In terms of social functioning, studies have indicated that patients report deterioration in the quality of their relationships with family and friends (Fresco et al., 1988). Estimates of sexual problems have varied greatly across studies, but the sexual function of men with a colostomy is more impaired than among patients with intact sphincters.

Few studies have evaluated quality of life among long-term survivors. Ramsey and colleagues (2000) conducted one of the few evaluations of quality of life among survivors. They studied 227 patients surviving at least five years from diagnosis using standardized measures of health-related quality of life and depression. Fourteen per cent of patients scored at or above the depression cutoff score. Depression was significantly more prevalent than among the general population. Depression was significantly higher among patients reporting comorbid health problems and low socioeconomic status. Mullens and colleagues (2004) evaluated risk perceptions and worry and anxiety in 81 survivors. They found that shorter-term survivors perceived the risk for recurrence to be higher and reported more intrusive worries about cancer. Overall levels of anxiety and worry about recurrence were low.

Issues

As described in the review above, the primary focus of research has been on physical symptoms and health-related quality of life. Much less attention has been paid to emotional distress and positive well-being, particularly among patients with gastric and oesophageal cancers. Because physical symptoms such as dysphagia and nausea are extremely troubling and likely to significantly interfere with quality of life, it is understandable why these aspects of quality of life are important targets for studies. However, greater attention should be paid to assessing emotional and social functioning.

The very small sample sizes of the majority of studies are noteworthy, particularly in evaluations of quality of life among patients with oesophageal, gastric and pancreatic tumours. Most studies are not powered sufficiently to test differences between patients undergoing different treatments or surgeries. Data regarding refusal rates are rarely presented, and thus it is not clear whether the samples are biased. Because most studies are cross-sectional, we do not have information about the course of distress responses over the illness trajectory. Both issues are likely due to the fact that the majority of patients with these cancers do not live very long, and thus it is difficult to follow patients for a significant period of time. Patients may be too ill to complete study surveys over a lengthy period of time. Another issue is the lack of knowledge regarding attitudinal factors contributing to differences in quality of life and distress outcomes in patients with gastrointestinal cancers. The dearth of information on this topic is probably due to the fact that health-related challenges; particularly pain, nausea, problems with eating and difficulties after meals; are the main contributors to distress responses in this very sick group of patients. However, psychological interventions could be informed by more knowledge about psychological vulnerabilities and strengths that contribute to wellbeing in this population. Given the major challenges these patients face, it is surprising to see that so few psychological interventions have been tested.

(See also 'Cancer: general', 'Coping with chronic illness', 'Coping with death and dying', and 'Quality of life'.)

REFERENCES

American Cancer Society. (2004). *Cancer Facts and Figures*. Atlanta, GA: American Cancer Society.

Baider, L., Perez, T. & De-Nour, A. K. (1989). Gender and adjustment to chronic disease. A study of couples with colon cancer. *General Hospital Psychiatry*, **11**, 1–8.

Cardoen, G., Daelen van Den, L., Boeckx, G. & Harton, F. (1982). Argumentatie-houding en resultaten in de behandeling van het rectumcarcinoom. *Acta Chirurgica Belgica*, **82**, 41–50.

Carney, C. P., Jones, L., Woolson, R. F. *et al.* (2003). Relationship between depression and pancreatic cancer in the general population. *Psychosomatic Medicine*, **65**, 884–8.

Collard, J., Otte, J., Reynaert, M. & Kestens, P. (1992). Quality of life three years or more after esophagectomy for cancer. *The Journal of Thoracic and Cardiovascular Surgery*, **104**(2), 391–4.

Fras, I., Litin, E. M. & Pearson, J. S. (1967). Comparison of psychiatric symptoms in carcinoma of the pancreas with those in some other intra-abdominal neoplasms. *American Journal of Psychiatry*, **123**(12), 1553–62.

Fresco, R., Hodoul Azema, D., Busso, M. *et al.* (1988). Les amputes du rectum: difficultes psychologiques, familiales et sexuelles. *Revue Medicale de la Suisse Romande*, **108**, 105–11.

Holland, J. C., Korzun, A., Tross, S. *et al.* (1986). Comparative psychological disturbance in patients with pancreatic and gastric cancer. *American Journal of Psychiatry*, **143**(8), 982–5.

Joffe, R. T., Rubinow, D. R., Denicoff, K. E., Maher, M. & Sindelar, W. F. (1986). Depression and carcinoma of the pancreas. *General Hospital Psychiatry*, **8**, 241–5.

Kelsen, D. P., Portenoy, R. K., Thaler, H. T. *et al.* (1995). Pain and depression in patients with newly diagnosed pancreas cancer. *Journal of Clinical Oncology*, **13**(3), 748–55.

van Knippenberg, F. C. E., Out, J. J., Tilanuis, H. W. *et al.* (1992). Quality of life in patients with resected oesophageal cancer. *Social Science & Medicine*, **35**(2), 139–45.

Loizou, L. A., Rampton, D., Atkinson, M., Robertson, C. & Bown, S. G. (1992). A prospective assessment of quality of life after endoscopic intubation and laser therapy for malignant dysphagia. *Cancer*, **70**(2), 386–91.

MacDonald, L. D. & Anderson, H. R. (1984). Stigma in patients with rectal cancer: a community study. *Journal of Epidemiology & Community Health*, **38**, 284–90.

Mullens, A. B., McCaul, K. D., Erickson, S. C. & Sandgren, A. K. (2004). Coping after cancer: risk perceptions, worry, and health behaviors among colorectal cancer survivors. *Psycho-oncology*, **13**(6), 367–76.

Piwonka, M. A. & Merino, J. (1999). A multidimensional modeling of predictors influencing the adjustment to a colostomy. *Journal of Wound, Ostomy, and Continence Nursing: official publication of The Wound, Ostomy and Continence Nurses Society/WOCN*, **26**(6), 298–305.

Ramsey, S. D., Andersen, M. R., Etzioni, R. *et al.* (2000). Quality of life in survivors of colorectal carcinoma. *Cancer*, **88**, 1294–303.

Sugimachi, K., Maekawa, S., Koga, Y., Ueo, H. & Inokuchi, K. (1986). The quality of life is sustained after operation for carcinoma of the esophagus. *Surgery, Gynecology & Obstetrics*, **162**, 544–6.

Svedlund, J., Sullivan, M., Liedman, B., Lundell, L. & Sjodin, I. (1997). Quality of life after gastrectomy for gastric carcinoma: controlled study of reconstructive procedures. *World Journal Surgery*, **21**, 422–33.

Svedlund, J., Sullivan, M., Sjodin, I., Liedman, B. & Lundell, L. (1996). Quality of life in gastric cancer prior to gastrectomy. *Quality of Life Research*, **5**, 255–64.

Thomas, C., Madden, F. & Jehu, D. (1984). Psychosocial morbidity in the first three months following stoma surgery. *Journal Psychosomatic Research*, **28**, 251–7.

Vernon, S.W., Perz, C.A., Gritz, E.R. *et al.* (1997). Correlates of psychologic distress in colorectal cancer patients undergoing genetic testing for hereditary colon cancer. *Health Psychology*, **16**, 73–86.

Vickery, C.W., Blazeby, J.M., Conroy, T. *et al.* (2001). Development of an EORTC disease-specific quality of life module for use in patients with gastric cancer. *European Journal of Cancer*, **37**, 966–71.

White, C.A. & Unwin, J.C. (1998). Postoperative adjustment to surgery resulting I the formation of a stoma: the importance of stoma-related cognitions. *British Journal of Health Psychology*, **3**, 85–93.

Williams, N.S. & Johnston, D. (1983). The quality of life after rectal excision for low rectal cancer. *British Journal of Surgery*, **70**, 60–2.

Wirsching, M., Druner, H.U. & Herrman, G. (1975). Results of psychosocial adjustment to long-term colostomy. *Psychotherapy and Psychosomatics*, **26**, 245–56.

Yaskin, J.C. (1931). Nervous symptoms as earliest manifestations of carcinoma of the pancreas. *Journal of the American Medical Association*, **96**, 1664–8.

Zabora, J., Brintzenhofeszoc, K., Curbow, B., Hooker, C. & Piantodosi, S. (2001). The prevalence of psychological distress by cancer site. *Psycho-oncology*, **10**(1), 19–28.

Cancer: general

Barbara L. Andersen and Laura E. Simonelli

The Ohio State University

Introduction

The human cost of cancer is staggering. Worldwide there were 10.9 million new cases, 6.7 million deaths and 24.6 million persons alive with cancer (within three years of diagnosis; Parkin *et al.*, 2005). In many countries cancer is the second leading cause of death, only outnumbered by heart disease. In the United States, it has been the leading cause of death for persons younger than 85 since 1999, and over 1 million new cancer cases and almost 600 000 deaths are expected in 2005 (Jemal *et al.*, 2005). However, there is striking variation across geographic locations. Research on the psychological and behavioural aspects of oncology began in the early 1950s; however, significant expansion has occurred in the last 25 years. This research has clarified biobehavioural factors in illness (Andersen *et al.*, 1994), including relations between psychological responses and factors (e.g. personality, mood, coping style) and behavioural variables (e.g. compliance with treatment, diet, exercise), with more recent research incorporating biologic systems (e.g. immune and endocrine) and examining the interaction of these variables and their relationship to disease course (Andersen *et al.*, 2004).

This chapter provides a brief overview of the central findings which have emerged on the psychological and behavioural aspects of cancer. Other chapters in this volume can be consulted for site-specific findings. By way of introduction, we will begin with data on cancer incidence, death rates and gender differences. Where data from the US are used, we note that they represent the same general trends found in other industrialized, western countries. The remainder of the chapter organizes the findings by disease-relevant time points, from diagnosis to recovery and/or death. We will conclude by highlighting psychological interventions which appear to be effective in aiding cancer patients.

Magnitude of the problem: incidence, death rates and gender differences

Cancers vary in their prevalence and mortality. Tables 1 and 2 display data from the USA on the incidence and death rates by specific sites and genders. Similarly, Tables 3 and 4 provide death rate data from other countries (Ferlay *et al.*, 2004).

Biobehavioural aspects

Diagnosis

An early clinical study suggested that the diagnosis of cancer produces an 'existential plight', meaning that the news brings shock, disbelief and emotional turmoil (Weisman & Worden, 1976). Today, we know that individuals even become anxious and alarmed at the time of medical screening. (French *et al.*, 2004; Wardle & Pope, 1992). When the diagnosis does come, the stress patients experience even relates to adverse biological consequences, such as a lowered immune response (Andersen *et al.*, 1998).

In the USA, as well as in most western countries, patients (including children) are told that their diagnosis is cancer (Krylov & Krylova, 2003). Cross-cultural research has indicated that the majority of patients want to be told their diagnosis

Table 1. Cancer incidence by site and gender in the United States (2005 estimates)

Cancer incidence					
Male (Total est. 710 040)			**Female (Total est. 662 870)**		
Site	Number	(%)	Site	Number	(%)
Prostate	232 090	(33%)	Breast	211 240	(32%)
Lung and bronchus	93 010	(13%)	Lung and bronchus	79 560	(12%)
Colon and rectum	71 820	(10%)	Colon and rectum	73 470	(11%)
Urinary bladder	47 010	(7%)	Uterine endometrial	40 880	(6%)
Melanoma of skin	33 580	(5%)	Lymphoma	27 320	(4%)
Lymphoma	29 070	(4%)	Melanoma of skin	26 000	(4%)
Kidney and pelvis	22 490	(3%)	Ovary	22 220	(3%)
Leukaemia	19 640	(3%)	Thyroid	19 190	(3%)
Oral cavity and pharynx	19 100	(3%)	Urinary bladder	16 200	(2%)
Pancreas	16 100	(2%)	Pancreas	16 080	(2%)

Adapted from *Cancer Facts and Figures – 2005*(2005), American Cancer Society. Inc.

Table 2. Cancer deaths by site and gender in the United States (2005 estimates)

Cancer deaths					
Male (Total est. 295 280)			**Female (Total est. 275 000)**		
Site	Number	(%)	Site	Number	(%)
Lung and bronchus	90 490	(31%)	Lung and bronchus	73 020	(27%)
Prostate	30 350	(13%)	Breast	40 410	(15%)
Colon and rectum	28 540	(10%)	Colon and rectum	27 750	(10%)
Pancreas	15 820	(4%)	Ovary	16 210	(6%)
Leukaemia	12 540	(4%)	Pancreas	15 980	(6%)
Esophagus	10 530	(3%)	Leukaemia	10 030	(4%)
Liver and bile duct	10 330	(3%)	Lymphoma	9050	(3%)
Lymphoma	10 150	(3%)	Uterine endometrial	7310	(3%)
Urinary bladder	8970	(3%)	Multiple myeloma	5640	(2%)
Kidney and pelvis	8020	(3%)	Brain and nervous system	5480	(2%)

Adapted from *Cancer Facts and Figures – 2005*(2005), American Cancer Society. Inc.

truthfully (e.g. Japan: Miyata *et al.*, 2004). However, in some countries, such as Turkey, cancer diagnoses are often viewed as death sentences leading to great distress, and poor physician–patient communication is considered one primary reason why many patients are not informed of their true diagnosis (Atseci *et al.*, 2004). These studies demonstrate the need for physicians and other health professionals to learn more effective means of communicating information (e.g. diagnosis, treatment, prognosis) to their patients (Atesci, 2004; Miyata *et al.*, 2004) (see 'Breaking bad news').

Patients experience a range of emotions, such as sadness, depression, hopelessness, fear, anxiety and anger, following their cancer diagnosis. It is not surprising that depression is the most common affective problem. Estimates of depressive symptoms vary from 5% to 50% in cancer patients, and it is thought that at least half of these patients would meet diagnostic criteria for clinical depression (Stommel *et al.*, 2004). There are several factors that affect the degree of emotional distress patients experience during this difficult time. Cancer site, stage, comorbidities, socio-demographic characteristics (i.e. age, education, gender), physical

functioning, symptom severity and treatment type have been identified as predictors of depressive symptoms in multiple cancer populations (Epping-Jordan *et al.*, 1999; Stommel *et al.*, 2004). For example, more advanced disease in cancer patients (e.g. breast) is related to poorer physical and mental health (Jacobsen *et al.*, 1998).

Psychosocial variables, such as coping (Epping-Jordan *et al.*, 1999), optimism (Andrykowski *et al.*, 2004), personality (Ranchor *et al.*, 2002) and social support (Varni & Katz, 1997) appear to be influential in psychological adjustment to cancer diagnosis and treatment. For example, low optimism moderated distress levels among women receiving abnormal transvaginal ultrasounds for ovarian cancer screening (Andrykowski *et al.*, 2004).

In addition to patient distress following diagnosis, several studies have addressed the emotional impact on patients' partners and families. Most studies have found that patients partners and offspring have comparable levels of anxiety and depressed mood throughout the various stages of cancer diagnosis and treatment (Edwards & Clarke, 2004). In addition, research suggests families that express feelings directly and solve problems effectively have lower levels of depression and anxiety (Edwards & Clarke, 2004).

Table 3. Age-adjusted death rates in adult males per 100 000 for disease sites and selected countries

Country	All sites	Colon/rectal	Lung	Prostate	Stomach
United States	152.6 (30)	5.2	48.7	15.8	4.0
Australia	147.1 (33)	18.7	34.7	17.7	5.7
Canada	156.6 (27)	16.1	48.5	16.6	5.9
Columbia	141.1 (36)	7.3	19.9	21.6	27.8
Denmark	179.2 (15)	23.3	45.2	22.6	5.4
England/Wales	162.3 (20)	17.5	42.9	17.9	8.7
France	191.7 (12)	18.2	47.5	18.2	7.0
Germany	161.8 (21)	19.9	42.4	15.8	10.3
Hungary	271.4 (1)	35.6	83.9	18.4	18.2
Israel	132.6 (42)	18.8	26.9	13.4	8.9
Japan	154.3 (29)	17.3	32.4	5.7	28.7
Netherlands	181.6 (14)	18.9	57.6	19.7	9.1
Poland	203.5 (7)	18.2	68.4	12.4	16.6
Russia	205.0 (6)	18.9	63.0	8.2	31.8
South Africa	163.6 (6)	7.9	23.0	22.6	7.6
Zimbabwe	183.6 (13)	6.5	12.0	23.5	10.4

Figures in parentheses are order of rank based on data from 50 countries in 2002. Adapted from J. Ferlay et al. (2004). GLOBOCAN 2002: Cancer Incidence, Mortality and Prevalence Worldwide IARC CancerBase No. 5. version 2.0, IARC Press, Lyon, 2004.

Table 4. Age-adjusted death rates in adult females per 100 000 for disease sites and selected countries

Country	All sites	Breast	Colon/rectal	Lung	Cervix	Endometrial
United States	111.9 (16)	19.0	11.6	26.8	2.3	2.6
Australia	99.0 (31)	18.4	13.3	13.8	1.7	1.6
Canada	114.3 (15)	21.1	11.7	25.6	2.5	1.9
Columbia	122.5 (8)	12.5	7.6	10.0	18.2	1.5
Denmark	148.1 (2)	27.8	19.2	27.8	5.0	2.9
England/Wales	122.7 (7)	24.3	12.4	21.1	3.1	1.8
France	96.3 (33)	21.5	11.8	8.0	3.1	2.2
Germany	110.4 (18)	21.6	15.7	10.8	3.8	1.9
Hungary	145.1 (3)	24.6	21.2	22.3	6.7	4.1
Israel	105.0 (24)	24.0	14.6	8.6	2.3	2.2
Japan	82.2 (44)	8.3	11.1	9.6	2.8	1.3
Netherlands	119.8 (10)	27.5	14.4	15.6	2.3	2.4
Poland	110.6 (17)	15.5	11.4	12.3	7.8	2.8
Russia	101.6 (27)	18.0	13.6	6.2	6.5	3.6
South Africa	107.6 (21)	16.4	6.4	6.9	21.0	1.5
Zimbabwe	165.4 (1)	14.1	6.2	5.8	43.1	2.8

Figures in parentheses are order of rank based on data from 50 countries in 2002. Adapted from J. Ferlay et al. (2004). GLOBOCAN 2002: Cancer Incidence, Mortality and Prevalence Worldwide IARC CancerBase No. 5. version 2.0, IARC Press, Lyon, 2004.

Nonetheless, it is clear that cancer diagnosis and its aftermath can be quite distressing for patients and their loved ones.

Treatment

A certain component of the emotional distress occurring at diagnosis is due to the anticipation of treatment. Current therapies include surgery, radiotherapy and radioactive substances, chemotherapy, hormonal therapy, immunotherapy and combination regimens and procedures (e.g. bone marrow transplantation, intra-operative radiotherapy). Some patients also undergo difficult diagnostic or treatment monitoring procedures (e.g. bone marrow aspirations), as well as physical examinations, radiology studies and/or laboratory work. Thus, the diagnostic process of selecting the appropriate therapy and the subsequent treatment events bring multiple occasions of medical stressors. The data are consistent in their portrayal of more distress (particularly fear and anxiety), and slower rates of emotional recovery for cancer patients than are found with healthy individuals also undergoing medical treatment. As cancer treatments (e.g. surgery, radiation, etc.) vary considerably in their intent, morbidity and mortality, we will review each of the major modalities separately and also discuss three clinical problems that are common across therapies: compliance; appetite and weight loss; and fatigue.

Surgery

There have been few investigations of cancer surgery, but there are numerous descriptive and intervention studies of the reactions of healthy individuals undergoing surgery for benign conditions (see 'Surgery'). The latter studies are consistent in their portrayal of (a) high levels of self-reported preoperative anxiety predictive of lowered postoperative anxiety and (b) postoperative anxiety predictive of recovery (e.g. time out of bed, pain reports). What may distinguish cancer surgery patients are higher overall levels of distress and slower rates of emotional recovery. For example, Gottesman and Lewis (1982) found greater and more lasting feelings of crisis and helplessness among cancer patients in comparison with benign surgery patients for as long as two months following discharge.

Interventions to reduce stress have been tested. Components of these interventions include procedural information (e.g. how the surgery is to be performed, description of postoperative recovery from the perspective of the patient, Wyatt et al., 2004), sensory information on the actual physical sensations of the surgery, behavioural coping instructions, cognitive coping interventions, relaxation and emotion-focused interventions. In a meta-analysis of this literature, Johnston and Vogele (1993) reported that procedural information and behavioural instructions show consistent and strong positive effects on postoperative recovery. Effects are significant for a broad band of measures, including ratings of negative affect and pain, amount of pain medication, length of stay and indices of recovery (see also 'Coping with stressful medical procedures').

Radiotherapy

At least 350 000 individuals receive radiation therapy each year. Clinical descriptions have noted patients' fears (e.g. being burned, hair loss, sterility): while such outcomes do occur, they are site- and dosage-dependent. To understand radiation fears, the surgical anxiety studies described above have been a paradigm. Here again, anxiety can often cause more overall distress than physical symptoms (Stiegelis et al., 2004). If interventions to reduce distress (especially anticipatory anxiety) are not conducted, heightened post-treatment anxiety can be found (Larsson & Starrin, 1992) and maintained post-therapy, particularly when treatment symptoms linger (e.g. diarrhoea, fatigue; King *et al.*, 1985). In addition to radiation fears, radiation related morbidities can lead to increased symptoms, such as appetite loss, fatigue and pain, and subsequently, a decrease in quality of life (Bansal *et al.*, 2004) (see 'Radiotherapy').

Chemotherapy

It is estimated that approximately 30% of cancer patients will develop anticipatory nausea, 80% will experience post-treatment nausea, and 55% will develop vomiting in response to cytotoxic treatments (Morrow *et al.*, 2002). The routine use of anti-emetic drugs has resulted in an overall lower incidence and severity of nausea and vomiting as a clinical problem. However, this change in clinical practice may have been somewhat offset by the use of more toxic regimens and the adjuvant treatment for disease types or stages which were previously not treated with chemotherapy (Andrykowski, 1993). It is clear that, in general, anti-emetics need to be used from the beginning not only to control nausea and vomiting, but to reduce the likelihood of the development of anticipatory reactions. Once anticipatory nausea and vomiting develops, anti-emetics are less effective (Morrow & Hickok, 1993), and patients may need behavioural treatment.

Psychological interventions have included the use of hypnosis, progressive muscle relaxation with guided imagery, self-administered stress management, systematic desensitization, cognitive distraction, self-care education and biofeedback (see 'Chemotherapy'). Overall, behavioural interventions can effectively control anticipatory nausea and vomiting in adult and pediatric cancer patients undergoing chemotherapy, but the effects on post-treatment nausea and vomiting are less clear (Redd *et al.*, 2001).

Bone marrow transplantation (BMT)

Over the past few decades, BMT has evolved from an experimental procedure performed as a last resort into an effective treatment for a variety of cancers (e.g. leukaemia, Hodgkin's disease and non-Hodgkin's lymphoma, breast cancer). However, it can also be an aggressive last course of treatment used when standard treatments have failed or a relapse of cancer occurs (Trask *et al.*, 2002).

BMT is a complex, toxic, and potentially fatal, treatment. The target of the treatment, the bone marrow, is destroyed with high dose chemotherapy, with or without whole body radiation afterwards. The transplanted bone marrow then comes from a donor (allogenic BMT) or from the patient him/herself (autologous BMT) after the marrow is removed and treated. Although allogenic BMT has a role, its expansion is limited by the need for a suitable donor and the subsequent risk of graft vs. host disease for the patient. In the case of autologous BMT, a variety of ex vivo procedures are used to destroy the malignant cells in the patient's marrow prior to re-infusion, including treatment with cytotoxic drugs, exposure to monoclonal antibodies which will attach tumour-associated antigens, or harvesting and introducing stem cells from the patient's peripheral blood.

Patients (and their families) are faced with a number of stressors: a life-threatening illness; locating a suitable donor (for allogeneic transplants; Phipps, 2002); and potentially fatal side effects. There are many other side effects as well (e.g. hair loss, mouth and gastrointestinal mucositis and infertility), and, of course, the treatment can fail and the disease persist or rapidly recur (Winer & Sutton, 1994). Hospitalization is prolonged (often four weeks or longer) and it is generally spent in isolation (Trask *et al.*, 2002).

The many difficulties can contribute to patients feeling out-of-control (helplessness), alone, anxious and depressed (Beanlands *et al.*, 2003). Psychological efforts have focused on providing support to patients, their families and healthcare staff (Phipps, 2002), and maximizing control for patients, such as making choices about the hospital environment whenever possible (see also 'Hospitalization in adults').

Cross-modality problems and efforts to reduce treatment distress

Important steps have also been made towards understanding the aetiology and prevention of at least three common disease/treatment-related complications. First, appetite and weight loss are significant clinical problems for cancer patients susceptible to tumour-induced metabolism or taste changes, having tumour-related obstructions (often diagnosed as primary cachexia/anorexia), or receiving gastrointestinal toxic chemotherapy or abdominal radiotherapy (secondary cachexia/anorexia). Research in this area has pointed the way, for example, to interventions employing novel tastes or 'scapegoat' foods (e.g. lemon-lime Kool-Aid, unusually flavoured hard sweets such as coconut; Schwartz *et al.*, 1996) to 'block' conditioning to familiar diet items, reducing food and beverage intake prior to drug administration, and ingesting carbohydrate rather than protein source meals. While food aversions may not result in appetite or weight loss, patients may become averse to their favourite foods which can, in turn, affect their daily routine and perceived quality of life (Berteretche *et al.*, 2004; Schwartz *et al.*, 1996) (see 'Quality of life').

Fatigue is another common problem reported by patients receiving radio- or chemotherapy (Schwartz *et al.*, 2001). Fatigue is described by patients as tiredness, lack of energy, confusion and poor concentration. Although a common experience, little systematic research has been conducted on the correlates of fatigue. However, research has demonstrated that pain and depression are often predictive of fatigue (Hwang *et al.*, 2003). Fatigue appears to reduce overall functional ability, but there is some hope from intervention research (Given *et al.*, 2002).

The expectation and/or experience of unpleasant side effects can comprise a patient's quality of life to the point that the patient may miss treatment appointments and/or be unwilling/unable to continue treatment, regardless if the treatment is curative or palliative (Morrow *et al.*, 2002). With non-compliance with chemotherapy, dosage reductions can lower the cure rate or hasten recurrence or death (Budman *et al.*, 1998) (see also 'Adherence to treatment').

In addition to interventions targeting physical symptom side effects and treatment compliance, interventions have been offered for the mood and anxiety problems which cancer patient often experience. Such interventions use multiple approaches including cognitive behaviour therapy, supportive counselling, education, relaxation procedures and supportive–expressive therapy, all of which are effective to some degree in reducing emotional distress (see 'Cognitive behaviour therapy', 'Relaxation training' and 'Counselling').

Choosing cancer treatments

Psychological and behaviour data have been important to patients and physicians alike for making choices among comparable treatments. Treatments that result in less quality-of-life disruption often become 'standard' treatment. The most obvious example of the importance of psychological data influencing cancer treatments was that documenting the more positive body image and sexuality outcomes for women treated with breast saving (lumpectomy plus adjuvant radiation and/or chemotherapy) procedures rather than modified radical mastectomy (Frierson & Andersen, 2006).

Recovery and long-term survival

The most important cancer endpoints have been treatment response rates, length of disease-free interval and survival. Yet, as the prognosis for some sites has improved, there has been increased attention to the quality of life, particularly for long-term survivors of cancer. The term 'survivor' typically refers to individuals surviving cancer at least five years, as the probability of late recurrence declines significantly after that time for most sites. As individuals recover and resume their life patterns, there may be residual emotional distress, other difficulties which require continued coping efforts, and even new problems (late sequelae) may occur.

An investigation by Helgeson, Snyder and Seltman (2004) sheds light on the various trajectories of adjustment to breast cancer over a period of four years. Helgeson *et al.* (2004) found that oldest patients had the lowest level of physical functioning and it deteriorated over time, while youngest patients had the highest physical functioning that substantially improved over time. In addition, personal resources, such as self-image and optimism, and social resources distinguished various courses of mental and physical functioning (see also 'Personality and health'). Lingering emotional distress from the trauma and consequences of diagnosis and treatment can occur for some cancer survivors (e.g. Gotay and Muraoka (1998)).

Sociodemographic variables may explain some differential outcomes in cancer survivors. For example, age at diagnosis has been found to be related to quality of life, with younger women experiencing more psychosocial difficulties and older women experiencing more physical difficulties (Bowman *et al.*, 2003). Furthermore, elderly cancer survivors with comorbidities (e.g. stroke, diabetes, hypertension and myocardial infarction) are at risk for impaired functional status (Garman *et al.*, 2003). Low socioeconomic status (SES) has been linked to higher rates of morbidity and mortality in cancer survivors (e.g. Zebrack *et al.*, 2002). Other SES markers such as years of education (Miller *et al.*, 2002) and employment status (Bloom *et al.*, 2004) have also been associated with poorer quality of life in gynaecologic and breast cancer survivors, respectively.

In addition to relevant sociodemographic variables; disease, treatment and psychosocial variables are also influential for outcomes in cancer survivors. For example, more advanced disease for breast cancer patients is related to poorer physical and mental health (Jacobsen *et al.*, 1998). Finally, several psychosocial factors appear to be relevant for adjustment in cancer survivors. First, regarding psychological variables, social support may influence physical symptoms and functioning, as well as distress in cancer survivors (Bloom *et al.*, 2004) (see also 'Social support and health'). Other psychosocial factors, such as coping, self-image, optimism and perceived control, have been identified as important influences on adjustment in longer-term survivors (Helgeson *et al.*, 2004).

Recurrence and death

Over 1.2 million individuals are diagnosed with cancer recurrence each year and over half will progress rapidly and die of their disease (Jemal *et al.*, 2005). Cancer recurrence and advanced cancer produce multiple psychological responses including depressive symptoms and difficulties with disability (Mahon & Casperson, 1997). At least at the time of recurrence diagnosis, stress is the predominant emotional response, and equivalent to that reported at the time of initial diagnosis (Andersen *et al.*, 2005). Later morbidities can include pain (Portenoy *et al.*, 1999), appetitive difficulties (e.g. anorexia, cachexia) and poor body image. It has been suggested that psychological factors, such as social support (Newsom *et al.*, 1996), emotional control (Classen *et al.*, 1996), or spirituality (Carr & Morris, 1996) may be moderators of patient distress.

At the time of cancer recurrence or advanced cancer, emotional turmoil and physical difficulty, psychological interventions appear to enhance the quality of life (e.g. Edelman *et al.*, 1999). Some interventions focus on management of pain, which is more common and less controllable for those with metastatic disease. The major cause of cancer pain in most cases is direct tumour involvement (i.e. metastatic bone disease, nerve compression), while other cases are due to medical therapy (e.g. postoperative, pain, radiation-induced pain). The remaining cases are individuals with pain problems unrelated to their cancer. The most difficult case is chronic pain associated with disease progression where combinations of anti-tumour therapy, anaesthetic blocks and behavioural approaches to pain control are considered. Behavioural research has focused on educational and assessment strategies and on pain reduction interventions, particularly hypnosis (for a review see Keefe *et al.*, 2005). When palliative therapy is of little use and/or brings further debilitation, psychological interventions may provide pain control and, secondarily, prevent or treat pain sequelae, such as sleep disturbances, reduced appetite, irritability and other behavioural difficulties.

Conclusion

Significant progress has been made in understanding the psychological and behavioural aspects of cancer. More is known about the psychological processes and reactions to the diagnosis and treatment of cancer than is known about any other chronic illness. Although most is known about the adjustment of breast cancer patients, other disease sites, men and children are becoming more commonly studied, but need further attention. Future research is likely to test the generalizability of these descriptive data and formulate general principles of adjustment to illness. While providing estimates of the magnitude of quality of life problems, these data can be used for models which predict which patients might be at greatest risk for adjustment difficulties (see Andersen (1994, 2002) for discussions). The latter is an important step towards designing interventions tailored to the difficulties and circumstances of cancer patients.

Literature on the use of psychological interventions to improve cancer patient's quality of life is growing (Andersen, 2002). The effectiveness of these interventions is robust, as they have reduced distress and enhanced the quality of life of many cancer patients. Despite the challenges of studying these patients, well-controlled investigations have been conducted and improvements in emotional distress have been found. In addition, change in other areas (e.g. self-esteem) have been found. Important for quality for life, psychological interventions can also lower or stabilize pain reports, which is particularly important in terminal patients considering their worsening pain and/or increasing debilitation.

Intervention components may be unique for different phases in the disease, but there are some commonalities. Therapy components have included: an emotionally supportive context to address fears and anxieties about the disease; information about the disease and treatment; behavioural coping strategies; cognitive coping strategies; and relaxation training to lower 'arousal' and/or enhance one's sense of control. There also appears to be a need for focused interventions for sexual functioning, particularly those treated for gynaecological, breast and prostate cancer, and previous intervention studies attest to the effectiveness of this specific component. It is important to understand how psychological interventions achieve these effects. In large measure, the psychological mechanisms may not be different from those operative from interventions designed for coping with other stressors. That is, confronting a traumatic stressor with positive cognitive states, active behavioural strategies and, eventually, lowered emotional distress may enhance one's sense of self-efficacy and one's feelings of control and provide realistic appraisals of stresses of the disease or treatment process. Similarly, for sexual interventions, information provides realistic expectations for sexuality and specific strategies to manage sexual activity when it is difficult or impossible.

Data suggests that the interventions produce more than situational improvement and may alter an individual's longer-term adjustment processes indicating that adjustment gains continue (and often increase) during the first post-treatment year. Immediate and longer-term psychological changes may, in turn, increase the likelihood of changes in behavioural mechanisms, such as increasing the likelihood of adaptive health behaviours (e.g. complying with medical therapy, improving diet exercise, etc.), to directly improve mental health, 'adjustment' and, possibly, medical outcomes. These data indicate that increasingly, issues of quality of life are being raised, and positive results have been achieved by behavioural sciences. However, as with most issues, further commitment and action is needed.

(See also other chapters on *Cancer*.)

REFERENCES

American Cancer Society. (2005). *Cancer Facts and Figures – 2005.*

Andersen, B. L. (2002). Psychological interventions for cancer patients. In A. Baum & B. L. Andersen (Eds.). *Psychosocial interventions for cancer* (pp. 179–216). Washington, DC: American Psychological Association.

Andersen, B. L., Farrar, W. B., Golden-Kreutz, D. M. *et al.* (2004). Psychological, behavioural, and immune changes after a psychological intervention: a clinical trial. *Journal of Clinical Oncology*, **22**, 3568–80.

Andersen, B. L., Kiecolt-Glaser, J. K. & Glaser, R. (1994). A biobehavioral model of cancer stress and disease course. *The American Psychologist*, **49**(5), 389–404.

Andersen, B. L., Shapiro, C. L., Farrar, W. B., Crespin, T. R. & Wells-DiGregorio, S. (2005). A controlled prospective study of psychological responses to cancer recurrence. *Cancer*, **104**, 1540–47.

Andersen, B. L., Turnquist, D., LaPolla, J. P. & Turner, D. (1988). Sexual functioning after treatment of in situ vulvar cancer: preliminary report. *Obstetrics and Gynecology*, **71**, 15–19.

Andrykowski, M. A. (1993). The Morrow/Hickok article reviewed: behavioral treatment of chemotherapy-induced nausea and vomiting. *Oncology*, **7**, 93–4.

Andrykowski, M. A., Boerner, L. M., Salsman, J. M. & Pavlik, E. (2004). Psychological response to test results in an ovarian cancer screening program: a prospective, longitudinal study. *Health Psychology*, **23**, 622–30.

Atesci, F. C., Baltalari, B., Oguzhanoglu, N. K. *et al.* (2004). Psychiatric morbidity among cancer patients and awareness of illness. *Supportive Care in Cancer*, **12**, 161–7.

Bansal, M., Mohanti, B. K., Shah, N. *et al.* (2004). Radiation related morbidities and their impact on quality of life in head and neck cancer patients receiving radical radiotherapy. *Quality of Life Research*, **13**, 481–8.

Beanlands, H. J., Lipton, J. H., McCay, E. A. *et al.* (2003). Self-concept as a "BMT patient", illness intrusiveness, and engulfment in allogenic bone marrow transplant recipients. *Journal of Psychosomatic Research*, **55**, 419–25.

Berteretche, M. V., Dalix, A. M., D'Ornano, A. M. C. *et al.* (2004). Decreases taste sensitivity in cancer patients under chemotherapy. *Supportive Care in Cancer*, **12**, 571–6.

Bloom, J. R., Stewart, S. L., Chang, S. & Banks, P. J. (2004). Then and now: quality of life of young breast cancer survivors. *Psycho-oncology*, **13**, 147–60.

Bowman, K. F., Deimling, G. T., Smerglia, V., Sage, P. & Kahana, B. (2003). Appraisal of the cancer experience by older long-term survivors. *Psycho-oncology*, **12**, 226–38.

Budman, D. R., Berry, D. A., Cirrincione, C. T., Henderson, I. C. *et al.* (1998). Dose and dose intensity as determinants of outcome in the adjuvant treatment of breast cancer. The Cancer and Leukemia Group B. *Journal of the National Cancer Institute*, **90**, 1205–11.

Carr, E. W. & Morris, T. (1996). Spirituality and patients with advanced cancer: a social work response. *Journal of Psychosocial Oncology*, **14**, 71–81.

Classen, C., Koopman, C., Angell, K. & Spiegel, D. (1996). Coping styles associated with psychological adjustment to advanced breast cancer. *Health Psychology*, **15**, 434–7.

Edelman, S., Bell, D. R. & Kidman, A. D. (1999). A group cognitive behaviour therapy programme with metastatic breast cancer patients. *Psycho-oncology*, **8**, 295–305.

589

Edwards, B. & Clarke, V. (2004). The psychological impact of cancer diagnosis on families: the influence of family functioning and patients' illness characteristics on depression and anxiety. *Psycho-oncology*, **13**, 562–76.

Epping-Jordan, J. E., Compas, B. E., Osowiecki, D. M. *et al.* (1999). Psychological adjustment in breast cancer: processes of emotional distress. *Health Psychology*, **18**, 315–26.

Ferlay, J., Bray, F., Pisani, P. & Parkin, D. M. (2004). GLOBOCAN 2002: Cancer Incidence, Mortality and Prevalence Worldwide IARC CancerBase No. 5. version 2.0, IARC Press, Lyon, 2004.

French, D. P., Maissi, E. & Marteau, T. M. (2004). Psychological costs of inadequate cervical smear results. *British Journal of Cancer*, **91**, 1887–92.

Frierson, G. F. & Andersen, B. L. (2006). Breast reconstruction. In D. B. Sarwer *et al.* (Eds.). *Psychological aspects of cosmetic and reconstructive plastic surgery* (pp. 173–188). Philadelphia: Lippincott, Williams, and Wilkens.

Garman, K. S., Pieper, C. F., Seo, P. & Cohen, H. J. (2003). Function in elderly cancer survivors depends on comorbidities. *The Journals of Gerontology. Series A, Biological Sciences and Medical Sciences*, **58**, M1119–24.

Given, B., Given, C. W., McCorkle, R. *et al.* (2002). Pain and fatigue management: results of a nursing randomized clinical trial. *Oncology Nursing Forum*, **29**, 949–56.

Gotay, C. C. & Muraoka, M. Y. (1998). Quality of life in long-term survivors of adult-onset cancers. *Journal of the National Cancer Institute*, **90**(9), 659–67.

Gottesman, D. & Lewis, M. (1982). Differences in crisis reactions among cancer and surgery patients. *Journal of Consulting and Clinical Psychology*, **50**, 381–8.

Helgeson, V. S., Snyder, P. & Seltman, H. (2004). Psychological and physical adjustment to breast cancer over 4 years: identifying distinct trajectories of change. *Health Psychology*, **23**, 3–15.

Hwang, S. S., Chang, V. T., Rue, M. & Kasimis, B. (2003). Multidimensional independent predictors of caner-related fatigue. *Journal of Pain and Symptom Management*, **26**, 604–14.

Jacobsen, P. B., Widows, M. R., Hann, D. M., Andrykowski, M. A. *et al.* (1998). Posttraumatic stress disorder symptoms after bone marrow transplantation for breast cancer. *Psychosomatic Medicine*, **60**, 366–71.

Jemal, A., Murray, T., Ward, E. *et al.* (2005). Cancer statistics, 2005. *CA: A Cancer Journal for Clinicians*, **55**, 10–30.

Johnston, M. & Vogele, C. (1993). Benefits of psychological preparation for surgery: a meta-analysis. *Annals of Behavioral Medicine*, **15**, 245–56.

Keefe, F. J., Aberneth, A. P. & Campbell, L. (2005). Psychological approaches to understanding and treating disease-related pain. *Annual Review of Psychology*, **56**, 601–30.

King, K. B., Nail, L. M., Kreamer, D., Strohl, R. A. & Johnson, J. E. (1985). Patients' descriptions of the experience of receiving radiation therapy. *Oncology Nursing Forum*, **12**, 55–61.

Krylov, A. A. & Krylova, G. S. (2003). Psychological and psychosomatic problems of oncology. *Klinicheskaia Meditsina*, **81**, 57–9.

Larsson, G. & Starrin, B. (1992). Relaxation training as an integral part of caring activities for cancer patients: effects on wellbeing. *Scandinavian Journal of Caring Sciences*, **6**, 179–85.

Mahon, S. M. & Casperson, D. M. (1997). Exploring the psychosocial meaning of recurrent cancer: a descriptive study. *Cancer Nursing*, **20**, 178–86.

Miller, B. E., Pittman, B., Case, D. & McQuellon, R. P. (2002). Quality of life after treatment for gynecological malignancies: a pilot study in an outpatient clinic. *Gynecologic Oncology*, **87**, 178–84.

Miyata, H., Tachimori, H., Takahashi, M., Saito, T. & Kai, I. (2004). Disclosure of cancer diagnosis and prognosis: a survey of the general public's attitudes towards doctors and families holding discretionary powers. *BMC Medical Ethics (electronic resource)*, **5**, E7.

Morrow, G. R. & Hickok, J. T. (1993). Behavioral treatment of chemotherapy-induced nausea and vomiting. *Oncology*, **7**, 83–9.

Morrow, G. R., Roscoe, J. A., Hickok, J. T., Andrews, P. L. R. & Matteson, S. (2002). Nausea and emesis: evidence for a biobehavioral perspective. *Supportive Care in Cancer*, **10**, 96–105.

Newsom, J. T., Knapp, J. E. & Schulz, R. (1996). Longitudinal analysis of specific domains of internal control and depressive symptoms in patients with recurrent cancer. *Health Psychology*, **15**, 323–31.

Parkin, D., Bray, F., Ferlay, J. & Pisani, P. (2005). Global cancer statistics, 2002. *CA: a cancer journal for clinicians*, **55**(2), 74–108.

Phipps, S. (2002). Reduction of distress associated with paediatric bone marrow transplant: complementary health promotion interventions. *Pediatric Rehabilitation*, **5**, 223–34.

Portenoy, R. K., Payne, D. & Jacobsen, P. (1999). Breakthrough pain: characteristics and impact in patients with cancer pain. *Pain*, **81**, 129–34.

Ranchor, A. V., Sanderman, R., Steptoe, A. *et al.* (2002). Pre-morbid predictors of psychological adjustment to cancer. *Quality of Life Research*, **11**, 101–13.

Redd, W. H., Montgomery, G. H. & DuHamel, K. N. (2001). Behavioral intervention for cancer treatment side effects. *Journal of the National Cancer Institute*, **93**, 810–23.

Schwartz, A. L., Mori, M., Gao, R., Nail, L. M. & King, M. E. (2001). Exercise reduces daily fatigue in women with breast cancer receiving chemotherapy. *Medicine and Science in Sports and Exercise*, **33**, 718–23.

Schwartz, M. D., Jacobsen, P. B. & Bovbjerg, D. H. (1996). Role of nausea in the development of aversions to beverage paired with chemotherapy treatment in cancer patients. *Physiology & Behavior*, **59**, 659–63.

Stiegelis, H. E., Ranchor, A. V. & Sanderman, R. (2004). Psychological functioning in cancer patients treated with radiotherapy. *Patient Education & Counseling*, **52**, 131–41.

Stommel, M., Kurtz, M. E., Given, C. W. & Given, B. A. (2004). A longitudinal analysis of the course of depressive symptomatology in geriatric patients with cancer of the breast, colon, lung, or prostate. *Health Psychology*, **23**, 564–73.

Trask, P. C., Paterson, A., Riba, M. *et al.* (2002). Assessment of psychological distress in prospective bone marrow transplant patients. *Bone Marrow Transplantation*, **29**, 917–25.

Varni, J. W. & Katz, E. R. (1997). Stress, social support and negative affectivity in children with newly diagnosed cancer: a prospective transactional analysis. *Psycho-oncology*, **6**, 267–78.

Wardle, J. & Pope, R. (1992). The psychological costs of screening for cancer. *Journal of Psychosomatic Research*, **36**, 609–24.

Weisman, A. D. & Worden, J. W. (1976). The existential plight in cancer: significance of the first 100 days. *International Journal of Psychiatry in Medicine*, **7**, 1–15.

Winer, E. P. & Sutton, L. M. (1994). Quality of life after bone marrow transplantation. *Oncology*, **8**, 19–31.

Wyatt, G. K., Donze, L. F. & Beckrow, K. C. (2004). Efficacy of an in-home nursing intervention following short-stay breast cancer surgery. *Research in Nursing and Health*, **27**, 322–31.

Zebrack, B. J., Zelter, L. K., Whitton, J. *et al.* (2002). Psychological outcomes in long-term survivors of childhood leukaemia, Hodgkin's disease, and non-Hodgkin's lymphoma: a report from the Childhood Cancer Survivor Study. *Pediatrics*, **110**(1), 42–52.

Cancer: gynaecologic

Kristen M. Carpenter and Barbara L. Andersen

The Ohio State University

Overview

Gynaecologic cancer cases account for approximately 12% of all new cancers in women; 49% of these involve the endometrium or uterus, 31% the ovary, 13% the cervix and 7% the vulva, vagina or other genital organs (Jemal *et al.*, 2004). Advances in screening techniques, (e.g. Pap smear for cervical cancer), and therapies have led to improved survival. Since the 1970s, death rates for gynaecologic cancers have significantly declined: currently a reduction of 49% for cervical cancer, 42% for endometrial, 27% for vaginal and vulvar and 11% for ovarian. See Table 1 for additional information by disease site. For the majority, gynaecologic cancer has become a survivable disease (Ries *et al.*, 2000). Thus, more women will survive and, necessarily, will be coping with the psychosocial morbidity associated with the disease and treatment.

Psychological reactions to diagnosis

The emotional reactions to gynaecologic cancer diagnosis are severe. In a review of studies using psychiatric (DSM-IV) criteria, Thompson and Shear (1998) reported that as many as 23% of patients might have major depressive disorder, an estimate four to five times higher than that for the general population (Spiegel, 1996). Anxiety symptoms are prevalent as well, particularly in women with poor physical functioning (Bodurka-Bevers *et al.*, 2000). In a sample of ovarian cancer patients ($n = 151$), a substantial portion of patients reported moderate to severe worry (55%), nervousness (40%) and irritability (34%) (Kornblith *et al.*, 1995). Psychological variables might also contribute; individuals who perceive their illness as severe tend to have greater mood disturbance (Marks *et al.*, 1986).

Physical & psychological sequelae of treatment

Gynaecologic cancer treatments have significant physiologic morbidities that affect both sexual and psychological adjustment. Hysterectomies, which are common treatments, result in vaginal shortening and dyspareunia (see 'Hysterectomy'). Extensive surgery damages pelvic nerves, threatening genital sensitivity and bladder control (Wilmoth & Botchway, 1999). In women over 40 and women with ovarian cancer, oopherectomy (removal of the ovaries) is also indicated. The resulting decrease in circulating sex steroid hormones can reduce sexual desire, vaginal elasticity and lubrication. Other surgical procedures include vulvectomy for vulvar cancer and pelvic exenteration for extensive disease at diagnosis or recurrence in the pelvis. Significant changes result in pelvic anesthesia, chronic difficulty with excretory functions, and severe body image disruption (Andersen & Hacker, 1983).

Radiotherapy is commonly used in regional or advanced cases (see 'Radiotherapy'). Acute morbidities include fatigue, diarrhoea, pelvic cramping, bleeding and painful urination. Long-term sequelae include fibrosis of the blood vessels, limited vaginal lubrication and reductions in vaginal elasticity. Other long-term effects include persistent bowel and bladder dysfunction, vaginal stenosis and vaginal shortening (Wilmoth & Botchway, 1999). Chemotherapy is often used adjuvant to surgery and/or radiation and is commonly accompanied by nausea and vomiting, fatigue, pain, hair loss and cognitive deficits, all of which impact short-term quality of life (see 'Chemotherapy'). Because oestrogen is implicated in gynaecologic cancers, anti-oestrogen agents are often utilized. The ovarian failure that results from chemotherapy and/or radiation leads to infertility, decreased sexual desire and lubrication and vaginal pain (Wilmoth & Botchway, 1999). This loss of reproductive capacity poses a particular concern for younger women who have not yet begun or completed childbearing (see 'Infertility').

Survivorship

The adverse effects of disease and treatment constitute a significant physical and emotional adjustment. Women with advanced and persistent disease tend to have the poorest adjustment (Lutgendorf *et al.*, 2002), possibly due to compromised physical functioning and poor prognosis (Guidozzi, 1993). Site-based

Table 1. Sociodemographic, prognostic, disease and treatment information for gynaecologic cancer

Site	Estimated new cases (U.S., 2004)[a]	Median age at diagnosis (1996–2000)[b]	5-year survival rate (1996–2000)[b]	Risk factors[c]	Presenting symptoms by extent of disease[d]	Common treatments[c]
Cervix	10 520	47	71%	Low socioeconomic status; multiple sexual partners; intercourse before age 20; several pregnancies; HPV; smoking	Localized: vaginal bleeding; excessive or purulent vaginal discharge; bladder or rectal fistulae Advanced: pelvic pain; urinary frequency; hematuria	Stage IB-IIA: radical hysterectomy with lymph node dissection; adjuvant radiotherapy for parametrial invasion, large/grade 3 lesions, nodal metastases Stage IIB-IV: hysterectomy with adjuvant radiotherapy; chemotherapy for distant metastases Locally advanced or recurrent disease: neoadjuvant chemotherapy with radical hysterectomy or pelvic exenteration
Endometrium	40 320	65	85%	Postmenopausal status; obesity; diabetes; hypertension; nulliparity; chronic anovulation; irregular menses; exogenous oestrogen consumption; pelvic irradiation; unopposed ERT; late menopause	Localized: irregular vaginal bleeding; pelvic pain; purulent vaginal discharge Advanced: ascites; pelvic/abdominal mass; bowel symptoms	Standard treatment: total abdominal hysterectomy with bilateral salpingo-oopherectomy; adjuvant radiotherapy recommended for high-grade lesions, myometrial involvement, or limited nodal involvement; adjuvant chemotherapy recommended with lymphadenopathy Advanced disease managed with combination of surgery, radiotherapy, chemotherapy and hormonal therapy
Ovary	25 580	59	53%	Family history of ovarian, breast, endometrial, or colon cancer; nulliparity; older age at first marriage or childbirth	Localized: abdominal pain, bloating, or swelling; dyspepsia; pelvic pressure; ascites; pelvic mass Advanced: anorexia; weight loss; nausea; vomiting; severe pelvic pain	Standard treatment: total abdominal hysterectomy with bilateral salpingo-oophorectomy and omenectomy; cytoreductive surgery, colectomy and bowel resection as indicated; adjuvant therapy Stage I: adjuvant radiotherapy, but not chemotherapy Advanced or recurrent disease:combination adjuvant or neoadjuvant chemotherapy; hormonal therapy
Vulva	3970	68	76%	Low socioeconomic status; multiple sexual partners; regular coffee consumption; vaginal dystrophy; leukoplakia; vulvar or vaginal inflammatory disease; HPV; cervical cancer	Localized: vulvar lesion, nodules, or masses; chronic pruritis; vulvar pain, burning, bleeding, or discharge; dysuria Advanced: large masses on the labia, urethra, vagina and/or rectum	Standard treatment: radical vulvectomy, bilateral groin lymphadenectomy; preoperative radiotherapy to debulk tumor and conserve vulvar tissue; adjuvant radiotherapy recommended for local nodal involvement Distant metastases: combination chemotherapy Advanced disease: pelvic exenteration

Notes: [a]Jemal *et al.*, 2004; [b]Reis et al., 2000; [c]Gusberg & Runowicz, 1991; [d]Averette & Nguyen, 1995.

comparisons indicate that women with cervical cancer are at increased risk for maladjustment, particularly early in treatment, possibly because they are younger than other patients at diagnosis (Griemel *et al.*, 2002). While subjective distress diminishes in the months following diagnosis, overall quality of life might be compromised. Further, specific cognitive (e.g. ability to concentrate) and social support deficits may continue long after treatment has ended (Klee *et al.*, 2000).

Results from studies of sexual functioning, most of which sample cervical patients, reveal chronic difficulties for patients. Studies comparing treatments are equivocal. Results from the only randomized treatment study to be conducted in this population indicate that surgery and radiation result in comparable disruptions in sexual desire and frequency of intercourse (Vincent *et al.*, 1975), however a non-randomized comparison suggests that inhibited desire, post-coital pain and bleeding are more common among radiotherapy patients (Schover *et al.*, 1989). Studies comparing gynaecologic cancer patients to healthy controls/norms demonstrate that women with cancer resume intercourse, but are more likely to report diminished sexual responsiveness (Weijmar-Schultz *et al.*, 1991) or to be diagnosed with inhibited desire, dyspareunia or inhibited orgasm (Andersen *et al.*, 1989). Studies indicate that, despite the grim picture painted by descriptive studies, psychosocial interventions may have a positive impact (Robinson *et al.*, 1999).

There is little data on the aspects of physical health that might influence quality of life for gynaecologic cancer survivors, but the available data suggest three trends. Firstly, side effects of treatment are persistent (Carlsson *et al.*, 2000; Matthews *et al.*, 1999). In fact, some patients rate the physical sequelae of treatment as the most significant challenge of survivorship (Wenzel *et al.*, 2002). Secondly, comparisons between normative samples and gynaecologic cancer survivors indicate few group differences in mood and quality of life. Still, a portion of patients, ranging from 20% to 63% across studies, have poor quality of life and persistent psychological maladjustment (Matthews *et al.*, 1999). Thirdly, there appears to be a relationship between physical impairment and psychological maladjustment, particularly for adjuvant therapy patients (Carlsson *et al.*, 2000). Ovarian patients might be at greater risk for difficulty, due in part to aggressive treatment regimens (Miller *et al.*, 2002). Thus, the primary difficulties in gynaecologic cancer survivorship include physical impairments and psychological outcomes, however physical health might pose a greater challenge. In addition, other data suggest that gynaecologic cancer patients are at higher risk for psychological maladjustment than other cancer survivors. Parker *et al.* (2003) interviewed breast, gastrointestinal, gynaecologic and urologic cancer survivors ($n = 351$) and assessed depressive symptoms, anxiety symptoms and psychological wellbeing. Depressive and anxiety symptoms were elevated for all survivors, but gynaecologic survivors reported significantly higher anxiety scores than all other patients, and higher depression scores and lower wellbeing scores than gastrointestinal and urologic survivors.

Psychosocial interventions

Psychosocial interventions can reduce distress, hasten resumption of routine activities and improve psychological and sexual outcomes. While a substantial literature examines the benefits of interventions in breast and other cancer patients (see Andersen, 2002), to date only six studies have examined the potential of psychosocial interventions in gynaecologic cancer samples.

Houts and colleagues (1986) used a peer counselling intervention for newly diagnosed patients ($n = 32$). Women were randomized to intervention ($n = 14$) or information-only ($n = 18$). All participants received a booklet containing information about effective coping strategies. Peer counselling was also delivered to intervention participants via telephone contacts with former cancer patients. Analyses indicated no between-group differences in emotional outcomes. Capone *et al.* (1980) provided brief, in-hospital counselling to newly diagnosed patients ($n = 56$). A non-equivalent control group included previously treated women. Analyses indicated no between-group differences in emotional distress; however intervention participants reported less confusion and self-image disruption and returned to work sooner.

Therapist-led interventions appear to be more effective. For instance, McQuellon *et al.* (1998) developed a brief clinic orientation to reduce anxiety, distress and uncertainty in newly diagnosed patients ($n = 150$). Participants were randomized into treatment and assessment-only groups. The programme lasted only 15–20 minutes and included a clinic tour, description of administrative procedures, provision of clinic information and a question-and-answer session. At follow-up, anxiety and mood disturbance decreased significantly for intervention subjects, whereas distress increased for assessment-only controls. Cain and colleagues (1986) compared individual and group intervention formats in a sample of 72 newly diagnosed patients ($n = 21$ individual, $n = 22$ group, $n = 29$ no-treatment controls). Both eight-session interventions included discussion of cancer aetiology, cancer treatment, body image, sexuality, relaxation and coping. Both formats were superior to the control group in reducing depression and anxiety, improving psychosocial adjustment and enhancing sexual functioning.

Three additional studies have addressed sexual outcomes. Capone *et al.* (1980) included a sexual therapy component, in which information about coping with and reducing sexual anxiety was provided. Intervention participants were twice as likely as controls to resume sexual activity within one year (84% vs. 43%). Robinson *et al.* (1999) evaluated a psychoeducational group for early-stage cervical and endometrial patients receiving radiotherapy ($n = 32$; $n = 15$ intervention, $n = 18$ controls). Use of vaginal dilators, which break fibrous adhesions as they develop, is recommended. The control condition included a brief counselling session in which subjects received a booklet on sexuality and cancer. The intervention comprised two 90-minute group sessions which included information about sexuality, discussion of sexual motivation and instruction on use of dilators, lubricants and Kegel exercises. Intervention participants had significantly less fear about sex after treatment and were significantly more likely to follow dilation recommendations. This was particularly true for younger women (<42 years), with intervention participants seven times more likely to comply with recommendations than controls. Caldwell *et al.* (2003) delivered a group intervention to 21 women (this study did not include a control group). Groups of three to five women attended weekly, 90-minute sessions for three months. Sessions focused on body image, sexuality, communication, infertility and other residual effects of adjuvant therapy. Results indicated improvement in sexual functioning following the intervention, with increased frequency of intercourse and enhanced pleasure and arousal sustained for up to three months (p < 0.10).

Summary

Significant physical, psychological and sexual morbidity occurs immediately following diagnosis and treatment. Broad-based psychosocial interventions appear to produce modest gains in psychological outcomes, and sexual functioning can be significantly enhanced with brief, cost-effective individual or group therapy. Additional research is needed to understand the experience of gynaecologic cancer patients and test quality of life enhancing interventions to help them recover and transition to survivorship.

(See also 'Cancer: general', 'Coping with chronic illness' and 'Coping with death and dying'.)

REFERENCES

Andersen, B. L. (2002). Biobehavioral outcomes following psychological interventions for cancer patients. *Journal of Consulting and Clinical Psychology*, **70**, 590–610.

Andersen, B. L., Anderson, B. & deProsse, C. (1989). Controlled prospective longitudinal study of women with cancer: I. Sexual functioning outcomes. *Journal of Consulting and Clinical Psychology*, **57**, 683–91.

Andersen, B. L. & Hacker, N. F. (1983). Psychosexual adjustment following pelvic exenteration. *Obstetrics & Gynecology*, **61**, 331–8.

Averette, H. E. & Nguyen, H. (1995). Gynaecologic cancer. In J. P. Murphy, W. Lawrence & R. E. Lenhard (Eds.). *Clinical oncology* (pp. 552–79). Washington, DC: American Cancer Society.

Bodurka-Bevers, D., Basen-Engquist, K., Carmack, C. L. *et al.* (2000). Depression, anxiety, and quality of life in patients with epithelial ovarian cancer. *Gynaecologic Oncology*, **78**, 302–8.

Bush, N., Haberman, M., Donaldson, G. & Sullivan, K. (1995). Quality of life of 125 adults surviving 6–18 years after bone marrow transplant. *Social Science & Medicine*, **40**, 479–90.

Cain, E. N., Kohorn, E. I., Quinlan, D. M., Latimer, K. & Schwartz, P. E. (1986). Psychosocial benefits of a cancer support group. *Cancer*, **57**, 183–9.

Caldwell, R., Classen, C., Lagana, L. *et al.* (2003). Changes in sexual functioning and mood among women treated for gynaecologic cancer who receive group therapy: a pilot study. *Journal of Clinical Psychology in Medical Settings*, **10**, 149–56.

Capone, M. A., Good, R. S., Westie, K. S. & Jacobson, A. F. (1980). Psychosocial rehabilitation of gynaecologic oncology patients. *Archives of Physical Medicine and Rehabilitation*, **61**, 128–32.

Carlsson, M., Strang, P. & Bjurstrom, C. (2000). Treatment modality affects long-term quality of life in gynaecologic cancer. *Anticancer Research*, **20**, 563–8.

Carver, C., Pozo-Kaderman, C., Harris, S. D. *et al.* (1994). Optimism versus pessimism predicts the quality of women's adjustment to early stage breast cancer. *Cancer*, **73**, 1213–20.

Chan, Y. M., Ngan, H. Y. S., Yip, P. S. F. *et al.* (2001). Psychosocial adjustment in gynaecologic cancer survivors: a longitudinal study of risk factors for maladjustment. *Gynaecologic Oncology*, **80**, 387–94.

Greimel, E., Thiel, I., Peintinger, F., Cegnar, I. & Pongratz, E. (2002). Prospective assessment of quality of life in female cancer patients. *Gynaecologic Oncology*, **85**, 140–7.

Guidozzi, F. (1993). Living with ovarian cancer. *Gynaecologic Oncology*, **50**, 202–7.

Gusberg, S. & Runowicz, C. (1991). Gynaecologic cancers. In A. Holleb, D. Fink & G. Murphy (Eds.). *Textbook of clinical oncology* (pp. 418–97). Atlanta, GA: American Cancer Society.

Hewitt, M., Rowland, J. & Yancik, R. (2003). Cancer survivors in the United States: age, health, and disability. *Journal of Gerontology: Medical Sciences*, **58**, 82–91.

Houts, P. S., Whitney, C. W., Mortel, R. & Bartholomew, M. J. (1986). Former cancer patients as counselors of newly diagnosed cancer patients. *Journal of the National Cancer Institute*, **76**, 793–6.

Jemal, A., Ram, T., Murray, T. *et al.* (2004). Cancer statistics, 2004. *CA: A Cancer Journal for Clinicians*, **54**, 8–29.

Klee, M., Thranov, I. & Machin, D. (2000). Life after radiotherapy: the psychological and social effects experienced by women treated for advanced stages of cervical cancer. *Gynaecologic Oncology*, **76**, 5–13.

Kornblith, A. B., Herndon, J. E., Weiss, R. B. *et al.* (2003). Long-term adjustment of survivors of early-stage breast carcinoma, 20 years after adjuvant therapy. *Cancer*, **98**, 679–89.

Kornblith, A. B., Thaler, H. T., Wong, G. *et al.* (1995). Quality of life in women with ovarian cancer. *Gynaecologic Oncology*, **59**, 231–42.

Lutgendorf, S. K., Anderson, B., Ullrich, P., Johnsen, E. L., Buller, R. E. *et al.* (2002). Quality of life and mood in women with gynaecologic cancer. *Cancer*, **94**, 131–40.

Marks, G., Richardson, J. L., Graham, J. W. & Levine, A. (1986). Role of health locus of control beliefs and expectations of treatment efficacy in adjustment to cancer. *Journal of Personality and Social Psychology*, **51**, 443–50.

Matthews, A. K., Aikens, J. E., Helmrich, S. P. *et al.* (1999). Sexual functioning and mood among long-term survivors of clear-cell adenocarcinoma of the vagina or cervix. *Journal of Psychosocial Oncology*, **17**, 27–45.

McQuellon, R. P., Wells, M., Hoffman, S. *et al.* (1998). Reducing distress in cancer patents with an orientation program. *Psycho-oncology*, **7**, 207–17.

Miller, B. E., Pittman, B., Case, D. & McQuellon, R. P. (2002). Quality of life after treatment for gynaecologic malignancies: a pilot study in an outpatient clinic. *Gynaecologic Oncology*, **87**, 178–84.

Parker, P. A., Baile, W. F., De Moor, C. & Cohen, L. (2003). Psychosocial and demographic predictors of quality of life in a large sample of cancer patients. *Psycho-oncology*, **12**, 183–93.

Reis, L. A. G., Eisner, M. P., Kosary, C. L. *et al.* (Eds.). (2000). *SEER cancer statistics review*, 1973–1997. Bethesda, MD: National Cancer Institute.

Robinson, J. W., Faris, P. D. & Scott, C. B. (1999). Psychoeducational group increases vaginal dilation for younger women and reduces sexual fears for women of all ages with gynaecologic carcinoma treated with radiotherapy. *International Journal of Radiation Oncology, Biology, & Physics*, **44**, 497–506.

Schover, L. R., Fife, M. & Gershenson, D. M. (1989). Sexual dysfunction and treatment for early stage cervical cancer. *Cancer*, **63**, 204–12.

Spiegel, D. (1996). Cancer and depression. *British Journal of Psychiatry*, **168**, 109–16.

Thompson, D. S. & Shear, M. K. (1998). Psychiatric disorders and gynaecological oncology: a review of the literature. *General Hospital Psychiatry*, **20**, 241–7.

Vincent, C. E., Vincent, B., Greiss, F. C. & Linton, E. B. (1975). Some marital-sexual concomitants of carcinoma of the cervix. *Southern Medical Journal*, **68**, 552–8.

Weijmar Schultz, W. C. M., van de Wiel, H. B. M. & Bouma, J. (1991). Psychosexual functioning after treatment for cancer of the cervix: a comparative and longitudinal study. *International Journal of Gynaecologic Cancer*, **1**, 37–46.

Wenzel, L. B., Donnelly, J. P., Fowler, J. M. *et al.* (2002). Resilience, reflection,

and residual stress in ovarian cancer survivorship: a gynaecologic oncology group study. *Psycho-oncology*, **11**, 142–53.

Wilmoth, M. C. & Botchway, P. (1999). Psychosexual implications of breast and gynaecologic cancer. *Cancer Investigation*, **17**, 631–6.

Cancer: head and neck

Gerry M. Humphris

University of St Andrews

Head and neck cancer is the sixth most common cancer worldwide and is ranked third in the developed world (Parkin *et al.*, 1999). The large majority (90%) of these cancers are of a similar type known as squamous cell carcinomas. They comprise 4% of all cancers in the United States and 5% in the United Kingdom. Central and eastern Europe currently show greater than double the incidence rates of either the UK or USA. An incidence of 10.2 lip, mouth and pharyngeal cancers per 100 000 population in the UK in 1996 was reported (2940 new cases) (Quin, 2001). Men contract the disease more than women in the ratio of approximately 3 to 1. About 50% will die of the disease.

Prognosis of small oral cancer lesions is better than large lesions. For instance, the median survival time of a patient with a lesion greater than 4 cm in diametre is 4 years less than a patient with a smaller lesion after controlling for age (Platz *et al.*, 1986). The overall health of head and neck cancer patients tends to be worse than that of the general public (Funk *et al.*, 1997). Recurrence rates for head and neck cancer are comparatively high and result in death for about 20% of patients. Approximately 40% have a relapse with further malignancy following initial treatment. Survival rates for head and neck cancer have hardly improved over the past 30 years (La Vecchia *et al.*, 1997) although they are dependent on severity. Early diagnosis improves survival significantly.

Treatment consists of surgery, radiotherapy or chemotherapy, either singly or in combination. Many head and neck (H&N) cancer patients are treated with high-dose radiotherapy (see 'Radiotherapy'). Associated sensitive tissues such as mucous membranes, nerves and circulatory structures are also irradiated. The increase of treatment intensity has produced significant improvements to outcome but raises side effects. Delay (greater than 6 weeks) in starting radiotherapy following surgery has been shown to be detrimental to 5-year local recurrence rate in head and neck cancer patients (Huang *et al.*, 2003).

Public health issues

The public are poorly informed about oral cancer. Some attempts have been made recently to improve public awareness especially for signs and symptoms (Cruz *et al.*, 2002) and to encourage recognition of the disease, highlight risk factors and encourage earlier seeking for advice and assessment of suspicious lesions (Conway *et al.*, 2002). There is some evidence that these interventions have stronger effects with people at higher risk, for example smokers (Humphris & Field, 2004). The benefits of these preventive approaches are indicated as early identification improves survival markedly.

The major risk factors for head and neck cancer include tobacco and alcohol use (see 'Tobacco use' and 'Alcohol abuse'). These substances continue to harm patients following treatment of the disease. About 30–40% of treated head and neck cancer patients continue to smoke following initial treatment (Allison, 2001). Those who continue to smoke after diagnosis of head and neck cancer show four times the recurrence rate compared to a control group (Stevens *et al.*, 1983) and treatment is less successful (Browman *et al.*, 1993). Alcoholism prior to diagnosis of a first head and neck cancer is correlated to increased mortality five years post-diagnosis (Deleyiannis *et al.*, 1996). The patients who drink heavily and smoke suffer an increased risk as 'tobacco synergizes with alcohol' (Johnson, 2001). This risk is 'super-multiplicative' for the mouth. Other risk factors that have been implicated including diet, oral hygiene and the human papilloma virus.

Psychological morbidity

Psychological distress (30% 'cases') has been found in long-term survivors (>6 years) (Bjordal & Kaasa, 1995). The impact of diagnosis and treatment has been a focus for longitudinal study. A high incidence of anxiety (35%) soon after diagnosis and peak levels of depression (30%) about 3 months following initial treatment have been reported in Scandinavia (Hammerlid *et al.*, 1999). One year following diagnosis both anxiety and depression returned to near pre-diagnosis levels. Comparable rates at 3 months following treatment adopting the same measures in the UK have been found (anxiety: 37%, depression: 28%) (Humphris, 2001).

Characteristics and course of treatment can have some influence on the patients' responses, however psychosocial variables have been clearly implicated in the development of anxiety and depression in this group.

Quality of life (QoL)

In the head and neck and oral cancer field there has been a rapid increase in the number of studies investigating patients' quality of life with eight specific measures developed (Ringash & Bezjak, 2001). For a recent description of the studies from 1980 up to 1998 see Rogers (Rogers *et al.*, 1999).

A 3-year longitudinal study in Sweden on the quality of life of 232 head and neck cancer patients from diagnosis used the EORTC QLQ-C30, which assesses core aspects and the EORTC QLQ H&N35 a specific module for head and neck cancer (Hammerlid *et al.*, 2001). After 3 years two-thirds (66%) of the patients were still alive. Their health-related quality of life was reduced to its lowest point immediately after treatment. However, virtually all of the sub-scales returned to pre-treatment levels after 12 months. Dry mouth, sexual responsiveness and dentition were significant problems that tended not to improve with time. There were very few changes occurring between the 1- and 3-year assessments. Mental distress made the strongest improvement after 3 years, whereas global quality of life increased as the next most significant change. Patients with advanced disease scored poorly on virtually all QoL measures. Other longitudinal studies assessing QoL, adopting standardized instruments, have reported a similar rise of QoL, on virtually all domains to pre-treatment levels after one year post-treatment (Rogers *et al.*, 1998).

The extensive work of de Graeff and de Leeuw with longitudinal assessment of quality of life and depression in head and cancer patients at the University Medical Centre of Utrecht, has shed light on the prediction of HRQoL. Raised depressive symptoms at pre-treatment predicted similar difficulties and difficulties in physical functioning at 6 and 12 months later (de Graeff *et al.*, 2000). The authors recommend the routine screening of psychosocial variables and physical symptoms before treatment may help to identify patients who may be susceptible to depression on recovery from surgery and/or radiotherapy for head and neck cancer (de Leeuw *et al.*, 2000*a*).

Recurrence fears

One study has reported the relationship of concerns with psychological disorder in 50 consecutive head and neck cancer patients in India (Chaturvedi *et al.*, 1996). These patients showed a significant relationship between the number of concerns and a screening measure for psychiatric 'caseness'. However, these investigators did not focus on recurrence fears specifically. One such study that has concentrated on patient recurrence fears was a cross-sectional survey of 100 patients with orofacial cancer. It found a high incidence of recurrence fears which were unrelated to the extent of the disease or when the diagnosis was made (Humphris *et al.*, 2003). Fifty patients were revisited successfully 2 years later, and these fears were found to be relatively stable ($r_s = 0.67$) (Lee-Jones, 1998). The point prevalence of concerns about the cancer returning was 65% in both the baseline and two-year follow-up samples. This is consistent with other reports of long-term survivors of head and neck cancer (Campbell *et al.*, 2000).

Patient reaction to recurrence

There are few research studies investigating the psychological reactions to recurrent cancer, and virtually none specific to head and neck cancer. An early report concludes that patients with a recurrence respond according to their reaction to their initial cancer diagnosis. (Schmale, 1976) For many patients their experience of a recurrence is a renewed sense of uncertainty for the future, grief and feelings of injustice (Chekryn, 1984).

Appearance

There is considerable variation in the concerns that patients express about appearance changes. An early study of 152 head and neck cancer patients showed that 82% had adapted to their disfigurement (West, 1977). Other investigators have alerted clinicians to unspoken distress at scarring and disfigurement resulting directly from surgery or radiotherapy. A Canadian study of 82 head and neck cancer patients showed a strong association between the level of disfigurement and depression (Katz *et al.*, 2003). Social support was shown to act as a buffer to women of their disfigurement (see 'Facial disfigurement and dysmorphology').

As previously mentioned, head and neck cancer patients express a variety of concerns which include recurrence fears and appearance. Many of these concerns are unresolved and coping strategies that tend to be employed include, avoidance, distraction and the use of alcohol (Chaturvedi *et al.*, 1996).

Social support

A statistically sophisticated study by the Utrecht group contributes some valuable findings in an under-researched area within the head and neck cancer specialty (de Leeuw *et al.*, 2000*b*). They studied 197 patients pre-treatment and followed them up 6 months later. Two competing models were tested, namely social support influenced depression or visa versa. Results were clear, as they showed that available support led to less depressive symptomology (see also 'Social support and health').

Psychological interventions

There have been a number of calls for introducing greater emotional support for head and neck cancer patients (Chaturvedi *et al.*, 1996). A psychosocial support programme was evaluated with head and neck cancer patients ($n = 144$) using a longitudinal, prospective, case-control study (Petruson *et al.*, 2003). The support programme consisted of visits from the cancer team, including a weekly visit during treatment and then once a month for the first 6 months following treatment, and then again 1 and 3 years after diagnosis. Of the 81 patients offered the support, 15 did not want to participate, 11 did not attend the first visit and three died, leaving 52 patients in the study group. The control group consisted of 232 patients of whom 92 were matched to the study group on tumour location, stage, gender and age. The dependent variables were assessed by the EORTC QoL measures at diagnosis, and at 3, 12 and 36 months after the start of treatment. At one-year follow-up the control group had a clinically and statistically better global quality of life score but this difference was not sustained at 3 years. One possible explanation for the lack of improvement in QoL was explained by the authors as a design problem as randomization was not possible (see also 'Social support interventions'). The authors stressed the need for improved training for hospital personnel to recognize patients with affective disorders.

A psychological intervention designed specifically for head and neck cancer patients, to identify and reduce patients' fears of recurrence following primary treatment has been reported (Humphris, 2001). The intervention consisted of 6 structured sessions featuring the encouragement of the patient to express their concerns over future disease and what prompted them (e.g. symptoms) to seek reassurance from self-checking or professional review.

The intervention demonstrated a short-term effect that reduced worries about cancer, anxious preoccupation and increased global quality of life. Some patients who participated in the intervention stated that they would have preferred to have the intervention sooner following their initial treatment (surgery or surgery and radiotherapy).

A recent feasibility study conducted in Montreal using the Nucare coping strategies programme demonstrated that global QoL and social and physical functioning improved immediately following the intervention phase. Although not a randomized controlled study some promising results were reported (Allison *et al.*, 2004).

Conclusion

The psychological care of the patient with head and neck cancer is a neglected research area and moreover is traditionally a less developed service compared to more common cancers. However, clear features of the disease and its treatment indicate the need to study and intervene with this patient group. Due to the natural progression of the disease and the likelihood of recurrence, healthcare personnel are encouraged to identify the key concerns expressed by patients and their carers.

(See also 'Cancer: general', 'Coping with chronic illness' and 'Coping with death and dying'.)

REFERENCES

Allison, P. (2001). Factors associated with smoking and alcohol consumption following treatment for head and neck cancer. *Oral Oncology*, **37**, 513–20.

Allison, P., Edgar, L., Nicolau, B. *et al.* (2004). Results of a feasibility study for a psycho-educational intervention in head and neck cancer. *Psycho-oncology*, **13**, 482–5.

Bjordal, K. & Kaasa, S. (1995). Psychological distress in head and neck cancer patients 7–11 years after curative treatment. *British Journal of Cancer*, **71**, 592–7.

Browman, G., Wong, G., Hodson, I. *et al.* (1993). Influence of cigarette smoking on the efficacy of radiation therapy in head and neck cancer. *New England Journal of Medicine*, **328**, 159–63.

Campbell, B., Marbella, A. & Layde, P. (2000). Quality of life and recurrence concern in survivors of head and neck cancer. *Laryngoscope*, **110**, 895–906.

Chaturvedi, S., Shenoy, A., Prasad, K., Senthilnathan, S. & Premlatha, B. (1996). Concerns, coping and quality of life in head and neck cancer patients. *Support Cancer Care*, **4**, 186–90.

Chekryn, J. (1984). Cancer recurrence: personal meaning, communication, and marital adjustment. *Cancer Nursing* (December 1984), 491–8.

Conway, D., Macpherson, L., Gibson, J. & Binnie, V. (2002). Oral cancer: prevention and detection in primary dental healthcare. *Primary Dental Care*, **9**, 119–23.

Cruz, G., Le Geros, R., Ostroff, J. *et al.* (2002). Oral cancer knowledge, risk factors and characteristics of subjects in a large oral cancer screening program. *Journal of the American Dental Association*, **133**, 1064–71.

de Graeff, A., de Leeuw, J., Ros, W., Hordijk, G., Blijham, G. & Winnubst, J. (2000). Pretreatment factors predicting quality of life after treatment for head and neck cancer. *Head and Neck*, **22**, 398–407.

de Leeuw, J., De Graeff, A., Ros, W. *et al.* (2000*a*). Prediction of depressive symptomatology after treatment of head and neck cancer: the influence of pre-treatment physical and depressive symptoms, coping, and social support. *Head and Neck*, **22**, 799–807.

de Leeuw, J., de Graeff, A., Ros, W. *et al.* (2000*b*). Negative and positive influences of social support on depression in patients with head and neck cancer: a prospective study. *Psycho-oncology*, **9**, 20–8.

Deleyiannis, F. W.-B., Thomas, D., Vaughan, T. & Davis, S. (1996). Alcoholism: independent predictor of survival in patients with head and neck cancer. *Journal of National Cancer Institute*, **88**, 542–9.

Funk, G., Karnell, L., Dawson, C. *et al.* (1997). Baseline and post-treatment assessment of the general health status of head and neck cancer patients compared with United States population norms. *Head and Neck*, **19**, 675–83.

Hammerlid, E., Ahlner-Elmqvist, M., Bjordal, K. *et al.* (1999). A prospective multicentre study in Sweden and Norway of mental distress and psychiatric morbidity in head and neck cancer patients. *British Journal of Cancer*, **80**, 766–74.

Hammerlid, E., Silander, E., Hornestam, L. & Sullivan, M. (2001). Health-related quality of life three years after diagnosis of head and neck cancer-a longitudinal study. *Head and Neck*, **23**, 113–25.

Huang, J., Barbara, L., Brouwers, M., Browman, G. & Mackillop, W. (2003). Does delay in starting treatment affect the outcomes of readiotherapy? A systematic review. *Journal of Clinical Oncology*, **21**, 555–63.

Humphris, G. (2001). *Fear of recurrence in orofacial cancer patients: the development and testing of a psychological intervention* (No. CP1031/0102). London: Cancer Research Campaign.

Humphris, G. & Field, E. (2004). Oral cancer information leaflet has benefit for smokers in primary care: results from two randomised control trials. *Community Dentistry and Oral Epidemiology,* **32**, 143–9.

Humphris, G., Rogers, S., McNally, D. *et al.* (2003). Fear of recurrence and possible cases of anxiety and depression in orofacial cancer patients. *International Journal of Maxillofacial Surgery,* **32**, 486–91.

Johnson, N. (2001). Tobacco use and oral cancer: a global perspective. *Journal of Dental Education,* **65**, 328–39.

Katz, M., Irish, J., Devins, G., Rodin, G. & Gullane, P. (2003). Psychosocial adjustment in head and neck cancer: the impact of disfigurement, gender and social support. *Head and Neck,* **25**, 103–12.

La Vecchia, C., Tavani, A., Francheschi, S. *et al.* (1997). Epidemiology and prevention of oral cancer. *Oral Oncology,* **33**, 302–12.

Lee-Jones, C. (1998). *A two year follow-up study investigating fear of recurrence in orofacial cancer patients.* Unpublished

Doctorate, University of Wales, Bangor, Lancashire.

Parkin, D., Pisani, P. & Ferlay, J. (1999). Estimates of the worldwide incidence of twenty-five major cancers in 1990. *International Journal of Cancer,* **80**, 827–41.

Petruson, K., Silander, E. & Hammerlid, E. (2003). Effects of psychological intervention on quality of life in patients with head and neck cancer. *Head and Neck,* **25**, 576–84.

Platz, H., Fries, R. & Hudec, M. (1986). *Prognoses of oral cavity carcinomas: results of a multicentre retrospective observational study.* Munich: Carl Hanser Verlag.

Quin, M. (2001). *Cancer trends in England and Wales 1950–1999* (Studies on medical and population subjects No. 66). London: Stationery Office.

Ringash, J. & Bezjak, A. (2001). A structured review of quality of life instruments for head and neck cancer patients. *Head and Neck,* **23**, 201–13.

Rogers, S., Fisher, S. & Woolgar, J. (1999). A review of quality of life assessment in oral cancer. *International Journal of Maxillofacial Surgery,* **28**, 99–117.

Rogers, S., Humphris, G., Lowe, D., Brown, J. & Vaughan, E. (1998). The impact of surgery for oral cancer on quality of life as measured by the Medical Outcomes Short Form 36. *European Journal of Cancer: Oral Oncology,* **34**, 171–9.

Schmale, A. H. (1976). Psychological reactions to recurrences, metastases or disseminated cancer. *International Journal of Radiation Oncology, Biology, Physics.,* **1**, 515–20.

Stevens, M., Gardner, J., Parkin, J. & Johnson, L. (1983). Head and neck cancer survival. *Archives of Otolaryngology,* **109**, 746–9.

West, D. (1977). Social adaptation patterns among cancer patients with facial disfigurements resulting from surgery. *Archives of Physical and Medical Rehabilitation,* **58**, 473–9.

Cancer: Hodgkin's and non-Hodgkin's lymphoma

Jennifer Devlen

Dickinson College

The lymphomas are a heterogenous group of neoplastic disorders of the lymphatic system of which there are two main types; Hodgkin's lymphoma (HL) and non-Hodgkin's lymphoma (NHL). Hodgkin's lymphoma was formerly called Hodgkin's disease after Thomas Hodgkin who first described it in 1832. It is rare, representing less than 1% of newly diagnosed cancers, with bimodal peaks in early adulthood and the elderly, and occurring slightly more frequently in males than females. The incidence of non-Hodgkin's lymphoma has been increasing steadily for the past 20 years for reasons that are as yet unclear (Evans & Hancock, 2003) and it currently accounts for approximately 4% of newly diagnosed cancers (Webster & Cella, 1998) in North America and western Europe where it is more common than in other regions of the world. Prevalence of NHL increases with age and there is a higher incidence in males (Evans & Hancock, 2003).

Treatment

Initial treatment of lymphoma generally involves chemotherapy often combined with involved-field radiotherapy. Courses of chemotherapy are spread out over several months, while radiotherapy is usually given five days a week for several weeks (see 'Chemotherapy' and 'Radiotherapy'). Most HL patients can be cured (overall survival rate greater than 80% at 10 years, and better survival rates for early stage HL) (Yung & Linch, 2003). Cure rates for NHL vary from approximately 50% to 90% depending on type and stage (Sweetenham, 2003). Overall, the prognosis for the lymphomas has improved significantly over the past three decades so one might reasonably expect that psychosocial morbidity in this group might be less than that in other forms of cancer that have a poorer prognosis or whose treatment entails the loss of a body part or function.

Psychological morbidity

At some time during the discovery of their disease or its treatment as many as two-thirds of patients are likely to be anxious, depressed or both (Devlen *et al.,* 1987*a*; Nerenz *et al.,* 1982). The onset of disease and referral to a cancer specialist is the period associated with the highest levels of emotional distress. Using standardized psychiatric interview schedules, Lloyd *et al.* (1984) identified 37.5% and Devlen *et al.* (1987*a*) found 36% of patients to be suffering clinically significant anxiety and/or depression during this time, rates consistent with cases of psychological distress obtained using the Brief Symptom Inventory (Zabora *et al.*, 2001), and similar to those found in patients with poorer prognosis diseases such as lung or pancreatic cancers (Zabora *et al.*, 2001). However, open and direct consultation with clinicians, a diagnosis and prognosis which may not be as terrible as they had feared, coupled with the commencement of treatment appears to resolve a great deal of the distress, and over one-third of those who were anxious or depressed during this time improved significantly once they started on chemotherapy or radiotherapy (Devlen *et al.*, 1987*a*).

At any point during treatment, the overall level of psychological morbidity is never as high as during the period surrounding diagnosis of the disease. However, morbidity persists in some patients, while others are at risk of developing a depressive disorder or anxiety state. A prospective study conducted by Devlen and colleagues (1987*a*) followed 120 newly diagnosed lymphoma patients over the first year, with in-depth interviews at diagnosis, then follow-up interviews at 2 months, 6 months and 12 months later. This allowed more detailed examination of the month-by-month prevalence, time of onset and duration of affective disorders. In total, 51% had clinical levels of psychiatric morbidity at some time during treatment with monthly levels of depression ranging from 8.3–15% for depression 5–12.5% for anxiety (Devlen, 1996). While the majority of this morbidity was found to occur in the first three months of treatment, new episodes, of depression especially, developed at any time up to one year after diagnosis.

Complications during treatment

Side effects of both chemotherapy and radiotherapy are very common in HL and NHL patients. Although the exact effects depend on the chemotherapeutic agents given, Devlen *et al.* (1987*a*) reported that 77.5% suffered nausea and 72% experienced vomiting, rates that are comparable to those recorded in other more recent samples of cancer patients receiving chemotherapy (Grunberg, 2004). In 27.5% of our sample, vomiting was severe, i.e. 6–10 episodes per day for 3 or more days post-treatment (Devlen *et al.*, 1987*a*). Nausea and vomiting are among the most troubling effects of treatment and can negatively impact patients' ability to function (Grunberg, 2004). There has been much speculation about the possibility of these effects prompting patients to withdraw from chemotherapy although there is little published data to indicate how much of a problem this really is. Up to 80% of patients may lose some or all of their hair (Devlen *et al.*, 1987*a*). Several patients who had wanted to keep their cancer private now had a publicly visible sign of their disease (Devlen, 1996). Less prevalent, but still significant complications of treatment include sore mouth, changes in perception of taste, sore skin, loss of or increase in appetite, constipation, diarrhoea, pain and peripheral neuropathy (Devlen *et al.*, 1987*a*; Nerenz *et al.*, 1982).

Conditioned nausea and vomiting

Like other cancer patients, those being treated for lymphoma experience pre-chemotherapy or anticipatory nausea (7–47%) and vomiting (20–28%) (Cameron *et al.*, 2001; Devlen *et al.*, 1987*a*). This phenomenon is commonly thought to result from classical conditioning (see 'Behaviour therapy'). Reminders of chemotherapy, such as the sight, smell or thought of the hospital, treatment or even the chemotherapy nurse can elicit nausea or vomiting. Although diminishing with time, these symptoms, nausea more so than vomiting, are not readily extinguished and have been reported to persist in a minority of patients (9–41%) many years post-treatment (Cameron *et al.*, 2001; Devlen *et al.*, 1987*b*). Decreased libido and sexual dysfunction whilst on treatment are common, and even after completion of treatment the prevalence of sexual dysfunction remains high (Devlen *et al.*, 1987*b*; Jonker-Pool *et al.*, 2004).

Cognitive impairments

Impairments in concentration (Cella & Tross, 1986) and memory have also been recorded. Although objective memory assessments indicate performance within normal ranges, Devlen *et al.* (1987*a*) and by Ahles *et al.* (2002) found significant differences in test scores for patients who reported such problems when compared with those who claimed no impairment. Mood disorders might account for some of these cognitive difficulties (Cull *et al.*, 1996) but not all (Brezden *et al.*, 2000; Devlen *et al.*, 1987*a*) and further investigation is warranted.

Predictors of morbidity

Psychological morbidity does not seem to be related to disease type (HL versus NHL) or stage (Devlen *et al.*, 1987*a*). There are no consistent gender differences in psychological morbidity in this group. Webster and Cella (1998) observed that older patients tend to report better emotional wellbeing than younger patients with equivalent objective health status. Greater distress was noted in HL patients who received combined-modality treatment when compared with those who were treated with only radiation (Ganz *et al.*, 2003). This may reflect the different levels of toxicity associated with these treatments, given that psychological morbidity has been related to treatment toxicity. Side effects involving the gastrointestinal tract: nausea, vomiting, diarrhoea, loss of appetite, sore mouth and taste changes were most likely to be correlated with both anxiety and depression (Devlen *et al.*, 1987*a,b*). Patients often stress the importance of eating well to maintain the strength necessary to endure treatment and combat the disease, and side effects that hinder this may explain some of this association. Patients may also misattribute treatment effects as being indicative of the recurrence of their disease, especially with vague effects such as tiredness and pain (Nerenz *et al.*, 1982) or when they occur some time after completion of treatment, as may be the case or post-radiation lethargy.

Long-term effects for survivors

As more lymphoma patients survive and residual problems become more apparent, attention has been directed toward investigating the long-term effects of these diseases and their treatments. Noted medical complications include second malignancies (the most common being lung cancer and breast cancer mainly attributable to radiotherapy that included those anatomical areas, and myeloid leukemia from chemotherapy agents), cardiac disease, endocrine disorders (particularly hypothyroidism after radiation) and dental caries and other oral diseases subsequent to neck irradiation (Parsa-Parsi et al., 1998; Wiedenmann et al., 2002; Yung & Linch, 2003). Furthermore, chemotherapeutic agents and gonadal radiation in the treatment can affect fertility: azoospermia in men and precocious menopause in women (Anselmo et al., 2001).

Numerous studies have reported fatigue as a significant long-term problem in this group. (Ganz et al., 2003; Loge et al., 1999; Wettergren et al., 2003), and there is some suggestion that it might be more prevalent in lymphoma patients than in other cancer survivors (Oldervoll et al., 2003). When compared with samples from the general population, HL survivors have reduced health-related quality of life, including impairments in social and role functioning (Loge et al., 1999). Problems with employment and difficulties with insurance and loan applications have also been recorded (Devlen et al., 1987b; Fletchtner et al., 1998). The two prospective studies that followed samples of lymphoma patients over time (Devlen et al., 1987a; Ganz et al., 2003) suggest that many of the symptoms and impairments evident at the time of diagnosis or during chemo- or radiotherapy tend to diminish quite quickly after completion of treatment. However, any impairments still evident one or two years later are not likely to show any further improvement (Ganz et al., 2003; Greil et al., 1999).

Conclusions and clinical implications

Treatments continue to improve cure rates in these diseases, and the ongoing goal is to reduce short- and long-term effects without compromising efficacy. In spite of an increasing body of literature on this patient group, many problems may go unrecognized in clinical practice. One study reports that oncology physicians and nurses may underestimate the incidence and impact of chemotherapy-induced nausea and vomiting (Grunberg, 2004). Anti-emetic regimens available for controlling nausea and vomiting will also help prevent anticipatory nausea/vomiting and the associated distress this causes. The publication of guidelines regarding anti-emetic prophylaxis has increased their use somewhat, but Grunberg claims there is still room for improvement.

Regular breast screening has recently been recommended for women who received radiotherapy that included the breast area and screening for other common malignancies in this group might also be advised.

Getting sufficient rest and limiting activity may be helpful whilst on active treatment, but Olderval and colleagues (2003) suggest this may be counterproductive for the chronic fatigue that persists after treatment has finished. They report significant benefits in HL survivors who participated in a 20-week home-based exercise programme. Future studies of interventions for fatigue might help to address this important problem.

Surveys of patients indicate significant levels of dissatisfaction with information and support concerning sexuality from the healthcare team, recommending that physicians initiate discussion of this topic at diagnosis and follow-up (Jonker-Pool et al., 2004). Prior to starting chemotherapy banking sperm, eggs or fertilized embryos might be options for patients (Anselmo et al., 2001). The post-menopausal uterus may still permit implantation and development of an embryo and Anselmo et al. (2001) report the use of egg donation in achieving successful full-term pregnancies in women previously treated for HL providing hope for this group that includes young adults who may want to start or complete a family.

A recent comprehensive review provides stronger evidence of cognitive changes related to chemotherapy in other cancers (Minisini et al., 2004). Future clinical trials and routine monitoring of cognitive function are needed to describe this phenomenon and the underlying mechanisms more clearly (Ahles, 2004).

On a more positive note, two-thirds of HL survivors interviewed by Wettergren et al. (2003) reported positive changes such as having become more mature, grateful and tolerant. In summary, advances in the treatment for lymphomas have meant that many will now be cured. Yet, despite this favourable prognosis considerable research indicates substantial physical, psychological and social problems, at least in the short term. The diagnosis of cancer, even one with an outcome that might ultimately be good, is still a time of considerable psychological distress and the ensuing aggressive treatments have significant impact on patient's functioning and wellbeing. There are some persistent problems, notably fatigue, but there is also evidence that many survivors adapt well in the long-term.

(See also 'Cancer: general', 'Coping with chronic illness' and 'Coping with death and dying.')

REFERENCES

Ahles, T. A., Saykin, A. J., Furstenberg, C. T. et al. (2002). Neuropsychologic impact of standard-dose systemic chemotherapy in long-term survivors of breast cancer and lymphoma. Journal of Clinical Oncology, 20, 485–93.

Ahles, T. A. (2004). Do systemic cancer treatment affect cognitive function? The Lancet Oncology, 5, 270–1.

Anselmo, A. P., Cavalieri, E., Aragona, C. et al. (2001). Successful pregnancies following an egg donation program in women with previously treated Hodgkin's disease. Haematologica, 86, 624–8.

Brezden, C. B., Phillips, K. A., Abdolell, M., Bunston, T. & Tannock, I. F. (2000). Cognitive function in breast cancer patients receiving adjuvant chemotherapy. Journal of Clinical Oncology, 18, 2695–701.

Cameron, C. L., Cella, D., Herndon, J. E. et al. (2001). Persistent symptoms among survivors of Hodgkin's disease: an explanatory model based on classical conditioning. Health Psychology, 20, 71–5.

Cella, D. F. & Tross, S. (1986). Psychological adjustment to survival from Hodgkin's disease. Journal of Consulting and Clinical Psychology, 54, 616–22.

Cull, A., Hay, C., Love, S. B. et al. (1996). What do cancer patients mean when they complain of concentration and memory problems? British Journal of Cancer, 74, 1674–9.

Devlen, J., Maguire, P., Phillips, P. & Crowther, D. (1987a). Psychological problems associated with diagnosis and treatment of lymphomas. II: Prospective study. *British Medical Journal*, **295**, 955–7.

Devlen, J., Maguire, P., Phillips, P., Crowther, D. & Chambers, H. (1987b). Psychological problems associated with diagnosis and treatment of lymphomas. I: Retrospective study. *British Medical Journal*, **295**, 953–4.

Devlen, J. (1996). Quality of life in Hodgkin's disease and lymphomas. In P. Selby & C. Bailey (Eds.). *Cancer and the adolescent*. London: BMJ Publishing Group.

Evans, L. S. & Hancock, B. W. (2003). Non-Hodgkin lymphoma. *The Lancet*, **362**, 139–46.

Fletchtner, H., Ruffer, J.-U., Henry-Amar, M. *et al.* (1998). Quality of life assessment in Hodgkin's disease: a new comprehensive approach. *Annals of Oncology*, **9**(Suppl. 5), S147–54.

Ganz, PA., Moinpour, C. M., Pauler, D. K. *et al.* (2003). Health status and quality of life in patients with early-stage Hodgkin's disease treated on Southwest Oncology Group study 9133. *Journal of Clinical Oncology*, **21**, 3512–19.

Greil, R., Holzner, B., Kemmler, G. *et al.* (1999). Retrospective assessment of quality of life and treatment outcome in patients with Hodgkin's disease from 1969 to 1994. *European Journal of Cancer*, **35**, 698–706.

Grunberg, S. M. (2004). Chemotherapy-induced nausea and vomiting: prevention, detection, and treatment – How are we doing? *Journal of Supportive Oncology*, **2**(Suppl. 1), 1–12.

Jonker-Pool, G., Hoekstra, H. J., van Imhoff, G. W. *et al.* (2004). Male sexuality after cancer treatment – needs for information and support: testicular cancer compared to malignant lymphoma. *Patient Education and Counseling*, **52**, 143–50.

Loge, J. H., Foss Abrahamsen, A., Ekeberg, O. & Kaasa, S. (1999). Reduced health-related quality of life among Hodgkin's disease survivors: a comparative study with general population norms. *Annals of Oncology*, **10**, 71–7.

Minisini, A., Atalay, G., Bottomley, A. *et al.* (2004). What is the effect of systemic anticancer treatment on cognitive function? *The Lancet Oncology*, **5**, 273–82.

Nerenz, D. R., Leventhal, H. & Love, R. R. (1982). Factors contributing to emotional distress during cancer chemotherapy. *Cancer*, **50**, 1020–7.

Oldervoll, L. M., Kaasa, S., Knobel, H. & Loge, J. H. (2003). Exercise reduces fatigue in chronic fatigued Hodgkin's disease survivors – results from a pilot study. *European Journal of Cancer*, **39**, 57–63.

Parsa-Parsi, R., Engert, A. & Diehl, V. (1998). An overview of the Fourth International Symposium on Hodgkin's disease. Recent advances in basic and clinical research. *Annals of Oncology*, **9**(Suppl. 5), S1–3.

Sweetenham, J. (2003). Fact file. Lymphoma classification - why does it matter? http://www.lymphoma.org.uk/support/Factfiles/lymphomaclassificationwhydoesitmatter.htm. (24 May 2005).

Webster, K. & Cella, D. (1998). Quality of life in patients with low-grade non-Hodgkin's lymhoma. *Oncology*, **12**, 697–717.

Wettergren, L., Bjorkholm, M., Axdorph, U., Bowling, A. & Langius-Eklof, A. (2003). Individual quality of life in long-term survivors of Hodgkin's lymphoma – a comparative study. *Quality of Life Research*, **12**, 545–54.

Wiedenmann, S., Wolf, J. & Diehl, V. (2002). An overview of the Fifth International Symposium on Hodgkin's lymphoma. Recent advances in basic and clinical research. *Annals of Oncology*, **13**(Suppl. 1), S1–3.

Yung, L. & Linch, D. (2003). Hodgkin's lymphoma. *The Lancet*, **361**, 943–51.

Zabora, J., Brintzenhofeszoc, K., Curbow, B., Hooker, C. & Piantadosi, S. (2001). The prevalence of psychological distress by cancer site. *Psycho-oncology*, **10**, 19–28.

Cancer: leukaemia

Janelle L. Wagner and Ronald T. Brown

Medical University of South Carolina

Overview

The leukaemias are a group of cancers of the blood forming tissues that are typically characterized by the type of white blood cells that is affected (lymphoid or myeloid) and the progressive nature of the abnormal cells (acute versus chronic). There are four common types of leukaemia: (i) acute lymphocytic leukaemia (ALL); (ii) chronic lymphocytic leukaemia (CLL); (iii) acute myeloid leukaemia (AML); and (iv) chronic myeloid leukaemia (CML). Specifically, ALL is defined as an abnormal white blood cell count and differential, abnormal haematocrit/haemoglobin and platelet counts, abnormal bone marrow with more than 5% blasts (immature cells), and signs and symptoms of the disease (http://cancer.gov). ALL and AML occur in both children and adults, although the chronic leukaemias (CLL, CML) affect primarily adults. Approximately 89% of leukaemia cases occur in adults over the age of 60 years (Lesko, 1998). The incidence of leukaemia in the United States is 10.9 per 100 000 individuals compared to 8.5 per 100 000 individuals in the United Kingdom (Parkin *et al.*, 1997).

The specific aetiology of leukaemia is unknown, although risk factors may consist of prenatal exposure to radiation and post-natal exposure to various toxins (see 'Toxins: environmental').

Treatments typically used in the management of specific neoplasms often place individuals at secondary risk for other malignancies including leukaemia. Down's syndrome and other genetic disorders, such as neurofibromatosis also pose significant risk factors for the development of leukaemia (NIH Publication number 02-3775 retrieved from http://cancer.gov).

Common presenting symptoms of leukaemia include fevers, frequent infections, fatigue, headaches, bleeding and bruising easily, joint and bone pain, abdominal swelling, lymphadenopathy and weight loss. These symptoms often are evaluated employing a series of diagnostic tests (e.g. blood tests, bone marrow aspiration or biopsy, spinal tap and/or chest X-ray). Once a diagnosis of leukaemia has been made, the standard treatment options typically include chemotherapy or radiation therapy or both, and transplantation, including bone marrow transplantation, particularly if there is a relapse.

Treatment for ALL is divided into induction, consolidation or intensification and maintenance therapy, with central nervous system (CNS) therapy provided at each stage, particularly if the individual has CNS involvement. Approximately 50–70% of children develop CNS leukaemia. For children with ALL, intensive therapy results in a favourable prognosis, though older children and adolescents (over the age of 10 years) often have a less favourable outcome (Pui & Evans, 1998). Treatment outcome for adults diagnosed with ALL is less favourable than for paediatric populations (Hoelzer et al., 2002). Typically, remission rates for adults are inversely associated with chronological age with older individuals having a more favourable prognosis than their younger counterparts (Keating et al., 1982). For individuals with leukaemia, frequently the adverse side effects associated with treatment cause the individual greater difficulties than the symptoms of the disease itself. Such adverse effects of chemotherapy include fatigue, alopecia, gastrointestinal distress, infertility, impairments in cognition (e.g. memory) and complications associated with the endocrine system (Hoelzer et al., 2002) (see 'Chemotherapy').

Psychosocial adjustment

Given the wide range of stressors (e.g. physical, social and financial) that individuals with leukaemia encounter, it is not surprising that studies have demonstrated significant adjustment difficulties in these individuals. For example, Montgomery and colleagues (2003) reported distress and mild to moderate depression in over half of their sample of adults with AML, and poor illness-specific adjustment in over 25% of the sample. Significant distress was predicted by two cognitive variables, namely helplessness/hopelessness and a 'fighting spirit'. In another study, 35% of patients undergoing induction and consolidation phases of treatment for leukaemia reported elevated levels of anxiety and depressive symptoms (Andrykowski et al., 1999). Thus, there is evidence to suggest that individuals with leukaemia have difficulty adjusting to their disease, treatment and associated adverse side effects. Unfortunately, in a significant number of cases, these high levels of anxiety and depressive symptoms may go undetected (Zittoun et al., 1999), despite evidence that depression is in fact associated with lower survival rates in individuals with cancer (Spiegel, 1996). Notably, cancer-related depression is not substantially different from depression in

other medical conditions, although psychological treatments should include components that directly address issues specific to cancer patients (Patrick et al., 2003) (see 'Cancer: general').

The physical and psychological impact of having a life threatening disease such as leukaemia, undergoing invasive medical procedures, and experiencing associated side effects such as nausea, pain and vomiting are recognized traumatic events (Stuber et al., 1994). Studies have demonstrated symptoms of post-traumatic stress disorder (PTSD) in survivors of leukaemia and their families (e.g. Best et al., 2001; Lesko et al., 1992). The severity of PTSD symptoms, such as levels of intrusive thoughts and imagery, are also associated with psychological distress (Lesko et al., 1992) (see also 'Post-traumatic stress disorder').

Demographic variables, including gender, age and socioeconomic status play a significant role in the above mentioned psychological symptoms often seen in individuals with leukaemia (i.e. Stark et al., 2002). To illustrate, men diagnosed with leukaemia reported increased general psychiatric distress while women reported poor social adjustment (Lesko et al., 1992). In another study, Greenberg and colleagues (1997) found that younger AML patients with less education were more likely to report increased psychological distress following treatment. Thus, men and women evidence different patterns of adjustment to leukaemia and younger, less educated patients are at increased risk for greater distress than are their older more educated counterparts.

Factors associated with adjustment

The literature has repeatedly demonstrated that medical, individual differences and social factors contribute to psychosocial adjustment in individuals with leukaemia (Holland, 1998). We now address specific psychosocial issues that are central to psychosocial adjustment in individuals with cancer and include quality of life, social support and coping skills.

Quality of life

Not surprisingly, given their invasiveness and adverse side effects, treatments for leukaemia have consistently been shown to affect health related quality of life (HRQL). According to Aaronson (1989), HRQL is comprised of four core domains: (i) disease state and physical symptoms; (ii) functional status; (iii) psychological and emotional functioning; and (iv) social functioning (Aaronson, 1989) (see 'Quality of life').

In a review of 21 studies assessing HRQL in individuals with AML, Redaelli and colleagues (2004) note consistent associations between both medical (physical symptoms, irradiation, illness duration) and demographic variables (education and gender) and quality of life. Studies have demonstrated decreased HRQL immediately following a diagnosis of the leukaemia and during the course of active therapies. However, long-term survivors of leukaemia report no significant differences in HRQL compared with their healthy peers, with the exception of sexual impairments that may include infertility, impotence and pain during intercourse.

HRQL is not stable across treatment phases, but may vary depending on the potency of prescribed treatments. For example, Schumacher and colleagues (2002) demonstrated improvements in quality of life over the course of inpatient chemotherapy treatment, and Stalfelt (1994) found differences in HRQL on a weekly basis that varied according to treatment regimen. Zittoun *et al.* (1997) also observed that individuals who experienced allogenic (allo) bone marrow transplants (BMT) reported more severe impairment in HRQL than those who underwent autologous (auto) BMT. In turn, individuals who received auto BMT reported worse HLRQ than their peers who were treated with chemotherapy only.

Social support

Social support has been demonstrated to be a resilience factor for both anxiety and depressive symptoms, and lack of social support may increase the risk for psychosocial difficulties (see 'Social support and health'). For example, poor social support during cancer treatment was associated with greater anxiety (Stark *et al.*, 2002). Alternatively, perceptions of the availability of social support in individuals with cancer also have been associated with fewer depressive symptoms (e.g. De Leeuw *et al.*, 2000) and better adjustment (for a review see Spiegel, 1997). Thus, it seems that an individual's perception of available social supports is critical to adjustment. Many individuals with leukaemia do report poor marital relations that in part may be due to several stressors, including financial strain and sexual impairments (Wellisch *et al.*, 1996).

Sources of social support typically derive from family or friendships; however, research suggests that communication and support from physicians also is associated with adjustment in individuals with leukaemia. For example, individuals who report distress are more likely to express dissatisfaction with information received by their healthcare provider and to indicate the need for additional time to discuss diagnostic and treatment issues (Montgomery *et al.*, 2003). Furthermore, over 90% of patients reported a preference for discussion of emotional issues with their physician, although over a quarter of the sample were of the notion that the physician should initiate the discussion (Detam *et al.*, 2000). Thus, unless physicians facilitate conversation of emotional adjustment, patients are unlikely to disclose such important information. When communication is open between patients and physicians, patients report greater use of adaptive coping styles and perceived autonomy in decision-making (Dermatis & Lesko, 1991) (see 'Healthcare professional–patient communication').

Coping skills

There are individual differences in the ways in which individuals with leukaemia cope with their illness. The use of adaptive coping strategies has been shown to be associated with decreased levels of distress in patients with leukaemia (Montgomery *et al.*, 2003). Various coping strategies may be modified over time and often correspond to the phases of cancer treatment (Caudell, 1996). Holland and Gooen-Piels (2000) have outlined three phases of 'normal responses' to cancer. Phase I is the initial response that may include disbelief, denial and shock. Phase II involves dysphoria, characterized by slow acknowledgment of the diagnosis, and significant distress, which may manifest as insomnia, anxiety, depression and recurrent thoughts of illness and death. Finally, Phase III is characterized by longer-term adaptation. This is the period in which individuals employ available resources and various coping strategies

(Holland & Gooen-Piels, 2000). Thus, depending on the stage of care, certain coping skills may be indicated and should be encouraged by health professionals. When faced with the stressors of a life-threatening disease such as leukaemia and its potential implications, including death, patients often explore the meaning of life and/or their beliefs of an afterlife. It is not uncommon for many individuals to consult religion or spirituality as a context for understanding their disease and promoting coping skills, such as prayer or meditation (Larson & Milano, 1995) (see also 'Coping with chronic illness' and 'Coping with death and dying').

Behavioural interventions

Intrusive and painful medical procedures associated with the experience of leukaemia, coupled with symptoms of anxiety and depression, as well as conditioned responses to treatment, create numerous stressors for an individual. Furthermore, individuals with leukaemia are often immunosuppressed, and for this reason, it is critical that they learn how to diminish arousal and enhance coping skills for the purpose of alleviating the effects of stress on their already compromised immune system (Caudell, 1996).

Behavioural interventions have long been employed to reduce pain in individuals with cancer as well as those with other chronic illnesses, and have repeatedly demonstrated beneficial effects on adjustment. For example, techniques such as relaxation, imagery and distraction have been shown to be effective in reducing pain, anxiety and nausea for individuals undergoing cancer treatment (for a review see Mundy *et al.*, 2003). When choosing a behavioural strategy, the clinician should attend to potential experiences of pain and fatigue and compromised functional status and to those techniques that are indicated for particular phases of care. Specifically, emotional support, stress management and cognitive restructuring are appropriate interventions for targeting fears and anxieties frequently common at diagnosis, while relaxation and imagery have been demonstrated to be effective in reducing pain, fear of procedures and nausea associated with the specific cancer treatments, including chemotherapy (for a review see Caudell, 1996) (see 'Behaviour therapy' and 'Relaxation training').

Burish and colleagues have conducted a series of randomized controlled studies to examine the effectiveness of relaxation and guided imagery techniques in reducing anxiety and nausea associated with chemotherapy. Specifically, Burish *et al.* (1987) found that progressive muscle relaxation and guided imagery were more effective than no behavioural treatment in either delaying or preventing nausea and vomiting. In another study, Carey and Burish (1987) demonstrated for individuals with leukaemia that relaxation training from a professional therapist was superior to no relaxation instruction or a relaxation audiotape at reducing anxiety associated with chemotherapy. Finally, Burish *et al.* (1991) provided data for a sample comprised in part of patients diagnosed with leukaemia to support the superiority of a coping preparation programme (e.g. information about procedure, tour of facility, etc.) compared with a relaxation training programme. Relaxation training alone was minimally effective in reducing anticipatory nausea associated with chemotherapy. Thus, these studies provide evidence supporting the efficacy of relaxation techniques and adaptive coping skills, when delivered by a trained therapist, in reducing distress related to leukaemia treatments.

Conclusions

In conclusion, the leukaemias are a group of blood cancers for which various invasive medical treatments with adverse side effects are indicated. Not surprisingly, studies have demonstrated symptoms of anxiety and depression in individuals with leukaemia. Factors such as quality of life, social support and coping skills are associated with psychosocial adjustment, and are often the target of behavioural interventions that have demonstrated efficacy in the reduction of anxiety and pain and promotion of healthy coping strategies for individuals with leukaemia. However, research with

adults has largely neglected examining post-traumatic stress symptoms, despite a growing body of research on this topic in the pediatric literature (for a summary see Vannatta & Gerhardt, 2003). Indeed, many individuals with leukaemia may experience these invasive medical procedures as traumatic. Future research should focus on a more in depth examination of PTSD symptoms in adults with leukaemia and the development of specific psychosocial interventions to target these symptoms. Finally, researchers and clinicians should diligently work towards dissemination of cognitive-behavioural interventions so they can more readily be available to patients and healthcare providers (see 'Cognitive behaviour therapy').

(See also 'Cancer: general', 'Coping with chronic illness' and 'Coping with death and dying'.)

REFERENCES

Aaronson, N. K. (1989). Quality of life assessment in clinical trials: methodological issues. *Controlled Clinical Trials,* **10**(4), 195S–208S.

Andrykowksi, M. A., Greinder, C. B., Altmaier, E. M. *et al.* (1995). Quality of life following bone marrow transplantation: findings from a multi-centre study. *British Journal of Cancer,* **7**(6), 1322–9.

Burish, T. G., Carey, M. P., Krozely, M. G. & Greco, F. A. (1987). Conditioned side effects induced by cancer chemotherapy: prevention through behavioral treatment. *Journal of Consulting and Clinical Psychology,* **55**, 42–8.

Burish, T. G., Snyder, S. L. & Jenkins, R. A. (1991). Preparing patients for cancer chemotherapy: effect of coping preparing and relaxation interventions. *Journal of Consulting and Clinical Psychology,* **59**, 518–25.

Carey, M. P. & Burish, T. G. (1987). Providing relaxation training to cancer chemotherapy patients: a comparison of three delivery techniques. *Journal of Consulting and Clinical Psychology,* **55**, 732–7.

Caudell, K. A. (1996). Psychoneuroimmunology and innovative behavioral interventions in patients with leukemia. *Oncology Nursing Forum,* **23**(3), 493–502.

De Leeuw, J. R., De Graeff, A., Ros, W. J. *et al.* (2000). Negative and positive influences of social support on depression in patients with head and neck cancer: a prospective study. *Psycho-oncology,* **9**(1), 20–8.

Dermatis, H. & Lesko, L. M. (1991). Psychosocial correlates of physician-patient communication at the time of informed consent for bone marrow transplantation. *Cancer Investigation,* **9**(6), 621–8.

Detmar, S. B., Aaronson, N. K., Wever, L. D., Muller, M. & Schornagel, J. H. (2000). How are you feeling? Who wants to know?

Patients' and oncologists' preferences for discussing health-related quality of life issues. *Journal of Clinical Oncology,* **18**(18), 3295–301.

Greenberg, D. B., Kornblith, A. B., Herndon, J. E. *et al.* (1997). Quality of life for adult leukemia survivors treated on clinical trials of Cancer and Leukemia Group B during the period 1971–1988: predictors for later psychologic distress. *Cancer,* **80**(10), 1936–44.

Hoelzer, D., Gokbuget, N., Ottmann, O. *et al.* (2002). Acute lymphoblastic leukemia. *American Society of Hematology,* 162–92.

Holland, J. C. (1998). *Psycho-oncology.* New York: Oxford University Press.

Holland, J. C. & Gooen-Piels, J. (2000). Principles of psycho-oncology. In J. C. Holland, E. Frei & B. C. Decker (Eds.). *Cancer Medicine,* (5th edn.). (pp. 943–58). Hamilton, Canada: BC Decker Inc.

Kazak, A. E. & Barakat, L. P. (1997). Brief report: parenting stress and quality of life during treatment for childhood leukemia predicts child and parent adjustment after treatment ends. *Journal of Pediatric Psychology,* **22**(5), 749–58.

Keating, M. J., McCredie, K. B., Bodey, G. P. *et al.* (1982). Improved prospects for long-term survival in adults with acute myelogenous leukemia. *Journal of the American Medical Assocation,* **248**(19), 2481–6.

Larson, D. B. & Milano, M. A. G. (1995). Are religion and spirituality clinically relevant in health care? *Mind/Body Medicine,* **1**(3), 147–57.

Lesko, L. M. (1998). *Hematopoietic dyscrasias.* In J. C. Holland (Ed.). *Psycho-oncology* (pp. 406–16). New York: Oxford University Press.

Lesko, L. M., Ostroff, J. S., Mumma, G. H., Mashberg, D. E. & Holland, J. C. (1992).

Long term psychological adjustment of acute leukemia survivors: impact of bone marrow transplantation versus conventional chemotherapy. *Psychosomatic Medicine,* **54**(1), 30–47.

Montgomery, C., Pocock, M., Titley, K. & Lloyd, K. (2003). Predicting psychological distress in patients with leukemia and lymphoma. *Journal of Psychosomatic Research,* **54**, 289–92.

Mundy, E. A., DuHamel, K. N. & Montgomery, G. H. (2003). The efficacy of behavioral interventions for cancer treatment-related side effects. *Seminars in Clinical Neuropsychiatry,* **8**(4), 253–75.

National Institute of Cancer. *Adult acute lymphoblastic leukemia.* Retrieved May 22, 2004, from http://cancer.org

National Institute of Cancer. (posted 3/31/2003). NIH Publication No. 02–3775. Retrieved May 22, 2004, from http://cancer.org

Noll, R. B., MacLean, W. E. Jr., Whitt, J. K. *et al.* (1997). Behavioral adjustment and social functioning of long-term survivors of childhood leukemia: parent and teacher reports. *Journal of Pediatric Psychology,* **22**(6), 827–41.

Parkin, D. M., Whelan, S. L., Ferlay, J., Raymond, L. & Young, J. (Eds.). (1997). *Cancer incidence in five continents,* Vol. **VII** (IARC Scientific Publications No. 143). Lyon, France: IARC.

Patrick, D. L., Ferketich, S. L., Frame, P. S. *et al.* (2003). National Institutes of Health State of the Science Conference statement: symptoms management in cancer: pain, depression, and fatigue, July 15–17, 2002. *Journal of the National Cancer Institute,* **95**(15), 1110–17.

Pui, C. H. & Evans, W. E. (1998). Acute lymphoblastic leukemia. *New England Journal of Medicine,* **339**, 605–15.

Redaelli, A., Stephens, J. M., Brandt, S., Botteman, M. F. & Pashos, C. L. (2004).

Short- and long-term effects of acute myeloid leukemia on patient health-related quality of life. *Cancer Treatment Reviews*, **30**, 103–17.

Schumacher, A., Wewers, D., Heinecke, A. *et al.* (2002). Fatigue as an important aspect of quality of life in patients with acute myeloid leukemia. *Leukemia Research*, **26**(4), 355–62.

Spiegel, D. (1996). Cancer and depression. *British Journal of Psychiatry*, **168**(30), 109–16.

Spiegel, D. (1997). Psychosocial aspects of breast cancer treatment. *Seminars in Oncology*, **24**(Suppl. 1), S1 36–S1 47.

Stark, D., Kiely, M., Smith, A. *et al.* (2002). Anxiety disorders in cancer patients: their nature, associations, and relation to quality of life. *Journal of Clinical Oncology*, **20**(14), 3137–48.

Stuber, M. L., Meeske, K., Gonzalez, S. (1994). Post-traumatic stress after childhood cancer: the role of appraisal. *Psycho-oncology*, **3**, 305–12.

Vannatta, K. & Gerhardt, C. A. (2003). Pediatric oncology. In M. Roberts (Ed.). *Handbook of Pediatric Psychology*, (3rd edn.). (pp. 342–57). New York: The Guilford Press.

Wellisch, D. K., Centeno, J., Guzman, J., Belin, T. & Schiller, G. J. (1996). Bone marrow transplantation vs. high-dose cytorabine based consolidation chemotherapy for acute myelogenous leukemia. A long-term follow-up study of quality of life measures of survivors. *Psychosomatics*, **37**(2), 144–54.

Zittoun, R., Achard, S. & Ruszniewski, M. (1999). Assessment of quality of life during intensive chemotherapy or bone marrow transplantation. *Psycho-oncology*, **8**(1), 64–73.

Zittoun, R., Suciu, S., Watson, M. *et al.* (1997). Quality of life in patients with acute myelogenous leukemia in prolonged first complete remission after bone marrow transplantation (Allogeneic or autologous) or chemotherapy: a cross-sectional study of the EORTC-GIMEMA AML 8A trial. *Bone Marrow Transplant*, **20**(4), 307–15.

Cancer: lung

Angela Liegey Dougall

University of Pittsburgh

Overview

Lung cancer is the most common cancer and the leading cause of cancer death worldwide, claiming more than one million lives annually (Stewart and Kleihues, 2003). Because patients with lung cancer usually do not experience symptoms until the disease has advanced, most patients are diagnosed in later stages of the disease with poor prognoses.

The leading cause of lung cancer is exposure to tobacco smoke. Smoking causes approximately 90% of lung cancer deaths in men and 80% in women (USDHHS, 2004). Non-smokers who are exposed to secondhand tobacco smoke at home, work, or in social settings are also at an increased risk.

Other risk factors for lung cancer have been identified, some of which are synergistic with smoking. Exposure to environmental carcinogens such as asbestos, radon, workplace chemicals and air pollution as well as diets low in fruits and vegetables increase risk (Boffetta, 2004; Miller *et al.*, 2004). A personal history of lung diseases such as chronic obstructive pulmonary disease and tuberculosis, a previous diagnosis of lung cancer, or a family history of lung cancer may also increase susceptibility (Ardies, 2003; Economou *et al.*, 1994).

Research evidence

The majority of patients are diagnosed with lung cancer after they start experiencing symptoms and have advanced disease. Physical symptoms include fatigue, difficulty in breathing, cough, pain, spitting blood and loss of appetite (Hollen *et al.*, 1999). The discomfort and distress associated with these symptoms are often high and several studies have reported that patients with lung cancer report more symptom distress than do patients with other cancers (Degner & Sloan, 1995). High levels of symptom distress have been found to predict decreased psychosocial functioning and shorter survival times (Degner & Sloan, 1995; Okuyama *et al.*, 2001).

Many patients with lung cancer report depressive symptomatology. One study found symptoms of depression in more than a third of the patients (Kramer, 1999). Depressive symptoms have been associated with poorer physical status, especially with difficulty in breathing and fatigue, as well as declines in social functioning and treatment status (Kurtz *et al.*, 2002; Okuyama *et al.*, 2001). Furthermore, use of depressive coping strategies, such as brooding and withdrawing from other people, have been found to predict shorter survival times (Faller & Schmidt, 2004).

The physical and psychosocial symptoms of lung cancer can interfere with daily functioning and quality of life (see 'Quality of life'). Reductions in quality of life have been associated with shorter survival times and with tumours that are less likely to respond to treatment (Montazeri *et al.*, 1998). Medical treatments for advanced lung cancer focus on controlling symptoms so that patients can maintain quality of life (Simmonds, 1999).

Clinical implications

Psychosocial interventions can complement traditional treatment for lung cancer by helping patients cope with symptoms, decrease distress and depression, and improve quality of life (McCorkle *et al.*, 1989). Families of patients with lung cancer also experience considerable distress (Haley *et al.*, 2001) and may benefit from psychosocial interventions that help them to cope with their loved one's disease, treatment and possible death.

Psychosocial interventions can also be used in prevention because many of the risk factors for lung cancer are behaviours that can be modified. Prevention efforts primarily focus on encouraging people not to start smoking and on smoking cessation because of the high risk associated with smoking and the reduction in risk attributed to smoking cessation (Peto *et al.*, 2000). Many efficacious and cost-effective smoking cessation programmes have been developed, but advances need to be made in the dissemination of these programmes as well as the achievement of long-term maintenance (Niaura & Abrams, 2002; see 'Tobacco use'). Other behavioural risk factors that could be targets of psychosocial interventions are dietary changes to increase consumption of fruits and vegetables and avoidance of situations that involve exposure to tobacco smoke.

Risk factors for lung cancer may be used to identify people who are at high risk for the disease. Spiral computed tomography (CT) scanning is being used in several screening trials to examine the feasibility and effectiveness of detecting lung cancer at earlier stages (Gohagan *et al.*, 2004). Long-term outcomes from these trials will help determine screening recommendations for people who are at high risk. Psychosocial interventions may help lessen the anxiety associated with screening and improve adherence to recommendations (see 'Screening: cancer').

Conclusions

Patients with lung cancer could benefit from psychosocial interventions that focus on maintaining quality of life and reducing distress. Psychosocial interventions could also be used to help people decrease their risk for lung cancer by modifying behaviours that put them at high risk such as smoking and poor diet.

(See also 'Cancer: general,' 'Coping with chronic illness' and 'Coping with death and dying.')

REFERENCES

Ardies, C.M. (2003). Inflammation as cause for scar cancers of the lung. *Integrative Cancer Therapies*, 2, 238–46.

Boffetta, P. (2004). Epidemiology of environmental and occupational cancer. *Oncogene*, 23, 6392–403.

Degner, L. & Sloan, J. (1995). Symptom distress in newly diagnosed ambulatory cancer patients and as a predictor of survival in lung cancer. *Journal of Pain Symptom Management*, 19, 423–31.

Economou, P., Lechner, J.F. & Samet, J.M. (1994). Familial and genetic factors in the pathogenesis of lung cancer. In J.M. Samet (Ed.). *Epidemiology of lung cancer* (pp. 353–96). New York: Marcel Dekker.

Faller, H. & Schmidt, M. (2004). Prognostic value of depressive coping and depression in survival of lung cancer patients. *Psycho-oncology*, 13, 359–63.

Gohagan, J., Marcus, P., Fagerstrom, R., Pinsky, P., Kramer, B., Prorok, P. & Writing Committee, Lung Cancer Screening Research Group. (2004). Baseline findings of a randomized feasibility trial of lung cancer screening with spiral CT scan vs. chest radiograph: the Lung Screening Study of the National Cancer Institute. *Chest*, 126, 114–21.

Haley, W.E., LaMonde, L.A., Han, B., Narramore, S. & Schonwetter, R. (2001). Family caregiving in hospice: effects on psychological and health functioning among spousal caregivers of hospice

patients with lung cancer or dementia. *Hospice Journal: Physical, Psychosocial, and Pastoral Care of the Dying*, 15, 1–18.

Hollen, P.J., Gralla, R.J., Kris, M.G., Eberly, S.W. & Cox, C. (1999). Normative data and trends in quality of life from the Lung Cancer Symptom Scale (LCSS). *Support Care Cancer*, 7, 140–8.

Kramer, J.A. (1999). Use of the Hospital Anxiety and Depression Scale (HADS) in the assessment of depression in patients with inoperable lung cancer. *Palliative Medicine*, 13, 353–4.

Kurtz, M.E., Kurtz, J.C., Stommel, M., Given, C.W. & Given, B. (2002). Predictors of depressive symptomatology of geriatric patients with lung cancer: a longitudinal analysis. *Psycho-oncology*, 11, 12–22.

McCorkle, R., Benoliel, J.Q., Donaldson, G. *et al.* (1989). A randomized clinical trial of home nursing care for lung cancer patients. *Cancer*, 64, 1375–82.

Miller, A.B., Altenburg, H., Bueno-De-Mesquita, B. *et al.* (2003). Fruits and vegetables and lung cancer: findings from the European Prospective Investigation into Cancer and Nutrition. *International Journal of Cancer*, 108, 269–76.

Montazeri, A., Gillis, C.R. & McEwen, J. (1998). Quality of life in patients with lung cancer: a review of literature from 1970 to 1995. *Chest*, 113, 467–81.

Niaura, R. & Abrams, D.B. (2002). Smoking cessation: progress, priorities, and

prospectus. *Journal of Consulting and Clinical Psychology*, 70, 494–509.

Okuyama, T., Tanaka, K., Akechi, T. *et al.* (2001). Fatigue in ambulatory patients with advanced lung cancer: prevalence, correlated factors, and screening. *Journal of Pain and Symptom Management*, 22, 554–64.

Peto, R., Darby, S., Deo, H. *et al.* (2000). Smoking, smoking cessation, and lung cancer in the UK since 1950: combination of national statistics with two case-control studies. *British Medical Journal*, 321, 323–9.

Simmonds, P. (1999). Managing patients with lung cancer. New guidelines should improve standards of care. *British Medical Journal*, 319, 527–8.

Stewart, B.W. & Kleihues, P. (Eds.). (2003). *World Cancer Report*. Lyon, France: International Agency for Research on Cancer Press.

United States Department of Health & Human Services (USDHHS). (2004). *The health consequences of smoking: a report of the Surgeon General*. Atlanta, GA.: US Department of Health and Human Services, Centers for Disease Control and Prevention, National Center for Chronic Disease Prevention and Health Promotion, Office on Smoking and Health.

Cancer: prostate

Stephen J. Lepore[1] and Katherine J. Roberts[2]

[1]Temple University
[2]Columbia University

Prostate cancer is one of the most common solid tumour malignancies in developed countries (Pisani *et al.*, 2002) and a leading cause of cancer death in American and European men (Bray *et al.*, 2002; American Cancer Society, 2005). This chapter highlights the effects of prostate cancer on quality of life and reviews the behavioural and psychosocial interventions designed to educate men about prostate cancer, enhance decision-making, or improve quality of life.

Quality of life

Prostate cancer and its treatments result in disease-specific and more general problems in quality of life (Eton & Lepore, 2002) (see 'Quality of Life'). The most common disease-specific problems are urinary and sexual dysfunction. Within a year after treatment, urinary problems often subside, but sexual problems tend to persist (e.g. Lubeck *et al.*, 1999). In men with localized disease, general problems, such as difficulties in social-, emotional- and physical-functioning are reported considerably less often than genito-urinary problems, and may not occur at all in some men (e.g. Lubeck *et al.*, 1999; Bisson *et al.*, 2002; Lepore *et al.*, 2003). Men with progressive disease are more likely to report social–emotional difficulties, as well as chronic pain and fatigue (e.g. Albertsen *et al.*, 1997). It is not yet clear how pharmacological and surgical control of progressive prostate cancer influences general quality of life outcomes.

Interventions

Informed decision-making about testing

Prostate cancer is often indolent and frequently affects men with other life-threatening illnesses, so it is difficult to evaluate the effects of screening and treatments on prostate cancer outcomes. This creates uncertainty over how best to detect and manage prostate cancer. Behavioural scientists have responded by creating decision support interventions that aim to increase men's knowledge about different screening and treatment options, assist them in clarifying their values for different outcomes related to screening and treatment, and improve decision quality.

Early prostate cancer is typically asymptomatic, so screening tests such as the digital rectal exam (DRE) and the prostate specific antigen (PSA) blood test provide the best methods of detection. Currently, screening populations for prostate cancer is not recommended by the US Preventive Services Task Force (US Preventive Services Task Force, 2002), mainly because there is no solid evidence that screening enhances survival odds. There is, however,

general agreement in the medical community about the need to educate patients to make individualized, informed choices about prostate cancer screening (e.g. Smith *et al.*, 2001).

In recent years, a spate of randomized controlled trials (RCTs) have evaluated the effects of decision-support interventions on screening decisions (for review, see Briss *et al.*, 2004). In one comprehensive trial (Davison *et al.*, 2002), men were randomly assigned to receive verbal and written information about the pros and cons of prostate cancer screening either prior to a periodic health exam (intervention group) or subsequent to the health exam and a follow-up interview (control group). Relative to controls, men in the intervention group took a more active role in the screening decision and had lower decisional conflict. The authors also found that the intervention did not create anxiety in men or alter their low rates of screening (see also 'Screening: cancer').

Research on decision-support interventions suggests that even minimal contact (e.g. an educational pamphlet) can increase knowledge (e.g. Volk *et al.*, 1999; Schapira & VanRuiswyk, 2000; e.g. Frosch *et al.*, 2001, 2003; Partin *et al.*, 2004). Intensive interventions may be warranted, however, because the knowledge gains tend to be modest, even though they are statistically significant in minimal interventions. One study showed that a decision support intervention led to more realistic beliefs about the benefits of prostate cancer screening (Schapira & VanRuiswyk, 2000). Several controlled trials (Volk *et al.*, 1999; Frosch *et al.*, 2001; Partin, Nelson *et al.*, 2004) showed lower screening interest among men who viewed a videotape, *PSA decision: what you should know*. The contrast between the results of these latter trials using the video and those of Davison *et al.*'s trial using verbal and written information raises questions about the specific factors that influence men's decisions in these studies. Given the controversial nature of prostate cancer screening, two important goals of these interventions should be to ensure that: (a) men's decisions are informed (i.e. they know their risk for prostate cancer, as well as potential benefits and limitations of testing), and (b) men's behaviours are congruent with their values or preferences (i.e. there are no barriers to testing if they want to test or undue pressure to test if they do not want to test). Further, there is a need to examine the effect of decision-support interventions on men at high-risk for prostate cancer, including first-degree relatives and men of African descent.

Informed decision-making about treatment

Medical uncertainties related to patient prognosis and responsiveness to different treatments makes treatment decisions very complex. In addition, there are no data from randomized trials that directly compare different types of treatment in men with similar stages of disease. Thus, it has been recommended that physicians use independent medical judgement when formulating treatment decisions and tailor the treatment to patients' values and preferences (Scherr *et al.*, 2003). In practice, therapeutic recommendations vary with the type of specialist a patient consults. In a United States nationwide random sample of urologists and radiation oncologists, most radiation oncologists (72%) believed that their therapy was just as good as radical prostatectomy for men with localized prostate cancer, whereas most urologists (93%) believed that radical prostatectomy was the treatment of choice (Fowler *et al.*, 2000).

Most men with prostate cancer are expected to and prefer to be involved in treatment decisions (Davison *et al.*, 2002). Their decision is influenced by many sources, including medical professionals, family and friends, and the media. The quality of the input from these different sources is highly variable. For example, in a review of 546 publicly available education materials on prostate cancer treatment, 502 did not describe all standard treatments and the rest did not provide sufficient information about side effects or other factors relevant to decision making (Fagerlin *et al.*, 2004). Physician input possibly has the greatest effect on patients' decisions but, here too, the quality of the input is not always adequate. Crawford *et al.* (1997) interviewed 1000 men with prostate cancer and 200 urologists and found that almost 100% of the urologists stated that they always discussed important considerations such as options for no therapy, life expectancy with and without therapy, patient preferences, costs and changes in sexual function, yet only about 20% of patients recalled similar discussions.

Quality of life interventions

Most psychosocial interventions for men with prostate cancer aim to improve quality of life by reducing symptoms, increasing knowledge, improving coping skills and creating supportive social ties. By increasing knowledge about the disease, interventions can help patients set realistic expectations about recovery and the causes of symptoms, and, perhaps, gain a sense of control over their thoughts, feelings and behaviours. Patients also can learn specific behaviours and coping skills for improving general health and functioning or dealing with stress and symptoms. Interventions that bring patients together in dyads or groups can facilitate the exchange of support and provide models of adaptive behaviour (see 'Support interventions').

There have been relatively few controlled, psychosocial interventions in men with prostate cancer. In one RCT, Lepore *et al.* (2003) compared quality of life outcomes in men recently treated for localized prostate cancer after they received either standard medical care or one of two types of multi-week, group education interventions – education alone or education plus facilitated peer discussion. Both intervention groups resulted in improved knowledge, physical functioning and health behaviours, but only the education-plus-discussion group resulted in more stable employment and reduction of sexual dysfunction. Both interventions tended to be more beneficial to persons with less formal education. In another study, Mishel *et al.* (2002) found that a nurse-delivered, multi-week telephone intervention, consisting of education and cognitive restructuring, improved problem-solving skills, enhanced appraisals of illness and improved urinary control among men treated for localized prostate cancer. Much work remains to be done in this area, including identifying the best type of intervention for men at different stages of disease.

Conclusions

Despite its prevalence, potential lethality and well-documented negative effects on men's genito-urinary functioning, there has been relatively little behavioural research aimed at reducing men's risk for prostate cancer, enhancing decision-making related to screening and treatment, or improving quality of life. Our review of the current literature suggests some promising directions for behavioural intervention, clinical care and future research.

In terms of quality of life, many side effects of treatments tend to subside within a year among men treated for localized disease, with the possible exception of sexual dysfunction. The impact on quality of life of men with metastatic disease may be greater, particularly with respect to symptom control and mental health. Descriptive research on quality of life outcomes will need to be updated continually, because medical treatment protocols evolve rapidly and may affect quality of life in ways that are as yet unknown. For example, hormonal therapy is increasingly being used in men with localized prostate cancer, but the literature provides scant information on how this therapy might affect quality of life.

Much of the current behavioural research is focused on decision-making related to screening or treatment. Interventions related to screening are effective at improving knowledge, yet the effects on screening behaviours and patient–physician communication are ambiguous. It also is not clear what effect decision-support interventions might have on men at high-risk for prostate cancer, including first-degree relatives and men of African descent. Interventions related to treatment also appear to be effective at increasing knowledge, but it is not entirely clear how they affect the decision-making process. It appears that most men rely on their physician's opinion, which may be biased toward his or her specialty (e.g. surgery, radiation), and does not necessarily take into account patients' values and preferences. It is critical for behavioural scientists to develop innovative, effective and economical ways to enhance informed and shared decision making related to treatment choices (see 'Medical decision-making'). There are new approaches on the horizon, such as a CD-ROM-based programme that uses a metaphor of rooms in a virtual health centre to organize information (Diefenbach & Butz 2004), but they have yet to be rigorously evaluated.

There are few high quality studies on the effectiveness of behavioural interventions aimed at quality of life. Early evidence suggests that these interventions can improve men's knowledge, coping skills and functional wellbeing. More work is needed to document the relative costs and benefits of different interventions, to respond to the needs of men with advanced disease and to address the potential needs of caregivers. Future research also should consider how to develop interventions that can be tailored to the unique needs of different individuals or groups. Intelligent computer-based systems may be a useful approach for men who will not attend groups or who want more information than they can feasibly get from a health educator or nurse during a brief telephone contact.

Finally, it should be noted that morbidity, mortality and quality of life endpoints are not equally distributed across social groups (American Cancer Society, 2005). Men of African descent, in particular, have an excess burden of morbidity and mortality due to prostate cancer. Less educated, poorer and minority men also suffer greater declines in their quality of life and take longer to recover from treatments (Lepore *et al.*, 2003; Litwin *et al.*, 1999). Poverty,

lower educational achievement and minority status tend to be associated with less knowledge about prostate cancer (Smith *et al.*, 1997; Lepore *et al.*, 2003), suggesting that education interventions should be especially fruitful with this population. However, we do not know whether the currently available approaches to educating men about prostate cancer or facilitating decision-making will be effective with poorer and minority men.

(See also 'Cancer: general', 'Coping with chronic illness' and 'Coping with death and dying'.)

REFERENCES

Albertsen, P. C., Aaronson, N. K., Muller, M. J., Keller, S. D. & Ware, J. E., Jr. (1997). Health-related quality of life among patients with metastatic prostate cancer. *Urology*, **49**, 207–16.

American Cancer Society. (2005). *Cancer Facts and Figures 2005*. Atlanta, GA: American Cancer Society, Inc.

Bisson, J. I., Chubb, H. L., Bennett, S. *et al.* (2002). The prevalence and predictors of psychological distress in patients with early localized prostate cancer. *BJU International*, **90**, 56–61.

Bray, F., Sankila, R., Ferlay, J. & Parkin, D. M. (2002). Estimates of cancer incidence and mortality in Europe in 1995. *European Journal of Cancer*, **38**, 99–166.

Briss, P., Rimer, B. Reilley, B. *et al.* (2004). Promoting informed decisions about cancer screening in communities and healthcare systems. *American Journal of Preventive Medicine*, **26**, 67–80.

Crawford, E. D., Bennett, C. L., Stone, N. N. *et al.* (1997). Comparison of perspectives on prostate cancer: analyses of survey data. *Urology*, **50**, 366–72.

Davison, B. J., Gleave, M. E., Goldenberg, S. L. *et al.* (2002). Assessing information and decision preferences of men with prostate cancer and their partners. *Cancer Nursing*, **25**, 42–9.

Diefenbach, M. & Butz, B. (2004). A multimedia interactive education system for prostate cancer patients: development and preliminary evaluation. *Journal of Medical Internet Research*, **6**, e3.

Eton, D. T. & Lepore, S. J. (2002). Prostate cancer and health-related quality of life: a review of the literature. *Psycho-oncology*, **11**, 307–26.

Fagerlin, A., Rovner, D., Stableford, S. *et al.* (2004). Patient education materials about the treatment of early-stage prostate cancer: a critical review. *Annals of Internal Medicine*, **140**, 721–8.

Fowler, F. J., Jr., McNaughton Collins, M., Albertsen, P. C. *et al.* (2000). Comparison of recommendations by urologists and radiation oncologists for treatment of clinically localized prostate cancer. *JAMA: Journal of the American Medical Association*, **283**, 3217–22.

Frosch, D. L., Kaplan, R. M., Felitti, V. (2001). The evaluation of two methods to facilitate shared decision making for men considering the prostate-specific antigen test. *Journal of General Internal Medicine*, **16**, 391–8.

Frosch, D. L., Kaplan, R. M. & Felitti, V. J. (2003). A randomized controlled trial comparing internet and video to facilitate patient education for men considering the prostate specific antigen test. *Journal of General Internal Medicine*, **18**, 781–7.

Lepore, S. J., Helgeson, V. S., Eton, D. T. & Schulz, R. (2003). Improving quality of life in men with prostate cancer: a randomized controlled trial of group education interventions. *Health Psychology*, **22**, 443–52.

Litwin, M. S., McGuigan, K. A., Shpall, A. I. & Dhanani, N. (1999). Recovery of health related quality of life in the year after radical prostatectomy: early experience. *The Journal of Urology*, **161**, 515–19.

Lubeck, D. P., Litwin, M. S., Henning, J. M. *et al.* (1999). Changes in health-related quality of life in the first year after treatment for prostate cancer: results from CaPSURE. *Urology*, **53**, 180–6.

Mishel, M. H., Belyea, M., Germino, B. B. *et al.* (2002). Helping patients with localized prostate carcinoma manage uncertainty and treatment side effects: nurse-delivered psychoeducational intervention over the telephone. *Cancer*, **94**, 1854–66.

Partin, M. R., Nelson, D., Radosevich, D. *et al.* (2004). Randomized trial examining the effect of two prostate cancer screening educational interventions on patient knowledge, preferences, and behaviors. *Journal of General Internal Medicine*, **19**, 835–42.

Pisani, P., Bray, F. & Parkin, D. M. (2002). Estimates of the world-wide prevalence of cancer for 25 sites in the adult population. *International Journal of Cancer*, **97**, 72–81.

Schapira, M. M. & VanRuiswyk, J. (2000). The effect of an illustrated pamphlet decision-aid on the use of prostate cancer screening tests. *The Journal of Family Practice*, **49**, 418–24.

Scherr, D., Swindle, P. W. & Scardino, P. T. (2003). National comprehensive cancer network guidelines for the management of prostate cancer. *Urology*, **61**(2 Suppl. 1), 14–24.

Smith, G. E., DeHaven, M. J., Grundig, J. P. & Wilson, G. R. (1997). African-American males and prostate cancer: assessing knowledge levels in the community. *Journal of the National Medical Association*, **89**, 387–91.

Smith, R. A., von Eschenbach, A. C., Wender, R. *et al.* (2001). American Cancer Society guidelines for the early detection of cancer: update of early detection guidelines for prostate, colorectal, and endometrial cancers. *CA: Cancer Journal for Clinicians*, **51**, 7–38.

US Preventive Services Task Force. (2002). *Prostate cancer screening*. Washington, DC: Department of Health and Human Services.

Volk, R. J., Cass, A. R. & Spann, S. J. (1999). A randomized controlled trial of shared decision making for prostate cancer screening. *Archives of Family Medicine*, **8**, 333–40.

Cancer: skin

Ron Borland and Suzanne Dobbinson

Victoria Health Centre for Tobacco Control

Epidemiology of skin cancer

Skin cancers can be broadly classified into two types, melanomas and non-melanomas. Melanomas are cancer of the melanocytes, which lie in the basal layer of the epidermis. Melanomas, unless detected at an early stage have a high fatality rate. Non-melanocytic skin cancers include two major types, basal cell carcinomas and squamous cell carcinomas (SCCs). Both of these forms of skin cancer are relatively benign; however, if neglected they can result in significant morbidity and, in some cases, death (especially from SCC).

The incidence of skin cancer is rising among fair-skinned populations throughout the world with the highest rates in Australia. People whose skin burns easily are at the highest risk. The principle aetiological factor for skin cancer is ultraviolet (UV) radiation, mainly from the sun's rays (Marks & Hill, 1992; IARC, 1992). Around two-thirds of daily UV radiation is transmitted in the two hours each side of true midday. In tropical areas, UV levels are high all year round. In temperate zones, UV levels only reach high levels in the summer months, except at high altitudes, or in reflecting environments where the levels can be much higher than normal. Nonetheless, some sun exposure is important for production of Vitamin D and total sun avoidance is not recommended. Vitamin D deficiency causes various bone diseases and may increase risk of immune disorders and even cancer (Vanchieri, 2004; Luca & Ponsonby, 2002).

There is no clear consensus on the mechanisms by which UV radiation leads to skin cancers. One major problem is the difficulty of measuring UV exposure across the lifespan. There is some evidence that melanoma may be a result of both acute episodic over-exposure, best indexed by sunburn and very high levels of cumulative exposure (such as is achieved in tropical and subtropical climates). By contrast, non-melanoma skin cancers, especially SCC (English et al., 1997), may be more closely linked to total UV exposure. Exposure in childhood and adolescence may be more important than adult exposure for later development of skin cancer. Regular use of sunscreen (which reduces UV exposure) can reduce squamous cell carcinoma (Green et al., 1999). Reliance on sunscreen alone is not considered adequate protection and may lead to extended exposure especially during intentional tanning (Autier et al., 1999).

Prevention

To reduce skin cancer risk involves reducing UV exposure, particularly acute over-exposure (or sunburn) and to focus these preventative activities on young people, while not neglecting the benefits that may come from appropriate exposure at all ages.

The most effective ways of reducing UV exposure are staying out of the sun when UV levels are high by staying indoors or seeking shade, covering up with clothing, wearing hats and using sunscreens. The sunscreens recommended vary from country to country, but generally a broad spectrum sun protection factor (SPF) 15 or greater is considered adequate, that is, sunscreens that block out around 94% of all UV radiation. In high UV exposure environments, SPF 30 sunscreen may be necessary.

The linchpin for the systematic scientific approach to melanoma control is good data: epidemiological data on the incidence and mortality from the disease, data on identified behavioural risk factors, data on the value of the risk behaviour to 'at risk' groups and data from the systematic evaluation of interventions.

Measuring sun protection

Strategies to measure sun protection fall into four broad categories: observation; diaries; recall of specific events; and reports of overall behaviour. Measuring sun protection behaviour is difficult because the need for it varies as a function of time of day, season of the year, time outside and prevailing weather conditions. Further, the extent to which extra protective action is required will vary as a function of the normal dress for the activities engaged in, e.g. swimmers need to rely more on sunscreen than golfers. This means that it is difficult for people to estimate what is usual across all kinds of activities and situations. Context-specific measures may be more valid. People tend to over-estimate the extent to which they take protective actions (at least in the context of a population who are well informed of the need to take such actions). This has been most clearly demonstrated in children. Estimates of sun protection based on overall reports should be treated with caution.

Direct observation, using observers or photographs can provide an accurate and potentially unbiased estimate of behaviour. However, it is restricted to visibly observable sun protection (thus excluding sunscreen use) and to public places (for practical and ethical reasons). It is also not practical to observe individuals over extensive periods, so data may not be representative of the people observed, though it can be of the situations observed.

Diaries of sun protective actions and outdoor experiences can be kept reliably (Girgis et al., 1993) and thus they have the potential to accurately describe individual behaviour. However, there are limits on how long people will keep them for, and demand characteristics associated with keeping them may lead to changes in sun protection behaviour, either for social desirability reasons or to minimize the amount of recording necessary.

Recall of specific events can only reasonably be done for a relatively short period (days). Measurement cannot change the actual behaviour, but recall can be selectively influenced by demand characteristics and may also vary with the salience of the activities. Attempts to validate specific recall with observational strategies suggest they are reasonably accurate, at least for behaviours in public places. Specific recall is likely to be representative for situations, although it may not be for individuals. It is probably the best method for monitoring population-wide trends.

It is also important to assess exposure. Monitoring sunburn incidence is useful as a marker of over exposure and risk, some measurement issues are reviewed by Shoveller and Lovato (2001). Polysulphone badges can help to quantify potential exposures for different body sites, or help to validate other estimates (Gies et al., 2004).

The challenge

Risk of UV exposure is related to lifestyle. Exposure can be incidental to outdoor activity or can be actively sought, as in sunbathing. There is limited capacity for getting people to spend less time outside, although it is possible to get people to schedule more of that time outside peak UV periods. The major focus needs to be on encouraging people to take suitable precautions when they are outside. Young people, especially males, spend more time out in the sun and expose more of their skin to the sun. Young people, especially women, are more likely to rely on sunscreens for sun protection. Men are more likely to wear sunhats than women, but women are more likely to avoid the sun or use sunscreens as protective measures. Both qualitative and quantitative research has identified a desire for a suntan as a major barrier to sun protection. Suntans are related to a self-image of being active, healthy and attractive, and others see suntanned individuals in a similar way (Arthey & Clarke, 1995). Other factors inhibiting sun protection include the perception that protective clothes and hats are unfashionable, particularly in the young; and, especially among men and older people, a reluctance to use sunscreen. Consistent with this, Hill et al. (1992) found that young people are more likely to get sunburnt than older people, and men are more likely to get burnt than women.men of African descent.

Behaviour change

The first stage of a prevention campaign involves informing the public about the risk; about strategies to reduce risk; and that risk reduction is worth considering (see 'Health promotion'). Health education programmes in schools and workplaces have been shown to produce improvements in sun protection, especially where they have used programmes that actively engaged participants. In many countries most, or all, of the population are at risk, so comprehensive mass-reach, population-based behaviour change strategies are required (Marks & Hill, 1992). These should include education and other activity directed at personal behaviour change, combined with activity directed at changing aspects of the physical or social context to make sun protection easier and/or more desirable.

One of the most extensive skin cancer prevention programmes has occurred in Victoria, Australia. In 1980, a small-scale campaign called 'Slip! Slop! Slap!' (Slip on a shirt!, Slop on sunscreen! And Slap on a hat!) was launched. By 1987 there was virtually total community awareness of the need for sun protection, but inadequate levels of behaviour change. In 1988, a more extensive campaign called 'SunSmart' was launched. At its peak it had a budget of about 30c US per person per year (for a population of around 4 million). The campaign aimed to change public perceptions of the acceptability of sun protection by linking it with fashionable images in TV and other advertising. The advertising also helped put skin cancer on the public agenda, which was important in encouraging community involvement both in education and in fostering appropriate structural change to support sun protection behaviour. For example, availability of fashionable sun protective hats and clothes, cheaper sunscreens, more appropriate outdoor policies in schools and workplaces, and increased provision of shade (Montague et al., 2001).

The early years of this campaign were associated with a marked increase in sun protection behaviour: hat use and sunscreen use increased markedly, as did the proportion of the population avoiding at least part of the peak UV radiation period of 11am–3pm (Hill et al., 1993). Furthermore, reported desire for a suntan fell as did personal beliefs about the desirability of a tan and beliefs that others preferred tans. Continual monitoring of community reactions revealed threats to good practice. People said that often sun protection took effort, and they wanted more good reasons to act. They asked for graphic images of the consequences of inaction. This was done and the motivation to act increased. While the campaign was well resourced it was able to improve or sustain good practice, but when it reduced in magnitude, there was some evidence of a drift back to less 'sun-smart' practices (Dobbinson et al., 2002; Dobbinson, 2004). This reversal provides extra evidence that the campaign had contributed to the community change. Keeping the public aware of the reasons why sun protection is important seems to be necessary for sustained attitudinal and behaviour change (for theories of health behaviour and behaviour change see 'Health belief model', 'Theory of planned behaviour' and 'Transtheoretical model of behaviour change').

Early detection

Because skin cancers grow in the skin, they are readily observable, particularly if they grow in easily visible areas. Thus it is potentially easy to detect them at an early stage of development when treatment is almost always successful. A variety of strategies have been used to encourage one-off self-screening. These can lead to an increase in melanoma detection through more people presenting to doctors with suspicious lesions (e.g. Doherty & MacKie, 1988) (see 'Screening: cancer'). Similar effects have occurred through increased community awareness of skin cancer. There is, however, still a need to improve people's understanding of what to look for. For example, most Australians believe melanomas are raised lesions even though virtually all early melanomas are flat (Borland et al., 1992), the exception being nodular melanomas (Kelly et al., 2003). Educational resources are needed that enable people to accurately distinguish potentially dangerous spots from those that are clearly benign.

There is increasing medical interest in instituting systematic programmes of self-screening or screening by professionals where all or most of the body could be checked on a regular basis. As yet there is no evidence about whether this would increase detection sufficiently to justify its adoption, even for high-risk groups. Behavioural research is needed to determine levels and frequencies of self-screening people will persist with. Efforts to maximize screening will involve developing strategies to minimize embarrassment, provide the skills to do the self-examination properly, ensure appropriate confidence in decisions to engender appropriate action, and ensure that people perform self-examinations regularly. A balance will need to be found between the potential benefits to health and what people are willing or able to do.

When people have identified spots which are of concern, it is crucial that they seek medical advice as quickly as possible. There is no good data available on the extent of delay in presenting, but some people do delay enough to affect their prognosis. Research is needed to identify modifiable determinants of delay (see 'Delay in seeking help').

A self-detection programme depends on more than an educated and willing public. It also requires doctors and other health practitioners who have the necessary knowledge and skills in accurate diagnosis and management, and who encourage the public to engage in appropriate self-screening.

(See also 'Cancer: general'.)

REFERENCES

Arthey, S. & Clarke, V. A. (1995). Suntanning and sun protection: a review of the psychological literature. *Social Science Medicine*, **40**, 265–74.

Autier, P., Dore, J. F., Negrier, S. *et al.* (1999). Sunscreen use & duration of sun exposure: a double-blind, randomized trial. *Journal of the National Cancer Institute*, **91**, 1304–9.

Borland, R., Marks, R. & Noy, S. (1992). Public knowledge about characteristics of moles and melanomas. *Australian Journal of Public Health*, **16**, 370–5.

Dobbinson, S. (2004). Reaction to the 2000/01 SunSmart Campaign: results from a telephone survey of Victorians. In *SunSmart Evaluation Studies No. 7*. Melbourne: The Cancer Council of Victoria. (www.sunsmart.com.au/s/facts/research.htm)

Dobbinson, S., Hill, D. & White, V. (2002). Trends in sun protection: use of sunscreen, hats and clothing over the past decade in Melbourne, Australia. In: *UV radiation and its effects – an update 2002*, Proceedings of a workshop held on 26–28 March 2002 in Christchurch New Zealand. Organized by the National Institute of Water and Atmospheric Research (NIWA) 2002.

Doherty, V. R. & MacKie, R. M. (1988). Experience of a public education programme on early detection of cutaneous malignant melanomas. *British Medical Journal*, **297**, 388–91.

English, D. R., Armstrong, B. K., Kricker, A. & Fleming, C. (1997). Sunlight, & Cancer. *Cancer Causes and Control*, **8**, 271–83.

Gies P., Roy, C. & Udelhofen, P. (2004). Solar and ultraviolet radiation. In D. Hill *et al.* (Eds.). *Prevention of skin cancer* (pp. 21–54). Dordrecht, Netherlands: Kluwer Academic Publishers.

Girgis, A., Sanson-Fisher, R. W., Tripodi, D. A. & Golding T. (1993). Evaluation of interventions to improve solar protection in primary schools. *Health Education Quarterly*, **20**, 275–87.

Green, A., Williams, G., Neal, R. *et al.* (1999). Daily sunscreen application and betacarotene supplementation in prevention of basal-cell and squamous-cell carcinomas of the skin: a randomised controlled trial. *The Lancet*, **354**, 723–9.

Hill, D., White, V., Marks, R. *et al.* (1992). Melanoma prevention: behavioral and nonbehavioral factors in sunburn among an Australian urban population. *Preventive Medicine*, **21**, 654–69.

Hill, D., White, V., Marks, R. & Borland, R. (1993). Changes in sun-related attitudes and behaviours, and reduced sunburn prevalence in a population at high risk of melanoma. *European Journal of Cancer Prevention*, **2**, 447–56.

International Agency for Research on Cancer (IARC). (1992). *Solar and ultraviolet radiation*. In World Health Organization (Ed.). Volume 55, Iarc Monographs on the Evaluation of Carcinogenic Risks to Humans. Lyon, France: IARC.

Luca, R. M. & Ponsonby, A. (2002). Ultraviolet radiation and health: friend and foe. *The Medical Journal of Australia*, **177**, 594–7.

Kelly, J. W., Chamberlain, A. J., Staples, M. P. & McAvoy, B. (2003). Nodular melanoma: no longer as simple as ABC. *Australian Family Physician*, **32**, 706–9.

Marks, R. & Hill, D. (1992). (Eds.). *The public health approach to melanoma control: prevention and early detection*. Geneva: International Union Against Cancer (UICC).

Montague, M., Borland, R. & Sinclair, C. (2001). Slip! Slop! Slap! and SunSmart, 1980–2000; Skin cancer control and 20 years of population-based campaigning. *Health, Education & Behavior*, **28**, 290–305.

Shoveller, J. A. & Lovato, C. Y. (2001). Measuring self-reported sunburn: challenges and recommendations. *Chronic Diseases in Canada*, **22**, 75–87.

Vanchieri, C. (2004). Studies shedding light on Vitamin D and cancer. *Journal of the National Cancer Institute*, **96**, 735–6.

Carotid artery disease and treatment

Jan Stygall and Stanton Newman

University College London

Thrombo-embolism and haemodynamic ischaemia secondary to atheromatous stenotic disease of the carotid and vertebral arteries are important causes of ischaemic stroke. In those patients with carotid stenosis the risk of stroke has been directly related to the severity of stenosis and the presence of symptoms (Inzitari et al., 2000). The average risk of stroke following a transient ischaemic attack (TIA) is about 8% in the first year and then 5% per annum, but, in patients with severe carotid stenosis, the risk even with medical treatment increases up to 28% over 2 years (NASCETC, 1991). Detection of significant carotid or vertebral artery stenosis after a TIA or stroke provides the opportunity for secondary preventive treatment of the stenosis to prevent a further stroke (see also 'Stroke').

Carotid endarterectomy (CEA), the surgical removal of the atheromatous plaque, was first performed fifty years ago and is, at present, still considered the gold standard in the treatment of severe symptomatic disease (Grace, 2004). The procedure usually involves the insertion of a silicon tube (shunt) directly into the opened internal and common carotid arteries. Blood then flows through the shunt from the carotid artery to the brain allowing the removal of the atherosclerotic plaque from the artery wall. A number of randomized clinical trials on selected groups of symptomatic and asymptomatic patients have indicated the benefits of CEA (NASCET, 1991; ACAS, 1995; ECST, 1998). However, it has been suggested by some investigators that there is insufficient evidence to recommend CEA in asymptomatic patients (Rabe & Sievert, 2004). Recently, the MRC Asymptomatic Carotid Surgery Trial (ASCT) Collaborative Group published a study indicating a positive effect of CEA in reducing stroke and death in asymptomatic patients over a 5-year period (MRC ASCT, 2004). However, in certain high risk patients (2–7%) CEA can in fact cause a stroke (NASCET, 1991; ECST, 1991). It has been suggested that perioperative risk of endarterectomy is higher in centres with surgeons of less experience (Alhaddad, 2004; Rabe & Sievert, 2004).

Factors which can lead to complications following CEA, include older age, female sex and the presence of co-morbidities such as obstructive pulmonary disease, advanced coronary artery disease and congestive heart failure (see 'Chronic obstructive pulmonary disease' and 'coronary heart disease: heart failure'). The majority of patients with carotid stenosis are older and have other co-morbidities. Various anatomical problems may also restrict the number of patients eligible for CEA. Due to these issues less invasive and potentially safer procedures have been explored.

Carotid artery balloon dilatation (angioplasty), and more recently carotid artery stenting (CAS) have become an alternative to CEA, especially for high risk sub-groups of patients. This technique involves the advancing of a balloon-tipped catheter into the carotid artery, the balloon is then inflated dilating the artery at which point a mesh tube (stent) which supports the artery is then opened to fill the artery and left in place. Five hundred and four patients with carotid artery stenosis were randomized to either CEA or angioplasty (26% with stents) in the Carotid and Vertebral Artery Transluminal Angioplasty Study (CAVATAS) similar major risks and efficacy of prevention of stroke were reported for both procedures, however CEA was associated with more minor complications such as cranial nerve injuries and haematomas (CAVATAS, 2001). The main complication of CAS is related to plaque fracture occurring in the carotid artery during balloon inflation. Some of this atherosclerotic material may become dislodged into the cerebral circulation potentially leading to a stroke. Several emboli protection devices (EPDs) have been developed to reduce the risk of embolization of atherosclerotic debris into the cerebral circulation during CAS to decrease the risk of stroke. Ongoing prospective randomized studies of lower-risk patients comparing the two procedures and the use of emboli protection devices are currently being performed.

Whilst frank stroke is an important cause of disability various studies have provided evidence that suggests that carotid stenosis is also associated with more subtle neuropsychological problems in both those with symptomatic and asymptomatic disease (e.g. Auperin et al., 1996; Kaplan et al., 1996; Rao, 2002). However, the majority of studies have been cross-sectional in design. Interestingly, Lloyd et al. (2004) found evidence of pre-existing cognitive deficits in patients who showed the generation of spontaneous microembolism prior to their CEA. A longitudinal study by Bakker et al. (2004) assessed 73 patients who had TIAs or moderately disabling cerebral ischaemic strokes that were proven by angiography to be attributable to carotid stenosis. Seventy per cent of these patients with a stroke and 39% of patients with a TIA were rated as being cognitively impaired at baseline. At one year, patients who had recurrent TIAs remained impaired whereas those with no recurrence of symptoms improved.

Researchers have also examined neuropsychological function pre- and post-CEA, with inconsistent findings being highlighted by two systematic reviews (Irvine et al., 1998). Improvement in performance following surgery was reported in over 50% of studies, no change in 43% with one study showing deterioration (Lunn et al., 1999). Methodological factors have often been cited as the cause of these discrepancies. There have also been suggestions that cognitive domains are differentially affected by the procedure. For example, Heyer et al. (1998) conducted a study of 112 patients undergoing CEA for symptomatic and asymptomatic carotid artery disease. They found that while 60% of patients showed an improvement in one or more test scores, 80% showed a decline in at least one test. Decline was detected most frequently in verbal memory tests whereas improvement was seen most commonly in psychomotor and executive function tests. However, more recently, Lloyd *et al.* (2004), defining cognitive deficit as a decline of one standard deviation or more on at least 2 tests, found that 45% of patients have cognitive deficits at 6 months post-procedure. In their study, patients were often poorer on tests of attention and word recognition and improvement was regularly seen in tests of delayed prose recall and non-verbal intelligence. Heyer *et al.* (1998) suggested that improvement in performance may be attributed to an increase in cerebral blood flow following surgery while decreased performance related to ischaemia from global hypoperfusion or microemboli. Unfortunately, unlike Lloyd *et al.* (2004), the occurrence of microemboli was not measured in the Heyer *et al.* study.

Transcranial Doppler (TCD) ultrasonography is the most commonly used technique to detect and monitor the occurrence of microemboli during various invasive procedures including CEA. Smith *et al.* (1998) have suggested that monitoring of the carotid artery during CEA is important in quality control and training. Studies have demonstrated that the number of emboli produced in the dissection stage of a CEA is related to the likelihood of infarcts as detected by MRI (Jansen *et al.*, 1994; Aackerstaff *et al.*, 1996). In a study by Gaunt *et al.* (1994) the incidence of microemboli was found to be related to changes in cognition: they also established that the detection of more than ten microemboli during the initial carotid dissection was associated with an increased likelihood of post-operative cognitive deterioration. Lloyd *et al.* (2004) also demonstrated intra-operative microemboli to be a significant predictor of cognitive decline.

A one centre study of a sub-group of patients in the CAVATAS trial showed substantially more microemboli detected during carotid angioplasty compared to CEA (Crawley *et al.*, 1997). However, two centres in the CAVATAS trial examined neuropsychological outcome following CEA compared to angioplasty and found no significant differences between the groups 6 months after treatment (Sivaguru *et al.*, 1999; Crawley *et al.*, 2000).

Quality of life (QoL) in patients with carotid artery occlusion has received relatively little attention. In a recent study by Bakker *et al.* (2004) self-perceived QoL remained affected 12 months after initial symptoms of a TIA or moderate stroke due to carotid occlusion even in the absence of further symptoms. Trudel *et al.* (1984) found that activities of daily living were not particularly affected following CEA. In contrast, there were marked restrictions in social and leisure activities. Salenius *et al.* (1990) examined the results of 44 surgically and 40 non-surgically treated patients with carotid stenosis documented by angiography in 1974–1976. During the follow-up period, the occurrence of cerebrovascular complications (death, stroke and/or TIA) was more frequent in the non-operated than in the operated group. No differences were found in the quality of life between the two groups, but the operated group expressed higher levels of satisfaction than the non-operated group. Sirkka *et al.* (1992) assessed patients 8–11 years after surgery and compared them with two control groups, one consisting of healthy individuals, the other group of patients having been considered for CEA approximately 11 years earlier, but not operated upon. The groups were matched on age, education, gender and, if applicable, duration of illness and lateralization of stenosis. They found that only those patients who had undergone two operations had a poorer quality of life than either of the control groups. Vriens *et al.* (1998) using the Sickness Impact profile to measure quality of life found no disruption 3 months after CEA. Lloyd *et al.* (2004) using the Short Form 36 (SF-36) also found that patients' self-reported health quality of life had not deteriorated at 6 months post-procedure. However, Dardik *et al.* (2001) also using the SF-36 found that patients with symptomatic carotid artery disease undergoing uncomplicated CEA reported an improved quality of life and overall health 3 months after the procedure. Conversely, those patients with postoperative complications reported a decline in both 'emotional health' and 'change in health' sub-scores. However, it has been suggested that generic quality of life measures do not tap all the factors which concern patients with carotid artery disease and that these measures should be supported by disease specific questionnaires (Hallin *et al.*, 2002) (see 'Quality of life' and 'Quality of life assessment').

REFERENCES

Aackerstaff, R. G., Jansen, C. & Moll, F. L. (1996). Carotid enderterectomy and intraoperative emboli detection: correlation of clinical, transcranial Doppler, and magnetic resonance findings. *Echocardiography*, **13**, 543–50.

Auperin, A., Berr, C., Bonithon-Kopp, C. *et al.* (1996). Ultrasonographic assessment of carotid wall characteristics and cognitive functions in a community sample of 59–71-year-olds: the EVA Study Group. *Stroke*, **27**, 1290–5.

Alhaddad, I. A. (2004). Carotid artery surgery vs stent: a cardiovascular perspective. *Catheterization and Cardiovascular Interventions*, **63**, 377–84.

Bakker, F. C., Klijn, C. J. M., van der Grond, J., Kappelle, L. J. & Jennekens-Schinkel, A. (2004). Cognition and quality of life in patients with carotid artery occlusion. A follow-up study. *Neurology*, **62**, 2230–5.

Bornstein, R., Benoit, B. G. & Trites, R. L. (1981). Neuropsychological changes following carotid endarterectomy *Canadian Journal of Neurological Science*, **8**, 127–32.

CAVATAS investigators. (2001). Endovascular versus surgical treatment in patients with carotid stenosis in the carotid and vertebral transluminal angioplasty study (CAVATAS): a randomised trial. *Lancet*, **357**, 1729–37.

Crawley, F., Clifton, A., Buckenham, T. *et al.* (1997). Comparison of hemodynamic cerebral ischemia and microembolic signals detected during carotid endarterectomy and carotid angioplasty. *Stroke*, **28**, 2460–4.

Crawley, F., Stygall, J., Lunn, S. *et al.* (2000). Comparison of microembolism detected by transcranial Doppler and neuropsychological sequelae of carotid surgery and percutaneous transluminal angioplasty. *Stroke*, **31**, 1329–34.

Dardik, A., Minor, J., Watson, C. & Hands L. J. (2001). Improved quality of life among patients with symptomatic carotid artery disease undergoing carotid endarterectomy. *Journal of Vascular Surgery*, **33**, 329–33.

European Carotid Surgery Trialists Collaboration Group (ECST). (1998). Randomized trial of endarterectomy for recently symptomatic carotid stenosis: final results of the MRC European Carotid Surgery Trial. *Lancet*, **351**, 1379–87.

Executive Committee for the Asymptomatic Carotid Atherosclerosis Study (ACAS). (1995). Endarterectomy for asymptomatic carotid artery disease. *JAMA: Journal of the American Medical Association*, **273**, 1421–8.

Gaunt, M. E., Martin, P. J., Smith, J. L. *et al.* (1994). Clinical revelance of intraoperative embolization detected by transcranial Doppler ultrasonography during carotid endarterectomy: a prospective study of 100 patients. *British Journal of Surgery*, **81**, 1435–9.

Grace, P. A. (2004). Fifty years of carotid surgery – hail and farewell? *Irish Journal of Medical Science*, **173**, 75–7.

Hallin, A., Bergqvist, D., Fugl-Meyer, K. & Holmberg, L. (2002). Areas of concern, quality of life and life satisfaction in patients with peripheral vascular disease. *European Journal of Vascular and Endovascular Surgery*, **24**, 255–63.

Heyer, E. J., Adams, D. C., Solomon, R. A. *et al.* (1998). Neuropsychometric changes in patients after carotid endarterectomy. *Stroke*, **29**, 1110–15.

Inzitari, D., Eliasziw, M., Gates, P. *et al.* (2000). The causes and risk of stroke in patients with asymptomatic internal carotid artery stenosis. *New England Journal of Medicine*, **342**, 1693–700.

Irvine, C. D., Gardner, F. V., Davies, A. H. & Lamont, P. M. (1998). Cognitive testing in patients undergoing carotid endarterectomy. *European Journal of Vascular and Endovascular Surgery*, **15**, 195–204.

Jansen, C., Ramos, L. M. P., van Heesewijk, M. D. *et al.* (1994). Impact of microembolism and hemodynamic changes in the brain during carotid endarterectomy. *Stroke*, **25**, 992–7.

Johnston, S. C., O'Mara, E. S., Manolio, T. A. *et al.* (2004). Cognitive impairment and decline are associated with carotid artery disease in patients without clinically evident cerebrovascular disease. *Anals of Internal Medicine*, **140**, 237–47.

Lloyd, A., Hayes, P. D., London, N. J. M., Bell, P. R. F. & Naylor, A. R. (2004). Does carotid endarterectomy lead to a decline in cognitive function or health related quality of life? *Journal of Clinical and Experimental Neuropsychology*, **26**, 817–25.

Lunn, S., Crawley, F., Harrison, M. J. G., Brown, M. M. & Newman, S. P. (1999). Impact of carotid endarterectomy upon cognitive functioning. A systematic review of the literature. *Cerebrovascular Diseases*, **9**, 74–81.

Mathiesen, E. B., Waterloo, K., Joakimsen, O. *et al.* (2004). Reduced neuropsychological test performance in asymptomatic carotid stenosis. *Neurology*, **62**, 695–701.

MRC Asymptomatic Carotid Surgery Trial (ASCT) Collaborative Group. (2004). Prevention of disabling and fatal strokes by successful carotid endarterectomy in patients without recent neurological symptoms: Randomised controlled trial. *Lancet*, **363**, 1491–1502.

North American Symptomatic Carotid Endarterectomy Trial Collaborators (NASCETC). (1991). Beneficial effect of carotid endarterectomy in symptomatic patients with high grade carotid stenosis. *New England Journal of Medicine*, **325**, 445–53.

Rabe, K. & Sievert, H. (2004). Carotid artery stenting: state of the art. *Journal of Interventional Cardiology*, **17**, 417–26.

Rao, R. (2002). The role of carotid stenosis in vasular cognitive impairment. *Journal of the Neurological Sciences*, **203–204**, 103–7.

Salenius, J. P., Harju, E., Kuukasjarvi, P., Haapanen, A. & Riekkinen, H. (1990). Late results of surgical and nonoperative treatment of carotid stenosis. Eighty-four patients documented by angiography in 1974–1976. *Journal of Cardiovascular Surgery: Torino*, **31**, 156–61.

Sivaguru, A., Gaines, P. A., Beard, J. & Venerables, G. S. (1999). Neuropsychological outcome after carotid angioplasty: a randomised control trial. *Journal of Neurology, Neurosurgery and Psychiatry*, **66**, 262 (Abstract).

Sirkka, A., Salenius, J. P., Portin, R. & Nummenmaa, T. (1992). Quality of life and cognitive performance after carotid endarterectomy during long-term follow-up. *Acta Neurologica Scandinavica*, **85**, 58–62.

Smith, J. L., Evans, D. H., Gaunt, M. E. *et al.* (1998). Experience with transcranial Doppler monitoring reduces the incidence of particulate embolization during carotid endarterectomy. *British Journal of Surgery*, **85**, 56–9.

Trudel, L., Fabia, J. & Bouchard, J. P. (1984). Quality of life of 50 carotid endarterectomy survivors: a long term follow up study. *Archives in Physical Medicine and Rehabilitation*, **65**, 310–12.

Vriens, E. M., Post, M. W., Jacobs, H. M. *et al.* (1998). Changes in health-related quality of life after carotid endarterctomy. *European Journal of Vascular and Endovascular Surgery*, **16**, 395–400.

Winslow, C. M., Solomon, D. H., Chassin, M. R. *et al.* (1988). The appropriateness of carotid endarterectomy. *New England Journal of Medicine*, **318**, 721–7.

Chemotherapy

Ingela Thuné-Boyle

University College London

'Chemotherapy' refers to treatment with drugs and can describe the treatment with drugs in any illness. It is however, mainly associated with the treatment of cancer where chemotherapy is short for 'cytotoxic chemotherapy'. Cytotoxic (cell poison) chemotherapy constitutes a group of drugs used to treat cancer by interfering with the process of cell reproduction.

Chemotherapy is a systemic therapy affecting the entire body. It is particularly toxic to rapidly dividing cells, a primary feature of tumour development, and it works by disrupting cellular function. Unlike radiotherapy, which is mainly used to treat local disease (see 'Radiotherapy'), the purpose of chemotherapy is to destroy cancer cells that may have spread from the primary site. It is therefore typically given to patients where there is evidence or suspicion of a regional disease spread (i.e. nodal involvement).

The goal of chemotherapy treatment may be (i) as a primary therapy with curative intent; (ii) as adjuvant therapy with curative or long term survival intent, i.e. by controlling the cancer, keeping it from spreading or by slowing its growth; (iii) as a neoadjuvant therapy with the aim of reducing tumour burden or to spare an organ; and (iv) as palliative therapy to relieve symptoms such as pain caused by advanced cancer, to help patients live more comfortably (Knobf *et al.*, 1998).

Side effects and the role of psychological factors

Although chemotherapy works best on rapidly dividing tumour cells, it may also damage healthy cells, especially those that also have a tendency to divide quickly such as cells in the blood, mouth, intestinal tract, nose, nails, vagina and hair. This can cause patients to experience a range of side effects such as nausea, vomiting, diarrhoea, hair loss, skin rash, sore mouth, loss of appetite, immunosuppression, weight gain, tingling and numbness, cessation of menstruation, neuropsychiatric effects and negative affects such as anxiety and depression (e.g. Holland and Lesko, 1990). In addition, 20% to 65% of patients may develop anticipatory nausea and vomiting (ANV) (Burish & Carey, 1984), (for more information on ANV, see 'Vomiting and nausea').

The number and severity of side effects vary widely depending on the drug combination, dosage, number of cycles and whether or not these drugs are given in combination with radiotherapy. However, there are also large variations in levels of side effects occurring in patients' receiving the same cytotoxic agents (e.g. Gralla *et al.*, 1981), suggesting that non-pharmacological factors may play a role (Haut *et al.*, 1991). It also suggests that toxicity ratings of chemotherapy do not reveal information about the actual experience of symptoms during treatment, or their influence on psychological wellbeing. Rather, they suggest an important role of psychological factors in response to chemotherapy treatment. For example, patient's pre-infusion expectations have been found to predict post-treatment nausea independent of pharmacological effects (e.g. Montgomery & Bovbjerg, 2000) and patient's expectations may also play an important role in the development of ANV separate to that of conditioning (Hickok *et al.*, 2001) (see 'Expectations and health'). Further, coping style such as the monitoring/blunting concept (Miller, 1995) and repressive coping (Byrne, 1961) may play a role in the number and severity of side effects experienced and/or reported by patients during and after treatment (e.g. Lehman *et al.*, 1990). Levels of anxiety have also been found to be associated with higher levels of symptom reporting during chemotherapy (e.g. Watson *et al.*, 1998) (see 'Symptom perception').

Cognitive functioning

Patients on chemotherapy often report difficulties with their abilities to remember, think and concentrate (e.g. Minisini *et al.*, 2004). There is evidence that chemotherapy can have an indirect effect on cognitive function caused by anaemia and through a reduction in hormone levels associated with chemotherapy induced menopause (e.g. Jacobsen *et al.*, 2004). It may also have a direct effect on the central nervous system. Problems with language, the visual–motor domains, memory, attention and concentration have been noted (e.g. Ahles *et al.*, 2002). However, a review by Minisini *et al.* (2004) found that most studies to date have suffered from methodological problems such as a small sample size, a lack of baseline measurement and many have also failed to control for other possible influential variables such as educational status and IQ. Further, factors such as age, ability to cope, anxiety, depression and fatigue can also influence cognitive ability and were often not controlled for in studies. Despite methodological limitations, current evidence to date nevertheless suggests that chemotherapy does cause cognitive dysfunction in a significant number of patients with cancer. Treatment-induced cognitive dysfunction may, in turn, affect the patient's ability to return to work, resume their previous activities and can therefore be detrimental on their quality of life.

Psychological impact

Chemotherapy engenders fear and uncertainty for many patients, as it is generally associated with upsetting side effects and distress. However, the prevalence of distress during chemotherapy varies across studies. Some have found clinical levels of distress in around a quarter of patients (e.g. Mooray *et al.*, 1991) while others have found as many as three quarters report moderate to severe levels of distress (Meyerowitz *et al.*, 1979). Distress has also been shown to increase during and up to a month following chemotherapy among patients with breast cancer and lymphoma (e.g. Buick *et al.*, 2000). End of treatment distress may occur as a result of patient's feelings of vulnerability to tumour recurrence as they are no longer monitored closely by hospital staff (Sinsheimer & Holland, 1987). However, a recent pilot study examining distress among males with testicular cancer before, during and after chemotherapy, found that initial anxiety before the start of treatment was highest and primarily anticipatory, but decreased over the course of chemotherapy (Trask *et al.*, 2003). This suggests that the course of distress during chemotherapy may be different in different cancers groups and that generalizations from one cancer group to another should be made with caution (see 'Cancer: general').

Some studies have also examined factors associated with psychological distress during chemotherapy treatment and have produced a range of different findings, even in the same cancer group. In breast cancer, Sinsheimer and Holland (1987) found that psychological distress was largely associated with hair loss, weight gain and fatigue. Knobf (1986) found fatigue to be the most distressing symptom in this cancer group, and Nerenz *et al.* (1984) found nausea and vomiting, fatigue, weakness and pain to have the strongest associations with distress in a sample of patients with breast cancer and lymphoma. What is common in these studies is the association of distress with fatigue, which is an increasingly recognized important symptom in many chronic conditions and treatments.

Some studies have also found that the number of side effects experienced by patients during chemotherapy to be associated with distress (e.g. Nerenz *et al.*, 1984). However, Thuné-Boyle *et al.* (2006) in a multivariate analysis, found that the number of symptoms was associated with patient's beliefs about the consequences of their illness and treatment and that these beliefs served as a mediator between symptoms and anxiety, and, to a lesser extent, depression. The aetiology of distress during chemotherapy is often complex and may also be influenced by other factors such as personality, coping style, age, type of cancer and prognosis (Knobf *et al.*, 1998).

Interventions

Physical symptoms during chemotherapy can be perceived as being so severe and so distressing that patients may delay or even stop treatment altogether (Carey & Burish, 1988). It is therefore important to find ways of reducing treatment-related distress, as poor adherence is likely to influence survival.

There are various medical interventions that are successful in reducing some of the unpleasant side effects during chemotherapy. For example, there has been a significant improvement in reducing nausea and vomiting with the development of new and more effective anti-emetic drugs during the last decade (Morganstern & Hesketh, 1999), and better ways of classifying emetogenic risk are now available (Hesketh *et al.*, 1997). Further, many cancer centres now administer erythropoietic agents to patients during chemotherapy to reduce anaemia and its associated fatigue. This, in turn, has been shown to improve quality of life during the treatment period (e.g. Iconomou *et al.*, 2003).

There are also scalp cooling methods that can be effective in preventing or reducing hair loss and its accompanying distress (e.g. Macduff *et al.*, 2003). They work by reducing the blood supply to the hair follicles and thereby decreasing the likelihood of the drugs reaching the area. They are however, not suitable when chemotherapy must be circulated through the body for longer periods of time or when very high doses are needed, and they vary in efficacy according to the chemotherapy drug used.

Many studies have examined the effectiveness of psychological interventions in reducing unpleasant side effects and the accompanying distress associated with these. A review by Carey and Burish (1988) investigating the usefulness of five such interventions: hypnosis, systematic desensitization; biofeedback; distraction; and relaxation and guided imagery, found that hypnosis was effective in reducing side effects associated with both pre- and post-chemotherapy and in reducing negative affects associated with cancer treatment (see 'Hypnosis'). The efficacy of systematic desensitization procedures appeared to be useful in reducing (ANV), while biofeedback, in combination with progressive muscle relaxation and guided imagery, showed promising results overall (see 'Biofeedback', 'Behaviour therapy' and 'Relaxation training'). Progressive muscle relaxation with guided imagery reduced physiological arousal and nausea as well as anxiety, and proved especially effective in reducing vomiting. Distraction techniques were found to be especially useful in children although it was not clear how long-lasting their effect was or whether the novelty of the distraction wore off over time. More recent reviews have found relaxation training alone or with guided imagery given during chemotherapy generally reduced treatment-related symptoms and improved emotional adjustment and quality of life (Luebbert *et al.*, 2001; Walker *et al.*, 1999).

A meta-analysis by Meyer and Mark (1995) investigated the effects of behavioural, educational, social support, counselling and therapy interventions found clear evidence that all of these had an effect on emotional and functional adjustment, and on treatment and disease-related symptoms, although the effect size was found to be relatively small. In fact, Dreher (1997) has argued for a need to develop and evaluate better interventions in order to minimize the psychological impact of cancer treatment. It is therefore important to identify other factors that may influence distress and how patients' experience and interpret their symptoms and their illness during the treatment phase (List & Butler, 1999). Examining the role of patient's beliefs about illness and treatment for example, may provide useful information in the design of interventions and may provide a focus for the content of interventions (see 'Lay beliefs about health and illness').

REFERENCES

Ahles, T. A., Saykin, A. J., Furstenberg, C. T. *et al.* (2002). Neuropsychologic impact of standard dose systemic chemotherapy in long-term survivors of breast cancer and lymphoma. *Journal of Clinical Oncology,* **20**, 485–93.

Buick, D. L., Petrie, K. J., Booth, R. *et al.* (2000). The emotional and functional impact of radiation and chemotherapy treatment for primary breast cancer. *Journal of Psychosocial Oncology*, **18** (1), 39–62.

Burish, T. G. & Carey, M. P. (1984). Conditioned response to chemotherapy: etiology and treatment. In B. Fox & B. Newberry (Eds.). *Impact of psychoendocrine systems in cancer and immunity* (pp. 311–20). New York: Hogrefe.

Byrne, D. (1961). The Repression–Sensitization scale: rational, reliability and validity. *Journal of Personality*, **29**, 334–49.

Carey, M. P. & Burish, T. G. (1988). Aetiology and treatment of the psychological effects associated with cancer chemotherapy: a critical review and discussion. *Psychological Bulletin*, **104**, 307–25.

Dreher, H. (1997). The scientific and moral imperative for broad-based psychosocial interventions for cancer. *Advances: the Journal of Mind–Body Health*, **13**, 38–49.

Gralla, R. J., Itri, L. M., Pisco, S. E. *et al.* (1981). Anti-emetic efficacy of high dose metoclopramide: randomised trials with placebo and pro-chlorperazine in patients with chemotherapy-induced nausea and vomiting. *New England Journal of Medicine*, **305**, 905–9.

Haut, M. W., Beckwith, B. E., Laurie, J. A. & Klatt, N. (1991). Post chemotherapy nausea and vomiting in cancer patients receiving out-patients chemotherapy. *Journal of Psychosocial Oncology*, **9**, 117–30.

Hesketh, P. J., Kris, M. G., Grunberg, S. M. *et al.* (1997). Proposal for classifying the acute emetogenicity of cancer chemotherapy. *Journal of Clinical Oncology*, **15**, 103–9.

Hickok, J. T., Roscoe, J. A. & Morrow, G. R. (2001). The role of patients' expectations in the development of anticipatory nausea related to chemotherapy for cancer. *Journal of Pain and Symptom Management*, **22**, 843–50.

Holland, J. C. & Lesko, L. M. (1990). Chemotherapy, endocrine therapy and immunotherapy. In J. C. Holland & J. H. Rowland (Eds.). *Handbook of psychooncology: psychosocial care for the patient with cancer* (pp. 145–62). New York: Oxford University Press.

Iconomou, G., Koutras, A., Rigopoulos, A., Vagenakis, A. G. & Kalofonos, H. A. (2003). Effect of recombinant human erythropoietin on quality of life in cancer patients receiving chemotherapy: results of a randomized, controlled trial. *Journal of Pain and Symptom Management*, **25**, 512–18.

Jacobsen, P. B., Garland, L. L., Booth-Jones, M. *et al.* (2004). Relationship of haemoglobin levels to fatigue and cognitive functioning among cancer patients receiving chemotherapy. *Journal of Pain and Symptom Management*, **28**, 7–18.

Knobf, M. T. (1986). Physical and psychological distress associated with adjuvant chemotherapy in women with breast cancer. *Journal of Clinical Oncology*, **4**, 678–84.

Knobf, M. T., Pasacreta, J. V., Valentine, A. & McCorkle, R. (1998). Chemotherapy, hormonal therapy, and immunotherapy. In J. C. Holland (Ed.). *Psycho-oncology* (pp. 277–88). Oxford University Press.

Lehman, C., Rimer, B., Blumberg, B. *et al.* (1990). Effects of coping style and relaxation on cancer chemotherapy side effects and emotional response. *Cancer Nursing*, **13**, 308–15.

List, M. A. & Butler, P. (1999). Measuring quality of life. In E. E. Vokes & H. M. Golomb (Eds.). *Oncologic therapies* (pp. 1171–85). Springer-Verlag. New York.

Luebbert, K., Dahme, B. & Hasenbring, M. (2001). The effectiveness of relaxation training in reducing treatment-related symptoms and improving emotional adjustment in acute non-surgical cancer treatment: a meta-analytical review. *Psycho-oncology*, **10**, 490–502.

Macduff, C., Mackenzie, T., Hutcheon, A., Melville, L. & Archibald, H. (2003). The effectiveness of scalp cooling in preventing alopecia for patients receiving epirubicin and docetaxel. *European Journal of Cancer Care*, **12**, 154–61.

Meyer, T. J. & Mark, M. M. (1995). Effects of psychosocial interventions with adult cancer patients: a meta-analysis of randomised experiments. *Health Psychology*, **14**, 101–8.

Meyerowitz, B. E., Sparks, F. C. & Spears, I. K. (1979). Adjuvant chemotherapy for breast carcinoma: psychosocial implications. *Cancer*, **43**, 1613–18.

Miller, S. M. (1995). Monitoring versus blunting styles of coping with cancer influence the information patients want and need about their disease. *Cancer*, **76**, 167–77.

Minisini, A., Atalay, G., Bottomley, A. *et al.* (2004). What is the effect of systemic anticancer treatment on cognitive function? *The Lancet Oncology*, **5**, 273–82.

Montgomery, G. H. & Bovbjerg, D. H. (2000). Pre-infusion expectations predict post-treatment nausea during repeated adjuvant chemotherapy infusion for breast cancer. *British Journal of Health Psychology*, **5**, 105–19.

Mooray, S., Greer, S., Watson, M. *et al.* (1991). The factor structure and factor stability of the hospital anxiety and depression scale in patients with cancer. *British Journal of Psychiatry*, **158**, 255–9.

Morganstern, D. E. & Hesketh, P. J. (1999). Chemotherapy induced nausea and vomiting. In E. E. Vokes & H. M. Golomb (Eds.). *Oncologic therapies* (pp. 1115–35). Springer-Verlag. New York.

Nerenz, D. R., Leventhal, H., Love, R. R. & Ringler, K. E. (1984). Psychological aspects of cancer chemotherapy. *International Review of Applied Psychology*, **33**, 521–9.

Sinsheimer, L. M. & Holland, J. C. (1987). Psychological issues in breast cancer. *Seminars in Oncology*, **14**, 75–82.

Thuné-Boyle, I. C. V., Myers, L. B. & Newman, S. P. (2006). The role of illness beliefs, treatment beliefs and perceived severity of symptoms in explaining distress in cancer patients during chemotherapy treatment. *Behavioural Medicine*, **32**, 19–29.

Trask, P. C., Paterson, A. G., Fardig, J. & Smith, D. C. (2003). Course of distress and quality of life in testicular cancer patients before, during and after chemotherapy: results of a pilot study. *Psycho-oncology*, **12**, 814–20.

Walker, L. G., Walker, M. B., Ogston, K. *et al.* (1999). Psychological, clinical and pathological effects of relaxation training and guided imagery during primary chemotherapy. *British Journal of Cancer*, **80**, 262–8.

Watson, M., Meyer, L., Thompson, A. & Osofsky, S. (1998). Psychological factors predicting nausea and vomiting in breast cancer patients on chemotherapy. *European Journal of Cancer*, **34**, 831–7.

Child abuse and neglect

Kevin D. Browne and Catherine Hamilton-Giachritsis

University of Birmingham

Introduction

Prevention of child maltreatment is traditionally classified into three levels: primary prevention (universal services aimed at the whole population); secondary prevention (targeted services for families identified as in need of further support); and tertiary prevention (services offered once difficulties have occurred). However, increasingly it has been argued that child maltreatment should be considered within the broader context of child welfare, families and communities (World Health Organization, 1998a,b). This approach assists in moving the focus away from child protection professionals to highlighting the role of the Health and Social Services in general. This has been termed the public health approach which promotes child care and protection within the broader context of child welfare, families and communities.

For example, the Health Service can look at areas of service provision for families and children, where good practice can impact on child welfare; specifically, pregnancy and childbirth-related services (primary prevention), targeting resources to families at risk of child maltreatment (secondary prevention) and the management of childhood health and illness (secondary and tertiary prevention). Families who come into contact with health and social services can be assessed in terms of need by considering the following three factors (Department of Health, 2000):

- Assessment of children's development needs in general
- Assessment of the parent(s) capacity to respond appropriately to their child's needs
- Assessment of the wider social and environmental factors that impact on the capacity to parent.

Most authors conclude that a multi-sector, inter-disciplinary approach is the most effective way of working together to promote children's rights to grow and develop in a safe family environment and provide care and protection to children (e.g. United Nations Convention on the Rights of the Child, 1989; Hallett & Birchell, 1992). In the UK, guidelines have been published by the Department of Health (1999; 2000) on how a range of professionals can work together to safeguard children. These guidelines have since been adopted by some other countries (e.g. Hungary, Romania) as they clearly define what is meant by child abuse and neglect.

Definitions

Child maltreatment is typically broken down into four different types. However, many children suffer more than one type of maltreatment at the same time and there are a minority of cases where the child is victimized in a ritualistic and terrorizing way.

Physical abuse

The child is physically hurt, injured, maimed or killed by a parent or caretaker, or the risk of such injury. This may include, but is not limited to, punching, beating, kicking, shaking, biting, strangulation, burning, or immersion in scalding water, with resulting bruises, welts, broken bones, burns, internal injuries or scars. Physical harm may also be caused when a parent or carer feigns the symptoms of, or deliberately causes ill health to a child whom they are looking after. This situation is commonly described using terms such as factitious illness by proxy or Munchausen syndrome by proxy.

Sexual abuse

Children are used to gratify adult sexual needs and fantasies by carers in position of responsibility, trust or power who force or coerce a child into sexual and/or pornographic (contact and/or non-contact) activities. These include: sexual penetration (rape, buggery, oral sex), sexual touching, fondling, voyeurism, exposure, frottage (rubbing against a person), child prostitution, production of pornographic materials. Children are incapable of providing informed consent to sexual interactions with adults.

Psychological/emotional abuse

The child is subject to threats, verbal attacks (belittling, humiliating, ridiculing, shouting), violent outbursts directed at others (e.g. spouse, sibling or elder abuse). S/he is threatened, frightened or placed in dangerous situations. Some level of emotional abuse is involved in all types of ill-treatment of a child, though it may occur alone.

Neglect

This is the failure of a parent or caretaker to provide their child with basic needs (such as food, clothes, shelter, warmth, education and healthcare), protection and supervision which may result in harm to health and development of the child. This also includes *Psychological neglect* – the consistent failure of a parent or caretaker to provide a child with appropriate support, attention, love and affection.

Incidence

The incidence of child abuse and neglect varies widely across different countries. This may be related to different reporting definitions and procedures. For example, reporting rates range from 43 per 1000 children in the USA to 3 per 1000 children in Belgium (Gilbert, 1997).

A survey of 50 States in the USA carried out by the National Center on Child Abuse Prevention Research (Wang, 1999) identified approximately three million cases (45 per 1000 children) of reported child abuse but only one third (15 per 1000) were later substantiated by a case worker, 54% of these were neglect cases, 20% were physical abuse, 10% sexual abuse and 3% emotional abuse. The remaining 14% were mixed and not easily categorized (Wang & Harding, 1999).

In England for the year ending 31 March 2004 (Department of Education and Skills, 2005) 72 100 children (6.5 per 1000) were subject to a child protection enquiry. Over half of these (38 500; 3.5 per 1000) were subject to a case conference and 80% of these resulted in the child being placed on a child protection register.

Therefore, 2.4 in 1000 children under 18 years were on child protection registers for actual or likely abuse and/or neglect. Of these, 41% were registered for neglect, 19% for physical abuse, 9% for sexual abuse, 18% for emotional abuse and 14% for cases of mixed abuse and/or neglect. The highest rates were found in very young children less than one year old (51 per 10 000, 11% of the total), with the likelihood of being on the register decreasing with age. Therefore, 68% of children on registers are aged less than 10 years. There were slightly more boys (2.4 per 1000) than girls registered overall (2.3 per 1000). However, 11% of girls were registered for 'sexual abuse' compared with 8% of boys, while more boys than girls were registered for 'physical abuse' (16% and 15% respectively). One in eight children registered in 2004 had previously been on the child protection register. In terms of placements, approximately 13% of those on the register (26 300) on 31 March 2004, were 'looked after' by local authorities (this figure represents 6% of all children in public care); of these, 79% were placed with foster parents, 5% were living in children's home or secure unit, 13% were placed with parents and 3% are placed for adoption or living independently.

Nevertheless it is claimed that the incidence figures for child abuse and neglect represent only a small proportion of those children who are victimized in childhood. Victim surveys and prevalence studies indicate that the number of people reporting that they have been abused in childhood is approximately ten times the incidence rate (Browne et al., 2002). Given the fact that infants are more at risk of maltreatment than any other age group, it is essential to intervene early with health and social services in order to prevent child abuse and neglect (Browne & Herbert, 1997).

Advantages of early intervention

The most important indicator that there is a need for early intervention is the level of fatal abuse and serious injury to children (Reder & Duncan, 2002). Child abuse and neglect is one of the most common causes of death and disability to children under five years, although children under one year are at greatest risk (Browne & Lynch, 1995). Parents are the most common offenders. It is estimated that in the United Kingdom that at least two children per week die from maltreatment (NSPCC, 2001), compared with 23 children per week in the USA (Wang & Harding, 1999). Therefore, these figures emphasize the need for timely interventions to reduce the number of children who continue to die or who are disabled for life because

interventions are either too late or the preventative services are inadequate. Although child protection systems have changed in the last 30 years, there has been little decline in the rate of child death (Creighton, 1995) which remains unacceptably high (NSPCC, 2001).

Early intervention is important from the perspective of the victim and the family, but also may significantly reduce the large financial cost of child abuse and neglect to society. These costs are both overt (e.g. medical care for victims, treatment of offenders, legal costs for public childcare) and less obvious (e.g. criminal justice and prosecution costs, specialist education). Over a decade ago, it was estimated that the total economic cost in the United Kingdom is £735 million per annum (National Commission for the Prevention of Child Abuse, 1996). Eastimates at the same time in the USA claimed $12 410 million dollars per annum (WHO, 1998b).

Alongside the impact on children, families and society, the cost of child protection once child abuse and neglect has occurred provides sufficient economic justification for more expenditure on preventative measures and services to support children and their families.

Primary prevention

Primary prevention techniques are aimed at the whole population and attempt to create a fundamental change across society. For example, public awareness campaigns that challenge misconceptions and aim to increase the public's understanding of the extent and nature of child maltreatment. Primary prevention services could include:

- maternity services (promoting safe pregnancy and childbirth)
- home visits by health workers
- school programmes on parenting and child development
- education of parents and caregivers
- community support
  - day nursery places
  - telephone helplines
  - drop-in community centres

Safe pregnancy and childbirth (maternity services)

Recommendations for pre-, peri- and antenatal care focus on providing safe pregnancy and childbirth (WHO, 1998b), which in turn impacts on the development of parental bonding and attachment formation (see also 'Pregnancy and childbirth').

During pregnancy, emphasis is placed on prenatal screening to identify potential disabilities, which (aside from the obvious implications for child and family) is also a known risk factor for child maltreatment (see 'Screening: antenatal'). Furthermore, maternal healthy lifestyle is vital for foetal development. Traditionally, this has focused on avoidance of alcohol, drug and cigarette use, as well as physical and mental wellbeing. However, a recent development is concern regarding mothers who are under-eating due to fears of weight gain.

During birth, the promotion of natural delivery and use of appropriate technology should be encouraged. Like other economically developed countries, in the UK the rate of Caesarean births has risen significantly in recent years and is an issue for discussion. Furthermore, significant evidence demonstrates the role of midwives in promoting a positive birth experience for mothers. Most importantly, perhaps, the presence of significant others (usually the father) during the birth and skin contact between mother and baby immediately following birth can impact on bonding between parent and child (Sluckin *et al.*, 1983).

Following birth, 24-hour access of significant others to the mother and child in the maternity unit reduces feelings of social isolation and promotes support and paternal involvement. Advice on appropriate neonatal care and practical parenting skills is essential (e.g. breast feeding, bathing, etc), assisting the parents to adjust to their new role (New & David, 1987) (see also 'Breastfeeding'). Overall, the aim is the promotion of sensitive parenting through positive post-birth experiences.

From first involvement with professionals due to pregnancy, midwives are best placed to provide continuity of care to expectant parents. A 'good practice' model is seen as the same midwife offering individualized support with pre-birth home visits, assistance in childbirth and infant care. In terms of child protection, positive birth experiences and bonding promote positive parenting and thereby limit the possibility of infant abandonment, poor parenting, insecure attachment and maltreatment (Browne & Saqi, 1988*a*; Roberts, 1988).

Home visits by health workers

Family doctors and community nurses (health visitors) in a number of countries (e.g. UK, France, New Zealand) make home visits and have ongoing contact with all children under five years. They are in a unique position to provide advice on practical parenting skills, health and wellbeing of the child and their parents and counsel parents to reinforce positive parenting and sensitive interactions with the child.

School programmes on parenting and child development

Professionals from health and education (e.g. nursery workers, teachers, school nurses and psychologists) are important in providing appropriate advice and education to parents as well as informing children about their rights and what it is like to be a parent. In addition they are well placed to monitor child development and family influences.

Education of parents and caregivers

Many initiatives aimed at promoting positive parenting now exist (Sure Start in England; Triple P in eight countries across the world). The advantage of Triple P (Positive Parenting Programme; Sanders & Cann, 2002) is the long-term evaluation that has taken place and its application in a variety of countries across the world (see Saunders, 1999). It is a multi-system approach, available for use by different professionals to promote positive parenting skills and sensitivity, e.g. raising awareness of verbal abuse and the implications of this on the development of a positive self-image in the child. Outcomes of such programmes implemented through home visits have shown improvements in parenting skills and the quality of the home

environment, a reduction in child behavioural problems and accidents, better management of postnatal depression and social support for mothers and improved rates of breastfeeding (Elkan *et al.*, 2000).

The overall purpose of any support is to assist positive parenting skills and to encourage the development of a secure attachment between child and parent (Bowlby, 1969; Cassidy & Shaver, 1999). Secure attachment is repeatedly referred to as the main aim of interventions, because of the significance of attachment formation both for long-term wellbeing (e.g. positive self-image) and in the early prevention of child maltreatment. In situations where a high number of risk factors for child maltreatment are present, child abuse and neglect are more likely to occur in the absence of positive interactions and secure attachments (Browne & Saqi, 1988*b*; Morton & Browne, 1998).

It is important, however, for professionals to remain aware that, whilst providing simple explanations to parents may assist in development of parental sensitivity to the child and infant attachment, the assessment of parenting and attachment is not simplistic and requires appropriate training. A common misperception is to refer to a child as 'attached'. Nearly all children are attached in some way; it is the quality of infant attachment which is of importance. This is dependent on the levels of acceptance, accessibility, consistency, sensitivity and co-operation of the primary caregiver (usually the natural mother; Maccoby, 1980). However, whilst maltreated children are more likely to show patterns of insecurity, it does not always follow that a maltreated child is insecurely attached or that a child who clings to their mother is securely attached. A meta-analysis of 13 studies showed three-quarters (76%) of maltreated samples were classified as having an insecure attachment to the mother compared to just one-third (34%) of non-maltreated samples (Morton & Browne, 1998).

Community support

When considering parenting, it is also very important to recognize that the transition to parenthood is a critical period in adult psychological development. Support should be provided to parents who are unable to cope. Again, these can be offered at a population level, such as via telephone helplines, drop-in centres, community support groups and voluntary groups, as well as at a secondary level where parents in difficulties are referred to specialist health and social services. Hence, multi-disciplinary training is required to enable primary care professionals to recognize and intervene with spouse abuse parental low self-esteem, anxiety, depression and alcohol/drug misuse. For example, a parent who has depression will struggle to respond to the child's needs on a consistent basis whilst dealing with his/her own difficulties (Roberts, 1988). All these factors strongly influence the quality of parental care and infant attachment which may have long-term effects on child development (Goldberg, 2000; Simpson & Rholes, 1998; Solomon & George, 1999) (see 'Postnatal depression').

Secondary prevention

Secondary prevention involves targeting resources to families identified as being 'high priority' for additional services. This can be achieved by identifying known 'risk' factors for child maltreatment in a family and offering additional services before maltreatment occurs. However, it is important to note that not all families who have the presence of these 'risk factors' will go on to maltreat their child. This screening is merely a means of ensuring that families who have additional needs are provided with support. Thus, whilst this approach can be seen as controversial, if the intervention following screening is positive and empowering, the effects of incorrectly identifying a family as 'high priority' or 'in need' of further services should be minimal. Furthermore, it has the potential to prevent victimization from ever beginning.

Numerous 'risk' factors have been identified through research. For example, Browne and Saqi (1988a) undertook a 5 year follow-up of 14 252 newborns in Surrey, England. A comparison of 106 abusing families with 14 146 non-abusing families identified from this population established 12 factors that distinguished between the two groups. These included:

- Child characteristics (i.e. infant premature and/or low birth weight; infant separate from mother at birth; infant mentally or physically disabled; twins or less than 18 months since last birth).
- Parental characteristics (i.e. step-parent or co-habitee; parent with history of childhood abuse; history of mental illness or substance misuse; parent less than 21 years of age at time of birth; parent indifferent, intolerant or over-anxious towards child)
- social and environmental characteristics (i.e. single or separated parent; history of family violence; socioeconomic difficulties).

However, using a one-off screening instrument based on a checklist of risk factors around the time of birth can create high numbers of false positives (i.e. identified high risk, but non-maltreating; Browne, 1995a). Therefore, it has been argued (Browne & Herbert, 1997; Hamilton & Browne, 2002) that additional assessment of the parent–child relationship should be undertaken. In England, this led to the development of the Child Assessment and Rating Evaluation (CARE) programme that is carried out over four home visits during the first year of the infant's life (Browne et al., 2000; Dixon et al., 2005a). Following the use of an initial screening checklist completed in association with parents (see Table 1), community nurses rate:

- parental perceptions
- parental attitudes
- indicators of attachment formation
- quality of parenting.

Initial evaluation on 1508 families in Essex showed that using Index of Need score (see Table 1) 4% of families were identified as a 'high priority' (with a score of 6 or more), 30% as low priority (with a score of 1–5) and 66% as having no risk factors at all. On follow-up it was found that 97% of all parents showed positive parenting skills and only 3% demonstrated insensitive, unrealistic and negative parenting. Those parents with poor skills were significantly more likely to have come from the high priority group. Where both a high number of risk factors and negative parenting existed, these families were regarded as requiring immediate interventions.

In the USA, the value of home visitation to families with newborns has been highlighted through the work of David Olds (Olds et al., 1993, 1997, 2002). The research was conducted over a 15-year period and on follow-up a number of significant differences were found between those families visited and those families with new-borns

Table 1. The prevalence of risk factors displayed by Abused Parent families (AP) and Non-abused Parent families (NAP) with a child 4 to 6 weeks of age (N = 4351)

Risk factors	Weighting[+]	AP (n = 135) n%	NAP (n = 4216) n%	Test statistic
Complications during birth/separated from baby at birth	1	23 (17%)	462 (11%)	$\chi^2_{1=4.875}$, $p < 0.05$*
Mother or partner under 21 years of age	1	23 (17%)	257 (6%)	$\chi^2_{1=25.995}$, $p < 0.0001$**
Mother or partner not biologically related to the child	1	1 (0.7%)	12 (0.3%)	Fishers Exact > 0.05
Twins, or less than 18 months between births	1	19 (14%)	299 (7%)	$\chi^2_{1=9.413}$, $p < 0.001$**
Child with physical or mental disabilities	1	4 (3%)	59 (1%)	Fishers Exact > 0.05
Feelings of isolation	1	17 (13%)	105 (3%)	Fishers Exact < 0.0001**
Serious financial difficulties	2	20 (15%)	143 (3%)	$\chi^2_{1 = 47.336}$, $p < 0.0001$**
Mother or partner treated for mental illness or depression	2	64 (47%)	303 (7%)	$\chi^2_{1 = 273.989}$, $p < 0.0001$**
Dependency for drugs and/or alcohol	2	7 (5%)	18 (0.4%)	Fishers Exact < 0.0001**
Infant seriously ill, premature or weighed under 2.5 kg at birth	2	17 (13%)	226 (5%)	$\chi^2_{1 = 12.975}$, $p < 0.0001$**
Single parent	3	13 (10%)	268 (6%)	$\chi^2_{1 = 2.319}$, $p = 0.128$
Adult in the household with violent tendencies	3	16 (12%)	33 (0.8%)	Fishers Exact < 0.0001**
Mother or partner feeling indifferent about their baby	3	64	441	Fishers Exact < 0.01**

*p <0.05; **p <0.01.

[+]Weighted Score summed to produce an Index of Need score for each family (Taken from Dixon et al., 2005a).

who were not. In summary, the visited families showed the following differences:

- Mothers
  - Less family aid received
  - 79% reduction in child abuse and neglect
  - 44% reduction in maternal alcohol/drug difficulties
  - 69% fewer arrests of mothers
- Teenagers
  - 54% fewer arrests of 15 year olds
  - 58% fewer sexual partners
  - 51% fewer days consuming alcohol
  - 28% fewer cigarettes smoked

Intervention with families that have been identified as maltreating children could be reduced if good primary and secondary prevention were available following the principles of a public health approach. This requires a shift in focus from child protection (usually seen as the responsibility of social services and law enforcement agencies) to safeguarding children through promoting child welfare and development. Therefore, health professionals need to focus on the psychological as well as the physical needs of children and their families with appropriate networks for referral and support. The health sector is the most appropriate agency for early prediction and prevention of child maltreatment (Browne, 1995b) but also has a significant role to play in identification and detection of child abuse and neglect in partnership with social services.

Tertiary prevention

Even in the presence of proactive primary and secondary prevention, the health professional's role in services that detect and identify child maltreatment is essential. The primary focus of healthcare professionals is the prevention of child disability, morbidity and mortality. However, children coming to the attention of health services through home or clinic visits also offer the potential to screen for the possibility of maltreatment alongside standard procedures for dealing with physical injuries and illnesses. To consider child maltreatment, history-taking by doctors and nurses should include components to promote identification of and protection from child abuse and neglect:

- History of family circumstances (e.g. presence of isolation, violence, addiction or mental illness)
- History of child's condition (e.g. story doesn't explain injury, delay in seeking help)
- Child's physical condition when undressed (e.g. presence of disability, lesions or genital discharge)
- Child's physical care (e.g. cleanliness, teeth, hair, nails, hygiene)
- Child's behaviour (e.g. frozen hyper-vigilance or aggressive hyperactivity)
- Parents/caretaker's behaviour and demeanour (e.g. low self-esteem, depressed, over-anxious, insensitive, careless, punishing, defensive).

Although abuse and/or neglect may already have occurred, an opportunity is available for healthcare professionals to recognize and respond to the situation. In the long-term this can prevent the child and sometimes the mother from experiencing further incidences of abuse and/or neglect which increase in severity with time (Browne & Hamilton, 1999; Hamilton & Browne, 1999).

Therefore, tertiary prevention offers services to children and families where abuse and/or neglect have already occurred. Reactive surveillance and identification of abused and/or neglected children leads to intervention both to stop the current maltreatment and to prevent recurrent victimization. The poor cost-effectiveness of tertiary prevention is highlighted by a study of police child protection units in England which showed that one in four children identified as victims of child maltreatment were referred again within a 27-month follow-up period, despite social service interventions following the initial referral (Hamilton & Browne, 1999).

Conclusion

Any involvement of health professionals in child protection must be seen in the broader context of multi-disciplinary networking and referral processes, preferably organized through a local child protection coordinating committee. The prevention of child abuse and neglect needs to take into account the United Nations Convention on the Rights of the Child (UNCRC, 1989). This requires all member states to offer effective child protection services placing the rights of the child and their best interests above those of adults, including the child's own parents. This notion is reflected in the UK Children Act (1989, 2004), which considers the child's welfare as paramount.

It is the child's right under international legislation to grow and develop in a family environment, preferably raised by their biological parents. Therefore, health and social services should be available to all parents in order to support those who are failing to cope with the demands of parenting. Where the child is in danger or their social, emotional and developmental needs are not being met, intervention is required. Family rehabilitation can be achieved often by working with the family in their home but sometimes short-term foster care is necessary where the foster carer acts as a role model to the parents. Only when the parent is assessed as not responding to intervention, or is unable to change within the developmental time frame of the child, should long-term alternatives (i.e. long-term fostering or adoption) be considered. Under no circumstances should young children (either with a disability or not) be placed in residential care institutions (including the use of maternity/paediatric units as a social care facility) without a primary caregiver as this has been shown, as with neglect situations, to have significantly detrimental effects on brain development (Glaser, 2000). Consequently, problems in the development of self and social relationships with others persist in those children who have grown up in institutional care (Browne et al., 2005). Ministries of Health are predominantly responsible for residential care of children less than three years old and currently there are 23 000 young children living in institutions within the European Union (including accession countries) for more than three months without their parents (Browne et al., 2005). Hence, the health sector has a large role to play in the prevention of child maltreatment both within families and within institutions.

REFERENCES

Bowlby, J. (1969). *Attachment and loss, Vol. 1. Attachment.* London: Hogarth.

Browne, K. D. (1995*a*). Preventing child maltreatment through community nursing. *Journal of Advanced Nursing*, **21**, 57–63.

Browne, K. D. (1995*b*). The prediction of child maltreatment. In P. Reder & C. Lucey (Eds.). *Assessment of parenting: psychiatric and psychological contributions.* London: Routledge.

Browne, K. D. & Hamilton, C. E. (1999). Police recognition of links between spouse abuse and child abuse. *Child Maltreatment*, **4**, 136–47.

Browne, K. D. & Lynch, M. (1995). The nature and extent of child homicide and fatal abuse (Editorial in Special Issue on Fatal Child Abuse), *Child Abuse Review*, **4**, 309–16.

Browne, K. D. & Saqi, S. (1988*a*). Approaches to screening families high-risk for child abuse. In K. D. Browne, C. Davies & P. Stratton (Eds.). *Early prediction and prevention of child abuse* (pp. 57–86). Chichester: Wiley.

Browne, K. D. & Saqi, S. (1988*b*). Mother–infant interactions and attachment in physically abusing families. *Journal of Reproduction and Infant Psychology*, **6**, 163–82.

Browne, K. D., Hamilton, C. E., Heggarty, J. & Blissett, J. (2000). Identifying need and protecting children through community nursing home visits. *Representing Children*, **13**(2), 111–23.

Browne, K. D. & Herbert, M. (1997). *Preventing family violence.* Chichester: J. Wiley.

Browne, K. D., Cartana, C., Momeu, L. *et al.* (2002). *Child abuse and neglect in Romanian families: a National prevalence study.* Copenhagen, Denmark: World Health Organization Regional Office for Europe.

Browne, K. D., Hamilton-Giacritsis, C. E., Johnson, R. *et al.* (2005). *Mapping the number and characteristics of children under three in institutions across Europe at risk of harm.* Birmingham, UK: University of Birmingham Press (in collaboration with EU/WHO).

Cassidy, J. & Shaver, P. R. (1999). *Handbook of attachment: theory, research and clinical applications.* New York: Guildford Press.

Creighton, S. J. (1995). Fatal child abuse: how preventable is it? *Child Abuse Review*, **4**, 318–28.

Department of Education and Skills (2005). *Statistics of education: referrals, assessments and children and young people on Child Protection Registers Year ending 31ˢᵗ March 2004, England.* London: The Stationery Office.

Department of Health (1999). *Working together to safeguard children.* London: Department of Health Children's Services Branch.

Department of Health, Department of Education and Employment and the Home Office (2000). *Framework for the assessment of children in need and their families.* London: The Stationery Office.

Dixon, L., Browne, K. D. & Hamilton-Giachritsis, C. E. (2005*a*). Risk factors of parents abused as children: a mediational analysis of the intergenerational continuity of child maltreatment (Part I). *Journal of Child Psychology and Psychiatry*, **46**, 47–57.

Dixon, L., Hamilton-Giachritsis, C. E. & Browne, K. D. (2005*b*). Behavioural measures of parents abused as children: a mediational analysis of the intergenerational continuity of child maltreatment (Part II). *Journal of Child Psychology and Psychiatry*, **46**, 58–68.

Elkan, R., Kendrick, D. Hewitt, M. *et al.* (2000). The effectiveness of domiciliary health visiting: a systematic review of international studies and a selective review of the British literature. *Health Technology Assessment*, **4**: 1–339.

Glaser, D. (2000). Child aubse and neglect and the brain – a review. *Journal of Child Psychology & Psychiatry*, **41**(1), 97–116.

Goldberg, S. (2000). *Attachment and development.* London: Arnold.

Gilbert, N. (1997). Conclusion: a comparative perspective. In N. Gilbert (Ed.). *Combating child abuse: international perspective and trends* (pp. 232–40). Oxford: Oxford University Press.

Hallet, C. & Birchall, E. (1992). *Co-ordination and child protection.* London: HMSO.

Hamilton, C. E. & Browne, K. D. (1999). Recurrent abuse during childhood: a survey of referrals to Police child protection units. *Child Maltreatment*, **4**, 275–86.

Hamilton, C. E. & Browne, K. D. (2002). Predicting physical maltreatment. In K. D. Browne, H. Hanks, P. Stratton & C. Hamilton (Eds.). *Early prediction and prevention of child abuse: a handbook* (pp. 41–56). Chichester: Wiley.

Maccoby, E. E. (1980). *Social development: psychology growth and the parent–child relationship.* New York: Harcourt Brace Jovanovich.

Morton, N. & Browne, K. D. (1998). Theory and observation of attachment and its relation to child maltreatment: a review. *Child Abuse and Neglect*, **22**(11), 1093–104.

National Commission of Enquiry in the Prevention of Child Abuse. (1996). *Childhood Matters, Vols 1 & 2.* London: NSPCC.

New, C. & David, M. (1987). *For the children's sake: making child care more than a women's business.* Harmondsworth: Penguin.

National Society for the Prevention of Cruelty to Children (2001). *Out of sight.* London: NSPCC.

Olds, D. L., Henderson, C. R., Phelps, C. *et al.* (1993). Effect of prenatal and infancy nurse home visitation on Government spending. *Medical Care*, **31**(2), 155–74.

Olds, D., Eckenrode, J., Henderson, C. *et al.* (1997). Long-term effects of home visitation on maternal life course and child abuse and neglect: fifteen year follow up of a randomized trial. *Journal of the American Medical Association*, **278**, 637–43.

Olds, D., Henderson, C. & Eckenrode, J. (2002). Preventing child abuse and neglect with prenatal infancy and home visiting by nurses. In K. D. Browne, H. Hanks, P. Stratton & C. Hamilton (Eds.). *Early prediction and prevention of child abuse: a handbook* (pp. 165–82). Chichester: Wiley.

Redar, P. & Duncan, S. (2002). Predicting fatal child abuse and neglect. In K. D. Browne, H. Hanks, P. Stratton & C. Hamilton (Eds.). *Early prediction and prevention of child abuse: a handbook* (pp. 23–40) Chichester: Wiley.

Roberts, J. (1988). Why Are some families more vulnerable to child abuse? In K. D. Browne, C. Davies & P. Stratton (Eds.). *Early prediction and prevention of child abuse* (pp. 43–56). Chichester: Wiley.

Saunders, M. R. (1999). The Triple-P positive parenting program: towards an empirically validated multi-level parenting and family support strategy for the prevention of behaviour and emotional problems in children. *Clinical Child and Famliy Psychology Review*, **2**, 71–90.

Saunders, M. R. & Cann, W. (2002). Promoting positive parenting as an abuse prevention strategy. In K. D. Browne, H. Hanks, P. Stratton & C. Hamilton (Eds.). *Early prediction and prevention of child abuse: a handbook* (pp. 145–64). Chichester: Wiley.

Simpson, J. A. & Rholes, W. S. (1998). *Attachment theory and close relationships.* New York: Guildford Press.

Sluckin, W., Herbert, M. & Sluckin, A. (1983). *Maternal bonding.* Oxford: Blackwell.

Solomon, J. & George, C. (1999). *Attachment disorganization.* New York: Guildford Press.

United Nations (1989). The convention on the rights of the child. New York: *United Nations High Commissioner of Human Rights* (http://www.ohchr.org/english/).

Wang, C. T. & Harding, K. (1999). *Current trends in child abuse reporting and fatalities: the results of the 1998 Annual fifty state survey.* Chicago: National Center on Child Abuse Prevention Research.

World Health Organization (1998a). *First meeting on strategies for child protection.* Padua, Italy, 29–31 October 1998. Copenhagen: WHO Regional Office for Europe.

World Health Organization (1998b). *Essential antenatal, perinatal and postpartum care.* Copenhagen: WHO Regional Office for Europe.

World Health Organization (1999). *Report of the consultation on child abuse prevention.* WHO, Geneva, 29–31 March 1999. Geneva: WHO.

Chromosomal abnormalities

Jeremy Turk

St. George's, University of London

Introduction

Genetic influences on psychological functioning are well established (McGuffin *et al.*, 2004). A multifactorial interactional model between polygenic inheritance and environmental experience is most commonly proposed. However, many single gene anomalies have characteristic psychological profiles.

The term 'behavioural phenotype' (O'Brien, 2002) describes aspects of psychological functioning attributable to a discrete underlying genetic anomaly, even when other contributors such as age, gender and social background are accounted for. The first published use of the term was by Nyhan in his proposal of an association between the inborn error of metabolism and severe self-mutilation in Lesch–Nyhan syndrome (Nyhan, 1972). Nyhan also reported behaviours characteristic of Cornelia de Lange syndrome including self-injury, hyperactivity and autistic features (Berney *et al.*, 1999).

Somewhat earlier, Langdon Down described characteristic personality traits in individuals with Down syndrome including strong powers of imitation, a lively sense of humour, obstinacy and amiability. Research confirms greater similarity of personality and temperament between people with Down syndrome than expected by chance (Nygaard *et al.*, 2002). It also confirms increased risks of Alzheimer's dementia (Holland *et al.*, 2000) and depression (Collacott *et al.*, 1998).

Clinical considerations

Information on psychiatric, psychological and behavioural functioning can be categorized into:

- intellectual functioning
- speech and language
- attentional deficits and impulse control
- social functioning and understanding
- other behavioural disturbances

Intellectual functioning

Intellectual abilities in those with a particular condition can vary widely. People with Down syndrome usually have moderate-to-severe intellectual disability, while those with fragile X syndrome usually have mild-to-moderate intellectual disability (Cornish *et al.*, 2004b). Profile of intellectual functioning varies too. Individuals with fragile X syndrome and Turner's syndrome commonly experience numeracy and visuospatial difficulties. Children with velocardiofacial (VCF) syndrome, caused by a chromosome 22 microdeletion (Murphy, 2004), also typically attain higher verbal than performance IQ scores. Individuals with Klinefelter's syndrome, who have one Y and two X sex chromosomes, usually have language problems.

Speech and language

Speech may be entirely absent as in Angelman syndrome (Clayton-Smith & Laan, 2003), of particular quality as in fragile X syndrome (jocular, litanic, perseverative, cluttered) (Cornish *et al.*, 2004a) or characterized by particular deficits such as the expressive language impairments in Klinefelter's syndrome (Mandoki *et al.*, 1991). Individuals with Williams syndrome are characteristically superficially grammatically correct with complex and fluent expressive language which may lead to over-estimation of general intellectual ability (Metcalfe, 1999).

Attentional deficits

Attentional deficits range from mild inattentiveness and distractibility through to severe hyperkinesis. Some conditions show specific associations, for example fragile X syndrome (Turk, 1998), Turner's

625

syndrome (Rovet & Ireland, 1994) and Sanfilippo syndrome (Bax & Colville, 1995).

Social impairments

Social difficulties are common in people with intellectual disability. They may present as shyness and social anxiety as in fragile X syndrome. Their significance is magnified when associated with language disorders and ritualistic/obsessional tendencies indicative of an autistic spectrum disorder. Autistic features are pronounced in many individuals with fragile X syndrome (Turk & Graham, 1997) and tuberous sclerosis (Baker et al., 1998).

Other behavioural disturbances

Self-injury is common and troublesome for many people with severe intellectual disability. Its nature ('topography') is surprisingly syndrome-specific. People with Lesch–Nyhan syndrome display skin scratching, lip biting and knuckle gnawing (Robey et al., 2003). Those with fragile X syndrome usually bite at the base of their thumb in response to anxiety or excitement (Symons et al., 2003). Smith–Magenis syndrome (17p11.2 deletion) is associated with usually mild-to-moderate intellectual disability, but particularly extreme self-mutilation including pulling out finger nails (onychotillomania) and inserting objects in to bodily orifices (polyemolokoilomania) (Sarimski, 2004). It is also associated with extreme sleep disturbance and hyperactivity (see 'Hyperactivity').

A general review of behavioural phenotypes

Behavioural phenotype syndromes can relate to anomalies throughout the human genome.

Sex chromosome anomalies

Turner's syndrome (45X)

Short stature and infertility are usually associated with average intellectual functioning, although IQ mean and distribution are shifted downwards slightly. There is a verbal/performance discrepancy with relative language strengths but special needs in numeracy and visuospatial abilities as well as social relationship and social competency problems and attentional deficits (McCauley et al., 2001).

Klinefelter's syndrome (47XXY)

Speech and language impairments belie relatively intact non-verbal skills. Characteristically speech and language development is delayed with visual–motor and sensory integration problems (Mandoki et al., 1991). Mean full scale IQ is in the low 90s (Bender et al., 1999).

XYY syndrome

Up to half of people with XYY syndrome have language and reading difficulties, delayed motor development and psychosocial problems (Geerts et al., 2003). Antisocial behaviour is rare though temper tantrums, impaired social relationships and oppositional or conduct disorders are common. Intelligence is usually average.

Fragile X syndrome

Fragile X syndrome is the most common identifiable inherited cause of intellectual disability (Hagerman & Hagerman, 2002). Abnormal DNA enlargement on the X chromosome expands transgenerationally, interfering with production of a protein critical for normal neurodevelopment. Mild to moderate intellectual disability (IQ 35–70) is usually associated with numeracy and visuospatial deficits. Rates of intellectual development parallel those of non-disabled peers until puberty when discrepancies widen, due to sequential information processing problems. Female 'carriers' may have a full mutation (greater than 200 DNA repeats) or a pre-mutation where repeat length is approximately 50–200. Intellectual anomalies occur in female carriers, being more severe with full mutations (Franke et al., 1996). Social, language and attentional deficits arise. Female carriers experience early menopause with premature ovarian failure and may also develop an adult tremor–ataxia syndrome (Hagerman & Hagerman, 2004). This also occurs in adult pre-mutation males.

Speech and language are usually delayed and distorted with echolalia, repetitive and perseverative utterances and cluttering; a combination of rapid and disrhythmic language. Talking often sounds humorous with up-and-down pitch swings.

Attentional deficits and overactivity are common and challenging. Comparison with non-fragile X intellectually disabled peers confirms higher levels of inattentiveness, restlessness and fidgetiness in boys with fragile X, even if gross motor activity levels are less remarkable (Turk, 1998). Unlike non-fragile X peers, those with fragile X do not tend to improve spontaneously with age, emphasizing the need for early identification and treatment.

Up to 30% of males have autism. Many more show communicatory and ritualistic impairments with a friendly and sociable, albeit shy and socially anxious, personality (Turk & Graham, 1997). Common features include delayed echolalia, repetitive speech, hand flapping, hand biting in response to anxiety or excitement, gaze aversion, preference for routine and sameness, sensory defensivenesses and delayed development of symbolic and imaginative play.

Autosomal chromosome disorders

Down syndrome

Down syndrome is the most common cause of intellectual disability. Apart from the rare translocation variety it always occurs as new mutations producing trisomy 21, the major risk factor being increasing maternal age. Given the mean level of intellectual functioning, in the moderate–severe intellectual disability range, rates of autistic spectrum disorder and attention deficit-hyperactivity disorder are surprisingly low. However autistic spectrum disorder does occur in as many as 10% of people with Down syndrome and diagnosis is often considerably delayed (Rasmussen et al., 2001). Hyperactive behaviours occur in up to 50%. Alzheimer's dementia has a markedly raised incidence and must be distinguished from depression (Collacott et al., 1998), 'challenging behaviour', and psychological reactions to life events.

Tuberous sclerosis

Tuberous sclerosis is a common and incapacitating cause of intellectual disability associated with three different genetic anomalies.

75–80% experience infantile spasms with a chaotic disorganized EEG ('hypsarrhythmia'). Number and size of pathological brain tubers are associated with degree of intellectual disability (O'Callaghan *et al.*, 2004). Their presence in temporal lobes is associated with autistic spectrum disorders (Baker *et al.*, 1998). Hyperactivity is common and relates to degree of cerebral damage and intellectual impairment.

Williams syndrome

Idiopathic hypercalcaemia is caused by a chromosome 7 microdeletion. Speech and language anomalies are universal, yet many show superior verbal skills compared to visuospatial and motor abilities (Atkinson *et al.*, 2001). Hyperacusis (dislike of loud or intense sounds) is common. Full scale IQ is usually in the 50s or 60s. Rates of behavioural disturbance are high, particularly hyperactivity, anxiety and eating and sleeping difficulties (Metcalfe, 1999).

Angelman and Prader–Willi syndromes

Angelman and Prader–Willi syndrome demonstrate the significance of chromosomal imprinting, whereby parental inheritance of the affected chromosome is all important. Both are caused by anomalies on the long arm of chromosome 15. Prader–Willi syndrome results from inheritance of a paternal chromosome 15 microdeletion, or from inheritance of two maternal chromosome 15s. The consequence is infantile floppiness, poor feeding, weak or absent cry and failure to thrive, with expressive language and articulation problems. Compulsive over-eating and gross obesity develop unless strict behavioural eating programmes and severe restrictions of food availability are maintained. There is absence of satiety and lack of the usual need to vary nature of food consumed in order to maintain interest in eating. Challenging behaviours include skin picking, stubbornness and temper outbursts in response to frustration combined with decreased pain sensitivity. Visuospatial skills are good, yet numeracy and short-term memory are areas of special need (Donaldson *et al.*, 1994). Intellectual functioning varies widely and there is liability to cyclical mood disorders (Descheemaeker *et al.*, 2002). Common sleep problems include sleep apnoea, snoring, early waking and excessive daytime sleepiness (see 'Sleep apnoea').

Angelman syndrome problems arise from inheritance of maternal chromosome 15 microdeletions, or inheritance of two paternal chromosome 15s. Individuals usually have severe intellectual disability with a happy disposition, paroxysmal laughter, jerky ataxic gait, sleep problems and tendency towards an open mouth (Clayton-Smith & Laan, 2003). Epilepsy occurs in over 80% and can take any form although atypical absences and myoclonic seizures are most common in adulthood (Laan *et al.*, 1997). Autistic features

with marked aloofness and passivity are common with substantially delayed social and communication skills (Peters *et al.*, 2004).

Disorders ascertained initially on basis of behavioural and developmental profiles

Many conditions have been described with developmental and behavioural profiles sufficiently characteristic to convince one of a behavioural phenotype's presence. Increasingly these are found to have underlying genetic anomalies. An example is Rett's syndrome where manifestation in females only was explained by X-linked inheritance with lethality for males who lack a healthy X chromosome (Colvin *et al.*, 2003). Following relatively unremarkable early development, intellectual and social decline commences at 6–12 months with subsequent levelling off of abilities. Autistic, social and communicatory impairments are common (Mount *et al.*, 2003). There is loss of purposeful hand movements, midline hand-wringing, hyperventilation, breath-holding, bruxism and tremulousness. The gene responsible (MECP2) is located on the X chromosome's long arm. Over 90% have epilepsy with frequent seizures (Steffenburg *et al.*, 2001).

Sotos syndrome (chromosome 5 long arm microdeletion) has behavioural associations with classic physical features of excessively rapid growth, and intellectual disability. Hyperactivity, clumsiness and poorly articulated speech occur (Rutter & Cole, 1991). There may also be social difficulties and emotional and behavioural disturbance including tantrums, sexual precocity, sleep problems, anxious behaviour, object phobias and attention deficits (Sarimski, 2003).

The importance of diagnosis (Turk, 2004)

Individuals and families have a right to know the exact natures and causes of their disabilities. Outdated notions that diagnosis produces negativism, inertia and suspension of efforts to overcome disadvantage have been superseded by awareness of how important such labels are in facilitating grief reactions, dissipating inappropriate guilt and anger, orientating families towards helpful and appropriate supports and interventions, and allowing them to relate to appropriate support groups (Carmichael *et al.*, 1999). Successful grief resolution enables focussing on the future, adjusting individual and family life accordingly, and planning ahead. Crucial genetic counselling can often be offered to extended families following successful diagnosis. Diagnostic awareness also allows for more rational interventions relevant to individuals' particular profiles of strengths and needs.

(See also 'Disability', 'Screening: genetic' and 'Screening: antenatal'.)

REFERENCES

Atkinson, J., Anker, S., Braddick, O. *et al.* (2001). Visual and visuospatial development in young children with Williams syndrome. *Developmental Medicine and Child Neurology*, **43**, 330–7.

Baker, P., Piven, J. & Sato, Y. (1998). Autism and tuberous sclerosis complex: prevalence and clinical features. *Journal of*

Autism and Developmental Disorders, **28**, 279–85.

Bax, M. C. O. & Colville, G. A. (1995). Behaviour in mucopolysaccharide disorders. *Archives of Disease in Childhood*, **73**, 77–81.

Bender, B. G., Harmon, R. J., Linden, M. G., Bucher-Bartelson, B. & Robinson, A.

(1999). Psychosocial competence of unselected young adults with sex chromosome abnormalities. *American Journal of Medical Genetics*, **88**, 200–6.

Berney, T. P., Ireland, M. & Burn, J. (1999). Behavioural phenotype of Cornelia de Lange syndrome. *Archives of Disease in Childhood*, **81**, 333–6.

Carmichael, B., Pembrey, M., Turner, G. & Barnicoat, A. (1999). Diagnosis of fragile X syndrome: the experiences of parents. *Journal of Intellectual Disability Research*, **43**, 47–53.

Clayton-Smith, J. & Laan, L. (2003). Angelman syndrome: a review of the clinical and genetic aspects. *Journal of Medical Genetics*, **40**, 87–95.

Collacott, R. A., Cooper, S.-A., Branford, D. & McGrother, C. (1998). Behaviour phenotype for Down's syndrome. *British Journal of Psychiatry*, **172**, 85–9.

Colvin, L., Fyfe, S., Leonard, S. et al. (2003). Describing the phenotype of Rett syndrome using a population database. *Archives of Disease in Childhood*, **88**, 38–43.

Cornish, K., Sudhalter, V. & Turk, J. (2004a). Attention & language in fragile X. *Mental Retardation and Developmental Disabilities Research Reviews*, **10**, 11–16.

Cornish, K. M., Turk, J., Wilding, J. et al. (2004b). Annotation: deconstructing the attention deficit in fragile X syndrome: a developmental neuropsychological approach. *Journal of Child Psychology and Psychiatry*, **45**, 1042–53.

Descheemaeker, M. J., Vogels, A., Govers, V. et al. (2002). Prader–Willi syndrome: new insights in the behavioural and psychiatric spectrum. *Journal of Intellectual Disability Research*, **46**, 41–50.

Donaldson, M. D. C., Chu, C. E., Cooke, A. et al. (1994). The Prader–Willi syndrome. *Archives of Disease in Childhood*, **70**, 58–63.

Franke, P., Maier, W., Hautzinger, M. et al. (1996). Fragile X carrier females: evidence for a distinct psychopathological phenotype? *American Journal of Medical Genetics*, **64**, 334–9.

Geerts, M., Steyaert, J. & Fryns, J. P. (2003). The XYY syndrome: a follow-up study on 38 boys. *Genetic Counselling*, **14**, 267–79.

Hagerman, P. J. & Hagerman, R. J. (2004). The fragile-X premutation: a maturing perspective. *American Journal of Human Genetics*, **74**, 805–16.

Hagerman, R. J. & Hagerman, P. J. (2002). *Fragile X syndrome: diagnosis, treatment and research*. Baltimore, London: Johns Hopkins University Press.

Holland, A. J., Hon, J., Huppert, F. A. & Stevens, F. (2000). Incidence and course of dementia in people with Down's syndrome: findings from a population-based study. *Journal of Intellectual Disability Research*, **44**, 138–46.

Laan, L. A., Renier, W. O., Arts, W. F. et al. (1997). Evolution of epilepsy and EEG findings in Angelman syndrome. *Epilepsia*, **38**, 195–9.

Mandoki, M. W., Sumner, G. S., Hoffman, R. P. & Riconda, D. L. (1991). A review of Klinefelter's syndrome in children and adolescents. *Journal of the American Academy of Child and Adolescent Psychiatry*, **30**, 167–72.

McCauley, E., Feuillan, P., Kushner, H. & Ross, J. L. (2001). Psychosocial development in adolescents with Turner syndrome. *Journal of Developmental and Behavioral Pediatrics*, **22**, 360–5.

McGuffin, P., Owen, M. J. & Gottesman, I. I. (2004). *Psychiatric genetics and genomics*. Oxford: Oxford University Press.

Metcalfe, K. (1999). Williams syndrome: an update on clinical and molecular aspects. *Archives of Disease in Childhood*, **81**, 198–200.

Mount, R. H., Hastings, R. P., Reilly, S., Cass, H. & Charman, T. (2003). Towards a behavioral phenotype for Rett syndrome. *American Journal on Mental Retardation*, **108**, 1–12.

Murphy, K. C. (2004). Review: the behavioural phenotype in velocardiofacial syndrome. *Journal of Intellectual Disability Research*, **48**, 524–30.

Nygaard, E., Smith, L. & Torgersen, A. M. (2002). Temperament in children with Down syndrome and in prematurely born children. *Scandinavian Journal of Psychology*, **43**, 61–71.

Nyhan, W. L. (1972). Behavioral phenotypes in organic genetic disease. *Pediatric Research*, **6**, 1–9.

O'Brien, G. (2002). *Behavioural phenotypes in clinical practice*. London: MacKeith Press.

O'Callaghan, F. J. K., Harris, T., Joinson, C. et al. (2004). The relation of infantile spasms, tubers and intelligence in tuberous sclerosis complex. *Archives of Disease in Childhood*, **89**, 530–3.

Peters, S. U., Beaudet, A. L., Madduri, N. & Bacino, C. A. (2004). Autism in Angelman syndrome: implications for autism research. *Clinical Genetics*, **66**, 530–6.

Rasmussen, P., Börjesson, O., Wentz, E. & Gillberg, C. (2001). Autistic disorders in Down syndrome: background factors and clinical correlates. *Developmental Medicine and Child Neurology*, **43**, 750–4.

Robey, K. L., Reck, J. F., Giacomini, K. D., Barabas, G. & Eddey, G. E. (2003). Modes and patterns of self-mutilation in persons with Lesch–Nyhan disease. *Developmental Medicine and Child Neurology*, **45**, 167–71.

Rovet, J. & Ireland, L. (1994). Behavioral phenotype in children with Turner syndrome. *Journal of Pediatric Psychology*, **19**, 779–90.

Rutter, S. C. & Cole, T. R. P. (1991). Psychological characteristics of Sotos syndrome. *Developmental Medicine and Child Neurology*, **33**, 898–902.

Sarimski, K. (2003). Behavioural and emotional characteristics in children with Sotos syndrome and learning disabilities. *Developmental Medicine and Child Neurology*, **45**, 172–8.

Sarimski, K. (2004). Communicative competence and behavioural phenotype in children with Smith–Magenis syndrome. *Genetic Counselling*, **15**, 347–55.

Steffenburg, U., Hagberg, G. & Hagberg, B. (2001). Epilepsy in a representative series of Rett syndrome. *Acta Paediatrica*, **90**, 34–9.

Symons, F. J., Clark, R. D., Hatton, D. D., Skinner, M. & Bailey, D. B. (2003). Self-injurious behavior in young boys with fragile X syndrome. *American Journal of Medical Genetics A*, **118**, 115–21.

Turk, J. (1998). Fragile X syndrome and attentional deficits. *Journal of Applied Research in Intellectual Disabilities*, **11**, 175–91.

Turk, J. (2004). The importance of diagnosis. In D. Dew-Hughes (Ed.). *Educating children with fragile X syndrome* (pp. 15–19). London: Routledge Falmer.

Turk, J. & Graham, P. (1997). Fragile X syndrome, autism and autistic features. *Autism*, **1**, 175–97.

Chronic fatigue syndrome

Ruth Cairns and Trudie Chalder

King's College London

Introduction and definitions

Fatigue is a very common complaint but is typically transient, self-limiting or explained by other circumstances. Chronic fatigue syndrome (CFS) is characterized by persistent or relapsing unexplained fatigue of new or definite onset lasting for at least six months. It is not a new condition and corresponds very clearly to an illness called neurasthenia, commonly seen in Europe around the turn of the twentieth century (Wessely et al., 1998). The terms 'myalgic encephalomyelitis' (ME) and 'post-viral fatigue syndrome' have also been used to describe CFS but are misleading and unsatisfactory: ME implies the occurrence of a distinct pathological process whereas post-viral fatigue syndrome wrongly suggests that all cases are preceded by a viral illness.

Operational criteria developed for research purposes by the US Centres for Disease Control and Prevention (CDC) (Fukuda et al., 1994) and from Oxford (Sharpe et al., 1991) are now widely used to define CFS. The American criteria require at least six months of persistent fatigue causing substantial functional impairment and at least four somatic symptoms (from a list of eight) occurring with the fatigue in a 6-month period. The presence of a medical disorder that explains the prolonged fatigue excludes a patient from a diagnosis of CFS, as do a number of psychiatric diagnoses. Although the British definition is similar it differs by requiring both physical and mental fatigue but no physical symptoms. By including a requirement for several physical symptoms, the American definition reflects the belief that an infective or immune process underlies the syndrome.

Aetiology

The prevalence of CFS has been reported as 0.1–2.6% in community and primary care-based studies, depending on the criteria used (Wessely et al., 1997). Women are at higher risk than men (Relative risk 1.3–1.7) (Wessely, 1995). In relation to aetiology, physiological and psychological factors are thought to work together to predispose an individual to CFS and to precipitate and perpetuate the illness (Afari & Buchwald, 2003). For example, many patients link the onset of their symptoms to infection and while it is unlikely that serious viral illness acts as a continuing focus of infection in CFS, it is known to trigger its onset in some individuals (Cleare & Wessely, 1996). Other risk factors for developing CFS include previous psychological illness (Wessely et al., 1998), and severe life events or difficulties in the months before onset (Hatcher & House, 2003; see 'Life events and health').

A wide range of factors may act to perpetuate chronic fatigue. Coping responses to acute fatigue are important determinants of prolonged fatigue: extreme physical activity after an acute illness may allow insufficient time for recovery whereas prolonged bed rest may cause physical deconditioning and further exacerbate symptoms. Illness beliefs and the attribution of symptoms to a physical cause, with minimization of psychological or personal contributions, are also important and have been related to increased symptoms and worse outcomes in CFS (Wilson et al., 1994; see 'Illness perceptions'). Similarly, catastrophic beliefs that exercise will be damaging or will worsen symptoms lead to the avoidance of physical and mental activities and greater disability (Petrie et al., 1995). Disrupted sleep patterns resulting from excessive daytime rest may contribute to fatigue, muscle pain and poor concentration.

The response and attitudes of others are also important in determining the course of fatigue. Overly concerned carers may reinforce patients' maladaptive beliefs and coping strategies by inadvertently encouraging disability. Sceptical or stigmatizing reactions from relatives, health professionals or work colleagues can cause frustration and leave the patient feeling isolated and unsupported (Deale & Wessely, 2001; Van Houdenhove et al., 2002; see 'Stigma').

Diagnosis

There are no diagnostic signs or symptoms of CFS. The clinical evaluation of chronically fatigued patients is aimed at excluding underlying medical or psychiatric causes of fatigue. In individuals with fatigue of more than six months duration a thorough history, physical examination, routine laboratory tests (full blood count, ESR, renal, liver and thyroid function and urinary protein and glucose) and mental state examination are sufficient to reach a diagnosis of CFS in most cases. Where abnormalities are revealed on physical or laboratory investigation, further investigations can be helpful to help establish alternative diagnosis but should otherwise be limited to avoid the risk of iatrogenic harm. Specialist referral should be limited to situations where there is an increased probability of an alternative diagnosis.

The relationship between CFS and psychiatric illness is more complex. Fatigue is a common symptom in mental illness and where an individual's fatigue is fully explained by a specific psychiatric disorder, a diagnosis of CFS should not be made. However, psychiatric co-morbidity (particularly with depressive, somatoform and anxiety disorders) is also common and when present should be diagnosed and treated in addition to the symptoms of CFS. This does not mean that psychiatric disorders are the cause of CFS and indeed a substantial minority of patients do not fulfil criteria for any psychiatric diagnosis (Wessely et al., 1998).

Treatment

The evidence suggests that the most effective treatments for CFS are cognitive behavioural therapy (CBT) and graded exercise therapy (see chapters on 'Cognitive behavioural therapy' and 'Exercise interventions'). The CBT model attempts to incorporate the heterogenous nature of the condition and stresses the role of perpetuating factors (Wessely *et al.*, 1991). The treatment for CFS therefore involves planned activity and rest, graded increases in activity, a sleep routine and cognitive restructuring of unhelpful beliefs and assumptions. One systematic review showed that CBT administered in specialist centres by skilled therapists led to improved physical functioning and quality of life compared with relaxation therapy or standard medical care (Price & Couper, 2002). In addition, a multi-centre randomized controlled trial (RCT) involving less experienced CBT therapists has reported improvements in fatigue severity and self-reported fatigue compared with guided support and no treatment (Prins *et al.*, 2001).

Graded aerobic exercise involves a structured exercise programme that is individually tailored to the patient's current level of activity and aims to gradually increase his or her aerobic activity. The exercise is usually walking and patients are advised not to exceed the prescribed exercise duration or intensity. RCTs evaluating graded exercise therapy have found that it improves measures of fatigue and physical functioning compared with flexibility training and relaxation training or general advice (Reid *et al.*, 2004).

There is insufficient evidence to suggest that antidepressants, corticosteroids or other pharmacological agents are beneficial in the treatment of CFS and no reliable evidence that dietary supplements, evening primrose oil or intra-muscular magnesium are helpful (Reid *et al.*, 2004). Prolonged rest cannot be recommended as a treatment for CFS and may actually perpetuate or increase fatigue in people recovering from a viral illness. A review of treatments for CFS reported both limited benefits and substantial adverse effects with immunoglobulin therapy (Rimes & Chalder, 2005). There is insufficient evidence for the use of interferon as an effective treatment for CFS.

Prognosis

CFS is not associated with an increased mortality rate and rarely constitutes a missed medical diagnosis when an attempt has been made to exclude organic illness prior to making the diagnosis. A recent systematic review of studies describing the prognosis of CFS identified 14 studies that used operational criteria to define cohorts of patients with CFS (Cairns & Hotopf, 2005). Full recovery from untreated CFS is rare and an improvement in symptoms is a more commonly reported outcome than full recovery. The median full recovery rate was 5% (range 0–31%) and the median proportion of patients who improved during follow-up was 39.5% (range 38–64%). Less fatigue severity at baseline, a sense of control over symptoms and not attributing illness to a physical cause were all associated with a good outcome. Psychiatric disorder was associated with poorer outcomes. The review looked at the course of CFS without systematic intervention but as reported above there is now increasing evidence for the effectiveness of cognitive behavioural and graded exercise therapies. Further research is necessary to explore the prognosis of CFS after such treatment has been given.

REFERENCES

Afari, N. & Buchwald, D. (2003). Chronic fatigue syndrome: a review. *The American Journal of Psychiatry*, **160**, 221–36.

Cairns, R. & Hotopf, M. (2005). Review article: the prognosis of chronic fatigue syndrome. *Occupational Medicine*, **55**, 20–31.

Cleare, A. J. & Wessely, S. C. (1996). Chronic fatigue syndrome: a stress disorder? *British Journal of Hospital Medicine*, **55**, 571–4.

Deale, A. & Wessely, S. (2001). Patients' perceptions of medical care in chronic fatigue syndrome. *Social Science and Medicine*, **52**, 1859–64.

Fukuda, K., Straus, S., Hickie, I. *et al.* (1994). The chronic fatigue syndrome: a comprehensive approach to its definition and study. *Annals of Internal Medicine*, **121**, 953–9.

Hatcher, S. & House, A. (2003). Life events, difficulties and dilemmas in the onset of chronic fatigue syndrome: a case-control study. *Psychological Medicine*, **33**, 1185–92.

Petrie, K., Moss-Morris, R. & Weinman, J. (1995). Catastophic beliefs and their implications in chronic fatigue syndrome. *Journal of Psychosomatic Research*, **39**, 31–7.

Price, J. R. & Couper, J. (2002). Cognitive behaviour therapy for CFS. In: *the cochrane library, Issue 2*. Oxford: Update Software.

Prins, J. B., Beijenberg, G., Bazelmans, E. *et al.* (2001). Cognitive behaviour therapy for chronic fatigue syndrome: a multicentre randomised trial. *The Lancet*, **357**, 841–5.

Reid, S., Chalder, T., Cleare, A., Hotopf, M. & Wessely, S. (2004). Chronic fatigue syndrome. *Clinical Evidence*, **11**, 1–3.

Rimes, K. A. & Chalder, T. (2005). Treatments for chronic fatigue syndrome. *Occupational Medicine*, **55**, 32–9.

Sharpe, M., Arcard, L. C., Banatvala, J. E. *et al.* (1991). A report – chronic fatigue syndrome: guidelines for research. *Journal of the Royal Society of Medicine*, **84**, 118–21.

Van Houdenhove, B., Neerinckx, E., Onghena, P. *et al.* (2002). *Psychotherapy and Psychosomatics*, **71**, 207–13.

Wessely, S., David, A., Butler, S. & Chalder, T. (1991). The cognitive behavioural management of the postviral fatigue syndrome. In: R. Jenkins, J. Mowbray (Eds.). *The postviral syndrome (ME)* (pp. 297–334). Chichester: John Wiley.

Wessely, S. (1995). The epidemiology of chronic fatigue syndrome. *Epidemiologic Reviews*, **17**, 139–51.

Wessely, S., Chalder, T., Hirsch, S., Wallace, P. & Wright, D. (1997). The prevalence and morbidity of chronic fatigue and chronic fatigue syndrome: a prospective primary care study. *American Journal of Public Health*, **87**, 1449–54.

Wessely, S., Hotopf, M. & Sharpe, M. (1998). *Chronic fatigue and its syndromes*, New York: Oxford University Press.

Wilson, A., Hickie, I., Lloyd, A. *et al.* (1994). Longitudinal study of outcome of chronic fatigue syndrome. *British Medical Journal*, **308**, 756–9.

Chronic obstructive pulmonary disease (COPD): chronic bronchitis and emphysema

Ad A. Kaptein and Klaus F. Rabe

Leiden University Medical Centre

Chronic bronchitis and (pulmonary) emphysema are two respiratory disorders with similar patterns of symptoms: shortness of breath (dyspnea), sputum production, coughing and chest tightness. The two disorders also share important aetiological and pathophysiological characteristics (smoking tobacco, inflammation and destruction of lung tissue). For these reasons, chronic bronchitis and emphysema increasingly are combined into the concept of chronic obstructive pulmonary disease: COPD.

Chronic bronchitis is defined in behavioural terms: 'the presence of cough and sputum production for at least three months in each of two consecutive years' (GOLD, 2001, p. 7). Emphysema is defined in pathological terms: 'destruction of the gas-exchanging surfaces of the lung (alveoli)' (GOLD, 2001, p. 7). Chronic obstructive pulmonary disease is defined as 'a disease state characterized by airflow limitation that is not fully reversible. The airflow limitation is usually both progressive and associated with an abnormal inflammatory response of the lungs to noxious particles or gases' (GOLD, 2001, p. 6; www.goldcopd.com).

The prevalence of physician-diagnosed COPD is about 2% for men and 1.5% for women. Differences in prevalence per country or region are attributable to a large extent to differences in the prevalence of cigarette smoking (see 'Tobacco use'). Morbidity in terms of hospitalization, physician visits, emergency department visits, is substantial. Socio-economic costs in terms of absenteeism from work, early retirement and medical care are impressive. The quality of life of COPD patients is severely impaired (Maillé et al., 1996). The Global Burden of Disease Study predicts that in 2020 COPD will reach fifth rank in terms of disability-adjusted life-years and third in leading causes of death (Murray & Lopez, 1997). Given its prevalence and impact, research on COPD is relatively underfunded, compared with such conditions as AIDS and breast cancer (Gross et al.,1999; Pauwels & Rabe, 2004).

Psychology and COPD

In contrast to patients with asthma (see 'Asthma'), patients with COPD have only recently become an object of study and care by psychologists. The first study by psychologists on COPD patients examined 'basic personality traits characteristic of patients with primary obstructive pulmonary emphysema' (Webb & Lawton, 1961). The issue of personality characteristics and trait-like phenomena continued to be the focus of early psychological and psychiatric research about patients with COPD. Agle & Baum (1977) used a psychiatric interview for that purpose within male patients enrolled in a pulmonary rehabilitation programme, and found relatively high levels of anxiety ('respiratory panic'), depression, body preoccupation, alcohol problems and sexual dysfunctions. Some thirty years later, similar results were reported: hospitalized COPD patients and a community-based COPD sample reported 58% and 43% prevalence of psychological distress, respectively, compared with 4% for a healthy control group and 14% for a sample with various chronic illnesses (Andenæs & Kalfoss, 2004).

A second line of research pertained to examining the neuropsychological consequences of COPD. Compared with age- and education-matched healthy controls, hypoxemia in COPD patients was found to be associated with neuropsychological deficits (e.g. complex perceptual motor performance, simple motor tasks and abstracting ability; Grant et al., 1982).

A third research line was developed on illness behaviour in COPD patients. Kinsman and his colleagues were the first to assess the emotional and cognitive responses in patients with chronic bronchitis and emphysema towards their disorder (Kinsman et al., 1983). They employed a symptom checklist, based on patient interviews. In descending order of frequency, the patients reported dyspnea, fatigue, sleep difficulties, congestion, irritability, anxiety, eating difficulties, helplessness/hopelessness, poor memory and alienation as consequences of their respiratory problems. These findings helped in extending earlier work (e.g. Agle & Baum, 1977) and refining psychological assessment in patients with COPD. They were also instrumental in informing the fourth line of psychological research in patients with COPD; i.e. quality of life.

Empirical and theoretical work about quality of life in patients with COPD became of age in the 1980s (see 'Quality of life'). In Canada, Guyatt and colleagues developed the Chronic Respiratory Disease Questionnaire (CRDQ; Guyatt et al., 1987), and, in the UK, Jones and colleagues developed the St. George's Hospital Respiratory Questionnaire (SGRQ; Jones et al., 1992). The CRDQ assesses dyspnea, fatigue, emotional function and mastery. The SGRQ has three component scores: symptoms; activity; and impacts on daily life; and a total score. The dimensions in both questionnaires reflect the dimensions identified by Kinsman and colleagues, and the functional effect of COPD and its consequent therapy upon a patient, as perceived by the patient. It is striking to observe the high number of biomedical publications on the topic of COPD that now include quality of life measures. 'Quality of life resources' is one of the components of the website of the American Thoracic Society (www.thoracic.org), and quality of life has become a secondary outcome measure in many studies, and a primary outcome measure in a few (Bateman et al., 2004). This would have been unheard of even ten years ago

(Kaptein *et al.*, 1993). Quality of life and patient reported outcomes are two concepts that have built bridges between biomedical respiratory scientists, respiratory clinicians and behavioural scientists (Curtis *et al.*, 1997).

Pharmacological treatment is in itself not always effective in controlling COPD. Pulmonary rehabilitation – the fifth topic of psychological research in the COPD field – is intended to supplement medical interventions. 'Pulmonary rehabilitation is a multidisciplinary programme of care for patients with chronic respiratory impairment that is individually tailored and designed to optimize physical and social performance and autonomy' (ATS, 1999, p. 1666). It combines pharmacological treatment with a set of other components, such as physical therapy that encourages exercise training and more effective breathing and coughing techniques, education (for patients, partners, family), together with psychosocial and behavioural interventions. It is only recently that psychologists have become involved with pulmonary rehabilitation. This coincides with psychology's emerging role in COPD research in general. Initially, physical rehabilitation was the focus in such programmes: exercise training; physical therapy; breathing exercises; pursed lip breathing; and smoking cessation. Patient education consisted of patients passively listening to classes about anatomy and physiology of lungs and breathing. Increasingly, components such as discussing the emotional impact of COPD, consequences for the partner, sexuality and coping skills training were added to pulmonary rehabilitation programmes. Meta-analyses indicate positive effects of pulmonary rehabilitation on exercise capacity, breathlessness, quality of life, number of hospitalizations, length of hospitalization and reductions in anxiety and depression (GOLD, 2001; Lacasse *et al.*, 2003).

A number of medical interventions in COPD patients have not yet been evaluated extensively. The effects of improving nutritional status in patients with more severe stages of COPD are currently being studied (Wouters, 2004). Psychological research on this topic is virtually lacking. Oxygen therapy is given to patients with severe COPD. A systematic review indicated that oxygen therapy can influence mortality positively in selected categories of patients (Crockett *et al.*, 2001). Lung volume reduction surgery (LVRS) intends to reduce the volume of lung tissue that is not involved with gas exchange, thereby improving oxygenation and exercise capacity. Its effects are still uncertain, although there is some evidence that LVRS positively affects exercise capacity and quality of life (GOLD, 2001). Large randomized controlled trials are in progress, with quality of life as a major outcome measure (Kaplan *et al.*, 2004). Increasingly, lung transplantation is perceived by patients with end-stage COPD as a form of miracle surgery. These perceptions, however, are not borne out yet; the number of donor organs is one major limiting factor. Moreover, long-term effects on survival, exercise capacity and quality of life are uncertain, and the costs are substantial (Studer *et al.*, 2004).

A sixth major area of psychological research in COPD pertains to smoking cessation. Although patients with COPD may prefer a technological and medical approach to their breathing problems, evidence points out that 'cigarette smoking is the major cause of COPD in the world, and smoking cessation is the only therapeutic intervention so far shown to reduce disease progression' (Barnes & Hansel, 2004, p. 985). Smoking cessation is the area where psychology's contribution to care for COPD patients

is clearly evident: the Transtheoretical Model of Behaviour Change and evidence-based smoking cessation intervention programmes are included in international guidelines on the management of COPD (see 'Transtheoretical model of behaviour change'). Intensive behavioural programmes (relapse prevention) combined with various types of pharmacotherapy (including antidepressants) and nicotine replacement products are usually part of stop smoking interventions (Wagena *et al.*, 2004) (see 'Tobacco use'). Relatively short-term (6–12 months) abstention rates are around 10% (Wagena *et al.*, 2004). COPD patients tend to be very resistant when it comes to giving up smoking. A COPD patient's plea is a strong reminder of this: 'I'll do whatever you say, take my medications every day, I'll exercise three times a week, practice my belly breathing technique – just don't take my cigarettes away' (Berry, 2001).

Therapeutic pessimism among physicians, psychologists and patients, about therapeutic gains from any intervention (except giving up tobacco use) has recently and gradually moved towards a cautiously more optimistic outlook. Psychological interventions in COPD patients contributed to this change (Kaptein, 2002). Self-management interventions for COPD patients represent the seventh major field of study, and it seems a promising line of research and intervention (Kaptein, 1997) (see 'Self-management'). The study by Atkins *et al.* (1984) was one of the very first studies in this area. Its theoretical and methodological standards are very high, and its results are encouraging. In the study, a cognitive–behavioural intervention was applied to outpatients with COPD. In a randomized controlled design, the intervention's effects were assessed on quality of life and exercise capacity, with various control conditions. The cognitive–behavioural intervention consisted of challenging pessimistic and passive cognitions, and replacing them by more positive and constructive self-statements, a physical exercise programme and home visits by trained psychology students. Results indicate the superiority of the cognitive–behavioural intervention condition over the other conditions on the major outcome variables (see 'Cognitive behaviour therapy'). Cochrane reviews of this area, however, indicate that more research is needed before generalizations about positive effects of self-management techniques can be made (Monninkhof *et al.*, 2003).

Closing remarks

In line with the groundbreaking work by Atkins *et al.* (1984) in COPD, further research is required on behavioural–cognitive interventions in COPD. Theoretical models such as the Self Regulation Model seem helpful in guiding empirical work on the identification of maladaptive illness perceptions and examining the effects of changing them (Scharloo *et al.*, 2000) (see 'Lay beliefs about health and illness'). Other areas of psychological research which need further exploration are smoking cessation programmes, refinements in assessment of psychological issues in COPD patients, for example, disease specific feelings of depression, sexuality and refinement of psychological assessment and interventions in the context of pulmonary rehabilitation.

A virtually neglected area is the image of COPD in the society at large (Viney, 1989). Work on illness cognitions seems to indicate a quite strong sense of self-blame among COPD patients about their own behaviour in relation to respiratory problems (Kaptein *et al.*, 2003). Not every smoker of cigarettes develops COPD, however, and not every COPD patient is, or was, a smoker. A better image of COPD may help boost feelings of self-esteem in afflicted patients and thereby improve their quality of life. The COPD initiative and the COPD alliance of the American Thoracic Society are excellent steps in this direction (www.goldcopd.com; www.thoracic.org).

REFERENCES

Agle, D. P. & Baum, G. L. (1977). Psychological aspects of chronic obstructive pulmonary disease. *Medical Clinics of North America*, **61**, 749–58.

ATS (American Thoracic Society). (1999). Pulmonary rehabilitation – 1999. *American Journal of Respiratory and Critical Care Medicine*, **159**, 1666–82.

Andenæs, R. & Kalfoss, M. H. (2004). Psychological distress in hospitalized patients with chronic obstructive pulmonary disease. *European Journal of Epidemiology*, **19**, 851–9.

Atkins, C. J., Kaplan, R. M., Timms, R. M., Reinsch, S. & Lofback, K. (1984). Behavioral exercise programs in the management of chronic obstructive pulmonary disease. *Journal of Consulting and Clinical Psychology*, **52**, 591–603.

Barnes, P. J. & Hansel, T. T. (2004). Prospects for new drugs for chronic obstructive pulmonary disease. *Lancet*, **364**, 985–96.

Bateman, E. D., Boushey, H. A., Bousquet, J. *et al.* (2004). Can guideline-defined asthma control be achieved? *American Journal of Respiratory and Critical Care Medicine*, **170**, 836–44.

Berry, M. J. (2001). Pleas from a pulmonary rehabilitation patient. *Chest*, **120**, 1427.

Crockett, A. J., Cranston, J. M., Moss, J. R. & Alpers, J. H. (2001). A review of long-term oxygen therapy for chronic obstructive pulmonary disease. *Respiratory Medicine*, **95**, 437–43.

Curtis, J. R., Martin, D. P. & Martin, T. R. (1997). Patient-assessed health outcomes in chronic lung disease. *American Journal of Respiratory and Critical Care Medicine*, **156**, 1032–9.

Global Initiative for Obstructive Lung Disease (GOLD) (2001). Global strategy for the diagnosis, management, and prevention of chronic obstructive pulmonary disease. NHLBI/WHO Workshop Report. Bethesda MD, NIH, 2001.

Grant, I., Heaton, R. K., McSweeny, A. J., Adams, K. M. & Timms, R. M. (1982). Neuropsychologic findings in hypoxemic chronic obstructive pulmonary disease. *Archives of Internal Medicine*, **142**, 1470–6.

Gross, C. P., Anderson, G. F. & Powe, N. R. (1999). The relation between funding by the national institutes of health and the burden of disease. *New England Journal of Medicine*, **340**, 1881–7.

Guyatt, G. H., Berman, L. B., Townsend, M., Pugsley, S. O. & Chambers, L. W. (1987). A measure of quality of life for clinical trials in chronic lung disease. *Thorax*, **42**, 773–8.

Jones, P. W., Quirk, F. H., Baveystock, C. M. & Littlejohns, P. (1992). A self-complete measure of health status for chronic airflow limitation. *American Review of Respiratory Disease*, **145**, 1321–7.

Kaplan, R. M., Ries, A. L., Reilly, J. & Mohsenifar, Z. for the NETT-group (2004). Measurement of health-related quality of life in the national emphysema treatment trial. *Chest*, **126**, 781–9.

Kaptein, A. A. (2002). Respiratory disorders and behavioral research. In A. A. Kaptein & T. L. Creer (Eds.). *Respiratory disorders and behavioral medicine* (pp. 1–17). London: Martin Dunitz Publishers.

Kaptein, A. A. (1997). Behavioural interventions in COPD: a pause for breath. *European Respiratory Review*, **7**, 88–91.

Kaptein, A. A. & Creer, T. L. (Eds.). (2002). Respiratory disorders and behavioral medicine. London: Martin Dunitz Publishers.

Kaptein, A. A., Brand, P. L. P., Dekker, F. W. *et al.* & the Dutch CNSLD Study Group (1993). Quality-of-life in a long-term multicentre trial in chronic nonspecific lung disease: assessment at baseline. *European Respiratory Journal*, **6**, 1479–84.

Kaptein, A. A., Scharloo, M., Helder, D. I. *et al.* (2003). Representations of chronic illnesses. In L. D. Cameron & H. Leventhal (Eds.). *The self-regulation of health and illness behaviour* (pp. 97–118). London: Routledge.

Kinsman, R. A., Yaroush, R. A., Fernandez, E. *et al.* (1983). Symptoms and experiences in chronic bronchitis and emphysema. *Chest*, **83**, 755–61.

Lacasse, Y., Brosseau, L., Milne, S. *et al.* (2003). Pulmonary rehabilitation for chronic obstructive pulmonary disease. (Cochrane Review). In: *the cochrane library, Issue 3*, 2003. Oxford: Update Software.

Maillé, A. R., Kaptein, A. A., de Haes, J. C. J. M. & Everaerd, W. T. A. M. (1996). Assessing quality of life in chronic non-specific lung disease: a review of empirical studies published between 1980 and 1994. *Quality of Life Research*, **5**, 287–301.

Monninkhof, E. M., van der Valk, P. D. L. P. M., van der Palen, J. *et al.* (2003). Self-management education for chronic obstructive pulmonary disease (Cochrane Review). In: *the cochrane library, Issue 2*, 2003. Oxford: Update Software.

Murray, C. J. L. & Lopez, A. D. (1997). Alternative projections of mortality and disability by cause 1990–2020: global burden of disease study. *Lancet*, **349**, 1498–504.

Pauwels, R. A. & Rabe, K. F. (2004). Burden and clinical features of chronic obstructive pulmonary disease (COPD). *Lancet*, **364**, 613–20.

Scharloo, M., Kaptein, A. A., Weinman, J. *et al.* (2000). Physical and psychological correlates of functioning in patients with chronic obstructive pulmonary disease. *Journal of Asthma*, **37**, 17–29.

Studer, S. M., Levy, R. D., McNeil, K. & Orens, J. B. (2004). Lung transplant outcomes: a review of survival, graft function, physiology, health-related quality of life and cost-effectiveness. *European Respiratory Journal*, **24**, 674–85.

Viney, L. L. (1989). *Images of illness*. Malabar, FL: Krieger.

Wagena, E. J., van der Meer, R. M., Ostelo, R. J. W. G., Jacobs, J. E. & van Schayck, C. P. (2004). The efficacy of smoking cessation strategies in people with chronic obstructive pulmonary disease: results from a systematic review. *Respiratory Medicine*, **98**, 805–81.

Webb, M. W. & Lawton, A. H. (1961). Basic personality traits characteristic of patients with primary obstructive pulmonary emphysema. *Journal of the American Geriatrics Society*, **9**, 590–610.

Wouters, E. F. M. (2004). Management of severe COPD. *Lancet*, **364**, 883–95.

Cleft lip and palate

Brent Collett and Matthew Speltz

University of Washington School of Medicine

Orofacial clefts are openings in the lip or roof of the mouth that result from arrested embryonic development in the first trimester. They are among the most common congenital malformations, with an incidence of 1 to 2 per 1000 live births (Derijcke *et al.*, 1996). Presentations include cleft lip only (CLO), cleft palate only (CPO) and cleft lip and palate (CLP). Clefts can also be categorized as 'unilateral' or 'bilateral' (involving one or both sides of the lip and/or palate), and 'incomplete' or 'complete' (involving only the soft palate versus both the soft and hard palates, and/or involving only the lip versus the lip and gumline). Most clefts are 'nonsyndromic', meaning that they are not associated with other malformations. Although aetiology remains unclear, most cases are believed to result from a combination of genetic vulnerability and prenatal exposures (e.g. tobacco, anticonvulsant medications), possibly interacting with maternal nutritional status (Prescott & Malcolm, 2002).

Clefts of the lip and palate can be detected by ultrasound in utero. Though this technology is developing rapidly, many cases are missed and often the diagnosis is not made until birth (see 'Screening: antenatal' and 'Foetal wellbeing'). During the neonatal period, most families are referred to a specialty hospital-based clinic for management of their child's care. Surgical repair of the cleft lip is typically undertaken by age 5 months, followed by cleft palate repair when children are 12–18 months old. Subsequent procedures and surgical revisions are scheduled according to patients' needs (see 'Reconstructive and cosmetic surgery'). Frequently encountered medical complications include difficulty in feedings, poor physical growth, velopharyngeal insufficiency (i.e. incomplete closure of the velopharyngeal sphincter, resulting in 'nasal' speech and/or regurgitation during feeding), chronic otitis media, orthodontic concerns and airway obstruction.

Psychological research with cleft populations dates back to the 1950s, with primary interest in social–emotional outcomes. The highly visible and stigmatizing nature of these conditions, in addition to the stress associated with multiple medical procedures during the early years, have prompted researchers to hypothesize that children with clefts have elevated risk for poor psychological and social adjustment. Research has focused on parents' emotional responses to having a child with a deformity; the quality of parent–child relationships; and children's social, emotional and behavioural functioning (see also 'Facial disfigurement'). Investigators have also studied the cognitive, language and academic development of youngsters with orofacial clefts and the related factors that contribute to these areas of functioning. The interdependent development of the face and central nervous system has generated interest in abnormal brain structures and/or functions that may predispose children with clefts to neuropsychological problems.

In this chapter, the research on parents' adjustment to their child's cleft diagnosis and the psychological and neurodevelopmental functioning of children with clefts will be reviewed. Implications of this research for clinical care and directions for future studies are also discussed.

Psychological and neurodevelopmental functioning

Parental adjustment

Qualitative studies have shown that many parents experience a period of bereavement after their child's birth, accompanied by a search for information about the cause and broader implications of their infant's cleft condition. Parents may develop idiosyncratic beliefs regarding the aetiology of the disorder including pseudo-medical explanations (e.g. pre-natal stress, medications used) and spiritual attributions (e.g. punishment for parental transgressions; Tisza & Gumpertz, 1962) (see also 'Attributions and health'). In survey studies, parents have expressed dissatisfaction with the manner in which their child's cleft diagnosis was provided and the information they received from medical providers in response to questions about the developmental and medical consequences of their child's condition (Strauss *et al.*, 1995).

In one study, the mothers of children with various craniofacial disorders (including orofacial clefts) reported higher levels of parenting stress, lower evaluations of self-competence, and higher levels of marital conflict than did the mothers of typical children (e.g. Speltz *et al.*, 1993). However, other studies have not supported the hypothesis that parents of children with clefts have more difficulties than do parents of non-cleft infants.

Parent–child relationships

Researchers have examined parents' and children's mutual responsiveness and social engagement during interaction, as well as the quality of the relationship as indexed by observations of attachment behaviours (e.g. using the Ainsworth 'Strange Situation'; see Speltz *et al.*, 1997). Some studies suggest that infants with clefts and their parents are less active, playful and responsive during parent–child interactions than are controls (Barden *et al.*, 1989). However, few differences in attachment behaviours between infants with clefts and control infants have been found.

Studies of toddler/preschooler–parent dyads have also produced variable findings, with some investigators reporting that the mothers of children with clefts show elevated levels of engagement and direction during interaction (e.g. Allen *et al.*, 1990). Although studies of parent–adolescent relationships in the cleft population are

634

lacking, this is a promising area of investigation, given the increasing involvement in medical decision-making of youth at this age (e.g. whether or not to pursue further cosmetic surgery) and its potential stress on the relationship.

Children's psychosocial functioning

Orofacial clefts have a stigmatizing social effect on children with this condition, as indicated by numerous studies of peer and adult perceptions. Children with clefts are consistently rated as less attractive and are described in less desirable terms than non-affected peers; findings that parallel those obtained in studies of typical children's physical attractiveness and observers' social perceptions. Even in the absence of a cleft lip, raters are able to detect the subtle craniofacial anomalies associated with 'invisible' clefts of the palate (e.g. mid-facial retrusion, orbital hypertelorism; Speltz et al., 1997). Studies have also investigated social attributions based on speech samples of children with clefts. Data on this issue are mixed, with early studies showing that children with clefts were rated as less preferred by peers based on their speech and more recent studies failing to show such an effect (Berry et al., 1997).

Research on the emotional and behavioural adjustment of children with clefts has produced conflicting results. The most commonly reported finding, based primarily on work by Richman et al. (e.g. Millard & Richman, 2001), is that children with clefts are more socially inhibited than controls, particularly in the classroom. Consistent with this description, findings from an observational study showed that preschoolers with clefts showed greater emotional restraint than non-cleft peers (Endriga et al., 2003). Adults with clefts have been found to report lower quality of life in multiple domains than comparison groups (e.g. Marcusson et al., 2001), an outcome often associated with a socially reclusive lifestyle.

It has been hypothesized that children with clefts are more likely than typical children to form negative self-perceptions, as they 'internalize' the presumably negative social responses of others (e.g. in relation to their anomalous physical appearance or speech). Commonly assessed domains of self-perception include appearance, friendships, problem-solving ability and intellectual competence. Children with 'visible' clefts (i.e. those with CLO and CLP) have reported poorer self-concept with regard to physical appearance than those with 'invisible' clefts of the palate only (Broder et al., 1994). However, few differences are found in other dimensions of self-perception. Indeed, in some studies children and adolescents with clefts have reported higher levels of self-concept in some domains (e.g. satisfaction with friendships, problem-solving and intellectual competence; Broder et al., 1994), a finding that may reflect a defensive response set.

Neuropsychological and academic outcomes

Research on early motor and mental development suggests that infants and toddlers with clefts lag slightly behind their peers on standardized measures, and have a higher than expected percentage score in the 'developmentally delayed' range (Kapp-Simon & Kruckeberg, 2000; Speltz et al., 2000). Comparisons among cleft groups suggest that those with CPO receive the lowest scores, followed by children with CLP and CLO, who tend to score roughly within the average range (Kapp-Simon & Kruckeberg, 2000). Children with associated malformations in addition to a cleft lip or palate appear to be at particular risk of developmental delay (Swanenburg De Veye et al., 2003).

Deficits in expressive and receptive language among children with orofacial clefts have been reported on the basis of standardized and observational measures (Morris & Ozane, 2003). Researchers have also shown that children with clefts score in the low average range on standardized measures of intelligence, with particular weakness in the verbal domain (Richman, 1980). However, differences are not consistently observed, and others have found that children with clefts score well within normal limits. An elevated rate of reading disabilities has been reported, with an estimated 30–40% of youth with clefts struggling in this area (Broder et al., 1998). When diagnostic sub-groups are compared, males with CPO tend to evidence the most notable cognitive, language and learning deficits in comparison with all other diagnosis–gender combinations (Broder et al., 1998). There is a paucity of neuropsychological and academic investigations of adolescents and adults, though it appears that deficits continue to be observed (Nopolous et al., 2002). Recent studies using neuroimaging suggest underlying differences in brain structure among individuals with clefts that may account for functional differences observed (Nopolous et al., 2002).

Clinical implications

The inconsistency and small magnitude of group differences in the preceding studies suggest that the majority of children with clefts show normal development. However, these studies also point to a significant minority of children with significant problems who need psychological assessment and treatment. Standards set forth by the American Cleft Palate–Craniofacial Association identify the need for childhood screening and assessment of developmental status, neuropsychological testing in older children, and various psychological interventions including pre-surgery anxiety reduction and social skills training. The elevated rates of reading disability among children with clefts indicate a particular need for routine screening and remediation of deficits in verbally mediated functions, including phonemic awareness and verbal fluency.

Research suggests that parents would benefit from psychological and educational interventions as well. During the first year of life, these services might target stress reduction; maternal feeding and teaching skills; and education regarding diagnosis and anticipated outcomes. A group format may be the most appropriate, and would promote social support among parents with similar experiences, in addition to providing education and training (see 'Social support interventions'). The anticipated effects of such interventions not only include better parental functioning, but also enhancement of the parent–child relationship. There is little doubt that the quality of parent–child interaction affects infant development. For example, in a cleft population, Speltz and colleagues (2000) found that quality of maternal teaching interactions in the first year predicted later cognitive functioning. Similarly, the quality of maternal feeding interactions was concurrently related to infants' physical growth (Coy et al., 2000) and their subsequent security of attachment (Speltz et al., 1997). In other high-risk infant groups, there is evidence that parent 'interaction coaching' can enhance infant development and preliminary evidence suggests that this approach is useful for cleft populations (Pelchat *et al.*, 1999).

Early childhood interventions in the cleft population should target parents and infants showing particularly high social and demographic risk. For example, in one study of infants with clefts, male infants of young, primiparous mothers reporting high depression (on a screening instrument) were at the highest risk of parent–child relationship difficulties (Speltz *et al.*, 1997), suggesting that this sub-group might especially be in need of assistance.

Conclusions and research recommendations

Research on the psychological aspects of clefts has yielded quite variable results. In part, this may reflect methodological limitations (e.g. use of small and diagnostically heterogeneous samples) and procedural differences across studies (e.g. lack of agreement on the most appropriate outcome measures). However, it is also likely that outcomes are diverse, depending on a host of medical and psychosocial factors. There is continuing need for well designed studies that examine the multifactorial context in which clefts are associated with better and worse outcomes. Cross-sectional, 'between-group' comparisons of cleft and non-cleft samples are numerous, but longitudinal, predictive analyses of developmental processes within cleft groups are rare and sorely needed. There is also need for randomized trials of the types of interventions already described (e.g. early reading interventions), which would advance theoretical understanding of developmental processes and provide clinically useful information that could improve the lives of individuals with orofacial clefts.

REFERENCES

Allen, R., Wasserman, G. A. & Seidman, S. (1990). Children with congenital anomalies: the preschool period. *Journal of Pediatric Psychology*, **15**, 327–45.

Barden, R. C., Ford, M. E., Jensen, A. G., Rogers-Salyer, M. & Salyer, K. E. (1989). Effects of craniofacial deformity in infancy on the quality of mother–infant interactions. *Child Development*, **60**, 819–24.

Berry, L. A., Witt, P. D., Marsh, J. L., Pilgram, T. K. & Eder, R. A. (1997). Personality attributions based on speech samples of children with repaired cleft palates. *Cleft Palate Craniofacial Journal*, **34**, 385–9.

Broder, H. L., Richman, L. C. & Matheson, P. B. (1998). Learning disability, school achievement, and grade retention among children with cleft: a two-center study. *Cleft Palate-Craniofacial Journal*, **35**, 127–31.

Broder, H. L., Smith, F. B. & Strauss, R. P. (1994). Effects of visible and invisible orofacial defects on self-perception and adjustment across developmental eras and gender. *Cleft Palate Craniofacial Journal*, **31**, 429–36.

Coy, K., Speltz, M. L., Jones, K., Hill, S. & Omnell, M. L. (2000). Do psychosocial variables predict the physical growth of infants with orofacial clefts? *Journal of Developmental and Behavioral Pediatrics*, **21**, 198–206.

Derijcke, A., Eerens, A. & Carels, C. (1996). The incidence of oral clefts: a review. *The British Journal of Oral & Maxillofacial Surgery*, **34**, 488–94.

Endriga, M. C., Jordan, J. R. & Speltz, M. L. (2003). Emotion self-regulation in preschool-aged children with and without orofacial clefts. *Journal of Developmental and Behavioral Pediatrics*, **24**, 336–44.

Kapp-Simon, K. A. & Kruckeberg, S. (2000). Mental development in infants with cleft lip and/or palate. *Cleft Palate Craniofacial Journal*, **37**, 65–70.

Marcusson, A., Akerlind, I. & Paulin, G. (2001). Quality of life in adults with repaired complete cleft lip and palate. *Cleft Palate Craniofacial Journal*, **38**, 379–85.

Millard, T. & Richman, L. C. (2001). Different cleft conditions, facial appearance, and speech: relationship to psychological variables. *Cleft Palate Craniofacial Journal*, **38**, 68–75.

Morris, H. & Ozanne, A. (2003). Phonetic, phonological, and language skills of children with a cleft palate. *Cleft Palate Craniofacial Journal*, **40**, 460–70.

Nopoulos, P., Berg, S., Canady, J. et al. (2002). Structural brain abnormalities in adult males with clefts of the lip and/or palate. *Genetics in Medicine*, **4**, 1–9.

Pelchat, D., Bisson, J., Ricard, N., Perreault, M. & Bouchard, J. M. (1999). Longitudinal effects of an early family intervention programme on the adaptation of parents of children with a disability. *International Journal of Nursing Studies*, **36**, 465–77.

Prescott, N. J. & Malcolm, S. (2002). Folate and the face: evaluating the evidence for the influence of folate genes on craniofacial development. *Cleft Palate Craniofacial Journal*, **39**, 327–31.

Richman, L. C. (1980). Cognitive patterns and learning disabilities in cleft palate children with verbal deficits. *Journal of Speech and Hearing Research*, **23**, 447–56.

Speltz, M. L., Endriga, M. C., Fisher, P. A. & Mason, C. A. (1997). Early predictors of attachment in infants with cleft lip and/or palate. *Child Development*, **68**, 12–25.

Speltz, M. L., Endriga, M. C., Hill, S. et al. (2000). Cognitive and psychomotor development of infants with orofacial clefts. *Journal of Pediatric Psychology*, **25**, 185–90.

Speltz, M. L., Morton, K., Goodell, E. W. & Clarren, S. S. (1993). Psychological functioning of children with craniofacial anomalies and their mothers: follow-up from late infancy to school entry. *Cleft Palate Craniofacial Journal*, **30**, 482–9.

Strauss, R. P., Sharp, M. C., Lorch, S. C. & Kachalia, B. (1995). Physicians and the communication of "bad news": parent experiences of being informed of their child's cleft lip and/or palate. *Pediatrics*, **96**, 82–9.

Swanenburg De Veye, H. F. N., Beemer, F. A., Mellenbergh, G. J., Wolters, W. H. G. & Heineman-De Boer, J. A. (2003). An investigation of the relationship between associated congenital malformations and the mental and psychomotor development of children with clefts. *Cleft Palate Craniofacial Journal*, **40**, 297–303.

Tisza, V. B. & Gumpertz, E. (1962). The parents' reaction to the birth and early care of children with cleft palate. *Pediatrics*, **30**, 86–90.

Cold, common

Anna L. Marsland[1], Sheldon Cohen[2] and Elizabeth Bachen[3]

[1]University of Pittsburgh
[2]Carnegie Mellon University
[3]Mills College

Upper respiratory infections (URI) as a group are responsible for 50% of all acute illnesses, with the common cold syndrome being most familiar. Colds are caused by over 200 viruses and are characterized by sore throat, congestion and mucus secretion. When exposed to viruses or other infectious agents, only a proportion of people develop clinical illness. Reasons for variability in response are not well understood and the possibility that psychological factors play some role in the aetiology and progression of infectious disease has received increased attention.

It is commonly believed that stressful life events influence the onset of URI by causing negative affective states (e.g. anxiety and depression) which, in turn, exert direct effects on biological processes or behavioural patterns that increase disease risk. The influence of stress on the immune system is considered the primary biological pathway through which stress can influence infectious disease susceptibility. While there is substantial evidence that stress is associated with changes in immune function (Herbert & Cohen, 1993; Segerstrom & Miller, 2004) (see 'Psychoneuroimmunology'), the implications of stress-induced immune changes for susceptibility to disease have not been established. To date, studies of stress and URI susceptibility have focused on establishing a link between stress and disease with little attention to pathways through which such an association might occur. The major findings of these studies are examined below.

There is consistent evidence that persons under stress report greater levels of URI symptoms and that stress results in greater health care utilization for URI (Cohen & Williamson, 1991). For example, Glaser et al. (1987) demonstrated that medical students report more infectious (mostly URI) illness during examination periods than at other times. Similarly, Stone et al. (1987) found that, for 79 married couples followed over three months, daily life events rated as undesirable increased three to four days prior to onset of self-reported symptoms of URI, close in time to the incubation period of many common cold viruses. The self-reported symptoms of URI measured in these studies may tap underlying pathology; however, it is also possible that they reflect a stress-induced misinterpretation of physical sensations without underlying illness. The latter interpretation is supported by studies in which effects of stress on symptoms, but not verified disease, are observed, and by evidence that stress is associated with increased symptom reporting in general, not only with symptoms directly associated with infectious pathology (Cohen & Williamson, 1991) (see 'Symptom perception').

Other investigators have verified the presence of pathology by physician diagnosis or biological methods. Several of these studies provide evidence that life stressors increase risk for verified upper respiratory disease. For example, Meyer and Haggerty (1962) followed 100 members of 16 families for a 12-month period. Daily life events that disrupted family and personal life were 4 times more likely to precede than to follow new streptococcal and non-streptococcal infections (as diagnosed by throat cultures and blood antibody levels) and associated symptomatology. Similar results were reported in a study of viral URIs in 235 members of 94 families (Graham et al., 1986). Here, high stress, as defined by scores on reported major stressful life events, daily events and psychological stress, was associated with more verified episodes and more symptom days of respiratory illness. Turner Cobb and Steptoe (1996) also found that higher levels of life event stress were associated with increased clinically-verified URI among 107 adults followed for 15 weeks. In sum, studies verifying infectious episodes suggest that stress increases risk for upper respiratory disease. However, community studies, like these, do not control for the possible effects of stressful events on exposure to infectious agents. Moreover, the literature on this topic is not entirely consistent; indeed, several studies have failed to find a relation between stress and upper respiratory disease (for review see Cohen & Williamson, 1991) (see also 'Life events and health').

Several prospective studies have eliminated the possible role of psychological effects on exposure by experimentally inoculating healthy individuals with common cold viruses (viral challenge studies). Here, volunteers are assessed for degree of stress and then experimentally exposed to a cold virus or placebo. They are then kept in quarantine and monitored for the development of infection and illness. Early viral challenge studies were limited by a range of methodological weaknesses (Cohen & Williamson, 1991), including insufficient sample sizes and lack of control for factors known to influence susceptibility to viral infection (including pre-existing antibodies to the infectious agent and age). Furthermore, the possible role of stress-elicited changes in health practices such as smoking and alcohol consumption was not considered. These limitations may account for initial failures to find consistent relations between stress and susceptibility to URI.

In contrast, recent viral challenge studies have included multiple controls for factors known to be independently associated with susceptibility to viral infection (e.g. Cohen et al., 1991, 1993, 1998; Stone et al., 1992). These studies consistently find a positive association between stress and susceptibility to URI. For example, among 394 healthy adults, stressful life events, perceptions of current stress and negative affect were all associated with an increased risk of developing biologically verified URI, with greater stress related linearly to susceptibility (Cohen *et al.*, 1991, 1993, 1998). Further examination of findings revealed that perceptions of stress and negative affect increased risk for illness through a different pathway than stressful life events. The former measures increased the probability of becoming infected (replicating virus), while the latter increased the probability of infected people developing clinical symptoms (Cohen *et al.*, 1995). More recent research from this group suggests that the longer the duration of stressful life events, the greater risk of becoming infected (Cohen *et al.*, 1998). A large group of control factors including age, sex, allergic status, body weight, season and virus-specific antibody status before challenge, could not explain the increased risk of colds for persons reporting greater stress. Smoking, alcohol consumption, diet, exercise and sleep quality also failed to explain the association between stress and illness.

In a similar study, Stone *et al.* (1992) examined development of symptoms among persons infected with rhinovirus. They found that those with more life events were more likely to develop clinical colds, although perceptions of current stress and negative affect were unrelated to symptom development. In contrast to studies described earlier, this investigation included only infected persons and hence could not assess susceptibility to infection where Cohen and colleagues found perceptions of stress and negative affect were related to susceptibility.

Recent attention has turned to an examination of psychosocial factors that may decrease susceptibility to URI by regulating emotion-sensitive biological systems and/or encouraging health-enhancing behaviours. These factors include dispositional positive affect and social engagement. Initial findings from viral challenge studies suggest that susceptibility to URI decreases in a dose-response manner with increased diversity of the social network and with trait sociability (Cohen *et al.*, 1997; Cohen *et al.*, 2003*a*) (see Social Support and Health). Furthermore, higher positive affect has been associated with decreased incidence of objective symptoms of upper respiratory illness among infected people (Cohen *et al.*, 2003*b*). These relationships appear to be independent of negative emotional styles, baseline immunity, demographics and health practices. Thus, there is some initial evidence that certain psychosocial factors are protective, being related to greater resistance to infection and the expression of fewer objective clinical symptoms.

In sum, well controlled studies support prospective studies of community samples in indicating that psychological stress is associated with increased susceptibility to the common cold. In addition, there is consistent evidence for increased symptom-reporting under stress. Recent studies also suggest that positive emotional styles, sociability and more diverse social networks are associated with greater resistance to developing colds. A number of potential pathways exist through which an association between psychosocial factors and infectious pathology might occur, including behavioral, hormonal and immune mechanisms. Future work is needed to explore these alternatives.

(See also 'Asthma' and 'Chronic obstructive pulmonary disease'.)

REFERENCES

Cohen, S., Doyle, W. J., Skoner, D. P. *et al.* (1995). State and trait negative affect as predictors of objective and subjective symptoms of respiratory viral infections. *Journal of Personality and Social Psychology*, **68**, 159–69.

Cohen, S., Doyle, W. J., Skoner, D. P. *et al.* (1997). Social ties and susceptibility to the common cold. *Journal of the American Medical Association*, **277**, 1940–44.

Cohen, S., Doyle, W. J., Turner, R. B., Alper, C. M. & Skoner, D. P. (2003*a*). Sociability and susceptibility to the common cold. *Psychological Science*, **14**, 389–95.

Cohen, S., Doyle, W. J., Turner, R. B., Alper, C. M. & Skoner, D. P. (2003*b*). Emotional style and susceptibility to the common cold. *Psychosomatic Medicine*, **65**, 652–7.

Cohen, S., Frank, E., Doyle, W. J. *et al.* (1998). Types of stressors that increase susceptibility to the common cold in healthy adults. *Health Psychology*, **17**, 214–23.

Cohen, S., Tyrrell, D. A. J. & Smith, A. P. (1991). Psychological stress and susceptibility to the common cold. *The New England Journal of Medicine*, **325**, 606–12.

Cohen, S., Tyrrell, D. A. J. & Smith, A. P. (1993). Negative life events, perceived stress, negative affect, and susceptibility to the common cold. *Journal of Personality and Social Psychology*, **64**, 131–40.

Cohen, S. & Williamson, G. M. (1991). Stress and infectious disease in humans. *Psychological Bulletin*, **109**, 5–24.

Glaser, R., Rice, J., Sheridan, J. *et al.* (1987). Stress-related immune suppression: health implications. *Brain, Behavior, and Immunity*, **1**, 7–20.

Graham, N. M. H., Douglas, R. B. & Ryan, P. (1986). Stress and acute respiratory infection. *American Journal of Epidemiology*, **124**, 389–401.

Herbert, T. B. & Cohen, S. (1993). Stress and immunity in humans: a meta-analytic review. *Psychosomatic Medicine*, **55**, 364–79.

Meyer, R. J. & Haggerty, R. J. (1962). Streptoccocal infections in families. *Pediatrics*, **29**, 539–49.

Segerstrom, S. C. & Miller, G. E. (2004). Psychological stress and the human immune system: a meta-analytic study of 30 years of inquiry. *Psychological Bulletin*, **130**, 601–30.

Stone, A. A., Reed, B. R. & Neale, J. M. (1987). Changes in daily event frequency precede episodes of physical symptoms. *Journal of Human Stress*, **13**, 70–4.

Stone, A. A., Bovbjerg, D. H., Neale, J. M. *et al.* (1992). Development of common cold symptoms following experimental rhinovirus infection is related to prior stressful life events. *Behavioral Medicine*, **Fall**, 115–20.

Turner Cobb, J. M. & Steptoe, A. (1996). Psychosocial stress and susceptibility to upper respiratory tract illness in an adult population sample. *Psychosomatic Medicine*, **58**, 404–12.

Complementary medicine

Felicity L. Bishop[1] and George T. Lewith[2]

[1]Aldemoor Health Centre
[2]University of Southampton

Introduction

Complementary and alternative medicine (CAM) includes a wide range of practices which do not fit in with the dominant biomedical model of health care and are not commonly provided within conventional medicine settings. In the 1960s CAM was on the fringe of the mainstream, in the 1970s it was positioned as alternative and in the 1990s it became complementary. In the new millennium, the position of CAM has changed again and is moving towards integration with conventional medicine, for example CAM therapies are commonly offered in palliative care and pain clinic contexts. Currently substantial numbers of people are turning to CAM. The prevalence of CAM use increased from 34% to 39% during the 1990s in the general population in the USA (Eisenberg *et al.*, 1998). In the UK 46% of the population can be expected to use one or more CAM therapies in their lifetime and 10% visited a practitioner of an established CAM therapy in 1998 (Thomas *et al.*, 2001). This chapter addresses the nature of these therapies which are proving so popular with patients, how are they regulated, whether they are seen as complementary or an alternative to conventional medicine and how conventional medicine is reacting to the rising popularity of other approaches to health care.

Popular CAM therapies

The most popular CAM therapies in the UK include acupuncture, osteopathy, chiropractic, herbal medicine and homeopathy. Descriptions of these therapies are provided in Table 1.

Patients perceive that CAM is effective, but within the context of evidence-based medicine there is substantial difference between efficacy and effectiveness. Patients perceive antidepressants to be effective, but the true efficacy of the chemical remedy versus placebo may confer only 15–20% of the overall effect of prescribing an antidepressant (see 'Placebos'). A similar situation may exist in acupuncture. It is known, for instance, that a single acupuncture point is effective for nausea. This may include post-anaesthetic nausea, chemotherapy-induced nausea and early morning sickness (Vickers, 1996) (see 'Nausea and vomiting'). However, the situation for the relative efficacy of acupuncture for pain is less clear (White *et al.*, 2002). There is evidence that herbs may be effective in certain specific conditions, for instance the use of St John's Wort in depression (Linde *et al.*, 1996), but while it is possible to accept that herbal extracts have real chemical efficacy, it is difficult to accept that homeopathy may work with no explicable mechanism, in spite of the available evidence which suggests that homeopathy is not simply a placebo (Linde *et al.*, 1997). CAM is a vast field that offers many challenges to researchers within both qualitative and quantitative research. Clearly there are some areas where it has proven efficacy, but these are relatively few and far more investigation is required before CAM can be fully integrated into an evidence-based framework.

The recent UK House of Lords' report (2000) highlighted the fact that much CAM practice was occurring without appropriate regulation. While the efficacy of each individual CAM treatment may be far from proven, it is a matter of public safety that CAM practitioners should be properly regulated, practising in an ethical and professional manner and providing treatments which are fundamentally safe. Osteopaths and chiropractors took the lead in the matter of statutory regulation and both are now regulated and have appropriate and elected general councils governing the profession, its processes and ethics. Acupuncture and herbal medicine are in the process of being regulated in the UK with discussions at an advanced stage, but no final decision on the exact form that this

Table 1. Popular forms of CAM

CAM Form	Description
Acupuncture	• Based on an energetic view of the body. • Stimulation of acupuncture points used to restore energy balance, promote healing and alleviate illness.
Osteopathy	• Holistic system of diagnosis and manual treatment for mechanical problems of the body. • Employs manipulation and massage of the soft tissue and joints to promote self-healing and treat musculoskeletal problems.
Chiropractic	• Manipulative technique founded on the idea that musculoskeletal problems are caused by the misalignment of vertebrae. • Spinal manipulations and adjustments are employed to improve alignment and alleviate musculoskeletal problems.
Herbal medicine	• Holistic model of health and illness, separate traditions include European, Chinese and Indian herbal medicines. • Plant-based herbal remedies are used to treat the cause of health problems and offer a cure beyond symptomatic relief.
Homeopathy	• Based on the Law of Similars (a substance that causes symptoms in a healthy person will alleviate those symptoms in a patient). • Treatment focuses on the whole person and tailors treatments to individuals, aiming to facilitate natural healing abilities through the prescription of remedies.

regulation may take. Furthermore, the manufacture, prescription and claims that can be made on various herbal products are in the process of review with the intention of harmonizing procedures on a European-wide basis.

Who uses CAM and why?

People who use CAM are more likely to be female, middle-aged, highly educated and have higher incomes. This picture is relatively consistent across population-based surveys (Astin, 1998), comparisons between users of CAM and conventional medicine (Furnham & Beard, 1995), and surveys of specific illness populations (Moore et al., 2000). CAM is used in the maintenance of current health, prevention of future problems and in relation to current illnesses. There is a tendency for CAM to be used by people with chronic, long-standing illnesses. For example Murray and Shepherd (1993) found that a higher proportion of CAM users (69%) than non-users (49%) had conditions such as anxiety, depression, asthma, eczema, hayfever, or musculoskeletal problems.

CAM use is associated with beliefs about medicine. People who use CAM are more likely than those who use conventional medicine to believe that:

1. They are able to have some control over the course of their health and that they should have a participatory role in treatments (Balneaves et al., 1999) (see 'Self-efficacy and health').
2. Health and illness are holistic in nature, for example psychological factors are important in the development of illness, and that treatments should involve the mind, body and soul (Astin, 1998).
3. Treatments should be natural and that natural treatments are more effective and less toxic than prescription medications (O'Callaghan & Jordan, 2003).

Thus people who use CAM hold beliefs which are broadly consistent with the philosophical ideas underlying certain forms of CAM. There is evidence that in addition to being attracted to CAM, people hold negative beliefs about conventional medicine. People who use CAM tend to be dissatisfied with a number of aspects of conventional medicine, including:

1. Failure of conventional medicine to offer cure or control over long-standing illness (McGregor & Peay, 1996).
2. Lack of time available and general communication and interpersonal skills of practitioners (Moore et al., 2000).
3. Side-effects and invasiveness of conventional medical treatments (Paterson & Britten, 1999).

Thus CAM use is related to dissatisfaction with conventional medicine. However, dissatisfaction is not equivalent to rejection. The majority of people who use CAM do so alongside conventional medicine, and CAM use has been associated with increased use of conventional medicine (Astin et al., 2000). People are attracted to certain features of CAM and are dissatisfied with, but have not rejected, conventional medicine. Future research needs to consider other possible reasons for CAM use and needs to investigate what happens once people have started to use CAM. There has been relatively little research so far on issues such as why people use specific CAM therapies and not others, and the factors that influence adherence to and ongoing use of CAM (see also 'Lay beliefs about health and illness').

CAM and conventional medicine

The recent increase in CAM popularity can be seen as a patient-initiated movement which is linked to a general increase in consumerism in western societies. Patients are taking their healthcare into their own hands, seeking out CAM therapies which are mostly still accessed through the private sector. At the same time as this increase in CAM use, paternalistic healthcare has fallen out of favour and is being replaced by a patient-centred model of care, which emphasizes patient autonomy and empowerment as ideals (see 'Patient-centred healthcare'). Furthermore, it is not only the general public who are turning to CAM: conventional healthcare professionals are now using CAM to a similar extent (Burg et al., 1998) and many refer patients to CAM practitioners or practice CAM themselves. This shift away from paternalism in conventional medicine combined with the increasing popularity of CAM has raised the profile of CAM therapies within the conventional medical community and so there are moves towards integration. For example, the teaching of CAM in medical schools is now commonplace (e.g. Owen & Lewith, 2001).

Despite this generally positive attitude of conventional practitioners towards CAM, the relationship between complementary and conventional medicine is far from unproblematic. Patients do not always disclose information to their doctors about their CAM use (Astin et al., 2000), and attempts to discuss CAM with medical doctors are not always successful. At a broader level, debates continue concerning appropriate methodological approaches to furthering the evidence base for CAM (Richardson, 2000). Recent moves towards integrated medicine have problematic issues for both conventional and complementary providers surrounding issues such as the evidence base, professional identity and conflicting ideologies. So, while there are movements towards integration there remain tensions between the dominant and complementary health care systems.

Looking to the future

There are no signs of the general interest in, and popularity of, complementary medicine decreasing. Research in CAM is still in its infancy and is a growing multidisciplinary area. The key issues now in CAM research are related to:

1. Understanding what the benefits and outcomes of CAM use are from the patient's perspective, in particular through the use of qualitative approaches and consulting expert patients.
2. Increasing research capacity through schemes such as those provided by the Department of Health (in the UK) and the NCCAM (in the USA). Such schemes will encourage and facilitate much needed quality research into many areas of CAM, including efficacy research and social science approaches to CAM.
3. Developing safe clinical approaches to the integration of CAM in appropriate clinical contexts. The position of CAM within a clinical framework needs to be formalized, and issues such as clinical governance, practitioner quality and regulation need to be negotiated within this context.

REFERENCES

Astin, J. A. (1998). Why patients use alternative medicine. Results of a national study. *Journal of the American Medical Association*, **279**, 1548–53.

Astin, J. A., Pelletier, K. R., Marie, A. & Haskell, W. L. (2000). Complementary and alternative medicine use among elderly persons: one year analysis of a Blue Shield medicare supplement. *Journal of Gerontology*, **55A**, M4–M9.

Balneaves, L. G., Kristjanson, L. J. & Tataryn, D. (1999). Beyond convention: describing complementary therapy use by women living with breast cancer. *Patient Education and Counseling*, **38**, 143–53.

Burg, M. A., Kosch, S. G., Neims, A. H. & Stoller, E. P. (1998). Personal use of alternative medicine therapies by health science center faculty. *Journal of the American Medical Association*, **280**, 1563.

Eisenberg, D. M., Davis, R. B., Ettner, S. L. et al. (1998). Trends in alternative medicine use in the United States, 1990–1997. *Journal of the American Medical Association*, **280**, 1569–75.

Furnham, A. & Beard, R. (1995). Health, just world beliefs and coping style preferences in patients of complementary and orthodox medicine. *Social Science and Medicine*, **40**, 1425–32.

House of Lords. (2000). *Complementary and alternative medicine*. Select Committee on Science and Technology – 6th Report, Session 1999–2000. London: HMSO.

Linde, K., Clausius, N., Ramirez, G. et al. (1997). Are the clinical effects of homoeopathy placebo effects? A meta-analysis of placebo-controlled trials. *Lancet*, **350**, 834–43.

Linde, K., Reamers, G., Mulrow, C. D. et al. (1996). St. John's Wort for depression – an overview and meta-analysis of randomised clinical trials. *British Medical Journal*, **313**, 253–8.

McGregor, K. J. & Peay, E. R. (1996). The choice of alternative therapy for health care: testing some propositions. *Social Science and Medicine*, **43**, 1317–27.

Moore, A. D., Petri, M. A., Manzi, S. et al. (2000). The use of alternative medical therapies in patients with systemic lupus erythematosus. *Arthritis and Rheumatism*, **43**, 1410–18.

Murray, J. & Shepherd, S. (1993). Alternative or additional medicine? An exploratory approach in general practice. *Social Science and Medicine*, **37**, 983–8.

O'Callaghan, F. V. & Jordan, N. (2003). Postmodern values, attitudes and the use of complementary medicine. *Complementary Therapies in Medicine*, **11**, 28–32.

Owen, D. & Lewith, G. (2001). Complementary and alternative medicine (CAM) in the undergraduate medical curriculum: the Southampton experience. *Medical Education*, **35**, 73–7.

Paterson, C. & Britten, N. (1999). "Doctors can't help much": the search for an alternative. *British Journal of General Practice*, **49**, 626–9.

Richardson, J. (2000). The use of randomized control trials in complementary therapies: exploring the issues. *Journal of Advanced Nursing*, **32**(2), 398–406.

Thomas, K. J., Nicholl, J. P. & Coleman, P. (2001). Use and expenditure on complementary medicine in England: a population based survey. *Complementary Therapies in Medicine*, **9**, 2–11.

Vickers, A. J. (1996). Can acupuncture have specific effects on health? A systematic review of acupuncture antiemesis trials. *Journal of the Royal Society of Medicine*, **89**, 303–11.

White, P., Lewith, G. T., Berman, B. & Birch, S. (2002). Reviews of acupuncture for chronic neck pain: pitfalls in conducting systematic reviews. *Rheumatology*, **41**, 1224–31.

Contraction

Beth Alder

Napier University

Introduction

Birth rates vary worldwide and are related to economic and social factors as well as contraceptive choice. In parts of Africa the birth rate is high (e.g. in Niger, 48.9 births per 1000 women and a fertility rate of 6.83 children born per woman). In Europe it is dramatically lower (in Germany 8.04 births per 1000 women and a fertility rate of 1.38 children born per woman) (CIA World Factbook, 2004). Although there is such gobal variation there is little cross-cultural evidence about psychological aspect of contraceptive choice and so this chapter will refer to evidence from western societies. In England and Wales, conceptions fell from over 850 000 in 1991 to 190 000 in 2002. In spite of the development of safe and effective contraceptive methods unintended pregnancies are common. In England and Wales, the percentage of conceptions terminated by abortion rose from 19.4% in 1991 to nearly 23% in 2002 with the highest percentages in those aged under 20 or over 40. The Total Fertility Rate (TFR) is the sum of age and specific fertility rates expressed per woman and controls for the changing age distribution over time. In 2002, the TFR in England and Wales was 1.65 per woman, which is similar to the rates between 1920 and 1940, before the widespread use and acceptability of contraception.

These observations mean that a simple relationship between knowledge and availability of contraception and its use is unlikely (Office of National Statistics, 2004*b,c*; http://www.statistics.gov.uk/).

The evidence for a contraceptive career suggests that young people use either condoms or no contraceptive method at all in their first sexual encounters. With increasing sexual and contraceptive experience they move to oral contraceptives. Once their family is considered to be complete they choose either male or female sterilization. Oddens (1996), in a population survey of contraceptive use in the UK and Germany, found that patterns of contraceptive use were closely related to variables such as age, parity, marital status and intention to have children. Age and the desire to have children are the major factors associated with contraceptive choice. The decline in the use of oral contraceptives with age has been related to perceptions of health risk.

The *UK General Household Survey* in 2002 included questions on the use of contraception for the first time since 1998. Since then, the most common methods for avoiding pregnancy used by women aged 16 to 49 have been the contraceptive pill, surgical sterilization (both male and female) and the male condom. In 2002, 72% of women aged 16 to 49 used at least one form of contraception, a figure that has remained relatively constant since it was first measured (Office of National Statistics, 2004*a*). In 2002/03 the contraceptive pill was used by 26% of women aged 16 to 49 in the UK. Sterilization, of either the woman or her partner was used by 21%, and the male condom by 19% (Office of National Statistics, 2004*a*).

After termination of pregnancy it might be expected that women would be highly motivated to use effective contraception. In a study of 100 women in Switzerland, 69% of women attending for termination of pregnancy claimed that they had used contraception in the cycle that had resulted in the pregnancy (Bianchi-Demicheli *et al.*, 2001). Most (83%) intended to use contraception to prevent another pregnancy. Most (60%) were using the pill 6 months later and fewer used condoms. After their termination most changed their method of contraception from their previous method, even though that method would have been recommended (Bianchi-Demicheli *et al.*, 2003) (see 'Abortion').

Oral contraception

Most pill users use the combined pill, which contains both oestrogen and progestogen. Oral contraceptives are easy to use, very effective, safe, inexpensive and readily available. They work by inhibiting ovulation with the progestogen component causing changes to the endometrium, which inhibits implantation, and to the cervical mucosa, which decreases sperm penetration. They do not interfere with the act of sexual intercourse and give women control over their fertility. There is evidence which shows that the more detached contraception is from sexual activity the more acceptable it is (Cramer, 1996). They also have the advantage that they reduce menstrual and premenstrual problems and give women the ability to time their menstruation (withdrawal bleeding). A recent study of Canadian university students found that only half had taken the pill, with an average length of use of 33.5 months (Fletcher *et al.*, 2001). Healthy, educated women showed a surprising lack of knowledge of the medication taken: 39% were unaware of the type of pill prescribed and 8% had not reviewed the risks and benefits with a health professional.

However, oral contraception is not without some disadvantages. Side effects reported with the early high oestrogen-dose oral contraceptive pills included reduced sexual interest and depression, but these are minimal in current low dose preparations (Oddens, 1999). Condon *et al.* (1995) carried out a retrospective study of 145 women and found that nearly half reported side-effects and most changes in wellbeing were perceived as negative. Fletcher *et al.* (2001) found that 43% attributed the following side-effects to the pill: weight gain (23%); nausea (16%); spotting (15%); depression (9%); headaches (7%); increased blood pressure (0.8%); and blood clots (0.8%). Few of these effects have been demonstrated in clinical trials. A survey of over 100 nursing students found that fear of side-effects or health risks were the most frequently cited reasons for stopping pill use, and the views of healthcare providers were influential (Gardner, 2001). It is difficult to carry out good prospective studies of pill users because of ethical difficulties and high attrition rates. Women who experience side-effects may stop using the pill, and those who continue are less likely to report side-effects. Women who take the pill probably do so because it is very important to them to have a very safe form of contraception and they may be more likely to tolerate side-effects.

Sterilization

Vasectomies in men and laparoscopic sterilizations in women are safe and effective. In the UK, the use of female sterilization has increased significantly from 35% in 1986 to 44% in 2002 (Office of National Statistics, 2004*a*). However, sterilization operations are effectively irreversible and so the decision to be sterilized means the couple need to be very sure that they will not want more children. Studies on long-term effect of vasectomy have found no evidence of adverse psychological effects. A study of 115 Chinese women who had been sterilized and were followed up over a year found that there was no adverse effect on sexual adjustment and that their mental health measured by the GHQ (Goldberg, 1972) significantly improved. The regret rate after one year was 3.4% (Tang and Chung, 1997). Women requesting sterilization appear to have no higher rates of psychiatric disorder than the general population.

Male condom use

There has been a steady rise in the proportion of women whose partners use condoms, from 13% in 1986 to 19% in 2002. Again, this trend was not observed across all age groups. Among women aged 45 to 49, condom use has declined since 1986. It has remained fairly constant among women aged 35 to 44 and increased among women under the age of 35.

Most recent research into psychological aspects of condom use has considered them as protecting against disease rather than pregnancy. Grimely *et al.* (1995) tested the Transtheoretical Model of Behaviour Change (Prochaska and DiClemente, 1984) on

248 American college students and found that it could predict patterns of condom use (see 'Transtheoretical model of behaviour change'). Mahoney et al. (1995) tested the Health Belief Model in college students in relation to condom use and HIV infection. Sporadic users differed from both consistent and non-users in the actual number of sex partners in the previous year and actual frequency of drunkenness during sexual intercourse; but only perceived susceptibility to infection and self-efficacy differed between the groups (see 'Health belief model' and 'Self-efficacy and health').

Other methods

The intrauterine device (IUD) is mainly used by parous women and confers good protection. Like the pill, it does not interfere with sexual activity. IUDs have been associated with heavier, prolonged and more painful menstruation but a positive impact on sex life (Oddens, 1999).

Emergency contraception is available on prescription in the USA and over the counter in over 30 countries. After unprotected intercourse it reduces the risk of pregnancy by 85%. Smith et al. (1996) carried out a population based survey of 1214 women in Grampian, Scotland (65% response rate). They found that although most women (94%) were aware of emergency contraception, only 39% knew the correct timing for its use. In a survey of attitudes in Scotland, Romania and Slovenia it was found that 72%, 81% and 94% of women respectively felt positive to the idea of a pill which inhibited ovulation. Over 50% thought that a pill which inhibited or interfered with implantation was an acceptable idea. Attitudes to abortion, availability of contraception and religious beliefs are likely to be important (Rimmer et al., 1992).

In the USA, a study of 371 low-income English- or Spanish-speaking women found that only 3% had used emergency contraception, 36% had heard of it and only 7% knew the correct timing for its use (Jackson et al., 2000). The lack of knowledge was associated with being older, multiparae and monolingual Spanish-speaking. One approach to increase its use is to provide supplies of emergency contraception to women in advance of need. It has been shown that this does not reduce the abortion rate (Fairhurst et al., 2004). Women were reluctant to ask for supplies and health professionals feared that women would overuse, abandon more reliable methods or might see this as sanctioning promiscuous behaviour. In the USA, the Food and Drug Administration (FDA) approved oral contraceptive pills as emergency contraceptives in 1997, but in 2004 the FDA rejected calls for over-the-counter status for emergency contraception and claimed that adolescent women had not been shown to understand the instructions (Tanne, 2004).

To try and understand women's use of emergency contraception Free et al. (2002) carried out an in-depth interview study of 30 sexually active women. Their attitudes and concerns included perceptions of low vulnerability to pregnancy, negative self-evaluation, knowledge and service barriers and concerns about what others think. These correspond well to variables identified in social cognition models such as the Health Belief Model and Theory of Planned Behaviour.

There is undoubtedly a demand for safe, effective and acceptable contraception and while there are new developments based on increased understanding of reproductive physiology (Baird and Glasier, 1999), the psychological aspects of acceptability and effective use remain important. The male pill is another possible development, but there is some doubt about whether women would trust men to take it regularly (Guillebaud, 1991). Large doses of testosterone can induce azoospermia but the side effects are intolerable and progress towards safe doses of androgens is slow. Sjogren and Gottlieb (2001) followed up 25 men during a year's use of testosterone contraception. Most rated the method as expected or better and the frequency of sexual intercourse and quality of sex life in general increased significantly. There was some evidence of increased aggression. The men were not blind to the therapy and their reports may have been influenced by their expectations, which might also have been a reason for accepting the therapy.

If, in spite of safe and effective methods, there are still unplanned pregnancies, then it is arguable that current methods of contraception are unacceptable. This has led to the search for new methods. Hormonal contraception was originally given orally but there are now contraceptive vaginal rings, transdermal patches and gels. It remains to be seen whether these are more acceptable.

Contraceptive choice

In a report based on surveys in 1992, Oddens (1996) suggests that attitudes towards the perceived medical nature of some contraceptive methods (oral contraceptives, sterilization and IUDs) influence contraceptive choice. Miller and Pasta (1996) carried out a study on 40 couples' contraceptive choice over a four-year period. They distinguished between method-choice and method-use in decision-making. Method-choice is about continuing with the present method or changing to a new one. Method-use is the actual use of the selected method, e.g. taking the oral contraceptive pill daily or inserting a diaphragm. They found that husbands and wives appeared to have equal influence on method-choice but intentions depended on their own preference.

(See also 'Sterilization and vasectomy'.)

REFERENCES

Baird, D. T. & Glasier, A. F. (1999). Contraception. *British Medical Journal*, **319**, 969–72.

Bianchi-Demicheli, F., Perrin, E., Bianchi, P. G. et al. (2003). Contraceptive practice before and after termination of pregnancy: a prospective study. *Contraception*, **67**(2), 107–113.

Bianchi-Demicheli, F., Perrin, E., Lüdicke, F. et al. (2001). Sexuality, partner relations and contraceptive practice after termination of pregnancy. *Journal of*

Psychosomatic Obstetrics and Gynecology, **22**, 83–90.

CIAWorld Factbook. (2004). http://www.photius.com/rankings/population/birth_rate_2004_0.html accessed 9 May 2005.

Condon, J. T., Need, J. A., Fitzsimmons, D. & Lucy, S. (1995). University students' subjective experiences of oral contraceptive use. *Journal of Psychosomatic Obstetrics and Gynecology*, **16**, 37–43.

Cramer, J. (1996). Compliance with contraceptives and other treatments. *Obstetrics and Gynecology*, **88**, 4S–12S.

Fairhurst, K., Ziebland, S., Wyke, S., Seaman, P. & Glasier, A. (2004). Emergency contraception: why can't you give it away? Qualitative findings from an evaluation of advance provision of emergency contraception. *Contraception*, **70**, 25–9.

Fletcher, P. C., Bryden, P. J. & Bonin, E. (2001). Preliminary examination of oral contraceptive use among university-aged females. *Contraception*, **63**, 229–33.

Free, C., Lee, R. M. & Ogden, J. (2002). Young women's accounts of factors influencing their use and non-use of emergency contraception: in-depth interview study. *British Medical Journal*, **325**, 1393–7.

Gardner, J. A. (2001). Perceptions of the use of oral contraception in female nursing students. Masters in research thesis, University of Dundee, UK.

Goldberg, D. (1972). *The detection of psychiatric illness by questionnaire*. Oxford: Oxford University Press.

Grimely, D. M., Prochaska, J. O., Velicer W. F. & Prochaska, G. E. (1995). Contraceptive and condom use adoption and maintenance: a stage paradigm approach. *Health Education Quarterly*, **22**, 20–35.

Guillebaud, J. (1991). *The pill*. Oxford: Oxford University Press.

Jackson, R., Schwarz, E. B., Freedman, L. & Darney, P. (2000). Knowledge and willingness to use emergency contraception among low-income post-partum women. *Contraception*, **61**, 351–7.

Mahoney, C. A., Thombs, D. L. & Ford, O. J. (1995). Health belief and self efficacy models: their utility in explaining college student condom use. *AIDS Education and Prevention*, **7**, 32–49.

Miller, W. B. & Pasta, D. (1996). The relationship of husbands and wives on the choice and use of contraception, a diaphragm and condoms. *Journal of Applied Social Psychology*, **26**, 1749–74.

Oddens, B. J. (1996). *Determinants of contraceptive use: national population-based studies in various West European countries*. Netherlands: Eburon.

Oddens, B. J. (1999). Women's satisfaction with birth control: a population survey of physical and psychological effects of oral contraceptives, intrauterine devices, condoms, natural family planning and sterilization among 1466 women. *Contraception*, **59**, 277–86.

Office of National Statistics (2004a). *Living in Britain – general household survey 2002*. London: HMSO.

Office of National Statistics (2004b). *Population trends 116*. London: HMSO.

Office of National Statistics (2004c). *Social trends 34*. London: HMSO.

Prochaska, J. O. & DiClemente, C. C. (1984). *The transtheoretical approach: crossing traditional boundaries of change*. Homewood, IL: Dow Jones-Irwin.

Rimmer, C., Horga, M., Cerar, V. et al. (1992). Do women want a once-a-month pill? *Human Reproduction*, **7**, 608–11.

Sheeran, P. (2002). Intention–behaviour relations: a conceptual and empirical review. In M. Hewstone & W. Stroebe (Eds.). *European review of social psychology* (pp. 1–36). Chichester, UK: John Wiley & Sons.

Sjogren, B. & Gottlieb, C. (2001). Testosterone for male contraception during one year: attitudes, well-being and quality of sex life. *Contraception*, **64**, 59–65.

Smith, B. H., Gurney, E. M., Aboulela, L. & Templeton, A. (1996). Emergency contraception: a survey of women's knowledge and attitudes. *British Journal of Obstetrics and Gynaecology*, **103**, 1106–9.

Tang, C. S. & Chung, T. K. (1997). Psychosexual adjustment following sterilization: a prospective study on Chinese women. *Journal of Psychosomatic Research*, **42**, 187–96.

Tanne, J. H. (2004). FDA rejects over the counter status for emergency contraceptive. *British Medical Journal*, **328**, 1219.

Coronary heart disease: impact

Paul Bennett

University of Cardiff

A myocardial infarction (MI) – potentially the most acute manifestation of coronary heart disease (CHD) – may be a devastating event. Its onset can be sudden, distressing and potentially life-threatening. Even if this is not the case, knowledge of disease status can trigger strong and frequently long-term emotional reactions as well as acting as a catalyst for risk behaviour change. As a consequence, it has been the focus of much of the psychological research in CHD.

Behavioural change

An infarction does seem to trigger appropriate behaviour change, although some changes may be relatively short-term. Hajek *et al.* (2002), for example, found that 6 weeks following MI, 60% of former smokers who did not intervention were reported to be not smoking. One year after MI, the figure had dropped to 37%.

Similarly, Dornelas *et al.* (2000) found 43% and 34% of patients not receiving any form of intervention were abstinent at 6 and 12 months respectively. Of note, here, was the finding by Scott and Lamparski (1985) that only patients who believed that smoking contributed to their cardiac problems were likely to maintain abstinence. Diet may also change in the short-term (Bennett *et al.*, 1999), although old habits may creep back over time. Leslie *et al.* (2004), for example, found the target of their nutritional programme of 5 portions of fruit and vegetables per day was achieved by 65% of participants involved. Thirty-one percent of their control group achieved this goal. The percentage of those eating healthily in the intervention group fell over a one-year follow-up period and did not differ from the control group by this time (see also 'Diet and health' and 'Tobacco use').

As with other risk behaviours, changes in exercise may be modest and fall over time. Bennett *et al.* (1999), for example, found significant spontaneous changes in mild to moderate exercise levels in the three months following MI. Levels in fitness may change markedly following participation in specific exercise programmes (e.g. Hevey *et al.*, 2003). However, how long such changes are maintained in the absence of continued follow-up is not clear. Lear *et al.* (2003) reported minimal changes from baseline on measures of leisure time exercise and treadmill performance one year following MI, despite participants taking part in a general rehabilitation programme (see 'Physical activity and health', 'Physical activity interventions' and 'Coronary heart disease: rehabilitation'). One final outcome is that of sexual activity. Wiklund *et al.* (1984) reported that compared with two months prior to MI, at one-year follow-up only 35% of the participants in their study claimed they had experienced no change in their sexual activity, while 60% 'had noted a decline'. Five percent reported that they had ceased sexual activity altogether. While fear was the predominant reason for reduced sexual activity at two-month follow-up, impotency and loss of interest were the most frequent explanations one year after MI. The use of beta-blockers, frequently used to stabilize and strengthen the cardiac function following MI (Ko *et al.*, 2002) would have contributed to these data. The incidence of erectile disorder after myocardial infarction ranges from 38–78% (Sainz *et al.*, 2004) (see also 'Sexual dysfunction').

Emotional distress

The psychological consequences of an MI may be profound and persistent. Wiklund *et al.* (1984), for example, interviewed a number of patients who had experienced an MI one year previously. Over a third of them thought about their heart disease frequently and 74% worried about their cardiac state. Fifty-eight percent reported that they were protected from physical exertion by friends and family, frequently as a consequence of anxiety rather than symptom severity. Psychometric measures or clinical interviews confirm these high levels of distress. Dickens *et al.* (2004), for example, reported the incidence of depression found by clinical interview as 20% in the period immediately following the infarction. Twenty-one percent of those not depressed at this time subsequently became depressed over the following year. Again using clinical interviews, Strik *et al.* (2004) found that 31% of a cohort of MI patients developed major or minor depression in the year following first MI.

The highest incidence rate was in the first month following their MI. Lane *et al.* (2002) found a 31% prevalence rate of elevated depression scores during hospitalization. The 4- and 12-month prevalence rates were 38% and 37%. The same group reported the prevalence of elevated state anxiety to be 26% in hospital, 42% at 4-month follow-up and 40% at the end of one year. They also reported high levels of co-morbidity between anxiety and depression. Grace *et al.* (2004) reported that one-third of patients experienced elevated anxiety at the time of their MI: 50% of their cohort remained anxious one year later. Interest in the rates of post-traumatic stress disorder as a consequence of MI has recently increased, with prevalence rates typically being around 8–10% up to one year following infarction (e.g. Bennett *et al.*, 2002).

Emotional benefits

Despite the consistent data suggesting the potential for negative emotional reactions to MI, the obverse may also be found. Petrie *et al.* (1999) reported that nearly two-thirds of people who had survived an MI reported some personal gains as a result of their illness some three months after its onset. The most highly endorsed positive outcome (endorsed by over 60% of respondents) was a change to a healthier lifestyle, although improvements in relationships, an appreciation of health and life, a change in life priorities and gains in empathy were also reported.

Predictors of emotional distress

Factors associated with distress may change over time. Dickens *et al.* (2004), for example, found that predictors of depression at the time of the MI were being a younger age, female, having a past psychiatric history, being socially isolated, experiencing other life problems and lacking a close confidant. Onset of depression over the year following the infarction was associated with having frequent angina. Strik *et al.* (2004) found similar associations between previous psychiatric history, depression, gender and age. Women and young men were most likely to be depressed. Post-traumatic stress disorder (PTSD) may be predicted by a number of factors, including neuroticism, the level of intrusive thoughts about the event while in hospital and lack of social support (Bennett *et al.*, 2002) (see 'Post-traumatic stress disorder').

Consequences of emotional distress

There is little doubt that the emotional reactions can influence important outcomes following MI. Depressed and anxious individuals are less likely to attend cardiac rehabilitation classes than those with less distress (Lane *et al.*, 2001). Paradoxically, they are more likely to contact doctors and to make and attend outpatient appointments, as well as have more re-admissions (Strik *et al.*, 2004) in the year following infarction. Many of these will be due to worry and health concerns rather than further validated cardiac problems. The impact of mood on health behaviour change is modest – although good quality longitudinal data addressing this issue are surprisingly lacking. Huijbrechts *et al.* (1996) reported that depressed and anxious patients were less likely to have stopped smoking five months after their MI than their less distressed counterparts. Similarly, Havik & Maeland (1988) reported that the MI patients who were least likely to quit smoking were those who had become increasingly depressed in the months immediately following their MI. Bennett *et al.* (1999) reported a modest association between low levels of exercise and depression, but no differences between depressed and non-depressed individuals on levels of smoking, alcohol consumption or diet. Finally, Shemesh *et al.* (2004) found that high levels of PTSD symptoms, but not depression or global distress scores, were significant predictors of non-adherence to aspirin.

Depression may also impact on important economic factors. Occupational factors mean that white-collar, male, and young workers are most likely to retain their jobs. However, mood and expectations about work will also significantly influence return to work. Depression has consistently been associated with delayed or failure to return to previous work after rehabilitation and low ratings of work or social satisfaction. Soderman *et al.* (2003), for example, found depression to predict low levels of resumption of full-time work and reduced working hours. Delay in returning to work was predicted by greater concerns about health and low social support. Resuming work at a lower activity level than before infarction was associated with older age, higher health concerns and patients' expectations of lower working capacity (independently of actual capacity).

Cognitive responses

The mechanisms through which depression and other negative emotions influence behaviour has not been fully investigated in cardiac patients. However, the likelihood is that any impact on behaviour is mediated by cognitive processes. One framework through which these have been investigated involves the Illness Perceptions Questionnaire (see 'Illness cognition assessment'). Using this, Petrie *et al.* (1996) found that attendance at cardiac rehabilitation was significantly related to a stronger belief during admission that the illness could be cured or controlled. Return to work within six weeks was significantly predicted by the perception that the illness would last a short time and have less grave consequences for the patient. Patients' belief that their heart disease would have serious consequences was significantly related to later disability in work around the house, recreational activities and social interaction. A strong illness identity was significantly related to greater sexual dysfunction at both three and six months. Although they did not

investigate it, these negative attributions and expectations are likely to be associated with depression and/or anxiety.

Impact and interaction with partners

The partners of patients also experience high levels of distress, often greater than that reported by the patient. Moser and Dracup (2004) also found that patients' adjustment to illness was worse when their partners were more anxious or depressed than themselves and was best when patients were more anxious or depressed than their partners. Stern and Pascale (1979) found that the women at greatest risk of depression or anxiety were those married to men who denied their infarction. In this situation, partners experienced high levels of anxiety when their partner engaged in what they may considered to be unsafe behaviours, such as high levels of physical exertion or continued smoking, which they are unable to control. In addition, many wives appear to inhibit angry or sexual feelings and become overprotective of their husbands (Stewart *et al.*, 2000). Bennett and Connell (1999) found two contrasting processes to influence anxiety and depression in patients' partners. The primary causes of partner anxiety was the physical health consequences of the MI, and in particular the perceived physical limitations imposed on their spouse by their MI. In contrast, the strongest predictors of partner depression were the emotional state of their spouse, the quality of the marital relationship and the wider social support available to them. Three disease factors were particularly associated with anxiety: the severity of the MI; the patients' perceptions of their health and physical limitations as a consequence of disease (see also 'Lay beliefs of health and illness'). Two patient coping responses to the MI, i.e. mental withdrawal and seeking instrumental social support, were also associated with partner anxiety.

Summary

While many people recover well from a myocardial infarction and make appropriate behavioural changes, many do not. In addition, a significant minority of individuals experience significant negative emotional effects. These may impact on all areas of life, from the social and sexual to the economic. Any of these changes may be mediated by cognitive processes, which may be responsive to relatively brief interventions at an early stage in the rehabilitation process (Petrie *et al.*, 2002).

(See also 'Coronary heart disease: cardiac psychology'; 'Coronary heart disease: heart failure'; 'Coronary heart disease rehabilitation' and 'Coronary heart disease: surgery'.)

REFERENCES

Bennett, P., Mayfield, T., Norman, P., Lowe, R. & Morgan, M. (1999). Affective and social cognitive predictors of behavioural change following myocardial infarction. *British Journal of Health Psychology*, **4**, 247–56.

Bennett, P., Owen, R., Koutsakis, S. & Bisson, J. (2002) Personality, social context, and cognitive predictors of post-traumatic stress disorder in myocardial infarction

patients. *Psychology and Health*, **17**, 489–500.

Bennett, P. & Connell, H. (1999). Dyadic responses to myocardial infarction. *Psychology, Health & Medicine*, **4**, 45–55.

Dickens, C. M., Percival, C., McGowan, L. *et al.* (2004). The risk factors for depression in first myocardial infarction patients. *Psychological Medicine*, **34**, 1083–92.

Dornelas, E. A., Sampson, R. A., Gray, J. F., Waters, D. & Thompson, P. D. (2000). A randomized controlled trial of smoking cessation counseling after myocardial Infarction. *Preventive Medicine*, **30**, 261–8.

Grace, S. L., Abbey, S. E., Irvine, J., Shnek, Z. M. & Stewart, D. E. (2004). Prospective examination of anxiety persistence and its relationship to cardiac symptoms and recurrent cardiac events. *Psychotherapy and Psychosomatics*, **73**, 344–52.

Hajek, P., Taylor, T. Z. & Mills, P. (2002). Brief intervention during hospital admission to help patients to give up smoking after myocardial infarction and bypass surgery: randomised controlled trial. *British Medical Journal*, **324**, 87–9.

Havik, O. E. & Maeland, J. G. (1988). Verbal denial and outcome in myocardial infarction patients. *Journal of Psychosomatic Research*, **32**, 145–57.

Hevey, D., Brown, A., Cahill, A. et al. (2003). Four-week multidisciplinary cardiac rehabilitation produces similar improvements in exercise capacity and quality of life to a 10-week program. *Journal of Cardiopulmonary Rehabilitation*, **23**, 17–21.

Huijbrechts, I. P., Duivenvoorden, H. J. & Deckers, J. W. (1996). Modification of smoking habits five months after myocardial infarction: relationship with personality characteristics. *Journal of Psychosomatic Research*, **40**, 369–78.

Ko, D. T., Hebert, P. R., Coffey, C. S. et al. (2002). Beta-blocker therapy and symptoms of depression, fatigue, and sexual dysfunction. *Journal of American Medical Association*, **288**, 351–7.

Lane, D., Carroll, D., Ring, C., Beevers, D. G. & Lip, G. Y. (2002). The prevalence and persistence of depression and anxiety following myocardial infarction. *British Journal Health Psychology*, **7**, 11–21.

Lear, S. A. Ignaszewski, A., Linden, W. et al. (2003). The extensive lifestyle management intervention (ELMI) following cardiac rehabilitation trial. *European Heart Journal*, **24**, 1920–7.

Leslie, W. S., Hankey, C. R., Matthews, D., Currall, J. E. & Lean, M. E. (2004). A transferable programme of nutritional counselling for rehabilitation following myocardial infarction: a randomised controlled study. *European Journal of Clinical Nutrition*, **58**, 778–86.

Moser, D. K. & Dracup, K. (2004). Role of spousal anxiety and depression in patients' psychosocial recovery after a cardiac event. *Psychosomatic Medicine*, **66**, 527–32.

Petrie, K. J., Buick, D. L., Weinman, J. & Booth, R. J. (1999). Positive effects of illness reported by myocardial infarction and breast cancer patients. *Journal of Psychosomatic Research*, **47**, 537–43.

Petrie, K. J., Cameron, L. D., Ellis, C. J., Buick, D. & Weinman, J. (2002). Changing illness perceptions after myocardial infarction: an early intervention randomized controlled trial. *Psychosomatic Medicine*, **64**, 580–6.

Petrie, K. J., Weinman, J., Sharpe, N. & Buckley, J. (1996). Role of patients' view of their illness in predicting return to work and functioning after myocardial infarction: longitudinal study. *British Medical Journal*, **312**, 1191–4.

Sainz, I., Amaya, J. & Garcia, M. (2004). Erectile dysfunction in heart disease patients. *International Journal of Impotence Research*, **16**(Suppl. 2), S13–S17.

Scott, R. R. & Lamparski, D. (1985). Variables related to long-term smoking status following cardiac events. *Addictive Behaviours*, **10**, 257–64.

Shemesh, E., Yehuda, R., Milo, O. et al. (2004). Posttraumatic stress, nonadherence, and adverse outcome in survivors of a myocardial infarction. *Psychosomatic Medicine*, **66**, 521–6.

Soderman, E., Lisspers, J. & Sundin, O. (2003). Depression as a predictor of return to work in patients with coronary artery disease. *Social Science and Medicine*, **56**, 193–202.

Stern, M. J. & Pascale, L. (1979). Psychosocial adaption postmyocardial infarction: the spouses' dilemma. *Journal of Psychosomatic Research*, **23**, 83–7.

Stewart, M., Davidson, K., Meade, D., Hirth, A. & Makrides, L. (2000). Myocardial infarction: survivors' and spouses' stress, coping, and support. *Journal of Advanced Nursing*, **31**, 1351–60.

Strik, J. J., Lousberg, R., Cheriex, E. C. & Honig, A. (2004). One year cumulative incidence of depression following myocardial infarction and impact on cardiac outcome. *Journal Psychosomatic Research*, **56**, 59–66.

Wiklund, I., Sanne, H., Vedin, A. & Wilhelmsson, C. (1984). Psychosocial outcome one year after a first myocardial infarction. *Journal of Psychosomatic Research*, **28**, 309–21.

Coronary heart disease: cardiac psychology

Robert Allan[1], Stephen Scheidt[1] and Christopher Smith[2]

[1]Weill Medical College, Cornell University
[2]Yeshiva University

'Cardiac psychology' and 'behavioural cardiology' are two new closely related sub-specialties in mental health and cardiology, respectively, informed by many hundreds of empirical studies conducted over nearly half a century. The fields have evolved with a unifying hypothesis that psychological and social variables, termed 'psychosocial factors', can affect the development and outcome from coronary heart disease (CHD), the leading cause of death and disability in the western world. Indeed, the recent case-control INTERHEART study of more than 15 152 cases and 14 820 controls in 52 countries reported that most risk factors for myocardial infarction (MI) have behavioural components that are modifiable, including cigarette smoking, regular physical activity, dietary lipids, abdominal obesity, daily consumption of fruits and vegetables and hypertension (Yusuf et al., 2004) (see also 'Diet and health', 'Physical activity and health', 'Tobacco use' and 'Hypertension'). A second INTERHEART study of psychosocial factors with 11 119 patients and 13 648 controls from 262 centres around the world determined that stress at work, at home and with finances, as well as major adverse life events, also increased the risk of acute MI (Rosengren et al., 2004).

In the late 1950s, some of the earliest research linked the Type A behaviour pattern with increased risk of MI. Since then, depression, social isolation, anger, anxiety and job strain, among others, have attained some degree of empirical validity as CHD risk factors. The as-yet unrealized 'holy grail' of cardiac psychology/behavioural cardiology is a reduction in cardiac morbidity and mortality with intervention to ameliorate negative behavioural or psychosocial characteristics. At this point in time, research linking some psychosocial factors with CHD onset and outcome is quite convincing. The intervention literature, however, is less consistent.

Psychosocial risk factors

Over the past few years, behavioural cardiology has attained substantial credibility in medicine. In 1999, Rozanski et al. (Rozanski et al., 1999) published a 'new frontiers' article in Circulation, the premier journal in cardiology, providing an exhaustive review of the literature. Since then, other comprehensive reviews have appeared (Allan & Scheidt, 2004); (Smith & Ruiz, 2002) as well as numerous reviews focused on specific psychosocial factors, including: depression (Smith & Ruiz, 2002); (Lett et al., 2004); (Barth et al., 2004); (van Melle et al., 2004) anxiety and depression; (Januzzi et al., 2000) psychosocial factors for sudden cardiac death; (Hemingway et al., 2001) for heart failure; (MacMahon & Lipp, 2002) and in women. (Bankier & Littman, 2002) See Eng et al. (Eng et al., 2002)

for the most recent database on social isolation in the introduction to their large-scale study of social ties and CHD.

Depression and social isolation are consistent and powerful risk factors, particularly for outcome after the diagnosis of CHD. A constellation of negative emotions (depression and anger) and one consequence of such negativity (social isolation) has emerged with striking predictive power from a number of studies. A recent, provocative twin study reported a possible genetic basis for the relationship between depression, anger and social isolation (Raynor et al., 2002).

An area of emerging importance is psychosocial adjustment in implantable cardioverter defibrillator patients. Many ICD patients are sudden death survivors and a significant percentage suffer from anxiety, depression and post-traumatic stress disorder (see 'Post-traumatic stress disorder') (Sears et al., 1999).

Autonomic imbalance is likely to be a major physiologic mechanism responsible for the harmful effects from psychosocial factors. Among many others, Curtis and O'Keefe (Curtis & O'Keefe, 2002) have discussed the hypothesis that heightened sympathetic and reduced parasympathetic nervous system activity are the major underlying links between mind, behaviour and CHD. In addition to direct effects of heightened sympathetic, or decreased parasympathetic activity, which include increased blood pressure, heart rate and myocardial contractility, there are indirect effects of autonomic imbalance, including increased platelet and clotting system reactivity, predisposition to thrombosis and atherosclerotic plaque rupture, as well as increased propensity to arrhythmia (see also 'Stress and health' and 'Psychoneuroimmunology').

Depression

A number of prospective studies have noted an increased relative risk (~1.5 to 2.0) of acute MI and cardiovascular mortality in depressed, but otherwise healthy individuals (Ferketich et al., 2000). The data linking depression with adverse events among patients with established cardiac disease are particularly striking, with a 1998 review noting that 11 of 11 studies reported worsened outcome (Glassman & Shapiro, 1998). The relative risk of future adverse cardiac events and cardiovascular mortality in depressed patients with established cardiac (usually coronary artery) disease is increased approximately three- to four-fold (Lett et al., 2004); (Barth et al., 2004); (van Melle et al., 2004). Between 35–45% of post-MI and post-coronary artery bypass graft surgery (CABG) patients suffer from some level of depression, ranging from a few symptoms to major depressive disorder. Results from two recent intervention trials suggest that much cardiac depression may remit spontaneously within a few months of the cardiac event (Glassman *et al.*, 2002); (Writing Committee for the ENRICHD investigators, 2003). Autonomic dysfunction is the physiologic mechanism most often cited as linking depression to increased cardiac mortality (Carney *et al.*, 2001).

Social isolation

In 1984, Ruberman *et al.* (Ruberman *et al.*, 1984) were among the first to provide evidence of increased mortality in socially isolated cardiac patients among 2320 male survivors of acute MI. In 1992, Case *et al.* (Case *et al.*, 1992) reported on 1234 patients six months after MI; the recurrent event rate for nonfatal MI or cardiac death was nearly double for those living alone compared with those living with a companion. Similarly, Williams *et al.* (Williams *et al.*, 1992) followed a consecutive sample of 1368 patients undergoing cardiac catheterization over 5 years. Unmarried individuals without a confidant had >3× increased risk of death compared with those who were married or had a close friend.

In a recent study of 430 CHD patients, Brummett *et al.* (Brummett *et al.*, 2001) reported that the most isolated individuals, those with 3 or fewer people in their social support network, had the worst outcome, with a relative risk of 2.43 for cardiac and 2.11 for all cause mortality. Once past a threshold of minimal support, additional social ties did not appear to provide extra benefit (see also 'Social support and health').

Hostility and anger

Free-floating or easily aroused anger, is one of the two major symptoms of the Type A behaviour pattern, one of the first psychosocial conditions suggested as a risk factor for CHD. A 1996 meta-analysis of 45 studies by Miller *et al.* (Miller *et al.*, 1996) suggested that chronic hostility is an independent risk factor for CHD as well as all-cause mortality, with the relationship strongest among younger patients.

More recently, J.E. Williams *et al.* (Williams *et al.*, 2000) studied 12 986 Americans without known CHD at baseline and reported a strong graded relationship between increasing 'trait anger' and subsequent MI and CHD mortality. Results were significant for only normotensive individuals, approximately two-thirds of the population under investigation. A similar relationship between scores on the Spielberger Trait Anger Scale and increased risk of haemorrhagic and ischaemic stroke was found in a sample of 13 851 men and women (Williams *et al.*, 2002). Eng *et al.* (Eng *et al.*, 2003) administered a slightly different measure of anger, the Spielberger Anger-Out Expression Scale, to 23 552 health professionals. Moderate, compared to low, expressed anger conferred a protective effect. It is remarkable that these three large studies have come to inconsistent conclusions about the expression of anger using similar anger measurement instruments (see 'Hostility, Type A behaviour and coronary heart disease').

In addition to depression, social isolation and hostility, there is limited evidence that several other psychosocial factors may increase risk of CHD, including job strain (Kivimaki *et al.*, 2002), 'phobic' anxiety (Kawachi *et al.*, 1994), Type D (distressed) personality (Denollet & Van Heck, 2001), and 'vital exhaustion' (Kop *et al.*, 1994).

Triggering of acute cardiac events

Within the past several decades, observational studies after both natural (Leor *et al.*, 1996) and man-made disasters (Meisel *et al.*, 1991) have reported higher rates of both MI and sudden cardiac death (SCD) than in normal times. We have also learned a great deal about 'triggering' from the recently completed Determinants of Time of Myocardial Infarction Onset Study. In the 'MI Onset study', most MIs could not be attributed to a specific cause. It is important to note that the absolute risk of MI in any given hour is quite low, only 1 in a million for a healthy 50-year-old male (Muller *et al.*, 1997). However, a number of behavioural 'triggers', some potentially avoidable, have been identified, including strenuous exertion (Mittleman *et al.*, 1993), intense anger (Mittleman *et al.*, 1995), sexual activity (Muller *et al.*, 1996), assuming the upright posture upon awakening (Muller *et al.*, 1997), use of marijuana (Mittleman *et al.*, 2001) and cocaine (Mittleman *et al.*, 1999). A small, but statistically significant Monday morning peak in MI, presumably related to beginning the work week, has also been noted (Willich *et al.*, 1992).

Triggers are suggested in approximately 17% of cases of MI (Muller *et al.*, 1997), with strenuous exertion the most potent. In the MI Onset Study, 4.4% of patients engaged in strenuous activity in the hour prior to their infarction (Mittleman *et al.*, 1993). However, the increased risk during and immediately following exercise is more than offset by a reduction in cardiac events during the rest of the week in active vs. sedentary people. In the MI Onset Study, 8% of patients reported an episode in which they were at least 'very angry' in the 24 hours prior to MI and 2.4% reported such anger in the 2 hours preceding their infarction (Mittleman *et al.*, 1995). Each time an individual becomes angry there is a 2.3× increased risk of triggering an MI during the angry episode and for a 2-hour hazard period afterwards.

Sexual activity is a modest trigger, accounting for fewer cases of MI than assuming the upright posture on awakening, reassuring information for cardiac patients with an active love life (Muller *et al.*, 1996).

A 1-hour hazard period has been identified after marijuana use with a 4.8 fold increased relative risk (Mittleman *et al.*, 2001). Similarly, cocaine elevated risk of MI 23.7 times over baseline for 1 hour after use (Mittleman *et al.*, 1999).

Two studies reported that physical and psychological stress, as well as anger, can serve as 'triggers' for ICD discharge (Fries *et al.*, 2002); (Lampert *et al.*, 2002). Intriguingly, 2 studies recently reported increased ICD discharge after the September 11, 2001 attack on the World Trade Center, both in the New York Metropolitan area (Steinberg *et al.*, 2004) and as far away from the disaster as Florida (Shedd *et al.*, 2004). Whether ICD discharge might be reduced with psychosocial intervention has not, to our knowledge, been reported.

Psychosocial interventions

A 1999 meta-analysis of 37 studies by Dusseldorp *et al.* (Dusseldorp *et al.*, 1999), concluded that psychosocial interventions provide a significant positive effect on cardiac risk factors, a 29% reduction in recurrent MI and a 34% reduction in cardiac mortality.

However, since then, clinical trials have produced mixed results. Following is a brief description of the trials that we consider most noteworthy (see also 'Coronary heart disease: rehabilitation').

The Recurrent Coronary Prevention Project (RCPP)

The Friedman and associates' Recurrent Coronary Prevention Project (RCPP) (Friedman *et al.*, 1986) was the first large-scale post-MI Type A behaviour modification programme, completed in 1987. After 4.5 years of group counseling, there was a 44% reduction in second MI, which was associated with reductions in Type A behaviour. The control group was subsequently offered Type A counselling and showed a similar reduction in MI recurrence rates over an additional year (Friedman *et al.*, 1987). The RCPP also determined that Type A counselling was most protective against cardiac death for patients with less severe MI (Powell & Thoresen, 1998), suggesting that psychosocial intervention is most effective when individuals are still relatively healthy. Further, there was a significant reduction in sudden, but not non-sudden, cardiac death (Brackett & Powell, 1988), providing support for the hypothesis that behavioural factors may precipitate lethal arrhythmias.

Enhancing Recovery In Coronary Heart Disease patients – 'ENRICHD'

The largest psychosocial intervention to date, ENRICHD was a randomized clinical trial of individual and group cognitive–behavioural psychotherapy vs. usual care for 2481 post-MI patients who met modified DSM-IV criteria for major or minor depression and/or low perceived social support (Writing Committee for the ENRICHD investigators, 2003). Cognitive–behavioural therapy is widely regarded as a well-researched and effective psychological treatment for depression (see 'Cognitive behaviour therapy') (Deckersbach *et al.*, 2000). Sertraline (Zoloft®) was provided for patients with high scores on the Hamilton Rating Scale for Depression or having less than a 50% reduction in Beck Depression Inventory scores after 5 weeks.

At 6 months, the cognitive–behavioural intervention reduced depression and social isolation in the treated groups compared with usual care controls. However, group differences diminished over time and became non-significant for depression at 30 months and for low perceived social support by 42 months. There were no reductions in recurrent MI or cardiac death rates with the intervention compared with usual care. Depression spontaneously improved to an unexpected degree in the usual care group, reducing the statistical power of the study design. A post hoc analysis of ENRICHD reported that white males, but not other sub-groups, had reduced recurrent nonfatal MI and cardiac mortality with the intervention compared to controls (Schneiderman *et al.*, 2004).

The Sertraline Antidepressant Heart Attack Randomized Trial - 'SADHART'

'SADHART' (Glassman *et al.*, 2002) was a drug trial, with no psychotherapy, for depression in post-MI and unstable angina patients, conducted to establish the safety and efficacy of sertraline in the cardiac population. Sertraline was found to be safe, with no reductions in ejection fraction. The incidence of major cardiovascular events was 14.5% in the sertraline treated group compared with 22.4% in the placebo group, a non-significant difference.

As with ENRICHD, SADHART found an unexpectedly high rate of improvement in depression in the control group. Nonetheless, sertraline-treated patients showed significantly greater improvement than controls on the Clinical Global Impression Improvement Scale, supporting a potential benefit of psychotropic intervention for depressed post-MI patients.

Intensive lifestyle change

The Lifestyle Heart Trial (Ornish *et al.*, 1990) achieved great national attention by demonstrating angiographic evidence for reversing coronary atherosclerosis with intensive lifestyle modification. Additionally, positron emission tomography (PET) scans have shown improved myocardial perfusion with such lifestyle changes (Ornish *et al.*, 1998).

In the Lifestyle Heart Trial, 48 CHD patients were randomized to intensive intervention or routine medical care. The intervention required a very low fat vegetarian diet, daily yoga and meditation, twice weekly support groups and regular exercise: approximately 14 hours per week of active participation (see also 'Physical activity interventions', 'Relaxation training' and 'Social support interventions'). After one year, 82% of experimental subjects showed regression of atherosclerotic lesions compared to 42% of controls (Ornish *et al.*, 1990). After four years, average stenosis diameter decreased in experimental patients but progressed in the control group (Ornish *et al.*, 1993).

Ornish's most recent work, the Multicenter Lifestyle Demonstration Project (Ornish, 1998), was a non-randomized study at 8 sites across the USA, designed to assess whether patients could avoid revascularization by making similar lifestyle changes. After 3 years, there were no significant differences in MI, stroke or deaths for treated vs. control subjects. The major finding of this demonstration project was an average cost savings of $29 529 per patient.

A most important unanswered question about Ornish's intensive lifestyle programme is whether a significant percentage of the population can be persuaded to live in ways so far from cultural norms. In addition, the number of patients studied in the Ornish programme is small and falls far short of the standards that warrant recommendations from respected authorities such as the Centers for Disease Control (CDC), National Cholesterol Education Program, American Heart Association or American College of Cardiology.

Psychological interventions

Jones and West (Jones & West, 1996) randomized 2328 post-MI patients to either routine medical care or 7 two-hour psychological interventions. Although there were encouraging reductions in angina and cardiac mortality at 6 months among intervention patients, after 1 year there were no significant differences in psychological factors, such as depression and anxiety or cardiac endpoints. One question posed by these results is that since the intervention was not successful at reducing psychosocial factors, why would it be expected to improve cardiac outcome? In our clinical experience, 14 hours of patient contact over a year would not be expected to have much of an impact. Additionally, patients were not pre-selected for any psychological condition, such as depression or distress: all patients, including those who did not need 'stress reduction' were included in the study.

In contrast, Blumenthal et al. (Blumenthal et al., 2002) randomly assigned 107 CHD patients with evidence of ambulatory or mental-stress-induced myocardial ischaemia to a 4-month programme of exercise or 'stress management'. The study was, in part, modelled after the RCPP. Psychosocial intervention consisted of 16 one-and-a-half-hour group sessions based a 'cognitive–social' model. After an average of 38 months, stress management was associated with a 0.26 relative risk ($p = 0.04$) of an adverse cardiac event compared with usual care control subjects who did not live near the medical centre. Follow-up after 5 years showed a similar reduction in adverse cardiac events as well as considerably reduced medical costs.

A number of clinical trials have been undertaken in Europe. In the Netherlands, Denollet and Brutsaert (Denollet & Brutsaert, 2001) studied 150 men with CHD who received either usual care or special intervention that added weekly two-hour group therapy sessions with a significant other to standard exercise cardiac rehabilitation for 3 months. In addition, 49% (38 of 78) of patients received weekly individual psychotherapy. At the end of 3 months, 43% of patients reported improvement and 15% worsening of distress. At 9 year follow-up, rate of death was 17% for control patients compared with 4% for intervention patients ($p = 0.009$).

Hamalainen and associates (Hamalainen et al., 1995) studied a group of 375 (74 women) acute MI patients in Finland who were provided with a comprehensive rehabilitation programme that included psychological discussion groups. Patients were followed for 15 years, after which there was a significantly lower incidence of sudden cardiac death (16.5% vs. 28.9%; $p = 0.006$) and cardiac mortality (47.9% vs. 58.5%; $p = 0.04$) in the intervention compared with the control group. The protective effects of the comprehensive cardiac rehabilitation programme were significant twelve years after all intervention had ceased.

In Sweden, Burell (Burell, 1996) randomized 268 non-smoking post-coronary artery bypass graft (CABG) patients to a group programme for modification of the TABP and cardiac risk factor education or a control group that received routine care. During the first year, intervention patients met for 17 three-hour sessions with 5–6 'booster sessions' in years two and three. At follow-up 4.5 years after surgery, there was a significant difference in total [7 vs. 16 ($p = 0.02$)] and cardiovascular [5 vs. 8 NS] deaths between treatment and control patients respectively. There were 14 fatal and non-fatal cardiovascular events in the intervention group compared with 19 in the control group ($p = 0.04$).

The current state of behavioural cardiology/cardiac psychology

Over the past several decades, the database linking psychosocial factors with the onset and outcome from CHD has been greatly expanded, with depression and social isolation strongly linked with worsened outcome. The intervention literature, however, has produced mixed results. Interventions to modify the TABP, the RCPP, Project New Life and Blumenthal's trial, have all reported improved outcome. Ironically, several large studies have reported that TABP is not a risk factor for CHD (Case et al., 1985); (Barefoot et al., 1989); (Ragland & Brand, 1988) and recent research on the global TABP has been largely abandoned in favour of a more specific focus on hostility, one of its core components (see 'Hostility, Type A behaviour and coronary heart disease'). The ENRICHD study, designed to treat depression and social isolation, essentially failed to improve both psychologic and cardiac outcome over the long term. Results strongly suggest that much post-MI depression remits spontaneously; important information for the design of future clinical trials.

Measurement of psychosocial variables is still a major issue. Most recent studies have relied on self-report questionnaires, which bias responses by limitations in subjects' self-awareness, as well as their willingness to acknowledge socially undesirable personality characteristics. At present, there are no agreed standards for assessment of any of the psychosocial risk factors, although some questionnaires, such as the Beck Depression Inventory, the Cook–Medley Hostility Scale and the Spielberger anger scales, have been used extensively.

A critical issue for intervention is its frequency and intensity. Ornish's programme requires great effort (14 hours a week), while Jones and West provided treatment of 14 hours over a year. We find that it is difficult for most cardiac patients to maintain heart healthy habits and after a 'honeymoon' of several months, most revert back to of their former unhealthy lifestyles. A 'healthy dose' of psychosocial intervention is likely needed for improved outcome.

Although the 'holy grail' of cardiac psychology/behavioural cardiology is the reduction of morbidity and morality, this has not yet been achieved. It should be noted, however, that most psychosocial interventions have reported improvements in quality of life, a worthy goal in its own right: it is not just how long one lives, but also how well (see 'Quality of life'). Many of the interventions in clinical cardiology, such as CABG (other than for 'left main coronary artery' and 'triple vessel' (disease) and percutaneous transluminal coronary angioplasty (PTCA), do not necessarily lead to reductions in morbidity and mortality either. Modern trials of new medical therapies increasingly include assessments of quality of life and cost-effectiveness, often measured as Quality Adjusted Years of Life (QAYL) [gained]. Although psychological or behavioural interventions have yet to definitely increase survival or decrease future cardiac events, it seems likely that the recent attention given to psychological issues in cardiac patients yields improved quality of life, and it is probably cost-effective.

(See also 'Coronary heart disease: rehabilitation', 'Coronary heart disease: heart failure', 'Coronary heart disease, impact', 'Coronary heart disease: surgery', 'Hostility, Type A behaviour and coronary heart disease' and 'Hypertension').

REFERENCES

Allan, R. & Scheidt, S. (2004). Cardiac psychology: psychosocial factors. In J.E. Manson, P.M. Ridker, J.M. Gaziano (Eds.). *Clinical Trials in Heart Disease: A Companion to 'Braunwald's Heart Disease'* (2nd edn.) (pp. 386–98). Philadelphia: Elsevier Saunders.

Bankier, B. & Littman, A.B. (2002). Psychiatric disorders and coronary heart disease in women – a still neglected topic: review of the literature from 1971–2000. *Psychotherapy and Psychosomatics*, **71**, 133–40.

Barefoot, J.C., Peterson, B.L. Harrell, F.E. *et al.* (1989). Type A behavior and survival: a follow-up study of 1,467 patients with coronary artery disease. *American Journal of Cardiology*, **64**, 427–32.

Barth, J., Schumacher, M. & Herrmann-Lingen, C. (2004). Depression as a risk factor for mortality in patients with coronary heart disease. *Psychosomatic Medicine*, **66**, 802–13.

Blumenthal, J.A., Babyak, M., Wei, J. *et al.* (2002). Usefulness of psychosocial treatment of mental stress-induced myocardial ischemia in men. *American Journal of Cardiology*, **89**, 164–8.

Brackett, C.D. & Powell, L.H. (1988). Psychosocial and physiological predictors of sudden cardiac death after healing of acute myocardial infarction. *American Journal of Cardiology*, **6l**, 979–83.

Brummett, B.H., Barefoot, J.C., Siegler, I.C. *et al.* (2001). Characteristics of socially isolated patients with coronary artery disease who are at elevated risk for mortality. *Psychosomatic Medicine*, **63**, 267–72.

Burell, G. (1996). Group psychotherapy in Project New Life: treatment of coronary-prone behavior for post coronary artery bypass patients. In R. Allan, S. Scheidt (Eds.). *Heart and mind: the practice of cardiac psychology* (pp. 291–310). Washington, D.C: American Psychological Association.

Carney, R.M., Blumenthal, J.A., Stein, P.K. *et al.* (2001). Depression, heart rate variability, and acute myocardial infarction. *Circulation*, **104**, 2024–8.

Case, R.B., Heller, S.S., Case, N.B. & Moss, A.J. (1985). Type A behavior and survival after acute myocardial infarction. *New England Journal of Medicine*, **312**, 737–41.

Case, R.B., Moss, A.J., Case, N., McDermott, M. & Eberly, S. (1992). Living alone after myocardial infarction: impact on prognosis. *Journal of the American Medical Association*, **267**, 515–19.

Curtis, B.M. & O'Keefe, J.H. (2002). Autonomic tone as a cardiovascular risk factor: the dangers of chronic fight or flight. *Mayo Clinic Proceedings*, **77**, 45–54.

Deckersbach, T., Gershuny, B.S. & Otto, M.W. (2000). Cognitive–behavioral therapy for depression: applications and outcomes. *Psychiatric Clinics of North America*, **23**, 795–809.

Denollet, J. & Brutsaert, D.L. (2001). Reducing emotional distress improves prognosis in coronary heart disease. *Circulation*, **104**, 2018–23.

Denollet, J. & Van Heck, G.L. (2001). Psychological risk factors in heart disease: what type D personality is (not) about. *Journal of Psychosomatic Research*, **51**, 465–8.

Dusseldorp, E., van Elderen, T., Maes, S. *et al.* (1999). A meta-analysis of psychoeducational programs for coronary heart disease patients. *Health Psychology*, **18**, 506–19.

Eng, P.M., Rimm, E.B., Fitzmaurice, G. & Kawachi, I. (2002). Social ties and change in social ties in relation to subsequent total cause-specific mortality and coronary heart disease incidence in men. *American Journal of Epidemiology*, **155**, 700–9.

Eng, P.M., Fitzmaurice, G., Kubzansky, L.D. *et al.* (2003). Anger expression and risk of stroke and coronary heart disease among male health professionals. *Psychosomatic Medicine*, **65**, 100–10.

Ferketich, A.K., Schwartzbaum, J.A., Frid, D.J., Moeschberger, M.L., for the National Health & Nutrition Examination Survey. (2000). Depression as an antecedent to heart disease among women and men in the NHANES I study. *Archieve of Internal Medicine*, **160**, 1261–8.

Friedman, M., Thoresen, C.E., Gill, J.J. *et al.* (1986). Alteration of Type-A behavior and its effect on cardiac recurrences in post myocardial infarction patients: summary results of the Recurrent Coronary Prevention Project. *American Heart Journal*, **112**, 653–65.

Friedman, M., Powell, L.H., Thoresen, C.E. *et al.* (1987). Effect of discontinuance of Type-A behavioral counseling on Type-A behavior and cardiac recurrence rate of post myocardial infarction patients. *American Heart Journal*, **114**, 483–90.

Fries, R., Konig, J., Schafers, H.J. & Bohm, M. (2002). Triggering effect of physical and mental stress on spontaneous ventricular tachyarrhythmias in patients with implantable cardioverter-defibrillators. *Clinical Cardiology*, **25**, 474–8.

Glassman, A.H. & Shapiro, P.A. (1998). Depression and the course of coronary artery disease. *American Journal of Psychiatry*, **155**, 4–11.

Glassman, A.H., O'Connor, C.M., Califf, R.M. *et al.* for the Sertraline Antidepressant Heart Attack Randomized Trial (SADHART) Group. (2002). Sertraline treatment of major depression in patients with acute MI or unstable angina. *Journal of the American Medical Association*, **288**, 701–9.

Hamalainen, H., Luurila, O.J., Kallio, V. & Knuts, L.R. (1995). Reduction in sudden deaths and coronary mortality in myocardial infarction patients after rehabilitation: 15-year follow-up study. *European Heart Journal*, **16**, 1839–44.

Hemingway, H., Malik, M. & Marmot, M. (2001). Social and psychological influences on sudden cardiac death, ventricular arrhythmia and cardiac autonomic function. *European Heart Journal*, **22**, 1082–101.

Januzzi, J.L., Stern, T.A., Pasternak, R.C. & DeSanctis, R.W. (2000). The influence of anxiety and depression on outcomes of patients with coronary artery disease. *Archieve of Internal Medicine*, **160**, 1913–21.

Jones, D.A. & West, R.R. (1996). Psychological rehabilitation after myocardial infarction: multicentre randomized controlled trial. *British Medical Journal*, **313**, 1517–21.

Kawachi, I., Colditz, G.A., Ascherio, A. *et al.* (1994). Prospective study of phobic anxiety and risk of coronary heart disease in men. *Circulation*, **89**, 1992–7.

Kivimaki, M., Leino-Arjas, P., Luukkonen, R. *et al.* (2002). Work stress and risk of cardiovascular mortality: prospective cohort study of industrial employees. *British Medical Journal*, **325**, 857–60.

Kop, W.J., Appels, A.P., Mendes de Leon, C.F. *et al.* (1994). Vital exhaustion predicts new cardiac events after successful coronary angioplasty. *Psychosomatic Medicine*, **56**, 281–7.

Lampert, R., Joska, T., Burg, M.M. *et al.* (2002). Emotional and physical precipitants of ventricular arrhythmia. *Circulation*, **106**, 1800–5.

Leor, J., Poole, W.K. & Kloner, R.A. (1996). Sudden cardiac death triggered by an earthquake. *New England Journal of Medicine*, **334**, 413–19.

Lett, H.S., Blumenthal, J.A., Babyak, M.A. *et al.* (2004). Depression as a risk factor for coronary artery disease, mechanisms, and treatment. *Psychosomatic Medicine*, **66**, 305–15.

MacMahon, K.M.A. & Lipp, G.Y. (2002). Psychological factors in heart failure. *Archieve of Internal Medicine*, **162**, 509–16.

Meisel, S.R., Kutz, I. & Davan, K.I. *et al.* (1991). Effect of the Iraqi missile war on incidence of acute myocardial infarction and sudden death in Israeli citizens. *Lancet*, **338**, 660–1.

Miller, T.Q., Smith, T.W., Turner, C.W. *et al.* (1996). A meta-analytic review of research on hostility and health. *Psychological Bulletin*, **119**, 322–48.

Mittleman, M.A., Maclure, M., Tofler, G.H. *et al.* (1993). Triggering of acute myocardial infarction by heavy physical exertion. *New England Journal of Medicine*, **329**, 1677–83.

Mittleman, M.A., Maclure, M., Sherwood, J.B. *et al.* for the Determinants of Myocardial Infarction Onset Study Investigators. (1995). Triggering of acute myocardial infarction onset by episodes of anger. *Circulation*, **92**, 1720–5.

Mittleman, M.A., Mintzer, D., Maclure, M. *et al.* (1999). Triggering of myocardial infarction by cocaine. *Circulation*, **99**, 2737–41.

Mittleman, M.A., Lewis, R.A., Maclure, M. *et al.* (2001). Triggering myocardial infarction by marijuana. *Circulation*, **103**, 2805–9.

Muller, J.E., Mittleman, M.A., Maclure, M. *et al.* for the Determinants of Myocardial Infarction Onset Study Investigators. (1996). Triggering of myocardial infarction by sexual activity. Low absolute risk and prevention by regular exercise. *Journal of the American Medical Association*, **275**, 1405–9.

Muller, J.E., Kaufmann, P.G., Luepker, R.V. *et al.* (1997). for the Mechanisms Precipitating Acute Cardiac Events Participants. Mechanisms precipitating acute cardiac events: review and recommendations of an NHLBI workshop. *Circulation*, **96**, 3233–9.

Ornish, D., Brown, S.E., Scherwitz, L.W. *et al.* (1990). Can lifestyle changes reverse coronary heart disease? *Lancet*, **336**, 129–33.

Ornish, D., Brown, S.E., Billings, J.H. *et al.* (1993). Can lifestyle changes reverse coronary atherosclerosis? Four-year results of the Lifestyle Heart Trial. *Circulation*, **88**, I-385 (Abstract).

Ornish, D., Scherwitz, L.W., Billings, J.H. *et al.* (1998). Intensive lifestyle changes for reversal of coronary heart disease. *Journal of the American Medical Association*, **280**, 2001–7.

Ornish, D. (1998). Avoiding revascularization with lifestyle changes: the multicenter lifestyle demonstration project. *American Journal of Cardiology*, **82**, 72T–76T.

Powell, L.H. & Thoresen, C.E. (1998). Effects of Type-A behavioral counseling and severity of prior acute myocardial infarction on survival. *American Journal of Cardiology*, **62**, 1159–63.

Ragland, D.R. & Brand, R.J. (1988). Type A behavior and mortality from coronary heart disease. *New England Journal of Medicine*, **318**, 65–9.

Raynor, D.A., Pogue-Geile, M.F., Kamarck, T.W., McCaffery, J.M. & Manuck, S.B. (2002). Covariation of psychosocial characteristics associated with cardiovascular disease: genetic and environmental influences. *Psychosomatic Medicine*, **64**, 191–203.

Rosengren, A., Hawken, S., Ounpuu, S. *et al.* for the INTERHEART Investigators. (2004). Association of psychosocial risk factors with risk of acute myocardial infarction in 11 119 cases and 13 648 controls from 52 countries (the INTERHEART study): case-control study. *Lancet*, **364**, 953–62.

Rozanski, A., Blumenthal, J.A. & Kaplan, J. (1999). Impact of psychological factors on the pathogenesis of cardiovascular disease and implications for therapy. *Circulation*, **99**, 2192–217.

Ruberman, W., Weinblatt, E., Goldberg, J.D. & Chaudhary, B.S. (1984). Psychosocial influences on mortality after myocardial infarction. *New England Journal of Medicine*, **311**, 552–9.

Schneiderman, N., Saab, P.G., Catellier, D.J. *et al.* for the ENRICHD Investigators. (2004). Psychosocial treatment within sex by ethnicity subgroups in the Enhancing Recovery in Coronary Heart Disease Clinical Trial. *Psychosomatic Medicine*, **66**, 475–83.

Sears, S.F., Todaro, J.F., Lewis, T.S., Sotile, W. & Conti, J.B. (1999). Examining the psychosocial impact of implantable cardioverter defibrillators: a literature review. *Clinical Cardiology*, **22**, 481–9.

Shedd, O.L., Sears, S.F., Harvill, J.L. *et al.* (2004). The World Trade Center attack: increased frequency of defibrillator shocks for ventricular arrhythmias in patients living remotely from New York City. *Journal of the American College of Cardiology*, **44**, 1265–7.

Smith, T.W. & Ruiz, J.M. (2002). Psychosocial influences on the development and course of coronary heart disease: current status and implications for research and practice. *Journal of Consulting and Clinical Psychology*, **70**, 548–68.

Steinberg, J.S., Arshad, A., Kowalski, M. *et al.* (2004). Increased incidence of life threatening ventricular arrhythmia in implantable defibrillator patients after the World Trade Center attack. *Journal of the American College of Cardiology*, **44**, 1261–4.

van Melle, J. P., de Jonge, P. & Spijkerman, T.A. *et al.* (2004). Prognostic association of depression following myocardial infarction with mortality and cardiovascular events: a meta-analysis. *Psychosomatic Medicine*, **66**, 814–22.

Williams, R.B., Barefoot, J.C. & Califf, R.M. (1992). Prognostic importance of social and economic resources among medically treated patients with angiographically documented coronary artery disease. *Journal of the American Medical Association*, **267**, 520–4.

Williams, J.E., Paton, C.C., Siegler, I.C. *et al.* (2000). Anger proneness predicts coronary heart disease risk: prospective analysis from the Atherosclerosis Risk in Communities (ARIC) Study. *Circulation*, **101**, 2034–9.

Williams, J.E., Nieto, F.J., Sanford, C.O. *et al.* (2002). The association between trait anger and incident stroke risk: the Atherosclerosis Risk in Communities (ARIC) Study. *Stroke*, **33**, 13–20.

Willich, S.N., Lowel, J., Lewis, M. *et al.* and the TRIMM Study Group. (1992). Increased Monday risk of acute myocardial infarction in the working population. *Circulation*, **86** (Suppl.1) 61.

Writing Committee for the ENRICHD investigators. (2003). Effects of treating depression and low perceived social support on clinical events after myocardial infarction: the enhancing recovery in coronary heart disease patients (ENRICHD) randomized trial. *Journal of the American Medical Association*, **289**, 3106–16.

Yusuf, S., Hawken, S., Ounpuu, S. *et al.* for the INTERHEART Investigators. (2004). Effect of potentially modifiable risk factors associated with myocardial infarction in 52 countries (the INTERHEART study): case-control study. *Lancet*, **364**, 937–52.

Coronary heart disease: heart failure

Kathleen Mulligan and Stanton Newman

University College London

Heart failure

Heart failure is a complex syndrome that can result from any structural or functional cardiac disorder which impairs the ability of the heart to pump (Cowie & Zaphiriou, 2002). Impairment in the pumping action of the heart can lead to a build-up of fluid in the lungs and extremities, causing symptoms of breathlessness and fatigue and signs of fluid retention in pulmonary congestion and peripheral oedema. It is primarily a disease of the elderly with an average age at diagnosis of 76 years and is more common in men than women. Heart failure is a major public health problem having an estimated prevalence of 0.4–2% in the general European population (Cowie et al., 1997). Recurrent prolonged hospital admissions are common and mortality is high. In the Framingham Heart Study, among a cohort with onset of heart failure between 1990–1999, one-year mortality was 28% in men and 24% in women; five-year mortality was 59% and 45% respectively (Levy et al., 2002).

Quality of life and mood

People with heart failure have reported poorer quality of life than that of the general population and those with a range of other chronic illnesses (Hobbs et al., 2002) (see 'Quality of life'). The extent to which their quality of life is impaired appears to be related to the extent of functional impairment as measured by the New York Heart Association classification (NYHA). Impairment in quality of life has been found to be related to both morbidity and mortality. In the Studies of Left Ventricular Dysfunction (SOLVD) trial, the quality of life dimensions of heart failure symptoms, impairment in activities of daily living and patients' assessment of their general health were found to be independent predictors of heart failure related hospitalizations and mortality (Konstam et al., 1996).

Depression is common in heart failure although reported prevalence varies, probably due to differences in the assessment and criteria for classification of depression and in the study populations. Most studies use questionnaire assessments which identify 'possible' or 'probable' depression but a diagnostic interview is required to confirm the presence of clinical depression (see 'Diagnostic interviews'). The percentage identified as depressed using clinical interview is therefore likely to be smaller than when using questionnaire assessment. Reported prevalence of depression in outpatient populations of heart failure has ranged from 11% who met the criteria for syndromal depression by diagnostic interview schedule (Turvey et al., 2002), to 48% who scored in the depressed range on the Beck Depression Inventory (Gottlieb et al., 2004). Prevalence of depression tends to be higher among inpatient populations. In one study, 13.9% of patients were diagnosed with major depressive disorder by clinical interview (Jiang et al., 2001). Using a questionnaire assessment Vaccarino et al. (2001) found that 77.5% scored within the depressed range. Depression appears in some studies to be more common in younger people and in women with heart failure (e.g. Freedland et al., 2003), although this finding is not consistent.

While it may be reasonable to hypothesize that higher rates of depression among inpatients result from greater illness severity this is generally not found. The absence of a correlation between depression and measures of severity of heart failure, such as left ventricular ejection fraction, indicates that in those with similarly severe disease, patients who are depressed report more severe symptoms than those who are not depressed (Freedland et al., 2003). There is evidence for a relationship between depression and the New York Heart Association (NYHA) classification of functional limitation, with higher rates of depression among those with greater functional limitation (Gottlieb et al., 2004). The direction of this relationship merits further examination; while the symptoms and functional limitations of heart failure may lead to depression, the presence of depression could also exacerbate symptoms and functional limitations (see 'Symptom perception').

Depression also appears to be associated with a poorer prognosis, although there are some conflicting findings. Hospital readmission has been found to be more frequent in depressed patients and depression has also been found to predict mortality (Faris et al., 2002). Vaccarino et al. (2001) found that after adjustment for demographic factors, medical history, baseline functional status and clinical severity, an increasing number of depressive symptoms was associated with a significantly higher risk of the combined endpoint of functional decline or death.

The important role of depression in heart failure extends to research which suggests that depression may increase the risk of developing heart failure. In a study of 4538 people aged 60 and over who were followed for an average of 4.5 years, people with depression were at more than twice the risk of developing heart failure as those without depression (Abramson et al., 2001). It has been suggested that the relationship between depression and heart failure may be due to a common pathophysiology. The neurohormonal activation, rhythm disturbances, inflammation and hypercoagulability that have been postulated to play a role in development and prognosis of heart failure are also seen in depressed patients (Joynt et al., 2004). Another study however, did not find that depression was an independent risk factor for subsequent development of heart failure (Chen et al., 1999), so further investigation is necessary in order to clarify the nature of the relationship.

The link between depression and heart failure raises the question of the extent to which heart failure patients receive treatment for depression. The evidence suggests that only a small proportion of those heart failure patients with depression receive treatment (Jacob *et al.*, 2003). A screening assessment for depression should be considered in all patients with heart failure.

In contrast to depression, there is little research on anxiety in heart failure. In a study of male inpatients, anxiety was not higher than in a group of healthy subjects but in the heart failure patients, those in NYHA class III reported higher anxiety than those in classes I and II (Majani *et al.*, 1999). No association between anxiety and mortality or hospitalization was found in the SOLVD trial (Konstam *et al.*, 1996). A link between anxiety and depression in heart failure was reported by Freedland and Carney (2000) who found anxious reactions to dyspnoea to be more common in depressed than non-depressed patients.

Self-management

Heart failure can worsen quickly so detection of early indicators of deterioration is important. One way to achieve this is for patients to self-monitor for signs of fluid retention such as shortness of breath, weight gain and oedema. In addition, self-management of the medication regimen and care over salt and fluid intake are important. Other lifestyle factors can have a significant impact and patients are encouraged to take regular exercise, give up smoking and abstain from alcohol if it was the cause of their heart failure (see 'Coronary heart disease: rehabilitation'). Many people with heart failure do not incorporate or maintain these self-management activities (Carlson *et al.*, 2001) and this can lead to rapid deterioration in their condition, often requiring hospital care. To date, most approaches to reduce the risk of hospital admission have involved more intensive follow-up at home or in clinic by multidisciplinary teams, or telephone follow-up; most programmes also include education. Many of these interventions have shown reductions in hospitalizations for heart failure and, in the case of multidisciplinary follow-up, all-cause hospitalization and mortality (McAlister *et al.*, 2004).

An interesting issue is the proportion of patients who, after these interventions, adopt the self-management behaviours that they have been taught. Uptake of self-management behaviours was examined in a study by Wright *et al.* (2003). Patients were randomized to either usual care or to a programme that included specialist and primary care follow-up, education, a diary and instructions for daily weighing. Of 100 patients in the intervention group, 76 used the diary, 51 of whom weighed themselves regularly (≥ once a week). Importantly those patients who weighed regularly were less likely to have a hospital admission and there was a trend for them to have

a longer time to first readmission and more days alive and out of hospital over the course of the study. Given the apparent benefits, studies need to examine ways of increasing the numbers of patients who adopt self-management behaviours (see 'Self-management').

In other illnesses, such as arthritis, asthma and diabetes, provision of information alone has been found to be insufficient to bring about behaviour change, leading to the incorporation into self-management interventions of psychological strategies such as motivational interviewing, problem-solving and cognitive–behavioural techniques (Newman *et al.*, 2004) (see 'Cognitive behaviour therapy' and 'Motivational interviewing'). In heart failure, few studies to date have gone beyond the provision of advice and instruction. Some do refer to the use of 'counselling' but the meaning of what is meant by counselling in this context and the theoretical approach used, if any, are unclear.

Interventions to improve people's self-management of their heart failure need to take account of cognitive, emotional and social factors which could act as barriers to behaviour change. The link between depression and outcomes in heart failure highlighted above may also involve behaviour in that depressed patients may be less likely to take their medication (Carney *et al.*, 1995) (see 'Adherence to treatment'). Other factors such as patients' beliefs about their illness and recommended treatment, as well as their cognitive capacity to follow advice, are also relevant. For example, one issue concerns the interpretation of symptoms and how they influence the taking of action. A qualitative study found that most patients did not accurately interpret worsening symptoms and act upon them promptly. Patients perceived heart failure as an acute, episodic condition and treated it as such, rather than as a chronic condition requiring ongoing monitoring and self-management (Horowitz *et al.*, 2004) (see 'Lay beliefs about health and illness' and 'Symptom perception').

Clinical implications of cognitive dysfunction were reported in a study by Ekman *et al.* which found that a low score on the Mini Mental State Exam was associated with non-participation in a nurse-directed outpatient programme (Ekman *et al.*, 2001). Research in this area is not well developed but studies to date suggest that cognitive impairment, particularly in memory and attention, is fairly widespread (Almeida & Flicker, 2001) and may be an influence on adherence to medication.

(See also 'Coronary heart disease: cardiac psychology', 'Coronary heart disease: impact', 'Coronary heart disease: rehabilitation', and 'Coronary heart disease: surgery'.)

REFERENCES

Abramson, J., Berger, A., Krumholz, H.M. & Vaccarino, V. (2001). Depression and risk of heart failure among older persons with isolated systolic hypertension. *Archieve of Internal Medicine*, **161**, 1725–30.

Almeida, O.P. & Flicker, L. (2001). The mind of a failing heart: a systematic review of the association between congestive heart failure and cognitive functioning. *Internal Medicine Journal*, **31**, 290–5.

Carlson, B., Riegel, B. & Moser, D.K. (2001). Self-care abilities of patients with heart failure. *Heart & Lung*, **30**, 351–9.

Carney, R.M., Freedland, K.E., Eisen, S.A., Rich, M.W. & Jaffe, A.S. (1995). Major depression and medication adherence in elderly patients with coronary artery disease. *Health Psychology*, **14**, 88–90.

Chen, Y.-T., Vaccarino, V., Williams, C.S. *et al.* (1999). Risk factors for heart failure

in the elderly: a prospective community-based study. *American Journal of Medicine*, **106**, 605–12.

Cowie, M.R., Mosterd, A., Wood, D.A. *et al.* (1997). The epidemiology of heart failure. *European Heart Journal*, **18**, 208–25.

Cowie, M. R. & Zaphiriou, A. (2002). Management of chronic heart failure. *British Medical Journal*, **325**, 422–25.

Ekman, I., Fagerberg, B. & Skoog, I. (2001). The clinical implications of cognitive impairment in elderly patients with chronic heart failure. *The Journal of Cardiovascular Nursing*, **16**, 47–55.

Faris, R., Purcell, H., Henein, M.Y. & Coats, A.J.S. (2002). Clinical depression is common and significantly associated with reduced survival in patients with non-ischaemic heart failure. *The European Journal of Heart Failure*, **4**, 541–51.

Freedland, K.E. & Carney, R.M. (2000). Psychosocial considerations in elderly patients with heart failure. *Clinics in Geriatric Medicine*, **16**, 649–61.

Freedland, K.E., Rich, M.W., Skala, J.A. *et al.* (2003). Prevalence of depression in hospitalized patients with congestive heart failure. *Psychosomatic Medicine*, **65**, 119–28.

Gottlieb, S.S., Khatta, M., Friedmann, E. *et al.* (2004). The influence of age, gender and race on the prevalence of depression in heart failure patients. *Journal of the American College of Cardiology*, **43**, 1542–9.

Hobbs, F.D., Kenkre, J.E., Roalfe, A.K. *et al.* (2002). Impact of heart failure and left ventricular systolic dysfunction on quality of life: a cross-sectional study comparing common chronic cardiac and medical disorders and a representative adult population. *European Heart Journal*, **23**, 1867–76.

Horowitz, C.R., Rein, S.B. & Leventhal, H. (2004). A story of maladies, misconceptions and mishaps: effective management of heart failure. *Social Science & Medicine*, **58**, 631–43.

Jacob, S., Sebastian, J.C. & Abraham, G. (2003). Depression and congestive heart failure: are antidepressants underutilized? *European Journal of Heart Failure*, **5**, 399–400.

Jiang, W., Alexander, J. & Christopher, E. (2001). Relationship of depression to increased risk of mortality and rehospitalization in patients with congestive heart failure. *Archives of Internal Medicine*, **161**, 1849–56.

Joynt, K.E., Whellan, D.J. & O'Connor, C.M. (2004). Why is depression bad for the failing heart? A review of the mechanistic relationship between depression and heart failure. *Journal of Cardiac Failure*, **10**, 258–71.

Konstam, V., Salem, D., Pouleur, H. *et al.* (1996). Baseline quality of life as a predictor of mortality and hospitalization in 5,025 patients with congestive heart failure. SOLVD Investigations. Studies of Left Ventricular Dysfunction Investigators. *American Journal of Cardiology*, **78**, 890–5.

Levy, D., Kenchaiah, S., Larson, M.G. *et al.* (2002). Long-term trends in the incidence of and survival with heart failure. *New England Journal of Medicine*, **347**, 1397–402.

Majani, G., Pierobon, A., Giardini, A. *et al.* (1999). Relationship between psychological profile and cardiological variables in chronic heart failure. The role of patient subjectivity. *European Heart Journal*, **20**, 1579–86.

McAlister, F.A., Stewart, S., Ferrua, S. & McMurray, J.J.V. (2004). Multidisciplinary strategies for the management of heart failure patients at high risk for admission. A systematic review of randomized trials. *Journal of the American College of Cardiology*, **44**, 810–19.

Newman, S., Steed, L. & Mulligan, K. (2004). Self-management interventions for chronic illness. *The Lancet*, **364** (9444), 1523–37.

Turvey, C.L., Schultz, K., Arndt, S., Wallace, R.B. & Herzog, R. (2002). Prevalence and correlates of depressive symptoms in a community sample of people suffering from heart failure. *Journal of American Geriatric Society*, **50**, 2003–8.

Vaccarino, V., Kasl, S.V., Abramson, J. & Krumholz, H.M. (2001). Depressive symptoms and risk of functional decline and death in patients with heart failure. *Journal of the American College of Cardiology*, **38**, 199–205.

Wright, S.P., Walsh, H., Ingley, K.M. *et al.* (2003). Uptake of self-management strategies in a heart failure management programme. *European Journal of Heart Failure*, **5**, 371–80.

Coronary heart disease: rehabilitation

Robert J. Lewin

University of York

History and ethos

Cardiac rehabilitation (CR) began in the 1960s. The rationale was that part of the heart muscle was no longer pumping but that a programme of exercise would strengthen the remaining muscle thereby restoring the patient's ability to lead a normal life. By the 1990s it was established that middle-aged, white males who had sustained a mild myocardial infarct (MI) could significantly increase their physical fitness, but that this had little impact on the poor psychosocial outcomes exhibited by approximately a third of patients. The term '*comprehensive* cardiac rehabilitation' was introduced to redefine CR as an activity that also attended to the psychosocial needs of patients (World Health Organization, 1993) and this is now widely accepted.

Content

The main tool for behaviour change is usually education in the form of group talks. It is unusual for psychosocial needs to be formally assessed and the only 'psychological' treatment provided in most centres is group relaxation classes. There is some evidence suggesting benefit from adding breathing retraining, (van Dixhoorn & Duivenvoorden, 1999) and stress management (Trzcieniecka-Green & Steptoe, 1996) (see 'Relaxation training' and 'Stress management').

Most national clinical guidelines have called for CR to move away from group programmes to an individualized programme based on assessment of need (including medical, psychological and social) and offering a 'menu' of treatment choices (Department of Health, 2002).

Delivery of cardiac rehabilitation

Social class, gender, area of domicile, ethnicity and age are all associated with low levels of uptake. Poor compliance is common, as many as 50% of patients will drop out of treatment (see 'Adherence to treatment'). A recent research monograph reviews these problems and the few published attempts to remedy them (Beswick et al., 2004). Services are mainly delivered by nurses and/or physiotherapists.

A large number of patients remain untreated, for example, in the UK each year only 60 000 of the 350 000 potential patients receive CR. The numbers involved suggest that delivering psychological interventions would in most cases have to be done by non-psychologists. An interesting possibility is to train laypeople or CHD patients to deliver the treatment. Using information technology (IT) may also reduce the demand on personnel: several research projects are underway assessing Internet- or computer-delivered CR programmes and at least one has reported results similar to traditional methods (Gordon et al., 2001).

Alternative methods

Two methods that use 'psychological' techniques and offer an alternative delivery method are in routine use. One used in the United States of America, is the MULTIFIT programme (Taylor et al., 1997). It is based on Banduras' theories of self-efficacy and involves self-recording and brief phone contacts with a facilitator for goal setting (see 'Self-efficacy and health'). The second, widely used in the UK, is the Heart Manual (HM) (Lewin et al., 1992). It is a six week, home-based, cognitive–behavioural (CB) intervention based around a patient-held workbook and audiotapes. Methods include reframing 'cardiac misconceptions', enhancing perceived global health and perceived control over the illness, self-recording, stress management, relaxation, breathing retraining and self-management advice for anxiety and depression (see 'Cognitive behaviour therapy'). It is administered by a 'facilitator' who has undertaken a 2-day training in the CB methods. Home-based programmes may improve uptake and compliance. In a choice trial offering the Heart Manual or hospital-based rehabilitation 44% of MI patients chose the HM and 87% completed it whereas 33% chose a hospital programme and 49% completed it (Dalal & Evans, 2003). Other studies have shown similar results (e.g. Smith et al., 2004).

Psychologically orientated individual counselling delivered by a nurse (Johnston et al., 1999) has also produced improvements in psychosocial outcomes and Petrie et al. have evaluated a pre-discharge, psychologist-led, 3-session (30–40 minutes each time) intervention designed to change illness beliefs and develop with the patient a post-discharge action plan. Scores on the Illness Perception Questionnaire changed inline with predictions and participants were more likely to have returned to work at 12 weeks post-discharge (Petrie et al., 2002) (see 'Lay beliefs about health and illness' and 'Illness cognition assessment').

Effect of cardiac rehabilitation on mortality and morbidity

A recent meta-analysis included 48 randomized trials (8940 patients) and showed a 20% reduction in all cause mortality at 2–5 years (odds ratio = 0.80; 95% CI: 0.68 to 0.93) (Taylor et al., 2004). It also showed an improvement in smoking but none in reinfarction rates, cholesterol (total and fractional), blood pressure or quality of life. A few trials have shown very significant benefits in all of these areas. A recent example is a study in Hong Kong that: improved anxiety and depression; improved scores on 6 of the 8 SF-36 quality of life dimensions and saved 640 US$ per patient through reducing the need for angioplasty (Yu et al., 2004). It was a long-term programme beginning in hospital and sustained over 2 years. It is probably fair to conclude that, when the standard UK 6–12 week outpatient model of CR is tested, there is improved exercise capacity but that quality of life and psychological factors are not improved (e.g. Bertie et al., 1992).

Taylor (2004) divided the studies in the meta-analysis into those regarded as being 'comprehensive' or exercise-based and found no advantage in survival for 'comprehensive' rehabilitation programmes. Three trials of psychosocial interventions have been powered to show a reduction in mortality. In the first, 2328 patients were randomized to usual care or to attend seven, 2-hour sessions with a clinical psychologist (Jones & West, 1996). The M-HART trial, randomized 1376 post-MI patients to monthly screening using the General Health Questionnaire or to routine care: patients scoring greater than 5, received one or more nurse visits aimed at 'reducing stress' (Frasure-Smith et al., 1997). Neither intervention had any effect on psychological outcomes or mortality. Both have been criticized for being atheoretical, having no detailed account of the therapeutic protocol or specific training for the 'therapist'. The third study, the ENRICHD trial, recruited and randomized 2481 patients to cognitive–behaviour therapy for depression. Depression improved but there was no reduction in mortality (Blumenthal et al., 2004).

The evidence reviewed above provides support to those who believe that psychology has little to contribute to CR. This, however, ignores the key tasks faced by most patients in returning to a normal or near normal life which are: changing an unhealthy lifestyle; adjusting to a frightening diagnosis; coping with anxiety and depression; relationship and sexual difficulties and the problems of managing a long-term chronic disease (see 'Coping with chronic illness').

Adjunctive psychological treatments

A recent systematic review of whether psychological interventions benefit CHD patients included 36 trials (12 841 patients). It concluded that any kind of psychological or stress management intervention caused small reductions in anxiety and depression and that there was a reduction of non-fatal reinfarctions (OR 0.78, 95% CI = 0.67, 0.90) but that publication bias made these conclusions 'insecure' (Rees et al., 2004). By way of contrast a review by Dusseldop et al. (1999) examined the effect of educational and psychological interventions on behavioural risk factors and showed that when interventions were successful there was an effect on mortality. Altogether there have been six systematic reviews of the same question and most were positive. However, despite the fact that each asked the same question, there is almost no agreement in the papers selected.

Cognitive–behavioural cardiac rehabilitation

The same lack of relationship between impairment and disability exists in CHD as in other chronic disease states. There is no significant relationship between ejection fraction (the efficiency of the pumping action of the heart) and functional ability, or between the extent of atheroma and angina. Or between impairment and psychological distress (except in end-stage disease when the symptom burden becomes overwhelming). There are moderate correlations between psychological predictors and functional performance, readmission to hospital, symptom report, quality of life, anxiety, depression, treatment costs and adherence to treatment.

The ways in which these factors interact in the case of angina suggested that CB chronic pain management techniques might be appropriate (Lewin, 1997) (see 'Pain management'). A hospital-based (Lewin *et al.*, 1995) and a home-based (Lewin *et al.*, 2002) Angina Management Programme has been developed and evaluated. Both forms had significant benefits showing a 70% and 40% reduction in angina respectively as well as improving aspects of disability. In addition to employing the common aspects of CB programmes this targets a set of symptom-specific and CHD-generic beliefs about heart disease which have been called 'cardiac misconceptions' (Maeland & Havik, 1989; Furze *et al.*, 2003). It is hypothesized that these lead to 'fear avoidance' of activity, leading to physical deconditioning and greater symptom load and further avoidance. There is evidence that a change in these beliefs predicts greater activity (Furze & Lewin, 2004).

Conclusions

Cardiac rehabilitation has a powerful effect in deferring death but little effect on reducing disability or improving a poor quality of life. Despite an obvious role, few psychologists are directly involved in delivery. There is evidence from systematic reviews that psychosocial interventions for CHD patients can have an effect on anxiety, depression and risk factors for CHD. Evidence of an effect on mortality is missing.

No conclusions can be drawn about the relative value of different treatments due to a lack of common outcome measures and failure to attempt independent replication. The psychologically malleable factors that predict disability in patients with CHD are the same as those in other chronic diseases. They include anxiety, depression, health beliefs and poor self-management strategies. A promising direction for research is to use CB chronic disease management methodology whilst paying attention to disease-specific beliefs. Psychological interventions in CR are most likely to be adopted if they can be delivered by other health professionals and in the future they may also be delivered by trained laypeople and the Internet.

(See also 'Coronary heart disease: cardiac psychology', 'Coronary heart disease: heart failure', 'Coronary heart disease, impact' and 'Coronary heart disease: surgery').

REFERENCES

Berkman, L.F., Blumenthal, J., Burg, M. *et al.* Effects of treating depression and low perceived social support on clinical events after myocardial infarction: the Enhancing Recovery in Coronary Heart Disease Patients (ENRICHD) trial. *Journal of the American Medical Association*, **289**, 3106–16.

Bertie, J., King, A., Reed, N., Marshall, A.J. & Ricketts, C. (1992). Benefits and weaknesses of a cardiac rehabilitation programme. *Journal of the Royal College of Physicians of London*, **26**, 147–51.

Beswick, A.D., Rees, K., Griebsch, I. *et al.* (2004). Provision, uptake and cost of cardiac rehabilitation programmes: improving services to under-represented groups. *Health Technology Assessment*, **8**, 1–152. (Available from http://www.ncchta.org/fullmono/mon841.pdf)

Blumenthal, J.A., Babyak, M.A., Carney, R.M. *et al.* (2004). Exercise, depression, and mortality after myocardial infarction in the ENRICHD trial. *Medicine Science Sports Exercise*, **36**, 746–55.

Burke, B.L., Arkowitz, H. & Menchola, M.J. (2003). The efficacy of motivational interviewing: a meta-analysis of controlled clinical trials. *Consulting and Clinical Psychology*, **71**, 843–61.

Dalal, H.M. & Evans, P.H. (2003). Achieving national service framework standards for cardiac rehabilitation and secondary prevention. *British Medical Journal*, **326**, 481–4.

Department of Health. (2002). *National service framework for coronary heart disease: chapter 7, cardiac rehabilitation. modern standards & service models.* London: Department of Health.

Dusseldorp, E., van Elderen, T., Maes, S., Meulman, J. & Kraaij, V. (1999). A meta-analysis of psychoeduational programs for coronary heart disease patients. *Health Psychology*, **18**, 506–19.

Frasure-Smith, N., Lesperance, F., Prince, R.H. *et al.* (1997). Randomised trial of home-based psychosocial nursing intervention for patients recovering from myocardial infarction. *The Lancet*, **350**, 473–9.

Furze, G., Bull, P., Lewin, R.J. & Thompson, D.R. (2003). Development of the York Angina Beliefs Questionnaire. *Journal of Health Psychology*, **8**, 307–15.

Furze, G. & Lewin, R.J.P. (2004). The effect of misconceptions about angina on physical activity (abstract). *European Journal of Cardiovascular Prevention and Rehabilitation*, **11**(Suppl.1), 16.

Gordon, N.F., Salmon, R.D., Mitchell, B.S. *et al.* (2001). Innovative approaches to comprehensive cardiovascular disease risk reduction in clinical and community-based settings. *Current Atherosclerosis Report*, **6**, 498–506.

Johnston, M., Foulkes, J., Johnston, D.W., Pollard, B. & Gudmundsdottir, H. (1999). Impact on patients and partners of inpatient and extended cardiac counselling and rehabilitation: a controlled trial. *Psychosomatic Medicine*, **61**, 225–33.

Jones, D.A. & West, R.R. (1996). Psychological rehabilitation after myocardial infarction: multicentre randomised controlled trial. *British Medical Journal*, **313**, 1517–21.

Lewin, B., Robertson, I.H., Cayol, E.L. *et al.* (1992). Effects of self-help post myocardial infarction rehabilitation on psychological adjustment and use of health services. *The Lancet*, **339**, 1036–40.

Lewin, B., Cay, E.L., Todd, I. *et al.* (1995). The Angina Management Programme: a rehabilitation treatment. *British Journal of Cardiology*, **2**, 221–6.

Lewin, B. (1997). The psychological and behavioural management of angina. *Journal of Psychosomatic Research*, **5**, 452–62.

Lewin, R.J., Furze, G., Robinson, J. *et al.* (2002). A randomised controlled trial of a self-management plan for patients with newly diagnosed angina. *British Journal of General Practice, 52*, 194–6, 199–201.

Lewin, R.J., Roebuck, A. & Thompson, D.R. (2004). *British Journal of Cardiology* (see also http://www.cardiacrehabilitation.org.uk/dataset.htm).

Maeland, J.G. & Havik, O.E. (1989). After the myocardial infarction. A medical and psychological study with special emphasis on perceived illness. *Scandinavian Journal of Rehabilitation Medicine, 22*(Suppl.), 1–87.

Petrie, K.J., Cameron, L.D., Ellis, C.J., Buick, D. & Weinman, J. (2002). Changing illness perceptions after myocardial infarction: an early intervention randomized controlled trial. *Psychosomatic Medicine, 64*, 580–6.

Rees, K., Bennett, P., West, R., Davey, S.G. & Ebrahim, S. (2004). Psychological interventions for coronary heart disease. *Evidence Based Nursing, 4*, 114.

Smith, K.M., Arthur, H.M., McKelvie, R.S. & Kodis, J. (2004). Differences in sustainability of exercise and health-related quality of life outcomes following home or hospital-based cardiac rehabilitation. *European Journal of Cardiovascular Prevention & Rehabilitation, 4*, 313–19.

Taylor, C.B., Miller, N.H., Smith, P.M. & DeBusk, R.F. (1997). The effect of a home-based, case-managed, multifactorial risk-reduction program on reducing psychological distress in patients with cardiovascular disease. *Journal of Cardiopulmonary Rehabilitation, 17*, 157–62.

Taylor, R.S., Brown, A., Ebrahim, S. *et al.* (2004). Exercise-based rehabilitation for patients with coronary heart disease: systematic review and meta-analysis of randomized controlled trials. *American Journal of Medicine, 116*, 682–92.

Trzcieniecka-Green, A. & Steptoe, A. (1996). The effects of stress management on the quality of life of patients following acute

myocardial infarction or coronary bypass surgery. *European Heart Journal, 17*, 1663–70.

Dixhoorn, J.J. & Duivenvoorden, H.J. (1999). Effect of relaxation therapy on cardiac events after myocardial infarction: a 5-year follow-up study. *Journal of Cardiopulmonary Rehabilitation, 19*, 178–85.

World Health Organization. (1993). *Needs and action priorities in cardiac rehabilitation and secondary prevention in patients with CHD*. Geneva: WHO Regional Office for Europe.

Yu, C.M., Lau, C.P., Chau, J. *et al.* (2004). A short course of cardiac rehabilitation program is highly cost effective in improving long-term quality of life in patients with recent myocardial infarction or percutaneous coronary intervention. *Archives of Physical & Medical Rehabilitation, 85*, 1915–22.

Coronary heart disease: surgery

Jan Stygall and Stanton Newman

University College London

Psychological responses to cardiac surgery

It has been suggested that a relatively high level of psychological morbidity follows cardiac surgery in contrast to other forms of surgery. However this view has not been borne out in formal research. Studies of general psychiatric morbidity, using standardized instruments, have shown a general reduction following cardiac surgery. Studies have also demonstrated that patterns of anxiety are similar to those found in other forms of surgery with a significant increase in anxiety in the days immediately before and after surgery followed by a significant drop in the weeks and months following surgery (Rymaszewska *et al.*, 2003). The prevalence of depression has been found to be the same before and after cardiac surgery, in the range of approximately 20–25% (Connerney *et al.*, 2001). Furthermore, studies have shown no differences in the emotional effects of either coronary bypass graft (CABG) surgery or valve replacement/repair (see also 'Stressful medical procedures' and 'Surgery').

Both anxiety and depression have been shown to predict adverse outcomes post-cardiac surgery (e.g. Connerney *et al.*, 2001; Rymaszewska *et al.*, 2003). Whereas early small studies (e.g. Connerney *et al.*, 2001) failed to find a relationship between depression and mortality after cardiac surgery, a large 12-year follow-up

study by Blumenthal *et al.* (2003) found depression to be an important independent predictor of mortality.

It is not surprising that the most potent predictor of mood state after cardiac surgery is mood prior to surgery. For example, Timberlake *et al.* (1997) found that 37% of patients were depressed pre-operatively, 50% at 8 days, 24% at 8 weeks and 23% 1 year after surgery. The pre-operative depression score was the best predictor of post-operative depression at all times of assessment.

Studies have demonstrated that depressed mood following surgery is influenced by a range of factors. For example, Coombs *et al.* (1989) found emotional social support to be highest in the days after surgery with higher social support at 5 days and 3 months being significantly associated with lower levels of depressed mood. This relationship, however, was not apparent at assessments conducted at 6 and 12 months post-surgery suggesting that perceived social support has an effect on mood only in the early period following CABG.

Patients' perceptions of their health have also been shown to be important in relation to mood state following cardiac surgery. Coombs *et al.* (1989) found that recurrence of chest pain and patient's perception of their overall health both contributed significantly to depressed mood when assessed 3 and 6 months after surgery. They attribute the importance of these findings to patients' increasing concerns regarding the success of the procedure (see also 'Lay Beliefs about health and illness' and 'Symptom perception').

The effect of pre-operative education programmes on outcome have been evaluated. In one of these, Shuldham *et al.* (2002) compared patients receiving a 1-day pre-operative education programme with patients undergoing normal care and found no differences in the groups on outcome measures of pain, anxiety, depression and wellbeing but, surprisingly, found that the programme was associated with increased hospital stay. In contrast, Arthur *et al.* (2000) found that patients who received exercise training, education and reinforcement were discharged from hospital earlier and had an improved quality of life 6 months post-surgery. It is as yet unclear what the key components should be for a pre-operative programme in cadiac surgery, but it is important to note that the latter study had a very intensive programme spread over a number of weeks.

Changes in cognitive function

Neuropsychological (NP) complications affecting memory, concentration, attention and speed of motor and mental response have been shown to occur in patients following cardiac surgery. However, the reported frequency of these changes varies widely between studies. Studies assessing participants 5–10 days post-operatively have reported the incidence of neuropsychological morbidity to range from 12.5% to 79%. Whereas, later assessments, conducted between 6 weeks and 6 months have detected neuropsychological dysfunction in 12–37% of participants (S. Newman & Stygall, 2000). Longer term consequences have shown a significant deterioration in a small number of patients up to five years post-surgery (e.g. M.F. Newman *et al.*, 2001; Selnes *et al.*, 2001; Stygall *et al.*, 2003).

This variation has been attributed in part to methodological factors which include differences in the number, type and sensitivity of neuropsychological tests used, the definition of dysfunction and the method of statistical analysis employed. These methodological issues have been addressed at international consensus conferences (Murkin *et al.*, 1995, 1997). Arguably, the most important factor is the timing of the assessment. Assessments conducted later in the recovery period (over 6 weeks) are considered to be more stable and to reflect a more persistent neuropsychological problem. However, although it has often been argued that pre-discharge assessments are likely to be contaminated by general surgical recovery (see, for example, 'Anaesthesia'), there is an indication that these assessments may predict longer-term decline (e.g. Stygall *et al.*, 2003; van Dijk *et al.*, 2004).

Studies examining NP decline and cardiac surgery have been conducted since the early 1980s. During this time major advances have been made in surgical and anaesthetic techniques, as well as the type of equipment used. Patients operated upon now tend to be older and have more co-morbid illness than those in the early studies and, as patient variables such as age and disease severity have been associated with post-operative cognitive decline, these issues further contribute to the variations seen.

Type of surgery

Some authors have suggested that valve replacement surgery, which is an open heart procedure, should show a higher incidence of neuropsychological problems than that observed in CABG. Although most studies comparing these two forms of surgery have found a higher risk of stroke in valve replacement patients (e.g. Burcerius *et al.*, 2003), very little research has been conducted comparing the more subtle NP changes. Those few studies that have been carried out have produced contradictory results, some reporting poorer NP outcome in valve patients (e.g. Andrew *et al.*, 2001) and others suggesting no difference (e.g. Browndyke *et al.*, 2002).

Factors associated with neuropsychological dysfunction

Studies have suggested a relationship between patient characteristics and NP decline following cardiac surgery. These include older age, diabetes, aortic atherosclerosis, cerebrovascular and peripheral vascular disease. Higher levels of education have been found to be protective (Ho *et al.*, 2004). In line with their higher morbidity and mortality (Edwards *et al.*, 1998) and increased risk of neurological events (Hogue *et al.*, 2001), it has been suggested that females may be more susceptible than males to NP decline following cardiac surgery. However, Bute *et al.* (2003) found that although women were more likely to report cognitive difficulties, objective NP assessments found no difference between men and women one year post-surgery.

Other studies have examined the effect of different surgical and anaesthetic techniques on NP outcomes. These include cardiopulmonary bypass (CPB), hypothermia and acid-base management. A number of studies have found a relationship between the duration of CPB and NP decline. Equipment used for CPB is constantly changing. A number of studies have examined whether newer forms of equipment lead to lower levels of neuropsychological problems. One example is the method of oxygenating the blood, where membrane oxygenators have been found to produce less decline than bubble oxygenators. A second has been the use of arterial line filters in the CPB circuit to filter out microscopic particles of debris and air where the use of a 40 micron filter was found to reduce the frequency of NP decline (see Newman & Stygall, 2000 review).

It is common for cardiac surgery using CPB to involve hypothermia. Hypothermia has been considered to be protective against ischaemic damage. However, studies using stroke or NP decline as an outcome measure have shown mixed results (Newman & Harrison, 2002). One possible explanation given is that any neuroprotection produced by hypothermia may be offset by damage that occurs during the rewarming process. A feasibility study by Bar-Yosef *et al.* (2004) has shown that limiting the maximum temperature during the rewarming phase of the operation can prevent cerebral hyperthermia and randomized controlled trials are currently being conducted to evaluate this approach.

Two techniques have been used to manage the effects of hypothermia on pH levels. In one, the fall in pH is corrected by adding CO_2 (pH stat); in the other, the CO_2 is kept constant (alpha stat). It has been demonstrated that alpha stat management leads to fewer individuals with cognitive deficits (e.g. Patel *et al.*, 1996).

Relationship between neuropsychological deficit and putative mechanism of damage

The mechanisms contributing to post cardiac surgery neuropsychological deficits are uncertain. However, two inter-related factors, microemboli and altered cerebral perfusion, have often been suggested. Although profound hypotension during surgery may cause severe cerebral consequences, there appears to be little relationship between less severe differences in blood pressure and NP dysfunction.

In recent years transcranial Doppler detection has been applied to detect high frequency signals that appear to reflect either air or particulate matter going into the brain (microemboli) during cardiac surgery. The candidates for particulate matter include artheromatous matter, fat and platelet aggregates. These microemboli are thought to originate from the CPB equipment and artheromatous plaque in the heart vessels. Some studies have reported an association between number of microemboli detected and NP decline, others have found no such relationship. The association between microemboli and NP dysfunction is problematical as, at present, the size, composition and ultimate location in the brain of the microemboli cannot be reliably determined.

The emergence of beating-heart (off-pump) surgery as a common technique for multi-vessel revascularization has opened up an avenue of research to isolate the role CPB plays in cognitive decline post cardiac surgery. Many of the early studies were biased as they were retrospective and used patients that were specially selected for off-pump surgery. Although these studies provided some evidence that off-pump surgery may lead to a reduction in the occurrence of microemboli and strokes, a more recent randomized controlled trial (Van-Dijk et al., 2002) found no difference in mortality, cardiac outcome or quality of life between patients receiving on or off-pump surgery at 1 month follow-up. At 3 months post surgery off-pump patients were found to have a better cognitive outcome compared to on-pump patients but these differences were not detected at 12 months. Further trials of this type are required to examine neurological and neuropsychological outcome following cardiac surgery.

Quality of life (QoL) following cardiac surgery

It would be expected that, without the constraints of chest pain and breathlessness associated with cardiac disease, increased levels of physical and social activity would occur after surgery. The advice given to the patient frequently includes a recommendation for increased physical activity. Consequently, it is not surprising that studies on both valve replacement and CABG surgery have found the majority of patients report increased levels of physical and social activity and improved QoL following cardiac surgery (e.g. Bute et al., 2003). However, these improvements are not experienced by all patients. Approximately, 25–49% of patients report decreased activity levels (Rymaszewska et al., 2003). Age, education, decline in NP functioning, pre-operative health status, co-morbid conditions and social isolation have all been shown to be important predictors of QoL outcome.

The research is less clear however with respect to gender differences. Various studies have suggested that women fare less well post-operatively, whilst others have found similar long-term outcomes for men and women. Women presenting for CABG tend to be older, less well educated, more likely to be single, living alone and unemployed. They are also more likely to have hypertension, diabetes and be overweight (see 'Diabetes mellitus' and 'Obesity'). It has therefore been argued that women do less well post-operatively due to pre-operative health status. A recent study by Bute et al. (2003) found that even when adjusting for pre-existing risk factors, women were more anxious, had a diminished ability to perform daily and work-related activities and lower exercise capacity in comparison to men. However, in another study looking at the impact of pre-operative health on QoL, Rumsfeld et al. (2001) found that whilst pre-operative health status was the major predictor of QoL following surgery it was those patients with poor pre-operative health that derived most QoL benefit from surgery. Various studies have found similar cardiac outcome and quality of life following off-pump compared to on-pump CABG (e.g. Ascione et al., 2004).

(See also 'Coronary heart disease: cardiac psychology', 'Coronary heart disease: heart failure'; 'Coronary heart disease: impact', 'Coronary heart disease: rehabilitation', and 'Carotid artery stenosis and treatment').

REFERENCES

Arthur, H.M., Daniels, C., McKelvie, R., Hirsh, J. & Rush, B. (2000). Effect of preoperative intervention on preoperative and postoperative outcomes in low-risk patients awaiting elective coronary artery bypass graft surgery. A randomized, controlled trial. *Annals of Internal Medicine*, 133, 253–62.

Ascione, R., Reeves, B.C., Taylor, F.C., Harpeet, K.S. & Angelini, G.D. (2004). Beating heart against cardioplegic arrest studies (BHACAS 1 and 2): qaulity of life at mid-term follow-up in two randomised controlled trials. *European Heart Journal*, 25, 765–70.

Andrew, M.J., Baker, R.A., Bennetts, J., Kneebone, A.C. & Knight, J.L. (2001). A comparison of neuropsychologic deficits after extracardiac and intracardiac surgery. *Journal of Cardiothoracic and Vascular Anesthesia*, 15, 9–14.

Bar-Yosef, S., Mathew, J.P., Newman, M.F., Landolfo, K.P. & Grocott, H.P. (2004). Prevention of cerebral hyperthermia during cardia surgery by limiting on-bypass rewarming in combination with post-bypass body surface warming: a feasibility study. *Anesthesia & Analgesia*, 99, 641–6.

Blumenthal, J.A., Lett, H.S., Babyak, M.A. et al. (2003). Depression as a risk factor for mortality after coronary artery bypass surgery. *Lancet*, 362(9362), 604–9.

Browndyke, J.N., Moser, D.J., Cohen, R.A. et al. (2002). Acute neuropsychological functioning following cardiosurgical interventions associated with the production of intraoperative cerebral microemboli. *The Clinical Neuropsychologist*, 16, 463–71.

Bucerius, J., Gummert, J.F., Borger, M.A. et al. (2003). Stroke after cardiac surgery: a risk factor analysis of 16,184 consecutive adult patients. *Annals of Thoracic Surgery*, 75, 472–8.

Bute, B.P., Mathew, J., Blumenthal, J.A. et al. (2003). Female gender is associated with impaired qaulity of life 1 year after coronary artery bypass surgery. *Psychosomatic Medicine*, 65, 944–51.

Connerney, I., Shapiro, P.A., McLaughlin, J.S., Bagiella, E. & Sloan, R.P. (2001). Relation between depression after coronary artery bypass surgery and 12-month outcome: a prospective study. *Lancet*, **358**, 1766–71.

Coombs, D., Roberts, R. & Crist, D. (1989). Effects of social support on depression following coronary artery bypass graft surgery. *Psychology and Health*, **3**, 29–35.

Edwards, F.H., Carey, J.S., Grover, F.L., Bero, J.W. & Hartz, R.S. (1998). Impact of gender on coronary bypass operative mortality. *Annals of Thoracic Surgery*, **66**, 125–31.

Ho, P.M., Arciniegas, D.B., Grigsby, J. *et al.* (2004). Predictors of cognitive decline following coronary artery bypass graft surgery. *Annals of Thoracic Surgery*, **77**, 597–603.

Hogue, C.W. Jr., Barzilai, B., Pieper, K.S. *et al.* (2001). Sex differences in neurological outcomes and mortality after cardai surgery: a society of thoracic surgery database report. *Circulation*, **103**, 2133–7.

Murkin, J.M., Newman, S.P., Stump, D.A. & Blumenthal, J.A. (1995). Statement of consnsus on assessment of neurobehavioral outcomes after cardiac surgery. *Annals of Thoracic Surgery*, **59**, 1289–95.

Murkin, J.M., Stump, D.A., Blumenthal, J.A. & McKhann, G. (1997). Defining dysfunction: group means versus incidence analysis – a statement of consensus. *Annals of Thoracic Surgery*, **64**, 904–5.

Newman, M.F., Kirchner, J.L., Phillips-Bute, B. *et al.* (2001). Longitudinal assessment of neurocognitive function after bypass surgery. *New England Journal of Medicine*, **344**, 395–402.

Newman, S.P. & Harrison, M.J.G. (2002). Coronary-artery bypass surgery and the brain: persisting concerns. *Lancet Neurology*, **1**, 119–25.

Newman, S.P. & Stygall, J. (2000). Neuropsychological outcome following cardiac surgery. In S. Newman & M.J.G. Harrison (Eds.). *The brain and cardiac surgery: causes of neurological complications and their prevention.* Amsterdam: Harwood.

Patel, R., Turtle, M.R.J., Chambers, D.J. *et al.* (1996). Alpha-stat acid-base regulation during cardiopulmonary bypass improves neuropsychologic outcome in patients undergoing coronary artery bypass grafting. *Journal of Thoracic and Cardiovascular Surgery*, **111**, 1267–79.

Rumsfeld, J.S., Migid, D.J., O'Brien, M. *et al.* (2001). Changes in health-related quality of life following coronary artery bypass graft surgery. *Annals of Thoracic Surgery*, **72**, 2026–32.

Rymaszewska, J., Kiejna, A. & Hadry, T. (2003). Depression and anxiety in coronary artery bypass grafting patients. *European Psychiatry*, **18**, 155–60.

Selnes, O.A., Royall, R.M., Borowicz, L.M. Jr. *et al.* (2001).Cognitive changes 5 years after coronary artery bypass grafting. *Archives of Neurology*, **58**, 598–604.

Shuldham, C.M., Fleming, S. & Goodman, H. (2002). The impact of pre-operative education on recovery following coronary artery bypass surgery. A randomised controlled clinical trial. *European Heart Journal*, **23**, 666–74.

Stygall, J., Newman, S.P., Fitzgerald, G. *et al.* (2003). Cognitive change 5 years after coronary artery bypass surgery. *Health Psychology*, **22**, 579–86.

Timberlake, N., Klinger, L., Smith, P. *et al.* (1997). Incidence and paterns of depression following coronary artery bypass following coronary artery bypass graft surgery. *Journal of Psychosomatic Research*, **43**, 197–207.

Van Dijk, D., Jansen, E.W.L., Hijman, R. *et al.* (2002). Cognitive outcome after off-pump and on-pump coronary artery bypass graft surgery: a randomized trial. *Journal of the American Medical Association*, **287**, 1405–12.

Van Dijk, D., Moons, K.G.M., Keizer, A.M.A. *et al.* (2004). Association between early and three month cognitive outcome after off-pump and on-pump coronary bypass surgery. *Heart*, **90**, 431–4.

Cystic fibrosis

Claire A. Glasscoe

Royal Liverpool Children's Hospital

The disease

Cystic fibrosis (CF) is the most common fatal hereditary disease in the Western world; although not confined to those of European ancestry, CF is rare in oriental and native African people (Tsui, 1990). The recessive gene is carried by 4% of the populations in the UK and US affecting 1:2000–3000 live births (Bobadilla *et al.*, 2002). The disease is characterized by generalized dysfunction of the exocrine glands. These produce excessively viscous mucus secretions that block ducts and are prone to infection. Lung infections are the most serious complication with 90% of those affected with CF eventually succumbing to pulmonary disease. Pancreatic insufficiency is present in 85–90% of patients with malabsorption of fat and protein. Sterility occurs in 98% of males whereas female fertility is near normal. Puberty is generally delayed by two years in both sexes reflecting the reduced height and weight potential.

During 1969–90 the median age of survival doubled in the US from 14 to 28 years (FitzSimmons, 1993) and was reported to be 30 years in the UK in 1994 (Dodge *et al.*, 1997). This improved prognosis is attributable to specialist multidisciplinary CF centres, early diagnosis and breakthroughs in management. Neonatal screening for CF has been piloted and implemented in some parts of Europe and in the US and Canada and scheduled to start nationally in the UK in 2006 (see 'Screening: antenatal').

Although discovery of the CF gene defect on the seventh chromosome (Kerem *et al.*, 1989), and its malfunction, brought real hope for an eventual cure, gene therapy has proved difficult to accomplish. Treatment is mainly palliative and aimed at slowing or preventing some of the secondary effects of the disease (Hodson & Geddes, 2000). The daily regimen typically includes:

- replacement of pancreatic enzymes and nutritional supplementation
- antibiotics administered orally and/or intravenously
- chest physiotherapy and postural drainage
- nebulization of bronchodilators and mucus thinning agents.

Psychosocial impact

Patients

Findings relating to psychological effect of CF for patients are inconsistent. Some researchers find no evidence of abnormality while others report symptoms of anxiety, depression and eating disorder. Thompson *et al.* (1990) compared children aged 7–14 years, with psychiatrically referred and non-referred children. Those with CF showed no more psychological disturbance than non-referred children, although they reported equivalent levels of worry, anxiety and poor self-image to children referred to child psychiatry.

Pearson *et al.* (1991) examined differences in two age groups, 8–15 years and 16–40 years and found elevated levels of disturbance. This was manifested by anorexic type eating disorder in younger patients (16.4%) and symptoms of anxiety (22.2%) and depression (42.4%) in the older age group. The developmental trend that emerged suggests that younger children may have expressed distress through oppositional behaviour with food consumption as a control issue. Adolescents and young adults showed more preoccupation with self-image perceptions and apprehension about the future (see 'Children's perceptions of illness and death').

Parents

Parenting a child with a chronic life-shortening condition poses unique challenges at every stage. Quittner *et al.* (1992) focused on the diagnosis phase and demonstrated that when stressors were linked to CF a strong association was found between role strain and depression for mothers. The same was not the case for fathers despite both parents reporting elevated levels of depression (64% of mothers, and 43% of fathers). Fathers were less involved in childcare and acknowledged more difficulty in carrying out treatment routines; their worries revolved around the financial burden associated with the disease. In this same study partners tended to rate their relationship between the norms for married and divorced couples, suggesting some degree of marital difficulty. A subsequent study at a later disease-stage with children aged 2–6 years by the same authors showed no significant differences in psychological distress or partner satisfaction from control parents (Quittner *et al.*, 1998).

Nevertheless, role strain represented by role frustration and conflict over child rearing continued to predict partnership dissatisfaction in mothers.

Families

Interplay between family lifecycle events, developmental processes in patients and siblings, and the course of the disease can be problematic. Families endeavour to contain the intrusion that CF makes into their lives by establishing routines for tasks, compartmentalizing information, redefining normality, reassessing priorities and the future and avoiding reminders of the disease (Bluebond-Langner, 1991). In a 2-year ethnographic study Bluebond-Langner observed these strategies being employed adaptively at salient points in the overall disease process allowing families to live as normal a life as possible. Wilson *et al.* (1996) found some support for the notion that family functioning operates in a compensatory way to avert the effects of physical decline. In this study increased symptoms mobilized a coping response and factors that undermined this homeostatic mechanism were extraneous life events such as loss of friends, change of school and house moves.

Psychological functioning and health status

Although earlier studies into the psychological aspects of families with a child with CF tended to emphasize dysfunction, recent research has focused more on resilience, coping strategies and adaptation. The work of Simmons and Goldberg (2001) suggests that the physical benefits of an early diagnosis may be tempered by potential disruption of the parent–child relationship, which may occasionally undermine the infant's physical growth. Patterson *et al.* (1990) used the Family Adjustment and Adaptation Response (FAAR) model to examine the effects of family functioning on health changes. The variables of family stress, family resources and parental coping combined explained 22% of the variance in height and weight changes over a 15-month period. Although the association is undoubtedly reciprocal this finding lends credence to the view that the whole family system needs to be considered with respect to children's health.

Treatment burden and adherence

As biomedical treatments become more complicated, physicians have expressed concern about the heavy burden of treatment families affected with CF are asked to carry. The involvement of both parents and the healthcare team in achieving a reasonable balance while ensuring adherence to core treatments is critical. Chest physiotherapy is crucial in preventing the onset of pulmonary disease, which is responsible for 90–95% of CF deaths, and yet it is the least adhered to aspect of treatment; only 40% completely adhering (Stark *et al.*, 1987) (see 'Adherence to treatment'). Dietary management is also necessary to prevent physical decline. The energy requirement needed to maintain optimum height and weight is 120–200% of the recommended dietary allowance (RDA) for healthy children, yet the average reported intake for children with CF is only 80% RDA (Stark *et al.*, 1990).

Koocher *et al.* (1990) argue that patients with CF do not all fail to follow medical advice for the same reasons. Three categories are outlined: those who for a variety of reasons are misinformed about treatment requirements; those who for emotional or psychological reasons are resistant to treatment and those who have arrived at a rational decision to refuse treatment. In the first instance a psychoeducational approach might be indicated, while in the second individual, group or family therapy may be more appropriate. In the final case the patient's wishes should be respected and accommodated as far as possible.

Psychological interventions

A systematic review (Glasscoe & Quittner, 2002) revealed genetic counselling, promotion of airway clearance, dietary management and moving towards independence as main targets for intervention trials. Interventions with specific relevance for CF include:

Biofeedback

In association with physiotherapy biofeedback may assist airway clearance and improve lung function (Delk *et al.*, 1994) (see 'Biofeedback').

Behavioural and cognitive therapy

Individual behavioural contracting and a group behavioural approach with parents and children can help promote adherence to chest physiotherapy and dietary requirements (Stark *et al.*, 1987; Stark *et al.*, 1990) (see 'Behaviour therapy' and 'Cognitive behaviour therapy').

Psychoeducation

Parents of children with CF are expected to perform complex medical tasks at home and monitor changes in their child's health. Such responsibility requires sound judgement and swift decision-making. A health education programme for the self-management of CF developed by Bartholomew *et al.* (1997) addresses these issues. The StarBright CD-ROM has a similar aim to promote knowledge and coping skills in children and adolescents (Davis *et al.*, 2004).

Family therapy

A CF diagnosis reverberates throughout the family, touching each individual and their relationships. Transitions during adolescence take on additional meaning in the context of CF and can be particularly difficult for families to negotiate (DeLambo *et al.*, 2004). A biopsychosocial systems perspective facilitating communication between family members can assist in these negotiations.

Conclusions

Cystic fibrosis is a chronic life-shortening disease with wide-reaching implications for patients and families. Although characterized more by resilience and coping than dysfunction this is a vulnerable group with sub-clinical levels of psychological distress. Most studies conclude that adequate family functioning is more important for psychological adjustment than illness severity. A fully integrated response considers the relationships between physical and psychological factors and views the disease and its management within a family context.

REFERENCES

Bartholomew, L.K., Czyzewski, D., Parcel, G.S. *et al.* (1997). Self-Management of cystic fibrosis: short-term outcomes for the Cystic Fibrosis Family Education Programme. *Health Education & Behaviour*, 25, 652–66.

Bluebond-Langner, M. (1991). Living with cystic fibrosis: a family affair. In J.D. Morgan (Ed.). *Young people and death* (pp. 46–62). Philadelphia: Charles Press.

Bobadilla, J.L., Macek Jr., M., Fine, J.P. & Farrell, P.M. (2002). Cystic fibrosis: a worldwide analysis of *CFTR* mutations – correlation with incidence data and application to screening. *Human Mutation*, 19, 575–606.

Davis, M.A., Quittner, A.L., Stack, C.M. & Yang, M.C.K. (2004). Controlled evaluation of the STARBRIGHT CD-ROM program for children and adolescents with cystic fibrosis. *Journal of Pediatric Psychology*, 29, 259–67.

Delk, K.K., Gevirtz, R., Hicks, D.A., Carden, F. & Rucker, R. (1994). The effects of biofeedback assisted breathing retraining on lung functions in patients with cystic fibrosis. *Chest*, 105, 23–8.

DeLambo, K.-E., Ievers-Landis, C.E., Drotar, D. & Quittner, A.L. (2004). Association between observed family relationship quality and problem-solving skills with treatment adherence in older children and adolescents with cystic fibrosis. *Journal of Pediatric Psychology*, 29, 342–53.

Dodge, J.A., Morison, S., Lewis, P.A. *et al.* (1997). Incidence, population and survival of cystic fibrosis in the UK, 1968–95. *Archives of Disease in Childhood*, 77, 493–6.

FitzSimmons, S.C. (1993). The changing epidemiology of cystic fibrosis. *The Journal of Pediatrics*, 122, 1–9.

Glasscoe, C.A. & Quittner, A.L. (2002). Psychological interventions for cystic fibrosis (Cochrane Review). *The cochrane library*, Issue 3. Oxford: Update Software.

Hodson, M.E. & Geddes, D.M. (2000). *Cystic fibrosis*. London: Arnold.

Kerem, B., Rommens, J.M., Buchanan, J.A. *et al.* (1989). Identification of the cystic fibrosis gene: genetic analysis. *Science*, 145, 1073–80.

Koocher, G.P., McGrath, M.L. & Gudas, L.J. (1990). Typologies of nonadherence in

cystic fibrosis. *Developmental and Behavioural Pediatrics*, 11, 353–8.

Patterson, J.M., McCubbin, H.I. & Warwick, W.J. (1990). The impact of family functioning on health changes in children with cystic fibrosis. *Social Science and Medicine*, 31, 159–64.

Pearson, D.A., Pumariega, A.J. & Seilheimer, D.K. (1991). The development of psychiatric symptomatology in patients with cystic fibrosis. *Journal of the American Academy of Child and Adolescent Psychiatry*, 30, 290–7.

Quittner, A.L., DiGirolamo, A.M., Michel, M. & Eigen, H. (1992). Parental response to cystic fibrosis: A contextual analysis of the diagnosis phase. *Journal of Pediatric Psychology*, 17, 683–704.

Quittner, A.L., Esplanage, D.L., Opipari, L.C. *et al.* (1998). Role strain in couples with and without a child with a chronic illness: associations with marital satisfaction, intimacy, and daily mood. *Health Psychology*, 17, 112–24.

Simmons, R.J. & Goldberg, S. (2001). Infants and preschool children. In M. Bluebond-Langner, B. Lask & D.B. Angst

(Eds.). *Psychosocial aspects of cystic fibrosis* (pp. 10–24). London: Arnold.

Stark, L.J., Bowen, A.M., Tyc, V.L., Evans, S. & Passero, M.A. (1990). A behavioral approach to increasing calorie consumption in children with cystic fibrosis. *Journal of Pediatric Psychology*, **15**, 309–26.

Stark, L.J., Millar, S.T., Plienes, A.J. & Drabman, R.S. (1987). Behavioral contracting to increase chest physiotherapy: a study of a young cystic

fibrosis patient. *Behavior Modification*, **11**, 75–86.

Thompson, R.J., Hodges, K. & Hamlett, K.W. (1990). A matched comparison of adjustment in children with cystic fibrosis and psychiatrically referred and nonreferred children. *Journal of Pediatric Psychology*, **15**, 745–59.

Tsui, L.-C. (1990). Population analysis of the major mutation in cystic fibrosis (Editorial). *Human Genetics*, **85**, 391–2.

Wilson, J., Fosson, A., Kanga, J.F. & D'Angelo, S.L. (1996). Homeostatic interactions: a longitudinal study of biological and family variables in children with cystic fibrosis. *Journal of Family Therapy*, **18**, 123–39.

Acquired hearing loss

Laurence McKenna and David Scott

Royal National Throat, Nose and Ear Hospital

Hearing loss that is acquired after the development of language is distinct from pre-lingual hearing loss in its psychological and social manifestations. This chapter is concerned with hearing loss that occurs after the development of language.

Audiological background

Hearing loss is categorized by the site of the lesion causing the loss. A lesion of the outer ear, ear drum or middle ear causes a conductive hearing loss, due to a reduction in hearing sensitivity. A cochlear hearing loss may lead to reduced auditory discrimination as well as reduced hearing sensitivity. A lesion affecting the auditory nerve may also cause reduced sensitivity and discrimination. Finally, a category of Central Auditory Processing Disorder (CAPD) has been identified in which cochlear function may be normal, but the person has auditory perceptual problems particularly in the presence of background noise. The categories of cochlear, retro-cochlear and central auditory dysfunction are referred to as sensori-neural hearing loss (SNHL). Most adults with an acquired hearing loss have cochlear dysfunction, with the most common aetiology being age-related hearing loss. Davis (1997) reported that 13.9% of the adult population (aged 18–80) have a SNHL equal to, or worse than, 25 dB (the level of a whisper) in the better ear. This prevalence rises with age such that 42% of elderly people have such a loss. This criterion of SNHL represents the point at which an individual might benefit from a hearing aid. Unfortunately, the shortfall in provision is such that millions of people in England and Wales who would benefit from a hearing aid do not have one (Davis, 1997).

Even in the presence of one normally hearing ear, a hearing impairment in the other may cause considerable hearing handicap. Acquired profound deafness is rare, but the consequences may be devastating. Conductive hearing loss is often amenable to surgical or medical treatment. In SNHL, surgical intervention is usually not possible, and those affected can only be offered hearing aids that

will not result in normal hearing abilities. In some cases of profound hearing loss, cochlear implantation is possible. Modern digital hearing aids and cochlear implants now help some people who previously could not benefit from older hearing aid equipment devices. Patients often fail to comply, however, with a technological approach to the management of hearing impairment and there is a risk of such advances producing technology-centred rather than patient-centred therapy.

Psychological profile of people with acquired hearing loss

A popular image of people with hearing impairment is that they suffer from psychological disturbances such as depression or paranoia; however, this idea is only partly supported by the literature (Andersson, 1995). The link between hearing loss and psychological status has been investigated in a number of ways. One approach has been to examine the prevalence of psychological problems among a population of hearing impaired people. For example, McKenna et al. (1991) reported that 27% of people attending a neuro-otology clinic with a main complaint of hearing loss were suffering from significant psychological disturbance. This is considerably higher than the prevalence of psychological disturbance among the general population but is lower than the prevalence rates associated with other audiological symptoms such as tinnitus or vertigo (McKenna et al., 1991; Asmundson et al., 1998). An alternative approach has been to examine the extent of hearing loss among populations of known psychiatric patients, but it has proved difficult to draw conclusions from this research as hearing loss can lead to misclassification of psychiatric morbidity (Kreeger et al., 1995). When other health problems are taken into consideration, the correlations between hearing loss and anxiety and depression are weaker. The presence of multiple audiological symptoms increases the likelihood of significant psychological distress. The high co-morbidity between hearing loss and tinnitus is particularly relevant in this respect (see 'Tinnitus').

A different approach to the study of hearing loss was taken by Kerr and Cowie (1997). They described the subjective experiences of people with acquired hearing loss in terms of six factors derived from a factor analysis of questionnaire responses. Only one of the factors obtained referred to the communication problems that one might expect to be associated with hearing loss. The others were concerned with psychological and social issues including a factor that referred to positive consequences such as increased social support and inner philosophical resources. The finding that hearing loss might be associated with positive consequences may seem surprising but there are other sources of evidence that the effects of hearing loss are not always those that one might suppose, e.g. not all cochlear implant users report a positive psychological outcome, even when the implant provides obvious acoustic benefit.

It is clear is that the relationship between hearing loss and psychological wellbeing is a complex one. Many people do not complain about their hearing loss and some people deny that they have a hearing problem even when confronted by the audiometric evidence (Gilhome Herbst & Humphrey, 1980). Audiological measures do not, however, predict the extent of psychological disturbance (Gilhome Herbst & Humphrey, 1980; Thomas & Gilhome Herbst, 1980; Kerr & Cowie, 1997). One study (Thomas & Gilhome Herbst, 1980), however, found that there was a higher degree of psychological disturbance among those with particularly severe hearing loss and poor speech discrimination who received little benefit from hearing aids. The ambiguous findings concerning the relationship between hearing loss and psychological wellbeing may be in part due to an overly simplistic assessment of psychological status. Many studies (e.g. Thomas & Gilhome Herbst, 1980; Singerman *et al.*, 1980) have classified people as either psychiatrically disturbed or not. Such a basic dichotomy excludes many distressed people who may fall short of the dysfunctional classification. Stephens and Kerr (2000) have suggested that the World Health Organization (WHO, 2000) classification of losses or abnormalities, limitations of activities, restrictions in participation and contextual factors may be useful in understanding the relationship between hearing loss and psychological disturbance. The WHO classification is set within the context of the social model of disability and suggests that disablement occurs within and by means of social and personal contextual factors (see 'Disability').

While the notion that social factors affect levels of hearing disability is now considered self-evident (e.g. a hearing impaired person is disabled by background noise), from a clinical point of view, it is also apparent that deafened people encounter psychological obstacles through factors such as anxiety and reduced motivation. Research from the field of cochlear implants adds to this picture. McKenna and Denman (1993) assessed a group of cochlear implant users' retrospective perceptions of changes in their psychological status and found that almost all believed that their lives were close to ideal prior to the onset of hearing loss, and that their lives were radically changed by deafness. It seems implausible that so many in any group would have had near perfect lives before losing their hearing. It is likely that this idealized view of their life as a hearing person represented a cognitive shift that increased the perception of loss and this reappraisal was, in turn, a determinant of the subsequent disability behaviour. To date, little work has been done to delineate the psychological processes that might be involved in this context, although the Theory of Planned Behaviour (Azjen, 1988) may have some resonance with the clinical observations made within audiology (see 'Theory of planned behaviour'). Skinner and Vaughan (1983) viewed hearing in behavioural terms. They suggested that hearing can be viewed as an operant, i.e. it is influenced by contingencies of reinforcement (see 'Behaviour therapy'). Skinner advocated that individuals should adopt an assertive approach to hearing difficulties while acknowledging that when it is impossible to hear: 'You do best to stop trying to hear things when you are having trouble. You are probably not enjoying what is said in a television programme if you are straining to hear it' (Skinner & Vaughan, 1983, p. 44).

It has also been suggested that auditory processing problems can affect cognitive functioning which itself may be compromised by stress (Pichora-Fuller, 2003; McKenna, 1997). The identification of this type of difficulty highlights the importance of including psychological factors in any model of hearing disability and rehabilitation.

Psychological treatment approaches

Although most people with a hearing loss will receive practical support and counselling from an audiologist, few will have their psychological needs identified or met via this route. For those who do receive psychological counselling, the emphasis is likely to be on working through a grief process, which is most relevant where the onset of hearing loss was sudden. Usually, it is only when a patient exhibits enduring distress that a referral to a psychologist is made. In such cases, difficulties adjusting to hearing loss are often associated with negative beliefs about the implications of the loss. In common with patients with other physical symptoms, patients with hearing loss may attach too much weight to beliefs concerning the adverse consequences of having a hearing impairment. Cognitive–behavioural therapy is often employed to address this source of distress (see 'Cognitive behaviour therapy').

A cognitive–behavioural approach to the management of hearing loss in elderly people has been described in a series of studies by Andersson and colleagues (Andersson *et al.*, 1995, 1997). This work focused on setting individualized treatment goals, behavioural tasks and communication strategies to assist the patient to employ hearing tactics, i.e. the methods used by hearing impaired people to solve everyday hearing problems such as facing the speaker, having the light shining on the speaker's face and asking the speaker to talk slowly and clearly. They found that patients treated in this way were better able to cope with their hearing loss and concluded that disability resulting from hearing impairment could be regarded as a behavioural problem which can form the focus of rehabilitation. They suggested that cognitive, and especially motivational, factors are of central importance in understanding hearing disability.

The work on hearing tactics has been reconsidered in the light of coping research. In a review, Andersson and Willebrand (2003) suggested that some of the benefits of hearing tactics may be a product of changes in appraisal rather than the application of the tactics themselves. They concluded that although coping research has much to add to our understanding of hearing loss, the concept of coping has usually been regarded as being simply equivalent to communication strategies or distress in relation to communication failure. This is in contrast with the more complex concept of coping endorsed by health psychologists (Lazarus, 1993). In a recent study (Andersson & Hägnebo, 2003), coping strategies were assessed using more standard coping measures (i.e. the Ways of Coping Questionnaire). The results showed that the participants with hearing loss ($N = 94$) used planned problem-solving and self-controlling coping strategies, whereas escape/avoidance responses were less frequently used than the other coping strategies.

REFERENCES

Andersson, G. (1995). *Hearing as behaviour. Psychological aspects of acquired hearing impairment in the elderly.* Doctoral Dissertation. Uppsala, Sweden: Acta Universitas Upsaliensis.

Andersson, G., Green, M. & Melin, L. (1997). Behavioural hearing tactics: a controlled trial of a short treatment programme. *Behavior Research and Therapy*, **35**, 523–30.

Andersson, G. & Hägnebo, C. (2003). Hearing impairment, coping strategies, and anxiety sensitivity. *Journal of Clinical Psychology in Medical Settings*, **10**, 35–9.

Andersson, G., Melin, L., Scott, B. & Lindberg, P. (1995). An evaluation of a behavioural treatment approach to hearing impairment. *Behaviour Research and Therapy*, **33**, 283–92.

Andersson, G. & Willebrand, M. (2003). What is coping? A critical review of the construct and its application in audiology. *International Journal of Audiology*, **42**, S97–103.

Asmundson, G.J.G., Larsen, D.K. & Stein, M.B. (1998). Panic disorder and vestibular disturbance: an overview of empirical findings and clinical implications. *Journal of Psychosomatic Research*, **44**, 107–20.

Azjen, I. (1988). *Attitudes, personality and behaviour.* Milton Keynes, UK: Open University Press.

Davis, A.C. (1997). Epidemiology. In D. Stephens, (Ed.). *Adult audiology, Volume 2, Scott Brown's Otolaryngology* (6th edn.) (pp. 2/3/1–2/3/38). Oxford: Butterworth-Heinemann.

Gilhome Herbst, K. & Humphrey, C. (1980). Hearing impairment and mental state in the elderly living at home. *British Medical Journal*, **281**, 903–5.

Kerr, P. & Cowie, R. (1997). Acquired deafness: A multidimensional experience. *British Journal of Audiology*, **31**, 177–88.

Kreeger, J.L., Raulin, M.L., Grace, J. & Priest, B.L. (1995). Effect of hearing enhancement on mental status ratings in geriatric psychiatric patients. *American Journal of Psychiatry*, **152**, 629–31.

Lazarus, R.S. (1993). Coping theory and research: past, present and future. *Psychosomatic Medicine*, **55**, 234–47.

McKenna, L. (1997). Audiological disorders: psychological state and cognitive functioning. Unpublished Doctoral Dissertation. London: The City University.

McKenna, L. & Denman, C. (1993). Repertory grid technique in the assessment of cochlear implant patients. *Journal of Audiological Medicine*, **2**, 75–84.

McKenna, L., Hallam, R.S. & Hinchcliffe, R. (1991). The prevalence of psychological disturbance in neuro-otology outpatients. *Clinical Otolaryngology*, **16**, 452–56.

Pichora-Fuller, M.K. (2003). Cognitive aging and auditory information processing. *International Journal of Audiology*, **42**, 2S26–32.

Singerman, B., Reidner, E. & Folstein, M. (1980). Emotional disturbance in hearing clinic patients. *British Journal of Psychiatry*, **137**, 58–62.

Skinner, B.F. & Vaughan, M.E. (1983). *Enjoy old age. A program for self-management.* London: Hutchinson.

Stephens, D. & Kerr, P. (2000). Auditory displacements: an update. *Audiology*, **39**, 322–32.

Thomas, A. & Gilhome Herbst, K. (1980). Social and psychological implications of acquired deafness for adults of employment age. *British Journal of Audiology*, **14**, 76–85.

World Health Organization. (2000). *International classification of functioning, disability and health. Pre-final draft. Full version.* Geneva: World Health Organization.

Dementias

Jenny Rusted

University of Sussex

Worldwide, we are currently witnessing an unprecedented demographic transformation, as life expectancy increases from the present 66 years of age to 77 years of age by 2050, and the proportion of the population over 60 doubles from 10 to 21%. A result of this increase in life expectancy is that the number of persons over the age of 60 years will rise from the current 600 million to around 1.5 billion by 2050. Britain will have over 6 million people over 75 years – double the 1985 figure, but significantly the great majority of older adults will reside in the less developed regions of the world (see also 'Ageing and health behaviour'). Currently around 60% of the world's older population live in less developed countries, i.e. an estimated 279 million: by 2050 this proportion is projected to increased to 88%. This explosion in numbers of the over-70s will bring higher incidences of age-related illness and infirmity. Longevity is one of humanity's major achievements, but it brings with it the challenge to adjust our societies to this new reality by changing attitudes, introducing new political, social, health and economic measures that shift us from the current youthful pyramidal structures that are becoming obsolete in most world regions, though at a significantly faster rate in the more industrialized countries. Many less developed countries are currently experiencing a significant downturn in natural population increase (births minus deaths), similar to the decline that occurred in industrialized nations a few decades earlier. Italy is currently the world's 'oldest' major country (around 20% of its population being over 65), and indeed, except for Japan (19% of population over 65), the 20 'oldest' countries are all in Europe, ensuring that it will remain the 'oldest' world region well into the twenty-first century. While the older share of the population is expected to more than double between 200 and 2030 in Asia, Latin America and the Caribbean (from around 5% to around 12%), ageing is occurring more slowly in sub-Saharan Africa, where relatively high birth rates, and the devastating power of the HIV/AIDs pandemic are keeping the population 'young' (current estimates of around 3% projected to increase by only 1% by 2030).

While an increasing body of evidence shows that ageing is not synonymous with gross deterioration in skills and abilities, there are, however, diseases for which incidence is age-related. Arguably the most devastating of these are the dementias. From the onset of the dementia, an individual is living with constant and growing sense of confusion. Idiosyncratic patterns of emergence of symptoms, and the essentially unpredictable slope of decline associated with the disease create an immensely difficult environment for both the patient and the carer. Because of the worldwide ageing phenomenon, existing in both developed and developing countries, dementia has a growing public health relevance. Indeed, international incidence and prevalence data for the dementias indicate little geographical variation across different countries.

Defining and characterizing the dementias

Dementia (of all types) affects 10% of the over-65s and some 20% of the over-85s. Worldwide, forecasts indicate a considerable increase in the number of demented elderly from 25 million in the year 2000 to 114 million in 2050 (84 million in less developed regions).

Technically speaking, dementia is a syndrome, a group of symptoms, that may vary significantly across sufferers. A number of disorders can produce the syndrome of dementia, and it is often hard to tell them apart. Of the dementias of organic origin, the three main types of dementia are vascular or multi-infarct dementia (VD, MID), dementia of the Alzheimer's type (DAT, SDAT, AD) and mixed MI/DAT. Vascular dementias result from multiple small strokes that ultimately produce sufficient tissue loss to produce cognitive and behavioural effects, often presenting as an uneven distribution of cognitive deficits, reflecting focal brain damage, and a stepwise deterioration of function, reflecting the temporal sequence of the brain infarcts. Less common dementias include Lewy body dementia (characterized by fluctuating and confused intellect; animated behaviour and intense visual hallucinations); Picks disease/frontotemporal dementias (characterized by early emergence of behavioural symptoms, slow loss of language/vocabulary and preserved

spatial orientation; disinhibition). Chronic conditions such as CJD and variant CJD, Parkinson's disease, HIV, Huntington's Chorea and Korsakoff's disease may induce a dementia in the later stages.

Over half of all dementias are of the Alzheimer type (DAT), characterized by insidious progressive and irreversible decline in cognitive function. Clinical diagnosis depends on a history of progressive cognitive impairments and personality change (once all other potential causes of problems are excluded), with memory impairment a central feature, and aphasia, apraxia, agnosia and disturbance of executive function all possible (see also 'Aphasia'). The patient is also likely to demonstrate significant decline in social and occupational functioning (Diagnostic and Statistical Manual of Mental Disorders, version IV, (2000)). A progression through five phases can be expected:

- Phase I (incipient dementia) is associated with repeated objective evidence of memory failures; decreased performance in demanding work or social settings; and moderate anxiety.
- Phase II (mild dementia) is associated primarily with memory deficits and mood disturbances; an inability to perform complex tasks previously achieved, a conscious withdrawal from challenging situations, and denial.
- Phase III (moderate dementia) brings a marked increase in language aphasias; difficulties recalling major events and memories; poor short-term recall, and repeated 'checking' behaviours; and the need for some assistance with what had previously been 'routine' tasks.
- Phase III (severe) involves pronounced language and motor disturbances, hallucinations and disturbed sleep patterns; a patient will have little memory for events/activities completed thirty minutes previous, will have gross failures of long established memories, and will require assistance with toileting, dressing and other routine activities of daily living.
- Phase IV (final stage) is associated with loss of all verbal abilities and memory for life events, though some recognition of key people can still be evidenced. Physically, the patient requires 24-hour care, exhibits uncontrollable behavioural disturbances, decreased arousal and loss of control of bodily functions.

Alzheimer-type dementia is familial in around 25–40% of cases, but is most likely to reflect complex interactive effects of genetic risk and environmental factors that increase diagnostic and prognostic heterogeneity. Indeed, only around 45% of MZ twins are concordant for DAT, and those that are show different patterns of expression, age of onset, severity and rate of decline (e.g. Welsh, 1993). The two biggest risk factors for DAT, in order, are age and a family history of Downs' syndrome or DAT. Identified genetic links include chromosome abnormalities at chr21, an ApoE connection via chr19, and a presenilin link via chr14 and chr1 (see Hardy, 2003).

Discriminating dementia from geriatric depression

An additional difficulty in the diagnosis of dementias is that of distinguishing early stages of dementia from geriatric depression. In the UK, for example, around 8% of patients admitted for dementia are in fact suffering from depression; geriatric depression is often referred to, indeed, as pseudodementia (see also 'Psychological care of the elderly'). Depressed individuals often complain of poor memory, poor concentration and poor short term memory, although there is usually little correlation between complaint and objective measures of memory performance. A more clinical assessment will in fact differentiate dementia from pseudodementia on an array of measures, including the more rapid onset of cognitive deficits in depressed elderly, the type and time course of mood disturbances, sleep/appetite disturbance, the specific pattern of short-term memory deficits and motivational indices on memory tasks (depressed elderly present with motivational deficits rather than actual decline in competence, but perception of difficulties results in frequent complaints of memory problems from depressed elderly).

There is some evidence for the co-existence of the two syndromes, but co-occurrence is neither necessary nor inevitable. Certainly it is unsurprising that early signs of dementia may lead an individual to feel depressed, but it remains unclear whether this response is a primary effect of the disease (associated with the fronto-temporal pathology, the brain structures responsible for mood), or a secondary reaction to awareness of an emerging condition. It is possible that a substantial number of individuals presenting with depression are in early stages of dementia, but there remains little consensus on the prognostic indicators that might distinguish between the progressors and the non-progressors (see Lee & Lyketsos, 2003).

Diagnosing a dementia

The presence of cognitive dysfunction reflecting a dementia can be assessed by administration of any of a number of very basic cognitive tests designed to provide a measure of current cognitive status. One of the most widely used cognitive assessment is the Mini Mental State Examination (Folstein *et al.*, 1975). This is a 30-item brief assessment of the client's orientation in time, place, short term memory registration, attention, working memory, language and hand dexterity. Despite its brevity, it is a robust and well established tool, picking up early stages of cognitive impairment quite accurately. The test does not claim to differentiate different forms of dementia, however, nor to discriminate between dementia and geriatric depression.

Improved accuracy of clinical diagnosis is most easily achieved by looking at the progressive nature of the impairment. Test–retest changes differentiate DAT from normal ageing, with a steeper slope of decline reflecting pathological over normal ageing. Longitudinal evaluation, however, presents no prospect for early intervention. Moreover, the dementias are characterized by large and idiosyncratic differences in rates of decline. With early diagnosis important both for treatment and resource management, factors that might predict rate of decline have generated particular interest, although again with very little consensus. Baseline cognitive status (educational level, opportunity for intellectual stimulation), gender, previous depression and lifestyle factors (associated with elevated blood pressure and high cholesterol, for example) have all been mooted as significant factors in prevalence and progression of dementia.

Difficulties associated with validation of clinical assessments of memory dysfunction lend further impetus to development of neurobiological measures for validating clinical results. In vivo CT scans and PET scans have established that the dementias are associated with reduced brain weight, cortical atrophy and ventricular enlargement. Measurement of cerebral blood flow and metabolism also indicate significant deficits in individuals with dementia. Other neuropathological markers such as CSF levels of amyloid or tau proteins are possible, but for all of these measures, the absence of clear boundaries between 'normal' and 'abnormal' brain measures remains a significant problem in dementia diagnosis (e.g. Blennow & Vanmechelan, 2003).

Clinical diagnosis alone is correct in about 75% of cases; if supplemented with neuroimaging of the medial temporal lobe or hippocampal regions, premorbid accuracy increases to around 90% of cases. The costs and limited availability of imaging facilities, however, have mitigated against their routine use in dementia diagnosis, at least in the over 65s, though newer 'reporter' molecules and development of technologies (e.g. SPECT) that provide 3D images of cerebral blood flow will reduce costs ain increase availability to psychogeriatricians (see 'Brain imaging and function').

Definitive diagnosis of a dementia depends upon examination of the brain pathology (neuropathological markers) and can only be confirmed at autopsy. Markers include significant atrophy of the brain, most importantly in the regions of the temporal lobe and frontal cortex, and specific neuropathological changes (for DAT, neurofibrillary tangles and senile plaques) (detailed in a seminal paper by Braak & Braak, 1995). In addition to neuropathological changes, there is a reduction in function in most brain neurotransmitters, and most significantly in the cholinergic system. Although neurotransmitter changes are probably secondary to the neuropathological changes in the cortex, reduced cortical choline acetyltransferease activity (the enzymatic marker for cholinergic system activity) provides a reliable correlate of clinical severity of the dementia (consistent with its vital role in memory encoding and retrieval).

Treatment

Recognising the documented role of the cholinergic system in learning and memory, therapeutic research in the past two decades has been aimed at treatments to correct the chronic deficiency in cholinergic activity, and thus to ameliorate the primary symptom, namely memory failure. All currently licensed cholinomimetics are cholinesterase inhibitors (ChEIs). Numerous studies document maintenance of baseline performance by ChEI treatment, particularly if the treatment programme is established early in the course of the dementia. This improvement may be maintained over a number of years (e.g. Rogers *et al.*, 2000). Vitamin E and the anti-oxidant drugs may also be of use for people who cannot tolerate cholinesterase inhibitors. Additional families of drugs that are currently under research include anti-inflammatory drugs, oestrogens, NMDA antagonists and anti-amyloid vaccines.

Supplementing the drug treatment, recent years have seen an increase in the development of cognitive rehabilitation programmes for people with dementia. These have focused on the value of memory training, cognitive orientation and on multimodal supplementation of verbal memory skills (see reviews by Rusted & Clare, 2004; Clare & Woods, 2004; Grandmaison & Simard, 2003).

In general, the evidence suggests that cognitive rehabilitation techniques produce short-term benefits for mildly impaired volunteers, over and above those that might be seen from general programmes of mental stimulation, but that they are time-consuming in their implementation, and may not generalize beyond those situations explicitly trained (see 'Neuropsychological rehabilitation').

Recognizing dementia

Dementia often only becomes apparent to the primary care physician when revealed in crisis situations such as the absence of the usual carer, or the onset of another medical problem (infection, or a household accident resulting in a hospital admission). Although symptoms may have been present for some time, loss of daily skills, forgetfulness or even confusion, are expected as part of normal ageing, and do not in the majority of elderly, constitute reasons for visiting their primary care physician. The lateness of identification, and therefore intervention, of an emerging dementia exacerbates problems of care management and treatment.

Iliffe (1997) suggested guidelines for good practice in dementia diagnosis that include provision of earlier diagnosis of dementia and anticipation of crises, improved diagnostic skills among primary workers, networks of responsive social, voluntary and medical agencies providing continuing care, improved symptomatic treatment and better family support. Unfortunately for the majority of families currently looking after a relative with dementia, the availability of such a well-rounded management programme is a long way off.

REFERENCES

Clare, L. & Woods, R.T. (2004). Cognitive training and cognitive rehabilitation for people with early-stage Alzheimer's disease: a review. *Neuropsychological Rehabilitation*, **14**, 385–401.

Blennow, K. & Vanmechelen, E. (2003). CSF markers for pathogenic processes in Alzheimer's disease: diagnostic implications and use in clinical neurochemistry. *Brain Research Bulletin*, **61**, 235–42.

Braak, H. & Braak, E. (1995). Staging of Alzheimer's disease-related neurofibrillary changes. *Neurobiology of Aging*, **16**, 271–8.

Diagnostic and Statistical Manual of Mental Disorders, version IV (2000).

Illife, S. (1997). Can delays in recognition of dementia in primary care be avoided? *Aging & Mental Health*, **1**, 7–10.

Lee, H.B. & Lyketsos, C.G. (2003). Depression in Alzheimer's disease: heterogeneity and related issues. *Biological Psychiatry*, **54**, 353–62.

Folstein, M.E., Folstein, S.E. & McHugh, P.R. (1975). Mini-mental state: a practical method for grading the cognitive state of patient by clinician. *Journal of Experimental Psychology*, **100**, 221–7.

Grandmaison, E. & Simard, M. (2003). A critical review of memory stimulation programs in Alzheimer's disease. *Journal of Neuropsychiatry and Clinical Neurosciences*, **15**, 130–44.

Hardy, J. (2003). The genetics of Alzheimer's disease. In Iqbal & Winblad (Eds.). *Alzheimer's disease and related disorders: research advances*. Bucharest: Ana Aslan.

Rogers, S.L., Doody, R.S., Pratt, R.D. & Ieni, J.R. (2000). Long-term efficacy and safety of donepezil in the treatment of Alzheimer's disease: final analysis of a US multicentre open-label study. *European Neuropsychopharmacology*, **10**, 195–203.

Rusted, J.M. & Clare, L. (2004). Cognitive approaches to the management of dementia. In Morris & Becker (Eds.). *The Cognitive Neuropsychology of Alzheimer-Type Dementia* (2nd edn.).

Diabetes mellitus

Alison Woodcock and Clare Bradley

Royal Holloway, University of London

Introduction

Diabetes mellitus is a chronic disorder, characterized by raised glucose levels in blood (hyperglycaemia) and urine (glycosuria). The cause may be inherited and/or acquired deficiency of insulin production by the pancreas, or insulin resistance, where the insulin produced is ineffective. Increased blood glucose concentrations can cause structural damage, particularly to blood vessels and nerves. Microvascular complications of diabetes (diabetic retinopathy, nephropathy and neuropathy) bring problems of blindness, kidney failure, foot ulcers, gangrene and erectile impotence. However, heart disease accounts for around 50% of deaths of people with diabetes. Management involves striving to maintain blood glucose at near-normal levels through behaviour change and medication, prevention or early detection and treatment of microvascular complications and reduction of cardiovascular risk, including hypertension, lipids and weight.

There are three main forms of diabetes. Type 1 diabetes usually develops in childhood or early adulthood. The pancreas stops producing insulin, so insulin by injection or infusion pump is essential for survival. Inhaled insulin is under evaluation. Type 2 diabetes typically begins in late adulthood, though maturity onset diabetes of the young (MODY) is increasing in children. Often, though not always, associated with high body mass index, insulin production and/or the body's response to insulin declines. Management initially involves diet and exercise, perhaps with tablets to increase insulin production or uptake. In time, insulin may be required. The third form, gestational diabetes, is not considered in detail here. Diabetes prevalence is increasing rapidly worldwide, with notable ethnic differences. For example, South Asians are particularly prone to Type 2 diabetes.

The landmark Diabetes Control and Complications Trial (DCCT) (1993) compared usual care of Type 1 diabetes with intensified management to tighten control. It provided clear evidence that chronic hyperglycaemia increases risk of microvascular complications. However, tight control increased episodes of severe hypoglycaemia (very low blood glucose levels). The influential United Kingdom Prospective Diabetes Study (UKPDS) (1998) demonstrated similar relationships between hyperglycaemia and microvascular complications in Type 2 diabetes. Additionally, intensified blood pressure management reduced macrovascular complications.

Because stabilizing blood glucose is a primary clinical goal of diabetes management, accurate measures are needed. At home, finger-prick samples and reagent strips can be used, with or without metres. The most commonly-used laboratory measure, haemoglobin A1c (HbA1c), measures average blood glucose over the previous 2–3 months. The normal range for HbA1c varies between assays but increasingly, laboratories provide 'DCCT-aligned' results. In the DCCT, normal HbA1c was below 6.05%, but in diabetes, HbA1c should probably not fall below 6; UK clinical guidelines for diabetes recommend keeping HbA1c between 6.5 and 7.5%, depending on cardiovascular risk (NICE, 2003). Although HbA1c is useful when making treatment decisions, the average may conceal episodes of hypoglycaemia. Hypoglycaemic symptoms are idiosyncratic and may include hunger, sweating, irritability, disorientation, concentration lapses or hallucinations. Mild symptoms can be resolved with quickly-absorbed carbohydrate (e.g. fruit juice or glucose tablet). More severe but conscious cases need help to administer oral carbohydrate. Hypoglycaemic coma may require a glucagon injection, to release glucose from the liver. At the other extreme, hyperglycaemia associated with lack of insulin in Type 1 diabetes can cause diabetic ketoacidosis and, if untreated, life-threatening coma.

The role of psychology

Diabetes management mostly occurs outside the medical setting and the daily life of someone with diabetes can involve many restrictions, as well as recommended activities including medication-taking and blood glucose monitoring. The knowledge, beliefs and behaviour of people with diabetes and their healthcare professionals may all affect diabetes control (see, for example, 'Lay beliefs about health and illness'). Psychological perspectives can therefore be valuable in enhancing self-care. Several important interventions have been devised and evaluated by multi-disciplinary teams that include psychologists (Norris *et al.*, 2001; Ismail *et al.*, 2004). Moreover, measurement of patient-reported psychological outcomes is becoming the norm in clinical trials of pharmacological interventions, including new insulin analogues. We will outline a few of the many ways in

which psychologists familiar with diabetes and its management have already made valuable contributions towards enhancing care of people with diabetes (for more, see Anderson & Rubin, 2002; Anderson & Wolpert, 2004; Bradley *et al.*, 1998; Glasgow *et al.*, 1999; Riazi & Bradley, 2000). Our brief overview of the role of psychology begins with measurement.

Measurement of psychological outcomes and processes

When only metabolic outcomes are measured, clinicians and pharmaceutical developers may value new treatments only if metabolic control improves. They may underestimate treatment benefits. This happened when an innovative diabetes education and training programme developed by Muhlhauser, Berger and colleagues in Germany was shown to improve glycaemic control. Psychological outcomes were not measured initially, but were later shown to improve markedly alongside glycaemic control when the programme was evaluated in the UK (DAFNE Study Group, 2002). It is important to aim for the best achievable profile of biomedical and psychological outcomes.

Questionnaires measuring psychological outcomes, developed with and for people with diabetes (e.g. Bradley, 1994; Bradley & Speight, 2002; Polonsky, 2000; Pouwer *et al.*, 2000) consider issues important and relevant to people with diabetes. In contrast, commonly used generic measures typically focus on health and illness, rather than the impact of diabetes, with the demands and restrictions of long-term self-care (Bradley, 2001). Measures of perceived health cannot be expected to detect diabetes-related quality of life impairments in someone without symptoms, who feels well (see also 'Quality of life assessment').

Where problems are identified in one or more biomedical or psychological outcome, measures of psychological processes such as diabetes-related knowledge, self-care skills and behaviour, locus of control and coping strategies can indicate what action might be appropriate. Thus, someone with poor glycaemic control, despite good diabetes-related knowledge, is unlikely to benefit from further information-giving. Patient-completed questionnaires can illuminate reasons for glycaemic control problems, preferences for different treatment regimens and for therapies such as relaxation training (Bradley, 1994).

Facilitating diabetes consultations

Psychologists can be most effective when sharing with healthcare professionals consultation skills such as negotiated target-setting, open questioning and listening to patients' perspectives and priorities. Although some cultures may still believe 'doctor knows best', the prevailing twenty-first century Western philosophy involves 'empowering' patients to manage their own diabetes (Glasgow & Anderson, 1999; Department of Health, 2003). Training health professionals in 'empowerment' and 'patient-centred consulting' can have significant patient benefits. In Sweden, Rosenqvist's team has developed patient-centred methods of working with patients and training interventions that encourage professionals to change how they work. For example, Holmström et al. (2004) have demonstrated that professionals can shift from a prescriptive, information-giving model to a reflective, supportive model or combined model of consulting (see also 'Patient-centred healthcare').

There has been limited success with brief interventions promoting patient participation in diabetes consultations. Kidd and colleagues (2004), aimed to encourage patient question-asking through brief interventions such as written encouragement to ask questions. Although intervention-group patients reported greater self-efficacy in asking questions, they asked no more questions than did controls. Although more satisfied, their glycaemic control was no different. It seems that some brief interventions may change beliefs without improving clinical outcomes, so there is still potential to develop feasible yet effective interventions. Unfortunately, wellbeing and quality of life have not always been included as outcomes in such studies.

By combining a short training intervention for primary care doctors and nurses with a booklet encouraging patients newly-diagnosed with Type 2 diabetes to prepare questions, Kinmonth and colleagues (1998) significantly improved wellbeing, treatment satisfaction and satisfaction with the doctor's consulting a year later, compared with controls. Although HbA1c did not differ, body mass index was higher in intervention patients. This illustrates the need to attend to the patient's concerns without losing sight of the medical agenda. Partnerships between psychologists and clinicians will be important in further developing feasible programmes to improve both psychological and biomedical outcomes.

Optimizing blood glucose monitoring

Most insulin-treated and some tablet-treated patients monitor their own blood glucose. If glycaemic control improves, and microvascular complications and hospital treatments are reduced, these benefits may far outweigh the costs of metres and reagent strips and the pain and inconvenience of self-testing. However, self-monitoring is not always performed optimally (see also 'Self-management'). Amongst children and adolescents, parental involvement predicts adherence to home monitoring and diabetes-related family conflict is related to poorer glycaemic control. Good practice needs to be established soon after diagnosis, through building positive family interaction and involvement in diabetes management (Anderson et al., 2002).

Glucose monitoring is cost-effective only when patients understand their readings and respond appropriately at the time, rather than seeking the doctor's verdict on a book of results, months later. Many patients with Type 2 diabetes who self-monitor do not even know their blood glucose targets. Problems may be overlooked when patients monitor at set times of day. If they learn to recognize how they feel when their blood glucose levels are outside the normal range and how their own body responds to medication, exercise, food, illness and stress, they can then test their blood at times likely to detect problems. Cox and colleagues developed a blood glucose awareness training (BGAT) programme and manual, subsequently refined as BGAT-2. Blood glucose monitoring is used, alongside symptom ratings, mood and environmental cues, to identify each patient's predictors of high and low blood glucose. An 'error grid' highlights error judgments that matter clinically, such as failure to detect extreme blood glucose levels. Efforts are then concentrated on reducing clinically important errors and learning when to take appropriate action, such as deciding not to drive. Impressive results have been demonstrated in several studies of people with Type 1 diabetes. The training improved not only estimation accuracy but also glycaemic control and occurrence of car accidents. BGAT-2 has been found to have multiple long-term benefits, over and above detection of hypoglycaemia and hyperglycaemia, including reduced fear of hypoglycaemia and improved diabetes knowledge a year later (Cox et al., 2001).

Psychological treatments of sexual dysfuction

Nowadays, erectile dysfunction (ED) is often treated as an organic, vasculogenic disease, with increasing focus on pharmacological treatments. Opinions vary on the importance of psychogenic causes (e.g. relationship issues, inadequate stimulation and performance anxiety) and the need to consider psychological as well as biomedical issues in treatment. Despite the 'blockbuster' status of sildenafil citrate oral medication for men with ED (Salonia et al., 2003), men with diabetes appear to respond less well long-term to a range of ED treatments than do those without (Penson et al., 2003). Diabetes is associated with sexual dysfunction for women too. Amongst men, ED is related to demographic and clinical factors (age, body mass index, diabetes duration and complications), but for women, psychological and social factors (depression and poor partner relationships) predict sexual dysfunction (Enzlin et al., 2003). To achieve more enduring treatment benefits, Heiman (2002) recommended combining pharmacological and psychological therapies for both men and women. Psychologists thus have an essential role in redressing the current imbalance in treatment perspectives (see also 'Sexual dysfunction').

Weight management programmes

In the 1980s and 90s, Wing and colleagues conducted studies evaluating various weight management programmes for people with Type 2 diabetes, where excess weight can obstruct diabetes control (see Wing's chapter in Anderson & Rubin, 2002). Programmes included combinations of nutrition education, behaviour modification, very low calorie diets and exercise, and resulted in some dramatic weight losses, with results improving as the programmes were developed and refined. The main problem is weight loss maintenance, suggesting a need for continuing support and encouragement. Clark (2004) reviewed obesity management in diabetes, highlighting the failure of any behavioural, dietetic or pharmacological treatment to achieve long-term weight loss. She questions the wisdom of encouraging eating restraint, with its many negative consequences, including self-blame, and suggests that encouraging weight *maintenance* rather than weight loss may be better for some individuals. A Cochrane review (Moore et al., 2004) considered 18 trials in which the main intervention was dietary advice and concluded that it was the adoption of regular exercise that appeared to improve glycaemic control.

Conclusion

Psychological perspectives are already evident in many innovative approaches to diabetes care in hospital and community settings, in policy documents such as the UK National Service Framework for Diabetes (Department of Health, 2003) and in clinical trial reports, demonstrating how psychologists can work with healthcare professionals to improve the lives of people with diabetes.

REFERENCES

Anderson, B.J. & Rubin, R.R. (Eds.). (2002). *Practical Psychology for Diabetes Clinicians* (2nd edn.). U.S.A.: American Diabetes Association.

Anderson, B.J. & Wolpert, H.A. (2004). A developmental perspective on the challenges of diabetes education and care during the young adult period. *Patient Education Counsel*, 53, 347–52.

Anderson, B.J., Vangsness, L., Connell, A. *et al.* (2002). Family conflict, adherence and glycaemic control in youth with short duration Type 1 diabetes. *Diabetic Medicine*, 19, 635–52.

Bradley, C. (Ed.). (1994). *Handbook of psychology and diabetes: a guide to psychological measurement in diabetes research and practice.* Chur Switzerland: Harwood Academic.

Bradley, C. (2001). Importance of differentiating health status from quality of life. *The Lancet*, 357, 7–8.

Bradley, C., Pierce, M.B., Hendrieckx, C., Riazi, A. & Barendse, S. (1998). Diabetes mellitus. In M. Johnston and D.W. Johnston (Eds.). *Health psychology* (pp. 277–304). (*Vol. 8* in A.S. Bellack and M. Hersen (Eds.). *Comprehensive clinical psychology.*) Oxford: Elsevier Science.

Bradley, C. & Speight, J. (2002). Patient perceptions of diabetes and diabetes therapy: assessing quality of life. *Diabetes Metabolism Research Reviews*, 18, S64–9.

Clarke, M. (2004). Is weight loss a realistic goal of treatment in type 2 diabetes? *Patient Education Counsel*, 53, 277–83.

Cox, D.J., Gonder-Frederick, L., Polonsky, W. *et al.* (2001). Blood glucose awareness training (BGAT-2): long-term benefits. *Diabetes Care*, 24, 637–42.

DAFNE study group. (2002). Training in flexible, intensive insulin management to enable dietary freedom in people with type 1 diabetes: the dose adjustment for normal eating (DAFNE) randomised controlled trial. *British Medical Journal*, 325, 746–9.

Department of Health. (2003). *National Service framework for diabetes.* London: Department of Health.

Diabetes Control and Complications Trial Research Group. (1993). The effect of intensive treatment of diabetes on the development and progression of long-term complications in insulin-dependent diabetes mellitus. *The New England Journal of Medicine*, 329, 977–86.

Enzlin, P., Mathiue, C., Van Den Bruel, A., Vanderschueren, D. & Demyttenaere, K. (2003). Prevalence and predictors of sexual dysfunction in patients with type 1 diabetes. *Diabetes Care*, 26, 409–14.

Glasgow, R.E. & Anderson, R.M. (1999). In diabetes care, moving from compliance to adherence is not enough: something else entirely different is needed. *Diabetes Care*, 22, 2090–2.

Glasgow, R.E., Fisher, E.B., Anderson, B.J. *et al.* (1999). Behavioural science in diabetes; contributions and opportunities. *Diabetes Care*, 22, 832–43.

Heiman, J.R. (2002). Sexual dysfunction: overview of prevalence, etiological factors, and treatments. *Journal of Sex Research*, 39, 73–8.

Holmström, I., Larsson, J., Lindberg, E. & Rosenqvist, U. (2004). Improving the diabetes-patient's encounter by reflective tutoring for staff. *Patient Education Counsel*, 53, 325–32.

Ismail, K., Winkley, K. & Rabe-Hesketh, S. (2004). Systematic review and meta-analysis of randomised controlled trials of psychological interventions to improve glycaemic control in patients with type 2 diabetes. *The Lancet*, 363(9421), 1569–70.

Kidd, J., Marteau, T.M., Robinson, S., Ukoumunne, O.C. & Tydeman, C. (2004). Promoting patients participation in consultations; a randomised controlled trial to evaluate the effectiveness of three patient-focused interventions. *Patient Education Counsel*, 52, 107–12.

Kinmonth, A.-L., Woodcock, A., Griffin, S., Spiegal, N. & Campbell, M.J. (1998). Randomised controlled trial of patient centred care of diabetes in general practice: impact on current well-being and future disease risk. *British Medical Journal*, 317, 1202–8.

Moore, H., Summerbell, C., Hooper, L. *et al.* (2004). Dietary advice for treatment of type 2 diabetes mellitus in adults. *Cochrane Database System Reviews.* (3): CD004097.

NICE (National Institute for Clinical Excellence). (2003). Management of Type 2 diabetes: management of blood glucose. London: National Institute for Clinical Excellence.

Norris, S.L., Engelau, M.M. & Venkat Narayan, K.M. (2001). Effectiveness of self-management training in type 2 diabetes: a systematic review of randomised controlled trials. *Diabetes Care*, 24, 561–87.

Penson, D.F., Latini, D.M., Lubeck, D.P. *et al.* (2003). Do impotent men with diabetes have more severe erectile dysfunction and worse quality of life than the general population of impotent patients? Results from the Exploratory Comprehensive evaluation of Erectile Dysfunction (ExCEED) database. *Diabetes Care*, 26, 1093–9.

Polonsky, W.H. (2000). Understanding and assessing diabetes-specific quality of life. *Diabetes Spectrum*, 13, 17–22.

Pouwer, F., Snoek, F.J., van der Ploeg, H.M., Adèr, H.J. & Heine, R.J. (2000). The Well-Being Questionnaire: evidence for a three-factor structure with 12 items (W-BQ12). *Psychological Medicine*, 30, 455–62.

Riazi, A. & Bradley, C. (2000). Diabetes, Type 1. In G. Fink (Ed.). *Encyclopedia of stress* (pp. 688–93). San Diego: Academic Press.

Salonia, A., Rigatti, P. & Montorsi, F. (2003). Sildenafil in erectile dysfunction: a critical review. *Current Medical Research and Opinion*, 19, 241–62.

UK Prospective Diabetes Study Group. (1998). Intensive blood-glucose control with sulphonylureas or insulin compared with conventional treatment and risk of complications in patients with type 2 diabetes (UKPDS 33). *The Lancet*, 352, 837–53.

Domestic violence, intimate partner violence and wife battering

Irene H. Frieze[1] and Maureen C. McHugh[2]

[1]University of Pittsburgh
[2]Indiana University of Pennsylvania

Partner violence occurs in all types of intimate relationships including marriages, cohabiting and dating. Estimates are that one-quarter to one-third of US marriages involve at least one incident of physical assault. Annually domestic violence will result in serious injury to more than 3.4 million US women. Dating violence is as extensive as marital violence, and violence is at similar levels in gay and lesbian relationships (McHugh et al., 1993).

Until recently, it was generally assumed that women were the only victims of battering, and many people referred to marital or domestic violence as 'wife battering'. Research has shown that, although women are more often injured by their partners, men can also be victims of violence from male partners and from their wives (Archer, 2000; Frieze, 2000). Because of this, researchers are beginning to use the term 'intimate partner violence' as a more neutral description (see Frieze, 2005). In the majority of cases of intimate partner violence, both partners use some level of violent behaviour toward the other. There are, however, different types of violent relationships, with some involving severe violence that is one-sided or mutual, and others involving only minor violence, either one-sided or mutual (Frieze, 2005; Williams & Frieze, 2005; McHugh & Bartoszek, 2000).

Intimate partner violence ranges from quite mild, involving actions such as slapping or shoving, with no resulting injury, to battering that can result in serious injury. Injuries typically involve bruises, lacerations and/or broken bones to the head, chest, abdomen and/or extremities and in some cases may extend to stab and/or bullet wounds. Certain types of partner violence can escalate in frequency and severity over time. In some cases a spouse/partner may be murdered. In other cases, partners may engage in low levels of violence over long periods of time and this does not become serious or create many injuries, except unintentionally. The timing of violence is not random, with more incidences at weekends, in the evenings and in the warm summer months. Over 60% of battered women report beatings during pregnancy.

Intimate partner violence is believed to be an under-reported crime, although women report the incidents to friends, family, police, lawyers, physicians, ministers, counsellors and social service agencies, such as shelters. In particular low-level violence is rarely reported to any authorities. Even when it is reported to formal authorities, there may be no effective way of reducing partner violence (Gondolf & Fisher, 1988). This is especially true for battered men and lesbians, who have few sources they can turn to for help, and whose concerns are rarely addressed.

Physicians are instructed to ask the woman about the origin of her injuries, document the injuries on her chart; determine the woman's safety; alert her to the danger of returning to the abuser; and make referrals to shelters or other agencies and programmes (Kurtz, 1987). Despite having such instructions, healthcare personnel do not identify a large proportion of battered women (Kurtz, 1987). There are many potential clues to the occurrence of battering. These include evidence of old injuries and injuries inconsistent with the 'story' given are clues to identification of battering. The battered woman may be depressed and/or suicidal, abuse alcohol and/or drugs and report psychosomatic complaints. Although less understood, it is now believed that battered men are even less likely to be identified than female victims of partner violence.

Although 65% of battered women have received psychiatric care, most of their therapists failed to inquire about violence. Advocates have called for a proactive approach by therapists to assess for violence, even when it is not the presenting complaint. Battered women frequently present with problems of anxiety, depression and somatic complaints. Intake interviews and schedules should include questions about interpersonal violence. Corroborating evidence, when available, suggests that battered women tend to under-report both the frequency and the severity of the violence they experience. Forgetting and minimizing are two coping strategies used by battered women (McHugh et al., 1993).

Research (Hansen & Harway, 1993) indicates that therapists often fail to identify the importance of reported physical violence and fail to generate appropriate interventions. Cessation of the violence should be the treatment goal. To date, most intervention strategies have focused on the victim. However, this perspective is increasingly seen as both victim-blaming and counter-productive (McHugh, 1993; Yllo & Bograd, 1988). Previously, much of the literature and treatment was based on the model proposed by Walker (1984) that battered women suffer from learned helplessness, a series of behavioural, cognitive and motivational deficits resulting from the randomness and aversiveness of the beatings. Newer approaches emphasize the help-seeking and coping mechanisms of battered women, viewing them as survivors rather than victims (e.g. Frieze, 2005; Gondolf & Fisher, 1988).

Psychotherapy for battered women typically addresses the following themes: isolation; self-esteem; expression of anger; life choices and decision-making; grief and loss; and termination issues. Alternatively, Hansen and Harway (1993) recommend that appropriate treatment for the battered woman include the following: an assessment including questions regarding the lethality of the situation and the client's safety; crisis intervention and provision of immediate protection to the victim; education including information about battering; and referrals (e.g. to shelters and to legal resources).

Research indicates that women remain at risk for violence and homicide even after terminating the abusive relationships and physically relocating. Also, men who batter in one relationship are likely to batter in subsequent relationships. There is also some evidence that some women are also violent toward more than one partner. Thus, it is imperative to intervene legally or therapeutically with the batterer.

Treatments for male batterers have been developed. These stress the need to challenge the abuser's rationalizations and excuses. Interventions with batterers frequently take the form of batterers' groups. Typically, batterer groups offer a combination of skills training and resocialization: group sessions address definitions of abuse; anger management; assertiveness training; challenging negative sex role stereotypes; communication skills and conflict resolution strategies. Research indicates that from one-half to three-quarters of men who complete such treatments are labelled non-violent at follow-up (McHugh & Bartoszek, 2000). When batterers are in treatment, their partners may be imperilled while falsely believing that the abuser is cured. It should be made clear to batterers and their partners that the risk of violence still exists. Therapists need to provide resources for safety and support of the partner, and monitor the situation for re-occurrence of violence. Indications of potentially lethal violence include serious depression, drug and alcohol use, threats and available firearms: these indications warrant warnings (to the spouse) and intervention (Hansen & Harway, 1993).

(See also 'Child abuse and neglect'.)

REFERENCES

Archer, J. (2000). Sex differences in aggression between heterosexual partners: a meta-analytic review. *Psychological Bulletin*, **126**, 651–80.

Frieze, I.H. (2000). Violence in close relationships – development of a research area: comment on Archer (2000). *Psychological Bulletin*, **126**, 681–4.

Frieze, I.H. (2005). *Hurting the one you love: violence in relationships*. Belmont, CA: Thompson/Wadsworth.

Gondolf, E. & Fisher, E. (1988). *Battered women as survivors: an alternative to treating learned helplessness*. Lexington, MA: Lexington Books.

Hansen, M. & Harway, M. (Eds.). (1993). *Battering and family therapy: a feminist perspective*. Newbury Park, U.S.A.: Sage.

Kurtz, D. (1987). Emergency department responses to battered women: resistance to medicalization. *Social Problems*, **34**, 69–81.

McHugh, M.C. (1993). Battered women and their assailants: a methodological critique. In M. Hansen & M. Harway (Eds.). *Battering and family therapy: a feminist perspective*. Newbury Park, U.S.A.: Sage, 54–68.

McHugh, M.C. & Bartoszek, T.A. (2000). Intimate violence. In M. Biaggio & M. Hersen (Eds.). *Issues in the psychology of women* (pp. 115–42). New York: Kluwer Academic.

McHugh, M.C., Frieze, I.H. & Browne, A. (1993). Battered women and their assailants. In F. Denmark & M. Paludi (Eds.). *Handbook on the psychology of women* (pp. 513–52). New York: Greenwood Press.

Walker, L.E. (1984). *The battered woman syndrome*. New York: Springer.

William, S. & Frieze, I.H. (2005). Patterns of violent relationships, psychological distress, and marital satisfaction in a national sample of men and women. *Sex Roles*, **52**, 771–84.

Yllo, K. & Bograd, M. (Eds.). (1988). *Feminist perspectives on wife abuse*. Beverly Hills, CA: Sage.

Drug dependency: benzodiazepines

Heather Ashton

University of Newcastle-upon-Tyne

Benzodiazepine tranquillisers were the most commonly prescribed drugs in the world in the 1970s and many patients took them regularly for years. Benzodiazepines include anxiolytics, such as diazepam, chlordiazepoxide, lorazepam, oxazepam and clonazepam; hypnotics, such as nitrazepam, temazepam, lormetazepam and loprazolam; and anticonvulsants such as clobazam. However, in the early 1980s long-term prescribed benzodiazepine users themselves realized that the drugs were associated with adverse effects. In particular, patients found it difficult to stop taking benzodiazepines because of withdrawal effects. Controlled trials of such patients (Petursson & Lader, 1981; Tyrer *et al.*, 1981) demonstrated beyond doubt that withdrawal symptoms in chronic users of 'therapeutic' doses of benzodiazepines were real and that such reactions indicated dependence on the drugs.

However, definitions of drug dependence have shifted in the last decade. A withdrawal syndrome is no longer considered sufficient evidence of dependence. The present criteria for a diagnosis of substance dependence include tolerance, escalation of dosage, continued use despite efforts to stop and knowledge of adverse effects and a withdrawal reaction (Table 1). Benzodiazepine dependence meets all these criteria and many long-term users develop a classic drug-dependence syndrome.

Table 1. Criteria for substance dependence[a]

A maladaptive pattern of substance use leading to significant impairment or distress, manifested by three or more of the following in the same 12-month period:

Tolerance
Withdrawal syndrome
Substance taken in larger amounts or for longer than intended
Persistent desire or unsuccessful attempts to decrease or control use
Excessive time spent obtaining, using or recovering from effects of substance
Important activities given up or reduced because of substance
Substance use continued despite knowledge of problem.

[a]Abridged from DSM-IV American Psychiatric Association (1994).

Table 2. Therapeutic actions of benzodiazepines

Actions	Clinical uses
Hypnotic	Short-term treatment of insomnia
Anxiolytic	Short-term treatment of anxiety
	Aid to alcohol withdrawal
	Acute treatment of agitated psychoses
Anticonvulsant	Epileptic and drug-induced convulsions
Amnesic	Premedication before surgery
Muscle relaxant	Muscle spasms, dystonias

Tolerance and dosage escalation

Benzodiazepines exert five therapeutic actions: hypnotic, anxiolytic, anticonvulsant, muscle relaxant and amnesic effects (Table 2). Tolerance develops at different rates and to different degrees for these various actions.

Tolerance to the hypnotic effects develops rapidly, within days or weeks of regular use, during which sleep profiles tend to return to pre-treatment levels. Recent evidence indicates that long-term benzodiazepine use no longer aids sleep (Curran et al., 2003). Although many poor sleepers report continued efficacy of benzodiazepine hypnotics, this is probably because they prevent withdrawal symptoms such as rebound insomnia. A considerable proportion of hypnotic users increase their dosage, sometimes to above recommended levels.

Tolerance to the anxiolytic effects of benzodiazepines develops more slowly. There is little evidence that benzodiazepines retain their anxiolytic efficacy after four months of regular treatment and clinical observations show that long-term benzodiazepine use does little to control, and may even aggravate anxiety. There is also evidence of dosage escalation in anxiolytic benzodiazepine users. In one clinical study over 25% of 50 patients were taking two prescribed benzodiazepines, the second having been added when the first ceased to be effective (Ashton, 1987). Tolerance to the anticonvulsant and muscle relaxant effects of benzodiazepines occurs within a few weeks of regular use in a high proportion of patients.

However, complete tolerance to the amnesic effects and other cognitive impairments does not appear to develop even after years of chronic use. Many studies of long-term benzodiazepine users have shown deficits in learning, memory, attention and visuospatial ability. These effects are most marked in the elderly in whom they may suggest dementia (see 'Dementias'). Improvement occurs when benzodiazepines are stopped (Curran et al., 2003), although it may be slow and perhaps incomplete.

Withdrawal effects and continued usage

Benzodiazepine withdrawal reactions include many symptoms common to anxiety states in general and some more characteristic of benzodiazepine withdrawal (Table 3). The syndrome, which includes both psychological and physical symptoms, can be mild and short-lived or severe and sometimes protracted. The incidence of acute withdrawal symptoms varies between 30–100% in different reports but many long-term users decline to participate in, or drop out from, studies because of withdrawal effects. Withdrawal symptoms prolong benzodiazepine use which often continues for years after the initial indication for taking the drugs has passed. Many long-term users, aware that the drugs are no longer effective and are causing adverse effects, have tried to stop or reduce dosage but have been unsuccessful because of the emergence of withdrawal symptoms.

Benzodiazepine-dependent populations

Therapeutic dose dependence

This population is large and consists of patients who have inadvertently become dependent on benzodiazepines prescribed by their doctors over months or years: estimates suggest that there are about one million long-term users in the UK, four million in the USA and several million worldwide. At least 50% of these are likely to be benzodiazepine dependent. A considerable proportion of such patients are elderly females taking benzodiazepine hypnotics, while other long-term users include patients with physical and psychiatric problems.

Prescribed high-dose dependence

A minority of patients who start on prescribed benzodiazepines may unintentionally begin to require higher and higher doses. Personality factors may contribute to this perceived need. At first their doctors may be compliant and some patients today are prescribed excessive doses, but on reaching the prescribed limit some may contact several doctors or hospital departments to obtain further supplies and may resort to 'street' benzodiazepines if other sources fail.

Recreational benzodiazepine abuse

Recreational abuse of benzodiazepines is a growing problem involving at least 140 000 individuals in the UK today. Illicit benzodiazepine abuse is common in polydrug users and alcoholics (Strang et al., 1993). Some people use them as their primary recreational drug, bingeing intermittently on high doses or injecting recreationally. Reasons given for taking benzodiazepines intravenously are that they enhance the 'high' obtained from illicit drugs (opiates,

Table 3. Some common benzodiazepine withdrawal symptoms

Symptoms common to anxiety states	Symptoms relatively specific to benzodiazepine withdrawal
Anxiety, panics	Perceptual disturbances, sense of movement
Agoraphobia	Depersonalization, derealization
Insomnia, nightmares	Hallucinations
Depression	Distortion of body image
Excitability	Tingling, numbness, altered sensation
Poor memory and concentration	Skin prickling
Dizziness	Sensory hypersensitivity
Weakness	Muscle twitches, jerks
Tremor	Tinnitus
Muscle pain, stiffness	Psychosis[a]
Night sweats	Confusion, delirium[a]
Palpitations	Convulsions[a]
Blurred or double vision	

[a] Usually only on rapid or abrupt withdrawal from high doses.

amphetamines, cocaine) and alcohol and also alleviate withdrawal effects from these drugs. Benzodiazepines can themselves produce a 'kick' when taken in high doses. Many illicit users of benzodiazepines become dependent and show typical withdrawal symptoms which can be severe (Seivewright & Dougal, 1993).

Pharmacological basis of benzodiazepine dependence

Positive and negative reinforcement

The reinforcement potential of a drug is judged by its ability to maintain or increase drug-taking or drug-seeking behaviour. Positive reinforcement is associated with rewarding effects directly exerted by the drug, while negative reinforcement is associated with the drug's ability to alleviate aversive states such as anxiety or withdrawal symptoms. Griffiths and Weerts (1997) argue that reinforcement is the major mechanism underlying both chronic long-term use and recreational use of benzodiazepines. These authors reviewed 26 studies showing reinforcing effects of benzodiazepines in man. Reinforcing effects, both positive and negative, of a number of benzodiazepines were clearly apparent in subjects with histories of drug or alcohol abuse, social alcohol drinkers, anxious subjects, insomniac subjects and patients undergoing abrupt benzodiazepine withdrawal.

Nearly all drugs that produce positive reinforcement (cocaine, amphetamine, nicotine, alcohol, opioids, cannabis and others) induce dopamine release in the limbic system (nucleus accumbens and/or prefrontal cortex) and it has been argued that dopamine activation in these rewarding areas is the final common pathway for all addictive drugs. High doses of benzodiazedpines may have a similar effect and it is noteworthy that recreational benzodiazepine abusers take doses many times greater than therapeutic dose users. By contrast, low doses of benzodiazepines do not release dopamine but act essentially as 'depunishing' drugs, providing negative reinforcement, possibly by decreasing activity in brain 'punishment systems'.

Mechanisms of tolerance and withdrawal

The basic mode of action of benzodiazepines is to enhance central gaba-aminobutyric acid (GABA) activity by interaction with specific sites on postsynaptic $GABA_A$ receptors. These contain multiple (at least 18) subunits and at present it seems that mainly α_1, and α_2 subtypes mediate benzodiazepine actions. It is proposed (Bateson, 2002) that chronic benzodiazepine use induces a chain of events in which uncoupling of the linkage between $GABA_A$ and benzodiazepine receptor sites leads to preferential degradation of these subunits which become internalized within the neurones. This provides a signal for changes in gene transcription, resulting in benzodiazepine tolerance. This pathway could operate on different time scales depending on the receptor subtypes and/or brain region involved, giving rise to differing rates of development of tolerance to various benzodiazepine actions.

Withdrawal of benzodiazepines once tolerance has developed would expose the recipient to all the drug-induced changes in GABA receptors. The result would be underactivity in the many central functions normally modulated by GABA-ergic mechanisms. Since GABA is a universal inhibitor of neural activity and decreases the release of many excitatory neurotransmitters, there would be a surge of excitatory nervous activity. Such activity, coupled perhaps with adaptive increases in sensitivity of excitatory receptors, may account for benzodiazepine withdrawal symptoms (Table 2). These changes may be slow to reverse and may do so at different rates, accounting for the variable duration and sometimes protracted nature of the benzodiazepine withdrawal syndrome (Ashton, 1995a).

Clinical implications

Adverse effects of long-term use

Apart from dependence, long-term benzodiazepine use is associated with many other adverse effects (Ashton, 1995b). These include psychomotor and cognitive impairment, interactions with other sedative drugs including alcohol, emotional clouding, depression, paradoxical excitement, aggressiveness and the insidious development of psychological and physical symptoms. Sociological costs include increased risk of traffic and other accidents, falls and fractures in the elderly, shoplifting (due to amnesia) and violent behaviour.

Prevention of dependence

These effects could largely be prevented by limiting prescriptions to short-term use (2–4 weeks only) in minimal dosage (Committee on Safety of Medicines, 1988). When used short-term, benzodiazepines can have great therapeutic value (Table 2) and dependence is not a problem, though care is needed in prescribing them to patients with a history of alcohol or drug abuse or dependent personality types. Although benzodiazepines are still the leading treatments for anxiety and are often initially helpful, long-term treatment is more appropriate with antidepressants and/or psychological intervention.

Management of dependence: benzodiazepine withdrawal

Unfortunately benzodiazepines are still prescribed long-term and there is a large population of long-term users who are already dependent. Withdrawal of benzodiazepines is a desirable option for many of these patients. The management of withdrawal consists essentially of gradual dosage reduction (usually over a period of several months) combined with psychological support (Ashton, 1994). The degree of support required varies from minimal intervention to formal psychological techniques. No adjuvant drugs have been found to be generally helpful, but antidepressants may be indicated if depression is severe. The success rate for withdrawal in motivated therapeutic dose users is good, up to 80–90% or more in some studies; physical and mental health improves after withdrawal or dosage reduction (Heather *et al.*, 2004; Curran *et al.*, 2003) and the relapse rate is low. Withdrawal failure and relapse rates may be higher in high-dose abusers.

The future

With rational prescribing, benzodiazepines are likely to remain useful drugs for short-term use. Prevalence of use should continue to decline as the number of chronic users decreases and fewer new patients become dependent. Caution is needed in prescribing non-benzodiazepine anxiolytics and hypnotics such as zopiclone (Zimovane, Imovane), zolpidem (Ambien) and zaleplon (Sonata), which have already been shown to have a dependence and abuse potential similar to that of benzodiazepines.

(See also 'Drug dependency: opiates and stimulants', 'Drugs: beta-blockers', 'Drugs: psychotropic medication' and 'Alcohol abuse').

REFERENCES

American Psychiatric Association. (1994). *Diagnostic & statistical manual of mental disorders (DSM-IV).* Washington, DC: APA.

Ashton, H. (1987). Benzodiazepine withdrawal: outcome in 50 patients. *British Journal of Addiction*, **82**, 665–71.

Ashton, H. (1994). The treatment of benzodiazepine dependence. *Addiction*, **89**, 1535–41.

Ashton, H. (1995*a*). Protracted withdrawal from benzodiazepines: the post-withdrawal syndrome. *Psychiatric Annals*, **25**, 174–9.

Ashton, H. (1995*b*). Toxicity and adverse consequences of benzodiazepine use. *Psychiatric Annals*, **25**, 158–65.

Bateson, A.N. (2002). Basic pharmacologic mechanisms involved in benzodiazepine tolerance and withdrawal. *Current Pharmaceutical Design*, **8**, 5–21.

Committee on Safety of Medicines. (1988). Benzodiazepines, dependence and withdrawal symptoms. *Current Problems*, **21**.

Curran, H.V., Collins, R., Fletcher, S. *et al.* (2003). Older adults and withdrawal from benzodiazepine hypnotics in general practice: effects on cognitive function, sleep, mood and quality of life. *Psychological Medicine*, **33**, 1223–37.

Griffiths, R.R. & Weerts, E.M. (1997). Benzodiazepine self-administration in humans and laboratory animals – implications for problems of long-term use and abuse. *Psychopharmacology*, **134**, 1–37.

Heather, N., Bowie, A., Ashton, H. *et al.* (2004). Randomised controlled trial of two brief interventions against long-term benzodiazepine use: outcome of intervention. *Addiction Research & Theory*, **12**, 141–54.

Petursson, H. & Lader, M.H. (1981). Withdrawal from long-term benzodiazepine treatment. *British Medical Journal*, **283**, 634–5.

Seivewright, N. & Dougal, W. (1993). Withdrawal symptoms from high dose benzodiazepines in polydrug users. *Drug and Alcohol Dependence*, **32**, 15–23.

Strang, J., Seivewright, N. & Farrell, M. (1993). Oral and intravenous abuse of benzodiazepines. In. C. Hallstrom (Ed.). *Benzodiazepine dependence* (pp. 128–42). Oxford: Oxford Medical Publications.

Tyrer, P., Rutherford, D. & Higgitt, T. (1981). Benzodiazepine withdrawal symptoms and propranolol. *Lancet*, **1**, 520–2.

Drug dependence: opiates and stimulants

Michael Gossop

Institute of Psychiatry

The nature of the disorder

Drug misuse is a complex and multifaceted phenomenon which can be understood in terms of three dimensions: consumption behaviours, problems; and dependence. Although conceptually distinct, in reality these dimensions tend to be related (sometime closely) in a number of ways.

Opiates and stimulants (predominantly heroin and crack cocaine) are among the drugs most commonly used by people presenting for treatment, and dependence upon these drugs is the most common reason for treatment. However, the classification of drug problems by specific substance can be misleading. Most drug misusers who require treatment are heavy and problematic users of more than one drug (Gossop, 2001).

Multiple drug use may involve the concurrent or sequential use of different substances. Among the reasons for multiple drug use are:

- *drug enhancement* (several drugs may be used at the same time to increase the desired effects)
- m*odification of effect* (e.g. to counteract the adverse or unwanted effects of one or more drugs as with cocaine and heroin used together so that either the heroin takes away some of the unpleasant overstimulation of the cocaine, or the stimulant offsets the sedation of the heroin)
- s*ubstitution* (taking a different drug as a substitute where the preferred drug is not available).

Assessment and setting treatment goals

Assessment is not an impersonal procedure to be completed prior to treatment. It is an important first stage of treatment. The therapist should use assessment as an opportunity to encourage the involvement of the drug user in their own recovery. It is more appropriate to regard this first stage of treatment as reaching mutual agreement about goals rather than simply setting goals.

For all types of drug misuse treatment, the intervention should be tailored to the needs and circumstances of the individual. This apparently simple and uncontentious statement turns out to have complex and far-reaching implications for policy and services if it is seriously applied in clinical practice. There is not, nor can there be expected to be, any single best treatment for these problems (Gossop, 2003). Both aetiology and outcome are influenced by a broad range of different factors. A thorough assessment should identify, for each individual case, the nature of the problem and appropriate and achievable goals for treatment. Also, the treatment process should identify as early as possible those particular factors (often outside the treatment setting) that will assist or hamper the achievement of the treatment goal(s).

It is important that both the therapist and the drug user should agree upon the goal(s) of treatment. This does not mean that the therapist cannot aspire to goals more ambitious than those set by the patient. However, it does imply that where the therapist seeks to attain some goal beyond that which is immediately acceptable to the patient, this may create certain tensions and require careful management.

Psychological treatments

There is a wide range of psychological treatment interventions. These differ in many respects, not least in the degree of emphasis given to cognitive, behavioural and social factors. In general, psychological treatments assume that addictive behaviours are substantially influenced by normal learning processes; that addictive behaviour is functional for the drug users; and that, as a learned behaviour, addictive behaviour can be modified or 'unlearned'.

Motivational Interviewing (MI) (see 'Motivational interviewing') has been popular and clinically influential in recent years (Miller, 1983; Miller & Rollnick, 1991). Its aim is to increase levels of cognitive dissonance until sufficient motivation is generated for consideration of the options and interventions for change. MI is primarily a counselling style concerned with the patient-therapist interaction, rather than an intervention procedure. The therapist initially adopts an empathic stance using techniques similar to those operationalized by Carl Rogers. This process is, however, modified to selectively reinforce statements of concern and elicit self-motivational statements.

One limitation of some addiction treatments is that they presume a prior commitment to change. MI has been found to be useful in many phases of treatment but it has been particularly useful in helping people who are still at an early stage of committing themselves to treatment or to changing their behaviour. However, motives do not translate directly into outcomes. Motivation alone is unlikely to be sufficient for change or the maintenance of change among many of the long-term, severely dependent drug users who seek treatment in addiction services.

An important distinction should be made between initial change and the maintenance of change. The factors and procedures which are most effective in inducing behaviour change may not be the most effective for producing generalization and maintenance of treatment effects. The problem of relapse is an important characteristic of all of the addictive disorders. A large proportion of people who have been treated for such problems tend to return to those behaviours within a short time of leaving treatment.

Marlatt and Gordon's (1985) Relapse Prevention (RP) model was the first major cognitive behavioural approach (see 'Cognitive behaviour therapy') to be used in the treatment of substance use disorders, and provides a straightforward conceptual model for understanding drug misuse problems. The primary goal of RP is to teach drug users who are trying to change their drug-taking behaviour how to identify, anticipate and cope with the pressures and problems that may lead towards a relapse. Two essential features are the identification of high-risk situations which increase the risk of relapse, and the development and strengthening of effective coping responses. High-risk situations may be events, objects, cognitions or mood states which have become associated with drug use and/or relapse. Many lapses are related to negative emotional states, social pressure and interpersonal conflicts, but antecedents to lapse may also include subjective experiences of 'urge' (sudden impulse to engage in an act) and 'craving' (Heather & Stallard, 1989). Risk factors often occur together, either in clusters or in sequence (Bradley et al., 1989) and they may operate in an additive or interactive manner (Shiffman, 1989).

Relapse Prevention requires an individualized assessment of high-risk situations for relapse involving a microanalysis of drug-related factors for each patient in terms of their social and environmental circumstances, and their cognitive appraisal of those situations. The effective delivery of RP requires a close inter-relationship between assessment and treatment planning.

Contingency management provides a system of incentives and disincentives according to which treatment delivery is organized by setting specific objective behavioural goals, and structuring the environment in a manner that is conducive to change (Stitzer et al., 1989) (see 'Behaviour therapy'). Contingency management has been found to be useful for extinguishing negative or undesirable behaviours, such as continued drug use or failure to comply with treatment requirements, and as a means of encouraging positive behaviours, such as engagement with treatment services. A persistent problem for addiction treatment services involves those patients who do not comply with the requirements of treatment programmes or who do not get better as a result of their contact with treatment. Contingency management has been found to be particularly useful as a treatment intervention for 'non-responsive' patients.

Twelve-step programmes and therapeutic communities

For more than six decades Alcoholics Anonymous (AA) has influenced the treatment of addiction problems. Together with its offshoot, Narcotics Anonymous (NA), this organization has been seen as the paradigm of the self-help movement for recovery from addiction, though many members tend to dislike the *self*-help label and prefer to see the fellowship as providing *mutual* support.

The programme consists of studying and following the Twelve Steps which emphasize two general themes: *spirituality* – belief in a 'higher power', which is defined by each individual and which represents faith and hope for recovery and *pragmatism* – doing 'whatever works' for the individual (Emrick, 1999).

Group meetings are one of the best known aspects of NA/AA. In groups, members share their experiences, achievements, their fears and their failures with peers whose advice supports the achievement

and maintenance of abstinence as well as the learning of new, prosocial behaviours (Brown et al., 2001). Role modelling can be further assisted by the sponsor. NA/AA also provides a structure for the member's free time and evening meetings may provide a supportive activity during a high-risk time of day. In these respects, NA/AA can serve as an effective aftercare resource (Ouimette et al., 1998).

In many countries, residential rehabilitation programmes are one of the longest established forms of treatment and in some countries, they remain one of the dominant treatment modalities. Many are based upon the principles of the Therapeutic Community (TC). With TCs the interaction between the individual and the community is itself seen as the treatment process, and the treatment ingredients are the programme structure, and the daily activities and social interactions in the TC. The primary staff members in many residential programmes are often recovering addicts who have themselves been rehabilitated in therapeutic communities.

The basic goal for residents in TCs in particular (but also in residential treatment programmes in general) involves a complete change in lifestyle involving abstinence from drugs, avoidance of antisocial behaviour, the development of prosocial skills and personal honesty. The specific objective of the TCs has been described as the treatment of individual disorders, 'but their larger purpose is to transform lifestyles and personal identities' (De Leon, 2000). Three psychological determinants of change within TCs are social role training, vicarious learning and efficacy training (see 'Self-efficacy and health').

At one time, traditional TCs worked with planned durations of stay of 2–3 years. Recent changes have led to modified residential TCs working with 6- to 9-month programmes, and short-term programmes with a 3- to 6-month programme (De Leon, 2000). Relatively short-stay, residential 'chemical dependency' programmes ('Minnesota Model', 'Hazelden' or 'chemical dependency' treatments) are often based upon the Twelve Steps. These programmes typically provide a highly structured 3–6 week package of residential care involving an intensive programme of daily lectures and group meetings designed to implement a recovery plan.

In an evaluation of Twelve-Step, cognitive–behavioural or combined Twelve-Step plus cognitive–behavioural treatments provided in 3–4 week inpatient programmes, all three treatments appeared to be effective in reducing substance use and psychological symptoms, and in reducing post-treatment arrests and imprisonment (Ouimette et al., 1997; Moos et al., 1999).

Pharmacotherapies

The most widely used form of pharmacotherapy involves methadone treatment. At the beginning of the 21st Century there were probably about half a million patients in methadone treatment worldwide. Methadone treatments are extremely diverse and programmes differ in doses prescribed, provision of counselling services, treatment policies and in drug use outcomes (Gossop & Grant, 1990; Ball & Ross, 1991; Stewart et al., 2000). In a meta-analysis of methadone treatment evaluations, Marsch (1998) reported consistent findings of reductions in illicit opiate use, HIV risk behaviours and crime. Methadone treatments are rarely restricted merely to the provision of methadone pharmacotherapy (Strain & Stoller (1999)) and additional counselling, medical and psychosocial services leads to improved efficacy of treatment compared to methadone alone (McLellan *et al.*, 1993).

Detoxification is a clearly delineated phase of treatment designed to eliminate or to reduce the severity of withdrawal symptoms when the physically dependent user stops taking drugs. The heroin withdrawal syndrome has been treated by methadone, other opioid agonists, clonidine, lofexidine, buprenorphine, opioid antagonists, as well as by hypnotic, anxiolytic, antidepressant and anti-psychotic drugs. Among the most commonly used treatments is gradually reducing doses of oral methadone.

Although there have been descriptions of withdrawal disturbances among regular stimulant users, the existence of a specific cocaine or amphetamine withdrawal syndrome is still uncertain (Lago & Kosten, 1994). Antidepressant drugs are sometimes given to counter dopamine depletion during cocaine withdrawal. Despite the theoretical rationale, the superiority of these drugs over a placebo in cocaine withdrawal has not been established (Kosten *et al.*, 1992). The use of substitute drugs for treatment of stimulant dependence is uncommon and of unknown effectiveness.

Opiate antagonist drugs such as naltrexone are also sometimes used to speed up withdrawal treatments or to help prevent relapse after detoxification. These substances bind to opiate receptors but without producing opiate type effects. They compete with opiate agonists such as heroin in such a way that opiates produce little or no effect. Antagonists appear to work well with highly motivated patients and when used under supervision (O'Brien, 1994). Because of their specific affinity for opiate receptors, such drugs have not been evaluated in the treatment of stimulant dependence.

Other interventions

The health risk behaviours of drug users have been the focus for various harm reduction activities. Dissemination of information about the transmission of HIV and other blood-borne infections is one of the least controversial prevention responses. This has been widely used and in some circumstances may be effective (Selwyn *et al.*, 1987).

Needle and syringe exchange schemes have been more controversial, though these have now been established in many countries (Stimson *et al.*, 1990). Many injecting drug users share needles, syringes, or other injecting equipment because of the lack of availability of sterile equipment.

Syringes have been supplied to users in a number of ways. Some services provide needles and syringes but make no requirement for the return of used equipment. The best known system involves the provision of needles and syringes to injectors on an exchange basis. This addresses public health concerns about used and possibly infected needles being left in public places, or disposed of in ways that may put others at risk. Attendance at exchange schemes has been found to be associated with reduced levels of sharing as well as increased contact with other treatment services (Stimson *et al.*, 1990).

Drug users may also be at risk through their sexual behaviour (see 'Sexual risk behaviour'). Many drug users engage in unprotected sex, often with multiple partners. Rates of prostitution tend to be higher among drug users (Hart *et al.*, 1989; Gossop *et al.*, 1993). Some drug users may be exposed to both drug risk and sexual risk through

having a sexual partner who injects drugs. Women may be at particular risk in this way (Gossop *et al.*, 1994*a*). In the United States, women infected with HIV by a drug using partner are the second largest group of women with AIDS (see also 'HIV and AIDS').

Since the earliest days of the HIV epidemic it has been known that homosexual activity may carry high risks of HIV transmission. Drug users may also be exposed to this form of risk. Gossop *et al.* (1994*b*) found that the factor most strongly associated with HIV seropositive status among a sample of heroin users was men having sex with men. Conversely, the strongest predictor of hepatitis infection was a drug risk factor, the number of years injecting drugs.

Treatment outcome

Early reviews of the effectiveness of treatments for addiction problems were often pessimistic about the impact of treatment upon outcome (e.g. Einstein, 1966; Clare, 1977). Such pessimism is no longer warranted. There is now an impressive accumulation of evidence to show that even people with severe dependence upon drugs can recover from their addictions and that treatment can play an important role in assisting recovery.

Large-scale, prospective, multi-site treatment outcome studies have played an important role in improving our understanding of treatment effectiveness (Simpson, 1997). Studies from both the United States and the UK have shown that patients who receive drug misuse treatment make improvements across a range of outcome measures (Simpson & Sells, 1990; Hubbard *et al.*, 1989, 1997). The results from the National Treatment Outcome Research Study (NTORS) showed substantial reductions after treatment in use of heroin, non-prescribed methadone and benzodiazepines, reduced injecting and sharing of injecting equipment, improvements in psychological health and reductions in crime, with improved outcomes still evident at 5-year follow-up (Gossop *et al.*, 2003).

However, a word of caution may be appropriate. For the therapist in the treatment setting it may be tempting to over-estimate the impact of treatment factors. The psychology of the individual and the social setting in which the individual lives exert powerful influences upon outcome. Hubbard *et al.* (1989) note that 'the role of treatment is to change behaviours and psychological states and to direct clients to community resources during and after treatment', and that 'programmes have no direct control on behaviour after clients leave treatment. Rather, treatment should influence post-treatment behaviour indirectly through changes in psychological states and behaviour during treatment' (p. 35). Effective treatments for drug problems look beyond the clinic to maintaining change in the real-life social environment.

There is broad agreement that many treatment and other factors may be related to outcome. Relatively little is known about what these factors are or how they affect outcome. An important question for clinicians and researchers is how to assess the impact of specific treatment process variables and identify 'active' and 'inert' components of treatment. The important developments in addiction treatments during the next decades may occur, not as a result of radical new discoveries, but through the improvement of existing interventions and through improved provision of treatments.

(See also 'Drug dependency: benzodiazapines', 'Drugs: beta-blockers', 'Drugs: psychotropic medication' and 'alcohol abuse'.)

Ball, J. & Ross, A. (1991). *The Effectiveness of methadone maintenance treatment.* New York: Springer.

Bradley, B., Phillips, G., Green, L. & Gossop, M. (1989). Circumstances surrounding the initial lapse to opiate use following detoxification. *British Journal of Psychiatry,* **154**, 354–9.

Brown, B., Kinlock, T. & Nurco, D. (2001). Self-help initiatives to reduce the risk of relapse. In F. Tims, C. Leukefeld & J. Platt (Eds.). *Relapse and recovery in addictions.* New Haven: Yale University Press.

Clare, A. (1977). How good is treatment? In G. Edwards & M. Grant (Eds.). *Alcoholism: new knowledge and new responses.* London: Croom Helm.

De Leon, G. (2000). *The therapeutic community: theory, model, and method.* New York: Springer.

Einstein, S. (1966). The narcotics dilemma: who is listening to what? *International Journal of the Addictions,* **1**, 1–6.

Emrick, C. D. (1999). Alcoholics Anonymous and other 12-step groups. In M. Galanter & H. D. Kleber (Eds.). *The American Psychiatric Press Textbook of Substance Abuse Treatment* (2nd edn.) (pp. 403–12). Washington, DC: American Psychiatric Press, Inc.

Gossop, M. (2001). A web of dependence. *Addiction,* **96**, 677–8.

Gossop, M. (2003). *Drug addiction and its treatment.* Oxford: Oxford University Press.

Gossop, M. & Grant, M. (1990). *The content and structure of methadone treatment programmes: a study in six countries.* Geneva: World Health Organization. (WHO/PSA/90.3).

Gossop, M., Griffiths, P. & Strang, J. (1994*a*). Sex differences in patterns of drug taking behaviour: a study at a London community drug team. *British Journal of Psychiatry,* **164**, 101–4.

Gossop, M., Marsden, J., Stewart, D. & Kidd, T. (2003). The National Treatment Outcome Research Study (NTORS): 4–5 year follow-up results. *Addiction,* **98**, 291–303.

Gossop, M., Powis, B., Griffiths, P. & Strang, J. (1993). Sexual behaviour and its relationship to drug taking among prostitutes in south London, *Addiction.*

Gossop, M., Powis, B., Griffiths, P. & Strang, J. (1994*b*). Multiple risks for HIV and hepatitis B infection among heroin users. *Drug and Alcohol Review,* **13**, 293–300.

Heather, N. & Stallard, A. (1989). Does the Marlatt model underestimate the importance of conditioned craving in the relapse process? In M. Gossop (Ed.). *Relapse and addictive behaviour.* London: Routledge.

Hubbard, R. L., Craddock, S. G., Flynn, P., Anderson, J. & Etheridge, R. (1997). Overview of 1-year outcomes in the Drug Abuse Treatment Outcome Study (DATOS). *Psychology of Addictive Behaviors,* **11**, 279–93.

Hubbard, R., Marsden, M., Rachal, V. *et al.* (1989). *Drug abuse treatment: a national study of effectiveness.* Chapel Hill, NC; London: University of North Carolina Press.

Kosten, T., Morgan, C., Falcione, J. & Schottenfeld, R. (1992). Pharmacotherapy for cocaine-abusing methadone-maintained patients using amantadine or desiprimine. *Archives of General Psychiatry,* **49**, 894–8.

McLellan, A. T., Arndt, I., Metzger, D., Woody, G. & O'Brien, C. (1993). The effects of psychosocial services in substance abuse treatment. *Journal of the American Medical Association,* **269**, 1953–9.

Marlatt, G. A. & Gordon, J. R. (1985). *Relapse prevention.* New York: Guilford Press.

Marsch, L. A. (1998). The efficacy of methadone maintenance interventions in reducing illicit opiate use, HIV risk behaviour and criminality: a meta-analysis. *Addiction,* **93**, 515–32.

Miller, W. R. (1983). Motivational interviewing with problem drinkers. *Behavioural Psychotherapy,* **1**, 147–72.

Miller, W. R. & Rollnick, S. (1991). *Motivational Interviewing.* New York: Guilford Press.

O'Brien, C. (1994). The treatment of drug dependence. *Addiction,* **89**, 1565–9.

Ouimette, P. C., Finney, J. W. & Moos, R. H. (1997). Twelve step and cognitive–behavioural treatment for substance abuse: a comparison of treatment effectiveness. *Journal of Consulting and Clinical Psychology,* **65**, 230–40.

Ouimette, P. C., Moos, R. H. & Finney, J. W. (1998). Influence of outpatient treatment and 12–step group involvement on one–year substance abuse treatment outcomes. *Journal of Studies on Alcohol,* **59**, 513–22.

Selwyn, P., Feiner, C., Cox, C., Lipshutz, C. & Cohen, R. (1987). Knowledge about AIDS and high–risk behavior among intravenous drug users in New York City. *AIDS,* **1**, 247–54.

Shiffman, S. (1989). Conceptual issues in the study of relapse. In M. Gossop (Ed.). *Relapse and addictive behaviour.* London: Routledge.

Simpson, D. D. (1997). Effectiveness of drug-abuse treatment: a review of research from field settings. In J. A. Egerton, D. M. Fox, A. I. Leshner (Eds.). *Treating drug abusers effectively.* Oxford: Blackwell.

Simpson, D. & Sells, S. (1990). *Opioid addiction and treatment.* Malabar: Krieger.

Stewart, D., Gossop, M., Marsden, J. & Strang, J. (2000). Variation between and within drug treatment modalities: data from the National Treatment Outcome Research Study (UK). *European Addiction Research,* **6**, 106–14.

Stimson, G., Donoghoe, M., Lart, R. & Dolan, K. (1990). Distributing sterile needles and syringes to people who inject drugs: the syringe exchange experiment. In J. Strang & G. Stimson (Eds.). *AIDS and drugs misuse.* London: Routledge.

Stitzer, M., Bigelow, G. & Gross, J. (1989). Behavioral treatment of drug abuse. In T. B. Karasu (Ed.). *Treatments of psychiatric disorders: a task force report of the American psychiatric association, Vol. 2.* Washington, DC: American Psychiatric Association.

Drugs: beta-blockers

Sari D. Holmes and David S. Krantz

Uniformed Services University of the Health Sciences

Beta-blockers are a class of drugs that selectively compete for and inhibit binding at the beta-adrenergic subset of receptors of the sympathetic nervous system (Middlemiss *et al.*, 1981; Patel & Turner, 1981). Beta-adrenergic receptors are primarily located in the heart and in the smooth muscle of the blood vessels and the lungs, but also exert metabolic and other effects. The beta-blockers are structurally similar to the body's adrenergic neurotransmitters, norepinephrine and epinephrine, and they exhibit their greatest effects during periods of intense sympathetic nervous system (SNS) activation. Therefore, the most common clinical use of these drugs is for the treatment of cardiovascular disorders, including hypertension and manifestations of ischaemic heart disease such as angina pectoris and cardiac arrhythmias (Frishman, 1980; Patel & Turner, 1981; Weiner, 1985).

However, since the introduction of these drugs and their wide therapeutic use, a variety of both desirable and unwanted psychological effects have been observed. One of the most frequently noted beneficial effects has been the reduction of reported anxiety by individuals in certain acutely stressful situations (e.g. performing before an audience or dental surgery) that are normally accompanied by several somatic manifestations of arousal (Frishman *et al.*, 1981; Noyes, 1982; Elman *et al.*, 1998). There have also been some reports that chronic beta-blocker therapy might lessen anger and irritability or 'coronary-prone' behaviour pattern (Schmeider *et al.*, 1983; Krantz & Durel, 1983; Fedorets *et al.*, 2004). In addition to these psychological effects (some of which may be considered beneficial) unwanted psychological and behavioural effects of beta-blockers have also been noted. These include side effects such as fatigue, depression, nightmares and disturbances of sleep and sexual function (Patel & Turner, 1981; Moss & Procci, 1982; Weiner, 1985; Head *et al.*, 1996; Keller & Frishman, 2003). This chapter will provide a brief overview of the psychological and behavioural effects of beta-blocking drugs.

Psychological effects

Reduction of chronic anxiety

The anxiolytic (anxiety-reducing) effects of beta-blockers in chronically anxious patients were first reported by Granville-Grossman and Turner (1966) for the drug propranolol. Beta-blockers have been shown to be effective in reducing symptoms of generalized anxiety disorder (Swartz, 1998), panic disorder (Hirschmann *et al.*, 2000), social anxiety disorder (Elliott & Reifler, 2000), obsessive compulsive disorder (Dannon *et al.*, 2000) and post-traumatic stress disorder (PTSD) (Taylor & Cahill, 2002; Vaiva *et al.*, 2003). In some studies beta-blockers were effective as adjunctive therapy with benzodiazepines or antidepressants (Dannon *et al.*, 2000; Hirschmann *et al.*, 2000), whereas other studies demonstrated the anxiolytic effects of beta-blockers alone (Swartz, 1998; Vaiva *et al.*, 2003).

Effects during situational stress

Considerable evidence has shown that beta-blockers can be useful in decreasing anxiety in certain acute stress situations. In healthy subjects, and in patients with cardiovascular disease, these drugs blunt the increases in cardiovascular activity and anxiety that accompany certain stressful activities such as public speaking, musical performance, parachute jumping, performing surgery and emotional upset (Middlemiss *et al.*, 1981; Neftel *et al.*, 1982; Benschop *et al.*, 1996; Elman *et al.*, 1998; Culic *et al.*, 2004). Anxiolytic effects have been reported for a variety of beta-blockers regardless of whether they have pharmacological properties that enable them to readily cross the blood–brain barrier. When situational stress leads to a decrement in performance, which in turn, increases anxiety further (e.g. tremor experienced by some musicians during public performance), reduction of anxiety or tremor by beta-blockade apparently leads to improved performance (Neftel *et al.*, 1982).

Other effects

In addition to their effects on anxiety, beta-blockers have been shown to influence depressed mood, anger, irritability and drug withdrawal. Reports of adverse mood state changes as a result of beta-blocker use have been confirmed, such that levels of tension, depression and total mood disturbance were higher on propranolol as compared to placebo (Head *et al.*, 1996). However, there is also evidence indicating that short-term, high-dose augmentation with pindolol is effective in SSRI (selective serotonin re-uptake inhibitor)-refractory patients (Brousse *et al.*, 2003; Sokolski *et al.*, 2004) and in reducing negative emotional states (Blumenthal *et al.*, 1988). Several studies (Schmeider *et al.*, 1983; Krantz *et al.*, 1982; Krantz & Durel, 1983; Fedorets *et al.*, 2004) suggest that, among patients with hypertension or coronary disease, chronic administration of beta-blockers may reduce anger and irritability or so-called 'coronary-prone behaviour' (see 'Hostility, Type A behaviour and coronary heart disease'). More recent studies suggest that these effects may be confined to beta-blockers that penetrate the brain, and are only evident among a sub-set of individuals (Krantz *et al.*, 1988). Furthermore, beneficial effects of propranolol have been found for cocaine dependence treatment, such that patients on the drug had lower cocaine withdrawal symptom severity than those on placebo (Kampman *et al.*, 2001).

Mechanism of beta-blocker effects on anxiety

It is not entirely clear whether the anti-anxiety effects of beta blockers result from their direct effects in the central nervous system or whether these effects result from the peripheral effects of these drugs. A central site of action is often assumed, especially when effects on mood or behavior are associated with a beta-blocker that readily penetrates into the brain (Cruickshank, 1980; Beversdorf *et al.*, 2002). Recent reported effects of beta-blockers relevant to SSRI efficacy (Brousse *et al.*, 2003; Sokolski *et al.*, 2004) and cocaine withdrawal (Kampman *et al.*, 2001) would be consistent with such an interpretation. However, various drugs in this class vary in the extent to which they penetrate the CNS, and anti-anxiety effects in acute stress situations are evident even for those beta-blockers that do not readily penetrate the brain (Neftel *et al.*, 1982).

It has been suggested that the peripheral effects of beta-blockers are sufficient to account for their anxiolytic effects, and that this involves the role of information processing concerning peripheral sympathetic responses on the subjective experience of emotion (Tyrer, 1976; Durel *et al.*, 1985). Peripheralist views of emotion (e.g. James–Lange, Schachter–Singer) suggest that the subjective experience of anxiety is a result of a sequence of physiological events beginning with sympathetic nervous system stimulation leading to arousal manifestations, such as palpitation and tremor. The perception, cognitive interpretation, or automatic processing of these responses acts to heighten the psychological aspects of anxiety based on this interpretation, beta-blockade inhibits peripheral psychological responses (e.g. rapid heart rate, tremor), interrupts the somatic psychic interaction, and thus reduces anxiety (Tyrer, 1976; Durel *et al.*, 1985; Elman *et al.*, 1998).

When compared with other anxiolytic drugs such as the minor tranquilizers (e.g. benzodiazepines), beta-blockers are probably most effective in patients whose anxiety is characterized by bodily complaints (Tyrer, 1976). In other words, when patients experience their anxiety more in terms of palpitations and tremor than as worry or mental tension, their anxiety is likely to be reduced by a beta-blocker. When psychic symptoms predominate, beta-blockers are considered much less effective than benzodiazipines.

Summary and conclusion

Beta-adrenergic blocking drugs, such as propranolol and atenolol, have utility in reducing the peripheral manifestations of anxiety and acute stress. These beneficial effects are most pronounced among individuals with somatic manifestations of anxiety. Effects of these drugs on mood are less consistent, and chronic use of these medications have occasionally been associated with unwanted side effects such as fatigue and depression.

(See also 'Drug dependency: opiates and stimulants', 'Drugs: benzodiazepines' and 'drugs: psychotropic medication'.)

REFERENCES

Benschop, R. J., Jacobs, R., Sommer, B. *et al.* (1996). Modulation of the immunologic response to acute stress in humans by beta-blockade or benzodiazepines. *FASEB Journal: Official Publication of the Federation of American Societies for Experimental Biology*, **10**, 517–24.

Beversdorf, D. Q., White, D. M., Chever, D. C. *et al.* (2002). Central beta-adrenergic modulation of cognitive flexibility. *Neuroreport*, **13**, 2505–7.

Blumenthal, J. A., Madden, D. J., Krantz, D. S. *et al.* (1988). Short-term behavioral effects of beta-adrenergic medications in men with mild hypertension. *Clinical Pharmacology and Therapeutics*, **43**, 429–35.

Brousse, G., Schmitt, A., Chereau, I. *et al.* (2003). Interest of the use of pindolol in the treatment of depression: review. *Encephale*, **29**, 338–50.

Cruickshank, J. M. (1980). The clinical importance of cardioselectivity and lipophilicity in beta blockers. *American Heart Journal*, **100**, 160–8.

Culic, V., Eterovic, D., Miric, D. *et al.* (2004). Triggering of ventricular tachycardia by meteorologic and emotional stress: protective effect of beta-blockers and anxiolytics in men and elderly. *American Journal of Epidemiology*, **160**, 1047–58.

Dannon, P. N., Sasson, Y., Hirschmann, S. *et al.* (2000). Pindolol augmentation in treatment-resistant obsessive compulsive disorder: a double-blind placebo controlled trial. *European Neuropsychopharmacology*, **10**, 165–9.

Durel, L. A., Krantz, D. S., Eisold, J. F. *et al.* (1985). Behavioral effects of beta blockers: reduction of anxiety, acute stress, and type A behavior. *Journal of Cardiopulmonary Rehabilitation*, **5**, 267–73.

Elliott, H. W. & Reifler, B. (2000). Social anxiety disorder. A guide for primary care physicians. *North Carolina Medical Journal*, **61**, 176–8.

Elman, M. J., Sugar, J., Fiscella, R. *et al.* (1998). The effect of propranolol versus placebo on resident surgical performance. *Transactions of the American Ophthalmological Society*, **96**, 283–91; discussion 291–4.

Fedorets, V. N., Radchenko, V. G. & Skoromets, A. A. (2004). Psychosomatic aspects of therapy in patients with ischemic heart disease of behavioral type A. *Klinicheskaia Meditsina*, **82**, 54–6.

Frishman, W. H. (1980). *Clinical pharmacology of the beta-adrenoreceptor blocking drugs.* New York: Appleton Century-Crofts.

Frishman, W. H., Razin, A., Swencionis, C. *et al.* (1981). Beta-adrenoreceptor blockade in anxiety states: New approaches to therapy? *Cardiovascular Reviews & Reports*, **2**, 447–59.

Granville-Grossman, K. & Turner, P. (1966). The effect of propranolol on anxiety. *Lancet*, **1**, 788.

Head, A., Kendall, M. J., Ferner, R. & Eagles, C. (1996). Acute effects of beta blockade and exercise on mood and anxiety. *British Journal of Sports Medicine*, **30**, 238–42.

Hirschmann, S., Dannon, P. N., Iancu, I. *et al.* (2000). Pindolol augmentation in patients with treatment-resistant panic disorder: a double-blind, placebo-controlled trial. *Journal of Clinical Psychopharmacology*, **20**, 556–9.

Kampman, K. M., Volpicelli, J. R., Mulvaney, F. *et al.* (2001). Effectiveness of propranolol for cocaine dependence treatment may depend on cocaine withdrawal symptom severity. *Drug and Alcohol Dependence*, **63**, 69–78.

Keller, S. & Frishman, W. H. (2003). Neuropsychiatric effects of cardiovascular drug therapy. *Cardiology in Review*, **11**, 73–93.

Krantz, D. S., Contrada, R. J., Durel, L. A. *et al.* (1988). Comparative effects of two beta-blockers on cardiovascular reactivity and type A behavior in hypertensives. *Psychosomatic Medicine*, **50**, 615–26.

Krantz, D. S. & Durel, L. A. (1983). Psychobiological substrates of the type A behavior pattern. *Health Psychology*, **2**, 393–411.

Krantz, D. S., Durel, L. A., Davia, J. E. *et al.* (1982). Propranolol medication among coronary patients: relationship to type A behavior and cardiovascular response. *Journal of Human Stress*, **8**, 4–12.

Middlemiss, D. N., Buxton, D. A. & Greenwood, D. T. (1981). Beta-adrenoceptor antagonists in psychiatry and neurology. *Pharmacological Therapy*, **12**, 419–37.

Moss, H. B. & Procci, W. R. (1982). Sexual dysfunction associated with oral hypertensive medications: a critical survey of the literature. *General Hospital Psychiatry*, **4**, 121–9.

Neftel, K. A., Adler, R. H., Kapelli, L. *et al.* (1982). Stage fright in musicians: a model illustrating the effect of beta-blockers. *Psychosomatic Medicine*, **44**, 461–9.

Noyes, R. (1982). Beta-blocking drugs and anxiety. *Psychosomatics*, **23**, 155–70.

Patel, I. & Turner, P. (1981). Central action of beta-adrenoceptor blocking drugs in man. *Medical Research Review*, **1**, 387–410.

Schmeider, R., Friedrich, G., Neus, H. *et al.* (1983). The influence of beta-blockers on cardiovascular reactivity and type A behavior pattern in hypertensives. *Psychosomatic Medicine*, **45**, 417–23.

Sokolski, K. N., Conney, J. C., Brown, B. J. & DeMet, E. M. (2004). Once-daily high-dose pindolol for SSRI-refractory depression. *Psychiatry Research*, **125**, 81–6.

Swartz, C. M. (1998). Betaxolol in anxiety disorders. *Annals of Clinical Psychiatry: Official Journal of the American Academy of Clinical Psychiatrists*, **10**, 9–14.

Taylor, F. & Cahill, L. (2002). Propranolol for reemergent posttraumatic stress disorder following an event of retraumatization: a case study. *Journal of Traumatic Stress*, **15**, 433–7.

Tyrer, P. J. (1976). *The role of bodily feelings in anxiety*. London: Oxford University Press.

Vaiva, G., Ducrocq, F., Jezequel, K. *et al.* (2003). Immediate treatment with propranolol decreases posttraumatic stress disorder two months after trauma. *Biological Psychiatry*, **54**, 947–9.

Weiner, N. (1985). Drugs that inhibit adrenergic nerves and block adrenergic receptors. In A. G. Goodman-Gilman, L. S. Goodman & A. Gilman (Eds.). *Goodman and Gilman's The Pharmacological Basis of Therapeutics* (7th edn.) (pp. 181–214). New York: Macmillan.

Drugs: psychotropic medication

Andrew Scholey[1], Andy Parrott[2] and David Kennedy[1]

[1]Northumbria University
[2]University of Wales Swansea

Introduction

Psychopharmacology offers a range of psychotropic medications to the medical practitioner. The decision to administer such medicines should be made in the context of evidence-based, realistic risk–benefits assessment and sound clinical judgement. With many psychotropics there is a potential for dependence. This can be manifest in two ways; tolerance, where an increased dose is required to produce the same effect, and withdrawal where negative psychological and/or physical consequences are associated with drug discontinuation. Such effects have been characterized in detail from studies of opiate addiction (see 'Drug dependency: opiates and stimulants'). The following sections summarizes specific health aspects of selected 'recreational' and prescription psychotropic agents.

Tobacco

Cigarette smoking leads to around 130 000 deaths annually in the UK. Part of the addictive potential of cigarettes lies in the delivery system; inhaled tobacco smoke generates a nicotine 'hit' within 10 seconds of inhalation, although nicotine dependence is also evident from other routes such as chewing tobacco. The behavioural effects are due to nicotine binding nicotinic acetylcholine receptors and in regular smokers cholinergic neuroadaptations probably underlie nicotine cravings during abstinence. These are transiently relieved by nicotine administration: indeed there is now strong evidence that while the regular smoker relieves negative effects of nicotine withdrawal they do not gain anything positive (Parrott *et al.*, 2004). Historically it was believed that smoking relieved stress: however there is now strong evidence that nicotine dependence itself causes stress (Parrott, 1999). This and other health risks associated with smoking are dramatically reduced following successful withdrawal from nicotine, which can be aided by the use of nicotine replacement systems (patches, inhalers, gum etc). The success of attempts to give up smoking is influenced by various factors (see meta-analysis by Viswesvaran & Schmidt, 1992). The highest abstention rates are achieved when nicotine substitution is combined with appropriate social support. (See also 'Tobacco use'.)

Alcohol

One in every 13 adults in the United Kingdom regularly drinks more than the recommended weekly levels of (21 units/week for males and 14 units/week for females) Alcohol use also increases in parallel with the use of psychoactive substances such as MDMA/ecstasy, amphetamine and cannabis (Parrott et al., 2001).

Following consumption, alcohol is distributed throughout the body but is more rapidly supplied to tissue that is dense in cells and has a good blood supply, such as the brain. Alcohol intoxication is associated with a number of detrimental behavioural effects including impaired memory, increased errors, disinhibition and a state sometimes described as 'alcohol myopia' (Steele & Josephs, 1990).

The terms alcohol abuse and alcohol dependence describe different levels of alcohol-related psychological problems (based, for example, on the DSM-IV criteria). For alcohol abuse one or more of the following criteria should have occurred for over a year: role impairment; hazardous use; legal problems related to alcohol use; social or interpersonal problems due to alcohol. To meet the criterion for alcohol dependence three of the following should have occurred for over a year: tolerance; alcohol withdrawal; drinking more than intended; unsuccessful attempts to cut down on use; excessive time related to alcohol; impaired social or work activities due to alcohol; use despite physical or psychological consequences.

Problem drinkers risk psychological dysfunction including anxiety and depression, and may experience physical withdrawal symptoms. There are also numerous medical problems related to heavy, chronic alcohol consumption including increased risk of coronary heart disease, liver cirrhosis, impotence and infertility, cancer and stroke. It is estimated that alcohol plays a part in up to 33 000 deaths per year in the UK (Department of Health, 2001). This represents 15.8 deaths per 100 000 for men and 7.6 per 100 000 in women. These figures are comparable with those for the United States and other European countries, although there is geographical variability within and between member states of both. In Europe there is traditionally a higher rate of alcohol-related mortality in areas such as Finland and the former East Germany with relatively fewer in countries such as The Netherlands and Sweden. Within the last year 1 in 4 adults in the UK will have experienced loss of memory following an alcoholic binge, injured themselves or another, or failed to carry out some task (National Statistics, 2001). Alcohol dependence may be treated by a number of behavioural and pharmacological interventions, the latter include acamprosate, ondansetron and sertraline. (See also 'Alcohol abuse'.)

Benzodiazepines

Like alcohol, benzodiazepines act as CNS (central nervous system) depressants; unlike alcohol they have been (and are) used as prescribed drugs for a range of disorders. The Royal College of Psychiatrists lists several psychiatric conditions that may respond to short-term benzodiazepine therapy (either as a primary or secondary treatment) including anxiety disorder, sleep disorder and depression. However they also warn against over-prescription of the drugs due to their potential for dependence and withdrawal, although some reviews have highlighted the inconsistency in the characterization of benzodiazepine dependence (e.g. Linsen et al., 1995). The cognitive impairment experienced while taking benzo-diazepines has been well documented (e.g. Thompson et al., 1999).

There is also evidence that cognitive dysfunction is a feature of long-term benzodiazepine use (Curran et al., 1994). Such function may be restored, though possibly not completely, following successful discontinuation and withdrawal (Barker et al., 2004). (See also 'Drug dependency: benzodiazepines'.)

Antipsychotics

The clinical aspects of schizophrenia include 'positive' symptoms such as auditory hallucinations, paranoid delusions and thought disorder, while 'negative' symptoms include social isolation and withdrawal (Walker et al., 2004). Traditional antipsychotic drugs such as chlorpromazine and haloperidol relieve positive symptoms in 70–80% of those with a diagnosis of schizophrenia. Recent years have seen the emergence of several newer antipsychotics, including risperidone, olanzapine and clozapine (Serretti et al., 2004). An advantage of these newer 'atypicals' is that they can often relieve negative symptoms, not only reducing the incidence and severity of hallucinations and delusions, but also facilitating greater social integration (Serretti et al., 2004). They also cause fewer adverse side effects, including dry mouth and Parkinsonian motor symptoms. Hence they are now the drugs of first choice, although the older typicals still remain widely used (Parrott, 1991; Parrott et al., 2004).

For clinical and health psychologists, the main function of antipsychotic drugs is to facilitate psychotherapeutic intervention. It has been confirmed that attempting therapy with unmedicated clients can be overarousing, and may lead to a heightening of 'positive' symptoms (Parrott et al., 2004). Since the advent of effective antipsychotic drugs, cognitive behavioural therapy, individual psychotherapy and many other forms of psychosocial intervention are now available (Marcinko & Read, 2004). Pharmcotherapy may reduce aberrant cortical and subcortical information processing. By reducing the incidence and/or severity of cortical hallucinations and delusions, new social–interpersonal skills can be learnt. This does however need a genuine psychotherapeutic programme and with therapeutic assistance (not necessarily by a professional), the client can become receptive to new ideas and suggestions on how to relearn and improve their social and interpersonal skills.

Antidepressants

Whereas schizophrenia affects 1% of the population, clinical depression occurs in 5–20%, depending upon definitions of severity and frequency. The majority are treated by an antidepressant, either a first generation drug such as imipramine or amitriptyline, or by a more modern psychopharmaceutical such as the Selective Serotonin Reuptake Inhibitor (SSRI) e.g. fluoxetine, or the Selective Noradrenaline Reuptake Inhibitor (SNRI) reboxotine (Parrott et al., 2004). Clinical guidelines for the therapeutic interventions in depression have been devised by Ellis (2004). In severe depression with psychosis, either electroconvulsive therapy (ECT) or a combination of antidepressant and antipsychotic drug, should be the first line of approach. The advantages of ECT are its rapid speed of action (via sub-chronic alterations in neurotransmitter activity), and higher overall clinical efficacy. Its main drawback is adverse cognitive–memory side effects. Transcranial Magnetic Stimulation may prove to offer clinical efficacy without adverse cognitive sequelae

(Lisanby, 2003). In moderate depression, cognitive behaviour therapy, interpersonal psychotherapy and antidepressant drug therapy, each demonstrate similar efficacy, but vary in availability and cost (Ellis, 2004). With mild depression, various psychological approaches might be attempted initially (e.g. book reading groups, exercise/jogging, hobbies, group sports). Any regular activity which reduces psychosocial isolation and increases feelings of self-efficacy, is likely to reverse the feelings of pressure and worthlessness which have become endemic to modern life.

Beta-blockers

Beta-blockers act by inhibiting the effects of noradrenaline at beta-adrenoreceptors which are present in a number of tissues, including the heart and smooth muscle of the bronchi and blood vessels. Their primary effect is to block activation of the sympathetic nervous system (the part of the autonomic nervous system responsible for preparing for 'fight-or-flight'). Thus they decrease heart rate and relax blood vessels, lowering blood pressure. These effects are seen primarily during heightened sympathetic activity (e.g. during exercise or stress) rather than at rest (Rang *et al.*, 1995). Beta-blockers are generally avoided in treating those with asthma and diabetes as their effects can exacerbate or mask the symptoms of these disorders (National Institute for Clinical Excellence guidelines 2001). (See also 'Drugs: beta-blockers'.)

Allergies to drugs and drug–drug interactions

Whilst adverse drug reactions are relatively common, including for psychotropic medicine, only 6–10% of these events are attributable to allergic reactions (Gruchalla, 2003). One of the major factors that characterizes allergic drug reactions is that they are generally unpredictable, and most often unrelated to the pharmacology of the drug in question. Theoretically, drug-related allergic reactions can be classified into one of four groups depending on immune system mechanisms involved (Coombs & Gell, 1975). However, a lack of knowledge of the mechanisms involved makes this identification process difficult in practice in many cases.

A related problem is that of drug–drug interactions. Presentation with co-morbid psychiatric problems is not uncommon and the specific combinations of drugs (e.g. mood stabilizers, antidepressants and antipsychotics) may produce unpredictable and unwanted interactions which the practitioner needs to be aware of and monitor vigilantly. (See also 'Allegies to drugs'.)

REFERENCES

Barker, M.J., Greenwood, K.M., Jackson, M. & Crowe, S.F. (2004). Persistence of cognitive effects after withdrawal from long-term benzodiazepine use: a meta-analysis. *Archives of Clinical Neuropsychology*, 19, 437–54.

Coombs, R. & Gell, P.G. (1975). Classification of allergic reactions responsible for clinical hypersensitivity and disease. In: P. Gell, R.R. Coombs & P.J. Lachman (Eds.). *Clinical aspects of immunology* (p. 761). Oxford, UK: Blackwell Scientific Publications.

Curran, H.V. (1992). Memory functions, alertness and mood of long-term benzodiazepine users: a preliminary investigation of the effects of a normal daily dose. *Journal of Psychopharmacology*, 6, 69–75.

Department of Health. (2001). Smoking, drinking and drug use among young people in 2000. *National Statistics*, www.doh.gov.uk/public/statspntables.htm

Ellis, P. (2004). Australian and New Zealand clinical practice guidelines for the treatment of depression. *Australian and New Zealand Journal of Psychiatry*, 38, 389–407.

Gruchalla, R.S. (2003). Drug allergy. *Journal of Allergy and Clinical Immunology*, 111, 548–59.

Linsen, S.M., Zitman, F.G. & Breteler, M.H.M. (1995). Defining benzodiazepine dependence: the confusion persists. *European Psychiatry*, 10, 306–11.

Lisanby, S.H. (2003). Focal brain stimulation with repetitive Transcranial Magnetic Stimulation (rTMS): implications for the neural circuitry of depression. *Psychological Medicine*, 33, 7–13.

Marcinko, L. & Read, M. (2004). Cognitive therapy for schizophrenia: treatment and dissemination. *Current Pharmaceutical Design*, 10, 2269–75.

National Statistics. (2001). *Psychiatric morbidity among adults*, 2000, www.statistics.gov.uk

Parrott, A.C. (1991). *Psychoactive drugs: efficacy and effects*. In M. Pitts & K. Phillips (Eds.). *The psychology of health*. London: Routledge.

Parrott, A.C. (1999). Does cigarette smoking cause stress? *American Psychologist*, 54, 817–20.

Parrott, A.C., Milani, R., Parmar, R. & Turner, J.J.D. (2001). Ecstasy polydrug users and other recreational drug users in Britain and Italy: psychiatric symptoms and psychobiological problems. *Psychopharmacology*, 159, 77–82.

Parrott, A., Morinan, A., Moss, M. & Scholey, A. (2004). *Understanding Drugs and Behaviour*. Chichester: John Wiley & Sons.

Rang, H.P. et al. (1995). *Pharmacology* (3rd edn.). New York: Churchill Livingstone.

Serretti, A., De Ronchi, D., Lorenzi, C. & Berardi, D. (2004). New antipsychotics and schizophrenia: a review on efficacy and side effects. *Current Medicinal Chemistry*, 11, 343–58.

Steele, C.M. & Josephs, R.A. (1990). Alcohol myopia: its prized and dangerous effects. *American Psychologist*, 45, 921–33.

Thompson, J.M., Neave, N., Moss, M.C. et al. (1999). Cognitive properties of sedation agents: comparison of the effects of nitrous oxide and midazolam on memory and mood. *British Dental Journal*, 187, 557–62.

Viswesvaran, C. & Schmidt, F.L. (1992). A meta-analytic comparison of the effectiveness of smoking cessation methods. *Journal of Applied Psychology*, 77, 554–61.

Walker, E., Kesler, L., Bollini, A. & Hochman, K.M. (2004). Schizophrenia: etiology and course. *Annual Review of Psychology*, 55, 401–30.

Dyslexia

Christine M. Temple

University of Essex

Dyslexia is a developmental disorder in the acquisition of reading skills, in children of otherwise normal intelligence, which cannot be explained on the basis of educational deprivation or sensory impairment. The child may have fluent speech and good communicative skills, yet has difficulty in mastering the formal written code employed for reading.

Historical perspectives

At the end of the nineteenth century, the term 'word blindness' was coined, first to refer to acquired disorders of reading resulting from brain damage, and then to refer to reading disabilities which occur developmentally. The angular gyrus was damaged in many cases of acquired word blindness and there was speculation that a congenital aplasia of the angular gyrus might underlie problems in learning to read. Early discussions of congenital word blindness can be found in Hinshelwood (1917).

Labelling

Throughout the twentieth century, there has been disagreement regarding the labelling of the disorder. This continues today, with the term 'developmental dyslexia' being accepted in most academic and medical settings but not in educational circles, where the terms 'specific reading disability', 'specific reading difficulty' and 'specific learning difficulty' are employed.

Incidence

Lewis and colleagues (1994) tested the population of 9- and 10-year-olds in a single education authority district in England, finding 6.2% with specific reading disabilities. It remains unclear whether these children represent a distinct group from the main distribution, or the lower tail of a normal distribution. Lewis *et al.* (1994) also reported a male to female ratio of 3.2:1, though Smith *et al.* (1991) suggest a lower ratio of 1.7:1–1.3:1.

Biological foundations

It has become evident that dyslexia is a heritable neurobiological syndrome. The concordance rate for dyslexia is 68% in monozygotic twins and 38% in dizygotic twins (De Fries & Alcaron, 1996). It is likely that several genes may be involved in the transmission of dyslexia with three possible sites implicated: chromosome 15q21 for single word reading (Smith *et al.*, 1983; Marino *et al.*, 2004),

chromosome 6p21.3 for phonemic segmentation and possibly single word reading (Cardon *et al.*, 1994; Grigorenko *et al.*, 1997; Gayan *et al.*, 1999) and chromosome 18p11.2 (Fisher *et al.*, 2002). Linkage has also been suggested to chromosomes 1, 2, 3 and other regions of 6 and 13.

Electrophysiological AEPs (auditory evoked potentials) at birth for speech and non-speech syllables discriminated those who eight years later would become dyslexic (Molfese, 2000). Specific EEG (electroencephalography) abnormalities have been reported, which have greater focus in temporo-parietal areas in some cases and in frontal areas in other cases (Duffy & McAnulty, 1985). Post-mortem analyses have revealed cyto-architectonic abnormalities, in the form of foci of ectopic neurons and microgyria, constellated in the left hemisphere (Galaburda *et al.*, 1985). A series of studies using PET and fMRI neuroimaging has demonstrated reduced activation of the left temporo-parietal region in adults with dyslexia, when carrying out rhyming and non-words reading tasks (e.g. Hagram *et al.*, 1992; Brunswick *et al.*, 1999). Reduced temporo-parietal activity has also been reported in fMRI studies of children with dyslexia doing a letter-rhyming task (Temple *et al.*, 2001) and MEG study of children reading (Simos *et al.*, 2000 a,b).

Cognitive neuropsychological analyses

Surface dyslexia

Cognitive neuropsychological analyses of the developmental dyslexias have delineated several different forms of the disorder, each of which is explicable in relation to models of normal reading. In developmental surface dyslexia (e.g. Coltheart *et al.*, 1983; Hanley *et al.*, 1992; Temple, 1997), words that conform to spelling-to-sound rules (e.g. beach) are read more easily than those that are not consistent with those rules (e.g. yacht). Errors indicate the application of a rule-based system (e.g. *bear→* 'beer'; *subtle→* 'subtill'). There is also homophone confusion, affecting words with the same pronunciations but different spellings (e.g. *pane* defined as 'something which hurts').

Surface dyslexia can be explained in relation to stage models of normal reading development, in terms of arrestment at an alphabetic stage, within which there is emphasis upon the use of letter-sound rules, with failure to progress to later orthographic/ hierarchical stages, which incorporate context sensitivity and analyses based upon meaningful sub-components of the target word.

In relation to models of normal adult reading, surface dyslexia reflects over-reliance upon a non-lexical, phonological reading route, which translates graphemes or letter clusters to phonemes or phonological segments and blends these to produce an integrated output (e.g. Coltheart *et al.*, 2001). The over-reliance upon the phonological reading route, leads to adequate ability to read non-words, but difficulty in reading irregular words. Homophone confusions arise because meaning is activated after the activation of pronunciation. Connectionist models, which represent relationships between orthography and phonology in a series of distributed connection weights, are also able to produce parallels to surface dyslexia, with emergent superiority in reading regular words. Early versions had difficulty in modelling the degree of accuracy in non-word reading (Seidenberg & McClelland, 1989). This was resolved in the subsequent dual route connectionist model of Plaut *et al.* (1996).

Possible underlying difficulties have been explored in surface dyslexia. Surface dyslexics have neither phonological difficulties nor general difficulties with visual memory (Castles & Coltheart, 1996) but have slower response times in reading (Seymour, 1986) and may have difficulties with rapid naming (Wolf & Bowers, 2000). Children with weak reading comprehension also demonstrate surface dyslexia (Nation & Snowling, 1998). Castles and Coltheart (1993) showed that 30% of developmental dyslexics display a surface dyslexic reading pattern. The syndrome has also been described following an early left occipital lesion in a child (Samuelsson, 2000).

Phonological dyslexia

In contrast to surface dyslexia, the major characteristic of developmental phonological dyslexia is a selective impairment of phonological reading processes. The term was first adopted by Temple and Marshall (1983) to refer to a teenage girl, who had significant difficulty in reading non-words aloud (e.g. *zan* → 'tan'; *chait* → 'chart'...'trait'). Reading errors included many paralexic responses (word substitutions), including morphological paralexias (in which the base morpheme is correct but an ending is altered, e.g. *image* → 'imagine'; *sickness* → 'sicken'). Phonological dyslexia has now been described in many languages.

Phonological dyslexia cannot be explained in relation to stage models of reading development. Orthographic skills are mastered, despite failure to master alphabetic skills, yet the acquisition of alphabetic skills is supposed to precede orthographic skills. One alternative is that there are different pathways to the acquisition of reading. Phonological dyslexia is explained with relative ease in relation to models of normal adult reading as follows. There is impaired development of the phonological reading route, but relatively normal development of lexico-semantic and direct reading routes, enabling recognition of a whole word and thereby activation of its meaning and then pronunciation, or its pronunciation directly. Both Coltheart *et al.*'s (2001) dual route cascade model and Plaut *et al.*'s (1996) dual route connectionist model can account for phonological dyslexia.

Some children with mixed dyslexia have impaired development of both reading systems, having difficulty with both non-words and irregular words.

Phonological processing

It has been suggested that a basic phonological processing deficit underlies many cases of developmental dyslexia though surface dyslexics have intact phonological skills. There is also dispute as to whether impaired phonological awareness causes or is a consequence of dyslexia, for example, Hatcher *et al.* (1994) reported that remediation, involving training in phonological awareness, only generalized to a significant improvement in reading when training in reading had also been involved. Other theories of single factor causes of developmental dyslexia include impaired magno-cellular pathways, impaired automization linked to cerebellar abnormality and impaired ocular dominance. None of these theories has yet proved convincing in accounting for the evidence.

REFERENCES

Brunswick, N., McCrory, E., Price, C.J., Frith, C.D. & Frith, U. (1999). Explicit and implicit processing of words and pseudowords by adult developmental dyslexics: a search for Wernicke's Wortschatz. *Brain*, **122**, 1901–17.

Castles, A. & Coltheart, M. (1993). Varieties of developmental dyslexia. *Cognition*, **47**, 149–80.

Castles, A. & Coltheart, M. (1996). Cognitive correlates of developmental surface dyslexia: a single case study. *Cognitive Neuropsychology*, **13**, 25–50.

Cardon, L.R., Smith, S.D., Fulker, D.W. et al. (1994). Quantitative train locus for reading diability on chromosome 6. *Science*, **266**, 276–9.

Coltheart, M., Masterson, J., Byng, S., Prior, M. & Riddoch, J. (1983). Surface dyslexia. *Quarterly Journal of Experimental Psychology*, **35**, 469–96.

Coltheart, M., Rastle, K., Perry, C., Langdon, R. & Ziegler, J.C. (2001). DRC: a dual route cascaded model

of visual word recognition and reading aloud. *Psychological Review*, **108**, 204–56.

De Fries, J.C. & Alarcon, M. (1996). Genetic of specific reading disability. *Mental Retardation & Developmental Disablities Research Review*, **2**, 39–47.

Duffy, F.H. & McAnulty, G.B. (1985). Brain electrical activity mapping (BEAM): the search for a physiological signature of dyslexia. In F.H. Duffy & N. Geschwind (Eds.). *Dyslexia: a neuroscientific approach to clinical evaluation*. Boston: Little, Brown and Co.

Fisher, S.E., Francks, C., Marlow, A.J. et al. (2002). Independent genome-wide scans identify chromosome 18 quantitative-trait locus influencing dyslexia. *Nature Genetics*, **30**, 86–91.

Galaburda, A.M., Sherman, G.F., Rosen, G.D., Aboitiz, F. & Geschwind, N. (1985). Developmental dyslexia: four consecutive cases with cortical anomalies. *Annals of Neurology*, **18**, 222–33.

Gayan, J., Smith, S.D., Cherny, S.S. et al. (1999). Quantitative-trait locus for specific language and reading deficits on chromosome 6p. *American Journal of Human Genetics*, **64**, 157–64.

Grigorenko, E.L., Wood, F.B., Meyer, M.S. et al. (1997). Susceptibility loci for distinct components of developmental dyslexia on chromosome 6 and 15. *Americal Journal of Human Genetics*, **60**, 27–39.

Hagram, J.O., Wood, F., Buchsbaum, M.S. et al. (1992). Cerebral brain metabolism in adult dyslexic subjects assessed with positron emission tomography during performance of an auditory task. *Archives of Neurology*, **49**, 734–9.

Hanley, J.R., Hastie, K. & Kay, J. (1992). Developmental surface dyslexia and dysgraphia: an orthographic processing impairment. *The Quarterly Journal of Experimental Psychology*, **44**, 285–319.

Hatcher, P.J., Hulme, C. & Ellis, A.W. (1994). Ameliorating early reading failure by integrating the teaching of reading and phonological skills: the phonological linkage hypothesis. *Child Development*, **65**, 41–57.

Hinshelwood, J. (1917). *Congenital word blindness*. Glasgow: H.K. Lewis.

Lewis, C., Hitch, G.J. & Walker, P. (1994). The prevalence of specific arithmetic difficulties and specific reading difficulties in 9- to 10-year old boys and girls. *Journal of Child Psychology and Psychiatry*, **35**, 283–92.

Marino, C., Giorda, R., Vanzin, L. *et al.* (2004). A locus on 15q15–15qter influences dyslexia: further support from a transmission/disequilibrium study in an Italian speaking population. *Journal of Medical Genetics*, **41**, 42–6.

Molfese, D.L. (2000). Predicting dyslexia at 8 years of age using neonatal brain responses. *Brain and Language*, **72**, 238–45.

Nation, K. & Snowling, M.J. (1998). Semantic processing and the development of word recognition skills: evidence from children with reading comprehension difficulties. *Journal of Memory & Language*, **39**, 85–101.

Plaut, D.C., McClelland, J.L., Seidenberg, M.S. & Patterson, K.E. (1996). Understanding normal and impaired word reading: computational principles in quasi-regular domains. *Psychological Review*, **103**, 56–115.

Samuelsson, S. (2000). Converging evidence for the role of occipital regions in orthographic processing: a case of developmental surface dyslexia. *Neuropsychologia*, **38**, 351–62.

Seidenberg, M. & McClelland, J. (1989). A distributed, developmental model of word recognition and naming. *Psychological Review*, **96**, 523–68.

Seymour, P. H. K. (1986). *Cognitive analysis of dyslexia*. London: Routledge and Kegan Paul.

Simos, P. G., Breier, J. L., Fletcher, J. M., Bergman, E. & Papanicolaou, A. C. (2000*a*). Cerebral mechanisms involved in word reading in dyslexic children: a magnetic source imaging approach. *Cerebral Cortex*, **10**, 809–16.

Simos, P. G., Breier, J. L., Fletcher, J. M. *et al.* (2000*b*). Brain activation profiles in dyslexic children during non-word reading; a magnetic source imaging study. *Neuroscience Letters*, **290**, 61–5.

Smith, S. D., Kimberling, W. J., Pennington, B. F. & Lubs, H. A. (1983). Specific reading disability: identification of an inherited form through linkage analysis. *Science*, **219**, 1345.

Smith, S. D., Kimberling, W. J. & Pennington, B. F. (1991). Screening for multiple genes influencing dyslexia. *Reading and Writing: an Interdisciplinary Journal*, **3**, 285–98.

Temple, C. M. (1997). *Developmental cognitive neuropsychology*. Hove, UK: Psychology Press.

Temple, C. M. & Marshall, J. C. (1983). A case study of developmental phonological dyslexia. *British Journal of Psychology*, **74**, 517–33.

Temple, E. (2001). Brain mechanisms in normal and dyslexic readers. *Current Opinion in Neurobiology*, **12**, 178–83.

Wolf, M. & Bowers, P. G. (2000). Naming-speed processes and developmental reading disabilities: an introduction to the special issue on the double-deficit hypothesis. *Journal of Learning Disabilties*, **33**, 322–4.

Eating disorders

Eric Stice and Heather Shaw

Oregon Research Institute

Eating disorders include a variety of psychiatric disturbances involving abnormalities in eating behaviours, maladaptive efforts to control shape and weight and disturbances in self-perception regarding body shape. The three eating disorder syndromes are anorexia nervosa, bulimia nervosa and binge eating disorder. This chapter will review research on the aetiology, prevention and treatment of these disorders.

Aetiology of eating disorders

Aetiological theories of anorexia nervosa have implicated numerous factors, including norepinephrine abnormalities, serotonergic abnormalities, childhood sexual abuse, low self-esteem, perfectionism, need for control, disturbed family dynamics, internalization of the thin-ideal, dietary restraint and mood disturbances (Wilson *et al.*, 2003). However, few prospective studies investigating factors predicting onset of anorexic pathology or increases in anorexic symptoms, and no prospective tests of multivariate aetiologic models have been conducted. Prospective studies are essential to determine whether a putative risk factor is a precursor, concomitant or consequence of eating pathology. The only prospective study that tested predictors of onset of threshold or sub-threshold anorexia nervosa found that girls with the lowest relative weight and with extremely low scores on a dietary restraint scale at baseline had increased risk for future onset of threshold and subthreshold anorexic pathology; non-significant effects were observed from early puberty, perceived pressure to be thin, thin-ideal internalization, body dissatisfaction and depressive symptoms (Stice, Presnell, & Bearman, 2004). All other studies collapsed across anorexic and bulimic pathology (e.g. McKnight Investigators, 2003). Thus, surprisingly little is known about the risk factors for anorexic pathology or how they work together to promote this pernicious eating disturbance.

Greater strides have been made toward understanding the risk factors for bulimic pathology. The sociocultural model posits that internalization of the thin-ideal for females combines with direct pressures for female thinness (e.g. weight-related teasing), promoting body dissatisfaction and increasing the risk for initiating dieting, negative affect and consequent bulimic pathology (Cattarin & Thompson, 1994). Body dissatisfaction is thought to lead females to engage in dietary restraint in an effort to conform to this thin-ideal, which paradoxically increases the likelihood of the initiation of binge eating. Dieting also entails a shift from a reliance on physiological cues to cognitive control over eating behaviours, resulting in vulnerability to over-eating when these cognitive processes are disrupted. Body dissatisfaction is also theorized to contribute to negative affect, which increases the risk that these individuals will turn to binge eating to provide comfort and distraction from these negative emotional states. Consistent with this model, thin-ideal internalization, perceived pressure to be thin, body dissatisfaction, dietary restraint and negative affect have been found to increase the risk for future onset of bulimic symptoms and bulimic pathology. Experiments have confirmed that reducing thin-ideal internalization, body dissatisfaction and negative affect produced decreases in bulimic symptoms, but have failed to support the dietary restraint model (see Stice, 2002 for a review).

To date there has been relatively little theory regarding the aetiologic processes that promote binge eating disorder, and theories that have been developed have conceptually overlapped with theories of bulimic pathology. Prospective studies suggest that initial elevations in body mass, body dissatisfaction, dietary restraint, negative affect and emotional eating increase the risk for future onset of binge eating (Vogeltanz-Holm et al., 2000; Stice, 2002).

It is likely that genetic factors also contribute to the development of eating disorders, although conflicting findings make it difficult to draw any firm conclusions. For example, in twin studies heritability estimates ranged from 0.0% to 70% for anorexia nervosa and from 0.0% to 83% for bulimia nervosa (Bulik et al., 1998; Fairburn et al., 1999). Further, one study found that the concordance rate for monozygotic twins was greater than for dizygotic twins (Treasure & Holland, 1989), but another had opposite findings (Walters & Kendler, 1995). Similarly, studies attempting to identify specific receptor genes associated with eating disorders have produced highly inconsistent results that have not been replicated (e.g. Hinney et al., 1998, 1999). The large range in parametre estimates suggests fundamental problems with sampling error resulting from small samples, the reliability of diagnostic procedures, or statistical models used to estimate genetic effects.

These aetiologic findings should be interpreted with some caution given several gaps in the literature. First, there appear to be no prospective studies testing whether any biological variable predicts onset of eating disorders, making it is impossible to determine whether biological abnormalities are a cause or consequence of eating pathology. Second, very few studies have predicted onset of anorexic pathology, bulimic pathology, or binge eating disorder, or focused on comparing and differentiating the risk factors for these three classes of eating disorders. Without these types of studies, it is impossible to differentiate the aetiologic processes that lead to eating disorders.

Prevention of eating disorders

Although initial eating disorder prevention programmes met with limited success, the effects from more recent trials are more promising. A recent meta-analytic review of 32 prevention programmes found that 53% of the programmes produced significant reductions in risk factors for eating pathology and that 25% produced significant effects for eating pathology (Stice & Shaw, 2004). For example, one intervention reduced the rate of threshold/sub-threshold eating pathology from 15% in the control condition to 6% in the intervention condition (Stice et al., 2004). The meta-analysis also identified several factors associated with larger intervention effects. Programmes which were directed at high-risk individuals, interactive (vs. didactic), targeted female adolescents over 15 years of age, had multiple sessions and used validated measures all produced larger effects. Programme content was less important than participant characteristics and research design in predicting intervention effects, though programmes with psychoeducational content were less effective. Results also suggested that the prevention programmes were more effective when they are not described as eating disorder prevention programmes per se (e.g. when they are described as body acceptance classes); in fact, 10 of the 15 prevention trials that significantly affected eating pathology were not presented as eating disorder prevention programmes.

Advances in eating disorder prevention programmes have been hindered by certain limitations, however. For instance, most prevention programmes have not been designed to reduce established risk factors for eating pathology; instead, most primarily provide information regarding eating pathology. In addition, a large proportion of prevention trials did not include a control group and therefore cannot disentangle true intervention effects from the effects of passage of time, regression to the mean, or measurement artifact. Moreover, because virtually no prevention trials have used placebo control conditions, it is not possible to rule out the possibility that any apparent intervention effects are due to demand characteristics or participant expectancies.

Treatment of eating disorders

There have been numerous randomized controlled trials of psychotherapy and pharmacotherapy in bulimia nervosa, and to a lesser extent binge eating disorder, but the research on the treatment of anorexia nervosa is very limited. Below, a brief overview of the treatment literature for each of the major eating disorders is provided. A more comprehensive overview can be found elsewhere (e.g. Wonderlich et al., 2003).

Generally two approaches have been used to treat adolescents with anorexia nervosa: individual psychodynamic therapy and family systems therapy (Wilson et al., 2003). There is an emerging consensus that family therapy is the best treatment option at this time for adolescent girls (Eisler et al., 1997). A type of family therapy, known as the 'Maudsley method' involves three stages: re-feeding the patient; negotiating a new pattern of relationships and adolescent issues; and termination (Lock et al., 2001). It appears to be most beneficial for anorexic individuals under age 19 who have been ill for a relatively short time (Wilson et al., 2003). Individual therapy for adult patients has also been used, and there is some research to support the notion that adult anorexic individuals benefit more from individual psychotherapy than from family therapy (Eisler et al., 1997). A variety of pharmacologic agents has also been evaluated in the treatment of anorexia nervosa, but due to the limited understanding of the biological basis of this disorder, trials have not been adequately grounded in aetiologic and maintenance theories and have therefore proven to be relatively ineffective (Steinglass & Walsh, 2004). Unfortunately, the consensus in the field is that treatments for anorexia nervosa have limited efficacy in reducing anorexic symptoms and behaviours. Clearly, there is a strong need for large scale, multi-centre trials for anorexia nervosa so that effective treatment strategies can be identified.

In contrast, great strides have been made in understanding both psychotherapeutic and pharmacotherapeutic treatments for bulimia nervosa. Cognitive behaviour therapy (CBT) (see 'Cognitive behaviour therapy') is considered the treatment of choice for bulimia nervosa (Wonderlich et al., 2004), due to its relatively rapid action and wealth of evidence suggesting reasonable efficacy. CBT focuses on decreasing restrictive dieting, addressing dysfunctional thoughts about shape and weight, interrupting binge–purge behaviours and enhancing self-esteem. Over 20 controlled trials of individual or group CBT for bulimia nervosa suggest that it is superior to minimal or wait list controls, as well as other interventions including behaviour therapy, psychodynamic therapy, supportive psychotherapy and pharmacotherapy (Wonderlich et al., 2004) (see also 'Behaviour therapy' and 'Psychodynamic psychotherapy').

Several other psychotherapeutic treatments for bulimia nervosa also appear promising, including interpersonal therapy targeting relationship issues and avoiding body shape and weight topics (Agras et al., 2000), and dialectical behaviour therapy (Safer et al., 2001). Trials of pharmacologic agents for bulimia nervosa have been more promising than similar trials for anorexia nervosa. However, it appears that adding drug therapy to CBT provides uncertain benefit beyond psychotherapy alone (Wilson et al., 2003).

Several psychotherapeutic treatments have also been used to treat binge eating disorder including CBT (e.g. Agras et al., 1997), interpersonal therapy (e.g. Wilfley et al., 2002) and dialectical behaviour therapy (Telch et al., 2001). All three of these psychotherapeutic approaches have been quite efficacious in reducing binge eating and promoting abstinence. The major limitation of these studies is that binge eating disorder subjects, who tend to be obese, do not lose substantial amounts of weight over long-term follow-up, even after reducing binge-eating behaviours. However, individuals who attain abstinence from binge eating are most likely to avoid further weight gain in longitudinal studies (Agras et al., 1995).

Binge eating disorder subjects have also been treated with simple dieting strategies, which have been slightly more effective in achieving weight loss than psychotherapeutic strategies, and have demonstrated a significant reduction in binge eating frequency (Goodrick et al., 1998). This is noteworthy, given predictions that dietary restriction in binge eating individuals would promote binge eating, rather than reduce it (Polivy & Herman, 1985). Low calorie diets have also been found to reduce bulimic symptoms (Presnell & Stice, 2003). These findings suggest that there may be fundamental problems with the restraint model of eating disorders.

Numerous pharmacologic therapies have also been tested in the treatment of binge eating disorder. However, similar to the evidence for bulimia nervosa, studies suggest that the addition of drugs adds little to CBT in treating binge eating disorder, and that drugs alone are not significantly more effective than placebo (Grilo et al., 2002).

Conclusions

Overall, it appears that anorexia nervosa is the least understood of the three eating disorders, and is in greatest need of studies that delineate risk factors that can be targeted in prevention programme and maintenance factors that can be targeted in treatment programmes. In contrast, more is known about the aetiology of both bulimia nervosa and binge eating disorder, as numerous studies have examined the individual and combined effects of various risk factors. Moreover, relatively effective treatments have been developed and evaluated for these latter two eating disorders. Nonetheless, a major priority for future research will be to investigate whether biological variables are risk factors for future onset of eating disorders and to investigate how biological and psychosocial factors work in concert to promote and maintain eating disorders. It is likely that increased understanding in these areas will yield major advances in terms of prevention and treatment programmes for these pernicious disorders.

(See also 'Diet and health' and 'Obesity'.)

REFERENCES

Agras, W. S., Telch, C. F., Arnow, B. et al. (1995). Does interpersonal therapy help patients with binge eating disorder who fail to respond to cognitive–behavioral therapy? Journal of Consulting and Clinical Psychology, 63, 356–60.

Agras, W. S., Telch, C. F., Arnow, B., Eldredge, K. & Marnell, M. (1997). One-year follow-up of cognitive–behavioral therapy for obese individuals with binge eating disorder. Journal of Consulting and Clinical Psychology, 65, 343–7.

Agras, W. S., Walsh, B. T., Fairburn, C. G., Wilson, G. T. & Kraemer, H. C. (2000). A multicenter comparison of cognitive–behavioral therapy and interpersonal therapy for bulimia nervosa. Archives of General Psychiatry, 57, 459–66.

Bulik, C. M., Sullivan, P. F. & Kendler, K. S. (1998). Heritability of binge-eating and broadly defined bulimia nervosa. Biological Psychiatry, 44, 1210–8.

Cattarin, J. A. & Thompson, J. K. (1994). A 3-year longitudinal study of body image, eating disturbance, and general psychological functioning in adolescent females. Eating Disorders, 2, 114–25.

Eisler, I., Dare, C., Russell, G. F. M. et al. (1997). Family and individual therapy in anorexia nervosa: a five-year follow-up. Archives of General Psychiatry, 54, 1025–30.

Fairburn, C. G., Cowen, P. J. & Harrison, P. J. (1999). Twin studies and the aetiology of eating disorders. International Journal of Eating Disorders, 26, 349–58.

Goodrick, G. K., Poston, W. S., Kimball, K. T., Reeves, R. S. & Foreyt, J. P. (1998). Nondieting versus dieting treatments for overweight binge-eating women. Journal of Consulting and Clinical Psychology, 66, 363–8.

Grilo, C. M., Masheb, R. M., Heninger, G. & Wilson, G. T. (2002). Psychotherapy and medication for binge eating disorder. Paper presented at the International Conference on Eating Disorders, Boston, MA.

Hinney, A., Bornscheuer, A., Depenbusch, M. et al. (1998). No evidence for involvement of the leptin gene in anorexia nervosa, bulimia nervosa, underweight or early onset extreme obesity: identification of two novel mutations in the coding sequence and a novel polymorphism in the leptin gene linked upstream region. *Molecular Psychiatry*, **3**, 539–43.

Hinney, A., Schmidt, A., Nottebom, K. *et al.* (1999). Several mutations in the melanocortin-4 receptor gene including a nonsense and a frameshift mutation associated with dominantly inherited obesity in humans. *Journal of Clinical Endocrinology and Metabolism*, **84**, 1483–6.

Lock, J., LeGrange, D., Agras, W. S. & Dare, C. (2001). *Treatment manual for anorexia nervosa: a family-based approach.* New York: Guilford Press.

McKnight Investigators. (2003). Risk factors for the onset of eating disorders in adolescent girls: results of the McKnight Longitudinal Risk Factor Study. *American Journal of Psychiatry*, **160**, 248–54.

Polivy, J. & Herman, C. P. (1985). Dieting and binge eating: a causal analysis. *American Psychologist*, **40**, 193–204.

Presnell, K. & Stice, E. (2003). An experimental test of the effect of weight-loss dieting on bulimic pathology: tipping the scales in a different direction. *Journal of Abnormal Psychology*, **112**, 166–70.

Safer, D. L., Telch, C. F. & Agras, W. S. (2001). Dialectical behavior therapy for bulimia nervosa. *American Journal of Psychiatry*, **4**, 632–4.

Steinglass, J. E. & Walsh, B. T. (2004). Psychopharmacology of anorexia nervosa,

bulimia nervosa, and binge eating disorder. In T. D. Brewerton (Ed.). *Clinical handbook of eating disorders: an integrated approach.* New York: Marcel Dekker.

Stice, E. (2002). Risk and maintenance factors for eating pathology: a meta-analytic review. *Psychological Bulletin*, **128**, 825–48.

Stice, E., Fisher, M. & Martinez, E. (2004). Eating disorder diagnostic scale: additional evidence of reliability and validity. *Psychological Assessment*, **16**, 60–71.

Stice, E., Presnell, K. & Bearman, S. K. (2004). Risk factors for onset of threshold and subthreshold bulimia nervosa: a 4-year prospective study of adolescent girls. Submitted.

Stice, E. & Shaw, H. (2004). Eating disorder prevention programs: a meta-analytic review. *Psychological Bulletin*, **130**, 206–27.

Telch, C. F., Agras, W. S. & Linehan, M. M. (2001). Dialectical behavior therapy for binge eating disorder. *Journal of Consulting and Clinical Psychology*, **69**, 1061–5.

Treasure, J. & Holland, A. (1989). Genetic vulnerability to eating disorders: evidence from twin and family studies. In H. Remschmidt & M. H. Schmidt (Eds.). *Child and youth psychiatry: European perspectives* (pp. 59–68). New York: Hogrefe & Huber.

Vogeltanz-Holm, N. D., Wonderlich, S. A., Lewis, B. A. *et al.* (2000). Longitudinal

predictors of binge eating, intense dieting, and weight concerns in a national sample of women. *Behavior Therapy*, **31**, 221–35.

Walters, E. E. & Kendler, K. S. (1995). Anorexia nervosa and anorexia-like syndromes in a population-based female twin sample. *American Journal of Psychiatry*, **152**, 64–71.

Wilfley, D. E., Welch, R. R., Stein, R. I. *et al.* (2002). A randomized comparison of group cognitive–behavioral therapy and group interpersonal psychotherapy for the treatment of overweight individuals with binge-eating disorder. *Archives of General Psychiatry*, **59**, 713–21.

Wilson, G. T., Becker, C. B. & Heffernan, K. (2003). Eating disorders. In E. J. Mash & R. A. Barkley (Eds.). *Child Psychopathology* (2nd edn.) (pp. 687–715). New York: Guilford.

Wonderlich, S. A., de Zwaan, M., Mitchell, J. E., Peterson, C. & Crow, S. (2003). Psychological and dietary treatments of binge eating disorder: conceptual implications. *International Journal of Eating Disorders*, **34**, 558–73.

Wonderlich, S. A., Mitchell, J. E. & Swan-Kremeier, L. (2004). An overview of cognitive–behavioral approaches to eating disorders. In T. D. Brewerton (Ed.). *Clinical handbook of eating disorders: an integrated approach.* New York: Marcel Dekker.

Eczema

David J. de L. Horne and Elizabeth A. Coombes

University of Birmingham and Cancer Centre

Introduction: prevalence and prognosis

Atopic eczema has been defined as 'an inflammatory disease, characterized by an itchy, erythmatous, poorly demarcated skin eruption, which has a predilection for the skin creases' (Williams, 1994, cited in Charman, 1999). Symptoms include intractable itching, skin damage and soreness. Where it lasts into adulthood it becomes a lifelong disease where the typical pattern is of a labile course resulting in some uncertainty and insecurity. Eczema or atopic dermatitis (AD) is a common childhood condition. It usually presents during the first year of life (Barnetson & Rogers, 2002) and in 60–70% of

cases clears up during teenage years, although relapses may occur (Charman, 1999). The remaining sufferers are older children, adolescents and adults with a chronic skin condition. Symptoms can be mild or severe, and if severe can have both physical and psychological repercussions for the sufferer and the whole family.

Eczema is probably the most common of the atopy diseases to come to the attention of psychologists and psychiatrists for treatment and may co-exist with other atopy disorders in up to 48% of cases (Diepgen & Fartasch, 1992). Eczema affects 15–20% of children in the United Kingdom and 2–3% of adults (Charman, 1999), with a rising trend of incidence of twofold to threefold over the past three decades (Barnetson & Rogers, 2002). A large cross-sectional survey of 715 033 children and adolescents, in 56 countries, revealed a range of prevalence rates from less than 2% in Iran to over 17% in Nigeria. When ethnicity was controlled for, environmental factors appeared to be of major importance (Williams *et al.*, 1999). There are difficulties, however, in accurately estimating prevalence due to a lack of consistency in measures of eczema, the use of varying age-groups and different sampling procedures (Charman, 1996).

Prognosis of eczema has been examined, mainly, via cross-sectional studies of risk factors, plus a limited number of longitudinal or follow-up studies. Vickers (1980) carried out a major study on 2000 children for 2 to 21 years, with excellent response rates to his surveys. He found that that eczema cleared up in about 90% of cases and only recurred in about 7%. Such factors as severity, birth order, method of infant feeding, ichthyosis, rhinitis or urticaria seemed to have no prognostic value. Conversely, early onset, seborrhaeic pattern and being male seemed to be good prognostic signs. Late onset, 'reversed pattern' (eczema in the antecubital and popliteal fossae, on the knees and elbows and perhaps the dorsum of the wrists and hands), co-morbid asthma and poor social environment seem to adversely affect prognosis. Why this should be so is not immediately apparent, and no adequate theoretical framework has been developed to account for such findings.

Specific features of the typical eczema patient on presentation are the itch, the erythema and sleeping problems. Itch is the main parametre and its effective control is a major prognostic sign. Various events, immunological and non-immunological, can affect the itch threshold. The scratching response has been well studied by Jordan and Whitlock (1974) who demonstrated that eczema sufferers develop conditioned itch–scratch responses more readily than controls and these responses were slow to extinguish. Emotional stress may initiate or exacerbate the itch–scratch cycle and stress management and relaxation techniques may be useful interventions (Koo & Lebwohl, 2001).

Sleep disturbances may be an issue in 'resistant' or 'severe' eczema and, certainly, itchy patients do tend to have a pattern of light, broken sleep. There has been debate as to why this is so. It can be argued that scratching behaviour itself (in response to the itch?) arouses eczema sufferers from deeper stages of sleep (Aoki *et al.*, 1991). On the other hand, the sleep pattern described is similar to that associated with depression and general inability to express a range of emotions (Tantum *et al.*, 1982) (see 'Sleep and health').

Causes of eczema

The causes of the eczema remain poorly understood (Williams, 1995). Certainly, both environmental factors (e.g. air pollution, smaller families with less exposure to infection, more pets, food allergies) and possible genetic factors (e.g. family history of atopy in two-thirds of cases (Rajka, 1986)) play significant roles.

Severity of eczema has been related to such factors as such as immunological status, level of cortisol, growth patterns, sleep patterns, family coping style, personality, etc. (e.g. Koblenzer & Koblenzer, 1988, in children; White, Horne & Varigos, 1980, in adults). Despite the difficulties in defining and quantifying

psychological stress there is some evidence linking it to exacerbation of conditions such as eczema (Koo & Lebwohl, 2001) and families with eczema sufferers have been reported as having more problems, regardless of number of life events, and a perceived lack of personal coping resources (Charman, 1996) (see 'Stress and health').

Psychological factors

Some eczema patients seem to 'over-value' some symptoms, e.g. a red face and some may describe their skin as though it had a 'mind of its own'! The need for control and frustration at the skin's unwillingness to respond may be significant factors in psychological treatment. Some patients may have difficulty in accepting that their emotions may affect the condition of their skin, but paradoxically, they may be hypersensitive to emotional issues, displaying higher levels than normal of anger (e.g. White *et al.*, 1980).

Self-monitoring of correlates with the condition of the skin is usually poor in both patients and their families, and hence recall of events associated with flare-ups can be scanty. However, recurrences are often coincidental with significant transition points in the lifespan, e.g. commencing school, marriage, a period of grief, etc. These stressful experiences may result in a reduction of the immunological system's ability to cope (e.g. Teshima *et al.*, 1982), and hence an increase in symptom severity.

Psychological variables may maintain, exacerbate or result from eczema. As a chronic disease, eczema has psychosocial implications. Having eczema, requiring special skin care can limit a child's ability to interact with peers (through restrictions or limits on physical activities such as sport or swimming). Sufferers can also feel unattractive and experience problems with self-image (Barnetson & Rogers, 2002). A general attitude of negative affectivity can make it difficult to develop and maintain rapport and adherence to treatments.

Little is known about protective factors. Why do so many young children get better (up to 90% by the age of 5 years) but a minority do not? Few, if any, medical explanations are proffered, but some psychological research suggests being male and absence of atopy in either parent may act as protective factors. Psychological factors may also influence adherence to treatment regimes. If a family is not familiar with eczema or chronic, illness they may be more inclined to attempt to actively seek treatment for eczema (e.g. Charman, 1996). Psychological considerations include maturational factors which may enable individuals to comprehend both how their disease is manifested and also how to learn better ways of coping with stress in their environment.

Medical treatment

Medical treatment (Charman, 1999) is multi-faceted and includes the use of both oral and topical steroids (sometimes in combination with antimicrobial steroids), emollient creams, wet dressings, phototherapy and allergen avoidance (e.g. dietary manipulation, or control of house-dust mites). Steroids are effective in the short-term but prolonged use is a problem because of unwanted side effects, such as general immunosuppression and damage to the skin.

However treatments are palliative rather than curative; and although around three-quarters of children may be clear of eczema by their teens, relapses do occur (McHenry *et al.*, 1995).

Psychological interventions

At this stage of our knowledge, the impact of psychosocial issues in terms of disease complexity and utilization of health facilities is limited, but they could be critical in determining effective long-term treatment (Charman, 1996).

Having eczema involves living with a chronic disease/illness, coping with the physical and emotional impact of unpleasant and aggressive treatment regimes, impact on family, self-image and ability to lead a 'normal' life. The challenge for psychology is to tailor interventions to the individual to address some or all of these phenomena.

There is beginning to be evidence that combining psychological interventions with conventional medical treatments can certainly ameliorate symptoms and enhance quality of life. However, most of the reported research has involved small groups of sufferers and lacks adequate controls.

A systemic perspective can consider factors relevant to where and when a patient opts to attend for treatment, probable compliance with treatment regimes and potential co-morbidities. Those who attend hospital-based specialty clinics and seek additional services have been reported as experiencing more stress, less emotional support and significantly more depression, anger, anxiety and subjective distress than those attending a general dermatology clinic or private practitioner.

Cognitive–behaviour therapy has been reported as useful in several studies of eczema sufferers (Halford & Miller, 1992; Horne *et al.*, 1989). Interventions include the use of biofeedback, relaxation, habit-reversal and so on (see 'Biofeedback', 'Cognitive behaviour therapy' and 'Relaxation training'). More recent research has shown that training in self-monitoring of symptom severity and change associated with environmental effects (both internal, such as the patient's own feelings (especially of itchiness) and thoughts; and external such as specific stressful situations at work or home) combined with habit-reversal (e.g. closing hands for three minutes to prevent scratching when feeling itchy) can be effective (Borge, 1994) (see 'Self-management'). Relaxation training also seems to be of benefit, especially when combined with self-monitoring and habit-reversal. One of the authors (DH) has used these three elements regularly in treating adult eczema patients and has found that patient-induced relaxing imagery of a soothing scene, such as a gentle breeze over water (such as a lake or the sea) can be more effective than relaxation without such autogenic imagery (Horne *et al.*, 1999).

Successfully counteracting the itch–scratch habit seems to be a key factor, especially for children. Sleep disturbance may trigger other physical, emotional and social problems and lead to irritability, poor concentration and less energy for play and other social activities (Fennessy *et al.*, 2000).

Some sufferers may have more profound emotional problems; for example, childhood sexual abuse. These effects may last into adulthood and require more intensive therapy (Horne *et al.*, 1989).

Family intervention may be effective to reduce the child's scratching behaviour by, for example, activity scheduling and non-contingent attention. Gil *et al.* (1988) found that parent responses, i.e. contingent physical touching and/or contingent attention to scratching behaviour in children, were important predictors of scratching behaviour even after controlling for demographic and medical status variables (see 'Behaviour therapy').

Psychological intervention allows patients to gain an important understanding of the relationships between stressors in their lives and flare-ups in their skin. This combined with the effective prevention of scratching the skin through habit-reversal, does seem to allow eczema patients to both lower their baseline levels of scratching and to take immediate, effective ameliorative measures when a flare-up does occur with consequent reduction in both oral steroid and more topical treatments (Horne *et al.*, 1989).

Recognition of the impact of psychosocial issues on eczema sufferers is a welcome step forward. But more good quality research is needed to explore the social, material and emotional impact of eczema on patients of all ages. Good communication between health professionals and patients is a key starting point. In addition, psychological interventions seem to have much to contribute: however, the majority of studies are small-scale and lack good controls.

Conclusions

Clinical judgements of disease severity tend to be contaminated by other clinical observations, based upon the patient's age, gender and estimated compliance. These judgements seem to influence decisions about treatment.

The first step in psychological therapy is to reassure the eczema sufferer that they have a real bodily illness with real discomfit, but also to help them realize that their thoughts, emotions and behaviours can be both a reaction to the illness but also influence its course.

Self-monitoring of factors leading to increased itchiness and scratching appears to be effective in increasing awareness of symptoms and their relationship to the patient's life. The addition of habit–reversal and relaxation training (particularly incorporating relaxing imagery), once a self-monitoring baseline has been established, appears to be an effective therapeutic intervention. However, for patients who do not respond to this 'package', more intensive psychological treatment may be warranted.

The role of psychological factors in understanding and treating people with eczema and other skin disorders has made some progress in recent years but generally the research is limited to case studies or small group studies, often with inadequate controls.

(See also 'Children's perceptions of illness and death' and 'Skin disorders'.)

Acknowledgements

The authors wish to acknowledge the ongoing collaboration and encouragement provided by Dr. George Varigos, the Senior Dermatologist at the Royal Melbourne Hospital, Australia, and also of Dr. Denise Charman of the Victoria University of Technology, Melbourne, Australia, whose Ph.D. studies greatly contributed to this chapter.

REFERENCES

Aoki, T., Kushimoto, H., Hishikawa, Y. & Savin, J. A. (1991). Nocturnal scratching and its relationship to the disturbed sleep of itchy subjects. *Clinical and Experimental Dermatology,* **16,** 268–72.

Barnetson, R. St. C. & Rogers, M. (2002). Childhood atopic eczema: clinical review. *British Medical Journal,* **324,** 1376–9.

Borge, A. (1994). *Behaviour therapy for skin disorders.* MSc thesis, University of Melbourne, Australia.

Charman, C. (1999). Atopic eczema: clinical review: clinical evidence. *British Medical Journal,* **318,** 1600–4.

Charman, D. P. (1996). *Patterns in atopic dermatitis: developing models to predict hospital utilization patterns in young children.* Unpublished PhD thesis, University of Melbourne. Australia.

Diepgen, T. L. & Fartasch, M. (1992). Recent epidemiological and genetic studies in atopic dermatitis. *Acta-Dermatologia Venerologia (Suppl.) Stockholm,* **176,** 13–18.

Fennessy, M., Coupland, S., Popsy, J. & Naysmith, K. (2000). The epidemiology and experience of atopic eczema during childhood: a discussion paper on the implications of current knowledge for health care, public health policy and research. *Journal of Epidemiology and Community Health,* **54,** 581–9.

Gil, K. M., Keefe, A., Sampson, H. A. *et al.* (1988). Direct observation of scratching behaviour in children with atopic dermatitis. *Behaviour Therapy,* **19,** 213–27.

Halford, K. & Miller, S. (1992). Cognitive behavioural stress management as treatment of atopic dermatitis: a case study. *Behaviour Change,* **9**(1), 19–24.

Horne, D. J. de L., Taylor, M. & Varigos, G. (1999). The effects of relaxation with and without imagery in reducing anxiety and itchy skin in patients with eczema. *Behavioural and Cognitive Psychotherapy,* **27,** 143–51.

Horne, D. J. de L., White, A. E. & Varigos, G. A. (1989). A preliminary study of psychological therapy in the management of atopic eczema. *British Journal of Medical Psychology,* **62,** 241–8.

Jordan, J. M. & Whitlock, F. A. (1974). Atopic dermatitis anxiety and conditioned scratch responses in cases of atopic dermatitis. *British Journal of Dermatology,* **86,** 574–85.

Koblenzer, C. S. & Koblenzer, P. J. (1988). Chronic intractable atopic eczema. *Archives of Dermatology,* **124,** 1673–7.

Koo, J. & Lebwohl, A. (2001). Psychodermatology: the mind and skin connection. *American Family Physician,* **64,** 1873–8.

McHenry, P. M., Williams, H. C. & Bingham, E. A. (1995). Management of atopic eczema. *British Medical Journal,* **310,** 843–53.

Rajka, G. (1986). Natural history and clinical manifestations of atopic dermatitis. *Clinical Review Allergy,* **4,** 650–5.

Tantum, D., Kalvey, R. & Brown, D. G. (1982). Sleep, scratching and dreams in eczema. *Psychotherapy Psychosomatic,* **37,** 26–35.

Teshima, H., Kubo, C., Kihara, H. *et al.* (1982). Psychosomatic aspects of skin diseases from the standpoint of immunology. *Psychotherapy Psychosomatic,* **37,** 165–75.

Vickers, C. H. F. (1980). The natural history of atopic eczema. *Acta Dermatologia Venercologia (Suppl.),* **92,** 113–15.

White, A., Horne, D. J. de L. & Varigos, G. A. (1980). The psychological profile of the atopic eczema patient. *Australasian Journal of Dermatology,* **31,** 13–16.

Williams, H. C. (1995). Atopic Eczema. *British Medical Journal,* **311,** 1241–3.

Williams, H., Robertson, C., Stewart, A. *et al.* (1999). Worldwide variations in the prevalence of symptoms of atopic eczema in the International Study of Asthma and Allergies in Childhood. *Journal of Allergy & Clinical Immunology,* **103,** 125–38.

Endocrine disorders

Eric A. Storch and Gary R. Geffken

University of Florida

Psychiatric symptomatology related to endocrine disorders

Psychiatric symptoms are commonly present during the course of endocrine disorders, which complicates diagnostic decisions. Common symptoms across endocrine diagnoses include affective disturbances (e.g. depression, anxiety), cognitive dysfunction, dementia, delirium and psychosis. This article provides a review of the psychiatric morbidity within endocrine disorders. Conditions associated with dysfunction of the pituitary, thyroid, parathyroid, adrenals and gonads are reviewed, as well as diabetes mellitus.

Disorders of the thyroid

Hypothyroidism

Hypothyroidism is the most common pathological hormone deficiency and can be classified on the basis of its time of onset (congenital or acquired), level of endocrine dysfunction responsible (primary or secondary) and severity (overt or mild). Overt hypothyroidism has been associated with symptoms such as energy loss, weight gain, slowed reflexes, cold intolerance, weight gain, constipation, dry skin, bradycardia, hoarseness and slowed cognitive processing. However, as many as 60–70% of newly diagnosed patients do not experience significant symptomatology (Ladenson et al., 1997). Those with mild hypothyroidism also often do not have symptoms.

Psychiatric and neurological manifestations can include depression (Ladenson et al., 1997), anxiety (Sait Gonen et al., 2004), psychosis (Alp et al., 2004), ataxia (Price & Netsky, 1966), seizures (Woods & Holmes, 1977) and coma (Nicoloff & LoPresti, 1993). Overt hypothyroidism commonly manifests itself with cognitive impairment and depression. Psychiatric symptoms progress in a gradual course of neurocognitive deficits beginning with mental slowing followed by cognitive disturbances (e.g. short-term memory problems) and depression. In most instances, psychiatric symptoms remit with thyroid hormone replacement, although improvement may take weeks or months.

Hyperthyroidism

Excessive amounts of circulating thyroid hormone result in thyrotoxicosis. Thyrotoxicosis may result from thyroid gland hyperactivity, ingestion of high levels of thyroid hormone or secretion of thyroid hormone for an ectopic site (Greenspan, 1997). Diffuse toxic goiter, also known as Grave's disease, is the most common form of hyperthyroidism. Generalized anxiety states, as well as symptoms similar to panic disorder, have been observed in hyperthyroidism (Sait Gonen et al., 2004). There are also links with mania and hypomania, depression, obsessive–compulsive symptoms and organic states such as delirium, although these presentations tend to be infrequent (Radanovic-Grguric et al., 2003). Other clinical manifestations include restlessness, fatigue, tremor, weight loss, irritability, emotional liability and insomnia (see also 'Hyperthyroidism').

Disorders of the parathyroid

Hyperparathyroidism

Primary hyperparathyroidism, a common cause of hypercalcaemia due to hypersecretion of parathyroid hormone (PTH), is typically linked to hypophosphatemia and elevated serum chloride levels. Hyperparathyroidism may also be secondary to renal failure. Symptomatic presentations of this disorder are characterized by the presence of kidney stones, bone disease and neuromuscular weakness (Bilezikian & Silverberg, 2004). However, as many as 60% of patients are asymptomatic (Takami et al., 2003). Weakness, fatigue, intellectual weariness, poor memory, decreased attention and depression, all of which are often difficult to detect or are mistaken for having different aetiologies, may present as initial signs of the disorder (Silverberg, 2002). Psychotic symptoms (e.g. paranoid delusions, hallucinations) and delirium have also been reported (Papa et al., 2003).

The type and severity of psychiatric symptoms have been related to serum calcium levels (Leigh & Kramer, 1984). Mood and cognitive symptoms have been linked to serum calcium levels of 12 to 16 mg/dL (normal levels range from 8.9 to 10.1 mg/dL). Delirium and psychotic symptoms are linked to levels of 16–19 mg/dL, and somnolence and coma develop in levels exceeding 19 mg/dL.

Hypoparathyroidism

The causes of hypoparathyroidism vary, representing disruptions of one or more of the steps in the development and maintenance of parathyroid hormone secretion. Injury to or removal of the parathyroid glands during neck surgery is the most common cause of acute or chronic hypoparathyroidism, although familial and autoimmune links have been reported (Marx, 2000). Dementia has been reported in cases of hypoparathyroidism (Levine & Gaoni, 1990). Cognitive disturbances and intellectual impairment have been reported as well (Kowdley et al., 1999) (see also 'Dementias').

Disorders of the adrenal system

Hypercortisolism

A chronic excess of glucocorticoids causes Cushing's syndrome. The pathogenetic mechanisms of Cushing's can be divided into corticotropin (adrenocorticotropic hormone)-dependent (from a pituitary or ectopic source) and corticotropin-independent (Boscaro et al., 2001). 'Cushing's disease', which accounts for 60–90% of the cases, is generally due to an over-production of corticotropin from a pituitary adenoma. As many as 85% of patients present with psychiatric symptoms and/or cognitive dysfunction. Common conditions include depression (Sonino & Fava, 2001), generalized anxiety disorder and panic disorder (Loosen et al., 1992). Bipolar disorder, including manic and hypomanic episodes, has been reported in 30% of patients with Cushing's syndrome (Sonino & Fava, 2001). Approximately 60% of patients have varying degrees of diffuse bilateral cerebral dysfunction, with overt impairment in nonverbal, visual–memory and graphomotor abilities (Mauri et al., 1993). Difficulties with concentration, forgetfulness, reasoning ability, comprehension and processing of new information have been also reported (Forget et al., 2000).

Hypocortisolism

The mechanisms involved in the development of hypocortisolism are unclear. Alterations on several levels of the hypothalamic–pituitary–adrenal (HPA) axis may contribute to the presence of hypocortisolism. Other factors, such as genetics, gender or early stress experiences, may also contribute to its development. Hypocortisolism for patients who have experienced a traumatic event and subsequently developed post-traumatic stress disorder has been reported (Yehuda, 1997). Hypocortisolism has also been reported in healthy individuals who endured ongoing stress (Caplan et al., 1979). Hypocortisolism has also been reported for patients suffering from bodily disorders, such as burnout with physical complaints, chronic fatigue syndrome, fibromyalgia and asthma among others (Demitrack et al., 1991; Crofford et al., 1994) (see 'Post-traumatic stress disorder', 'Chronic fatigue syndrome' and 'Asthma'). Other clinical symptoms include weakness, fatigue, loss of appetite, depression, apathy, irritability, anhedonia, poverty of thought and social withdrawal (Brown, 1975). Although psychotic symptoms and delirium have been reported, some psychotropic medications tend to exacerbate hypotension symptoms and thus, are contraindicated (Stern & Prange, 1991).

Diabetes mellitus

Diabetes mellitus (DM) is a highly prevalent, chronic disease with a prevalence of diagnosed and undiagnosed cases to be approximately 16 million cases (Harris et al., 1998). Of these people, approximately 90–95% have Type II diabetes (Harris, 1995). DM is a complex and challenging disease due to the necessary integration of daily medical tasks (e.g. blood glucose monitoring) and lifestyle modifications. The stress of having a serious chronic illness, taken with the rigorous nature of the diabetic treatment protocol, predisposes some to adjustment difficulties (Cox & Gonder-Frederick, 1992) (see 'Diabetes mellitus').

Although some inconsistencies exist, studies have generally shown an increased psychiatric morbidity among individuals with Types I and II diabetes (see Geffken et al., 1998 for a review), particularly with regard to individuals in poor metabolic control (Lustman et al., 1986). The most common psychiatric diagnosis is depression, with reports in adults estimating rates between 8.5% to 27.3% (Goldney et al., 2004). However, the aetiological nature of this condition is unclear and it is probably multi-determined. Anxiety disorders, particularly specific phobias (e.g. needle phobia), are also commonly found (Dantzer et al., 2003). Again, anxiety is likely due to multiple causes, including neuronal and structural damage secondary to hypoglycaemia (Auer, 1986), classical conditioning (Sheehan & Sheehan, 1982) and stress related to chronic disease management.

Disorders of growth

Growth hormone (GH) is produced by the anterior pituitary gland and impacts physical stature. In children, GH excess is linked to gigantism, whereas deficiency produces short stature or dwarfism. In adults, GH excess causes acromegaly; GH deficiency is not linked to specific physical stigmata.

In childhood clinic-referred samples, numerous psychological problems have been related to short stature, including low self-esteem (Csapo, 1991), increased rates of externalizing (e.g. impulsive, easily distracted, attention-seeking; Storch et al., 2005) and internalizing behaviours (e.g. anxiety, somatic complaints; Holmes et al., 1985) and poor social competency (Downey et al., 1997). Among non-referred children, however, data have failed to support the hypothesis that short stature is related to psychosocial adjustment (Downie et al., 1997). The effects of short stature are thought to extend to later life as adults who were diagnosed with short stature during childhood report greater psychological problems (e.g. depression, social withdrawal, social phobia; Stabler et al., 1996) and academic, occupational and social impairment related to their short stature (Crowne et al., 1990). Pituitary gigantism has been linked to depression by some (Margo, 1981), but not others (Abed et al., 1987).

Reproductive disturbances

Hyperprolactinaemia

Hyperprolactinaemia is a common endocrine disorder of the hypothalamic-pituitary axis (Petty, 1999). Common causes of hyperprolactinaemia include pituitary adenomas, chronic renal failure primary and dopamine receptor antagonists such as antipsychotic drugs. There are a range of clinical consequences of chronic hyperprolactinaemia including, sexual dysfunction (e.g. diminished libido, decreased arousal, orgasmic dysfunction, impotence), reproductive dysfunction (e.g. anovulation, irregular menstrual cycles, subfertility, decreased oestrogen, decreased testosterone) and psychiatric and cognitive symptoms including depression, memory deficits and psychosis. Hyperprolactinaemia development and exacerbation has been linked with the use of conventional antipsychotic medications (Kinon et al., 2003) and risperidone (Tran et al., 1997) (see also 'Sexual dysfunction').

Gonadal dysfunction

Hypogonadism in men can be of a primary (directly involving the testes) or secondary (involving the hypothalamic–pituitary axis) nature. Prior to puberty, hypogonadism is linked to failure to develop male sex characteristics; after puberty, it may result in decreased libido, muscle mass and sexual dysfunction. Klinefelter's syndrome, the most common cause of primary gonadal failure, has been associated with a range of psychiatric disturbances including personality changes, and mood and psychotic disorders (Wakeling, 1972). Turner's syndrome, a sex chromosome abnormality with a female phenotype, has been linked with factors that may interfere with healthy psychosocial adjustment (e.g. short stature, sexual infantilism) (Downey et al., 1989) (see also 'Chromosomal abnormalities').

REFERENCES

Abed, R. T., Clark, J., Elbadawy, M. H. F. *et al.* (1987). Psychiatric morbidity in acromegaly. *Acta Psychiatrica Scandinavia*, **75**, 635–9.

Alp, R., Saygin, M., Ucisik, M. *et al.* (2004). Initial presentation of Hashimoto's thyroiditis with psychotic symptoms: a case report. *Bulletin of Clinical Psychopharmacology*, **14**, 83–7.

Auer, R. N. (1986). Progress review: hypoglycemic brain damage. *Stroke*, **17**, 699–708.

Bilezikian, J. P. & Silverberg, S. J. (2004). Asymptomatic primary hyperparathyroidism. *New England Journal of Medicine*, **350**, 1746–51.

Boscaro, M., Barzon, L., Fallo, F. *et al.* (2001). Update on Cushing's syndrome. *Lancet*, **357**, 783–91.

Brown, G. M. (1975). Psychiatric and neurologic aspects of endocrine disease. *Hospital Practice*, **10**, 71–9.

Caplan, R. D., Cobb, S. & French, J. R. (1979). White collar work load and cortisol: disruption of a circadian rhythm by job stress? *Journal of Psychosomatic Research*, **23**, 181–92.

Cox, D. J. & Gonder-Frederick, L. (1992). Major developments in behavioral diabetes research. *Journal of Consulting and Clinical Psychology*, **60**, 628–38.

Crofford, L. J., Pillemer, S. R., Kalogeras, K. T. *et al.* (1994). Hypothalamic-pituitary-adrenal axis perturbations in patients with fibromyalgia. *Arthritis Rheumatoid*, **37**, 1583–92.

Crowne, E. C., Shalet, S. M., Wallace, W. H. B. *et al.* (1990). Final height in boys with untreated constitutional delay in growth and puberty. *Archives of Disorders in Children*, **65**, 1109–12.

Csapo, M. (1991). Psychosocial adjustment of children with short stature (achondroplasia): social competence, behavior problems, self-esteem, family functioning, body image, and reaction to frustrations. *Behavior Disorders*, **16**, 219–24.

Dantzer, C., Swendsen, J., Maurice-Tison, S. *et al.* (2003). Anxiety and depression in juvenile diabetes. A critical review. *Clinical Psychology Review*, **23**, 787–800.

Demitrack, M. A., Dale, J. K., Straus, S. E. *et al.* (1991). Evidence for impaired activation of the hypothalamic–pituitary–adrenal axis in patients with chronic fatigue syndrome. *Journal of Clinical Endocrinology and Metabolism*, **73**, 1224–34.

Downey, J., Ehrhardt, A. A., Gruen, R. *et al.* (1989). Psychopathology and social functioning in women with Turner syndrome. *Journal of Nervous and Mental Disease*, **177**, 191–201.

Downie, A. B., Mulligan, J., Stratford, R. J. *et al.* (1997). Are short normal children at a disadvantage? The Wessex Growth Study. *British Medical Journal*, **314**, 97–100.

Forget, H., Lacroix, A., Somma, M. *et al.* (2000). Cognitive decline in patients with Cushing's syndrome. *Journal of the International Neuropsychological Society*, **6**, 20–9.

Geffken, G. R., Ward, H. E., Staab, J. P. *et al.* (1998). Psychiatric morbidity in endocrine disorders. *The Psychiatric Clinics of North America*, **21**, 473–80.

Goldney, R. D., Phillips, P. J., Fisher, L. J. *et al.* (2004). Diabetes, depression, and quality of life: a population study. *Diabetes Care*, **27**, 1066–70.

Greenspan, F. S. (1997). The thyroid gland. In F. S. Greenspan, G. J. Strewler (Eds.). *Basic and Clinical Endocrinology* (5th edn.). Stamford, CT: Appleton & Lange.

Harris, M. I. (1995). *Diabetes in america* (2nd edn.) NIH Publication No. 95–1468, pp. 1–14. National Diabetes Data Group, National Institutes of Health, National Institute of Diabetes and Digestive and Kidney Diseases.

Harris, M. I., Flegal, K. M., Cowie, C. C. *et al.* (1998). Prevalence of diabetes, impaired fasting glucose, and impaired glucose tolerance in US adults: the Third National Health and Nutrition Examination Survey, 1988–1994. *Diabetes Care*, **21**, 518–24.

Holmes, C. S., Karlsson, J. A. & Thompson, R. G. (1985). Social and school competencies in children with short stature: longitudinal patterns. *Journal of Developmental and Behavioral Pediatrics*, **6**, 263–7.

Kowdley, K., Coull, B. M. & Orwoll, E. S. (1999). Cognitive impairment and intracranial calcification in chronic hypoparathyroidism. *American Journal of Medical Science*, **317**, 273–7.

Kinon, B. J., Gilmore, J. A., Liu, H. *et al.* (2003). Prevalence of hyperprolactinemia in schizophrenic patients treated with conventional antipsychotic medications or risperidone. *Psychoneuroendocrinology*, **28** (S2), 55–68.

Ladenson, P. W., Braverman, L. E., Mazzaferri, E. L. *et al.* (1997). Comparison of recombinant human thyrotropin administration to thyroid hormone withdrawal for radioactive iodine scanning in patients with thyroid carcinoma. *New England Journal of Medicine*, **337**, 888–96.

Leigh, H. & Kramer, S. I. (1984). The psychiatric manifestation of endocrine disorders. *Advances in Internal Medicine*, **29**, 413–45.

Levine, Y. & Gaoni, B. (1990). The hypoparathyroid syndrome: psychiatric observations and case description. *Israel Journal of Psychiatry and Related Sciences*, **27**, 242–6.

Loosen, P. T., Chanbliss, B., DeBold, C. R. *et al.* (1992). Psychiatric phenomenology in Cushing's disease. *Pharmacopsychiatry*, **25**, 192–8.

Lustman, P. J., Griffith, L. S., Clouse, R. E. *et al.* (1986). Psychiatric illness in diabetes mellitus: relationship to symptoms and glucose control. *Journal of Nervous and Mental Disease*, **174**, 735–42.

Margo, A. (1981). Acromegaly and depression. *British Journal of Psychiatry*, **139**, 467–8.

Marx, S. J. (2000). Hyperparathyroid and hypoparathyroid disorders. *New England Journal of Medicine*, **343**, 1863–75.

Mauri, M., Sinforiani, E., Bono, G. *et al.* (1993). Memory impairment in Cushing's disease. *Acta Neurological Scandinavia*, **87**, 52–5.

Nicoloff, J. T. & LoPresti, J. S. (1993). Myxedema coma: a form of decompensated hypothyroidism. *Endocrinology Metabolic Clinics of North America*, **22**, 279–90.

Papa, A., Bononi, F., Sciubba, S. *et al.* (2003). Primary hyperparathyroidism: acute paranoid psychosis. *American Journal of Emergency Medicine*, **21**, 250–1.

Petty, R. G. (1999). Prolactin and antipsychotic medications: mechanism of action. *Schizophrenia Research*, **35**, S67–S73.

Price, T. R. & Netsky, M. G. (1966). Myxedema and ataxia: cerebellar alterations and "neural myxedema bodies". *Neurology*, **16**, 957–62.

Radanovic-Grguric, L., Filakovic, P., Jelena, B. *et al.* (2003). Depression in patients with thyroid dysfunction. *European Journal of Psychiatry*, **17**, 133–44.

Sait Gonen, M., Kisakol, G., Savas Cilli, A. *et al.* (2004). Assessment of anxiety in subclinical thyroid disorders. *Endocrinology Journal*, **51**, 311–15.

Sheehan, D. V. & Sheehan, K. H. (1982). The classification of anxiety and hysterical states: towards a more heuristic classification. *Journal of Clinical Psychopharmacology*, **2**, 386–93.

Silverberg, S. J. (2002). Non-classical target organs in hyperparathyroidism. *Journal of Bone and Mineral Research*, **17** (Suppl. 2), N117–125.

Sonino, N. & Fava, G. A. (2001). Psychiatric disorders associated with Cushing's syndrome. Epidemiology, pathophysiology, and treatment. *CNS Drugs*, **15**, 361–73.

Stabler, B., Clopper, R. R., Siegel, P. T. *et al.* (1996). Links between growth hormone deficiency, adaptation, and social phobia. *Hormone Research*, **45**, 30–3.

Stern, R. & Prange, A. (1991). Neuropsychiatric aspects of endocrine disorders. In H. Kaplan & B. Sadock (Eds.). *Comprehensive textbook of psychiatry*. Baltimore: Williams and Wilkins.

Storch, E. A., Lewin, A., Silverstein, J. H. *et al.* (2005). Psychological adjustment of children with short stature: a comparison of children with short stature and type one diabetes. *Journal of Pediatric Endocrinology and Metabolism*, **18**, 395–401.

Takami, H., Ikeda, Y., Okinaga, H. *et al.* (2003). Recent advances in the management of primary hyperparathyroidism. *Endocrine Journal*, **50**, 369–77.

Tran, P. V., Hamilton, S. H., Kuntz, A. J. *et al.* (1997). Double-blind comparison of olanzapine versus risperidone in the treatment of schizophrenia and other psychotic disorders. *Journal of Clinical Psychopharmacology*, **17**, 407–18.

Wakeling, A. (1972). Comparative study of psychiatric patients with Klinefelter's syndrome and hypogonadism. *Psychological Medicine*, **3**, 139–54.

Woods, K. L. & Holmes, G. K. (1977). Myxoedema coma presenting in status epilepticus. *Postgraduate Medicine Journal*, **53**, 46–8.

Yehuda, R. (1997). Sensitization of the hypothalamic-pituitary-adrenal axis in posttraumatic stress disorder. *Annals of the New York Academy of Science*, **821**, 57–75.

Enuresis

Martin Herbert

Exeter University

Diagnosis

The term 'enuresis' is used when a child, beyond the age of antici- pated bladder control and socially correct toileting behaviour, uri- nates into clothing or other inappropriate places. The defining age is usually considered to be five years. Whether the urinating is inten- tional or involuntary is not relevant to the general diagnosis. However, involuntary urination during the night, in a child who has never ceased to wet the bed (or has lost a previously acquired skill) is referred to as 'nocturnal enuresis', and colloquially as 'bed- wetting'. Nocturnal enuresis is one of the commonest reasons for families seeking help from primary care physicians. The problem was referred to as early as the sixteenth century in *The boke of chyldren* by Thomas Phaire, in a chapter entitled 'Of pissing in the bedde'.

'Diurnal enuresis' is the term for involuntary daytime urination. It occurs in approximately 1 in 10 of the children with nocturnal enuresis. A distinction is also made between children who are 'reg- ular' and those who are 'intermittent' bedwetters. Most enuretic children have what is called 'primary' nocturnal enuresis, meaning that they have wet their beds since toddlerhood. 'Secondary' enure- sis is the term applied to children who revert to bedwetting after a sustained period of dry beds. Although urinary tract infections or diabetes may play a role in secondary enuresis, it is often impossible to identify any specific medical cause. It may, however, be asso- ciated with psychological causes such as problems at home (e.g. a divorce) school (e.g. bullying), or other life stresses that precipitate a regression.

Assessment

Although most children with enuresis are physically normal, they will usually (and preferably) be physically examined by a primary care physician or paediatrician to exclude medical conditions. The doctor may arrange for urine tests to check for infections or other abnormalities, if any disorders are suspected. Constipation is some- times associated with enuresis, occasionally involving soiling of underwear ('encopresis') in serious cases. Usually, mild constipation is remedied by simple dietary measures, but severe cases of consti- pation may require intensive treatment before the enuresis can be tackled. Primary enuresis may be associated with other disorders such as attention deficit hyperactivity disorder (ADHD) and sickle cell anaemia (Herbert, 2003) (see 'Hyperactivity' and 'Sickle cell disease').

Children with enuresis are at risk of having, or developing emo- tional and behaviour problems. Clinical psychologists have the par- ticular behavioural skills that are needed for assessing and treating

enuresis, and (if required) encopresis. Some cases continue (if untreated) into late adolescence and even adulthood.

Toilet training: incidence of bedwetting

A child might be considered toilet trained when s/he is able to use the toilet (or potty) reasonably independently, perhaps with assis- tance over adjusting clothing. There is much variation in the age at which children achieve control between and within different cul- tures. Knowledge of the norms (averages) in typical development, while bearing in mind that there is a wide range of individual differ- ences, might help parents feel more relaxed about the 'implicit' timetable for the development of continence. There is no one age at which children cease to wet the bed (see Murphy & Carr, 2000).

Control of the bowels is attained before bladder control. The developmental sequence is generally as follows:

1. bowel control at night
2. bowel control during the day
3. bladder control during the day
4. bladder control at night.

The sequence may vary for children; some achieve bowel and bladder control 'simultaneously'. Girls tend to be quicker than boys in becoming continent. Lack of control is frequently seen in children in residential establishments.

Causation

Causation in enuresis is multifactorial, involving medical, develop- mental, psychosocial, or genetic causes factors (see Butler, 1998; Clayden *et al.*, 2002):

1. *Medical causes* of enuresis might include (*inter alia*), urinary tract infection, diabetes, urinary tract obstruction, or neurogenic blad- der (i.e. a bladder with impaired nerve function). Physiological causes may involve small functional bladder capacity, or a deficit in the amount of antidiuretic hormone (ADH) produced. The presence of this hormone concentrates urine and prevents the bladder from filling up during sleep. Among uncommon physical causes are chronic renal or kidney disease, diabetes, tumours and seizures. Such potentially important causes should make an expert physical examination a matter of routine.
2. *Developmental influences*: some enuretic children suffer from developmental delays other than incontinence; also an above average likelihood of a learning disability. (Herbert, 2003). A high level of 'skill' is needed before the bladder can be controlled

during sleep, so it is perhaps not surprising that some children do not achieve it with ease, especially when disabled or under stress.

3. *Psychosocial causes* (see Herbert, 2003): enuresis may have its origins in faulty learning. Some cases of enuresis are related to toilet training that was begun too early, or carried out in a very forcible manner. Young children lack a sufficiently mature signalling mechanism between the bladder and the brain to become aware of a full bladder. Consequently, they fail to wake up and wet the bed. Punishment is inappropriate. In fact, children with enuresis are most likely to have their toilet training initiated late. Enuresis may be an adjustment problem (notably in the sensitive period when the child is trying to learn control) as a result of high levels of life-stress. Both harsh 'pressurizing' of the child, or (conversely) complacent neglect of training, may lead to the failure of this development. Parents who are very controlling and quick to find fault may also trigger problems with bladder control (Table 1) (Herbert, 1996). Emotional problems may be superimposed when the child is made to feel acute shame at his or her 'babyish' ways. Children at risk of becoming bedwetters (mainly girls) tend to come from lower socioeconomic groups, and from large families living in overcrowded conditions. Mothers who give birth as teenagers constitute a further predisposing factor. In most cases, the causal mechanisms that underlie the risk factors (causal associations) are not known.

4. *Genetics*: enuresis often runs in families. Of children with nocturnal enuresis, 70% have a parent who was late in becoming dry. About twice as many boys as girls suffer from enuresis. The concordance rate for identical twins is 68% and 36% for fraternal (non-identical) twins. Molecular genetic evidence has not yet implicated a single gene. The most likely conclusion in our present state of knowledge is that the genetic influence in nocturnal enuresis is heterogeneous. (Clayden et al., 2002).

Enuresis in adults

Nocturnal enuresis in adulthood is probably related to a nerve problem that affects bladder function, or a problem with the hormonal secretion by a gland at the base of the brain. A urological examination is likely to include an evaluation for a structural (anatomic) abnormality. There are medications (depending upon the cause of the problem) that can remedy the incontinence, treatment that may possibly have to be taken for a lifetime in order to remain effective. Young adults (teenagers) with enuresis often have a parent who had the same problem at about the same age.

Table 1. Frequency of bedwetting

Age in years	Approximate number of children in every 100 who wet the bed
2	75
3	40
4	30
5	20
6–9	12
10–12	5
15	1–2

Treatment

The treatment of enuresis falls into three categories: counselling; behavioural methods; and medication. Often, more than one treatment is used at the same time (see reviews of methods and their effectiveness by Butler, 1998; Clayden et al., 2002; Doleys, 1977a,b; Murphy & Carr, 2000; Ondersma & Walker, 1998; Shaffer, 1994; Walker, 1995). The evidence suggests that:

(i) counselling: alone this is rarely effective.

(ii) behavioural treatments are generally effective; these include:

    a. incentives (tangible and symbolic rewards) for achieving bladder control;

    b. bladder training such as graduated delay of bladder emptying to increase bladder control;

    c. conditioning methods, such as a urine alarm that wakens the child when s/he wets a pad to which it is connected;

    d. decreasing fluids taken at night;

    e. teaching the child to attend and respond to bladder sensations at night.

The most successful treatments available are the 'urine alarm' and 'dry bed' systems. The urine alarm system attaches a moisture sensor attached to the child's night-time underwear, and a small speaker on a bedside table or on the shoulder of the child. A very small amount of urine activates a loud alarm that causes the child to tense reflexly, thus inhibiting the flow of urine. The parent escorts the younger child to the toilet in order to complete the urinating. Adherence to this programme should produce a positive outcome, with the child waking up 'unprompted' after 4 to 6 weeks of treatment. Reliable bladder control is usually achieved after around 12 weeks of training. At such a time the backup alarm is no longer required. Many clinicians prefer to begin treatment with the use of incentive sticker (reward) charts, adding a urine alarm if the child does not respond to this so-called 'operant method'.

The evidence for the superiority of the urine alarm method (with rates of remission between 80 and 90%) over no-treatment and other-treatment control procedures, is well documented for nocturnal enuresis (e.g. Doleys, 1977a,b). Although there was an average relapse rate of 40%; nearly 60% of these returned to continence after booster sessions. In another study of 127 enuretic children (Van Londen et al., 1995), 97% in a urine alarm programme which was supplemented with immediate contingency (operant/rewards) management, were continent compared with 84% of the group that received delayed contingency management and 73% who received a routine enuresis alarm programme. Only 8% of the first group had deteriorated after two-and-a half years (see 'Behaviour therapy').

A meta-analysis of 78 studies by Houts et al. (1994), while reporting that the highest success rates for psychological programmes were those using urine alarms, also found the alarm method to be no more effective than the medical treatments (tricyclics and desmopressin) at post-treatment. However, they were significantly superior at follow-up.

(iii) medication: Tricyclic drugs (somewhat out of favour because of adverse side effects and poor results) and desmopressin are used in the treatment of enuresis. Desmopressin is available as a nasal spray administered before bedtime. Continence is achieved relatively quickly in 70% of children; another 10% show significant improvement. It is only effective while the child is on medication; relapse occurs when it is discontinued. Children require a behavioural intervention before they can be taken off desmopressin.

Medication alone is often the first treatment of choice by physicians, a preference not supported by the evidence. Clayden *et al.* (2002, p. 804) state, in an extensive review, that 'it is puzzling that medication is so often preferred to the alarm when the latter is more effective, safer and less expensive'. It has to be said that despite the potential of urine alarm methods, problems of a technical nature can reduce their success. For example, sweat may trigger the alarm; batteries go flat; the child's clothing and bedding are not prepared properly; inconsistency on the part of exhausted parents; insufficient expert monitoring of the programme; premature withdrawal of therapy and so on. Butler (1998) provides an excellent review of the advantages of the enuresis alarm, and some of the practical difficulties that can hinder the usual expectation of success.

Conclusions

The findings on enuresis reviewed above suggest that:

(i) Urine alarm-based methods (the so-called 'bell-and-pad' apparatus) is the most effective treatment for enuresis.

(ii) A contingency management programme, where children obtain rewards for avoiding bedwetting (see 'Behaviour therapy') can be effective used alone, but is more successful when applied in combination with the urine alarm procedure.

(iii) Such programmes require a psycho-educational element so that parents (of necessity involved in their implementation) receive adequate explanations and rationales for the procedures, as well as painstaking instructions for their correct use.

(iv) To meet these objectives, a detailed guide describing behavioural and combined methods of treating nocturnal and diurnal enuresis has been prepared for practitioners and parents (by Herbert, 1996).

(See also 'Children's perceptions of illness and death' and 'Incontinence'.)

REFERENCES

Butler, R. J. (1998). Annotation: night wetting in children – psychological aspects. *Journal of Child Psychology & Psychiatry*, **39**, 453–63.

Clayden, G., Taylor, E., Loader, P. *et al.* (2002). Wetting and soiling in childhood. In M. Rutter & E. Taylor (Eds.). *Child and Adolescent Psychiatry* (4th edn.) (p. 804). Oxford: Blackwell Science.

Doleys, D. M. (1977*a*). Behavioural treatments for nocturnal enuresis in children: a review of the recent literature. *Psychological Bulletin*, **8**, 30–54.

Doleys, D. M. (1977*b*). Effectiveness of psychological and pharmacological treatments for nocturnal enuresis.

Journal of Child Psychological and Psychiatry, **39**, 307–22.

Herbert, M. (1996). *Toilet training, bedwetting and soiling.* Leicester: BPS Books (The British Psychological Society).

Herbert, M. (2003). *Typical and atypical behaviour: from conception to adolescence.* Leicester/Oxford: BPS/Blackwell Publications.

Ondersma, S. J. & Walker, C.E. (1998). Elimination disorders. In T.H. Ollendick & M. Hersen (Eds.). *Handbook of Child Psychopathology* (3rd edn.). New York: Plenum Press.

Shaffer, D. (1994). Enuresis. In M. Rutter, E. Taylor & L. Hersov (Eds.). *Child and*

Adolescent Psychiatry: Modern Approaches (3rd edn.). Oxford: Blackwell Scientific Publications.

Van Londen, A., Van Londen, B., Monique, W. *et al.* (1995). Relapse rate and subsequent parental reaction after successful treatment of children suffering from nocturnal enuresis: A 21/2-year follow-up of bibliotherapy. *Behaviour Research & Therapy*, **33**, 309–11.

Walker, C. E. (1995). Elimination disorders: Enuresis and encopresis. In M.C. Roberts (Ed.). *Handbook of Pediatric Psychology* (2nd edn.). New York: Guilford Press.

Epilepsy

Graham Scambler

University College London

Definition, prevalence and incidence

An epileptic seizure is the result of an abnormal paroxysmal discharge of cerebral neurones. Epilepy itself is often defined as a continuing tendency to epileptic seizures. The form of the seizure depends on the site of the neuronal discharge in the brain. There are as many causes of epilepsy as there are seizure types. Rare genetic disorders like Tay–Sachs disease, congenital malformations, anoxia, trauma, brain tumours, infectious diseases, acquired metabolic diseases, degenerative disorders and chronic alcoholism can all lead to epilepsy. There is evidence too that a low convulsive threshold can be inherited.

If the neuronal discharge remains confined to one part of the brain, the resultant seizure is described as 'partial'. If the discharge begins in one part of the brain but subsequently spreads to all parts, the seizure is said to be 'partial with secondary generalization'. Sometimes the abnormal discharge originates in the mesodiencephalic system and spreads more or less simultaneously to all parts of the brain, in which case the reference is to a 'primary generalized' seizure. Since it is generally understood that all partial seizures arise from some focal area of structural abnormality in the brain, all partial seizures, plus those seizures which are secondarily generalized from some focal onset, can be described as 'symptomatic epilepsy'. Primary generalized epilepsy is never symptomatic of underlying brain damage, and can thus be described as 'idiopathic epilepsy'.

Epilepsy is more common than many realize, although rates depend on the definition used and on case ascertainment. The prevalence of epilepsy is generally estimated to be between 5 and 10 cases per 1000 persons, and the overall incidence to be about 50 cases per 100 000 persons. The highest incidence is at the two extremes of life, with 50% of cases being under age 1 or over age 60. The prognosis varies with such factors as number of seizures at presentation, seizure type and use of anti-epileptic drugs (AEDs). In one recent review of the evidence (Bell & Sander, 2002), four prognostic groups were identified:

1. Excellent prognosis (20–30%): usually only a few seizures occur and spontaneous remission is the rule.
2. Good prognosis (30–40%): seizures are easily controlled by AEDs and, once remission is achieved, it is usually permanent.
3. AED-dependant prognosis (10–20%): AEDs suppress seizures and remission may be achieved, but relapse is likely if AEDs are stopped.
4. Bad prognosis (up to 20%): AEDs are palliative rather than suppressive of seizures. A few might respond to novel AEDs or surgery.

The mortality rate is slightly but significantly increased in those with epilepsy. In newly diagnosed epilepsy, death is commonly attributed to the underlying pathology, while in chronic epilepsy a familiar cause of death is Sudden Unexpected Death in Epilepsy (SUDEP) (the rate of sudden unexpected death being 20 times higher in those with epilepsy than in the general population).

Epilepsy services

In a contemporary survey of evidence-based standards of care for adults with epilepsy (Rajpura & Sethi, 2004), the authors conclude that although epilepsy services appear to be fairly standard throughout the UK, there is a need for more methodologically robust studies to determine the most clinically effective model of service provision for people with epilepsy. The existing quality of care, they add, is generally poor. Contributions to the World Epilepsy Day Symposium in November, 2004 established that the situation in the UK is the norm rather than the exception. In fact it is estimated that 70–90% of people with epilepsy in developing countries are not receiving any treatment or are not treated effectively (Ahmad, 2005). In a systematic review of specialist epilepsy services

in the UK (Meads *et al.*, 2002), no evidence was found either that specialist epilepsy clinics improved outcomes when compared with general outpatient neurology clinics, or that specialist epilepsy nurses improved outcomes when compared to usual care in an inpatient, outpatient or primary care physician/general practice (GP) setting. There was good evidence, however, that the 'process' of treatment and care was enhanced in the epilepsy nurse groups. In a study of the management of people with epilepsy in general practice, Goodwin and colleagues (2002) highlighted a number of deficiencies. Of the 116 participants, 71 were identified as requiring specialist review: 31 of these had experienced no seizures for five years. The authors judged that many were taking unnecessary medication and suffering unnecessary side effects.

Psychosocial sequelae of epilepsy

Approximately one in three people with epilepsy experience difficulties in addition to the physical impact of their conditions, including cognitive and psychosocial problems. Herman and Whitman (1986) have assessed the evidence for causal linkages between sets of 'neuroepilepsy', 'medication' and 'psychosocial' variables and measures of impairment. The results reflect the funding research bias towards neuroepilepsy and medication variables. Neuroepilepsy variables thought to be associated with psychiatric or psychological impairment include age at onset, aetiology, seizure control, duration of epilepsy, multiple seizure types, type of aura and neuropsychological status. Medication variables coming into this category are polypharmacy, serum levels of AEDs, type of medication and folic acid levels. The list of psychosocial variables is longer but each is less well researched: fear of seizures, perceived stigma, perceived discrimination, adjustment to epilepsy, locus of control, life events, social support, socioeconomic status and childhood home environment. The relative neglect of psychosocial factors in research is ironic given the prima facie plausibility of causal links between these and impairment. The psychosocial factors can be discussed under four subheadings.

Professional care

It is the physician who is empowered to make the diagnosis of epilepsy and to apply the diagnostic label. To communicate a diagnosis of epilepsy is to transform a 'normal person' into 'an epileptic' (Scambler & Hopkins, 1986). There is clear evidence that this new, unwanted status or identity can be more distressing and disruptive of lives than the anticipation or fact of recurrent seizures (see 'Coping with chronic illness').

However, if the communication of the diagnosis is often the most dramatic episode in relationships with physicians, it is generally but one moment in relationships beginning with the initial consultation and ending only with the cessation of AEDs or death. During these relationships people look to physicians, and increasingly to specialist epilepsy nurses, to replace uncertainty with expert accounts of tests, aetiology, therapy and prognosis. They also aspire to be treated effectively and with consideration of the full range of psychosocial sequelae of epilepsy. Occasionally their demands may be unrealistic: for all the lapses exposed by the growing number of audits, it remains the case that many of the uncertainties surrounding epilepsy cannot be alleviated, given the current state of medical knowledge. But, interestingly, one common finding in Britain and in the United States relates to physicians' 'disinterest' in the day-to-day problems of coping with epilepsy (Schneider & Conrad, 1983; Scambler, 1989).

Personal identity

People perceive the status or identity of 'epileptic' to be discrediting through their association of epilepsy with stigma (Scambler, 2004) (see 'Stigma'). Often it is accompanied by a sense of shame and, more saliently perhaps, a fear that others will reject, exclude or otherwise discriminate against them. This fear of discrimination has been termed 'felt stigma', and actual discrimination 'enacted stigma'. Felt stigma can predispose people to conceal their condition if they can, this being the strategy of choice for many, within as well as outside their families. Nor is felt stigma a function of seizure frequency, as is commonly supposed. Concealment reduces opportunities for enacted stigma; paradoxically, felt stigma typically causes more distress than enacted stigma. Other strategies than concealment include minimizing risks through avoidance of others; pragmatic or selective disclosing; or, more rarely, a defiant 'avowal of normality'. Strategies in fact vary by role and over time.

Family management

Epilepsy often begins in childhood, and children's understanding of their circumstances is conditioned by parents' explanations and behaviour. Parents, like doctors, may act as 'stigma coaches', training their offspring to feel ashamed and apprehensive about their epilepsy, prescribing concealment by advice or example (Schneider & Conrad, 1980). This is a form of over-protection, and over-protection is a key source of anger and resentment among young people with epilepsy, which may be associated with behavioural and adjustment problems later.

In adolescence and adulthood felt stigma typically leads to concealment (see also 'Children's perceptions of illness and death'). Boy-or girlfriends tend not to be told, and even engagements may not provoke openness. The same fear of rejection that proscribes mention of the word 'epilepsy' makes for a persistent sense of unease in case one day a seizure or other cue might lead to or precipitate exposure. There is little evidence that open disclosure, or even unwitting 'exposure' (e.g. a witnessed seizure), are likely to be followed by the termination of relationships, although it can happen. Uncertainty and bewilderment and occasionally conflict, tend to be succeeded by new, 'negotiated' equilibria (Scambler, 1989).

Work opportunities

Epilepsy is still associated with higher than average rates of unemployment and under-employment, although it must be borne in mind that epilepsy is sometimes one symptom of conditions much more disabling. Estimates of the proportion of British adults with epilepsy experiencing employment problems vary from 25–70%, depending on the criteria used. Difficulties may be the product of either enacted stigma or more legitimate forms of discrimination, for example banning driving. Felt stigma too can lead to disadvantage: people occasionally avoid or withdraw from the labour market, or decline opportunities for advancement, through felt stigma.

A wide range of studies have shown that felt stigma also leads to policies of non-disclosure to employers, at least when seizure frequency renders this strategy viable. While concealment reduces the prospects of meeting with enacted stigma or legitimate discrimination, it can prompt severe daily anxiety and tension in 'information management'.

Conclusions

There are implications here for improved quality of care. There is a need for patients' own perspectives to be elicited and taken seriously. Typically these perspectives are characterized by: (1) 'felt stigma': the perception of epilepsy as stigmatizing and a social and psychological burden; (2) 'rationalization': an urge to make sense of what is happening in order to restore cognitive order; and (3) 'action strategy': a need to develop ways of coping with epilepsy and its concomitant psychosocial problems. Doctors tend to be interested in those aspects of rationalization which facilitate diagnosis and management, but not in the process per se. Neither felt stigma nor action strategy tend to make it onto medical agendas for consultations, and are often handled badly when raised by patients. Physicians do not merely need to manage, inform and advice, but also to listen, which can be therapeutic in its own right. These are qualities which research studies are beginning to reveal in specialist epilepsy nurses.

REFERENCES

Ahmad, K. (2005). Improvements needed in care for patients with epilepsy. *Lancet Neurology*, **4**, 16.

Bell, G. & Sander, J. (2002). The epidemiology of epilepsy: the size of the problem. *Seizure*, **11** (Suppl. A), 306–16.

Goodwin, M., Wade, D., Luke, B. & Davies, P. (2002). A survey of a novel epilepsy clinic. *Seizure*, **11**, 519–22.

Hermann, B. & Whitman, S. (1986). Psychopathology in epilepsy: a multietiologic model. In S. Whitman & B. Hermann (Eds.). *Psychopathology in epilepsy: social dimensions.* Oxford: Oxford University Press.

Meads, C., Burls, A. & Bradley, P. (2002). Systematic reviews of specialist epilepsy services. *Seizure*, **11**, 90–8.

Rajpura, A. & Seth, S. (2004). Evidence-based standards of care for adults with epilepsy – a literature review. *Seizure*, **13**, 45–54.

Scambler, G. (1989). *Epilepsy.* London: Tavistock.

Scambler, G. (2004). Re-framing stigma: felt and enacted stigma and challenges to the sociology of chronic and disabling

conditions. *Social Theory and Health*,
2, 29–46.

Scambler, G. & Hopkins, A. (1986).
'Being epileptic': coming to terms with
stigma. *Sociology of Health and Illness*,
8, 26–43.

Schneider, J. & Conrad, P. (1980). In the
closet with illness: epilepsy, stigma
potential and information control. *Social
Problems*, **28**, 32–44.

Schneider, J. & Conrad, P. (1983). *Having
epilepsy: the experience and control of*

illness. Philadelphia: Temple University
Press.

Epstein–Barr virus infection

Rona Moss-Morris[1] and Meagan Spence[2]

[1]University of Southampton
[2]The University of Auckland

The Epstein–Barr virus (EBV) is a tumourogenic herpes virus that has been implicated in a wide range of human illnesses such as Hodgkin's disease and B lymphoproliferative disease; however it most commonly causes infectious mononucleosis (IM) often referred to as glandular fever (Macsween & Crawford, 2003). Primary infection with EBV typically occurs subclinically between the ages of one and six, after which the virus latently inhabits B lymphocyte cells. Previous infection with EBV is indicated by the presence of EBV antibody titres in the serum, while lack of these antibodies indicates vulnerability to EBV infection (Kasl *et al.*, 1979). In the Western world, a second peak of EBV infection occurs between 14 and 20 years of age. Estimates suggest that 90% of the world's population are seropositive for EBV by the age of 30 and carry the virus as a lifelong latent infection (Papesch and Watkins, 2001).

Epstein–Barr virus and infectious mononucleosis

When people get infected with EBV, a number seroconvert without developing the clinical signs of IM. Those who develop the clinical syndrome experience an acute illness characterized by fatigue, sore throat, tender lymph nodes and fever, which usually resolves within two to four weeks (Rea *et al.*, 2001). The puzzle is why some infected individuals develop clinical IM while others do not.

In an attempt to answer this question, Kasl and colleagues (1979) investigated 432 young American cadets over a four-year period. They monitored when the cadets became infected with EBV for the first time and found that those who had a high level of motivation combined with poor academic achievement were significantly more likely to develop clinical IM than those who did not. These results suggest that the development of clinical signs following infection with EBV is dependent in part on psychological factors. More work is needed to investigate other possible psychological risk factors and the biological sequelae associated with these factors.

Psychoneuroimmunology and elevated Epstein–Barr virus titres

A larger body of research within the area of psychoneuroimmunology has investigated antibody titres to EBV as a measure of immune system competence. Psychoneuroimmunology (PNI) is the study of how psychological factors may impact on the immune and neuroendocrine systems (see 'Psychoneuroimmunology'). Because EBV infection is largely ubiquitous and the virus remains in the body in a latent form, levels of elevated titres of EBV antibodies are seen to reflect a possible reactivation of the latent virus associated with a down regulation of cellular immunity (Van Rood *et al.*, 1993). Studies have shown that higher antibody levels to EBV are associated with a range of diverse stressors such as divorce, loneliness, marital dissatisfaction, care giving for a relative with Alzheimer's disease, space flight and university exams (Burleson *et al.*, 2002; Kiecolt-Glaser *et al.*, 1988; Sarid *et al.*, 2001; Stowe *et al.*, 2001). Personality and coping styles including high levels of emotional suppression, defensiveness and trait anxiety have also been significantly linked to elevated EBV antibody titres (Esterling *et al.*, 1993) (see 'Personality and health' and 'Emotional expression and health'). In addition, psychological interventions designed to reduce stress have significantly decreased these antibody titres (Van Rood *et al.*, 1993).

The relationship between stress and raised antibody titres may not be as straightforward as these early results suggest, however. Glaser and colleagues (1999) compared antibody levels in a homogeneous population of students attending a military academy before and after basic training, during a semester break and during examination week and found that only during the exam week were levels significantly raised. These results suggest that certain stressors may have a more profound effect on the down regulation of the immune system than others.

Are elevated Epstein–Barr virus antibody titres clinically relevant?

Although elevated EBV antibody titres have been taken as a measure of the down regulation of the immune system, how, or if, this relates to clinical outcome remains a moot point. In the 1980s, elevated antibody titres were implicated as causal factors in conditions such as depression and chronic fatigue syndrome (CFS) and received much media attention (Moss-Morris & Petrie, 2000). Subsequent well designed studies comparing depressed and CFS patients with matched healthy controls found no significant differences in EBV antibody titres between these groups (Buchwald & Komaroff, 1991). Longitudinal studies have also failed to find sustained evidence of EBV infection in CFS patients, and improvement in symptoms and the clinical features of the disorder appear unrelated to changes in EBV titres (Buchwald & Komaroff, 1991; Matthews *et al.*, 1991).

Infectious mononucleosis as a risk factor for the development of chronic fatigue syndrome

The weight of evidence suggests that elevated EBV titres play little role in CFS. However, the clinical manifestation of EBV (i.e. an acute episode of IM) appears to be a relevant risk factor. A number of prospective studies have tracked the natural history of IM in order to determine the likelihood of developing chronic problems such as fatigue, fibromyalgia and depression. Estimates of fatigue post-IM range from 9–22%, in comparison with 0–6% of patients who experience fatigue six months after an upper respiratory tract infection (URTI) (White *et al.*, 1998). A study of the incidence of fibromyalgia following IM, however, found no greater risk of this condition than would be found in the general population (Rea *et al.*, 1999). With regard to depression, White and colleagues (2001) found that whilst new episodes of depression were triggered in the acute stages of IM, six months post-illness there was no greater incidence of depression than was found before onset of IM. We can conclude then, that for a group of predisposed individuals, the experience of IM places them at greater risk of developing chronic fatigue, but not other related conditions such as fibromyalgia or depression (see 'Chronic fatigue syndrome').

Patients with an acute episode of IM therefore provide an ideal group with which to prospectively examine other factors which may interact with the virus in causing the onset of chronic fatigue. White and colleagues (White *et al.*, 2001) followed patients who had experienced either IM or an URTI. At six months they compared those who had developed fatigue with those who had recovered on a large number of demographic, clinical and laboratory factors and on a range of psychosocial measures. They found that the most reliable predictors of fatigue at six months were: IM as opposed to URTI; a lower extroversion score; and lower laboratory tested physical fitness at two months post-illness.

Another study found that of 150 patients with IM, 12% reported significant ongoing fatigue and disability six months later (Buchwald *et al.*, 2000). These patients were more likely to be female, to have

experienced more life events in the six months prior to IM, and to have received greater family support during their illness (see also 'Life events and health'). Candy and colleagues (2003) demonstrated that female gender and negative illness beliefs most reliably predicted fatigue cases six months post-IM. Finally, Spence and Moss-Morris (in preparation) followed up a large cohort of people who had experienced a severe acute infection; including 758 people with *Campylobacter* gastroenteritis and 260 with IM. Whilst IM was a significant predictor in the development of fatigue at three months, this was not the case at six months, with a similar proportion of gastroenteritis patients developing fatigue as IM patients. A number of psychological predictors were significantly related to chronic fatigue at six months, including anxiety, depression, somatization, perfectionism, negative illness beliefs and 'all-or-nothing' behaviour. Multivariate analysis indicated that the strongest predictor of fatigue six months post-IM was negative perceptions of the initial acute illness (see 'Lay beliefs about health and illness' and 'Symptom perception').

Commonalties emerge from the findings of the IM studies. Each has confirmed IM as a significant risk factor for the development of chronic fatigue in the short term; however, the extent of this influence may be less significant from six months post-illness. All found that their predictors differed according to the time point that outcome was measured; with biological predictors, such as higher levels of atypical lymphocytes (Katon *et al.*, 1999) and activated CD4 and CD8 (Candy *et al.*, 2003), perhaps more likely to predict fatigue at two or three months, whilst psychological predictors become more significant at six months post-illness.

The psychological factors shown to predict chronic fatigue or CFS following IM provide some support for the cognitive–behavioural model of this illness (Surawy *et al.*, 1995). Levels of psychopathology, such as anxiety and depression, together with personality characteristics, such as perfectionism and low extroversion, may act as predisposing factors. When such individuals are faced with needing to ease back from their commitments because of IM, they may respond in characteristic ways which help to perpetuate their fatigue. Initially, they may take some time off to recover. However, inactivity conflicts with their need to achieve in order to feel good about themselves or to please others, so they rush back to their commitments before they are fully well. This generates more symptoms as well as stress; the symptoms are interpreted as signs of the original illness, rather than signs of stress or recovery, and they return to bed. If this cycle continues, patients may develop the belief that they have a serious ongoing illness which does not seem to go away. They may develop a pattern of accommodating to their symptoms, which ultimately results in deconditioning and ongoing fatigue.

The fact that studies have shown that negative illness beliefs, 'all-or-nothing' behaviour in response to symptoms, and lack of physical fitness predict chronic fatigue post-IM, provide good support for the cognitive–behavioural aspects of the model (Candy *et al.*, 2003; Spence and Moss-Morris in preparation; White *et al.*, 2001). Furthermore, a simple behavioural intervention during the recovery phase of IM, where patients were encouraged to slowly, but surely, increase their levels of activity was shown to reduce the incidence of CFS post-IM (Candy *et al.*, 2004) (see 'Behaviour therapy' and 'Cognitive behaviour therapy').

In summary, the EBV provides intriguing avenues for the exploration of the relationship between psychology and biology. Psychological factors have been shown to predict who develops clinical signs of IM after EBV infection, and who goes on to develop ongoing fatigue after IM. The latent nature of the virus means that antibody titres can be used to measure activity of the immune system and how this may be influenced by factors such as stress.

(See also 'Herpes virus infection'.)

REFERENCES

Buchwald, D. & Komaroff, A. L. (1991). Review of laboratory findings for patients with chronic fatigue syndrome. *Reviews of Infectious Disease*, **13**, S12–18.

Buchwald, D. S., Rea, T. D., Katon, W. J., Russo, J. E. & Ashley, R. L. (2000). Acute infectious mononucleosis: characteristics of patients who report failure to recover. *American Journal of Medicine*, **109**, 531–7.

Burleson, M. H., Poehlmann, K. M., Hawkley, L. C. *et al.* (2002). Stress-related immune changes in middle-aged and older women: 1-year consistency of individual differences. *Health Psychology*, **21**, 321–31.

Candy, B., Chalder, T., Cleare, A. J. *et al.* (2003). Predictors of fatigue following the onset of infectious mononucleosis. *Psychological Medicine*, **33**, 847–55.

Candy, B., Chalder, T., Cleare, A. J., Wessely, S. & Hotopf, M. (2004). A randomised controlled trial of a psycho-educational intervention to aid recovery in infectious mononucleosis. *Journal of Psychosomatic Research*, **57**, 89–94.

Esterling, B. A., Antoni, M. H., Kumar, M. & Schneiderman, N. (1993). Defensiveness, trait anxiety, and Epstein–Barr viral capsid antigen antibody titers in healthy college students. *Health Psychology*, **12**, 132–9.

Glaser, R., Friedman, S. B., Smyth, J. *et al.* (1999). The differential impact of training stress and final examination stress on herpes virus latency at the United States Military Academy at West Point. *Brain, Behavior, & Immunity*, **13**, 240–51.

Kasl, S. V., Evans, A. & Niederman, J. C. (1979). Psychosocial risk factors in the development of infectious mononucleosis. *Psychosomatic Medicine*, **41**, 445–66.

Katon, W., Russo, J. E., Ashley, R. L. & Buchwald, D. S. (1999). Infectious mononucleosis: psychological symptoms during the acute and subacute phases of illness. *General Hospital Psychiatry*, **21**, 21–9.

Kiecolt-Glaser, J. K., Kennedy, S., Malkoff, S. *et al.* (1988). Marital discord and immunity in males. *Psychosomatic Medicine*, **50**, 213–29.

Macsween, K. F. & Crawford, D. H. (2003). Epstein–Barr virus – recent advances. *The Lancet Infectious Diseases*, **3**, 131–40.

Matthews, D. A., Lane, T. J. & Manu, P. (1991). Antibodies to Epstein–Barr virus in patients with chronic fatigue. *Southern Medical Journal*, **84**, 832–40.

Moss-Morris, R. & Petrie, K. (2000). *Chronic fatigue syndrome*, London: Routledge.

Papesch, M. & Watkins, R. (2001). Epstein–Barr virus infectious mononucleosis. *Clinical Otolaryngology and Allied Sciences*, **26**, 3–8.

Rea, T., Russo, J., Katon, W., Ashley, R. L. & Buchwald, D. (1999). A prospective study of tender points and fibromyalgia during and after an acute viral infection. *Archives of Internal Medicine*, **159**, 865–70.

Rea, T. D., Russo, J. E., Katon, W., Ashley, R. L. & Buchwald, D. S. (2001). Prospective study of the natural history of infectious mononucleosis caused by Epstein–Barr virus. *Journal of the American Board of Family Practice*, **14**, 234–42.

Sarid, O., Anson, O., Yaari, A. & Margalith, M. (2001). Epstein–Barr virus specific salivary antibodies as related to stress caused by examinations. *Journal of Medical Virology*, **64**, 149–56.

Spence, M. & Moss-Morris, R. (in preparation). The path from glandular fever to chronic fatigue syndrome: can the cognitive behavioural model provide map?

Stowe, R. P., Pierson, D. L. & Barrett, A. D. (2001). Elevated stress hormone levels relate to Epstein–Barr virus reactivation in astronauts. *Psychosomatic Medicine*, **63**, 891–5.

Surawy, C., Hackmann, A., Hawton, K. & Sharpe, M. (1995). Chronic fatigue syndrome: a cognitive approach. *Behaviour Research Therapy*, **33**, 535–44.

Van Rood, Y. R., Bogaards, M., Goulmy, E. & van Houwelingen, H. C. (1993). The effects of stress and relaxation on the *in vitro* immune response in man: a meta-analytic study. *Journal of Behavioural Medicine*, **16**, 163–81.

White, P. D., Thomas, J. M., Amess, J. *et al.* (1998). Incidence, risk and prognosis of acute and chronic fatigue syndromes and psychiatric disorders after glandular fever. *British Journal of Psychiatry*, **173**, 475–81.

White, P. D., Thomas, J. M., Kangro, H. O. *et al.* (2001). Predictions and associations of fatigue syndromes and mood disorders that occur after infectious mononucleosis. *Lancet*, **358**, 1946–54.

Facial disfigurement and dysmorphology

Nichola Rumsey

University of the West of England

Disfigurement

Introduction

The UK Office of Population Censuses and Surveys (OPCS) (1988/1989) has defined a disfigured person as someone who 'suffers from a scar, blemish or deformity which severely affects (their) ability to lead a normal life'. Macgregor (1990) has described facial disfigurement as a 'psychological and social death'. Disfigurement can result from many causes including congenital conditions (e.g. a cleft of the lip), from trauma (e.g. burns), surgical intervention (e.g. treatment for cancer), strokes and skin conditions (e.g. acne). Current estimates suggest that 10% of the population have some kind of facial 'difference' that sets them apart from the norm (Changing Faces, 2001). Recent research, however, suggests that the extent to which a visible difference results in social disability involves a complex interplay of psychological and social factors (Rumsey & Harcourt, 2004) (see also 'Disability').

The importance of the face in social interaction has long been recognized in the academic disciplines of psychology, history and anthropology. In a society that places a high premium on physical attractiveness and 'wholeness', it is not surprising that a sizeable research literature attests to the benefits of having a physically attractive facial appearance. When compared with the first impressions formed of those with an unattractive facial appearance, good-looking people are perceived to be more intelligent, popular, honest and socially desirable. Research also indicates that attractiveness is positively related to expectations of future success, happiness and marital satisfaction (Thompson et al., 1999). Relatively little research and funding has been devoted to examining the effects of having an unattractive or disfigured facial appearance. However, common themes emerge from the research and writings that are available.

Difficulties experienced by disfigured people

Facial disfigurement can have far-reaching psychosocial consequences. The most common problems experienced by those with facial disfigurements, whether congenital or acquired, involve negative self-perceptions and difficulties in social interaction, with problems particularly apparent at times of change, for example, moving to a new neighbourhood, starting new school, or beginning a new job (Rumsey & Harcourt, 2004). First encounters can be problematic, with difficulties reported in situations such as meeting new people, making friends, developing relationships and succeeding in job interviews.

Many disfigured people attribute the problems they experience to the negative reactions of others, complaining that they are avoided or rejected by the general public. Studies of the process of social interaction have shown that avoidance does occur. However, this avoidance is not necessarily the result of 'rejection' (Rumsey & Harcourt, 2005). A first meeting with a facially disfigured person is potentially problematic, as the normal rules of social interaction may not apply. The other party may be concerned that conventional patterns of non-verbal communication will be misconstrued (for example, eye contact might be interpreted as staring). Avoidance can feel preferable to the risk of embarrassment for either or both parties. Social encounters may also be thrown off-balance by the behaviour of the person with the disfigurement. Unconventional verbal or non-verbal communication can result from the inability to use facial musculature in the usual ways. Anticipating negative reactions from others, the affected person may adopt a shy or defensive interaction style (Macgregor, 1990), increasing the likelihood of negative reactions from others. Spirals of unhelpful emotions (e.g. social anxiety), maladaptive thought processes (e.g. fear of negative social evaluations), unfavourable self-perceptions (e.g. lowered self-esteem) and negative behaviour patterns (e.g. excessive social avoidance) may result.

Lansdown et al. (1991) characterized a visible difference as an underlying stressor throughout the lifespan, maintaining that life is likely to be appreciably harder for those with a face which is out of the ordinary. For children and adolescents, the majority of problems focus on teasing by others, on fear of going to new places and on problems associated with negative feelings about the self (Frances, 2003). However, disfigurements in children are not associated with any identifiable personality pattern, reports of delinquency, raised incidence of bad behaviour or lack of educational success (see also 'Children's perceptions of illness and death'). The intensified focus on physical appearance during adolescence can present difficulties. Image counts in the dating game, and joining social groups can be difficult if social confidence is eroded. Lansdown (1990) and others believe that problems in adolescence and adulthood are under-reported, as most data are collected in response to questions asked in medical settings, when the atmosphere is frequently not conducive to open discussion of social and psychological issues. Research involving older people is scarce: however, Spicer (2002) found that compared with middle-aged and younger adults, a smaller proportion of older adults affected by skin conditions reported high levels of appearance concerns, yet many still experienced considerable distress.

Factors playing a part in adjustment

Although the evidence suggests that people with facial differences are at risk for psychosocial problems, not all are equally affected.

Rumsey *et al.* (2002) found levels of anxiety, depression, social anxiety and social avoidance and perceptions of quality of life were unfavourable compared to published norms in 33–50% of a sample of over 600 outpatients attending for treatment of a variety of disfiguring conditions. What factors account for the differences in distress? Contrary to the expectations of many, the extent, type and severity of a disfigurement consistently fail to predict levels of adjustment. A person's subjective perception of how noticeable their difference is to others has been found to be a better indicator of psychological disturbance than an 'objective' rating provided by others (Rumsey *et al.*, 2004). In some cases, the cause of the disfigurement can exacerbate distress. As an example, the circumstances surrounding a burn injury may engender a variety of negative emotions such as guilt or blame in those affected (see 'Burns'). However, generalizations based on broad aetiological categories of disfigurement, (e.g. congenital as opposed to acquired) have limited utility as predictors of adjustment and distress and should be avoided (Newell, 2000).

Despite the common assumption that females experience more distress as the result of disfigurement than men, findings relating to gender effects are mixed (Rumsey & Harcourt, 2004). The considerable impact of social factors such as the current societal obsession with physical appearance and the prevailing images of attractiveness in all forms of media have been widely noted (see for example, Thompson *et al.*, 1999), however, the nuances of experiencing disfigurement in different cultural contexts remain largely uninvestigated.

Models of adjustment, (see for example, Newell, 2000; Kent, 2002) have placed increasing emphasis on cognitive processes to explain variations in adjustment. These include the emphasis placed on physical appearance in self-perceptions (e.g. self-esteem, body image), biases in information processing (e.g. vulnerability to media messages relating to attractiveness), the processing of social information (Moss & Carr, 2004) and processes of social comparison. In recent years, there have been calls to move away from an exclusive focus on the problems and difficulties associated with disfigurement, towards a broader research agenda that includes the strengths of people who cope well (Strauss, 2001). Research relating to protective factors is still in its infancy: however mounting evidence suggests that these include effective social interaction skills, good quality social support and a positive family environment which stresses the importance of a broad range of personal qualities (other than appearance) in self-esteem and self-worth (Rumsey & Harcourt, 2004).

Endriga and Kapp-Simon (1999) have highlighted the multiple domains of risk and protection in adjustment to craniofacial conditions. Researchers are only just beginning to unravel the complex interplay of factors affecting adjustment to disfigurement, motivation to seek treatment and responses to the outcome of treatment (see 'Reconstructive Surgery').

Meeting the needs of people with facial differences

Expanding the biomedical model of care

The assumption underlying treatment offered within the UK National Health Service is that improvements in physical appearance will reduce psychological distress and improve quality of life. Normalizing a person's appearance can clearly offer

benefits: however, the problems experienced by facially disfigured people are predominantly social and psychological. Although changes in appearance may be beneficial for many, they rarely provide the complete answer (Wallace & Lees, 1988; Hughes, 1998; Sarwer, 2002). Given the multifaceted nature of adjustment, the prevailing biomedical model of care needs to be expanded to include psychosocial support and intervention as routine adjuncts or alternatives to appearance enhancing treatment.

Interventions are likely to be particularly appropriate at key points, including following the birth (or prenatal diagnosis) of an infant with a disfiguring anomaly, times of transition during childhood, adolescence and adulthood (for example, starting or changing school; changing neighbourhoods or social groups; seeking and starting a new job) (Hearst & Middleton, 1997). Ideally, in order to promote a preventive rather than a reactive approach, and to avoid the stigmatizing nature of a referral for psychological 'treatment', support and intervention should be offered as part of routine care.

Providing information and support

If full multidisciplinary care cannot be offered, alternative methods of support should be explored. Clarke and Cooper (2001) have reported that many healthcare professionals would like to address the concerns of their patients, but feel they lack the appropriate training to deal with the psychosocial consequences of disfigurement. In response, the authors described the development and successful implementation of condition-specific information packs and training courses. An appreciation of common psychosocial difficulties should be achieved by all members of the care team, and routine screening for psychosocial difficulties should be implemented (see Rumsey *et al.*, 2002). Information and specialist resource materials should be readily available (see Changing Faces www.changingfaces.org.uk). Appropriate referral routes for more complex difficulties should be identified.

Cognitive–behavioural interventions

Kleve *et al.* (2002) reported significant improvements following an average of six individual cognitive–behavioural therapy sessions on measures of social anxiety, appearance-related distress, general anxiety and depression in adults with a range of disfiguring conditions. These improvements were maintained six months post-intervention. As many of the problems associated with facial disfigurement are associated with social interaction, some researchers have focused their attention on packages that aim to develop effective social interaction skills. These have been used successfully with children and adolescents with craniofacial conditions (Kapp-Simon, 1995), burns (Blakeney *et al.*, 2005) and with adults with disfigurements resulting from a variety of conditions (Robinson *et al.*, 1996). However, the relative efficacy of the many components of these interventions has yet to be clarified (see 'Cognitive behaviour therapy').

Conclusion

Facial disfigurement can have far-reaching social and psychological consequences. To date, insufficient resources have been devoted either to understanding the consequences of the pressures exerted by the tidal wave of media and societal attention on physical appearance, or to developing healthcare provision to more closely meet the needs of those affected.

Dysmorphology

Definition and typical features

The term dysmorphobia comes from *dysmorfia*, a Greek work meaning ugliness, specifically of the face. In body dysmorphic disorder (BDD), the affected person experiences excessive self-focused attention and a preoccupation with an imagined defect, or exaggerates a minor physical anomaly, often of the face, hair or skin (Phillips, 2002). The feature is felt to be unbearably ugly and is regarded with loathing, repugnance and shame (Birtchnell, 1988). In DSM-IV (Diagnostic and Statistical Manual of Mental Disorders. 4th edn.), BDD is classified as a somatoform disorder, with its delusional variant considered to be a psychotic disorder. Associated behaviours are time-consuming, and typically include frequent mirror checking (though some avoid mirrors altogether), avoidance of social situations and excessive camouflage. There are high levels of co-existing conditions including depression, suicidal ideation, obsessive compulsive disorder and social phobia. Social, academic and occupational functioning are frequently impaired. In a study of 188 patients with BDD, Phillips and Diaz (1997) found that more that 25% had been completely housebound for a minimum of a week, nearly 30% had attempted suicide and more than half had been hospitalized at least once.

The origins of BDD are thought to be multifactorial and to include neurobiological, genetic, sociocultural and psychological factors.

The exact prevalence of BDD is unknown. Estimates of 0.7% in the general population, rising to 12% of those attending dermatology clinics have been reported (Phillips, 2002). However, as the condition involves both secrecy and shame, these figures are likely to be under-estimates. The age of onset is typically from early adolescence through to the late twenties, and the condition is often chronic. Research findings relating to gender differences in incidence are inconsistent (Veale, 2004).

Treatment decisions and intervention

Uncertainty about the aetiology of BDD is reflected in the diversity of recommendations for treatment, which include antidepressant medication, psychotherapy, cognitive–behavioural therapy and cosmetic surgery (Veale, 2004) (see 'Cognitive behaviour therapy' and 'Reconstructive surgery'). Evidence for the effectiveness of interventions is currently limited. In the first instance, people suffering from BDD will probably approach a plastic surgeon, maxillofacial surgeon or dermatologist for treatment, highlighting the need for collaboration and a skilful assessment of psychological factors involved in requests for surgery. Although the majority of people with BDD believe surgical alteration is the only way to effectively address their problems, expectations of outcome are often unrealistic. Surgery, if performed, is often perceived by the patient as unsuccessful, leading to further requests for operations, or the shifting of dissatisfaction to another part of the body. The consensus in the literature is to avoid surgical intervention, referring sufferers instead for psychiatric assessment and treatment.

REFERENCES

American Psychiatric Association (1994). *Diagnostic and Statistical Manual of Mental Disorders*, (4th edn.) (DSM-IV). Washington, DC: American Psychiatric Association.

Birtchnell, S. (1988). Dysmorphobia: a centenary discussion. *British Journal of Psychiatry*, **153**, 41–3.

Blakeney, P., Thomas, C., Holzer, C., Rose, M., Berniger, F. & Meyer, W. (2005). Efficacy of a short-term, intensive social skills training program for burned adolescents. *Journal of Burn Care Rehabilitation*, **26**(6), 546–55.

Changing Faces. (2001). *Facing disfigurement with confidence*. London: Changing Faces. (Changing Faces, www.changingfaces.org.uk).

Clarke, A. & Cooper, C. (2001). Psychological rehabilitation after disfiguring injury or disease: investigating the training needs of specialist nurses. *Journal of Advanced Nursing*, **34**, 18–26.

Endriga, M. & Kapp-Simon, K. A. (1999). Psychological issues in craniofacial care: state of the art. *Cleft Palate Craniofacial Journal*, **36**, 3–11.

Frances, J. (2003). *Educating children with facial disfigurements*. London: Taylor & Francis.

Grossbart, T. & Sherman, C. (1986). *Skin deep: a mind/body program for healthy skin*. New York: William Morrow.

Hearst, D. & Middleton, J. (1997). Psychological intervention and models of current working practice. In R. Lansdown, N. Rumsey, E. Bradbury, A. Carr & J. Partridge (Eds.). *Visibly different: coping with disfigurement* (pp. 158–71). Oxford: Butterworth-Heinemann.

Hughes, M. (1998). *The social consequences of facial disfigurement*. Aldershot: Ashgate Publishing.

Kapp-Simon, K. (1995). Psychological interventions for the adolescent with cleft lip and palate. *Cleft Palate Craniofacial Journal*, **32**, 104–8.

Kent, G. (2002). Testing a model of disfigurement: effects of a skin camouflage service on well being and appearance anxiety. *Psychology and Health*, **17**, 377–86.

Kleve, L., Rumsey, N., Wyn-Williams, M. & White, P. (2002). The effectiveness of cognitive–behavioural interventions

provided at outlook: a disfigurement support unit. *Journal of Evaluation of Clinical Practice*, **8**, 387–95.

Lansdown, R. (1990). Psychological problems of patients with cleft lip and palate: a discussion paper. *Journal of the Royal Society of Medicine*, **83**, 448–50.

Lansdown, R., Lloyd, J. & Hunter, J. (1991). Facial deformity in childhood: severity and psychological adjustment. *Child Care, Health and Development*, **17**, 165–71.

Macgregor, F. (1990). Facial disfigurement: problems and management of social interaction and implications for mental health. *Aesthetic Plastic Surgery*, **14**, 249–57.

Moss, T. & Carr, A. (2004). Understanding adjustment to disfigurement: the role of self concept. *Psychology and Health*, **19**, 737–48.

Newell, R. (2000). *Body image and disfigurement care*. London: Routledge.

Office of Population Censuses & Surveys (1988/1989). *The disability survey*. London: OPCS.

Partridge, J. (1990). *Changing faces: the challenge of facial disfigurement*. Harmondsworth: Penguin.

Phillips, K. (2002). Body Image & Body Dysmorphic Disorder. In T. Cash & T. Pruzinsky (Eds.). *Body image: a handbook of theory, research & clinical practice* (Chapter 36). New York: The Guilford Press.

Phillips, K. & Diaz, S. (1997). Gender differences in body dysmorphic disorder. *The Journal of Nervous and Mental Disease,* **185**, 570–7.

Robinson, E., Rumsey, N. & Partridge, J. (1996). An evaluation of the impact of social interaction skills training for facially disfigured people. *British Journal of Plastic Surgery,* **49**, 281–9.

Rumsey, N., Clarke, A. & Musa, M. (2002). Altered body image: the psychosocial needs of patients. *British Journal of Community Nursing,* **7**, 563–6.

Rumsey, N., Clarke, A., White, P., Wyn-Williams, M. & Garlick, W. (2004). Altered body image: auditing the appearance-related concerns of people with visible disfigurement. *Journal of Advanced Nursing,* **48**, 1–11.

Rumsey, N. & Harcourt, D. (2004). Body image & disfigurement: issues & interventions. *Body Image,* **1**, 83–97.

Rumsey, N. & Harcourt, D. (2005). *The psychology of appearance.* Maidenhead: Open University Press.

Sarwer, D. (2002). Cosmetic surgery and changes in body image. (Chapter 48). In T. Cash & T. Pruzinsky (Eds.). *Body image: a handbook of theory, research & clinical practice.* New York: Guilford Press.

Spicer, J. (2002). Appearance-related concern in older adults with skin disorder: an exploratory study. Unpublished Doctoral Thesis, Exeter University, UK.

Strauss, R. (2001). "Only skin deep". *Cleft Palate Craniofacial Journal,* **22**, 56–62.

Thompson, K., Heinberg, L., Altabe, M. & Tantleff-Dunn, S. (1999). *Exacting beauty: theory, assessment and treatment of body image disturbance.* Washington DC: American Psychological Association.

Veale, D. (2004). Advances in a cognitive behavioural model of body dysmorphic disorder. *Body Image,* **1**,113–25.

Wallace, L. & Lees, J. (1988). A psychological follow up study of adult patients discharged from a British burn unit. *Burns,* **14**, 39–45.

Fetal wellbeing: monitoring and assessment

Peter G. Hepper[1], James C. Dornan[2] and Dan McKenna[2]

[1]Queen's University
[2]Royal Jubilee Maternity Service

The main aim of obstetric practice is to ensure that mothers and babies remain healthy during pregnancy and birth. A variety of techniques may be employed to monitor and assess fetal health. This chapter concentrates upon techniques available to assess the health of the fetus. However it should be noted that the mother's health and wellbeing is inextricably linked to that of the fetus and a key element of antenatal care is the careful monitoring and management of the mother's health (see 'Antenatal care').

Key issues in assessing fetal wellbeing

The high-risk fetus in the low-risk population

Some mothers are classed as high-risk, i.e. at increased risk of having a baby with a problem due to some known factor, e.g. maternal age and Down's syndrome. Such mothers are relatively easy to identify and offered tests to assess the condition of their fetus (see 'Screening: antenatal'). However the majority of fetal problems arise in the low-risk population of mothers, who present no obvious signs of having a fetus with an abnormality. A reduction in the incidence of fetal problems rests with advances in identifying the high-risk fetus in the low-risk population (McKenna *et al.*, 2003).

Screening and diagnosis

Diagnostic techniques, whilst providing a definitive answer regarding the presence of a particular problem, can be expensive in time and money and carry a serious risk to the fetus, e.g. amniocentesis, which may result in a miscarriage. These tests are thus unsuitable for widespread use with the low-risk population. This has lead to the development of screening tests that do not carry a risk to the fetus. Such tests do not definitively indicate the presence of a particular problem but rather assess the probability that the fetus is affected. Where a fetus is identified as having a high probability of an abnormality, further, diagnostic, tests can be offered. Screening tests are not without their problems. Mothers have to interpret the risk factor, e.g. 1 in 50, to determine whether they will avail themselves of further testing. Some mothers consider 1:50 a low risk, whereas others consider 1:5000 a very high risk (see 'Risk perception'). Screening tests also create significant anxiety. For a risk of 1:50, 49 of the mothers who undergo further testing will not have a fetus with that problem. It is essential that mothers are supported through these tests and the limitations of the test explained.

Validation of screening tests

A number of screening tests have been developed to assess elements of fetal health (NICE, 2003). However there has been little examination of their efficacy and thus decisions on their routine application during pregnancy await appropriate trials.

Improving fetal health

Whilst new techniques and screening tools are developed, effective treatments for the 'abnormal' fetus are scarce. For many years the only option, and still the main option, to deal with fetal compromise was early delivery. However, new possibilities for treatment are being developed. Pre-conceptually, taking folic acid as a dietary supplement reduces the incidence of neural tube defects (Fraser & Fisk, 2003). Fetal surgical techniques have been developed to treat diagnosed conditions, e.g. spina bifida (Olutoye & Adzick, 1999) but research is needed to assess their success. The future will undoubtedly witness pioneering techniques to 'treat' diagnosed problems in the fetus.

Assessing fetal health

What can be monitored or assessed?

There are a number of different measures that can provide information on the status of the fetus. These are:

- fetal cells – for chromosomal and genetic analysis
- fetal growth – comparison against norms
- physical structure – presence, absence or deformity of body parts or organs
- biochemical products – e.g. human chorionic gonadotrophin as part of screening test for Down's syndrome
- fetal environment – amniotic fluid volume
- fetal heart rate and circulation
- fetal behaviour.

Technology to monitor the fetus

The oldest 'technology' is that of palpation of the abdomen and this still has a role in assessing fetal health. Ultrasound provides detailed pictures of the fetus enabling assessment of fetal size, structure, environment and behaviour. Ultrasound also offers the means for monitoring fetal heart rate and Doppler assessment of the circulatory system. MRI (Magnetic resonance imaging) scans have been used to obtain pictures of the fetus (Glastonbury & Kennedy, 2002) but this technology is not routinely used to monitor the fetus.

Routine fetal monitoring

The health of the low-risk fetus is routinely assessed using a combination of ultrasound, and screening tests offered for Down's syndrome and the presence of specific diseases.

At the first antenatal visit, usually before 14 weeks gestation, ultrasound is used to assess gestational age and fetal viability, to detect multiple fetuses and gross abnormalities. Screening tests based on a maternal blood sample are offered to assess, e.g. rhesus and rubella status, anaemia, hepatitis B virus, HIV and syphilis. Screening for Down's syndrome will be offered. It is recommended (NICE, 2003) that screening for Down's syndrome uses the 'integrated test' based on measurement of pregnancy associated plasma protein A; human chorionic gonadotrophin; alpha-fetoprotein; unconjugated estrodial; inhibin A obtained from a maternal blood sample; and the measurement of nuchal translucency (the subcutaneous space between cervical spine and skin) observed by ultrasound. It is essential that the woman is given full information about the particular test and her right to accept or decline the test should be made clear (see 'Informed consent' and 'Screening: general issues').

Women will be offered an anomaly ultrasound scan between 18–20 weeks gestation. The role of a scan at this gestation is now well established. In the hands of trained operator and with a modern ultrasound machine 98–99% of open neural tube defects will be detected (Smith & Hau, 1999).

The size of the fetus is assessed at each antenatal visit, usually by ultrasound guided measurement. Fetal growth occurs almost linearly in normal pregnancy. Of particular concern is the fetus whose growth slows down during the course of pregnancy (intrauterine growth restriction, (IUGR)): such fetuses are considered compromised and may require early delivery.

Clinical assessment in late pregnancy determines whether the fetus is in the correct and safe position to deliver normally and is undertaken by abdominal palpation.

Monitoring during labour

It is customary to monitor fetal heart rate during labour. If the fetus is low-risk, i.e. singleton, at term (37–42 weeks), cephalic presentation, appropriately grown, in spontaneous labour with clear liquor and no major antenatal events having occurred and the mother is healthy, the fetal heart rate may be auscultated. If antenatal complications have occurred or the mother has a medical condition, e.g. pre-eclampsia, diabetes or a problem has arisen during labour such as unexpected bleeding, then, electronic monitoring of the fetal heart rate (cardiotocography) is traditionally applied. The fetal heart rate trace is assessed for its rate, the presence of long-term and short-term variability, accelerations and decelerations. If the decelerations occur after the contraction has reached the nidus they are known as late decelerations and are indicative of impending fetal compromise. In these situations a blood sample may be obtained from the fetal scalp and a pH of <7.2 may be indicative of severe hypoxia and warrant timely delivery.

Non-routine assessment of fetal health

The majority of pregnancies are uneventful and require little intervention. Indeed it is important to recognize the normality of this physiological event. In some cases, however, the fetus may be considered at high risk of an anomaly, e.g. Down's syndrome in women over 35, or routine monitoring reveals an abnormality. In these cases additional tests may be offered to monitor the fetus's health.

Chromosomal and genetic analysis

Women may be offered amniocentesis or chorionic villus sampling to obtain a sample of fetal cells for chromosomal or genetic analysis. Usually undertaken before 18 weeks gestation these tests provide a definitive diagnosis on the presence of chromosomal or genetic defects.

Fetal heart rate monitoring

Antenatal cardiotocography (CTG) is used to assess the health of the fetus at a specific instant in time. A heart-rate trace showing a normal rate, the presence of accelerations of fetal movement, variability of >5 bpm and absence of decelerations is usually indicative of a healthy fetus at that moment in time. A CTG alone is not however predictive of how the fetus may be beyond 12 or 24 hours.

Umbilical artery waveforms measured using Doppler

Blood flow through the arteries and veins in the umbilical cord can be measured using ultrasound to provide an assessment of the fetal circulatory systems. Abnormalities in blood flow assessed by Doppler can predict IUGR, and the absence of end diastole flow is indicative of severe compromise (Baschat et al., 2000). Doppler ultrasound of the fetal middle cerebral artery revealing increased blood flow may be indicative of fetal compromise (Bahado-Singh et al., 1999).

The biophysical assessment of the fetus

Eight biophysical features, identifiable on ultrasound, are commonly observed in the high-risk pregnancy. Four reflect the acute wellbeing of the fetus: movements; tone; breathing; and changes in heart-rate patterns. Four reflect the chronic state of the fetus: umbilical artery Doppler measurements; placental architecture; amniotic fluid volume; and fetal weight estimation. Although some of these tests have not been subjected to rigorous scientific or clinical scrutiny, emerging evidence suggests that ultrasound assessment of the fetus's environment and growth should become part of the 'routine' antenatal visit. In one study, 2000 low-risk patients were randomized to receive traditional antenatal care or traditional antenatal care *plus an ultrasound examination* at 30–32 weeks and at 36–37 weeks gestation (McKenna et al., 2003). The ultrasound scan assessed placental maturity, amniotic fluid volume and estimated fetal weight. This study showed that the introduction of an ultrasound scan increased antenatal intervention, did not increase admissions to neonatal intensive care, and importantly reduced the chances of delivering a growth restricted fetus by about a third. The perinatal mortality rate in growth-restricted fetuses is four to ten times higher than that of normally grown infants (Chiswick, 1985). Furthermore, growth restricted fetuses

that do not die in utero are more likely to suffer other complications e.g. birth hypoxia, neonatal complications in the neonatal period, impaired neurodevelopment and cerebral palsy in childhood and non-insulin-dependent diabetes and hypertension in later life (Barker et al., 1993). In light of this evidence, the routine ultrasound assessment of the fetal environment in British obstetric practice may soon be considered the norm. It is already part of routine obstetric practice in North America.

Neurobehavioural assessment of the fetus

Whilst ultrasound may be used to visualize structural abnormalities, assessment of fetal CNS functioning has remained elusive to traditional obstetric techniques. Recent attention has focussed on the behaviour of the fetus as a means of assessing neural integrity. Since behaviour is a reflection of neural functioning and it has been argued that the assessment of the fetus's behaviour will provide information on its wellbeing. Fetal behaviour, observed using ultrasound, may be defined as any action or reaction of the fetus and may be divided into two main categories; spontaneous (under the volition of the fetus) or elicited (contingent upon the presentation of a stimulus, e.g. sound). Both have been used to assess wellbeing.

Differences in behaviour have been found in fetuses with abnormalities, e.g. anencephaly (Visser et al., 1985), Trisomy 18 (Hepper & Shahidullah, 1992a), maternal diabetes (Mulder et al., 1987). Environmental influences may also be observed, e.g. low doses of alcohol alter the fetus's startle behaviour (Little et al., 2002).

The fetus's response to an auditory stimulus has been developed as a prenatal test of deafness (Shahidullah & Hepper, 1993). One technique which may prove useful in assessing neural integrity is that of habituation (Hepper & Leader, 1996). Differences in habituation have been observed in fetuses with Down's syndrome (Hepper & Shahidullah, 1992b). Fetal habituation performance has been found to predict postnatal development as assessed on Bayley's scale of neurobehavioural development (Ratcliffe et al., 2002a,b).

Summary

It is unlikely that a single test will provide a complete assessment of fetal health. A combination of the above approaches will enable a comprehensive assessment of fetal wellbeing but much work needs to be undertaken to evaluate the effectiveness of individual tests and new tests need to be developed to further advance our ability to monitor and assess the health of the fetus.

(See also 'Pregnancy and childbirth', 'Screening: antenatal', 'Screening: general issues and premature babies').

REFERENCES

Bahado-Singh, R. O., Kovanci, E., Jeffres, A. et al. (1999). The Doppler cerebroplacental ratio and perinatal outcome in intrauterine growth restriction. *American Journal of Obstetrics and Gynecology*, **180**, 750–6.

Baschat, A. A., Gembruch, U., Reiss, I. et al. (2000). Relationship between arterial and venous Doppler and perinatal outcome in fetal growth restriction. *Ultrasound in Obsterics and Gynecology*, **16**, 407–13.

Barker, D. J., Gluckman, P. D., Godfrey, K. M. et al. (1993). Fetal nutrition and cardiovascular disease in adult life. *Lancet*, **341**, 938–41.

Chiswick, M. (1985). Intrauterine growth retardation. *British Medical Journal*, **291**, 845–7.

Fraser, R. B. & Fisk, N. M. (2003). *Periconceptional folic acid and food fortification in the prevention of neural tube defects. Scientific advisory committee opinion paper 4.* London: Royal College of Obstetricians and Gynaecologists.

Glastonbury, C. M. & Kennedy, A. M. (2002). Ultrafast MRI of the fetus. *Australasian Radiologist*, **46**, 22–32.

Hepper, P. G. & Leader, L. R. (1996). Fetal habituation. *Fetal and Maternal Medicine Review*, **8**, 109–23.

Hepper, P. G. & Shahidullah, S. (1992*a*). Trisomy 18: behavioural and structural abnormalities: an ultrasonographic case study. *Ultrasound in Obstetrics and Gynaecology*, **2**, 48–50.

Hepper, P. G. & Shahidullah, S. (1992*b*). Habituation in normal and Down syndrome fetuses. *Quarterly Journal of Experimental Psychology*, **44B**, 305–17.

Little, J. F., Hepper, P. G. & Dornan, J. C. (2002). Maternal alcohol consumption during pregnancy and fetal startle behaviour. *Physiology and Behavior*, **76**, 691–4.

McKenna, D., Tharmaratnam, S., Mahsud, S. *et al.* (2003). A randomized trial using ultrasound to identify the high-risk fetus in a low-risk population. *Obstetrics and Gynaecology*, **101**, 626–32.

Mulder, E. J. H., Visser, G. H. A., Bekedam, D. J. & Prechtl, H. F. R. (1987). Emergence of behavioural states in fetuses of type-1-diabetic women. *Early Human Development*, **15**, 231–51.

NICE. (2003). *Antenatal care. Routine care for the healthy pregnant woman.* London: National Institute of Clinical Excellence.

Olutoye, O. O. & Adzick, N. S. (1999). Fetal surgery for myelomeningocele. *Seminars in Perinatology*, **23**, 462–73.

Ratcliffe, S. J., Leader, L. R. & Heller, G. Z. (2002*a*). Functional data analysis with application to periodically stimulated foetal heart rate data. 1: Functional regression. *Statistics in Medicine*, **21**, 1103–14.

Ratcliffe, S. J., Heller, G. Z. & Leader, L. R. (2002*b*). Functional data analysis with application to periodically stimulated foetal heart rate data. 2: Functional logistic regression. *Statistics in Medicine*, **21**, 1115–27.

Shahidullah, S. & Hepper, P. G. (1993). Prenatal hearing tests? *Journal of Reproductive and Infant Psychology*, **11**, 143–6.

Smith, N. C. & Hau, C. (1999). A six year study of the antenatal detection of fetal abnormality in six Scottish health boards. *British Journal of Obstetrics and Gynaecology*, **106**, 206–12.

Visser, G. H. A., Laurini, R. N., de Vries, J. I. P., Bekedam, D. J. & Prechtl, H. F. R. (1985). Abnormal motor behaviour in anencephalic fetuses. *Early Human Development*, **12**, 173–82.

Gastric and duodenal ulcers

Paul Bennett

University of Cardiff

Gastric ulcers are ulceration of the lining of the stomach. As their name suggests, duodenal ulcers occur in the duodenum, which is the part of the small intestine immediately following the stomach in the gastrointestinal tract. Collectively, they are referred to as peptic ulcer disease. Their most common symptom is abdominal discomfort or pain. These symptoms typically come and go for several days or weeks, occur two to three hours after eating, and are relieved by eating. Symptoms may at their worst during the night, when the stomach is empty following a meal. Other symptoms include poor appetite, weight loss, bloating, nausea and vomiting. If the disease process is not treated, the ulcer may erode through the entire stomach wall, resulting in the potentially fatal outflow of its contents into the abdomen.

Until relatively recently, peptic ulcers were thought to be the result of stress, which was thought to increase acid secretion within the stomach and hence also the duodenum. More recently, this psychological explanation has been largely superseded by a biological model. This suggests that a bacterium known as *Helicobacter pylori* (*H. pylori*) is responsible for the disorder. *Helicobacter pylori* infection is thought to weaken the protective mucous coating of the stomach and duodenum, allowing acid to get through to the sensitive lining beneath. Both the acid and the bacteria irritate the lining and cause the ulcer. This biological model of ulceration has increasingly been seen as the primary model of ulceration (e.g. Centers for Disease Control and Prevention: http://www.cdc.gov/ulcer/md.htm), although there remains the possibility of other routes to ulcers, including stress.

The stress hypothesis has drawn on a number of strands of evidence (see Levenstein, 2000). These suggest, firstly, that while the evidence for *H. pylori* as a casual factor is strong, there is no reason to assume that it is the only factor which may contribute to the development of ulcers. Secondly, there is consistent evidence that stress may increase risk for ulcers in both animals and humans, prolong their duration and that reductions in stress may result in improvements in disease status. Stress therefore does seem to be involved in the aetiology of ulcers. One principal way in which stress may influence disease is through its impact on gastric acids. An alternative pathology in which stress mediates the immunological response to *H. pylori* infection has not been investigated. However, given our present understanding of psychoneuroimmunology, this possibility cannot be excluded (see 'Psychoneuroimmunology'). Stress may also have an indirect role by stimulating other behaviours known to effect ulceration, including cigarette smoking (e.g. Shigemi *et al.*, 1999), lack of sleep (Segawa *et al.*, 1987) and increased alcohol consumption (Levenstein *et al.*, 1997)

More than *H. pylori*

The first evidence supporting the possibility of alternative routes to ulceration lies in findings that most people who carry the *H. pylori* bacteria never have ulcers, and that *H. Pylori* infection is not present in all cases of ulcers. Ciociola *et al.* (1999) calculated that 29% of duodenal ulcer patients have no active *H. pylori* infection. The most frequent alternative route is through the ingestion of non-steroidal anti-inflammatory drugs, but other causes cannot be excluded.

Stress as a precipitating factor

A number of well designed and executed studies have shown a relationship between stress (defined in a variety of ways) and ulceration. The National Health and Nutrition Epidemiologic Survey (Anda *et al.*, 1992), for example, found a 60% additional rate of medically confirmed ulceration among people with high stress in comparison with those with low stress. Individuals in the highest quintile for stress were nearly three times as likely to develop peptic ulcers than those reporting low levels of stress even after adjustment for ulcer-related factors, including aspirin use and smoking. In the Alameda County Study longitudinal study (Levenstein *et al.*, 1997), participants with high levels of distress at baseline were over twice as likely (odds ratio, 2.2) to develop ulcers over a nine-year period than those with low levels of distress after adjustment for levels of smoking, alcohol consumption, skipping breakfast and lack of sleep. The raw odds ratio between high and low distress groups was 2.8. In a second longitudinal study using confirmed diagnoses, Medalie *et al.* (1992) followed a cohort of 8458 men aged over 40 years with no history of ulcers for 5 years. Multivariate logistic regression revealed a significant independent association between radiologically confirmed duodenal ulcers and baseline measures of family problems (odds ratio, 1.6), low levels of intimacy and social support (odds ratio, 2.06) and internalization of negative affect (odds ratio, 1.89). By comparison, the odds ratio between smokers and non-smokers was 1.64. Animal studies confirm the role of stress in the aetiology of ulcers with stressors such as early separation from mothers, cold water immersion and bodily restraint all being associated with the high levels of ulceration (e.g. Ackerman *et al.*, 1975; Kim *et al.*, 2002).

Stress as a maintaining factor

Once peptic ulcer disease has been diagnosed, stress may impede ulcer healing. Hui *et al.* (1992), for example, followed a total of 122 endoscopically validated duodenal ulcer patients either in the active or remission phase for a period of 6 months. Patients who experienced a relatively high number of adverse life events or who remained stressed over the follow-up period were less likely to heal than those whose stress remitted. In a much larger population of over 2000 duodenal ulcer patients, Holtmann *et al.* (1992) found

healing rates and relapse were significantly associated with physician ratings of patient stress over a one-year period. In a further longitudinal study of 75 patients with endoscopically confirmed duodenal ulcer Levenstein *et al.* (1996) found that over a period of 14 months, a poor prognosis was predicted by low-status occupation, low education, depression, stressful life events. Of note were their findings that factors including smoking, alcohol consumption, use of anti-inflammatory drugs and *H. pylori* levels did not predict outcome.

Treating stress improves prognosis

Perhaps as a result of the rapid response to medical treatments (often using a combination of antibiotics and drugs which inhibit the production of stomach acid), studies of the psychological treatment of peptic ulcers are rare. However, the evidence they provide does bear on the stress–ulcer relationship. Despite its low number of participants ($n = 22$), the study reported by Brooks and Richardson (1980) remains the key study of this approach. They randomly allocated patients with radiologically confirmed diagnoses of duodenal ulcers into either an intensive psychological intervention comprising an educative phase, relaxation training, cognitive restructuring and coping injury or an attention placebo condition (see 'Cognitive behaviour therapy' and 'Relaxation training'). All participants received antacid medication. Over a follow-up period of 60 days, patients in the active intervention experienced significantly fewer symptomatic days, and consumed less medication, although X-rays revealed similar levels of healing in both groups. It was in the longer term follow-up, however, that the strength of the intervention proved most beneficial. Significantly fewer participants in the active intervention (1 in 9) than in the placebo group (5 in 8) reported a recurrence of the disorder. Participants in the active intervention also attended hospital less frequently and none required surgery, compared to two in the placebo intervention. Without radiological or endoscopic confirmation of differences in disease state, these differences should be treated with some caution. However, they admit the possibility that changes in stress may influence disease processes.

Stress mechanisms

Not only is there empirical evidence of a role of stress in peptic ulcer disease, there are also plausible disease mechanisms. The most frequently cited psychobiological mechanism suggests that stress increases levels of gastric acids, which in turn increase erosion and ulceration of the gut wall. The model gains support from a number of relatively small naturalistic studies that have found stress and gastric acid levels to co-vary. In one study, Feldman *et al.* (1992) found that gastric acid output is correlated with levels of psychological distress, measures of tension, conflict and anxiety, in individuals with no ulceration. In addition, personality traits such as impulsivity and social isolation are also implicated in more labile acid secretion rates. Ocktedalen *et al.* (1984) followed a group of men participating in an intensive five-day training programme, involving heavy exercise and sleep deprivation. Levels of acid output rose by 300% among participants not given drugs to reduce acid secretion among whom there was no increase in acid secretion. A second pathway that has received even less research involves the interaction between *H. pylori* and stress. One study in humans suggested the possibility that stress may moderate immunological responses to *H. pylori* infection. Levenstein *et al.* (1995) found that among patients with peptic ulcers, levels of *H. pylori* antibodies were lower among anxious patients than among less anxious individuals, suggesting stress may suppress the production of these antibodies and adversely influence levels of *H. pylori* within gut. By contrast, Kim *et al.* (2002) found *H. pylori* and stress were independent predictors of ulceration in rates exposed to *H. pylori* and water immersion-restraint stress (see also 'Stress and health').

Conclusions

Helicobacter pylori infection appears to be the most frequent cause of peptic ulceration, and its treatment the most effective way of curing the condition. However, stress may also be implicated in its development and maintenance either as an independent factor, one which influences other risk behaviours such as smoking or alcohol consumption, or through moderating effect on levels of *H. pylori* within the gut. Accordingly, some people with peptic ulcers may still benefit from interventions designed to reduce stress, particularly in the longer-term, where this reduction may have a preventive role.

REFERENCES

Ackerman, S. H., Hofer, M. A. & Weiner, H. (1975). Age at maternal separation and gastric erosion susceptibility in the rat. *Psychosomatic Medicine*, **37**, 180–4.

Anda, R. F., Williamson, D. F., Escobedo, L. G. *et al.* (1992). Self-perceived stress and the risk of peptic ulcer disease: a longitudinal study of US adults. *Archives of Internal Medicine*, **152**, 829–33.

Brooks, G. R. & Richardson, F. C. (1980). Emotional skills training: a treatment program for duodenal ulcer. *Behavior Therapy*, **11**, 198–207.

Ciociola, A. A., McSorley, D. J., Turner, K. *et al.* (1999). *Helicobacter pylori* infection rates in duodenal ulcer patients in the United States may be lower than previously estimated. *American Journal of Gastroenterology*, **94**, 1834–40.

Feldman, M., Walker, P., Goldschmiedt, M. *et al.* (1992). Role of affect and personality in gastric acid secretion and serum gastrin concentration: comparative studies in normal men and in male duodenal ulcer patients. *Gastroenterology*, **102**, 175–80.

Holtmann, G., Armstrong, D., Poppel, E. *et al.* (1992). Influence of stress on the healing and relapse of duodenal ulcers. *Scandinavian Journal of Gastroenterology*, **27**, 917–23.

Hui, W. M., Shiu, L. P., Lok, A. S. F. *et al.* (1992). Life events and daily stress in duodenal ulcer disease. *Digestion*, **52**, 165–72.

Kim, Y. H., Lee, J. H., Lee, S. S. *et al.* (2002). Long-term stress and *Helicobacter pylori* infection independently induce gastric mucosal lesions in C57BL/6 mice. *Scandinavian Journal of Gastroenterology*, **37**, 1259–64.

Levenstein, S. (2000). The very model of a modern aetiology: a biopsychosocial view of peptic ulcer. *Psychosomatic Medicine*, **62**, 176–85.

Levenstein, S., Kaplan, G. A. & Smith, M. W. (1997). Psychological predictors of peptic ulcer incidence in the Alameda County study. *Journal of Clinical Gastroenterology*, **24**, 140–6.

Levenstein, S., Prantera, C., Scribano, M. L. *et al.* (1996). Psychologic predictors of

duodenal ulcer healing. *Journal of Clinical Gastroenterology*, **22**, 84–9.

Levenstein, S., Prantera, C., Varvo, V. *et al.* (1995). Patterns of biologic and psychologic risk factors for duodenal ulcer. *Journal of Clinical Gastroenterology*, **21**, 110–17.

Medalie, J. H., Stange, K. C., Zyzanski, S. J. *et al.* (1992). The importance of biopsychosocial factors in the development of duodenal ulcer in a cohort of middle-aged men. *American Journal of Epidemiology*, **136**, 1280–7.

Oektedalen, O., Guldvog, I., Opstad, P. K. *et al.* (1984). The effect of physical stress on gastric secretion and pancreatic polypeptide levels in man. *Scandinavian Journal of Gastroenterology*, **19**, 770–8.

Shigemi, J., Mino, Y. & Tsuda, T. (1999). The role of perceived job stress in the relationship between smoking and the development of peptic ulcers. *Journal of Epidemiology*, **9**, 320–6.

Segawa, K., Nakazawa, S., Tsukamoto, Y. *et al.* (1987). Peptic ulcer is prevalent among shift workers. *Digestive Diseases and Sciences*, **32**, 449–53.

Growth retardation

Michael Preece

Institute of Child Health

Definition

Variation in the growth of children occurs in two dimensions. The easiest to understand is the simple variation in height at any given age including full maturity. Less obvious is the variation that occurs in the timing of events during the growth process such as the

age at which puberty commences or adult height is reached: this is usually referred to as tempo.

In the case of boys, the average age of attaining adult height is 18 years but this may vary by as much as three years in either direction. Thus a perfectly healthy boy may not stop growing until 21 years of age and this would be an example of growth retardation

(Preece, 1998). In the case of girls, the same degree of variation is seen, but, on average, adult height is achieved some two years earlier than for boys.

Once the child reaches mature height, tempo has no more effect and the variation in height amongst adults is not dependent upon it. The major influence on adult height, assuming the individuals are all healthy, is heredity with a typical correlation coefficient between the mid-parental height and the height of the subject being 0.7 (Tanner, 1966). This is in keeping with a polygenic mode of inheritance for stature. During childhood the hereditary element still applies but variation in tempo will also contribute to the total variance in height. For example, a child of parents of average height might be relatively short simply because of delayed tempo of growth; this is more commonly referred to as growth retardation. It should be clear that growth retardation should not be used to describe short stature unless there is clear evidence of delayed tempo.

Using the above strict definition, it is possible for growth retardation to be present in a child of normal height. This would apply when the child has tall parents, but the delayed tempo makes the child appear shorter than would be expected from the parents. This effect is temporary and resolves as maturity is reached and the influence of the delayed tempo ends and, unless the delay is very severe, seldom leads to clinically relevant problems.

Clinical indicators

Short stature for a given chronological age will usually be part of the clinical picture unless the child is from a very tall family. In a child of peripubertal age there will be evidence of delay in other milestones such as the events of puberty. In many cases there will be as much concern about the latter as about the short stature. Similarly to the attainment of adult height there is a range of normal variation of about three years either side of the average age of attaining each stage of puberty. It is a convenient quirk of nature that the standard deviation of the age of attaining most pubertal events is one year (Tanner, 1962) and therefore a total range of six years around the average should include about 99% of healthy individuals.

In younger children, the assessment of tempo is much more difficult on clinical grounds although dental maturation can sometimes be used. If clinically relevant, skeletal maturation can be assessed from an X-ray of the left hand and wrist and provides a useful tool. From this a 'bone-age' is calculated which is equal to the chronological age of a healthy child with the same physical appearance on the X-ray. Thus a 10-year-old patient with tempo delayed two years will have a bone-age of eight 'years'. Using this technique a reasonable estimate of mature height may be obtained.

Clinical relevance

Some degree of growth retardation is very common and is responsible for a large number of referrals. It appears to be much more common in boys than in girls, but it is not clear whether this is due to a truly lower incidence in girls or whether it reflects social attitudes to height or a combination of both these factors. In many cases there is a combination of delayed growth and familial short stature which presumably reflects a selection bias, in that children who are delayed and from short families are more likely to cause concern and present clinically. In contrast, those from tall families will only present if the delay is extreme such that they appear short when compared to their peers or that the delay in puberty is sufficient to cause distress in its own right.

The importance of the condition lies in the psychological distress that can result. This is not usually a great problem before the age when adolescence usually commences (about 10 years in girls and 11 years in boys) and is not usually a permanent problem if handled sympathetically (Voss & Mulligan, 1994; Sandberg, & Voss, 2002). However, adolescence is a time of much anxiety even when it proceeds uneventfully, and children with severe pubertal and growth delay experience many additional problems particularly in their relationships with their peers (Gordon et al., 1982). For this reason the condition needs serious treatment and sympathy even though it is effectively an extension of normal development and by its nature, temporary. Management generally involves reassurance along with active intervention to accelerate the attainment of puberty and the adolescent growth spurt. The latter is usually achieved with a short course of low dose anabolic steroids (Stanhope & Preece, 1988).

REFERENCES

Gordon, M., Crouthamel, C., Post, E. M. & Richman, R. A. (1982). Psychosocial aspects of constitutional short stature: social competence, behaviour problems, self-esteem and family functioning. *Journal of Paediatrics*, **101**, 477–80.

Preece, A. M. (1998). Principles of normal growth: auxology and endocrinology. In A. Grossman (Ed.). *Clinical Endocrinology*, (2nd edn.) (pp. 845–54). Oxford: Blackwell Scientific Publications.

Sandberg, D. E. & Voss, L. D. (2002). The psychosocial consequences of short stature: a review of the evidence. *Best Practice and Research. Clinical and Endocrinology Metabolism*, **16**, 449–63.

Stanhope, R. & Preece, M. A. (1988). Management of constitutional delay of growth and puberty. *Archives of Diseases of Childhood*, **63**, 1104–10.

Tanner, J. M. (1962). *Growth at adolescence*. Oxford: Blackwell.

Tanner, J. M. (1966). Galtonian eugenics and the study of growth. *Eugenics Review*, **58**, 122–35.

Voss, L. D. & Mulligan, J. (1994). The short normal child in school: self-esteem, behaviour, and attainment before puberty (The Wessex Growth Study). In B. Stabler & L. E. Underwood (Eds.). *Growth, stature and adaptation* (pp. 47–64). Chapel Hill, NC: University of North Carolina.

Haemophilia

Ivana Marková

University of Stirling

'Haemophilia' is a term referring to a group of genetically transmitted life-long blood clotting disorders which are caused by a defect in one or more of the plasma clotting factors. The most common are sex-linked recessive disorders, haemophilia A (classic haemophilia) and haemophilia B (Christmas disease), which are due to an isolated deficiency of the clotting activity of factor VIII or of factor IX, respectively. People with these disorders suffer bleeding into soft tissues, for example, joints, muscles or internal organs, which can happen after trauma or spontaneously. These bleeds can be very painful, and repeated episodes lead to weakening and crippling of joints. Bleeds into internal organs and the brain can be life-threatening. There is no cure for haemophilia.

Another common blood disorder is von Willebrand's disease or vascular haemophilia. It is an autosomal dominant genetic disorder, i.e. it is not sex-linked and affects both men and women. It is due to a combination of an abnormal factor VIII molecule with abnormal platelet function. Many problems related to treatment and its complications, as well as social and psychological problems are similar to those found in haemophilia A and B.

Genetics and clinical manifestation

Haemophilias A and B are genetically transmitted as follows: an affected woman carries a defective gene on one of her X chromosomes, which she can pass to any of her children. This means that there is a 50% chance that any of her sons will have haemophilia and a 50% chance that any of her daughters will be a carrier. None of the sons of a haemophilic male will have the disease but all of his daughters will be obligatory carriers. In the majority of families with haemophilia (approximately 70%) the evidence of transmission of a defective gene can be established and family trees indicating such transmission can be constructed. In the remaining 30% of families, haemophilia might have been transmitted for generations through female carriers who themselves did not suffer the disease, or it might have occurred as a result of a spontaneous mutation (see also 'Screening: genetic').

The clinical manifestations of haemophilias A and B are identical and only blood tests can differentiate between them. Haemophilia affects approximately 1 in 5000 of the male population; it can be found in all human races and also in a variety of animal species. The incidence of haemophilia B is approximately 1/6 to 1/10 of that of haemophilia A.

Haemophilia occurs in different degrees of severity and these are related to the level of deficiency of the relevant clotting factors(s) in the blood. It is common to classify the disease as mild (more than 5% of the normal activity of the factor), moderate (between 1–2% and 5%) and severe (less than 1–2%). People with mild haemophilia usually need special care only when having surgery, while those with severe haemophilia may bleed spontaneously, either for no obvious reason or after emotional trauma. If haemophilia is known to be in a family, it can be diagnosed prenatally from a fetal blood sample (see 'Screening: antenatal' and 'Fetal wellbeing: monitoring & assessment'). Alternatively, it will be diagnosed in the child as a result of bruising, cutting teeth, surgery or injury. Mild haemophilia might not be diagnosed until adulthood.

Treatment of haemophilia

Haemophilias A and B are treated by replacing the missing clotting factor. During the last 50 years there has been a systematic technological effort to simplify and purify the treatment. Treatment by transfusion of full blood was replaced in the 1920s by injecting blood plasma and this was a standard treatment until the late 1960s. The patient had to go to hospital for this treatment and, if necessary, stay there over a period of time. Technological advancements in the late 1960s led to the production of various kinds of factor concentrates. As these products became safe and stable, they could be kept in home freezers. Programmes of home treatment were introduced enabling self-infusion or infusion to be given by a suitably trained relative or friend. Since this treatment can be administered either prophylactically or immediately after the bleeding occurs, it reduces long-lasting crippling of joints and painful bleeding. Thanks to the introduction of home treatment people with haemophilia have regained their independence and can take part in various kinds of physical activity without constant worries about injuries.

Since factor concentrates are blood products, there has always been a danger of viral contamination. While in recent years there have been tremendous advances in the development of pure and safer plasma-derived concentrates, simultaneously, genetically engineered recombinant DNA factors VIII and IX have been developed and are used as a treatment for children. The latest development in the treatment of haemophilia involves the possibility of gene therapy, now being in the stage of clinical trials. This treatment, which involves introducing a normal copy of the defective gene into a cell, produces the protein that was missing or defective. This, again, is a treatment of the affected individual but not a cure; the individual will pass the defective gene to the next generation. As with any genetically based treatments today, gene therapy for haemophilia is widely discussed and controversial due to its perceived ethical and psychological concerns.

Treatment and care of people with haemophilia remains highly specialized and is carried out, in wealthy countries, in specialist haemophilia centres. Monitoring of the progress in treatment and of all haemophilia related issues in national haemophilia organizations is made through the World Federation of Hemophilia, which was founded in 1963 and has headquarters in Montréal, Canada.

There are two types of specialized centres. First, there are comprehensive care centres, which provide a broad range of medical and related services offering a wide range of diagnoses and treatments. Their staff consists of specialists with high expertize, like haematologists, dentists, nurses, physiotherapists, orthopaedic surgeons, geneticists and counsellors. People with haemophilia should be registered with, and regularly reviewed at, a comprehensive care centre. Secondly, there are haemophilia centres, which tend to have a smaller number of patients and do not offer the comprehensive range of services. They provide care, information and support for patients and their families.

The World Federation of Hemophilia also offers haemophilia training programmes and care workshops in developing countries. Moreover, people with haemophilia and local centres can consult the World Federation of Hemophilia website, which provides the news, advice and support.

Treatment-related complications

While the treatment by factor concentrates introduced in the late 1960s has led to a dramatic improvement in the quality of life of patients and their families, by the mid-1970s it was apparent that chronically treated patients had developed a variety of serious complications (e.g. inhibitors to treatment, hepatitis and chronic liver disease). Inhibitors to treatment are caused by the inability of the body to distinguish between treatment clotting factors and harmful foreign invaders, e.g. bacteria. As a result, the body produces antibodies, i.e. inhibitors that destroy the clotting factor which is supposed to treat the bleeding. Inhibitors constitute a long-term clinical problem for up to 20% of people with severe haemophilia A, and they are less of a problem for people with haemophilia B.

Other treatment-related problems are due to several hepatitis viruses transmitted through blood products and causing liver disease. Among these, hepatitis C is of particular concern, as there is not as yet a vaccine for hepatitis C. Hepatitis C affects most people with haemophilia who received clotting factor concentrates before 1986, that is, before effective heat treatment was first introduced in wealthy countries of the world, including the UK.

Finally, in the 1970s and early 1980s many people with haemophilia were infected with HIV through contaminated blood products. Unfortunately, by the time the problem came to awareness, in some parts of the world as many as 90% of severely affected patients with haemophilia B, and a small percentage of those with haemophilia A, had become infected and many have died. In order to alleviate suffering of patients affected by HIV, the World Federation of Hemophilia and national haemophilia organizations launched substantial efforts to speed up blood donation screening and to physically treat blood and blood products. Moreover, governments of wealthy countries approved plans for financial assistance to patients who were infected by HIV during the epidemic (see also 'HIV and AIDS').

By the mid-1980s, blood donors were screened for the presence of HIV, and concentrates of clotting factors used for the treatment of bleeds, were heat-treated to destroy HIV. In order to destroy any harmful viruses, apart from being heated, concentrates are now treated in a number of other ways during manufacture, e.g. by adding to them solvent and detergent mixtures. All patients are vaccinated against hepatitis A and B.

Psychosocial problems of haemophilia

Throughout history, haemophilia has always presented a wide spectrum of psychological and behavioural challenges to patients, carriers and their relatives. The nature of these challenges keeps changing with the advances in diagnosis and treatment and with dealing with treatment complications. All these changes have a profound effect on social and psychological problems of patients and their families, as well as on social representations of haemophilia in the general public.

Haemophilia, like other chronic disorders, is a family matter. Moreover, being a sex-linked genetic disorder, it imposes different kinds of trauma on women and men and on the related family decisions. Prospective parents must decide whether to undergo diagnostic procedures in order to discover whether the fetus is affected with haemophilia and, if it is, whether they wish to undergo a termination of the pregnancy (see 'Screening: antenatal' and 'Abortion'). No matter how accurate and safe fetal diagnosis may become, it is perception and acceptance of such procedures and ethical concerns of the involved individuals that determine the subsequent course of action. There are several stages in bringing up a child with haemophilia that parents may find particularly difficult: coping with the diagnosis, teaching the pre-school child to look after himself, overcoming anxiety about the child's starting school and solving the problem of the child's career. The parents might find it difficult to strike a balance between the necessary and unnecessary restrictions imposed on the child. With the development of factor concentrates in the last four or five decades, the aim for a person with haemophilia at school, at work and in the family, has been 'to be as normal as possible'. However, adults with haemophilia, attempting to find employment, are faced with the problem of whether or not to tell their future employers about their disease. This of course also depends on how severe their haemophilia is. Getting life assurance has always been a problem for severely affected patients, and this problem has been aggravated as a result of haemophilia's association with AIDS.

The psychosocial impact of HIV and AIDS on patients and their families has been unprecedented and they have experienced two main kinds of problem. First, there is the problem of coping with the physical and mental trauma due to HIV and AIDS. While HIV infection in men with haemophilia is no longer due to blood products, new cases of HIV infection include women infected by their spouses and children who were infected by HIV presumably during pregnancy.

The second problem is related to the general public's social representations of haemophilia and HIV/AIDS. Throughout history, haemophilia has always been surrounded by mysteries of bleeding as well as by misconceptions, e.g. that a person with haemophilia can bleed to death from a needle prick. Misconceptions on the part of the general public, the fear of stigma and the fear of being rejected by employers or by intimate friends have often led to patients concealing their haemophilia (see 'Stigma'). The problem of HIV/AIDS has only amplified these problems. The public misunderstanding of haemophilia and misconceptions about the transmission of HIV/AIDS in people with haemophilia has been experienced as a double stigma. While public education is essential to diminish social and psychological problem experienced by people with haemophilia and their families, equally important to consider are the rapid technological advancements in treatment and eventually for 'cure' of haemophilia which offer good prospects for the future.

REFERENCES

Behring, L. L. C., Lusher, J. M. & Kessler, C. M. (Eds.). (1991). *Hemophilia and von Willebrand's disease in the 1990's,* Elsevier Science Publishers.

Bloom, A. L., Forbes, C. D., Thomas, D. & Tuddenham, E. G. D. (Eds.). (1994). *Haemostasis and thrombosis.* Edinburgh: Churchill-Livingstone.

Bussing, R. & Johnson, S. B. (1992). Psychosocial issues in hemophilia before and after the HIV crisis: a review of current research. *General Hospital Psychiatry,* **14,** 387–403.

Forbes, C. D., Adedort, L. & Madhok, R. (Eds.). (1997). *Haemophilia.* London: Chapman & Hale.

Jones, P. (2002). *Living with Haemophilia.* (5th edn.). Oxford: Oxford University Press.

Kelley, L. A. (2000). *Raising a child with hemophilia.* King of Prussia, PA: Aventis-Behring L. L. C.

Markova, I. (1997). The family and haemophilia. In C. D. Forbes, L. Adedort & R. Madhok (Eds.). *Haemophilia* (pp. 335–46). London: Chapman & Hale.

Mason, P. J., Olson, R. A. & Parish, K. L. (1988). AIDS, hemophilia, and prevention efforts within a comprehensive care program, *American Psychologist,* **43,** 971–6.

Miller, R., Fields, P. A., Goldspink G. *et al.* (2002). Somatic gene therapy for haemophilia: some counselling issues for today and tomorrow. *Psychology, Health and Medicine,* **7,** 163–72.

Ratnoff, O. D. & Forbes, C. D. (Eds.). (1994). *Disorders of Hemostasis* (2nd edn.). Philadelphia: Saunders.

Head injury

Erin D. Bigler

Brigham Young University

Head injuries are generally divided into two types: closed and open or penetrating (Graham *et al.,* 2002). In open or penetrating injuries, the skull is breached, most commonly struck with violent force by foreign objects during an assault or from a gun shot or as a result of the head impacting some part of the vehicle in a motor vehicle accident (MVA). Part of the damage from penetrating injuries often includes bone fragments and other debris associated with the trauma that directly injures the brain. In addition to the mechanical damage to brain tissue, there is typically local haemorrhaging that also damages the brain, since the forces that penetrate the brain usually tear blood vessels in the region of penetration. The pathological consequences of open or penetrating injuries to the brain are most likely to produce focal brain injuries, although often generalized damage may also occur. Open head injuries are less common than closed and some, like gunshot wounds (GSW) to the head, are associated with very high mortality.

The most common head injury associated with survival is a closed head injury (CHI), where the brain is injured by the mechanical, concussive and movement forces within the cranium, secondarily through impact to the head and/or acceleration/deceleration forces. Either regional or global, such forces place what are referred to as tensile or shear-strain effects throughout the brain. These effects have the potential to stretch neural tissue, particularly axons, which in turn damages either their structure or function. Because of the vulnerability of the axon in CHI, the effects of trauma are often thought of in terms of a diffuse axonal injury (DAI, Graham *et al.,* 2002). These same shear-strain forces may also damage, disrupt or shear blood vessels, which may also be a major source of residual damage from trauma. This is often referred to as a haemorrhagic shear injury and can often be readily visualized by neuroimaging techniques (Tong *et al.,* 2004) (see 'Brain imaging and function'). Obviously, anything that disrupts the integrity of the vasculature has the potential to damage brain tissue either directly or through the secondary effects of disrupting blood flow; the brain has no capacity to store oxygen or glucose and needs a constant blood supply. Another aspect of brain injury is referred to as the neurotoxic cascade (Hatton, 2001; Kaminska *et al.,* 2004). As brain cells are injured, there is often an abnormal release of neurotransmitters or a disruption in synaptic function which can result in biochemical changes that damage or kill brain cells. As brain cells die, volume loss occurs, resulting in either focal or generalized reduction in a specific brain region or in the brain overall. In CHI, generalized cerebral atrophy, as measured by neuroimaging, is proportional to the severity of injury and relates to outcome (Bigler, 2005).

Because it is the most common, this chapter will focus primarily on CHI, review current definitional standards, epidemiology, how to assess and treat brain injury and the long-term outcome.

Definition of brain injury and brain injury severity

Brain injury is defined by some alteration or impairment in normal neurological homeostasis or presence of a distinct abnormality caused by trauma, such as experiencing a brain contusion in a fall as shown by neuroimaging studies (Bigler, 1990) (see 'Brain imaging and function'). The mildest form of injury is that which results from a concussion, wherein the mildest form is but a brief, transient disruption in neurological function as described in Table 1. The most well-studied concussions are those associated with sports injury, the majority of which are likely to have a benign course (Guskiewicz et al., 2003; McCrea et al., 2003). As the level of concussion increases so do the potential sequelae, particularly after what is referred to as a complicated concussion, where, for example, there is neuroimaging evidence of a brain contusion or presence of a skull fracture. Severity of head injuries are often graded by the Glasgow Coma Scale (GCS, Teasdale & Jennett, 1974), which is a scale from

Table 1. Concussion grading systems

Grade	Cantu	Colorado	Roberts	American Academy of Neurology
0				'Bell ringer'; no LOC; no PTA
1	No LOC; PTA <30 min	No LOC; confusion without amnesia	No LOC; PTA <30 min	No LOC; transient confusion; concussion symptoms or mental status abnormality resolve in <15 min
2	LOC <5 min; PTA >30 min and <24 h	No LOC; confusion with amnesia	LOC <5 min; PTA >30 min and <24 h	No LOC; transient confusion; concussion symptoms or mental status abnormality last >15 min
3	LOC >5 min or PTA >24 h	LOC	LOC >5 min or PTA >24 h	Any LOC, either brief or prolonged

LOC = loss of consciousness; PTA = post-traumatic amnesia
Adapted with permission from Leclerc et al. (Leclerc, Lassonde, Delaney, Lacroix & Johnston, 2001).

3 (deep coma, unresponsive) to 15 (no alteration in level of consciousness). Typically, GCS scores in the 13–15 range are considered mild; 9–12 is moderate, while 8 and below are moderate-to-severe traumatic brain injuries (TBI). Two other defining characteristics of brain injury are duration of loss of consciousness (LOC) and post-traumatic amnesia (PTA). Memory is the most commonly disrupted cognitive function in TBI and the length of time between the accident and the re-establishment of continuous memory for immediate past events, or the degree of PTA is predictive of outcome (Dikmen et al., 2003; Katz & Alexander, 1994). As shown in Figure 1 regardless of which measure of injury severity is examined, duration of LOC, length of PTA or level of GCS are all associated with the development of cerebral atrophy.

Epidemiology

Bruns and Hauser (2003) review the epidemiology of TBI wherein estimates vary, depending on the minimal definition used to define TBI, but safely conclude that the annual incidence rate in North American and Europe exceeds 200 per 100 000 population (see also Center for Disease Control website: www.cdc.gov. for up-to-date epidemiological statistics). This makes TBI one of the leading causes of death and disability in the world.

Assessment

Brain injury and its severity are defined by the events that cause the injury and by clinical findings during the initial medical assessment of the patient after the injury. As already stated, presence and duration of LOC and/or PTA, as well as GCS, define the severity of injury and some of its sequela. Most patients with moderate or worse CHI will be hospitalized, whereas those in the mild range are less likely to be hospitalized other than to be assessed in the accident and emergency department/emergency room. The majority with grade II or less concussion (see Table 1) may not even be initially medically assessed. The Diagnostic and Statistical Manual, 4th edn (DSM-IV) of the American Psychiatric Association (1994) as shown in Table 2, lists the common core neurobehavioural sequelae associated with head injury.

From the perspective of evaluating the cognitive and neurobehavioural deficits in the patient who has sustained a head injury, there are typically three general areas of assessment; neuropsychological, neuropsychiatric and neuroimaging. Each will be addressed below.

Neuropsychological

From a neuropsychological standpoint, the most common neurocognitive changes occur in the domain of short-term memory, attention/concentration and executive function (i.e. novel problem-solving skills, planning, organizational abilities, etc.). Guidelines by Lezak et al. (2004) provide a framework to assess these types of deficits. Neurobehaviourally, the changes that typically occur do so within the framework of mood- and anxiety-based disorders as well as potential changes in personality and temperament (Silver et al., 2005), although damage to frontal and temporal brain regions often results in significant personality changes, the so-called frontal lobe

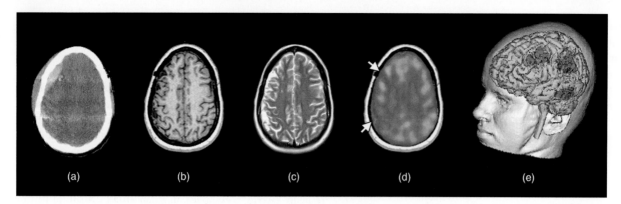

Fig 1 (A) Day-of-injury computerized tomography (DOI CT) scan taken within an hour of this patient sustaining a severe head injury when a delivery truck collided with the patient's vehicle. Her head struck the door frame and computerized tomography (CT) imaging shows a prominent cerebral haematoma with underlying contusion (bruising) to the brain. Two years after injury, magnetic resonance imaging (MRI) studies show generalized atrophy of the left hemisphere in the MRI sequences shown in (B) and (C). Atrophy is indicated by increased amounts of cerebral spinal fluid visualized on the surface of the brain. (D) represents the results of single photon emission tomography (SPECT) imaging where the darker image involving most of the left hemisphere (see arrows) represents less perfusion or uptake of the radiopharmaceutical as shown. Finally (E), the three dimensional (3-D) image of the patient's brain shows where the greatest amounts of cerebral atrophy could be detected.

Table 2. Research criteria for post-concussional disorder

A. A history of head trauma that has caused significant cerebral concussion.
   Note: The manifestations of concussion include loss of consciousness, post-traumatic amnesia and less commonly, post-traumatic onset of seizures. The specific method of defining this criterion needs to be established by further research.

B. Evidence from neuropsychological testing or quantified cognitive assessment of difficulty in attention (concentrating, shifting focus of attention, performing simultaneous cognitive tasks) or memory (learning or recalling information).

C. Three (or more) of the following occur shortly after the trauma and last at least three months:
   1. becoming fatigued easily
   2. disordered sleep
   3. headache
   4. vertigo or dizziness
   5. irritability or aggression on little or no provocation
   6. anxiety, depression, or affective lability
   7. changes in personality (e.g. social or sexual inappropriateness)
   8. apathy or lack of spontaneity

D. The symptoms in Criteria B and C have their onset following head trauma or else represent a substantial worsening of pre-existing symptoms

E. The disturbance causes significant impairment in social or occupational functioning and represents a significant decline from a previous level of functioning. In school-age children, the impairment may be manifested by a significant worsening in school or academic performance dating from the trauma.

F. The symptoms do not meet criteria for Dementia due to Head Trauma and are not better accounted for by another mental disorder (e.g. Amnestic Disorder due to Head Trauma, Personality Change due to Head Trauma).

From DSM-IV-™, pp. 705–6. Diagnostic and Statistical Manual of Mental Disorders 4th edn. (American Psychiatric Association, 1994).

syndrome (Cato *et al.*, 2004). (See 'Neuropsychological assessment' chapter for more information.)

Neuropsychiatric

As mentioned above, disorders that centre on changes in personality, mood and emotional regulation are commonplace in TBI and are the primary reason behind neuropsychiatric consultation and treatment of the patient with a head injury (Silver *et al.*, 2005). Large-scale epidemiological studies of neuropsychiatric outcome have clearly shown the increased lifetime prevalence of depression and anxiety-based disorders in those who have sustained a TBI (Dikmen *et al.*, 2004; Fann *et al.*, 2004; Holsinger *et al.*, 2002; Jorge *et al.*, 2004; Oquendo *et al.*, 2004). Some of the neurobehavioural

sequela listed in Table 2 may be amenable to various pharmacotherapies following neuropsychiatric assessment.

Neuroimaging

Tremendous advances in neuroimaging have provided various methods for detailed analyses of structural and functional deficits associated with brain injury (see Bigler, 2005). Figure 1 shows what residual damage from a severe TBI looks like on initial computerized tomography (CT) and on follow-up magnetic resonance imaging (MRI) in a patient who sustained a significant head injury. A consequence of this more lateralized left hemisphere damage, as visualized on the imaging studies, was that the patient had significant language and memory deficits on neuropsychological testing, as well as requiring neuropsychiatric treatment for post-TBI depression. Additional details of the type of neuroimaging possible are provided in the chapter '*Brain imaging and function*'.

Treatment

Depending on the residual neurological and neurobehavioural deficits and brain regions injured, a variety of potential treatment options exists for the individual who sustain a CHI. When neuropsychological tests demonstrate cognitive deficits; various cognitive rehabilitation strategies may be available (see Borgaro *et al.*, 2003; Miller *et al.*, 2003) (see 'Neuropsychological rehabilitation'). Likewise, cognitive behaviour therapies and other forms of psychotherapy may be beneficial in treating a variety of behavioural changes which accompany head injury (Salmond *et al.*, 2005) (see 'Cognitive behaviour therapy'). Additionally, psychotherapeutic techniques may help address adjustment and stress related problems that often attend an individual with a brain injury. In concussion, the mildest form of TBI, immediate educational and psychotherapeutic intervention may minimize the occurrence and development of the so-called post-concussive syndrome (Millis *et al.*, 2001). Also, medications for memory, mood, sleep and related functions may be necessary. As shown by Annegers and Coan (2000) there is a significant increase in the incidence of post-traumatic epilepsy and anticonvulsant medication may be part of the treatment regime (see also 'Epilepsy'). There is considerable psychiatric morbidity associated with having a head injury (Fann *et al.*, 2004; Holsinger *et al.*, 2002; Jorge *et al.*, 2004), as already discussed.

Long-term outcome

Moderate-to-severe TBI is associated with increased levels of impaired social, personal and vocational outcome (Colantonio *et al.*, 2004). Individuals who have experienced a significant TBI have an increased risk of dementia later in life (Plassman *et al.*, 2000) (see 'Dementias'). As already mentioned, having a TBI also increases the risk of post-traumatic epilepsy (Annegers & Coan, 2000) and a variety of neuropsychiatric disorders. There is greater psychosocial stressors in families where an individual has sustained a TBI and individuals with moderate-to-severe TBI are more likely to be disabled (Colantonio *et al.*, 2004).

Summary

Cognitive and neurobehavioural sequela are commonplace in head injury, especially in moderate-to-severe injury where high levels of permanent disability exist. Significant improvements in the assessment and treatment of head injury have occurred over the last decade, particularly in the area of neuroimaging findings in detecting brain abnormalities associated with trauma.

Acknowledgments

Supported in part by the Ira Fulton Foundation. The technical assistance of Tracy Abildskov and Craig Vickers and the editorial assistance of Jo Ann Petrie are gratefully acknowledged.

REFERENCES

American Psychiatric Association (APA). (1994). *DSM-IV: Diagnostic and Statistical Manual of Mental Disorders*, (4th edn.). Washington, DC: American Psychiatric Association.

Annegers, J. F. & Coan, S. P. (2000). The risks of epilepsy after traumatic brain injury. *Seizure*, **9**, 453–7.

Bigler, E. D. (2005). Structural imaging. In J. M. Silver, S. C. Yudofsky & R. E. Hales (Eds.). *Textbook of Traumatic Brain Injury*, (2nd edn.). Washington, DC: American Psychiatric Association.

Bigler, E. D. (Ed.). (1990). *Traumatic brain injury*. Austin, TX: Pro-Ed.

Blatter, D. D., Bigler, E. D., Gale, S. D. *et al.* (1995). Quantitative volumetric analysis of brain MR: normative database spanning 5 decades of life. *American Journal of Neuroradiology*, **16**, 241–51.

Blatter, D. D., Bigler, E. D., Gale, S. D. *et al.* (1997). MR-based brain and cerebrospinal fluid measurement after traumatic brain injury: correlation with neuropsychological outcome. *American Journal of Neuroradiology*, **18**, 1–10.

Borgaro, S., Caples, H. & Prigatano, G. P. (2003). Non-pharmacological management of psychiatric disturbances after traumatic brain injury. *International Review of Psychiatry*, **15**, 371–9.

Bruns, J., Jr. & Hauser, W. A. (2003). The epidemiology of traumatic brain injury: a review. *Epilepsia*, **44**(Suppl. 10), 2–10.

Cato, M. A., Delis, D. C., Abildskov, T. J. & Bigler, E. (2004). Assessing the elusive cognitive deficits associated with ventromedial prefrontal damage: a case of a modern-day Phineas Gage. *Journal of the International Neuropsychological Society*, **10**, 453–65.

Colantonio, A., Ratcliff, G., Chase, S. *et al.* (2004). Long-term outcomes after moderate to severe traumatic brain injury. *Disability and Rehabilitation*, **26**, 253–61.

Dikmen, S. S., Bombardier, C. H., Machamer, J. E., Fann, J. R. & Temkin, N. R. (2004). Natural history of depression in traumatic brain injury. *Archives of Physical Medicine & Rehabilitation*, **85**, 1457–64.

Dikmen, S. S., Machamer, J. E., Powell, J. M. & Temkin, N. R. (2003). Outcome 3 to 5 years after moderate to severe traumatic brain injury. *Archives of Physical Medicine and Rehabilitation*, **84**, 1449–57.

Fann, J. R., Burington, B., Leonetti, A. *et al.* (2004). Psychiatric illness following traumatic brain injury in an adult health maintenance organization population. *Archives of General Psychiatry*, **61**, 53–61.

Graham, D. I., Gennarelli, T. A. & McIntosh, T. K. (2002). Trauma. In D. I. Graham & P. L. Lantos (Eds.). *Greenfield's Neuropathology*, (7th edn.) (pp. 823–98). New York: Arnold.

Guskiewicz, K. M., McCrea, M., Marshall, S. W. *et al.* (2003). Cumulative effects associated with recurrent concussion in collegiate football players: the NCAA concussion study. *Journal of the American Medical Association*, **290**, 2549–55.

Hatton, J. (2001). Pharmacological treatment of traumatic brain injury: a review of agents in development. *CNS Drugs*, **15**(7), 553–81.

Holsinger, T., Steffens, D. C., Phillips, C. *et al.* (2002). Head injury in early adulthood and the lifetime risk of depression. *Archives of General Psychiatry*, **59**, 17–22.

Jorge, R. E., Robinson, R. G., Moser, D. *et al.* (2004). Major depression following traumatic brain injury. *Archives of General Psychiatry*, **61**, 42–50.

Kaminska, B., Gaweda-Walerych, K. & Zawadzka, M. (2004). Molecular mechanisms of neuroprotective action of immunosuppressants – facts and hypotheses. *Journal of Cellular and Molecular Medicine*, **8**, 45–58.

Katz, D. I. & Alexander, M. P. (1994). Traumatic brain injury. Predicting course of recovery and outcome for patients admitted to rehabilitation. *Archives of Neurology*, **51**, 661–70.

Leclerc, S., Lassonde, M., Delaney, J. S., Lacroix, V. J. & Johnston, K. M. (2001). Recommendations for grading of concussion in athletes. *Sports Medicine*, **31**, 629–36.

Lezak, M. D., Howieson, D. B. & Loring, D. W. (2004). *Neuropsychological Assessment*, (4th edn.). New York: Oxford University Press.

McCrea, M., Guskiewicz, K. M., Marshall, S. W. *et al.* (2003). Acute effects and recovery time following concussion in collegiate football players: the NCAA concussion study. *Journal of the American Medical Association*, **290**, 2556–63.

Miller, M. A., Burnett, D. M. & McElligott, J. M. (2003). Congenital and acquired brain injury. 3. Rehabilitation interventions: cognitive, behavioral, and community reentry. *Archives of Physical Medicine & Rehabilitation*, **84**(3 Suppl. 1), S12–17.

Millis, S. R., Rosenthal, M., Novack, T. A. *et al.* (2001). Long-term neuropsychological outcome after traumatic brain injury. *Journal of Head Trauma Rehabilitation*, **16**, 343–55.

Oquendo, M. A., Friedman, J. H., Grunebaum, M. F. *et al.* (2004). Suicidal behavior and mild traumatic brain injury in major depression. *The Journal of Nervous and Mental Disease*, **192**, 430–4.

Plassman, B. L., Havlik, R. J., Steffens, D. C. *et al.* (2000). Documented head injury in early adulthood and risk of Alzheimer's disease and other dementias. *Neurology*, **55**, 1158–66.

Salmond, C. H., Menon, D. K., Chatfield, D. A., Pickard, J. D. & Sahakian, B. J. (2005). Deficits in decision-making in head injury survivors. *Journal of Neurotrauma*, **22**, 613–22.

Silver, J. M., McAllister, T. W. & Yudofsky, S. C. (Eds.). (2005). *Textbook of Traumatic Brain Injury*, (2nd edn.). Washington, DC: American Psychiatric Publishing, Inc.

Teasdale, G. & Jennett, B. (1974). Assessment of coma and impaired consciousness: a practical scale. *Lancet*, **2**, 81–4.

Tong, K. A., Ashwal, S., Holshouser, B. A. *et al.* (2004). Diffuse axonal injury in children: clinical correlation with hemorrhagic lesions. *Annals of Neurology*, **56**, 36–50.

Headache and migraine

Bjørn Ellertsen

University of Stavanger

Introduction

Headache is one of the most common nuisances known to man. The pain may be secondary, as in fever or hypertension, or primary, as in migraine. It has been estimated that about 30% of people in the western world suffer from one or more severe headache episodes per year. In the UK, more than 3 million workdays are estimated lost per year due to headache. The majority of headache patients have migraine, tension-type headache (TTH) or combinations of these. About 65% of the patients seen in headache clinics suffer from migraine, 25% from TTH and about 10% from other types of headache. Although such samples are selective, the relative proportions of types of headache are probably representative of the population. The causes of headache syndromes like migraine, cluster headache and TTH are largely unknown. However, knowledge about clinical, physiological, biochemical and psychological characteristics is substantial.

The definitions of headache syndromes lacked precision in the past, making it problematic to compare studies. Therefore, the International Headache Society (IHS) formed a Classification Committee which published diagnostic criteria in 1988 (IHS, 1988). Most research published after 1988 adheres to these criteria.

Pathophysiology

In the field of psychophysiology, psychological variables are manipulated while physiological variables are measured as dependents. The field has yielded important information about the pathophysiology of headache. When reviewing the literature on response characteristics of patients, it becomes evident that the earlier distinction between migraine as vascular, and TTH as myalgic is oversimplified. Abnormal vasomotor responses have been observed in migraine patients in a number of studies. In general, data suggest labile autonomic nervous system activity. In an early study, non-medicated female migraine patients were found to show slower habituation to strong auditory stimuli than controls. They also showed more pronounced pulse wave amplitude reduction in the temporal arteries during stressful stimulation, and a pronounced pulse wave amplitude increase while resting afterwards (Ellertsen & Hammerborg, 1982). Surface EMG levels in the frontal muscles were higher in migraine patients than controls. In non-medicated TTH patients, significantly less pronounced heart rate responses were observed, as compared with controls. Further, TTH patients showed pulse wave amplitude increases in response to stimulation, whereas controls showed a slight decrease (Ellertsen *et al.*, 1987*a*).

TTH patients showed significantly higher frontal EMG levels than controls, but not higher than migraine patients. Thus, vascular abnormalities occur in both types of headache but they appear to have different vascular response patterns.

There is by now no doubt that central nervous processes play a central part in migraine attacks. The vascular hypothesis of migraine has been superseded by a more integrated theory which involves both vascular and neuronal components. It has been demonstrated that the visual aura experienced by some migraine sufferers arises from cortical spreading depression (CSD), and that this neuronal event also may activate perivascular nerve afferents, leading to vaso-dilatation and neurogenic inflammation of the meningeal blood vessels and, thus, throbbing pain (Silberstein, 2004). There is com-pelling evidence accumulated to support the concept that CSD is responsible for migraine aura (Parsons, 2004). Thus, it has been demonstrated that migraine attacks are associated with both parox-ysmal vascular and electrical changes, caused by centrally triggered brainstem mechanisms. The electrical changes have been studied using both evoked potentials (EP) and SCP. Measurement of SCP in migraine patients has indicated a habituation deficit caused by brainstem-related dysfunction. Habituation shows systematic variation around a migraine attack. After an attack, habituation is normal (Kropp et al., 2002). Many patients with migraine develop more chronic TTH over the years and TTH patients are often seen to develop more severe and short-lasting migraine type attacks. It is therefore always important to look into the history of each headache patient when diagnosing and planning treatment.

Personality and psychopathology

The question of psychopathology and characteristic personality traits in patients with recurring or chronic headache has been discussed in a number of publications (e.g. Philips, 1976; Adler, Adler & Packard, 1987; Ellertsen, 1992; Mongini et al., 2000; Lanzi et al., 2001; Waldie & Poulton, 2002; Huber & Henrich, 2003; Mongini et al., 2003). A review of this literature on migraine and TTH shows that a main area of discussion revolves around the ques-tion of cause and effect. Although most studies report an increased prevalence of emotional and psychological disturbances, the ques-tion of predisposing personality factors remains unanswered. Waldie and Poulton (2002) reported from a 26-year longitudinal study and concluded that migraine and TTH seem to be distinct disorders with different developmental characteristics. Migraine was associated with maternal headache, anxiety symptoms in childhood, anxiety during adolescence and stress reactivity person-ality traits at the age of 18. TTH was associated with neck or back injury before the age of 13. More prospective studies are needed in order to shed light on these important questions, but there are few truly longitudinal studies available (see also 'Personality and health').

The Minnesota Multiphasic Personality Inventory (MMPI and the revision MMPI-2) has been used in a number of studies of head-ache patients. One issue is whether MMPI profiles obtained in pain patients actually reflect neurotic traits, since items concerning bodily symptoms contribute to the scales in question. However, affirmative responses to MMPI items concerning bodily symp-toms are insufficient to drive any clinical MMPI scale into the abnormal range. Prognosis and planning of treatment is dependent on a number of variables. Some of these are undoubtedly reflected in the MMPI and other personality measures. Most MMPI studies of headache patients have demonstrated characteristic profiles in these groups. In general, patients show 'neurotic' MMPI profiles, where the clinical scales reflecting health concerns, depression and somatization are elevated.

In their classic study, Kudrow and Sutkus (1979) found that patients with 'vascular headache' (migraine and cluster headache) scored lowest, TTH and 'combination headache' intermediate and post-traumatic and 'conversion' headache patients highest on the neuroticism scales of the MMPI. One possible interpretation of these data is that a continuum of increased stress and pressures, or an interaction between stressors and predisposing personality characteristics, was reflected in the MMPI. It has been maintained that the relationship between certain personality traits and head-ache becomes more pronounced as the chronicity of the headache problem develops. DeDomini et al. (1983) found that MMPI elevations were more pronounced in patients with 'daily headache', as compared with patients with headache attacks. Thus, combina-tions of intensity, severity and duration of pain problems seem to be strongly related to the degree of neuroticism found in personality tests. Zwart et al. (1996) found normal MMPI-2 profiles in migraine and cluster headache patients. Significant depression and somatiza-tion was found in TTH and cervicogenic headache patients. When all groups were analysed together, there was a strong relationship between headache duration per month and scale elevations. Comparable personality data from boys with migraine, using the Personality Inventory for Children (PIC), yielded no significant differences between patients and controls. (Ellertsen & Troland, 1989). There was, however, a relationship between duration of head-ache problems and PIC factor scales indicating social withdrawal and social incompetence within the patient group.

Significant lowering of MMPI scales has been reported in groups of migraine and TTH patients who responded favourably to biofeed-back treatment (see 'Biofeedback'). In one study, MMPI profiles were compared in female migraine before and after biofeed-back treatment in a 2-year follow-up study (Ellertsen et al., 1987c). There were no differences between most and least improved patients before start of treatment. However, the least improved group showed unchanged profiles, whereas most improved patients showed significant changes on 5 MMPI scales. Decreased somatic complaints, less tension, improved interpersonal relationships and more energy was indicated. Similar changes in MMPI profiles after therapeutic intervention were reported by Fan et al. (1999). They concluded that management of migraine should include psychological intervention. In summary, the research discussed shows that depression, anxiety and somatization are found in chronic headache syndromes, whereas mild anxiety levels seem to be characteristic in recurring headache.

Applied psychophysiology

Hand temperature biofeedback has been used routinely in treat-ment of migraine patients since Sargent and Green (1972) first published their promising data on this method. The objective is to achieve learned control of peripheral vasomotor tonus, which in turn is assumed to contribute to normalization of autonomic lability, and hence reduced headache problems. Electromyographic (EMG) biofeedback treatment of TTH was originally described by Budzynski *et al.* (1970). Obviously, the two different treatment approaches were inspired by the aetiological distinction between vascular and muscular mechanisms in the headache syndromes. Few biofeedback studies have combined clinical trials and psychophysiological evaluation. In one study, heart rate and pulse wave amplitude response patterns predicted biofeedback treatment outcome (Ellertsen *et al.*, 1987). This pointed to a potential utility of psychophysiology in identifying patients who respond favourably to this type of treatment. Migraine patients showing most pronounced clinical improvement also showed a normalization of pulse wave amplitude response patterns after treatment (Ellertsen *et al.*, 1987).

Biofeedback treatment effects are well documented in adult and child migraine patients (Hermann & Blanchard, 2002;

Andrasik, 2003). In general, meta-analyses of clinical trials show that biofeedback, relaxation training and hypnosis treatment all yield effects comparable to prophylactic medication, i.e. an average reduction of attacks around 45%, as compared with 14% placebo effects (e.g. Holroyd & Penzien, 1990) (see 'Biofeedback', 'Relaxation training' and 'Hypnosis'). More recent treatment of migraine using EEG biofeedback (neurofeedback) has yielded promising results. Thus, it has been demonstrated that migraine patients can learn to control their SCPs and learn to habituate through the use of neurofeedback, which in turn leads to a reduction in the numbers of attacks (Kropp *et al.*, 2002).

In summary, the fields of psychophysiology, abnormal psychology and applied psychophysiology have made important contributions to our understanding of headache syndromes and also contributed to improved diagnostic and treatment procedures.

REFERENCES

Adler, C. S., Adler, S. M. & Packard, R. C. (1987). *Psychiatric aspects of headache.* Baltimore: Williams & Wilkins.

Andrasik, F. (2003). Behavioral treatment approaches to chronic headache. *Neurological Sciences,* **24**(Suppl. 2), 280–5.

Budzynski, T., Stoyva, J. & Adler, C. (1970). Feedback-induced muscle relaxation: application to tension headache. *Journal of Behavioural Therapy and Experimental Psychiatry,* **1**, 205.

DeDomini, P., DelBene, E., Gori-Savellini, S. *et al.* (1983). Personality patterns of headache sufferers. *Cephalalgia,* (Suppl. 1), 195–220.

Ellertsen, B. (1992). Personality factors in recurring and chronic pain. *Cephalalgia,* **12**, 129–32.

Ellertsen, B. & Hammerborg, D. (1982). Psychophysiological response patterns in migraine patients. *Cephalalgia,* **2**, 19–21.

Ellertsen, B., Nordby, H. & Sjaastad, O. (1987*a*). Psychophysiologic response patterns in tension headache: effects of tricyclic antidepressants. *Cephalalgia,* **7**, 55–63.

Ellertsen, B., Nordby, H., Hammerborg, D. & Thorlacius, S. (1987*b*). Psychophysiologic response patterns in migraine before and after temperature biofeedback. *Cephalalgia,* **7**, 109–24.

Ellertsen, B., Troland, K. & Kløve, H. (1987*c*). MMPI profiles in migraine before and after biofeedback treatment. *Cephalalgia,* **7**, 101–8.

Ellertsen, B. & Troland, K. (1989). Personality characteristics in childhood migraine. *Cephalalgia,* **9**(Suppl. 10), 238–9.

Fan, A. Y., Gu, R. J. & Zhou, A. N. (1999). MMPI changes associated with therapeutic intervention: a migraine control study. *Headache,* **39**(8), 581–5.

Hermann, C. & Blanchard, E. B. (2002). Biofeedback in the treatment of headache and other childhood pain. *Applied Psychophysiology and Biofeedback,* **27**, 143–62.

Holroyd, K. A. & Penzien, D. B. (1990). Pharmacological versus non-pharmacological prophylaxis of recurrent migraine headache: a meta-analytic review of clinical trials. *Pain,* **42**, 1–13.

Huber, D. & Henrich, G. (2003). Personality traits and stress sensitivity in migraine patients. *Journal of Behavioral Medicine,* **29**, 4–13.

International Headache Society (1988). Classification and diagnostic criteria for headache disorders, cranial neuralgias and facial pain. *Cephalalgia,* **8**(Suppl. 7).

Kropp, P., Siniatchkin, M. & Gerber, W. (2002). On the pathophysiology of migraine – links for "Empirically based treatment" with neurofeedback. *Applied Psychophysiology and Biofeedback,* **27**, 203–13.

Kudrow, L. & Sutkus, B. J. (1979). MMPI pattern specificity in primary headache disorders. *Headache,* **19**, 18–24.

Lanzi, G., Zambrino, C. A., Ferrari-Ginevra, O. *et al.* (2001). Personality traits in childhood and adolescent headache. *Cephalalgia,* **21**, 53–60.

Mongini, F., Ibertis, F., Barbalonga, E. & Raviola, F. (2000). MMPI-2 profiles in chronic daily headache and their relationship to anxiety levels and accompanying symptoms. *Headache,* **40**, 466–72.

Mongini, F., Keller, R., Deregibus, A. *et al.* (2003). Personality traits, depression and migraine in women: a longitudinal study. *Cephalalgia,* **23**, 186–92.

Parsons, A. A. (2004). Cortical spreading depression: its role in migraine pathogenesis and possible therapeutic intervention. *Current Pain and Headache Reports,* **8**, 410–16.

Philips, C. (1976). Headache and personality. *Journal of Psychosomatic Research,* **20**, 535–42.

Sargent, J. D. & Green, E. E. (1972). The use of autogenic feedback training in a pilot study of migraine and tension headache. *Headache,* **12**, 120–4.

Silberstein, S. D. (2004). Migraine pathophysiology and its clinical implications. *Cephalalgia,* **24**(Suppl. 2), 2–7.

Waldie, K. E. & Poulton, R. (2002). Physical and psychological correlates of primary headache in young adulthood: a 26 year longitudinal study. *Journal of Neurology, Neurosurgery and Psychiatry,* **72**, 86–92.

Zwart, J. A., Ellertsen, B. & Bovim, G. (1996). Psychosocial factors and MMPI-2 patterns in migraine, cluster headache, tension-type headache, and cervicogenic headache. *New Trends in Experimental & Clinical Psychiatry,* **12**, 167–74.

Herpes

John Green

St. Mary's Hospital

Background

Genital herpes is an extremely common infection caused by one of the two related Herpes simplex viruses, HSV-1 and HSV-2. HSV-1 is the cause of cold sores around the mouth but can infect the genitals and be transmitted either oro–genitally or by genital–genital contact. HSV-2 is mainly a genital infection although orolabial infection can occur. Both viruses establish lifelong infections in the nerve roots and can be periodically reactivated causing recurrent episodes. During episodes small blisters appear which are itchy or painful and which break down in about a day to leave an open sore, which usually heals in about a week in those who are immunocompetent. However inapparent lesions are common and asymptomatic shedding, production of virus in the absence of lesions, also occurs in the absence of frank episodes. Most infections are believed to result from inapparent lesions or asymptomatic shedding since avoidance of sex during obvious episodes is common.

Genital recurrence rates are higher on average for HSV-2 than for HSV-1. Some individuals have only a single obvious episode, others can have episode rates up to one per fortnight. While episodes usually diminish in frequency over the years there is considerable variation. Infection is lifelong and cannot be eliminated. Treatment is by antivirals which, when used on a continuing basis, largely or completely suppress episodes during active treatment but do not affect natural history.

Most people with genital herpes have never been diagnosed and are unaware that they are infected. Estimates of incidence are based on serology but are limited because they are based on HSV-2 antibodies only. Orolabial HSV-1 infection is very common and serology cannot distinguish the site of infection. Since in many countries HSV-1 accounts for half or more of clinical cases, as a rough rule of thumb rates for HSV-2 might to be doubled to estimate overall genital infection rates. On this basis the incidence of genital infection with the HSV viruses in the USA and Europe in adults under 35 is probably in the 15–25% range with some populations showing rates in excess of 50%. HSV infection is a common cause of genital ulcer disease in developing countries. Rates are rising worldwide, particularly rapidly for HSV-1.

Fortunately the disease causes little in the way of long-term physical morbidity. The main risk is transmission to the neonate at birth where disseminated herpes of the neonate can cause blindness, brain damage or death. Transmission to neonates is unusual except where the mother is infected late in pregnancy. Cases of disseminated herpes of the neonate are rare in Western Europe although they are more common in areas of social and relationship instability, for instance some inner city areas of the USA.

Risk of transmission can probably be reduced by antiviral treatment of the mother (RCOG, 2002). Caesarian section is sometimes used where risk or transmission is thought particularly high. Otherwise the main problem is psychological morbidity and reduced quality of life.

Psychological effects

Psychological morbidity is very common at the time of diagnosis with half of patients being clinically anxious and about a tenth clinically depressed on the HADS (Carney et al., 1994). In those who do not get an (apparent) recurrence these symptoms usually resolve over a few months. In those with recurrences, psychological distress remains high for several months or even years. Distress does usually resolve eventually and by 5–6 years most patients report that their sexual and interpersonal function are similar to before they were infected and their levels of anxiety and depression are not different from population norms (Brookes et al., 1993; Cassidy et al., 1997). A few patients however fail to adjust over many years.

There is little systematic information on non-adjusters. There is no way at present to predict who will have difficulty in adjusting. Such evidence as is available suggest that non-adjusters are more likely to be women, although not exclusively so. Possibly this is in part because episodes are usually more painful in women. Frequency and severity of episodes are related to level of psychological distress and hence those with higher levels of reported distress might be more likely to be women. Higher initial levels of distress might be associated with more problems adjusting, although this is not established. However the infection may also feed into negative societal stereotypes of women's genitalia as 'contaminated'. Additionally there is some evidence that even amongst adjusters the experience of a chronic condition outside the patient's control may have a broader impact on the patient's thinking about the world (Green & Kocsis, 1997).

Data on the impact of antiviral treatment on psychological well-being is surprisingly limited as most early drug trials used episode frequency as their endpoint. However available evidence suggests that suppression of episodes can reduce psychological distress and improve quality of life. (Carney et al., 1993; Patel et al., 1999). Clinical experience suggests that the effects may persist after treatment cessation, possibly because stopping episodes allows patients space to adjust psychologically.

While many patients report unfounded concerns about casual household transmission and transfer to other sites on their own bodies (very rare and then probably only shortly after infection) and concerns surrounding pregnancy their main concern is usually how to deal with current and future sexual relationships.

Genital herpes can lead to suspicion between partners. Diagnosis may be delayed and misdiagnosis outside specialist clinics is not uncommon. A tenth or more of 'first' episodes are actually recurrences of infection that may in some cases have been acquired some time prior to current relationship. Infection can occur from an apparently uninfected partner by asymptomatic shedding or during inapparent episodes. Orogenital transmission, particularly by HSV-1 from asymptomatic shedding in the saliva is probably common. It can be difficult to establish who gave it to whom and under what circumstances and, in the case of HSV-1 transmission, the source partner may have acquired orolabial infection non-sexually and then passed it on through oral sex.

Herpes is a heavily stigmatized disease which has received extensive, grossly misleading press coverage. Consequently many of those who are infected are unwilling to confide in friends or family. Most patients, at the time of diagnosis, are unable to think of anyone they know who has the disease, leading to a sense of loneliness and having been 'picked out' (see 'Stigma').

While standard advice is to disclose to sexual partners before first intercourse most patients delay informing partners until they are sure of the relationship, often when moving in with a partner or otherwise making a psychological commitment (Green et al., 2003). There are also practical reasons for delayed disclosure at this time. It can be difficult to hide recurrent infection or ongoing treatment when living with someone. The usual tactic adopted by those planning to disclose to a partner is to 'test out' their attitudes to the disease before disclosure. Depending on the response disclosure may or may not occur. Individuals frequently fail to inform casual partners, in part because of fears that they may tell others.

Condoms provide some protection against transmission but this is less than for bacterial infections. Antiviral medication reduces but does not eliminate infectivity (Corey et al., 2004). It is thought likely that individuals usually become less infectious over time, at least those whose episodes decline in frequency, and that the chances of transmission in a discordant couple reduce with length of relationship. Unfortunately transmissions can, and do, occur in couples who have engaged in unprotected sexual intercourse for many years without any problem.

There has been considerable interest in the utility and psychological impact of type-specific antibody tests for HSV (Mullan & Munday, 2003; Page et al., 2003). The availability of type-specific antibody tests for genital herpes has meant that it is possible to establish whether couples where one partner has episodes and the other does not are truly discordant, or whether the partner without episodes is infected but asymptomatic. The tests are acceptable to most couples under these circumstances since they have implications for their use of prophylaxis to prevent transmission. Under these circumstances serological tests do not appear to have a high incidence of adverse psychological sequelae. Discussion of the issues with the couple prior to testing is, however, likely to be important in clinical practice. The tests are also acceptable to many, but by no means all, patients as a routine screen for possible infection in genitourinary medicine (GUM) clinics, although the utility of serological tests for an infection so common in the general population and where there is no obvious treatment is uncertain. There have been suggestions in some countries that population screening, for instance in young people, might be appropriate as a measure to control spread. However existing tests do not have perfect specificity and sensitivity and there are grounds for concern over the likely proportion of false positives in low incidence populations.

A great deal of effort has been expended on trying to establish whether there is a link between stress and recurrences, as many patients believe. In part this has been motivated by the idea that the disease might be a good model on which to test psychoneuroimmunological hypotheses, although in fact the disease is probably a poor model since it would recur anyway regardless of stress and ongoing recording of episodes and asymptomatic shedding is fraught with practical difficulties. Green and Kocsis (1997) found the evidence for stress causing recurrences unconvincing. The issue is complicated because the episodes cause stress in themselves and because higher levels of distress may affect recognition of, and retrospective reporting of, episodes as happens in ocular herpes infections (Kip et al., 2001). Additionally viral replication starts some days prior to the frank episode and it is possible that the immunological response to replication in itself may raise stress levels, generating a spurious apparent linkage.

There have been a number of studies seeking to intervene psychologically in individuals with recurrent genital herpes. In most the target has been to reduce the frequency of episodes rather than to encourage adjustment. With few exceptions these studies have been small and have had methodological problems, particularly the use of retrospective accounts of episode frequency, which can make them difficult to interpret. Although demonstrating a reliable and consistent impact of psychological interventions on recurrences would be of considerable theoretical interest it is not clear how achievable this is. Antivirals already offer considerable control over episodes. Demonstrating an improvement in the speed and extent of psychological adjustment through psychological intervention would seem of greater practical importance currently, and clinical experience and what is known about psychological aspects of the disease suggest that this is likely to be an achievable goal.

(See also 'Epstein–Barr virus infection' and 'Sexually transmitted infections'.)

REFERENCES

Brookes, J. L., Haywood, S. & Green, J. (1993). Adjustment to the psychological and social sequelae of recurrent gential herpes simplex infection. *Genitourinary Medicine*, **69**, 384–7.

Carney, O., Ross, E., Ikkos, G. & Mindel, A. (1993). The effect of suppressive oral acyclovir on the psychological morbidity associated with recurrent genital herpes. *Genitourinary Medicine*, **69**, 457–9.

Carney, O., Ross, E., Bunker, C., Ikkos, G. & Mindel, A. (1994). A prospective study of the psychological impact on patients with a first episode of genital herpes. *Genitourinary Medicine*, **70**, 40–5.

Cassidy, L., Meadows, J., Catalan, J. & Barton, S. (1997). Are reported stress and coping style associated with frequent recurrence of genital herpes. *Genitourinary Medicine*, **73**, 263–6.

Corey, L., Wald, A., Patel, R. *et al.* (2004). Once-daily valocyclovir to reduce the risk of transmission of genital herpes. *New England Journal of Medicine*, **350**, 11–20.

Green, J. & Kocsis, A. (1997). Psychological factors in recurrent genital herpes. *Genitourinary Medicine*, **73**, 253–9.

Green, J., Ferrier, S., Kocsis, A. *et al.* (2003). Determinants of disclosure of genital herpes to partners. *Sexually Transmitted Infection*, **79**, 42–4.

Kip, K. E., Cohen, F., Cole, S. R. *et al.* (2001). Recall bias in a prospective cohort study of acute time-varying exposures: example from the herpetic eye disease study. *Journal of Clinical Epidemiology*, **54**, 482–7.

Mullan, H. M. & Munday, P. E. (2003). The acceptability of the introduction of a type specific herpes antibody screening test into a genitourinary medicine clinic in the United Kingdom. *Sexually Transmitted Infection*, **79**, 129–33.

Page, J., Taylor, J., Tideman, R. L. *et al.* (2003). Is HSV serology useful for the management of first episode genital herpes? *Sexually Transmitted Infection*, **79**, 276–9.

Patel, R., Tyring, S., Strand, A., Price, M. J. & Grant, D. M. (1999). Impact of suppressive antiviral therapy on the health related quality of life of patients with recurrent genital herpes infection. *Sexually Transmitted Infection*, **75**, 398–402.

RCOG, Royal College of Obstetricians and Gynaecologists. (2002). *Management of Genital Herpes in Pregnancy, Clinical Guideline No 30*.

HIV/AIDS

Michael H. Antoni and Adam W. Carrico

University of Miami

Individuals infected with Human Immunodeficiency Virus (HIV) endure a chronic disease which requires behaviour changes and psychosocial adaptation (see 'Coping with chronic illness'). Health psychologists are in a position to make a unique contribution to the care of HIV-infected persons by designing and implementing behavioural interventions capable of facilitating these adjustments. Here we review many of the challenges facing HIV-infected persons as well as highlight potential targets for behavioural interventions.

A revolution with HAART

Due to the substantial reductions in morbidity and mortality associated with the advent of Highly Active Anti-Retroviral Therapy (HAART), HIV infection is now commonly conceptualized as a chronic illness (Bangsberg *et al.*, 2001). By directly suppressing HIV replication, HAART-treated individuals may attenuate T-helper (CD4+) cell decline and delay the onset of Acquired Immune Deficiency Syndrome (AIDS). However, not all HIV-infected patients treated with HAART display adequate viral suppression which may be due in large part to suboptimal adherence as well as the emergence of drug-resistant strains of the virus (Bangsberg *et al.*, 2001; Tamalet *et al.*, 2003). Questions also remain regarding the appropriate time to initiate HAART in HIV-infected patients due to variability in the extent immune reconstitution, increased incidence of opportunistic infections in the months following initiation and reports of profound drug-related toxicities (Yeni *et al.*, 2002). As a result, the current state of medical treatment for HIV infection dictates that healthcare providers take into account the dynamic interplay among contextual, patient-related and treatment-related factors in order to deliver the best possible patient care.

HAART is a demanding regimen that requires unprecedented levels of patient adherence, greater than or equal to 95% to maximize the clinical benefits. Further complicating adherence to HAART are the special indications (e.g. taking medications with food) which accompany many medications in order to attenuate the severity of side effects, maximize bioavailability and ensure a constant therapeutic dose. Much of the research in this area continues to focus on what methods are most reliable and valid in the measurement of patient adherence to antiretroviral medications. Drawing upon a larger existing literature in a variety of medical populations, adherence has been examined using numerous methods including physician ratings, pharmacy refills, measuring medication levels in peripheral venous blood samples, patient self-report and electronic monitoring (Dunbar-Jacob *et al.*, 2002). It is likely that patient-reported HAART adherence is an over-estimate on average. On the other hand, more 'objective' measures (i.e. medication event monitoring system; MEMS) may underestimate adherence due to the lack of fit between the technology and the patient lifestyle factors (Samet *et al.*, 2001). As a result, investigations of adherence to HAART should employ multiple measures that utilize different methods of assessment (Llabre *et al.*, 2006). Investigations that employ the MEMS should also include assessments of participant experiences using this technology, and those that utilize only self-report measures of adherence to HAART would do well to examine the influence of socially desirable responding. Finally, regardless of the chosen measure(s), investigations should establish validity by examining the relationship of adherence with HIV viral load and HIV medication resistance genotyping where possible (see also 'Adherence to treatment').

Adherence to HAART is influenced by a host of variables such as experiences with the treatment regimen, access to resources, patient psychosocial functioning and social/cultural factors (Fogarty *et al.*, 2002). One treatment-related factor which appears to be a significant obstacle to continuing HAART is the side effects many patients experience. In fact, medication intolerance is the most commonly cited reason among patients for termination of HAART (Park *et al.*, 2002). Greater knowledge of possible side effects from antiretroviral medications, younger age and prescription of four or more antiretroviral drugs with Ritonavir have also been associated with premature termination of HAART (Park *et al.*, 2002). In addition, a number of psychosocial factors such as depressed mood and poor emotional functioning have been related to non-adherence to HAART (Catz *et al.*, 2000). The effects of psychosocial factors on HAART adherence and subsequent HIV disease progression are especially salient given the illness experience of persons living with HIV/AIDS.

Psychosocial adjustment to HIV/AIDS

In the face of social stigma, HIV-infected persons must manage the multiple demands of a life-threatening illness as well as financial hardships, bereavement and other personal losses (see also 'Stigma'). Possibly due to the high prevalence rates of these stressors, HIV-infected individuals are at increased risk for developing an affective or adjustment disorder across the disease spectrum (Bing *et al.*, 2001). In fact, results from a meta-analysis of 10 published studies indicate that the risk of developing major depressive disorder is two times higher in HIV-infected samples when compared with HIV-negative peers (Ciesla & Roberts, 2001). While increased levels of distress may be observed across the HIV disease spectrum, patient illness burden has been identified as a potent predictor of psychosocial adjustment as AIDS develops (Lyketsos *et al.*, 1996) and progresses (Siegel *et al.*, 1997).

To varying degrees, patients with an AIDS-related condition (ARC) are subject to elevated levels of stigma/discrimination, grapple with existential concerns, must cope with the physical disfigurement or disability (see 'Facial disfigurement' and 'Disability') and experience greater treatment burden associated with a 'disease within a disease' (De Moore *et al.*, 2000). Thus, the emergence of various ARCs may have dramatically different implications for patient psychosocial adjustment depending on the extent of illness burden and stigma experienced. For example, unlike many other ARCs, Kaposi's Sarcoma (KS) lesions may be readily visible and are commonly recognized (particularly in the gay community). As a result, individuals with KS may experience discrimination across a number of domains as well as increased levels of depression, anxiety and social isolation when compared to other individuals with AIDS. These observations are supported by qualitative data indicating that fear of KS ranks as high as fears of death, neurological deficits and pain among HIV-infected patients (Bor, 1993). In addition, physical disfigurement may

be a common concern in patients with KS (De Moore *et al.*, 2000). Thus, there is compelling clinical and qualitative evidence to indicate that examining distress and illness-related concerns within AIDS-defined populations will provide a deeper understanding of the diverse experiences of individuals living with AIDS.

A number of investigations have examined the role of depressed mood in CD4+ cell decline, progression to AIDS and mortality (Leserman, 2003). Because of observations that clinically significant changes in HIV viral load (Kalichman *et al.*, 2002) and increased symptom burden have both been associated with reactive depressed mood, the directionality of the relationship between depression and HIV disease progression has been hotly debated. Therefore, longitudinal investigations with repeated measurements of psychosocial and immunologic data provide the most reliable findings examining the role of depression in HIV disease progression. Future investigations examining of the putative mechanisms will undoubtedly lend further support to the role of depression in HIV disease progression.

Depressed mood may influence HIV disease progression via a number of pathways. First, depressed mood may be associated with increases in a variety of health-risk behaviours (e.g. non-adherence to HAART, substance use and sexual risk-taking) that in turn impact HIV disease progression. In particular, research examining the mediational role of HAART adherence remains an area for further study (Leserman, 2003). Neuroendocrine dysregulation represents another plausible pathway whereby depressed mood influences immune status and longevity. Elevations in cortisol and catecholamines (e.g. norepinephrine; NE) are commonly observed in depressed persons, and have been demonstrated to impact HIV replication, immune function and disease progression (Leserman *et al.*, 2000). Cortisol influences maturational selection of CD4+ cells in these lymphoid organs (Norbiato *et al.*, 1997), facilitates HIV infection of CD4+ cells (Markham *et al.*, 1986) and is associated with high rates of apoptosis in CD4+ cells and accessory cells in the lymphoid tissue (Clerici *et al.*, 1997). Release of NE at sympathetic nervous system terminals provides opportunities for this catecholamine to influence the progression of HIV infection at the primary site of viral replication. By binding with beta-2 adrenergic receptors on the lymphocyte membrane, NE induces cellular changes via the G protein linked adenyl cyclase-cAMP-protein kinase A signaling cascade. In vitro data have observed that cellular changes of this nature are associated decrements in interferon-gamma and interleukin-10 which in turn are associated with elevations in HIV viral load over an 8-day period (Cole *et al.*, 1998). Taken together, it is likely that both behavioural and neuroendocrine mechanisms make unique contributions to HIV disease progression.

Although a number of investigations have examined the association between psychosocial adjustment and HIV disease progression (Cole & Kemeny, 2001; Leserman, 2003), there is a general consensus that these effects have not been reliably observed (Kopinsky *et al.*, 2004). These discrepancies may be due in large part to the heterogeneity of patient populations across samples and utilization of multiple outcome measures as indicators of HIV disease progression. Researchers have indicated that this literature may benefit from investigations that examine patient subgroups at both extremes of the disease spectrum. Specifically, the most vulnerable populations may hold promise for future investigations of the effects of psychosocial factors on HIV disease progression. Examining a more homogenous group of patients with respect to HIV disease stage may also provide useful information regarding the putative mechanisms of the effects of psychosocial variables on HIV disease progression and may provide some interesting data on the most beneficial time frame(s) for psychological intervention (Kopinsky *et al.*, 2004). We propose that investigations of persons living with KS appear to meet these criteria and provide unique opportunities to examine the dynamic interactions among psychosocial factors, viruses, glucocorticoids, cytokines and angiogenesis that are relevant to this ARC (Miles, 2000) (see also 'Psychoneuroimmunology').

Behavioural interventions

A variety of behavioural interventions have been developed as adjuncts to medical treatment for HIV-infected persons at various disease stages to decrease distress, enhance coping skills and encourage health-promoting behaviours with the hope of enhancing quality of life as well as slowing disease progression (Antoni, 2003). Components of these treatments such as relaxation, cognitive restructuring and coping skills may account for some of the psychosocial, neuroendocrine and immunologic changes observed (Antoni, 2003) (see 'Cognitive behaviour therapy' and 'Relaxation training'). Although it appears that conducting these interventions in a group format may offer optimal efficacy and cost-efficiency, future work needs to address the various components of these multi-modal interventions to better understand their mechanisms of action. By gaining a better understanding of the most potent mechanisms of change in these treatments, a new generation of interventions can be developed that more effectively capitalizes on these factors to maximize the benefits derived by patients. It is also plausible that different stress management components are more efficacious in different populations. However, the ultimate test of the efficacy of these interventions will require long-term follow-up to assess effects on ongoing psychosocial adjustment and clinical health course. Ultimately, by understanding those factors influencing psychosocial adjustment to HIV infection, behavioural interventions may be refined to address the array of challenges that are experienced by persons living with HIV/AIDS.

(See also 'Sexual risk behaviour' and 'Sexually transmitted infections'.)

REFERENCES

Antoni, M. H. (2003). Stress management and psychoneuroimmunology in HIV infection. *CNS Spectrums*, **8**, 40–51.

Bangsberg, D. R., Perry, S., Charlebois, E. D. *et al.* (2001). Non-adherence to highly active antiretroviral therapy predicts progression to AIDS. *AIDS*, **15**, 1181–3.

Bing, E. G., Burnam, M. A., Longshore, D. *et al.* (2001). Psychiatric disorders and drug use among human immunodeficiency virus-infected adults in the United States. *Archives of General Psychiatry*, **58**, 721–8.

Bor, R. (1993). Counseling patients with AIDS-associated Kaposi's Sarcoma. *Counselling Psychology Quarterly*, **6**, 91–9.

Catz, S. L., Kelly, J. A., Bogart, L. M. *et al.* (2000). Patterns, correlates, and barriers to medication adherence among persons prescribed new treatments for HIV disease. *Health Psychology*, **19**, 124–33.

Cielsa, J. A. & Roberts, J. E. (2001). Meta-analysis of the relationship between HIV infection and the risk for depressive disorders. *The American Journal of Psychiatry*, **158**, 725–30.

Clerici, M., Trabattoni, D., Piconi, S. *et al.* (1997). A possible role for the cortisol/anticortisols imbalance in the progression of Human Immunodeficiency Virus. *Psychoneuroendocrinology*, **22**, S27–31.

Cole, S. W. & Kemeny, M. E. (2001). Psychosocial influences on the progression of HIV infection. In R. Ader, D. L. Felten & S. Cohen (Eds.). *Psychoneuroimmunology*, (3rd edn.). San Diego, CA: Academic Press.

Cole, S. W., Korin, Y. D., Fahey, J. L. & Zack, J. A. (1998). Norepinephrine accelerates HIV replication via protein kinase A-dependent effects on cytokine production. *Journal of Immunology*, **161**, 610–16.

De Moore, G. M., Hennessey, P., Kunz, N. M., Ferrando, S. J. & Rabkin, J. G. (2000). Kaposi's Sarcoma: the scarlet letter of AIDS. *Psychosomatics*, **41**, 360–3.

Dunbar-Jacob, J., Schlenk, E. A. & Caruthers, D. (2002). Adherence in the management of chronic disorders. In A. J. Christensen & M. H. Antoni (Eds.). *Chronic physical disorders: behavioral medicine's perspective*. Malden, MA: Blackwell Publishers.

Fogarty, L., Roter, D., Larson, S. *et al.* (2002). Patient adherence to HIV medication regimens: a review of published and abstract reports. *Patient Education and Counseling*, **46**, 93–108.

Kalichman, S. C., Difonzo, K., Austin, J., Luke, W. & Rompa, D. (2002). Prospective study of emotional reactions to changes in HIV viral load. *AIDS Patient Care and STD's*, **16**, 113–20.

Kopinsky, K. L., Stoff, D. M. & Rausch, D. M. (2004). Workshop report: the effects of psychological variables on the progression of HIV-1 disease. *Brain, Behavior, and Immunity*, **18**, 246–61.

Leserman, J. (2003). HIV disease progression: depression, stress, and possible mechanisms. *Biological Psychiatry*, **54**, 295–306.

Leserman, J., Petitto, J. M., Golden, R. N. *et al.* (2000). Impact of stressful life events, depression, social support, coping, and cortisol on progression to AIDS. *The American Journal of Psychiatry*, **157**, 1221–8.

Llabre, M., Weaker, K., Duran, R. *et al.* (2006). A measurement model of medication adherence to highly active antiretroviral therapy and its relation to viral load in HIV+ adults. *AIDS Patient Care and STDs*, **20**, 701–10.

Lyketsos, C. G., Hoover, D. R., Guccione, M. *et al.* (1996). Changes in depressive symptoms as AIDS develops. *The American Journal of Psychiatry*, **153**, 1430–7.

Markham, P. D., Salahuddin, S. Z., Veren, K. *et al.* (1986). Hydrocortisone and some other hormones enhance the expression of HTLV-III. *International Journal of Cancer*, **37**, 67–72.

Miles, S. A. (2000). Cytokines, viruses, and angiogenesis: new therapies for Kaposi's Sarcoma. In E. G. Fiegal (Ed.). *AIDS-related* cancers and their treatment: basic and clinical oncology. New York, NY: Marcel Dekker, Inc.

Norbiato, G., Bevilacqua, M., Vago, T. *et al.* (1997). Glucocorticoids and immune function in Human Immunodeficiency Virus infection: a study of hypercortisolemic and cortisol-resistant patients. *Journal of Clinical Endocrinology and Metabolism*, **82**, 3260–3.

Park, W., Laura, Y., Scalera, A., Tseng, A. & Rourke, S. (2002). High rate of discontinuations of highly active

antiretroviral therapy as a result of antiretroviral intolerance in clinical practice: missed opportunities for support? *AIDS*, **16**, 1084–6.

Samet, J. H., Sullivan, L. M., Traphagen, E. T. & Ickovics, J. R. (2001). Measuring adherence among HIV-infected persons: is MEMS consummate technology? *AIDS and Behavior*, **5**, 21–30.

Siegel, K., Karus, D. & Raveis, V. H. (1997). Correlates of change in depressive symptomatology among gay men with AIDS. *Health Psychology*, **16**, 230–8.

Tamalet, C., Fantini, J., Tourres, C. & Yashi, N. (2003). Resistance of HIV-1 to multiple antiretroviral drugs in France: a 6-year survey (1997–2002) based on an analysis of over 7000 genotypes. *AIDS*, **17**, 2383–8.

Yeni, P. G., Hammer, S. M., Carpenter, C. C. J. *et al.* (2002). Antiretroviral treatment for adult HIV-infection in 2002. *Journal of the American Medical Association*, **288**, 137–42.

Hormone replacement therapy

Christine Stephens

Massey University

With an unprecedented number of women living beyond midlife in western countries, the impact of menopause is an important public health issue. Middle-aged women are one of the largest single age groups in these populations, and every middle-aged woman must inevitably experience menopause. Since the 1950s, exogenous hormones known as hormone replacement therapy (HRT) have been increasingly prescribed to women to counteract adverse symptoms at menopause (McPherson, 2004). More recently it was suggested that long term HRT was beneficial and use by middle-aged women in Britain, increased substantially, from under 5% in the 1980s to 33% in 1998 (Kmietowicz, 2000). In the US, 38% of menopausal women were taking HRT in 2002 (Minelli *et al.*, 2004). In New Zealand, HRT use among middle-aged women increased from 12% in 1991 to 20% in 1997 (North & Sharples, 2001). However, the findings of the Women's Health Initiative (WHI) study (Rossouw *et al.*, 2002) received much media attention, changed perceptions of the risks and benefits and were associated with an immediate change in use. In the United States, Haas *et al.* (2004) reported a drop in use among women undergoing mammography of 18% per quarter. In New Zealand, 58% of 998 women initially stopped taking HRT (Lawton *et al.*, 2003). These dramatic changes reflect the problems involved in making a decision about HRT for many women. Generally, the decision making issues focussed on by medical and psychological research, are understandings of the changing knowledge about benefits and risks of HRT use, and the broader social context in which women must make their decisions about HRT.

Medical benefits and risks

Physical and psychological symptoms of menopause

HRT has been prescribed for middle-aged women to alleviate menopausal symptoms such as hot flushes, night sweats, atrophy of the vagina and skin changes. Hot flushes are the most common experience, occurring in up to 75% of menopausal women (Joffe *et al.*, 2003). In the 1990s, the benefits of oestrogen in reducing the incidence of osteoporosis and heart disease were emphasized (McKinney & Thompson, 1998). This change in focus, from the treatment of specific menopausal symptoms to prophylactic and possibly long-term treatment, changed the potential role of HRT in middle-aged women's lives, and added to the complexity of decision making about HRT. In 2002 the WHI reported that the effects of oestrogen plus progestin (for women with intact uteruses) on healthy post-menopausal women increased risk of breast cancer, CHD, stroke and venous thromboembolism and, despite decreased risk of hip fracture and colorectal cancer, concluded that this combination is not suitable for prevention of chronic diseases (Rossouw *et al.*, 2002). These and other recent findings support previous evidence of the risks of HRT such as breast cancer, the benefits in regard to osteoporosis and completely counteracted previous epidemiological findings that suggested cardiovascular benefits.

Depressed mood is often cited as a symptom of menopause, and the use of HRT to treat dysphoria has been widely accepted (Barlow, 1992). It is clear that hormone changes are not related to major depressive disorder (Schmidt & Rubinow, 1991), and extensive research has provided only equivocal support for an association between hormones and mood. Clinical trials have provided some support for enhancement of mood through the administration of oestrogen to healthy non-depressed women (e.g. Klaiber *et al.*, 1997; Derman *et al.*, 1995). However, others (e.g. Girdler *et al.*, 1999) found that HRT was not associated with changes in mood. Prospective studies of HRT in surgically menopausal non-depressed women have also demonstrated a positive effect (e.g. Sherwin & Gelfand, 1985) but Phillips and Sherwin (1992) also found no effect of HRT on mood. It has been suggested that clinical samples are biased and certainly, population studies of menopausal women generally indicate that emotional wellbeing is not affected by menopause (Hunter, 1990). Studies using population samples to examine psychological distress or mood have shown no differences between HRT users and non-users in Australian (Slaven & Lee, 1998) and New Zealand (Stephens & Ross, 2000) samples. The WHI trial included a sample of 1511 women randomly assigned to oestrogen plus progestin or placebo. After three years there were no differences in depressive symptoms, mental health or vitality. In the light of such findings, alternative treatment strategies are being explored for mood disturbances that occur in menopausal women (Joffe *et al.*, 2003).

Cognitive functioning and hormones

Changes in cognitive functioning, particularly memory problems, are also complained of by women at menopause. Basic research indicates that oestrogen has multiple effects on brain function (Cutter *et al.*, 2003) and, among middle-aged women, the most promising effect of oestrogen has been observed on verbal memory. Observational and experimental studies have found a positive relationship between oestrogen and verbal memory, in both post-surgical and naturally menopausal women. However, there have been studies of equal merit which have failed to find such a link (Stephens *et al.*, 2003). Oestrogens are also implicated in Alzheimer's disease (Waring *et al.*, 1999) but the most recent findings of clinical trials (e.g. Mulnard *et al.*, 2000) show that HRT treatment of older women has no effect on the progress of such neuropsychological disorders. Again, the findings of the WHI trials have added weight to these conclusions. Among women over 65 it was found that random assignment to oestrogen had no effect on mild cognitive impairment, but the group taking HRT was actually at higher risk of developing dementia (Shumaker *et al.*, 2003).

Thus, information that is available to middle-aged women from multiple sources (such as primary care physicians, pharmaceutical companies, literature or the Internet) is rapidly changing, and often conflicting in regard to the risks and benefits of HRT use and the nature of menopause (Breheny & Stephens, 2001; Daley, 1999). These factors contribute to the difficulties for women deciding about HRT (Stephens *et al.*, 2001), without taking into account the wider social context in which these decisions must be made.

The social context of HRT decision-making

Lay understandings of health

The information presented to women about disease risks and benefits is inclined to cause extreme anxiety or confusion, or may be simply ignored as outside everyday concerns. It is difficult for women to see their 'self' in terms of risk ratios provided by medical research (unless they see themselves as candidates for disease, for example because of a family history). Some explanation for this difficulty comes from research showing that medical discourses are part of, but do not encompass all of, understandings of health. Firstly, attitudes towards menopause have been found to predict HRT use more strongly than experiencing symptoms (Breheny & Stephens, 2001). Furthermore, narrative researchers such as Blaxter (1993) demonstrate how health is understood in terms of biography and social relations. Work with middle-aged women has shown that it is this wider social world, beyond medical discourse, that enables women to position themselves as users of HRT or not (Stephens *et al.*, 2004) (see also 'Lay beliefs about health and illness' and 'Risk perception').

Competing constructions of HRT

Our social world includes controversy over virtually every aspect of HRT use. The last few decades have seen publicly contested changes in the meanings of menopause (e.g. Bell, 1987; Goldstein, 2000). The construction of menopause as a deficiency disease requiring medical treatment has been strongly contested in sociological literature (Griffiths, 1999) and this debate carried into the media where constructions of menopause as a medical or natural change compete (e.g. Lupton, 1996). When analyzing women's talk to identify the use of these discourses in practice, Hunter and O'Dea, (1997) determined that biomedical discourses do not include the complexity of women's experiences, and Griffiths (1999) highlighted contradictions in women's talk about HRT. Women resisted the medicalization of menopause and were critical of doctors, yet made use of a medical model of risk to make their decisions about HRT. Stephens *et al.* (2004) noted that women drew upon a common range of discourses which construct HRT in different ways (such as support for a threatening change, as a biomedical aid, as a 'drug' to be avoided by the virtuous or as unnatural). The women used different constructions according to the social function of their talk at the time, like accounting for their use of HRT or to discuss concerns about the choices available to them. The researchers concluded that different contexts such as a doctor's surgery or discussion with a friend, would lead to the use of different (apparently contradictory) constructions.

Embodied experience

Such analyses highlight the discursive aspects of the social world but can neglect the importance of embodied experience. Goldstein (2000) described women's distress in the face of constructions of menopause which dismiss the very somatic nature of their experiences. An emphasis on the psychosocial aspects of bodily changes is not helpful to women who are suffering from heavy bleeding, sleepless nights or incontinence. To understand the complexities of having and being a body in a social world, Stephens (2001) used women's accounts to show the importance of physical experiences such as hot flushes in terms of their experiential and social meanings together. For example, the discomfort of a flushed face has quite different import at home or at work, in the company of males or females or among those of different social status.

The experience of symptoms also has important moral meanings in a social world in which it is virtuous to 'get on with it', or the use of HRT is seen as a crutch for the weak (Breheny & Stephens, 2003). Women would benefit from understandings, applied in medical settings, which include the complex interactions of the physical and social aspects of menopause and HRT use.

Clinical implications

Although longitudinal studies have somewhat clarified the medical risks and benefits of HRT, the difficulties of the decision have not been ameliorated for women and many questions are unresolved (Rymer et al., 2003; Wang-Cheng & Rosenfeld, 2003). The current results are already being subjected to various interpretations, and although most recommend that HRT is beneficial for immediate symptoms and unsuitable for long-term use (e.g. Minelli et al., 2004), other commentators are pointing to the low real risk ratio, the benefits for osteoporosis or to remaining questions about the prophylactic use of oestrogen (McPherson, 2004). All women should have access to accurate unbiased information about the benefits, risks and side effects of using HRT. However, the ongoing problem is multiple conflicting interpretations and the personal relevance of risk/benefit ratios (Bond & Bywaters, 1998). Current recommendations have also brought to the fore the problem of when and how to cease HRT use; an issue commonly discussed by women on Internet sites. When we also consider the social and moral milieu in which women experience menopausal changes or use HRT, the dilemmas for women are clearly ongoing. It is apparent that the HRT decision should be made on an individual basis in discussion between a woman and her doctor (Griffiths, 2003).

These sorts of recommendations accord well with shared decision making in medical practice (Griffiths, 1999; Mort, 1996). One result is that women are being offered increasing levels of personal responsibility with which they may not be comfortable (Budge et al., 2000) and this aspect deserves more attention. McLellan (2002) asked women about their preferred decision making style and most wished for a shared final decision. However, this balance changed across the decision process during which many women preferred that the doctor decide about providing information, and wanted their doctors' help when considering their choices (see also 'Patient-centred healthcare').

Conclusion

The results of research in regard to the positive and negative aspects of HRT use continue to be a source of confusion to women who expect to take more personal responsibility for such decisions. Health practitioners who are responsible for prescribing HRT must be aware of the complexities of the decision for each woman and the importance of the social context, beyond the medical consultation, in which she must cope with her physical experiences or account for her use of pharmaceuticals. It is important to develop our understandings of how the medical information may be integrated with the psychosocial implications of making these decisions.

(See also 'Menopause and Post-menopause'.)

REFERENCES

Barlow, D. H. (1992). Hormone replacement therapy and other menopause associated conditions. *British Medical Bulletin*, **48**, 356–67.

Bell, S. E. (1987). Changing ideas: the medicalization of menopause. *Social Science and Medicine*, **24**, 535–42.

Bond, M. & Bywaters, P. (1998). Working it out for ourselves: women learning about hormone replacement therapy. *Women's Studies International Forum*, **21**, 65–76.

Blaxter, M. (1993). Why do the victims blame themselves? In A. Radley (Ed.). *Worlds of illness* (pp. 92–108). London: Routledge.

Breheny, M. & Stephens, C. (2003). Healthy living and keeping busy: a discourse analysis of mid-aged women's attributions for menopausal experience. *Journal of Language and Social Psychology*, **22**, 169–89.

Breheny, M. & Stephens, C. (2001). The importance of attitudes in predicting Hormone replacement therapy use by mid-aged women in a New Zealand community sample. *Women and Health*, **29**, 29–43.

Budge, R. C., Stephens, C. & Carryer, J. (2000). Decision making: New Zealand women speak about doctors and HRT. *New Zealand Family Physician*, **27**, 41–7.

Cutter, W. J., Norbury, R. & Murphy, D. G. M. (2003). Oestrogen, brain function, and neuropsychiatric disorders. *Journal of Neurology, Neurosurgery and Psychiatry*, **74**, 837–40.

Daley, J. (1999). Medical uncertainty and practice variation get personal: what should I do about Hormone replacement therapy? *Annals of Internal Medicine*, **130**, 602–4.

Derman, R. J., Dawood, M. Y. & Stone, S. (1995). Quality of life during sequential hormone replacement therapy: a placebo-controlled study. *International Journal of Fertility*, **40**, 73–8.

Gindler, S. S., O'Briant, C., Steege, J., Grewen, K. & Light, K. C. (1999). A comparison of the effect of estrogen with or without progesteron on mood and physical symptoms in postmenopausal women. *Journal of Women's Health & Gender-Based Medicine*, **8**, 637–46.

Goldstein, D. E. (2000). 'When ovaries retire': contrasting women's experiences with feminist and medical models of menopause. *Health*, **4**, 309–23.

Griffiths, F. (1999). Women's control and choice regarding HRT. *Social Science and Medicine*, **49**, 469–81.

Griffiths, F. (2003). Taking hormone replacement therapy. *British Medical Journal*, **327**(7419), 820–1.

Haas, J. S., Kaplan, C. P., Gerstenberger, E. P. & Kerlikowske, K. (2004). Changes in the use of postmenopausal hormone therapy after the publication of clinical trial results. *Annals of Internal Medicine*, **140**, 184–8.

Hunter, M. S. (1990). Somatic experience of the menopause: a prospective study. *Psychosomatic Medicine*, **52**, 357–67.

Hunter, M. S. & O'Dea, I. (1997). Menopause: bodily changes and multiple meanings. In J. Ussher (Ed.). *Body talk: the material and discursive regulation of sexuality, madness and reproduction* (pp. 199–222). London: Routledge.

Joffe, H., Soares, C. N. & Cohen, L. S. (2003). Assessment and treatment of hot flushes and menopausal mood disturbance. *Psychiatric Clinics of North America*, **26**, 563–80.

Klaiber, E. L., Broverman, D. M., Vogel, W., Peterson, L. G. & Snyder, M. B. (1997). Relationships of serum estradiol levels, menopausal duration, and mood during hormonal replacement therapy. *Psychoneuroendocrinology*, **22**, 549–58.

Kmietowicz, Z. (2000). Women's health study signs up millionth woman. *British Medical Journal*, **321**(7267), 981.

Lawton, B., Rose, S., McLeod, D. & Dowell, A. (2003). Changes in use of hormone replacement therapy after the report from the women's health initiative: cross sectional survey of users. *British Medical Journal*, **327**(7419), 845–6.

Lupton, D. (1996). Constructing the menopausal body: the discourses on hormone replacement therapy. *Body and Society*, **2**, 91–7.

McKinney, K. A. & Thompson, W. (1998). A practical guide to prescribing hormone replacement therapy. *Drugs*, **56**, 49–57.

McLellan, T. (2002). New Zealand women's preference for treatment decision-making when considering hormone replacement therapy. Unpublished Masters Thesis, Massey University, Palmerston North, New Zealand.

McPherson, K. (2004). Where are we now with hormone replacement therapy? *British Medical Journal*, **328**(7436), 357–8.

Minelli, C., Abrams, K. R., Sutton, A. J. & Cooper, N. J. (2004). Benefits and harms associated with hormone replacement therapy: clinical decision analysis. *British Medical Journal*, **328**, 371. doi: 10.1136/bmj.328.7436.371.

Mort, E. A. (1996). Clinical decision-making in the face of scientific uncertainty: hormone replacement therapy as an example. *The Journal of Family Practice*, **42**, 147–51.

North, F. M. & Sharples, K. (2001). Changes in the use of hormone replacement therapy in New Zealand from 1991–1997. *New Zealand Medical Journal*, **114**(1133), 250–3.

Phillips, S. M. & Sherwin, B. B. (1992). Effects of estrogen on memory function in surgically menopausal women. *Psychoneuroendocrinology*, **17**, 485–95.

Rossouw, J. E., Anderson, G. L., Prentice, R. L. *et al.* Writing Group for the Women's Health Initiative Investigators (2002). Risks and benefits of estrogen plus progestin in healthy postmenopausal women: principal results from the women's health initiative randomized controlled trial. *Journal of the American Medical Association*, **288**, 321–33.

Rymer, J., Wilson, R. & Ballard, K. (2003). Making decisions about hormone replacement therapy. *British Medical Journal*, **326**(7384), 322–6.

Schmidt, P. J. & Rubinow, D. R. (1991). Menopause-related affective disorders: a justification for further study. *The American Journal of Psychiatry*, **148**, 844–52.

Sherwin, B. B. & Gelfand, M. M. (1985). Sex steroids and affect in the surgical menopause: a double-blind, cross-over study. *Psychoneuroendocrinology*, **10**, 325–35.

Shumaker, S. A., Legault, C., Rapp, S. R. *et al.* WHIMS Investigators (2003). Estrogen plus progestin and the incidence of dementia and mild cognitive impairment in postmenopausal women: the women's health initiative memory study: a randomized controlled trial. *Journal of the American Medical Association*, **289**, 2651–62.

Slaven, L. & Lee, C. (1997). Mood and symptom reporting among middle-aged women: the relationship between menopausal status, hormone replacement therapy, and exercise participation. *Health Psychology*, **16**, 203–8.

Slaven, L. & Lee, C. (1998). A cross-sectional survey of menopausal status, symptoms and psychological distress in a community sample of Australian women. *Journal of Health Psychology*, **3**, 117–23.

Stephens, C. (2001). Women's experience at the time of menopause: accounting for biological, cultural and psychological embodiment. *Journal of Health Psychology*, **6**, 651–64.

Stephens, C., Carryer, J. & Budge, R. C. (2001). Decisions about starting and ceasing HRT use: information needs for women. *Nursing Praxis in New Zealand*, **17**, 33–43.

Stephens, C., Carryer, J. & Budge, C. (2004). To have or to take: discourse, positioning, and narrative identity in women's accounts of HRT. *Health: An Interdisciplinary Journal for the Social Study of Health, Illness and Medicine*, **8**, 329–50.

Stephens, C., Hamilton, Y. M. & Pachana, N. A. (2003). Hormone replacement therapy and everyday memory in mid-aged New Zealand women. *New Zealand Journal of Psychology*, **32**, 13–21.

Stephens, C. & Ross, N. (2000). The relationship between hormone replacement therapy use and psychological symptoms: no effects found in a New Zealand sample. *Health Care for Women International*, **23**, 408–14.

Wang-Cheng, R. & Rosenfeld, J. A. (2003). Hormone replacement therapy. *British Medical Journal USA*, **327**, E139–E140. doi: 10.1136/bmjusa.02090003.

Waring, S. C., Rocca, W. A., Petersen, R. C. *et al.* (1999). Postmenopausal estrogen replacement therapy and risk of AD. *Neurology*, **52**, 965–70.

Hospital acquired infection

Jan Stygall and Stanton Newman

University College London

Any infection not present or incubating at the time of admission into hospital is classified as a nosocomial infection and is often referred to as a hospital acquired infection (HAI). Approximately 1 in 10 patients acquire an infection after admission into hospital of which it has been estimated that 30% or more could be prevented (Gastmeier, 2004).

Urinary tract infection (usually catheter-associated), surgical-site infection, bloodstream infections and pneumonia (usually ventilator-associated) account for more than 80% of all HAIs. The most frequently occurring infections are urinary tract accounting for approximately 35% of HAIs however they are associated with the lowest mortality and cost (see 'Urinary tract symptoms'). Surgical-site infections account for around 20% and are third in cost whereas bloodstream infections and pneumonia are less common, explaining about 15% each; however these are linked with much higher mortality and costs. While the rates of both urinary tract and surgical-site infections have recently declined slightly, bloodstream infections and methicillin-resistant *Staphylococcus aureus* (MRSA) infections are rapidly rising. Patients in intensive care units account for 25% of HAI cases with nearly 70% being attributed to micro-organisms that are resistant to one or more antibiotics (Burke, 2003).

Among the factors that promote HAI are underlying diseases and decreased patient immunity, invasive diagnostic and therapeutic techniques, widespread antimicrobial resistance, lack of infection control measures and environmental hygiene (Lazzari *et al.*, 2004). However, the exact extent to which the environment plays a part is largely unknown. Recently concerns have been raised regarding the perceived falling standards of cleanliness in hospitals in the UK, which has been linked with the rise in HAIs. However, Dancer (2004) argues that although there may well be a connection between dirty hospitals and HAI, there is, at present little evidence to confirm this claim. Evaluating the quality of 'cleanliness' is not an easy task and usually, unless an infection has already occurred, the only method employed is visual assessment. Dancer (2004) suggests there are internationally agreed microbiological standards for air, water and food preparation surfaces in the food industry, which should be mirrored in hospitals. A recent World Health Organization consultation on the 'Prevention and Control of HAI' called for an international strategy to establish standards, procedures and methods for HAI surveillance, prevention and control and to promote their implementation at a national level.

As organisms have to be transmitted from the environment to the patient one likely route is via the hands of healthcare workers (HCWs). It has been argued that hand hygiene is the simplest and most effective measure for preventing hospital-acquired infections. Hand hygiene behaviour includes both handwashing and hand rubbing with alcohol-based solutions. Recommendations have been issued to guide HCWs practice, however adherence with hand hygiene recommendations is usually estimated at below 50%. Another method of transmission via the hands is the misuse of gloves. Girou *et al.*, (2004) in a study of 120 HCWs found improper gloving in 64.4% of instances and in 18.3% of contacts gloves were not removed before performing strict aseptic precautions. This non-adherence is seen in a wide range of different types of HCW, e.g. nurses, doctors, physiotherapists etc. (Jenner *et al.*, 2002). There is also evidence that adherence rates vary not only with type of HCW, i.e. nurses have higher adherence rates than physicians, but also by speciality such as doctors in anaesthetics, accident and emergency etc. (Pittet *et al.*, 2004) (see also 'Healthcare work environments').

Although guidelines regarding hand hygiene are widely available, a survey reported in 1999 found that in 90% of infection control programmes handwashing education was not provided (see McGuckin *et al.*, 2001). In common with other health behaviour intervention studies, providing information only, appears to have limited effect on behaviour with various studies reporting little relationship between knowledge and hand hygiene (e.g. Kennedy *et al.*, 2004). The most frequently implemented intervention has been education and training where HCWs have explained to them why and when hand hygiene should be practised and also shown the appropriate techniques to adopt. Studies involving education have also been shown, however, to have minimal long-term effects on handwashing behaviour although, there is an indication that surveillance and feedback to HCWs of infection rates can enhance adherence to policies (e.g. Stone *et al.*, 2000). There is also evidence that different types of HCWs respond differently to differing methods of education (Seto, 1995). Pillet *et al.* (2004) suggest that infection control professionals should learn from the behavioural sciences and become 'agents of change'. They identified multiple predictors of handwashing hygiene, and therefore suggested a move away from the purely knowledge-based programmes of infection control to a more behavioural approach which may incorporate a variety of different methods.

O'Boyle *et al.* (2001, p. 352) suggest 'although the hand hygiene procedure itself is simple, HCW's behaviour related to hand hygiene is a complex phenomenon that is not easily understood, explained or changed'. Various barriers to adhering to hand hygiene have been suggested such as: skin irritation; inaccessibility of hand hygiene supplies; interference with HCW–patient relationship; patient needs perceived as priority; wearing of gloves; forgetfulness; lack of knowledge of guidelines; insufficient time for hand hygiene; high workload; understaffing; and lack of evidence of impact of hand hygiene on infection rates.

The handwashing hygiene of other HCWs, especially those perceived as role models, has been shown to impact upon handwashing behaviour both positively and negatively. Perceived role models who show good handwashing behaviour will elicit good behaviour from other HCWs; conversely a senior member of staff who takes little notice of handwashing procedures can produce the opposite effect (e.g. Jenner *et al.*, 2002; Pittet *et al.*, 2004).

Although theoretical models have often been employed to examine the impact of beliefs on various health behaviours, very few studies have applied these models to investigate HCW's perceptions regarding infection control. O'Boyle *et al.* (2001) used the Theory of Planned Behaviour (TPB; Ajzen & Fishbein, 1980) as an explanatory model for adherence to hand hygiene recommendations in a longitudinal study involving 120 nurses (see 'Theory of planned behaviour'). Although the TPB motivational variables predicted 'intention to handwash' and intention was related to 'self-reported adherence' the TPB model did not predict actual adherence. Actual adherence was predicted by nursing activity which included type of ward, shift, patient to nurse ratio etc. Jenner *et al.* (2002) also using TPB included the concept of 'barriers' from the Health Belief Model (HBM; Rosenstock, 1966) with a single item as a measure of 'personal responsibility' to explore health behaviours of 104 hospital-based HCWs in relation to hand hygiene (see 'Health belief model'). They found that attitudes and personal responsibility were significant predictors of intention with perceived behavioural control and intention being significant predictors of behaviour. Two barriers to hand washing (availability and number and location of sinks) were found to correlate with both behaviour and perceived behavioural control. Barriers were also found to significantly influence infection control adherence in two other studies employing the HBM (Osbourne, 2003; Williams *et al.*, 1994). Levin (1999) examined TPB, TPB plus perceived risk and Theory of Reasoned Action (TRA; Ajzen & Fishbein, 1980) in identifying predictors of HCWs' intention and self-reported use of gloves. They found that intention, attitude and perceived risk were significant predictors of behaviour. Intention was the best predictor of glove use with perceived control contributing most. Although the predictive potential of 70% using TRA in relation to HCWs' reported glove use could not be improved by either TPB or TPB with perceived risk, the authors argue that these variables provided an important insight into HCWs' intention regarding the use of gloves.

A patient education behavioural model was employed in studies by McGurkin and colleagues. In their UK study conducted in 2001, patients were requested to ask 'Did you wash your hands?' of any HCW who had direct contact with them. Adherence to the programme was measured by soap/alcohol usage and handwashing per bed. Handwashing increased on average by 50%. However, HCWs washed their hands significantly more often when dealing with surgical patients than with medical ones. Sixty-two per cent of patients felt at ease when asking HCWs if they had washed their hands. Seventy-eight per cent of HCWs said they had washed their hands. Interestingly all patients asked nurses, but only 35% asked doctors. Similar findings were reported in an earlier study conducted by McGuckin *et al.* (1999) in the USA with 57% of patients reporting they had asked the HCW about handwashing and soap usage increased by 34%. Another study conducted in the UK (Sen *et al.*, 1999) found that patients were reluctant to enquire whether HCWs had washed their hands. However, the major difference between these two studies was that the patient participants in the McGuckin *et al.* study were told specifically that the HCW would expect to be asked about handwashing and that the HCWs were supportive of the study.

Most research into the study, and enhancing, of infection control practices have concluded that future programmes need to employ both an integrated and multidisciplinary approach.

(See also 'Patient safety and iatrogenesis'.)

REFERENCES

Ajzen, I. & Fishbein, M. (1980). The theory of planned behaviour. *Organization Behavior and Human Decision Processes*, **50**, 179–211.

Burke, J. P. (2003). Infection control – a problem for patient safety. *New England Journal of Medicine*, **348**, 651–6.

Dancer, S. J. (2004). How do we assess hospital cleaning? A proposal for microbiological standards for surface hygiene in hospitals. *Journal of Hospital Infection*, **56**, 10–15.

Gastmeier, P. (2004). Nosocomial infection surveillance and control policies. *Current Opinion in Infectious Diseases*, **17**, 295–301.

Girou, E., Chai, S. H., Oppein, F. *et al.* (2004). Misuse of gloves: the foundation for poor compliance with hand hygiene and potential for microbial transmission? *Journal of Hospital Infection*, **57**, 162–9.

Godin, G., Naccache, H. & Fortin, C. (1998). Understanding physicians' intentions to use a simple infection control measure: wearing gloves. *American Journal for Infection Control*, **26**, 413–17.

Jenner, E. A., Watson, P. W. B., Miller, L., Jones, F. & Scott, G. M. (2002). Explaining hand hygiene practice: an extended application of the Theory of Planned Behaviour. *Psychology, Health & Medicine*, **7**, 311–26.

Kennedy, A. M., Elward, A. M. & Fraser, V. J. (2004). Survey of knowledge, beliefs, and practices of neonatal intensive care unit healthcare workers regarding noscomial infections, central venous catheter care, and hand hygiene. *Infection Control and Hospital Epidemiology*, **25**, 747–52.

Lazzari, S., Allegranzi, B. & Concia, B. (2004). Making hospitals safer: the need for a global strategy for infection control in health care settings. *World Hospital Health Service*, **40**, 36–42.

Levin, P. F. (1999). Test of the Fishbein and Ajzen models as predictors of health care workers' glove use. *Research in Nursing & Health*, **22**, 295–307.

McGuckin, M., Waterman, R., Storr, J. *et al.* (2001). Evaluation of patient-empowering

hand hygiene programme in the UK. *Journal of Hospital Infection*, **48**, 222–7.

O'Boyle, C. A., Henly, S. J. & Larson, E. (2001). Understanding adherence to hand hygiene recommendations: the theory of planned behavior. *American Journal of Infection Control*, **29**, 352–60.

Osborne, S. (2003). Influences on compliance with standard precautions among operating room nurses. *American Journal of Infection Control*, **31**, 415–23.

Pittet, D., Simon, A., Hugonnet, S. *et al.* (2004). Hand hygiene among physicians: Performance, beliefs, and perceptions. *Annals of Internal Medicine*, **141**, 1–8.

Rosenstock, I. M. (1966). Why people use health services. *Millbank Memorial Fund Quarterly*, **44**, 94–124.

Sen, R., Keaney, M., Trail, A., Howard, C. & Chadwick, P. (1999). Healthcare workers washed their hands on only a third of occasions. *British Medical Journal*, **319**, 518.

Seto, W. H. (1995). Training the work force – models for effective education in infection control. *Journal of Infection Control*, **30**(Suppl.) 241–7.

Stone, S., Kibbler, C., How, A. & Balestrini, A. (2000). Feedback is necessary in

strategies to reduce hospital acquired infection. *British Medical Journal*, **321**, 302.

Williams, C. O., Campbell, S., Henry, K. & Collier, P. (1994). Variables influencing

worker compliance with universal precautions in the emergency department. *American Journal of Infection Control*, **22**, 138–48.

Huntington's disease

Maurice Bloch

University of British Columbia

Huntington's disease (HD) is a genetic disease which is transmitted as an autosomal dominant trait. It is a chronic degenerative disease of the CNS characterized by movement disorder, cognitive deterioration and personality change. While found in all parts of the world HD is most commonly found in Caucasians of whom about 1:10 000 individuals are affected. Onset is subtle and insidious and occurs most frequently between 30 and 50 years of age. Juvenile onset is seen in about 10% of cases and about 20% have onset at over 50 years of age with diagnoses as late as the eighth decade reported. The disease progresses inexorably, culminating in death usually 15 to 25 years after observed onset. Late onset HD tends to progress more slowly than early onset forms of the disease. There is thus far no effective treatment or cure for the disease.

HD is commonly known for its jerky, dance-like (choreic) movements. Movement may, however, also be rigid, especially in the juvenile form and the later stages of the adult form. Cognitive deficits (dementia) commonly associated with HD include difficulty with memory (primarily a retrieval problem), attention and concentration. While the dementia of HD is primarily subcortical and is non-aphasic, it includes many additional cognitive functions such as cognitive speed and fluency verbal fluency, difficulty persisting with, or initiating, a task and with change of set (see also 'Dementias').

Becoming affected with HD may have a tremendous impact on the psyche. Organic change is compounded with psychological trauma. High rates of schizophrenia, anxiety disorders, alcoholism and other psychiatric illnesses are reported. Irritability, poor impulse control, angry and hostile behaviour are observed in many sufferers of HD during circumscribed periods of the illness. While insight and orientation remain relatively intact throughout the illness, judgement is often impaired. This may be observed in bad business decisions, inappropriate sexual behaviour and impaired social judgement. Depression is the most common psychiatric illness seen in HD and is associated with a higher rate of suicide. Harper *et al.* (1991) have surveyed the literature and have found studies reporting suicide rates which range between 0.5% and 12.7%.

It is difficult to separate out the aetiology of a mental illness when biological, psychological and social factors are all contributing. This is the case with affective disorders associated with HD. There is, however, growing evidence that affective disorders are related to the pathophysiology of HD. A prevalence rate of affective disorder, of between 9% and 44% has been reported (Harper *et al.*, 1991). Peyser and Folstein (1990) found that about 10% of all HD patients have manic episodes, some have delusions and hallucinations. Many respond to appropriate pharmacological treatment. Affective disorder is more common in some families, in persons of Caucasian ancestry and in those with later onset.

Irrespective of the aetiology of the psychiatric problems or of the dyskinesia and dementia associated with HD, the impact on the individual and the family is profound. However, textbooks on HD (Folstein, 1989; Harper *et al.*, 1991) in citing over 500 publications related to HD rarely refer to the psychosocial impact of the disease.

The psychosocial adaptation of the individual living at risk for HD and to the onset and diagnosis of the disease is described in a Model of Psychological Response Stages (Bloch *et al.*, 1993). During the warning stage, asymptomatic individuals become aware of their risk status for HD and develop adaptive psychological defensive strategies. In response to the early signs and symptoms of HD (incipient stage) unconscious working through of this realization occurs while it is kept out of conscious awareness. When symptoms can no longer be ignored, the possibility of diagnosis of HD is acknowledged (breakthrough stage). After the delivery of the diagnosis short- and long-term adaptive responses to living with HD occur (adjustment stage).

Living with an individual affected with HD will have serious ramifications for family members, for their roles and for the family system. The caregiver may take over the role functions of the affected person while maintaining his/her previous roles and at the same time providing care for the affected person. In the case of a genetic disease the caregiving spouse lives with the awareness that any number of the children may have inherited the gene and may develop the disease. The burden is multiplied for those families in which multiple members are concurrently affected. The caregiving spouse, who has no genetic loading for the disease, is pivotal in maintaining the integrity of family functioning. The needs of the caregiver are, however, often neglected. Time taken to fulfil social and personal needs is frequently accompanied by strong feelings of guilt. Attrition over the years wears the caregiver down and may culminate in family breakdown or increased vulnerability to mental health problems.

The attitude of the affected person and of the caregiver toward the disease may have substantial influence on the attitude to the disease of any children in the family. Children are more likely to view the disease as catastrophic if the parents treat it as such (see 'Children's perceptions of illness and death'). This will happen in those families where the affected individual is perceived as not accepting the disease, is rejected by the family or behaves in ways destructive and embarrassing for family members. A less threatened and more wholesome relationship to the disease is more likely to develop in those families where there is a positive attitude of challenge and struggle in a context of love and support. Nevertheless, the child too must bear a great deal. The burden of being thrust, perhaps, into a quasi-parenting role vis-a-vis the affected parent and the negative impact of the shadow of this incurable disease hanging over the at risk children may be immense. Anxiety and uncertainty must be borne and may influence important decisions about marriage, childbearing and career.

In 1983 a polymorphic DNA marker for the HD gene was discovered (Gusella *et al.*, 1983). This lead to the offering of predictive testing for HD using linkage analysis. Ten years later the cloning of the gene for HD was reported (The Huntington Disease Collaborative Research Group, 1993). The mutation in the HD gene was identified to be an unstable CAG-trinucleotide expansion. Persons affected with HD have a CAG repeat length over 36 and are considered at 'increased risk' for developing HD should they live long enough. However, some individuals with repeat lengths between 36–41 may never develop HD in their lifetime. CAG repeats between 27–35 are referred to as intermediate alleles and will not result in the development of clinical HD in their lifetimes. However, the CAG expansion is unstable and may lead to an expansion in the progeny of the carrier of the intermediate allele especially if this carrier is a male (Goldberg *et al.*, 1993).

There is a significant inverse relationship between CAG repeat length and age of onset of HD. A greater CAG expansion is associated with an earlier age of onset. However, caution must be exercised when predicting age of onset for a particular CAG repeat length as the precision of predictions is relatively low, with wide confidence limits. (Langbehn *et al.*, 2004).

The discovery of the HD gene has overturned some of the previous dogma about HD. It is now accepted that new mutations of the HD gene are not uncommon (Falush *et al.*, 2001); that the penetrance of the HD gene is not complete and that, in particular, there is a range of trinucleotide repeats sizes at which the disease may or may not manifest (Goldberg *et al.*, 1993). There is evidence that not all apparent HD phenotypes are caused by an abnormality in the HD gene (Goizet *et al.*, 2002). Consequently direct gene testing has become important not only to provide testing for at risk individuals and to definitively diagnosis late onset cases where the symptoms may be more subtle and the diagnosis more difficult to ascertain but also as a definitive diagnostic test for individuals with no family history of HD.

Earlier linkage testing was less than 100% accurate and could not be carried out at all if blood (DNA) was not available from crucial family members. It is now possible to offer predictive testing by direct gene analysis, at a level of much greater accuracy, and testing can now include persons for whom the previous linkage test had been uninformative or who did not have any blood samples from crucial family members. Direct testing also allows persons at less than 50% risk (such as grandchildren of affected persons) to be tested even while their parent (at 50% risk) is still alive. This creates the dilemma of indirectly providing predictive testing for the parent when the CAG expansion is detected in the child (Creighton *et al.*, 2003; Lindblad, 2001; Brinkman *et al.*, 1997). Questions concerning the use of the test for the purposes of testing minor children must be addressed. (Bloch & Hayden, 1990) (see 'Screening: genetic').

In surveys undertaken prior to the availability of the predictive test 57–84% of at risk individuals indicated an interest in the test (Evers-Kieboom *et al.*, 1987; Kessler *et al.*, 1987). Actual uptake of the test worldwide, at between 5–24% has been significantly lower than anticipated (Creighton *et al.*, 2003). The reasons for this may include the cost of testing in countries where the test is not covered by universal health plans; the increasing hope for future treatment in the context of a late onset disease; the perceived burden of the disease in the family; and fear of discriminatory practices in areas of insurance or employment.

The uptake of prenatal predictive testing has been very low (Simpson & Harper, 2001; Maat-Kievit *et al.*, 1999; Creighton *et al.*, 2003). This low uptake may be attributed to the emotional trauma of abortion and to the hope that there would be a cure for the child in the future (see also 'Screening: antenatal').

The impact of predictive testing on individuals has been extensively reported. In a worldwide study of 4527 individuals who had undergone predictive testing the frequency of catastrophic events (defined as suicide, suicide attempts and psychiatric hospitalization) was estimated to be 0.97% (Almqvist *et al.*, 1999). Half of these individuals were noted to already be affected with HD. An increased risk result, psychiatric history prior to the predictive testing and being unemployed were identified as factors associated with an increased likelihood of a catastrophic event following predictive testing. A five-year follow-up study identified persons who had experienced a clinically significant adverse event since receiving their predictive test result (clinical depression; psychiatric hospitalization; planned, attempted or successful suicide; marked increase in alcohol consumption; breakdown of a primary relationship or scoring significantly high level of distress on the Global Severity Index of the Symptom Checklist 90(R) reported a frequency of 6.9% (14 of 202 individuals) (Almqvist *et al.*, 2003). The most frequent adverse event was clinical depression (6 individuals) and attempted suicides (3 individuals). The study found that psychological distress was significantly reduced for both the increased and decreased risk groups after receiving predictive test results.

HD is the first disease for which a test to modify genetic risk has been available. The counselling protocols developed for HD predictive testing have been adopted as a blueprint for counselling persons entering genetic testing for other diseases such as breast cancer and polycystic kidney disease. The basic protocol includes at least two sessions of pre-results counselling, the preference that a supportive companion accompany the candidate to the results session and that ongoing follow-up be provided and be available on demand. (Went, 1994). Nevertheless predictive testing has created new counselling challenges, ethical and moral dilemmas. Issues of third party interest, social cost and patient confidentiality have arisen (see also 'Screening: general issues').

REFERENCES

Almqvist, E. W., Bloch, M., Brinkman, R., Craufurd, D. & Hayden, M. R., on behalf of an **International Huntington Disease Collaborative Group**. (1999). A worldwide assessment of the frequency of suicide, suicide attempts or psychiatric hospitalization after predictive testing for Huntington disease. *American Journal of Human Genetics*, **64**, 1293–304.

Almqvist, E. W., Brinkman, R., Wiggins, S. & Hayden, M. R., on behalf of the **Canadian Collaborative Study of Predictive Testing**. (2003). Psychological consequences and predictors of adverse events for five years after testing for Huntington disease. *Clinical Genetics*, **64**, 300–9.

Bloch, M. & Hayden, M. R. (1990). Opinion: predictive testing for Huntington disease in childhood: challenges and implications. Editorial. *American Journal Medical Genetics*, **46**, 1–4.

Bloch, M., Adam, S., Wiggins, S., Huggins, M. & Hayden, M. R. (1992). Predictive testing for Huntington disease in Canada: the experience of those receiving an increased risk. *American Journal Medical Genetics*, **42**, 499–507.

Bloch, M., Adam, S., Fuller, A. *et al.* (1993). Diagnosis of Huntington disease: a model for the stages of psychological response based on experience of a predictive testing program. *American Journal Medical Genetics*, **47**, 368–74.

Brinkman, R. R., Mezei, M. M., Theilmann, J., Almqvist, E. & Hayden, M. R. (1997). The likelihood of being affected with Huntington disease by a particular age, for a specific CAG size. *American Journal of Human Genetics*, **60**, 1202–10.

Creighton, S., Almqvist, E. W., MacGregor, D. *et al.* (2003). Predictive, pre-natal and diagnostic genetic testing for Huntington's disease: the experience in Canada from 1987–2000. *Clinical Genetics*, **63**, 462–75.

Evers-Kiebooms, G., Cassiman, J. J. & van den Berghe, H. (1987). Attitudes toward predictive testing for Huntington's disease: a recent survey in Belgium. *Journal of Medical Genetics*, **24**, 275–9.

Falush, D., Almqvist, E., Brinkman, R. R., Iwasa, Y. & Hayden, M. R. (2001). Measurement of mutational flow implies a high new mutation rate for Huntington disease and substantial under-ascertainment of late onset cases. *American Journal of Human Genetics*, **68**, 373–85.

Folstein, S. E. (1989). *Huntington's disease: a disorder of families*. Baltimore: The Johns Hopkins University Press.

Goizet, C., Lesca, G. & Durr, A. (2002). Presymptomatic testing in Hungtington's disease and autosomal dominant cerebellar ataxias. *Neurology*, **59**, 1330–6.

Goldberg, Y. P., Kremer, B., Andrew, S. E. *et al.* (1993). Molecular analysis of new mutations for Huntington's disease: intermediate alleles and sex of origin effects. *Nature Genetics*, **5**, 174–9.

Gusella, J., Wexler, N. S., Conneally, P. M. *et al.* (1983). A polymorphic DNA marker genetically linked to Huntington's disease. *Nature*, **306**, 234–8.

Harper, P. S., Morris, M. J., Quarrell, O. *et al.* (1991). *Huntington's* disease. Philadelphia: W. B. Saunders.

Huntington Disease Collaborative Research Group. (1993). A novel gene containing a trinucleotide repeat that is expanded and unstable on Huntington's disease chromosomes. *Cell*, **72**, 971–83.

Kessler, S., Field, T., Worth, L. & Mosberger, H. (1987). Attitudes of persons at risk for Huntington disease toward predictive testing. *American Journal of Medical Genetics*, **26**, 259–70.

Kessler, S. & Bloch, M. (1989). Social system response to Huntington disease. *Family Process*, **28**, 59–68.

Langbehn, D. R., Brinkman, R. R., Falush, D. *et al.* (2004). A new model for prediction of the age of onset and penetrance for Huntington's disease based on CAG length. *Clinical Genetics*, **65**, 267–77.

Lindblad, A. N. (2001). To test or not to test: an ethical conflict with presymptomatic testing of individuals at 25% risk for Huntington's disorder. *Clinical Genetics*, **60**, 442–6.

Maat-Kievit, A., Vegter-van der Vlies, M. Zoeteweij, M. *et al.* (1999). Predictive testing of 25 percent at-risk individuals for Huntington's disease (1987–97). *Amerian Journal of Medical Genetics (Neuropsychiatric Genetics)*, **88**, 662–8.

Peyser, C. E. & Folstein, S. E. (1990). Huntington's disease as a model for mood disorders. Clues from neuropathology and neurochemistry. *Molecular and Chemical Neuropathology*, **12**, 99–119.

Simpson, S. A. & Harper, P. S. on behalf of the **UK Huntington's Disease Prediction Consortium**. (2001). Prenatal testing for Huntington's disease: experience within the UK 1994–98. *Journal of Medical Genetics*, **38**, 333–5.

Went, L. J. (1994). Guidelines for the molecular genetics predictive test in Huntington's disease. International Huntington's Association (IHA) and the World Federation of Neurology (WFN) Research Group on Huntington's Chorea. *Neurology*, **44**, 1533–6.

Hyperactivity

Bjørn Ellertsen and Ine M. Baug Johnsen

University of Stavanger

In 1902, a paper published in *The Lancet* pointed to the fact that 'abnormal physical conditions in children' could be caused by diseases of the central nervous system (CNS). This conclusion was based on observations of children developing hyperactive, antisocial behaviour after encephalitis (Still, 1902). Kahn and Cohen further discussed the clinical picture in 1934, introducing the concept 'organic driveness' (Kahn & Cohen, 1934). Bradley (1937) reported clinical efficacy of CNS stimulants in hyperactive children a few years later.

The concept of minimal brain dysfunction (MBD) was used for many years to describe children with hyperactivity and attention problems. However, this concept was used differently both between and within countries, thus making comparison of research reports problematic and clinical evaluations different. Accordingly, the MBD concept has been abandoned in clinical practice and research, whereas Attention Deficit Hyperactivity Disorder (ADHD) has become the internationally accepted term and diagnosis for the group of children described as MBD or hyperactive in older publications (APA, 1994).

Hyperactivity is regarded as a predominant symptom in ADHD children, but the relative importance of this symptom has been discussed extensively over the years. In *The Diagnostic and Statistical Manual-III of* The American Psychiatric Association (DSM-III), the syndrome was subdivided into attention deficit disorder with or without hyperactivity. The DSM-III revision broke this down into ADHD only, thus demanding that hyperactivity should be present in order to diagnose ADHD. In the DSM-IV (APA, 1994), the sub-division reappeared (predominantly inattentive, predominantly hyperactive or both). It is important to underscore that hyperactive behaviour also occurs as part of other clinical syndromes than the typical ADHD syndrome and therefore must be excluded through differential clinical evaluation. It is equally important to be aware of the high proportion of co-morbidity between ADHD and other developmental disorder such as learning disabilities (Ghelani *et al.*, 2004) and developmental coordination disorder (DCD) (Kaplan *et al.*, 1998; Kadesjø & Gillberg, 2003).

Hyperactive children diagnosed as ADHD in present clinical practice seldomly present a history of encephalitis or other CNS diseases. Genetic factors have been found to play a central role in the syndrome (Swanson & Castellanos, 2002), as well as prenatal factors. Reported findings from multiple methods of brain imaging suggest that specific abnormalities may be associated with ADHD. These abnormalities seem to affect neural networks related to attention, information processing, alerting, orienting, working memory and executive functions (Swanson & Castellanos, 2002). There are, however, no biological diagnostic markers of ADHD. The diagnosis is based on behavioural characteristics only. Hyperactivity has been vividly described in a large number of publications and textbooks. The DSM-IV requires that a minimum of 6 out of 9 symptoms of hyperactivity–impulsivity have persisted for more than 6 months, and to a degree that is maladaptive and inconsistent with developmental level. In addition, at least 6 out of 9 symptoms of inattention are required.

The hyperactivity symptoms include behaviours such as fidgeting, leaving the classroom seat when inappropriate, running about or climbing in situations where this is inappropriate, difficulties in playing quietly, often 'on the go' as if 'driven by a motor', excessive talking, blurting out answers before questions are completed, difficulties in awaiting turn and interrupting or intruding on others. When evaluating behaviours like these, it is of crucial importance to take into account the chronological and mental age level of the child (APA, 1994). The clinician must therefore be trained both in normal developmental psychology as well as psychopathology. The incidence of ADHD has ranged considerably between epidemiological studies, depending on diagnostic criteria employed, but international consensus seems to place it between 3 and 5% in school-aged children when the DSM-IV criteria are employed (Barkley, 1998). The picture becomes far more complicated when 'pure' Attention Deficit Disorder (ADD) is added and it may be argued that clinical and diagnostic criteria and procedures regarding ADD, with no hyperactivity, are in need of further thorough clinical research. As it is now, the question of ADD is often raised in children, adolescents and adults where other psychopathology is obvious. This is, however, not the topic of the present chapter.

An extensive evaluation is required with regard to ADHD. The evaluation should comprise clinical observation, paediatric neurological and psychiatric examination, neuropsychological assessment, motor coordination evaluation and personality testing, in order to sort out the individual problem profile in ADHD. In cases where the referred child does not meet the criteria for ADHD, this extensive and multi-disciplinary evaluation usually provides sufficient information to arrive at alternative diagnoses and treatment planning. Important differential diagnoses are mental retardation, anxiety disorders, depression, coping failure, Tourette's syndrome, psychopathology and side effects of medication. A number of rating scales and observation guides are available for ADHD (e.g. Barkley, 1998).

Co-morbidity may be the rule rather than the exception in children with ADHD. Up to 44% of ADHD children may have at least one other psychiatric disorder, 32% two others and 11% at least three (Barkley, 1998). Psychiatric co-morbidities in question are oppositional and defiant behaviour, aggressiveness, conduct disorder, anxiety and mood disorders. There is also a well established co-morbidity between ADHD and DCD (Harvey & Reid, 2003; Kadesjø & Gillberg, 2003; Kaplan *et al.*, 1998). For this reason it is important that all children assessed for possible ADHD also are assessed with regard to motor coordination difficulties. The motor coordination problems in question should be assessed using standardized and norm-based methods, such as the Movement-ABC test (Henderson & Sugden, 1992). Children who are found to have such problems may show significant and long-lasting improvement after high-dosage, task-specific motor training (Iversen *et al.*, in press). There is also co-morbidity between ADHD and reading/writing problems. Such problems will, however, normally be identified by the school system and are not further discussed here.

The clinical efficacy of CNS stimulant treatment, such as methylphenidate, in children with ADHD is indisputable. In spite of this well established fact, this type of intervention is repeatedly and at times heavily debated. Ignorance about the pharmacological and clinical effects of the medication is one reason for this, and less than optimal diagnostic procedures leading to incorrect treatment another. However, we advocate that other treatment procedures are tried out before medication is considered. The reasons for this go back to the co-morbidities, particularly the defiant and conduct dimensions. One useful approach is to use behaviour modification programmes as the first step in ADHD children with such co-morbidities in order to see how many ADHD problems 'are left' after such intervention (see 'Behaviour therapy'). There are a number of studies of the efficacy of behaviour modification procedures in ADHD. Hinshaw *et al.* (2002) present a discussion of findings from such studies and conclude that multimodal treatment, combining intensive behavioural intervention with well delivered pharmacological agents, typically ranks better than either treatment component alone. A similar discussion regarding the treatment of adolescents with ADHD, for which there is far less research data, has been presented by Barkley (2004). Central stimulants can contribute by facilitating effects of behavioural modification procedures, but there is always a risk of state dependent learning. Learning that took place on medication may deteriorate when medication is withdrawn. In any case, we advise against pure pharmacological treatment.

The question of prognosis in ADHD is controversial. Until the late 1980s, ADHD was generally considered a childhood disorder that was typically outgrown by adolescence and always by adulthood.

A number of studies have shown that this is not the case. It has been demonstrated that from 50% to 80% continue to experience significant ADHD symptoms into their adult lives (Murphy & Gordon, 1998). Although many cope with this, there is reason to believe that the symptoms may cause self-medication, problems holding a job, marital distress, juvenile delinquency and adult criminality. In addition, co-morbidities such as mood disturbances are also present in adult ADHD. There is reason to believe that there is a significant proportion of untreated ADHD among adult substance abusers and criminals. Thus, early intervention and proper treatment is of great importance in order to prevent such developments.

REFERENCES

APA, American Psychiatric Association. (1994). *Diagnostic and Statistical Manual of Mental Disorders*, (4th edn.). Washington, DC: American Psychiatric Association.

Barkley, R. A. (1998). *Attention Deficit Hyperactivity Disorder. A handbook for diagnosis and treatment.* New York: The Guilford Press.

Barkley, R. A. (2004). Adolescents with attention deficit/hyperactivity disorder: an overview of empirically based treatment. *Journal of Psychiatric Practice.* **10**(1), 39–56.

Bradley, C. (1937). The behavior of children receiving benzedrine. *American Journal of Psychiatry*, **94**, 577–85.

Ghelani, K., Sidhu, R., Jain, U. & Tannock, R. (2004). Reading comprehension and reading ability in adolescents with reading disability and Attention Deficit/ Hyperactivity Disorder. *Dyslexia*, **10**(4), 364–84.

Harvey, W. J. & Reid, G. (2003). Attention Deficit Hyperactivity Disorder: a review of research on movement skill performance

and physical fitness. *Adapted Physical Activity Quarterly*, **20**(1), 1–25.

Henderson, S. E. & Sugden, D. A. (1992). *Movement Assessment Battery for Children.* Kent: The Psychological Corporation.

Hinshaw, S. P., Klein, R. G. & Abikoff, H. B. (2002). Childhood attention-deficit disorder: nonpharmacological treatments and their combinations with medication. In J. M. Gorman & P. Nathan (Eds.). *A Guide to Treatments that Work*, (2nd edn.). London: Oxford University Press.

Iversen, S., Ellertsen, B., Tytlandsvik, A. & Nødland, M. (in press). Intervention for 6 year-old children with motor coordination difficulties: parental perspectives at follow-up in middle childhood. *Advances in Physiotherapy.*

Kadesjø, B. & Gillberg, C. (2003). Developmental Coordination Disorder in Swedish 7-year-old children. In E. Farber & M. Hertzig (Eds.). *Annual progress in child psychiatry and child development: 2000–2001.* New York: Brunner-Routledge.

Kahn, I. & Cohen, L. H. (1934). Organic driveness: a brainstem syndrome and an experience. *New England Journal of Medicine*, **210**, 748–56.

Kaplan, B., Wilson, B. N., Dewey, D. & Crawford, S. G. (1998). DCD may not be a discrete disorder. *Human Movement Science*, **17**(4–5), 471–90.

Murphy, K. R. & Gordon, M. (1998). Assessment of adults with ADHD. In R. A. Barkley (Ed.). *Attention deficit hyperactivity disorder. A handbook for diagnosis and treatment.* New York: The Guilford Press.

Still, G. F. (1902). Some abnormal physical conditions in children. *The Lancet*, **1**, 1077–82.

Swanson, J. M. & Castellanos, F. X. (2002). Biological Bases of ADHD – Neuroanatomy, Genetics, and Pathophysiology. In P. S. Jensen & J. R. Cooper (Eds.). *Attention deficit hyperactivity disorder: state of the science, best practices.* Kingston: Civic Research Institute.

Hypertension

Katherine Joekes and Sandra N. Boersma

Leiden University

The term 'essential hypertension' is used when there is no clear identified medical reason for raised blood pressure. Blood pressure (BP) is determined by cardiac output (i.e. blood ejected by the left ventricle of the heart), peripheral resistance (i.e. force against which

blood moves during circulation) and blood volume. An increase in one of these factors will give rise to increased BP if the other influences remain constant. Systolic blood pressure (SBP) is associated with contraction of the heart, whilst diastolic blood pressure (DBP) refs to the force between contractions. Most experts agree on the definition of hypertension, i.e. above 140 mm Hg SBP and/or above 90 mm Hg DBP. Hypertension is a known risk factor for stroke and other cardiovascular events, as well as end-stage renal disease (see Coronary heart disease chapters and 'Stroke'). In the western world approximately 20% of middle-aged adults suffer from hypertension, with higher prevalence in the elderly (80% of >65-year-old group) and in Afro-Caribbeans (50% in middle age). Hypertension is asymptomatic, and therefore often remains undetected and untreated. In the UK, the state-run health service spent around £840 million ($1.5 billion) in 2001 on prescriptions for antihypertensive drugs, nearly 15% of the total annual cost of all primary care drugs (NoEHGDG, 2004). Certain psychological and behavioural factors have long been associated with the aetiology of hypertension. In fact, only 30%–60% of the variation in essential hypertension in the population can be accounted for by genetic factors (Levy et al., 2000). In addition to pharmacotherapy, psychological and behavioural interventions tend to be aimed at prevention or aiding reduction of existing hypertension.

Aetiology of hypertension

Physiological mechanisms have been proposed linking psychological factors with long term BP regulation. The mechanisms are thought to involve a complex interaction between central and sympathetic nervous system activity and neurohormonal regulation. One of the models that has received much attention in recent decades focuses on cardiovascular reactivity to stress (Lovallo & Gerin, 2003). It has long been recognized, both from animal and human research, that acute stress provokes raised BP (Obrist, 1981). Studies of laboratory stressors (reviewed by Treiber et al., 2003) supply reasonable evidence that cardiovascular reactivity to stress can predict increased risk for the development of hypertension. Care should be taken not to simply extrapolate findings from laboratory studies to 'real life' stressors. One area of research that has tried to overcome this shortcoming has focused on occupational stress. For example, Ming and colleagues (2004) followed air traffic controllers for a period of 20 years, and identified that increased BP reactivity in response to job stress was associated with long term risk of hypertension, after controlling for age, body mass index and baseline BP readings. It remains unclear, however, to what extent moderating or confounding variables (e.g. age, gender, pre-existing disease, health behaviours or genetic characteristics) play a role (see 'Stress and health'). These findings, combined with the fact that descendants of hypertensives tend to show greater cardiovascular reactivity to stress than children whose parents do not suffer from hypertension (Fredrikson & Matthews, 1990), intimate that cardiovascular reactivity is partly genetically determined. This would mean that prolonged stress is only a risk factor for hypertension for those people who are predisposed to respond with greater cardiovascular reactivity. The availability of ambulatory BP monitors has provided further insight into the relationship between 'real life' job stress and elevated BP which may result in long term hypertension (Schnall et al., 1998).

Psychological factors other than stress have also been linked with hypertension. In a quantitative review of 15 prospective studies, Rutledge and Hogan (2002) found moderate support that psychological factors such as anger, anxiety and depression predicted hypertension development in the long term. Although these authors are critical of the various measures used to assess psychological factors and BP, they conclude that these overall findings have clinical relevance. Schum and colleagues (2003) identified similar findings regarding a positive relationship between trait anger and raised ambulatory BP in a meta-analysis. It is not immediately obvious how these studies relate to the findings cited above with respect to cardiovascular reactivity to stress. An underlying mechanism has been suggested, namely perseverative cognition, such as rumination and worry. This would be responsible for prolonged duration of cardiovascular reactivity to a discrete stressor, as well as for the psychophysiological activation associated with negative emotional states, including anger, anxiety and depression (Brosschot & Thayer, 2004) (see also 'Hostility, Type A behaviour and coronary heart disease'). Further to the psychological factors, issues related to behaviours such as diet, obesity, exercise habits, and alcohol abuse have shown stronger links with development of hypertension (Shapiro & Goldstein, 1982). It is likely that physiological, psychological and lifestyle factors operate interactively rather than independently to promote hypertension.

Assessment

Within both clinical and research settings the use of ambulatory or home BP monitoring is now recommended for the assessment of sustained hypertension, in favour of solely clinic based measures. These methods deal with the common 'white-coat' hypertension phenomenon, which is the presence of BP values higher than normal when measured by a physician in the medical environment (Celis & Fagard, 2004).

Psychological and behavioural interventions aimed at prevention and reduction of hypertension

Psychological or behavioural components have been added to interventions aimed at the prevention or reduction of hypertension through enhancing adherence to anti-hypertensive medication, reducing stress or encouraging health behaviour change.

The main treatment for hypertension consists of pharmacotherapy. However, Benson and Britten (2004) found that four in five people had reservations about taking antihypertensive medication, and nearly one in five suffered adverse side effects. These findings, in combination with the asymptomatic character and lifelong nature of hypertension, may explain the high levels of non-adherence with antihypertensive medication. Adherence (also called compliance) is estimated to be around 50%, which has serious implications for BP control (Kroesel-Wood et al., 2004) (see also 'Adherence to treatment'). In a review of 58 different interventions aimed at enhancing adherence, explored in randomized controlled trials, Schroeder and colleagues (2004) identified that interventions which contain motivational or behavioural components show promising, albeit modest, results. Further to this, interventions related to hypertension can be aimed either at changing health behaviour or stress management. Considering the role of stress in the development of hypertension, there were high hopes for stress-reducing interventions in the 1970s, including meditation, relaxation, biofeedback and cognitive–behavioural therapies (see 'Biofeedback', 'Cognitive behaviour therapy' and 'Relaxation training'). On reviewing such interventions, however, they have generally not been effective in the management of high blood pressure (Dubbert, 1995; Blumenthal, 2002), although an individualized stress management programme has shown more promising results (see Blumenthal, 2002). Although it is suggested that stress management might usefully supplement other behavioural interventions (e.g. aiding behaviour modification such as smoking cessation), it is no longer seen as a viable single approach to reducing BP.

Being overweight, high-sodium diets and alcohol abuse are known risk factors for the development of hypertension, and to a lesser degree lack of exercise and smoking (No EHGDG, 2004). All these behaviours are susceptible to change, and have been the targets of simple or complex interventions. When reviewing these behavioural factor individually, the benefits of weight loss on BP reduction are most clear cut, with reductions of 7–10 mm Hg SBP and 6–7 mm Hg DBP following weight loss of around 8–10 kg in both normotensive and hypertensive individuals who are overweight, whilst sodium reduction and increased exercise show smaller effects (Blumenthal et al., 2002). Behaviour change interventions will implicitly make use of psychotherapeutic strategies. Explicit use of such strategies in behaviour change interventions has also been examined. In a review of patient-centred behavioural interventions, Boulware and colleagues (2001) located 15 studies which offered, in addition to the usual pharmacotherapy, either self-monitoring of BP, counselling or structured training courses. The latter two generally focused on multidimensional lifestyle changes (i.e. weight loss, healthy diet, exercise and tobacco cessation). They conclude that adding counselling to usual care produced additional reductions of 5–6 mm Hg in both SBP and DBP. Although the mechanisms for this improvement are not immediately obvious (did the intervention improve health behaviours, or did it improve adherence to medication, patient awareness, regular check-ups?) this review does suggest the potential benefits of such behavioural interventions. A recent randomized controlled trial aimed at achieving behaviour modification in a healthy population with above optimal BP (including borderline hypertensives) consisted of a combination of counselling and behavioural strategies without pharmacotherapy. They found promising results, with improvements in health behaviours and associated reduction in BP after six months, and 30–35% of the participants returning to optimal BP levels (Writing Group of the Premier Collaborative Research Group, 2003).

It can be concluded that behaviour-related lifestyle factors, in particular being overweight, lead to hypertension. Furthermore, individuals who respond to prolonged stress with greater cardiovascular reactivity are also at risk of suffering from elevated BP. Psychological and behavioural interventions aimed at preventing or reducing hypertension may primarily strive towards increasing adherence with antihypertensive medication and facilitating healthy lifestyle.

(See also Coronary Heart Disease chapters.)

REFERENCES

Bensen, J. & Britten, N. (2004). Patients' views about taking anti-hypertensive drugs: questionnaire study. *British Medical Journal*, **326**, 1314–15.

Blumenthal, J. A., Sherwood, A., Gullette, E. C. D., Georgiades, A. & Tweedy, D. (2002). Behavioral approaches to the treatment of essential hypertension. *Journal of Consulting and Clinical Psychology*, **7**, 569–89.

Boulware, L. E., Daumit, G. L., Frick, K. D. *et al.* (2001). An evidence-based review of patient-centred behavioral interventions for hypertensives. *American Journal of Preventive Medicine*, **21**, 221–32.

Brosschot, J. F. & Thayer, J. F. (2004). Worry, perseverative thinking and health. In I. Nyklicek, L. R. Temoshok & A. J. J. M. Vingerhoets (Eds.). *Emotional expression and health: advances in theory, assessment and clinical applications* (pp. 99–114). London: Brunner-Rutledge.

Celis, H. & Fagard, R. H. (2004). White-coat hypertension: a clinical review. *European Journal of Internal Medicine*, **15**, 348–57.

Dubbert, P. M. (1995). Behavioral (life-style) modification in the prevention and treatment of hypertension. *Clinical Psychology Review*, **15**, 187–216.

Fredrikson, M. & Matthews, K. A. (1990). Cardiovascular responses to behavioral stress and hypertension: a meta-analytic review. *Annals of Behavioral Medicine*, **12**, 30–9.

Kroesler-Wood, M., Thomas, S., Muntner, P. & Morisky, D. (2004). Medication adherence: a key factor in achieving blood pressure control and good clinical outcomes in hypertensive patients. *Current Opinion in Cardiology*, **19**, 357–62.

Levy, D., DeStefano, A. L., Larson, M. G. *et al.* (2000). Evidence for a gene influencing blood pressure on chromosome 17. Genome scan linkage results for longitudinal blood pressure phenotypes in subjects from the Framingham Heart Study. *Hypertension*, **36**, 477–83.

Lovallo, W. R. & Gerin, W. (2003). Psychophysiological reactivity: mechanisms and pathways to cardiovascular disease. *Psychosomatic Medicine*, **65**, 36–45.

Ming, E. E., Adler, G. K., Kessler, R. C. *et al.* (2004). Cardiovascular reactivity to work stress predicts subsequent onset of hypertension: the air traffic controller health change study. *Psychosomatic Medicine*, **66**, 459–65.

North of England Hypertension Guideline Development Group (NoEHGDG). (2004). *Essential hypertension: managing adult patients in primary care. Evidence-based clinical practice guideline.* Centre for Health Services Research, Newcastle-upon-Tyne. National Institute of Clinical Excellence (NICE) Clinical Guideline 18.

Obrist, P. A. (1981). *Cardiovascular psychophysiology.* New York: Academic Press.

Rutledge, T. & Hogan, B. (2002). Quantitative review of prospective evidence linking psychological factors with hypertension development. *Psychosomatic Medicine*, **64**, 758–66.

Schnall, P. L., Schwartz, J. E., Landsbergis, P. A., Warren, K. & Pickering, T. G. (1998). A longitudinal study of job strain and ambulatory blood pressure. Results from a three-year follow up. *Psychosomatic Medicine*, **60**, 697–706.

Schroeder, K., Fahey, T. & Ebrahim, S. (2004). How can we improve adherence to blood pressure-lowering medication in ambulatory care? *Archives of Internal Medicine*, **164**, 722–32.

Schum, J. L., Jorgenson, R. S., Verhaeghen, P., Sauro, M. & Thibodeau, R. (2003).

Trait anger, anger expression, and ambulatory blood pressure: a meta-analytic review. *Journal of Behavioral Medicine*, **26**, 395–415.

Shapiro, D. & Goldstein, I. B. (1982). Biobehavioral perspectives on hypertension. *Journal of*

Consulting & Clinical Psychology, **50**, 841–58.

Treiber, F. A., Kamarck, T., Schneiderman, N. *et al.* (2003). Cardiovascular reactivity and development of preclinical and clinical disease states. *Psychosomatic Medicine*, **65**, 46–62.

Writing Group of the Premier Collaborative Research Group. (2003). Effects of comprehensive lifestyle modification on blood pressure control. *Journal of the American Medical Association*, **289**, 2083–93.

Hyperthyroidism

Nicoletta Sonino[1] and Giovanni A. Fava[2]

[1]University of Padova
[2]University of Bologna

The term 'hyperthyroidism' refers to disorders which result from overproduction of hormone by the thyroid gland. The term 'thyrotoxicosis' is broader and denotes the clinical, physiological and biochemical findings that occur when the tissues are exposed to, and respond to excess thyroid hormone, thyroxine (T_4) and triiodothyroxine (T_3), not necessarily originating from the thyroid gland. Common symptoms include nervousness, sleep disturbances, tremors, frequent bowel movements, excessive sweating and heat intolerance. Weight loss is usual despite a normal appetite and food intake. Graves' disease, also known as Basedow's disease, is the most common form of hyperthyroidism in patients younger than 40 years. It is a disorder which has a complex pathogenesis (with involvement of autoimmune factors) and is characterized by these major manifestations: thyrotoxicosis associated with diffuse goitre, ophthalmopathy and dermopathy. Other relatively common forms include toxic adenoma, toxic multinodular goitre and subacute thyroiditis.

A large body of literature on psychosocial aspects of hypherthyroidism is available

Life events

The notion that stressful life events may be followed by hyperthyroidism has been a common clinical observation. Bram (1927) reviewed 3343 cases of exophthalmic goitre. In 85% of cases he detected 'a clear history of psychic traumas as the exciting cause of the disease'. Several retrospective controlled studies (Winsa *et al.*, 1991; Sonino *et al.*, 1993*a*; Kung, 1995; Radosavljevic *et al.*, 1996; Yoshihuchi *et al.*, 1998; Matos-Santos *et al.*, 2001) have substantiated these clinical observations. All these studies used valid and reliable methods for life events collection. In controlled studies, stressful life events have been found to be significantly more frequent in the year preceding the onset of Graves' disease than in controls

and patients with non autoimmune thyrotoxicosis (toxic nodular goitre). Daily hassles were also associated with hyperthyroidism and were found to affect the short-term outcome of antithyroid drug therapy (Yoshihuchi *et al.*, 1998) (see also 'Life events and health'). Stress may affect the regulatory mechanism of immune function in a number of ways (see 'Psychoneuroimmunology'). Within the complex pathogenesis of autoimmune thyroid hyperfunction, these studies emphasize the role of emotional stress.

Psychological disturbances

Hyperthyroidism is commonly associated with depression, anxiety and irritability. Major depression is a common complication. It was reported to occur in about a quarter of patients with untreated Graves' disease (Kathol & Delahunt, 1986; Sonino *et al.*, 1993*b*). Psychomotor agitation, weight loss and insomnia were found to be common symptoms (Demet *et al.*, 2002). The association between hyperthyroidism and bipolar disorder (with occurrences of mania) has been also described (Nath & Sagar, 2001). Anxiety disorders (and particularly panic attacks) are another common manifestation of hyperthyroidism (Kathol & Delahunt, 1986).

A survey study of neuropsychiatric complaints of patients with Graves' disease (Stern *et al.*, 1996) found that irritability was the most frequent symptom, occurring in nearly 80% of patients. Antithyroid treatment leads to a significant improvement in depressive and anxiety symptoms in most patients (Kathol *et al.*, 1986). Affective disturbances may be precipitated by hyperthyroidism but may also antedate its clinical manifestations or predispose to its onset.

Quality of life

Functional capacity (the ability to perform daily life activities, social interactions, intellectual and cognitive function and economic status), perceptions (levels of wellbeing and illness attitudes) and effects of symptoms of disease (with resulting general impairment, which are often subsumed under the rubric of quality of life) have become the focus of increased attention in hyperthyroidism (see also 'Quality of life'). Psychiatric symptoms (and particularly depression) may considerably affect quality of life and influence how the endocrine disease process is experienced. However, psychological wellbeing is not simply a lack of distress, and a compromised quality of life may occur also when significant psychopathology does not occur (Sonino & Fava, 1998). Graves' ophthalmopathy has attracted particular attention as a source of compromised quality of life in patients with hyperthyroidism (Terwee *et al.*, 1998).

Psychological symptoms following treatment

An improvement in psychological disturbances and quality of life frequently occurs with successful endocrine treatment. However, this is not always the case. In a recent study (Sonino *et al.*, 2004), a sample of patients with remitted endocrine disease (including hyperthyroidism) was found to present high prevalence of psychological distress. Quality of life may thus also be compromised when the patient is apparently doing well from a hormonal viewpoint. Indeed, long-term residual complaints and psychosocial sequelae were found to be common after remission of hyperthyroidism (Fahrenfert *et al.*, 2000). Over one-third of patients with a full-time job were unable to resume the same work after treatment.

Clinical implications

Many patients with hyperthyroidism are in need of psychological support. Patients have become more aware of these issues. Their difficulties in coping with thyroid disease have led to the development of several patients' associations (Wood, 1998). Normalization of thyroid hormones values does not always result in re-establishment of a satisfactory quality of life.

Psychological help appears to be particularly important after endocrine treatment has been provided, to facilitate changes of lifestyle and maladaptive attitudes which may hinder recovery.

(See also 'Endocrine disorders'.)

REFERENCES

Bram, I. (1927). Psychic traumas in pathogenesis of exophthalmic goiter. *Endocrinology*, **11**, 106–16.

Demet, M. M., Ozmen, B., Deveci, A. *et al.* (2002). Depression and anxiety in hyperthyroidism. *Archives of Medical Research*, **33**, 552–6.

Fahrenfort, J. J., Wilterdirk, A. M. L. & van der Veen, E. A. (2000). Long-term residual complaints and psychosocial sequelae after remission of hyperthyroidism. *Psychoneuroendocrinology*, **25**, 201–11.

Kathol, R. G. & Delahunt, J. W. (1986). The relationship of anxiety and depression to symptoms of hyperthyroidism using operational criteria. *General Hospital Psychiatry*, **8**, 23–8.

Kathol, R. G., Turner, R. & Delahunt, J. W. (1986). Depression and anxiety associated with hyperthyroidism. Response to antithyroid therapy. *Psychosomatics*, **27**, 501–5.

Kung, A. W. C. (1995). Life events, daily stresses and coping in patients with Graves' disease. *Clinical Endocrinology*, **42**, 303–8.

Matos-Santos, A., Lacarda Nobre, E., Costa, J. G. E. *et al.* (2001). Relationship between the number and impact of stressful life events and the onset of Graves' disease and toxic nodular goitre. *Clinical Endocrinology*, **55**, 15–19.

Nath, J. & Sagar, R. (2001). Late-onset bipolar disorder due to hyperthyroidism. *Acta Psychiatrica Scandinavica*, **104**, 72–5.

Rodosavljevic, V. R., Jakovic, S. M. & Marinkovic, J. M. (1996). Stressful life events in the pathogenesis of Graves' disease. *European Journal of Endocrinology*, **134**, 699–701.

Sonino, N. & Fava, G. A. (1998). Psychological aspects of endocrine disease. *Clinical Endocrinology*, **48**, 1–7.

Sonino, N., Fava, G. A., Belluardo, P., Girelli, M. E. & Boscaro, M. (1993*b*). Course of depression in Cushing's syndrome: response to treatment and comparison with Graves' disease. *Hormone Research*, **39**, 202–6.

Sonino, N., Girelli, M. E., Boscaro, M. *et al.* (1993*a*). Life events in the pathogenesis of Graves' disease. *Acta Endocrinologica*, **128**, 293–6.

Sonino, N., Navarrini, C., Ruini, C. *et al.* (2004). Persistent psychological distress in patients treated for endocrine disease.

Psychotherapy and Psychosomatics, **73**, 78–83.

Stern, R. A., Robinson, B., Thorner, A. R. *et al.* (1996). A survey of neuropsychiatric complaints in patients with Graves' disease. *Journal of Neuropsychiatry and Clinical Neuroscience*, **8**, 181–5.

Terwee, C. B., Gerding, M. N., Dekker, F. W., Prummel, M. F. & Wiersinga, W. M. (1998). Development of a disease specific quality of life questionnaire for patients with Graves' ophthalmopathy: the GO-QOL. *British Journal of Ophthalmology*, **82**, 773–9.

Winsa, B., Adami, H. O., Bergstrom, R. *et al.* (1991). Stressful life events and Graves' disease. *Lancet*, **338**, 1475–9.

Wood, L. C. (1998). Support groups for patients with Graves' disease and other thyroid conditions. *Endocrinology and Metabolism Clinics of North America*, **27**, 101–7.

Yoshihuchi, K., Kumano, H., Nomura, S. *et al.* (1998). Psychological factors influencing the short-term outcome of antithyroid drug therapy in Graves' disease. *Psychosomatic Medicine*, **60**, 592–6.

Hyperventilation

David K.B. Nias

University of London

Hyperventilation is over-breathing or breathing in excess of metabolic requirements. It usually involves rapid high thoracic rather than diaphragmatic breathing. Typically it occurs during an asthma attack or when a predisposed person is feeling anxious or in a state of shock such as following surgery or severe injury (see also 'Asthma'). From a clinical perspective it is important to distinguish between acute or transient over-breathing and chronic or persistent hyperventilation. It is the latter type that has generated a lot of interest especially in connection with anxiety disorders. Controversially the chronic form has even been given the status of a syndrome, namely hyperventilation syndrome or HVS. Attempts have been made to attribute it as a cause of various disorders and panic disorder in particular. Clinical accounts, together with proposed treatments, have appeared for more than 100 years. This history provides a good example of the interaction of physical (e.g. asthma) and mental (e.g. anxiety) factors and the inherent difficulty of differentiating between cause and effect.

Over-breathing occurs as part of the classic 'fight or flight' response as the body involuntarily prepares for action (see 'Stress and health'). Such breathing soon removes sufficient carbon dioxide from the lungs to lead to a significant fall in the blood level of carbon dioxide, a state known as 'hypocapnia'. There is also a loss of carbonic acid that leads to buffer depletion as the body compensates. These changes set in train a number of somatic sensations that typically are misinterpreted by the patient as serious, such as sudden chest pain. Paradoxically there is also a sense of breathlessness that, combined with the resulting emotional arousal, leads to more over-breathing and so the symptoms tend to continue (Barlow, 2002).

Historical perspective

The immediate or acute effects of over-breathing were demonstrated to the Physiological Society in 1908, when selected members of the audience were asked to deliberately over-breathe. Many and varied symptoms (such as muscle spasm) soon became dramatically apparent. It was recorded that 'even observers became distressed'. A good example of the possible relevance of psychological factors in aetiology was highlighted in a widely publicized account of an over-breathing epidemic in a girl's school in the 1960s. Following a three-hour school parade in which some girls had actually fainted, many complained the next day of 'feeling dizzy and peculiar'. By the afternoon, 85 girls had been taken to hospital and the school closed; a similar pattern occurred as soon as the school was reopened. Physical examinations at the hospital were essentially negative, and detective work at the school ruled out food poisoning and leaking gas. Conversion hysteria was considered because of altered sensations in the limbs (e.g. pins and needles), but in the end it was

claimed that hyperventilation was to blame (Moss & McEvedy, 1966).

Because of the 'downward spiral' mechanism of anxiety, over-breathing, somatic symptoms and then more anxiety, chronic over-breathing has been proposed as having aetiological significance in the development of both physical and psychological disorders. Links with physical disorders have ranged from heart disease to spontaneous pneumothorax (collapsed lung). Links with exhaustion and 'battle fatigue' were made during World War I. Similarly it has been linked with many psychosomatic conditions such as hypochondriasis, conversion disorder (somatization type) and chronic fatigue syndrome (see 'Psychosomatics' and 'Chronic fatigue syndrome'). Most research has been directed at the link with panic disorder, a condition often associated with rapid breathing. However, although over-breathing can worsen or even bring on symptoms, it is now regarded more as a reaction to or a symptom of an underlying physical or psychogenic condition. Even if it is not a fundamental cause of other disorders, what is becoming apparent is that treatment for hyperventilation can help as part of a broader programme for other disorders generally.

Symptoms and diagnosis

Patients who habitually over-breathe complain of a variety of symptoms and are often referred for numerous tests before an experienced clinician recognizes the abnormal breathing. Instead of obvious signs such as rapid breathing it is more subtle respiratory signs, such as yawning, that are characteristic of habitual over-breathing. Neurological signs include dizziness and headache; gastrointestinal signs include dry throat and acid regurgitation; musculoskeletal signs include tension and weakness; and cardiovascular signs include palpitations and chest pain. The latter naturally are often of extreme concern to patients. Psychological symptoms include anxiety, anger and associated problems such as sleep loss and fatigue, all of which can in turn lead to a worsening of symptoms (Lum, 1987).

Although acute attacks may be obvious, chronic hyperventilation is difficult to diagnose and its prevalence is unknown with estimates ranging up to a quarter of patients who have been tested for this chronic form of the condition. It is particularly common in patients with panic and other anxiety disorders. Hyperventilation often comes to light only after extensive testing for other symptoms that patients typically present with such as fatigue or chest pain. Acute over-breathing, as may occur in a panic attack, is usually obvious when the characteristic rapid breathing is accompanied by the symptoms of hypocapnia. Chronic hyperventilation, as may occur in patients who present with a variety of symptoms, is much harder to diagnose. Because of their various somatic complaints, patients may be referred to different specialists before attempts are made to test for hyperventilation. Although a variety of breathing tests can be given, including vital capacity, there is no critical diagnostic test in spite of many attempts to find one.

Because of buffer depletion, people who chronically hyperventilate find it difficult to hold their breath and so one test is 'breath holding time'. Such people are found able to hold their breath comfortably for only a few seconds. Another is the 'voluntary' or 'hyperventilation provocation test' in which people are asked to over-breathe and then to rate any symptoms experienced. At the same time, levels of blood carbon dioxide can be measured by the non-invasive technique of a rapid infrared carbon dioxide analyser. A variation is the 'imagery' or 'think' test in which people are asked to recall episodes of emotional arousal (e.g. anger) while testing for hypocapnia. Similarly, an exercise test in the form of a cycle ergometer is used to test how soon hypocapnia develops following leg ache. However, when rigorously researched these various tests, whether conducted in response or at rest, give inconclusive and unreliable results (Lindsay et al., 1991).

In a double-blind trial of the 'hyperventilation provocation test', patients with suspected hyperventilation tended to recognize their symptoms during both this test and during a placebo condition in which carbon dioxide levels were maintained by manual titration. A sub-group of patients also underwent ambulatory monitoring and was found to over-breathe after rather than before spontaneous symptom attacks (Hornsveld, et al., 1996). This latter finding, in particular, was put forward as casting doubt on the validity of hyperventilation as a syndrome. Instead it provides evidence that hyperventilation is a consequence rather than a cause of anxiety and related disorders.

Treatment

One of the simplest and best known techniques for sudden attacks of over-breathing is the 'paper bag' method. Using a paper bag, patients are instructed to re-breathe the air they have just breathed out. By taking in less oxygen this helps to restore their blood level of carbon dioxide. When there is also a reduction in their symptoms, patients can be reassured that their symptoms are associated with (if not caused by) over-breathing and not something more sinister. However, carbon dioxide levels may increase too quickly causing problems and so this method is not recommended for general use. Also while it can work for acute attacks (it also helps for hiccups), it is of limited use in chronic cases. Controlled trials for the paper bag method, and indeed other techniques, aimed at correcting habitual breathing patterns have been disappointing with little more than a placebo effect being apparent (Garssen et al., 1992). This is consistent with hyperventilation being a manifestation, albeit a complex one, of an underlying disorder rather than a syndrome in its own right.

More advanced techniques have been researched with the finding that a combination of methods works best. For example, medication (e.g. beta-blockers) is often prescribed in combination with relaxation training (e.g. autogenic training or yoga, see 'Relaxation training'). Even better is to combine such methods with in vivo exposure to the circumstances that lead to over-breathing. Graded desensitization to the events that typically trigger over-breathing for that individual seem to help. Similarly, in another study patients with panic disorder experienced how their symptoms could be created or made worse by deliberately over-breathing. They were then encouraged to re-attribute the cause of these symptoms using a cognitive therapy approach (Clark et al., 1985) (see 'Cognitive behaviour therapy'). Applications of the biofeedback method, such as how to recognize tension and over-breathing, have also been developed with promising results (Meuret, Wilhelm & Roth, 2004) (see 'Biofeedback'). Finally because slow breathing is better than rapid, exercises to develop slow diaphragmatic breathing are a useful part of an overall treatment programme.

Interest in this topic has helped in our understanding of how mental and physical factors interact. Research has helped to improve the management of acute attacks of over-breathing, such as in cases of severe shock or head injury (Diringer, 2002). For chronic cases of hyperventilation, it is apparent that treatment should focus on the underlying cause (what is causing the over-breathing in the first place) as well as on other symptoms (such as anxiety). Training in how to develop normal breathing patterns is then more likely to help.

REFERENCES

Barlow, D. H. (Ed.). (2002). Anxiety and its Disorders: The Nature and Treatment of Anxiety and Panic, (2nd edn.). New York: Guilford Press.

Clark, D. M., Salkovskis, P. M. & Chalkley, A. J. (1985). Respiratory control as a treatment for panic attacks. Journal of Behavior Therapy and Experimental Psychiatry, 16, 23–30.

Diringer, M. (2002). Hyperventilation in head injury: what have we learned in 43 years? Critical Care in Medicine, 30, 2142–3.

Garssen, B., de Ruiter, C. & van Dyck, R. (1992). Breathing retraining: a rational placebo? Clinical Psychology Review, 12, 141–53.

Hornsveld, H. K., Garssen, B., Fiedeldij Dop, M. J. C., van Spiegel, P. I. & de Haes, J. C. J. (1996). Double-blind placebo-controlled study of the hyperventilation provocation test and the validity of the hyperventilation syndrome. Lancet, 348, 154–8.

Lindsay, S. J. E., Saqi, S. & Bass, C. (1991). The test–retest reliability of the hyperventilation provocation test. Journal of Psychosomatic Research, 35, 155–62.

Lum, L. C. (1987). Hyperventilation syndromes in medicine and psychiatry: a review. Journal of the Royal Society of Medicine, 80, 229–31.

Meuret, A. E., Wilhelm, F. H. & Roth, W. T. (2004). Respiratory feedback for treating panic disorder. Journal of Clinical Psychology, 60, 197–207.

Moss, P. D. & McEvedy, C. P. (1966). An epidemic of over-breathing among schoolgirls. British Medical Journal, 2, 1295–300.

Hysterectomy

Susan Ayers

University of Sussex

Introduction

Hysterectomy is the most common major gynaecological operation in the UK and the USA. Prevalence rates vary in different countries and range from 8% in France, 10% in the UK and 22% in Australia to approximately one-third of women in the Netherlands and the USA. Hysterectomies are usually carried out for benign conditions, such as abnormal menstrual bleeding, fibroids and endometriosis and are therefore elective operations. In the USA, for example, approximately 90% of hysterectomies are elective operations. However, approximately 10% of hysterectomies are carried out for malignant conditions such as cancer of the cervix or uterus (see 'Cancer: gynaecological').

There are three main types of hysterectomy: a subtotal hysterectomy, in which only the uterus is removed; a total hysterectomy, in which both the uterus and the cervix are removed; and a radical hysterectomy, in which the uterus, cervix, surrounding tissue, upper vagina and sometimes the pelvic lymph nodes are removed. Radical hysterectomies are usually only done in extreme circumstances such as cancer of the uterus or cervix. In addition, some women will have their fallopian tubes and ovaries removed at the same time, which initiates menopause. In these cases women have to decide about whether or not to use hormone replacement therapy (see 'Hormone replacement therapy'). Currently, the most common hysterectomy carried out is the total hysterectomy, which is thought to be preferable for benign conditions because it avoids later complications with the cervix such as cervical cancer. However, recent evidence suggests that total hysterectomies are associated with more physical complications, a longer recovery time and poorer sexual functioning compared to subtotal hysterectomies, although this remains contentious (Thakar et al., 2002).

Preparation for hysterectomy

Hysterectomy is a major operation and, as such, women are likely to be anxious and benefit from psychological preparation, which can improve postoperative recovery (see 'Stressful medical procedures' and 'Surgery'). Research looking more specifically at preparation for gynaecological procedures indicates that women judge procedural information to be most important but prefer a combination of procedural, sensory, coping and reassuring information (Wallace, 1984).

Psychosocial impact of hysterectomy

In common with many other medical procedures, the psychosocial impact of hysterectomy often bears little relationship with the medical assessment of the severity of the symptoms which warranted the hysterectomy. A number of explanations for the impact of hysterectomy on women have been put forward and focus on different contributory factors. For example, biological explanations emphasize the role of hormonal changes or disruption to pelvic anatomy. Psychodynamic explanations emphasize the symbolic role of the womb in women's self-concept. Cognitive–behavioural approaches emphasize the role of information, anxiety, stress and illness behaviour. These different explanations are not necessarily conflicting and may be more or less important in individual cases. However, they have obvious implications for intervention, which will be discussed.

Research into the experience and psychosocial impact of hysterectomy has looked at a range of outcomes; primarily physical recovery, mood, psychiatric disorder, sexual function and quality of life. There are many inconsistent findings, which can be attributed to methodological differences. Early cross-sectional, or retrospective, research found that hysterectomy was associated with sexual problems, emotional problems and decreased quality of life. For example, early research looking at mood and psychiatric disturbances established that a higher proportion of women who have had a hysterectomy suffer from mood disturbances or psychiatric disorders compared with women of a similar age in the general population (Richards, 1974). However, later prospective studies showed that these problems are present in women before hysterectomy and that, following hysterectomy, there is either an improvement or no change in psychological wellbeing (Khastgir et al., 2000). The outcome of hysterectomy therefore needs to be placed in the context of the symptoms that precede it, as well as individual, interpersonal and social factors both before and after hysterectomy. This is consistent with the diathesis–stress approach to life events and illness (see 'Stress and health'). This makes the outcome of hysterectomy difficult to examine in practice, as it requires large prospective studies of women with gynaecological problems in order to measure a wide range of clinical and psychosocial factors. A few well designed prospective trials have been carried out in the last two decades and this chapter briefly summarizes findings from some of these trials with reference to mood, quality of life and sexual functioning.

As previously mentioned, women with symptoms which warrant hysterectomy already have a higher prevalence of mood disorders than comparative norms. The most common mood disorder is depression with up to a third of women having clinical depression before the hysterectomy. For example, a prospective study of 1101 women in the USA found that 28% of women who undergo hysterectomy are depressed before the operation (Rhodes et al., 1999). The prevalence of clinical depression after hysterectomy varies widely in different research studies. However, there is evidence to suggest that over a half of women with psychiatric morbidity before hysterectomy no longer fulfil criteria for psychiatric disorder after hysterectomy (Gath *et al.*, 1995). Despite the recovery of a substantial proportion of women, depression prior to hysterectomy is associated with poorer outcomes in terms of physical symptoms (e.g. pain), quality of life (e.g. activity limitation, social functioning) and sexual functioning (see 'Sexual dysfunction' and 'Quality of life'). For example, Hartmann *et al.* (2004) found that women with preoperative depression were three to five times more likely to have impaired quality of life, physical functioning, mental health and social functioning two years after the hysterectomy.

Studies of quality of life following hysterectomy find a similar pattern to the effect of hysterectomy on mood. Quality of life is generally improved after hysterectomy compared with preoperation levels (Hartmann *et al.*, 2004), but remains poorer than population norms for women of a similar age group (Thakar *et al.*, 2004).

The impact of hysterectomy on sexual function has been increasingly studied in recent decades, with inconsistent results. This is unsurprising when it is considered that sexual function is also associated with age, ethnicity, mental health, relationship problems and a range of socioeconomic conditions (Laumann *et al.*, 1999). Reviews of research into sexual function after hysterectomy have concluded there is either no change or an improvement in frequency and quality of sexual function for the majority of women after hysterectomy (Farrell & Kieser, 2000; Katz 2002; Maas, Weijenborg & ter Kuile, 2003). Individual studies suggest that sexual function after hysterectomy is predicted by sexual functioning before the operation (Rhodes *et al.*, 1999), emotional wellbeing and relationship with partner (Bancroft *et al.*, 2003). Physical aspects of sexual function, such as arousal, vaginal lubrication and orgasm are poor predictors of sexual functioning post-hysterectomy.

Intervention

When looking at psychosocial interventions for hysterectomy there are a number of issues that need to be considered, such as what type of intervention is most appropriate, when should it be applied (pre- or post-operatively), efficacy and effectiveness. The type of intervention provided is partly dependent upon the explanation one adopts

for the psychosocial outcome of hysterectomy. For example, if a biological explanation is adopted then HRT may be the preferred form of intervention (see 'Hormone replacement therapy'). If a cognitive–behavioural explanation is adopted then the intervention may comprise of information provision, techniques to reduce anxiety or increase adaptive coping strategies (see 'Cognitive behaviour therapy').

There is, however, little research on the provision of psychological intervention specifically for women with hysterectomy. Research that has been done tends to focus on the provision of preoperative information and coping techniques, which are usually found to have a positive effect on outcome. For example, Miro and Raich (1999) carried out a controlled trial of the provision of relaxation techniques preoperatively and found this was associated with less reported pain after surgery and with more activity three weeks after surgery compared with controls. The chapter on 'Surgery' gives more information on psychological preparation for surgery in non-specific surgical groups. As yet, little research has looked at provision of psychotherapy to women before or after hysterectomy, despite the higher than usual prevalence of psychiatric morbidity in women at these times. Some researchers have suggested that psychotherapy before hysterectomy could serve as a 'clinical filter' to identify patients for whom psychotherapy may be more useful than hysterectomy (Kincey & McFarlane, 1984). In addition, it seems likely that psychotherapy could be a useful adjunctive therapy for women undergoing hysterectomy who have psychiatric morbidity.

Conclusion

Women undergoing hysterectomy have increased psychiatric morbidity, decreased quality of life and poorer sexual function than women of a similar age in the population. Prospective studies have now established that after hysterectomy mood, quality of life and sexual function improve for the majority of women although levels still remain worse than norms. Intervention studies have concentrated on provision of information and coping techniques preoperatively, with largely beneficial results. Psychotherapy interventions have not been examined but may be useful in cases of psychiatric morbidity.

REFERENCES

Bancroft, J., Loftus, J. L. & Long, J. S. (2003). Distress about sex: a national survey of women in heterosexual relationships. *Archives of Sexual Behavior*, **23**, 193–208.

Gath, D., Rose, N., Bond, A. *et al.* (1995). Hysterectomy and psychiatric disorder: are the levels of psychiatric morbidity falling? *Psychological Medicine*, **25**, 277–83.

Farrell, S. A. & Kieser, K. (2000). Sexuality after hysterectomy. *Obstetrics and Gyecology*, **95**, 1045–51.

Hartmann, K. E., Ma, C., Lamvu, G. M. *et al.* (2004). Quality of life and sexual function after hysterectomy in women with preoperative pain and

depression. *Obstetrics and Gynecology*, **104**, 701–9.

Hoogendoorn, D. (1984). The odds on hysterectomy and estimation of the number of cancer deaths prevented by hysterectomies in their current incidence. *Ned Tijdschr Geneeskd*, **128**, 1937–40.

Katz, A. (2002). Sexuality after hysterectomy. *Journal of Obstetric, Gynecologic, and Neonatal Nursing*, **31**, 256–62.

Khastgir, G., Studd, J. W. & Catalan, J. (2000). The psychological outcome of hysterectomy. *Gynecological Endocrinology*, **14**, 123–31.

Kincy, J. & McFarlane, T. (1984). Psychological aspects of hysterectomy. In A. Broome & L. Wallace (Eds.). *Psychology and gynaecological problems* (pp. 142–60). London: Tavistock Publications.

Laumann, E. O., Paik, A. & Rosen, R. C. (1999). Sexual dysfunctions in the United States: prevalence and predictors. *Journal of the American Medical Association*, **281**, 537–44.

Maas, C. P., Weijenborg, P.Th.M. & ter Kuile, M. M. (2003). The effect of hysterectomy on sexual functioning. *Annual Review of Sex Research*, **14**, 83–113.

Miro, J. & Raich, R. M. (1999). Effects of a brief and economical intervention in preparing patients for surgery: does coping style matter? *Pain*, **83**, 471–5.

Rhodes, J. C., Kjerulff, K. H., Langenberg, P. W. & Guzinski, G. M. (1999). Hysterectomy and sexual functioning. *Journal of the American Medical Association*, **282**, 1934–41.

Richards, D. H. (1974). A post-hysterectomy syndrome. *Lancet*, **ii**, 983–5.

Thakar, R., Ayers, S., Clarkson, P., Stanton, S. & Manyonda, I. (2002). Outcomes after total versus subtotal abdominal hysterectomy. *New England Journal of Medicine*, **347**, 1318–25.

Thakar, R., Ayers, S., Georgakapolou, A. et al. (2004). Hysterectomy improves quality of life and decreases psychiatric symptoms: a prospective and randomised comparison of total versus subtotal hysterectomy. *British Journal of Obstetrics & Gynaecology*, **111**, 1115–20.

Immunization

Roger Booth

The University of Auckland

Overview

Immunization is designed to stimulate immune responses against antigens of infectious agents (e.g. bacteria or viruses) and generate specific immunological memory such that successfully immunized individuals, when exposed to the infectious agent later in life, will respond with protective immunity. When this response was first being elucidated, the cellular and molecular interactions involving T and B lymphocytes (main cells of the immune system), antibodies (antigen-specific effector molecules) and cytokines (immune regulatory hormones) were thought to operate virtually autonomously within the body, influenced predominantly by the internal state of the immune network and the characteristics of antigens (foreign shapes derived from infectious agents). However, individual differences in susceptibility to infection and effectiveness of immunity following vaccination, led to exploration of non-physiological factors.

Research using laboratory animals demonstrated that 'lifestyle' factors such as overcrowding (Edwards & Dean, 1977) and exposure to physically stressful conditions (Sheridan, 1998) reduced immune responses to immunization often to the point that the animals become susceptible to infection. Such studies extended into the human arena have confirmed that many aspects of human psychology affect immune responses to vaccination and should be considered as significant factors in vaccine effectiveness.

Research evidence

Stress and immunization

When healthy women were immunized with a novel antigen, keyhole limpet haemocyanin (KLH), those reporting more stressful events had lower baseline and post-immunization lymphocyte proliferation (Snyder *et al.*, 1993) and anti-KLH antibody levels in their blood, while those reporting more social support had higher responses (Snyder *et al.*, 1990; Snyder *et al.*, 1993). In medical students immunized with KLH either at the time of an important examination or during examination-free term-time, the likelihood of developing delayed-type hypersensitivity (DTH) skin responses to KLH was reduced in the more distressed subjects independently of behavioural and demographic variables, but anti-KLH antibodies and the proliferation of KLH-specific T lymphocytes in culture were not related to levels of distress suggesting that, in this model, cellular rather than humoral immune responses appear susceptible to the influence of distress (Smith *et al.*, 2004).

Other research, has focused on clinically relevant vaccines. For example, hepatitis B vaccines administered to medical students at examination time yielded poorest responses in those students who were the most stressed and anxious, while those reporting greater social support demonstrated stronger vaccine-specific responses (Glaser *et al.*, 1992). In another study, anti-hepatitis B antibody concentrations were negatively related to stress scores but not to coping styles nor to loneliness during the first two months after immunization (Jabaaij *et al.*, 1993). Such stress effects early in the generation of the response may be due, at least in part, to effects on hypothalamic–pituitary–adrenocortical activity and sympathetic nervous system activation, as variations in levels of activation of these systems in response to an acute laboratory stress test (i.e. stress reactivity) was associated with individual differences in immune response to hepatitis B vaccine (Burns *et al.*, 2002*b*).

Several studies have found significant associations between psychological stress and responses to influenza virus vaccination.

Elderly people caring for relatives with dementia are considered to be living under conditions of chronic stress (consistent with activation of their hypothalamic–pituitary–adrenocortical axis, as measured by salivary cortisol was elevated (Vedhara *et al.*, 1999)). When groups of such people were immunized with influenza vaccine, their resulting anti-influenza antibody responses and antigen-specific production of various cytokines were significantly lower than age-, sex- and socioeconomically-matched control groups (Kiecolt-Glaser *et al.*, 1996; Vedhara *et al.*, 1999). Kohut and colleagues (2002) found that two weeks after immunization, anti-influenza antibody concentrations were greater in exercising elderly people than in a sedentary group, and perceived stress and optimism and social activity were predictors of immune cytokine levels.

Mild levels of daily perceived stress have also been found to influence responses to influenza vaccines in healthy young adults. Five months after immunization, participants who reported significantly more life events and perceived stress had lower levels of anti-influenza antibodies and were more likely to be in the 'vaccine failure' category (Burns *et al.*, 2003). The timing of psychological stress relative to immunization is also important as shown be the recent work of Miller and colleagues (2004). Stress ratings on the two days before the vaccine and the day it was given were not associated with antibody response, but ten days afterward appeared to shape the long-term antibody response.

Perceived stress effects are not confined to viral vaccines, and can also affect antibody responses to bacterial vaccines against pneumococcal pneumonia (Glaser *et al.*, 2000) and meningitis (Burns *et al.*, 2002*a*) (see also 'Stress and health' and 'Psychoneuroimmunology').

Negative affect, anxiety and depression

There are associations among stress reactivity, trait negative affect and antibody response to hepatitis B immunization in healthy young adults (Marsland *et al.*, 2001). In a double-blind study of rubella vaccination, low concentrations of rubella antibodies following immunization were predicted by high neuroticism scores, and by low self-esteem (Morag *et al.*, 1999). As outlined in the chapter 'Symptom perception', because negative affect is strongly associated with symptom reporting, Diefenbach and colleagues (1996) explored the relationship between these variables and symptom experience following immunization in a group of elderly volunteers before and after three inoculations (influenza, tetanus toxoid and KLH). Negative affect was related to cross-sectional symptom reporting as expected but not to increases in symptom reporting from before to after the symptom-producing inoculation procedure. In contrast, in elderly people following influenza vaccination, those with high anxiety or depression scores were more likely to suffer from side effects (Allsup & Gosney, 2002). Because depression is associated with enhanced production of inflammatory cytokines that influence various conditions associated with ageing, Glaser and colleagues (2003) assessed the relationship between depressive symptoms and changes in inflammatory response after an influenza virus vaccination. Even modest depressive symptoms appeared to sensitize the inflammatory system in older adults and to produce amplified and

prolonged inflammatory responses after infection and other immunological challenges, which could accelerate a range of age-related diseases.

Gulf War syndrome

Following the Gulf War, many soldiers claimed to be suffering from a wide variety of incapacitating symptoms (Jamal, 1998). During the conflict these soldiers were exposed to many potentially damaging risk factors including environmental adversities and multiple vaccinations. Multiple vaccinations in themselves did not seem to be harmful, but when combined with the stresses of Gulf War deployment, appeared to be associated with adverse health outcomes (Hotopf *et al.*, 2000). Although some investigators have questioned the validity of this finding (Shaheen, 2000; Bolton *et al.*, 2001), a large cohort study of Gulf War veterans concluded that 'consistent, specific, and credible relations, warranting further investigation, were found between health indices and two exposures, the reported number of inoculations and days handling pesticides' (Cherry *et al.*, 2001). Pertussis was often used as an adjuvant in the vaccines administered to soldiers and this, in combination with stress or neurotoxic chemicals, may have triggered neurodegeneration through sustained induction of the inflammatory cytokines in the brain (Tournier *et al.*, 2002).

Conclusions and clinical implications

Responses to immunization are influenced by a variety of factors – the vaccine itself, vaccination procedure, capacity of the recipient to respond to the vaccine (dependent on genetic factors, sex, age and nutrition), behaviour (sleep, smoking, substance abuse, diet) – as well as stress, anxiety, depression and negative affect. In a recent critical review, Cohen and colleagues (2001) concluded that there is a relationship between psychological stress and antibody responses to immunizations in humans (convincing in the case of secondary responses but less convincing for primary responses) and that more attention needs to be paid to the kinetics of stress and antibody response and their inter-relations. Moreover, health practices did not mediate relations between stress and antibody responses, but elevated cortisol levels among stressed individuals may play a role.

Because the inhibitory impact of perceived stress on responses to immunization can be partially predicted in individuals by acute stress reactivity (i.e. stress-induced sympathetic nervous system activation) (Marsland *et al.*, 2002), the opportunity exists for interventions to diminish the effect. As an example, Klingman (1985) assessed the effectiveness of a brief preparatory cognitive–behavioural intervention in a school population undergoing mass inoculation against rubella. Girls in the intervention group reported less anxiety and exhibited more cooperative behaviour during inoculation than did those in the control group. Whether there were also significant differences between the groups in immune response to the vaccine is an intriguing question yet to be investigated. Distress during childhood immunization is a common phenomenon and may affect the immune response. Consequently, identifying factors that influence or ameliorate this distress may well improve the efficacy of childhood immunization. Moreover, interventions, such as exercise in elderly people undergoing influenza immunization (Kohut *et al.*, 2002) may also be more generally effective by reducing perceived stress and anxiety.

Finally, although most of the research into psychological factors relating to immunization have focused on immune compromise associated with 'negative' psychological constructs, Hayney and colleagues (2003), studying a cohort of healthy individuals, found significant positive correlations between psychological wellbeing and quality relationships and the production of key cytokines one month after influenza and hepatitis A immunizations.

(See also 'MMR vaccine'.)

REFERENCES

Allsup, S. J. & Gosney, M. A. (2002). Anxiety and depression in an older research population and their impact on clinical outcomes in a randomised controlled trial. *Postgraduate Medical Journal*, **78**, 674–7.

Bolton, J. P., Lee, H. A. & Gabriel, R. (2001). Vaccinations as risk factors for ill health in veterans of the Gulf war. Conclusion may be flawed by inadequate data. *British Medical Journal*, **322**, 361–2.

Burns, V. E., Carroll, D., Drayson, M., Whitham, M. & Ring, C. (2003). Life events, perceived stress and antibody response to influenza vaccination in young, healthy adults. *Journal of Psychosomatic Research*, **55**, 569–72.

Burns, V. E., Drayson, M., Ring, C. & Carroll, D. (2002*a*). Perceived stress and psychological well-being are associated with antibody status after meningitis C conjugate vaccination. *Psychosomatic Medicine*, **64**, 963–70.

Burns, V. E., Ring, C., Drayson, M. & Carroll, D. (2002*b*). Cortisol and cardiovascular reactions to mental stress and antibody status following hepatitis B vaccination: a preliminary study. *Psychophysiology*, **39**, 361–8.

Cherry, N., Creed, F., Silman, A. *et al.* (2001). Health and exposures of United Kingdom Gulf war veterans. Part II: The relation of health to exposure. *Occupational and Environmental Medicine*, **58**, 299–306.

Cohen, S., Miller, G. E. & Rabin, B. S. (2001). Psychological stress and antibody response to immunization: a critical review of the human literature. *Psychosomatic Medicine*, **63**, 7–18.

Diefenbach, M. A., Leventhal, E. A., Leventhal, H. & Patrick-Miller, L. (1996). Negative affect relates to cross-sectional but not longitudinal symptom reporting: data from elderly adults. *Health Psychology*, **15**, 282–8.

Edwards, E. A. & Dean, L. M. (1977). Effects of crowding of mice on humoral antibody formation and protection to lethal antigenic challenge. *Psychosomatic Medicine*, **39**, 19–24.

Glaser, R., Kiecolt-Glaser, J. K., Bonneau, R. H. *et al.* (1992). Stress-induced modulation of the immune response to recombinant hepatitis B vaccine. *Psychosomatic Medicine*, **54**, 22–9.

Glaser, R., Robles, T. F., Sheridan, J., Malarkey, W. B. & Kiecolt-Glaser, J. K. (2003). Mild depressive symptoms are associated with amplified and prolonged inflammatory responses after influenza virus vaccination in older adults. *Archives of General Psychiatry*, **60**, 1009–14.

Glaser, R., Sheridan, J., Malarkey, W. B., Maccallum, R. C. & Kiecolt-Glaser, J. K. (2000). Chronic stress modulates the immune response to a pneumococcal pneumonia vaccine. *Psychosomatic Medicine*, **62**, 804–7.

Hayney, M. S., Love, G. D., Buck, J. M. *et al.* (2003). The association between psychosocial factors and vaccine-induced cytokine production. *Vaccine*, **21**, 2428–32.

Hotopf, M., David, A., Hull, L. *et al.* (2000). Role of vaccinations as risk factors for ill health in veterans of the Gulf war: cross sectional study. *British Medical Journal*, **320**, 1363–7.

Jabaaij, L., Grosheide, P. M., Heijtink, R. A. *et al.* (1993). Influence of perceived psychological stress and distress on antibody response to low dose rDNA hepatitis B vaccine. *Journal of Psychosomatic Research*, **37**, 361–9.

Jamal, G. A. (1998). Gulf War syndrome – a model for the complexity of biological and environmental interaction with human health. *Adverse Drug Reactions and Toxicology Reviews*, **17**, 1–17.

Kiecolt-Glaser, J. K., Glaser, R., Gravenstein, S., Malarkey, W. B. & Sheridan, J. (1996). Chronic stress alters the immune response to influenza virus vaccine in older adults. *Proceedings of the National Academy of Science USA*, **93**, 3043–7.

Klingman, A. (1985). Mass inoculation in a community: the effect of primary prevention of stress reactions. *American Journal of Community Psychology*, **13**, 323–32.

Kohut, M. L., Cooper, M. M., Nickolaus, M. S., Russell, D. R. & Cunnick, J. E. (2002). Exercise and psychosocial factors modulate immunity to influenza vaccine in elderly individuals. *Journal of Gerontology, Ageing, Biological Science and Medical Science*, **57**, M557–62.

Marsland, A. L., Bachen, E. A., Cohen, S., Rabin, B. & Manuck, S. B. (2002). Stress, immune reactivity and susceptibility to infectious disease. *Physiology and Behavior*, **77**, 711–16.

Marsland, A. L., Cohen, S., Rabin, B. S. & Manuck, S. B. (2001). Associations between stress, trait negative affect, acute immune reactivity, and antibody response to hepatitis B injection in healthy young adults. *Health Psychology*, **20**, 4–11.

Miller, G. E., Cohen, S., Pressman, S. *et al.* (2004). Psychological stress and antibody response to influenza vaccination: when is the critical period for stress, and how does it get inside the body? *Psychosomatic Medicine*, **66**, 215–23.

Morag, M., Morag, A., Reichenberg, A., Lerer, B. & Yirmiya, R. (1999). Psychological variables as predictors of rubella antibody titers and fatigue – a prospective, double blind study. *Journal of Psychiatric Research*, **33**, 389–95.

Shaheen, S. (2000). Shots in the desert and Gulf war syndrome. Evidence that multiple vaccinations during deployment are to blame is inconclusive. *British Medical Journal*, **320**, 1351–2.

Sheridan, J. F. (1998). Norman Cousins Memorial Lecture 1997. Stress-induced modulation of anti-viral immunity. *Brain, Behavior and Immunity*, **12**, 1–6.

Smith, A., Vollmer-Conna, U., Bennett, B. *et al.* (2004). The relationship between distress and the development of a primary immune response to a novel antigen. *Brain, Behavior and Immunity*, **18**, 65–75.

Snyder, B. K., Roghmann, K. J. & Sigal, L. H. (1990). Effect of stress and other biopsychosocial factors on primary antibody response. *Journal of Adolescent Health Care*, **11**, 472–9.

Snyder, B. K., Roghmann, K. J. & Sigal, L. H. (1993). Stress and psychosocial factors: effects on primary cellular immune response. *Journal of Behavioral Medicine*, **16**, 143–61.

Tournier, J. N., Jouan, A., Mathieu, J. & Drouet, E. (2002). Gulf War syndrome: could it be triggered by biological warfare-vaccines using pertussis as an adjuvant? *Medical Hypotheses*, **58**, 291–2.

Vedhara, K., Cox, N. K., Wilcock, G. K. *et al.* (1999). Chronic stress in elderly carers of dementia patients and antibody response to influenza vaccination. *Lancet*, **353**, 627–31.

Incontinence

Siobhan Hart

Colchester General Hospital

Incontinence, that is the uncontrolled voiding of urine or faeces (or both), is a common problem which, contrary to many assumptions, is not restricted to the extremes of the lifespan. Amongst children it is more common in boys (see 'Enuresis'), but at all other ages it is more prevalent in women. Widely quoted UK figures put the prevalence of urinary incontinence at about 1.6% of men and 8.5% of women in the age range 15–64 while the corresponding figures for those aged over 65 are 6.9% and 11% respectively (Thomas *et al.*, 1980). Figures from a postal survey into faecal or double (i.e. faecal and urinary) incontinence carried out by the same team (Thomas *et al.*, 1984) suggest prevalences of 4.2% and 1.7% for men and women respectively in the age range 15–64 and 10.9% and 13.3% for men and women older than 64. However, precise figures are very difficult to obtain and many cases go unreported because of shame and embarrassment (incontinence has been dubbed 'the last taboo') or because many believe that some degree of incontinence is part of the normal ageing process or the inevitable consequence of childbirth. All too many cases only come to light during the course of investigation of some other condition that requires attention. Predictably the incidence of both urinary and faecal incontinence is very much higher amongst elderly institutionalized individuals. This is hardly surprising as incontinence is one of the major factors that leads to institutionalization in this section of the population.

Apart from its obvious implications for personal hygiene and general health, the psychosocial consequences of incontinence can be devastating for victims and their families, causing much personal distress, as well as disrupting patterns of everyday living and interpersonal relationships. Recent years have seen growing interest in documenting and quantifying these psychosocial consequences. A number of incontinence specific health-related quality of life questionnaires have been developed and their psychometric properties evaluated (Naughton *et al.*, 2004, Rockwood, 2004) (see 'Quality of life' and 'Quality of life assessment').

The causes of incontinence are many and complex and include congenital abnormalities, damage to the peripheral sensory and motor neural networks and/or to the complex urino-rectal musculature brought about by disease or physical trauma. In addition, incontinence can be caused by damage to the central nervous system, either to the spinal cord or to the brain. Psychological factors can also play a causal role, perhaps most prominently in cases of juvenile incontinence, but also indirectly in adults where emotional distress, such as following bereavement, may serve as a trigger. Psychological distress, including that generated by incontinence itself can also serve to exacerbate the situation. It follows that the first step in treatment must be a detailed investigation to determine the relevant factors and their relative importance. Only then can the most appropriate intervention be determined. This may range from surgery through pharmacological treatment to psychological and behavioural management. Most often the treatment involves a combination of approaches.

This initial investigation must include the sensitive and empathic exploration of the broader psychosocial and contextual issues to establish the meaning of incontinence for affected individuals and their families as well as helping them develop realistic expectations regarding treatment procedures and their outcomes.

Successful applications of psychological interventions have been documented in a wide variety of client groups, including those with head injury, stroke, multiple sclerosis and neurodegenerative conditions (including those which lead to cognitive impairment and dementia) as well as individuals with learning difficulties (see Smith & Smith, 1987) (see also 'Head Injury', 'Stroke' and 'Dementias'). Treatment approaches include classical and operant conditioning, pelvic floor exercises, biofeedback, anxiety management, interventions to treat depression as well as approaches aimed at wider systemic issues which might be causing or compounding incontinence and leading to excess disability.

The use of classical conditioning is exemplified by the 'bell and pad' method of treating enuresis. An alarm triggered by urine release causes awakening and constriction of the sphincter muscle. After a number of nights the interoceptive cues of bladder distension that precede urine release come to be associated with the alarm and in time will trigger wakening prior to urination. Originally developed as an intervention with children it has also proved effective with other client groups (see 'Enuresis').

Many successful treatments of incontinence have incorporated operant conditioning principles whereby behaviours which are positively reinforced tend to become more frequent while those which are not are gradually extinguished. Although specific details vary from case to case such approaches generally share common elements. Firstly, complex sequences of behaviour, such as toileting, are broken down into their component parts. Secondly, detailed observation establishes the frequencies of various behaviours as well as determining their antecedents and consequences. Thirdly, specific target behaviours are identified and reinforcement schedules used to alter their frequency. Fourthly, the efficacy of the intervention is regularly assessed and the programme adjusted as necessary. Behavioural modification programmes are very resource intensive and require high levels of commitment from patients and their families. A key element in the success of any operant programme is the consistency of reinforcement schedules; something that is not always appreciated. While there is no doubt that behaviour modification techniques can significantly improve continence, surprisingly little work has been carried out to optimize treatments, identify those who are most/least likely to benefit or evaluate how well continence is maintained in the absence of intensive input from health professionals (Burgio, 2004, Goode, 2004, Whitehead, 2004) (see 'Behaviour therapy').

Pelvic floor muscle rehabilitation focuses less on voiding habits per se and instead concentrates upon improving the strength and control of pelvic floor muscles. Originally developed as a method of treating urinary stress incontinence, it has been successfully applied to other forms of urinary incontinence and indeed to faecal incontinence.

A number of studies have incorporated biofeedback techniques as a key element in pelvic floor muscle rehabilitation programmes. Essentially biofeedback techniques provide people with continence problems with information about pressure in the bowel or bladder, or about the activity in key muscle groups. This is presented in the form of an audio or visual signal that changes as a function of changes in the physiological parameter being measured. It is particularly useful when the intrinsic kinaesthetic feedback is diminished or distorted. Although biofeedback has been used with considerable success there has been very little in the way of standardization of procedures or investigations aimed at optimizing the effectiveness of the procedure, especially when there are reports of alterations of physiological parametres that are only loosely coupled with improvements in continence (Tries, 2004). The choice of physiological parametre to be the signal source, the number and duration of treatment sessions would appear to be a matter of local custom and practice rather than being based on any theory or empirical evidence. Moreover evaluations must also take account of the contributions of other aspects of the treatment programme as biofeedback is generally only one element in a more extensive treatment package that will typically include relaxation techniques and patient/family education (see 'Biofeedback' and 'Relaxation Training').

Incontinence draws together many of the key themes that run through other chapters in this book, for example, the need to take a holistic approach that incorporates biological, psychological and social elements; the absolute necessity for good communication between healthcare providers and patients and their families; education; compliance; the need for theoretically driven approaches which identify key factors in specific cases and tailor treatment approaches to match these as well as the need for empirical evidence of efficacy. Incontinence is not the most glamorous aspect of healthcare. However it is always treatable even if it cannot be cured and there is usually much that can be done to improve the quality of life of those afflicted.

REFERENCES

Burgio, K. (2004). Behavioural treatment options for urinary incontinence. *Gastroenerology*, **126**, S82–9.

Goode, P. S. (2004). Predictors of treatment response to behavioural therapy and pharmacotherapy. *Gastroenterology*, **126**, S141–5.

Naughton, M. J., Donovan, J., Badia, X. *et al.* (2004). Symptom severity and QOL scales for urinary incontinence. *Gastroenterology*, **126**, S114–23.

Rockwood, T. H. (2004). Incontinence symptom severity and QOL scales for fecal incontinence. *Gastroenterology*, **126**, S106–13.

Smith, P. S. & Smith, I. J. (1987). *Continence and incontinence: psychological approaches to development and treatment.* London: Croom Helm.

Thomas, T. M., Egan, M., Walgrove, A. & Meade, T. W. (1984). The prevalence of faecal and double incontinence. *Community Medicine*, **6**, 216–20.

Thomas, T. M., Plymat, K. R., Balannin, J. & Meade, T. W. (1980). Prevalence of urinary incontinence. *British Medical Journal*, **281**, 1243–5.

Tries, J. (2004). Protocol- and therapist-related variables affecting out comes of behavioural interventions for urinary and fecal incontinence. *Gastroenterology*, **126**, S152–8.

Whitehead, W. E. (2004). Control groups appropriate for behavioural interventions. *Gastroenterology*, **126**, S159–3.

Infertility

Annette L. Stanton[1] and Julia T. Woodward[2]

[1]University of California
[2]Duke University Medical Center

Introduction

The substantial majority of young adults intend to become parents, but not all achieve a goal of conceiving easily when pregnancy is desired. The 1995 National Survey of Family Growth interviews conducted with 10 847 women suggested that 7.1% of married couples (2.1 million) in the United States met criteria for infertility (i.e. no contraceptive use and no pregnancy for 12 months or more; Abma et al., 1997), and 15% of women of reproductive age reported a past infertility-associated healthcare visit. In the United Kingdom, one in six couples has a fertility problem (Human Fertilisation and Embryology Authority, 2004). The American Society for Reproductive Medicine (ASRM, 1997) estimates that infertility affects females and males with almost equal frequency. Sources of female infertility commonly include ovulatory disorders and tubal or pelvic problems. Male infertility typically involves problems with sperm production (e.g. abnormal sperm density, motility or morphology) or impaired sperm delivery. Infertility remains unexplained following diagnostic work-up in approximately 20% of couples.

Approximately 44% of those with impaired fecundity (i.e. difficulty conceiving or carrying a pregnancy to term) seek medical services, with higher rates among those who are white, older, married, childless and more affluent (Chandra & Stephen, 1998). Over 50% of infertile couples who pursue treatment become pregnant (ASRM, 1997). Among the available infertility treatments, a dramatic rise in the use of assisted reproductive technology (ART; i.e. fertility treatments in which both eggs and sperm are handled in the laboratory) occurred in recent years, with a 66% rise in the number of ART procedures performed in the United States from 1996 to 2001 (Wright et al., 2004). Although the high cost of ART has limited its use to a small minority of infertile couples, the live birth rate from ART also increased substantially during that time – from 28% in 1996 to 33% in 2001 for the most common ART procedure of using freshly fertilized embryos from the patient's own eggs (Wright et al., 2004). These rates vary markedly, however, as a function of patient and treatment factors; for example, the 33% rate quoted above subsumed a 41% rate in women under 35 years of age and a 7% rate among women over 42 years. An escalation in multiple births has accompanied the increase in ART use. Infants conceived through ART accounted for 1% of total births in the US in 2001, but the proportion of twins and triplets or more attributed to ART were 14% and 42%, respectively (Wright et al., 2004), posing greater health risk to mother and infant.

Research in psychology and related fields pertinent to infertility has centred on four questions: (1) can psychological and behavioural factors cause infertility or influence response to medical treatment? (2) what is the impact of infertility on psychological adjustment? (3) can we identify psychosocial risk and protective factors with regard to the adjustment of infertile couples? (4) can psychosocial interventions alter the course of infertility or enhance adjustment?

Behavioural and psychological factors in the aetiology of infertility

A number of health behaviours and their consequences are involved in the aetiology of infertility. Unsafe sexual practices can transmit diseases (e.g. pelvic inflammatory disease) which are a frequent and preventable cause of infertility (see 'Sexual risk behaviour'). Both being overweight and underweight are associated with infertility in women (Rich-Edwards et al., 2002), and a recent dietary intervention trial revealed significant weight loss and improvement in reproductive abnormalities in obese women with polycystic ovary syndrome who were seeking fertility treatment (Stamets et al., 2004). Cigarette smoking, a behaviour practised by approximately 30% of reproductive age women and 35% of reproductive age men, also has been associated with a greater likelihood of infertility (with stronger evidence for women than men), as well as with lower conception rates in ART (The Practice Committee of the American Society for Reproductive Medicine, 2004). Provision of information regarding the link between smoking and infertility along with exhaled carbon monoxide monitoring, with or without a brief, stage-of-change intervention, were associated with an increased rate of maintained smoking cessation from 4% at baseline to 24% after 12 months in one trial with infertile women (Hughes et al., 2000).

The contention that psychological features contribute to infertility has a long history, beginning with psychoanalytic views and continuing in much modified form in investigations of stress-related determinants of fertility problems and of response to infertility treatments. Strong experimental evidence demonstrates that a variety of stressors can induce reproductive problems in nonhuman animals (e.g. deCatanzaro & Macniven, 1992), and physical stressors, such as intense and enduring physical activity, can contribute to menstrual disturbances and compromised fertility in humans (Chen & Brzyski, 1999). The biological pathways through which stress might affect reproduction and response to infertility treatments, including neuroendocrine and autonomic routes, are increasingly well understood (Domar & Seibel, 1997). However, no comprehensive theory has been advanced to specify the relations among specific psychological and stress-related factors, biological processes and reproductive outcomes. Further, research has not demonstrated that psychological factors play a definitive aetiological role in infertility, although interest in the role of stress and associated psychological variables in infertility treatment response has increased in recent years (e.g. see Gallinelli et al., 2001; Klonoff-Cohen et al., 2001) (see also 'Stress and health').

Psychological adjustment to infertility

Certainly, the experience of infertility can disrupt one's cherished life goals and affect multiple life domains; moreover, undergoing what are often invasive, prolonged and costly medical treatments for infertility, without a guarantee of the desired outcome, may compound the challenges of infertility. However, reviewers of the empirical literature on psychological adjustment to infertility find little evidence that global psychological functioning or marital satisfaction is impaired in infertile couples on average compared to fertile couples or normative data (e.g. Eugster & Vingerhoets, 1999; Greil, 1997; Stanton & Danoff-Burg, 1995). As an example, Edelmann and Connolly (1998) followed couples upon referral to an infertility clinic and at seven months. Couples also completed weekly diary ratings of distress over 22 weeks during diagnosis and medical treatment. Little evidence of psychopathology, including depressive symptoms and anxiety, emerged. The weekly diaries also revealed a general lack of distress, although they evidenced wide interindividual variation. As found in a number of other studies, women reported greater distress connected to infertility than did men. In general, findings in this literature reveal both the psychological resilience of most individuals who face infertility and the substantial individual variability in response. Such variation renders it important to identify risk and protective factors for adjustment to infertility.

Predictors of adjustment to infertility

The environmental, social and personal contexts, as well as situation-specific cognitive appraisal and coping processes, have been investigated with regard to their associations with psychological adjustment to infertility (see Stanton et al., 2002, for a brief review and relevant citations). Several demographic factors (e.g. high socioeconomic status, having other children) and personality attributes (e.g. optimism, high self-esteem) have been associated with more favourable adjustment in infertile couples (see also 'Socioeconomic status and health' and 'Personality and health'). Research on relations of medical factors (e.g. diagnosed cause, infertility duration) with psychological function has yielded mixed results, but engaging in a greater number of medical treatments and incurring more expense are related to greater perceived stress from infertility.

Because a minority of couples experience infertility and because particular cultural influences can render not having children socially stigmatizing, infertility often presents social challenges. Couples undergoing infertility typically must attempt to manage questions from others regarding their own parental status and look on as multiple friends and family members get pregnant and have children. Interpersonal support, both within the dyad experiencing infertility and from close others, is associated with more favourable psychological adjustment (see also 'Social support and health').

With regard to cognitive appraisals, couples typically perceive infertility both as carrying the potential for harm (e.g. loss of a desired role) and benefit (e.g. strengthening the marriage). Finding some positive meaning in infertility predicts better adjustment. Greater perceived control also is related to more positive adjustment, when the relevant life domain is indeed potentially controllable (e.g. pursuing medical treatment, managing negative emotions regarding fertility problems) (see 'Perceived control').

A consistent finding regarding coping processes is that coping through attempting to avoid thoughts and feelings surrounding infertility predicts poor adjustment. In contrast, such approach-oriented strategies as problem-focused coping and emotional expression regarding infertility predict more favourable psychological status. Further, one partner's coping has been shown to affect the other's adjustment.

Psychosocial intervention in infertility

Controlled intervention research targeting factors shown to predict infertility-related adjustment is accumulating. These experimental trials often test cognitive–behavioural techniques for stress management and typically are delivered to women (or couples) in a group format (see 'Cognitive behaviour therapy'). In general, findings are promising with regard to enhancing adjustment (e.g. reducing depressive symptoms; Domar et al., 2000b; McQueeney et al., 1997). Although findings require cautious interpretation, some evidence suggests that such interventions also are associated with increased pregnancy rates in the intervention versus the control group (Domar et al., 2000a; Hosaka et al., 2002). However, mechanisms through which psychosocial interventions might influence pregnancy rates have not been demonstrated empirically.

Directions for research and application

It is important to move beyond the descriptive, cross-sectional methodologies that characterize much of the psychosocial research on infertility to investigation of determinants of psychological and reproductive outcomes in individuals and couples with fertility problems within longitudinal and experimental designs. Both predictive research and randomized, controlled trials of psychosocial interventions are essential. Given that psychologists and other mental health professionals are working in infertility clinics to perform psychological evaluations of patients (e.g. gamete donors and those seeking donor services) and to provide psychological interventions, research is needed to establish the evidence base for the effectiveness of such services. In the light of the expanding use of ART, theoretically grounded research on decision-making, stress and coping in couples as they elect various medical procedures will be of value, as will studies that examine psychological and biological outcomes of these treatments. Study of the psychosocial implications of ethical issues surrounding ART also is warranted. Finally, psychosocial research in infertility primarily has involved women and couples who are married, relatively affluent, white and participating in specialized fertility treatments. Research is needed with individuals who do not or cannot elect specialized medical services, as are studies to examine the generalizability of extant findings to diverse groups.

In their capacities as researchers and clinicians, psychologists certainly can play a valuable role in addressing the challenges of infertility. They can aid in identifying and intervening with biopsychosocial contributors to and consequences of infertility. For example, the area will benefit from development of effective prevention programmes that target biopsychosocial contributors (e.g. smoking, unsafe sexual practices) to infertility and associated treatment outcomes. The demonstration of marked diversity in response to infertility implies that many individuals will not need psychological assessment or counselling, although psychosocial intervention may prove invaluable to the health and wellbeing of some individuals and couples who confront fertility problems.

REFERENCES

Abma, J. C., Chandra, A., Mosher, W. D., Peterson, L. S. & Piccinino, L. J. (1997). Fertility, family planning, and women's health: new data from the 1995 National Survey of Family Growth. National Center for Health Statistics. *Vital and Health Statistics*, **23**(19), 1–114.

American Society for Reproductive Medicine. (1997). *Patient's fact sheet: Infertility*. Birmingham, AL: American Society for Reproductive Medicine.

Chandra, A. & Stephen, E. H. (1998). Impaired fecundity in the United States: 1982–1995. *Family Planning Perspectives*, **30**, 34–42.

Chen, E. C. & Brzyski, R. G. (1999). Exercise and reproductive dysfunction. *Fertility and Sterility*, **71**, 1–6.

deCatanzaro, D. & Macniven, E. (1992). Psychogenic pregnancy disruptions in mammals. *Neuroscience and Biobehavioral Research*, **16**, 43–53.

Domar, A. D., Clapp, D., Slawsby, E. A. *et al.* (2000*a*). Impact of group psychological interventions on pregnancy rates in infertile women. *Fertility and Sterility*, **73**, 805–12.

Domar, A. D., Clapp, D., Slawsby, E. A. *et al.* (2000*b*). The impact of group psychological interventions on distress in infertile women. *Health Psychology*, **19**, 568–75.

Domar, A. & Seibel, S. (1997). The emotional aspects of infertility. In M. Seibel (Ed.). *Infertility: a comprehensive text* (2nd edn.). East Norwalk, CT: Appleton-Lange.

Edelmann, R. J. & Connolly, K. J. (1998). Psychological state and psychological strain in relation to infertility. *Journal of Community and Applied Social Psychology*, **8**, 303–11.

Eugster, A. & Vingerhoets, A. J. J. M. (1999). Psychological aspects of in vitro fertilization: a review. *Social Science & Medicine*, **48**, 575–89.

Gallinelli, A., Roncaglia, R., Matteo, M. L. *et al.* (2001). Immunological changes and stress are associated with different implantation rates in patients undergoing in vitro fertilization–embryo transfer. *Fertility and Sterility*, **76**, 85–91.

Greil, A. L. (1997). Infertility and psychological distress: a critical review of the literature. *Social Science and Medicine*, **45**, 1679–704.

Hosaka, T., Hidehiko, M., Sugiyama, R. N., Izumi, S. & Makino, T. (2002). Effect of psychiatric group intervention on natural-killer cell activity and pregnancy rate. *General Hospital Psychiatry*, **24**, 353–6.

Hughes, E. G., Lamont, D. A., Beecroft, M. L. *et al.* (2000). Randomized trial of a "stage-of-change" oriented smoking cessation intervention in infertile and pregnant women. *Fertility and Sterility*, **74**, 498–503.

Human Fertilisation and Embryology Authority. (2004). *Facts and figures*. (http://www.hfea.gov.uk/PressOffice/Factsandfigures). Website accessed 7/7/04.

Klonoff-Cohen, H., Chu, E., Natarajan, L. & Sieber, W. (2001). A prospective study of stress among women undergoing in vitro fertilization or gamete intrafallopian transfer. *Fertility and Sterility*, **76**, 675–87.

McQueeney, D. A., Stanton, A. L. & Sigmon, S. (1997). Efficacy of emotion-focused and problem-focused group therapies for women with fertility problems. *Journal of Behavioral Medicine*, **20**, 313–31.

Rich-Edwards, J. W., Spiegelman, D., Garland, M. *et al.* (2002). Physical activity, body mass index, and ovulatory disorder infertility. *Epidemiology*, **13**, 184–90.

Stamets, K., Taylor, D. S., Kunselman, A. *et al.* (2004). A randomized trial of the effects of two types of short-term hypocaloric diets on weight loss in women with polycystic ovary syndrome. *Fertility and Sterility*, **81**, 630–7.

Stanton, A. L. & Danoff-Burg, S. (1995). Selected issues in women's reproductive health: psychological perspectives. In A. L. Stanton & S. Gallant (Eds.). *Psychology of women's health: progress and challenges in research and application* (pp. 261–305). Washington, DC: American Psychological Association.

Stanton, A. L., Lobel, M., Sears, S. & DeLuca, R. S. (2002). Psychosocial aspects of selected issues in women's reproductive health: current status and future directions. *Journal of Consulting and Clinical Psychology*, **70**, 751–70.

The Practice Committee of the American Society for Reproductive Medicine. (2004). Smoking and infertility. *Fertility and Sterility*, **81**, 1181–6.

Wright, V. C., Schieve, L. A., Reynolds, M. A., Jeng, G. & Kissin, D. (2004). Assisted reproductive technology surveillance – United States, 2001. *Morbidity and Mortality Weekly Report*, **53**(SS-1), 1–20.

Inflammatory bowel disease

Paul Bennett

University of Cardiff

Inflammatory bowel disease (IBD) refers to two disorders: Crohn's disease and ulcerative colitis. Both are remitting diseases, with alternating periods of exacerbation and remission with symptoms of pain, diarrhoea and anorexia. Ulcerative colitis usually affects the large colon and results from inflammation of its inner lining. Crohn's disease results from an inflammation of the entire thickness of the intestinal wall, and may occur anywhere in the gastrointestinal tract, although it most frequently occurs in the small intestine. Complications of both disorders include the development of fistulas and scarring which may lead to obstruction and distension and, potentially fatal, rupture of the bowel. Both are thought to result from immune dysfunction and carry a high risk for the development of cancer (see 'Cancer: digestive tract').

Aetiology and impact

Initial aetiological theories suggested both ulcerative colitis and Crohn's disease to be psychosomatic in origin (see 'Psychosomatics'). Early analytical work by Alexander provided clinical evidence of this relationship, while a number of uncontrolled studies found a high percentage of IBD patients to report adverse life events prior to symptom exacerbation. However, controlled studies have shown little consistent evidence that IBD patients experience more stress preceding exacerbation than is typically encountered by healthy controls. Indeed, Von Wietersheim et al. (1992) found the number of life events reported in the previous six months by ulcerative colitis patients to be lower than those reported by patients undergoing surgery for minor injuries. However, they listed more feelings of being under pressure.

More pertinent, however, may be studies examining the impact of daily hassles. Duffy et al. (1991) followed a large cohort of IBD patients for approximately six months, and found that major life events and daily strains independently prospectively contributed to the variance in both self-reported and medically verified symptoms of IBD. The combined stress and demographic variables explained a total of 47% of the variance in disease activity. In a smaller study involving a more fine-grain analysis, Greene et al. (1994) followed 11 patients for a period of one year. A daily diary of stress, coping and mood provided a measure of psychosocial stress and its emotional responses. Pooled time series analysis revealed a prospective effect of stress on the self-reported signs and symptoms of IBD. Daily and monthly stress were positively associated with disease activity.

The symptoms of IBD may also contribute to distress. Porcelli et al. (1996), for example, reported prospective data on a large cohort of IBD patients, evaluating the relationship between psychological distress and disease activity. Patients were evaluated at baseline and six-month follow-up, and grouped as 'unchanged', 'improved' and 'worsened'. The clinical course of IBD affected the extent of psychological distress. An improvement in disease activity over time was related to a decrease in the anxiety scores. A worsening in disease activity over time was related to increase in anxiety scores.

Interventions

Interventions with IBD patients have been of two types: those targeted primarily at symptom reduction, and those at reducing distress resulting from symptom exacerbation. Unfortunately, few satisfactory studies of either type have been conducted, limiting the conclusions which may be drawn from the research. In one of the first such studies, Karush et al. (1977) allocated IBD patients to either medical treatment alone or in combination with supportive psychotherapy. Over the eight-year period of the study, patients in the combined treatment group experienced shorter and less severe exacerbations and longer periods of remission. However, the study was seriously compromised by non-random allocation to condition and a failure to control for the use of steroids and antibiotics. Subsequently, Milne et al. (1986) reported significant improvements on measures of symptomatology over a follow-up period of one year in patients assigned to a stress management protocol relative to those assigned to a standard treatment control group. No differential changes in medication which may explain these differences occurred. However, patients in the intervention condition reported significantly more symptoms and psychological stress at baseline, and their relative improvement on both types of measure may be attributable to regression to the mean. One final study examined the relationship between stress management and symptoms. Schwarz and Blanchard (1991) reported the only failure of IBD patients to benefit from psychological therapy in comparison to a symptom monitoring condition. Participants in the active condition reported significant reductions in five symptoms following an intervention comprising progressive muscle relaxation, thermal biofeedback and cognitive stress management techniques (see 'Biofeedback', 'Cognitive behaviour therapy' and 'Relaxation training'). Over the same period of time, patients in the symptom monitoring group reported decreases in all eight of the symptoms being monitored. When this group subsequently received the intervention, their symptoms increased.

More positively, a number of studies suggest that psychological distress resulting from symptom flare up may be reduced through the use of psychological techniques. Despite the lack of symptomatic change, patients in the active intervention of Schwarz and Blanchard (1991) reported less symptom-related stress, less depression and less anxiety than those in the control group. Mussell *et al.* (2003) also found a cognitive behavioural group treatment to reduce levels of depression, and disease-related worries and concerns. Finally, Shaw and Ehrlich (1987) found evidence that psychological interventions may help patients cope better with the pain associated with IBD. They allocated 40 patients with IBD to either a relaxation training or attention control condition. Immediately following the intervention and at six-week follow-up, patients in the active intervention reported significantly less frequent and intense pain, and were more able to control their pain. In addition, significantly fewer patients were taking anti-inflammatory drugs (see also 'Pain management').

Conclusions

There is some evidence of a modest relationship between everyday levels of stress and IBD symptomatology. It is not clear, however, whether psychological interventions can impact on the symptoms of IBD, although there is more evidence that such interventions may help patients cope better with them.

(See also 'Irritable bowel syndrome', 'Gastric and duodenal ulcers' and 'Cancer: digestive tract'.)

REFERENCES

Duffy, L. C., Zielezny, M. A., Marshall, J. R. *et al.* (1991). Relevance of major stress events as an indicator of disease activity prevalence in inflammatory bowel disease. *Behavioral Medicine,* **17**, 101–10.

Greene, B. R., Blanchard, E. B. & Wan, C. K. (1994). Long-term monitoring of psychosocial stress and symptomatology in inflammatory bowel disease. *Behaviour Research and Therapy,* **32**, 217–26.

Karush, A., Daniels, G. E., Flood, C. & O'Connor, J. F. (1977). *Psychotherapy in chronic ulcerative colitis.* Philadelphia: W. B. Saunders and Co.

Milne, B., Joachim, G. & Niedhart, J. (1986). A stress management programme for inflammatory bowel disease patients. *Journal of Advanced Nursing,* **11**, 561–7.

Mussell, M., Bocker, U., Nagel, N., Olbrich, R. & Singer, M. V. (2003). Reducing psychological distress in patients with inflammatory bowel disease by cognitive–behavioural treatment: exploratory study of effectiveness. *Scandinavian Journal of Gastroenterology,* **38**, 755–62.

Porcelli, P., Leoci, C., Guerra, V., Taylor, G. J. & Bagby, R. M. (1996). A longitudinal study of alexithymia and psychological distress in inflammatory bowel disease. *Journal of Psychosomatic Research,* **41**, 569–73.

Schwarz, S. P. & Blanchard, E. B. (1991). Evaluation of a psychological treatment for inflammatory bowel disease. *Behaviour Research and Therapy,* **29**, 167–77.

Shaw, L. & Ehrlich, A. (1987). Relaxation training as a treatment for chronic pain caused by ulcerative colitis. *Pain,* **29**, 287–93.

Von Wietersheim, J., Köhler, T. & Feiereis, H. (1992). Relapse – precipitating life events and feelings in patients with Inflammatory Bowel Disease. *Psychotherapy and Psychosomatics,* **58**, 103–12.

Intensive care unit

Christina Jones and Richard D. Griffiths

University of Liverpool

Overview

A critical illness is a major life event for patients and their relatives and happens within the confines of an intensive care unit (ICU). The ICU is where you will find some of the sickest patients in the hospital, with very intensive medical and nursing interventions and monitoring being undertaken around the clock. In the UK each patient has a dedicated nurse looking after them as they may require support for different failed organs, such as artificial ventilation, dialysis or drugs to raise their blood pressure.

The psychological impact of a critical illness is now recognized to go well beyond the confines of the ICU. The patients admitted to an ICU vary in age, illness type and severity and this differs considerably between hospitals depending on the population they serve. Patients undergoing major surgery who know before they go to theatre that they will be admitted to ICU afterwards may experience a strong sense of security because they have been prepared for their admission beforehand (Shi *et al.*, 2003). However, for the many patients who develop an illness needing an admission to ICU as an emergency such preparation is simply not possible. The reasons for admission to ICU may vary greatly, from a major car crash to severe pneumonia. However the majority of these patients will be so ill that they will need a ventilator to do their breathing for them for varying periods of time, from hours to months. Their perception of their surroundings and comprehension of information may be clouded as they wake from the sedation and analgesia, which has been given to keep them comfortable with the ventilator. Patients in ICU are completely emotionally and physically dependent on the staff looking after them. Keeping patients informed and giving them a sense of security and hope is a real challenge, but providing emotional support may be sufficient to help many patients cope with this dependence. A recent study found that feelings of vulnerability were reduced when patients were well informed; received care which was personalized to their own needs; and had a family member present (McKinley *et al.*, 2002).

In the past when patients left the ICU they were discharged to their admitting speciality, for example surgery, and follow-up was left to this team. This follow-up therefore had a tendency to concentrate on the problem as identified at admission. But since the introduction of formal follow-up and specialized ICU outpatient clinics, awareness of the longer-term psychological impact on patients of such a severe multi-system illness has been growing (Jones & Griffiths, 2002). Anxiety; depression; panic attacks; new phobias, such as agoraphobia, and high levels of symptoms of post-traumatic stress disorder (PTSD) have all been reported in ICU patients (see 'Post-traumatic stress disorder'). One particular challenge in this patient group is the fragmentary nature of patients' recall for their illnesses and the high incidence of delusional memories, such as hallucinations, paranoid delusions and nightmares. These delusional memories are described by patients as being very vivid, as if they really happened to them. Although patients may recognize intellectually that these memories cannot be true, the frightening emotional content make them hard to ignore.

Research evidence

In the past, the myriad of psychological and behavioural disturbances occurring within ICU have been unhelpfully called 'ICU psychosis or syndrome'. It is now recognized that most patients suffer delirium at some stage in ICU. This may or may not be accompanied by agitation but increasingly is recognized to be associated with delusions and hallucinations. It is not surprising, given the serious medical conditions, metabolic derangements and numerous drugs that the incidence of delirium varies considerably, dependent on the patient population. It is described ranging from between 19% (Dubois *et al.*, 2001) to over 80% (Ely *et al.*, 2001*a*) within intensive care. A validated, practical and reliable assessment tool to diagnose delirium in ICU is available. Called the Confusion Assessment Method for the ICU (CAM-ICU) (Ely *et al.*, 2001*b*) it is recommended for routine use by the practice guidelines for sedation of the American Society of Critical Care Medicine (Jacobi *et al.*, 2002). Further clues to the aetiology of delirium come from the recognition that neuropathological changes, especially during severe sepsis may be common (Sharshar *et al.*, 2003).

While the patient is in ICU and once the effects of sedation and illness have lessened, symptoms of anxiety and depression have been reported (Goldman & Kimball, 1987; Chlan, 2003; Bardellini *et al.*, 1992) but reliably establishing these diagnoses within ICU where patients cannot freely talk due to oral or tracheal intubations is contentious. The criteria used to assess depression, in particular, are somewhat unclear. A withdrawn patient may be labelled as depressed when they are actually delirious. In this case the administration of an antidepressant should be avoided until clear diagnostic criteria are available as they may further cloud cognition in this acute setting.

Following serious illness, anxiety, panic attacks and depression are common in other patient groups (House *et al.*, 1995). ICU patients are no exception to this and anxiety and depression are common in both patients and their families after discharge. For close family members, high levels of anxiety symptoms are predictive of developing the symptoms of PTSD (Jones *et al.*, 2004). One large study involving 3655 patients reported problems with emotional behaviour, sleep and alertness, particularly with the younger patients aged between 30–50 years (Tian and Reis Miranda, 1995). The delusional memories that patients can recall from their stay in ICU can be vivid and can precipitate PTSD-related symptoms. The memory of patients may be disturbed with some suffering amnesia for the ICU stay (Jones *et al.*, 2000). Where delusional memories are the sole recollections of ICU, with no factual memories being recalled at all, the risk of developing high levels of PTSD-related symptoms is even higher (Jones *et al.*, 2001). In addition, there seems to be a strong correlation between symptom levels in family members and patients (Jacobi *et al.*, 2002). This may be because the patient and relatives are unable to support each other.

Although physical recovery can be improved by the use of a self-directed rehabilitation package, the ICU Recovery Manual, early in the convalescent phase, psychological recovery may not be as simple (Jones *et al.*, 2003). While depression may be improved, the self-directed package had less impact on anxiety and PTSD-related symptoms. This is particularly so when patients report having delusional memories, so emphasizing the importance of recognizing such patients and ensuring an appropriate referral for further treatment.

In addition to psychological distress critical illness can also have an impact on cognitive function, particularly on strategic thinking and memory, possibly reflecting frontal lobe problems. At this present time it is unclear if the cognitive deficits noted so far are permanent due to neurological damage or may recover with time (Ambrosino *et al.*, 2002; Hopkins *et al.*, 1999; Jackson *et al.*, 2003).

Clinical implications

For ICU treatment

It has been the tradition in the UK and many Northern European countries to sedate patients to ensure the patients' compliance with the ventilator. This practice has been defended in terms of the patients' comfort and to reduce anxiety while in ICU. Clearly such drugs have significant impact of the patients' cognitive function and may affect the ability to understand and remember information given to them (see 'Anaesthesia'). Research has not, until recently, been undertaken to examine the ideal depth of sedation to ensure that patients are not traumatized by their experience of ICU. Sedation may have a role to play in the formation of delusional memories by clouding cognition. In a recent retrospective study the impact of waking the patient daily while on ICU from their continuous sedation was evaluated in terms of their later psychological distress (Kress *et al.*, 2003). There was a trend towards those patients who were woken daily being less distressed and less likely to develop PTSD than those who were kept continuously sedated and only woken up to get them to breathe on their own without a ventilator.

This may have major clinical implication for the way patients are cared for on ICU.

Psychological services after discharge

At present, once ICU patients are discharged home, even where follow-up services exist, there may be little provision for counselling or referral to clinical psychology. A few hospitals around the UK have dedicated counsellors and/or clinical psychologists with sessional time for ICU. For the majority of patients the first person they may tell about their problems will be their GP (primary care physician). While some GPs now have counsellors attached to the surgery, the waiting list can be lengthy. Little research has been undertaken on particular therapeutic approaches to address psychological distress in this patient group.

Interventions

A simple intervention, which has been imported from Sweden and is well received by patients, is to keep a patient diary with photographs whilst on ICU (Bäckmann & Walther, 2001). This can be written by staff and family and is given to the patient afterwards. The language used is everyday and any medical words are explained. Periods of confusion or agitation are also written about with a possible reason for this. A small pilot study in Sweden showed that patients felt that the diary helped them come to terms with their illness and recall what had happened (Bergbom et al., 1999). For those who could not remember ICU, the diary seemed to fill in the lost time. This intervention needs formal evaluation to ensure that some patients are not made more distressed by reading a diary and seeing photographs of themselves in ICU.

Conclusion

Further research is needed to understand the processes behind the formation of delusional memories on ICU and to examine the impact of therapeutic interventions undertaken within the ICU, such as altering sedation practice, on later psychological health.

The growth of counselling services for patients diagnosed with cancer is in recognition of the psychological impact of severe illness. At present only about a third of ICUs in the UK follow up their patients in a dedicated clinic. The provision of counselling or psychology services specifically for this patient group is sparse. Psychological services for post-ICU patients are required so that each patient is appropriately assessed and given the necessary support. Physical recovery after critical illness is on the whole good, although it is a lengthy process. If psychological services are not available for some patients their optimal quality of life may never be achieved.

REFERENCES

Ambrosino, N., Bruletti, G., Scala, V., Porta, R. & Vitacca, M. (2002). Cognitive and perceived health status in patients with chronic obstructive pulmonary disease surviving acute on chronic respiratory failure: a controlled study. *Intensive Care Medicine*, **28**, 170–7.

Bäckmann, C. G. & Walther, S. M. (2001). Use of a personal diary written on the ICU during critical illness. *Intensive Care Medicine*, **27**, 426–9.

Bardellini, S., Servadio, G., Chiarello, M. & Chiarello, E. (1992). Sleep disorders in patients in recovery. Preliminary results in 20 patients. *Minerva Anestesiol*, **58**, 527–33.

Bergbom, I., Svensson, C., Berggren, E. & Kamsula, M. (1999). Patients' and relatives' opinions and feelings about diaries kept by nurse in an intensive care unit: pilot study. *Intensive and Critical Care Nursing*, **15**, 185–91.

Chlan, L. L. (2003). Description of anxiety levels by individual differences and clinical factors in patients receiving mechanical ventilatory support. *Heart Lung*, **32**, 275–82.

Dubois, M.-J., Bergeron, N., Dumont, M., Dial, S. & Skrobik, Y. (2001). Delirium in an intensive care unit: a study of risk factors. *Intensive Care Medicine*, **27**, 1297–304.

Ely, E. W., Gautam, S., Margolin, R. et al. (2001a). The impact of delirium in the intensive care unit on hospital length of stay. *Intensive Care Medicine*, **27**, 1892–900.

Ely, E. W., Margolin, R., Francis, J. et al. (2001b). Evaluation of delirium in critically ill patients: validation of the confusion assessment method for the intensive care unit (CAM-ICU). *Critical Care Medicine*, **29**, 1370–9.

Goldman, L. S. & Kimball, C. P. (1987). Depression in intensive care units. *International Journal of Psychiatry Medicine*, **17**, 201–12.

Hopkins, R. O., Weaver, L. K., Pope, D. et al. (1999). Neuropsychological sequelae and impaired health status in survivors of severe acute respiratory distress syndrome. *American Journal of Respiratory and Critical Care Medicine*, **160**, 50–6.

House, A., Mayou, R. & Mallinson, C. (1995). *Psychiatric aspects of physical disease*. London: Royal College of Physicians and Royal College of Psychiatrists.

Jackson, J. C., Hart, R. P. Gordon, S. M. et al. (2003). Six month neuropsychological outcome from medical intensive care unit patients. *Critical Care Medicine*, **31**, 1226–34.

Jacobi, J., Fraser, G. L., Coursin, D. B. et al. (2002). Clinical practice guidelines for the sustained use of sedatives and analgesics in the critically ill adult. *Critical Care Medicine*, **30**, 119–41.

Jones, C. & Griffiths, R. D. (2002). Physical and psychological recovery. In R. D. Griffiths & C. Jones (Eds.). *Intensive care after care* (pp. 53–6). Oxford, UK: Butterworth & Heinemann.

Jones, C., Griffiths, R. D. & Humphris, G. (2000). Disturbed memory and amnesia related to intensive care. *Memory*, **8**, 79–94.

Jones, C., Griffiths, R. D., Humphris, G. H. & Skirrow, P. M. (2001). Memory, delusions, and the development of acute posttraumatic stress disorder-related symptoms after intensive care. *Critical Care Medicine*, **29**, 573–80.

Jones, C., Skirrow, P., Griffiths, R. D. et al. (2003). Rehabilitation after critical illness: a randomised, controlled trial. *Critical Care Medicine*, **31**, 2456–61.

Jones, C., Skirrow, P., Griffiths, R. D. et al. (2004). Post traumatic stress disorder-related symptoms in relatives of patients following intensive care. *Intensive Care Medicine*, **30**, 456–60.

Kress, J. P., Gehlbach, B., Lacy, M. et al. (2003). The long-term psychological effects of daily sedative interruption on critically ill patients. *American Journal of Respiratory and Critical Care Medicine*, **168**, 1457–61.

McKinley, S., Nagy, S., Stein-Parbury, J., Bramwell, M. & Hudson, J. (2002). Vulnerability and security in seriously ill patients in intensive care. *Intensive and Critical Care Nursing*, **18**, 27–36.

Sharshar, T., Gray, F., Lorin de la Grandmaison, G. *et al.* (2003). Apoptosis of neurons in cardiovascular autonomic centres triggered by inducible nitric oxide synthase after death from septic shock. *Lancet*, **362**, 1799–805.

Shi, S. F., Munjas, B. A., Wan, T. T. *et al.* (2003). The effects of preparatory sensory information on ICU patients. *Journal of Medical Systems*, **27**, 191–204.

Tian, Z. M. & Reis Miranda, D. (1995). Quality of life after intensive care with the sickness impact profile. *Intensive Care Medicine*, **21**, 422–8.

Intimate examinations

Penelope Cream

Royal Free Hospital

Any medical examination that involves unusually close contact with a comparative stranger may be termed intimate. The degree of intimacy is subjective, and may depend on factors such as previous experience of similar medical contact, cultural and social norms and related life events, such as abuse or childbirth.

Examinations that are generally described as intimate include breast, pelvic, genital and rectal or anal examinations. However, procedures such as urodynamic investigations (Shaw *et al.*, 2000) and physiotherapy treatment can also prove intimate for many patients, as can undressing for any type of medical examination. Nearly every specialty within medicine and surgery involves intimate examination, and particularly primary care, sexual health, gynaecology and obstetrics, gastroenterology, emergency medicine, genito-urinary medicine and dermatology. Even the less classically intimate specialties, such as cardiology, involve procedures such as femoral artery catheterization through the groin that may be embarrassing to the patient.

Psychological impact of intimate examination

There are significant clinical implications of negative reactions to examination. Patients may be less likely to seek help or delay treatment for health problems or fail to attend screening, such as for mammography, cervical smears or colonoscopy (see 'Delay in seeking help'). Patients may feel unable to disclose the full extent of their concerns or difficulties. The level of self-efficacy (Bandura, 1977), in this case the ability to recognize and act on the need to seek medical care, that a patient holds is an important factor in determining compliance with intimate examination (see 'Self-efficacy and health behaviour'). This helps the patient to overcome instinctive psychological reactions to the procedure, such as embarrassment, fear and anxiety (Marshall, 1994). Patients' health beliefs can be influenced by their examination experiences and a traumatic experience when young could have a long-lasting impact on a patient's future help-seeking behaviour (Bodden-Heidrich *et al.*, 2000).

Factors that affect comfort during intimate examination

Both clinician and patient comfort are important: embarrassment and anxiety tend to be 'contagious'. If the clinician can contain the patient's emotions and concerns, the examination will progress more easily and will be less likely to deter attendance at future appointments. In turn, the awkward or nervous practitioner may make a previously unembarrassed patient feel uncomfortable and worried.

Patient factors

The patient may experience a range of reactions on attending for an intimate examination. These include individual variation in characteristics such as coping style, shame, embarrassment and fear. Other factors include feelings of vulnerability, awkwardness, humiliation and pain. These are more likely to be present if the patient has had a distressing experience in a previous intimate examination, has suffered sexual abuse or feels unable to communicate effectively with staff. Patients attending for a routine test that they have had many times before are likely to be less affected by the procedure than those admitted as an emergency or who cannot understand what is happening to them, for instance. In this case the level of perceived control is an effective indicator of psychological discomfort; the more control the patient feels he or she has over the situation, the lower the embarrassment and anxiety tend to be (e.g. Stattin *et al.*, 1991) (see also 'Perceived control').

Cultural or religious factors play a part in the patient's level of comfort during the intimate examination (Dean, 1998). It may not be appropriate for a male clinician to examine women from certain ethnic backgrounds, for instance, nor to have male chaperones, interpreters or other observers present. Equally, the female practitioner should be mindful of whether a male patient finds it unacceptable to be examined by a woman.

763

Clinician factors

P. Cream

Sensitive and effective communication is of the utmost importance, and may facilitate both the examination itself and subsequent disclosure of other matters, such as digestive or sexual difficulties (Berman *et al.*, 2003), body image problems, abuse and trauma experiences (Wijma *et al.*, 2003), treatment compliance issues and psychological conditions. A considerable number of patients attending gynaecological clinics, for example, have been found to have co-morbid psychological difficulties (Byrne, 1984) and practitioners carrying out intimate examinations are well placed to elicit further information and prompt referrals for additional problems.

Factors that have been found to relate directly to communication include gender congruency, trust in the clinician and the patient's level of perceived control over the situation. Communication and education about the procedure work most effectively when tailored to the individual patient's coping style: some people prefer more or less information before the procedure, depending on whether they are avoidant or active copers (Miller, 1987). If they are very anxious, extra time may be needed to explain what is happening because of the slowing of the ability to take in information when anxious or under stress (see also 'Healthcare professional–patient communication').

Characteristics of the clinician contribute to the ease of examination. Embarrassment, awkwardness and shame can touch both parties in an examination; the sensitive practitioner can benefit by being aware of his or her own reactions to the nervous or embarrassed patient, and decide in advance how to reassure and normalize distress. Good interpersonal skills can alleviate discomfort considerably (Hall *et al.*, 1994). A lack of confidence on the part of the doctor or nurse can lead to awkwardness or mistrust for the patient. Training issues may contribute to this lack of confidence. In many medical schools it is difficult to find sufficient examination opportunities to feel proficient, and doctors have reported avoiding carrying out breast (Desnick *et al.*, 1999) and rectal examinations (Lurie *et al.*, 1998) because of a fear of causing pain or embarrassment to the patient. A lack of skill in perceiving patients' attitudes and feelings towards pelvic examination may influence how and whether the procedure is carried out (Fiddes *et al.*, 2003). This reluctance can result in unnecessary referrals to specialists (Turner & Brewster, 2000). Pilot schemes using lay teaching associates are being tested in the UK, and have already been found to be successful in Scandinavia, North America and Australia in increasing trainees' skills and examination opportunities (Pickard *et al.*, 2003).

Although respect for the patient is of the utmost importance in all medical settings, intimate procedures require particular care in both interpersonal and environmental terms to help the patients feel that they are retaining as much dignity as possible. Guidelines exist in many settings to guide intimate examination procedures. In the UK, the Royal College of Obstetricians and Gynaecologists (1997), for instance, suggests that a clinician should never comment on the patient's body or functioning while performing the examination, while research on shame and dignity indicates that fears of how one's body appears to a doctor or nurse can contribute considerably to distress (Lazare, 1987).

Gender congruency effects have been found in the literature, although in certain populations these tend to be less important, such as with women who have had a child and who may have extensive experience of examination. Derose *et al.* (2001) found that women clinicians were perceived by both male and female patients as being more sensitive, more empathic and thought to possess better communication and technical skills than their male colleagues. However, patients who had had satisfactory examinations with a male clinician were happy to continue seeing a man and tended not to express a preference of practitioner gender when asked (Lodge *et al.*, 1997). The age of the patients has an effect on practitioner preference: young male patients undergoing genital examination in the US showed a strong preference towards having a female doctor (Van Ness & Lynch, 2000), while older patients tend to prefer a more senior doctor.

Some reports have shown that the position in which intimate examinations are carried out can influence patient comfort and reduce distress. Women's preference for either a supine or semi-sitting position has been found to be influenced by the gender of the examiner and previous experience of intimate examination, with semi-sitting position being linked to a reduction in anxiety with a male clinician. Women have been found to prefer a semi-sitting over supine position for pelvic examination if the clinician were male or if they were being examined for the first time (Seymore *et al.*, 1986). Research into male prostate rectal examinations has found that a variation in position can reduce pain associated with the examination but does not decrease embarrassment (Frank *et al.*, 2001).

The environment in which the examination is carried out is important in maintaining privacy and respect for the patient. Teaching environments need to be handled particularly sensitively, and consideration should be given to the effect of third parties, whether trainees, students, family members or chaperones. The majority of women in Webb and Opdahl's (1996) study indicated a preference for a chaperone if being examined by a male doctor; other studies have shown that female patients prefer to be alone with a female clinician. While the majority of patients prefer privacy when undressing, opinion is more divided on the necessity of a blanket or gown, although this depends on the nature of the procedure. Designs for new gowns for victims of sexual abuse have been trialled successfully, and have been found to reduce anxiety during the examination (Smith & Smith, 1999). One of the strongest factors in patient distress is a lack of privacy and a fear of or actual interruption during the examination, and this contributed considerably to dissatisfaction with the procedure.

Overall, the successful intimate examination or procedure depends on a combination of components: effective and empathic communication; privacy and mutual respect; dignity; and trust for both patient and clinician. These factors, together with clinical confidence and sensitivity, will help a potentially difficult and emotionally charged procedure to go smoothly, and facilitate help-seeking and screening behaviours in the future.

REFERENCES

Bandura, A. (1977). Self-efficacy: toward a unifying theory of behavior change. *Psychological Review*, **84**, 191–215.

Berman, L., Berman, J., Felder, S. *et al.* (2003). Seeking help for sexual function complaints: what gynecologists need to know about the female patient's experience. *Fertility and Sterility*, **79**, 572–6.

Bodden-Heidrich, R., Walter, S., Teutenberger, S. *et al.* (2000). What does a young girl experience in her first gynecological examination? Study on the relationship between anxiety and pain. *Journal of Pediatric and Adolescent Gynecology*, **13**, 139–42.

Byrne, P. (1984). Psychiatric morbidity in a gynaecology clinic: an epidemiological survey. *British Journal of Psychiatry*, **144**, 28–34.

Dean, J. (1998). Examination of patients with sexual problems. *British Medical Journal*, **317**, 1641–3.

Derose, K., Hays, R. D., McCaffrey, D. R. & Baker, D. W. (2001). Does physician gender affect satisfaction of men and women visiting the emergency department? *Journal of General Internal Medicine*, **16**, 218–26.

Desnick, L., Taplin, S., Taylor, V., Coole, D. & Urban, N. (1999). Clinical breast examination in primary care: perceptions and predictors among three specialties. *Journal of Women's Health*, **8**, 389–97.

Fiddes, P., Scott, A., Fletcher, J. & Glaiser, A. (2003). Attitudes towards pelvic examination and chaperones: a questionnaire survey of patients and providers. *Contraception*, **67**, 313–17.

Frank, J., Thomas, K., Oliver, S. *et al.* (2001). Couch or crouch? Examining the prostate: a randomized study comparing the knee-elbow and the left-lateral position. *BJU International*, **87**, 331–4.

Hall, J. A., Irish, J. T., Roter, D. L., Ehrlich, C. M. & Miller, L. H. (1994). Satisfaction, gender, and communication in medical visits. *Medical Care*, **32**, 1216–31.

Lazare, A. (1987). Shame and humiliation in the medical encounter. *Archives of International Medicine*, **147**, 1653–8.

Lodge, N., Mallett, J., Blake, P. & Fryatt, I. (1997). A study to ascertain gynaecological patients' perceived levels of embarrassment with physical and psychological care given by female and male nurses. *Journal of Advanced Nursing*, **25**, 893–907.

Lurie, N., Margolis, K., McGovern, P. G. & Mink, P. (1998). Physician self-report of comfort and skill in providing preventive care to patients of the opposite sex. *Archives of Family Medicine*, **7**, 134–7.

Marshall, G. (1994). A comparative study of re-attenders and non-re-attenders for second triennial national breast screening programme appointments. *Journal of Public Health Medicine*, **16**, 79–86.

Miller, S. (1987). Monitoring and blunting: validation of a questionnaire to assess styles of information seeking under threat. *Journal of Personality and Social Psychology*, **52**, 345–53.

Pickard, S., Baraitser, P., Rymer, J. & Piper, J. (2003). Can gynaecology teaching associates provide high quality effective training for medical students in the United Kingdom? Comparative study. *British Medical Journal*, **327**, 1389–92.

The Royal College of Obstetricians and Gynecologists (1997). *Intimate examinations: report of a working party.* London: RCOG Press.

Seymore, C., DuRant, R. H., Jay, M. S. *et al.* (1986). Influence of position during examination, and sex of examiner on

patient anxiety during pelvic examination. *Journal of Pediatrics*, **108**, 312–17.

Shaw, C., Williams, K., Assassa, P. R. & Jackson, C. (2000). Patient satisfaction with urodynamics: a qualitative study. *Journal of Advanced Nursing*, **32**, 1356–63.

Smith, M. S. & Smith, M. T. (1999). A stimulus control intervention in the gynecological exam with sexual abuse survivors. *Women's Health*, **30**, 39–51.

Stattin, H., Magnusson, D., Olah, A., Kassin, H. & Yadagiri-Reddy, N. (1991). Perception of threatening consequences of anxiety-provoking situations. *Anxiety Research*, **4**, 141–66.

Turner, K. J. & Brewster, S. F. (2000). Rectal examination and urethral catheterization by medical students and house officers: taught but not used. *BJU International*, **86**, 422–6.

Van Ness, C. J. & Lynch, D. A. (2000). Male adolescents and physician sex preference. *Archives of Pediatric and Adolescent Medicine*, **154**, 49–53.

Webb, R. & Opdahl, M. (1996). Breast and pelvic examinations: easing women's discomfort. *Canadian Family Physician*, **42**, 54–8.

Wijma, B., Schei, B., Swahnberg, K. *et al.* (2003). Emotional, physical, and sexual abuse in patients visiting gynaecology clinics: a Nordic cross-sectional study. *Lancet*, **361**, 2107–13.

Irritable bowel syndrome

Paul Bennett

University of Cardiff

Irritable bowel syndrome (IBS) is a disorder of the large bowel. There are number of diagnostic criteria for diagnosis of the condition, but the Rome criteria (Drossman, 1999) are perhaps the most often used. These state that the disorder involves three months of continuous or recurrent symptoms of abdominal pain or discomfort that is relieved by defecation and/or associated with a change in frequency of stool matter and/or associated with a change in consistency of stool. In addition, two or more of the following are present for at least three days a week: altered stool frequency; altered stool form; passage of mucous; and feelings of bloating or abdominal distension. These symptoms are relatively common, with estimates of the prevalence of IBS within the general population varying between 3 and 18%, with women being about twice as likely as men to experience IBS symptoms (e.g. Drossman *et al.*, 1993)

Early aetiological models suggested IBS was a primary psycho-physiological disorder. Latimer (1981) even suggested that its symptoms and aetiology are synonymous with those of anxiety, with symptom choice (anxiety or IBS) being determined by social learning. This strong theory is no longer tenable, and more support is given to a weaker 'stress' hypothesis, which suggests that IBS symptoms are multi-causal and can result from a variety of factors, including gut infection, food intolerance and stress (see 'Psychosomatics').

Linkages with stress

There is consistent evidence linking IBS to high levels of stress. Firstly, IBS patients have higher levels of co-morbidity with psychiatric conditions than among comparison groups. Walker *et al.* (1990), for example, found that 93% of IBS patients met the diagnostic criteria for at least one short-term psychiatric disorder. This compared with 19% of patients with inflammatory bowel disease. Secondly, IBS patients have higher levels of psychometrically measured stress than other populations. Schwarz *et al.* (1993), for example, reported IBS patients scored more highly than 'normal' controls on a variety of measures of depression and anxiety. Unfortunately, the dependence of these studies on patients who actively sought medical treatment for their symptoms renders interpretation of their findings difficult. Up to 80% of people with IBS do not consult a physician as a result of their symptoms. In addition, those who do visit their doctor more for other minor or vague symptoms than the average, and report higher levels of stress than non-attenders (e.g. Drossman *et al.*, 1988). Thus, the apparently high levels of psychological co-morbidity found among patients with IBS may be the result of studying people with high levels anxiety or depression who seek medical help more readily for relatively minor symptoms than people with lower levels of distress (see 'Symptom perception'). This process would inflate the apparent relationship between IBS and stress.

Despite this caveat, there is evidence to suggest that among IBS patient populations, levels of IBS activity do co-vary, to some extent, with levels of stress. Bennett *et al.* (1998) followed a cohort of 117 patients with IBS, and found that chronic life stress predicted 97% of symptom intensity between baseline and 16-month follow-up. No one exposed to even one chronic stressor improved clinically over the period of the study. All those who did improve, did so in the absence of such a stressor. Whitehead *et al.* (1992) reported another such study, examining the relationship between the occurrence of life events and IBS symptoms over a series of three-month periods in a group of 39 women. Changes in life events accounted for 10% of the variance in symptoms. In a third longitudinal study, Dancey *et al.* (1998) found that daily hassles contributed to increased symptoms up to two days following their occurrence.

Aetiology

Two pathways have been identified through which stress may influence the symptoms of IBS. The autonomic stress model of IBS

suggests that people with the condition respond to stressful events with high levels of gut motility as a result of either autonomic or enteric nervous system over-activity or the gut responds to similar levels of activity in a more vigorous manner than in people without the disorder. This may be compounded by decreased thresholds for pain and rectal sensations at times of stress (Murray *et al.*, 2004). Thus, people with IBS may have a gut that is highly responsive to stress, and from which there may be more sensations indicating a need to defecate, than other individuals. A second pathway may involve the onset of the disorder as a result of infection, for example, with the *Campylobacter* bacteria, with stress contributing to its maintenance. This may be the result of a stress-mediated inability to down-regulate the initial inflammatory stimulus efficiently (Barbara *et al.*, 2004) (see also 'Stress and health').

Stress is generally seen as external to the individual, but there is some evidence that some stress may be self-generated or be the result from past stressful experiences. Negative perfectionism may contribute to the symptoms. Somatic perceptions may also be cognitively exaggerated in some IBS patients, contributing to the perception of pain severity (Lackner *et al.*, 2004). Drossman *et al.* (1990) suggested that previous sexual or physical abuse may account for the high levels of distress among female patients with IBS. They found higher levels of pre-adolescent sexual and physical abuse among female patients with IBS disorders than among comparable female patients with organic gastrointestinal diseases. These findings, however, have not always been replicated (e.g. Hobbis *et al.*, 2002). Further, the theory does not explain the mechanisms through which such an association may be manifest.

Treating IBS

IBS may usefully be treated with drug medication including smooth muscle relaxants and bulking agents (see Poynard *et al.*, 2001). Dietary interventions involving supplementary dietary fibre may also be of value (Bijkerk *et al.*, 2004). However, here we focus on the impact of psychological interventions.

Perhaps the most widely used intervention to treat IBS involves the use of cognitive behaviour therapy, which seems to compare well with medical interventions (e.g. Bennett & Wilkson, 1985) (see 'Cognitive behaviour therapy'). In an interesting development of the potential interplay between medical and psychological treatments, Darnley *et al.* (2002) examined whether stress management could add to the effectiveness of medical treatment in non-responders to the initial intervention. All the people in her study were first given drug treatment. Those that continued to have IBS symptoms some six weeks later received either a stress management programme or continued on the drug regime, in the hope that additional time on the drug would improve their symptoms. Among the non-responders, patients in the cognitive behavioural programme fared best, reporting significant improvements in a variety of measures of IBS symptoms as well as reductions in measures of emotional distress. Data from Keefer *et al.* (2002), who found long-term reductions in abdominal pain, diarrhoea and bloating following instruction in meditation, suggests that even relatively simple interventions may be of benefit.

Although later studies have provided confirmatory evidence, the most substantial study of the effectiveness of psychotherapy remains that of Svedlund (1983). He evaluated the effectiveness of medication alone or in combination with an intervention comprising up to ten hours of sessions aimed at helping participants modify maladaptive behaviour, find new solutions to problems, and to cope more effectively with stress and emotional problems. In this, it appears very close to the cognitive–behavioural interventions previously described. At one-year follow-up, the combined treatment group maintained significantly greater improvements on a variety of measures of IBS symptoms, including pain and bowel dysfunction. Finally, Gonsalkorale et al. (2003) found 71% of IBS patients initially responded to hypnotherapy. Of these, 81% maintained their improvement over five years (see 'Hypnosis').

Conclusions

Although not all cases of IBS will be the result of stress, and some may result from a combination of stress and other insults to the gut, the role of stress in the aetiology of IBS is now well established, at least among the specific populations that attend medical clinics. Stress may influence gut motility, perceptions of gut activity and immunological changes in the gut that result in the initiation or maintenance of symptoms. It may also moderate emotional and cognitive responses to somatic sensations within the gut and rectum. People who do have stress-related IBS may benefit from a variety of interventions designed to moderate stress levels and change their cognitive content.

(See also 'Inflammatory bowel disease', 'Gastric and duodenal ulcers' and 'Cancer: digestive tract'.)

REFERENCES

Barbara, G., De Giorgio, R., Stanghellini, V. et al. (2004). New pathophysiological mechanisms in irritable bowel syndrome. *Alimentary Pharmacology & Therapeutics*, **20**(s2), 1–9.

Bennett, E. J., Tennant, C., Piesse, C., Badcock, C.-A. & Kellowab, J. E. (1998). Level of chronic life stress predicts clinical outcome in irritable bowel syndrome. *Gut*, **43**, 256–61.

Bennett, P. & Wilkinson, S. (1985). A comparison of psychological and medical treatment of the irritable bowel syndrome. *British Journal of Clinical Psychology*, **24**, 215–16.

Bijkerk, C. J., Muris, J. W., Knottnerus, J. A., Hoes, A. W. & de Wit, N. J. (2004). Systematic review: the role of different types of fibre in the treatment of irritable bowel syndrome. *Alimentary Pharmacology & Therapeutics*, **19**, 245–51.

Dancey, C. P., Taghavi, M. & Fox, R. J. (1998). The relationship between daily stress and symptoms of irritable bowel: a time-series approach. *Journal of Psychosomatic Research*, **44**, 537–45.

Darnley, S. E., Kennedy, T., Jones, R., Chalder, T. & Wessley, S. (2002). A randomised controlled trial of the addition of cognitive behavioural therapy (CBT) to antispasmodic therapy for irritable bowel syndrome (IBS) in primary care. *Gastroenterology*, **122**, A-69.

Drossman, D. A. (1999). The functional gastrointestinal disorders and the Rome II process. *Gut*, **45**(Suppl. 2), 1–5.

Drossman, D. A., Leserman, J., Nachman, G. et al. (1990). Sexual and physical abuse in women with functional or organic gastrointestinal disorders. *Annals of Internal Medicine*, **113**, 828–33.

Drossman, D. A., Leserman, J., Nachman, G., Li, Z., Zagami, E. A. & Patrick, D. L. (1998). Psychosocial factors in the irritable bowel syndrome. A multivariate study of patients and non-patients with irritable bowel syndrome. *Gastroenterology*, **95**, 701–8.

Drossman, D. A., Li, Z., Andruzzi, E. et al. (1993). U. S. householder survey of functional gastrointestinal disorders. Prevalence, sociodemography, and health impact. *Digestive Diseases and Science*, **38**, 1569–80.

Drossman, D. A., Sanders, R. S., McKee, D. C. & Lovitz, A. J. (1982). Bowel patterns among subjects not seeking medical care: use of a questionnaire to identify a population with bowel dysfunction. *Gastroenterology*, **83**, 529–34.

Gonsalkorale, W. M., Miller, V., Afzal, A. & Whorwell, P. J. (2003). Long term benefits of hypnotherapy for irritable bowel syndrome. *Gut*, **52**, 1623–9.

Hobbis, I. C., Turpin, G. & Read, N. W. (2002). A re-examination of the relationship between abuse experience and functional bowel disorders. *Scandinavian Journal of Gastroenterology*, **37**, 423–30.

Keefer, L. & Blanchard, E. B. (2002). A one year follow-up of relaxation response meditation as a treatment for irritable bowel syndrome. *Behaviour Research and Therapy*, **40**, 541–6.

Lackner, J. M., Quigley, B. M. & Blanchard, E. B. (2004). Depression and abdominal pain in IBS patients: the mediating role of catastrophizing. *Psychosomatic Medicine*, **66**, 435–41.

Latimer, P. (1981). Irritable bowel syndrome: a behavioral model. *Behaviour Research and Therapy*, **19**, 475–83.

Murray, C. D., Flynn, J., Ratcliffe, L. et al. (2004). Effect of acute physical and psychological stress on gut autonomic innervation in irritable bowel syndrome. *Gastroenterology*, **127**, 1695–703.

Poynard, T., Regimbeau, C. & Benhamou, Y. (2001). Meta-analysis of smooth muscle relaxants in the treatment of irritable bowel syndrome. *Alimentary Pharmacology & Therapeutics*, **15**, 355–61.

Schwarz, S. P., Blanchard, E. B., Berreman, C. F. et al. (1993). Psychological aspects of irritable bowel syndrome: comparisons with inflammatory bowel disease and nonpatients controls. *Behaviour Research and Therapy*, **31**, 297–304.

Svedlund, J. (1983). Psychotherapy in irritable bowel syndrome. A controlled outcome study. *Acta Psychiatrica Scandinavica* **306**(Suppl.), 1–86.

Walker, E. A., Roy-Byrne, P. P., Katon, W. J. et al. (1990). Psychiatric illness and irritable bowel syndrome: a comparison with inflammatory bowel disease. *American Journal of Psychiatry*, **147**, 1656–61.

Whitehead, W. E., Crowell, M. D., Robinson, J. C., Heller, B. R. & Schuster, M. M. (1992). Effects of stressful life events on bowel symptoms: subjects with irritable bowel syndrome compared with subjects without bowel dysfunction. *Gut*, **33**, 825–30.

Lymphoedema

Anne Williams

Napier University

Lymphoedema, the chronic accumulation of fluid in the interstitial tissues, is due to an insufficiency in the lymphatic system (British Lymphology Society, 2001). Most commonly, it involves one or more limb/s but an oedema of the trunk, head and neck or genitalia may also occur. Lymphoedema affects over 1.33 per 1000 of the population (Moffatt et al., 2003) and can have significant physical, psychosocial and economic implications. This chapter overviews relevant pathophysiology, outlines the causes of lymphoedema, explores the psychosocial impact and describes management strategies for lymphoedema.

Underlying pathophysiology

The lymphatic system is composed of a vast network of lymphatic vessels and over 700 lymph nodes, many of which are sited in regional groups at the neck, axillary and inguinal areas. The system transports excess fluid and proteins from the interstitial tissues to the blood circulation (Stanton, 2000) and also has an important immunological function. Networks of thin-walled lymphatic vessels lie in the dermis, supported by elastic fibres and anchoring filaments. Stimulated by local tissue movement, these lymphatics open, allowing fluid to pass into the system and drain via precollector and collector vessels through lymph nodes and into larger lymphatics, such as the thoracic duct, finally returning to the blood circulation (Földi & Földi, 2003). Lymph flow is influenced by contractions in the muscular wall of the collectors and ducts. Variations in local pressures due to pulsation of adjacent blood vessels and the skeletal muscle pump, along with changes in intra-thoracic and intra-abdominal pressures during breathing, also enhance lymph flow.

Table 1. Lymphoedema staging criteria

Stages of lymphoedema	Features of lymphoedema
Stage 0	Latent or sub-clinical stage that can exist for many years: impaired lymph transport occurs but swelling is not evident.
Stage 1	Excess volume is less than 20%; fluid accumulates but reduces with elevation.
Stage 2	Excess volume of 20–40%; initially skin is pitting but becomes non-pitting and swelling does not reduce on elevation.
Stage 3	Excess volume of >40%; non-pitting swelling with persistent skin and tissue changes.

International Society of Lymphologists (2003).

The accumulation of protein-rich fluid leads to increased limb volume, changes in limb shape, skin and tissue damage and inflammation. The epidermis becomes stretched and dry. Eventually, the tissues become hard, fibrotic and vulnerable to recurrent infection or cellulitis (Table 1). A positive Stemmer's sign (an inability to pinch the skin at the base of the second toe) is a differential diagnostic sign for lymphoedema.

Epidemiology

Primary lymphoedema is characterized by lymph vessel aplasia (absence), dysplasia (reduction) or other intrinsic abnormalities in lymph vessels or lymph nodes; it may also be associated with genetic abnormalities (Burnand & Mortimer, 2003). The prevalence of primary lymphoedema is unclear although it affects around 8–12% of all patients referred to specialist lymphoedema clinics (Williams et al., 1996; Sitzia et al., 1998; Cleave, 2002).

Secondary lymphoedema results from damage to the lymphatic system due to various cancer- or non-cancer-related changes. Recent studies indicate that up to 38% of women experience problems such as arm swelling and restricted arm movement following breast cancer (Engel et al., 2003; Querci della Rovere et al., 2003), despite the use of more conservative treatment approaches. Lymphoedema has also been reported in 41% of those treated for invasive cervical cancer (Werngren-Elgstrom & Lidman, 1994) with a 29% incidence following lymph node dissection for malignant melanoma (Serpell et al., 2003) (see chapters on 'Cancer').

Non-cancer-related causes of lymphoedema include trauma, limb dependency, chronic venous disease and infection. Oedema has been identified in 35% of those with leg ulceration (Moffatt et al., 2004). Lymphatic filariasis, a tropical disease spread by mosquitos and caused by infection with the organism Wuchereria bancrofti, a worm that enters the lymphatic system, is the most common cause of secondary lymphoedema worldwide but rarely seen in the developed world (Bernhard et al., 2003).

Psychosocial issues

The literature mainly focuses on breast cancer-related swelling. An early study of women with breast cancer-related lymphoedema reported greater psychological morbidity, impaired physical functioning and impaired adjustment to illness in those with lymphoedema as compared to a non-lymphoedema control group (Tobin et al., 1993). Woods (1993) also described altered sensations in women with breast cancer-related lymphoedema and suggested that levels of psychological distress were not directly related to severity of swelling. High levels of psychological, social, sexual and functional morbidity have been further identified in women with upper limb swelling, exacerbated by poor social support, pain and a passive and avoidant coping style (Passik & McDonald, 1998).

Johansson *et al.* (2003) interviewed 12 women with mild-to-moderate lymphoedema describing problem-focussed or emotion-focussed approaches to coping and highlighting their difficulties with the reactions of other people. Beaulac *et al.* (2002) used the FACT-B tool and identified lower scores in those with increased limb volume. Coster *et al.* (2001) have also described the validation of a quality of life scale based on the FACT-B questionnaire and incorporating additional questions pertaining to arm swelling.

Studies of other lymphoedema groups are limited. Ryan *et al.* (2006) studied 82 women with lower limb swelling related to gynaecological cancer, describing altered sensations in the swollen leg and identifying the impact on appearance, mobility and finances. A phenomenological study of people with various types of lymphoedema reported difficulties with self-image (Williams *et al.*, 2004) and highlighted the problems experienced by people with non-cancer-related lymphoedema in accessing treatment. In particular, it described their isolation, prolonged anxiety and feelings of depression due to misdiagnosis of the condition by health professionals.

The psychological morbidity of lymphoedema and its relationship with quality of life has not been adequately evaluated (Rietman *et al.*, 2003). The association between lymphoedema and other common physical symptoms such as pain, restricted movement and numbness and their influence on psychological distress also remains unclear. Problems with pain and discomfort in lower limb swelling have been reported (Sitzia & Sobrido, 1997; Moffatt *et al.*, 2003) but quality of life and psychological assessment tools for lymphoedema are inadequate (Sitzia & Sobrido, 1997; Poole & Fallowfield, 2002) and further validation of condition specific tools is required (see 'Quality of life' and 'Quality of life assessment').

Management strategies

Lymphoedema treatment aims to reduce swelling, improve limb shape, promote healthy skin and tissues and enhance quality of life. A comprehensive initial assessment is vital and provides the baseline for individualized treatment planning and long-term monitoring of this chronic condition. Detailed medical history and assessment is undertaken to include skin and tissue condition, physical difficulties, psychosocial and information needs and factors that may affect outcome. Limb circumferential measurements are used to calculate the volume of the limb and provide a comparison with the unaffected side in a unilateral oedema.

Of central importance is the need to maintain good skin condition and prevent complications through various measures:

- Keeping the skin supple and healthy with daily hygiene and moisturizing with bland emollients
- Avoiding any cuts, scratches, bites or burns; applying antiseptic if they occur and prescribing antibiotics to treat cellulitis
- Avoiding restrictive clothing, having blood pressure taken or injections on the affected limb

- Using the limb normally but avoiding heavy or repetitive activities that exacerbate swelling.

Treatment consists of a two-phased approach using a combination of treatment modalities. Phase one, often called intensive treatment or Decongestive Lymphatic Therapy (DLT), combines daily skin care, manual lymphatic drainage (MLD) massage, multi-layer lymphoedema bandaging (MLLB) and isotonic exercises over a 2–4 week period. A therapist (often a nurse or physiotherapist) provides the treatment, commonly as an outpatient.

Manual lymphatic drainage is a specialized massage following the Vodder, Földi, Casley-Smith or Leduc methods. It increases lymph drainage and enhances the uptake of proteins into the lymphatics, helping to establish collateral routes to redirect fluid to unaffected areas. It is specifically indicated for treating breast, genital and head and neck oedema.

Multi-layer lymphoedema bandaging is usually reapplied daily, after MLD, to reduce swelling and reshape the limb. The pressure from the bandages forces fluid towards the root of the limb. A stockinette lining and soft padding or foam are used to protect and reshape the limb prior to application of layers of short stretch bandages. The digits are often bandaged.

Phase two is a maintenance period of independent care and is suitable for those with those with mild lymphoedema or following intensive treatment. This requires a considerable degree of commitment and lifestyle adjustment, incorporating skincare, specific exercises, self-massage and the wearing of compression hosiery garments within the daily routine. Specialized lymphoedema compression garments are worn daily to prevent fluid accumulation and support the muscle pump. These should be measured and fitted by an experienced practitioner to ensure comfort and efficacy. Exercises are used to improve posture, develop muscle tone and enhance lymph drainage. Careful positioning of the limb and wearing of appropriate clothing and footwear are also important in optimizing mobility and function.

Treatments are modified depending on the severity of the lymphoedema, health and age of the patient. Additional problems such as recurrent cancer, cardiac or renal failure may complicate treatment outcome. Equally, care must be taken to ensure that quality of life is not unnecessarily compromised by the treatment regime.

Diuretics have limited use for lymphoedema and can lead to electrolyte imbalance in the long term. However, they may be used to treat co-existing conditions such as ascites or congestive cardiac failure (see 'Coronary heart disease: heart failure'). Intermittent compression pumps such as the *'flowtron'* should also be used with caution as they can produce a fibrotic band at the root of the limb and may increase the risk of genital oedema in people with lower limb swelling (Boris *et al.*, 1995).

Evidence base

The evidence base for lymphoedema treatment is developing. A randomized controlled trial of 83 patients with chronic limb oedema showed that 18 days of bandaging followed by hosiery achieved a significantly greater effect on limb volume than hosiery alone (Badger *et al.*, 2000). Manual lymphatic drainage has also resulted in significant changes in limb volume and some quality of life domains, as measured by the EORTC QLQ-C30, in women with breast cancer-related lymphoedema (Williams *et al.*, 2002).

Other authors have reported significant improvements in quality of life following treatment (Mirolo *et al.*, 1995; Weiss & Spray, 2002; Mondry *et al.*, 2004) although further work is required to explore the efficacy and cost effectiveness of lymphoedema treatment in different groups.

Conclusion

Lymphoedema is an under-recognized condition that requires long-term intervention but can be successfully controlled. Assessment of quality of life and psychological changes is important in identifying those requiring additional support or referral, although valid and reliable tools are lacking. Individuals should be assessed by practitioners with appropriate knowledge and skills and may require referral for specialist lymphoedema treatment.

REFERENCES

Badger, C. M. A., Peacock, J. L. & Mortimer, P. S. (2000). A randomised, controlled, parallel-group clinical trial comparing multi-layer bandaging followed by hosiery versus hosiery alone in the treatment of patients with lymphoedema of the limb. *Cancer*, **88**, 2832–7.

Bealac, S. M., McNair, L. A., Scott, T. E., LaMorte, W. W. & Kavanah, M. T. (2002). Lymphedema and quality of life in survivors of early-stage breast cancer. *Archieves of Surgery*, **137**, 1253–7.

Bernhard, L., Bernhard, P. & Magnussen, P. (2003). Management of patients with lymphedema caused by filariasis in north-eastern Tanzania. *Physiotherapy*, **89**, 743–9.

Boris, M., Weindorf, S. & Lasinski, B. B. (1998). The risk of genital edema after external pump compression for lower limb lymphedema. *Lymphology*, **31**, 15–20.

British Lymphology Society (2001). *Clinical definitions*. Caterham, UK: British Lymphology Society.

Burnand, K. G. & Mortimer, P. S. (2003). Lymphangiogenesis and the genetics of lymphoedema. In N. Browse, K. G. Burnand & P. S. Mortimer (Eds.). (Chapter 5). *Diseases of the lymphatics*. London: Arnold.

Cleave, N. (2002). *Meeting the need in a defined population*. Presentation to the British Lymphology Society Conference, Milton Keynes.

Coster, S., Poole, K. & Fallowfield, L. J. (2001). The validation of a quality of life scale to assess the impact of arm morbidity in breast cancer patients post-operatively. *Breast Cancer Research and Treatment*, **68**, 273–82.

Engel, J., Kerr, J., Schlesinger-Raab, A., Sauer, H. & Holzel, D. (2003). Axilla surgery severely affects quality of life: results of a 5-year prospective study in breast cancer patients. *Breast Cancer Research and Treatment*, **79**, 47–57.

Földi, M. & Földi, E. (2003). Physiology and pathophysiology of the lymphatic system. In M. Földi, E. Földi & S. Kubik (Eds.).

Textbook of lymphology for physicians and lymphedema therapists. Munich, Amsterdam and New York: Urban and Fischer, Elsevier.

International Society of Lymphology (2003). The diagnosis and treatment of peripheral lymphedema. Consensus document of the international society of lymphology. *Lymphology*, **36**, 84–91.

Johansson, K., Holström, H., Nilsson, I. *et al.* (2003). Breast cancer patients' experiences of lymphoedema. *Scandinavian Journal of Caring Sciences*, **17**, 35–42.

Mirolo, B. R., Bunce, I. H., Chapman, M. *et al.* (1995). Psychosocial benefits of postmastectomy lymphoedema therapy. *Cancer Nursing*, **18**, 197–205.

Moffatt, C. J., Franks, P. J., Doherty, D. C. *et al.* (2003). Lymphoedema: an underestimated health problem. *Quarterly Journal of Medicine*, **96**, 731–8.

Moffatt, C. J., Franks, P. J., Doherty, D. C. *et al.* (2004). Prevalence of leg ulceration in a London population. *Quarterly Journal of Medicine*, **97**, 431–7.

Mondry, T. E., Riffenburgh, R. H. & Johnstone, P. A. (2004). Prospective trial of complete decogesative therapy for upper extremity lymphedema after breast cancer therapy. *Cancer Journal*, **10**, 42–8.

Passik, S. D. & McDonald, M. V. (1998). Psychosocial aspects of upper extremity lymphedema in women treated for breast carcinoma. *Cancer*, **83**, 2817–20.

Poole, K. & Fallowfield, L. J. (2002). The psychological impact of post-operataive arm morbidity following axillary surgery for breast cancer: a critical review. *The Breast*, **11**, 81–7.

Querci della Rovere, R. G., Ahmad, I., Singh, P. *et al.* (2003). An audit of the incidence of arm lymphoedema after prophylactic level I/II axillary dissection without division of the pectoralis minor muscle. *Annals of the Royal College of Surgeons of England*, **85**, 158–61.

Reitman, J. S., Dijkstra, P. U., Hoekstra, H. J. *et al.* (2003). Late morbidity after treatment of breast cancer in relation to activities and quality of life: a systematic

review. *European Journal of Surgical Oncology*, **29**, 229–38.

Ryan, M., Stainton, M. C., Jaconelli, C. *et al.* (2003). The experience of lower limb lymphoedema for women after treatment for gynaecologic cancer. *Oncology Nursing Forum*, **30**, 417–23.

Serpell, J. W., Carne, P. W. & Bailey, M. (2003). Radical lymph node dissection for melanoma. *ANZ Journal of Surgery*, **73**, 294–9.

Sitzia, J., Woods, M., Hine, P. *et al.* (1998). Characteristics of new referrals to twenty-seven lymphoedema treatment units. *European Journal of Cancer Care*, **7**, 255–62.

Sitzia, J. & Sobrido, L. (1997). Measurement of health-related quality of life of patients receiving conservative treatment for limb lymphoedema using the Nottingham Health Profile. *Quality of Life Research*, **6**, 373–84.

Stanton, A. (2000). How does tissue swelling occur? The physiology and pathophysiology of interstitial fluid formation. In R. Twycross, K. Jenns & J. Todd (Eds.). *Lymphoedema* (Chapter 2). Oxford, UK: Radcliffe Medical Press.

Tobin, M. B., Lacey, H. J., Meyer, L. & Mortimer, P. S. (1993). The psychological morbidity of breast-cancer-related swelling. *Cancer*, **72**, 3248–52.

Weiss, J. M. & Spray, B. J. (2002). The effect of complete decongestive therapy on the quality of life of patient with peripheral lymphedema. *Lymphology*, **35**, 46–58.

Werngren-Elgstrom, M. & Lidman, D. (1994). Lymphoedema of the lower extremities after surgery and radiotherapy for cancer of the cervix. *Scandinavian Journal of Plastic Reconstructive Surgery and Hand Surgery*, **28**, 289–93.

Williams, A. E., Bergel, S. & Twycross, R. G. (1996). A 5-year review of a lymphoedema service. *European Journal of Cancer Care*, **5**, 56–9.

Williams, A. F., Vadgama, A., Franks, P. J. & Mortimer, P. S. (2002). A randomized controlled crossover study of manual lymphatic drainage therapy in women with breast cancer-related lymphoedema.

European Journal of Cancer Care, **11**, 154–261.

Williams, A. F., Moffatt, C. J. & Franks, P. J. (2004). A phenomenological study of the lived experiences of people with lymphoedema. *International Journal of Palliative Nursing*, **10**, 279–86.

Woods, M. (1993). Patients perceptions of breast cancer-related lymphoedema. *European Journal of Cancer Care*, **2**, 125–8.

Malaria

Julie A. Carter

University College London and Kenya Medical Research Institute/Wellcome Trust Research Laboratories

Malaria is defined as an acute febrile illness with parasitaemia (presence of parasites in the blood), although this may not be detectable, depending upon local capability for parasitologic confirmation. Four species of protozoal plasmodia: *Plasmodium falciparum*; *P. vivax*; *P. ovale*; and *P. malariae* can cause human malaria, transmitted by the female *Anopheles* mosquito when biting for a blood meal. The clinical features of uncomplicated malaria, i.e. fever, diarrhoea, headache, generalized aching and vomiting are non-specific and describe the symptoms of a variety of febrile illnesses prevalent in malaria-endemic areas.

Overview

Over 40% of the world's population from more than 90 countries lives with the risk of malaria. The World Health Organization (WHO) estimates that there are over 300 million clinical cases of malaria each year, resulting in the deaths of over 1 million people, 90% of whom are children under 5 years in sub-Saharan Africa. An estimated 3 million children are admitted to hospital with malaria each year in endemic regions of sub-Saharan Africa, although this represents only a minority of clinical cases, as more than 80% of patients have no contact with formal health services. Many deaths from malaria occur at home, making the establishment of reliable health statistics difficult.

In endemic areas, almost every child is infected with the malaria parasite but most carry it asymptomatically. Approximately 1–2% of clinical infections result in severe disease, which is characterized by the presence of life-threatening complications, operationally defined as any malaria syndrome associated with high mortality (>5%) despite appropriate hospital treatment (Newton & Krishna, 1998). The majority of severe disease and mortality is due to *P. falciparum*. Cerebral malaria (CM) is the most severe complication of the disease, presenting as a diffuse encephalopathy. Alterations in level of consciousness, ranging from drowsiness to deep coma, are often precipitated by seizures, which are reported in the histories of 50–80% of children (Molyneux *et al.*, 1989).

The morbid consequences of malaria have, until recently, been overlooked in the face of high mortality rates and the limited means of detecting such problems in many less developed countries. Children surviving severe falciparum malaria were traditionally considered to make a full recovery. However, research in the past two decades has indicated that severe malaria is associated with persisting neurological and cognitive impairments in survivors. CM is the defined end of the spectrum of severe malaria: clinically discrete and comparatively easy to identify, it has been the subject of most studies, with up to 24% of African children surviving the disease reported to have neurological and/or cognitive deficits (Carter *et al.*, 2005a). Estimates of the prevalence of impairments have varied according to the definition of the disease, length of follow-up and nature of the assessment techniques. However, the data consistently suggest persisting impairments in a proportion of childhood survivors of CM.

The burden of severe disease is borne by children, so the majority of studies investigating neurological and cognitive impairments have involved this population group. Adults living in endemic areas with exposure to repeated malaria infections since birth generally attain a degree of immunity from severe disease. Conversely, travellers from non-endemic areas are highly susceptible to malaria: if the disease is contracted, the outcome depends on factors such as chemoprophylaxis (drugs taken to prevent malaria), exposure to mosquito bites and the genotype (genetic constitution) of the individual. The few studies involving adult survivors of severe malaria have reported that the risk of long-term neurological or cognitive impairment is minimal (Dugbartey *et al.*, 1998), although a study of Vietnam veterans reported some neuropsychological deficits (Richardson *et al.*, 1997).

Research evidence and clinical implications

Early studies

The first studies investigating impairments associated with CM generally used neurological discharge examinations to detect deficits up to 18 months after the acute episode. In consequence, they tended to identify gross deficits, most commonly, ataxia, paresis, cortical blindness and severe speech and language deficits (Bondi, 1992; Brewster *et al.*, 1990; Carme *et al.*, 1993; Meremikwu *et al.*, 1997; Molyneux *et al.*, 1989; van Hensbroek *et al.*, 1997). Children with severe neurological impairments such as spastic tetraparesis or vegetative states often die at home within months of discharge, thus do not present at follow-up (Newton *et al.*, 2000).

Impairments generally fall into two categories; transient and persisting. For example, ataxia is commonly reported at discharge but usually resolves rapidly. Cortical blindness and hemiparesis often improve within the first six months but may not completely resolve (see 'Blindness and visual disability'). Speech and language deficits are reported to be among the most commonly occurring impairments and may present as complete mutism at first, usually improving over time (Bondi, 1992; Brewster *et al.*, 1990). Neurological disorders such as epilepsy may develop after discharge (see 'Epilepsy'). A recent study reported that more than 9% of children assessed up to 9 years after recovery from CM had epilepsy (Carter *et al.*, 2004).

Risk factors

Neurological impairment following CM has been associated with prolonged or focal seizures (Bondi, 1992; Brewster *et al.*, 1990; Meremikwu *et al.*, 1997; van Hensbroek *et al.*, 1997); deep coma (van Hensbroek *et al.*, 1997); prolonged coma (Bondi, 1992; Brewster *et al.*, 1990; Meremikwu *et al.*, 1997; van Hensbroek *et al.*, 1997); raised intracranial pressure (Newton *et al.*, 1997); hypoglycaemia (Bondi, 1992; Brewster *et al.*, 1990) and severe anaemia (Brewster *et al.*, 1990), although the latter finding has not been replicated in other studies (Bondi, 1992). van Hensbroek and colleagues (1997) found that hypoglycaemia and lactic acidosis, strong predictors of fatality, were not independently predictive of neurological impairment. Depth and length of coma and multiple convulsions were the only independent risk factors for subsequent neurological deficits, suggesting that morbidity and mortality may not share a common pathologic pathway.

Studies of persisting impairments

By developing more detailed, culturally-appropriate assessment tools, researchers have started to investigate the prevalence of persisting or subtle impairments in the past decade, often concentrating on neuropsychological functioning (see 'Neuropsychological assessment'). Muntendam and colleagues (1996), in one of the earliest studies of this type, found no impairments in 36 Gambian children assessed an average of 3 years after hospitalization, except in the balance task of a sensory–motor development test. In a larger case control series, Holding and colleagues (1999) administered a detailed battery of cognitive and behavioural assessments, adapted from the Kaufman Assessment Battery for Children (K-ABC), and a brief language assessment to Kenyan children with a history of severe malaria with impaired consciousness. They found a significant sub-group (14%) with impairments in cognitive functions, language and behaviour. Group differences were found on measures of attention, syntax, articulation and behaviour, suggestive of possible impairments in higher order (executive) functions. Boivin (2002) also administered an adapted version of the K-ABC to 29 Senegalese children and matched controls but reported contrasting results, with group differences in performance on aspects of sequential and simultaneous processing, non-verbal performance and attentional capacity.

Carter and colleagues recruited a large, unselected group of Kenyan children with a history of CM and administered a broad spectrum of developmental assessments up to 9 years after the initial insult. These children performed significantly poorer than children unexposed to severe malaria on measures of vocabulary, pragmatics, higher level language and non-verbal functioning (Carter *et al.*, 2005*b*). The presence of long-term epilepsy significantly increased the risk of problems in language, memory, attention, behaviour and motor skills. This study also suggested the existence of a group of children with particularly poor performance on assessments in which there was average group performance. Twenty-four per cent of children with previous CM had impaired cognition, behaviour, motor skills, hearing or vision, in comparison with 10% of the unexposed group (Carter *et al.*, 2005*a*).

Academic performance may be affected by repeated episodes of *P. falciparum* or *P. vivax*, particularly mathematical and language performance (Fernando *et al.*, 2003). Language deficits may cause particular difficulties at school, as much of what is taught is encoded in literate language and most basic academic skills are conveyed through verbal expression. Carter and colleagues concluded that the level of performance shown by children in their study suggested that they would have difficulties in an educational environment without specific support (Carter *et al.*, 2005*a*), although such support is rarely available in rural Africa. In addition, difficulties may only become apparent as children progress and face more complex cognitive and linguistic demands, both socially and educationally, raising the possibility that the number of children with problems may increase over time.

Impairments associated with other manifestations of falciperum malaria

Falciparum malaria produces a range of other neurological manifestations, such as multiple, prolonged or focal seizures with rapid recovery of consciousness after the seizure, which are more common than CM. Despite this, the prevalence and characteristics of acquired neurological impairment following such manifestations have received little attention. Children with a history of severe malaria with complicated seizures (either prolonged, repetitive or focal) have been found to have significantly reduced performance on measures of phonology, pragmatics and behaviour relative to children unexposed to severe malaria (Carter *et al.*, 2005*b*). Twenty-four per cent of children surviving severe malaria and complicated seizures are reported to have a neurological or cognitive impairment (Carter *et al.*, 2005*a*). These results suggest that severe malaria with complicated seizures may be associated with a different pattern of deficits than CM, yet may still cause problems for children, particularly in the educational environment.

Healthcare workers and educators working with children with neurological or cognitive impairments associated with any form of severe malaria should consider the other challenges these children may face, including stigma and reduced opportunities in education, marriage and employment (Kisanji, 1995) (see 'Children's perceptions of illness and death' and 'Stigma'). The negative consequences of impairments may also extend to the child's family, who rely on each family member for help in the home: for example, in most African homes, girls cook, clean the house and look after younger siblings as early as 7 to 8 years of age. On the other hand, Kisanji (1995) argues that children with impairments and their families experience fewer problems in less developed compared to more developed countries, particularly in the extended family situation in which responsibility for care can be shared amongst family members.

Conclusions

The pattern emerging from research on neurological and cognitive impairments associated with severe malaria is of a problem affecting many more children than initially realized. Evidence of persisting deficits following CM and impairments associated with other neurological manifestations of severe malaria suggest a major public health problem in terms of education and development in malaria-endemic areas.

Child health and survival is considered to be the most important public health issue in less developed countries. However, the WHO reports that malaria constitutes 10% of Africa's overall disease burden. While the burden of malaria continues to be so high, the number of children with neurological or cognitive deficits associated with the disease will remain a significant (although perhaps under-recognized) problem. Recent research emphasizes the importance of identifying children at risk of impairment following malaria and making provision for follow-up after the disease. The search for effective and affordable interventions in the acute phase of malaria and primary prevention clearly remain high priorities.

REFERENCES

Boivin, M. J. (2002). Effects of early cerebral malaria on cognitive ability in Senegalese children. *Journal of Developmental and Behavioral Pediatrics*, **23**(5), 353–64.

Bondi, F. S. (1992). The incidence and outcome of neurological abnormalities in childhood cerebral malaria: a long-term follow-up of 62 survivors. *Transactions of the Royal Society of Tropical Medicine and Hygiene*, **86**, 17–19.

Brewster, D. R. Kwiatkowski, D. & White, N. J. (1990). Neurological sequelae of cerebral malaria in children. *Lancet*, **336**, 1039–43.

Carme, B., Bouquety, J. C. & Plassart, H. (1993). Mortality and sequelae due to cerebral malaria in African children in Brazzaville, Congo. *American Journal of Tropical Medicine and Hygiene*, **48**, 216–21.

Carter, J. A., Mung'ala-Odera, V., Neville, B. G. R. et al. (2005a). Persistent neuro-cognitive impairments associated with severe falciparum malaria in Kenyan children. *Journal of Neurology Neurosurgery and Psychiatry*, **76**, 476–81.

Carter, J. A., Neville, B. G. R., White, S. et al. (2004). Increased prevalence of epilepsy associated with severe falciparum malaria in children. *Epilepsia*, **45**(8), 978–81.

Carter, J. A., Ross, A. J., Neville, B. G. R. et al. (2005b). Developmental impairments following severe falciparum malaria in

children. *Tropical Medicine and International Health*, **10**, 3–10.

Dugbartey, A. T., Dugbartey, M. T. & Apendo, M. Y. (1998). Delayed neuropsychiatric effects of malaria in Ghana. *Journal of Nervous and Mental Disease*, **186**(3), 183–6.

Fernando, S. D., Gunawardena, D. M., Bandara, M. R. S. S. et al. (2003). The impact of repeated malaria attacks on the school performance of children. *American Journal of Tropical Medicine and Hygiene*, **69**, 582–8.

Holding, P. A., Stevenson, J., Peshu, N. & Marsh, K. (1999). Cognitive sequelae of severe malaria with impaired consciousness. *Transactions of the Royal Society of Tropical Medicine and Hygiene*, **93**, 529–34.

Kisanji, J. (1995). Growing up disabled. In P. Zinkin & H. McConachie (Eds.). *Disabled children and developing countries*, London: MacKeith Press.

Meremikwu, M. M., Asindi, A. A. & Ezedinachi, E. (1997). The pattern of neurological sequelae of childhood cerebral malaria among survivors in Calabar, Nigeria. *Central African Journal of Medicine*, **43**, 231–4.

Molyneux, M. E., Taylor, T. E., Wirima, J. J. & Borgstein, A. (1989). Clinical features and prognostic indicators in paediatric cerebral malaria: a study of 131 comatose Malawian

children. *Quarterly Journal of Medicine*, **71**, 441–59.

Muntendam, A. H., Jaffar, S., Bleichrodt, N. & van Hensbroek, M. B. (1996). Absence of neuropsychological sequelae following cerebral malaria in Gambian children. *Transactions of the Royal Society of Tropical Medicine and Hygiene*, **90**, 391–4.

Newton, C. R., Crawley, J., Sowumni, A. et al. (1997). Intracranial hypertension in Africans with cerebral malaria. *Archives of Disease in Childhood*, **76**, 219–26.

Newton, C. R., Hien, T. T. & White, N. (2000). Cerebral malaria. *Journal of Neurology Neurosurgery and Psychiatry*, **69**, 433–41.

Newton, C. R. & Krishna, S. (1998). Severe falciparum malaria in children: current understanding of pathophysiology and supportive treatment. *Pharmacology and Therapeutics*, **79**, 1–53.

Richardson, E. D., Varney, N. R., Roberts, R. J., Springer, J. K. & Woods, P. S. (1997). Long-term cognitive sequelae of cerebral malaria in Vietnam veterans. *Applied Neuropsychology*, **4**, 238–43.

van Hensbroek, M. B., Palmer, A., Jaffar, S., Schneider, G. & Kwiatkowski, D. (1997). Residual neurologic sequelae after childhood cerebral malaria. *Journal of Pediatrics*, **131**, 125–9.

Mastalgia (breast pain)

Antonio V. Millet[1] and Frederick M. Dirbas[2]†

[1]Valencia School of Medicine
[2]†Stanford University

Introduction

Most women consider premenstrual mild cyclic breast pain (mastalgia) lasting for one to four days as normal. For some, however, mastalgia can be moderate-to-severe and last over five days each month, causing a great discomfort. Women with mastalgia are generally reluctant to consult medical personnel and those who do will often report recent quantitative or qualitative increases in their pain (Dixon, 1999). Because of increased awareness of breast cancer, more women than ever before are seeking professional advice (Klimberg, 1998) (see also 'Cancer: breast'). Subjective by nature, mastalgia is difficult to quantify and, at present, few physicians adopt a systematic diagnostic approach. Available treatments are few and limited by low efficacy and multiple side effects.

Prevalence and classification

Mastalgia is the most common breast complaint for which women consult their healthcare providers: up to 70% of women under 55 years old experience it (Arona, 1998; Dixon, 1999). Many patients with mastalgia consult once (36%) or more (5%) (Ader & Shriver, 1997). Neither marital status, household income, education, nor race appears to influence these rates (Ader et al., 2001). Breast pain is usually classified as cyclical mastalgia (CM) and non-cyclical mastalgia (NCM). CM occurs in a predictable pattern, often premenstrually, while NCM is described as a constant or intermittent breast pain with no relationship to menstruation. Chest wall pain accounts for 7% of the consulting women.

Natural history and impact on daily activities

Both CM and NCM run a chronic relapsing course: persistence over a decade is not infrequent (Davies et al., 1998). Severe mastalgia accounts for important costs and interferes with sexual activity (48% of the patients), physical activity (36%), social activity (13%) and working/school activity (6%) (Ader & Browne, 1997; Ader & Shriver, 1997). Some patients with CM engage in some form of non-harmful self-medication (e.g. vitamin supplements) and others initiate self-treatments that may be associated with serious adverse effects such as dieting, using over-the-counter medication, diuretics (Ader & Browne, 1997). A higher use of mammography among women under 35 years with mastalgia has been reported (Ader & Browne, 1997; Ader & Shriver, 1997; Ader et al., 2001).

Associated health and behavioural factors

Mastalgia has been associated with smoking, caffeine intake, low levels of physical activity and perceived stress although some of these associations are controversial (Ader et al., 2001). However, nutrition and alcohol consumption are not associated with mastalgia (Ader et al., 2001). Although CM is a well known component of premenstrual syndrome (PMS), over 80% of women with CM do not meet criteria for PMS in either retrospective (Ader et al., 1997) or prospective studies (Ader et al., 1999) (see 'Premenstrual syndrome'). Oral contraceptives have been found in some studies to decrease moderate-to-severe CM (RR 0,45) and somatic symptoms of PMS (Ader et al., 2001; Unruh, 1996).

Attitudes of healthcare providers towards mastalgia

Healthcare providers consulted are commonly gynaecologists (72%), family physicians (10%) and nurses (10%). Responses to questions about pain are not associated with the specialty of healthcare providers (Ader & Browne, 1997). In general, when faced with chronic pain for which they are unable to identify any organic origin physicians tend to conclude that the pain is psychogenic, especially when patients are female (Unruh, 1996) (see 'Psychosomatics'). Common responses are that CM is 'normal' (58%) and due to 'fibrocystic changes' (14%) or 'hormone disturbances' (4%). Less than 10% of providers ordered tests, referred the patient to a breast clinic, advised breast self-examination, suggested avoiding caffeine (4%) or prescribed treatment (4%) (Ader et al., 2001) (see also 'Attitudes of health professionals').

Risk of subclinical cancer

No increased risk of breast cancer has been clearly associated with mastalgia so far (Klimberg, 1998). Cancer has to be considered seriously in any patient with unilateral, localized and persistent mastalgia (Klimberg, 1998).

Mastalgia aetiology

Mastalgia is poorly understood and we can only speculate on its causes.

Histological abnormality

Most of the patients with mastalgia have also breast nodularity and tenderness. There is, however, no relationship between histology and symptoms and it is now accepted that fibrocystic changes are associated with normal breast involution.

Hormonal

Hormonal cause of CM is suggested by its natural history and it has been noted that women with CM are more likely to be premenopausal, nulliparous or be very young when they have their first baby. However, hormone levels are similar in women with and without mastalgia. An increased sensitivity to normal levels of hormones might account for CM but this hypothesis has not been proved.

Other physiological explanations

Mastalgia has been related to an upward shift in the circadian PRL profile, an increased PRL response to TRH and anti-dopaminergic drugs and to a loss of seasonal variations. In addition, there is some evidence suggesting that women with mastalgia have increased levels of saturated fatty acids and reduced proportions of essential fatty acids.

Neurosis

Recent studies have shown increased anxiety and depression among mastalgia patients compared to controls. In addition, women with severe breast pain have had a greater incidence of significant life events than women without severe mastalgia (Colegrave et al., 2001). However, the data is cross-sectional so it is likely that emotional distress is a result of mastalgia rather than a cause. Somatic and emotional distress in patients with mastalgia is likely to influence the care they need (Colegrave et al., 2001). Some people are unlikely to be helped unless their anxiety and fears (about breast cancer and others) are addressed (Colegrave et al., 2001). In states of acute stress, prolactin release may form a physiological basis for mastalgia.

Management

History-taking and pain characterization

Any woman who presents with mastalgia should undergo a careful history-taking (enabling the physician to classify mastalgia) and a thorough physical examination. Prospective daily recording of pain characteristics for at least 2 months using scales such as the Cardiff Breast Pain Chart, or other visual analogue scales, provides the physician with very accurate data (Dixon, 1999; Klimberg, 1998; Ader et al., 1999; Tavaf-Motamen et al., 1998); 20% of the patients will find spontaneous remission of mastalgia (Ader, 2001). Although over-used in women with mastalgia, mammography should be considered in some patients (Ader & Browne, 1997; Ader & Shriver, 1997; Ader et al., 1999; Dujim et al., 1998; Goodwin et al., 1997; Royal College of Physicians, 1998). After completion of history-taking and PE/imaging, most patients can be reassured and only a few will require any other treatment (Barros et al., 1999).

Lifestyle measures and dietary changes

Numerous lifestyle interventions have been proposed to relieve breast pain. Results must be interpreted with caution due to high rate of responses to placebo (20%) (Khanna et al., 1997) (see 'Placebos').

For women who exercise vigorously, a well-fitting support bra can provide substantial pain relief (Abdel Hadi, 2000). Sedentary life has been reported in up to 80% of women with mastalgia: for them, increasing exercise levels may improve pain via release of endorphins (see 'Physical activity interventions').

The association between methylxanthine consumption (coffee, tea, chocolate, cola beverages) and mastalgia is controversial and results of methylxanthines avoidance are controversial (Goodwin et al., 1997) but given the well-known health benefits of caffeine avoidance, a methylxanthine-restricted diet may be recommended.

Evening Primrose Oil (EPO) is rich in gamma-linolenic acid (GLA), a precursor of prostaglandin E1. It is a well tolerated and effective treatment of mastalgia, although mechanism of action is unknown (Goodwin et al., 1997). Long courses (over 4 months) are recommended by most authors. EPO is considered the first-line treatment in young, potentially long-term, patients with milder symptoms as well as in those who desire pregnancy, who choose to continue using oral contraceptives (OC) or who want to avoid hormonal therapies (see also 'Complementary medicine').

Endocrine therapy

Bromocriptine, danazol and tamoxifen have been shown to be effective in treating cyclical mastalgia (Ader, 2001). With and unknown mechanism of action, Danazol is currently the only medication approved by the United States. FDA for this indication. Low-dose regimens are recommended to minimize side effects. Unfortunately, relapse rates after termination of treatment are high (about 70%). It is not recommended as a first-line drug and should be reserved for patients whose pain is strongly affecting their lifestyle.

Use of tamoxifen (10 mg/day) is currently limited, under close supervision, to patients with severe symptoms and in whom all standard first-line therapies have failed. Success rates of tamoxifen in treatment of CM are around 80–90% (GEMB Group, 1997; Kontostolis et al., 1997). Bromocriptine is used as a second line therapy when danazol is not tolerated; response rates to bromocriptine are about 50–65%.

Non-hormonal options

Analgesics taken when pain occurs are often effective (response rate: 90%) (Arona, 1998). Anxiety and other psychological disorders have been found to be more frequent among patients with mastalgia (Fox et al., 1997). Although mastalgia does not represent a psycho-neurotic problem, emotions can function as aggravating factors and some women are unlikely to be helped unless their anxiety is addressed. Whether distress is secondary to, or causal of, mastalgia is part of the presenting problem and requires careful management. Psychiatric evaluation and a trial of antidepressants might be beneficial in patients who fail to respond to 'standard pharmacological interventions'. If mastalgia is persistently localized to a small area, excision may be curative in exceptional cases.

(See also: 'Pain management.')

REFERENCES

Abdel Hadi, M. S. (2000). Sports brassiere: is it a solution for mastalgia? *The Breast Journal*, **6**, 407–9.

Ader, D. N. (2001). Mastalgia. In I. Jatoi (Ed.). *Manual of breast diseases, Vol. 1* (pp. 77–94). Philadelphia: Lippincott, Williams and Wilkins.

Ader, D. N. & Browne, M. W. (1997). Prevalence and impact of cyclic mastalgia in a United States clinic-based sample. *American Journal of Obstetrics and Gynecology*, **177**, 126–32.

Ader, D. N. & Shriver, C. D. (1997). Relationship of cyclical mastalgia to PMS. *Journal of the American College of Surgeons*, **185**, 466–7.

Ader, D. N., Shriver, C. D. & Browne, M. W. (1999). Cyclical mastalgia: premenstrual syndrome or recurrent pain disorder? *Journal of Psychosomatic Obstetrics and Gynecology*, **20**, 198–202.

Ader, D. N., South-Paul, J., Adera, T. & Deuster, P. A. (2001). Cyclical mastalgia: prevalence and associated health and behavioral factors. *Journal of Psychosomatic Obstetrics and Gynecology*, **22**, 71–6.

Arona, A. J. (1998). Mastalgia. In W. H. Hindel (Ed.). *Breast care* (pp. 152–65).

Barros, A. C., Mottola, J., Ruiz, C. A. *et al.* (1999). Reassurance in the treatment of mastalgia. *The Breast Journal*, **5**, 162–5.

Colegrave, S., Holcombe, C. & Salmon, P. (2001). Psychological characteristics of women presenting with breast pain. *Journal of Psychosomatic Research*, **50**, 303–7.

Davies, E. L., Gateley, C. A., Miers, M., Mansel, M. E. *et al.* (1998). The long-term course of mastalgia. *Journal of the Royal Society of Medicine*, **91**, 462–4.

Dixon, J. M. (1999). Managing breast pain. *The Practitioner*, **243**, 484–6, 488–9, 491.

Dujim, L. E., Guilt, G. L. & Hendriks, J. H. (1998). Value of breast imaging in women with painful breasts: observational follow-up study. *British Medical Journal*, **317**, 1492–5.

Fox, H., Walker, R. G., Heys, S. D., Ah-See, A. K. & Eremin, O. (1997). Are patients with mastalgia anxious, and does relaxation therapy help? *Breast*, **6**, 138–42.

GEMB Group. (1997). Tamoxifen therapy for cyclical mastalgia: a controlled trial. *Breast*, **5**, 212.

Goodwin, P. J., Miller, A., Del Giudice, M. E. *et al.* (1997). Breast health and associated premenstrual symptoms in women with severe cyclic mastalgia.

American Journal of Obstetrics and Gynecology., **176**, 998–1005.

Khanna, A. K., Tapodar, J. & Misra, M. K. (1997). Spectrum of benign breast disorders in a university hospital. *Journal of the Indian Medical Association*, **95**, 5–8.

Klimberg, S. V. (1998). Etiology and management of breast pain. In K. I. Bland & E. M. Copeland (Eds.). *The breast: comprehensive management of benign and malignant diseases, Vol. 1* (pp. 247–60). Philadelphia: WB Saunders Company.

Kontostolis, E., Stefanidis, K., Navrozoglou, I. & Lolis, D. (1997). Comparison of tamoxifen with Danazol for treatment of cyclical mastalgia. *Gynecological Endocrinology*, **11**, 393.

Royal College of Physicians. (1998). *Making the best use of a department of clinical radiology: guidelines for doctors.* London: author.

Tavaf-Motamen, H., Ader, D. N., Brown, M. W. & Shriver, C. D. (1998). Clinical evaluation of mastalgia. *Archives of Surgery*, **133**, 211–13.

Unruh, A. M. (1996). Gender variations in clinical pain experience. *Pain*, **65**, 123–67.

Meningitis

Julie A. Carter

University College London and Kenya Medical Research Institute/Wellcome Trust Research Laboratories

Meningitis is an acute infectious disease, arising from infection of the membranes surrounding the brain and spinal cord by one of several microorganisms, such as bacteria, viruses, parasites and fungi. Recovery from meningitis has long been associated with severe neurological and/or cognitive deficits, including hearing impairment, epilepsy, motor impairments and learning disability. Those surviving without obvious or severe deficits have traditionally been considered to make a complete recovery. This view has recently been challenged by evidence that subtle cognitive, academic or behavioural problems may persist years after recovery from the disease.

Overview

Most research studies on impairments associated with meningitis have examined bacterial meningitis. Acute bacterial meningitis is one of the most common infections of the central nervous system (CNS). In more developed countries, *Streptococcus pneumoniae* and *Neisseria meningitides* are the most common pathogens responsible for community-acquired bacterial meningitis. *Haemophilus influenzae* meningitis has almost been eliminated due to the Hib vaccination. Bacterial meningitis is 10 times more common in children from less developed than more developed countries and the case fatality rate is higher, partly due to the prevalence of HIV infection, which makes children more prone to invasive bacterial infections (Molyneux *et al.*, 2003). In sub-Saharan Africa, the 'meningitis belt', an area stretching from Senegal in the west to Ethiopia in the east with a population of 300 million people, is also subject to recurring epidemics of meningococcal disease, primarily due to the serogroups *N. meningitidis* A, C and W135. A systematic review of 26 reports of neurological and cognitive impairments in survivors of bacterial meningitis indicated that up to 57% of children are left with deficits at least six months after recovery (Carter *et al.*, 2003).

Tuberculous meningitis is usually caused by the spread of *Mycobacterium tuberculosis* from the primary site of infection. In high-incidence geographic areas, tuberculous meningitis usually affects young children several months after primary infection, whereas in low-incidence areas, adults are more often affected, frequently after the reactivation of a dormant subcortical or meningeal focus. In sub-Saharan Africa, tuberculous meningitis is now the most common form of bacterial meningitis due to the impact of HIV/AIDS (Donald & Schoeman, 2004). Despite antituberculosis chemotherapy, tuberculous meningitis continues to cause death or severe neurocognitive deficits in more than half of those affected (Thwaites *et al.*, 2004).

Viral meningitis is the most common cause of acute aseptic meningitis. The most common causes are enteroviruses, herpes viruses, arboviruses and mumps and measles viruses. The disease is usually benign and self-limiting, making the prevalence difficult to estimate because many cases do not present to medical facilities. There are few data on impairments subsequent to aseptic meningitis: reports suggest it has the lowest rate of impairments of any form of meningitis, affecting between 2.2% and 9.1% of children (Carter *et al.*, 2003).

Other forms of meningitis such as fungal meningitis and parasitic meningitis are uncommon in more developed countries. However, *Cryptococcus neoformans*, which usually affects the immuno-incompetent, is now the second leading cause of death among HIV-positive patients worldwide. Neurological deficits, particularly severe visual impairment, are reported to be common in survivors (Day & Lalloo, 2004). Eosinophilic meningitis may be caused by prolonged schistosomiasis infection or ingestion of raw or pickled fish, shellfish, snake or amphibian. Again, severe neurological deficits may occur in those who recover, related to the physical damage caused by the parasites (Day & Lalloo, 2004).

Research evidence and clinical implications

The risk of neurological or psychological impairment in survivors of bacterial meningitis is correlated with factors such as age; time and clinical stability before effective treatment; type of microorganism; bacterial load in the cerebrospinal fluid (CSF); intensity of the patient's inflammatory response and time elapsed to sterilize CSF cultures (Saez-Llorens & McCracken Jr, 2003). Patients at the extremes of age (neonates and the elderly) tend to have the poorest prognosis. Neonatal meningitis is commonly caused by Group B Streptococci and *Escherichia coli*. A prospective study from the USA reported impairments in 68% of survivors

(Franco *et al.*, 1992), although another study, in which data were derived from medical notes, reported a lower rate of 16% (Klinger *et al.*, 2000).

Bacterial aetiology has a substantial impact on the outcome of ABM: pneumococcal meningitis usually results in higher levels of impairment in children, followed by *Haemophilus* and meningococcal meningitis (Baraff *et al.*, 1993). Pneumococcal meningitis also has a devastating effect on morbidity in adults. Van de Beek and colleagues (2004*a*) reported a higher prevalence of cranial nerve palsy, aphasia, hemiparesis and quadriparesis in adult survivors of pneumococcal meningitis compared to meningococcal meningitis. Tuberculous meningitis is also associated with high levels of impairment in adults: 29% of survivors are reported to have cranial nerve palsy; 16%, hemiparesis and 7%, paraparesis (Thwaites *et al.*, 2004).

Hearing impairment is reported in 2% to 38% of children surviving bacterial meningitis, the variation in reported prevalence due to heterogeneity in study populations, baseline disease severity, methods of assessment, types of impairment investigated and duration of follow-up (Carter *et al.*, 2003). Cochlear dysfunction is considered to be the reason for the hearing impairment: Richardson and colleagues (1997) reported that all children with sensori-neural hearing loss as a result of meningitis failed to produce otoacoustic emissions. The cochlear dysfunction causing the hearing loss is generally thought to be the result of labyrinthitis or the effects of bacterial toxins or inflammatory mediators on the hair cells of the Organ of Corti. Other possible mechanisms include similar processes acting on the endocochlear potential, metabolic defects secondary to low CSF glucose and the effects of changes in intra-cranial pressure (ICP) transmitted through the cochlear aqueduct (Richardson *et al.*, 1997). Meningitic hearing loss has been found to be a risk factor for poor school progress but is not considered to be the cause of the academic and behavioural problems often reported in children following meningitis (Koomen *et al.*, 2003; see also 'Deafness and hearing loss').

Between 2% and 40% of children are reported to have a cognitive and/or language impairment at least six months after recovery from bacterial meningitis (Carter *et al.*, 2003). Deficits, listed in order of frequency, are described as learning disability, speech disorder or delay, developmental delay, language disorder or delay, poor speech or minimal brain dysfunction. Few studies provide information on the neuropsychological impairments underlying learning, speech or language problems. A recent study that investigated the neuropsychological profile of childhood survivors of bacterial meningitis reported generic problems in cognitive functioning, speed and motor steadiness, rather than impairments in specific neuropsychological domains (Koomen *et al.*, 2004*a*).

Behavioural deficits are reported in 2% to 18% of children, often in the areas of social and school adjustment (Carter *et al.*, 2003). Reported problems, again listed in order of frequency, include hyperactivity, school behaviour problems, irritability, nervousness and temper tantrums (see 'Hyperactivity').

Multiple impairments are reported in the most severely affected survivors: for example, 15% of children in Grimwood and colleagues' (1995) study had more than one impairment. These children often require high levels of rehabilitative and educational support.

At the other end of the spectrum of severity, it is becoming clear that even children who seem to have recovered completely may have residual problems. One-third of Dutch children who survived bacterial meningitis without severe impairments were found to have academic and/or behavioural problems an average of seven years later (Koomen *et al.*, 2004*a*). Parental reports highlighted problems in school achievement, concentration and mood. Academic limitations were in the areas of mathematics, reading and writing; a high proportion of children had repeated classes at school or had been placed in schools for children with special needs.

The cause of academic and cognitive deficits post-meningitis is still debated, with some suggesting that bacterial meningitis causes a developmental delay and others stating that the illness irreparably impairs cognition (Koomen *et al.*, 2004*a*). Koomen and colleagues (2004*b*) identified nine independent risk factors for impairment: sex; birthweight; father's educational level; S. *pneumoniae* as the causative pathogen; CSF leukocyte count; delay between admission and antibiotic therapy; dexamethasone use; anticonvulsant therapy for seizures; and prolonged fever. Risk factors for mortality or morbidity in adults are reported to be those indicative of systemic compromise, a low level of consciousness and infection with S. *pneumoniae* (van de Beek *et al.*, 2004*a*). A meta-analysis of clinical trials indicated that dexamethasone has a protective effect on hearing in pneumococcal meningitis if administered before the start of antibiotic therapy (McIntyre *et al.*, 1997). Conversely, its use is not reported to prevent severe deficits in adolescents and adults with tuberculous meningitis (Thwaites *et al.*, 2004). Adjunctive corticosteroid therapy has also been associated with a reduction in the frequency of neurological impairments in adult survivors of bacterial meningitis (van de Beek *et al.*, 2004*b*).

Neurological or cognitive impairments may be transient in nature. Pikis and colleagues (1996) state that five children with motor impairments and one child with hearing loss recovered, although four of the children were left with other impairments. Salih and colleagues (1991) report a similar pattern with two children with hemiplegia recovering but later developing epilepsy. The prevalence of epilepsy after bacterial meningitis increases over time and may develop years after the initial insult (Pikis *et al.*, 1996; Pomeroy *et al.*, 1990; see also 'Epilepsy'). Health workers and educators need to remain aware of the child's medical history, even years after recovery.

Conclusions

Despite advances in treatment and improvements in mortality rates, the risks of long-term impairment following bacterial and tuberculous meningitis have not been greatly reduced. Survivors may have hearing deficits, cognitive deficits, behaviour problems or seizures. In less developed countries, the toll of meningitis will continue to be more pronounced because of the lack of prompt and adequate treatment and the impact of HIV/AIDS. Children with HIV are more likely to develop impairments subsequent to meningitis than children not infected with HIV, although the types of impairment are similar (Molyneux *et al.*, 2003).

There is increasing recognition of more subtle cognitive deficits in apparently unaffected survivors of meningitis (Grimwood *et al.*, 1995; Koomen *et al.*, 2004*a*). These deficits, although difficult to detect on formal assessment, may still adversely affect the child's social and educational functioning and suggest that the burden of impairment and disability as a result of meningitis, particularly in less developed countries, is probably much greater than has previously been recognized. With the increasing number of studies examining risk factors for impairment, it may in the future become possible to identify people at higher risk of developing deficits. This would enable more concentrated follow-up of this subgroup of survivors and early detection and adequate rehabilitation of impairments.

(See also 'Children's perceptions of illness and death'.)

REFERENCES

Baraff, L. J., Lee, S. I. & Schriger, D. L. (1993). Outcomes of bacterial meningitis in children: a meta-analysis. *Pediatric Infectious Disease Journal*, **12**, 389–94.

Carter, J. A., Neville, B. G. R. & Newton, C. R. J. C. (2003). Neuro-cognitive sequelae of acquired central nervous system infections in children: a systematic review. *Brain Research Reviews*, **43**, 57–69.

Day, J. N. & Lalloo, D. G. (2004). Neurological syndromes and the traveler: an approach to differential diagnosis. *Journal of Neurology Neurosurgery and Psychiatry*, **75** (suppl. 1), i2–9.

Donald, P. R. & Schoeman, J. F. (2004). Tuberculous meningitis. *New England Journal of Medicine*, **351**, 1719–20.

Franco, S. M., Cornelius, V. E. & Andrews, B. F. (1992). Long-term outcome of neonatal meningitis. *American Journal of Diseases of Children*, **146**, 567–71.

Grimwood, K., Anderson, V. A., Bond, L. *et al.* (1995). Adverse outcomes of bacterial meningitis in school-age survivors. *Pediatrics*, **95**, 646–56.

Klinger, G., Chin, C. N., Beyene, J. & Perlman, M. (2000). Predicting the outcome of neonatal bacterial meningitis. *Pediatrics*, **106**, 477–82.

Koomen, I., Grobbee, D. E., Jennekens-Schinkel, A., Roord, J. J. & van Furth, A. M. (2003). Parental perception of educational, behavioural and general health problems in school-age survivors of bacterial meningitis. *Acta Paediatrica*, **92**, 177–85.

Koomen, I., Grobbee, D. E., Roord, J. J. *et al.* (2004*b*). Prediction of academic and behavioural limitations in school-age survivors of bacterial meningitis. *Acta Paediatrica*, **93**, 1378–85.

Koomen, I., van Furth, A. M., Kraak, M. A. C. *et al.* (2004*a*). Neuropsychology of academic and behavioural limitations in school-age survivors of bacterial meningitis. *Developmental Medicine and Child Neurology*, **46**, 724–32.

McIntyre, P. B., Berkey, C. S., King, S. M. *et al.* (1997). Dexamethasone as adjunctive therapy in bacterial meningitis. A meta-analysis of randomized clinical trials since 1988. *Journal of the American Medical Association*, **278**, 925–31.

Molyneux, E. M., Tembo, M., Kayira, K. *et al.* (2003). The effect of HIV infection on paediatric bacterial meningitis in Blantyre, Malawi. *Archives of Disease in Childhood*, **88**, 1112–18.

Pikis, A., Kavaliotis, J., Tsikoulas, J. *et al.* (1996). Long-term sequelae of pneumococcal meningitis in children. *Clinical Pediatrics*, **35**, 72–8.

Pomeroy, S. L., Holmes, S. J., Dodge, P. R. & Feigin, R. D. (1990). Seizures and other neurologic sequelae of bacterial meningitis in children. *New England Journal of Medicine*, **323**, 1651–7.

Richardson, M. P., Reid, A., Tarlow, M. J. & Rudd, P. T. (1997). Hearing loss during bacterial meningitis. *Archives of Disease in Childhood*, **76**, 134–8.

Saez-Llorens, X. & McCracken Jr., G. H. (2003). Bacterial meningitis in children. *Lancet*, **361**, 2139–48.

Salih, M. A., Khaleefa, O. H., Bushara, M. *et al.* (1991). Long term sequelae of childhood acute bacterial meningitis in a developing country.

A study from the Sudan. *Scandinavian Journal of Infectious Diseases*, **23**, 175–82.

Thwaites, G. E., Nguyen, D. B., Nguyen, H. D. *et al.* (2004). Dexamethasone for the treatment of tuberculous meningitis in adolescents and adults. *New England Journal of Medicine*, **351**, 1741–51.

van de Beek, D., de Gans, J., McIntyre, P. & Prasad, K. (2004*b*). Steroids in adults with bacterial meningitis: a systematic

review. *Lancet Infectious Diseases*, **3**, 139–43.

van de Beek, D., de Gans, J., Spanjaard, L. *et al.* (2004*a*). Clinical features and prognostic factors in adults with bacterial meningitis. *New England Journal of Medicine*, **351**, 1849–59.

Menopause and postmenopause

Myra S. Hunter

King's College London

The menopause literally refers to a woman's last menstrual period occurring, on average, between 50 and 51 years of age. Cessation of menstruation is preceded by a gradual reduction in output of oestrogen by the ovaries and fewer ovulatory cycles (see Richardson, 1993). The menopause transition is characterized by hot flushes and night sweats, or vasomotor symptoms, which are experienced by between 50 and 70% of women in western cultures. For the majority of women these are not seen as problematic. It is estimated that between 10 and 15% of women find them difficult to cope with, mainly because of their frequency or their disruptive effects upon sleep. The average duration of the menopause transition, assessed by menstrual changes and hot flushes, is estimated to be four years but there is considerable variation between women (McKinlay *et al.*, 1992).

The menopause has for centuries been associated with emotional and physical pathology, and myths about its impact upon sexual function, femininity, ageing and women's sanity abound. Menopause was even once postulated to cause psychosis (involutional melancholia) but there is no evidence to support this. The commonly used term 'change of life' reflects the view that the menopause is closely associated with general emotional and social adaptations of mid-life.

The development of hormone replacement or oestrogen therapy (HRT) has had a major impact upon definitions of the menopause and the development of health services. The menopause is now seen as a cluster of symptoms caused by hormone deficiency and treatable with HRT. While initially recommended for the treatment of hot flushes, HRT has been advocated for the alleviation of symptoms, as well as the prevention of osteoporosis, cardiovascular

disease and even dementia in postmenopausal women. However, claims for long-term health benefits have been modified by the results of recent prospective trials of hormone treatments, particularly the Women's Health Initiative (WHI) (Rossouw *et al.*, 2002) and the Million Women Study (MWS) (Manson *et al.*, 2003). Together these studies suggest that HRT does not protect against cardiovascular disease (and in fact was associated with small but increased risks of strokes and blood clots in the WHI trial) and is associated with a small but increased risk of breast cancer. Moreover, claims that HRT might protect against mild cognitive impairment or dementia were not supported (Tanne, 2004). These findings have impacted upon hormone therapy use, with many women discontinuing or reducing the doses of HRT (Hersh *et al.*, 2004) and an increased interest in non-medical treatments (see 'Osteoporosis' and 'Hormone replacement therapy').

Psychologists and other social scientists have attempted to understand the nature of changes across the menopause transition. Early studies suffered from methodological problems, such as reliance upon clinical samples and use of unstandardized measures. Cross-sectional studies produced mixed results, but several prospective studies carried out in the 1980s and '90s together provide fairly strong evidence that, on average, the menopause does not have a negative effect upon mood or wellbeing for the majority of middle-aged women (Avis *et al.*, 1994; Dennerstein *et al.*, 1999). Similarly, qualitative studies have revealed that the menopause can have benefits, such as the end of menstrual periods and the need for contraception, as well as challenges, such as hot flushes and night sweats and perceiving the menopause as a marker of ageing (Hunter & O'Dea, 1997; Busch *et al.*, 2003). Studies comparing the experience of the menopause in different cultures tend to reveal a diversity of experience, suggesting that the meaning ascribed to it and women's reactions to it are, in part, culturally determined (Lock, 1986).

Psychologists have examined the influence of psychosocial factors such as life stresses, beliefs and expectations, as well as sociodemographic variables as predictors of menopausal experience. In general, psychosocial factors have been found to account for a greater proportion of the variation in measures of mood and psychological symptoms than stage of menopause. For example, predictors of depressed mood during the menopause include a history of depressed mood, low socioeconomic status, life stress (particularly that involving losses or exits of people from the social network) and negative beliefs, for example, that the menopause is likely to bring emotional and physical problems (Hunter, 1993). The results of a large prospective study of a cohort of women followed since birth in 1946 provides evidence of risk factors across the lifespan, such as parental divorce and prior experience of physical or emotional problems as adults, for psychological distress in midlife (Kuh et al., 2002). Interestingly menopausal status was not associated with levels of distress. Women who have an early menopause, those who have severe hot flushes and those who have undergone surgical menopause have been found to be more likely to experience emotional reactions. Correlational studies have failed to find a significant relationship between oestrogen levels and depressed mood. However, it is possible that the rapid withdrawal of hormones, as occurs with removal of the ovaries, might have impact upon mood.

The implications of this research have been an increased awareness of the need to provide balanced information about the menopause, as well as the need to develop a choice of clinical interventions for those women who do experience problems during this time of life. For example, a health promotion intervention offered to premenopausal women was found to increase knowledge and reduce negative attitudes to the menopause (Liao & Hunter, 1998). For menopausal symptoms, there is a growing interest in complementary therapies and herbal remedies but the evidence for their effectiveness to date is not very strong (Kronenberg & Fugh-Berman, 2002; Moyad, 2002). The extent to which the symptoms are perceived as a problem is less associated with hot flush frequency or duration, but more with cognitions (perceptions of ability to cope), mood (depressed mood, anxiety) and lower self-esteem (Hunter & Liao, 1996; Reynolds, 1997). There is growing evidence that treatments involving relaxation therapy can effectively reduce hot flushes (Stevenson & Delprato, 1983; Freedman & Woodward, 1992; Irvin et al., 1996). A four-session cognitive–behavioural treatment (CBT) including relaxation has been developed that incorporated stress management, psychoeducation, moderating precipitants of hot flushes and relaxation (Hunter & Liao, 1996). Using a patient preference design (comparing no treatment (monitoring) vs. HRT vs. CBT), women experiencing hot flushes and night sweats during the menopause transition reported comparable improvements following either CBT or HRT. There were no significant changes in the monitoring group but both active treatments resulted in a 50% reduction in hot flush frequency (see 'Cognitive behaviour therapy' and 'Relaxation training').

Given that women who do seek help for menopausal problems tend to have higher levels of distress than non-attenders at clinics, it has been suggested that they may be attributing distress resulting from life problems to the menopause. Problem clarification using a biopsychosocial framework might enable a range of possible influences to be considered. There is some evidence to suggest that psychological interventions might be beneficial in helping women to find appropriate solutions to their problems (Hunter & Liao, 1995; Greene, 2003).

REFERENCES

Avis, N., Brambrilla, D. & McKinlay, S. (1994). A longitudinal analysis of the association between menopause and depression: results from the Massachusetts women's health study. *Annals of Epidemiology*, **4**, 214–20.

Busch, H., Barth-Olofsson, A. S., Rosenhagen, S. & Collins, A. (2003). Menopausal transition and psychological development. *Menopause*, **10**, 179–87.

Dennerstein, L., Lehert, P., Burger, H. & Dudley, E. (1999). Mood and the menopause transition. *Journal of Nervous and Mental Diseases*, **187**, 685–91.

Freedman, R. R. & Woodward, S. (1992). Behavioral treatment of menopausal hot flushes: evaluation by ambulatory monitoring. *American Journal of Obstetrics and Gynecology*, **167**, 436–9.

Greene, J. G. (2003). Has psychosocial research on the menopause any clinical relevance? *Climacteric*, **6**, 23–30.

Hersh, A. L., Stefanick, M. L. & Stafford, R. S. (2004). National use of postmenopausal hormone therapy: annual trend and response to recent evidence. *Journal of the American Medical Association*, **291**, 47–53.

Hunter, M. S. (1993). Predictors of menopausal symptoms: psychological aspects. In H. G. Burger (Ed.). *The menopause: clinical endocrinology and metabolism* (pp. 33–46). London: Baillière Tindall.

Hunter, M. S. & Liao, K. L. M. (1995). Problem-solving groups for mid-aged women in general practice: a pilot study. *Journal of Reproductive and Infant Psychology*, **13**, 147–51.

Hunter, M. S. & Liao, K. L. M. (1996). An evaluation of a four-session cognitive behavioural intervention for menopausal hot flushes. *British Journal of Health Psychology*, **1**, 113–25.

Hunter, M. S. & O'Dea, I. (1997). Menopause: bodily changes and multiple meanings. In J. M. Ussher (Ed.). *Body talk: the material and discursive regulation of sexuality, madness and reproduction* (pp. 199–222). London: Routledge.

Irvin, J. H., Domar, A. D., Clark, C., Zuttermeister, P. C. & Friedman, R. (1996). The effects of relaxation response training on menopausal symptoms. *Journal of Psychosomatic Obstetrics and Gynaecology*, **17**, 202–7.

Kronenberg, F. & Fugh-Berman, A. (2002). Complementary and alternative medicine for menopausal symptoms: a review of randomised controlled trials. *Annals of Internal Medicine*, **137**, 806–13.

Kuh, D., Hardy, R., Rodgers, B. & Wadsworth, M. E. J. (2002). Lifetime risk factors for women's psychological distress in midlife. *Social Science & Medicine,* **55**, 1957–73.

Liao, K. L. M. & Hunter, M. S. (1998). Preparation for the menopause: prospective evaluation of a health education intervention for mid-aged women. *Maturitas,* **29**, 215–24.

Lock, M. (1986). Ambiguities of ageing: Japanese experience and perceptions of the menopause. *Culture, Medicine and Psychiatry,* **10**, 23–46.

McKinlay, S. M., Brambrilla, D. J. & Posner, J. (1992). The normal menopause transition. *Maturitas,* **14**, 103–16.

Manson, J. E., Hsia, J., Johnson, K. C. *et al.* (2003). Estrogen plus progestin and the risk of coronary heart disease.

New England Journal Medicine, **349**, 523–34.

Moyad, M. A. (2002). Complementary therapies for reducing hot flashes in prostate cancer patients: reevaluating the existing indirect data from studies of breast cancer and postmenopausal women. *Urology,* **59**, 20–33.

Reynolds, F. A. (1997). Perceived control over menopausal hot flushes: exploring the correlates of a standardised measure. *Maturitas,* **27**, 215–21.

Richardson, S. (1993). The biological basis of the menopause. In H. G. Burger (Ed.). *The menopause: clinical endocrinology and metabolism* (pp. 1–16). London: Baillière Tindall.

Rossouw, J. E., Anderson, G. L., Prentice, R. L. *et al.* (2002). Risks and

benefits of oestrogen plus progestin in health postmenopausal women: principal results from the Women's Health Initiative randomised controlled trial. *Journal of the American Medical Association,* **288**, 321–33.

Stevenson, D. W. & Delprato, D. J. (1983). Multiple component self control programme for menopausal hot flushes. *Journal of Behaviour Therapy & Experimental Psychiatry,* **14**, 137–40.

Tanne, J. H. (2004). Oestrogen doesn't protect mental function in older women. *British Medical Journal,* **328**, 1514.

MMR vaccine

Emily Buckley

Staffordshire University

The MMR triple vaccine provides protection from measles, mumps and rubella (German measles). These diseases can have serious complications such as convulsions, temporary or permanent deafness, meningitis, brain damage and even death. However, since the introduction of the MMR vaccine in 1988, these once common diseases have become rare in the Western World.

In the United Kingdom, children are expected to receive two doses of the combined vaccine, the first at 12–15 months of age and the second between three and five years. In 1997/8 MMR vaccination coverage was at its highest level with 91% of all children being vaccinated by their second birthday. However MMR coverage is now at its lowest for over ten years with only 82% of all children being immunized with MMR in 2003, and in some areas such as London, uptake has fallen to only 72%. This is far below the current Government targets which advocate that 95% of all children should be immunized by the age of two in order to maintain herd immunity. In 2002 the UK had the first measles outbreaks for a decade (Office of National Statistics, 2004). Worldwide 890 000 children die as a result of measles each year, mainly in countries with poor immunization coverage (Owens, 2002), and as

such, the reasons for falling immunization rates need to be addressed.

Non-immunization has been attributed to a number of factors including parental attitudes to immunization (such as unfamiliarity with diseases) and unsatisfactory provision of services. Furthermore, media coverage of possible side effects of the MMR vaccine (namely Crohn's disease and autism, see 'Parental attitudes' section below for more details) has been credited with undermining the Governments position on the safety and efficacy of the vaccine (see also 'Immunization').

Parental attitudes

Public perception of the severity of diseases has changed substantially in recent years, largely as a result of the success of vaccination in reducing the morbidity and mortality of disease. In Western countries parents tend to be unaware of the risks that these diseases pose and often report differential opinions regarding the severity of the three diseases, with measles perceived to be far more serious than mumps or rubella (Smailbegovic *et al.*, 2003). This belief in itself undermines parents' belief in the need for the combined vaccine in light of its potential side effects (see 'Risk perception').

However, the view that parents who refuse the MMR are ill-informed is not justified. Parents who have concerns about vaccination have often read widely in both medical and non-medical literature to try to settle their concerns (Agbley & Campbell, 1998). The majority of parents who refuse vaccinations have very strong views about vaccination, and appear to have received plenty of advice from professionals as well as other sources such as friends, family and the media before making their decisions (New & Senior, 1991).

Adverse publicity in the early 1990's (Wakefield *et al.*, 1993) which linked the MMR vaccine to Crohn's disease led to 2000 fewer children being vaccinated in the following three months. More recently, Wakefield *et al.* (1998) suggested links between the MMR vaccine and autism in children. Recent research has shown that as a result of media coverage, parents want more information to be available to them about the risks and benefits of MMR. Although a large number of studies have failed to find an association between the MMR vaccine and autism (Fombonne & Chakrabarti, 2001; Meldgaard Madsen *et al.*, 2002; Peltola *et al.*, 1998) and despite continued assurances by the Government, MMR uptake rates have continued to fall. Parents still feel that the information available to them about the diseases and vaccine safety is insufficient and unreliable, and that health professionals are not easily available to support them (Bond *et al.*, 1998; Gill & Sutton, 1998). Health professionals have a duty to provide accurate information to enable parents to make an informed decision about whether to have their children vaccinated, and parents' concerns should be treated seriously and sympathetically. Parental confidence in the Government and NHS positions on MMR has declined, and has resulted in great parental anxiety (Begg *et al.*, 1998), not only for the parents who refuse MMR immunization, but also in those who accept the vaccine (Roberts *et al.*, 2002).

Healthcare professionals and government

UK government policy dictates that payments to primary care practices for immunizing children are dependent upon the percentage of the practice immunized, in order to maintain high vaccination levels within the population. Many parents are sceptical of health professionals' motives as a result of this system of payment, and feel that they cannot trust health professionals' opinions due to a perceived vested interest (Evans *et al.*, 2001). Doctors are also becoming increasingly dissatisfied with this payment system, and are aware that it is undermining primary care physicians (GPs) in the eyes of their patients, and so they have requested that the Government changes the payment system.

Furthermore, there resides in the UK a general feeling of mistrust within the public regarding the Government's position on matters of public health which stems from the handling of the BSE (bovine spongiform encephalopathy) crisis (Kmietowicz, 2002).

The public were reassured on numerous occasions over a ten-year period that there was no risk to humans from consumption of meat products from BSE-infected cattle, until in March 1996 it was announced that BSE was likely to have been transmitted to humans causing a variant form of the neurodegenerative Creutzfeldt–Jakob Disease (Phillips *et al.*, 2000). The Government continues to maintain that the combined MMR vaccine is the safest and most effective way to protect children, and that harm will come to children if they do not receive two doses of MMR. However a substantial minority of people would like their children to receive three separate vaccines, and if faced with the option of the combined vaccine or none, will opt for none. The Department of Health's uncompromising position risks alienating the public by failing to respect parent's autonomy (Jewell, 2001).

The Government is in a difficult position because they do not want a repeat of the pertussis (whooping cough) debacle in the 1970's, when the media publicized a possible link between the pertussis vaccine and brain damage. An alternative vaccine was offered to parents, which led the public to believe that the Government had doubts about the vaccine's safety and coverage fell to 30% (Vernon, 2003).

Research also suggests that some health professionals may lack confidence in the need for MMR. Some health professionals are sceptical of the need for MMR in light of the media controversy, and this is likely to affect the advice that they provide to parents. Smith *et al.* (2001) found that the confidence of primary care physicians (GPs), practice nurses and health visitors in the MMR vaccine fell following the publication of Wakefield's two papers. Forty per cent of respondents were unsure about the need for a second dose of the MMR, and more than one in ten felt that a second dose was unnecessary. Providers of complementary and alternative medicine have also been shown to have negative attitudes towards the MMR (Schmidt & Ernst, 2003). These researchers argue that the reduced confidence in the safety of MMR and professional uncertainty about the need for MMR vaccination will have contributed to the decline in MMR uptake, and suggest that more professional as well as public education is needed.

Conclusion

MMR uptake rates have been falling since the early 1990s as a result of speculation regarding potential side effects of the vaccine, and rates will continue to fall if the public confidence in MMR is not restored. The majority of research suggests that parents want more information to be available to them, along with the opportunity to discuss concerns with health professionals, and that this is likely to result in an increase in MMR uptake if parents' anxieties are dealt with effectively. Many health professionals' confidence in MMR has also been undermined, and there is a need to re-educate professionals regarding the need for immunization, and to provide them with all available evidence regarding safety of the vaccine so that they can provide fully informed advice to parents (Smith *et al.*, 2001). Providing parents with more and better information, and involving them in decisions regarding vaccination, moving to a policy of concordance rather than compliance, is likely to increase confidence in the vaccine, and lead to an increase in MMR uptake. (Bellaby, 2003). However, we must also acknowledge the fact that vaccination is not compulsory in the UK, and therefore parents have the right to refuse to have their children immunized, whether it be for philosophical or scientific reasons. In the main, parents are acting conscientiously, and do what they perceive to be in the best interests of their children (Bradley, 1999).

REFERENCES

Agbley, D. & Campbell, H. (1998). Summary of factors affecting immunisation uptake levels. In V. Hey (Ed.). *Immunisation research: a summary volume*. London: HEA.

Begg, N., Ramsay, M., White, J. & Bozoky, Z. (1998). Media dents confidence in the MMR vaccine. *British Medical Journal*, **361**, 561.

Bellaby, P. (2003). Communication and miscommunication of risk: understanding UK parents' attitudes to combined MMR vaccination. *British Medical Journal*, **327**, 725–8.

Bond, L., Nolan, T., Pattison, P. & Carlin, J. (1998). Vaccine preventable diseases and immunisations: a qualitative study of mothers' perceptions of severity, susceptibility, benefits and barriers. *Australian and New Zealand Journal of Public Health*, **22**(4), 441–6.

Bradley, P. (1999). Should childhood immunisation be compulsory? *Journal of Medical Ethics*, **25**, 330–4.

Evans, M., Stoddart, H. *et al.* (2001). Parent's perspectives on the MMR immunisation: a focus group study. *British Journal of General Practice*, **51**, 904–10.

Fombonne, E. & Chakrabarti, S. (2001). No evidence for a new variant of measles-mumps-rubella-induced autism. *Pediatrics*, **108**, 4, E58.

Gill, E. & Sutton, S. (1998). Immunisation uptake: the role of parental attitudes. In V. Hey (Ed.). *Immunisation research: a summary volume*. London: HEA.

Jewell, D. (2001). MMR and the age of unreason. Editorial. *British Journal of General Practice*, **51**, 901–3.

Kmietowicz, Z. (2002). Government launches intensive media campaign on MMR. *British Medical Journal*, **324**, 383.

Meldgaard Madsen, K., Hviid, A., Vestergaard, M. *et al.* (2002). A population-based study of measles, mumps and rubella vaccination and autism. *New England Journal of Medicine*, **347**(19), 1477–82.

New, S. J. & Senior, M. L. (1991). "I don't believe in needles": qualitative aspects of a study into the uptake of infant immunisation in two English health authorities. *Social Science and Medicine*, **33**(4), 509–18.

Office of National Statistics (2004). MMR immunisation of children by their second birthday: by region, 2002/3: Social Trends 34. www.statistics.gov.uk

Owens, S. R. (2002). Injection of confidence. *EMBO Reports*, **3** (5), 406–9.

Peltola, H., Patja, A. *et al.* (1998). No evidence for measles mumps and rubella vaccine-associated inflammatory bowel disease or autism in a 14-year prospective study. *The Lancet*, **351**, 1327–8.

Phillips, Bridgeman, J. & Ferguson-Smith, M. (2000). *The BSE Inquiry*. London, UK: The Stationery Office. Accessed from www.bseinquirg.gov.uk

Roberts, K. A., Dixon-Woods, M. *et al.* (2002). Factors affecting uptake of childhood immunisation: a Bayesian synthesis of qualitative and quantitative evidence. *The Lancet*, **360**, 1596–9.

Schmidt, K. & Ernst, E. (2003). MMR vaccination advice over the internet. *Vaccine*, **21**, 1044–7.

Smith, A., McCann, R. & McKinlay, I. (2001). Second dose of MMR vaccine: health professionals' level of confidence in the vaccine and attitudes towards the second dose. *Communicable Disease and Public Health*, **4**, 273–7.

Smailbegovic, M. S., Laing, G. J. & Bedford, H. (2003). Why do parents decide against immunisation? The effect of health beliefs and health professionals. *Child: Care, Health and Development*, **29**(4), 303–11.

Vernon, J. G. (2003). Immunisation policy: from compliance to concordance? *British Journal of General Practice*, **53**, 399–404.

Wakefield, A. J., Pittilo, R. M., Sim, R. *et al.* (1993). Evidence of persistent measles virus infection in Crohn's disease. *Journal of Medical Virology*, **39**, 345–53.

Wakefield, A. J., Murch, S. H., Anthony, A. *et al.* (1998). Ileal-lymphoid-nodular hyperplasia, non-specific colitis, and pervasive developmental disorder in children: an early report. *The Lancet*, **351**, 637–41.

Motor neurone disease

Laura H. Goldstein

King's College London

Introduction

Motor Neurone Disease (MND), is a terminal, progressive neurodegenerative disease of the central nervous system. The most common form of MND is amyotrophic lateral sclerosis (ALS) involving both upper and lower motor neurones (UMNs, LMNs). Less common are primary lateral sclerosis (involving only UMNs) progressive muscular atrophy (involving only LMNs) and progressive bulbar palsy (PBP) where there is predominant involvement of the motor systems of the brainstem (Leigh & Ray-Chaudhuri, 1994). Peak age at onset is in the sixth decade of life. Incidence is around 1–2: 100 000 per year and prevalence 5–6:100 000. Median survival in ALS is 3.5 years from diagnosis, death commonly resulting from respiratory failure. Disease progression is generally variable but prognosis is poorest in those presenting with bulbar signs (about 25% of cases). Typically the disease presents with limb muscle weakness. Overall 90–95% of cases are sporadic, but 5–10% are familial in nature. At present there is no cure for MND. However the glutamate release antagonist, riluzole, has been shown to improve survival at 18 months (Lacomblez et al., 1996).

Psychological research concerning people with MND has predominantly involved investigations of the neuropsychological profile associated with ALS and of emotional and psychosocial issues (Goldstein & Leigh, 1999).

Neuropsychological aspects of MND

Increasing evidence that MND involves extra-motor cerebral regions is provided by findings of mild cognitive impairment occurring in up to 35–40% of non-demented patients with ALS, and by reports that a fronto-temporal dementia may also be seen in ~5% of sporadic cases (see 'Dementias'). Cognitive testing in MND patients, with or without dementia, may be complicated by the dysarthria or motor impairment associated with the disease. Whilst cognitive impairment is not exclusively associated with bulbar impairment, they may be associated (e.g. Abrahams et al., 1997; Massman et al., 1996).

MND without dementia

In non-demented MND patients, neuropsychological deficits have been elicited most consistently on executive function tests of orthographic or semantic verbal fluency (e.g. Abrahams et al., 1997, 2000). Executive dysfunction has been shown in studies using the Wisconsin Card Sorting Test (e.g. Abrahams et al., 1997; David & Gillham, 1986; Massman et al., 1996), picture sequencing (Talbot et al., 1995) as well as measures of response inhibition and focussed attention (e.g. Abrahams et al., 1997).

Memory deficits are more variable and are generally thought to reflect poor encoding. They may occur in tasks of word recognition, learning of object line drawings, recall of prose passages and verbal learning (Abrahams et al., 1997; David & Gillham, 1986). Memory dysfunction may occasionally reflect the consequences of respiratory weakness and can respond to treatment (Newsom-Davis et al., 2001).

Some non-demented ALS patients may demonstrate language impairments (e.g. Abrahams et al., 2004; Rakowicz & Hodges, 1998) although data are contradictory (Abrahams et al., 2000). It has yet to be determined how these cases relate to the dementia that may be associated with ALS (e.g. Bak et al., 2001). In general, more posterior functions are intact.

MND-dementia

In ~5% of sporadic cases and ~15% of familial cases of MND (see Barson et al., 2000 who suggest a higher prevalence rate), a frontal-type dementia occurs, characterized by a breakdown of social and personal behaviour and change in personality. Cognitive impairment usually precedes physical difficulties (e.g. Neary et al., 1990). Where neuropsychological assessment has been possible, impaired abstract reasoning, mental inflexibility, reduced verbal fluency, poor response inhibition, impaired attention, deficient confrontation naming and a non-fluent dysphasia have been reported (e.g. Neary et al., 1990). Memory is variably affected but visuospatial and posterior functions appear intact.

Psychological and psychosocial factors in MND

Mood

Studies have generally reported relatively low levels of anxiety and depression in people with MND (e.g. Goldstein et al., 1998; Hogg et al., 1994; Moore et al., 1998; Rabkin et al., 2000). Anxiety and/or depression scores on questionnaires are variably correlated with functional impairment (e.g. Goldstein et al., 1998; Hogg et al., 1994). Identifying the emotional concomitants of MND is important in view of the reported prognostic role of mood in this illness (Johnston et al., 1999).

About 20% of MND patients experience pathological laughing and crying (emotional lability; EL) which is more common in patients with bulbar symptoms. Measures exist for its evaluation (e.g. Newsom-Davis et al., 1999) and EL may be correlated with aspects of executive dysfunction (McCullagh et al., 1999).

Quality of life (QoL)

Whilst illness characteristics may influence perceived QoL in people with MND (e.g. Nelson *et al.*, 2003), when measured in other than health status terms this has been found to have little direct relationship to illness severity, but more to factors such as social support, existential factors, everyday cognitive functioning and spiritual and religious aspects of the person's life (e.g. Ganzini *et al.*, 1999; Goldstein *et al.*, 2002; Simmons *et al.*, 2000). Studies investigating the impact and nature of caring for a person with MND indicate the need for psychological support to be provided for carers as well as people with MND (e.g. Goldstein *et al.*, 1998, 2000; Rabkin *et al.*, 2000; Trail *et al.*, 2003). Psychological and psychosocial factors may be important determinants of treatment choices (e.g. ventilation) and end-of-life options (Ganzini *et al.*, 2002; Trail *et al.*, 2003) (see Quality of Life).

and care of people with MND and how this relates to treatment choices and QoL. In addition psychological factors related to having the familial form of the disease require consideration. At present most of the care provided to patients and their families relates to the physical impact of the disease, but since existential issues are clearly important to people with MND, greater clarity concerning how best to address such matters within a medical and psychological setting would be of value. In addition the adoption of theoretical models of coping with illness would assist in both understanding the factors that influence people's adjustment to MND and how best to intervene when adjustment is poor.

(See also 'Coping with chronic illness' and 'Neuropsychological rehabilitation'.)

Conclusions

As a progressive, disabling and life-limiting disease, MND poses several clinical challenges. Research is needed to describe how cognitive impairment impacts on the everyday functioning

Acknowledgements

Much of our group's work has been supported by the Wellcome Trust, the Medical Research Council and the Motor Neurone Disease Association, UK.

REFERENCES

Abrahams, S., Goldstein, L.H., Al Chalabi, A. *et al.* (1997). Relation between cognitive dysfunction and pseudobulbar palsy in amyotrophic lateral sclerosis. *Journal of Neurology, Neurosurgery and Psychiatry*, **62**, 464–72.

Abrahams, S., Goldstein, L.H., Simmons, A. *et al.* (2004). Word retrieval in amyotrophic lateral sclerosis: a functional magnetic resonance imaging study. *Brain*, **127**, 1507–17.

Abrahams, S., Leigh, P.N., Harvey, A. *et al.* (2000). Verbal fluency and executive dysfunction in amyotrophic lateral sclerosis (ALS). *Neuropsychologia*, **38**, 734–47.

Bak, T.H., O'Donovan, D.G., Xuereb, J.H., Boniface, S. & Hodges, J.R. (2001). Selective impairment of verb processing associated with pathological changes in Brodmann areas 44 and 45 in the motor neurone disease–dementia–aphasia syndrome. *Brain*, **124**, 1–20.

Barson, F.P., Kinsella, G.J., Ong, B. & Mathers, S.E. (2000). A neuropsychological investigation of dementia in motor neurone disease (MND). *Journal of the Neurological Sciences*, **180**, 107–13.

David, A.S. & Gillham, R.A. (1986). Neuropsychological study of motor neuron disease. *Psychosomatics*, **27**, 441–5.

Ganzini, L., Johnston, W.S. & Hoffman, W.F. (1999). Correlates of suffering in amyotrophic lateral sclerosis. *Neurology*, **52**, 1434–40.

Ganzini, L., Silveira, M.J. & Johnston, W.S. (2002). Predictors and correlates of interest in assisted suicide in the final month of life among ALS patients in Oregon and Washington. *Journal of Pain and Symptom Management*, **24**, 312–17.

Goldstein, L.H., Adamson, M., Barby, T., Down, K. & Leigh, P.N. (2000). Attributions, strain and depression in carers of partners with MND: a preliminary investigation. *Journal of the Neurological Sciences*, **180**, 101–6.

Goldstein, L.H., Adamson, M., Jeffrey, L. *et al.* (1998). The psychological impact of MND on patients and carers. *Journal of the Neurological Sciences*, **160**(Suppl. 21).

Goldstein, L.H., Atkins, L. & Leigh, P.N. (2002). Correlates of quality of life in people with motor neuron disease (MND). *ALS and Other Motor Neuron Disorders*, **3**, 123–9.

Goldstein, L.H. & Leigh, P.N. (1999). Motor neurone disease: A review of its emotional and cognitive consequences for patients and its impact on carers. *British Journal of Health Psychology*, **4**, 193–208.

Hogg, K.E., Goldstein, L.H. & Leigh, P.N. (1994). The psychological impact of motor neurone disease. *Psychological Medicine*, **24**, 625–32.

Johnston, M., Earll, L., Giles, M. *et al.* (1999). Mood as a predictor of disability and survival in patients diagnosed with ALS/MND. *British Journal of Health Psychology*, **4**, 127–36.

Lacomblez, L., Bensimon, G., Leigh, P.N. *et al.* (1996). A confirmatory dose-ranging study of riluzole in ALS. ALS/Riluzole Study Group-II. *Neurology*, **47**(Suppl. 4), S242–250.

Leigh, P.N. & Ray-Chaudhuri, K. (1994). Motor neuron disease. *Journal of Neurology, Neurosurgery and Psychiatry*, **57**, 886–96.

Massman, P.J., Sims, J., Cooke, N. *et al.* (1996). Prevalence and correlates of neuropsychological deficits in amyotrophic lateral sclerosis. *Journal of Neurology, Neurosurgery and Psychiatry*, **61**, 450–5.

McCullagh, S., Moore, M., Gawel, M. & Feinstein, A. (1999). Pathological laughing and crying in amyotrophic lateral sclerosis: an association with prefrontal cognitive dysfunction. *Journal of the Neurological Sciences*, **169**, 43–8.

Moore, M.J., Moore, P.B. & Shaw, P.J. (1998). Mood disturbances in motor neurone disease. *Journal of the Neurological Sciences*, **160**, S53–6.

Neary, D., Snowden, J.S., Mann, D.M. *et al.* (1990). Frontal lobe dementia and motor neuron disease. *Journal of Neurology, Neurosurgery and Psychiatry*, **53**, 23–32.

Nelson, N.D., Trail, M., Van, J.N., Appel, S.H. & Lai, E.C. (2003). Quality of life in patients with amyotrophic lateral sclerosis: perceptions, coping resources, and illness characteristics. *Journal of Palliative Medicine*, **6**, 417–24.

Newsom-Davis, I.C., Abrahams, S., Goldstein, L.H. & Leigh, P.N. (1999). The emotional lability questionnaire: a new measure of emotional lability in amyotrophic lateral sclerosis. *Journal of the Neurological Sciences*, **169**, 22–5.

Newsom-Davis, I.C., Lyall, R.A., Leigh, P.N., Moxham, J. & Goldstein, L.H. (2001). The effect of non-invasive positive pressure ventilation (NIPPV) on cognitive function in amyotrophic lateral sclerosis (ALS): a prospective study. *Journal of Neurology, Neurosurgery & Psychiatry*, **71**, 482–7.

Rabkin, J.G., Wagner, G.J. & Del Bene, M. (2000). Resilience and distress among amyotrophic lateral sclerosis patients

and caregivers. *Psychosomatic Medicine*, **62**, 271–9.

Rakowicz, W.P. & Hodges, J.R. (1998). Dementia and aphasia in motor neuron disease: an underrecognised association? *Journal of Neurology, Neurosurgery & Psychiatry*, **65**, 881–9.

Simmons, Z., Bremer, B.A., Robbins, R.A., Walsh, S.M. & Fischer, S. (2000). Quality of life in ALS depends on factors other than strength and physical function. *Neurology*, **55**, 388–92.

Talbot, P.R., Goulding, P.J., Lloyd, J.J. *et al.* (1995). Inter-relation between "classic"

motor neuron disease and frontotemporal dementia: neuropsychological and single photon emission computed tomography study. *Journal of Neurology, Neurosurgery & Psychiatry*, **58**, 541–7.

Trail, M., Nelson, N.D., Van, J.N., Appel, S.H. & Lai, E.C. (2003). A study comparing patients with amyotrophic lateral sclerosis and their caregivers on measures of quality of life, depression, and their attitudes toward treatment options. *Journal of the Neurological Sciences*, **209**, 79–85.

Multiple sclerosis

Rona Moss-Morris[1], Kirsten van Kessel[2] and Emma L. Witt[2]

[1]University of Southampton
[2]The University of Auckland

Multiple Sclerosis (MS) is a chronic disease of the central nervous system (CNS) for which there is no known cause or cure. The disease is characterized by the destruction of the myelin sheath surrounding the nerves resulting in the formation of plaques. These plaques disrupt the transmission of nerve impulses leading to the symptoms of the illness which include, but are not limited to, spasticity, loss of balance and co-ordination, blurred or double vision, numbness, speech distortions, bladder and bowel problems, fatigue and cognitive dysfunction (Robinson, 1988). Plaques can occur in a variety of different sites resulting in substantial variation in the type and nature of the symptoms across individuals.

The course of the illness is also highly variable and unpredictable (Robinson, 1988). A small percentage of patients have a relatively benign course, characterized by an abrupt onset, little disease activity and no permanent disability. The majority have either a relapsing-remitting or a relapsing-progressive course. Patients experience periods of partial or total remission where the illness is inactive, interspersed with symptom relapses. Finally, MS can have a chronic-progressive course, in which there is a progressive worsening of symptoms and disability. Patients may be initially diagnosed with one type of MS, but over time progress to another.

There is substantial variation in the worldwide distribution of MS, with prevalence rates greater than 100 cases per 100 000 of population identified in many areas of the United Kingdom, Europe and North America. In contrast, considerably lower prevalence rates are found in Africa, the Middle East and Asia (Compston, 1998). MS is more common in females than males, with a gender ratio approaching 2:1 (Compston, 1998).

The onset of MS is typically between 20 and 40 years of age. These relatively young individuals are faced with a lifetime of uncertainty and in a minority of cases, a shortened lifespan. They have to cope with an unpredictable illness, loss of function, alteration of life roles and the experience of a range of debilitating, changeable and sometimes embarrassing symptoms. Consequently, adapting to MS can be particularly arduous. A number of factors are associated with poorer adjustment in MS including the length of the prediagnosis period, illness uncertainty, cognitive impairment, remission status, incontinence and sexual dysfunction (Aikens *et al.*, 1997; Franklin *et al.*, 1988; Mushlin *et al.*, 1994; Rao *et al.*, 1991) (see 'Coping with chronic illness', 'Incontinence' and 'Sexual dysfunction'). However, many of these factors are inherent within the illness and provide few indicators as to how health professionals may be able to assist patients in adjusting to MS. This chapter will focus on psychosocial factors which may provide potential avenues for assisting the adjustment process, and in some instances, possibly attenuate the disease process.

Emotional responses

Emotional states have been linked with MS onset or exacerbation throughout the history of the disease. In the late nineteenth century Charcot related experiences such as grief and anger to MS onset. In the early twentieth century it was widely held that an MS-prone personality increased susceptibility in the face of emotional stress (LaRocca, 1984). Although more recent research has found no evidence of a premorbid MS personality profile (VanderPlate, 1984), the role of emotions in MS is clearly important.

MS patients report a range of emotions in response to experiencing an unpredictable, degenerative and debilitating illness including depression, anger and anxiety (Mohr & Cox, 2001). Emotional responses may also be associated with neurological changes and a small percentage of patients experience pathological laughing and crying and euphoria (Mohr & Cox, 2001).

Depression is the most commonly studied emotional state in MS. Around 50% of MS patients report a lifetime prevalence of major depression (Mohr & Cox, 2001). Depression may be due to a number of factors including the psychosocial consequences of the illness or the neurological changes associated with the disease process. In some instances, depression may be an iatrogenic effect of MS disease-modifying drugs.

Rates of anxiety also appear to be high with reported point prevalence rates ranging between 19% to 34% (Mohr & Cox, 2001). However, anxiety and other emotional responses in MS have received less attention in the literature. More work is needed in this area because not only do patients' psychological responses impact on their quality of life, but preliminary evidence suggests that they impact on the MS disease process itself. Psychological distress and depression has been shown to affect levels of T-helper cells implicated in the immune system's attack on the CNS, and to increase levels of the cytokine interferon-gamma (Mohr *et al.*, 1998; Foley *et al.*, 1992) (see 'Psychoneuroimmunology').

Stress

Further evidence that emotional states may play an important role in the exacerbation of MS disease comes from the stress literature. A meta-analysis of 14 studies found that stressful life events were associated with MS exacerbation, with a weighted average effect size of $d = 0.53$. The results were not affected by differences in study design, method and sample characteristics, and were significant for exacerbation at onset and during the course of disease (Mohr *et al.*, 2004*b*). These results are particularly pertinent when one takes into account that interferon beta, the class of drugs used to moderate the disease process in MS, show an average effect size in exacerbation reduction of $d = 0.36$, and this effect reduces after the first year (Filippini *et al.*, 2003).

How stress contributes to disease activity is less clear. One possibility is that stress impacts on the immune system, but to date there is no specific biological model to explain the effect of stress on individuals with MS disease. It is also not known whether different types of stressors have a differential impact on the disease process, or whether it is the nature of the emotional response to the stressor that is most important.

A model of stress and MS also needs to take into account a bi-directional relationship, where stress is both a result of living with the condition and a contributor to disease progression (Schwartz *et al.*, 1999). MS itself may be a source of considerable stress and adjustment to the illness has been shown to be related to disease characteristics (McReynolds *et al.*, 1999). However, there are a number of factors that may moderate the stressful effects of the illness such as the way in which patients cope with their illness, their social resources and their illness perceptions. These are discussed in turn.

Coping

Much of the work on coping in MS has adopted the Folkman and Lazarus (1984) coping framework, which suggests that the impact of a potentially stressful event is moderated by the person's appraisals of the event as threatening, their available coping resources and the actual strategies put in place to deal with the stressor (see 'Stress and health'). In support of this model is the preliminary evidence that coping strategies may moderate the relationship between stress and disease activity. Mohr and colleagues (2002) found that greater use of distraction was associated with less stress and fewer new brain lesions eight weeks later. Furthermore, coping strategies have been shown to be better predictors of adjustment to MS than level of physical impairment (McCabe *et al.*, 2004). Poorer adjustment has been consistently associated with a greater reliance on passive, avoidant emotion-focused coping (Mohr & Cox, 2001). Research on the use of problem-focused coping is more mixed, with some studies finding a significant correlation with better adjustment outcomes, and others reporting no relationship. It may be that certain problem-focused strategies are more effective at different stages of the disease (Mohr & Cox, 2001).

Social support

Social support is also important for adjustment to chronic illness. In MS, low levels of social support and less use of social support seeking are associated with higher levels of psychological distress and depression (Mohr *et al.*, 2004*a*). Peer support from other people with MS is often proposed as an effective means of reducing MS-related distress and is frequently used by MS support groups. However, intervention studies provide inconsistent evidence of a beneficial effect of peer support on adjustment (Messmer Uccelli *et al.*, 2004). It may be that peer support is more appropriate at certain stages of the disease process, and for coping with particular issues. Alternatively, it may be that the most beneficial effects of social support are experienced when people actively seek the type of support they need. Messmer Uccelli and colleagues (2004) suggest that social support interventions that aim to teach people with MS methods of accessing support, as well as coping skills, may be more effective in enhancing adjustment. Further research is needed on the roles and interaction between social support and coping strategies in adjustment to MS (see 'Social support and health').

Caregivers

Partners and family members often play a key caregiving or social support role to people with MS. This can be a demanding task as caregivers are often the main source of emotional and physical support, sometimes for many years. They may also face their own adjustment issues in relation to their partners' or family members' MS, including psychological distress, reduced social and recreational opportunities and financial strain. Caregivers of people with MS report less social support than the general population, with lower levels of support associated with greater distress (McKeown *et al.*, 2003). This suggests that caregivers should also be considered when looking at interventions aimed at helping patients with MS adjust to their condition.

Illness and symptom perceptions

Although most of the studies investigating psychosocial aspects of adjustment to MS have focused on the coping literature, there is a growing body of evidence that patients' beliefs are also important in adjusting to MS. The illness representations framework refers to the thoughts and beliefs a person has about their illness, and the way he/she understands and makes sense of the disease (Leventhal *et al.*, 1997). Illness representations influence how someone will respond or behave, and in turn these behaviours affect adaptation to the condition.

Studies which have looked at illness representations in patients with MS have shown that believing a wide range of symptoms are associated with the condition and that MS has many negative effects on one's life is associated with increased social dysfunction, poor self-esteem, depression and anxiety, higher level of illness intrusiveness and greater impairment in physical functioning (Jopson & Moss-Morris, 2003; Vaughan *et al.*, 2003). These effects are independent of the severity of the illness itself. The only domain of adjustment more closely associated with the severity of the illness is physical dysfunction. There is also evidence of an association between illness beliefs and fatigue in MS, and that fatigue in MS may in part develop because of a feeling of helplessness in the face of symptoms and a tendency to focus unduly on bodily sensations (Jopson & Moss-Morris, 2003; Vercoulen *et al.*, 1996, 1998) (see 'Lay beliefs about health and illness' and 'Symptom perception').

Psychological interventions

The evidence reviewed above suggests that psychological interventions may be useful in helping patients to develop skills to cope with emotions and to adjust to the MS diagnosis and symptoms. To date, there have been few randomized controlled trials evaluating the efficacy of psychological interventions with MS patients. In their review of the empirical literature, Mohr and Cox (2001) note that most studies have focused on the treatment of depression in MS evaluating cognitive–behavioural therapies (CBT), relaxation, supportive group therapy and antidepressant medications (see 'Cognitive behaviour therapy', 'Relaxation training' and 'Social support interventions'). One recent comparative trial found that CBT and setraline were more effective than supportive–expressive group psychotherapy at reducing depression in MS (Mohr *et al.*, 2001). However, only small numbers of patients made significant improvements, and the authors of this study recommend more aggressive strategies such as a combination of treatment modalities. Another study found that telephone-administered CBT decreased depressive symptoms in MS patients (Mohr *et al.*, 2000), offering an alternative treatment delivery method for patients who are unable to attend clinic appointments.

Future interventions for MS patients need to focus on a broader range of adjustment variables, such as coping with symptoms like fatigue and pain, levels of social adjustment and generalized distress. The fact that illness representations contribute to outcome suggests that it might be important to provide MS patients with skills to develop accurate beliefs about their illness and modify those illness cognitions that have been shown to relate to poorer outcome. Similarly, more work needs to be done on finding alternatives to passive coping strategies in MS and to test the efficacy of stress reduction techniques on slowing MS progression.

REFERENCES

Aikens, J.E., Fischer, J.S., Namey, M. & Rudick, R.A. (1997). A Replicated prospective investigation of life stress, coping, and depressive symptoms in multiple sclerosis. *Journal of Behavioral Medicine*, **20**, 433–45.

Compston, A. (Ed.). (1998). *McAlpine's multiple sclerosis*. London: Churchill Livingstone.

Filippini, G., Munari, L., Incorvaia, B. *et al.* (2003). Interferons in relapsing remitting multiple sclerosis: a systematic review. *Lancet*, **361**, 545–52.

Foley, F.W., Traugott, U., LaRocca, N.G. *et al.* (1992). A prospective study of depression and immune dysregulation in multiple sclerosis. *Archives of Neurology*, **49**, 238–44.

Folkman, S. & Lazarus, R. (1984). If it changes it must be a process: a study of emotion and coping during three stages of a college examination. *Journal of Personality and Social Psychology*, **48**, 150–70.

Franklin, G.M., Heaton, R.K., Nelson, L.M., Filley, C.M. & Seibert, C. (1988).

Correlation of neuropsychological and MRI findings in chronic/progressive multiple sclerosis. *Neurology*, **38**, 1826–9.

Jopson, N.M. & Moss-Morris, R. (2003). The role of illness severity and illness representations in adjusting to multiple sclerosis. *Journal of Psychosomatic Research*, **54**, 503–11.

LaRocca, N.G. (1984). Psychosocial factors in multiple sclerosis and the role of stress. *Annals of the New York Academy of Sciences*, **436**, 435–42.

Leventhal, H., Benyamini, Y., Brownlee, S. *et al.* (1997). Illness representations: theoretical foundations. In K.J. Petrie & J.A. Weinman (Eds.). *Perceptions of health and illness* (pp. 19–45). London: Harwood Academic Publishers.

McCabe, M.P., McKern, S. & McDonald, E. (2004). Coping and psychological adjustment among people with multiple sclerosis. *Journal of Psychosomatic Research*, **56**, 355–61.

McKeown, L., Porter-Armstrong, A. & Baxter, G. (2003). The needs and

experiences of caregivers of individuals with multiple sclerosis: a systematic review. *Clinical Rehabilitation*, **17**, 234–48.

McReynolds, C.J., Koch, L.C. & Rumrill, Jr. (1999). Psychosocial adjustment to multiple sclerosis: implications for rehabilitation professionals. *Journal of Vocational Rehabilitation*, **12**, 83–91.

Messmer Uccelli, M., Mancuso Mohr, L., Battaglia, M.A., Zagami, P. & Mohr, D.C. (2004). Peer support groups in multiple sclerosis: current effectiveness and future directions. *Multiple Sclerosis*, **10**, 80–4.

Mohr, D.C., Boudewyn, A.C., Goodkin, D.E., Bostrom, A. & Epstein, L. (2001). Comparative outcomes for individual cognitive–behavior therapy, supportive–expressive group psychotherapy, and sertraline for the treatment of depression in multiple sclerosis. *Journal of Consulting & Clinical Psychology*, **69**, 942–9.

Mohr, D.C., Classen, C. & Barrera, M.J. (2004*a*). The relationship between social support, depression and treatment for depression in people with multiple sclerosis. *Psychological Medicine*, **34**, 533–41.

Mohr, D.C. & Cox, D. (2001). Multiple sclerosis: empirical literature for the clinical health psychologist. *Journal of Clinical Psychology*, **57**, 479–99.

Mohr, D.C., Goodkin, D.E., Nelson, S., Cox, D. & Weiner, M. (2002). Moderating effects of coping on the relationship between stress and the development of new brain lesions in multiple sclerosis. *Psychosomatic Medicine*, **64**, 803–9.

Mohr, D.C., Goodkin, D.E., Marietta, P. *et al.* (1998). Relationship between treatment of depression and interferon-gamma in patients with multiple sclerosis. Paper presented at American Academy of Neurology, Minneapolis.

Mohr, D.C., Hart, S.L., Julian, L., Cox, D. & Pelletier, D. (2004*b*). Association between stressful life events and exacerbation in multiple sclerosis:

a meta-analysis. *British Medical Journal*, **328**, 731.

Mohr, D.C., Likosky, W., Bertagnolli, A. *et al.* (2000). Telephone-administered cognitive-behavioral therapy for the treatment of depressive symptoms in multiple sclerosis. *Journal of Consulting & Clinical Psychology*, **68**, 356–61.

Mushlin, A., Mooney, C., Grow, V., Phelps, C. (1994). The value of diagnostic information to patients with suspected multiple sclerosis. *Archives of Neurology*, **51**, 67–72.

Rao, S., Leo, G., Bernardin, L. & Unverzagt, F. (1991). Cognitive dysfunction in multiple sclerosis. I. Frequency, patterns, and prediction. *Neurology*, **41**, 685–91.

Robinson, I. (1988). *Multiple Sclerosis*, London: Routledge.

Schwartz, C.E., Foley, F.W., Rao, S.M. *et al.* (1999). Stress and course of disease in multiple sclerosis. *Behavioral Medicine*, **25**, 110–16.

VanderPlate, C. (1984). Psychological aspects of multiple sclerosis and its

treatment: toward a biopsychosocial perspective. *Health Psychology*, **3**, 253–72.

Vaughan, R., Morrison, L. & Miller, E. (2003). The illness representations of multiple sclerosis and their relations to outcome. *British Journal of Health Psychology*, **8**, 287–301.

Vercoulen, J.H., Hommes, O.R., Swanink, C.M. *et al.* (1996). The measurement of fatigue in patients with multiple sclerosis. A multidimensional comparison with patients with chronic fatigue syndrome and healthy subjects. *Archives of Neurology*, **53**, 642–9.

Vercoulen, J., Swanink, C., Galama, J. *et al.* (1998). The persistence of fatigue in chronic fatigue syndrome and multiple sclerosis: development of a model. *Journal of Psychosomatic Research*, **45**, 507–17.

Myasthenia gravis

Ruth Epstein

Royal National Throat, Nose & Ear Hospital

Myasthenia gravis

Myasthenia gravis is a neurological disease which is characterized by abnormal muscle fatigability. It may affect any group of muscles; head and neck muscles are initially most affected, with extraocular muscles most commonly involved (Stell, 1987). The disease is relatively rare, with an incidence between 2 and 10 per 100 000 (Garfinkle & Kimmelman, 1982). This condition occurs in all ages, but is usually seen in young adults and is twice as common in women as men. Onset for females is reported in the third decade of life, while in males it is during the sixth decade (Garfinkle & Kimmelman, 1982). Aetiology is unknown, but current evidence suggests that it is an autoimmune disease attributed to a decrease in the number of acetylcholine receptors in the motor end plate (Fritze *et al.*, 1974).

Patients with myasthenia gravis tend to show bulbar symptoms, with the initial and most common being drooping of the eyelids or ptosis (Grob, 1961). They also report dysarthria characterized by hypernasality, reduced loudness, increased breathiness and articulatory imprecision (Aronson, 1990), dysphagia, diplopia,

weakness of the legs and blurred vision. The unique features of myasthenia gravis are fatigability, fluctuation of function and restoration of function after rest (Colton & Casper, 1990). Diagnosis depends on the typical clinical picture and can be confirmed by intravenous administration of edrophonium (Tensilon Test), laryngeal electromyographic measurements or detection of anti-acetylcholine receptor antibodies in the blood. If the patient is asked to count aloud, the voice gets progressively less distinct and more nasal.

A common diagnostic pitfall is the interpretation of symptoms of myasthenia gravis as being psychogenic, especially if the patient has a history of psychiatric illness. Furthermore, physical signs in early myasthenia gravis are often precipitated by emotional stress, accounting for the possibility of mistaking this disease for a conversion reaction (Ball & Lloyd, 1971) (see also 'Psychosomatics').

A number of recent studies have examined the psychosocial impact of myasthenia gravis. On the whole, the results suggest that patients with this condition experience depression at a higher rate than the general population and at a similar rate as patients with other chronic illnesses (Fisher *et al.*, 2003; Magni *et al.*, 1988;

Knieling *et al.*, 1995). Furthermore, patients with myasthenia gravis who attributed their illness to psychosocial factors proved to be more depressive, insecure and excitable at the time of diagnosis. Interestingly, six months later, they demonstrated a psychological stabilization and decreased depression, which was attributed to using an emotionally centred coping process (Knieling *et al.*, 1995).

Medical management of myasthenia gravis consists of administration of anticholinesterase drugs (e.g. pyridostigmine) with steadily increased dosage, until the desirable effect is obtained. Steroids are used for severe cases (Smith & Ramig, 2003). The effectiveness of thymectomy (removal of the thymus gland) remains debatable.

Most remissions occur in the first few years of the disease, but relapses are common. Neonatal myasthenia is occasionally seen in infants of affected mothers, but usually resolve in a few weeks.

REFERENCES

Aronson, A.E. (1990). *Clinical Voice Disorders* (3rd edn.). New York: Thieme Medical.

Ball, J.R.B. & Lloyd, J.H. (1971). Myasthenia gravis as hysteria. *Medical Journal of Australia*, **1**, 1018–20.

Colton, R.H. & Casper, J.K. (1990). *Understanding voice problems.* Baltimore: Williams & Williams.

Fisher, J., Parkinson, K. & Kothari, M. (2003). Self-reported depressive symptoms in myasthenia gravis. *Journal of Clinical Neuromuscular Disease*, **4**, 105–8.

Fritze, D., Hermann, C., Naiem, F., Smith, G.S. & Walford, R.L. (1974). HL-A antigens in myasthenia gravis. *The Lancet*, **1**, 240.

Garfinkle, T. & Kimmelman, C. (1982). Neurologic disorders: amyotrophic lateral sclerosis, myasthenia gravis, multiple sclerosis and poliomyelitis. *American Journal of Otolaryngology*, **3**, 204–12.

Grob, W. (1961). Myasthenia gravis. *Archives of Internal Medicine*, **108**, 615–38.

Knieling, J., Weiss, H., Faller, H. & Lang, H. (1995). Psychological causal attributions by myasthenia gravis patients: a longitudinal study of the significance of subjective illness theories after diagnosis and in follow-up. 1. *Psychotherapy, Psychosomatics, Medicine. Psychology*, **45**, 373–80.

Magni, G., Micaglio, G.F., Lalli, R. *et al.* (1988). Psychiatric disturbances associated with myasthenia gravis. *Acta Psychiatrica Scandinavica*, **77**, 443–5.

Smith, M. & Ramig, L.O. (2003). *Neurologic disorders and the voice.* In: Rubin, J., Sataloff, R. & Korovin, G. (Eds.). USA, 409–33.

Sataloff, R. & Korovin, G. (Eds.). (2003). *Diagnosis and treatment of voice disorders* (p. 409). Delmar Learning.

Stell, P.M. (Ed.). (1987). *Scott-Brown's Otolaryngology* (5th edn.). London: Butterworth & Co.

Neurofibromatosis

Rosalie E. Ferner

Guy's Hospital

Neurofibromatosis 1 (NF1) is a common autosomal dominant disease with an estimated birth incidence of 1 in 2500 and a prevalence of 1 in 4000 (Huson *et al.*, 1991). The principal and defining clinical features are café au lait patches, skinfold freckling, cutaneous neurofibromas (benign peripheral nerve sheath tumours), iris Lisch nodules (hamartomas) and characteristic bony dysplasia (Huson *et al.*, 1988; National Institutes of Health Consensus Development Conference, 1988) (Table 1). The majority of patients are diagnosed by the age of three years. NF1 arises as a spontaneous mutation in 50% of individuals and there is a wide variety of disease expression in patients with NF1, even within families. Neurofibromatosis 1 is clinically and genetically distinct from the rare condition neurofibromatosis 2, which is characterized by bilateral vestibular schwannomas (benign tumours of the eighth cranial nerve), schwannomas involving other cranial nerves, spinal nerve roots and peripheral nerves and by central nervous system meningiomas and gliomas (Evans *et al.*, 1992).

The gene for NF1 has been identified on chromosome 17q11.2 by positional cloning (Viskochil *et al.*, 1990; Wallace *et al.*, 1990) and the protein product is neurofibromin, which has high levels of expression in the brain and acts as a tumour suppressor (Gutmann *et al.*, 1991). Neurofibromin reduces cell proliferation by promoting the inactivation of the protooncogene p21RAS, which has a major role in mitogenic intracellular signalling

Table 1. Diagnostic criteria for neurofibromatosis 1

Two or more criteria are needed for diagnosis:
- Six or more café au lait patches $>15\,mm$ in adults and $>5\,mm$ in children
- Two or more neurofibromas or one plexiform neurofibroma
- Axillary or groin freckling
- Lisch nodules (iris hamartomas)
- Optic pathway glioma
- A first degree relative with NF1
- A distinctive osseus lesion such as sphenoid wing dysplasia or thinning of the long bone cortex with or without pseudoarthrosis

Source: National Institutes of Health Consensus Development Conference, 1988.

pathways. Neurofibromin also has a function in adenylate cyclase control and microtuble binding, which could be crucial for normal brain function (Guo et al., 2000; Xu, 1990).

The neurological complications of NF1 arise from tumours and malformations, as a result of deformities of the skull and skeleton and as a consequence of neurofibromas compressing peripheral nerves, spinal nerve roots and the spinal cord (Ferner, 1998). Cognitive impairment is a common and clinically important complication of NF1 and patients may present with low IQ, specific learning problems, behavioural difficulties or a combination of these manifestations (Ferner et al., 1996; North et al., 1997).

The majority of individuals with NF1 have an IQ in the low average range and the mean full scale IQ is between 89 and 94 (Ferner et al., 1996; Legius et al., 1995; North et al., 1997). Profound cognitive deficit in unusual and an IQ less than 70 occurs in 4.8% to 8% of patients, only slightly higher than in the general population (North et al., 1997). Some researchers have reported lower performance IQs than verbal IQs in children with NF1, but this discrepancy is not evident in most assessments of children or adults (North et al., 1997). There is no indication that cognitive impairment in NF1 improves with age in either cross-sectional or longitudinal studies (Hyman et al., 2003; Ferner et al., 1996).

A child with a specific learning disability, fails to attain his or her academic potential, regardless of cultural or socioeconomic background and in the absence of overt neurological, genetic or general medical problems. The disorder may be evident despite a normal or more rarely, above-average intelligence. Specific learning difficulties have been documented in 30% to 65% of children with NF1 and include visual spatial impairment, incoordination, handwriting and language difficulties, poor reading, spelling and mathematical skills (Lorch et al., 1999; Schrimsher et al., 2003). Individuals with NF1 have slower reaction times and higher error rates on continuous attention and divided attention tasks, compared with matched controls (Ferner et al., 1996).

Children with NF1 exhibit disruptive behaviour, misinterpret social cues and attention deficit hyperactivity disorder (ADHD) has been observed in 50% of young NF1 patients (Mautner et al., 2002) (see 'Hyperactivity'). In a recent study on personality, NF1 children and adolescents were less conscientious and more emotionally unstable and irritable than their peers in the general population (Prinzie et al., 2003). Poor social skills have been described in NF1 children, particularly those with ADHD. NF1 individuals have a reduced capacity for planning and organization, display inflexibility and have difficulty in selecting appropriate strategies to cope with unfamiliar and complex tasks, consistent with impaired executive function (Ferner et al., 1996).

The aetiology of the cognitive deficit in NF1 has not been elucidated. Psychiatric problems including depression, anxiety, psychosis, alcoholism and anorexia nervosa have been observed. These problems do not account for cognitive dysfunction in NF1, but, as might be anticipated, patients with anxiety and depression have slower reaction times and motor coordination (Ferner et al., 1996). Autism has been reported in NF1 individuals, but epidemiological studies do not indicate that this disorder occurs with increased frequency in NF1 (Mouridsen et al., 1992). Socio-demographic factors, macrocephaly, age and gender differences do not contribute to learning problems (Ferner et al., 1996; North et al., 1997). The presence of neurological and/or medical complications is weakly

associated with a lower mean full scale IQ in NF1 patients (Ferner et al., 1996).

A neuropathological study considered the anatomical basis of intellecutal impairment and the authors hypothesized that cognitive problems in NF1 are related to underlying migrational abnormaliites in the developing brain (Rosman & Pearce, 1967). Unidentified bright objects (UBOs) have been identified as focal areas of high signal intensity on T2 weighted MRI, predominantly in the basal ganglia, brainstem and cerebellum (Bognanno et al., 1988; Ferner et al., 1993; North et al., 1997). The lesions do not cause obvious neurological deficit and develop in the majority of children with NF1, but tend to disappear in adulthood. Their nature and significance is unclear, but they may represent aberrant myelination or gliosis (Di Paulo et al., 1995). There have been reports that the presence of UBOs is associated with cognitive dysfunction, and in some cases this was related to the site and volume of the UBOs (Joy et al., 1995; Moore et al., 1996). A recent study suggested that UBOs represent a marker for impaired fine motor performance in individuals with NF1 (Feldmann et al., 2003). However, other studies have found no association between the number, size and sites of T2-weighted hyperintensities and cognitive problems in NF1 (Ferner et al., 1993; Legius et al., 1995). In a longitudinal study, a significant decrease in the number size and intensity of UBOs on brain MRI over an eight-year period, was not mirrored by a commensurate improvement in cognitive performance in NF1 children (Hyman et al., 2003).

Mice with heterozygous mutations of the NF1 gene have exhibited similar cognitive deficits to those encountered in humans. Visual spatial problems, impaired motor coordination and attention deficit have been documented and improve with remedial training (Silva et al., 1997). Mouse models of learning problems in NF1 have suggesed that the cognitive dysfunction is due to excessive Ras activity leading to impaired long-term potentiation, in turn caused by increased GABA-mediated inhibition (Silva et al., 1997).

An increased frequency of structural brain abnormalities has been demonstrated in NF1 individuals with severe learning probems in whom there is a deletion of the whole NF1 gene (Korf et al., 1999). The authors conjecture that intellectual impairment in these patients arises from abnormal brain development as opposed to a defect of brain function associated with haploinsufficiency of the NF1 gene product.

Currently there is no specific treatment for individuals with cognitive impairment and NF1. Prompt educational assessment is advocated with appropriate remedial help and one to one tuition where possible. Children with an ADHD profile respond to judicious treatment with methylphenidate and cognitive behavioural therapy is helpful in some instances (Mautner et al., 2002) (see 'Cognitive behaviour therapy'). Recent research has demonstrated a reversal of cognitive deficits in mice when Ras activation is blocked by farneysl transferase inhibitors (Costa et al., 2002). Lovostatin, a specific inhibitor of HMG-CoA improves learning difficulties in a mouse model and has a potential therapeutic role in NF1 patients (Li et al., 2005). These latest findings have brought us a step closer to an understanding of the molecular basis for cognitive impairment in NF1, and coupled with longitudinal clinical studies and functional imaging should prepare the way for future therapy in humans.

REFERENCES

Bognanno, J.R., Edwards, M.K., Lee, T.A. *et al.* (1988). Cranial MR imaging in neurofibromatosis. *American Journal of Radiology*, **151**, 381–8.

Chapman, C.A., Waber, D.P., Bassett, N., Urion, D.K. & Korf, B.R. (1996). Neurobehavioural profiles of children with neurofibromatosis 1 referred for learning disabilities are sex-specific. *American Journal of Medical Genetics*, **67**, 127–32.

Costa, R.M., Federov, N.B., Kogan, J.H. *et al.* (2002). Mechanism for the learning deficits in a mouse model of neurofibromatosis 1. *Nature*, **415**, 526–3.

DiPaolo, D.P., Zimmerman, R.A., Rorke, L.B. *et al.* (1995). Neurofibromatosis type 1: pathologic substrate of high-signal-intensity foci in the brain. *Radiology*, **195**, 721–4.

Evans, D.G.R., Huson, S.M., Donnai, D. *et al.* (1992). A clinical study of type 2 neurofibromatosis. *Quarterly Journal of Medicine*, **84**, 603–18.

Feldman, R., Denecke, J., Grenzebach, M., Schuierer, G. & Weglage, J. (2003). Motor and cognitive function and T2-weighted MRI hyperintensities. *Neurology*, **61**, 1725–8.

Ferner, R.E., Chaudhuri, R., Bingham, J., Cox, T. & Hughes, R.A.C. (1993). MRI in neurofibromatosis 1. The nature and evolution of increased intensity T2 weighted lesions and their relationship to intellectual impairment. *Journal of Neurology, Neurosurgery, and Psychiatry*, **56**, 492–5.

Ferner, R.E., Hughes, R.A.C. & Weinman, J. (1996). Intellectual impairment in neurofibromatosis 1. *Journal of the Neurological Sciences*, **138**, 125–33.

Ferner, R.E. (1998). Clinical aspects of neurofibromatosis. In M. Upadhyaya & D.N. Cooper (Eds.). *Neurofibromatosis 1: from genotype to phenotype* (pp. 21–38). Oxford: Bios.

Guo, H.F., Tong, J., Hannan, F., Luo, L. & Zhong, Y. (2000). A neurofibromatosis 1-regulated pathway is required for learning in drosophila. *Nature*, **403**, 895–8.

Gutmann, D.H., Wood, D.L. & Collins, F.S. (1991). Identification of the neurofibromatosis type 1 gene product. *Proceedings of the National Academy of Sciences*, **88**, 9658–62.

Huson, S.M., Harper, P.S. & Compston, D.A.S. (1988). von Recklinghausen neurofibromatosis: clinical and population study in South East Wales. *Brain*, **111**, 155–81.

Huson, S.M., Clark, P., Compston, D.A.S. *et al.* (1991). A genetic study of von Recklinghausen neurofibromatosis in South East Wales. 1: Prevalence, fitness, mutation rate, and effect of parental transmission on severity. *Journal of Medical Genetics*, **26**, 704–11.

Hyman, S.L., Gill, D.S., Shores, E.A. *et al.* (2003). Natural history of cognitive deficits and their relationship to MRI T2-hyperintensities in NF1. *Neurology*, **60**, 1139–45.

Joy, P., Roberts, C., North, K. & deSilva, M. (1995). Neuropsychological function and MRI abnormalities in neurofibromatosis type 1. *Development Medicine and Child Neurology*, **37**, 906–14.

Korf, B.R., Schneider, G. & Poussaint, T.Y. (1999). Structural anomalies revealed by neuroimaging studies in the brains of patients with neurofibromatosis type 1 and large deletions. *Genetics in Medicine*, **1**, 136–40.

Legius, E., Descheemaeker, M.J., Steyaert, J. *et al.* (1995). Neurofibromatosis type 1 in childhood: correlation of MRI findings with intelligence. *Journal of Neurology, Neurosurgery, and Psychiatry*, **59**, 638–40.

Li, W., Cui, Y., Kushner, S.A. *et al.* (2005). The HMG-CoA reductase inhibitor lovostatin reverses the learning and attention deficits in a mouse model of neurofibromatosis 1. *Current Biology*, **15**, 1961–70.

Lorch, M., Ferner, R., Golding, J. & Whurr, R. (1999). The nature of speech and language impairment in adults with neurofibromatosis 1. *Journal of Neurolinguistics*, **12**, 157–65.

Mautner, V.F., Kluwe, L., Thakker, S.D. & Leark, R.A. (2002). Treatment of attention deficit hyperactivity disorder in neurofibromatosis 1. *Development Medicine and Child Neurology*, **44**, 164–70.

Moore, B.D., Slopis, J.M., Schomer, D., Jackson, E.F. & Levy, B.M. (1996). Neuropsychological significance of areas of high signal intensity on brain MRIs of children with neurofibromatosis. *Neurology*, **46**, 1660–8.

Mouridsen, S.E., Andersen, L.B., Sorensen, S.A., Rich, B. & Isager, T. (1992). Neurofibromatosis in infantile autism and other types of childhood psychoses. *Acta Paedopsychiatrica*, **55**, 15–18.

National Institutes of Health Consensus Development Conference. (1988). National Institutes of Health Consensus Development Conference Statement Neurofibromatosis. *Archieves of Neurology (Chicago)*, **45**, 575–8.

North, K.N., Riccardi, V., Samango-Sprouse, C. *et al.* (1997). Cognitive function and academic performance in neurofibromatosis. 1: consensus statement from the NF1 Cognitive Disorders Task Force. *Neurology*, **48**, 1121–7.

Ozonoff, S. (1999). Cognitive impairment in neurofibromatosis type 1. *American Journal of Medical Genetics*, **89**, 45–52.

Prinzie, P., Descheemaeker, M.J., Vogels, A. *et al.* (2003). Personality profiles of children and adolescents with neurofibromatosis type 1. *American Journal of Medical Genetics*, **118A**, 1–7.

Rosman, N.P. & Pearce, J. (1967). The brain in multiple neurofibromatosis (von Recklinghausen's disease): a suggested neuropathological basis for the associated mental defect. *Brain*, **90**, 829–38.

Schrimsher, G.W., Billingsley, R.C., Slopis, J.M. & Moore, B.D. (2003). Visual spatial performance deficits in children with neurofibromatosis 1. *American Journal of Medical Genetics*, **120A**, 326–30.

Silva, A.J., Frankland, P.W., Marowitz, Z. *et al.* (1997). A mouse model for the learning and memory deficits associated with neurofibromatosis type 1. *Nature Genetics*, **15**, 281–4.

Viskochil, D., Buchberg, A.N., Xu, G. *et al.* (1990). Deletions and a translocation interrupt a cloned gene at the neurofibromatosis type 1 locus. *Cell*, **62**, 1887–92.

Wallace, M.R., Marchuk, D.A., Anderson, L.B. *et al.* (1990). Type 1 neurofibromatosis gene: indentification of a larger transcript disrupted in three NF1 patients. *Science*, **249**, 181–6.

Xu, G.F., O'Connell, P., Viskochil, D. *et al.* (1990). The neurofibromatosis type 1 gene encodes a protein related to GAP. *Cell*, **62**, 599–608.

Xu, H. & Gutmann, D.H. (1997). Mutations in the GAP-related domain impair the ability of neurofibromin to associate with microtubules. *Brain Research*, **759**, 149–52.

Non-cardiac chest pain

Christopher Bass

John Radcliffe Hospital

Introduction

Non-cardiac chest pain (henceforth referred to as NCCP) has attracted an enormous amount of both clinical and research interest in the last five years. This has been accompanied by the publication of a number of major reviews by gastroenterologists (Botoman, 2002) as well as psychiatrists and psychologists (Thurston et al., 2001). More recently Accident and Emergency (A&E) physicians have also shown an interest in the topic (Goodacre et al., 2002), whereas cardiologists have been more concerned with rapid access chest pain clinics (Wood, 2001). What has provoked the resurgence of interest in this topic?

There are a number of possible explanations. First, the establishment of rapid access chest pain clinics in the UK has revealed that between one-half and three-quarters of patients attending these clinics do not have coronary heart disease. Second, high rates of patients with 'undifferentiated' or non-cardiac chest pain have been detected in chest pain observation units established both in the USA and the UK. Finally, there is evidence that these patients are not only a significant economic burden (Eslick et al., 2002) but also that certain interventions can reduce chest pain, consultation rates and disability (Mayou et al., 1997).

In this chapter the prevalence, diagnosis, pathophysiology, economic burden and management of patients with non-cardiac chest pain will be discussed. It is important to emphasize that the cause of NCCP is often multifactorial and that eliciting the interaction between each patients' symptom experience and interpretation is a key part of the clinical interview.

Prevalence

Non-cardiac chest pain (NCCP) occurs frequently within the general population. A recent population based survey based in the USA found that 23% of adults aged 25–74 years had NCCP, (defined as 'those who reported chest pain but did not have a history of cardiac disease' Lock et al., 1997). In an Australian population-based study of 672 residents aged 18 years or more asked to complete a validated chest pain questionnaire, 39% had experienced chest pain at some time. Of these, only 77% had a history of MI and 8% of angina (Eslick et al., 1999). Of those classified as having NCCP, most (77%) had not presented for medical care in the past 12 months.

Non-cardiac chest pain accounts for 2–5% of all admissions to accident and emergency departments, although the proportion of patients with NCCP presenting to A&E departments depends to a large extent on referral criteria. Over 50% of patients referred to cardiologists with chest pain are diagnosed as having non-cardiac

chest pain (Mayou et al., 2000). Significantly, these patients continue to report symptoms and disability six months after discharge from the clinics. More recent findings from rapid access chest pain clinics (RACPC) have revealed that between 50 to 75% of all patients seen in these clinics have NCCP. Furthermore, when RACPC is offered to all patients of any age there is a threefold increase in the patients assessed for chest pain. This suggests that increasing numbers of patients with NCCP are being referred to secondary care services.

Aetiology/pathophysiology

In all likelihood NCCP is the consequence of a combination of minor physical and psychological factors that interact. Most clinical accounts of NCCP include a variety of causes including muscloskeletal, gastro-oesophageal (mainly reflux and oesophageal dysmotility), 'micro vascular' angina and psychological causes.

Gastroenterological causes

It should be appreciated that a variety of common gastroenterological conditions usually associated with abdominal pain can occasionally present with chest pain. These include peptic ulcers, gallstones and irritable bowel syndrome (see 'Gastric and duodenal ulcers' and 'Irritable bowel syndrome'). If the history is suggestive these can be investigated using appropriate techniques (de Caestecker, 2002). This having been said, the oesophagus is the more usual focus of gastroenterological scrutiny.

Gastro oesophageal reflux remains the single commonest disorder resulting in atypical chest pain. Treatment with acid suppressive agents results in a significant improvement in chest pain in the majority of patients, and in a recent double-blind placebo controlled trial of omeprazole versus placebo a significant clinical response was noted in the patients receiving omeprazole (Achem et al., 1997), although a large placebo effect was seen, common in therapeutic trials in patients with functional upper GI disorders (see 'Placebos').

Musculoskeletal disorders

There is no doubt that musculoskeletal disorders can cause chest pain but their overall prevalence is difficult to estimate. Musculoskeletal causes of chest pain have been implicated in 13 to 19% of patients with negative cardiac studies (Wise et al., 1992). In this study 69 of 100 patients with chest pain but normal coronary angiograms had chest wall tenderness compared to none of the 25 control arthritic patients. Of particular interest in this study is that reproduction of typical chest pain occurred in only 16 of these patients. Furthermore, the exact origin of muscloskeletal pain remains obscure, but it should be appreciated that chest wall tenderness may simply be a reflection of convergence of visceral and somatic nociceptors at spinal level, in a similar fashion to the well-recognized phenomenon of abdominal tenderness elicited in painful abdominal visceral disorders.

Cardiovascular factors

In some cases the cause of pain may be related to functional abnormalities of blood flow at a microvascular level, although the clinical relevance of these remains controversial.

Psychosocial factors

Although anxiety disorders (with or without panic attacks) have been shown to be associated with non-cardiac chest pain (Katon, 1996; Fig. 2), not all patients with non-cardiac chest pain have conspicuous psychiatric disorder. The importance of identifying panic attacks or panic disorder is that these patients tend to report persistent medically unexplained symptoms and place an undue financial burden on outpatient services and hospitals as well as have a negative impact on social and vocational function if the diagnosis is not made. There are a number of useful screening questions for panic attacks that should be asked. These are shown in Box 1.

The patient may report psychological problems such as abnormal health beliefs, e.g. exaggerated fears of death, marked conviction of disease despite negative findings and intense bodily preoccupation. These abnormal illness beliefs and worries can act as maintaining factors in patients with non-cardiac pain whatever the initial cause (see also 'Lay beliefs about health and illness' and 'Symptom perception').

Pathophysiological mechanism such as hyperventilation can also contribute to symptoms (Cooke *et al.*, 1996) and, in some patients, cardio-respiratory symptoms can be provoked by using simple provocation tests. For example the breath-holding test and hyperventilation provocation test (where the patient is asked to over-breathe for 60 seconds) can reproduce chest discomfort in some patients (see 'Hyperventilation').

In addition for looking for physical signs, such as chest wall tenderness, by palpating the chest wall, it is important to examine the patient for evidence of physiological arousal involving the respiratory symptom, such as gasping or sighing respirations as well as very short breath-holding time (less than 20 seconds).

When enquiring about psychological abnormalities it is important to ask patients about experience of distressing life events as precipitants of anxiety and depressive disorders. These should be routinely sought by physicians, i.e. asking about events signifying loss, threat and rejection in the six to nine months before the

onset on the symptoms. For example, asking questions such as 'tell me about any changes or set backs that occurred in the months before your symptoms began' are useful. A component of life stress; severe and chronic threat, has been shown to have a large and consistent effect on symptom intensity over time in patients with irritable bowel syndrome (Bennett *et al.*, 1998). This and other research (e.g. Bradley *et al.*, 1993) suggests that the experience of the stressor, and efforts to deal with it, constitute the primary link between prolonged exposure to threat and changes in symptom intensity and reporting (see also 'Life events and health' and 'Stress and health').

An interactive model

Research findings therefore suggest that a multitude of somatic factors interact to produce chest-localized sensations that it may act as a stimulus to misinterpretation and pain. Thus, gastro-oesophageal reflux and occasionally oesophageal spasm are common triggers, as are hyperventilation, chronic obstructive airways disease and intercostal muscle spasm. All these factors can cause chest discomfort. A crucial factor for determining the way in which these sensations are interpreted are previous experience, e.g. exposure to family members or others with heart disease, and previous illness experience, e.g. heart or lung disease as a child. Recent distressing life events may act as factors to provoke increased arousal and low mood, which may lead to physiological changes and bodily sensations such as palpitations and chest discomfort. These may then become a focus for somatic preoccupation and concern about underlying heart disease. Subsequent sensations of chest pain, from whatever cause, may then be interpreted by the patient as signs of disease, especially in the presence of adverse and ongoing psychosocial circumstances.

The importance of iatrogenic or physician-induced factors should never be under estimated. For example, in one-third of patients in one well-known study the discovery of a systolic murmur or tachycardia by physicians was ascribed incorrectly to heart disease, yet these patients with normal hearts were advised to restrict activity (Wood, 1941). Inappropriate treatment of non-cardiac chest pain with anti-anginal medication is also ill-advised, and it is worth noting that it is very difficult to 'undiagnose' angina (Dart *et al.*, 1983).

Management

The aim for early and effective intervention is crucial, but patients vary not only in terms of the frequency and severity of symptoms and associated disability but also in their needs for explanation and treatment of their physical and psychological problems. For this reason management needs to be flexible. Patients may find a factsheet helpful (see Price *et al.*, in press).

Avoiding iatrogenic worries

A consultation for chest pain is inherently worrying. Inevitably, many patients assume that they have severe heart disease that will have major adverse effects on their life. These concerns may be greatly increased by delays in investigation, by comments or behaviours by doctors and by contradictory and inconsistent comments.

Communication

Problems in the care of patients with chest pain often arise from failures in communication between primary and secondary care. Lack of information and contradictory and inconsistent advice makes it less likely that patients and their families will gain a clear understanding of the diagnosis and treatment plan. It is important to make sure that information is passed on to and understood by patients and relatives (see 'Healthcare professional–patient communication').

Effective reassurance

Those with mild or brief symptoms may improve after negative investigation and simple reassurance. Further hospital attendance may then be unnecessary. Others with more severe symptoms and illness concerns will benefit from a follow-up visit four to six weeks after the cardiac clinic visit (or A&E/emergency room visit), which allows time for more discussion and explanations. This may be with either a gastroenterology or cardiac nurse in the outpatient clinic or with a doctor in primary care. It also provides a valuable opportunity to identify patients with recurrent or persistent symptoms who may require further help (see below) (see 'Reassurance').

Specialist treatments

Psychological and psychopharmacological treatment should be considered for patients with continuing symptoms and disability, especially if these are associated with abnormal health beliefs, depressed mood, panic attacks, or other symptoms, fatigue or palpitations. Both cognitive–behavioural therapy (Mayou *et al.*, 1997; van Peski-Oosterban *et al.*, 1999) and selective serotonin re-uptake inhibitors (Varia *et al.*, 2000) have been shown to be effective. A recent systematic review of psychological interventions in the management of non-specific chest pain suggested a modest benefit, particularly for those using a cognitive behavioural framework (Kisely *et al.*, 2005) (see 'Cognitive behaviour therapy').

Tricyclic antidepressants are helpful in reducing reports of pain in patients with chest pain and normal coronary arteries (Cannon *et al.*, 1994). However, patients often find them unacceptable in the context of NCCP because of side effects, even at low dosage. Sertraline may be an effective alternative according to one randomized trail in NCCP and certainly appears to cause fewer side effects.

Organizing care

Because of the heterogeneity of the needs of patients with non-cardiac chest pain, a 'stepped' approach to care has been proposed. The cardiologist working in a busy outpatient clinic may require access to additional resources if he nor she is to provide adequate management for the large numbers of patients with non-cardiac chest pain, some of whom may have co-existing angina or be recovering from coronary artery bypass graft surgery. One way of doing this is to employ a specialist cardiac nurse who has received additional training in the management of these problems. The nurse can provide patient education, simple psychological intervention and routine follow-up in a separate part of the cardiac outpatient clinic. For those patients who require more specialist psychological help it is important for the cardiac department (possibly the cardiac nurse) to collaborate with the clinical psychology or liaison psychiatry service.

Some departments may prefer to offer treatment as an out patient using a group cognitive behavioural approach. In this way more patients can be managed with fewer treatment resources. Potts *et al.* (1999) demonstrated that a psychological treatment package (education, relaxation, breathing training, graded exposure to activity and challenging automatic thoughts about heart disease) was not only feasible, but also reduced pain, psychological morbidity and disability, and improved exercise tolerance.

Long-term management

In many patients the symptoms can become chronic and difficult to manage, and in this group psychological factors are likely to be important (Miller *et al.*, 2001). There is evidence that a strong clinician–patient interaction leads to not only greater compliance and satisfaction, but also to a reduced number of return visits for IBS-related symptoms (Owens *et al.*, 1995). A key component of this 'physician–patient interaction' is the physician's awareness of the patient's psychosocial history, which includes enquiry about relevant life events, exploring psychosocial history and eliciting patients' concerns. Moreover, patient's complaints improve more when they visit the same clinician throughout the outpatient consultations and when they are satisfied with the consultations (van Dulmen *et al.*, 1997). In some patients several consultations may be required to help them make tentative connections between psychological factors, life stresses and the pain (Guthrie & Thomson, 2002). Even in the absence of conspicuous mood disorder, low dose tricyclic antidepressants are effective long-term treatments in patients with functional chest pain (Prakash & Clouse, 1999).

REFERENCES

Achem, S., Kolts, B., Macmath, T. *et al.* (1997). Effects of omeprazole versus placebo in treatment of non cardiac chest pain and gastroesphageal reflux. *Digestive Diseases and Sciences,* **42,** 2138–45.

Bass, C. & Mayou, R. (2002). Chest pain. *British Medical Journal,* **325,** 588–91.

Bennett, E.J., Tennant, C.C., Piesse, C., Badcock, C.A. & Kellow, J.E. (1998). Level of chronic life stress predicts clinical outcome in irritable bowel syndrome. *Gut*, **43**, 256–61.

Botoman, V.A. (2002). Non-cardiac chest pain. *Journal of Clinical Gastroenterology*, **34**, 6–14.

Bradley, L.A., Richter, J., Pulliam, T. *et al.* (1993). The relationship between stress and symptoms of gastrooesophageal reflux: the influence of psychological factors. *American Journal of Gastroenterology*, **88**, 11–19.

Cannon, R.O., Quyyumi, A.A., Mincemoyer, R. *et al.* (1994). Imipramine in patients with chest pain despite normal coronary angiograms. *New England Medical Journal*, **330**, 1411–17.

Cooke, R.A., Auggiansah, A., Wang, J., Chambers, J.B. & Owen, W. (1996). Hyperventilation and oesophageal dysmotility in patients with non-cardiac chest pain. *American Journal of Gastroenterology*, **91**, 480–4.

Clouse, R., Lustman, P., Eckert, T. *et al.* (1987). Low dose trazodone for symptomatic patients with oesophageal contraction abnormalities: a double blind, placebo controlled trial. *Gastroenterology*, **92**, 1027–36.

Dart, A.M., Davies, H.A., Griffith, J. & Henderson, A.H. (1983). Does it help to undiagnosed angina? *European Heart Journal*, **4**(7), 461–2.

de Caestecker, J. (2002). Diagnosis and management of gastrointestinal causes of chest pain of uncertain origin. *Clinical Medicine*, **2**, 402–5.

Eslick, G., Coulshed, D.S. & Tally, N.J. (2002). The burden of illness of non-cardiac chest pain. *Ailmentary Pharmacology and Therapeutics*, **16**, 1217–23.

Eslick, G.D., Talley, N.J., Young, L.J. & Jones, M.P. (1999). Non-cardiac chest pain in the population prevalence and impact (abstract). *Journal of Gastroenterology and Hepatology*, **14**, A214.

Goodacre, S., Morriss, F.M., Campbell, S., Arnold, J. & Angelini, K. (2002). A propspective, observational study of a chest pain observation unit in a British hospital. *Emergency Medicine Journal*, **19**, 117–21.

Guthrie, E. & Thompson, D. (2002). Abdominal pain and functional gastro-intestinal disorders. *British Medical Journal*, **325**, 701–3.

Katon, W. (1996). Panic disorder; relationship to high medical utilisation, unexplained physical symptoms, and medical costs. *Journal of Clinical Psychiatry*, **57**, (suppl.) 10, 11–18.

Kisely, S., Campbell, L. & Skerritt, P. (2005). Psychological interventions for symptomatic management of non-specific chest pain in patients with normal coronary anatomy. *Cochrane Database Systematic Review Jan 25*, **1**: CD004101.

Lock, G.R., Talley, N.J., Rett, S. *et al.* (1997). Prevalence and clinical spectrum of gastro oesophageal reflux in the community. *Gastroenterology*, **112**, 1448–52.

Mayou, R., Bryant, B., Sanders, D. *et al.* (1997). A controlled trial of cognitive behavioural therapy for non-cardiac chest pain. *Psychological Medicine*, **27**, 1021–31.

Mayou, R., Bass, C., Hart, G., Tyndel, S. & Bryant, B. (2000). Can clinical assessment of chest pain be made mopre therapeutic? *Quarterly Journal of Medicine*, **93**, 805–11.

Mayou, R., Bass, C. & Bryant, B. (1999). Management of non-cardiac chest pain: from research to clinical practice. *Heart*, **81**, 387–92.

Miller, A., North, C., Clouse, R. *et al.* (2001). The associations of irritable bowel syndrome and somatisation disorder. *American Journal of Clinical Psychiatry*, **13**, 25–30.

Owens, D., Nelson, D. & Talley, N. (1995). The irritable bowel syndrome: long-term prognosis and the physician–patient interaction. *Annals of Internal Medicine*, **122**, 107–12.

Potts, S., Lewin, R., Fox, K. & Johnstone, E. (1999). Group psychological treatment

for chest pain with normal coronary arteries. *Quarterly Journal of Medicine*, **92**, 81–6.

Prakash, C. & Clouse, R. (1999). Long-term outcome from tricyclic antidepressant treatment of functional chest pain. *Digestive Diseases and Sciences*, **44**, 2373–9.

Price, J. *et al.* (in press). Developing a rapid access chest pain clinic: qualitative studies of patients' needs and experiences. *Journal of Psychosomatic Research*.

Sutcliffe, S.J., Fox, K.F. & Wood, D.A. (2000). How to set up and run a Rapid Access Chest Pain Clinic. *British Journal of Cardiology*, **11**, 692–702.

Thurston, R.C., Keefe, F.J., Bradley, L., Krishnhan, K. & Caldwell, D.S. (2001). Chest Pain in the absence of coronary artery disease: a biopsychosocial perspective. *Pain*, **93**, 95–100.

Van Dulmen, A., Fennis, J., Mokkink, H. *et al.* (1997). Persisting improvement in complaint-related cognitions initiated during medical consultations in functional abdominal complaints. *Psychological Medicine*, **27**, 725–9.

van Peski-Oosterbaan, A. S., Spinhoven, P., van Rood, Y. *et al.* (1999). Cognitive behavioural therapy for non-cardiac chest pain: a randomised trial. *American Journal of Medicine*, **132**, 424–9.

Varia, I., Logue, E., O'Connor, C. *et al.* (2000). Randomized trial of sertraline in patients with unexplained chest pain of non-cardiac origin. *American Heart Journal*, **140**, 367–72.

Wise, C.M., Semble, E.L. & Dalton, C.B. (1992). Musculoskeletal Chest Wall Syndrome in patients with non-cardiac chest pain: a study of 100 patients. *Archives of Physical Medicine and Rehabilitation*, **73**, 147–9.

Wood, S. (2001). Rapid assessment of chest pain. *British Medical Journal*, **323**, 586–7.

Wood, P. (1941). De Costa's Syndrome (or effort syndrome). *British Medical Journal*, I, 767–72, 805–11, 845–51.

Obesity

Jennifer J. Thomas and Kelly D. Brownell

Yale University

Introduction

A critical turning point in the history of human food consumption has become evident. With famine and undernutrition the central food issues for much of human history, we now face the opposite: overnutrition and obesity. The number of individuals who are overnourished now equals or exceeds the number undernourished (WHO, 1998), and the prevalence of obesity is increasing in every corner of the world. The percentage of individuals in the USA who are either overweight or obese rose from 55.9% in 1994 to 65.7% in 2002 (Flegal *et al.*, 2002; Hedley *et al.*, 2004) leading the Centers for Disease Control and Prevention to apply the word 'epidemic' (CDC, 2004).

The most widely used index of obesity is the body mass index (BMI), which is calculated as weight in kilograms divided by height in meters squared (i.e. kg/m^2). The World Health Organization defined obesity as a BMI $\geq 30\,kg/m^2$, given epidemiological data showing that mortality at this weight is increased by 30% (Manson *et al.*, 1995). Premature deaths associated with obesity are primarily attributable to cardiovascular disease, Type II diabetes and several cancers (Pi-Sunyer, 1993) (see chapters on 'Coronary heart disease' and 'Diabetes mellitus'). Obesity also carries many additional complications including hypertension, sleep apnoea, gall bladder disease and osteoarthritis (see 'Hypertension', 'Sleep apnoea' and 'Osteoarthritis'). Some, but not all, data suggest that obesity is associated with increased risk for psychological distress, including binge eating and depression. Because obese individuals are considered personally responsible for their condition, psychosocial complications include prejudice and discrimination in important areas of living such as education, employment and healthcare (Puhl & Brownell, 2001). The annual cost of obesity to society in the USA alone, calculating direct costs such as preventative and treatment services and indirect costs such as the value of lost wages due to disability and early mortality, is estimated to be $70 billion annually (Colditz, 1999), which constitutes 9.4% of the national healthcare expenditure. Beyond these costs are the realities of human suffering produced by the physical and psychosocial impact of being overweight.

Aetiology: the toxic environment

Body weight is determined by a complex interaction of biological and environmental factors. Genetic predisposition makes weight gain more likely in some people than others, and helps account, to some extent, for a host of factors such as susceptibility to related diseases. Heritability estimates of obesity range from 25–40% (Bouchard, 1994; Price, 2002). A landmark study found that weights of adult adoptees more closely resembled the weights of their biological than their adoptive parents (Stunkard *et al.*, 1986). Investigators have recently identified at least five single-gene defects which produce obesity in laboratory animals, perhaps most notably the leptin deficiency marked by the ob/ob genotype in mice (Zhang *et al.*, 1994). However, it is unlikely that most human obesity results from simple Mendellian determinism. Research suggests that genes confer a wide range of 'obesigenic' vulnerabilities, including differences in food preferences, resting metabolic rate, weight gain in response to overfeeding and body distribution of excess adipose tissue.

Genes, however, are not the cause of the obesity epidemic. Even the highest heritability estimates (in the range of 40%) leave the majority of population variance in weight to be explained by non-genetic factors. In addition, genes cannot explain why people from less obese countries gain weight when moving to more obese countries or why the prevalence of obesity in many countries has increased year by year. The most parsimonious explanation for the recent upsurge in obesity is the modern environment. Strong environmental forces converge to make unhealthy food choices almost inevitable. Unhealthy foods taste good and connect with biological preferences for sugar and fat, but are also convenient, highly accessible, promoted heavily and inexpensive; exactly the factors that should apply to healthy foods but do not. The confluence of these characteristics is so troubling that one of us (KB) has labelled modern conditions a 'toxic environment' (Brownell, 1994).

Human preferences for energy-dense foods (such as those high in sugar and fat) are either inborn or learned very early in life (Birch, 1999). The palatability of highly caloric foods may have bestowed an evolutionary advantage on our hunter-gatherer ancestors, who needed to consume as much as possible when food was plentiful to avoid starvation. In addition to being appetizing, calorie-dense foods are available as never before, not only in convenience stores, vending machines and fast food restaurants, but also in locations previously unrelated to food retailing, such as schools, pharmacies, hospitals and petrol (gas) stations. Even small changes in accessibility can alter consumption volume: in one experiment, secretaries given candy jars to keep on their desks ate nearly three times as many candies as secretaries who had the jars placed on another desk just two meters away (Painter *et al.*, 2002).

The promotion of unhealthy foods is stunning. In 1998 alone, soft drinks companies spent $115.5 million on advertising, and fast food giant McDonald's spent more than $1 billion. These figures tower over the mere $1 million spent by the National Cancer Institute to promote the '5 a day' fruit and vegetable campaign (Nestle & Jacobson, 2000). The average American child views

10 000 food advertisements annually on television alone; nearly all are for foods such as sugared cereals, soft drinks, fast foods heavily processed snacks and sweets/candy. Joining this traditional marketing are high levels of 'guerrilla marketing' (e.g. product placements in movies and video games, virtual placements of products in re-runs of television shows and infiltration of schools).

The economics of food also conspire to create unhealthy eating. Heavy and selective subsidies of the agriculture industry (especially the corn industry) have many effects, including artificial support of a meat-based diet and low costs for sweetening foods with high fructose corn syrup. The low cost of unhealthy foods compared with better alternatives creates an inverse relationship between energy density and cost and a positive and unfortunate relationship between nutrient density and cost, making it difficult for poor individuals to buy healthy foods. Price disparities are so great that some experts have equated dietary recommendations aimed at low income families to 'economic elitism' (Drewnowski & Barratt-Fornell, 2004).

It is probably no coincidence that meals and waistlines are being 'supersized' in parallel; an increase in portion size has coincided with the increase in obesity. Current marketplace portions of ready-to-eat foods such as bagels, hamburgers, muffins and soft drinks exceed US Food and Drug Administration serving size recommendations by two- to eight-fold (Young & Nestle, 2003). The original Hershey's chocolate bar weighed 0.6 oz.; current versions range from 1.6 to 8 oz. Studies show that consumption increases with increasing portion size. Individuals presented with increasingly large servings of potato chips on succeeding days ate more chips when served larger portions and did not compensate by altering their caloric intake at dinnertime three hours later (Rolls *et al.*, 2004). This phenomenon has been demonstrated in both children and adults and applies to many foods eaten under many circumstances. There is some evidence that people compensate less well at subsequent meals when between meal snacks come in liquid rather than solid foods (Almiron-Roig *et al.*, 2003), making soft drinks a logical target for change.

In addition to the convergence of factors encouraging a high calorie diet, the tacit promotion of sedentary behaviour is yet another manifestation of the toxic environment. Despite experts' exercise recommendations of 30 minutes per day, 28% of US adults do not engage in any physical activity and another 28% are not regularly active (Mokdad *et al.*, 2001). For much of history, individuals survived by being physically active (acquiring food was necessary and demanding). People were then paid to be active because work required physical labour. Today, energy-saving devices ranging from tractors to computers mean that individuals must expend leisure time and financial resources to join health clubs or purchase exercise equipment in order to be active. Additionally, unsafe, busy streets and suburban sprawl discourage pedestrian traffic. Although 25% of all trips are shorter than one mile, three-quarters of these are made by automobile (Koplan & Dietz, 1999).

In sum, genetic factors may predispose individuals to weight gain, but aggregate environmental pressures promoting an increasingly energy-dense diet and sedentary lifestyle bring that vulnerability to fruition. Put more succinctly, 'genes load the gun, the environment pulls the trigger' (Bray, 1998).

Overcoming obesity: the tension between treatment and prevention

Given the negative health impact of excess weight, it is imperative that individuals who are already obese receive adequate care. Research supports a stepped approach in which treatment intensity and expense is proportional to degree of overweight (NIH/NHLB, 1998). Obese individuals are encouraged to reduce weight by increasing physical activity and consuming an appropriate diet, but those at higher BMIs may require increasingly structured interventions to that end. For example, individuals with a BMI < 27 may benefit from self-directed diet and exercise efforts or brief weight-management counselling from a primary care physician. Those somewhat heavier could consider embarking on a self-help or behavioural weight loss programme. At BMI ≥ 30, individuals may benefit from pharmacotherapy or a very low-calorie diet, and, at BMI ≥ 40, bariatric surgery becomes an option. Utilizing this treatment-matching algorithm, it is hoped that maximum health benefits can be achieved at minimum risk to the patient. It must be noted, however, that longitudinal studies comparing treatments across BMI categories are necessary to validate this approach.

Within the stepped care paradigm, behavioural treatments are among the most conservative and produce modest but perhaps the most sustainable weight losses. Well replicated findings suggest that a 20-week course of group behavioural treatment induces a 9% reduction in initial body weight; without further treatment, individuals typically regain one-third of their lost weight in the ensuing year (Wadden & Foster, 2000). Very low calorie diets (400–800 calories/day) result in double the weight loss of the 1200–1500 calories/day meal plan of traditional behavioural approaches, but are associated with such rapid weight regain that there is no significant difference between the two treatments at two-year follow-up (Torgerson *et al.*, 1997). One of the more robust findings of the behavioural literature is that physical activity is the best predictor of sustained losses (Pronk & Wing, 1994) (see 'Physical activity and health' and 'Physical activity interventions').

Pharmacotherapy represents the next most intensive approach. Two primary medications are approved by the US Food and Drug Administration for weight reduction and maintenance. Combined with improved diet, both drugs produce modest weight losses. Sibutramine, which acts on receptors in the hypothalamus to increase satiety, produced a 7% reduction in initial weight at one year compared with a 2% reduction in patients assigned to placebo (Lean, 1997). Orlistat, which partially blocks the absorption of dietary fat, produced a 10% loss in contrast to 6% with placebo (Davidson *et al.*, 1999). Neither medication alone has been shown to be superior to behavioural interventions, although it is possible that the combination of behaviour therapy and pharmacotherapy may improve outcome.

For people double their ideal body weight or more, obesity surgery can be impressive. Different surgical methods have been used over the years, moving from the intestine initially to the stomach at the present time. Surgical advances have greatly reduced complications, improved weight losses and reduced costs (e.g. laparoscopic surgery has decreased hospital stays). Obesity surgery produces striking weight losses (100 pounds or more in many cases), good maintenance and clear changes in risk factors.

Initial treatments set the goal of helping patients achieve ideal weight (Foster, 1995), but large weight losses are rare and difficult to maintain. In addition, it is now clear that even small reductions of 5–15% of initial body weight may help reduce (but certainly not eliminate) the health complications of obesity such as hypertension and Type II diabetes (Blackburn, 1995). Unfortunately, such small improvements are seldom satisfying to patients and often lead to unhappiness and abandonment of the diet and exercise regimen. Thus, given that current treatments are either not very effective (e.g. behaviour therapy, pharmacotherapy) or too expensive to implement broadly (e.g. surgery), they should be conceptualized as needed care for the afflicted but not sufficient to reduce prevalence. Prevention must become the priority and environmental change the means to that end.

Public policy approaches

Public policy has a profound impact on diet and activity patterns of the population. There are countless examples, including the following: (1) agriculture subsidies that affect the prices of healthy and unhealthy foods; (2) trade policy that affects the availability and price of particular foods in different countries; (3) a failure to regulate food advertising, thus offering food companies unfettered access to children; (4) education policy that fails to connect healthy eating and physical activity with academic performance; and (5) community planning policies in which neighbourhoods are constructed in ways that discourage physical activity.

The environment conspires to damage eating, inhibit movement and overwhelm personal responsibility. Policy change is a powerful means for improving the environment, but only recently has this concept been considered in the realm of obesity prevention. Relatively little research has evaluated the impact of policy change, hence it is difficult to establish priorities. Based on what is known about the determinants of obesity, combined with experience in areas such as tobacco control, it is possible to propose certain approaches as a beginning.

Policy interventions span a wide range of possibilities affecting issues as broad as economic policy to local issues such as selling soft drinks in schools. These have been discussed in detail elsewhere (Brownell, 1986; Brownell & Horgen, 2004; Nestle, 2002; Nestle & Jacobson, 2000; Schmitz & Jeffery, 2000). Examples will be given here.

The first two examples pertain to creating a healthier food environment for children. One is to restrict children's food advertising. The high exposure, combined with research showing that such advertising has a negative impact on eating, suggests that reduction would be helpful (Brownell & Horgen, 2004; Horgen et al., 2001; Story & French, 2004). Young children do not have the cognitive ability to distinguish between advertising and regular programming, placing them at particular risk.

Banning soft drinks from schools would be another potential public policy solution to protect children. A single 20 oz bottle of a typical cola drink contains 15 teaspoons of sugar. Soft drink consumption is associated with weight gain, displacement of milk consumption and dental cavities (American Academy of Pediatrics, 2004). Unfortunately, many school districts turn to 'pouring rights' contracts with soft drink companies to raise money for academic needs and extra-curricular activities. Unhealthy eating is then both promoted and modelled in the school environment. Replacing soft drinks with healthier beverages might help reverse this troubling trend.

A third potential public policy approach would be to tax unhealthy foods. Given the inverse relationship between energy density and cost, current pricing schemes encourage the consumption of high-calorie, processed foods to the exclusion of fresh fruits and vegetables. A tax on poor foods could work not only to decrease consumption of these foods but also to raise funds for public health programmes. One comprehensive review suggested that even small levies, such as one penny per can of soda drink, could raise substantial revenues (Jacobson & Brownell, 2000).

A final public policy solution would be to invest in community improvements that would promote the integration of physical activity into everyday life. For example, municipal funds could be directed towards building parks and sidewalks. New urban developments could eliminate homogenizing zoning requirements which discourage walking. Indeed, even simple, inexpensive interventions such as posting signs encouraging the use of stairs rather than escalators have demonstrated some effectiveness (Brownell et al., 1980) (see also 'Health promotion').

Conclusion

By any standard, obesity is a global crisis. The death, disability and personal suffering attributed to poor diet, physical inactivity, and weight gain are startling. Extrapolating ahead from the condition of today's children, the picture becomes even more grim.

Society's response, particularly in individualist cultures like that of the United States, has been to blame obesity on the individual, ascribe negative personal characteristics as the cause, and resist changing conditions which make it so difficult for people to eat better and increase activity. The resistance to change is profound because of the political influence of massive food and agriculture businesses.

Treatments for obesity may help those in need but show no promise as a public health intervention. Lack of effectiveness and high cost limit the impact and number of people who can be treated, thus making prevention a priority. The default approach, to count on education in the hope that people will be persuaded to change, has thus far demonstrated limited impact. Public policy change, beginning with the concept of protecting children from a toxic environment, is likely to have the largest and most rapid influence. Courageous action, based in science and buffered from special interests, will be necessary to reverse the troubling deterioration in diet, physical activity and weight seen around the world.

(See also 'Diet and health' and 'Physical activity and health'.)

Almiron-Roig, E., Chen, Y. & Drewnowski, A. (2003). Liquid calories and the failure of satiety: how good is the evidence? *Obesity Reviews*, **4**, 201–12.

American Academy of Pediatrics. (2004). Soft drinks in schools. *Pediatrics*, **113**, 152–4.

Birch, L.L. (1999). Development of food preferences. *Annual Nutrition Review*, **19**, 41–62.

Blackburn, G.L. (1995). Effect of degree of weight loss on health benefits. *Obesity Research*, **3**(Suppl.), 211–16.

Bouchard, C.B. (1994). Genetics of obesity: Overview and research direction. In C.B. Bouchard (Ed.). *The genetics of obesity* (pp. 223–33). Boca Raton, FL: CRC Press.

Bray, G.A. (1998). *Contemporary diagnosis and management of obesity*. Newton, PA: Handbooks in Healthcare.

Brownell, K.D. (1986). Public health approaches to obesity and its management. *Annual Review of Public Health*, **7**, 521–33.

Brownell, K.D. (1994). Get slim with higher taxes (Op Ed.). *New York Times*, **December 15**, A-29.

Brownell, K.D., Stunkard, A.J. & Albaum, J.M. (1980). Evaluation and modification of exercise patterns in the natural environment. *American Journal of Psychiatry*, **137**, 1540–5.

Brownell, K.D. & Horgen, K.B. (2004). *Food fight: the inside story of the food industry, America's obesity crisis, and what we can do about it*. New York: McGraw-Hill.

Centers for Disease Control and Prevention. Obesity and overweight. Retrieved November 18, 2004, from www.cdc.gov/nccdphp/dnpa/obesity/index.htm.

Colditz, G.A. (1999). Economic costs of obesity and inactivity. *Medicine and Science in Sports and Exercise*, **31**(Suppl. 1), S663–7.

Davidson, M.H., Hauptman, J., DiGirolamo, M. et al. (1999). Weight control and risk factor reduction in obese subjects treated for 2 years with Orlistat: A randomized controlled trial. *Journal of the American Medical Association*, **281**, 235–42.

Drewnowski, A. & Barratt-Fornell, A. (2004). Do healthier diets cost more? *Nutrition Today*, **29**, 161–8.

Flegal, K.M., Carroll, M.D., Ogden, C.L. & Johnson, C.L. (2002). Prevalence and trends in obesity among U.S. adults, 1999–2000. *Journal of the American Medical Association*, **288**, 1723–7.

Foster, G.D. (1995). Reasonable weights: determinants, definition, and practice. In D.B. Allison & F.X. Pi-Sunyar (Eds.). *Obesity treatment: establishing goals, improving outcomes, and reviewing the research agenda* (pp. 35–44). New York: Plenum.

Hedley, A.A., Ogden, C.L., Johnson, C.L. et al. (2004). Prevalence of overweight and obesity among U.S. children, adolescents, and adults, 1999–2002. *Journal of the American Medical Association*, **291**, 2847–50.

Horgen, K.D., Choate, M. & Brownell, K.D. (2001). Television and children's nutrition. In D.G. Singer & J.L. Singer (Eds.). *Handbook of children and the media* (pp. 447–61). San Francisco: Sage.

Jacobson, M.F. & Brownell, K.D. (2000). Small taxes on soft drinks and snack foods to promote health. *American Journal of Public Health*, **90**, 854–7.

Koplan, J.P. & Dietz, W.H. (1999). Caloric imbalance and public health policy. *Journal of the American Medical Association*, **282**, 1579–81.

Lean, M.E.J. (1997). Sibutramine – A review of clinical efficacy. *International Journal of Obesity*, **21**(Suppl.), 30–6.

Manson, J.E., Willett, W.C., Stampfer, M.J. et al. (1995). Body weight and mortality among women. *New England Journal of Medicine*, **333**, 677–85.

Mokdad, A.H., Bowman, B.A., Ford, E.S. et al. (2001). The continuing epidemics of obesity and diabetes in the United States. *Journal of the American Medical Association*, **286**, 1195–1200.

National Institutes of Health/National Heart, Lung, and Blood Institute. (1998). Clinical guidelines on the identification, evaluation, and treatment of overweight andobesity in adults: the evidence report. *Obesity Research*, **6**(Suppl.), 5–210.

Nestle, M. (2002). *Food politics: how the food industry influences nutrition and health*. Berkeley, CA: University of California Press.

Nestle, M. & Jacobson, M.F. (2000). Halting the obesity epidemic: a public health policy approach. *Public Health Reports*, **115**, 12–24.

Painter, J.E., Wansink, B. & Hieggelke, J.B. (2002). How visibility and convenience influence candy consumption. *Appetite*, **33**, 237–8.

Pi-Sunyer, F.X. (1993). Medical hazards of obesity. *Annals of Internal Medicine*, **119**, 655–60.

Price, R.A. (2002). Genetics and common obesities: background, current status, strategies and future prospects. In T.A. Wadden & A.J. Stunkard (Eds.). *Handbook of obesity treatment* (pp. 73–94). New York: Guilford Press.

Pronk, N.P. & Wing, R.R. (1994). Physical activity and long-term maintenance of weight loss. *Obesity Research*, **2**, 587–99.

Puhl, R. & Brownell, K.D. (2001). Bias, discrimination, and obesity. *Obesity Research*, **9**, 788–805.

Rolls, B.J., Roe, L.S., Kral, T.V.E., Meengs, J.S. & Wall, D.E. (2004). Increasing the portion size of a packaged snack increases energy intake in men and women. *Appetite*, **42**, 63–9.

Schmitz, M.K. & Jeffery, R.W. (2000). Public health interventions for the prevention and treatment of obesity. *Medical Clinics of North America*, **84**, 491–512.

Story, M. & French, S. (2004). Food advertising and marketing directed at children and adolescents in the U.S. *International Journal of Behavioral Nutrition and Physical Activity*, **1**, 1–17.

Stunkard, A.J., Sorensen, T.I., Hanis, C. et al. (1986). An adoption study of human obesity. *New England Journal of Medicine*, **314**, 193–8.

Torgerson, J.S., Lissner, L., Lindross, A.K., Kruijer, H. & Sjostrom, L. (1997). VLCD plus dietary and behavioral support versus support alone in the treatment of severe obesity: a randomised two-year clinical trial. *International Journal of Obesity*, **21**, 987–94.

Wadden, T.A. & Foster, G.D. (2000). Behavioral treatment of obesity. *Medical Clinics of North America*, **84**, 441–61.

World Health Organization. (1998). Obesity: preventing and managing the global epidemic. Geneva, Switzerland: World Health Organization.

Young, L.R. & Nestle, M. (2003). Expanding portion sizes in the US marketplace: implications for nutrition counseling. *Journal of the American Dietetic Association*, **103**, 231–4.

Zhang, Y., Proenca, R., Maffei, M. et al. (1994). Positional cloning of the mouse obese gene and its human homologue. *Nature*, **372**, 425–32.

Oral care and hygiene

Gerry Humphris

University of St Andrews

Oral diseases and prevention

Virtually without parallel, individual action can successfully prevent the onset of two major oral diseases; dental caries and periodontal disease. Dental caries is a localized progressive decay of the tooth, marked by the demineralization of the enamel by organic acids. These acids develop owing to the fermentation of carbohydrates in the diet by plaque bacteria. A cavity is produced by the continued destruction of the tooth mineral and protein, resulting eventually in the tooth pulp and the surrounding tissues becoming infected. Periodontal disease is an inflammatory condition of the connective tissues which support the tooth and gums (gingivae). It is the result of toxins produced from bacterial plaque which initiates an inflammatory reaction. The tissue breakdown which ensues is due to the inflammatory response being left unchecked. The bone supporting the tooth atrophies leading to high tooth mobility and eventual tooth loss. Although the two diseases are not ordinarily life-threatening, they do influence the quality of life (Locker, 2004; McGrath & Bedi, 2004) and the economic efficiency of nations through the loss of millions of working hours each year, costs associated with treating the diseases and debilitating pain from the diseases themselves (Miller *et al.*, 1975).

Caries and periodontal disease are ubiquitous. The World Health Organization report on oral health presents a comprehensive picture of the extent of both diseases, especially in industrialized countries. (Petersen, 2003). Approximately 60–90% of school children have been affected and almost all adults (above 95%). Most children worldwide show evidence of early signs of periodontal disease. Severe periodontitis is found in about 5–15% of the global population. This condition is often responsible for premature tooth loss. It is clear that lifestyle has a major impact on the incidence of both these diseases, especially, frequent intake of sugary foods and drinks, tobacco and alcohol consumption. A good example is smoking behaviour and its link with periodontal diseases (see, for example, 'Cancer: head and neck'). Over half of the incidence of this disease in adults is attributable to smoking. (Tomar & Asma, 2000) From an international perspective, models are being developed which include behavioural risk factors to understand caries levels across varied communities. (Pine *et al.*, 2004)

There are a number of other conditions which are typically seen in oral medicine units such as lichen planus, burning mouth syndrome, candida and oral cancer. Malfunctioning saliva glands can produce dry mouth (Sjogen's syndrome). Craniofacial conditions require psychological issues to be explored such as temporo mandibular dysfunction and body dysmorphic disorder. A review of the psychological factors implicated in nine oral health disorders encourages psychologists and other social scientists to collaborate with oral health specialists (Albino, 2002). The major emphasis of a great deal of this work has been to develop and evaluate a variety of methods of changing individual preventive health behaviours. These behaviours can be divided into two main groups. First, those that improve oral hygiene and include tooth brushing, flossing (and other mechanical aids to remove plaque) and dieting to reduce sugar intake and, secondly, those behaviours that are seeking professional advice, such as attendance to oral screening programmes and dental check-ups. Two sections below summarize some of the important psychological findings associated with each of the two groups of preventive health behaviours. A short section will follow noting some of the changes in oral health and how psychologists are responding.

Psychological approaches to oral hygiene

The encouragement of new preventive health behaviours such as the use of fluoride mouth rinses, has demonstrated the limited positive effect of informative campaigns with young people (Kegeles & Lund, 1982). The success of these approaches may be limited as many of these behaviours have a strong habitual element to them, therefore previous behaviour may help to explain current behaviour (Humphris & Weinman, 1990). Theory of Planned Behaviour constructs (Tedesco *et al.*, 1993) have successfully predicted flossing and tooth brushing behaviour (see 'Theory of planned behaviour'). Interventions which have introduced modelling and reinforcement procedures rather than concentrating solely on attitude change paradigms (for a review, see Blount *et al.* (1989)) have shown substantial impact. These behavioural approaches have clearly demonstrated the benefit of analyzing the consequences of the behaviour to the individual (see 'Behaviour therapy'). However, the problems of maintenance and generalization outside the limits of the programme intervention still have to be overcome, as well as resource implications.

Psychological approaches in oral care

There are many examples of applying psychology in the dental office or surgery. They can be categorized into differentiating the psychological profiles of people who enter the care system and the psychological factors responsible for adherence to advice. Oral health disorders are typically chronic and therefore require continued care over extensive periods. These areas will be briefly discussed under the next three subsections.

Entrance into the care system

Numerous studies, consisting of national and regional cross-sectional surveys have investigated the variables believed to be responsible for the public's utilization of dental services. Three factors, other than the system variables associated with geographical location and the supply of dental personnel includes cost, perception of need for treatment and anxiety or fear. A large literature now exists on understanding the aetiology, maintenance and treatment of dental anxiety (Kvale *et al.*, 2004). The great advantage of studying this psychological construct in the dental context is that it is common (Kent, 1997) and most people are not embarrassed to discuss their worries unless their fears are very severe (Moore *et al.*, 2004). Attempts to reduce dental anxiety by the use of explanatory and advisory leaflets, modelling films and introductory preparatory sessions have shown proven benefits in increased attendance especially for moderately dentally anxious people (Gatchel, 1986). Even the completion of a brief formal dental anxiety assessment instrument has been found to confer benefit in certain circumstances (Dailey *et al.*, 2002)

Acceptance of treatment

Avoidance of certain dental procedures such as the local anaesthetic injection and the use of the high-speed drill is a common psychological phenomena, which causes considerable distress to the patient and concern for the dentist. Technological advances in dental technology are changing traditional treatment approaches however. These include the use of laser hand pieces removing the dread of the high-speed drill's whine. Minimal invasive approaches, which are also of low cost, have been developed, especially for less developed countries (Frencken & Holmgren, 2004). One such procedure (atraumatic restorative treatment) consists of the decayed tooth material being literally scooped out from the tooth cavity and an anti-bacterial lining introduced, followed by an airtight filling material which caps the tooth. Dental clinicians may help their patients by attending carefully to their patients' concerns through listening; providing patients the opportunity to control aspects of the timing of their treatment (e.g. stop signals); and giving advice on pain management. Other procedures found to be effective include relaxation and distraction. (Humphris & Ling, 2000) (see 'Relaxation training' and 'Pain management').

Maintenance of care

To encourage care over longer periods, the psychological issues discussed above for oral hygiene practices are important. The outcomes for dental visitors from utilizing screening and treatment services have been found to be important determinants for repeated appointments. Patient satisfaction scales have shown the importance of dental personnel attending not only to the technical quality of their service but also to the personal aspects of dealing with individuals, each with unique concerns and wishes. Clinicians may improve the strong associations that patients make to a particular practice by attending closely to appropriate communication skills designed to set the patient at ease, to make the dental environment predictable and introduce a relaxed and friendly personal style (Sondell *et al.*, 2004). It is widely recognized that dentists are prone to occupational stress and burnout (see 'Burnout in health professionals'). These unpleasant psychological states are known to influence quality of care and appear to be linked to significant changes in the design of health service organizations. Research continues to identify those individuals most at risk at the start of their careers (Humphris *et al.*, 2002) and ways to prevent staff developing severe burnout (Brake *et al.*, 2001).

The future

The trend of caries reduction, some improvements in periodontal health and increased personal longevity bring the possibility of major changes in the oral health of western industrialized populations, so that the problems experienced in the future may focus on the attrition of tooth enamel and its repair. Individuals' responses to a chronic reduction in the effectiveness and aesthetics of worn teeth will become an important area for the future. A related topic is the increasing technology of prosthetics and provision of implants to replace teeth lost through infection, traumatic accident or malignancy. The employment of psychological models of disability and distress have contributed to the careful evaluation of some of these procedures (Lindsay *et al.*, 2000). What is not often appreciated by the public that these new advanced prostheses, possible because of dramatic improvements in bio-materials will require life long maintenance including annual inspections to ensure the implant's viability. Oral-facial cancer appears to be increasing in some populations especially in countries where tobacco consumption has shown a rapid increase (e.g. China and Eastern Europe). Interest is growing in attempting to prevent this particularly aggressive cancer. The field of food selection and its importance in modifying preferences to a non-carcogenic diet, the beliefs of individuals about fluoride additives in water supplies and the public's views towards water quality, are areas to which psychologists are making increasing contributions. The common risk factor approach will become an important consideration in the implementation of future oral health promotion programmes. The benefits of reducing sugar intake will impact not only on the incidence of caries but also on body mass index and obesity concentrating coordinated efforts to improve a spectrum of health improvements.

REFERENCES

Albino, J. (2002). A psychologist's guide to oral diseases and disorders and their treatment. *Professional Psychology: Research and Practice*, **33**, 176–82.

Blount, R., Santilli, L. & Stokes, T. (1989). Promoting oral hygiene in pediatric dentistry: a critical review. *Clinical Psychology Review*, **9**, 737–46.

Brake, H., Gorter, R., Hoogstraten, J. & Eijkman, M. (2001). Burnout intervention among Dutch dentists: long-term effects. *European Journal of Oral Science*, **109**, 380–7.

Dailey, Y., Humphris, G. & Lennon, M. (2002). Reducing patients' state anxiety in general dental practice: a randomized controlled trial. *Journal of Dental Research*, **81**, 319–22.

Frencken, J. & Holmgren, C. (2004). ART: minimal intervention approach to manage dental caries. *Dental Update*, **31**, 295–8.

Gatchel, R. (1986). Impact of a videotaped dental fear-reduction program on people who avoid dental treatment. *Journal of* *the American Dental Association*, **112**, 218–21.

Humphris, G. & Weinman, J. (1990). Development of dental health beliefs and their relation to dental health behaviour. In L. Schmidt, J. Schwenkmezger, J. Weinman & S. Maes (Eds.), *Theoretical and applied aspects of health psychology.* London: Harwood Academic.

Humphris, G. & Ling, M. (2000). *Behavioural sciences for dentistry.* Edinburgh: Churchill Livingstone.

Humphris, G., Blinkhorn, A., Freeman, R. *et al.* (2002). Psychological stress in undergraduate dental students: baseline results from seven European dental schools. *European Journal of Dental Education*, **6**, 22–9.

Kegeles, S. & Lund, A. (1982). Adolescents' health beliefs and acceptance of a novel preventive dental activity. *Health Education Quarterly*, **9**, 96–111.

Kent, G. (1997). Dental phobias. In G. Davey (Ed.). *Phobias – a handbook of theory, research and treatment.* London: John Wiley and Sons Ltd.

Kvale, G., Berggren, U. & Milgrom, P. (2004). Dental fear in adults: a meta-analysis of behavioural interventions. *Community Dental Oral Epidemiology*, **32**, 250–64.

Lindsay, S., Millar, K. & Jennings, K. (2000). The psychological benefits of dental implants in patients distressed by untolerated dentures. *Psychology and Health*, **15**, 451–66.

Locker, D. (2004). Oral Health and quality of life. *Oral Health and Preventive Dentistry*, **2**(Suppl.1), 247–53.

McGrath, C. & Bedi, R. (2004). A national study of the importance of oral health to life quality to inform scales of oral health related quality of life. *Quality of Life Research*, **13**, 13–18.

Moore, R., Brodsgaard, I. & Rosenberg, N. (2004). The contribution of embarrassment to phobic dental anxiety: a qualitative research study. *BMC Psychiatry*, **19**, 10.

Petersen, P. (2003). The World Oral Health Report 2003: continuous improvement of oral health in the 21st century – the approach of the WHO Global Oral Health

Programme. *Community Dentistry and Oral Epidemiology*, **31**(Suppl.1), 3–24.

Pine, C., Adair, P., Petersen, P. *et al.* (2004). Developing explanatory models of health inequalities in childhood dental caries. *Community Dental Health*, **21**(Suppl. 1), 86–95.

Sondell, K., Soderfeldt, B. & Palmqvist, S. (2004). Underlying dimensions of verbal communication between dentists and patients in prosthetic dentistry. *Patient Education and Counselling*, **50**, 157–65.

Tedesco, L., Keffer, M., Davis, E. & Christersson, L. (1993). Self-efficacy and reasoned action: predicting oral health status and behaviour at one, three and six month intervals. *Psychology and Health*, **8**, 105–22.

Tomar, S. & Asma, S. (2000). Smoking-attributable periodontitis in the United States: findings from NHANES III. National Health and Nutrition Examination Survey. *Journal of Periodontology*, **71**, 743–51.

Osteoarthritis

Isidro Villanueva and Alex Zautra

Arizona State University

Osteoarthritis (OA) is the most common rheumatic disease and most prevalent form of arthritis (Centers for Disease Control and Prevention, 1990). OA is described as a degenerative non-inflammatory type of arthritis that mainly affects the joint cartilage; however, in a proportion of subjects, some mild inflammation can occur. OA is characterized by softening and disintegration of articular cartilage, with reactive phenomena such as vascular congestion and osteoblastic activity in the subarticular bone, new growth of cartilage and bone (i.e. osteophytes) at the joint margins and capsular fibrosis.

Epidemiology of osteoarthritis

Moderate-to-severe OA affects more than 12% of the adults between the ages of 25 and 74 years (CDC, 1990). Estimates of the prevalence of OA based on radiographic evidence range from 30–90%, depending on age group (Lawrence *et al.*, 1998). In women, for example, OA is currently the most prevalent chronic condition and the rate of self-reported cases is projected to increase in the next decades. A population-based study showed incident rates of 2/1000 per year for knee OA (Wilson *et al.*, 1990). Advancing age, female gender and obesity constitute some of the identified risk factors for OA (see 'Obesity'). Symptomatic OA affects roughly 6% of the adult population, 10% of persons over 65 years of age (Felson *et al.*, 1987). Among those individuals between the ages of 55–64, the rate is estimated at 7.5% for women and 4.3% for men (Davis *et al.*, 1991).

Estimated medical care costs for individuals with arthritis in the US were $15 billion and total costs were $65 billion in 1992 (Yelin & Callahan, 1995). It has also been estimated that OA is responsible for 75–80% of the total cost of arthritis (Felts & Yelin, 1989). The management of the risks of gastrointestinal complications of non-steroidal anti-inflammatory drugs (NSAIDs) may add a substantial amount to the cost of treatment (Straus, 2001).

Clinical features of osteoarthritis

The principal clinical features of OA are pain, stiffness, decreased function, joint instability, muscle weakness and fatigue. Pain worsens with use of the affected joint and is alleviated with rest. Morning stiffness lasting less than 30 minutes is common. In advanced stages of arthritis most patients show profound structural articular changes, including the impairment of muscles and other peri-articular tissues. These structural changes, accompanied by co-morbidities and age-related regression in physical conditioning, determines further impairment and disability at advanced ages (Manek, 2000).

Impact of arthritis on physical function

Arthritis, in general, is a principal cause of disability, as compared to several other chronic health conditions and after adjustment for age, gender and co-morbidity (Guccione et al., 1994). Functional tasks, such as ascending stairs, walking, transfer from seated to standing position and daily activities, are reported to be severely impaired in arthritis patients. There are multiple interrelated biomechanical and psychological factors which have been reported to influence the pathways that lead to physical disability in people with arthritis (O'Reilly et al., 1998; Salaffi et al., 1991; van Baar et al., 1998a). Quadriceps weakness has often been found to be the greatest single predictor of lower limb functional limitation (Slemenda et al., 1997). Neurological deficits, impaired propioception, laxity, restricted range of motion and aerobic deconditioning have all been correlated with worse scores on physical function tests (Sharma et al., 1999; Van Baar et al., 1998). Psychological factors such as self-efficacy, coping, depression and anxiety have also been shown to be independent predictors of disability among individuals with knee OA (Lorig & Holman, 1993; Rejeski et al., 1998; Summers et al., 1988) (see 'Self-efficacy and health' and 'Coping with chronic illness').

Management of arthritis

The development of new drugs for OA is hampered by, among other factors, the lack of surrogate markers of disease activity. New information on the role of inflammation in OA has increased our awareness of the disease process and suggested potentially valuable new treatment targets; however, a great deal of clinical research remains until effective new treatments for OA are available. Analgesics and NSAIDs are the most commonly used medications, yet they provide only partial relief. The use of analgesics and, especially, NSAIDs results in high incidence of side effects, with increased risk of major gastrointestinal complications (i.e. ulcers, bleeding, perforation. The prevalence of NSAID-induced ulcers is 10–30% and 15–35% of all peptic ulcer complications are caused by NSAIDs (Tenenbaum, 1999).

The goals for managing arthritis are reduction of pain, prevention or reduction of disability and improvement of quality of life. For many arthritis patients, pain, disability and reduced quality of life persist in spite of treatment (see 'Quality of life'). There is clearly a need to develop new approaches to enhance the effectiveness of therapeutic strategies.

Health interventions in arthritis

Many guidelines recommend patient education and exercise as complements to medication (Hochberg et al., 1995; Lane & Thompson, 1997). Results with these interventions vary across individuals, regardless of disease activity or medication use.

Exercise therapy

Regular physical activity is associated with better health for people of all ages (Pate et al., 1995) (see 'Physical activity and health'). Current recommendations for the accumulation of 30 minutes of moderate physical activity on most days of the week provide a feasible and effective treatment for persons with arthritis (Department of Health and Human Services, 1996). Many of the factors that lead to disability in arthritis can be improved with exercise (i.e. muscle strength, propioception, range of motion, cardiovascular fitness and co-morbidities associated with arthritis, such as diabetes, hypertension and obesity) (Baker & McAlindon, 2000; O'Grady et al., 2000).

Muscle dysfunction may be implicated in the pathogenesis and progression of knee OA (Sharma, 2001). Strong quadriceps can decrease impulse loading on the lower limb, which has been identified as a potential factor contributing to onset and progression of knee OA (Radin et al., 1991). Rehabilitation programs have shown a decrease in joint pain and disability without exacerbation of arthritis pain (Schilke et al., 1996; Slemenda et al., 1997).

Regular exercise can also have an impact on psychological status. Affect, effective coping and perception of self-efficacy, have been reported to improve (Bell et al., 1998; Hurley et al., 2003; Keefe et al., 1996). Rejeski et al. (1998) found that aerobic and resistance exercise increased self-efficacy, which in turn mediated the effect that such programmes had on disability (see 'Physical activity interventions'). Studies in arthritis have shown beneficial effects of exercise therapy on outcomes (Bautch et al., 1997; Borjesson et al., 1996; King et al., 1991; Kovar et al., 1992); however, psychological characteristics, which are shown to be potential mediators, have rarely been measured.

Psycho-educational interventions

Patient education, defined as any set of planned educational activities designed to improve patients' health behaviours and/or health status (Lorig et al., 1993), is thought to be beneficial in helping patients to cope and co-operate with their disease and its management. Although improvements in pain, functional ability, psychological wellbeing and health status have been shown (Goeppinger & Lorig, 1997; Lorig et al., 1993; Mazzuca et al., 1999), analytic reviews are ambiguous about the effect on these outcomes in arthritis patients (Hawley, 1995; Hirano et al., 1994; Superio-Cabuslay et al., 1996). A recent review found moderate effect sizes for pain and low for functional ability (Hawley, 1995).

The Arthritis Self-Help Course (ASHC) has proven to be effective for patients with arthritis on aspects such as behaviour changes, self-efficacy and health status (Lorig *et al.*, 1993). It focuses on increasing the participant's perception of being able to cope with pain and other symptoms. The intervention has shown to have a positive effect on the frequency of exercise and relaxation behaviours while reducing pain (Lorig *et al.*, 1985). It has been reported that changes in outcomes obtained with this intervention are not related to changes in behaviours (Lorig *et al.*, 1989), but to changes in self-efficacy (Lorig & Gonzalez, 1992). The ASHC has been shown to be effective in the long-term with improvements in pain and self-efficacy maintained after four years while reducing physicians' visits (Lorig *et al.*, 1993). The reported data do not, however, support the existence of a strong link between changes in self-efficacy and improvement in health outcomes. Thus, it is important to investigate additional psychological dimensions as potential predictors or mediators of this effect.

Emotion-regulation interventions

On the horizon are psychosocial interventions with a new emphasis on emotional regulation (Zautra, 2003, pp. 117–31; Zautra *et al.*, in press). These approaches focus directly on the quality of the emotional life of the patient, and introduce methods through which the patient is better able to regulate their emotional state. Mindfulness meditation, for example, has been used with increasing frequency in pain management (Kabat-Zinn, 1990). In this approach the emphasis is placed not on cognitive–behavioural approaches of pain reduction, but rather on acceptance and 'letting-go' of suffering associated with pain and other stressors. These approaches do not target negative affective states exclusively. More sophistical emotion-regulation models address the preservation and enhancement of positive states, and the value of emotion complexity rather than simply dampening negative emotions (Davis *et al.*, in press). Once we recognize pain as an emotional process (Craig, 2003) which is influenced by central mechanisms, there can be little doubt but that integrative approaches such as these will be valuable additions to the clinician and his/her osteoarthritis patient (Hamilton *et al.*, in press; van Puymbreck *et al.*, 2004) (see also 'Pain' and 'Pain management').

Traditional physiopathological vs. biopsychosocial model

The vast majority of treatment decisions in rheumatology are driven by the traditional physiopathological model (Hurley *et al.*, 2003). According to this model OA is the consequence of a lifetime of mechanical (ab)use that causes joint damage, physiological disfunction and impairment. Clearly, this model is too simplistic to explain the complexities of a chronic condition such as arthritis. For example, the biomedical model cannot explain why people with advanced joint damage frequently report less pain than people with minimal structural damage, whereas others with low levels of damage often report severe pain (Creamer *et al.*, 1999). Nor can it explain why some people receive considerable benefit from a particular intervention, whereas other people with similar disease activity obtain little or no benefit (Hurley *et al.*, 2003).

Alternatively, the assumptions of the biopsychosocial model for arthritis suggest that there is a biological cause of nociception that is perceived as painful, but the model takes a broader view of pain and disability stating that people's 'pain behaviour' is a product of their beliefs, understandings, experiences and emotions, which may be modulated by their social environment (Turk, 1996). This model emphasizes the role people's beliefs and use of specific coping strategies play in adjustment to living with arthritis. Consequently, this model views arthritis as the result of complex interactions between joint damage, muscle dysfunction, obesity, pain, disability, psychological profile, social support and economic resources (Hurley *et al.*, 2003).

The identified psychological dimensions, however, still explain only a small percentage of the variance of different outcomes in studies with arthritis patients (Persson *et al.*, 1999). Identifying further predictive or mediating factors in emotion regulation may increase understanding of the dynamics of treatment response in the context of different health interventions. Targeting these characteristics in the design of better psychosocial interventions could result in better health outcomes for patients with arthritis or other chronic diseases. Also, the ability to predict outcomes based on psychological profiles may potentially be used for the identification of subjects that could most benefit from psychosocial and complementary health interventions. To date, most studies investigating these issues have been cross-sectional and have studied differences between patients instead of changes over time in the same individuals. A longitudinal design would permit a more thorough examination of potential causal relationships between psychological dimensions and health status change.

(See also 'Rheumatoid arthritis').

REFERENCES

American Physical Therapy Association. (1997). Guide to physical therapist practice. *Physical Therapy*, **77**, 1163–5.

Baker, K. & McAlindon, T.E. (2000). Exercise for knee osteoarthritis. *Curr Op Rheum*, **12**, 456–63.

Bell, M.J., Lineker, S.C., Wilkins, A.L., Goldsmith, C.H. & Badley, E.M. (1998). A randomized controlled trial to evaluate the efficacy of community based physical therapy in the treatment of people with rheumatoid arthritis. *The Journal of Rheumatology*, **25**, 231–7.

Centers for Disease Control and Prevention. (1995). Estimated number of US population with physician-diagnosed osteoarthritis, 1990. Atlanta, USA: Centers for Disease Control and Prevention.

Craig, A.D. (2003). Pain mechanisms: labeled lines versus convergence in central processing. *Annual Review of Neuroscience*, **26**, 1–30.

Creamer, P., Lethbridge-Cejku, M. & Hochberg, M.C. (1999). Determinants of pain severity in knee osteoarthritis: effect of demographic and psychosocial variables using 3 pain measures. *The Journal of Rheumatology*, **26**, 1785–92.

Davis, M.E., Zautra, A.J. & Smith, B.W. (2004). Dynamic model of affect relationships within interpersonal relation. *Journal of Personality*, **72**, 1133–60 .

Davis, M.A., Ettinger, W.H., Neuhaus, J.M. & Mallon, K.P. (1991). Knee osteoarthritis and physical functioning: evidence from the NHANES I epidemiologic follow-up study. *The Journal of Rheumatology*, **18**, 591–8.

Department of Health and Human Services. (1996). *Physical activity and health: a*

Report of the Surgeon General, US Department of Health and Human Services Center for Disease Control and Prevention. Atlanta, Ga: National Center for Chronic Disease Prevention and Health Promotion.

Felson, D.T., Naimark, A., Anderson, J.J. et al. (1987). The prevalence of knee osteoarthritis in the elderly: the Framingham Osteoarthritis Study. *Arthritis and Rheumatism*, **30**, 914–18.

Felts, W. & Yelin, E. (1989). The economic impact of the rheumatic diseases in the United States. *The Journal of Rheumatology*, **16**, 867–84.

Guccione, A.A., Felson, D.T., Anderson, J.J. et al. (1994). The effects of specific medical conditions on the functional limitations of elders in the Framingham study. *American Journal of Public Health*, **84**, 351–8.

Hamilton, N., Zautra, A.J. & Reich, J. (in press). Affect and pain in rheumatoid arthritis: do individual differences in affective regulation and affective intensity predict emotional recovery from pain. *Annals of Behavioral Medicine*.

Hawley, D. (1995). Psycho-educational interventions in the treatment of arthritis. *Bailliere's Clinical Rheumatology*, **9**, 803–23.

Hirano, P., Laurent, D. & Lorig, K. (1994). Arthritis patient education studies, 1987–1991: a review of the literature. *Patient Ed Couns*, **24**, 49–54.

Hochberg, M.C., Altman, R.D., Brandt, K.D. et al. (1995). Guidelines for the Medical Management of Osteoathritis Part II. Osteoarthritis of the Knee. *Arthritis and Rheumatism*, **38**, 1541–6.

Hurley, V.M., Mitchell, H.L. & Walsh, N. (2003). In osteoarthritis, the psychosocial benefits of exercise are as important as physiological improvements. *Exercise and Sport Sciences Reviews*, **31**, 138–43.

Kabat-Zinn, J. (1990). *Full catastrophe living: using the wisdom of your body and mind to face stress, pain, and illness.* New York: Dell.

Keefe, F.J., KashikarZuck, S. & Opiteck, J. (1996). Pain in arthritis and musculoskeletal disorders: the role of coping skills training and exercise interventions. *The Journal of Orthopedic and Sports Physical Theraphy*, **24**, 279–90.

Lane, N.E. & Thompson, J.M. (1997). Management of osteoarthritis in the primary-care setting: an evidence-based approach to treatment. *The American Journal of Medicine*, **103**, 25–30.

Lawrence, R.C., Helmick, C.G., Arnett, F.C. et al. (1998). Estimates of the prevalence of arthritis and selected musculoskeletal disorders in the United States. *Arthritis and Rheumatism*, **41**, 778–99.

Lorig, K. & Gonzalez, V. (1992). The integration of theory with practice: a twelve year case study. *Health Ed Q*, **19**, 355–68.

Lorig, K. & Holman, H. (1993). Arthritis self-management studies: a twelve years review. *Health Ed Q*, **20**, 17–28.

Lorig, K., Mazonson, P. & Holman, H. (1993). Evidence suggesting that health education for self-management in patients with chronic arthritis has sustained health benefits while reducing health care costs. *Arthritis and Rheumatism*, **36**, 439–46.

Manek, N.J. (2000). Osteoarthritis: current concepts in diagnosis and management. *American Family Physician*, **61**, 1795–804.

Mazzuca, S.A., Brandt, K.D., Katz, B.P., Hanna, M.P. & Melfi, C.A. (1999). Reduced utilization and cost of primary care clinic visits resulting from self-care education for patients with osteoarthritis of the knee. *Arthritis and Rheumatism*, **42**, 1267–73.

O'Grady, M., Fletcher, J. & Ortiz, S. (2000). Therapeutic and physical fitness exercise prescription for older adults with joint disease: an evidence-based approach. *Rheumatic Disease Clinics of North America*, **26**, 617–46.

O'Reilly, S.C., Muir, K.R. & Doherty, M. (1998). Knee pain and disability in the Nottingham community: association with poor health status and psychological distress. *British Journal of Rheumatology*, **37**, 870–3.

Pate, R.R., Pratt, M., Blair, S.N. et al. (1995). Physical activity and Public Health – a Recommendation from the Centers for Disease Control And Prevention and the American College of Sports Medicine. *The Journal of the American Medical Association*, **273**, 402–7.

Persson, L.O., Berglund, K. & Sahlberg, D. (1999). Psychological factors in chronic rheumatic diseases – a review: the case of rheumatoid arthritis, current research and some problems. *Scandinavian Journal of Rheumatology*, **28**, 137–44.

Radin, E.L., Yang, K.H., Riegger, C., Kish, V.L. & O'Connor, J.J. (1991). Relationship between lower limb dynamics and knee joint pain. *Journal of Orthopedic Research*, **9**, 398–405.

Rejeski, W.J., Ettinger, W.H., Martin, K. & Morgan, T. (1998). Treating disability in knee osteoarthritis with exercise therapy: a central role for self-efficacy and pain. *Arthritis Care and Research*, **11**, 94–101.

Salaffi, F., Cavalieri, F., Nolli, M. & Ferraccioli, G. (1991). Analysis of disability in knee osteoarthritis. Relationship with age and psychological variables but not with radiographic score. *The Journal of Rheumatology*, **18**, 1581–6.

Schilke, J.M., Johnson, G.O., Housh, T.J. & O'Dell, J.R. (1996). Effects of muscle-strength training on the functional status of patients with osteoarthritis of the knee joint. *Nursing Research*, **45**, 68–72.

Sharma, L., Lou, C., Felson, D.T. et al. (1999). Laxity in healthy and osteoarthritic knees. *Arthritis and Rheumatism*, **42**, 861–70.

Slemenda, C., Heilman, D.K. & Brandt, K.D. (1998). Reduced quadriceps strength relative to body weight. *Arthritis and Rheumatism*, **41**, 1951–9.

Summers, M.N., Haley, W.E., Reveille, J.D. & Alarcon, G.S. (1988). Radiographic assessment and psychological variables as predictors of pain and functional impairment in osteoarthritis of the knee or hip. *Arthritis and Rheumatism*, **31**, 204–8.

Superio-Cabuslay, E., Ward, M. & Lorig, R. (1996). Patient education interventions in osteoarthritis and rheumatoid arthritis: a meta-analytic comparison with nonsteroidal anti-inflammatory drug treatment. *Arthritis Care and Research*, **9**, 292–301.

Tenenbaum, J. (1999). The epidemiology of nonsteroidal anti-inflammatory drugs. *Canadian Journal of Gastroenterology*, **13**, 119–22.

Turk, D.C. (1996). Biopsychosocial perspectives on chronic pain. In R.J. Gatchel & D.C. Turk (Eds.). *Psychological approaches to pain management: a practitioner's handbook* (pp. 3–32). New York: Guilford Press.

Van Baar, M.E., Dekker, J., Lemmens, J.A., Oostendorp, R.A. & Bijlsma, J.W. (1998*a*). Pain and disability in patients with osteoarthritis of hip or knee: the relationship with articular, kinesiological, and psychological characteristics. *The Journal of Rheumatology*, **25**, 125–33.

Van Baar, M.E., Dekker, J., Oostendorp, R. et al. (1998*b*). The effectiveness of exercise therapy in patients with osteoarthritis of the hip or knee: a randomized clinical trial. *The Journal of Rheumatology*, **25**, 2432–9.

Van Puymbroeck, C., Zautra, A.J. & Harakas, P. (2004). Chronic pain and depression: twin burdens of adaptation. In A. Steptoe (Ed.). *Depression and physical illness*. Cambridge, UK: Cambridge University Press.

Wilson, M.G., Michet, C.J., Ilstrup, D.M. & Melton, L.J. (1990). *Idiopathic symptomatic osteoarthritis of the hip* and knee – a population-based incidence study. *Mayo Clinic Proceeding*, **65**, 1214–21.

Yelin, E. & Callahan, L.H. (1995). The economic cost and social and psychological impact of musculoskeletal conditions. National Arthritis Data Work Groups. *Arthritis and Rheumatism*, **38**, 1351–62.

Zautra, A.J., Fasman, R., Reich, J.W., Harakas, P., Johnson, L.M., Olmstead, M. & Davis, M.C. (2005). Fibromyalgia: evidence for deficits in positive affect regulation. *Psychosomatic Medicine*, **67**, 147–55.

Zautra, A.J., Johnson, L.M. & Davis, M.C. (2005). Positive affect as a source of resilience for women in chronic pain. *Journal of Consulting and Clinical Psychology*, **73**, 212–20.

Osteoporosis

Myra S. Hunter

King's College London

Osteoporosis is an age-related condition characterized by decreased bone mass and increased susceptibility to fractures. It does affect men but is more common in women after the menopause, predisposing older women particularly to fractures of the wrist, spine and hip (see 'Menopause and postmenopause'). Osteoporosis is considered a major health problem and is increasing in prevalence due to changes in lifestyle, increasing longevity and the greater proportion of older people in the population. The prevalence of osteoporosis in women in the UK was 8.1% in 2002. Therefore, approximately 2.6 million women in England and Wales would have osteoporosis (NICE, 2004) and in the United States this figure would reach at least 20 million women (Turner *et al.*, 2003).

Osteoporosis is usually defined, somewhat arbitrarily, by bone density measures (BDM) of bone mass lower than age-matched norms (typically BDM below -2.5 SD). However, fractures may not develop until the seventieth decade. Peak bone mass occurs at the age of 35, after which time bone repair becomes gradually less efficient. After the menopause, bone is lost more rapidly for about 3 to 5 years, and then slows down again. In women over 50 the risk of osteoporosis is estimated to be about one in three and approximately one in six for hip fracture. Risk factors for osteoporosis include low body mass index, current smoking, early menopause, family history of maternal hip fracture and long term systemic corticosteriod use and conditions affecting bone metabolism.

'Primary prevention' aims to increase bone mass during years of bone maturation in the general population by promoting adequate calcium intake (800–1000 mg per day), regular weight-bearing exercise (e.g. brisk walks) and reduction in tobacco, alcohol and caffeine use. There is evidence from large scale cross-sectional general population surveys that knowledge about osteoporosis is limited and that women are not taking adequate preventative measures (Silver Wallace, 2002; Terrio & Auld, 2002). Primary prevention programmes, targeting women of all ages, have produced rather mixed results. For example, Sedlack *et al.* (2000) evaluated three osteoporosis educational programmes of varying levels of intensity and found that while all programmes increased knowledge there were no corresponding changes in beliefs or behaviours. Similarly, Blalock *et al.* (2000) compared an information pack (information about osteoporosis) with an action pack (how to increase exercise and calcium intake). Those having the information pack increased knowledge but in neither group were there effects upon behaviours. Increasing knowledge amongst young people and producing lifestyle changes for a condition that may, or may not, develop in the future is a problem for primary prevention. Klohn and Rogers (1991) examined young women's intentions to prevent osteoporosis by increasing calcium intake and exercise. They manipulated descriptions of osteoporosis along dimensions of visibility, time of onset and rate of onset. Their results indicated that informing young women that osteoporosis can result in visible or disfiguring consequences increased the appraisal of severity of the condition and also increased intentions to comply with a regimen of increased calcium and exercise. Further prospective research is needed to examine the relationships between intentions and behavioural change in younger women.

'Secondary prevention' refers to efforts to minimize bone loss due to ageing and postmenopausal changes and includes assessment of risk and advice, mainly about diet, exercise and hormone use, for middle-aged and older women. The main focus of medical research has been on the use of oestrogen, or hormone replacement therapy (HRT), which can reduce the risk of spine, hip and other osteoporotic fractures (Lees & Stevenson, 2001). However, recent epidemiological evidence suggests that, for HRT to be an effective method of preventing fractures, continuous and lifelong use is required, which is problematic since only a small proportion of women are prepared to take HRT long term (see 'Hormone replacement therapy').

Although there are conflicting reports, it is generally considered that increasing calcium alone has minimal impact upon reducing bone loss, unless levels are unduly low initially. However, adequate calcium is essential for benefits to be gained from exercise (Smith, 1990). Exercise, and physical activity, has been associated with a positive influence on bone mass in a range of cross-sectional studies, but the effects of exercise interventions have been less consistent. Exercise regimes have been variable between studies, as has the duration of the intervention (Smith & Gilligan, 1991). In a randomized trial of weight-bearing exercise among women treated with HRT after a surgical menopause, the addition of exercise was associated with a highly significant 8% increase in spinal bone density in one year, compared with HRT alone (Notelovitz *et al.*, 1991). In addition to strengthening bones, physical activity may reduce the risk of fractures by improving muscle strength and balance, which may act to prevent falls, especially in the elderly (see 'Physical activity interventions').

Community studies focusing on middle-aged and older women appear to be more promising than those targeting younger women. In a UK study two 2-hour health promotion workshops were offered to 45-year-old women, which increased knowledge about the menopause and lifestyle changes (Liao & Hunter, 1994). Five years later the women, then aged 50, were reassessed in order to examine the long-term impact of the intervention (Hunter & O'Dea, 1999). The intervention group had retained their higher levels of knowledge compared with the controls. Smoking prevalence reduced in both groups by 7% across the five years; while exercise levels increased in the intervention group from 44% to 56% but remained the same at 39% for the controls. Turner *et al.* (2003) developed an osteoporosis prevention programme, which produced changes in behaviours, particularly weight-bearing physical activity, dairy product intake and decreases in caffeine. Whereas a similar community based

programme was less successful (Blalock *et al.*, 2002). Further research is needed to examine the optimum methods of producing behaviour change.

'Treatment' refers to efforts to maintain and prevent fractures and further bone loss, as well as orthopaedic interventions and rehabilitation, in those suffering from osteoporosis. Drug therapies include HRT, bisphosphonates, selective oestrogen receptor modulators, parathyroid hormone, calcium and vitamin D. The choice of interventions is influenced by factors such as BMD, stage of disease, nature and site of fracture, age, co-morbidities and side effects. Another approach that warrants attention in the prevention of osteoporotic fractures, particularly hip fractures, is the avoidance of falls. Strategies to reduce the incidence of falls in the elderly might include the elimination of environmental hazards, increasing muscle strength, use of hip protectors and avoidance of drugs which impair balance. For example, a 30-minute educational programme provided for women aged 60 plus in several community settings increased intentions to take calcium and to use strategies to reduce falls (Curry *et al.*, 2002). For those who develop fractures that cause pain and reduce mobility, research is needed to explore ways of improving quality of life (Cook *et al.*, 1993).

REFERENCES

Blalock, S.J., Smith, S.S., DeVellis, R.F. *et al.* (2000). Effects of educational materials concerning osteoporosis on women's knowledge, beliefs and behaviour. *American Journal of Health Promotion, 14*, 161–9.

Blalock, S.J., DeVellis, R.F., Patterson, B.M. *et al.* (2002). Effects of an osteoporosis prevention program incorporating educational materials. *American Journal of Health Promotion, 16*, 146–56.

Cook, D.J., Guyatt, G.H., Adachi, J. *et al.* (1993). Quality of life issues in women with vertebral fractures due to osteoporosis. *Arthritis and Rheumatism, 36*, 750–6.

Curry, L.C., Hogstel, M.O., Davis, G.C. & Frable, P.J. (2002). Population-based osteoporosis education for older women. *Public Health Nursing, 19*, 460–9.

Hunter, M.S. & O'Dea, I. (1999). An evaluation of a health education intervention for mid-aged women: five year follow-up of effects upon knowledge, impact of menopause and health. *Patient Education & Counselling, 38*, 249–55.

Klohn, L.S. & Rogers, R.W. (1991). Dimensions of the severity of a health

threat: the persuasive effects of visibility, time of onset and rate of onset on young women's intentions to prevent osteoporosis. *Health Psychology, 10*, 323–9.

Lees, B. & Stevenson, J.C. (2001). The prevention of osteoporosis using sequential low-dose hormone replacement therapy with estradiol-17 beta and dydrogesterone. *Osteoporosis International, 12*, 251–8.

Liao, K.L.M. & Hunter, M.S. (1994). The women's midlife project: an evaluation of psychological services for mid-aged women in general practice. *Clinical Psychology Forum, 65*, 19–22.

National Institute for Clinical Excellence. (2004). Appraisal consultation document – Secondary prevention of osteoporotic fragility fractures in postmenopausal women. http://www.nice.org.uk

Notelovitz, M., Martin, D., Tesar, R. *et al.* (1991). Estrogen therapy and variable resistance weight training increase bone mineral in surgically menopausal women. *Journal of Bone Mineral Research, 6*, 583–90.

Sedlack, C.A., Doheny, M.O. & Jones, S.L. (2000). Osteoporosis edcation programmes: changing knowledge and

behaviours. *Public Health Nursing, 17*, 398–402.

Silver Wallace, L. (2002). Osteoporosis prevention in college women: application of the expanded health belief model. *American Journal of Health Behaviour, 26*, 163–72.

Smith, R. (1990). *Osteoporosis*. London: Royal College of Physicians.

Smith, E.L. & Gilligan, C. (1991). Physical activity effects on bone metabolism. *Calcified Tissue International, 49*, 50–4.

Terrio, K. & Auld, G.W. (2002). Osteoporosis knowledge, calcium intake and weight-bearing physical activity in three age groups of women. *Journal of Community Health, 27*, 307–19.

Turner, L.W., Wallace, L.S., Hunt, S.B. & Gray, A.S. (2003). Changes in behavioural intentions among middle-aged women: results form an osteoporosis prevention program. *Psychological Reports, 93*, 521–6.

Parkinson's disease

Marjan Jahanshahi

Institute of Neurology, University College London

This progressive neurological disorder is named after James Parkinson who first described it in 1817 under the label of 'shaking palsy'. The major symptoms are resting tremor, slowness of movement initiation and execution, muscular rigidity and postural abnormality. About 1 in 1000 of the population suffer from it. It is a disorder of old age, with the average age of onset in the sixties, although in hospital-based series 10 to 20% of cases started before the age of 40. The disorder is related to degeneration of dopamine-producing cells in the substantia nigra pars compacta resulting in depletion of striatal dopamine. Parkinson's disease provides a model of basal ganglia dysfunction, through which the contribution of the striatum to movement, cognition, affect and motivation can be studied. Dopamine replacement therapy is the main medical treatment, which initially controls the motor symptoms but after prolonged use is associated with side effects such as dyskinesias and on-off fluctuations. Since the mid 1990s, surgical techniques such as pallidotomy and high frequency deep brain stimulation of the internal segment of the globus pallidus or the subthalamic nucleus have been increasingly used and shown to be effective treatments of chronic Parkinson's disease.

Psychological features

Cognitive impairment

Dementia, that is a loss of intellectual abilities and memory impairment of sufficient severity to interfere with social or occupational functioning, when present develops late in the course of the illness (see also 'Dementias'). The rate of dementia in Parkinson's disease has been estimated to be 15–20% (Brown & Marsden, 1984). It has been suggested that the nature of dementia in Parkinson's disease and other subcortical disorders such as Huntington's disease and Progressive Supranuclear Palsy may be different from the cortical dementia of Alzheimer's disease (Albert et al., 1974). Instead of the amnesic, aphasic, apraxic and agnosic features of cortical dementia, subcortical dementia is characterized by forgetfulness, slowing of thought processes, alterations in personality and mood and a reduced ability to manipulate acquired knowledge. However, the validity of the distinction between cortical and subcortical dementia has been questioned on the basis of the neuropathological and neuropsychological evidence (Whitehouse, 1986; Brown & Marsden, 1988).

Cognitive impairment in non-demented patients with Parkinson's disease is more prevalent, affecting about 40% of patients (Cummings, 1988). Impairment on cognitive tasks requiring effortful processing, internal control of attention, self-directed planning, sequencing and temporal ordering have been described in these patients. The basal ganglia are intimately linked with the prefrontal cortex and since the general picture of cognitive dysfunction in non-demented patients with Parkinson's disease has similarities to that shown by patients with damage to the prefrontal cortex, many refer to the 'frontal deficit' in Parkinson's disease (see Brown & Jahanshahi, 1991). The striatum is also considered to be a substrate for certain types of procedural learning (Soliveri et al., 1992). Consistent with this, implicit learning on tasks such as the serial reaction time task and the weather prediction task is impaired in Parkinson's disease.

Psychiatric problems and psychosocial functioning

The rate of depression in Parkinson's disease is estimated to be between 30 to 50% (Cummings, 1992). Depression in Parkinson's disease may be a result of the alteration of brain monoamines that are implicated in the aetiology of both Parkinson's disease and depression. Alternatively, depression may be a reaction to the onset and experience of living with the progressive illness which entails disability in daily activities, alteration of social and occupational roles, financial concern and dependence on others (see 'Coping with chronic illness' and 'Disability'). Although physical disability is a major contributor to depression, psychological factors such as low self-esteem and use of maladaptive coping strategies are also important determinants of depression in Parkinson's disease. Certain subgroups of Parkinson's disease patients may be more vulnerable to depression: patients in the earliest as well as those in the most advanced stages of illness, those with an early age of onset and those with rapid progression (see Brown & Jahanshahi, 1994).

The unpredictability of function associated with on-off fluctuations, the impairment of balance and risk of falls when walking are among the symptoms likely to contribute to development of anxiety and particularly 'fear of falling' which are quite common and can lead to avoidance of leaving the house and eventually social isolation. Hallucinations and delusions are other psychiatric symptoms experienced in Parkinson's disease which are typically drug-induced. Apathy characterized by reduced motivation and lack of affect, and fatigue described as an overwhelming sense of tiredness and lack of energy, are common in the mid to late stages of the illness and can result in patients remaining inactive most of the day. Sexual problems are relatively common but often overlooked in Parkinson's disease because of the advanced age of most sufferers (see 'Sexual dysfunction'). Sleep disturbance and pain are common complaints, both with multiple causes, but often secondary to the motor symptoms such as rigidity that can make turning in bed difficult or result in aching of the neck and back (see 'Sleep and health').

Management

The course of this progressive disorder varies across patients, with some showing little disability, cognitive impairment or depression after many years, while others becoming severely disabled, demented or depressed. The approach to management should, therefore, be tailored to the needs of the individual patient.

Neuropsychological assessment may aid in differential diagnosis of idiopathic Parkinson's disease from other akineto-rigid Parkinsonian syndromes. In patients who become demented, behavioural techniques can be used to manage the behavioural problems associated with dementia and the carer/family's need for support should not be ignored (see 'Behaviour therapy').

It has been recommended that in chronic neurological disorders such as Parkinson's disease, the focus of medical management should be on ensuring the best 'quality of life' for the patient and their family (see 'Quality of life'). As result, in recent years quality of life has become an important outcome measure in evaluating medical or surgical interventions for the illness. Depression, disability, postural instability and cognitive impairment have been found to be predictors of quality of life in Parkinson's disease, accounting for 72% of variance of quality of life scores in one study (Schrag et al., 2000). Therefore, to enhance the quality of life of the patients, depression and disability could be targets for management efforts of the multidisciplinary team.

The natural history of depression in Parkinson's disease is not linear or parallel to the progression of the physical illness. Therefore, it can not be assumed that symptomatic improvement of Parkinson's disease would result in a parallel improvement of depression. Depression in Parkinson's disease needs to be treated directly. Evidence suggests that depression in Parkinson's disease is undertreated (Cummings, 1992). One reason for this may be a failure to detect depression because of the similarity of some of the symptoms of the two disorders (e.g. psychomotor retardation, lack of facial expression). Another reason for a failure to detect and treat depression in Parkinson's disease may relate to the fact that adaptation to chronic illness is a dynamic process which shows many variations across time and individuals. Thus, the peak time of psychological distress and depression may differ across sufferers: for some it may be early on in relation to accepting the diagnosis, for others it may be later in the course of illness as it becomes more disabling or when dopaminergic medication lose some of their efficacy and medication-related complications such as on-off fluctuations, end-of-dose akinesia, and dyskinesias develop. Individually tailored therapeutic programmes should be on offer throughout the course of the disease from the point of diagnosis to allow the patient and the family to adjust to the changing demands of the disease. Cognitive–behavioural techniques are useful in the management of these patients (Ellgring et al., 1990). Antidepressant medication is effective in the treatment of depression in Parkinson's disease (Cummings, 1992).

Similarly, given their multifactorial nature, it cannot be assumed that anxiety, sexual problems, sleep disturbances or pain in Parkinson's disease can be 'cured' simply by treating the motor symptoms. Direct treatment of anxiety, sleep problems and pain may be necessary. Sex therapy, taking account of the added stresses of chronic illness and the interfering effect of the motor symptoms and medication, may be appropriate.

REFERENCES

Albert, M.L., Feldman, R.G. & Willis, A.L. (1974). The 'subcortical dementia' of progressive supranuclear palsy. *Journal of Neurology, Neurosurgery, and Psychiatry,* **37**, 121–30.

Brown, R.G. & Jahanshahi, M. (1991). Neuropsychology of Parkinsonian syndromes. In T. Caraceni & G. Nappi (Eds.). *Focus on Parkinson's disease* (pp. 121–33). Milan: Masson.

Brown, R.G. & Jahanshahi, M. (1994). Depression in Parkinson's disease - A psychosocial viewpoint. In W.J. Weiner & A.E. Lang (Eds.). *Behavioural neurology of movement disorders. Advances in Neurology, Vol. 65* (pp.61–84). New York: Raven Press.

Brown, R.G. & Marsden, C.D. (1984). How common is dementia in Parkinson's disease? *Lancet,* **ii**, 1262–5.

Brown, R.G. & Marsden, C.D. (1988). 'Subcortical dementia': the neuropsychological evidence. *Neuroscience,* **25**, 363–87.

Cummings, J.L. (1988). Intellectual impairment in Parkinson's disease: clinical, pathologic, and biochemical correlates. *Journal of Geriatric Psychiatry and Neurology,* **1**, 24–36.

Cummings, J.L. (1992). Depression in Parkinson's disease: a review. *American Journal of Psychiatry,* **149**, 443–54.

Ellgring, H., Seiler, S., Nagel, U. et al. (1990). Psychosocial problems of Parkinson patients: approaches to assessment and treatment. In M.B. Streifler, A.D. Korcyzn, E. Melamed & M.H.H. Youdim (Eds.). *Parkinson's disease: anatomy, pathology and therapy, Advances in Neurology, Vol. 53* (pp. 349–53). New York: Raven Press.

Schrag, A., Jahanshahi, M. & Quinn, N.P. (2000). What contributes to quality of life in patients with Parkinson's disease? *Journal of Neurology, Neurosurgery, and Psychiatry,* **69**, 308–12.

Soliveri, P., Brown, R.G., Jahanshahi, M. & Marsden, C.D. (1992). Procedural memory in neurological disease. *European Journal of Cognitive Psychology,* **4**, 161–93.

Whitehouse, P.J. (1986). The concept of subcortical dementia: another look. *Annals of Neurology,* **19**, 1–6.

Pelvic pain

Robert R. Edwards and Jennifer A. Haythornthwaite

Johns Hopkins University School of Medicine

Introduction

Because of the dearth of research examining the involvement of psychosocial factors in acute pelvic pain, this chapter focuses on chronic pain in the pelvic region, excluding abdominal pain. Although remarkably common in the female population, chronic pelvic pain (CPP) constitutes a broad and poorly-defined diagnostic category. Indeed, a recent survey of published studies noted that over 90% of investigators did not specify anatomical locations of pain beyond noting that it was 'in the pelvic region', and approximately three-quarters of published CPP studies included no information on whether physical pathology was present (Williams et al., 2004).

The most commonly utilized definition of CPP; 'recurrent or constant pain in the lower abdominal region that has lasted for at least 6 months', ignores aetiology (Zondervan & Barlow, 2000). The International Association for the Study of Pain (IASP) has also promulgated a definition for CPP without obvious pathology, but such terms have been criticized for drawing an artificial distinction between organic and non-organic pain (Grace, 2000). Current conceptualizations of pain generally utilize the IASP's definition of pain as 'an unpleasant sensory and emotional experience associated with actual or potential tissue damage or described in terms of such damage' (International Association for the Study of Pain, 1979). This inclusion of affect in the definition of pain has largely abolished old distinctions between 'organic' and 'functional' pain. It is now widely accepted that psychological factors such as affect and cognitions are intimately tied to the experience of pain these factors influence the perception and report of pain and are in turn modulated by the experience of pain (Turk & Okifuji, 2002) (see 'Pain' and 'Pain Management'). This biopsychosocial model of the experience of pain (Nielson & Weir, 2001) has spurred much investigation into the psychosocial underpinnings and consequences of chronic pain, including CPP.

CPP is predominantly a women's health problem, affecting approximately one in seven US women (Mathias et al., 1996), though estimated rates vary widely depending on the setting studied. Although epidemiological studies estimate a community prevalence of 15% in women aged 18–50 (Mathias et al., 1996), surveys in gynaecologists' offices/consulting rooms yield estimates of 39% among women aged 18–45 who reported CPP, with even greater prevalence noted in younger women and African-Americans (Jamieson & Steege, 1996). In primary care settings, rates are comparable to asthma and back pain, and the lifetime prevalence is estimated to be around 33% (Zondervan et al., 1998). In the mid-1990s, total annual direct costs of CPP in the USA were estimated at $3 billion (Mathias et al., 1996).

In approximately two-thirds of cases, the cause of CPP is unknown (Mathias et al., 1996). Because of the frequent lack of physical findings, women with CPP are often suspected of having a psychological aetiology to their illness, contributing to feelings of demoralization and frustration (Grace, 2000). Compared with their pain-free counterparts, women with CPP use three times more medications, have four times more non-gynaecologic operations and are five times more likely to have a hysterectomy (Williams et al., 2004). Patients diagnosed with CPP have a higher prevalence of first-degree relatives also diagnosed with CPP than in the general population, and CPP is often co-morbid with inflammatory bowel disease, irritable bowel syndrome and fibromyalgia (Marshall, 2003). Moreover, women diagnosed with CPP are at greater risk for dysmenorrhea and dyspareunia, both of which are associated with diminished quality of life (see 'Quality of Life').

Risk factors

The aetiology of CPP is quite variable and can include gynaecological, urinary, musculoskeletal, neuropathic, immunological and gastrointestinal factors. For example, a woman with endometriosis and a woman with post-herpetic neuralgia (i.e. shingles) affecting the pelvic region would both be diagnosed with CPP and could be included together in a CPP research study (Williams et al., 2004). In spite of this aetiological variability, a number of factors have been shown to be associated with an elevated risk of CPP. Medically, the presence of another chronically painful condition such as irritable bowel syndrome or fibromyalgia appears to confer increased risk (see 'Irritable bowel syndrome'). The presence of endometriosis is a reliable predictor of the development of CPP (2004). A history of abdominal or pelvic surgery, or of a Caesarean delivery, are also risk factors for the future development of CPP (2004).

Non-medical risk factors for CPP include being female or African-American (Kjerulff et al., 1996; Jamieson et al., 1996). The majority of women with CPP are of reproductive age, suggesting that postmenopausal and premenarchal women may be at lower risk (2004). A recent investigation also noted that lower educational achievement increased the likelihood of CPP (Roth et al., 2001). Additionally, several cross-sectional findings indicate that women with CPP are more likely than pain-free controls to be separated or divorced (2004). Multiple studies have identified the number of past sexual partners as a risk factor (Reed et al., 2000). Perhaps the most widely-recognized risk factor, aside from female sex, is a history of physical or sexual abuse, described in detail below.

811

Sexual and physical abuse

Many have hypothesized that a history of abuse may be a primary aetiological factor in women's complaints of CPP (Ehlert, Heim & Hellhammer, 1999). However, methodological limitations in existing studies, including retrospective cross-sectional designs and non-standardized screening questions, necessitate caution in drawing firm conclusions. In spite of these limitations, the existing literature does suggest that patients with CPP show elevated rates of sexual and physical abuse history. In controlled studies, the prevalence of childhood sexual victimization of CPP patients has been rated at around 50–60%, compared to 20–30% for gynaecological controls (Fry et al., 1997; Reed et al., 2000). CPP patients have also demonstrated higher lifetime rates of sexual abuse compared to patients with low back pain (Lampe et al., 2000) or chronic headaches (Walling et al., 1994). This latter study also found increased risk when major sexual abuse was reported in both childhood and adulthood (Walling et al., 1994), a finding replicated in a much larger sample of non-pregnant women surveyed in a primary care setting (Jamieson & Steege, 1997). A recent study revealed that while childhood physical abuse was predictive of the later development of chronic pain generally, childhood sexual abuse was specifically related to the development of CPP (Lampe et al., 2003). However, we should also note that a recent prospective study of abuse in chronic pain found that while retrospective self-report of childhood abuse was greater in chronic pain patients relative to controls, objectively documented physical or sexual abuse was not associated with the later development of any type of chronic pain, suggesting that abuse–pain relationships are complex (Raphael et al., 2001).

Psychological and psychiatric sequelae of CPP

Failure to identify clear organic precipitants to CPP has spurred many investigators to consider the influence of psychological factors (Grace, 2000). Clear differences emerge when women with and without CPP are compared, although the cross-sectional methodologies make causal interpretations impossible. For example, the lifetime prevalence of major depression in women with CPP has been reported at 64%, compared to 17% of pain-free control women presenting to a gynaecological clinic (Harrop-Griffiths et al., 1988). Women with CPP, both with and without identified organic pathology, have been shown to have greater scores on the Beck Depression Inventory than gynaecological patients without CPP (Fry et al., 1997). Interestingly, there is some evidence that the aetiology of CPP does not impact on women's psychological status; a recent meta-analysis found that CPP groups with and without identified organic pathology did not differ from one another on measures of depression, anxiety, or psychopathology (Mcgowan et al., 1998), though both groups differed consistently from healthy controls. Since psychological and psychiatric co-morbidity are common across many chronic pain conditions (Turk et al., 2002), the most informative studies compare CPP with other pain groups. Pelvic pain may produce more negative sequelae than pain in other locations, independent of pain severity (Wesselmann et al., 1997). The pelvic region has important personal significance, and, in an analogue study, subjects asked to imagine genital pain appraised themselves as being more ill, more worried, more irritable, more depressed and more likely to be experiencing an emergency than when asked to imagine pain in other locations (Klonoff et al., 1993).

As in many chronic pain conditions, women with CPP have been shown to demonstrate diminished quality of life, with greater pain severity being associated with reduced functioning (Rannestad et al., 2000) (see 'Quality of Life'). Women with endometriosis and CPP describe poorer health, greater interference in activities and greater pain during intercourse compared to women with no diagnosis or other non-gynaecological pains (Mathias et al., 1996). Although women with CPP describe much of the pain-related interference common to most chronic pain conditions (e.g. reduced social activities, impaired work performance), pain during intercourse and the resulting sexual interference appears to be a particularly significant problem. Eighty-eight percent of CPP respondents describe having pain during or after intercourse at least some of the time in the past month (Mathias et al., 1996). Women with CPP report sexual interference that is similar to those with vulvodynia, which is significantly greater than pain-free controls (Reed et al., 2000) and women presenting for infertility treatment. However, studies have yet to fully examine the impact of this sexual interference on interpersonal relationships; moreover, little research has examined the possibility that sex therapy reduces pain during or after intercourse (see also 'Sexual Dysfunction').

Alterations in pain processing

Several laboratory studies have examined pain sensitivity in women with pain in the pelvic region. Women with dysmenorrhea reported higher levels of anxiety and higher ratings of pain in response to calibrated noxious stimuli presented in the laboratory (Granot et al., 2001). The authors concluded that enhanced pain sensitivity might partially contribute to the symptoms of dysmenorrhea. Similar findings were demonstrated in women with vulvar vestibulitis, who also showed higher increases in blood pressure during painful stimulation (Granot et al., 2002). Women with vulvar vestibulitis who were most sensitive to laboratory pain stimulation also obtained the least benefit from surgical and non-surgical treatments (Granot et al., 2004), These findings suggest the possibility that central nervous system processing of pain may be abnormal in patients with CPP, as has been found in fibromyalgia patients (Gracely et al., 2003). Whether this sensitization precedes or is consequent to the development of CPP is not known; however, the fact that greater laboratory pain sensitivity was associated with reduced treatment benefit highlights the importance of considering dysregulation of central pain processing in treating CPP.

Treatments

Research on the efficacy of treatments for CPP is still in its infancy (Stones et al., 2000); while many treatment approaches have been recommended, the majority have not been rigorously tested. The following treatments have been recommended for CPP patients solely on the basis of their effectiveness in alleviating pain in patients with other chronic conditions: non-steroidal anti-inflammatory medications, oral contraceptives, exercise and physical therapy (2004) (see also 'Contraception' and 'Physical activity interventions'). For certain conditions such as interstitial cystitis, additional pharmacological treatments also include antibiotics and antihistamines. Surgical approaches may also be recommended, depending on the presumed cause of the pain. There are some encouraging data for hysterectomy: women with CPP who underwent hysterectomy experienced greater pain relief than women treated medically, with approximately 75% of surgically-treated women obtaining some pain relief at 1-year follow-up (see 'Hysterectomy'). Clinical trials of acupuncture and acupressure demonstrate superiority over placebo treatments in the reduction of pain (ACOG, 2004), and these treatments may represent a viable, less invasive intervention before proceeding with surgery (see 'Complementary medicine').

Psychological and psychiatric treatments

Although psychological assessment and treatment are frequently recommended for CPP, very few studies have examined the efficacy of psychological or psychiatric interventions in comparison to a control group. Tricyclic antidepressants (TCAs) have been repeatedly shown in other pain disorders to improve pain, sleep and mood (Salerno et al., 2002). Open-label trials (Walker et al., 1991) and clinical reviews (Reiter, 1998) suggest that the use of TCAs may be helpful for women with CPP, although systematic clinical trials have yet to be completed. One small, randomized, double-blind crossover trial of sertraline revealed no improvement in pain or disability compared to placebo (Engel, Jr. et al., 1998). Larger, clinical trials examining the efficacy of antidepressants in this population are clearly needed. Biofeedback has shown impressive results for women with vulvodynia, with a substantial reduction in pain intensity, improved sexual functioning, and improvements in psychological adjustment (Bergeron et al., 2001) (see 'Biofeedback'). Supportive therapy, encompassing patient education and promotion of effective self-care strategies, is mildly effective in CPP; stress and anxiety reduction have been found to be beneficial to some extent in most patients (see 'Cognitive behaviour therapy'). The multidisciplinary care that has been consistently successful in treating other chronic pain conditions (Flor et al., 1992) has been adapted for the treatment of CPP (see 'Pain management'). Significantly more women randomized to receive an integrated approach of combined medical evaluation, psychological treatment and physical therapy improved on measures of pain and disability compared to those receiving standard care (Peters et al., 1991). In other studies of multi-modal treatment, outcomes are generally improved using a multi-disciplinary approach. For example, disabled patients treated multi-modally are almost twice as likely to return to work (Dinoff et al., 2003). Surprisingly however, randomized clinical trials have not continued to examine psychological interventions for CPP or its combination with other treatment modalities.

Summary

CPP is a highly prevalent and costly condition, with a variable aetiology and uncertain treatment course. CPP has long been associated clinically with psychiatric comorbidity, a history of sexual abuse and severe psychological sequelae. Since longitudinal studies are rare, we have little information on whether psychological disturbance precedes CPP, or is consequent to the development of pain. Although preliminary work and several randomized, controlled, studies of psychological interventions are promising, future work examining the efficacy of multidisciplinary care, empirically-validated psychological treatments such as cognitive–behavioural therapy and biofeedback is necessary to develop optimal intervention strategies.

REFERENCES

American College of Gynaecologists (ACOG) (2004). Practice Bulletin No. 51. Chronic pelvic pain. *Obstetrics and Gynecology*, **103**, 589–605.

Bergeron, S., Binik, Y. M., Khalife, S. *et al.* (2001). A randomized comparison of group cognitive-behavioral therapy, surface electromyographic biofeedback, and vestibulectomy in the treatment of dyspareunia resulting from vulvar vestibulitis. *Pain*, **91**, 297–306.

Dinoff, B. L., Meade-Pruitt, S. M. & Doleys, D. M. (2003). Mental health care providers: resource rather than last resort in patients with chronic pelvic pain. *Clinical Obstetrics & Gynecology*, **46**, 804–10.

Ehlert, U., Heim, C. & Hellhammer, D. H. (1999). Chronic pelvic pain as a somatoform disorder. *Psychotherapy and Psychosomatics*, **68**, 87–94.

Engel, C. C. Jr., Walker, E. A., Engel, A. L., Bullis, J. & Armstrong, A. (1998). A randomized, double-blind crossover trial of sertraline in women with chronic pelvic pain. *Journal of Psychosomatic Research*, **44**, 2003–7.

Flor, H., Fydrich, T. & Turk, D. C. (1992). Efficacy of multidisciplinary pain treatment centers: a meta-analytic review. *Pain*, **49**, 221–30.

Fry, R. P. W., Crisp, A. H. & Beard, R. W. (1997). Sociopsychological factors in chronic pelvic pain: a review. *Journal of Psychosomatic Research*, **42**, 1–15.

Grace, V. M. (2000). Pitfalls of the medical paradigm in chronic pelvic pain. *Baillièr's best practice & research. Clinical obstetrics & gynaecology*, **14**, 525–39.

Gracely, R. H., Grant, M. A. & Giesecke, T. (2003). Evoked pain measures in fibromyalgia. *Best Practice & Research Clinical Rheumatology*, **17**, 593–609.

Granot, M., Friedman, M., Yarnitsky, D. & Zimmer, E. Z. (2002). Enhancement of the perception of systemic pain in women with vulvar vestibulitis. *BJOG: An International Journal of Obstetrics and Gynaecology*, **109**, 863–6.

Granot, M., Yarnitsky, D., Itskovitz-Eldor, J. *et al.* (2001). Pain perception in women with dysmenorrhea (1). *Obstetrics and Gynecology*, **98**, 407–11.

Granot, M., Zimmer, E. Z., Friedman, M., Lowenstein, L. & Yarnitsky, D. (2004). Association between quantitative sensory testing, treatment choice, and subsequent pain reduction in vulvar vestibulitis syndrome. *The Journal of Pain*, **5**, 226–32.

Harrop-Griffiths, J., Katon, W., Walker, E., Holm, L., Russo, J. & Hickok, L. (1988). The association between chronic pelvic pain, psychiatric diagnoses and childhood sexual abuse. *Obstetrics and Gynecology*, **71**, 589–94.

International Association for the Study of Pain (1979). Pain terms: a list with definitions and notes on usage. *Pain*, **6**, 249–52.

Jamieson, D. J. & Steege, J. F. (1996). The prevalence of dysmenorrhea, dyspareunia, pelvic pain, and irritable bowel syndrome in primary care practices. *Obstetrics and Gynecology*, **87**, 55–8.

Jamieson, D. J. & Steege, J. F. (1997). The association of sexual abuse with pelvic pain complaints in a primary care population. *American Journal of Obstetrics and Gynecology*, **177**, 1408–12.

Kjerulff, K. H., Langenberg, P., Seidman, J. D., Stolley, P. D. & Guzinski, G. M. (1996). Uterine leiomyomas. Racial differences in severity, symptoms and age at diagnosis. *The Journal of Reproductive Medicine*, **41**, 483–90.

Klonoff, E. A., Landrine, H. & Brown, M. (1993). Appraisal and response to pain may be a function of its bodily location. *Journal of Psychosomatic Research*, **37**, 661–70.

Lampe, A., Doering, S., Rumpold, G. *et al.* (2003). Chronic pain syndromes and their relation to childhood abuse & stressful life events. *Journal of Psychosomatic Research*, **54**, 361–7.

Lampe, A., Solder, E., Ennemoser, A. *et al.* (2000). Chronic pelvic pain and previous sexual abuse. *Obstetrics and Gynecology*, **96**, 929–33.

Marshall, K. (2003). Interstitial cystitis: understanding the syndrome. *Alternative Medicine Review*, **8**, 426–37.

Mathias, S. D., Kuppermann, M., Liberman, R. F., Lipschutz, R. C. & Steege, J. F. (1996). Chronic pelvic pain: prevalence, health-related quality of life, and economic correlates. *Obstetrics and Gynecology*, **87**, 321–7.

Mcgowan, L. P. A., Clark-Carter, D. D. & Pitts, M. K. (1998). Chronic pelvic pain: a meta-analytic review. *Psychology and Health*, **13**, 937–51.

Nielson, W. R. & Weir, R. (2001). Biopsychosocial approaches to the treatment of chronic pain. *The Clinical Journal of Pain*, **17**, S114–27.

Peters, A. A., van Dorst, E., Jellis, B. *et al.* (1991). A randomized clinical trial to compare two different approaches in women with chronic pelvic pain. *Obstetrics and Gynecology*, **77**, 740–4.

Rannestad, T., Eikeland, O. J., Helland, H. & Qvarnstrom, U. (2000). Quality of life, pain, and psychological well-being in women suffering from gynecological disorders. *Journal of women's health & gender-based medicine*, **9**, 897–903.

Raphael, K. G., Widom, C. S. & Lange, G. (2001). Childhood victimization and pain in adulthood: a prospective investigation. *Pain*, **92**, 283–93.

Reed, B. D., Haefner, H. K., Punch, M. R. *et al.* (2000). Psychosocial and sexual functioning in women with vulvodynia and chronic pelvic pain. A comparative evaluation. *Journal of Reproductive Medicine*, **45**, 624–32.

Reiter, R. C. (1998). Evidence-based management of chronic pelvic pain. *Clinical obstetrics and gynecology*, **41**, 422–35.

Roth, R. S., Punch, M. R. & Bachman, J. E. (2001). Educational achievement and pain disability among women with chronic pelvic pain. *Journal of Psychosomatic Research*, **51**, 563–9.

Salerno, S. M., Browning, R. & Jackson, J. L. (2002). The effect of antidepressant treatment on chronic back pain: a meta-analysis. *Archives of Internal Medicine*, **162**, 19–24.

Stones, R. W., Selfe, S. A., Fransman, S. & Horn, S. A. (2000). Psychosocial and economic impact of chronic pelvic pain. *Baillièr's best practice & research. Clinical obstetrics & gynaecology*, **14**, 415–31.

Turk, D. C. & Okifuji, A. (2002). Psychological factors in chronic pain: evolution and revolution. *Journal of consulting clinical psychology*, **70**, 678–90.

Walker, E. A., Roy-Byrne, P. P., Katon, W. J. & Jemelka, R. (1991). An open trial of nortriptyline in women with chronic pelvic pain. *International journal of psychiatry in medicine*, **21**, 245–52.

Walling, M. K., Reiter, R. C., O'Hara, M. W. *et al.* (1994). Abuse history and chronic pain in women: I. Prevalences of sexual abuse and physical abuse see comments. *Obstetrics and Gynecology*, **84**, 193–9.

Wesselmann, U., Burnett, A. L. & Heinberg, L. J. (1997). The urogenital and rectal pain syndromes. *Pain*, **73**, 269–94.

Williams, R. E., Hartmann, K. E. & Steege, J. F. (2004). Documenting the current definitions of chronic pelvic pain: implications for research. *Obstetrics and Gynecology*, **103**, 686–91.

Zondervan, K. & Barlow, D. H. (2000). Epidemiology of chronic pelvic pain. *Baillièr's best practice & research. Clinical obstetrics & gynaecology*, **14**, 403–14.

Zondervan, K. T., Yudkin, P. L., Vessey, M. P. *et al.* (1998). The prevalence of chronic pelvic pain in women in the United Kingdom: a systematic review. *British journal of obstetrics and gynaecology*, **105**, 93–9.

Post-traumatic stress disorder

Donna Posluszny[1], Stacie Spencer[2] and Andrew Baum[1]

[1]University of Pittsburgh Medical Center
[2]University of Pittsburgh

The history of medicine, occupational health and psychiatry has been punctuated by recurring themes related to what is now called post-traumatic stress disorder (PTSD). For several centuries, aversions to, and maladies from, extremely stressful events have been described, but clues to their causes have only recently been discovered. Previously called 'railway spine', 'battle fatigue' and 'shellshock', post-traumatic stress syndromes have been a topic for speculation and diagnosis when no other label will suffice.

Over the past 30 years, investigation of traumatic stress has exploded and a substantial mass of research evidence has been gathered. Initially, this was primarily due to an interest in the uniquely pervasive symptoms of Vietnam veterans. However, tragedy is not limited to war and the development of PTSD is not limited to soldiers. The recent proliferation of PTSD research in diverse populations has added to the understanding of PTSD as a mental health disorder, to our understanding of human reactions to stress, and to knowledge about possible links between mental and physical health.

PTSD first appeared in the third version of the Diagnostic and Statistical Manual of the American Psychiatric Association (APA, 1980) and was clarified in DSM-IIIR (APA, 1987). Prior to this time, it was believed that prolonged reaction to a traumatic event was due to pre-existing personal weakness (McFarlane, 1990; Tomb, 1994). However, with the accumulation of data indicating a consistency in reactions to combat and non-combat traumatic events, it became apparent that the nature of the traumatic event plays an important role in the reaction to that event. Thus, the severity of the event was one of the criteria for a diagnosis of PTSD and was defined as that which would be 'markedly distressing to almost anyone'. This tautological definition was challenging to operationalize. In DSM-IV, the focus shifted from the severity of the event to exposure and reaction to the event.

PTSD is best described as an anxiety disorder that often follows exposure to an extreme stressor that causes injury, threatens life, or threatens physical integrity (APA, 1994). Characteristics of PTSD include persistent re-experiencing of the traumatic event or situation through intrusive distressing thoughts and dreams, acting or feeling like the event is recurring and intense psychological and physiological reactions to cues that are associated with the event. Also characteristic of PTSD are the avoidance of thoughts, feelings, people, places and activities related to the event, difficulty remembering important aspects of the event, restricted range of affect, feeling detached, and a sense of a shortened life-expectancy. The signs and symptoms of PTSD can be either acute, lasting for less than three months or more chronic, lasting for several years. In some cases, the onset of symptoms is delayed for six months or more.

Incidence of PTSD

Family and relationship abuse, criminal assault, rape, motor vehicle accidents, airplane crashes, natural disasters (e.g. floods, earthquakes and hurricanes), human-caused disasters (e.g. the Buffalo Creek Dam collapse), exposure to noxious agents (e.g. Three Mile Island) or pathogens (e.g. HIV) have also been associated with PTSD symptoms. Though variable, approximately 10–30% of people who are exposed to an extreme stressor appear to develop PTSD and 9% of the population in the United States, overall, experiences symptoms of PTSD in their lifetime (Breslau et al., 1991; Tomb, 1994). Incidence rates vary with the event: incidence of PTSD following rape is estimated at 80%, after tragic death at 30%, after motor vehicle accidents with injury at 23%, long after childhood molestation (23%) and after serious accidents at 13% (Breslau et al., 1991; Green, 1994). PTSD rates in firefighters following a serious bushfire were as high as 36% (McFarlane, 1992), and PTSD rates for male and female Vietnam veterans are as high as 31% and 27%, respectively (Fairbanks et al., as cited in Green, 1994; Kulka et al., 1990). These rates reflect lifetime rates for PTSD and are considerably larger than current rates at any given time. Dissecting incidence in Vietnam veterans, for example, shows that of the 31% or 27% with lifetime PTSD, only approximately 15% and 9% showed current PTSD from 1990–1994 (Fairbanks et al., as cited in Green, 1994; Kulka et al., 1990).

PTSD following specific events

As suggested above, a number of highly stressful events have been identified that can cause people to experience symptoms of PTSD. Typically, these events involve life threat or otherwise compromise victims' sense of safety and control. We briefly consider a few major areas of investigation focused on well-established causes of the disorder.

Criminal assault and rape

Rates of PTSD are high immediately following domestic violence or rape (e.g. Rothbaum et al., 1992; Jones et al., 2001). In about half of these cases, symptoms gradually improve in a few months. Specific crime features have been associated with the onset of PTSD symptoms in rape victims. If rape was by a stranger, involved use of weapons, was perceived as life-threatening, or resulted in actual injury or completed rape, victims appear to be more likely to develop symptoms of PTSD (Bownes et al., 1991; Resnick et al., 1992).

Perceptions of control are important in the development of PTSD following criminal assault, and general perception of control over aversive events predict PTSD symptom severity (Kushner et al., 1993) (see 'Perceived control'). Intrusive thoughts also play a significant role in maintaining PTSD symptoms following rape. Victims with PTSD symptoms take longer to process or respond to high-threat words than do rape victims without PTSD and no-rape controls (Cassidy et al., 1992; Foa et al., 1991). Interference on this task has been correlated with intrusive thoughts (Cassidy et al., 1992).

Disasters

Research on disaster-related PTSD covers a wide range of events including earthquakes (Yang et al., 2003) tornadoes (North et al., 1989), volcanic eruptions (Adams & Adams, 1984), floods (Green et al., 1990a; North et al., 2004), airplane crashes (Perlberg, 1979; Smith et al., 1989) and nuclear accidents (Baum et al., 1983; Wert, 1979). It is difficult to summarize findings regarding PTSD across these disasters because of methodological differences in research and differences in stressors or context (Smith & North, 1993). This variability across studies may help explain why symptom rates reported in disaster studies range from 2–100% and why there is no apparent pattern of symptoms by disaster event (Smith & North, 1993).

There are specific features of disasters which are related to PTSD. One distinguishing characteristic is whether the disaster is 'natural' or 'technological'. Results suggest that natural disasters are associated with more chronic stress (e.g. Baum et al., 1983). For example, symptoms of PTSD persisted for as long as 6 years following the radioactive gas leak at Three Mile Island and for as long as 14 years following the Buffalo Creek Dam collapse (Baum et al., 1993; Green et al., 1990b. Symptoms of stress appear to be more prevalent and to last longer following technological disasters, although exposure to both kinds of disasters is often brief (Smith et al., 1989). Perceptions of control also reflect important differences between natural and technological disasters (Baum et al., 1993; Davidson et al., 1982). Both are uncontrollable, but technological disasters reflect a loss of control. Natural disasters are distressing, but human-made disasters threaten peoples' assumptions about order and control. For example, one study compared flood victims and a no-disaster control group with a group of neighbours of a leaking hazardous waste dump and found that the latter were more alienated, physiologically aroused and performed less well on challenging tasks nine months after finding out about the leak (Baum *et al.*, 1992).

Combat veterans

As noted above, PTSD was not uncommon among Vietnam veterans, and research from other conflicts has been consistent with these studies. Up to 38% of survivors of the siege of Sarajevo in Bosnia Herzegovina had measurable PTSD three years later and up to half of Gulf War veterans seeking care for unexplained medical problems had PTSD (Hikmet *et al.*, 2004; Natelson *et al.*, 2001; Rosner *et al.*, 2003). More recent studies of PTSD in more proximal conflicts are important in filling in gaps in the existing literature and expanding on some of these key differences. War-related PTSD is not unique in Vietnam veterans. There is evidence of PTSD among World War II and Korean War veterans, but more cases have been reported from the Vietnam War. The most obvious reason for the difference in reported rates may simply be that researchers were alerted to, and looking for, PTSD in Vietnam veterans. At the same time, there appear to have been characteristics of the Vietnam conflict that may have contributed to unexpectedly high rates of distress. There is also evidence of PTSD among both male and female veterans (e.g. McTeague *et al.*, 2004; Monnier *et al.*, 2004; Pereira, 2002). The persistence of PTSD symptoms is associated with intrusive memories of combat events (Davidson & Baum, 1993). Vietnam combat veterans also exhibit interference for combat-trauma related stimuli but not for neutral, positive, or other threat stimuli (McNally *et al.*, 1993).

Terrorism

Recent studies have targeted terrorism as a potential cause of psychological trauma. Research on this topic has been limited by logistic factors and the nature and frequency of these stressors. There is evidence that people exposed to the bombing of the Murrah Federal Building that was bombed in Oklahoma City experienced significant trauma and PTSD (Tucker *et al.*, 1999). Susceptibility to terrorism is affected by proximity (i.e. whether an individual was there and directly affected; Fullerton *et al.*, 2004) but people far from the epicentre of the attack can experience important psychological syndromes (Schuster, M.A., Stein, B.D., Jaycox, L.H., Collins, R.L., Marshall, G.N. *et al.*, 2001). Media exposure may play a significant role in this phenomenon, contributing to distress experienced far from the point of attack (e.g. Dougall *et al.*, 2005). Other susceptibility factors for response to terrorism remain to be studied but appear to include history of PTSD (e.g. Qin *et al.*, 2003).

PTSD and physical health

Interest in PTSD is 'bidirectional' if you will, with investigators of the effects of PTSD on mental and physical health and on medical procedures and illnesses on PTSD. A recent text (Schnurr &

Green, 2004) summarizes a good deal of work on the former and research is increasingly addressing the latter (Tedstone & Tarrier, 2003). Serious medical illnesses, such as cancer and heart disease, are stressful and expose people to a broad range of threats, burdens and potential losses. They often pose sudden and intense life threat, introducing the possibility of psychological trauma and many aspects of their treatment are stressful as well. They also challenge one's fundamental outlook on life and may evoke existential anxiety and fear.

Symptoms of PTSD have been documented in a variety of medical illnesses, although the general incidence of PTSD tends to be lower than that associated with more traditional types of traumatic events. Cancer has been a main area of focus, as the life-threatening nature of the illness, suddenness of diagnosis and severe impact on life brought on by treatment requirements lend themselves to possible traumatic reactions (for review, see Kangas *et al.*, 2002). Most of this work has targeted breast cancer patients with early stage disease, and finds that 3–12% of the sample meet PTSD criteria, although many more report symptoms of PTSD (e.g. Alter *et al.*, 1996; Cordova *et al.*, 1995; Green *et al.*, 1998; Tjemsland *et al.*, 1998). PTSD has also been documented in lymphoma survivors (Lella & Tross, 1986), gynaecologic cancer patients (Posluszny *et al.*, 2003), lung cancer patients (Dougall *et al.*, 2004) prostate cancer patients and cancer patients undergoing bone marrow transplants (Jacobsen *et al.*, 1998; Mundy *et al.*, 2000). Studies of other disease populations suggest similar evidence patterns (e.g. 8–20% of heart attack survivors report clinically significant PTSD symptoms; Doerfler *et al.*, 1994; Ginzburg *et al.*, 2003; Shemesh *et al.*, 2001) (see 'Coronary heart disease: impact'). PTSD symptoms have also been documented in patients undergoing trauma surgery or seeking treatment for a traumatic injury (Glynn *et al.*, 2003; Zatzick *et al.*, 2003), as well as patients experiencing severe burn injuries (Patterson *et al.*, 1990; Perry *et al.*, 1992; Roca *et al.*, 1992) (see 'Burns').

Predictors of PTSD

Not all of those exposed to traumatic stressors develop PTSD afterwards. In fact, most do not. Other variables, including childhood trauma, early separation from parents, abnormal adolescent development, pre-existing personality disorders (e.g. depression and anxiety disorders), or family history of anxiety may make some people more susceptible to developing PTSD (Astin *et al.*, 1995; Brady *et al.*, 1994; Green *et al.*, 1990a). Factors that precede exposure to traumatic factors and interactions among past, present and anticipated events appear to be important as well (Breslau *et al.*, 1991; Hendin *et al.*, 1983; Holloway & Ursano, 1984). However, evidence does not support the notion that premorbid factors alone determine development of the disorder (e.g. Boman, 1986; Foy *et al.*, 1984; Green *et al.*, 1990a; Green & Berlin, 1987; Ursano *et al.*, 1981) (see 'Stress and health').

It is possible that the more powerful, sensual and evocative the event, the more likely the survivor will be to develop PTSD. This is consistent with data that indicate that higher rates of PTSD are observed following severe, horrific and grotesque events (e.g. Green, 1990; Green *et al.*, 1990a). While evidence from WWII prisoners of war suggests that the severity of the trauma (e.g. amount of weight lost, amount of torture) can predict PTSD

(Speed *et al.*, 1989), for most traumatic events PTSD is predicted by the individual's appraisal of the event as severe rather than the objective severity of the stressor (Perry *et al.*, 1992). In fact, intrusive thoughts about combat in Vietnam was a better predictor of current distress than was severity of combat exposure (Davidson & Baum, 1993). A longitudinal study of burn survivors, measured PTSD symptoms at 2, 6 and 12 months following the traumatic event (Perry *et al.*, 1992). Rates of PTSD at 2 months were predicted by lower perceptions of social support. At 6 months, PTSD was predicted by negative affect and intrusive thoughts experienced at 2 months and at 12 months PTSD was predicted by negative affect and avoidant thoughts experienced at 6 months.

Biobehavioural factors

While the extent to which PTSD and more common forms of distress share common pathways and origins is not clear, some have argued that PTSD can be considered an extreme consequence of stress (e.g. Davidson & Baum, 1986). As such, several biological substrates for the disorder have been proposed. Some have investigated 'trauma centres' in the brain, focusing on noradrenergic activity (e.g. Krystal, 1990). Noradrenergic activity has been implicated as a key component of stress responding, and inhibition of central noradrenergic activity with drugs decreases the stress response (Redmond & Krystal, 1984). Manipulation of norepinephrine and other catecholamines also affects fear-enhanced startle responses, and enhanced startle reactions are symptomatic of PTSD (Davis, 1980; Orr, 1990). Alternatively, some have argued that helplessness is an important aspect of PTSD and the biological effects of inescapable shock in animals have been used as the basis for a model of the profound changes associated with PTSD (e.g. van der Kolk *et al.*, 1985).

Some investigators have found that post-traumatic stress syndromes reflect decreases in some hormones while increasing others; in one study mean urinary cortisol in male inpatients with PTSD were comparable to those of paranoid schizophrenics but lower than those exhibited by other schizophrenics or patients with bipolar or major depressive disorders (Kosten *et al.*, 1987). At the same time, PTSD patients showed norepinephrine levels that were greater than those of the other patient groups and more epinephrine than all but bipolar (manic) patients. These findings have been replicated and extended and the norepinephrine/cortisol rations have been used as a diagnostic tool for PTSD (Mason *et al.*, 1988). Irregularities in the cortisol-producing hypothamamic–pituitary–adrenal cortical axis have been investigated in more detail and appear to be a likely factor in the development and/or maintenance of PTSD (e.g. Yehuda *et al.*, 1990; Yehuda, 2002) (see also 'Psychoneuroimmunology').

REFERENCES

Adams, P. R. & Adams, G. R. (1984). 'Mount St Helen's ashfall: evidence for a disaster stress reaction'. *American Psychologist*, **39**, 252–60.

Adler, A. (1943). Neuropsychiatric complications in victims of Boston's Coconut Grove disaster. *Journal of the American Medical Association*, **123**, 1098–101.

Allodi, F. A. (1994). Post-traumatic stress disorder in hostages and victims of torture. *Psychiatric Clinics of North America*, **17**, 279–88.

American Psychiatric Association (APA) (1980). *Diagnostic and Statistical Manual of Mental Disorders* (3rd edn.). Washington, DC: American Psychiatric Association.

American Psychiatric Association (APA) (1987). *Diagnostic and Statistical Manual of Mental Disorders* (3rd edn.). Revised. Washington, DC: American Psychiatric Association.

American Psychiatric Association (APA) (1994). *Diagnostic and Statistical Manual of Mental Disorders* (4th edn.). Washington, DC: American Psychiatric Association.

Astin, M. C., Ogland-Hand, S. M., Coleman, E. M. & Foy, D. W. (1995). Posttraumatic stress disorder and childhood abuse in battered women: comparisons with mentally distressed women. *Journal of Consulting and Clinical Psychology*, **63**, 308–12.

Alter, C., Pelcovitz, D., Axelrod, A. *et al.* (1996). Identification of PTSD in cancer survivors. *Psychosomatics*, **37**, 137–43.

Baum, A., Cohen, L. & Hall, M. (1993). Control and intrusive memories as possible determinants of chronic stress. *Psychosomatic Medicine*, **55**, 274–86.

Baum, A., Fleming, R. & Davidson, L. M. (1983). Natural disaster and technological catastrophe. *Environment and Behavior*, **15**, 333–5.

Baum, A., Fleming, I., Israel, A. & O'Keefe, M. K. (1992). Symptoms of chronic stress following a natural disaster and discovery of a human-made hazard. *Environment and Behavior*, **24**, 347–65.

Boman, B. (1986). Combat stress, post-traumatic stress disorder, and associated psychiatric disturbance. *Psychosomatics*, **27**, 567–73.

Bownes, L. T., O'Gorman, E. C. & Sayers, A. (1991). Psychiatric symptoms, behavioural responses and post-traumatic stress disorder in rape victims. *Issues in Criminological and Legal Psychology*, **1**, 25–33.

Brady, K. T., Killeen, T., Saladin, M. S. & Dansky, B. (1994). Comorbid substance abuse and posttraumatic stress disorder: characteristics of women in treatment. *American Journal on Addictions*, **3**, 160–4.

Bremner, J. D., Scott, T. M., Delaney, R. C. & Southwick, S. M. (1993). Deficits in short-term memory in posttraumatic stress disorder. *American Journal of Psychiatry*, **150**, 1015–19.

Breslau, N., Davis, G., Andreski, P. & Peterson, E. (1991). Traumatic events and post-traumatic stress disorder in an urban population of young adults. *Archives of General Psychiatry*, **48**, 216–22.

Cameron, C. (1994). Veterans of a secret war: survivors of childhood sexual trauma compared to Vietnam war veterans with PTSD. *Journal of Interpersonal Violence*, **9**, 117–32.

Cassidy, K. L., McNally, R. J. & Zeitlin, S. B. (1992). Cognitive processing of trauma cues in rape victims with posttraumatic stress disorder. *Cognitive Therapy and Research*, **16**, 283–95.

Davidson, L. M. & Baum, A. (1986). Chronic stress and posttraumatic stress disorders. *Journal of Consulting and Clinical Psychology*, **54**, 303–8.

Davidson, L. M. & Baum, A. (1993). Predictors of chronic stress among Vietnam veterans: stress exposure and intrusive recall. *Journal of Traumatic Stress*, **6**, 195–212.

Davidson, L. M., Baum, A. & Collins, D. L. (1982). Stress and control-related problems at Three Mile Island. *Journal of Applied Social Psychology*, **12**, 349–59.

Davis, M. (1980). Neurochemical modulation of sensory-motor reactivity: acoustic and tactile startle reflexes. *Neuroscience Biobehavioral Review*, **4**, 241–63.

Doerfler, L., Pbert, L. & DeCosimo, D. (1994). Symptoms of posttraumatic stress disorder following myocardial infarction and coronary artery bypass surgery. *General Hospital Psychiatry*, **16**, 193–9.

Engdahl, B., Eberly, R. E. & Blake, J. D. (1997). Assessment of posttraumatic stress disorder in World War II veterans. *Psychological Assessment*. **8**, 445–9.

Foa, E. B., Feske, U., Murdock, T. B. & Kozak, M. J. (1991). Processing of threat-realted information in rape victims. *Journal of Abnormal Psychology*, **100**, 56–62.

Foy, D. W., Sipprelle, R. C., Rueger, D. B. & Carroll, E. M. (1984). Etiology of posttraumatic stress disorder in Vietnam veterans: analysis of preliminary, military, and combat exposure influences. *Journal of Consulting and Clinical Psychology*, **52**, 79–87.

Fullerton, C. S., Ursano, R. J. & Leming, Wang, M. S. (2004). Acute stress disorder, posttraumatic stress disorder, and depression in disaster or rescue workers. *American Journal of Psychiatry*, **161**, 1370–6.

Ginzburg, K., Solomon, Z., Koifman, B. *et al.* (2003). Trajectories of posttraumatic stress disorder following myocardial infarction: a prospective study. *Journal of Clinical Psychiatry*. **64**, 1217–23.

Glynn, S. M., Asarnow, J. R. *et al.* (2003). The development of acute post-traumatic stress disorder after orofacial injury: a prospective study in a large urban hospital. *Journal of Oral and Maxillofacial Surgery*, **61**, 785–92.

Goodwin, F. & Bunney, W. E. (1971). Depression following reserpine: a reevaluation. *Seminars in Psychiatry*, **3**, 435–48.

Green, B. L. (1990). Defining trauma: terminology and generic stressor dimensions. *Journal of Applied Social Psychology*, **20**, 1632–42.

Green, B. L. (1994). Psychosocial research in traumatic stress: an update. *Journal of Traumatic Stress*, **7**, 341–62.

Green, B. L., Grace, M. C., Lindy, J. D., Gleser, G. C. & Leonard, A. (1990*a*). Risk factors for PTSD and other diagnoses in a general sample of Vietnam veterans. *American Journal of Psychiatry*, **147**, 729–33.

Green, B. L., Lindy, J. D. & Grace, M. C. (1985). Posttraumatic stress disorder. *Journal of Nervous and Mental Disease*, **173**, 406–11.

Green, B. L., Lindy, J. D., Grace, M. C. & Gleser, G. C. (1990*b*). Buffalo Creek survivors in the second decade: stability of stress symptoms. *American Journal of Orthopsychiatry*, **60**, 43–54.

Green, B. L., Lindy, J. D., Grace, M. C. & Leonard, A. C. (1992). Chronic posttraumatic stress disorder and

diagnostic comorbidity in a disaster sample. *Journal of Nervous and Mental Disease*, **180**, 760–6.

Green, B., Rowland, J. H., Krupnick, J. L. *et al.* (1998). Prevalance of post-traumatic stress disorder in women with breast cancer. *Psychosomatics*, **39**, 102–11.

Helzer, J. E., Robins, L. M. & McEvoy, L. (1987). Posttraumatic stress disorder in the general population: findings of the epidemiologic catchment area survey. *New England Journal of Medicine*, **317**, 1630–4.

Hendin, H., Hass, A. P., Singer, P., Gold, F. & Trigos, G. G. (1983). The influence of precombat personality on posttraumatic stress disorder. *Comprehensive Psychiatry*, **24**, 530–4.

Holloway, H. C. & Ursano, R. J. (1984). The Vietnam veteran: memory, social context, and metaphor. *Psychiatry*, **47**, 103–8.

Jacobsen, P. B., Widows, M. R., Hanna, D. M. *et al.* (1998). Post-traumatic stress disorder symptoms after bone marrow transplantation for breast cancer. *Psychosomatic Medicine*, **60**, 366–71.

Jacobsen, L. K., Southwick, S. M. & Kosten, T. R. (2001). Substance use disorders in patients with posttraumatic stress disorder: a review of the literature. *American Journal of Psychiatry*, **158**, 1184–90.

Jones, L., Hughes, M. & Unterstaller, U. (2001), Post-traumatic stress disorder (PTSD) in victims of domestic violence: a review of the research. *Trauma Violence & Abuse*. **2**, 99–19.

Kangas, M., Henry, J. L. & Bryant, R. A. (2002). Posttraumatic stress disorder following cancer: a conceptual and empirical review. *Clinical Psychology Review*, **22**, 499–524.

Keane, T. M. & Wolfe, J. (1990). Comorbidity in post-traumatic stress disorder: an analysis of community and clinical studies. *Journal of Applied Social Psychology*, **20**, 1776–88.

Keane, T. M., Fairbank, J. A., Caddell, J. M., Zimering, R. T. & Bender, M. E. (1985). a behavioral approach to assessing and treating posttraumatic stress disorder in Vietnam veterans. In C. R. Figley (Ed.). *Trauma and its wake* (pp. 257–94). New York: Brunner/Mazel.

Kilpatrick, D. G., Best, C. L., Saunders, B. E. & Veronen, L. J. (1987). Rape in marriage and in dating relationships: how bad is it for mental Health? *Annals of the New York Academy of Sciences*, **528**, 335–44.

Kosten, T. R., Mason, J. W., Giller, E. L., Ostroff, R. B. & Harkness, L. (1987). Sustained urinary norepinephrine and epinephrine elevation in posttraumatic

stress disorder. *Psychoneuroendocrinology*, **12**, 13–20.

Krystal, J. H. (1990). Animal models for post-traumatic stress disorder. In E. Giller (Ed.). *Biological assessment and treatment of P. T. S. D.* (pp. 3–26). Washington DC: APA Press, Inc.

Kulka, R. A., Schlenger, W. E., Fairbank, J. A. *et al.* (1990). *Trauma and the Vietnam war generation*. New York: Brunner/Mazel.

Kushner, M. G., Riggs, D. S., Foa, E. B. & Miller, S. M. (1993). Perceived controllability and the development of posttraumatic stress disorder (PTSD) in crime victims. *Behaviour Research and Therapy*, **31**, 105–10.

Lella, D. & Tross, S. (1986). Psychological adjustment to survival from Hodgkin's disease. *Journal of Consulting and Clinical Psychology*, **54**, 616–22.

Lordova, M., Andrykowski, M., Kenady, D. *et al.* (1995). Frequency and correlates of posttraumatic-stress-disorder-like symptoms after treatment for breast cancer. *Journal of Consulting and Clinical Psychology*, **63**, 981–6.

McFarlane, A. C. (1986). Posttraumatic morbidity of a disaster: study of cases presenting for psychiatric treatment. *Journal of Nervous and Mental Disease*, **174**, 4–13.

McFarlane, A. C. (1990). Vulnerability to posttraumatic stress disorder. In M. E. Wolf & A. D. Mosnaim (Eds.). *Posttraumatic stress disorder: etiology, phenomenology, and treatment*. Washington, DC: American Psychiatric Press, Inc.

McFarlane, A. C. (1992). Avoidance and intrusion in posttraumatic stress disorder. *Journal of Nervous and Mental Disease*, **180m**, 439–45.

Maida, C. A., Gordon, N. S., Steinberg, A. & Gordon, G. (1989). Psychosocial impact of disasters; victims of the Baldwin Hills fire. *Journal of Traumatic Stress*, 37–48.

Mason, J. W., Giller, E. L., Kosten, T. R. & Harnkess, L. (1988). Elevation of urinary norepinephrine/cortisol ration in posttraumatic stress disorder. *Journal of Nervous and Mental Disease*, **176**, 498–502.

McNally, R. J., English, G. E. & Lipke, H. J. (1993). Assessment of intrusive cognition in PTSD: use of the modified Stroop paradigm. *Journal of Traumatic Stress*, **6**, 33–41.

McNew, J. A. & Abell, N. (1995). Posttraumatic stress symptomatology: similarities and differences between Vietnam veterans and adult survivors of childhood sexual abuse. *Social Work*, **40**, 115–26.

McTeague, L. M., McNally, R. J. & Litz, B. T. (2004). Prewar, war-zone, and postwar predictors of posttraumatic stress in female

Vietnam veteran health care providers. *Military Psychology*, 16, 99–114.

Mellman, T. A., Randolph, C. A., Brawman-Mintzer, O., Flores, L. P. & Milanes, F. J. (1992). Phenomenology and course of psychiatric disorders associated with combat-related posttraumatic stress disorder. *American Journal of Psychiatry*, 149, 1568–74.

Miller, J. A., Turner, J. G. & Kimball, E. (1981). Big Thimpson Flood victims: one year later. *Family Relations*, 30, 111–16.

Monnier, J., Grubaugh, A. L., Knapp, R. G., Magruder, K. M. & Frueh, B. C. (2005). US female veterans in VA primary care: post traumatic stress disorder symptoms and functional status. *Primary Care Psychiatry*. 9, 145–50.

Mundy, E. A., Blanchard, E. B., Cirenza, E. *et al.* (2000). Posttraumatic stress disorder in breast cancer patients following autologous bone marrow transplantation or conventional cancer treatments. *Behavioral Research Therapeutic* 38, 1015–27.

Mundy, E. & Baum, A. (2004). Medical disorders as a cause of psychological trauma and posttraumatic stress disorder. *Current Opinion in Psychiatry*, 17, 123–7.

Natelson, B. H., Tiersky, L. & Nelson, J. (2001). The diagnosis of posttraumatic stress disorder in Gulf veterans with medically unexplained fatiguing illness. *Journal of Nervous and Mental Disease*. 189, 795–6.

North, C. S., Smith, E. M., McCool, R. E. & Lightcap, P. E. (1989). Acute postdisaster coping and adjustment. *Journal of Traumatic Stress*, 2, 353–60.

North, C. S., Kawasaki, A., Spitznagel, E. L. & Hong, B. A. (2004). The course of PTSD, major depression, substance abuse, and somatization after a natural disaster. *The Journal of Nervous and Mental Disease*. 192, 823–9.

Orr, S. P. (1990). Psychophysiologic studies of posttraumatic stress disorder. In E. L. Giller, Jr. (Ed.). *Biological assessment and treatment of posttraumatic stress disorder*. Washington, DC: American Psychiatric Press.

Patterson, D. R., Carrgian, L., Questad, K. A. & Robinson, R. (1990). Posttraumatic stress disorder in hospitalized patients with burn injuries. *Journal of Burn Care & Rehabilitation*, 11, 181–4.

Pereira, A. (2002). Combat trauma and the diagnosis of post-traumatic stress disorder in female and male veterans. *Military Medicine*, 167, 23–7.

Perlberg, M. (1979). Trauma at Tenerife: the psychic aftershocks of a jet disaster. *Human Behavior*, 49–50.

Perry, S., Difede, J., Musngi, G., Frances, A. J. & Jacobsberg, L. (1992). Predictors of

posttraumatic stress disorder after burn injury. *American Journal of Psychiatry*, 149, 931–5.

Posluszny, D., Edwards, R., Comerci, J. *et al.* (2003). Longitudinal analysis of traumatic stress in gynecologic cancer patients. Paper presented at the annual meeting of the association for advancement of behavior therapy, Boston, MA.

Qin, J., Mitchell, K. J., Johnson, M. K. *et al.* (2003). Reactions to and memories for the September 11, 2001 terrorist attacks in adults with posttraumatic stress disorder. *Applied Cognitive Psychology*. 17, 1081–97.

Reaves, M. E., Callen, K. E. & Maxwell, M. J. (1993). Vietnam veterans in the general hospital: seven years later. *Journal of Traumatic Stress*, 6, 343–50.

Redmond, E. D. & Krystal, J. H. (1984). Multiple mechanisms of withdrawal from opioid drugs. *Annual Review of Neuroscience*, 7, 443–78.

Resnick, H. S., Kilpatrick, D. G., Best, C. L. & Kramer, T. L. (1992). Vulnerability-stress factors in development of posttraumatic stress disorder. *Journal of Nervous and Mental Disease*. 180, 424–30.

Roca, R., Spence, R. & Munster, A. (1992). Posttraumatic adaptation and distress among adult burn survivors. *American Journal of Psychiatry*, 149, 1234–8.

Rosner, R., Powell, S. & Butollo, W. (2003). Posttraumatic stress disorder three years after Sarajevo. *Journal of Clinical Psychology*, 59, 41–55.

Rothbaum, B. O., Foa, E. B., Riggs, D. S. Murdock, T. & Walsh, W. (1992). A prospective examination of post-traumatic stress disorder in rape victims. *Journal of Traumatic Stress*, 5, 455–75.

Shemesh, E., Rudnick, A., Kaluski, E. *et al.* (2001). A prospective study of posttraumatic stress symptoms and nonadherence in survivors of a myocardial infarction (MI). *General Hospital Psychiatry*, 23, 215–22.

Sierles, F. S., Chen, J., McFarland, R. E. & Taylor, M. A. (1983). Posttraumatic stress disorder and concurrent psychiatric illness: a preliminary report. *American Journal of Psychiatry*, 140, 1177–9.

Sierles, F. S., Chen, J., Messing, M. L., Besyner, J. K. & Taylor, M. A. (1986). Concurrent psychiatric illness in non-Hispanic outpatients diagnosed as having posttraumatic stress disorder. *Journal of Nervous and Mental Disease*, 174, 171–3.

Smith, E. M. & North, C. S. (1993). Post traumatic stress disorder in natural disasters and technological accidents. In J. P. Wilson & B. Raphael (Eds.). *International handbook*

of traumatic stress syndromes (pp. 405–19). New York: Plenum Press.

Smith, E. M., North, C. S., McCool, R. E. & Shea, J. M. (1989). Acute post-disaster psychiatric disorders: identification of those at risk. *American Journal of Psychiatry*, 146, 202–6.

Smith, E. M., Robins, L. N., Przybeck, T. R., Goldring, E. & Solomon, S. D. (1986). Psychosocial consequences of a disaster. In J. H. Shore (Ed.). *Disaster stress studies: new methods and findings* (pp. 50–76). Washington, DC: American Psychiatric Press.

Speed, N., Engdahl, B., Schwartz, J. & Eberly, R. (1989). Posttraumatic stress disorder as a consequence of the POW experience. *Journal of Nervous and Mental Disease*, 177, 147–53.

Tedstone, J. E. & Tarrier, N. (2003). Posttraumatic stress disorder following medical illness and treatment. *Clinical Psychology Review*, 23, 409–48.

Tjemsland, L., Soreide, J. A. & Malt, U. F. (1998). Post-traumatic distress symptoms in operable breast cancer: III. Status one year after surgery. *Breast Cancer Research & Treatment*, 47, 141–51.

Tomb, D. A. (1994). The phenomenology of post-traumatic stress disorder. *Psychiatric Clinics of North America*, 17, 237–50.

Tucker, P., Pfefferbaum, B., Nixon, S. J. & Foy, D. W. (1999). Trauma and recovery among adults highly exposed to a community disaster. *Psychiatric Annals*, 29, 78–83.

Uddo, M., Vasterling, J. J., Brailey, K. & Sutker, P. B. (1993). Memory and attention in combat-related post-traumatic stress disorder (PTSD). *Journal of Psychopathology and Behavioral Assessment*, 15, 43–52.

Ursano, R. J., Boydstan, J. A. & Wheatly, R. P. (1981). Psychiatric illness in U. S. Air Force Vietnam prisoners of war: a five-year follow-up. *American Journal of Psychiatry*, 138, 310–13.

Van der Kolk, B., Greenberg, M., Boyd, J. & Krystal, J. (1985). Inescapable shock, neurotransmitters and addiction to trauma: towards a psychobiology of post traumatic stress. *Biological Psychiatry*, 20, 314–25.

Wert, B. J. (1979). Stress due to nuclear accident: a survey of an employee population. *Occupational Health Nursing*, 27, 16–24.

Yang, Y. K., Yeh, T. L., Chen, C. C. *et al.* (2003). Psychiatric morbidity and posttraumatic symptoms among earthquake victims in primary care clinics. *General Hospital Psychiatry*, 25, 253–61.

Yehuda, R., Southwick, S. M., Perry, B. D., Mason, J. W. & Giller, E. L. (1990). Interactions of the hypothalamic-pituitary-adrenal axis and the catecholaminergic system in posttraumatic stress disorder. In E. L. Giller, Jr. (Ed.). *Biological assessment and treatment of posttraumatic stress disorder.* Washington DC: American Psychiatric Press.

Yehuda, R. (2002). Current status of cortisol findings in poet-traumatic stress disorder. *Psychiatric clinics of North America*, 341–68.

Zatzick, D. F., Russo, J. E. & Katon, W. (2003). Somatic, posttraumatic stress, and depressive symptoms among injured patients treated in trauma surgery. *Psychosomatics: Journal of Consultation Liaison Psychiatry*, **44**, 479–84.

Postnatal depression

Sandra A. Elliott

St. Thomas' Hospital

'Postnatal depression' is the term applied to depression in the postnatal year (Elliott, 2000). Prevalence studies suggest that up to 30% of postnatal women have symptoms of depression and between 10% and 15% fulfil diagnostic criteria for depressive disorder (O'Hara & Swain, 1996). These figures do not include the 'blues' (emotional lability for a day or two around days 3 to 5) or puerperal psychosis (severe, but rare, disorders with onset typically within 14 days and usually requiring hospitalization). There is no space to address postnatal depression in men (Matthey *et al.*, 2000). The text also relates only to English-speaking women in cultures similar to the indigenous population of the UK. Whilst there have been a few studies in other cultures (e.g. Clifford *et al.*, 1999) and countries (e.g. Cooper *et al.*, 2002), the transcultural approach to the study of perinatal mental health is still in the early stages (Marks *et al.*, 2004).

Experience and consequences

Controlled studies have demonstrated marked differences in prevalence between postnatal women and appropriate controls for both blues and puerperal psychoses but not for postnatal depression. However, postnatal women do report higher levels of depressive symptoms and social maladjustment, particularly marital adjustment (O'Hara *et al.*, 1990). Research is therefore consistent with clinical experience that postnatal depression has a greater psychosocial impact than depression at other times. Many women are very distressed about the depression itself when it occurs at this critical time in their life and relationships. Postnatal depression can place considerable extra strain on partners and close family members, affecting social and leisure activities and causing financial problems within the family (Boath *et al.*, 1998).

Infants of mothers who experienced postnatal depression are more likely to be insecurely attached to their mothers, to have behavioural problems and deficits in cognitive functioning and these problems may still be present at school age (Hay *et al.*, 2003; Murray *et al.*, 2003). Detailed ratings of videotaped mother–infant interactions have revealed differences between depressed and non-depressed women, suggesting that this may be one mechanism by which postnatal depression influences subsequent infant development. The characteristics of interaction which are typical of parent–child communication, and which attract infant attention, are the very characteristics most disrupted by depression. Murray *et al.* (2003) postulated four processes by which postnatal depression could be connected with later difficulties in the child. Firstly, the lack of contingency in the parent's response could affect the child's learning about its own agency. Secondly, insensitive or unresponsive parental behaviour may fail to develop the infant's ability to sustain attention. Thirdly, any hostility or markedly intrusive behaviour may cause infant distress, creating problems with cognition and memory. Finally, self/other distinctions may not be learnt if the parent has a reduced level of imitation of the infant's expressions. However, it is also possible that the association between postnatal depression and developmental difficulties in the child is a result of a third factor not yet accounted for.

Vulnerability factors and precipitants

Almost every conceivable factor has been postulated as a cause for postnatal depression. Few have proved consistently associated (O'Hara & Swain, 1996). The biggest surprise is the lack of evidence for an association with progesterone or other hormones. However, there are significant methodological problems with trying to map peripheral measures of fluctuating hormones with mood, so it is not possible to state with confidence that hormonal dysfunction plays no part in the aetiology of postnatal depression. Hormones may play a significant part in a minority of depressed women (Gregoire *et al.*, 1996; Harris, 1996; Lee, 2000).

Research is broadly consistent with psychosocial models, which view childbirth as a significant life event at a time of increased physical and emotional vulnerability, with the same potential for precipitating depression as other major events (see 'Life events and health'). Though many academic disputes continue about whether childbirth has specific effects which distinguishes postnatal depression from depression at other times (e.g. Elliott, 1990, 2000; Nicolson, 1998; Whiffen & Gotlib, 1993) most researchers agree that postnatal depression is related to similar predisposing factors as is depression at other times, i.e. a previous psychiatric history; previous consultation with a doctor for depression, anxiety or 'nerves'; depression or anxiety during pregnancy; a poor marital relationship; and inadequate social support (O'Hara & Swain, 1996).

Life events, both independent such as the death of a parent before the arrival of the baby, and related such as premature birth and admission to a Neonatal Intensive Care Unit, may precipitate depression in the postnatal period. Most psychological models of depression propose diathesis–stress aetiology (see 'Stress and health'), which acknowledges the role of pre-existing vulnerability and stressful events in the aetiology of depression. Research findings are broadly consistent with such models (O'Hara et al., 1991). However, there have been surprisingly few papers specifically addressing psychological models for postnatal depression (Hipwell et al., 2004; Moorhead et al., 2003; Warner et al., 1997), which may be because evidence suggests that aetiologically it is the same as depression at other times. It is the context and consequences that differ, so the task would be to adapt psychological models developed for depression in general. Grazioli and Terry (2000) found some evidence of support for the diathesis-stress component of Beck's cognitive theory (see 'Cognitive behaviour therapy'), since dysfunctional attitudes about performance evaluation had a greater impact on postnatal depressive symptoms at high levels of parental stress. They propose that future studies specific to the postnatal period should develop measures specific to that context.

Leverton devised questions to assess vulnerability factors in pregnancy, which were predictive of psychiatric status in the first three months postpartum (Elliott et al., 2000). However, no one has yet been able to produce an antenatal measure with sufficient predictive power to identify 'high risk' individuals (Austin & Lumley, 2003). Such instruments are valuable for research purposes, but ethical and practical difficulties seriously limit their use in clinical practice (Henshaw & Elliott, 2005).

Detection

Women may be reluctant to report depressive symptoms for fear of stigma through illness labelling and/or because they believe (incorrectly) that postnatal depression per se can lead to the removal of their baby by health or social workers. Many undiagnosed depressions improve with time and the help of family or friends. However, some do not, and untreated can last past the baby's first birthday. Cox and colleagues therefore developed a screening questionnaire for use at the 6-week postnatal check and at specified intervals thereafter (Cox & Holden, 2003). Given that dysphoria lies on a continuum (Green, 1998), the positive predictive value of this questionnaire, known as the Edinburgh Postnatal Depression Scale (EPDS), is surprisingly high, though it varies with the population under test and the type of criterion psychiatric interview. All validations have been in research contexts rather than routine clinical practice

(Murray et al., 2004). Postnatal screening questionnaires share the ethical dilemmas of invasion of privacy, labelling and practical problems for large-scale administration with antenatal vulnerability questionnaires (Henshaw & Elliott, in press). Many using the questionnaire may not be aware that the EPDS will also produce raised scores with anxiety (Ross, 2003) or other disorders which include depressed mood or anxiety (Czarnocka and Slade, 2000; Leverton and Elliott, 2000). However, when used by properly trained health professionals they can form part of early intervention programmes (Elliott et al., 2001).

Prevention and treatment

In accordance with the research on aetiology, prevention programmes focus on psychological vulnerability and psychosocial stress rather than the biological changes after delivery (Elliott et al., 2000; Zlotnick et al., 2001). A common theme to these programmes is demystifying the experience of depression (Elliott, 1990). Unhappy feelings are expected, accepted and understood. Previously 'invisible' stresses in women's lives become visible, enabling women to come to terms with or change the aspects of their lives that depress them. Pregnant women are also discouraged from having 'superwoman' expectations or perfectionist beliefs about their performance in the motherhood role (Grazioli & Terry, 2000). The idea is that expecting some adjustment difficulties and negative moods as the norm will mean that these are not catastrophized to produce 'depression about depression' (Teasdale, 1985).

Unfortunately, there is inconsistent evidence about the efficacy of prevention programmes. Debates continue about whether certain programmes are ineffective or whether positive results in other trials are a statistical artefact or of insufficient clinical significance to be cost effective (Stuart et al., 2003).

In contrast, various treatments appear to be effective, including primary care interventions based on non-directive counselling (Holden et al., 1989, Wickberg & Hwang, 1996) as well as specialist psychological therapies such as cognitive behaviour therapy and psychodynamic approaches (Cooper et al., 2003) and interpersonal psychotherapy (O'Hara et al., 2000) (see 'Cognitive behaviour therapy' and 'Psychodynamic psychotherapy'). Three pilot trials suggest group treatments may also be beneficial (Honey et al., 2002; Meager & Milgrom, 1996 and Fleming et al., 1992). There has been only one controlled trial of antidepressants for postnatal depression (Appleby et al., 1997), which showed no added benefit over counselling and high rates of women declining to take part in the trial because of concerns about antidepressants. The lack of evidence on the effects of antidepressants on breastfeeding infants makes psychological interventions the first-line treatment for many postnatal women (Stuart et al., 2003).

Healthcare systems

Multilevel, multidisciplinary systems are required to make the most effective use of the high levels of health professional contact (Elliott et al., 2003; Henshaw and Elliott, 2005). The first requirement is for midwives to make sensitive enquiries about previous and current mental health problems. It is particularly important that those with previous bipolar disorder or puerperal psychosis are referred to a psychiatrist to develop a care plan because of their greatly increased risk of a rapid relapse after the birth (Oates, 2005).

Even though antenatal groups are unlikely in themselves to prevent postnatal depression, they can provide a context for preparing primiparae for their new lives and to learn about resources available if they experience psychological difficulties postnatally. Early detection may ensure that a few non-directive counselling based visits by a primary care professional will be sufficient to halt and reverse the

spiral. Such visits may reveal complex issues such as abuse in childhood, neglect or difficult relationship with mother, previous pregnancy loss or cot death, bereavement or marital problems. Alternatively, visits may identify other mental health problems such as obsessions and compulsions or post traumatic stress symptoms following a difficult birth experience (Czarnocka & Slade, 2000) (see 'Post-traumatic stress disorder'). Referral on to cognitive or psychodynamic psychotherapy from a psychologist or other psychological therapist should then be suggested to the mother.

REFERENCES

Appleby, L., Warner, R. W., Whitton, A. L. & Faragher, B. (1997). A controlled study of fluoxetine and cognitive–behavioural counselling in the treatment of postnatal depression. *British Medical Journal*, **314**, 932–6.

Austin, M. P. & Lumley, J. (2003). Antenatal screening for postnatal depression: a systematic review. *Acta Psychiatrica Scandinavica*, **107**, 10–17.

Boath, E. H., Pryce, A. J. & Cox, J. L. (1998). Postnatal depression: The impact on the family. *Journal of Reproductive and Infant Psychology*, **16**, 199–203.

Clifford, C., Day, A., Cox, J. L. & Werrett, J. (1999). A cross-cultural analysis of the Edinburgh postnatal depression scale (EPDS) in health visiting practice. *Journal of Advanced Nursing*, **30**, 655–64.

Cooper, P. J., Landman, M., Tomlinson, M. *et al.* (2002). Impact of a mother–infant intervention in an indigent peri-urban South African context: pilot study. *British Journal of Psychiatry*, **180**, 76–81.

Cooper, P. J., Tomlinson, M., Swartz, L. *et al.* (1999). Postpartum depression and the mother–infant relationship in a South African peri-urban settlement. *British Journal of Psychiatry*, **175**, 126–34.

Cooper, P. J., Murray, L., Wilson, A. & Romaniuk, H. (2003). Controlled trial of the short- and long-term effect of psychological treatment of postpartum depression: I. Impact on maternal mood. *British Journal of Psychiatry*, **182**, 412–19.

Cox, J. L. & Holden, J. (Eds.). (2003). *Perinatal mental health: a guide to the Edinburgh postnatal depression scale*. London: Gaskell Press.

Czarnocka, J. & Slade, P. (2000). Prevalence and predictors of post-traumatic stress symptoms following childbirth. *British Journal of Clinical Psychology*, **39**, 35–52.

Elliott, S. A. (1990). Commentary on 'childbirth as a life event'. *Journal of Reproductive and Infant Psychology*, **8**, 147–59.

Elliott, S. A. (2000). Report on the Satra Bruk Workshop on Classification of Postnatal

Mental Disorders. *Archives of Women's Mental Health*, **3**, 27–33.

Elliott, S. A., Leverton, T. J., Sanjack, M. *et al.* (2000). Promoting mental health after childbirth: a controlled trial of primary prevention of postnatal depression. *British Journal of Clinical Psychology*, **39**, 223–41.

Elliott, S. A., Ashton, C., Gerrard, J. & Cox, J. L. (2003). Is trainer training an effective method for disseminating evidence-based practice for postnatal depression? *Journal of Reproductive and Infant Psychology*, **21**, 219–28.

Elliott, S. A., Gerrard, J., Ashton, C. & Cox, J. L. (2001). Training health visitors to reduce levels of depression after childbirth: an evaluation. *Journal of Mental Health*, **10**, 613–25.

Fleming, A. S., Klein, E. & Corter, C. (1992). The effects of a social support group on depression, maternal attitudes and behaviour in new mothers. *Journal of Child Psychology and Psychiatry*, **33**, 685–98.

Grazioli, R. & Terry, D. J. (2000). The role of cognitive vulnerability and stress in the prediction of postpartum depressive symptomatology. *International Review of Psychiatry*, **8**, 37–54.

Green, J. M. (1998). Postnatal depression or perinatal dysphoria? Findings from a longitudinal community-based study using the Edinburgh postnatal depression scale. *Journal of Reproductive and Infant Psychology*, **16**, 143–55.

Gregoire, A. J., Kumar, R., Everitt, B., Henderson, A. F. & Studd, J. W. (1996). Transdermal oestrogen for treatment of severe postnatal depression. *Lancet*, **6**, 930–3.

Harris, B. (1996). Hormonal aspects of postnatal depression. *International Review of Psychiatry*, **8**, 27–36.

Hay, D. F., Pawlby, S., Angold, A., Harold, G. T. & Sharp, D. (2003). Pathways to violence in the children of mothers who were depressed postpartum. *Developmental Psychology*, **39**, 1083–94.

Henshaw, C. & Elliott, S. A. (Eds.). (2005). *Screening for perinatal depression*. London: Jessica Kingsley.

Hipwell, A. E., Reynolds, S. & Pitts Crick, E. (2004). Cognitive vulnerability to postnatal depressive symptomatology. *Journal of Reproductive and Infant Psychology*, **22**, 211–27.

Holden, J. M., Sagovsky, R. & Cox, J. L. (1989). Counselling in a general practice setting: controlled study of health visitor's intervention in treatment of postnatal depression. *British Medical Journal*, **298**, 223–6.

Honey, K. L., Bennett, P. & Morgan, M. (2002). A brief psycho-educational group intervention for postnatal depression. *British Journal of Clinical Psychology*, **41**, 405–10.

Lee, D. T. S. (2000). Review: progestogens do not resolve postnatal depression but oestrogens may improve depression scores. *Evidence Based Mental Health*, **3**, 9.

Leverton, T. J. & Elliott, S. A. (2000). Is the EPDS a magic wand?: 1. A comparison of the Edinburgh postnatal depression scale and health visitor report as predictors of diagnosis on the present state examination. *Journal of Reproductive and Infant Psychology*, **18**, 279–96.

Marks, M. N., O'Hara, M., Glangeaud-Freudenthal, N. *et al.* (Eds.). (2004). Transcultural study of postnatal depression (TCS-postnatal depression): development and testing of harmonised research methods. *British Journal of Psychiatry*, **184**(Suppl. 46).

Matthey, S., Barnett, B., Ungerer, J. & Waters, B. (2000). Paternal and maternal depressed mood during the transition to parenthood. *Journal of Affective Disorders*, **60**, 75–85.

Meager, I. & Milgrom, J. (1996). Group treatment for postpartum depression: a pilot study. *Australian and New Zealand Journal of Psychiatry*, **30**, 852–60.

Moorhead, S. R. J., Owens, J. & Scott, J. (2003). Development and piloting of the pregnancy related beliefs questionnaire (PRBQ). *Behavioural and Cognitive Psychotherapy*, **31**, 207–13.

Murray, L., Cooper, P. J. & Hipwell, A. (2003*a*). Mental health of parent's caring for infants. *Archives of Women's Mental Health*, **6**(suppl. 2), s71–7.

Murray, L., Cooper, P. J., Wilson, A. & Romaniuk, H. (2003). Controlled trial of the short- and long-term effect of psychological treatment of postpartum depression: II impact on the mother child relationship and child outcome. *British Journal of Psychiatry*, **182**, 420–7.

Murray, L., Woolgar, M. & Cooper, P. J. (2004). Detection and treatment of postpartum depression. *Community Practitioner*, **77**, 13–17.

Nicolson, P. (1998). *Postpartum depression: psychology, science and the transition to motherhood*. London: Routledge.

Oates, M. R. (2003). Perinatal psychiatric disorders: a leading cause of maternal morbidity and mortality. *British Medical Bulletin*, **67**, 1, 219–29.

Oates, M. (2005). Screening for serious mental illness: the confidential enquiries into maternal deaths. In C. Henshaw & S. A. Elliott (Eds.). *Screening for perinatal depression*. London: Jessica Kingsley.

O'Hara, M. W. & Swain, A. M. (1996). Rates and risk of postpartum depression – a meta-analysis. *International Review of Psychiatry*, **8**, 37–54.

O'Hara, M. W., Zekoski, E. M., Philipps, L. H. C. & Wright, E. S. (1990). Controlled prospective study of postpartum mood disorders; comparison of childbearing and non-childbearing women. *Journal of Abnormal Psychology*, **99**, 3–15.

O'Hara, M. W., Schlechte, J. A., Lewis, D. A. & Varner, M. W. (1991). Controlled prospective study of postpartum mood disorders. Psychological, environmental and hormonal variables. *Journal of Abnormal Psychology*, **100**, 63–73.

O'Hara, M. W., Stuart, S., Gorman, L. L. & Wenzel, A. (2000). Efficacy of interpersonal psychotherapy for postpartum depression. *Archives of General Psychiatry*, **57**, 1039–45.

Ross, L. E., Gilbert Evans, S. E., Sellers, E. M. & Romach, M. K. (2003). Measurement issues in postpartum depression: anxiety as a feature of postpartum depression. *Archives of Women's Mental Health*, **6**, 51–7.

Stuart, S., O'Hara, M. W. & Gorman, L. L. (2003). The prevention and psychotherapeutic treatment of postpartum depression. *Archives of Women's Mental Health*, **6**(suppl. 2), s57–s69.

Teasdale, J. D. (1985). Psychological treatments for depression. How do they work? *Behavioural Research and Therapy*, **23**, 157–65.

Warner, R., Appleby, L., Whitton, A. & Faragher, B. (1997). Attitudes towards motherhood in postnatal depression: development of the maternal attitudes questionnaire. *Journal of Psychosomatic Research*, **43**, 351–8.

Whiffen, V. E. & Gotlib, I. H. (1993). Comparison of postpartum and nonpostpartum depression: clinical presentation, psychiatric history and psychosocial functioning. *Journal of Consulting and Clinical Psychology*, **61**, 485–94.

Wickberg, B. & Hwang, C. P. (1996) Counselling of postnatal depression: a controlled study on a population-based Swedish sample. *Journal of Affective Disorders*, **39**, 209–16.

Zlotnick, C., Johnson, S. L., Miller, I. W., Pearlstein, T. & Howard, M. (2001) Postpartum depression in women receiving public assistance: pilot study of an interpersonal therapy-oriented group intervention. *American Journal of Psychiatry*, **158**, 638–40.

Pregnancy and childbirth

Lyn Quine[1] and Liz Steadman[2]

[1]University of Kent
[2]Canterbury Christ Church University

Over six hundred thousand children will be born in England and Wales in 2005. While the huge majority of these will be healthy, some 6000 will die before their first birthday and some 45 000 will be of low birthweight, placing them at risk. Still others will be disabled as a result of complications during the pregnancy or birth. For some mothers the quality of the birth experience will be poor and their satisfaction with antenatal services low. In this review we examine the principal social and psychological variables that may affect these outcomes and consider the contribution that psychological theory has made to our understanding of the epidemiological factors of pregnancy and childbirth.

In the following brief overview, we argue that risk factors are not distributed randomly in society and independent of living and working conditions, but are disproportionately prevalent among lower socioeconomic groups. We suggest some of the pathways by which risk factors may mediate social inputs and outcomes.

Early childhood mortality

Infant mortality in England and Wales has fallen from 9.4 per 1000 live births in 1984 to 5.6 per 1000 in 2000. Improvements in absolute social conditions played a major role in reducing mortality in the last century, along with increased medical knowledge and improved services, but marked effects of relative social and economic disadvantage are still present. For example, there are noticeable regional differences across the country, and large differences between district authorities within the same region, associated with their prevailing social and economic conditions (see 'Socioeconomic status and health').

The significance of social class is extremely marked: mortality rates during the first year are strongly class related even when age and parity are controlled. In the United Kingdom, the Office for National Statistics publishes data based on the father's occupation, and for each of the indices there is a steady gradient from low mortality in Social Class I to high mortality in Social Class V. For 1998–2000, mortality in Social Class V was twice that of Social Class I, and in fact showed a very slight widening, by 0.5%, between the three-yearly figures for 1997–1999 and 1998–2000. However, for births registered by mother only, many of whom will be teenage mothers, the infant mortality rate in 1998–2000 was 7.6 per 1000 births, which is approximately a third higher than the overall national rate. The steepest gradient in infant mortality occurs for the postneonatal period: 2.7:1 for postneonatal mortality against 1.6:1 for neonatal mortality. Postneonatal mortality is of particular importance because the child who dies after the first month of life will normally have been discharged from hospital and therefore domestic, social and environmental factors are more likely to be implicated than quality of neonatal medical care.

Low birthweight

Another index of pregnancy outcome is low birthweight, now normally defined as 2500 g or less. As with early childhood mortality, there is a sharp difference between the top and bottom of the social scale in England and Wales. For babies born into Social Class V, the infant mortality rate is 68% higher than those born into Social Class I, and when children up to age of four are included, the mortality rate in Class V is double that of Class I (Schuman, 1998). However, there has been a sharp decline in both perinatal and infant mortality among low birthweight children over the years. Despite this, low birthweight children who survive have high rates of medical and developmental problems (e.g. Barker, 2004) though whether these too are class related is not known.

Complications of pregnancy

National Health Service (NHS) Maternity Statistics provide the most important measure of complications in pregnancy in England, as they estimate total maternity discharges (of delivered women only) by complications. This includes a very wide range of complications.

The figures indicate a slight trend towards fewer reported complications. In 1994–1995, for example, hypertension was a complication for 7% of women, and fetal problems reported in 25% of deliveries, whereas in 2002–2003 the figures had dropped to 6% and 20% respectively. In 2002–2003 the principal recorded complications were prolonged second stage labour and prolonged pregnancy (Department of Health, 2004). Although the figures are not broken down by social class, the literature indicates that there is evidence for an association between pre-term delivery and socio-economic factors, including social class (e.g. Peacock *et al.*, 1995) (see 'Premature babies').

Social and psychological factors affecting pregnancy and childbirth

The preceding review of epidemiological data has shown that one of the most important social inputs affecting pregnancy outcome is social class. There is a downward trend towards adverse pregnancy outcomes through the social classes, a pattern that has been reported many times throughout the health literature on children and adults alike. Our next concern is to examine whether social and psychological risk factors are disproportionately prevalent among lower socioeconomic groups and whether such factors might act as mediators between social class and outcome, thus providing a psychological explanation for some of the statistics.

Psychosocial factors: life events and social support

Studies have found that a high frequency of life events during pregnancy is associated with pre-term delivery and other adverse pregnancy outcomes. For example, Newton and Hunt (1984) found that both pre-term delivery and other adverse pregnancy outcomes were associated with life events and that life events were more common among working class women (see also 'Life events and health'). An even better predictor of low birthweight was smoking during pregnancy, which the authors suggested was a mediator of stress. Many other studies have reported similar findings (e.g. Peacock *et al.*, 1995).

The literature also suggests that a woman can be protected or buffered from the effects of severe life events if she has good support networks, and again it has been suggested that working class women are less likely to have good social support networks (Oakley & Rajan, 1991) (see *Social support and health*).

However, the problems in disentangling the effects of social support and life events are well documented. Many life events, such as bereavement, also include loss of social support. In addition, there are problems in disentangling the effects of personality variables such as neuroticism and self-esteem (see 'Personality and health'). Intervention studies that have manipulated social support are therefore instructive. Social support throughout the pregnancy has been shown in some studies to reduce the incidence of low birthweight and pregnancy complications, hospital admissions in pregnancy and use of neonatal intensive care. Furthermore, the effects of social support can be maintained well after the birth has taken place. In a longitudinal intervention study in England, Oakley *et al.* (1996) found that factors such as the child's and mother's health, and the child's development were not only enhanced during and after the birth, but that these advantages were still evident at 1-year and 7-year follow-ups.

Simply having another woman present at the birth has been shown to reduce women's use of analgesia, pain during labour and assessments of how well they coped during labour (Hofmeyr *et al.*, 1991). Support can also have a positive effect on fetal heart rate and birthweight: fetuses of women in labour with poor social support can show a higher incidence of abnormal heart rate, as well as lower birth weight (Lidderdale & Walsh, 1998) (see 'Social support interventions').

Emotional factors: maternal distress, anxiety and depression

A number of authors have found a significant relationship between emotional factors and a variety of pregnancy outcomes from complications of pregnancy and satisfaction with the birth experience to fetal and neonate behaviour (e.g. Van den Bergh, 1990). Other literature has focused on the role of psychological rather than physiological processes. A classic longitudinal study on pregnancy and mothering in the East End of London carried out by Wolkind and Zajicek (1981), for example, found that the average weight of children born to mothers with a diagnosed psychiatric condition was significantly lower than for children with psychiatrically healthy mothers. The disturbed mothers were on average younger, attended antenatal classes less frequently and smoked more; and it was smoking that predicted low birthweight best of all. The evidence thus begins to suggest a complex pattern of relationships between social class and outcome, with psychosocial risk factors acting as mediators.

Other studies have explored a variety of related concepts, including trait and state anxiety, psychodynamic defences, maternal distress and emotional state (e.g. Mulder *et al.*, 2002). Some writers argue that psychological and life stress variables do not function independently but work in synergy.

Cognitive factors: knowledge, beliefs and attitudes to pregnancy

Much of the work on the role of knowledge has been by the use of intervention studies. The main interest has been to test whether increasing knowledge, for example through antenatal classes, leads to more appropriate behaviours and more positive outcomes. The effects of antenatal classes and outcome as a form of social support on behaviour have been studied by Dragonas and Christodoulou (1998), while Renkert and Nutbeam (2001) examine what women really learn through antenatal education. The evidence is not entirely consistent in either area, but the overall trend is towards positive relationships.

According to Becker's Health Belief Model (Janz & Becker, 1984), whether a woman takes action to avoid complications in pregnancy, by making full use of antenatal services, smoking less and changing her diet, for example, is predicted by three main variables: how vulnerable she perceives herself to be to the complications; how severe or important she believes them to be; and her evaluation of the benefits and costs of taking action (see 'Health belief model').

It has been suggested by Becker that, in order for health beliefs to be translated into action, a trigger is necessary to reinforce their personal relevance. In a study by Reading *et al.* (1982), this idea was applied to the role of ultrasound scanning. Of two groups of women who were scanned at their first antenatal visit, one group were given high feedback, in which they were shown the size and shape of the fetus and its movements were pointed out, and the other group were given no picture and no specific verbal description or comments. Both groups were given advice about smoking and drinking. At follow-up, adherence with this advice was significantly higher in the women who had been given feedback than in those who had not.

Other studies of beliefs during pregnancy have used Ajzen's model, the Theory of Planned Behaviour (Ajzen, 1991) (see 'Theory of Planned Behaviour'). For example, this model has been used successfully to predict breastfeeding intention and duration (Duckett *et al.*, 1998), and smoking cessation during pregnancy (Bennett & Clatworthy, 1999). In each case, the model showed that beliefs played an important role.

Findings concerning the relationship between women's beliefs and attitudes towards pregnancy and pregnancy outcome suggest that beliefs do have an impact on subsequent behaviour. For example, Owen and Penn (1999) report that 80% of women who quit smoking during pregnancy believed that smoking was very dangerous to their baby, compared to only 30% of those who continued to smoke. It has been argued that attitudes may influence a woman's behaviour during pregnancy through posture, diet, smoking, drinking, how early she visits a doctor for antenatal care, how well she takes care of herself and so on, all of which, in turn, may affect the outcome of the pregnancy.

Coping resources and strategies

It is in the way that women cope with their pregnancy that many of the psychosocial mediators are drawn together. Coping has been defined as the problem-solving efforts made by an individual when the demands of a given situation tax adaptive resources (Lazarus *et al.*, 1974) (see 'Stress and health'). The central process is cognitive appraisal, which is a mental process by which people assess whether a demand threatens their wellbeing (primary appraisal), appraise their resources for meeting the demand, formulate solutions and select strategies (secondary appraisal). For a number of women, lack of material resources may reduce their choice of coping strategies: lack of physical resources may mean that pre-existing physical or psychological ill-health will impede the process of coping; lack of social resources may mean that fewer people can be called upon to help; lack of psychological and intellectual resources may produce cognitive problems including an inability to respond to difficulties in optimistic, persistent and flexible ways, an explanatory style that focuses on the internal, stable and global factors of negative events (see 'Attributions and health') and low self-efficacy (see 'Self-efficacy and health'). Pregnancy care will be seen as the responsibility of outside professionals, and internal locus of control will be weak. This may lead, in turn, to the selection and use of ineffectual coping strategies and the likely result will be an increased willingness to take dangerous behavioural risks, whether failing to carry out positive measures, such as taking up antenatal services, or continuing to pursue negative behaviours, such as smoking and drinking in pregnancy. The central issue is whether such women can be identified and classified, and the answer appears to be that many are from lower socioeconomic groups where maternal deprivation is prevalent (e.g. Quine *et al.*, 1993).

Behavioural factors: smoking

As an example of behavioural factors associated with pregnancy outcome we select just one, that of smoking. A summary of research on smoking and pregnancy outcome, also covering the effects of 'passive smoking', can be found in Cornelius and Day

(2001). Smoking during pregnancy has been shown many times to be associated with fetal and neonatal mortality, low birthweight and developmental retardation and indeed the first evidence appeared as early as 1957. More recently, the St George's Hospital birth weight study has investigated prospectively the association between pregnancy outcome and a large number of socioeconomic, psychological and behavioural variables, including smoking. Results so far from the St George's data show that smoking is related to foetal growth and that for women who smoke there is a twofold increase in the risk of preterm delivery (e.g. Peacock et al., 1995). All the reported effects increase with the number of cigarettes smoked but, if the mother changes her behaviour before the end of the fourth month of pregnancy, the risk to the baby is determined by the new pattern of behaviour and not the original one. Although these studies provide evidence that the association is causal and serious, some researchers (e.g. Oakley, 1989) argue that smoking in pregnancy is linked to various aspects of women's material and social position. Working class women experience poorer material conditions and lower social support, which makes negative life events and chronic long term difficulties more likely. These, in turn, lead to stress. Smoking is a coping strategy used in response both to stress and to impoverished material and social conditions.

However, an important point to emerge from the research is that the effects of smoking during pregnancy appear to operate independently of potentially confounding factors, such as social class, parity, the mother's age and height and the sex of the child, though there are, of course, marked differences in the incidence of smoking by social group. For example, 31% of women from the manual classes smoke as against 21% in the non-manual classes, and data from the 2000 Infant Feeding Survey conducted by the Department of Health indicate that 4% of pregnant women in Class I continued to smoke during pregnancy against 26% in Class V. The implication is that many women who smoke continue to do so during pregnancy: pregnancy does not stop them and, again, the problem is more prevalent in the lower socioeconomic groups (see 'Tobacco use').

Finally, what has been established is that maternal smoking during pregnancy is not only associated with an increased risk during gestation and delivery, but also for the offspring to later develop childhood or adult behavioural or medical conditions, such as early onset adult diabetes (Montgomery & Ekbom, 2002) and tobacco dependence (Buka et al., 2003).

Pregnancy outcome: a summary

In this review we have seen that social class has marked effects on pregnancy outcome. We have examined the psychosocial and behavioural risk factors for poor outcome and concluded that they, also, are distributed disproportionately among the lower socioeconomic groups. The most important aspect of lower social class appears to be impoverished material and social conditions and resources, which lead, we argue, to two principal effects. On the one hand, they produce an increase in negative life events and chronic long-term difficulties, often with an absence of social support. On the other, they lead to a reduction in the level of access to information, in part through lack of education. Life events and lack of support may lead in turn to emotional problems, including lowered self-esteem, stress, anxiety and depression, while poor education and lack of access to information produce a corresponding range of cognitive problems, including a lack of knowledge and a set of beliefs and attitudes that lead the woman to see herself as vulnerable to illness and complications but helpless to prevent them. The emotional and cognitive effects combine to produce a set of coping styles and strategies that are characterized by hopelessness and a willingness to take potentially serious risks. From there, it is a short step to inappropriate behaviours, poor uptake of maternity services and attendance at antenatal care, smoking, drinking, poor diet and self-care and thence to negative outcomes. The brief review presented here is essentially a framework for integrating past findings and guiding future research. However it suggests that further examination of psychosocial and behavioural factors offers promise for understanding the underlying processes linking deprivation to pregnancy outcome.

(See also 'Antenatal care', 'Screening: antenatal', 'Fetal wellbeing' and 'Premature babies'.)

REFERENCES

Ajzen, I. (1991). The theory of planned behaviour. Organizational Behavior and Human Decision Processes, 50, 179–211.

Barker, D. J. (2004). Developmental origins of adult health and disease. Journal of Epidemiology and Community Health, 58(2), 114–15.

Bennett, P. & Clatworthy, J. (1999). Smoking cessation during pregnancy: Testing a psycho-biological model. Psychology, Health and Medicine, 4(3), 319–26.

Buka, S., Shenassa, E. & Niaura, R. (2003). Elevated risk of tobacco dependence among offspring of mothers who smoked during pregnancy: a 30-year prospective study. American Journal of Psychiatry, 160(11), 1978–84.

Cornelius, M. D. & Day, N. L. (2001). The effects of tobacco use during and after pregnancy on exposed children. Alcohol Research and Health, 24(4), 242–9.

Department of Health. (2004). NHS Maternity Statistics, England: 2002–03. Bulletin 2004/10.

Dragonas, T. & Christodoulou, G. N. (1998). Prenatal care. Clinical Psychology Review, 18(2), 127–42.

Duckett, L., Henley, S., Avery, M. et al. (1998). A theory of planned behavior-based structural model for breast-feeding. Nursing Research, 47(6), 325–36.

Hofmeyr, G. I., Nikodem, V. C., Wolman, W. L., Chalmers, B. E. & Kramer, T. (1991). Companionship to modify the clinical birth environment: effects on progress and perceptions of labour and breast feeding. British Journal of Obstetrics and Gynaecology, 98, 756–64.

Janz, N. K. & Becker, M. H. (1984). The health belief model: a decade later. Health Education Quarterly, 11, 1–47.

Lazarus, R. S., Averill, J. R. & Opton, E. M. (1974). The psychology of coping: issues of research and assessment. In G. V. Coehio,

D. A. Hamburg & J. E. Adams (Eds.). *Coping and adaptation*. New York: Basic Books.

Lidderdale, J. M. & Walsh, J. J. (1998). The effects of social support on cardiovascular reactivity and perinatal outcome. *Psychology and Health*, **13**(6), 1061–70.

Montgomery, S. M. & Ekbom, A. (2002) Smoking during pregnancy and diabetes mellitus in a British longitudinal birth cohort. *British Medical Journal*, **324**, 26–7.

Mulder, E. J. H., de Medina, P. G., Huizink, A. C. *et al.* (2002). Prenatal maternal stress: effects on pregnancy and the (unborn) child. *Early Human Development*, **70**(1–2), 3–14.

Newton, R. W. & Hunt, L. P. (1984). Psychosocial stress in pregnancy and its relation to low birthweight. *British Medical Journal*, **288**, 1191–4.

Oakley, A. (1989). Smoking in pregnancy smokescreen or risk factor? Towards a materialist analysis. *Sociology of Health and Illness*, **11**, 311–35.

Oakley, A., Hickey, D., Rajan, L. & Rigby, A. S. (1996). Social support in pregnancy: does it have long-term effects? *Journal of Reproductive and Infant Psychology*, **14**(1), 7–22.

Oakley, A. & Rajan, L. (1991). Social class and social support – the same or different? *Sociology*, **25**(1), 31–59.

Owen, I. & Penn, G. (1999). *Smoking and pregnancy: a survey of knowledge, attitudes and behaviour, 1992–9*. London: Health Development Agency.

Peacock, J. L., Bland, J. M. & Anderson, H. R. (1995). Preterm delivery: effects of socioeconomic factors, psychological stress, smoking, alcohol, and caffeine. *British Medical Journal*, **311**, 531–5.

Quine, L., Rutter, D. R. & Gowen, S. D. (1993). Women's satisfaction with the quality of the birth experience: a prospective study of social psychological predictors. *Journal of Reproductive and Infant Psychology*, **11**, 107–13.

Reading, A. E., Campbell, S., Cox, D. M. & Sledmere, C. M. (1982). Health beliefs and health care behaviour in pregnancy. *Psychological Medicine*, **12**, 79–83.

Renkert, S. & Nutbeam, D. (2001). Opportunities to improve maternal health literacy through antenatal education: an exploratory study. *Health Promotion International*, **16**(4), 381–8.

Schuman, J. (1998). *Childhood, infant and perinatal mortality, 1996; social and biological factors in deaths of children aged under 3*. London: Office for National Statistics/Stationery Office.

Van den Bergh, B. R. (1990). The influence of maternal emotions during pregnancy on fetal and neonatal behaviour. *Journal of Prenatal and Perinatal Psychology and Health*, **5**(2), 119–30.

Wolkind, S. & Zajicek, E. (Eds.). (1981). *Pregnancy: a psychosocial and social study*. London: Academic Press.

Premature babies

Heather Mohay

Queensland University of Technology

Definition of prematurity

The World Health Organization (1993) classifies infants on the basis of gestational age with those born at <37 weeks gestation classed as preterm, those born at <32 weeks as very preterm and those at <28 weeks as extremely preterm. Birthweight is also frequently used to classify infants. Those with birthweights of <2500 g are classed as low birthweight (LBW), those <1500 g as very low birthweight (VLBW) and those <1000 g as extremely low birthweight (ELBW). The latter are generally born at <28 weeks gestation and have the highest mortality and morbidity rates (Draper *et al.*, 1999). Lubchenco (1976) argued that both birthweight and gestational age need to be considered when classifying infants. She classified infants with a birthweight <10th percentile for their gestational age, i.e. those exhibiting intrauterine growth retardation, as small for gestational age (SGA). These infants may be born at term or earlier in pregnancy and as they require somewhat different medical management and are at greater risk for perinatal death or adverse developmental outcomes than appropriately grown infants of the same gestational age (Lubchenco, 1976) it is important for them to be accurately identified.

Preterm birth occurs in approximately 7% of confinements with infants with birthweights of <1000 g accounting for less than 1% of all deliveries (Australian Institute of Health and Welfare National Perinatal Statistics Unit, 2003).

Survival rates

Nowadays, providing they are cared for in a neonatal intensive care unit (NICU), over 95% of preterm and very preterm infants survive as do more than half of those born as early as 24 weeks gestation and weighing around 500 g. Advances in neonatal care have particularly affected the survival of ELBW infants however the medical interventions necessary to keep these infants alive may cause complications which are associated with adverse developmental outcomes

(Hack & Fanaroff, 1999). Survival alone is not therefore an adequate measure of success. The health, development and quality of life of survivors along with the impact of their survival on their families and on health and education services must also be considered.

Developmental outcomes for preterm infants

Many of the follow-up studies of preterm infant have been marred by poor research design. In addition wide variations exist in the selection of study populations, the age of follow-up, the outcome measures used and the definition of disability adopted (Aylward, 2002; Bhutta *et al.*, 2002) (see 'Disability assessment'). These shortcomings make it difficult to compare studies, but preterm infants are clearly at increased risk of adverse developmental outcomes.

Developmental disabilities

Variations in the criteria used to define severity of disability and to select the conditions and level of disability to be reported, have resulted in wide disparities in the disability rates reported by different studies. However, the consensus is that preterm infants are at higher risk for disabilities than term infants and that ELBW infants are at greater risk than their larger preterm counterparts. In the general population approximately 4% of children have major childhood disabilities. In VLBW infants this rises to about 14% and in ELBW infants it is at least 25%. Most of these disabilities are mild to moderate rather than severe with intellectual impairment and cerebral palsy being the most common disabilities reported. (Vohr *et al.*, 2000).

Correcting for prematurity when assessing growth and development

A correction is normally applied to the age of preterm infants to allow for their shorter gestation. This involves subtracting the number of weeks they were born preterm from their chronological age. Conventionally this correction has been made until children reach two years of age but there is some evidence of continued catch-up, suggesting that correction for gestational age should continue into school years (Ment *et al.*, 2003; Rickards *et al.*, 1989). When age is corrected for prematurity the development of preterm and full-term infants is comparable although preterm infants are, on average, somewhat behind in all domains of development, with the smaller more preterm infants faring worse than their larger preterm age-mates.

Growth

Children born preterm are more likely than those born at term to have growth parametres <10th percentile in the first two years of life (O'Callaghan *et al.*, 1995) Some catch-up growth occurs during childhood (Hack *et al.*, 1996) but they tend to remain shorter and lighter than their full-term counterparts even in adolescence (Saigal *et al.*, 2001) (see *Growth retardation*).

Health

In the NICU preterm infants may have many medical problems and they continue to experience more illness and hospital admissions than full-term infants during the first two years of life (Hack & Fanaroff, 1999). However, as they get older they become more robust and suffer no more health problems than other children (Saigal *et al.*, 2001; Stjernqvist & Svenningsen, 1999).

Movement and motor development

Cerebral palsy is diagnosed in approximately 14% of preterm infants with those having a birthweight of <1000 g being at higher risk than the larger preterm infants. In addition a significant number of preterm infants have other neurological abnormalities or minor movement problems which may interfere with educational progress (Burns *et al.*, 1999; Powls *et al.*, 1995). Nonetheless most premature infants reach the major motor milestones at very similar (corrected) ages to full-term infants.

Cognitive development

Intellectual impairment occurs in at least four times more children born preterm than those born at term with smaller preterm infants at greater risk than those born closer to term. However, when children who have a disability are excluded, the mean developmental quotient of preterm infants in the first two years of life and their subsequent IQ, have generally been found to be within the average range, although below those of term infants (Bhutta *et al.*, 2002). Despite these relatively optimistic finding with regards to IQ, more detailed studies have identified problems in specific abilities such as perceptual organization, even in neurologically intact preterm infants. Furthermore over 40% of VLBW infants and 50% of ELBW infants have learning problems at school and more than 20% have attention deficits (Anderson *et al.*, 2003; Saigal *et al.*, 2003; Stjernqvist & Svenningsen, 1999) (see *Hyperactivity*). Indeed these have been identified as the two most common problems affecting children born preterm.

Infant assessments provide only global measures of development and do not identify more subtle cognitive deficits. Executive dysfunction has been shown to be associated with learning problems and attention disorders in school-aged children (Jarvis & Gathercole, 2003) and there is some evidence that children who were born preterm display deficits in executive function even before they enter school (Harvey *et al.*, 1999). Measures of executive function may therefore provide a means of early identification of children who will later experience learning or attention difficulties. Differences in the brain structure of preterm infants shown in Magnetic Resonance Imagery may also be linked to these subtle abnormalities in cognition and attention (Peterson *et al.*, 2000).

Language development

Approximately 3% of preterm infants have a sensorineural hearing loss requiring the use of hearing aids and many others have intermittent conductive hearing loss due to recurrent middle ear infections (Vohr *et al.*, 2000) (see 'Deafness and hearing loss'). Hearing impairment is associated with delayed language development but if these children are excluded, preterm infants show little delay in their early language acquisition (McAllister *et al.*, 1993) although subtle problems, particularly in expressive language, may become apparent at school age (Jennische, 1999).

Social/emotional development

Parents frequently report that preterm infants are irritable and fussy and have irregular feeding and sleeping patterns, but their scores on temperament measures differ very little from those of full-term infants (Oberklaid *et al.*, 1986). Furthermore, apart from attention deficits and overactivity, they do not have more behaviour problems, delinquency or psychiatric disorders than their peers during childhood and adolescence (Hille *et al.*, 2001). Nor do they have poorer global self-esteem despite being smaller, more poorly co-ordinated and having lower school achievements (Saigal *et al.*, 2002) but they do appear to have some difficulties with peer relationships (Wolke, 1998).

Influence of preterm birth on parents

The development of preterm infants is not only influenced by the adverse circumstances surrounding their birth and early weeks of life but also by the long-term environment in which they live. A supportive and stimulating home environment may offset the problems associated with early medical complications. Unfortunately a disproportionate number of preterm infants live in socially disadvantaged families where parents have limited resources. Hence the children's development may be compromised by both medical and psychosocial adversity (see 'Socioeconomic status and health' and 'Pregnancy and childbirth').

Preterm birth and the ensuing anxiety about their infant's well-being in the NICU are stressful for parents. Postnatal depression, anxiety about the infant's survival and development, guilt that they may have caused the early birth and helplessness in the face of complex technology and staff expertise, are common emotions experienced by mothers of preterm infants (Davis *et al.*, 2003) (see 'Postnatal depression').

The transition from hospital to home can also be anxiety provoking as parents question their ability to care for the infant. A situation in which the infant is immature, behaviourally disorganized and medically vulnerable and the parents feel anxious, incompetent and financially stressed, is ripe for the establishment of inappropriate interaction patterns and poor attachment which can have long-term detrimental effects on the parent–child relationship and the child's development.

Conclusions

The survival rate for preterm infants has increased dramatically and many of these children show normal patterns of development. Nevertheless the risk of disability is increased and their development in all domains is likely to be inferior to that of full-term infants. This becomes particularly apparent at school age when children born preterm are at high risk for learning difficulties, attention disorders and overactivity.

The risk for disability and poor developmental outcome is inversely related to birthweight and gestational age.

Both medical complications associated with prematurity, and psychosocial disadvantage contribute to adverse developmental outcomes for preterm infants. The medical care and subsequent education of these children places a substantial burden on health and education services as well as an emotional and financial strain on the family.

To reduce the frequency of negative sequelae and the costs associated with them it is necessary to:

1. improve medical management to avoid the complications associated with poor developmental outcomes
2. establish reliable methods for the early identification of infants who have behavioural or cognitive deficits which will interfere with their educational progress and develop intervention programmes to reduce these problems
3. support parents in the NICU and at home to enable them to provide optimal environments to promote their infants' development.

(See also 'Pregnancy and childbirth', 'Antenatal care', 'Screening: antenatal' and 'Fetal Well-being'.)

REFERENCES

Anderson, P., Doyle, L. W. & Victorian Infant Collaborative Study Group (2003). Neurobehavioural outcomes of school-age children born extremely low birth weight or very preterm. *Journal of the American Medical Association*, **289**, 3264–72.

Australian Institute of Health and Welfare National Perinatal Statistics Unit (2003). Australia's mothers and their babies 2000. Sydney: Australian Institute of Health and Welfare National Perinatal Statistics Unit.

Aylward, G. P. (2002). Methodological issues in outcomes studies of at-risk infants. *Journal of Pediatric Psychology*, **27**, 37–45.

Bhutta, A. T., Cleves, M. A., Casey, P. H., Craddock, M. M. & Anand, S. (2002).

Cognitive and behavioural outcomes of school age children who were born preterm: a meta-analysis. *Journal of the American Medical Association*, **288**, 728–37.

Burns, Y., Ensbey, R. & O'Callaghan, M. (1999). Motor abilities at eight and ten years of children born weighing less than 1,000 g. *Physiotherapy*, **85**, 360–9.

Davis, L., Edwards, H., Mohay, H. & Wollin, J. (2003). The course of depression in mothers of premature infants in hospital and at home. *Australian Journal of Advanced Nursing*, **21**, 20–7.

Draper, E. S., Manktolow, B., Field, D. J. & James, D. (1999). Prediction of survival for preterm birth by weight and gestational

age: retrospective population based study. *British Medical Journal*, **319**, 1093–7.

Hack, M., Weissman, B. & Borawski, C. E. (1996). Catch-up growth during childhood among very low-birth-weight children. *Archives of Pediatrics and Adolescent Medicine*, **150**, 1122–9.

Hack, M. & Fanaroff, A. A. (1999). Outcomes of children of extremely low birthweight and gestational age in the 1990s. *Early Human Development*, **53**, 193–218.

Harvey, J., O'Callaghan, M. J. & Mohay, H. (1999). Executive function at preschool of children who weighed 500–999 grams at birth: a case control study. *Developmental Medicine and Child Neurology*, **41**, 292–7.

Hille, E. T., den Ouden, A. L., Saigal, S. *et al.* (2001). Behavioural problems in children who weigh 1000 g or less at birth in four countries. *Lancet*, **357**, 1641–3.

Jarvis, H. L. & Gathercole, S. E. (2003). Verbal and nonverbal working memory and achievements on national curriculum tests at 11 and 14 years of age. *Educational and Child Psychology*, **20**, 123–40.

Jennische, M. (1999). Speech and language skills in children who required neonatal intensive care: linguistic skills at 6½ years of age. *Acta Paediatrica*, **88**, 371–82.

Lubchenco, L. O. (1976). *The high risk infant.* Philadelphia: Saunders.

McAllister, L., Masel, C., Tudehope, D. *et al.* (1993). Speech and language outcomes in preschool-aged survivors of neonatal intensive care. *European Journal of Disorders of Communication*, **28**, 383–94.

Ment, L. R., Vohr, B. R., Allen, W. & Katz, K. H. (2003). Changes in cognitive function over time in very low birth weight infants. *Journal of the American Medical Association*, **289**, 705–11.

Oberklaid, F., Prior, M. & Sanson, A. (1986). Temperament of pre-term versus full-term infants. *Journal of Behavioural Pediatrics*, **7**, 159–62.

O'Callaghan, M. J., Burns, Y., Gray, P. *et al.* (1995). Extremely low birth weight and control infants at 2 years corrected age: a comparison of intellectual abilities motor performance, growth and health. *Early Human Development*, **40**, 115–25.

Peterson, B. S., Vohr, B. R., Staib, L. H. & Cannistraci, C. J. (2000). Regional brain volume abnormalities and long term cognitive outcome in preterm infants. *Journal of the American Medical Association*, **284**, 1939–48.

Powls, A., Botting, N., Cooke, R. W. & Marlow, N. (1995). Motor impairment in children 12–13 years old with a birthweight of less than 1,250 g. *Archives of Diseases in Childhood*, **72**, 62–6.

Rickards, A. L., Kitchen, W. H., Doyle, L. W. & Kelly, E. A. (1989). Correction of developmental and intelligence test scores for premature birth. *Australian Paediatric Journal*, **25**, 127–9.

Saigal, S., Stoskopf, B. L., Streiner, D. L. & Burrows, E. (2001). Physical growth and current health status of infants who were of extremely low birthweight and controls at adolescence. *Pediatrics*, **108**, 407–15.

Saigal, S., Lambert, M., Russ, C. & Hoult, L. (2002). Self-esteem of adolescents who were born prematurely. *Pediatrics*, **109**, 429–34.

Saigal, S., den Ouden, A. L., Wolke, D. *et al.* (2003). School-age outcomes in children who were extremely low birth weight from four international population based cohorts. *Pediatrics*, **112**, 943–8.

Stjernqvist, K. & Svenningsen, N. W. (1999). Ten-year follow-up of children born before 29 gestational weeks: health, cognitive development, behaviour and school achievement. *Acta Paediatrica*, **88**, 557–62.

Vohr, B. R., Wright, L. L., Dusick, A. M. *et al.* (2000). Neurodevelopmental and functional outcomes of extremely low birthweight in the National institute of child health and human development neonatal research network, 1993–1994. *Pediatrics*, **105**, 1216–26.

Wolke, D. (1998). Psychological development of prematurely born children. *Archieves of Diseases in Childhood*, **78**, 567–70.

World Health Organization (1993). *International Statistical Classification of Diseases and Related Health Problems (ICD-10).* Geneva: World Health Organization.

Premenstrual syndrome

Jane M. Ussher

University of Western Sydney

Premenstrual distress is now widely recognized to be a major social and health problem, with epidemiological surveys estimating that 95% of women experience physical and psychological changes premenstrually. Up to 40% experience moderate distress, categorized by clinicians and researchers as Premenstrual Syndrome (PMS) and 11–13% experience severe distress and disruption to their lives, categorized as Premenstrual Dysphoric Disorder (PMDD) (Steiner & Born, 2000). However, ever since discussions of premenstrual distress first appeared contemporaneously in the medical and psychoanalytic literature in 1931, this has been a research field dogged by controversy and disagreement.

Initially described as 'premenstrual tension', and attributed to either hormonal imbalances (Frank, 1931), or to intrapsychic conflict exacerbated by women's social role (Horney, 1931), it was renamed 'Premenstrual Syndrome' in 1953, 'Late Luteal Phase Dysphoric disorder in the DSM III-R and 'Premenstrual Dysphoric Disorder' in the DSM-IV. Regardless of the diagnostic classification adopted, the divide between biomedical and psychological explanations continues to this day, with a range of competing theories associating PMS with a single causal factor. Biological theories of PMS can be divided into six categories: gonadal steroids and gonadoptrophins; neurovegetive signs (sleep, appetite changes); neuroendocrine factors; serotonin and other neurotransmitters; β-endorphin; and other potential substrates (including prostaglandins, vitamins, electrolytes and CO_2) (Parry, 1994, p.47). The psychosocial theories include: personality; cognitions associated with femininity and menstruation; the influence of stress and life events; and propensity for psychological illness (Walker, 1997). Following controlled clinical trials, the mostly widely advocated theories at the current time are serotonin imbalance, leading to the prescription of selective serotonin reuptake inhibitors (SSRIs) (Mortola *et al.*, 2002); or cognitive schemas, linked to life stress, leading to the adoption of cognitive–behaviour therapy (CBT) (Blake *et al.*, 1998; Hunter *et al.*, 2002*a*) (see 'Cognitive behaviour therapy').

One limitation of existing research is that aetiological assumptions are erroneously made on the basis of statistically significant relationships between reporting of symptoms and the particular dependant variable of interest, or on the basis of treatment efficacy. Aspirin is an effective cure for headache, and inhalation of CO_2 an effective treatment for panic attacks, yet we would not propose that either aspirin or CO_2 are implicated in the aetiology of either disorder. The very premise of a causal relationship is also flawed, as the discovery of a correlation between premenstrual distress and a particular hormone does not mean that the hormone caused the distress. Each may be related to a third variable, such as stress, or not related at all (Gannon, 1988).

Equally, conducted within a positivist epistemological framework (Ussher, 1996), existing research reifies PMS as a disorder, implicitly conceptualizing it as a static or fixed entity, with the occurrence (or non-occurrence) of symptoms as the end-point of analysis (Ussher, 2002*a*). The cultural construction of 'PMS' or 'PMDD', women's ongoing appraisal and negotiation of changes in emotion, behaviour, or bodily sensations, the meaning of PMS in their lives and the role of relationships in the development of premenstrual symptoms are issues that are marginalized or negated.

Women's negotiation of PMS in a cultural and relational context

The bodily functions we understand as a sign of 'illness' vary across culture and across time (Sedgewick, 1987). Women's interpretation of psychological and bodily changes as being 'symptoms' of PMS cannot be understood outside of the social and historical context in which they live, influenced by the meaning ascribed to these changes in a particular cultural context. In cultures where PMS does not circulate as a discursive category, women do not take up the position of PMS sufferer, and do not blame PMS, or the premenstrual body, for psychological distress (Chandra & Chaturvedi, 1992). This has led feminist critics to argue that PMS and PMDD are merely the latest in a line of diagnostic categories which act to pathologise the reproductive body (Parlee, 1991; Nash & Chrisler, 1997). However, we also need to acknowledge the vulnerability experienced by women premenstrually, the role of the body or social stressors in premenstrual experiences and women's subjective evaluation and negotiation of psychological and bodily changes (see also 'Cultural and ethnic factors in health').

Recent research has demonstrated that the development of premenstrual symptoms, and the construction of these symptoms as 'PMS', is a shifting process of negotiation and coping, which occurs in a relational context. For example, in research conducted in the UK and Australia, three inter-related processes of appraisal and coping were found to be central to the experience and construction of PMS. These were, awareness of premenstrual changes in emotion, ability to cope, or reactivity to others; expectations and perceptions of these changes; and mode of response or coping (Ussher, 2002*a*). At each stage in this process, women could resist, or take up, the position of 'PMS sufferer': the construction of premenstrual change as PMS was not inevitable. Relational issues were a major predictor of self-diagnosis and coping. Feeling out of control and unable to

tolerate negative emotional or bodily change, particularly in situations where there were overwhelming demands from partner or children, was the most common description of PMS given by women in narrative interviews (Ussher, 2003*a*). The most problematic 'symptoms' were anger or depression in the context of family relationships, leading to the desire to be alone and to eschew responsibility, followed by shame or guilt (Ussher, 2003*b*). Women, and their families, attributed these 'symptoms' to PMS, even when alternative explanations could be found and thus through a process of splitting, disassociated negative emotions or behaviours from the woman. Many women also reported self-silencing and self-sacrifice in relation to their families during the non-premenstrual phase of the cycle, with grievances in relationships coming to the fore and being expressed premenstrually (Ussher, 2004*b*). This rupture in self-silencing appears to function to allow the expression of both day-to-day frustrations, and anger associated with more substantial relationship issues, which are repressed during the rest of the month as women attempt to be 'good' (Ussher, 2004*a*). This supports previous findings that women who report premenstrual symptoms also report higher levels of relationship dissatisfaction or difficulties (Ryser & Feinauer, 1992) and that constructions of femininity are tied to experiences of premenstrual distress (Cosgrove & Riddle, 2003) (see also 'Gender issues and women's health').

There is evidence from previous research that that many women do experience increased vulnerability or sensitivity to external stress during the premenstrual phase of the cycle, resulting from a combination of hormonal or endocrine changes, sensitivity to changes in autonomic arousal and differential perceptions of stress premenstrually, linked to cultural constructions of 'PMS' as negative and debilitating. Experimental research has also demonstrated that dual or multiple task performance is more difficult premenstrually, and whilst women can compensate with increased effort, this can result in increased levels of anxiety. It is thus not surprising that many women report reacting to the stresses and strains of daily life with decreased tolerance premenstrually, particularly when they carry multiple responsibilities. This is the one time in the month that they cannot live up to internalized idealized expectations of femininity, with increased vulnerability, or reduced tolerance, leading to a rupture in self-silencing.

A material–discursive–intrapsychic model of premenstrual distress

In order to understand these different aspects of women's premenstrual experience, we need to adopt a multi-factorial perspective. This can be achieved through adopting a Material–Discursive–Intrapsychic (MDI) model, which posits that an ongoing interaction of material (e.g. changes in hormones, physiological arousal, neurotransmitters, or life stresses), discursive (e.g. cultural constructions and representations of PMS, reproduction and gender) and intrapsychic factors (e.g. mode of evaluating and coping with changes, expectations of self, defence mechanisms) combine to produce emotions, bodily sensations and behaviours, which come to be diagnosed as 'PMS' or 'PMDD' by the woman herself, or by a clinician (Ussher, 1999).

Multifactorial models for PMS, within a biopsychosocial framework, have previously been put forward (Walker, 1995; Blake,

1995; Ussher, 1992; Bancroft, 1993). However, MDI does not position either psychological or biological aetiological factors as the point of origin of PMS; it develops the analysis of psychological processes involved in PMS beyond the cognitive–behavioural; and is the first to explicitly engage with constructionist and discursive accounts of PMS, through acknowledging the role of discursive representations of 'PMS' and femininity in analyses of the development and course of premenstrual symptoms. In using the MDI model as the basis of prevention and intervention for PMS, a combination of approaches would be suggested as optimum. This would include: the challenging of negative cultural constructions of the reproductive body and of PMS; couple therapy, if relationship issues are a significant factor in women's distress; individual psychological interventions which take material, discursive and intrapsychic factors on board (e.g. Ussher *et al.*, 2002*b*); and if necessary, biomedical treatments (such as SSRIs) to alleviate severe symptoms. Such a multifactorial approach to PMS is common practice when clinicians are working with individual women; this approach can be justified on the basis of the research literature and now needs to appear as a legitimate focus in theoretical analyses of PMS, heralding a move away from narrow unilinear models of aetiology and treatment.

REFERENCES

American Psychiatric Association (APA) (1987). *Diagnostic and statistical manual of mental disorders*, Edition IIIR Washington DC: American Psychiatric Association.

American Psychiatric Association (APA) (2000). *Diagnostic and statistical manual of mental disorders*, Edition IV Washington DC: American Psychiatric Association.

Bancroft, J. (1993). The premenstrual syndrome: a reappraisal of the concept and the evidence. *Psychological Medicine*, **241**(suppl.), 1–47.

Blake, F. (1995). Cognitive therapy for premenstrual syndrome. *Cognitive and Behavioral Practice*, **2**, 167–85.

Blake, F., Salkovskis, P., Gath, D., Day, A. & Garrod, A. (1998). Cognitive therapy for premenstrual syndrome: a controlled trial. *Journal of Psychosomatic Research*, **45**, 307–18.

Chandra, P. S. & Chaturvedi, S. K. (1992). Cultural variations in attitudes toward menstruation. *Canadian Journal of Psychiatry*, **37**, 196–8.

Cosgrove, L. & Riddle, B. (2003). Constructions of femininity and experiences of menstrual distress. *Women & Health*, **38**, 37–58.

Frank, R. (1931). The hormonal causes of premenstrual tension. *Archives of Neurological Psychiatry*, **26**, 1053.

Gannon, L. (1988). The potential role of exercise in the alleviation of menstrual disorders and menopausal symptoms: a theoretical synthesis of recent research. *Women and Health*, **14**, 105–27.

Horney, K. (1931). Die Pramenstruellen Verstimmungen. *Zeitscher. f. Psychoanalytische Padagogik*, **5**, 1–17.

Hunter, M. S., Ussher, J. M., Browne, S. *et al.* (2002). A randomised comparison of psychological (cognitive behaviour therapy), medical (fluoxetine) and combined treatment for women with Premenstrual Dysphoric Disorder. *Journal of Psychosomatic Obstetrics and Gynaecology*, **23**, 193–9.

Mortola, J. F., Brunswick, D. J. & Amsterdam, A. J. (2002). Premenstrual syndrome: cyclic symptoms in women of reproductive age. *Psychiatric Annals*, **32**, 452–62.

Nash, H. C. & Chrisler, J. C. (1997). Is a little (psychiatric) knowledge a dangerous thing? The impact of premenstrual dysphoric disorder on perceptions of premenstrual women. *Psychology of Women Quarterly*, **21**, 315–22.

Parlee, M. (1991). The social construction of PMS: a case study of scientific discourse as cultural contestation., Paper presented at '*The good body: asceticism in contemporary culture*' conference. Institute for the Medical Humanities, Texan University, Galveston, April 12–13.

Parry, B. (1994). Biological correlates premenstrual complaints. In J.Gold, H., & S.Severino, K. (Eds.). Premenstrual dysphoria: myths and realities. (pp. 47–66) London: American Psychiatric Press.

Ryser, R. & Feinauer, L. L. (1992). Premenstrual syndrome and the marital relationship. *American Journal of Family Therapy*, **20**, 179–90.

Sedgewick, P. (1987). *Psychopolitics*. London: Pluto Press.

Steiner, M. & Born, L. (2000). Advances in the diagnosis and treatment of premenstrual dysphoria. *CNS Drugs*, **13**, 287–304.

Ussher, J. M. (1992). Research and theory related to female reproduction: implications for clinical psychology. *British Journal of Clinical Psychology*, **31**, 129–51.

Ussher, J. M. (1996). Premenstrual syndrome: reconciling disciplinary divides through the adoption of a material–discursive epistemological standpoint. *Annual Review of Sex Research*, **7**, 218–51.

Ussher, J. M. (1999). In A. Kolk, M. Bekker & K. Van Vliet (Eds.). *Advances in women and health research* (pp. 47–64). Tilburg: Tilburg University Press.

Ussher, J. M. (2002*a*). Processes of appraisal and coping in the development and maintenance of Premenstrual dysphoric disorder. *Journal of Community and Applied Social Psychology*, **12**, 1–14.

Ussher, J. M. (2003*a*). The role of Premenstrual dysphoric disorder in the subjectification of women. *Journal of Medical Humanities*, **24**, 131–46.

Ussher, J. M. (2003*b*). The ongoing silencing of women in families: an analysis and rethinking of premenstrual syndrome and therapy. *Journal of Family Therapy*, **25**, 387–404.

Ussher, J. M. (2004). Blaming the body for distress: Premenstrual dysphoric disorder and the subjectification of woman. In A. Potts, N. Gavey, & A. Watherall (Eds.). *Sex and the body* (pp. 183–202). Palmerstone North, NZ: Dunmore Press.

Ussher, J. M. (2004*b*). Premenstrual syndrome and self-policing: ruptures in self-silencing leading to increased self-surveillance and blaming of the body, *Social Theory and Health*, **2**, 1–19.

Ussher, J. M., Hunter, M. & Cariss, M. (2002*b*). A woman-centred psychological intervention for premenstrual symptoms, drawing on cognitive–behavioural and narrative therapy. *Clinical Psychology and Psychotherapy*, **9**, 3319–31.

Walker, A. (1995). Theory and methodology in Premenstrual syndrome research. *Social Science and Medicine*, **41**, 793–800.

Walker, A. (1997). *The menstrual cycle*. London: Routledge.

Psoriasis

Catherine J. O'Leary

Guy's Hospital

Psoriasis

Psoriasis is a chronic, non-contagious skin condition affecting between 1% and 2% of the populations of industrialized countries (Russo *et al.*, 2004). It is characterized by lesions of skin which are inflamed, itchy and scaly. Severity can range from lesions on the elbows alone to extensive body coverage. The most common form of psoriasis is chronic plaque, characterized by lesions round in shape, a few centimetres in diameter, raised and covered in a silvery scale. Any part of the skin may be affected including the scalp. Psoriasis can also result in pitting, discolouration and separation from the nail bed of both finger and toe nails. In addition, 1 in 20 psoriasis sufferers have psoriatic arthritis of the joints. Many people with psoriasis experience the Koebner phenomenon in which lesions occur in areas where there has been skin trauma or injury, such as a cut, an injection site or burn.

The severity of psoriasis is rarely static. The majority of individuals cycle between differing levels of severity throughout their lifetime, experiencing 'spontaneous' remissions and flare-ups during the course of their condition. There is no cure for psoriasis and instead treatment is aimed at reducing symptoms and improving the appearance of the skin. Medical treatments include topical ointments and creams, phototherapy and systemic treatments. These can be unpleasant to use and time-consuming, often involving frequent hospital visits.

In recent years, it has become clear that in addition to the physical problems such as pain, itching and flaky skin, psoriasis also causes a great deal of psychological disability. There is evidence to suggest that people with psoriasis experience high levels of anxiety (Fortune *et al.*, 2000) and depression (Akay *et al.*, 2002), suicidal ideation (Gupta & Gupta, 1998), reduced quality of life (Scharloo *et al.*, 1998) and sexual dysfunction (Gupta & Gupta, 1997) (see 'Quality of life' and 'Sexual dysfunction').

Interestingly, research has suggested that increased levels of emotional distress are not directly related to the severity of psoriasis (Stern *et al.*, 2004). Instead several factors appear to contribute to such distress, one of the main contributing factors being a fear of negative evaluation. Leary *et al.* (1998) found that a strong fear of negative evaluation was significantly correlated with poorer social life, family relationships, recreation and leisure and emotional wellbeing. Similarly, Fortune *et al.* (1997) found that anticipating negative reactions from others and a fear of being rejected were strongly related to psychosocial disability and a poor quality of life. Common stressors experienced by Fortune *et al.*'s (1997) sample included feeling the need to wear inconvenient or unattractive clothes in order to cover up and strangers making insensitive or rude remarks (see also 'Facial disfigurement').

In one survey, individuals rated the stigma associated with psoriasis as being the worst aspect of the condition and reported feeling the need to hide their skin from others, avoiding many daily activities such as swimming, wearing short sleeves or going to the hairdressers (Stankler, 1981) (see 'Stigma'). In one study, 19% of the sample reported incidents where they had been asked to leave a public place such as a swimming pool because of the appearance of their skin (Ginsburg & Link, 1993).

The location of the psoriasis also appears to be a significant contributor to psychological distress and this ties in with a fear of negative evaluation. Psoriasis occurring in areas that are not so easily covered up such as the face, neck and hands, results in poorer levels of quality of life (Heydendael *et al.*, 2004). The way in which psoriasis interferes with day to day chores or one's ability to work has also been found to influence the amount of psychological distress experienced (Ginsburg & Link, 1989).

Rapp *et al.* (2001) found that the coping strategies used by many psoriasis sufferers actually impaired quality of life. More specifically, telling others about psoriasis, covering the lesions and avoiding people was associated with poorer levels of health-related quality of life. In contrast, telling people that psoriasis is not contagious was related to smaller decreases in quality of life. Scharloo *et al.* (2000) found that people who coped by expressing emotions, seeking social support and distraction were less anxious and depressed and had a better physical health at a 1-year follow-up (see 'Emotional expression and health' and 'Social support and health'). In contrast, the belief that psoriasis causes many symptoms was associated with more visits to the outpatient clinic and worse levels of quality of life and depression one year later.

Recent studies have examined illness perceptions; that is individuals' common sense understanding of their psoriasis, and how these beliefs affect quality of life and psychological wellbeing (see 'Lay beliefs about health and illness'). Scharloo *et al.* (1998) found that beliefs about the diagnosis and the symptoms associated with psoriasis were important factors in explaining the variance in quality of life. Fortune *et al.* (2000) found that if psoriasis sufferers believed that they were to blame for having psoriasis then they were more likely to experience pathological worry. Worry was associated with a stronger belief that psoriasis had an emotional cause and the belief that psoriasis would be chronic or recurring (see also *Attributions and health*).

Although it is unclear why psoriasis develops, it is often suggested that psychological stress in the individual's life may cause the condition to flare and worsen. There have been a number of studies looking at the role stress plays in the onset and exacerbation of psoriasis (see 'Stress and health'). However, the findings have been mixed and this may be the result of numerous methodological difficulties such as small samples sizes, retrospective design and psychometric invalidity (for example Arntez *et al.*, 1985; Gaston *et al.*, 1987; Payne *et al.*, 1985). In addition, these studies have been hampered by difficulties regarding the definition of stress. Overall there is a lack of firm evidence linking stress to the onset or worsening of psoriasis (O'Leary *et al.*, 2004; Picardi & Abeni, 2001).

Much of the evidence suggesting a relationship between stress and psoriasis has arisen from self-report studies, with high proportions of individuals with psoriasis reporting stress as the major precipitating factor in the onset and exacerbation of their condition (Mazzetti *et al.*, 1994; Zachariae *et al.*, 2004). Al'Abadie *et al.* (1994) found that people with psoriasis were more likely to report a stressful experience as pre-dating the onset or exacerbation than those with other skin conditions (for example acne, alopecia, basal cell carcinoma). In a large survey of Nordic sufferers ($n > 5000$) 35% reported that the onset of their psoriasis occurred during a period of worry, whilst over 65% of the sample reported that their condition was exacerbated by stress (Zachariae *et al.*, 2004). The authors of this survey suggest that there may be a sub-group of individuals who are more psychologically reactive to their psoriasis.

It is important to note that many individuals with psoriasis have been informed by their practitioners or through self-help books (e.g. Marks, 1981) that psoriasis is related to stress. This is likely to lead to a cognitive bias in the remembering and reporting of stressful events. In a recent study examining causal beliefs in psoriasis (O'Leary *et al.*, 2004), a strong belief in stress as a causal factor was found in over 60% of the sample. This belief was significantly associated with higher levels of anxiety, depression and perceived stress. However, there was no association between perceived stress and measures of psoriasis severity. This suggests that the perception that stress as a causal factor may in fact be detrimental to emotional wellbeing.

A number of psychological interventions for people with psoriasis have been developed and these tend to be based on two basic assumptions: (i) that psychological stress is related to the exacerbation of the condition and (ii) that much of the psychological morbidity in psoriasis is related to factors such as the anticipation of others' reactions, feelings of shame or embarrassment and not the severity of psoriasis.

The efficacy of such psychological interventions has generally been reported in the form of case studies. Winchell *et al.* (1988) reviewed four case studies in which relaxation and suggestions of improvement resulted in actual improvements in severity. In one case, the intervention resulted in complete remission. Whilst case studies can be a useful source of information, controlled trials with larger samples provide more conclusive evidence.

Zacharie *et al.* (1996) have examined the efficacy of a stress-management programme using a randomized control trial design.

In this study, 51 patients were assigned to a treatment group or a control. The intervention consisted of cognitive–behavioural stress management, relaxation training and imagery training (see 'Cognitive behaviour therapy' and 'Relaxation training'). The results demonstrated small but significant improvements in psoriasis severity in the treatment group from baseline to end of treatment. There were no changes in the control group. Interestingly there was no change in perceived stress for either group throughout the trial. This suggests that an improvement in levels of daily stress cannot account for the change.

Kabat-Zinn *et al.* (1998) applied a meditation-based stress reduction programme to 37 patients with psoriasis undergoing photo(chemo)therapy (UVB or PUVA). Patients were assigned to either the treatment condition (audiotaped instructions played during photo(chemo)therapy) or a control condition (no taped instructions). The patients were not blinded but were told that the tapes would make treatment more pleasant. Nothing was said to create expectations of an improvement due to the tapes. There was a trend towards faster clearance of plaques in the treatment group, although the results did not reach statistical significance. Due to the lack of significance this study presents only tentative evidence for the efficacy of a stress-reduction approach to intervention.

Main *et al.* (2000) have developed a biopsychosocial approach to the treatment of psoriasis, The Psoriasis Symptom Management Programme (PSMP). The PSMP is a 6-week group programme, and involves cognitive–behavioural techniques aimed at modifying unhelpful thoughts and beliefs and relaxation, alongside traditional medical management. Whilst their preliminary results appear to be encouraging (Richards *et al.*, 1999), less than 10% of those offered the PSMP accepted a place questioning the requirement for such psychological therapy (Fortune *et al.*, 1998). A recent outcome study (Fortune *et al.*, 2004) has shown that at 6-month follow-up, the PSMP had been successful in modifying some illness perceptions, namely perceptions relating to the number of symptoms associated with the condition, the strength of belief in the severity of the condition and in attributions for emotional causes. However, perceptions relating to cure or control of psoriasis or beliefs about physical causes did not change. Similarly the use of coping strategies did not change.

In summary, current research suggests that psoriasis can result in psychological disturbance. Furthermore, someone with relatively mild psoriasis may be more distressed than someone with severe psoriasis if that psoriasis occurs in visible places, stops them from working or socialising or if they expect people to judge them harshly. The implications of these research findings are that clinicians cannot estimate the psychological impact of psoriasis simply by looking at the extent and severity of the condition. There is preliminary evidence to suggest that psychological treatments aimed at reducing social anxiety and modifying unhelpful beliefs (for example the belief that one is being evaluated negatively) help people to cope with this chronic skin condition.

(See also 'Skin disorders', 'Acne' and 'Eczema'.)

REFERENCES

Akay, A., Pekcanlar, A., Bozdag, K. E., Altintas, L. & Karaman, A. (2002). Assessment of depression in subjects with psoriasis vulgaris and lichen planus. *Journal of European Academy of Dermatology and Venereology*, **16**(4), 347–52.

Al'Abadie, M. S., Kent, G. G. & Gawkrodger, D. J. (1994). The relationship between stress and the onset and exacerbation of psoriasis and other skin conditions. *British Journal of Dermatology*, **130**, 199–203.

Arnetz, B. B., Fjellner, B., Eneroth, P. & Kallner, A. (1985). Stress and psoriasis: psychoendocrine and metabolic reactions in psoriatic patients during a standardized stressor exposure. *Psychosomatic Medicine*, **47**(6), 528–41.

Fortune, D. G., Richards, H. L., Main, C. J. & Griffiths, C. E. (2000). Pathological worrying, illness perceptions and disease severity in patients with psoriasis. *British Journal of Health Psychology*, **5**, 71–82.

Fortune, D. G., Richards, H. L., Griffiths, C. E. & Main, C. J. (2004). Targeting cognitive–behaviour therapy to patients' implicit model of psoriasis: results from a patient preference controlled trial. *British Journal of Clinical Psychology*, **43**(1), 65–82.

Fortune, D. G., Main, C. J., O'Sullivan, T. M. & Griffiths, C. E. M. (1997). Quality of life in patients with psoriasis: the contribution of clinical variables and psoriasis-specific stress. *British Journal of Dermatology*, **137**, 755–60.

Fortune, D. G., Richards, H. L., Main, C. J., O'Sullivan, T. M. & Griffiths, C. E. (1998). Developing clinical psychology services in an outpatient dermatology specialty clinic: what factors are associated with non-uptake of the service? *Clinical psychology Forum*, **115**, 34–6.

Gaston, L., Lassonde, M., Bernier-Buzzanga, J., Hodgins, S. & Crombez, J. (1987). Psoriasis and stress: a prospective study. *Journal of the American Academy of Dermatology*, **17**, 82–6.

Ginsburg, I. H. & Link, B. G. (1993). Psychosocial consequences of rejection and stigma feelings in psoriasis patients. *International Journal of Dermatology*, **32**, 587–91.

Gupta, M. A. & Gupta, A. K. (1997). Psoriasis and sex: a study of moderately to severely affected patients. *International Journal of Dermatology*, **36**(4), 259–62.

Gupta, M. A. & Gupta, A. K. (1998). Depression and suicidal ideation in dermatology patients with acne, alopecia areata, atopic dermatitis and psoriasis. *British Journal of Dermatology*, **139**(5), 846–50.

Heydendael, V. M., de Borgie, C. A., Spuls, P. I. *et al.* (2004). The burden of psoriasis is not determined by disease severity only. *The Journal of Investigative Dermatology. Symposium Proceedings*, **9**(2), 131–5.

Jowett, S. & Ryan, T. (1985). Skin disease and handicap: an analysis of the impact of skin conditions. *Social Science and Medicine*, **20**(4), 425–9.

Kabat-Zin, J., Wheeler, E., Light, T. *et al.* (1998). Influence of mindfulness mediation-based stress reduction intervention on rates of skin clearing in patients with moderate to severe psoriasis undergoing phototherapy (UVB) and photochemotherapy (PUVA). *Psychosomatic Medicine*, **60**, 625–32.

Leary, M. R., Rapp, S. R., Herbst, K. C., Exum, M. L. & Feldman, S. R. (1998). Interpersonal concerns and psychological difficulties of psoriasis patients: effects of disease severity and fear of negative evaluation. *Health Psychology*, **17**(6), 530–6.

Main, C. J., Richards, H. L. & Fortune, D. G. (2000). Why put new wine in old bottles: the need for a biopsychosocial approach to the assessment, treatment and understanding of unexplained and explained symptoms in medicine. *Journal of Psychosomatic Research*, **48**, 511–14.

Marks, R. (1981). *Coping with psoriasis* (pp. 26–33). London: Sheldon Press.

Mazzetti, M., Mozzetta, A., Soavi, G. *et al.* (1994). Psoriasis, stress and psychiatry: psychodynamic characteristics of stressors. *Acta Dermato-Venereologica. Supplementum*, **186**, 62–4.

Payne, R. A., Rowland Payne, C. M. E. & Marks, R. (1985). Stress does not worsen psoriasis? A control study of 32 patients. *Clinical Experimental Dermatology*, **10**, 239–45.

O'Leary, C. J., Creamer, D., Higgins, E. & Weinman, J. (2004). Perceived stress, stress attributions and psychological distress in psoriasis. *Journal of Psychosomatic Research*, **57**(5), 465–71.

Picardie, A. & Abeni, D. (2001). Stressful life events and skin diseases: disentangling evidence from myth. *Psychother Psychosom*, **70**(3), 118–36.

Rapp, S. R., Cottrell, C. A. & Leary, M. R. (2001). Social coping strategies associated with quality of life decrements among psoriasis patients. *British Journal of Dermatology*, **145**, 610–16.

Richards, H. L., Fortune, D. G., Bowcock, S. *et al.* (1999). Cognitive–behavioural management of psoriasis (abstract). *British Journal of Dermatology*, **141**, 979.

Russo, P. A., Ilchef, R. & Cooper, A. J. (2004). Psychiatric morbidity in psoriasis: a review. *Australasian Journal of Dermatology*, **45**(3), 155–61.

Scharloo, M., Kaptein, A., Weinman, J. *et al.* (1998). Illness perceptions, coping and functioning in patients with rheumatoid arthritis, chronic obstructive pulmonary disease and psoriasis. *Journal of Psychosomatic Research*, **44**(5), 573–85.

Scharloo, M., Kaptein, A., Weinman, J. *et al.* (2000). Patients' illness perceptions and coping as predictors of functional status in psoriasis: a 1-year follow-up. *British Journal of Dermatology*, **142**, 899–907.

Stankler, L. (1981). The effect of psoriasis on the sufferer. *Clinical and Experimental Dermatology*, **6**, 303–6.

Stern, R. S., Nijsten, T., Feldman, S. R., Margolis, D. J. & Rolstad, T. (2004). Psoriasis is common, carries a substantial burden even when not extensive, and is associated with widespread treatment dissatisfaction. *The Journal of Investigative Dermatology. Symposium Proceedings*, **9**(2), 136–9.

Winchell, S. A. & Watts, R. A. (1988). Relaxation therapies in the treatment of psoriasis and possible pathophysiologic mechanisms. *Journal of the American Academy of Dermatology*, **18**, 101–4.

Zacharie, R., Oster, H., Bjerring, P. & Kragballe, K. (1996). Effects of psychologic intervention on psoriasis: a preliminary report. *Journal of the American Academy of Dermatology*, **34**, 1008–15.

Zachariae, R., Zachariae, H., Blomqvist, K. *et al.* (2004). Self-reported stress reactivity and psoriasis-related stress of Nordic psoriasis sufferers. *Journal of the European Academy of Dermatology and Venereology*, **18**(1), 27–36.

Radiotherapy

Sara Faithfull

University of Surrey

Radiotherapy is a common treatment modality for cancer with over 50% of individuals receiving radiation at some time during the course of their disease. Despite the extent of its use and the length of time it has been available our knowledge is limited in how it affects individuals not only physically but also emotionally and socially. Radiotherapy can cause problems through side effects of treatment. These can be temporary symptoms (acute effects) that occur during or in the months following treatment, but also longer lasting effects (late effects) that can develop many months to years following radiotherapy. Much of the knowledge that exists as to how people react or cope with radiation treatment is focused on the physical effects and much less on the psychological responses. However radiation reactions can often exacerbate existing functional or emotional difficulties that can be as a result of the disease, age or a combination of therapies. This chapter explores the incidence and specific psychological problems identified as a result of radiotherapy treatment for cancer. The evidence is reviewed for psychosocial interventions for those undergoing or completing radiotherapy.

The need to include information representing patients' views of their condition has become more important as survival from cancer has gradually increased. Evaluations of treatment modalities have psychological and social consequences. Clearly, with cancer treatment, a person's physical health status contributes much to the psychological impact of a treatment modality. However, factors that should also be considered are the emotional impact and the effect cancer treatment has on social and personal relationships.

Incidence of psychosocial problems

Assessing the psychological impact of cancer treatment on patients is expressed in terms of current definitions of anxiety and depression. Early studies of psychological morbidity suggest that 20 to 35% of all individuals with cancer experience anxiety and/or depression during the course of their therapy (Fallowfield, 1990) (see 'Cancer: general'). Many studies have identified the emotional and physical distress associated with radiotherapy (Forester et al., 1978; Christman, 1990; King et al., 1985). However, the proportion of people who experience distress or have psychological problems is unclear. Peck and Boland's (1977) much quoted work first identified that patients fear and misunderstand the use of radiation treatment and have negative attitudes to its effectiveness as cancer therapy. They interviewed people ($n=50$) undergoing radiotherapy and found most experienced mild to moderate anxiety. They determined that at the start of treatment 60% experienced anxiety. This rose to 80% after treatment was completed. However, much has changed in health care since this study was conducted, with greater openness

about cancer diagnosis and information-giving prior to treatment. Maraste et al. (1992) identified that 15% of women undergoing adjuvant breast irradiation experienced distress as anxiety rather than as depression or other psychological states. More recent work has identified that individuals still fear radiation and consider it negatively (Hammick et al., 1998). However, Hammick et al.,'s small study does not identify whether this attitude influences people's experiences or distress more widely. Young & Maher (1992), in an audit of a counselling service, found that 44% of those attending a British radiotherapy centre had abnormal levels of anxiety. Beyond this there has been little systematic study of the social or psychological reactions to radiation treatment and the proportion of people who experience specific problems.

Emotional distress is not limited to just the time of radiotherapy; it is recognized in several studies that it changes over the course of treatment. Physical symptoms may persist or worsen over several weeks and, therefore, the period of delivery of treatment may not represent the true time course of the impact of therapy. Holland et al. (1979), in a study of women with breast cancer having adjuvant radiotherapy, found that they had higher overall anxiety scores than women not having therapy. As women neared the end of their treatment, they became more depressed and were less hopeful about being cured. Forester et al. (1978) also found that patients reported restlessness, anxiety, apprehension, social isolation and feelings of withdrawal at the end of treatment. Ward et al. (1992), in a small study of women's reactions to completion of radiotherapy, acknowledge that the end of treatment does not always bring relief. Out of the 38 women interviewed, 11 (30%) found termination of treatment upsetting, and this was frequently connected to a worsening of side effects and not just the completion of the course of treatment. Women who were most anxious or depressed at the beginning of treatment were those most upset at treatment completion. This is also reflected in work by Graydon (1988) who suggests that emotional distress at the beginning of treatment is predictive of post-treatment functioning. Anderson and Tewfik (1985), in a sample of 45 women treated with external beam radiotherapy, found significant changes in anxiety between pre- and post-treatment assessments. As treatment progressed, patients with an initially high level of anxiety reported a significant reduction, those with moderate anxiety reported no change and those with low levels of anxiety reported significant increases. Several studies identify that fear at the outset of treatment is predictive of how well individuals adapt to radiotherapy. However, given the complexity of the radiotherapy treatment context, it is not surprising that a wide range of stresses can affect individuals at different times during the treatment trajectory (Lamszus & Verres, 1995).

Many of the studies discussed focus on specific populations and it is not clear how they can be generalized or whether disease specific determinants influence distress. These studies are focused within narrow parametres of distress and psychological morbidity, which may not reflect the everyday difficulties experienced with radiotherapy treatment (Fitch et al., 2003). Munro et al., who explored broader perceptions of distress in radiotherapy, found that men and women interviewed within the first 24 hours of starting radiotherapy had concerns that were different from their concerns at the end of treatment. Twenty people were asked to rank cards giving details of treatment related sequelae or concerns in order of severity of distress caused. It was found that concerns at the end of treatment were practical in nature, for example not being able to wash. Lower down the list were concerns that the treatment might not work. Distress was also caused by physical symptoms: fatigue ranked second both at the beginning and end of radiotherapy. However, Munro et al. (1989) only investigated distress at two time points, the beginning and end of treatment, which meant any distress experienced in the period following treatment remained undiscovered. Assessments that focus specifically on psychological morbidity, such as depression or anxiety, may not capture these other issues and therefore may not be particularly helpful in clinical practice, or address aspects of service delivery that result in distress. With a broader perspective, identifying what patients themselves feel as distressing, different elements may be identified that influence the impact of treatment. In the absence of a large-scale study looking prospectively at psychological problems, distress, physical symptoms and quality of life in cancer, it is impossible to draw meaningful conclusions. The emotional impact of treatment is not simple to assess and few centres routinely screen patients undergoing radiotherapy (Faithfull, 2003).

Clinical implications

Information provision and reduction of anxiety

Studies exploring strategies for the provision of information in radiotherapy have mainly been conducted in North America. The literature highlights that individuals undergoing radiotherapy have little knowledge or insight into what to expect with regard to the potential side effects of radiotherapy. Research has shown that preparatory information prior to receiving radiotherapy helps improve coping and has been shown to significantly reduce emotional distress and improve functioning following treatment (Johnson et al., 1989). Rainey (1985), in an evaluation of the provision of audiovisual educational material, found that the intervention used improved knowledge of treatment but that differences between the control and intervention groups diminished as treatment progressed. Those having the intervention had less emotional distress.

Porock (1995), in a prospective study, found that those who received structured information experienced less anxiety and had higher levels of satisfaction during and after treatment (see also 'Patient satisfaction'). Dodd and Ahmed (1987) looked at differences in preference for information and found people preferred a more cognitive style of information. Studies of different types of information have shown that regardless of the style of patient education, all forms help improve the knowledge of radiation treatment for those having therapy (Israel and Mood, 1988; Johnson et al., 1989).

The assumption is that by making people better informed they will feel less anxious and be able to cope more effectively throughout treatment. Although this has been demonstrated in surgical and coronary care (Mumford et al., 1982), the exact mechanism and time scales may be different for radiotherapy.

There is a problem in these studies in that evaluations of the effectiveness of information provision are often based on knowledge recall. Understanding or being able to recount facts about radiotherapy is not equivalent to the benefits that such information may have in terms of outcomes. Information and patient education had greater impact at the start of radiotherapy than when therapy was completed (Rainey, 1985). This may be because those who felt less prepared for treatment were able, as treatment progressed, to improve their knowledge. It has been suggested that information improves self-care ability and the use of strategies by patients themselves (Dodd, 1984, 1988). Self-care strategies have not been shown to have significant benefits in terms of symptom control or reducing emotional distress (Johnson et al., 1988, 1989). One possible reason for this is that effective self-care strategies may depend on the socio-economic status and social support mechanisms from family and friends, which may vary widely between different people (Hanucharurnkul, 1989). Evidence is now available in the literature that suggests that not only do different cancer groups require different levels of information, but, also, the type and timing of information are also important (Campbell-Forsyth, 1990; Frith, 1991). Few studies have identified how informational interventions have an impact on psychological distress (see, for example, 'Stressful medical procedures' and 'Surgery'). However a study by Steigelis et al. (2004) identified that radiotherapy information provision has a correlation between individuals feelings of control and the level of illness uncertainty and that this is especially important for high-risk patients who perceive little control and more uncertainty (see 'Perceived control'). Therefore, targeted information giving has been shown to be most effective where it is given in combination with emotional support and pre treatment visit to the radiotherapy department.

Counselling and psychotherapy interventions

Studies have identified that radiotherapy treatment results in high levels of anxiety and emotional distress (Peck & Boland, 1977; Forester et al., 1978) and, therefore, researchers have tried to reduce these sequelae by offering psychotherapy or counselling services. Forester et al. (1985), in a randomized trial, used a psychotherapeutic approach to try to reduce distress. The intervention was not a specific type of psychotherapy but reflected the individuals' emotional needs (see 'Counselling'). Thirty minutes of psychotherapy were given weekly over 10 weeks to provide emotional support. A significant reduction was found in both emotional and physical signs of distress in the intervention group, compared with those having conventional medical follow-up. Criticisms of this study were the feasibility of offering such intensive counselling to all those undergoing radiotherapy and the potential cost. In response, a further study using group psychotherapy showed that this decrease in emotional distress was also achieved using a group approach (Forester et al., 1993) (see 'Group therapy'). Interestingly, subjects who had the lowest baseline distress scores seemed unaware of their cancer diagnosis and were found by the end of therapy to have higher distress levels. The overall conclusion was that psychotherapy was able to enhance the quality of life for those undergoing radiotherapy treatments. The degree to which individuals acknowledge their cancer was considered an important factor in their initial distress level and subsequent response to radiotherapy.

More recently there has been an increasing awareness of the psychosocial needs of those undergoing cancer treatments and this has been reflected in the provision of counselling services for radiotherapy. However, there are few constructive reviews of their effectiveness. Young and Maher (1992), in an audit of the work of a radiographer counsellor, provide insight into the dilemmas of providing such a service. Young and Maher felt that counselling had been of benefit in 50% of those who had received it. They believed counselling had reduced emotional distress, but pointed out that this was a subjective assessment at one time point that had not been evaluated in a randomized trial. They reported that the work was stressful and that the counsellor was deluged with referrals, but that overall such a service did have benefits.

Conclusion

Radiotherapy as a cancer therapy has clearly a level of psychosocial morbidity. Routinely screening for morbidity may be problematic in terms of referral ability and capacity in busy radiotherapy departments. However it is imperative to identify those undergoing radiotherapy in need of intervention and concentrate limited resources on those who would most benefit. The research evidence identifies that existing radiotherapy assessment tools that assess morbidity may not reflect emotional concerns. There are indications that the broader spectrum of radiotherapies impact is being overlooked, and that concerns about adapting to the effects of treatment, worry about every day concerns such as travel and the bother factor of physical symptoms are underrepresented. With a broader perspective, identifying what patients themselves feel as distressing, different elements may be identified that influence the impact of radiotherapy. People often have misunderstandings as to the effects or why they are having radiotherapy, and improved informed consent and information provision has made progress in reducing some of this anxiety prior to radiotherapy. What should be remembered is that psychosocial distress changes over the course of radiotherapy and, although information is often targeted at the start of therapy, anxiety can be just as high at the completion of treatment. The provision of combination interventions such as counselling and information are beneficial to patient outcomes and have been shown to reduce anxiety. With new radiotherapy treatments emerging and more combination therapies the impact of radiotherapy is harder to entangle for the whole effect of cancer therapy. Defining what causes distress and how it changes over time are important issues for clinical practice, with implications for decisions about when care or support is required and who should receive it.

(See also 'Cancer', 'Stressful medical procedures' and 'Chemotherapy').

REFERENCES

Anderson, B. & Tewfik, H. (1985). Psychological reactions to radiation therapy: reconsideration of the adaptive aspects of anxiety. *Journal of Personality and Social Psychology*, **48**, 1024–32.

Campbell-Forsyth, L. (1990). Patients' perceived knowledge and learning needs concerning radiation therapy. *Cancer Nursing*, **13**, 81–9.

Christman, N. (1990). Uncertainty and adjustment during radiotherapy. *Nursing Research*, **39**, 17–20.

Dodd, M. (1984). Patterns of self-care in patients receiving radiation therapy. *Oncology Nursing Forum*, **11**, 23–30.

Dodd, M. (1988). Patterns of self care in patients with breast cancer. *Western Journal of Nursing Research*, **10**, 7–24.

Dodd, M. & Ahmed, N. (1987). Preference for type of information in cancer patients receiving radiation therapy. *Cancer Nursing*, **10**, 244–51.

Faithfull, S. (2003). Assessing the impact of radiotherapy. In S. Faithfull & M. Wells (Eds.). *Supportive care in radiotherapy*. Churchill Livingstone: Edinburgh.

Fallowfield, L. (1990). *The quality of life: the missing measurement in health care*. Human Horizons. London, Souvenir Press.

Fitch, M., Gray, R., McGowan, T. *et al.* (2003). Travelling for radiation cancer treatment: patient perspectives. *Psycho-oncology*, **12**, 664–74.

Forester, B., Cornfield, D., Fless, J. & Thompson, S. (1993). Group psychotherapy during radiotherapy: effects on emotional and psychosocial distress. *American Journal of Psychiatry*, **150**, 1700–6.

Forester, B. M., Kornfield, D. & Fleiss, J. (1978). Psychiatric aspects of radiotherapy. *American Journal of Psychiatry*, **135**, 960–3.

Forester, B., Kornfield, D. & Fleiss, J. (1985). Psychotherapy during radiation: effects on emotional and physical distress. *American Journal of Psychiatry*, **142**, 22–7.

Frith, B. (1991). Giving information to radiotherapy patients. *Nursing Standard*, **5**, 33–5.

Graydon, J. (1988). Factors that predict patients' functioning following treatment for cancer. *International Journal of Nursing Studies*, **25**, 117–24.

Hammick, M., Tutt, A. & Tait, D. (1998). Knowledge and perception regarding radiotherapy and radiation in patients receiving radiotherapy: a qualitative study. *European Journal of Cancer Care*, **7**, 103–12.

Hanucharurnkul, S. (1989). Predictors of self care in cancer patients receiving radiotherapy. *Cancer Nursing*, **1**, 21–7.

Holland, J., Rowland, A., Lebovitz, A. & Rusalem, R. (1979). Reactions to cancer treatment: assessment of emotional response to adjuvant radiotherapy as a guide to planned intervention. *Psychiatric Clinics North America*, **2**, 347–58.

Israel, M. & Mood, D. (1988). Three media presentations for patients receiving radiation therapy. *Cancer Nursing*, **5**, 57–63.

Johnson, J., Lauver, D. & Nail, N. (1989). Process of coping with radiation therapy. *Journal of Consulting and Clinical Psychology*, **57**, 358–64.

Johnson, J., Nail, L., Lauver, D., King, K. & Keys, H. (1988). Reducing the negative impact of radiation therapy on functional status. *Cancer*, **61**, 46–51.

King, K., Nail, L., Kreamer, K., Strohl, R. & Johnson, J. (1985). Patients' descriptions of the experience of receiving radiation therapy. *Oncology Nursing Forum*, **12**, 55–61.

Lamszus, K. & Verres, R. (1995). Social support of radiotherapy patients in emotional stress and crisis situations. *Strahlenther Onkol*, **171**, 408–14.

Maraste, R., Brandt, L., Olsson, H. & Ryde-Brandt, B. (1992). Anxiety and depression in breast cancer patients at start of adjuvant radiotherapy. *Acta Oncologica*, **31**, 641–3.

Mumford, E., Schlesinger, H. & Glass, G.
(1982). The effects of psychological
intervention on recovery from surgery and
heart attacks: an analysis of the literature.
Americal Journal of Public Health, **72,**
141–57.

**Munro, A., Biruls, R., Griffin, A., Thomas, H.
& Vallis, K.** (1989). Distress associated with
radiotherapy for malignant disease: a
quantitative analysis based on patients
perceptions. *British Journal Cancer,* **60,**
370–4.

Peck, A. & Boland, J. (1977). Emotional
reactions to radiation treatment. *Cancer,*
40, 180–4.

Porock, D. (1995). The effect of preparatory
patient education on the anxiety and
satisfaction of cancer patients receiving
radiation therapy. *Cancer Nursing,* **18,**
206–14.

Rainey, L. (1985). Effects of preparatory
patient education for radiation oncology
patients. *Cancer,* **56,** 1056–61.

Stiegelis, H., Hagedoorn, M., Sanderman, R.
et al. (2004). The impact of an
informational self management
intervention on the association between
control and illness uncertainty before and
psychological distress after radiotherapy.
Psycho-oncology, **13,** 248–59.

**Ward, S., Viergutz, G., Tormey, D.,
DeMuth, J. & Paulen, A.** (1992).
Patients reactions to completion of
adjuvant breast cancer therapy. *Nursing
Research,* **41,** 362–6.

Young, J. & Maher, E. (1992). The role of
a radiographer counsellor in a large centre
for cancer treatment: a discussion
paper based on an audit of the work of
a radiographer counsellor. *Clinical
Oncology,* **4,** 232–5.

Rape and sexual assault

Irene H. Frieze[1] and Maureen C. McHugh[2]

[1]University of Pittsburgh
[2]Indiana University of Pennsylvania

Rape is one of the most feared events in the lives of many women
(Rozee & Koss, 2001). There is no clear definition of rape (Frieze,
2005). It is seen differently by those who have experienced various
types of forced sex and by therapists, other helpgivers and those in
the legal fields (Kahn & Mathie, 2000). In one large US study of
college women, only 46% of the women defined by the researchers
as being raped thought of their own experiences as 'rape' (Fisher
et al., 2000). However, even those who do not define what happened
to them as 'rape' may suffer psychological or physical symptoms.

Rape is defined in various ways by different legal codes, but basically involves forced sexual contact. The most common form of rape
involves a male perpetrator and a female victim, but other forms
also exist. The rapist may be a complete stranger, someone who
casually knows the victim, or someone who is well known. Marital
rape is increasingly being recognized as a crime.

Studies attempting to determine the prevalence of rape provide
widely varying estimates, depending on the specific definition of
'rape', the sample questioned and the methodologies used. Acts
that are legally defined as rape may not be perceived as such by
the victim. And, many rapes are never reported to authorities. In a
national random sample of adults in the United States who were
surveyed about various sexual experiences, 23% of women said they
had been raped (forced to have sex) at some point in their lives,
while 4% of men reported being forced to have sex (Laumann
et al., 1994).

Younger women and adolescents and African-American women
are the most common victims of reported rapes in the USA. Rates
vary greatly across the world. Rape is used during wartime as an act
of aggression by one group against the women associated with the
'enemy'.

Researchers have debated whether rape is primarily a sexual
crime or an aggressive crime. It is generally believed that both can
be true, and that some rapists are more motivated by sex and others
by aggressive feelings. Some rapists appear to believe that their victims enjoy being forced to have sex and may even seek out the same
victim again. Others clearly intend to physically injure or even kill
their victims (Groth, 1979).

The large majority of the rapes found in anonymous surveys
involve acquaintance rapes. Rapes involving strangers are more
likely to be violent and are more often reported to authorities, but
they are relatively rare, compared to forced sex involving people
known to each other. Forced sex occurring in ongoing relationships
is often accompanied with other forms of partner violence, but not
always (see 'Domestic violence'). When the assailant is known to the
victim, and especially if the assailant is a regular partner, forced sex
is often not defined as 'rape' by the victim. Researcher opinions
differ about whether or not any form of unwanted sexual activity
should be classified as 'rape,' especially in cases where the 'victim'
does not classify it as rape.

Those who have been raped may show reactions to that event for
many years, although many who are forced to have sex do not
appear to be traumatized. Typical reactions of those who do react
strongly vary over time, and a number of stage models have been
proposed to describe these changing reactions (e.g. Burgess &
Holmstrom, 1985). The victim of rape, similar to victims of other
traumatic events, typically has an immediate emotional reaction

which may take the form of denial, disbelief, numbness, or disorientation (Frieze *et al.*, 1987). The specific reactions of rape victims have been labeled as 'Rape Trauma Syndrome' (Burgess & Holmstrom, 1985). After the initial shock, rape victims might experience any of a variety of emotions including anger, anxiety, helplessness and psychosomatic and other physical symptoms. Unlike other crime victims, rape victims often experience difficulties in sexual functioning. There may also be difficulties in relating to men in general, and to a husband or boyfriend, for the female who has been raped. These short-term reactions are followed by more long-term effects which may include nervous breakdown, attempted suicide and other effects labeled as post-traumatic stress disorder (American Psychiatric Association, 1980; Kilpatrick *et al.*, 1985) (see 'Post-traumatic stress disorder'). Not all rape victims follow this sequence, though.

The strong psychological reactions of some rape victims appear to be greater than one might expect by analyzing only the physical injury resulting from the rape (Frieze *et al.*, 1987). One reason for this is that rape and other forms of victimization lead the victim to question or reassess basic assumptions about the world. People generally believe that they are safe and are not potential rape victims. Many women fear rape, and even those women who do fear rape attempt to live their lives in ways that they feel will protect them. When someone does become a rape victim, they must cope not only with the direct consequences of whatever happened to them, but also with the violation of their belief in a safe world. The fear and anxiety so commonly found in rape victims results from a fear of what could happen again even more than from what has already happened.

A number of coping mechanisms have been identified that characterize rape victim responses. These include redefining what happened so that it provides a sense of meaning to the victim. Reactions such as self-blame can be dysfunctional if they add to guilt feelings in the victim or cause her to withdraw from normal activities (Burt & Katz, 1987). It is not uncommon for rape victims to move their residences and to stop seeing old friends. This may be done to protect themselves from the possibility of another rape or because previous social interactions have become uncomfortable.

Rape victims may hesitate in seeking help from the medical or therapeutic communities, police, or even from friends, because they have found that other people have negative beliefs about victims generally and rape victims in particular. A set of stereotypic beliefs ('rape myths') that blame women for tempting men or being in the wrong place at the wrong time are widely held (Burt, 1980). Such feelings may be communicated to the help-seeking victim, resulting in a 'second injury' of a psychological nature (Symonds, 1976).

The first form of treatment for rape victims is often medical. The physician must look for signs of physical injury and for signs of sexually transmitted disease or pregnancy. Once these medical needs are taken care of, the rape victim may then seek psychological counselling (Allison & Wrightsman, 1993). Although this may be one-to-one therapy, treatment often occurs in self-help groups. Many clinicians and others working with women who have been raped feel that they should be labeled as 'rape survivors' rather than 'rape victims' once they have begun to cope with their trauma. Medical staff and therapists need to be careful to avoid blaming the rape victim and causing a 'second injury'.

Other forms of sexual assault tend to have similar consequences for their victims, but are generally less traumatic. These include exhibitionism, voyeurism and forced touching.

REFERENCES

Allison, J. A. & Wrightsman, L. S. (1993). *Rape: the misunderstood crime.* Newbury Park, CA: Sage.

American Psychiatric Association (APA) (1980). *Diagnostic and statistical manual of mental disorders* (3rd edn.). Washington, DC: American Psychiatric Association.

Burgess, A. W. & Holmstrom, L. L. (1985). Rape trauma syndrome and post-traumatic stress response. In A. W. Burgess (Ed.). *Research handbook on rape and sexual assault* (pp. 46–61). New York: Garland.

Burt, M. R. (1980). Cultural myths and supports for rape. *Journal of Personality and Social Psychology,* **38,** 217–30.

Burt, M. R. & Katz, B. L. (1987). Dimensions of recovery from rape: focus on growth outcomes. *Journal of Interpersonal Violence,* **2,** 57–81.

Fisher, B. S., Cullen, F. T. & Turner, M. G. (2000). *The sexual victimization of college women.* Washington, DC: National Institute of Justice.

Frieze, I. H. (2005). *Hurting the one you love: violence in relationships.* Belmont, CA: Thompson/Wadsworth.

Frieze, I. H., Hymer, S. & Greenberg, M. S. (1987). Describing the crime victim: psychological reactions to victimization. *Professional Psychology: Research and Practice,* **18,** 299–315.

Groth, N. (1979). *Men who rape: the psychology of the offender.* New York: Plenum.

Kahn, A. S. & Mathie, V. A. (2000). Understanding the unacknowledged rape victim. In C. B. Travis & J. W. White (Eds.). *Sexuality, society, and feminism* (pp. 377–403). Washington, DC: American Psychological Association.

Kilpatrick, D. C., Best, C. L., Veronen, L. J. *et al.* (1985). Mental health correlates of criminal victimization: a random community survey. *Journal of Consulting and Clinical Psychology,* **53,** 866–73.

Laumann, E. O., Gagnon, J. H., Michael, R. T. & Michaels, S. (1994). *The social organization of sexuality.* Chicago: University of Chicago Press.

Rozee, P. D. & Koss, M. P. (2001). Rape: a century of resistance. *Psychology of Women Quarterly,* **25,** 295–311.

Symonds, M. (1976). The rape victim: psychological patterns of response. *American Journal of Psychoanalysis,* **35,** 27–34.

Reconstructive and cosmetic surgery

Nichola Rumsey

University of the West of England

Introduction

Reconstructive surgery to normalize congenital abnormalities or repair injuries following trauma has a long and venerable history (Harris, 1997), however, until relatively recently, elective plastic surgery for cosmetic purposes was often sought covertly (Macgregor, 1979) and was considered an option accessible only to the wealthy. Currently, cosmetic surgery is considered a boom industry, and is increasingly accepted as an additional tool in the armoury of beauty enhancement techniques in Western societies. In the USA, the rates for procedures such as breast augmentation and rhinoplasties have increased by 700% in the past decade (Sarwer, 2002) and figures for the UK also show a dramatic increase in uptake. The increased popularity is fuelled by greater levels of disposable income amongst segments of the population, ever increasing media coverage of appearance-enhancing techniques and advertisers promoting myths and dreams associated with beauty.

The jury is still out in relation to whether people derive significant long-term psychological benefits from cosmetic surgery (Sarwer & Crerand, 2004). Most seek surgery as a solution to social and psychological problems. In addition, it is widely accepted that psychological factors play a significant role in every stage of treatment, including the decision to seek surgery, coping in the postoperative phase and in longer-term adjustment to changes in appearance (Pruzinsky, 2004), yet the input of psychologists into preoperative assessment and postoperative support is very much the exception rather than the rule.

Preoperative assessment

Pruzinsky (2002) recommends that a preoperative assessment of prospective patients for both reconstructive and cosmetic surgery should include an exploration of the motivation for surgery, the expectation of outcome, the extent of current dissatisfaction with the feature in question and body image in general, the impact of patients' concerns on daily functioning and their current and past psychological functioning.

Motivation for reconstructive surgery

The problems reported by those seeking reconstructive surgery frequently involve difficulties in social situations. Feelings of self-consciousness, social anxiety, negative self-perceptions and evidence of behavioural avoidance are common (Rumsey & Harcourt, 2005). Despite the prevalence of assumptions of a relationship between the severity of the disfigurement and the degree of preoperative distress, research has consistently shown these to be unfounded. Increasing numbers of patients are undergoing reconstructive surgery following the surgical excision of malignant tumours. In these cases, the decision of whether and when to undergo reconstructive surgery can be complicated by issues of life threat. Harcourt *et al.* (2003) have illustrated that the uptake rates for breast reconstruction following mastectomy vary considerably between treatment teams, and are influenced by information and advice given by the surgeon (see 'Cancer: breast').

Treatment decision-making

The involvement of prospective patients in treatment decision-making should be encouraged, with pressure from families and significant others to undergo surgery assessed and minimized. Surgical procedures should be carefully planned to take account relevant physical (e.g. growth) and social (e.g. transition to a new social group) factors. For children and adolescents with very visible disfigurements which are causing distress, the balance between waiting for physical growth to be completed to optimise the chances of a good long-term result and the potential psychological problems associated with a long wait for surgery, can be a precarious one. Patients' wishes should be given as much weight as possible, with treatment decisions kept under regular review (Hearst & Middleton, 1997) (see also 'Cleft lip and palate' and 'Facial disfigurement').

Undue influence exerted by prevailing surgical protocols should be avoided (for example, the expectation that surgery will take place at a particular age). Prospective patients should be able to feel free to decline treatment if they wish.

Care providers may have to curb their enthusiasm to intervene, and remind themselves that psychological reactions to disfigurements vary considerably. They should also bear in mind that the aspiration of people with disfigurements is often to look unremarkable, rather than perfect (Pruzinsky, 2004).

In the preoperative phase, the psychologist should assess whether another intervention, for example, counselling, cognitive–behavioural intervention or social skills training would be an appropriate forerunner, adjunct or alternative to surgery (see 'Cognitive behaviour therapy'). If the person is experiencing significant additional life stressors, appearance concerns may become a 'hook' on which to hang other problems. If surgery is planned on the UK National Health Service, there may be a long wait before the procedure takes place. In such cases it would also be appropriate to consider additional interventions during the wait (for example, coping strategies designed to reduce the person's avoidance of social situations).

Motivation for cosmetic surgery

Sarwer and Crerand (2004) have noted that the results of studies exploring the motivation to seek cosmetic surgery appear to have been influenced by the assessment method used, with interview studies reporting higher rates of psychopathology than studies employing psychometric measures. Research carried out in the 1960s relied heavily on interviews, and suggested that potential patients were frequently neurotic, with a substantial proportion suffering from a discernible psychiatric diagnosis (for example, disturbances of body image such as eating disorders or body dysmorphic disorder (see 'Eating disorders' and 'Facial disfigurement'). Research in the 1970s and 80s made more frequent use of standardized measures, and reported more modest levels of psychopathology. Most commentators agree that those suffering from body image disorders should be referred for psychiatric assessment and treatment, rather than accepted for surgery. An exception has been a study by Edgerton et al. (1991) which concluded that combined surgical-psychological rehabilitation provided relief for 83% of a sample of 67 cases, who were judged preoperatively to have moderate or severe psychological disorders.

A raft of psychological factors have been proposed to explain the motivation to seek cosmetic surgery of those in whom psychopathology is absent. These include perceptual processes (e.g. self-esteem, body image and the relationship between the two), developmental factors (e.g. maturational timing and history of appearance related teasing), cognitive processes (e.g. social comparisons; biases in the processing of information during social interactions) and sociocultural processes (e.g. the influence of media images). However, no clear psychological profile is yet apparent.

While some prospective patients seek surgery merely as a confidence booster, others are seeking solutions to more debilitating concerns. Feelings of self-consciousness and social anxiety are common, with frequent complaints that personal, social or occupational functioning is affected in a detrimental way by appearance-related distress. As in reconstructive surgery, the decision to undergo a cosmetic procedure should be a personal one and not the result of pressure from family or friends (Rumsey & Harcourt, 2005). The majority of prospective patients will have been experiencing distress for some time. It is therefore relevant to explore the timing of the decision to seek surgery as there may be a significant precipitating factor.

Expectations of outcome

In all forms of appearance enhancing surgery, care should be taken that expectations of outcome are realistic (see also 'Expectations and health'). In what ways does the prospective patient anticipate that life will be different post-surgery? There should be a realization that despite messages to the contrary in media articles and advertising, surgical intervention will not provide a 'magical' cure for problems experienced presurgery. With reconstructive surgery, it is rarely possible to restore an appearance to its pre-disfigured state (Pruzinsky, 2002) and many patients (for example, those undergoing breast reconstruction) will require a series of operations over a lengthy time period. The question of 'when to stop' in the quest for a normal appearance can be complex.

Surgeons should endeavour to make the changes the patient wants, resisting any temptation to produce a technically more attractive result (Macgregor, 1979).

Clear information should also be provided to ensure that patients are prepared for postoperative bruising and swelling and for the often distressing early postoperative appearance of surgical wounds. This is particularly important when procedures are likely to result in an unusual level of post-surgical discomfort. In orthognathic surgery for example, patients may be required to endure some degree of mechanical restraint of the jaw for a period of several weeks and may be restricted to a liquid diet. Some patients experience distress and feelings of panic resulting from the restriction. In all forms of plastic surgery, there is often a significant period before the final outcome can be assessed.

Emergency admissions

Many psychological factors are relevant in the acute and postoperative phases for plastic surgery patients admitted as emergencies. For example, Wisely and Tarrier (2001) and others have highlighted the potential of psychological interventions to relieve the difficulties experienced by burns patients, their families and by the staff treating them. In the acute phase, distress frequently relates to the experience of pain, to sleep deprivation, to anxiety associated with unplanned hospitalization and emotions relating to the cause of the injury. Patients may display post traumatic stress symptoms (Pruzinsky, 2002) (see 'Post-traumatic stress disorder'). In the reconstructive phase, intervention may be helpful in order to establish realistic expectations of the outcome of surgery (for example the relationship of the likely outcomes to a person's original appearance and function). Interventions can be provided in the form of play therapy for children, or individual treatment or support groups for adolescents, adults and families. In the later phases of treatment, liaison with schools or the workplace has been shown to be beneficial, both in terms of preparing the patients for a return to school or the workplace and also for peers or colleagues who may be uncertain of how best to behave (Frances, 2003).

The postoperative period

Pruzinsky (2002) has pointed out that in the immediate postoperative period following reconstructive surgery, patients often experience depression, anxiety and doubts concerning the eventual outcome of the surgical procedure. Reactions to changes in appearance are by no means universally positive. Buffone, for example, (1989) estimated that 30% of patients undergoing orthognathic procedures experience a reactive depression. Effective preparation for surgery may reduce post operative levels of psychological morbidity and reassurance and empathy from a psychologist or healthcare professional who has established rapport with the patient in the preoperative stage is likely to be well received.

The benefits of surgery

The benefits of plastic surgery are widely proclaimed in the media, but have yet to be established through research. Sarwer et al. (2002)

reported significant reductions in dissatisfaction with a specific feature in female cosmetic surgery patients, but could find no improvements to overall body image or to the importance ascribed to physical appearance in evaluations of the self. Although systematic research is lacking, there are anecdotal reports that some experience unwelcome feelings of change to their 'identity' as the result of their changed appearance (Macgregor, 1979). Some tell of difficulties in dealing with increased attention from other people to their enhanced appearance, others, particularly those whose appearance has been 'normalized' may have problems coping with the lack of attention afforded to anyone with an unremarkable appearance. In cases where disappointment is evident, psychological support and appropriate intervention have the potential to improve adjustment. A minority of patients display a seemingly insatiable desire for further surgery. In such cases, a psychiatric referral is widely considered more appropriate than offers of further surgery (Veale, 2004).

Conclusion

More research is needed to understand fully the factors involved in the motivation of people to seek appearance enhancing surgery, and in influencing postoperative outcomes. The numbers of people undergoing cosmetic and reconstructive surgery are increasing rapidly year on year. Given that psychological factors play a significant part in all stages of both elective cosmetic and reconstructive surgery, the participation of psychologists in the evaluation, treatment and follow-up of patients has the potential to significantly improve the quality of care provision.

REFERENCES

Buffone, G. (1989). Consultations with oral surgeons: new roles for medical psychotherapists. *Medical Psychotherapy: An International Journal*, **2**, 33–48.

Edgerton, M., Langman, M. & Pruzinsky, T. (1991). Plastic surgery and psychotherapy in the treatment of one hundred psychologically disturbed patients. *Plastic and Reconstructive Surgery*, **88**, 594–608.

Frances, J. (2003). *Educating children with facial disfigurements*. London: Taylor & Francis.

Hearst, D. & Middleton, J. (1997). Psychological intervention and models of current working practice. In R. Lansdown, N. Rumsey, E. Bradbury, A. Carr & J. Partridge (Eds.). *Visibly different: coping with disfigurement* (pp. 158–71). Oxford: Butterworth-Heinemann.

Harcourt, D., Rumsey, N., Ambler, N. *et al.* (2003): The psychological impact of mastectomy with or without breast reconstruction: a prospective, multi-centred study. *Plastic and Reconstructive Surgery*, **111**(3), 1060–8.

Harris, D. (1997). Types, causes and physical treatment of visible differences. In R. Lansdown, N. Rumsey, E. Bradbury, T. Carr & J. Partridge (Eds.). *Visibly different: coping with disfigurement* (pp. 79–90). Oxford: Butterworth-Heinemann.

Macgregor, F. (1979). *After plastic surgery: adaptation and adjustment*. New York: Praeger.

Pruzinsky, T. (2002). Body image adaptation to reconstructive surgery for acquired disfigurement. In T. Cash & T. Pruzinsky (Eds.). *Body image: a handbook of theory, research & clinical practice* (Chapter 50). New York: The Guilford Press.

Pruzinsky, T. (2004). Enhancing quality of life in medical populations: a vision for body image assessment and rehabilitation as standards of care. *Body Image Journal*, **1**, 71–81.

Rumsey, N. & Harcourt, D. (2005). Body image and disfigurement: issues and interventions. *Body Image Journal*, **1**, 83–97.

Rumsey, N. & Harcourt, D. (2005). *The psychology of appearance*. Maidenhead: Open University Press.

Sarwer, D. B. (2002). Cosmetic Surgery and Changes in Body Image. In T. Cash & T. Pruzinsky (Eds.). *Body image: a handbook of theory, research & clinical practice* (Chapter 48). New York: The Guilford Press.

Sarwer, D. B. & Crerand, C. E. (2004). Body image and cosmetic medical treatments. *Body Image Journal*, **1**, 99–111.

Sarwer, D. B., Wadden, T. A. & Whitaker, L. A. (2002). An investigation of changes in body image following cosmetic surgery. *Plastic and Reconstructive Surgery*, **109**, 363–9.

Veale, D. (2004). Advances in a cognitive behavioural model of body dysmorphic disorder. *Body Image Journal*, **1**, 113–25.

Wisely, J. & Tarrier, N. (2001). A survey of the need for psychological input in a follow-up service for adult burn-injured patients. *Burns*, **27**, 801–7.

Renal failure, dialysis and transplantation

Keith J. Petrie

The University of Auckland

The treatment of chronic renal failure

A chronic loss of kidney function may be caused by a number of factors, these commonly include diabetes, glomerulonephritis, chronic hypertension and familial polycystic renal disease (see 'Diabetes mellitus' and 'Hypertension'). A decline in renal function causes a gradual accumulation of the body's waste products and this is indicated by increasing levels of urea and creatinine in the blood. The metabolic disturbance accompanying renal failure leads to a number of physical symptoms, most notably lethargy and drowsiness, nausea and vomiting, as well as anorexia (see 'Vomiting and nausea').

The point at which patients are offered dialysis as a treatment for renal failure can vary according to the different policies of renal units, but treatment is typically instituted when the patient's renal symptoms reach a level that interferes with their ability to carry out their work or normal daily functions. Earlier treatment is associated with better survival and a preservation of nutrition. Some patients with a particularly poor medical prognosis, or with other major health problems that interfere with successful adaptation to a life on dialysis, may be advised against treatment.

Haemodialysis and continuous ambulatory peritoneal dialysis (CAPD) are the two types of dialysis treatment used to correct the on-going effects of kidney failure. In haemodialysis, the patient's blood is passed through an artificial kidney machine that removes waste products by passing the blood across a semi-permeable membrane. Most patients on haemodialysis must dialyse three times a week for between four and six hours. Often this can be done independently by the patient in their own home or through coming in to a dedicated hospital haemodialysis unit.

CAPD works according to the same general principle as haemodialysis but the whole process is conducted inside the body. In CAPD, dialysis fluid is run into the peritoneal cavity via a surgically implanted catheter. The peritoneum is a large semi-permeable membrane that lines the cavity, and once the dialysis fluid has been run in, it is left to exchange substances with the patient's blood. The fluid is drained after about 4–6 hours and the whole cycle is repeated each day, on three or four occasions. Improved rates of survival and correction of anaemia, as well as a more liberal diet, are features of CAPD. The choice between haemodialysis and CAPD is an important one for patients with each treatment having both advantages and disadvantages that have to be set against the patient's social and occupational circumstances.

The transplantation of a kidney from a cadaver or a living relative is the other treatment option for renal failure patients. The introduction of a new generation of immunosuppressive drugs has resulted in improved rates of graft function; now, with these drugs, 90% of kidney transplants from a deceased donor are successful. Transplantation is generally recognized as the best treatment available for end-stage renal failure. Freed from the drudgery of dialysis and the symptoms of kidney failure, transplant patients report significantly higher quality of life and have lower rates of psychological problems (Gudex, 1995) (see 'Quality of life'). However, there are some disadvantages to transplantation in terms of the need to take long-term medication and increased rates of malignancy. The possibility of coping with a failed graft for patients is a significant psychological blow, and one some patients do not want to risk facing again. A failed graft is often particularly traumatic when the kidney has been donated by a relative. Unfortunately, the demand for kidneys is outstripped by their availability, which consigns a sizeable proportion of patients to long-term dialysis. The impending arrival of successful xeno-grafts may overcome the current shortage of kidneys but will undoubtedly bring with it additional psychological adjustment problems.

Psychological problems and quality of life

The difficulties inherent in renal disease are a function of the physiological consequences of kidney failure, the restrictions imposed by a relentless dialysis regimen and the ongoing psychological adjustments required by a chronic illness. One of the most disabling effects of end-stage renal disease (ESRD) is lethargy and tiredness. This interferes not only with daily work function, but also with family relationships, as the patient often lacks the energy to engage in previously enjoyed social activities. A reduction in sexual activity is also common in ESRD (see 'Sexual dysfunction'). Patients on dialysis also complain of a variety of other physical symptoms such as itchy skin and sleep problems that interfere with their daily life (see 'Sleep disorders'). The recent development of recombinant human erythropoietin that acts to raise the oxygen-carrying capacity of the blood has had a major impact on treatment of ESRD by reducing tiredness and other symptoms due to anaemia.

The process of dialysis treatment also creates difficulties that compromise wellbeing. Most common among these are problems with the fluid and diet restrictions required, the development of needle stick fears in haemodialysis patients, and trouble with dialysis technique that can result in periodic infections. Often patients' frustrations with their condition and ongoing dialysis show themselves in compliance problems with the treatment, diet and fluid restrictions. Non-compliance is a major problem in patients on dialysis as the regimen has many of the characteristics that work to decrease compliance (see 'Adherence to treatment'). The treatment is complex, long-lasting and directly impacts on the patient's lifestyle. Non-compliance can also lead to conflict between staff and patients. Staff may become aggravated with patients who are perceived as not doing their share in managing their condition and, conversely, patients can come to see staff as representing an enforcement rather than a therapeutic role. This can result in patients feeling unable to bring up their personal difficulties and problems with staff. There is some evidence that behavioural programmes utilizing self-monitoring and reinforcement can improve the level of adherence to fluid restrictions among haemodialysis patients (Christensen *et al.*, 2002) (see 'Behaviour therapy').

Given this combination of physiological and psychological problems it is not surprising to find higher rates of psychiatric problems and impaired wellbeing in dialysis groups when compared to renal transplant patients and general population groups (Gudex, 1995). Uncertainty about the future and a lack of energy seem to be important factors in contributing to the differences in reported quality of life between patients on dialysis and the general population. Compared with transplant patients, patients on dialysis report a poorer quality of life, more problems with activities of daily living and significantly more negative emotions such as anxiety and depression (Cameron *et al.*, 2000; Gudex, 1995; Petrie, 1989). Despite the difficulties in assessing depression in dialysis patients because of the overlap in somatic symptomotology, high levels of depression have been consistently found in dialysis patients (Kimmel, 2002; Levenson & Glocheski, 1991).

Adjustment to treatment

The adjustment to treatment for renal failure shares similar characteristics to other chronic illnesses. The first part of this process involves coping with a loss of body function and an awareness of the need for long-term treatment. The next phase is learning the techniques associated with dialysis and dealing with the restrictions that this routine places on daily life and relationships. The final phase is an incorporation of the changes in appearance, function and lifestyle necessary with treatment into a new self-image and identity. The ability of patients to deal with each of these stages varies quite significantly depending on their own psychological resources. Difficulties in the early stages can have considerable impact on eventual adjustment to dialysis. A common emotional reaction is that of denial. This may range from a reluctance to accept that dialysis is really necessary to a casualness in using proper dialysis technique, or frequent breaking of dietary and fluid restrictions later in the treatment process (see also 'Coping with chronic illness').

A number of psychosocial factors have been shown to be associated with adherence to dialysis and dietary restrictions. These include lower levels of social support, the patient's negative perception of their illness and lower patient satisfaction with the care from their medical specialist (Kimmel *et al.*, 1998; Kovac *et al.*, 2002) (see 'Social support and health', 'Lay beliefs about health and illness' and 'Patient satisfaction'). Recent work also suggests patients' own ideas about the cause of renal failure and the effectiveness of treatment may be promising areas for future research on adherence to dietary and fluid restrictions (Krespi *et al.*, 2004).

The treatment of renal failure creates considerable difficulties for patients and their families. They must adapt to the loss of a bodily function and the accompanying energy-sapping symptoms. Given the demands and restrictions of life on dialysis as well as the psychological issues of dependency and an uncertain future, the surprising aspect is perhaps not how many patients become depressed but how resilient the majority are to the demands and restrictions of renal disease.

REFERENCES

Cameron, J. I., Whiteside, C., Katz, J. & Devins, G. M. (2000). Differences in quality of life across renal replacement therapies: a meta-analytic comparison. *American Journal of Kidney Disease*, **35**, 629–37.

Christensen, A. J., Moran, P. J., Wiebe, J. S., Ehlers, S. L. & Lawton, W. J. (2002). Effect of a behavioural self-regulation intervention on patient adherence in hemodialysis. *Health Psychology*, **21**, 393–7.

Gudex, C. M. (1995). Health-related quality of life in endstage renal failure. *Quality of Life Research*, **4**, 359–66.

Kimmel, P. L., Peterson, R. A., Weihs, K. L. *et al.* (1998). Psychosocial factors,

behavioural compliance and survival in urban haemodialysis patients. *Kidney International*, **54**, 245–54.

Kimmel, P. L. (2002). Depression in patients with chronic renal disease: What we know and what we need to know. *Journal of Psychosomatic Research*, **53**, 951–6.

Kovac, J. A., Patel, S. S., Peterson, R. A. & Kimmel, P. L. (2002). Patient satisfaction with care and behavioural compliance in end-stage renal disease patients treated with haemodialysis. *American Journal of Kidney Diseases*, **39**, 1236–44.

Krespi, R., Bone, M., Ahmad, R., Worthington, B. & Salmon, P. (2004).

Haemodialysis patients' beliefs about renal failure and its treatment. *Patient Education and Counseling*, **53**, 189–96.

Levenson, J. L. & Glocheski, S. (1991). Psychological factors affecting end-stage renal disease: a review. *Psychomsomatics*, **32**, 382–9.

Petrie, K. J. (1989). Psychological well-being and psychiatric disturbance in dialysis and renal transplant patients. *British Journal of Medical Psychology*, **62**, 91–6.

Repetitive strain injury

Gerard P. van Galen

Nijmegen Institute for Cognition and Information

Repetitive strain injury (RSI) is a syndrome in the upper extremities (hands, arms, shoulder and/or neck) and is characterized by sensations of pain, stiffness, fatigue, heat and cold, tingling, numbness, redness of the skin, cramps and loss of fine movement control, eventually leading to general disability. Usually pain, fatigue and stiffness, especially in the neck and shoulder region, are early symptoms, whereas functional loss and disability are mostly seen in advanced states. Initial, temporary episodes of pain and fatigue during repetitive tasks are defined as phase I severity. In phase II the pain has become more persistent and has generalized to other everyday movements. In phase III, pain and functional loss are continuous and unrelated to repetitious movements.

Since symptoms primarily develop in people whose work involves repetitious movements during long shifts, RSI is considered a typical occupational disorder with overuse of upper extremity muscles as a common denominator, although excessive computer gaming has been known to cause RSI complaints as well ('Nintendo arm'). Alternative terms are 'occupational overuse syndrome', 'work-related upper extremity disorder' (WRUED) and sometimes 'focal dystonia', although the latter term essentially refers to a different, neurological disorder.

Specific and non-specific forms of RSI

RSI complaints generally do not relate to any known biological disorder. Only in a minority of cases (<15%) does standard medical examination reveal tendomyogene or peripheral neuro-conductive abnormalities (Kiesler & Finholt, 1988). To allow a differential diagnosis of specific or non-specific RSI a protocol has been developed with discriminating provocative tests (Sluiter et al., 2001). Today, it is standard practice to distinguish the specific types of RSI from the nonspecific varieties where examination cannot uncover a biological cause. These non-specific forms of RSI include carpal and cubital tunnel syndrome, Guyon channel syndrome, trigger finger, epicondylitis, rotator cuff syndrome, thoracic outlet syndrome and tendonitis and arthrosis of the upper limbs.

Incidence

RSI complaints are widespread in the occupational population of industrialized countries. In the Netherlands, for example, 20–40% of the working population suffer from RSI, with higher incidence rates in industrial workers (e.g. agribusiness) than in office workers (National Health Council of the Netherlands, 2000). Other risk groups are hairdressers, plumbers, musicians, cleaning and laundry personnel. The impact of RSI on sick leave is high:

annually, 8% of all employees are absent for shorter or longer periods and between 5 and 10% of incapacity benefit claims are RSI-related. Other countries have similar statistics (Dembe, 1999; Levenstein, 1999).

Aetiology

Risk factors

Epidemiological, predominantly retrospective, studies have analyzed self-reports and medical files on complaints, work conditions and personal characteristics to identify correlations between complaints and risk factors. Authoritative reviews have been published by the US Department of Health and Human Services (Bernard, 1997), the USA National Research Council (2001) and Bongers et al. (2002). There is strong evidence that primary factors in the aetiology of RSI are excessive, repetitious and/or forceful motions accompanied by static postures. Apart from these primary workplace factors, epidemiological studies also indicate an association with negative psychosocial factors such as high workload, low appreciation and deviating self-control mechanisms.

Parallel to the epidemiological findings, comparative descriptive research, comparing patients and healthy controls, has revealed pathophysiological abnormalities such as hyper-algesia and loss of kinaesthetic sensitivity in RSI patients. Also, higher levels of muscular co-contraction and limb stiffness have been observed during motor tasks (see below). The problem with such findings, however, is that symptoms may well be the result of the syndrome and not the cause.

Poor ergonomics

From an ergonomic perspective, the design of most computer keyboards and visual display units (VDUs) elicit unsupported, pronated postures of the hands and an anterior position of head and shoulders. The VDU is often awkwardly placed (not at eye level, too far or too close). Although, thus far, there has been little well-controlled research into better designed tools, designers have tried to reduce the inherent awkward hand and wrist posture of conventional keyboards by constructing a vertically tilted or upright keyboard. Evidence suggests that this can lower muscular tension while keying (Rempel et al., 1999; Tittiranonda et al., 1999).

Personality

There is hardly any evidence for a typical RSI personality. Although some studies have found correlations between RSI and anxiety and

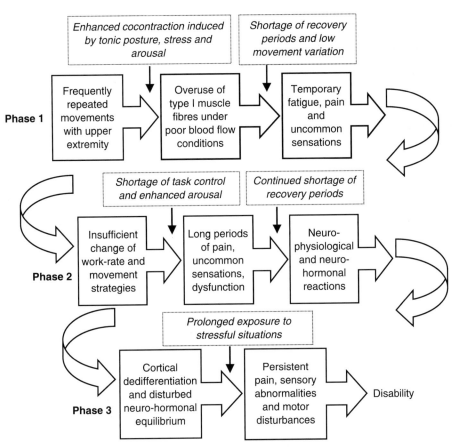

Fig 1 Model representing the three consecutive phases in the development of RSI complaints. Pathophysiological processes are positioned according to temporal evolution from phase1 to phase 2 and 3. Environmental factors are given in italics.

depression or internal locus of control, it should be stressed that these were weak correlations and only present in advanced states of the syndrome. Moreover, these results may be due to the pain (Vlaeyen & Linton, 2000) (see 'Pain' and 'Pain management'). None of the studies has uncovered any psychiatric conditions in RSI patients when measured after the onset of RSI (Windgassen & Ludolph, 1991).

Pathophysiological accounts

Divergent pathophysiological mechanisms have been proposed for the aetiology of the syndrome. Explanations can be divided into three categories. First, there are the more peripheral theories on tissue damage caused by overuse. A second group, which is more behaviourally oriented, centres on findings of high degrees of muscle tension associated with precise, repeated movements and task-related stress. A third group focuses on neurological and neuro-hormonal changes resulting from pain and distress due to exposure to prolonged repeated movements. In recent accounts RSI is described as a multi-factorial syndrome starting with peripheral muscular dysfunction, exaggerated by stress factors, leading to a hampered blood flow, pain and dysfunction. In more advanced states this eventually causes central neurological dysfunction. Figure 1 summarizes this view in a three-phase model.

Tissue damage and the Cinderella hypothesis

Although imaging techniques have failed to detect unequivocal tissue damage in RSI patients, there is evidence from animal research that repeated movements at least have temporary negative effects on type I muscle fibres and indirectly on stapling of $Ca++$ ions in muscle tissue that may cause pain and cell damage. Pain, in turn, may lead to enhanced muscle tension, initiating a cycle of hampered blood flow, more pain and more tension. Specifically in repetitive fine movements, the smallest type I muscle fibres are continuously active and are, therefore, like Cinderella in the fairy tale, more exposed to overuse. Electromyographic studies have indeed found evidence of type I deficits (Westgaard & DeLuca, 1999; Sogaard et al., 2001).

A less well-documented proposal claims that repeated movements lead to friction and temperature damage in tendons. The problem here again is that such damage has rarely been detected in human and animal models. However, from a theoretical viewpoint, it may well be possible that, especially for abnormal, non-neutral joint postures, friction and pulling strain on tendons is high.

Muscle tension and co-contraction

The second, behavioural explanation starts from the observation that RSI patients have less effective movement strategies (Bloemsaat et al., 2004). Hughes and McLellan (1985) measured the EMG of fore- and upper-arm muscles in patients and controls during tapping and handwriting tasks. The patients exhibited higher levels of muscular co-contraction, i.e. the fine-tuning in their agonist–antagonist muscle combinations was inferior to that found in the controls. Gomer *et al.* (1987) reported analogous outcomes in postal workers: the introduction of a complicated postal address coding system led to enhanced distress and hand tremors, changing the EMG spectral density function, all indicative of a disturbed muscle metabolism. A common denominator in co-contraction research is that repeated movement, high precision demands and mental load all lead to enhanced levels of muscular tension and co-contraction (Laursen *et al.*, 2002; Visser *et al.*, 2004). High muscle tension makes movements more fatiguing and finally less precise, again leading to still higher levels of contraction. Van Galen and Van Huygevoort (2000) propose a stress and human performance theory in which they postulate that all human movement is the product of noisy neuromuscular recruitment and servomechanisms. Different biomechanical degrees of freedom allow humans to control their inherently noisy movements. Amongst these are using optimal force levels (approximating 28% of the maximum force), feedback and feedforward control and applying friction and support with the work plane. A particular useful degree of freedom is limb stiffness, achieved by installing optimal levels of co-contraction between antagonist muscle pairs. Varying stiffness through co-contraction or by applying higher friction with work planes, however, has its limitations in that higher levels of stiffness make movement energetically less efficient. Several investigations have indeed provided evidence that stiffness and co-contraction is enhanced in conditions of stress and mental load and in RSI patients and the elderly extra sensitivity has been demonstrated (Bloemsaat *et al.*, 2004; Gribble *et al.*, 2003). In the proposed model (see Figure 1) it is assumed that non-neutral and inflexible postures during repetitive tasks interact with mental load and other physical stressors, such as auditory noise, poor illumination, vibration, etc. All of these have an impoverishing effect on neuromotor output signals, leading to higher tension and poor metabolic conditions for muscles, tendons and joints.

Neurological processes

Some of the research on RSI has focused on central neurological changes specifically during distal movements. In animal studies with owl monkeys, Byl *et al.* (1996) measured receptive fields in the cortex after prolonged exposure to a repetitious squeezing task. They found deterioration and dedifferentiation in cortical area 3b. This condition coincided with a loss of sensorimotor discrimination, which has also been found in patients. An alternative theory about a central neurological component in the persistence of pain in advanced states of RSI is of neuroendocrine origin. Clauw and Chrousos (1997) hypothesized that continuous coping with pain and stress in advanced states of pain may eventually lead to a lowered pain threshold following an initial increase. Their explanation focuses on the pituitary and adrenal glands, which normally work together in stress coping but may be exhausted

after long exposures to stress (see 'Stress and health' and 'Psychoneuroimmunology'). Patients thus become highly sensitive to even very common pain stimuli.

Towards an integrative model

In Figure 1 the three explanatory theories of RSI and their ingredients overuse, bad postures, task stressors, social pressures, central neurological deformation, all leading to sub-optimal stiffness regulation, pain and dysfunction, have been integrated in a comprehensive model.

Treatment and prevention

There is a profusion of preventive measures for the workplace and rehabilitation techniques for RSI patients, but only a few have been tested in methodologically sound trials (for overviews of rehabilitation studies, see Karjalainen *et al.*, 2003*a,b*; Konijnenberg *et al.*, 2001; Verhagen *et al.*, 2004; for studies on preventive interventions see Lincoln, 2001). Ergonomic training in situ has not yet delivered long-lasting positive results but there is some evidence that working with vertically oriented keyboards and less sideward forearm postures for mouse-handling have positive effects on muscle tension and complaints. Alleviation of complaints through software inducing controlled pauses during VDU work are very limited and reductions in sick leave non-existent (Van den Heuvel *et al.*, 2003). Behavioural programmes targeting muscular relaxation through biofeedback from surface electromyography (Nord *et al.*, 2001; Faucett *et al.*, 2002) have proved more effective (see 'Biofeedback' and 'Behaviour therapy'). Apart from ergonomic measures and direct muscle-training techniques there is a wide variety of physiotherapeutic interventions aimed at a more general enhancement of stress-coping skills. They include exercise training, fitness, massage and concurrent cognitive training and counselling (see 'Counselling' and 'Cognitive behaviour therapy'). To date, however, there is little or contradictory evidence for their efficacy.

Conclusion

Although still only partly understood, the syndrome of repetitive strain injury can be defined as complaints due to muscular overuse, non-neutral static postures, high muscle tension and task-related stress. In advanced states central neurological dysfunction is likely to play a role. A full understanding of the syndrome can only be attained if we consider both peripheral and physiological mechanisms and the more behavioural and emotional components as elements which exaggerate each other's effects in motor processes. Although further treatment and prevention research is required, it is assumed that reorganizing work schedules, improving tools and work environments and training workers to apply more relaxed movement strategies will help us to master RSI, at present one of the most prevalent occupational hazards.

REFERENCES

Bernard, B. P. (Ed.). (1997). *Musculoskeletal disorders and workplace factors: A critical* review of epidemiologic evidence for work-related musculoskeletal disorders of the neck, upper extremity, and low back. (2nd printing). Cincinnati, OH: US

Department of Health and Human Services.

Bloemsaat, J. G., Ruijgrok, J. M. & Van Galen, G. P. (2004). Patients suffering from nonspecific work related upper extremity disorders exhibit insufficient movement strategies. *Acta Psychologica*, **115**, 17–33.

Bongers, P. M., Kremer, A. M. & Ter Laak, J. (2002). Are psychosocial factors, risk factors for symptoms and signs of the shoulder, elbow, or hand/wrist? A review of the epidemiological literature. *American Journal of Industrial Medicine*, **41**, 315–42.

Byl, N. N., Merzenich, M. M. & Jenkins, W. M. (1996). A primate genesis model of focal dystonia and repetitive strain injury: I. Learning-induced dedifferentiation of the representation of the hand in the primary somatosensory cortex in adult monkeys. *Neurology*, **47**, 508–20.

Clauw, D. J. & Chrousos, G. P. (1997). Chronic pain and fatigue syndromes: overlapping clinical and neuroendocrine features and potential pathogenic mechanisms. *Neuroimmunomodulation*, **4**, 134–53.

Dembe, A. E. (1999). The changing nature of office work: effects on repetitive strain injuries. *Occupational Medicine State of the Art Reviews*, **14**, 61–72.

Faucett, J., Garry, M., Nadler, D. & Ettare, D. (2002). A test of two training interventions to prevent work-related musculoskeletal disorders of the upper extremity. *Applied Ergonomics*, **33**, 337–47.

Gomer, F. E., Silverstein, L. D., Berg, W. K. & Lassiter, D. L. (1987). Changes in electromyographic activity associated with occupational stress and poor performance in the workplace. *Human Factors*, **29**, 131–43.

Gribble, P. L., Mullin, L. I., Cothros, N. & Mattar, A. (2003). Role of cocontraction in arm movement accuracy. *Journal of Neurophysiology*, **89**, 2396–405.

Hughes, M. & McLellan, D. L. (1985). Increased co-activation of the upper limb muscles in writer's cramp. *Journal of Neurology, Neurosurgery, and Psychiatry*, **48**, 782–7.

Karjalainen, K., Malmivaara, A., Van Tulder, M. *et al.* (2003a). *Multidisciplinary rehabilitation for fibromyalgia and musculoskeletal pain in working age adults.* (Cochrane Review). In: The Cochrane Library, Issue 4. Chichester, UK: John Wiley & Sons, Ltd.

Karjalainen, K., Malmivaara, A., Van Tulder, M. *et al.* (2003b). *Multidisciplinary biopsychosocial rehabilitation for neck and shoulder pain among working age adults.* (Cochrane Review). In: The Cochrane Library, Issue 4. Chichester, UK: John Wiley & Sons, Ltd.

Kiesler, S. & Finholt, T. (1988). The mystery of RSI. *American Psychologist*, **43**, 1004–15.

Konijnenberg, H. S., De Wilde, N. S., Gerritsen, A. A. *et al.* (2001). Conservative treatment for repetitive strain injury. *Scandinavian Journal Work Environment & Health*, **27**, 299–310.

Laursen, B., Jensen, B. R., Garde, A. H. & Jorgensen, A. H. (2002). Effect of mental and physical demands on muscular activity during the use of a computer mouse and keyboard. *Scandinavian Journal of Work Environment & Health*, **28**, 215–21.

Levenstein, C. (1999). Economic losses from repetitive strain injuries. *Occupational Medicine State of the Art Reviews*, **14**, 149–61.

Lincoln, A. E. (2001). A summary of 'Interventions for the primary prevention of work-related carpal tunnel syndrome'. In A. C. Bittner, P. C. Champney & S. J. Morrissey (Eds.). *Advances in occupational ergonomics and safety*, (pp. 47–54). Amsterdam: IOS Press.

National Health Council of the Netherlands. (2000). *RSI*. The Hague: National Health Council. (Publication number 2000/22.)

National Research Council and the Institute of Medicine. (2001). *Musculoskeletal disorders and the workplace: low back and upper extremities*. Washington, DC: National Academy Press.

Nord, S., Ettare, D., Drew, D. & Hodge, S. (2001). Muscle learning therapy: efficacy of a biofeedback based protocol in treating work-related upper extremity disorders. *Journal of Occupational Rehabilitation*, **11**, 23–31.

Rempel, D., Tittiranonda, P., Burastero, S., Hudes, M. & So, Y. (1999). Effect of keyboard keyswitch design on hand pain. *Journal of Occupational and Environmental Medicine*, **41**, 111–19.

Sluiter, J. K., Rest, K. M. & Frings-Dresen, M. H. W. (2001). Criteria document for evaluating the work-relatedness of upper-extremity musculoskeletal disorders. *Scandinavian Journal of Work Environment & Health*, **27**, Suppl. 1, 1–102.

Sogaard, K., Sjøgaard, G., Finsen, L., Olsen, H. B. & Christensen, H. (2001). Motor unit activity during stereotyped finger tasks and computer mouse work. *Journal of Electromyography & Kinesiology*, **11**, 197–206.

Tittiranonda, P., Rempel, D., Armstrong, T. & Burastero, S. (1999). Effect of four computer keyboards in computer users with upper extremity musculoskeletal disorders. *American Journal of Industrial Medicine*, **35**, 647–61.

Van den Heuvel, S., De Looze, M. P., Hildebrandt, V. H. & Thé, K. H. (2003). The effects on work-related neck and upper limb disorders of software programs that stimulate regular breaks and excercises – a randomized controlled trial. *Scandinavian Journal of Work Environment & Health*, **29**, 106–16.

Van Galen, G. P. & Van Huygevoort, M. A. (2000). Error, stress the role of neuromotor noise in space oriented behaviour. *Biological Psychology*, **51**, 151–71.

Verhagen, A. P., Bierma-Zeinstra, S. M. A., Karels, C. *et al.* (2004). *Ergonomic and physiotherapeutic interventions for treating upper extremity work related disorders in adults Cochrane Database Syst Rev*; (1):CD003471.

Visser, B., De Looze, M. P., De Graaff, M. P. & Van Dieën, J. H. (2004). Effects of precision demands and mental pressure on muscle activation and hand forces in computer mouse tasks. *Ergonomics*, **47**, 202–17.

Vlaeyen, J. W. S. & Linton, S. J. (2000). Fear-avoidance and its consequences in chronic musculoskeletal pain. A state of the art. *Pain*, **85**, 317–32.

Westgaard, R. H. & DeLuca, C. J. (1999). Motor unit substitution in long-duration contractions of the human trapezius muscle. *Journal of Neurophysiology*, **82**, 501–4.

Windgassen, K. & Ludolph, A. (1991). Psychiatric aspects of writer's cramp. *European Archive of Psychiatry and Clinical Neuroscience*, **241**, 170–6.

Rheumatoid arthritis

Kathleen Mulligan and Stanton Newman

University College London

Rheumatoid arthritis (RA) is a chronic inflammatory disease that affects the synovial tissue surrounding the joints. This inflammation is associated with swelling and pain. As the disease progresses, joint tissue may become permanently damaged. The combined effects of inflammation and joint damage result in progressive disability. The causes of RA are, as yet, unknown but it is generally considered an autoimmune disease, although there is no clear evidence of what factors trigger this destructive response of the body's immune system. The onset of symptoms is gradual and insidious in most instances, although a small proportion of individuals (10–15%) may have a more rapid progression.

Joint pain, swelling and stiffness are the main symptoms of the disease, but individuals also report fatigue and general malaise. Individuals with RA describe their pain as throbbing and burning, but not as scalding, drilling or cutting (Wagstaff *et al.*, 1985). They describe their pain differently from individuals with osteoarthritis; in particular they are likely to refer to 'heat' (see 'Osteoarthritis'). Stiffness has always been harder to define and may be difficult for patients to distinguish from pain, but individuals with RA refer to resistance to movement, limited range and lack of movement (Helliwell & Wright, 1991). Clinically important levels of fatigue have been reported in over 40% of patients (Wolfe *et al.*, 1996). A multidimensional assessment of fatigue in RA found higher levels of general and physical fatigue as opposed to mental fatigue and different aspects of fatigue selectively explained variance in different dimensions of quality of life (Rupp *et al.*, 2004).

The impact of RA on individuals' lives is considerable. Using the SF-36, a generic measure of health-related quality of life, studies (e.g. Picavet & Hoeymans, 2004) have shown that RA is associated with impaired quality of life, especially on dimensions of physical functioning (see 'Quality of life' and 'Quality of life assessment'). A small minority of people with RA are wheelchair- or bed-bound and, for the rest, walking may be both difficult and tiring. Individuals with RA also report being concerned about falling (Jamison *et al.*, 2003), so they may further restrict their mobility. The net effect of RA on individuals' quality of life is considerable and is compounded by its impact on capacity to work and reduced income (Wolfe & Hawley, 1998). It can also reduce social and leisure activities and ability to perform domestic roles.

Studies which have compared individuals with RA to the general population have found raised levels of depression (Dickens *et al.*, 2002) which is frequently accompanied by anxiety (Van Dyke *et al.*, 2004). It is important, however, to recognize that RA does not lead to higher levels of depression than other chronic clinical conditions (DeVellis, 1993). Studies have failed to find a direct relationship between the physical markers of the extent or activity of the disease and depression. Evidence has, however, been accumulating that the impact of RA is mediated through a number of psychological factors. Notable amongst these are self-efficacy, coping responses and illness beliefs (see 'Lay beliefs about health and illness' and 'Self-efficacy and health').

Self-efficacy refers to the self-confidence people have in their ability to perform a particular behaviour. The Arthritis Self-Efficacy Scales (Lorig *et al.*, 1989) assess people's self-efficacy to perform a number of everyday activities of daily living but also other elements of managing arthritis, such as the ability to reduce pain and deal with the psychological demands of the illness. The results of several studies indicate that self-efficacy may be an important concept for our understanding of functioning in arthritis. For example, it has been found to be related to daily ratings of pain, mood, coping and coping efficacy (Lefebvre *et al.*, 1999), to changes in health status over two years (Brekke, Hjortdahl & Kvien, 2001) and to outcomes in intervention studies (Smarr *et al.*, 1997).

The strategies people use to try to limit the impact of their arthritis are also important. Studies may be divided into those that have focused on the way people cope with specific symptoms of RA, such as pain, and those that have considered coping with RA in general. Studies on coping with pain in RA have assessed whether particular coping strategies lead to better psychological wellbeing. The general finding is that the use of active coping strategies is associated with better outcomes than more passive coping strategies (see 'Pain' and 'Pain management'). Smith *et al.* (1997) found a relationship between coping strategies and a number of measures of psychological adjustment. For example, using the active coping strategy of positive reappraisal of pain was associated with greater life satisfaction and positive affect whereas the passive coping strategy of disengagement was associated with poorer adjustment. The use of passive pain coping strategies, such as catastrophizing and praying and hoping, has been found, along with helplessness, to mediate between disability and pain and between disability and depression (Covic *et al.*, 2003). Studies that have examined how individuals cope with RA in general have also found the use of passive coping strategies to be associated with poorer outcomes, for example, poorer social functioning (Scharloo *et al.*, 1998). The strategy of wishful thinking has been associated with poorer wellbeing, while the coping strategy of cognitive restructuring (rethinking the cognitions around the illness and its implications) tends to be associated with better psychological wellbeing (Newman & Revenson, 1993). It is important to be aware, also, that the way people cope with RA may change over the course of the disease, for example, denial appears to be greater in the early stages (Treharne *et al.*, 2004).

The way people think about their RA may be another important influence on outcome. Groarke *et al.* (2004) assessed the illness beliefs and coping strategies of women with RA and found that illness identity was associated with poorer outcomes in that people who attributed more symptoms to RA reported poorer physical function and more pain and depression (for more information on illness beliefs see 'Illness cognition assessment'). More serious perceived illness consequences were associated with poorer physical function and more pain. In this same study, patients who perceived their illness as more controllable reported less physical impairment, pain and depression, while those who thought that their RA would last a long time reported poorer physical function. The importance of coping strategies was also apparent in that depression was associated with high use of coping by denial and with less frequent use of the active coping strategies of planning, seeking instrumental social support, positive reinterpretation and growth and acceptance.

These studies have established that how one thinks about and what one does to confront RA has an impact on outcome and have spawned a number of approaches to intervention which aim to alter how individuals manage their RA in order to improve psychological wellbeing and reduce symptoms and disability.

Psychological interventions

The interventions developed and applied to individuals with RA have involved a variety of components, drawn from different theoretical approaches. One of the most widely used psychological interventions in RA and other chronic painful disorders is cognitive–behaviour therapy (CBT) (see 'Cognitive behaviour therapy'). CBT includes a number of components such as relaxation training, cognitive coping strategies, goal-setting with self-reinforcement, communications training, assertiveness training and problem-solving. One of the objectives of CBT is to enable individuals to perceive themselves to have more personal control over symptoms such as pain (Keefe & Caldwell, 1997) and over the course of their disease (see also 'Perceived control'). Because increased perceptions of control have been found to have a positive effect on mood and other aspects of wellbeing (Rhee *et al.*, 2000), CBT can also help to address any accompanying depression. The concept of self-efficacy has also been an important influence on the development of interventions in RA. The widely used Arthritis Self-Management Programme (Lorig, 1986), for example, aims to enhance participants' self-efficacy to manage pain and other aspects of their arthritis by teaching skills such as problem-solving, cognitive symptom management and communication with healthcare professionals.

There can be considerable overlap between interventions in the components (or combination of components) that they include, making evaluating the efficacy of individual components difficult. Studies also measure several different outcomes such as psychological wellbeing and reductions in pain and disability. Consequently, it has proved difficult to ascertain which component has the most effect on the outcome variables under study (Newman *et al.*, 2001). A Cochrane review grouped studies according to their main approach and found that those which focused mainly on strategies to facilitate behaviour change appeared to produce more favourable outcomes than those which used primarily information provision or counselling (Riemsma *et al.*, 2002). The number of studies in each category was small suggesting that further research is necessary to investigate the comparable efficacy of different approaches. It is important to note that a particular approach may be more beneficial for some outcomes than others; for example, self-management interventions seem to be particularly successful in changing behavioural outcomes (Newman *et al.*, 2004) (see 'Self-management').

REFERENCES

Brekke, M., Hjortdahl, P. & Kvien, T. K. (2001). Self-efficacy and health status in rheumatoid arthritis: a two-year longitudinal observational study. *Rheumatology (Oxford)*, **40**, 387–92.

Covic, T., Adamson, B., Spencer, D. & Howe, G. (2003). A biopsychosocial model of pain and depression in rheumatoid arthritis: a 12-month longitudinal study. *Rheumatology (Oxford)*, **42**, 1287–94.

DeVellis, B. M. (1993). Depression in rheumatological diseases. In S. Newman & M. Shipley (Eds.). *Psychological aspects of rheumatic disease Baillière's Clinical Rheumatology* (pp. 241–58). London: Baillière-Tindall.

Dickens, C., McGowan, L., Clark-Carter, D. & Creed, F. (2002). Depression in rheumatoid arthritis: a systematic review of the literature with meta-analysis. *Psychosomatic Medicine*, **64**, 52–60.

Groarke, A., Curtis, R., Coughlan, R. & Gsel, A. (2004). The role of perceived and actual disease status in adjustment to rheumatoid arthritis. *Rheumatology (Oxford)*, **43**, 1142–9.

Helliwell, P. S. & Wright, V. (1991). Stiffness – a useful symptom but an elusive quality. *Proceedings of the Royal Society*, **84**, 95–8.

Jamison, M., Neuberger, G. B. & Miller, P. A. (2003). Correlates of falls and fear of falling among adults with rheumatoid arthritis. *Arthritis and Rheumatism*, **49**, 673–80.

Keefe, F. J. & Caldwell, D. S. (1997). Cognitive behavioral control of arthritis pain. *Medical Clinics of North America*, **81**, 277–90.

Lefebvre, J. C., Keefe, F. J., Affleck, G. *et al.* (1999). The relationship of arthritis self-efficacy to daily pain, daily mood, and daily pain coping in rheumatoid arthritis patients. *Pain*, **80**, 425–35.

Lorig, K. (1986). Development and dissemination of an arthritis patient education course. *Family & Community Health*, **9**, 23–32.

Lorig, K., Chastain, R. L., Ung, E., Shoor, S. & Holman, H. R. (1989). Development and evaluation of a scale to measure perceived self-efficacy in people with arthritis. *Arthritis and Rheumatism*, **32**, 37–44.

Newman, S., Mulligan, K. & Steed, L. (2001). What is meant by self-management and how can its efficacy be established? *Rheumatology (Oxford)*, **40**, 1–4.

Newman, S. & Revenson, T. A. (1993). Coping with rheumatoid arthritis. In S. Newman & M. Shipley (Eds.). *Psychological aspects of rheumatic disease Baillière's Clinical Rheumatology* (pp. 259–80). London: Baillière-Tindall.

Newman, S., Steed, L. & Mulligan, K. (2004). Self-management interventions for chronic illness, *The Lancet*, **364**, 1523–37.

Picavet, H. S. & Hoeymans, N. (2004). Health related quality of life in multiple musculoskeletal diseases: SF-36 and EQ-5D in the DMC3 study. *Annals of the Rheumatic Diseases*, **63**, 723–9.

Rhee, S. H., Parker, J. C., Smarr, K. L. *et al.* (2000). Stress management in rheumatoid arthritis: what is the underlying mechanism? *Arthritis Care and Research*, **13**, 435–42.

Riemsma, R. P., Taal, E., Kirwan, J. R. & Rasker, J. J. (2002). Patient education programmes for adults with rheumatoid arthritis. *British Medical Journal*, **325**, 559.

Rupp, I., Boshuizen, H. C., Jacobi, C. E., Dinant, H. J. & Van Den Bos, G. A. M. (2004). Impact of fatigue on health-related quality of life in rheumatoid arthritis. *Arthritis Care and Research*, **51**, 578–85.

Scharloo, M., Kaptein, A. A., Weinman, J. *et al.* (1998). Illness perceptions, coping and functioning in patients with rheumatoid arthritis, chronic obstructive pulmonary disease and psoriasis. *Journal of Psychosomatic Research*, **44**, 573–85.

Smarr, K. L., Parker, J. C., Wright, G. E. *et al.* (1997). The importance of enhancing

self-efficacy in rheumatoid arthritis. *Arthritis Care and Research*, **10**, 18–26.

Smith, C. A., Wallston, K. A., Dwyer, K. A. & Dowdy, S. W. (1997). Beyond good and bad coping: a multidimensional examination of coping with pain in persons with rheumatoid arthritis. *Annals of Behavioral Medicine*, **19**, 11–21.

Treharne, G. J., Lyons, A. C., Booth, D. A. Mason, S. R. & Kitas, G. D. (2004). Reactions to disability in patients with early versus established rheumatoid arthritis. *Scandinavian Journal of Rheumatology*, **33**, 30–8.

Van Dyke, M. M., Parker, J. C., Smarr, K. L. *et al.* (2004). Anxiety in rheumatoid

arthritis. *Arthritis and Rheumatism*, **51**, 408–12.

Wagstaff, S., Smith, O. V. & Wood, P. H. N. (1985). Verbal pain descriptors used by patients with arthritis. *Annals of Rheumatic Disease*, **44**, 262–5.

Wolfe, F., Hawley, D. J. & Wilson, K. (1996). The prevalence and meaning of fatigue in rheumatic disease. *The Journal of Rheumatology.*, **23**, 1407–17.

Wolfe, F. & Hawley, D. J. (1998). The longterm outcomes of rheumatoid arthritis: work disability: a prospective 18 year study of 823 patients. *The Journal of Rheumatology*, **25**, 2108–17.

Road traffic accidents: human factors

Frank P. McKenna

University of Reading

Although the term accident is in general use it has some important drawbacks. In the English language the term implies that the event was unintended and that it was random with no apparent cause. No great issue will be taken with the unintended part of the definition (though driver suicides do play a small part, Hernetkoski & Keskinen, 1998). The reader should, however, not operate with the assumption that these events are random with no apparent cause. Although the disadvantage of the term accident is commonly voiced, one advantage of the term is rarely considered. Unlike alternative terms such as 'crash' the term 'accident' offers the opportunity (not taken up on this occasion) to examine behaviour across a wide variety of domains including occupational settings, home environment, aviation and maritime environments. While the term crash does not have much credence in domains such as occupational settings, the term accident can readily be applied and may offer the possibility that similar processes (such as inexperience, fatigue and violations) may operate across domains. Despite the clear flaws in the term it will, on balance, be retained for the present purposes.

An interesting feature of the study of traffic accidents is that they are relatively rarely considered in the context of health. This is most unfortunate.

The magnitude of the problem

Across the world the major cause of death among 1 to 40 year-olds is road accidents (World Health Organization, 2004). For high income countries the casualty trends are decreasing, but, for low to middle income countries, the casualties are increasing. Overall, between the years 2000 and 2020, the forecast is that worldwide traffic deaths will

increase by 66% (Kopits & Cropper, 2003). In terms of hospital use in low and middle income countries, road traffic casualties are the most frequent users of operating theatres and intensive care units (Odero *et al.*, 1997). Even in high income countries with relatively good safety records the casualties are considerable. For example, Evans (1991) calculated that in the USA there were more traffic deaths in the years 1977–1988 than in all US battle deaths in all wars from the revolutionary war through to the Vietnam war. Road accidents are, therefore, a major public health issue for most countries in the world.

Demographics

Across the world the fatality rate for age and gender presents a consistent pattern. Younger drivers have a higher fatality risk than older drivers and men have a higher fatality risk than women (Peden *et al.*, 2002). Even when the relative numbers of drivers and their mileage is taken into account the same conclusion is reached (Evans, 1991).

Violations

Parker *et al.* (1995) note that the term human error has been used rather imprecisely to describe very different ways in which behaviour can contribute to accidents. In a factor analysis of self-reports, three distinct factors emerge (Reason *et al.*, 1990). These factors have been labelled errors, lapses and violations. Errors have been defined as deviations from planned actions; lapses as failures of attention; and violations as deliberate infringements of safe practices. Although it is often argued that it is only violations that are related to accident involvement (e.g. Lawton *et al.*, 1997) there is evidence for a role for both errors and lapses.

The relationship between violations and accident involvement is well established. Gerbers and Peck (2003) found that those drivers who have violated have a subsequent accident rate that is more than three times higher than those with no violations. Violations that have been shown to be important are speed choice, close following and drunk driving. The link between speed choice and accident involvement has been shown by work demonstrating that casualties track speed limit changes (Rock, 1995); those observed to drive faster have more accidents (Wasielewski, 1984) and those who choose faster speeds on a video test have more speed-related accidents (Horswill & McKenna, 1999). Close following is implicated by the work of Evans and Wasielewski (1983) who found that observed following distance was associated with accident involvement. The relationship between drunk driving and accident involvement has been known for some time. A recent challenge for most societies is to determine the maximum level of alcohol that is permitted for drivers. Mann (2002) has noted that different societies might consider different criteria. For example, if research is considered that examines the decrement produced by alcohol on skilled performance then a level of 20 mg% would be justified. However, if research on elevated collision risk is considered then a level of 50 mg% would be justified.

Driving skill/experience

One obvious thought is that those who are more skilled have fewer accidents. Williams and O'Neill (1974) found that, contrary to prediction, those who were more skilled (race drivers) had more accidents on normal roads. Logically, some basic skill is required otherwise the vehicle would frequently be out of control. In learning to drive the relationship between driving test errors and accident involvement can be examined. Here the pattern is not entirely clear. Maycock (1995) reports that the one consistent finding across gender was that a higher order skill, awareness and anticipation was related to accident involvement. Although Baughan and Sexton (2002) found that awareness was implicated, they also found that general test errors were a better predictor of accident involvement, but, critically, these relationships were dependent on taking other factors into account. High-fault drivers drive less often and less in the dark, to the extent that they do not actually have more accidents. It is only when driving experience and driving at night are taken into account that there is a statistical relationship.

Maycock *et al.* (1991) examined the effects of age versus driving experience and found that experience dominated. In the first year of driving there was a 30% reduction in accident liability irrespective of age. In moving from age 17 to 18, drivers could expect a 6% reduction in accident liability. More particularly, McCartt *et al.* (2003) have shown that the accident rate is very high in the first few

months or 1000 miles of driving and then decreases. Clearly, drivers are learning, but what? One candidate is hazard perception, which refers to the ability of drivers to detect potential threats. It has been shown that new drivers are slow to detect hazards, but with experience and/or training hazard perception improves (McKenna & Horswill, 1999).

Fatigue

Horne and Reyner (1999) have argued that not only are sleep-related accidents more common than generally realized, but, also, they are more liable to be serious. The increased severity is a function of the fact that little avoidance action takes place in the form of steering or braking. Fatigue-related accidents are difficult to quantify and, in part, determining that an accident is fatigue-related relies on a process of elimination. To label an accident as fatigue-related, the general approach is to eliminate such factors as alcohol, medical disorder, suicide, and vehicle defects and then to determine whether avoidance behaviour (such as steering and braking) is absent. On this basis it has been estimated that sleep-related factors account for between 9 and 16% of all accidents and between 15 and 20% on motorways (Horne & Reyner, 1995; Maycock, 1996). Clearly, some proportion of these accidents may be due to sleep disorders. While it has been found that those with a sleep disorder, such as sleep apnoea (see 'Sleep apnoea') are more than six times more likely to have had a traffic accident (Teran-Santos *et al.*, 1999), it might be thought that the prevalence in the general population would be low. However, epidemiological investigation of the prevalence of sleep apnoea indicates that this may occur, often unrecognized, in 1 in 20 adults and in a milder, normally unrecognized form in 1 in 5 adults (Young *et al.*, 2002).

Maycock (1996) reported that 29% of drivers indicated that they had come close to falling asleep at the wheel at least once. In my own work I have found that, in a survey of over 10 000 drivers who were attending a speed awareness course, 16% indicated that they had fallen asleep at the wheel in the last two years. Acute sleep loss would appear to play a part in causing road accidents. Both Hartley (2004) and Stutts *et al.* (2003) report that having less than six hours of sleep the night before is a risk factor. It has also been found that those on night shift are at higher risk of a sleep-related accident (Stutts *et al.*, 2003). It would appear, therefore, that any factor that delays or disrupts sleep may be a risk factor (see 'Shiftwork and health' and 'Sleep and health').

Conclusion

Road traffic accidents are a major public health problem that is increasing. Tackling this problem will include finding methods to deliver new drivers with safe learning experiences, reducing driving violations and reducing the number of sleepy drivers.

(See also 'Accidents: psychological influences' and 'Patient safety and iatrogenesis').

REFERENCES

Baughan, C. J. & Sexton, B. (2002). Do driving test errors predict accidents? Yes and no. In Behavioural Research in

Road Safety: Eleventh seminar proceedings, 197–209. London: Department for Transport.

Evans, L. (1991). *Traffic safety and the driver*, 405. New York: Van Nostrand Reinhold.

Evans, L. & Wasielewski, P. (1983). Risky driving related to driver and vehicle characteristics. *Accident Analysis and Prevention*, **15**, 121–36.

Gerbers, M. A. & Peck, R. C. (2003). Using traffic conviction correlates to identify high accident-risk drivers. *Accident Analysis and Prevention*, **35**, 903–12.

Hartley, L. R. (2004). Fatigue and driving. In T. Rothengatter & R. D. Huguenin (Eds.). *Traffic & transport psychology*. Amsterdam: Elsevier.

Hernetkoski, K. & Keskinen, E. (1998). Self-destruction in Finnish motor traffic accidents in 1974–1992. *Accident Analysis and Prevention*, **30**, 697–704.

Horne, J. & Reyner, L. (1995). Sleep-related vehicle accidents. *British Medical Journal*, **310**, 565–7.

Horne, J. & Reyner, L. (1999). Vehicle accident related to sleep: a review. *Occupational and Environmental Medicine*, **56**, 289–94.

Horswill, M. S. & McKenna, F. P. (1999). The development, validation, and application of a video-based technique for measuring an everyday risk-taking behaviour: drivers' speed choice. *Journal of Applied Psychology*, **84**, 977–85.

Kopits, E. & Cropper, M. (2003). *Traffic fatalities and economic growth. Policy Working Paper, no. 3035*. Washington, DC: The World Bank. http://econ.worldbank.org/files/25935_wps3035.pdf.

Lawton, R., Parker, D., Manstead, A. S. R. & Stradling, S. G. (1997). The role of affect in predicting social behaviours: the case of road of traffic violations. *Journal of Applied Social Psychology*, **27**, 1258–76.

Mann, R. E. (2002). Choosing a rational threshold for the definition of drunk driving: what research recommends. *Addiction*, **97**, 1237–8.

Maycock, G. (1995). Novice driver accidents in relation to learning to drive, the driving test, and driving ability and behaviour. In G. B. Grayson (Ed.). *Behavioural research in road safety, 5* (pp. 1–13). Crowthorne: Transport Research Laboratory.

Maycock, G. (1996). Sleepiness and driving: the experience of UK car drivers. *Journal of Sleep Research*, **5**, 229–37.

Maycock, G., Lockwood, C. R. & Lester, J. F. (1991). *The accident liability of car drivers. Transport and Road Research Laboratory. Research report 315*. Crowthorne: Transport Research Laboratory.

McCartt, A. T., Shabanova, V. I. & Leaf, W. A. (2003). Driving experience, crashes and traffic citations of teenage beginning drivers. *Accident Analysis and Prevention*, **35**, 311–20.

McKenna, F. P. & Horswill, M. (1999). Hazard perception and its relevance for driver licensing. *IATTS Research*, **23**, 36–41.

Odero, W., Garner, P. & Zwi, A. (1997). Road traffic injuries in developing countries: a comprehensive review of epidemiological studies. *Tropical Medicine and International Health*, **2**, 445–60.

Parker, D., Reason, J. T., Manstead, A. S. R. & Stradling, S. G. (1995). Driving errors, driving violations and accident involvement. *Ergonomics*, **38**, 1036–48.

Peden, M., McGee, K. & Sharma, G. (2002). *The injury chart book: a graphical overview of the global burden of injuries*. Geneva: World Health Organization.

Reason, J. T., Manstead, A. S. R., Stradling, S. G., Baxter, J. S. & Cambell, K. (1990). Errors and violations on the road: a real distinction. *Ergonomics*, **33**, 1315–32.

Rock, S. M. (1995). Impact of the 65mph speed limit on accidents, deaths and injuries in Illinois. *Accident Analysis and Prevention*, **27**, 207–14.

Stutts, J. C., Wilkins, J. W., Osberg, J. S. & Vaughn, B. V. (2003). Driver risk factors for sleep-related crashes. *Accident Analysis and Prevention*, **35**, 321–31.

Teran-Santos, J., Jimenez-Gomez, A. & Cordero-Guevaro, J. (1999). The association between sleep apnea and the risk of traffic accidents. *New England Journal of Medicine*, **340**, 847–51.

Young, T., Peppard, P. E. & Gottlieb, D. J. (2002). Epidemiology of obstructive sleep apnea. *American Journal of Respiratory and Critical Care Medicine*, **165**, 1217–39.

Wasielewski, P. (1984). Speed as a measure of driver risk: observed speeds versus driver and vehicle characteristics. *Accident Analysis and Prevention*, **16**, 89–103.

Williams, A. F. & O'Neill, B. (1974). On-the-road driving records of licensed race drivers. *Accident Analysis and Prevention*, **6**, 263–70.

World Health Organization. (2004). *World report on traffic injury prevention*. Geneva: World Health Organization.

Screening: antenatal

Elizabeth Dormandy

King's College London

Antenatal screening is an important part of antenatal care as practised across the world (see 'Antenatal care'). Pregnant women and their partners are routinely offered a range of screening tests to identify those who are at increased risk of a fetal anomaly including chromosomal abnormalities, structural abnormalities or haemoglobin disorders. Recently there has been a policy shift regarding the aim of antenatal screening, from reducing the incidence of conditions to facilitating informed choices for those offered screening (National Screening Committee, 2000) (see also 'Screening: general issues'). This chapter describes the choices available for pregnant women and considers the extent to which informed choice is realized.

Screening Choices

Women are offered screening tests which differ according to the condition screened for, the time in pregnancy, the detection rates and the safety of associated diagnostic tests. This section describes the choices available to women about antenatal screening.

Screening for chromosomal abnormalities

Down's syndrome (Trisomy 21) is the most common chromosomal abnormality screened for and affects about 1 in 700 live births in the UK. A variety of screening tests using different markers have been introduced during the last twenty years. These include ultrasound measurement of nuchal translucency and measurements in maternal serum of alpha-fetoprotein, pregnancy associated plasma protein, human chorionic gonadotrophin, oestriol or inhibin. Screening tests use different combinations of markers, with the name reflecting characteristics of the test such as the number of markers assessed (Double or Triple), the type of marker assessed (nuchal translucency), where it was developed (Bart's or Leeds) or the way the risk assessment was performed (Integrated). As markers alter during gestation, reliable screening requires ultrasound dating of pregnancy and tests to be taken at specific times in gestation. The reported detection rates for antenatal screening tests for Down's syndrome vary between about 50 and 95% with a 5% false positive rate. The most cost effective screening test at the moment is reported to have a 95% detection rate with a 5% false positive rate (Gilbert et al., 2001) (see 'Fetal well being').

Screening results are usually reported as the risk of having a baby affected by the condition. Women are identified as being at increased risk in comparison either to a specified cut-off or other risk, such as age-related risk. Health professionals and women find communicating and understanding risk results difficult (see 'Risk perception' and 'Communicating risk'). Women at increased risk are offered diagnostic tests such as amniocentesis or chorionic villus sampling (CVS). These identify with virtual certainty if a fetus is affected, but are associated with a risk of miscarriage, which is greater for CVS than for amniocentesis.

If Down's syndrome is diagnosed in the fetus, women are offered the choice of continuing or terminating the pregnancy. This is a complex and tough area for women and their partners to deal with. Most women with a diagnosis of Down's syndrome terminate the pregnancy (Mansfield et al., 1999) (see 'Abortion'), but little empirical work has been done to explore how best to inform and support women and their partners making decisions following a diagnosis of chromosomal abnormality.

There has been much discussion between health professionals about which test characteristics are most valued by women. A recent study has shown that pregnant women and health professionals both valued safe tests, conducted early in pregnancy with higher detection rates, but that health professionals placed greater emphasis on earlier tests than did women (Bishop et al., 2004).

Screening for structural abnormalities

Women are offered ultrasound scans to screen for structural anomalies and UK guidelines recommend an ultrasound scan between 18 and 20 weeks gestation. A recent systematic review reported that ultrasound screening detected about half of the structural abnormalities and that detection rates varied according to the organ or system studied, with higher detection rates for central nervous

system abnormalities than for skeletal or cardiac abnormalities (Bricker et al., 2000). Some structural anomalies may also indicate an increased risk of chromosomal abnormality. Ultrasound screening can also identify markers of uncertain significance, so called 'soft-markers', that often resolve within a short period of time. Diagnostic tests following ultrasound screening are usually more detailed ultrasound scans.

Women place a high value on ultrasound scans and perceive ultrasound scans as a social occasion to 'see' their baby, rather than as an opportunity to screen for fetal anomalies (Bricker et al., 2000). These differences in the perceived aims of ultrasound scan between pregnant women and healthcare professionals can leave women and their partners shocked if anomalies are suspected or identified (Baillie et al., 2000).

Screening for sickle cell or thalassaemia

Sickle cell disorders and thalassaemia are inherited disorders that affect haemoglobin and are most common among people of African and Caribbean descent and among people of Mediterranean and South Asian descent respectively (see 'Sickle cell disease'). Although screening for these conditions has been available in the UK for 30 years, evidence suggests that women have not made informed choices about these tests. Some women are not offered tests in a timely manner to allow a reproductive choice (Modell et al., 2000). Screening is offered inappropriately, for example on the basis of family name or skin colour (Atkin & Ahmad, 1998) and women are poorly informed about the screening test (Ahmed et al., 2002). The poor quality of the screening service offered to women at risk for sickle cell and thalassaemia may be associated with the ethnicity of the at risk groups (see 'Cultural and ethnic factors in health').

Choices about diagnostic tests

Samples for diagnostic testing are taken by CVS between about 10 and 14 weeks or by amniocentesis after 14 weeks. Samples can be analysed either by karyotyping or by molecular methods such as FISH (fluorescent in situ hybridization) or PCR (polymerase chain reaction). Karyotyping and molecular methods differ in the number of chromosomes examined and the time taken for analysis. Karyotyping requires the cells to be cultured and examines all 23 pairs of chromosomes present in a cell, whereas molecular tests examine specific chromosomes. Reporting time takes up to three weeks for karyotyping, and two to three days for molecular tests.

The choice between CVS and amniocentesis is usually determined by the time the screening test result is known, with CVS offered earlier in pregnancy. In the UK the predominant method of analysis is karyotyping, but the method of analysis and the selection of those to whom it is made available varies across the country (Grimshaw et al., 2003). A recent survey has shown that about two-thirds of pregnant women, about half of their partners and just over half of healthcare professionals prefer molecular to karyotypic analysis (Grimshaw et al., 2003).

Informed choice

Research on the factors associated with making informed choices has tended to assess one dimension only, usually knowledge about a procedure. It is now widely acknowledged that informed choice is more complex than this and involves several dimensions. A consensus is emerging that an informed choice has two core characteristics: first, it reflects an individual's values, and second, it is made in the context of good knowledge (Bekker et al., 1999). An informed choice has been defined as: 'a decision based on relevant knowledge, consistent with the decision-maker's values and behaviourally implemented' (Marteau et al., 2001). A recent study reported that about half the women offered antenatal Down syndrome screening made an informed choice (Dormandy et al., 2002) (see also 'Informed consent').

Women's experience of screening

Women place great value on information about antenatal screening tests, and there is some evidence to suggest that women prefer to discuss screening with a health professional rather than receiving written information (Stapleton et al., 2002). Women's level of knowledge about screening tests is low and interventions to increase knowledge about antenatal screening tests have not been effective.

Women who receive increased risk results from screening are anxious, with anxiety levels returning to normal following a normal diagnostic test result, but for some women anxiety remains after a normal diagnostic test result (Green et al., 2004). Concerns have been raised that providing information will result in increased anxiety but evidence suggests this is not the case (Green et al., 2004), and there is some evidence that information may reduce anxiety (Rowe et al., 2002).

The influence of healthcare professionals

There is limited and conflicting evidence about the extent to which healthcare professionals may influence individuals' choices about antenatal screening tests. It is known that health professionals present information differently in different contexts. For example, health professionals provide more negative information about a condition in the context of antenatal screening than in the context of a baby born with a condition (Loeben et al., 1998). There is some evidence that health professionals' attitudes may be associated with the uptake of screening tests. A descriptive study of antenatal HIV testing indicated an association between health professionals' attitudes towards HIV testing and uptake in women who consulted them, but this was not found in a study in the context of antenatal Down's syndrome screening (Simpson et al., 1999; Dormandy & Marteau, 2004). One small study has examined the association between health

professionals' attitudes and women's decisions about termination in the context of fetal sex chromosome abnormality. Health professionals reported providing more negative information about the condition to a group of parents who subsequently terminated the pregnancy than did health professionals to a group of parents who decided to continue with the pregnancy (Hall et al., 2003) (see 'Attitudes of health professionals').

The social context of informed choice

Concern has been expressed that offering antenatal screening for fetal anomalies represents a eugenic policy, and may undermine the role of disabled people in society (Alderson, 2001). Facilitating informed choice has been seen as a way of separating antenatal screening programmes from eugenic aims (Kerr et al., 1998): that is it enables women to act in line with their own values and attitudes rather than the values of others. An alternative interpretation is that informed choice is an ideology rather than reality because of the difficulties health professionals experience when providing non-directive counselling (Williams et al., 2002): that is women are likely to act in line with society's values rather than their own.

Screening programmes

The low levels of women's knowledge is perhaps not surprising given the poor written information available and the low levels of health professionals' knowledge about screening tests (Murray et al., 2001; Sadler, 1997). Screening is often poorly implemented with a lack of guidelines or awareness of guidelines and tests offered inappropriately or tests not offered. In the UK, national programmes for Down's syndrome screening, ultrasound screening and haemoglobinopathy screening have been implemented, in part to address these problems. The success of these programmes at improving women's experiences and rates of informed choice has yet to be evaluated.

(See also 'Antenatal care', 'Fetal wellbeing' and other chapters on Screening.)

Conclusion

Screening for fetal anomalies is widely offered to pregnant women and their partners but the evidence suggests that rates of informed choice are low. For screening programmes to achieve their aim of offering informed choices to all women, three objectives need to be met. First, empirical evidence on how to facilitate informed choice is required. Second, evidence-based standards for facilitating informed choice need to be set. Third, rates of informed choice need to be monitored.

REFERENCES

Ahmed, S., Bekker, H., Hewison, J. & Kinsey, S. (2002). Thalassaemia carrier testing in Pakistani adults: Behaviour, knowledge and attitudes. Community Genetics, 5, 120–7.

Alderson, P. (2001). Prenatal screening, ethics and Down's syndrome: a literature review. Nursing Ethics, 8, 360–74.

Atkin, K. & Ahmad, W. (1998). Genetic screening and haemoglobinopathies:

ethics, politics and practice. Social Science and Medicine, 46, 445–58.

Baillie, C., Smith, J., Hewison, J. & Mason, G. (2000). Ultrasound screening for chromosomal abnormality: women's reactions to false positive results. *British Journal of Health Psychology*, **5**, 377–94.

Bekker, H., Thornton, J. G., Airey, C. *et al.* (1999). Informed decision making: an annotated bibliography and systematic review. *Health Technology Assessment*, **3**, 1.

Bishop, A. J., Marteau, T. M., Armstrong, D. *et al.* (2004). Women and health care professionals' preferences for Down syndrome screening tests: a conjoint analysis study. *British Journal of Obstetrics and Gynaecology*, **111**, 775–9.

Bricker, L., Garcia, J., Henderson, J. *et al.* (2000). Ultrasound screening in pregnancy: a systematic review of the clinical effectiveness, cost effectiveness and women's views. *Health Technology Assessment*, **4**, 16.

Dormandy, E., Hooper, R., Michie, S. & Marteau, T. M. (2002). Informed choice to undergo prenatal screening: a comparison of two hospitals conducting testing either as part of a routine visit or requiring a separate visit. *Journal of Medical Screening*, **9**, 109–14.

Dormandy, E. & Marteau, T. M. (2004). Uptake of an antenatal screening test: the role of healthcare professionals' attitudes towards the test. *Prenatal Diagnosis*, **24**, 864–8.

Gilbert, R. E., Augood, C., Gupta, R. *et al.* (2001). Screening for Down's syndrome: effects, safety, and cost effectiveness of first and second trimester strategies. *British Medical Journal*, **323**, 425.

Green, J. M., Hewison, J., Bekker, H., Bryant, L. & Cuckle, H. S. (2004).

Psychosocial aspects of genetic screening of pregnant women and newborns: a systematic review. *Health Technology Assessment*, **8**, 33.

Grimshaw, G., Szczepura, A., Hulton, M. *et al.* (2003). Evaluation of molecular tests for prenatal diagnosis of chromosome abnormalities. *Health Technology Assessment*, **7**, 10.

Hall, S., Abramsky, L. & Marteau, T. M. (2003). Health professionals' reports of information given to parents following the prenatal diagnosis of sex chromosome anomalies and outcomes of pregnancies: a pilot study. *Prenatal Diagnosis*, **23**, 535–8.

Kerr, A., Cunningham-Burley, S. & Amos, A. (1998). Eugenics and the new genetics in Britain: examining contemporary professionals' accounts. *Science, Technology and Human Values*, **23**, 175–98.

Loeben, G., Marteau, T. M. & Wilfond, B. (1998). Mixed messages: presentation of information in cystic fibrosis screening pamphlets. *American Journal of Human Genetics*, **63**, 1811–19.

Mansfield, C., Hopfer, S. & Marteau, T. M. (1999). Termination rates after prenatal diagnosis of Down syndrome, spina bifida, anencephaly and Turner and Klinefelter syndromes: a systematic literature review. *Prenatal Diagnosis*, **19**, 808–12.

Marteau, T. M., Dormandy, E. & Michie, S. (2001). A measure of informed choice. *Health Expectations*, **4**, 99–108.

Modell, B., Harris, R., Lane, B. *et al.* (2000). Informed choice in genetic screening for thalassaemia during pregnancy:

audit from a national confidential inquiry. *British Medical Journal*, **320**, 337–41.

Murray, J., Cuckle, H. S., Sehmi, I., Wilson, C. & Ellis, A. (2001). Quality of written information used in Down syndrome screening. *Prenatal Diagnosis*, **21**, 138–42.

National Screening Committee. (2000). *Second Report of the UK National Screening Committee*, London: Department of Health.

Rowe, R., Garcia, J., Macfarlane, A. & Davidson, L. (2002). Improving communication between health professionals and women in maternity care: a structured review. *Health Expectations*, **5**, 63–83.

Sadler, M. (1997). Serum screening for Down's syndrome: how much do health professionals know? *British Journal of Obstetrics and Gynaecology*, **104**, 176–9.

Simpson, W., Johnstone, F. D., Boyd, F. *et al.* (1998). Uptake and acceptability of antenatal HIV testing: randomised controlled trial of different methods of offering the test. *British Medical Journal*, **316**, 262–7.

Stapleton, H., Kirkham, M. & Thomas, G. (2002). Qualitative study of evidence based leaflets in maternity care. *British Medical Journal*, **324**, 639.

Williams, C., Alderson, P. & Farsides, B. (2002). Too many choices? Hospital and community staff reflect on the future of prenatal screening. *Social Science and Medicine*, **55**, 743–53.

Screening: cancer

Kevin D. McCaul and Amber R. Koblitz

North Dakota State University

Secondary prevention, or the early discovery of cancer through screening, is based on the idea that identifying a disease before symptoms develop will enable early treatment and extended survival. Screening tests to detect cancer have increased in number over the last decade, and technological advances are certain to produce many more such tests in the decade ahead. In fact, the development of technologies useful for cancer detection has outpaced research demonstrating the value of those new technologies. As a consequence, different screening tests are associated with different levels of uncertainty about whether they can accurately detect cancer and reduce deaths from cancer.

Reducing cancer deaths is an important goal. Cancer is the second leading cause of death in industrialized countries (ACS, 2004a), cancer treatment often creates significant psychological and physical suffering, and survivors continue to show poorer health outcomes compared to people who have not experienced cancer for years after treatment (Yabroff *et al.*, 2004) (see 'Cancer: general'). Given the potential importance of cancer screening in reducing mortality, we raise four questions: (a) What effective cancer screening tests are available? (b) How can we encourage people to adopt cancer screening behaviours? (c) What are the psychological consequences of cancer screening? and (d) What are the important directions for future psychological research concerning cancer screening?

Cancer screening technologies

An ideal cancer screening technique is reliable and accurate, carries little or no risk, allows for early detection which can lead to cancer prevention, and is inexpensive. Not surprisingly, no such test exists, and all screening technologies differ in the extent to which they meet these different criteria. Given imperfect screening tests, it is worth considering the value of screenings most commonly performed to detect the following (most frequently diagnosed) cancers: breast; prostate; colon; and cervical (see Curry *et al.*, 2003).

Three common screening modalities are available to identify breast cancer in patients; clinical breast examination (CBE), mammography and breast self-examinations (BSE). We will not deal with BSE in any detail here, because of a more complete discussion in the present volume (see 'Self-examination'); suffice it to say, however, that many researchers are unconvinced that BSE is a worthwhile screening technique. CBEs are typically performed in a health care setting by a health professional who simply searches the breast tissue for abnormalities, and (similar to BSE), it is also unclear whether CBEs have a mortality benefit, although they are easy to perform and inexpensive. Mammograms are a more intrusive screening in which the breast is scanned by low-dose X-rays. Mammography is the best (albeit imperfect) screening test currently available, showing a significant effect in reducing mortality for older women (see also 'Cancer: breast').

Two controversial screenings are available for prostate cancer; digital rectal examination (DRE) and prostate-specific antigen (PSA) detection. DREs are inexpensive, involving only a brief exam by a health professional, but the exam may have little value in terms of contributing to reduced mortality. PSAs are also relatively inexpensive, involving only tests for PSA concentrations in blood. PSA detection is much more sensitive (more likely to detect cancer) than DRE, but its specificity (degree to which it also does not identify men without cancer as having cancer; that is, false positives) differs for men of different ages. More problematic, though, are lingering doubts about the necessity of treating all prostate cancers and potentially serious treatment complications (e.g. impotence). Thus, much uncertainty surrounds the value of PSA, sparking researchers to study how best to provide information to men so they can make an informed decision about the test (see Myers, 2005) (see also 'Cancer: prostate').

Health professionals can use several tests to detect colorectal cancer; faecal occult blood test (FOBT), flexible sigmoidoscopy, double contrast barium enema and colonoscopy. The FOBT test faecal specimens for the presence of occult blood. Flexible sigmoidoscopy relies on a small digital camera to identify polyps and cancer in the descending colon. Double contrast barium enema is a radiological exam that looks for polyps or cancer in the rectum and colon. Colonoscopy, a more expensive test, is nevertheless the 'gold' standard test used to identify colorectal cancer, allowing the physician to examine the entire colon and to remove polyps to actually prevent cancer from occurring (Mandel *et al.*, 1993). Recent studies have revealed a relationship between screening and decreased incidence of colorectal cancer, although identification of the best screening test remains a contentious issue (Curry *et al.*, 2003) (see also 'Cancer: digestive tract').

The Pap smear is the screening test of choice for cervical cancer, even though the test lacks sensitivity and has considerable inter-observer disparities. If a Pap smear detects the presence of abnormal cells, cervical cancer can often be prevented, making this screening test a high priority (see also 'Cancer: gynaecological').

Encouraging people to screen

Screening levels

Adoption of different screening techniques differs widely by cancer type and screening methodology (ACS, 2004*b*). Most women in the USA, for example, are adherent to recommended screening for cervical (82%) and breast cancer (70%). Rates are meaningfully lower for colon cancer (39% of people older than 50 in the last year) and prostate cancer (54% of men having a PSA test in the previous year). Because of the uncertainty surrounding screening for prostate cancer and because colon cancer can be prevented, colon screening rates should be higher than for prostate cancer (Sirovich *et al.*, 2003). Moreover, the overall screening rates obscure an important fact: Screening levels are significantly lower for people of lower socio-economic status, and the disparity has increased in the USA since 1987 (Swan *et al.*, 2003). Socioeconomic disparities are also observed in countries with national screening programmes, such as the United Kingdom (McCaffery *et al.*, 2002).

Most of the screening data concern whether people have 'ever' or recently been screened, and we know much less about repeated screening. The latter question is especially important because the determinants of repeated screening may be distinct from those of initial screening. Rothman (2000) theorizes that beliefs about the costs and benefits of screening determine initial testing, but one's experience with screening itself (e.g. was it painful?; Elwood *et al.*, 1998) determine whether people will return. Answering the question about repeated screening will take longitudinal designs (see Rakowski *et al.*, 2004) and, as far as we are aware, the Rothman hypothesis has not been tested in the cancer screening context.

Understanding screening

Researchers interested in the determinants of screening have often correlated a long list of variables with screening behaviour, often using multiple regression. Although such research may be valuable initially for uncovering relationships, it is an atheoretical approach – a better strategy is to test variables based on an overall model of the process; best of all is to compare different models (Weinstein, 1993). The latter strategy says that some theoretically driven variables will predict screening better than others and these variables might differ across screening types. Too little of this sort of comparative research has been conducted.

Most theoretical models used to understand screening behaviour have been based on some version of subjective utility theory. This theoretical approach (see Kahneman & Tversky, 2000) suggests that in considering whether to act, people consider the likely costs and benefits, weight those outcomes by how personally important they are, and implicitly perform an algebraic computation to arrive at an overall decision. Of course, people rarely make decisions in precisely this way (Simon, 1955), but, nevertheless, costs and benefits predict whether or not people will get screened (Zapka & Lemon, 2004). Costs and benefits (barriers) are at the heart of the Health Belief Model (HBM; Strecher et al., 1997), and variables drawn from this model have routinely been shown to correlate, though modestly, with screening (Yarbrough & Braden, 2001) (see 'Health belief model').

More recently developed theoretical approaches add several features to the rational sorts of 'belief' models. Leventhal's Illness Representations Model, for example, introduces illness beliefs not typically represented in the HBM (for example, 'when does colon cancer start to appear?'; 'what causes colon cancer?'; 'Can I control whether or not I get colon cancer?'). Leventhal et al. (2001) also point out that emotional responses to cancer, such as fear, can motivate screening adoption or avoidance (see 'Lay beliefs about health and illness').

A second type of theoretical model suggests that people go through discrete decision-making stages before engaging in screening (Rakowski et al., 1992). Weinstein's (1988) Precaution Adoption Model, for example, emphasizes perceptions of personal vulnerability to cancer, and risk judgments have been shown to predict screening (e.g. Katapodi et al., 2004; McCaul et al., 1996).

Finally, Miller et al. (1996) developed a model emphasizing the potential importance of individual differences as screening determinants. The Cognitive-Social Health Information Processing Model (C-SHIP) provides a framework that emphasizes the beliefs, expectations, feelings, and goals that a person brings to the situation. The model suggests that people differ in how they process information and that these differences will interact with situations. The C-SHIP model nicely accounts for a number of findings related to BSE and mammography screening for breast cancer, and this model deserves additional research.

Most models of health-protective behaviour at least acknowledge situational determinants, although they differ in their emphasis on such variables. However, contextual variables are likely to have large effects on screening. Indeed, physician recommendation is well known as the best predictor of breast cancer screening in the USA. Women who have been screened are much more likely to report that their doctor 'suggested' they have a mammogram (Fox & Stein, 1991), for example, and physician advice predicts both first-time and repeated mammograms (Lerman et al., 1990). A second important contextual variable is whether or not screening is centralized. In the UK, for example, the national healthcare system pays for screening after defining who is eligible. In the USA, payment for screening is highly dependent on individual insurance providers. In the latter case, individual beliefs and feelings may predict more variance in screening behaviours, whereas contextual factors are likely to play a much larger role in national healthcare systems (see 'Screening: general issues').

Increasing screening

Many researchers have taken the variables predicting screening and incorporated them into screening interventions. And many different strategies have shown some success. Decreasing barriers by lowering costs is important, for example, especially for under-served populations (e.g. Legler et al., 2002; Skaer et al., 1996). Similar system changes have been made within the medical environment, to ensure appropriate recommendations are made and reminders integrated within surgery/office systems (Costanza et al., 2000). At the individual level, researchers have focused on tailoring interventions to the particular attributes of each individual. So, for example, one message might be used for a man who fears the colonoscopy procedure; a completely different message would be used for a woman who says she is not at all at risk for colon cancer. Although tailored messages attract more attention than those which are not tailored (Skinner et al., 1999), we do not know if the impact in terms of increased screening is worth the extra costs of tailoring (e.g. Clark et al., 2002).

The consequences of screening

Given that we are recommending screening, it is important to remember that screening is not cost-free. Cancer screening can be stressful: for example, Pap smears are uncomfortable; so, too, is preparation for a colonoscopy. More importantly, screening results are sometimes in error, and an important problem is a false-positive result. The jury is still out on the overall effects of false positives, but two tentative conclusions seem warranted. First, false-positive results are upsetting and create increases in anxiety (Aro et al., 2000; Cunningham et al., 1998). However, it is also important to note that (a) distress is relatively short-lived (Wardle et al., 1993) and (b) false positive results do not generally inhibit people from obtaining a follow-up screening or from continuing to engage in screenings; indeed, some data suggest that false-positive screenings produce *better* subsequent adherence (Burman et al., 1999; Lerman et al., 1991 but also see Ford et al., 2003).

Conclusions and questions to ask

We have learned much from research to date; indeed, a recent special issue of the journal *Cancer* includes many empirically tested 'lessons learned' (Meissner et al., 2004). However, here are things we still need to know with much more precision than at present:

- How do we best communicate the uncertainty often surrounding imperfect screening tools so that people are 'fully informed' (Rimer et al., 2004)?
- Why do persons identified as of 'lower socioeconomic status' show lower rates of screening and how can we change this important disparity?
- How do theories compare in their power to predict screening? (Weinstein, 1993).
- What determines repeat as opposed to initial screening?

- Are the consequences of imperfect screening tools minimal that result in false positives small enough that they are easily offset by the benefits?

(See also 'Screening in healthcare', 'Screening: antenatal', 'Screening: cardiac', 'Screening: genetic' and 'Self-examination: breasts, testicles'.)

REFERENCES

American Cancer Society, Inc. (2004*a*). *Cancer facts & figures 2004*. Retrieved December 2, 2004, from http://www.cancer.org/downloads/STT/CAFF_finalPWSecured.pdf.

American Cancer Society, Inc. (2004*b*). *Cancer prevention & early detection facts & figures 2004*. Retrieved December 2, 2004, from http://www.cancer.org/downloads/STT/CPED2004PWSecured.pdf.

Aro, A. R., Absetz, S. P., van Elderen, T. M. *et al.* (2000). False-positive findings in mammography screening induces short-term distress – breast cancer-specific concern prevails longer. *European Journal of Cancer*, **36**, 1089–97.

Burman, M. L., Taplin, S. H., Herta, D. F. & Elmore, J. G. (1999). Effect of false-positive mammograms on interval breast cancer screening in a health maintenance organization. *Annals of Internal Medicine*, **131**, 1–6.

Clark, M. A., Rakowski, W., Ehrich, B. *et al.* (2002). The effect of a stage-matched and tailored intervention on repeat mammography (1). *American Journal of Preventive Medicine*, **22**, 1–7.

Costanza, M. E., Stoddard, A. M., Luckmann, R. *et al.* (2000). Promoting mammography: results of a randomized trial of telephone counseling and a medical practice intervention. *American Journal of Preventive Medicine*, **19**, 39–46.

Cunningham, L. L., Andrykowski, M. A., Wilson, J. F. *et al.* (1998). Physical symptoms, distress, and breast cancer risk perceptions in women with benign breast problems. *Health Psychology*, **17**, 371–5.

Curry, S. J., Byers, T. & Hewitt, M. (Eds.). (2003). *Fulfilling the potential of cancer prevention and early detection*. Washington, DC: The National Academies Press.

Elwood, M., McNoe, B., Smith, T., Bandaranayake, M. & Doyle, T. C. (1998). Once is enough – why some women do not continue to participate in a breast cancer screening programme. *The New Zealand Medical Journal*, **111**, 180–3.

Ford, M. E., Havstad, S. L., Flickinger, L. & Johnson, C. C. (2003). Examining the effects of false positive lung cancer screening results on subsequent lung cancer screening adherence. *Cancer Epidemiology, Biomarkers and Prevention*, **12**, 28–33.

Fox, S. A. & Stein, J. A. (1991). The effect of physician-patient communication on mammography utilization by different ethnic groups. *Medical Care*, **29**, 1065–82.

Kahneman, D. & Tversky, A. (2000). Prospect theory: an analysis of decision under risk. In D. Kahneman & A. Tversky (Eds.) *Choices, values, and frames*. (pp. 17–43). New York: Cambridge University Press.

Katapodi, M. C., Lee, K. A., Facione, N. C. & Dodd, M. J. (2004). Predictor of perceived breast cancer risk and the relation between perceived risk and breast cancer screening: a meta-analytic review. *Preventive Medicine*, **38**, 388–402.

Legler, J., Meissner, H. I., Coyne, C. *et al.* (2002). The effectiveness of interventions to promote mammography among women with historically lower rates of screening. *Cancer Epidemiology Biomarkers, and Prevention*, **11**, 59–71.

Lerman, C., Rimer, B., Trock, B., Balshem, A. & Engstrom, P. F. (1990). Factors associated with repeat adherence to breast cancer screening. *Preventive Medicine*, **19**, 279–90.

Lerman, C., Trock, B., Rimer, B. K. *et al.* (1991). Psychological and behavioral implications of abnormal mammograms. *Annals of Internal Medicine*, **114**, 657–61.

Leventhal, H., Leventhal, E. A. & Cameron, L. (2001). Representations, procedures, and affect in illness self-regulation: a perceptual–cognitive model. In A. Baum, T. A. Revenson & J. E. Singer (Eds.). *Handbook of health psychology*, Mahwah, NJ: Lawrence Erlbaum Associates.

Mandel, J. S., Bond, J. H., Church, T. R. *et al.* (1993). Reducing mortality from colorectal cancer by screening for fecal occult blood. Minnesota Colon Cancer Control Study. *New England Journal of Medicine*, **328**, 1365–71.

McCaffery, K., Wardle, J., Nadel, M. & Atkin, W. (2002). Socioeconomic variation in participation in colorectal cancer screening. *Journal of Medical Screening*, **9**, 104–8.

McCaul, K. D., Branstetter, A. D., Schroeder, D. M. & Glasgow, R. E. (1996). What is the relationship between breast cancer risk and mammography screening? A meta-analytic review. *Health Psychology*, **15**, 1–8.

Meissner, H. I., Smith, R. A., Rimer, B. K. *et al.* (2004). Promoting cancer screening: learning from experience. *Cancer*, **101**, 1107–17.

Miller, S. M., Shoda, Y. & Hurley, K. (1996). Applying cognitive–social theory to health-protective behavior: breast self-examination in cancer screening. *Psychological Bulletin*, **119**, 70–94.

Myers, R. (in press). Decision counseling in cancer prevention and control. *Health Psychology*. Special Issue: Basic and Applied Decision Making in Cancer Control. 24(4 suppl.), S71–7.

Rakowski, W., Breen, N., Meissner, H. *et al.* (2004). Prevalence and correlates of repeat mammography among woman aged 55–79 in the Year 2000. National Health Interview Survey. *Preventive Medicine*, **39**, 1–10.

Rakowski, W., Dube, C. E., Marcus, B. H. *et al.* (1992). Assessing elements of women's decisions about mammography. *Health Psychology*, **11**, 111–18.

Rimer, B. K., Briss, P. A., Zeller, P. K., Chan, E. C. & Woolf, S. H. (2004). Informed decision making: what is its role in cancer screening? *Cancer*, **101**, 1214–28.

Rothman, A. J. (2000). Toward a theory-based analysis of behavioral maintenance. *Health Psychology*, **19**, 64–9.

Sirovich, B. E., Schwartz, L. M. & Woloshin, S. (2003). Screening men for prostate and colorectal cancer in the United States: does practice reflect the evidence? *Journal of the American Medical Association*, **289**, 1414–20.

Simon, H. A. (1955). A behavioral model of rational choice. *The Quarterly Journal of Economics*, **69**, 99–119.

Skaer, T. L., Robison, L. M., Sclar, D. A. & Harding, G. H. (1996). Financial incentive and the use of mammography among Hispanic migrants to the United States. *Health Care for Women International*, **17**, 281–91.

Skinner, C. S., Campbell, M. K., Rimer, B. K., Curry, S. & Prochaska, J. O. (1999). How effective is tailored print communication? *Annals of Behavioral Medicine*, **21**, 290–8.

Strecher, V. J., Champion, V. L. & Rosenstock, I. W. (1997). In D. S. Gochman (Ed.). *Handbook of health behavior research I: Personal and social determinants* (pp. 71–91). Plenum Press, New York.

Swan, J., Breen, J., Coates, R. J., Rimer, B. K. & Lee, N. C. (2003). Progress in cancer screening practices. *Cancer*, **97**, 1528–40.

Wardle, F. J., Collins, W., Pernet, A. L. *et al.* (1993). Psychological impact of screening for familial ovarian cancer. *Journal of the National Cancer Institute*, **85**, 653–7.

Weinstein, N. D. (1988). The precaution adoption process. *Health Psychology*, **7**, 355–86.

Weinstein, N. D. (1993). Testing four competing theories of health-protective behavior. *Health Psychology*, **12**, 324–33.

Yabroff, K. R., Lawrence, W. F., Clauser, S., Davis, W. W. & Brown, M. L. (2004). Burden of illness in cancer survivors: findings from a population-based national sample. *Journal of the National Cancer Institute*, **96**, 1322–30.

Yarbough, S. S. & Braden, C. J. (2001). Utility of health belief model as a guide for

explaining or predicting breast cancer screening behaviours. *Journal of Advances in Nursing*, **33**, 677–88.

Zapka, J. G. & Lemon, S. C. (2004). Interventions for patients, providers, and health care organizations. *Cancer* (Suppl.), **101**, 1165–87.

Screening: cardiac

Alethea F. Cooper

St. Thomas' Hospital

Cardiac risk factors

Cardiac screening is a focus of attention because cardiovascular diseases are responsible for the deaths of 16.7 million people worldwide each year (World Health Organization, 2003), but 50% of deaths and disability from cardiovascular disease (CVD) can be reduced through reduction of major coronary risk factors (World Health Organization, 2002). Population-based studies, such as the well known Framingham Heart Study, demonstrated several major risk factors to be independent predictors of coronary heart disease (CHD) although the studies were based on a mainly White population in Massachusetts, USA. Major risk factors include cigarette smoking, hypertension, high serum low-density lipoprotein cholesterol, low levels of high-density lipoprotein cholesterol, diabetes mellitus and advancing age. Data from the Framingham Heart Study form the basis of internationally used coronary prediction algorithms (Wilson *et al.*, 1998), two dimensional risk charts (Wood *et al.*, 1998) and a Cardiac Risk Assessor computer programme (The Framingham Risk Equation; Anderson *et al.*, 1991) for calculating risk in patients without known existing CHD. Psychological factors are absent from risk calculation instruments, although recent reviews have detailed the role of psychological factors in manifestation of CHD (Rozanski *et al.*, 2005).

Cardiac screening is generally based on a 'high risk' approach in which individuals in the general population at particularly high risk are identified for provision of advice, further diagnostic investigation, or treatment in order to reduce their risk of manifestation of CHD or CVD. A reduction of risk factors is important because people with multiple risk factors for heart disease are three to five times more likely to die, suffer a heart attack, or other major cardiovascular event than people without such conditions or risk factors (DoH, NSF, 2000). Modifiable behavioural risk factors include smoking, diet, physical inactivity and overweight/obesity. The Nurses Health Study (Stampfer *et al.*, 2000) demonstrated that women in whom these risk factors are low carry 84% less risk for heart disease

and stroke. Risk factors such as hypertension, hypercholesterolaemia and diabetes are usually modified through pharmacological management if behavioural interventions (increasing exercise, dietary changes) have proved to be ineffective.

Although not addressed specifically within this chapter, it should be remembered that there are inequalities in cardiac risk that are manifest between countries, social classes and ethnic groups.

Psychological reaction to screening

An adverse reaction to a screening programme was first described by Haynes (Haynes *et al.*, 1978) in steelworkers, whose levels of absenteeism rose on receiving a diagnosis of hypertension. The most direct adverse psychological response to health screening is increased anxiety, which may occur not only in patients who receive positive results but also on invitation to attend for screening and also on receiving a negative result. Studies investigating the results of screening in relation to these possible outcomes are described in detail below.

Response to information about increased risk

A systematic review examining the psychological impact of risk assessment for various illnesses identified 21 studies investigating the impact of informing individuals about CVD risk (Shaw *et al.*, 1999). Sixteen of these studies examined the impact of screening for hypertension, two looked at the effect of screening for total cholesterol, one compared receiving a label of low risk vs. high risk and two investigated the impact of screening vs. no screening (one study involved screening plus an intervention). Outcome measures in the CVD studies were emotional (anxiety, depression, distress), cognitive (health perceptions) and behavioural (absenteeism from work), and were evaluated according to short-term (within one month of risk assessment) and/or long-term (greater than one month after risk assessment) impact. The results of the studies specific to CVD risk are consistent with the overall results of the review, which are based on a total of 54 studies.

Quantitative analysis of a small selection of the 54 studies, including one or two investigating CVD risk, indicated that receiving a positive adverse test result was associated in the short-term with increased anxiety (Irvine *et al.*, 1989), but not in the long-term for anxiety or for depression (Ambrosio *et al.*, 1984; Rudd *et al.*, 1986). Quantitative evaluation of risk assessment on short-term depression was not conducted.

A descriptive analysis was undertaken for all studies. Eight CVD studies investigated absenteeism which increased in just two. A negative impact on perceptions of health was revealed in three out of five studies (one short-term impact, one long-term, one not specified). It should be noted that the quality of these cross-sectional studies received a low grade by the review authors. In two more highly graded prospective studies, no long term effect was found in one and in the other perceptions of current health improved.

A recently published randomized controlled trial confirms the results of the review. Christensen *et al.* (2004) investigated psychological distress, in relation to receiving a low, moderate, elevated, or high risk label, in 1507 people aged 30–49 in Denmark. Four elements of psychological distress: anxiety/insomnia; depression; social impairment/hyochondria; and social dysfunction were measured before screening, then again one and five years later, using the GHQ-12 (Goldberg, 1978). Participants were randomized to a control group (no screening) or one of two intervention groups involving health screening and written feedback but with either an optional or planned follow-up visit with the primary care physician. No differences were found in GHQ-12 scores during the follow-up period according to group randomization or according to self-report baseline risk (current smoker or overweight). This result confirmed results of an earlier, smaller study by Christensen (1995) in 273 men aged 40–49 where there were no changes in GHQ scores at six months following identification of increased/high risk for CHD on screening.

In a non-randomized study, Connelly *et al.* (1998) examined the impact of receiving a high, moderate, or low risk score in 5000 middle-aged (45–69 years) men. The 28-item GHQ (Goldberg & William, 1988) was completed prior to initial screening, immediately following risk factor labelling, and three months later. Receiving a label of 'above average risk' of heart disease did not appear to lead to increased psychological symptoms, although men receiving a 'moderate risk' label were at immediate increased risk.

Response to information about minimal risk

Few studies have examined the impact of receiving a 'low risk' screen result in a between-group design where the control group underwent no screening. However, when examining within-group data in studies where a 'low risk' label is compared with 'high risk', there is little evidence of a short or long-term effect (Connelly *et al.*, 1998; Shaw *et al.*, 1999). A separate issue related to receiving 'minimal risk' feedback is that of false reassurance. In a study of 428 men between 30 and 33 years of age it has been suggested that men who

screened negative for CVD risk may have used the result to justify their health behaviour; importantly, these men did not exhibit healthier behaviour with regard to smoking, diet, or physical inactivity when compared to those who screened positive for CVD risk (Tymstra & Bieleman, 1987).

The response to receiving a negative result has been more extensively investigated in relation to patients undergoing diagnostic coronary angiography for symptoms of chest pain, although this test is not strictly a screening procedure. Between 34 and 56% of patients undergoing coronary angiography have either normal coronary arteries (NCA) or mild non-obstructive atherosclerosis (Beitman *et al.*, 1989; Carter *et al.*, 1994). However, a substantial body of evidence suggests that such individuals may continue to report symptoms and are compromised with regard to emotional, social and physical functioning. In one prospective study 46 patients undergoing coronary angiography on the basis of symptoms were told they had insignificant lesions and should not limit activities. However, at one year, 29 patients continued to consult a doctor for cardiac-related symptoms (Bass *et al.*, 1983). After one decade up to three-quarters of patients continued to report chest pain, had undergone further hospital treatment and were using cardiac medication. One-third were unable to work for medical reasons (Potts & Bass, 1993).

Patients with non-cardiac chest pain have a good outcome in relation to cardiac mortality, but it is recommended that in order to prevent such morbidity, an 'early and confident diagnosis of non-cardiac chest pain should be made' with an emphasis on the psychological aspects of medical management (Bass & Mayou, 2002). Bass and Mayou (2002) suggest that following a diagnosis of NCA, symptoms of depression and association of the chest pain with anxiety or panic attacks should be sought, as should the presence of possible precipitating stressful life events; patients' beliefs about their chest pain should also be elicited. Effective, consistent communication between healthcare professionals and the patient as well as between healthcare professionals in primary and secondary care should help to minimize the concerns of the patient and reassurance, education and information may be sufficient in 30–40% of patients. However, in the 60–70% of patients with continuing symptoms and limitation of physical activity, specialist management and treatment is recommended and may necessitate pharmacological treatment for oesophageal disorders or antidepressants, psychological support and intervention (e.g. cognitive behavioural therapy and/or further medical investigation such as referral to a gastroenterologist (Bass & Mayou, 2002).

The association between psychosocial factors and chest pain associated with NCA was investigated in a case-control study by Cheng *et al.* (2003). Compared with patients with rheumatism or healthy individuals, individuals with NCA were less likely to receive social support in times of stress, more likely to show a monitoring perceptual style, and to demonstrate inflexible problem-focused coping with poor management of stress-related emotions. The authors point out both are potentially anxiety-provoking mechanisms which could increase tension in the thoracic muscles and worsen breathing patterns, thus provoking chest pain and reinforcing perceptions of cardiac pain. The role for psychological intervention and management posited by Bass and Mayou (2002) is thus reinforced.

Approaches to cardiac screening

The possible psychological consequences of screening for CHD should not be considered in isolation from the impact of interventions to reduce high risk in cases where this is identified. A recent review showed little impact of primary prevention population-based interventions (Ebrahim & Davey Smith, 2001). Marteau and Kinmouth (2002) suggest the current strategy of population based targeting of individuals rather than recruitment through an informed choice paradigm may influence the success of interventions. The authors argue for debate regarding shifting towards an informed choice approach to cardiac screening and summarise succinctly the argument for conducting cardiovascular screening within an informed choice paradigm (Marteau & Kinmouth, 2002). Informed choice involves the provision of high quality, personally relevant information and, as such, the ultimate choice of the individual reflects his or her values. Although informed choice is imperative in circumstances such as antenatal screening it is suggested that this approach may be more cost effective than a traditional public health approach to cardiac screening because it may result in participants who are more motivated to take action to reduce their risks. The authors acknowledge that such an approach may result in an increase in health inequalities and stress that written material be comprehensible and should also be of a nature that does not induce high levels of fear.

The role of risk perception and consequences of interventions

Illness perceptions have been shown to be of paramount importance in relation to management and coping with CHD, as well as response to acute symptoms. Perceptions of risk of heart disease have also been assessed along with the importance attached to individual risk factors prior to screening and intervention in the British Family Heart Study in 3725 patients by Marteau et al. (1995). Although there were strong associations between perceived risk and levels of individual risk factors, as well as overall risk score calculated using epidemiologically derived data, a third of people held views of heart disease risk that were different to the overall risk score. Study participants ascribed less importance to blood pressure and cholesterol and more to smoking and parental death from heart disease. Patients were categorized as 'optimists', 'realists' or 'pessimists' according to the relationship between their perceived risk of CHD and actual risk score: the reported presence of personal and family related risk factors accounted for significant differences between the three groups. The study authors suggest that possible differences between an individual's perceived risk and a calculated risk score should be considered by health professionals prior to intervention to address cardiovascular risk, in order to improve communication and, thus, optimize likelihood of engagement in lifestyle behaviour change.

This raises another important issue. Although it would appear that cardiac screening and/or participation in an intervention does not result in long-term psychological distress, an unexpected finding in the British Heart Study suggests that intervention participants, when successfully achieving modest risk reduction specifically with regard to weight loss and smoking cessation, may be likely to perceive a diminution in their ability to further lessen their cardiac risk (Marteau et al., 1996). Such 'false reassurance' could be harmful for such individuals in the presence of continued raised risk.

Result of interventions to reduce adverse effect of screening

There is evidence that interventions that aim to reduce the adverse psychological consequences of receiving a positive test result following screening are effective (Shaw et al., 1999). Such interventions have included information provision (vs. no information) reassurance (vs. typical counselling), and cognitive behavioural stress management (vs. no intervention; see 'Stress management' and 'Cognitive behavioural therapy'). Required elements of an effective screening intervention include information regarding the condition, and the likelihood, meaning and implications of possible test results.

Summary and avenues for future work

Whilst a result indicating increased risk following cardiac screening may be associated with an immediate increase in psychological distress, it appears this is unlikely to remain the case at follow-up as little as one month later. This is probably dependent on the manner in which risk information is provided because interventions to negate adverse outcome have been shown to be effective. The result of screening and receiving a 'minimal risk' label has received little investigation although the concept of false reassurance should be considered.

More recently, it has been suggested that other psychological sequelae may occur as a result of screening and intervention programmes, such as reduced perception of ability to make changes following intervention participation. It is suggested this may be a result of disempowerment in those who have been unable to achieve change or false reassurance in those who have implemented small changes, particularly in visible risk factors such as weight loss and smoking cessation; but this needs to be understood more fully.

The use of an informed choice paradigm for cardiac screening may be subject to future debate and the amount of information provided before and following screening and how it is communicated are issues that warrant careful consideration with further evaluation.

(See also 'Coronary heart disease: impact', 'Coronary heart disease: cardiac psychology', 'Coronary heart disease: rehabilitation', and 'Screening in healthcare: general issues'.)

REFERENCES

Anderson, K. M., Wilson, P. W. F., Odell, P. M. & Kannel, W. B. (1991). An updated coronary risk profile: a statement for health professionals. *Circulation*, **83**, 357–63.

Bass, C., Clyde, W., Hand, C. & Jackson, G. (1983). Patients with angina with normal and near normal coronary arteries: clinical and psychosocial state 12 months after angiography. *British Medical Journal*, **287**, 1505–8.

Bass, C. & Mayou, R. (2002). ABC of psychological medicine: chest pain. *British Medical Journal*, **325**, 588–91.

Beitman, B. D., Mukerji, V., Lamberti, J. W. *et al.* (1989). Panic disorder in patients with chest pain and angiographically normal coronary arteries. *American Journal of Cardiology*, **63**, 1399–403.

Carter, C., Maddock, R., Zoglio, M. *et al.* (1994). Panic disorder and chest pain: a study of cardiac stress scintigraphy patients. *Americal Journal of Cardiology*, **74**, 296–8.

Cheng, C., Wong, W., Lai, K. *et al.* (2003). Psychosocial factors in patients with noncardiac chest pain. *Psychosomatic Medicine*, **65**, 443–9.

Christensen, B. (1995). Psychological reactions to information about risk of ischaemic heart disease in practice. *Scandinavian Journal of Primary Health Care*, **13**, 164–7.

Christensen, B., Engberg, M. & Lauritzen, T. (2004). No long-term psychological reaction to information about increased risk of coronary heart disease in general practice. *European Journal of Cardiovascular Prevention and Rehabilitation*, **11**, 239–43.

Connelly, J., Cooper, J., Mann, A. & Meade, T. W. (1998). The psychological impact of screening for risk of coronary heart disease in primary care settings. *Journal of Cardiovascular Risk*, **5**, 185–91.

Department of Health. (2000). *National Service Framework for Coronary Heart Disease, Chapter Two: Preventing coronary heart disease in high risk patients*. London: Stationery Office.

Goldberg, D. (1978). *Manual of the General Health Questionnaire*. Windsor, UK: NFER Publishing.

Goldberg, D. & Williams, P. (1988) *A user's guide to the General Health Questionnaire*. Windsor, UK: NFER Nelson.

Haynes, R. B., Sackett, D. L., Taylor, W., Gibson, E. S. & Johnson, A. L. (1978). Increased absenteeism from work after detection and labeling of hypertensive patients. *New England Journal of Medicine*, **299**, 741–4.

Irvine, M. J., Garner, D. M., Olmsted, M. P. & Logan, A. G. (1989). Personality differences between hypertensive and normotensive individuals: influence of knowledge of hypertension status. *Psychosomatic Medicine*, **51**, 537–49.

Marteau, T. M. & Kinmonth, A. L. (2002). Screening for cardiovascular risk: public health imperative or matter for individual informed choice? *British Medical Journal*, **325**, 78–80.

Marteau, T. M., Kinmonth, A. L., Pyke, S. & Thompson, S. on behalf of the British Family Heart Study Group. (1995). Readiness for lifestyle advice: self-assessment of coronary risk prior to screening in the British family heart study. *British Journal of General Practice*, **45**, 5–8.

Marteau, T. M., Kinmonth, A. L., Thompson, S. & Pyke, S. on behalf of the British Family Heart Study Group. (1996). The psychological impact of cardiovascular screening and intervention in primary care: a problem of false reassurance? *British Journal of General Practice*, **46**, 577–82.

Potts, S. G. & Bass, C. M. (1993). Psychosocial outcome and use of medical resources in patients with chest pain and normal or near-normal coronary arteries. *Quarterly Journal of Medicine*, **86**, 583–93.

Rozanski, A., Blumenthal, J. A., Davidson, K. W., Saab, P. G. & Kubzansky, L. (2005). The epidemiology, pathophysiology, and management of psychosocial risk factors in cardiac practice. *Journal of the American College of Cardiology*, **45**, 637–51.

Shaw, C., Abrams, K. & Marteau, T. M. (1999). Psychological impact of predicting individuals' risks of illness: a systematic review. *Social Science and Medicine*, **49**, 1571–98.

Stampfer, M. J., Hu, F. B., Manson, J. E., Rimm, E. B. & Willet, W. C. (2000). Primary prevention of coronary heart disease in women through diet and lifestyle. *New England Journal of Medicine*, **343**, 16–22.

Tymstra, T. & Bieleman, B. (1987). The psychosocial impact of mass screening for cardiovascular risk factors. *Family Practice*, **4**, 287–90.

Wilson, P. W. F., D' Agostino, R. B., Levy, D. *et al.* (1998). Prediction of coronary heart disease using risk factor categories. *Circulation*, **97**, 1837–47.

Wood, D. A., De Backer, G., Faergeman, O., Graham, I., Marcia, G. & Pyorala, K. with members of the Task Force. (1998). Prevention of coronary heart disease in clinical practice. Recommendations of the Second Joint Task Force of the European Society of Cardiology, European Atherosclerosis Society and European Society of Hypertension. *European Heart Journal*, **19**, 1434–503.

World Health Organization (WHO). (2003). *World Health Report*. Geneva: WHO.

World Health Organization (WHO). (2002). Integrated Management of Cardiovascular Risk. *Report of a WHO Meeting*, Geneva, July.

Screening: genetic

Shoshana Shiloh

Tel Aviv University

Screening tests are medical tests carried out on presumably healthy people to identify an existing illness or pre-disease condition. They comprise a sub-category of health protective behaviours, sometimes labelled detection behaviour or secondary prevention. Screening is advocated as a cost-effective means of identifying individuals at a very early, pre-symptomatic stage of a disease when treatment is more effective and less costly. Identifying people at risk for disease enables health services to target those most likely to benefit from early intervention (see 'Screening in healthcare').

Psychologically, screening is different from other health behaviours. In contrast to 'true' preventive behaviours (e.g. exercising) that reduce the likelihood of future disease and provide a sense of safety, screening behaviours detect the presence of a serious illness and can be frightening. For this reason, conclusions gained from studying the former might not apply to screening behaviours. Despite these observations, there is still no specific theoretical framework for screening behaviour.

Four dimensions of screening have meaningful psychological implications:

1. *Screening for disease versus risk factors.* Detecting a risk factor for an illness (e.g. high cholesterol levels) is likely to be less fear-provoking than disease detection, since a positive test indicates only an increased chance of future harm. However, the recent completion of the sequencing of the human genome has brought predictive genetic testing to learn about one's risk to develop many common medical conditions (cancers, diabetes) later in life, for which there is little, or no prevention. Screening for such risk factors raises concerns about possible adverse social and psychological impacts of knowing one's risks, and is one of the major challenges facing health psychology in the twenty-first century.

2. *Screening individuals at-risk versus population screening.* Most people undergoing population-based screening programmes are certain their health is fine. For them, the very act of screening may introduce doubts about their health, and a positive result shifts them from certainty into an upsetting state of uncertainty. On the other hand, testing for those already identified as being at increased risk for a disease, regardless of the outcome, provides some certainty. Given that uncertainty about one's health is an aversive state, the psychological implications of screening for at-risk and the general population may be considerably different.

3. *Prenatal versus pre-symptomatic screening.* Many screening tests can be performed prenatally by procedures such as amniocentesis and ultrasound (see 'Screening: antenatal' and 'Fetal well-being'). Unlike pre-symptomatic testing, many prenatal tests have become routine and are afforded less deliberation and intentional action. However, procedures like amniocentesis carry a small risk to the fetus and thus, involve stress both from the procedure and the test result. Moreover, prenatal diagnosis implicates an option of abortion, which provides a complete relief from the health threat but elicits ethical dilemmas and additional distress.

4. *Genetic versus somatic testing.* Unlike somatic pre-symptomatic testing, genetic information has implications not only for the tested individuals but also for their families and future generations. Guilt, shame, stigma and intricate family dynamics are involved. Carriers of genetic predisposing mutations for hereditary cancer experience difficulty divulging the result to family members, and receive both supportive and unsupportive responses from extended family members related to their carrier status. Thus, the genetic revolution in medicine that makes available many new screening tests is expected to affect the lives of large populations and require more involvement of psychologists.

Some of these dimensions may partly overlap, like genetic testing and screening for risk factors. But, some genetic testing identifies an existing condition (e.g. Down's syndrome), and some somatic testing identifies risk factors (e.g. HIV antibody testing). Thus, the four-dimensional representation of screening results in $2 \times 2 \times 2 \times 2 = 16$ combinations of screening tests that will have different psychological implications for the same medical condition being tested. For example, a screening test for breast cancer may be experienced differently if it is somatic (mammography) or genetic (testing for mutations carrying an increased risk for developing the disease in the future). These tests may be experienced differently by women of the general population compared to women at high risk because of family history of the disease. The same genetic screening test can (potentially) be performed pre-natally, among at-risk families and the general population, and raise completely different ethical, social and psychological concerns.

Psychological research on screening behaviour has addressed two main questions. First, What motivates healthy individuals to be tested? Second, What are the psychological impacts of being tested? Most studies were conducted on one screening test and one population. In view of the multidimensionality of screening behaviours, over-generalization from any single study to other screening situations with different dimensional features should be avoided. Following is an overview of some of the pertinent findings.

Motivations for genetic screening

The bulk of the research has identified four categories of factors: cognitions; information/communication; emotions and individual differences.

Cognitions

Many studies of screening were theoretically based on health behaviour models like the Health Belief Model (HBM) (Maiman & Becker, 1974), and the Theory of Planned Behavior (Ajzen, 1998) (see 'Health belief model' and 'Theory of planned behaviour'). These models outline several general belief categories associated with health behaviour: beliefs about the disease threat, about benefits and costs of the specific behaviour, control beliefs and beliefs about social norms. Findings from numerous studies on a variety of populations and screening tests have supported the idea that beliefs explain screening intentions and behaviour.

The Health Belief Model was used as a framework for understanding differences between tested and untested persons among populations at-risk for severe hereditary conditions (Evers-Kiebooms & Decryuenaere, 1998). Perceived benefits of testing predicted most of the variance in parents' intentions to use prenatal diagnosis (Sagi *et al.*, 1992), attitudes and subjective norms were the best predictors of intentions to participate in genetic testing for hereditary cancers (Braithwaite *et al.*, 2002), and perceived risk was found related to greater readiness to undergo genetic testing for breast cancer susceptibility (Jacobsen *et al.*, 1997).

Perceived preventability of the disease was found especially important for predictive genetic testing (Shiloh *et al.*, 1999). The distinction between unpreventable diseases like Huntington's disease (HD) (see 'Huntington's disease'), and diseases for which there are strategies that can reduce risk, like breast cancer, can explain the differences between uptake of predictive genetic testing for those two diseases among at-risk populations: 15% for HD (Bloch *et al.*, 1989) and 43–80% for breast cancer mutation (Loader *et al.*, 1998).

Information/communication factors

Cognitions are largely formed by information, hence a separate but related body of research focused on communication and doctor–patient issues. Media coverage of genetic testing has been extensive in recent years, but this coverage is often not useful and may even be misleading for individuals at risk for genetic disease (Stockdale, 1999). Healthcare providers play a major role in genetic screening tests: their recommendation or referral of patients to cancer genetic susceptibility testing was found related to their beliefs about factors that affect cancer risk, and the practice environment (Sifri *et al.*, 2003).

The guidelines of the UK General Medical Council (1999) state that information provided prior to consent for a screening test should include the purpose of screening, the likelihood of positive and negative findings, the possibility of false positive and false negative findings, the uncertainties and risks attached to the screening process, any significant medical, social or financial implications of screening and follow-up plans. These guidelines emphasize the risks and benefits of both the procedure and the results.

The information given before screening is important in producing responses to test results. Despite this, screening tests, especially in pregnancy care, are sometimes presented as routine procedures with little attendant explanation of the purpose of the test, the likelihood of being recalled, the meaning of positive or negative results, or probable action following a positive result. More knowledge about genetic testing does not simply lead to unambiguous acceptance. While those with a low level of knowledge had difficulty taking a stance on testing, those with the highest level of knowledge were both more enthusiastic and more sceptical about testing (Jallinoja & Aro, 2000).

How the information is framed and presented is also important. The same information communicated in positive terms would be less motivating than a negative frame. For example, women receiving a negatively framed prenatal risk-factor test result were more likely to opt for amniocentesis than women receiving a positively framed test result (Shiloh *et al.*, 2001). Michie *et al.* (2004*a*) found that even small changes within an information leaflet can change attitudes towards genetic testing. For example, attitudes towards testing were more positive when the information leaflet was glossy and in colour vs. black and white. These authors raised the concern that form and method of presentation may unintentionally change attitudes, and eventually behaviour, and they emphasized the need for evaluation studies about genetic information leaflets before they are used clinically.

Emotions

Emotional motivations exist as well. In contrast to policymakers, for whom the primary goal of screening programmes is to reduce disease prevalence, many participants perceive these programmes as a way to regulate emotions, to be reassured.

Reassurance-seeking can explain uptake of predictive genetic testing for conditions for which no preventive treatment is available, like HD, and seeking prenatal diagnosis with no intention to abort an affected fetus. Women's opinions about genetic testing for breast cancer risk also showed a greater attention to the emotional and social consequences of positive test results than to physical outcomes (Vuckovic *et al.*, 2003).

Worry and anxiety are clearly related to screening behaviour, but the strength and direction of the relationship are uncertain. Cancer worry (but not perceived risk) predicted greater interest and more favourable beliefs about the benefits of genetic testing for breast cancer risk (Cameron & Diefenbach, 2001) (see 'Screening: cancer'). But, women with extremely high levels of cancer anxiety were also reported to reject genetic testing (Shiloh *et al.*, 1998). These contradictory findings can be explained by a curvilinear relationship, with increasing levels of worry predicting higher screening levels up to a point, and trailing off when worry gets too great.

In addition to emotions experienced when a screening decision is made, a range of affects have been addressed lately, like regret, guilt, anger, surprise and disappointment, anticipated by individuals as a result of different choices and test results. Intentions to pursue genetic testing were significantly affected by anticipated emotions and concerns about the ability to handle them (Hadley *et al.*, 2003).

Emotional factors may also explain the 'intention-attendance gap' observed in many screening programmes. Most individuals express very favourable attitudes toward a wide range of screening tests, but this does not translate into similarly high rates of utilization. A goal conflict may exist between utility considerations and fear of obtaining positive test results, and between a desire to reduce uncertainty and hopes to receive good news. This corresponds with the possible conflict delineated in the self-regulatory model (Leventhal, 1971) between two parallel action plans elicited in reaction to health threats: to reduce the danger and to reduce the fear experienced (see 'Lay beliefs about health and illness').

Demographic and individual differences

There is evidence that beyond process level factors, cultural and individual differences are also associated with genetic screening behaviour. For example, African American and Latino women undergo prenatal diagnostic testing less often than White and Asian women, possibly because the potential acceptance of a child with Down's syndrome was found highest among African-Americans and Latinos, who were also more likely than Asians and Whites to state that their faith/religion would influence the prenatal testing decision (Learman *et al.*, 2003) (see also 'Cultural and ethnic factors in health').

Individual differences were also found positively related to screening intentions for genetic risk factors for breast cancer among women of the general population. Women who were more interested in being tested were characterized by higher levels of desire for control, more external (powerful others) health locus of control, less preference for self-treatment, more preference for medical information and stronger need for closure (Shiloh *et al.*, 1998) (see 'Perceived control'). Among relatives of carriers of breast cancer genes, those who chose to undergo genetic testing following an educational counselling programme were more likely to be older, to have lower levels of optimism and to report higher levels of cohesiveness in their families (Biesecker *et al.*, 2000).

Summary

Cognitive, communicational, emotional, cultural and personal factors combined additively and interactively explain much of the variance in screening behaviours. Empirical evidence supports combinations of predictors. Such combinations are consistent with self-regulatory theories of health behaviour like the Cognitive-Social Health Information Processing theory (C-SHIP), which maintains that interpretations and expectancies, beliefs, affects, goals and values activated together during cognitive affective processing determine individuals' reactions to health threats (Miller *et al.*, 1996).

Outcomes of genetic screening

Apart from medical outcomes, reactions to screening after receiving positive and negative test results were studied extensively. Most studies focused on cognitive, emotional and behavioural outcomes.

Cognitive outcomes

Laboratory studies using the TAA paradigm[1] showed that screening test results were interpreted within a cognitive frame of beliefs about illnesses, initiated biased information-processing and stimulated self-protective cognitive processes such as minimization (Ditto & Croyle, 1995). The results provided clear support for denial reactions to unfavourable medical test results, especially when individuals perceived no possibility of a preventive action to reduce the threat. Despite this, individuals were ultimately responsive to risk factor information, but the evidential requirements they demanded for accepting an unfavourable result were stricter than for accepting a favourable diagnosis. A false consensus bias in risk factor appraisals was also revealed: subjects told that they have TAA deficiency estimated its prevalence in the general population to be higher than did subjects told they do not. Appraisals of test results were also found to involve social comparisons and to be sensitive to social influences.

Similar cognitive processes were reported among women undergoing genetic screening tests for carrying the fragile X mutation. After receiving test results, non-carriers perceived fragile X syndrome to be more serious than before testing than carriers. Coping strategies activated by participants were minimization, acceptance of the possibility of being a carrier, a sense of being able to deal with the outcomes, positive comparison, problem solving and positive interpretation (McConkie-Rosell *et al.*, 2001).

Experimental studies showed that the availability of genetic testing also activates hindsight bias and responsibility attributions. After reading a scenario in which a woman declined to take a genetic screening test and had an affected baby, retrospective judgments

of the likelihood that the child would have had a genetic disorder were higher. Moreover, the more likely a negative outcome was perceived to be, the more responsible the mother was held for not taking the genetic screening test (Menec & Weiner, 2000) (see 'Attributions and health').

Emotional outcomes

Prenatal genetic screening tests influence the emotional experience of pregnancy. The genetic test itself induces considerable stress independent of the invasiveness of the testing procedure. Significant reductions in stress from pre-screening to post-screening were found among women and their partners upon receiving a normal test result (Kowalcek *et al.*, 2002). However, receiving an abnormal prenatal diagnosis, or experiencing pregnancy loss as a result of the diagnostic testing was extremely distressing and required extensive psychological counselling and support (Bourguignon *et al.*, 1999) (see 'Screening: antenatal' and 'Abortion'). Gender differences were also observed. Following screening for carriers of cystic fibrosis, women responded more positively than men to a negative test result and less positively than men to a positive test result. These differences were attributed to women's greater appraisals of threats to reproduction compared to men's, and men's greater use of a minimization coping strategy with threat (Marteau *et al.*, 1997).

Pre-implantation genetic diagnosis (PGD) is a new and exciting technology, that may alleviate much of the emotional burden involved in prenatal diagnosis and termination of affected pregnancies by using in vitro fertilization and genetically screened healthy embryos to establish a pregnancy. The psychological effects of these new procedures are still unknown.

Both negative and positive emotional consequences of screening for disease risk were also found. Unaffected individuals in cancer-predisposition testing programmes were generally accurate in anticipating emotional reactions to test results. However, cancer patients participating in genetic testing experienced higher levels of anger and worry than they had anticipated, and underestimation of subsequent distress emotions related to increase in general psychological distress after six months (Dorval *et al.*, 2000). Some buffers may attenuate adverse emotional effects of a positive test result. For example, increased levels of distress during the waiting period between testing and disclosure of results for breast cancer genetic risk were found associated with an unoptimistic personality and a tendency to suppress emotions (Lodder *et al.*, 1999).

A systematic review of the literature about screening for individuals' genetic risk of disease (Shaw *et al.*, 1999) showed that receiving a positive test result was likely to cause anxiety, depression, poorer perceptions of health and psychological distress in the first four weeks after testing. But, there was no evidence of severe or persistent adverse psychological effects in the long term. Feared extreme reactions like suicide were not found even among people informed with certainty that they will develop an untreatable fatal disease like HD.

Surprisingly, there were even reports of decreased distress following positive results in testing for HD (Wiggins *et al.*, 1992).

---

[1] A research procedure in which study participants are 'tested' for the presence of a fictitious risk factor they believe is real, are randomly assigned to receive either a positive or a negative test result, and complete questionnaires about the fictitious condition, the test and their actual health.

These findings were explained by various factors, including providing certainty to high-risk populations in a state of uncertainty prior to testing, pre-selection of those who undergo the test, pre-test expectations, minimization coping strategies and the effects of pre-testing counselling (Marteau & Croyle, 1998).

Behavioural outcomes

Being detected in screening as a carrier of a genetic mutation is expected to result in behavioural changes. Most pregnant women detected in screening tests as carriers of the cystic fibrosis mutation came for counselling, had their partner tested, and, if he was also a carrier, had prenatal diagnosis (Levenkron et al., 1997). Moreover, in screening programmes carried out in high schools for detecting recessive gene carriers of various genetic diseases, test results were recalled and resulted in testing of partners and requests for prenatal diagnosis even 20 years after screening (Mitchell et al., 1996).

The evidence with regard to genetic screening for personal disease risk is more complex. A literature review (Marteau, 1995) concluded that people seem to make few, if any, changes in behaviour following screening from which they learn about their health risks. In studies that found behavioural changes following screening, the direction of change was inconsistent. For example, informing smokers about their genetic susceptibility for cancer made them more depressed and fearful, but did not enhance their attempts to quit smoking (Lerman et al., 1997). In one study, positive test results even led to increased smoking when combined with fatalistic views (McNeil et al., 1988).

On the other hand, among individuals at hereditary risk for colon cancer, mutation-negative individuals decreased and mutation-positives increased their use of colonoscopy (Hadley et al., 2004). Genetic testing and identification of women at increased risk for breast and ovarian cancers increased surveillance and risk-reducing operations among mutation carriers, including oophorectomy (Schwartz et al., 2003), which may ultimately impact ovarian cancer mortality. However, in another study, decline in screening for breast cancer was attributed to a false sense of over-reassurance following a favourable result in testing for hereditary cancer (Meiser et al., 2001).

How and what health professionals communicate with patients about genetic testing may explain variance in behaviours following testing. For example, worries and the desire for inappropriate screening following negative genetic testing results for genetic colon cancer risk can be avoided by emphasizing high accuracy and low residual risk in communicating test results (Michie et al., 2004b).

Clinical implications

Beyond the theoretical interest, much of the research in the field deals with practical public health questions, such as how to promote screening behaviour and how to prevent adverse effects of testing. Concern about the psychological effects of notification of positive screening results for severe conditions prompted the call that all such screening programmes be accompanied by informed consent and counselling services.

Optimal decision making about genetic screening requires a personal, reasoned evaluation of positive and negative consequences of testing. Simple educational and counselling strategies can be successful in reducing distress and improving adherence in screening programmes. Studies assessing the effectiveness of interventions designed to prevent adverse psychological reactions to screening tests reported favourable results. Interacting with a genetic counsellor was found preferred for its personal, individualized nature, but computer educational programmes were also found accepted or preferred for being self-paced, private and informative (Green et al., 2001). Interventions guided by research findings and theory were suggested with the goal of preparing the individual for predictive genetic testing by cognitively and emotionally activating potential reactions to test results, facilitating accurate appraisal of cognitive and emotional reactions and enabling successful processing of those reactions (Shoda et al., 1998). Caution was raised, however, against interventions reducing anxiety too much, below the appropriate dose necessary for adequate continuing protective behaviour (Shaw et al., 1999).

(See also 'Screening in healthcare', 'Screening: antenatal', 'Screening: cardiac' and 'Screening: cancer'.)

REFERENCES

Ajzen, I. (1998). Models of human social behavior and their application to health psychology. *Psychology and Health*, **13**, 735–9.

Biesecker, B. B., Ishibe, N., Hadley, D. W. et al. (2000). Psychological factors predicting BRCA1/BRCA2 testing decisions in members of hereditary breast and ovarian cancer families. *American Journal of Medical Genetics*, **93**, 257–63.

Bloch, M., Fahy, M., Fox, S. & Hayden, M. R. (1989). Predictive testing for Huntington's disease: II. Demographic characteristics, life-style patterns, attitudes, and psychosocial assessments of the first fifty-one test candidates. *American Journal of Medical Genetics*, **32**, 217–24.

Bourguignon, A., Briscoe, B. & Nemzer, L. (1999). Genetic abortion: considerations for patient care. *Journal of Perinatal & Neonatal Nursing*, **13**, 47–58.

Braithwaite, D., Sutton, S. & Steggles, N. (2002). Intention to participate in predictive genetic testing for hereditary cancer: the role of attitude toward uncertainty. *Psychology and Health*, **17**, 761–72.

Cameron, L. D. & Diefenbach, M. A. (2001). Responses to information about psychosocial consequences of genetic testing for breast cancer susceptibility: influences of cancer worry and risk perceptions. *Journal of Health Psychology*, **6**, 47–59.

Ditto, P. H. & Croyle, R. T. (1995). Understanding the impact of risk

factor test results: insights from a basic research program. In R. T. Croyle (Ed.). *Psychosocial effects of screening for disease prevention and detection* (pp. 144–81). New York: Oxford University Press.

Dorval, M., Patenaude, A. F., Schneider, K. A. et al. (2000). Anticipated versus actual emotional reactions to disclosure of results of genetic tests for cancer susceptibility: findings from p53 and BRCA1 testing programs. *Journal of Clinical Oncology*, **18**, 2135–42.

Evers-Kiebooms, G. & Decruyenaere, M. (1998). Predictive testing for Huntington's disease: a challenge for persons at risk and for professionals. *Patient Education and Counseling*, **35**, 15–26.

General Medical Council. (1999). *Seeking patients' consent: the ethical considerations.* London: General Medical Council.

Green, M. J., McInerney, A. M., Biesecker, B. B. & Fost, N. (2001). Education about genetic testing for breast cancer susceptibility: Patient preferences for a computer program or genetic counselor. *American Journal of Medical Genetics,* **103**, 24–31.

Hadley, D. W., Jenkins, J., Dimond, E. *et al.* (2003). Genetic counseling and testing in families with hereditary nonpolyposis colorectal cancer. *Archives of Internal Medicine,* **163**, 573–82.

Hadley, D. W., Jenkins, J., Dimond, E. *et al.* (2004). Colon cancer screening practices after genetic counseling and testing for hereditary nonpolyposis colorectal cancer. *Journal of Clinical Oncology,* **22**, 39–44.

Jacobsen, P. B., Valdimarsdottir, H. B., Brown, K. L. & Offit, K. (1997). Decision-making about genetic testing among women at familial risk for breast cancer. *Psychosomatic Medicine,* **59**, 459–66.

Jallinoja, P. & Aro, A. R. (2000). Does knowledge make a difference? The association between knowledge about genes and attitudes toward gene tests. *Journal of Health Communication,* **5**, 29–39.

Kowalcek, I., Muhlhoff, A., Bachmann, S. & Gembruch, U. (2002). Depressive reactions and stress related to prenatal medicine procedures. *Ultrasound in Obstetrics & Gynecology,* **19**, 18–23.

Learman, L. A., Kuppermann, M., Gates, E. *et al.* (2003). Social and familial context of prenatal genetic testing decisions: are there racial/ethnic differences? *American Journal of Medical Genetics Part C – Seminars in Medical Genetics,* **119C**, 19–26.

Lerman, C., Gold, K., Audrain, J. *et al.* (1997). Incorporating biomarkers of exposure and genetic susceptibility into smoking cessation treatment: effects on smoking-related cognitions, emotions, and behavior change. *Health Psychology,* **16**, 87–99.

Levenkron, J. C., Loader, S. & Rowley, P. T. (1997). Carrier screening for cystic fibrosis: test acceptance and one year follow-up. *American Journal of Medical Genetics,* **73**, 378–86.

Leventhal, H. (1971). Fear appeals and persuasion: the differentiation of a motivational construct. *American Journal of Public Health,* **61**, 1208–24.

Loader, S., Levenkron, J. C. & Rowley, P. T. (1998). Genetic testing for breast-ovarian cancer susceptibility: a regional trial. *Genetic Testing,* **2**, 305–13.

Lodder, L. N., Frets, P. G., Trijsburg, R. W. *et al.* (1999). Presymptomatic testing for

BRCA1 and BRCA2: how distressing are the pre-test weeks? *Journal of Medical Genetics,* **36**, 906–13.

Maiman, L. A. & Becker, M. H. (1974). The health belief model: origins and correlates in psychological theory. *Health Education Monograph,* **2**, 336–53.

Marteau, T. M. (1995). Toward an understanding of the psychological consequences of screening. In R. T. Croyle. (Ed.). *Psychosocial effects of screening for disease prevention and detection* (pp. 185–99). New York: Oxford University Press.

Marteau, T. M. & Croyle, R. T. (1998). Psychological responses to genetic testing. *British Medical Journal,* **316**, 693–6.

Marteau, T. M., Dundas, R. & Axworthy, D. (1997). Long term cognitive and emotional impact of genetic testing for carriers of cystic fibrosis: the effects of gender and test result. *Health Psychology,* **16**, 51–62.

McConkie-Rosell, A., Spiridigliozzi, G. A., Sullivan, J. A., Dawson, D. V. & Lachiewicz, A. M. (2001). Longitudinal study of the carrier testing process for fragile X syndrome: perceptions and coping. *American Journal of Medical Genetics,* **98**, 37–45.

McNeil, T. F., Sveger, T. & Thelin, T. (1988). Psychosocial effects of screening for somatic risk: the Swedish alpha-1-antitripsin experience. *Thorax,* **43**, 505–7.

Meiser, B., Butow, P. N., Barratt, A. L. *et al.* **(The Psychological Impact Collaborative Group).** (2001). Long-term outcomes of genetic counseling in women at increased risk for developing hereditary breast cancer. *Patient Education and Counseling,* **44**, 215–25.

Menec, V. H. & Weiner, B. (2000). Observers' reactions to genetic testing: the role of hindsight bias and judgments of responsibility. *Journal of Applied Social Psychology,* **30**, 1670–90.

Michie, S., DiLorenzo, E., Lane, R., Armstrong, K. & Sanderson, S. (2004*a*). Genetic information leaflets: Influencing attitudes towards genetic testing. *Genetics in Medicine,* **6**, 219–25.

Michie, S., Thompson, M. & Hankins, M. (2004*b*). To be reassured or to understand? A dilemma in communicating normal cervical screening results. *British Journal of Health Psychology,* **9**, 113–23.

Miller, S. M., Shoda, Y. & Hurley, K. (1996). Applying cognitive–social theory to health-protective behavior: breast self-examination in cancer screening. *Psychological Bulletin,* **119**, 70–94.

Mitchell, J. J., Capua, A., Clow, C. & Scriver, C. R. (1996). Twenty-year outcome

analysis of genetic screening programs for Tay—Sachs and beta-thalassemia disease carriers in high schools. *American Journal of Human Genetics,* **59**, 793–8.

Sagi, M., Shiloh, S. & Cohen, T. (1992). Application of the health belief model in a study on parents' intentions to utilize prenatal diagnosis of cleft lip and/or palate. *American Journal of Medical Genetics,* **44**, 326–33.

Schwartz, M. D., Kaufman, E., Peshkin, B. N. *et al.* (2003). Bilateral prophylactic oophorectomy and ovarian cancer screening following BRCA1/BRCA2 mutation testing. *Journal of Clinical Oncology,* **21**, 4034–41.

Shaw, C., Abrams, K. & Marteau, T. M. (1999). Psychological impact of predicting individuals' risks of illness: a systematic review. *Social Science & Medicine,* **49**, 1571–98.

Shiloh, S., Ben-Sinai, R. & Keinan, G. (1999). Effects of controllability, predictability, and information-seeking style on interest in predictive genetic testing. *Personality and Social Psychology Bulletin,* **25**, 1187–95.

Shiloh, S., Eini-Jaffe, N., Ben-Neria, Z. & Sagi, M. (2001). Framing of prenatal screening test results and women's health-illness orientations as determinants of perceptions of fetal health and approval of amniocentesis. *Psychology and Health,* **16**, 313–25.

Shiloh, S., Petel, Y., Papa, M. & Goldman, B. (1998). Motivations, perceptions and interpersonal differences associated with interest in genetic testing for breast cancer susceptibility among women at high and average risk. *Psychology and Health,* **13**, 1071–86.

Shoda, Y., Mischel, W., Miller, S. M. *et al.* (1998). Psychological interventions and genetic testing: Facilitating informed decisions about BRCA1/2 cancer susceptibility. *Journal of Clinical Psychology in Medical Settings,* **5**, 3–17.

Sifri, R., Myers, R., Hyslop, T. *et al.* (2003). Use of cancer susceptibility testing among primary care physicians. *Clinical Genetics,* **64**, 355–60.

Stockdale, A. (1999). Public understanding of genetics and Alzheimer disease. *Genetic Testing,* **3**, 139–45.

Vuckovic, N., Harris, E. L., Valanis, B. & Stewart, B. (2003). Consumer knowledge and opinions of genetic testing for breast cancer risk. *American Journal of Obstetrics and Gynecology,* **189**, S48–53.

Wiggins, S., Whyte, P., Huggins, M. *et al.* (1992). The psychological consequences of predictive testing for Huntington's disease. *The New England Journal of Medicine,* **327**, 1401–5.

Self-examination: breasts, testicles

R. Glynn Owens

The University of Auckland

Technological advances have provided the means whereby several cancers can be screened by a range of devices. These include the use of automated cytology scanning for abnormal cells in cervical smears, mammographic techniques for the early detection of breast tumours, and the use of genetic screening methods to detect various cancers which are to a greater or lesser degree genetically determined (e.g. some breast and colonic cancers) (see 'Screening: cancer'). Such developments notwithstanding, there remains a potential role for self-examination procedures since (a) there remain many cancers for which technological procedures are not available (b) some procedures involve elements of risk, for example, the use of ionizing radiation in mammography, which limit the frequency with which they can be applied and (c) practical constraints may limit the applicability of the procedures to only a subset of those at risk.

For example, in the UK some 1 in 12 women will have breast cancer at some point in their lives, but for a number of reasons, (including logistical reasons and variation in the characteristics of the disease in women of different ages), screening by invitation is currently available only once every three years, and only to women in the 50–64 age group (with plans for extension up to age 70 in the near future). Yet breast cancer is far from unknown in younger women, and nor is it unknown for a tumour to grow to a significant size in less than the three-year time interval between successive examinations. Even the best screening by invitation programmes have take-up rates below 100%, and of course for many cancers no routine screening programme exists. Thus testicular cancer, the most common cancer in young men in the European Union, and malignant melanoma, a cancer whose incidence is one of the fastest rising in many countries, are both seriously dependent on early detection and treatment. Despite this, no routine screening programme exists, and self-detection and reporting remains the main route to presentation.

Self-examination differs from technological approaches in a number of important ways. On the positive side, the cost of such programmes is minimal, they can be made available to the whole of the population at risk, and the inherent risk to the individuals is (arguably) minimal. Despite these advantages, however, self-examination strategies have disadvantages that have led some commentators to decry their use altogether. Chief among these disadvantages are (a) the difficulty of producing self-examination procedures that can be easily and effectively learned by those at risk (b) the difficulty of persuading individuals to perform self-examination with sufficient regularity and (c) the added problem that once a potential symptom is discovered, it remains the responsibility of the individual to present for diagnosis and treatment without significant delay.

Such problems reveal a number of respects in which a better understanding of psychological processes may increase the effectiveness of self-examination procedures, and psychologists have been active in researching many of these aspects.

Self-examination in practice

Psychological research into self-examination dates back many years. With respect to the problems outlined above, the main areas of study have concerned take-up of the procedure and delay in presentation, both of which are critical if any programme of self-examination is to be effective. As regards take-up, there are several aspects including the need to increase the number of people who undertake self-examination and the need to ensure that those who do practise self-examination do so correctly, with the appropriate frequency and throughout the period of life for which it is acknowledged to be relevant. For the most part, results of such research have not been encouraging, generally indicating that few people perform such self-examination and that of those who do, only a minority perform the procedure with appropriate regularity. Thus Duffy and Owens (1984) in a UK study found only 10% of women claiming to perform monthly breast self-examination. For testicular self-examination (TSE) figures as low as 2% have been reported (Sheley et al., 1991). Given that studies of frequency of self-examination typically rely on self-report data, there is the additional possibility that even these low figures are inflated by recall biases and social desirability effects.

The role of knowledge on likelihood and effectiveness of self-examination has been assessed in a number of studies. Ivaz (2002) conducted a questionnaire survey of boys aged 14–16 in inner London, finding that although a large proportion knew about the age group most affected and that testicular cancer was curable if treated early, less than half were aware of how to perform TSE and only 8% did so regularly. Even lower rates of TSE were reported by Lechner et al. (2002), finding only 2% of a sample of young men (aged 15–19) in Holland reporting regular TSE. The effect of specific training in breast self-examination (BSE) was investigated by Philip et al. (1984), who conducted a longitudinal study of a group of women who had been taught BSE with a control group; when followed-up no significant difference in staging was found between experimental and control groups, although the tumours presented by the former were significantly smaller.

Such discouraging findings have prompted several researchers to identify psychological factors which distinguish those who perform self-examination from those who do not. Such studies have often drawn on established health psychology perspectives such as Becker's (1974) Health Belief Model or Ajzen and Fishbein's (1980)

Theory of Reasoned Action (see 'Health belief model' and 'Theory of planned behaviour'). Whilst these models have been considered with respect both to BSE and TSE (e.g. Umeh & Rogan-Gibson, 2001; Brubaker & Wickersham, 1990), results have generally been of varying consistency. Some studies which have investigated the variables directly have found significant relationships; for example Reno (1988) found that perceived benefits and perceived susceptibility (dimensions of the Health Belief Model) correlated significantly with TSE practice, and Gil et al. (2003) noted that rates of BSE were higher in women with a family history of breast cancer and associated higher perceived susceptibility. It is notable however that in the latter study, although those with a family history substantially overestimated their own risk as around 50%, only a third of the women performed regular BSE. Other psychological variables such as self-efficacy have also been investigated, with some evidence suggesting their relationship to self-examination practice (e.g. Luszczynska & Schwarzer, 2003). Actual knowledge of the disease has been reported as a significant predictor of both TSE (Rudolf, 1988) and BSE (Owens et al., 1985).

An encouraging sign in recent research has been the wider recognition of cultural and sub-cultural factors in determining self-examination and similar behaviours, with Sadler et al. (2003) and Petro-Nustus and Mikhail (2002) investigating self-examination practices among Japanese-American women and Jordanian women respectively, while Fish and Wilkinson (2003) looked at lesbians' accounts of why they do not perform BSE. Such recognition of varying perceptions amongst different societal groups seems likely to enhance understanding of variation in take-up and continued practice (see also 'Cultural and ethnic factors in health').

It must be remembered, of course, that self-examination, unlike screening by health professionals, leaves an additional responsibility with the individual; once a suspected symptom has been found, this needs to be presented without delay for diagnosis and (if necessary) treatment. Whilst a simplistic 'commonsense' perspective might expect that if someone takes the trouble to self-examine, they will therefore take appropriate action on discovery of a symptom, research suggests that this is not necessarily the case, with Duffy and Owens (1984) for example, finding no correlation between BSE practice and promptness of reporting. As with self-examination practice, there is also the possibility that reporting of delay is subject to recall and social desirability bias, although a study using a guided-recall procedure concluded that there was little evidence of such bias in reports of delay (Owens & Heron, 1990).

Conclusions

Given the practical limitations of technological screening, or screening by health professionals, effective self-examination procedures remain highly desirable. As yet, however, evaluations of such procedures have failed to provide encouraging evidence of their efficacy, although this may result at least in part from the failure of researchers to recognize the additional role of delay of presentation when symptoms are discovered through self-examination. There remains a need for effective psychological strategies that will enhance take-up of effective self-examination and prompt reporting of detected symptoms.

(See also 'Screening: cancer' and 'Screening: general issues'.)

REFERENCES

Ajzen, I. & Fishbein, M. (1980). *Understanding attitudes and predicting behaviour.* Englewood Cliffs: Prentice-Hall.

Becker, M. H. (1974). The Health Belief Model and sick role behaviour. *Health Education Monographs*, **2**, 409–19.

Brubaker, R. G. & Wickersham, D. (1990). Encouraging the practice of testicular self-examination: a field application of the theory of reasoned action. *Health Psychology*, **9**, 154–63.

Duffy, J. E. & Owens, R. G. (1984). Factors affecting promptness of reporting in breast cancer patients. *Hygie: International Journal of Health Education*, **2**, 29–32.

Fish, J. & Wilkinson, S. (2003). Understanding lesbians' healthcare behaviour: the case of breast self-examination. *Social Science and Medicine*, **56**, 235–45.

Gil, F., Mendez, I., Sirgo, A. et al. (2003). Perception of breast cancer risk and surveillance behaviours of women with family history of breast cancer. *Psycho-Oncology*, **12**, 821–7.

Ivaz, S. (2002). Testicular cancer awareness. *Family Practice*, **19**, 707.

Lechner, L., Oenema, A. & de Nooijer, J. (2002). Testicular self-examination (TSE) among Dutch young men aged 15–19: determinants of the intention to practice TSE. *Health Education Research*, **17**, 73–84.

Luszczynska, A. & Schwarzer, R. (2003). Planning and self-efficacy in the adoption and maintenance of breast self-examination: a longitudinal study on self-regulatory cognitions. *Psychology and Health*, **18**, 93–108.

Owens, R. G., Duffy, J. E. & Ashcroft, J. J. (1985). Women's responses to detection of breast lumps: a British study. *Health Education Journal*, **44**, 69–70.

Owens, R. G. & Heron, K. (1990). Accuracy of estimates of delay by women seeking breast cancer treatment. *Journal of Psychosocial Oncology*, **7**, 193–7.

Petro-Nustus, W. & Mikhail, B. I. (2002). Factors associated with breast self-examination among Jordanian women. *Public Health Nursing*, **19**, 263–71.

Philip, J., Harris, W. G., Flaherty, C. et al. (1984). Breast self-examination; clinical results from a population-based prospective study. *British Journal of Cancer*, **50**, 7–12.

Reno, D. R. (1988). Men's knowledge and health beliefs about testicular cancer and testicular self-examination. *Cancer Nursing*, **11**, 112–17.

Rudolf, V. M. (1988). The practice of TSE among college men: effectiveness of an educational program. *Oncology Nursing, Forum*, **15**, 45–8.

Sadler, G. R., Takahashi, M. & Nguyen, T. (2003). Japanese-American women: behaviors and attitudes toward breast cancer education and screening. *Health Care for Women International*, **24**, 18–26.

Sheley, J. F., Kinchen, E. W., Morgan, D. H. & Gordon, D. F. (1991). Limited impact of testicular self-examination promotion. *Journal of Community Health*, **16**, 117–24.

Umeh, K. & Rogan-Gibson, J. (2001). Perceptions of threat, benefits, and barriers in breast self-examination amongst young asymptomatic women. *British Journal of Health Psychology*, **6**, 361–72.

Sexual dysfunction

Patricia J. Morokoff

University of Rhode Island

Sexual functioning in men and women encompasses behaviours, physiological responses and subjective states of awareness. These phenomena are influenced by personal and relationship histories as well as cultural expectations. A linear sexual response cycle was hypothesized by Masters and Johnson (1966), in which desire precedes initiation of sexual activity, followed by arousal, orgasm and resolution. The psychosexual diagnostic categories of the American Psychiatric Association's *Diagnostic and statistical manual of mental disorders* (DSM) (third edition and onwards) are based on this model. In general, a sexual *dysfunction* is a physiological response and/or state of awareness contrary to these expectations for normative sexual functioning. This chapter will summarize issues relating to sexual dysfunctions including prevalence, risk factors and treatments.

Sexual dysfunctions in men

Definitions and prevalence

Erectile dysfunction (ED) has been defined as 'the persistent inability to attain and maintain a penile erection adequate for sexual performance' (NIH Consensus Panel, 1993). Knowledge of the epidemiology of this condition has been facilitated by two large population/community based studies, the National Health and Social Life Survey (NHSLS) (Laumann *et al.*, 1999) and the Massachusetts Male Aging Study (MMAS) (Feldman *et al.*, 1994). In the NHSLS study, the percentage of men reporting difficulties maintaining or achieving an erection ranged from 7% for those aged 18–29 to 18% for those aged 50–59. In the MMAS baseline study, complete ED was reported by less than 10%, moderate by 25% and mild by 17%. The likelihood of complete ED tripled from 5 to 15% between the ages of 40 and 70. Over 52% of men reported some level of ED. However, in neither the NHSLS or MMAS study were men asked if their erectile functioning was a problem. It is generally agreed (see DSM-IV-TR) that a psychosexual functioning diagnosis should not be made unless the symptom is viewed as a problem. Therefore these studies cannot be said to provide data on the prevalence of the diagnosis of ED, but rather on erectile symptoms (see 'Men's health').

In addition, other symptoms of sexual dysfunction were reported in the NHSLS study, including premature ejaculation (approximately 30%), hypoactive sexual desire (approximately 15%) and difficulty achieving orgasm (less than 10%). Overall, 31% of men reported some type of sexual problem.

Risk factors for erectile dysfunction

There are numerous behavioural and lifestyle risk factors, including smoking and being overweight, that predict future ED (Feldman *et al.*, 2000), while initiation of physical activity lowers risk (Derby *et al.*, 2000). In addition being unmarried, the victim of childhood sexual abuse, or a perpetrator of abuse is associated with erectile problems as is emotional distress and declining income (Laumann *et al.*, 1999) (see 'Risk perception', 'Sexual risk behaviour', 'Tobacco use', 'Obesity', 'Rape and sexual assault', 'Domestic violence: intimate partner violence and wife battering'). Medical conditions and associated treatments create risk for ED. Diabetes mellitus; heart disease; hypertension; decreased HDL; medications for diabetes, hypertension and cardiovascular disease; and prostate cancer treatment have all been found to be associated with ED (Kubin *et al.*, 2003) (see 'Diabetes mellitus' and 'Hypertension'). Depression is associated with ED, especially among younger men (Nicolosi *et al.*, 2004). Other related psychological characteristics include low levels of dominance and increased anger (Feldman *et al.*, 1994). Finally, there is significant comorbidity among symptoms of sexual dysfunction in men (Cameron *et al.*, 2005). Men who report symptoms of ED also report lower orgasmic function, sexual desire, less mutual initiation of sex and sexual satisfaction. Men without ED reported greater relationship satisfaction, sexual self-confidence and sexual spontaneity.

Assessment and treatment

Since erectogenic medications, such as Viagra, came on the market, the number of men seeking treatment for ED and other sexual dysfunctions has increased dramatically (Skaer *et al.*, 2001). Before 1998 male sexual dysfunctions were typically treated by urologists or mental health specialists, but now primary care physicians are most likely to be consulted. This dramatic shift in provider utilization prompted publication of guidelines for optimal assessment and treatment of men's sexual problems (Lue *et al.*, 2004; The Process of Care Consensus Panel, 1999). An interview to determine sexual, medical and psychosocial history is the first step in assessment with sensitivity to cultural, religious and ethnic factors. Physical examination is necessary to corroborate aspects of the medical history as well as potentially revealing unexpected physical conditions. Further diagnostic evaluation is often recommended. The Process of Care Consensus Panel (1999) identified first, second and third line treatment options. First line options include oral erectogenic drugs (e.g. Viagra), vacuum constriction devices and psychosexual therapy. A comparative study